Volume 2

Hepatology

A TEXTBOOK OF LIVER DISEASE

Second Edition

David Zakim, M.D.

Vincent Astor Distinguished Professor of
  Medicine
Cornell University Medical College
Professor of Cell Biology and Genetics
Cornell University Graduate School of
  Medical Sciences
Director, Division of Digestive Diseases
New York Hospital-Cornell University
  Medical Center
New York, New York

Thomas D. Boyer, M.D.

Professor of Medicine
University of California
San Francisco, California
Chief, Gastroenterology
Veterans Administration Hospital
San Francisco, California

1990
W. B. SAUNDERS COMPANY
Harcourt Brace Jovanovich, Inc.
Philadelphia ○ London ○ Toronto
Montreal ○ Sydney ○ Tokyo

W. B. SAUNDERS COMPANY
Harcourt Brace Jovanovich, Inc.

The Curtis Center
Independence Square West
Philadelphia, PA 19106

Library of Congress Cataloging-in-Publication Data

Hepatology / [edited by] David Zakim, Thomas D. Boyer.
—2nd ed.

      p.   cm.

Includes bibliographies and index.

ISBN 0-7216-2108-2

1. Liver—Diseases. I. Zakim, David.   II. Boyer, Thomas D.

[DNLM: 1. Liver Diseases.   WI 700 H5292]

RC845.H46   1989

616.3′62—dc19

DNLM/DLC   89–6018

Editor: William Lamsback
Designer: Terri Siegel
Production Manager: Carolyn Naylor
Manuscript Editors: Lorraine Zawodny, Jodi von Hagen and Kathleen Mason
Illustration Coordinator: Lisa Lambert
Indexer: Dennis Dolan
Cover Designer: Michelle Maloney

Hepatology

0–7216–3380–5 Volume I
0–7216–3381–1 Volume II
ISBN 0–7216–2108–2 Set

Last digit is the print number: 9   8   7   6   5   4   3   2   1

To two of our teachers:
Eric Kao and Telfer Reynolds

CONTRIBUTORS

GILBERT ASHWELL, M.D.
NIH Institute Scholar, National Institute of Diabetes and Digestive and Kidney Diseases, National Institutes of Health, Bethesda, MD
Receptor-Mediated Endocytosis: Mechanisms, Biologic Function, and Molecular Properties

BRUCE R. BACON, M.D.
Associate Professor of Medicine and Physiology and Biophysics, Louisiana State University School of Medicine in Shreveport; Chief, Section of Gastroenterology and Hepatology, Louisiana State University School of Medicine, Shreveport, LA
Hemochromatosis: Iron Metabolism and the Iron Overload Syndromes

PHILIP S. BARIE, M.D., F.A.C.S.
Assistant Professor of Surgery, Cornell University Medical College; Attending Surgeon and Director, Surgical Intensive Care Unit, The New York Hospital-Cornell Medical Center, New York, NY
Gallbladder Disease; Diseases of the Bile Ducts

NATHAN M. BASS, M.D., PH.D.
Assistant Professor of Medicine, University of California, San Francisco, School of Medicine; Attending Physician, University of California, San Francisco, Hospitals and Clinics, San Francisco, CA
Hepatic Function and Pharmacokinetics; Drug-Induced Liver Disease

DANIEL D. BIKLE, M.D., PH.D.
Associate Professor of Medicine, University of California, San Francisco, School of Medicine; Codirector, Special Diagnostic and Treatment Unit, Veterans Administration Medical Center, San Francisco, CA
Metabolism and Functions of Vitamins A, D, and K

D. MONTGOMERY BISSELL, M.D.
Professor of Medicine, University of California, San Francisco, School of Medicine; Attending Physician, University of California Hospitals and San Francisco General Hospital Medical Center, San Francisco, CA
Connective Tissue Metabolism and Hepatic Fibrosis

NORBERT BLANCKAERT, M.D., PH.D.
Professor of Clinical Pathology, Catholic University of Leuven; Coordinator of Clinical Laboratories, University Hospital St. Rafael, Leuven, Belgium
Physiology and Pathophysiology of Bilirubin Metabolism

HERBERT L. BONKOVSKY, M.D.
Professor of Medicine and Associate Professor of Biochemistry, Emory University School of Medicine; Attending Physician and Chief of Digestive Disease Laboratory and the Liver Study Unit, Emory University

Hospital; Attending Physician, Grady Memorial Hospital, Atlanta, GA
Porphyrin and Heme Metabolism and the Porphyrias

LLOYD L. BRANDBORG, M.D.
Clinical Professor of Medicine, Emeritus, University of California, San Francisco, School of Medicine, San Francisco, CA
Parasitic Diseases of the Liver; Bacterial and Miscellaneous Infections of the Liver

FRANCESCO CALLEA, M.D., PH.D.
Head, Department of Pathology, G. Gaslini Institute, Genova Quarto, Italy
Cholestatic Syndromes of Infancy and Childhood

JOSE L. CAMPRA, M.D.
Adjuvant Professor of Internal Medicine, National University of Cordoba School of Medicine; Deputy Chief, Centro de Endoscopia Diagnostico e Investigacion en Gastroenterologia, Hospital San Roque, Cordoba, Argentina
Hepatic Granulomata

JOHN P. CELLO, M.D.
Professor of Medicine, University of California, San Francisco, School of Medicine; Chief, Gastroenterology, San Francisco General Hospital, San Francisco, CA
The Liver in Systemic Conditions

ALLEN D. COOPER, M.D.
Associate Professor of Medicine and Physiology, Stanford University, Stanford, CA; Director, Research Institute, Palo Alto Medical Foundation, Palo Alto, CA
Hepatic Lipoprotein and Cholesterol Metabolism

VALEER J. DESMET, M.D., PH.D.
Professor of Histology and Pathology, Faculty of Medicine, Catholic University of Leuven; Head, Department of Pathology II, University Hospital St. Rafael, Leuven, Belgium
Cholestatic Syndromes of Infancy and Childhood

DANIEL DEYKIN, M.D.
Professor of Medicine and Public Health, Boston University School of Medicine; Chief, Cooperative Studies Program, Boston Veterans Administration Medical Center, Boston, MA
Alterations of Hemostasis in Patients with Liver Disease

TERRENCE M. DONOHUE, JR., PH.D.
Assistant Professor of Internal Medicine and Biochemistry, University of Nebraska College of Medicine; Research Chemist, Veterans Administration Medical Center, Omaha, Nebraska
Synthesis and Secretion of Plasma Proteins by the Liver

MURRAY EPSTEIN, M.D., F.A.C.P.
Professor of Medicine, University of Miami School of
Medicine; Attending Physician, Nephrology Section, VA
Medical Center and Division of Nephrology, James M.
Jackson Memorial Medical Center, Miami, FL
*Functional Renal Abnormalities in Cirrhosis:
Pathophysiology and Management*

GEOFFREY C. FARRELL, M.D., F.R.A.C.P.
Associate Professor of Medicine, The University of
Sydney, Sydney, Australia; Head, Gastroenterology Unit,
Westmead Hospital, Westmead, New South Wales,
Australia
Postoperative Hepatic Dysfunction

NELSON FAUSTO, M.D.
Professor and Chairman, Department of Pathology and
Laboratory Medicine, Division of Biology and Medicine,
Brown University, Providence, RI
Hepatic Regeneration

JOHAN FEVERY, M.D., PH.D.
Professor of Medicine, Catholic University of Leuven;
University Hospital Gasthuisberg, Leuven, Belgium
Physiology and Pathophysiology of Bilirubin Metabolism

LOUIS D. FIORE, M.D.
Assistant Professor of Medicine, Boston University School
of Medicine; Director, Thrombosis Service, Boston
Veterans Administration Medical Center, Boston, MA
Alterations of Hemostasis in Patients with Liver Disease

JAMES H. FOSTER, M.D.
Professor of Surgery,
University of Connecticut School of Medicine; Attending
Surgeon, University of Connecticut Health Center, John
Dempsey Hospital, Farmington, CT
*Surgical Management of Primary Hepatocellular
Carcinoma and Metastatic Liver Cancer; Liver Trauma*

FAYEZ K. GHISHAN, M.D.
Professor of Pediatrics and Professor of Molecular
Physiology and Biophysics; Director, Division of
Gastroenterology-Nutrition, Department of Pediatrics,
Vanderbilt Medical School; Attending Physician,
Vanderbilt Children's Hospital, Nashville, TN
*Inborn Errors of Metabolism That Lead to Permanent
Liver Injury; Alpha₁-Antitrypsin Deficiency*

NORMAN GITLIN, M.D.
Professor of Medicine, University of California, San
Francisco, School of Medicine, San Francisco, CA; Chief
of Gastroenterology, Veterans Administration Medical
Center, Fresno, CA
*Clinical Aspects of Liver Diseases Caused by Industrial
and Environmental Toxins*

HENRY I. GOLDBERG, M.D.
Professor of Radiology, University of California, San
Francisco, Department of Radiology, University of
California, San Francisco, Medical Center,
San Francisco, CA
*Radiologic Evaluation of Disorders of the Liver and
Biliary System*

IRA S. GOLDMAN, M.D.
Assistant Professor of Medicine, Cornell University
Medical College, New York, NY; Assistant Attending
Physician, Division of Gastroenterology, North Shore
University Hospital, Manhasset, NY
*Parasitic Diseases of the Liver; Bacterial and
Miscellaneous Infections of the Liver*

LEONARD I. GOLDSTEIN, M.D.
Assistant Clinical Professor, University of California, Los
Angeles, School of Medicine; Attending Physician,
UCLA Medical Center, Los Angeles, CA
Liver Transplantation

JOHN L. GOLLAN, M.D., PH.D., F.R.A.C.P.,
F.R.C.P.
Associate Professor of Medicine, Harvard Medical
School; Director, Gastroenterology Division, and
Attending Physician, Brigham and Women's Hospital;
Consultant Physician, Children's Hospital Medical Center,
Boston, MA; Consultant Physician, Brockton-West
Roxbury Veterans Administration Medical Center,
Brockton, MA
*Copper Metabolism, Wilson's Disease, and Hepatic
Copper Toxicosis*

HARRY L. GREENE, M.D.
Professor, Pediatrics, Associate Professor, Biochemistry
Vanderbilt University Medical School; Director, Clinical
Nutrition Research Unit, Vanderbilt University Hospital,
Nashville, TN
*Inborn Errors of Metabolism That Lead to Permanent
Liver Injury; Alpha₁-Antitrypsin Deficiency*

JAMES H. GRENDELL, M.D.
Associate Professor of Medicine and Physiology,
University of California, San Francisco; Attending
Physician, San Francisco General Hospital,
San Francisco, CA
The Liver in Systemic Conditions

D. M. HEUMAN, M.D.
Assistant Professor of Medicine, Division of
Gastroenterology, Medical College of Virginia School of
Medicine, Virginia Commonwealth University; Assistant
Professor of Medicine, Gastroenterology Section,
McGuire Veterans Administration Medical Center,
Richmond, VA
*Physiology and Pathophysiology of Enterohepatic
Circulation of Bile Acids; Pathogenesis and Dissolution of
Gallstones*

ROBERT S. HILLMAN, M.D.
Professor of Medicine, University of Vermont School of
Medicine, Burlington, VT; Chairman, Department of
Medicine, Maine Medical Center, Portland, ME
The Liver and Hematopoiesis

P. B. HYLEMON, PH.D.
Professor of Microbiology and Medicine, Medical College
of Virginia School of Medicine, Virginia Commonwealth
University, Richmond, VA
*Physiology and Pathophysiology of Enterohepatic
Circulation of Bile Acids*

IRA M. JACOBSON, M.D.
Assistant Professor of Medicine, Cornell University
Medical College; Assistant Attending Physician,
New York Hospital, New York, NY
*Gallbladder Disease; Diseases of the Bile Ducts;
Nonsurgical Treatment of Biliary Tract Disease*

RICHARD B. JENNETT, M.D.
Assistant Professor of Internal Medicine, University of
Nebraska College of Medicine; Research Associate and
Attending Physician, Omaha Veterans Administration
Medical Center, Omaha, NE
Synthesis and Secretion of Plasma Proteins by the Liver

ALBERT L. JONES, M.D.
Professor of Medicine and Anatomy, University of
California, San Francisco; Associate Chief of Staff for
Research and Development, San Francisco Veterans
Administration Medical Center, San Francisco, CA
Anatomy of the Normal Liver

E. ANTHONY JONES, M.D., F.R.C.P.
Professor of Medicine, George Washington University
Hospital, Washington, D.C.; Chief, Liver Diseases
Section, Digestive Diseases Branch, National Institute of
Diabetes and Digestive and Kidney Diseases, National
Institutes of Health, Bethesda, MD
Fulminant Hepatic Failure

NEIL KAPLOWITZ, M.D.
Professor of Medicine, University of California, Los
Angeles, School of Medicine; Chairman, Division of
Gastroenterology, Wadsworth Veterans Administration
Medical Center, Los Angeles, CA
Biochemical Tests for Liver Disease

MICHAEL C. KEW, M.D., D.Sc., F.R.C.P.
Professor of Medicine, Witwatersrand University Medical
School; Senior Physician, Johannesburg and Hillbrow
Hospitals; Attending Hepatologist, Baragwanath and
Rand Mutual Hospitals; Honorary Research Associate,
South African Institute for Medical Research,
Johannesburg, South Africa
Tumors of the Liver

MICHAEL J. KROWKA, M.D.
Assistant Professor of Medicine, Mayo Medical School,
Rochester, MN; Consultant, Thoracic Diseases and
Internal Medicine, Mayo Clinic, Jacksonville, FL
*Cardiovascular and Pulmonary Complications of Liver
Diseases*

JAY H. LEFKOWITCH, M.D.
Professor of Clinical Pathology, College of Physicians and
Surgeons, Columbia University; Attending Pathologist,
Columbia-Presbyterian Medical Center, New York, NY
Pathologic Diagnosis of Liver Disease

JAMES LEVINE, M.D.
Assistant Professor of Medicine, Harvard University
School of Medicine; Attending Physician, Division of
Hematology-Oncology, New England Deaconess Hospital,
Boston, MA
Alterations of Hemostasis in Patients with Liver Disease

CHARLES J. LIGHTDALE, M.D.
Associate Professor of Clinical Medicine, Cornell
University Medical College; Director, Gastrointestinal
Endoscopy, Memorial Sloan-Kettering Cancer Center,
New York, NY
Laparoscopy

WILLIS C. MADDREY, M.D.
Magee Professor of Medicine and Chairman of the
Department, Jefferson Medical College of Thomas
Jefferson University, Philadelphia, PA
Chronic Hepatitis

CAROLYN MONTGOMERY, M.D.
Professor in Residence, Department of Anatomic
Pathology, University of California, San Francisco, School
of Medicine; Acting Chief, Anatomic Pathology Service,
San Francisco Veterans Administration Medical Center,
San Francisco, CA
Alcoholic Liver Disease

EDWARD W. MOORE, M.D.
Professor of Medicine, Physiology, and Pathology and
Director of Gastrointestinal Research, Medical College of
Virginia School of Medicine, Virginia Commonwealth
University; Attending Physician, Medical College of
Virginia Hospitals and McGuire Veterans Administration
Medical Center, Richmond, VA
Pathogenesis and Dissolution of Gallstones

ROBERT K. OCKNER, M.D.
Professor of Medicine and Director, Liver Center,
University of California, San Francisco; Chief, Division of
Gastroenterology, Moffitt-Long Hospitals; Attending
Physician, San Francisco General Hospital and San
Franscisco Veterans Administration Medical Center;
Consultant, Letterman Army Medical Center, San
Francisco, CA
Drug-Induced Liver Disease

GUSTAV PAUMGARTNER, M.D.
Professor of Medicine and Chairman, Department of
Medicine II, University of Munich, Munich, Federal
Republic of Germany
Extracorporeal Shock-Wave Lithotripsy of Gallstones

ROBERT L. PETERS, M.D.*
Formerly Professor of Pathology, University of Southern
California School of Medicine, Los Angeles, CA; and
Chief Pathologist, Rancho Los Amigos Medical Center,
Downey, CA
Hepatic Granulomata

NEVILLE R. PIMSTONE, M.D., F.C.P.(S.A.)
Professor of Internal Medicine, University of California,
Davis, School of Medicine, Davis, CA; Chief, Division of
Gastroenterology, University of California, Davis,
Medical Center, Sacramento, CA
Liver Transplantation

JORGE RAKELA, M.D.
Associate Professor of Medicine, Mayo Medical School;
Consultant, Division of Gastroenterology and Internal
Medicine, Mayo Medical Center, Rochester, MN
*Cardiovascular and Pulmonary Complications of Liver
Diseases*

---

*Deceased 2-16-85

DONALD REED, Ph.D.
Professor of Biochemistry, Department of Biochemistry and Biophysics, Oregon State University; Director, Environmental Health Sciences Center, Oregon State University, Corvallis, OR
Chemical Mechanisms in Drug-Induced Liver Injury

TELFER B. REYNOLDS, M.D.
Clayton G. Loosli Professor of Medicine, University of Southern California School of Medicine; Chief, Hepatology Division, Los Angeles County-University of Southern California Medical Center, Los Angeles, CA
Hepatic Granulomata

PETER D. I. RICHARDSON, Ph.D.
Head of Clinical Research, Astra Pharmaceuticals, Ltd., Kings Langley, Hertfordshire, U.K.
Liver Blood Flow

WILLIAM S. ROBINSON, M.D.
Professor, Department of Medicine, Stanford University School of Medicine; Attending Physician and Consultant in Infectious Diseases, Stanford University Hospital, Stanford, CA; Consultant in Infectious Diseases, Palo Alto Veterans Administration Medical Center, Palo Alto, CA
Biology of Human Hepatitis Viruses

JOSEPH ROLL, M.D.
Assistant Professor of Medicine, University of California, San Francisco, School of Medicine; Attending Physician, San Francisco General Hospital Medical Center
Connective Tissue Metabolism and Hepatic Fibrosis

BORIS H. RUEBNER, M.D.
Professor of Pathology, University of California, Davis, School of Medicine, Davis, CA; Attending Physician, University of California, Davis, Medical Center, Sacramento, CA
Liver Transplantation

TILMAN SAUERBRUCH, M.D.
Professor of Medicine, Department of Medicine II, University of Munich, Munich, Federal Republic of Germany
Extracorporeal Shock-Wave Lithotripsy of Gallstones

DANIEL F. SCHAFER, M.D.
Associate Professor of Internal Medicine, University of Nebraska College of Medicine; Investigator, Liver Study Unit, Omaha Veterans Administration Medical Center, Omaha, NE
Hepatic Encephalopathy; Fulminant Hepatic Failure

BRUCE F. SCHARSCHMIDT, M.D.
Professor of Medicine, University of California, San Francisco, School of Medicine; Attending Physician, University of California, San Francisco, Affiliated Hospitals, San Francisco, CA
Bile Formation and Cholestasis

LEONARD B. SEEFF, M.D.
Professor of Medicine, Georgetown University School of Medicine; Chief, Gastroenterology and Hepatology Section, Veterans Administration Medical Center, Washington, D.C.
Diagnosis, Therapy, and Prognosis of Viral Hepatitis

DAVID A. SHAFRITZ, M.D.
Professor of Medicine and Cell Biology, Albert Einstein College of Medicine, Yeshiva University; Attending Physician, Bronx Municipal Hospital Center, Bronx, NY
Hepatitis B Virus Persistence, Chronic Liver Disease, and Primary Liver Cancer

MORRIS SHERMAN, M.B., B.Ch., Ph.D.
Assistant Professor of Medicine, Division of Gastroenterology, University of Toronto; Staff Gastroenterologist, Toronto General Hospital, Toronto, Ontario, Canada
Hepatitis B Virus Persistence, Chronic Liver Disease, and Primary Liver Cancer

MICHAEL F. SORRELL, M.D.
Henry J. Lehnhoff Professor and Chairman, Department of Internal Medicine, University of Nebraska College of Medicine; Attending Physician, University of Nebraska Medical Center and Omaha Veterans Administration Hospital, Omaha, NE
Synthesis and Secretion of Plasma Proteins by the Liver

CLIFFORD J. STEER, M.D.
Professor of Medicine and Cell Biology and Member, Institute of Human Genetics, University of Minnesota School of Medicine, Minneapolis, MN
Receptor-Mediated Endocytosis: Mechanisms, Biologic Function, and Molecular Properties

STEPHEN E. STEINBERG, M.D.
Associate Professor of Medicine, Division of Gastroenterology-Hepatology, State University of New York at Stony Brook Health Sciences Center School of Medicine; Attending Physician, University Hospital at Stony Brook, Stony Brook, NY; Attending Physician, Veterans Administration Medical Center, Northport, NY
The Liver and Hematopoiesis

ANDREW STOLZ, M.D.
Assistant Professor of Medicine, University of California, Los Angeles, School of Medicine; Research Associate Investigator, Wadsworth Veterans Administration Medical Center, Los Angeles, CA
Biochemical Tests for Liver Disease

ANTHONY S. TAVILL, M.D., F.R.C.P.
Professor of Medicine and Academic Director of Gastroenterology, Case Western Reserve University School of Medicine; Director, Division of Gastroenterology, Cleveland Metropolitan General Hospital, Cleveland, OH
Hemochromatosis: Iron Metabolism and the Iron Overload Syndromes

RUEDI F. THOENI, M.D.
Associate Professor of Radiology, University of California, San Francisco; Chief of CT/GI Section, Attending Physician, Medical Center at the University of California, San Francisco, and Moffitt-Long Hospitals, San Francisco, CA
Radiologic Evaluation of Disorders of the Liver and Biliary System

HOWARD C. THOMAS, B.Sc., Ph.D., M.D., F.R.C.P.
Professor and Chairman of Medicine, St. Mary's Medical

School, Imperial College of Science, Technology and Medicine, London University; Consultant Hepatologist, St. Mary's Hospital, London, U.K.
Immunologic Mechanisms in Chronic Liver Disease

DAVID R. TRIGER, M.A., B.M., B.CH., D.PHIL., F.R.C.P.
Reader in Medicine, University of Sheffield Medical School; Honorary Consultant Physician, Royal Hallamshire Hospital, Sheffield, U.K.
Evaluation of Liver Disease by Radionuclide Scanning

DEAN J. TUMA, PH.D.
Professor of Internal Medicine and Biochemistry, University of Nebraska College of Medicine; Associate Career Scientist, Omaha Veterans Administration Medical Center, Omaha, NE
Synthesis and Secretion of Plasma Proteins by the Liver

RAN TUR-KASPA, M.D.
Assistant Professor (Senior Lecturer) of Medicine, Department of Medicine A, Hadassah Medical School of Hebrew University; Permanent Chief Physician, Department of Medicine A, Hadassah University Hospital, Jerusalem, Israel
Hepatitis B Virus Persistence, Chronic Liver Disease, and Primary Liver Cancer

REBECCA W. VAN DYKE, M.D.
Assistant Professor of Medicine, University of California, San Francisco, School of Medicine; Attending Physician, Moffitt-Long Hospitals, San Francisco, CA
The Liver in Pregnancy

DAVID H. VAN THIEL, M.D.
Professor of Medicine, University of Pittsburgh School of Medicine; Chief of Gastroenterology at the University of Pittsburgh and Presbyterian-University Hospital, Pittsburgh, PA
Disorders of the Hypothalamic-Pituitary-Gonadal and Thyroidal Axes in Patients with Liver Disease

DONALD A. VESSEY, PH.D.
Professor of Medicine and Pharmacology, University of California, San Francisco, School of Medicine; Co-Chief, Liver Study Unit, San Francisco Veterans Administration Medical Center, San Francisco, CA
Metabolism of Drugs and Toxins by the Human Liver

JOHN M. VIERLING, M.D.
Associate Professor of Medicine, University of Colorado School of Medicine; Director, Transplantation Hepatology, University of Colorado Health Sciences Center; Attending Physician, Denver Veterans Administration Medical Center, Denver, CO
Hepatobiliary Complications of Ulcerative Colitis and Crohn's Disease; Primary Biliary Cirrhosis

Z. R. VLAHCEVIC, M.D.
Professor and Chairman, Division of Gastroenterology, Virginia Commonwealth University Medical College of Virginia; Chief, Gastroenterology Section, McGuire Veterans Administration Medical Center, Richmond, VA
Physiology and Pathophysiology of Enterohepatic Circulation of Bile Acids, Pathogenesis and Dissolution of Gallstones

RICHARD WARD, M.D.
Professor of Surgery, University of California, Davis, Medical Center, Sacramento, CA
Liver Transplantation

ROGER L. WILLIAMS, M.D.
Associate Professor of Medicine and Pharmacy, University of California, San Francisco, Schools of Medicine and Pharmacy; Director, Drug Studies Unit, School of Pharmacy, University of California, San Francisco, San Francsico, CA
Hepatic Function and Pharmacokinetics

PETER G. WITHRINGTON, PH.D.
Associate Professor, The Medical College of St. Bartholomew's Hospital, University of London; Attending Physician, Saint Bartholomew's Hospital, London, U.K.
Liver Blood Flow

CAMILLUS L. WITZLEBEN, M.D.
Professor of Pathology, University of Pennsylvania School of Medicine; Pathologist-in-Chief, Children's Hospital of Philadelphia, Philadelphia, PA
Cystic Diseases of the Liver

TERESA L. WRIGHT, B.M., B.S.
Assistant Professor of Medicine, University of California, San Francisco, School of Medicine; Attending Physician, San Francisco Veterans Administration Medical Center, San Francisco, CA
Diagnosis and Management of Cirrhotic Ascites

PREFACE TO SECOND EDITION

The goal of the first edition of *Hepatology* was to provide a framework of pathophysiology as a basis for understanding liver function and liver disease in addition to authoritative, up-to-date descriptions of the clinical and laboratory manifestations of liver diseases and the diagnostic and therapeutic strategies for managing them. Half of the first edition thus comprised discussions of hepatic morphology, physiology, and biochemistry; mechanisms of injury to the liver; and the impact of disordered hepatic function on the physiology of other systems. The interval of seven years between the first and second editions of *Hepatology* has not weakened our belief that the practice of medicine is most effective when based on an understanding of the fundamental pathophysiologic events that lead to disordered function. The philosophy determining the organization and content of the second edition hence is the same as it was for the first. But there have been major changes in *Hepatology* because of new knowledge about liver function and about the causes and treatments of liver disease.

Thirty-seven contributors to the second edition were not represented in the first. Several new chapters have been added, and there is expanded coverage in many of the revised chapters. Changes in authorship have been made to infuse the book with new perspectives, even in well-established aspects of liver disease. Sadly, however, Dr. Robert Peters, who was an important contributor to the first edition, has died. His skill as a pathologist and dedication to scholarship in medicine will be missed by everyone with an interest in liver disease.

Section I of the current edition continues to discuss normal morphology and function. New chapters have been added here on receptor-mediated endocytosis, collagen and lymphokine metabolism, and the metabolism of bile acids. The problem of cirrhotic ascites in Section II (Manifestations of Liver Disease) is now a separate chapter. Section IV, which is devoted to the clinical aspects of liver disease, contains the largest number of completely new chapters, providing new information on the chemical mechanisms of drug-induced liver injury, the molecular biology of persistent infection with hepatitis B virus, surgical management of liver trauma, surgical management of liver tumors, and liver disease in pregnancy. The single chapter on diseases of the biliary tract in the first edition has been expanded to five chapters, including one on lithotripsy.

As was true seven years ago, there remain unresolved problems in patients with liver disease and controversies about the application of therapies. Areas of uncertainty and controversy are delineated in the text so that the reader will discern not only where we are in the progressive struggle to change the natural course of liver disease but also where we need to go.

Finally, we continue to hope that *Hepatology*, by defining areas of insufficient knowledge and controversy, will stimulate students and investigators to pursue definitive answers to the important problems that remain unsolved.

DAVID ZAKIM
THOMAS D. BOYER

CONTENTS

15

Connective Tissue Metabolism and Hepatic Fibrosis

D. Montgomery Bissell, M.D.
Joseph Roll, M.D.

II Manifestations of Abnormal Liver Function

16

Hepatic Encephalopathy

Daniel F. Schafer, M.D.
E. Anthony Jones, M.D., F.R.C.P

17

Fulminant Hepatic Failure

E. Anthony Jones, M.D., F.R.C.P.
Daniel F. Schafer, M.D.

18

Functional Renal Abnormalities in Cirrhosis: Pathophysiology and Management

Murray Epstein, M.D., F.A.C.P.

19

Disorders of the Hypothalamic-Pituitary-Gonadal and Thyroidal Axes in Patients with Liver Disease

David H. Van Thiel, M.D.

20

Cardiovascular and Pulmonary Complications of Liver Diseases

Jorge Rakela, M.D.
Michael J. Krowka, M.D.

21

The Liver and Hematopoiesis

Stephen E. Steinberg, M.D.
Robert S. Hillman, M.D.

22

Alterations of Hemostasis in Patients with Liver Disease

Louis Fiore, M.D.
James Levine, M.D.
Daniel Deykin, M.D.

III   Evaluation of Hepatic Function

IV   Clinical Characteristics, Etiologies, and Management of Specific Diseases of the Liver

IV

Clinical Characteristics, Etiologies, and Management of Specific Diseases of the Liver

IV A. Toxic Injury to the Liver

30

Chemical Mechanisms in Drug-Induced Liver Injury

Donald Reed, Ph.D.

ABBREVIATIONS

BCNU = 1,3-bis(2-Chloroethyl)-1-nitrosurea
DQ = diquat
F-actin = filamentous actin
G-actin = globular actin
GSH = glutathione
GSSG = glutathione disulfide
NADP⁺ = nicotinamide-adenine dinucleotide phosphate (oxidized)
NADPH = nicotinamide-adenine dinucleotide phosphate (reduced)

Basic research on the mechanisms of drug-induced liver injury has shown that metabolism of a drug to a reactive intermediate is usually the basis for toxic injury. Sometimes such a process, which is known as bioactivation, occurs in a minor metabolic pathway that often involves only a small part of the administered dose. At least two hypotheses exist (Fig. 30–1) for drug-induced liver injury.[1] One suggests that covalent binding of reactive intermediates to thiol and other functional groups in protein initiates drug-induced hepatotoxicity. The other hypothesis suggests that drug-induced hepatotoxicity results from oxidative stress: oxidation of thiols, peroxidation of lipids, and alterations in calcium homeostasis. These events are reversible per se until there is loss of cellular integrity by additional damage such as extensive blebbing of cellular membranes. This causes irreversible damage and nearly free exchange between intracellular constituents and the surrounding milieu. Bioactivation, however, is not the only factor determining whether an agent is toxic. All tissues contain mechanisms for detoxifying reactive intermediates. The status of these mechanisms also influences whether a given amount of a specific agent will be toxic. We review in this chapter the pathways by which chemicals are metabolized to proximate toxins, the mechanism by which toxic intermediates damage cells, and mechanisms for preventing or limiting this damage.

The pioneering studies by Miller and Miller established that bioactivation of foreign compounds gave reactive intermediates and metabolites that were capable of chemical interaction with cellular constituents.[2] These interactions, whether enzymatic or nonenzymatic, may yield adducts of cellular macromolecules that make major contributions to the overall degree of cell injury. The formation of electrophiles (electron-deficient molecules), which are called alkylating agents, and free radicals by bioactivation of drugs and foreign chemicals is well documented, as illustrated by reviews on bioactivation and metabolism of 15 classes of chemicals.[3] In contrast, certain cancer chemotherapeutic agents of the nitrogen mustard class are direct-acting drugs that do not require bioactivation for either pharmacologic action or toxicity. The metabolism of these drugs and reactions between them and cellular components have been reviewed recently.[4] The direct-acting cancer chemotherapeutic drugs are also referred to as alkylating agents, as are those such as cyclophosphamide that require bioactivation. Enzymatic mechanisms for detoxication of drugs and other xenobiotics are reviewed in Chapter 9.

The dynamics of drug metabolism—for example, competition within detoxication pathways, pool sizes, and rates of conjugate formation in vivo—are not understood clearly. As might be expected, the viability and survival of cells depend on the status of "built-in" protective mechanisms. Chemically induced liver injury can occur because systems for protection are depleted. Even molecular oxygen, during its normal physiologic functions, is transformed to some extent into chemically reactive intermediates, including superoxide anion radical (O·) and hydrogen peroxide. Glutathione, a unique tripeptide, provides antioxidant reducing equivalents and is a substrate for formation of glutathione (GSH) conjugates.

COVALENT BINDING OF REACTIVE INTERMEDIATES

Both the extent and the molecular targets of covalent binding by reactive intermediates vary with the properties of the intermediates, especially chemical reactivity and, to some extent, sites of formation. The liver, because it is a primary site of drug metabolism, is also a major source of chemically reactive intermediates.

The half-life of a reactive intermediate determines, in part, the site of the molecular targets with which it reacts. Some reactive intermediates possess sufficient stability to be transported throughout the body (for a review see reference 5). Also, there are threshold doses for toxicity of certain chemicals. Above these levels, covalent binding increases greatly for relatively small increases in dose of the chemical. The importance of a threshold for safe use of drugs has been discussed in detail by Gillette.[6] Dose-response for the toxicity of bromobenzene, a noncarcinogenic chemical, illustrates the threshold effect. The concentration of GSH in liver decreases after the administration of toxic doses of bromobenzene. The basis for this is the conjugation of the oxidative product, an epoxide of bromobenzene, with GSH. Eventually, the rate of formation of the conjugate of the reactive epoxide becomes limited

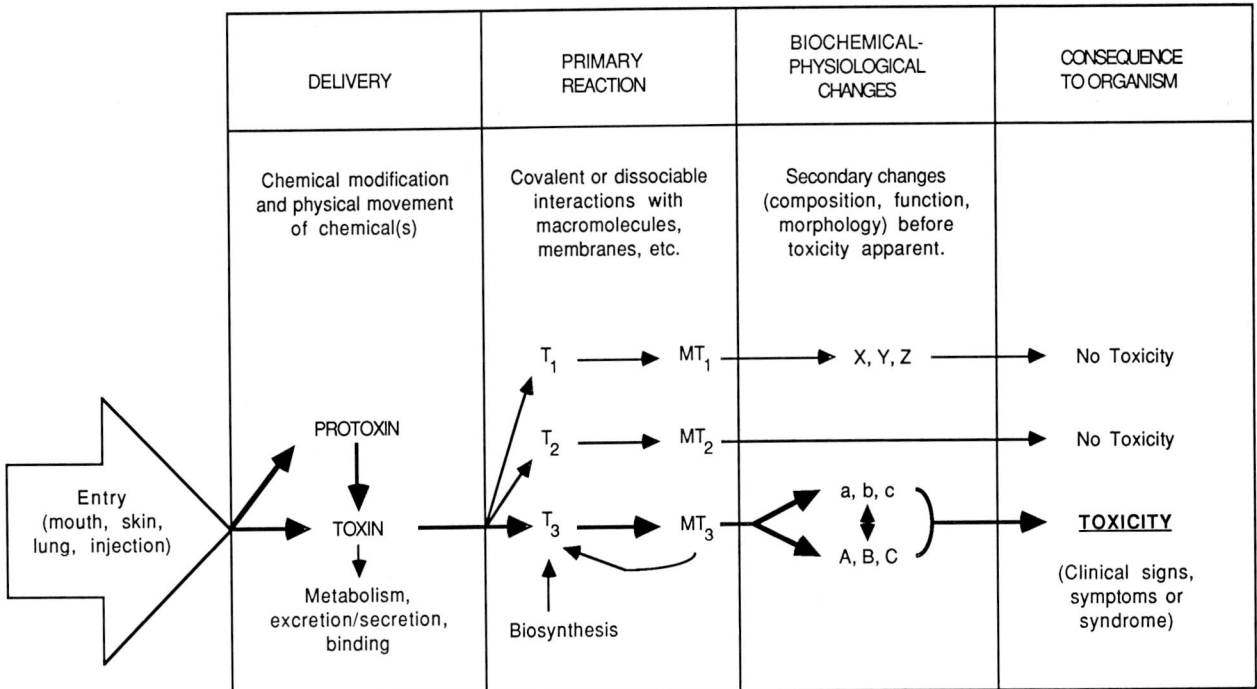

DELIVERY	PRIMARY REACTION	BIOCHEMICAL-PHYSIOLOGICAL CHANGES	CONSEQUENCE TO ORGANISM
Chemical modification and physical movement of chemical(s)	Covalent or dissociable interactions with macromolecules, membranes, etc.	Secondary changes (composition, function, morphology) before toxicity apparent.	

Figure 30–1. Scheme illustrating phases of developing toxicity following entry of drugs into an organism. Heavy lines and letters lead to toxicity, whereas light lines are events that are unproductive. T_1, T_2, T_3 and MT_1, MT_2, MT_3 are targets before and after modification by the drug, respectively, and A, B, C; X, Y, Z; and a, b, c represent an undefined and often unconnected number of changes that may or may not be sequential. Acute and chronic toxicity may be differentiated by the time in one or several of the phases. Recovery from changes in function or morphology can occur by regeneration of T_3 and by disposal and repair of modified tissue. (Modified from Aldridge WN. Trends Pharmacol Sci 2:228, 1981, with permission.)

by the availability of GSH, which in turn is limited by its rate of synthesis, and the rate of reaction between reactive intermediates of bromobenzene and macromolecules in the liver increases markedly as GSH is depleted.[7] Thus, the rate of replenishment of GSH, as well as the rate of depletion, is a critical factor in acute hepatotoxicity by bromobenzene.

Acetaminophen (paracetamol, 4-hydroxyacetanilide) causes centrilobular hepatic necrosis upon overdosage.[8] The drug mainly undergoes sulfation and glucuronidation at normal dose levels in most species (Fig. 30–2). However, at dose levels that begin to saturate the pathways of sulfation and glucuronidation, bioactivation occurs to an increasing extent, forming the reactive intermediate *N*-acetyl-*p*-benzoquinone imine (NAPQI) (Fig. 30–3).[9] NAPQI is a highly reactive compound. It reacts with cell components if not detoxified by conjugation with GSH, which depletes GSH and diminishes the efficiency of cytoprotective mechanisms. Thus, overdosage with acetaminophen causes depletion of cellular GSH, followed by oxidation, alkylation (covalent binding), or both of cysteinyl residues in cellular proteins. Another mechanism of acetaminophen-induced cell injury is oxidative stress.[10, 11] NAPQI-induced cytotoxicity is accompanied by oxidation of thiol groups in proteins, and cytotoxicity of NAPQI can be prevented by a reducing agent for disulfides, e.g., dithiothreitol (DTT). There is uncertainty, however, about the relative contributions of oxidative stress and injury mediated by covalent binding of NAPQI during overdosage of acetaminophen (Fig. 30–4).

Large doses of morphine in rats also deplete hepatic glutathione and are associated with threefold elevation in activities of glutamic oxaloacetic transaminase (SGOT) and glutamic pyruvic transaminase (SGPT) in serum.[12–14] Prior treatment of rats with phenobarbital enhances the morphine-elicited rise in SGOT and SGPT.[15] The bioactivation of morphine involves a cytochrome P450–dependent oxidation at the benzylic C-10 position to form an electrophilic species that can react with nucleophilic thiols such as GSH.[16] Thus, metabolism of morphine can deplete thiols and cause liver damage. Overdosage or use of morphine in combination with other drugs that require GSH for detoxification therefore will increase the risk of toxicity to either agent. Alkylation of critical cellular targets by a metabolic intermediate appears to be important in the heptotoxicity of morphine.

Furosemide shows negligible covalent binding and little nephro- or hepatotoxicity below a threshold dose of about 150 mg/kg.[17, 18] Metabolism of furosemide does not deplete the liver of glutathione, except by oxidative stress, nor apparently of any other protective nucleophiles. These results suggest that the relative reactivity of nucleophiles in the cell, including GSH and thiol groups of proteins, is important in the unusually selective covalent binding of furosemide to proteins.

Chemically reactive intermediates produced during metabolism of xenobiotics can bind to proteins in endoplasmic reticulum,[19, 20] to nuclear proteins,[21–23] cytosolic proteins,[24–26] and to DNA.[23, 27] Covalent binding to DNA has been proposed as a quantitative indicator for genotoxicity.[27] The correspondence of covalent binding to proteins and the cytotoxic properties of drugs and foreign chemicals remains uncertain, because there is only a general understanding of how adduct formation alters the function of

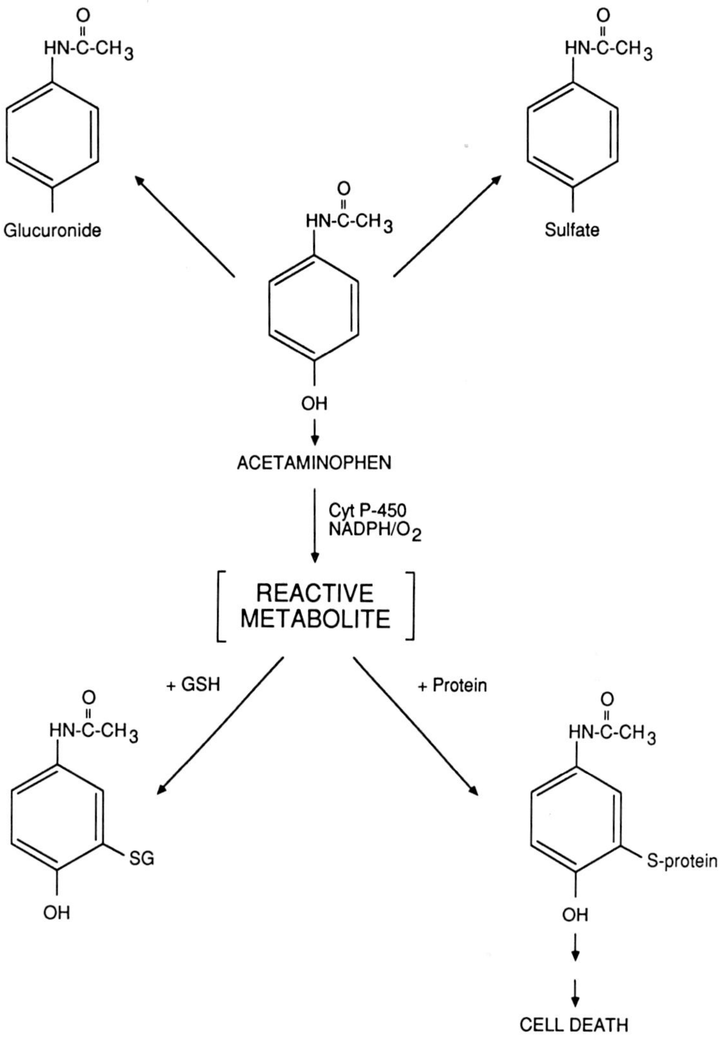

Figure 30–2. Proposed metabolism of acetaminophen in the liver. (From van de Straat R. In: van de Straat R, ed. Paracetamol-Induced Hepatotoxicity and Prevention by Structural Modification. Amsterdam, Free University Press, 1987, with permission.)

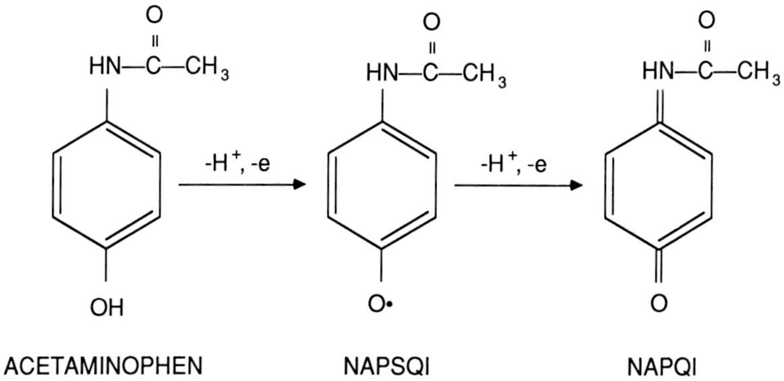

Figure 30–3. Structures of acetaminophen and its proposed reactive metabolites N-acetyl-p-semiquinone imine (NAPSQI) and N-acetyl-p-benzoquinone imine (NAPQI). (From van de Straat R. In: van de Straat R, ed. Paracetamol-Induced Hepatotoxicity and Prevention by Structural Modification. Amsterdam, Free University Press, 1987, with permission.)

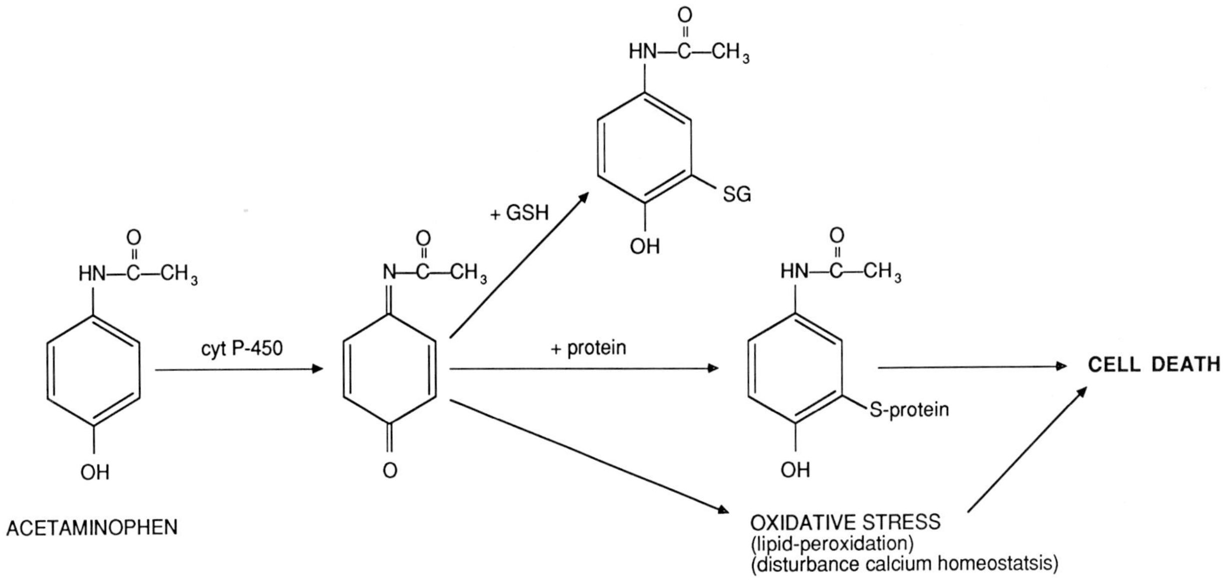

Figure 30–4. Proposed mechanisms for the hepatotoxicity induced by the reactive metabolite of acetaminophen. (From van de Straat R. In: van de Straat R, ed. Paracetamol-Induced Hepatotoxicity and Prevention by Structural Modification. Amsterdam, Free University Press, 1987, with permission.)

specific proteins. Also, little attention has been given to the significance of damage to DNA for acute hepatocellular toxicity.

HOMEOSTASIS OF GLUTATHIONE

Depending on the cell type, the intracellular concentration of GSH is in the range of 0.5 to 10 mM.[28] Concentrations in the liver are 4 to 8 mM. Nearly all the glutathione is present in the reduced form of GSH. Less than 5 per cent of the total is present as glutathione disulfide (GSSG). Continual endogenous production of reduced oxygen species, including hydrogen peroxide and lipid hydroperoxides, causes constant production of some GSSG, however (Fig. 30–5). The GSH content of various organs and tissues represents at least 90 per cent of the total nonprotein, low-molecular weight thiols. The liver content of GSH is nearly twice that in kidneys and testes and more than threefold greater than in the lungs. The importance of hepatic GSH for protection against reactive intermediates has been reviewed extensively.[29, 30] However, additional information about the status of GSH in mammalian tissues continues to

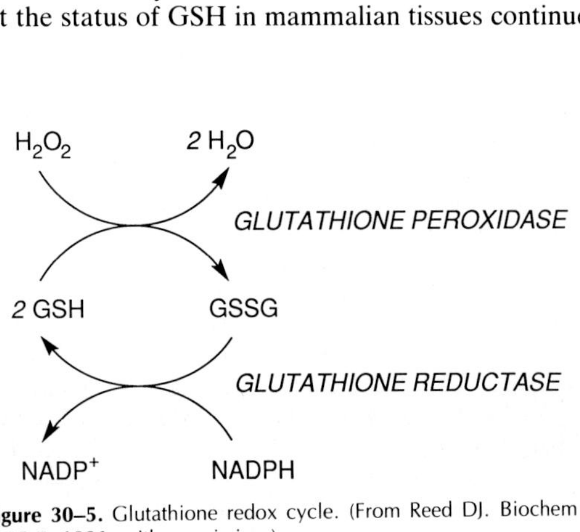

be reported. The high concentration (up to 7 to 8 mM) of GSH in the glandular tissue of the stomach compared with the squamous portion or other portions of the gastrointestinal tract has been suggested to account for the resistance of the glandular portion of the stomach to certain carcinogens as compared with the squamous portion, which is highly susceptible to induction of tumors by polycyclic aromatic hydrocarbons.[31]

Cystine has a sparing effect on the requirement of the essential amino acid methionine in the rat.[32] This observation is in agreement with the unidirectional process of transsulfuration in which methionine sulfur and serine carbon are used in cysteine biosynthesis by way of the cystathionine pathway (for a review, see reference 29).

The cystathionine pathway in the liver is of major importance among pathways of drug metabolism that involve GSH or cysteine or both. Depletion of GSH by rapid conjugation can increase synthesis of GSH to rates as high as 2 to 3 μmol/hour/g wet liver tissue.[33] The cysteine pool in the liver, which is about 0.2 μmol/g, has an estimated half-life of 2 to 3 minutes at such high rates of synthesis of GSH.[29] Although the cystathionine pathway appears to be highly responsive to the need for cysteine biosynthesis in the liver, the organ distribution of the pathway may be limited. Recent evidence indicates that in mammals such as rats the liver may be the main site of cysteine biosynthesis, which occurs via the cystathionine pathway. Maintenance of high concentrations of GSH in the liver in association with high rates of secretion into plasma and extensive extracellular degradation of GSH and GSSG supports the concept that liver GSH is a physiologic reservoir of cysteine.[34, 35]

Liver has two pools of GSH. One has a fast (2-hour) and the other a slow (30-hour) turnover.[35, 36] The mitochondrial pool of GSH (about 10 per cent of the total cellular pool) has a half-life of 30 hours; the half-life of the cytoplasmic pool is 2 hours, suggesting that the mitochondrial pool represents the stable pool of GSH in whole animals.[37]

The concentration of GSH in the liver is altered in rats

Figure 30–5. Glutathione redox cycle. (From Reed DJ. Biochem Pharmacol 35:7, 1986, with permission.)

by diurnal or circadian variations and starvation. The highest levels of GSH occur at night and early morning and the lowest levels in the late afternoon. The maximum variation is as much as 25 to 30 per cent.[31, 38, 39] Starvation limits the availability of methionine for synthesis of GSH in the liver and decreases the concentration of GSH by about 50 per cent of the level in fed animals.[38, 40, 41] Assuming GSH is a physiologic reservoir for plasma cysteine,[35] efflux of GSH from liver will continue during starvation, and the released cysteine will help maintain levels of GSH in organs other than the liver.

Treatment of rats with an inhibitor of γ-glutamyl transpeptidase (AT-125) prevents degradation of GSH in plasma, leading to massive excretion of GSH in the urine.[42] This treatment also lowers the hepatic content of GSH because it inhibits recycling of cysteine to the liver.[37] A physiologic decrease in interorgan recycling of cysteine to the liver for synthesis of GSH could account in part for the decrease of hepatic GSH during starvation and for the marked diurnal variation in concentrations of GSH in liver.

The efflux of GSH from the liver and metabolism of GSH and GSSG in plasma appears to ensure a continuous supply of cysteine in plasma. This pool of cysteine should minimize in turn the fluctuation of GSH concentrations within the various organs that require only cysteine or cystine or both rather than methionine for synthesis of GSH.

DEPLETION OF GSH AND DRUG-INDUCED INJURY

Fasting enhances the hepatotoxicity of many drugs and other xenobiotics. One of the earliest studies of this phenomenon compared the effects of fasting and various diets on chloroform-induced hepatotoxicity.[43] Increased hepatotoxicity in association with fasting occurred with chemicals that depleted GSH, including carbon tetrachloride,[44-50] 1,1-dichloroethylene,[51] acetaminophen,[50, 52, 53] and bromobenzene.[50, 52] Decreases in the hepatic concentration of GSH as observed in fasted mice[50] and rats[51-54] could account for the enhanced toxicity of these chemicals in fasted animals. Thus, depletion of GSH in the liver secondary to pretreatment with diethyl maleate, also increased the hepatotoxicity of acetaminophen, bromobenzene, carbon tetrachloride, and anthracyclines.[55, 56] Interestingly, the hepatotoxicity of thioacetamide, a substrate for the flavin-dependent mono-oxygenase present in microsomes,[57] is enhanced after fasting[50] but not after pretreatment with diethyl maleate.[56] In a review of the toxicologic implications of drug metabolism, Welch suggested that depletion of GSH could be a useful toxicologic tool for the early detection of toxic metabolites.[58]

The activation of oxygen by reduction to superoxide anion radical (O_2^-), hydrogen peroxide (H_2O_2), and possibly hydroxyl free radical (·OH), and singlet oxygen ($^1O_2$), can be important for the toxicity of drugs and chemicals that are reduced or oxidized enzymatically by one-electron transfers. After a one-electron redox reaction, the resulting intermediate transfers the extra single electron to molecular oxygen to yield the superoxide anion radical and the parent drug or chemical, which can undergo repeated one-electron reductions, oxidations, or both to then provide one electron to molecular oxygen. The generation of reactive oxygen species in this way is termed redox cycling and is involved in the toxicity of many hydroquinones, quinones, metal chelates, nitro compounds, amines, and azo compounds.[59]

Formation of hydrogen peroxide by redox cycling consumes GSH in a reaction catalyzed by glutathione peroxidase. The hydrogen peroxide is metabolized to water and GSH, to GSSG, which is then reduced by NADPH-dependent glutathione reductase.

The enhancement of hepatotoxicity by depletion of GSH has been noted during the metabolism of bromobenzene.[60-62] When hepatocytes were pretreated with diethyl maleate, which reduced intracellular levels of GSH by about 70 per cent, added bromobenzene caused levels of GSH to fall to 5 per cent of initial levels, and cell death (75 per cent by 5 hours) was noted. Addition of cysteine, methionine or N-acetyl-cysteine prevented bromobenzene-induced toxicity,[63] but it did not prevent depletion of GSH. Bromobenzene, in the presence of a cysteine source, reduced initial levels of GSH to about 40 per cent of control.[61] The presence of metyrapone, an inhibitor of cytochrome P450-dependent mono-oxygenase reactions, eliminated bromobenzene-induced toxicity. These data are consistent with a requirement for P450-mediated activation of bromobenzene before conjugation with GSH. They do not indicate significant oxidative stress due to redox cycling of a metabolite of bromobenzene.

The intracellular concentration of GSH in isolated hepatocytes has been examined under conditions of oxidative stress. Production of malondialdehyde, which is an index of lipid peroxidation and occurs during oxidative stress, could be stimulated by addition of diethyl maleate (which reacts with GSH). This observation suggests that intracellular concentrations of GSH are important for the integrity of membranes.[64] That is, GSH protects against oxidative damage to unsaturated fatty acids in biologic membranes. The metal chelates, ADP·Fe^{3+} and PP_i·Fe^{3+}, which stimulate malondialdehyde production, caused iron-induced peroxidation of lipids and decreased the level of cellular GSH by about 40 per cent.[64]

GLUTATHIONE COMPARTMENTATION AND DRUG-INDUCED INJURY

Since the depletion of hepatocellular GSH by diethyl maleate never exceeds 90 to 95 per cent of total cell GSH, a pool of GSH appears unavailable to conjugate with diethyl maleate. This pool of GSH appears to be in the mitochondria.[37, 67] Hepatocytes depleted of GSH by reaction with diethyl maleate can remain viable for several hours, eventually resynthesizing the original complement of GSH. Without additional stress, such as acetaminophen[65] or ADP·Fe^{3+},[64] lipid peroxidation and cell death are not observed. Studies in this laboratory have shown that no formation of malondialdehyde above control levels was noted during 5 hours of incubation in hepatocytes partially depleted of GSH by 1,3-bis(2-chloroethyl)-1-nitrosourea (BCNU).[66] However, if adriamycin was included to enhance oxidative stress by redox cycling, GSH levels were decreased to less than 10 per cent by 3 hours, coincident with a dramatic increase in production of malondialdehyde and leakage of lactate dehydrogenase from the cells. Like diethylmaleate, there is a pool of GSH in mitochondria that is unaffected by treatment with BCNU.[37, 67] However, accessibility of BCNU to the mitochondrial matrix was shown by inhibition of mitochondrial glutathione reductase. In contrast to the effects of BCNU, a GSH S-transferase–dependent reaction with ethacrynic acid occurred in association with a rapid leakage of lactate dehydrogenase.[67]

Since the mitochondrial pool of GSH has a half-life of

about 30 hours,[37] it is expected that fasting will not deplete it. Fasting, in fact, does not increase the spontaneous rates or carbon tetrachloride-induced rates of lipid peroxidation. Hence, it may be that lipid peroxidation events are related to the size of the mitochondrial pool of GSH in liver. Moreover, perhaps certain "antioxidant" proteins in the mitochondria participate with GSH in preventing lipid peroxidation.

A controversial approach to assessing the potential for drugs to cause lipid peroxidation in vivo is to treat an intact animal with a drug or drug combination and subsequently to measure products of lipid peroxidation in microsomes. In this manner, the depletion of glutathione in vivo with agents that form glutathione conjugates enhances subsequent lipid peroxidation in vitro. Results from such experiments show consistently that an in vivo threshold of 1 μmol GSH/g liver is associated with spontaneous lipid peroxidation in microsomes.[68] This critical value of GSH is about 20 per cent of the initial concentration of GSH. Addition of exogenous GSH inhibited the lipid peroxidation in vitro in a concentration-dependent manner; 1 μM GSH yielded 50 per cent inhibition.

GLUTATHIONE REDUCTASE AND GLUTATHIONE PEROXIDASE

Glutathione reductase, which is important in the regulation of the bioreductive activation of drugs by GSH, is itself regulated by the redox status of the cell. Being similar to other reductases such as nitrate, nitrite, and $NADP^+$ reductase, GSH reductase is inactivated upon reduction by its own electron donor, NADPH. It has been proposed that this auto-inactivation of glutathione reductase by NADPH and the protection as well as reactivation by GSSG regulates the enzyme in vivo.[69] The activity of glutathione reductase may reflect the physiologic needs of the cell, especially during oxidative stress. For example, 40 to 50 μM intracellular NADPH inactivates glutathione reductase in the absence of GSSG and decreases glucose metabolism via the hexose monophosphate pathway. The physiologic ratio of GSSG:GSH should provide sufficient GSSG at this level of NADPH to permit retention of significant glutathione reductase activity by preventing inactivation.[69]

GLUTATHIONE REDOX CYCLE

It is apparent that a major protective role against the reactive drug intermediates, which are generated by bioreduction and cause oxidative stress by redox cycling, is provided by the ubiquitous glutathione redox cycle (Fig. 30–5). This cycle utilizes NADPH and, indirectly, NADH-reducing equivalents in the mitochondrial matrix as well as the cytoplasm to provide GSH by the glutathione reductase–catalyzed reduction of GSSG. The rates of NADPH consumption in liver by the various NADPH-dependent enzymes indicate that glutathione reductase has by far the highest rate (Table 30–1). Therefore, when the glutathione redox cycle is functioning at maximum capacity to eliminate hydrogen peroxide, a major regulatory effect is imposed on other NADPH-dependent pathways.

The mitochondrial glutathione redox cycle has a role in regulating mitochondrial oxidations in liver. Various oxidants decrease O_2 uptake by isolated mitochondria and cause a complete turnover of GSH via glutathione peroxi-

TABLE 30–1. ESTIMATION OF THE RATES OF NADPH CONSUMPTION IN LIVER

Activity	Rate (μmol/min/g Liver)	Reference
Fatty acid synthesis	1–2	71
Mixed function oxidase	1–2	72
t-Butyl hydroperoxide reduction	1.5	73
Glutathione reductase*	8–10	74

Source: Reed DJ. Biochem Pharmacol 35:7, copyright 1986, Pergamon Press plc.

*The estimated maximal rate of glutathione peroxidase activity is 40 μmol/min/g liver.[75]

dase every 10 minutes.[76] It appears that a continuous flow of reducing equivalents through the glutathione redox cycle is balanced by a continuous formation of mitochondrial NADPH, which is needed for glutathione reductase activity. In addition, metabolism of hydrogen peroxide in mitochondria poses a regulatory function in regard to the oxidation of substrates by lipoamide-dependent ketoacid oxidases,[76] which generate NADPH-reducing equivalents. The entire $NADPH:NADP^+$ pool may turn over at least once every minute during a maximum oxidant challenge.[76]

HEPATOCELLULAR INJURY BY REDOX CYCLING

Diquat (DQ) (Fig. 30–6), a bipyridyl herbicide that is hepatotoxic, is a model compound for redox cycling. It generates large amounts of superoxide anion radical and hydrogen peroxide within cells (Fig. 30–7). Evidence to support the protective role of the glutathione redox cycle is that the toxicity of diquat in vivo and in vitro appears to be mediated by redox cycling and is greatly enhanced by prior treatment with BCNU,[77] which is an inhibitor of glutathione reductase.[78] Ebselen, a synthetic compound possessing glutathione peroxidase–like activity, protects against diquat cytotoxicity when extracellular glutathione is present in the medium.[79] Superoxide anion radical, which can reduce ferric iron to ferrous iron, is produced during diquat toxicity. Desferrioxamine, which chelates intracellular iron in the ferric state with an affinity constant of 10^{31},[80] provides considerable protection against diquat-induced toxicity. Therefore, hydrogen peroxide and transition metals have been suggested as major contributors to diquat toxicity.[80] Even though the hydroxyl radical or a related species seems the most likely ultimate toxic product of the hydrogen peroxide–ferrous iron interaction, scavengers of hydroxyl radical afford only minimal protection.[80] However, the high degree of reactivity of hydroxyl radicals assures

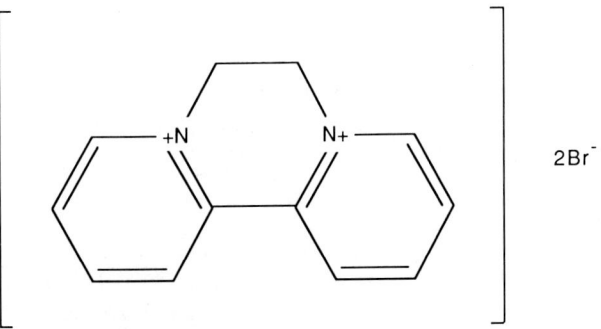

Figure 30–6. Diquat.

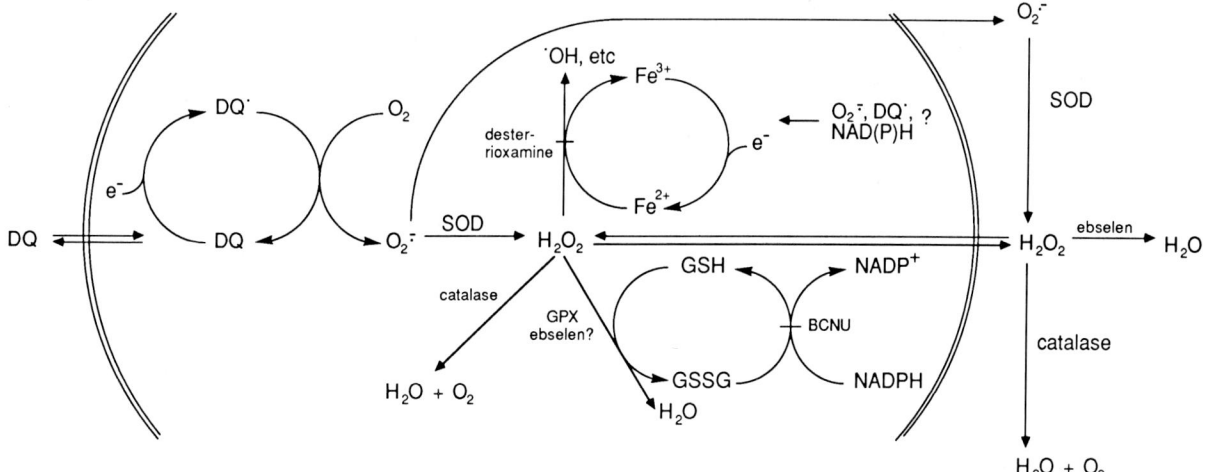

Figure 30–7. Scheme of postulated interactions between diquat, diquat-derived active oxygen species, internal and external enzymes, and transition metals. DQ = diquat; DQ• = diquat radical; GPX = glutathione peroxidase; SOD = superoxide dismutase.

that the site of interaction with cellular components is within close proximity (a few angstroms) of the site of generation of the radical. Much remains to be understood about the mechanism of cytotoxicity by the various redox cycling agents, including the quinones, menadione, and adriamycin, which are discussed in more detail later.

LIPID PEROXIDATION AND OXIDATIVE CELL INJURY

Oxidative stress, which is based on activated molecular species of oxygen is a complex process that can result in the peroxidative damage of all major classes of biochemicals, including amino acids, carbohydrates, lipids, proteins, and nucleic acids (Fig. 30–8).[82, 83] However, damage to membrane lipids and the associated alterations in bulk properties of membranes frequently have been considered to be the basis for drug-induced hepatocellular injury and loss of cell viability (for a review see reference 81).

Oxidative stress has been characterized in terms of the sequence of events that appear early in development of cell injury with the hepatocyte model system (Fig. 30–9).[83] Depletion of intracellular GSH is suggested to be critical if not a prerequisite for subsequent alterations in protein thiol and calcium homeostasis. In addition, a combination of calcium release from intracellular stores and inhibition of calcium efflux appears to result in a marked and sustained increase in cytosolic concentration of calcium associated with surface blebbing and increased activity of certain

calcium-dependent enzymes.[83] GSH appears to exert a protective effect by preventing oxidation and loss of function of protein thiol groups, which appear critical for calcium transport by the endoplasmic reticulum.[83]

DRUG-INDUCED BIOREDUCTION, THE RATE OF GLUTATHIONE CONSUMPTION, AND ITS REGULATION

The bioreduction reactions in the activation of drugs can consume a significant fraction of the reducing equivalents in the cell that are derived from NADPH. The availability of reducing equivalents consumed via NADPH and glutathione quickly provides the reducing equivalents for bioreduction of drugs. Bioreduction in the activation of drugs appears to incur the potential hazards of "prodrugs." Prodrugs undergo conversion to active drugs essentially by two mechanisms: (1) direct conversion or (2) the formation of an unstable intermediate that undergoes a reaction, usually spontaneous, to yield the active drug.[70, 85] These processes are not exclusive, and the intermediates may have the potential for greater toxicity than the drug itself.

The glutathione redox cycle (see Fig. 30–5) is the major pathway providing the reducing equivalents for bioreduction of drug-induced formation of superoxide anion radical and hydrogen peroxide (Fig. 30–10). The maximum rate of GSSG reduction by glutathione reductase appears to be about 8 to 10 μmol/min/g of liver.[74] Glutathione peroxidase, a selenium-dependent enzyme that is highly

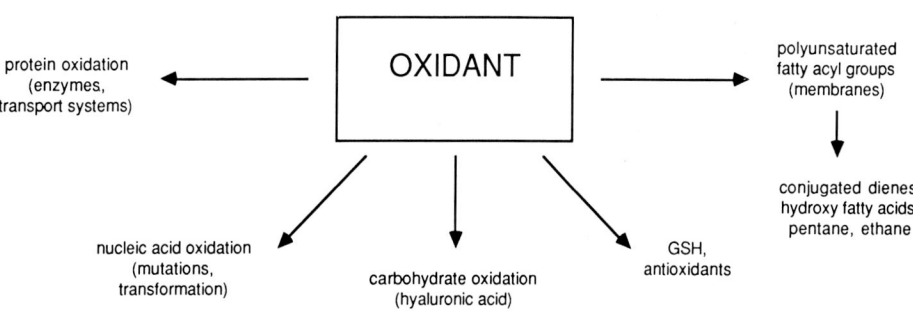

Figure 30–8. Molecular targets of oxidative injury. GSH = reduced glutathione. (From Keberle H. Ann NY Acad Sci 119:758, 1964, with permission.)

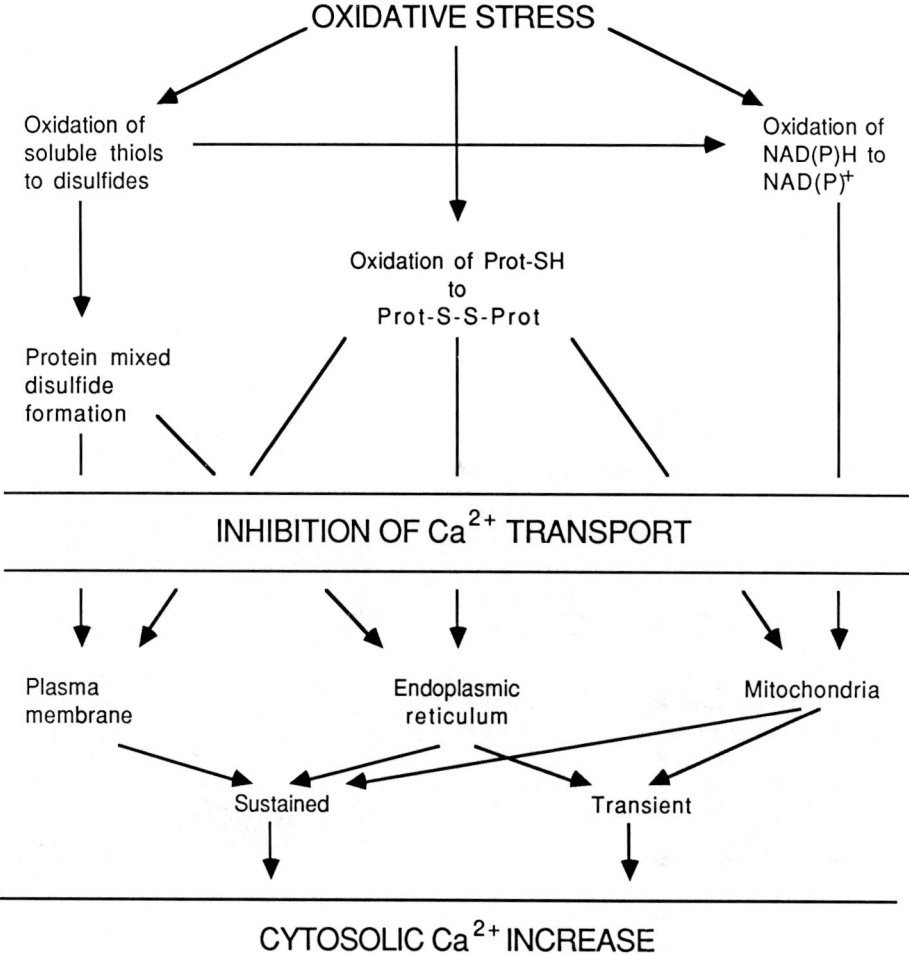

Figure 30–9. Mechanisms contributing to the increase in cytosolic Ca^{2+} level during oxidative stress in isolated hepatocytes. (From Bellomo G, Orrenius S. Hepatology 5:876, 1985, © by Am. Assoc. for The Study of Liver Diseases.)

NITROAROMATIC REDOX CYCLING

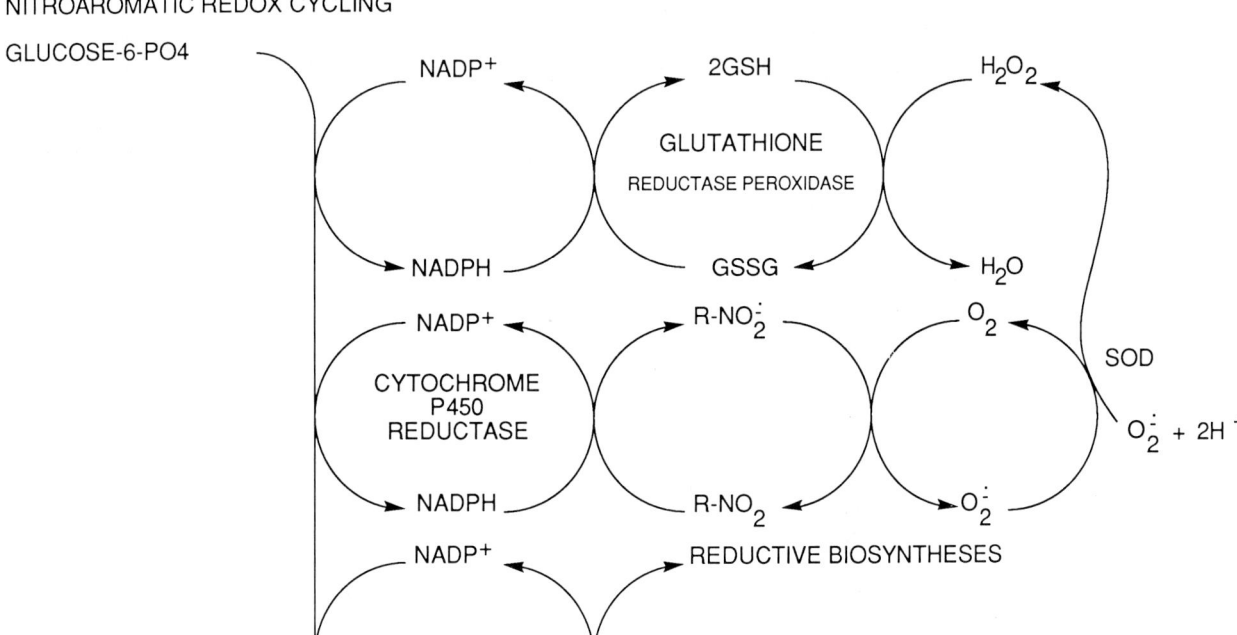

Figure 30–10. Nitro aromatic reduction and redox cycling SOD = superoxide dismustase. (From Reed DJ. Biochem Pharmacol 35:7, 1986, with permission.)

specific for glutathione, is capable of rapidly detoxifying hydrogen peroxide and certain hydroperoxides. The maximal rate of GSSG oxidation by glutathione peroxidase is 40 μmol/min/g liver.[75] Since the maximum rate of NADP+ reduction to NADPH by the hexose monophosphate pathway in the liver appears to be about 1 to 2 μmol/min/g liver,[71, 72, 87] the glutathione redox cycle, when functioning at maximum capacity, can impose a major regulating effect on fatty acid synthesis, the activities of mixed-function oxidases, and other NADPH-dependent functions.

The extent to which bioreduction uses mitochondrial-reducing equivalents is uncertain, but evidence is increasing that such effects are important and relate to both calcium and protein thiol homeostasis of mitochondria. For example, the loss of NADPH, which occurs following addition of menadione to isolated mitochondria, is not related to its consumption via the glutathione redox cycle but more likely to bioreductive metabolism by NADH-ubiquinone oxidoreductase.[88, 89]

NAPQI, a reactive metabolite of acetaminophen (discussed earlier in the section Covalent Binding of Reactive Intermediates), undergoes a nonenzymatic, two-electron reduction in the presence of glutathione to yield stoichiometric amounts of acetaminophen and GSSG.[90] BCNU-induced inactivation of glutathione reductase prevents the reduction of NAPQI-generated GSSG and increases cytotoxicity but has no effect on the covalent binding of NAPQI to cellular proteins. A competing reaction at physiologic pH is the formation of an acetaminophen-GSH conjugate. Incubation of NAPQI with hepatocytes yields the same reaction products in control and in BCNU-treated hepatocytes. The thiol dithiothreitol protects against cytotoxicity even after covalent binding has occurred. It has been

speculated that the toxicity of NAPQI for isolated heptocytes results primarily from its oxidative effects on cellular proteins.[90]

Bioreductive activation of aromatic and heterocyclic nitro compounds occurs by reduction of the nitro moiety to unstable intermediates, including free radicals (Fig. 30–11).[91, 92] The production of superoxide anion radicals and nitrone anion free radicals during metabolism of nitrazepam is a typical example of secondary formation of hydrogen peroxide via NADPH cytochrome P450 reductase that is capable of stimulating the consumption of both GSH and NADPH-reducing equivalents.[93]

The antitumor agent adriamycin (benzanthraquinone) undergoes rapid bioreduction by NADPH-dependent cytochrome P450 reductase with concomitant consumption of oxygen.[94] Adriamycin cytotoxicity may be the result of free radicals formed by bioreduction that overwhelm the cellular antioxidant capacity, including that proportion provided by the glutathione redox cycle. Inactivation of glutathione reductase with BCNU has permitted the demonstration of the protective role of the glutathione redox cycle against an adriamycin-mediated challenge.[66, 67] Depletion of GSH concurrently with inactivation of glutathione reductase can enhance the cellular injury mediated by adriamycin-generated radicals in isolated hepatocytes.[67]

BIOREDUCTION BY GLUTATHIONE S-TRANSFERASES

GSH-dependent protection against lipid peroxidation has been demonstrated in mitochondria,[95–97] nuclei,[98] microsomes,[95, 97–101] and cytosol of rat liver.[102–105] Lipid peroxida-

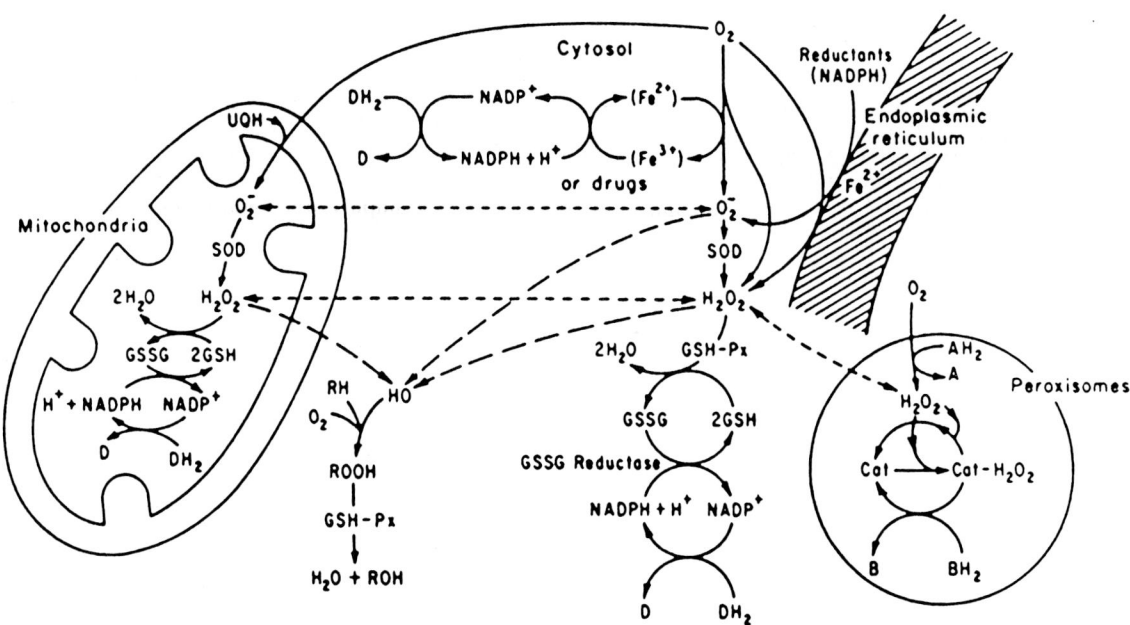

Figure 30–11. Schematic diagram of cellular protection against oxygen-mediated toxicity. UQH: semiquinone of ubiquinone. D, DH, AH_2, B, BH_2: various cellular substrates involved in enzymatic redox reactions. SOD, superoxide dismutase; CAT, catalase. (Modified by permission of the publisher from Hepatic hydroperoxide metabolism, by Sies H, et al. In: Isolation, Characterization, and Use of Hepatocytes, p. 341. Copyright 1983 by Elsevier Science Publishing Co, Inc.)

tion induced in mitochondria also is inhibited by respiratory substrates such as succinate, which leads indirectly to reduction of ubiquinone to ubiquinol. The latter is a potent antioxidant.[106–108] However, the essential factor in preventing accumulation of lipid peroxides and lysis of membranes in mitochondria is glutathione peroxidase.[109] Although the prevention of free radical attack on membrane lipids may occur by an electron shuttle that utilizes vitamin E and GSH in microsomes, similar activity may not be capable of inhibiting peroxidation in mitochondria.[99, 110] Instead, mitochondrial GSH S-transferase(s) may prevent lipid peroxidation in mitochondria by a nonselenium glutathione–dependent peroxidase activity. Three GSH S-transferases have been isolated from the mitochondrial matrix,[111] and

TABLE 30–2. PROFILES OF GSH S-TRANSFERASES AND GSH PEROXIDASES IN RAT LIVER

Location		GSH S-transferase (CDNB)	Substrate	GSH Peroxidase
Mitochondria	Whole	Distribution of total activity (Cyt, 90%; Mit, 7%)[113]	CHP	Distribution of total activity (Cyt, 60%; Mit, 28 percent; Mic, 7%[114]
	Matrix	Isolation of three enzymes[111]	tBH	Se-independent, 5 percent activity Se-dependent Mit activity[76]
			CHP and tBH H_2O_2	Purification of Se-dependent[115]
	Innermem		CHP and H_2O_2	Se-independent, available both substrates*[116]
	Outermem	N-ethylmaleimide–activatable, immunochemical identity with microsomal enzyme[112]		
Microsomes		N-ethylmaleimide–activatable, purification distinct from cytosolic enzymes[117, 118, 119]	CHP	N-ethylmaleimide–activatable, purification, associated with GSH S-transferase activity[120]
		Distribution of specific activity (Cyt, 91%; Mic, 9%;[121] no activity toward BSP,[119] inhibition by BSP[122]		
Cytosol		Presence of at least 7 enzymes distinct from cytosolic enzymes[123, 124, 125]	CHP and H_2O_2	Presence of Se-dependent (CHP and H_2O_2) and Se-independent (CHP)[126]
		Inhibition by BSP[127]	CHP and tBH	Identity of GSH S-transferase B and Se-independent, and inhibition by BSP[128]
Cumene hydroperoxide			CHP CHP	35% of Se-independent activity[129]

Source: Yonaha M, Tampo Y. Biochem Pharmacol 36:2831, copyright 1987, Pergamon Press plc.)
*Data in mice (such activity is detectable in mitochondrial intermembrane space of rat livers). Unpublished work.
DNB = dinitrobenzene; tBH = t-butylhydroperoxide; CHP = cumene hydroperoxide.

nearly 5 per cent of the mitochondrial outer membrane protein consists of microsomal glutathione S-transferase.[112] GSH S-transferase in the outer mitochondrial membrane could provide the GSH-dependent protection of mitochondria by scavenging lipid radicals by a mechanism that requires vitamin E and is abolished by bromosulfophthalein.[112] Some properties of the GSH S-transferases and glutathione peroxidases in the rat liver are summarized in Table 30–2.[113–129]

MITOCHONDRIAL CALCIUM AND DRUG-INDUCED HEPATOTOXICITY

Mitochondria can sequester large amounts of calcium.[130] This process is driven by the membrane potential (Fig. 30–12). Recent studies of this process, which is sensitive to ruthenium red,[131] have led to the proposal that mitochondria may be a major regulator of cytosolic concentrations of calcium under pathologic conditions. Storage sites for calcium in mitochondrial membranes can apparently maintain extramitochondrial calcium at levels 5 to 10 times higher than normal cytosolic levels.[132] It appears that under normal physiologic conditions, these sites are responsible solely for regulating intramitochondrial calcium homeostasis.[133] Although mitochondrial regulation of cytosolic calcium appears unlikely, recent observations show that ruthenium red can prevent oxidative stress and associated cell injury under certain conditions.[134] A variety of hepatotoxins, including acetaminophen[135] and menadione,[136] can deplete soluble and protein thiols and disrupt calcium homeostasis. A partial explanation for the loss of calcium homeostasis under these conditions is a decrease in the activity of calcium-ATPase in plasma membranes secondary to oxidation of essential thiols in the protein or by formation of covalent adducts.[86, 136]

PROTEIN THIOLS AND HEPATOTOXICITY

Thiol groups are known to be important for normal protein functions, and increasing evidence supports their vital importance for cell viability during cytotoxic events. Protein inactivation by oxidation of protein cysteinyl thiols occurs in more than 240 enzymes.[137, 138] Membrane-bound enzymes are damaged during lipid peroxidation, and evidence of vitamin E protection strongly supports a free radical mechanism for protein damage via oxidative stress.[139] Oxidative stress can cause loss of protein functions by damaging amino acid residues other than cysteine, including methionine, tryptophan, and histidine. An important aspect of such damage is that lipid peroxidative events can amplify free radical processes that propagate chain reactions. Failure to terminate free radical processes with a chain-breaking antioxidant, such as vitamin E, can lead to 4 to 10 propagation events occurring per initiation, and thus each initiation is amplified.[96] Products of lipid peroxidation can also compromise detoxication systems. Since the reduction of lipid hydroperoxides by GSH utilizes NADPH for the regeneration of GSH from GSSG, the rate of NADPH production can be limiting during oxidative stress.[70] Therefore, GSSG may be transported from the liver when reduction is limited by low levels of NADPH.[140] Decreased availability of NADPH and GSH can impair GSH-dependent detoxication pathways for hydrogen peroxide[75] and free radicals[100] and can decrease protection of thiols in protein.[141] Thus, energy-dependent processes involving NADPH, GSH, and thiols in proteins, appear to be critically involved in cellular homeostasis during drug-induced toxicity.

ALTERATION OF CALCIUM HOMEOSTASIS

Of major interest is the question of whether a unifying mechanism exists for drug-induced liver injury. Necrotic tissues accumulate calcium.[142] It has been proposed that the accumulation of calcium represents an influx of extracellular calcium from interstitial spaces into injured cells.[143] Since such an influx was thought to occur regardless of the mechanism of toxication, this extracellular calcium-dependent mechanism was termed the final common pathway for cell death.[144] For example, a variety of hepatotoxins, including ethyl methanesulfonate, phallodin, and the calcium ionophore A23187 are known to require extracellular calcium for the expression of toxicity in cultured hepatocytes.[144, 145] In contrast, the toxicity of carbon tetrachloride, bromobenzene, and ethyl methanesulfonate for freshly isolated hepatocytes was not dependent upon extracellular calcium but was potentiated by the absence of calcium in

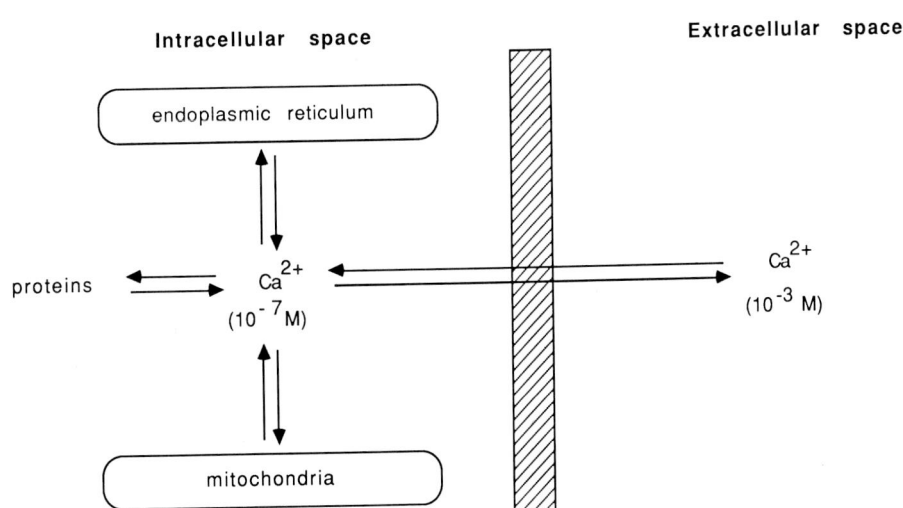

Figure 30–12. Ca^{2+}-compartmentation in the hepatocyte, which is regulated by various active transport systems in the mitochondria, endoplasmic reticulum, and plasma membrane. (From van de Straat R. In: van de Straat R. Paracetamol-Induced Hepatotoxicity and Prevention by Structural Modification. Amsterdam, Free University Press, 1987, with permission.)

the medium.[146–148] Insight into these kinds of discrepancies came from the observation that cell viability was closely associated with the antioxidant status of the cells—especially in the absence of extracellular calcium.[141, 149–152] Differences in the antioxidant composition of the media appear critical for the differential effects of calcium on cell toxicity.

THE CALCIUM OMISSION MODEL OF OXIDATIVE INJURY

A model for hepatocellular injury based on omission of calcium from the medium shows extensive oxidative injury to freshly isolated rat hepatocytes by alteration in calcium homeostasis (Fig. 30–13). Hepatocytes incubated in the absence of calcium form increased products of lipid peroxidation and have a marked loss of mitochondrial and cytosolic GSH concomitant with increased formation of GSSG and efflux of GSH and GSSG.[153] In addition, vitamin E is depleted rapidly and leakage of potassium and lactate dehydrogenase are increased during calcium omission.[154] The presence of antioxidants such as vitamin E (succinate ester), N,N'-diphenyl-p-phenylenediamine, and the iron chelators [desferrioxamine and edetic acid (EDTA)] prevents the loss of GSH, vitamin E, and thiols in proteins and prevents lipid peroxidation as measured by formation of malondialdehyde. Calcium omission resulted in a marked decline of the mitochondrial membrane potential, which

could be prevented by ruthenium red–induced blockage of calcium uptake into the mitochondria through the uniport system (Fig. 30–14).[134] Ruthenium red in fact abolished completely the oxidative stress and cell injury associated with the absence of extracellular calcium. From these results, Thomas and Reed concluded that cycling of calcium into and out of mitochondria may be an essential component of oxidative stress that is provoked by calcium deprivation.[134, 154] On the other hand, the oxidative stress and severe cell damage generated by paraquat and BCNU, which had only a slight effect on mitochondrial membrane potential, were not prevented by ruthenium red. Thus, the oxidative stress generated by redox active chemicals is distinct from that generated by the absence of extracellular calcium. The absence of calcium appears to induce calcium cycling in and out of the mitochondria by way of the calcium transport processes to amplify the effects of oxidative stress. Cell injury and cell death do not result solely from a decline of mitochondrial membrane potential, but impairment of endogenous antioxidant defense mechanisms appears to predispose cells to oxidative damage.

An important feature of the injury caused by calcium omission is the massive blebbing of isolated hepatocytes.[155] The blebbing is reversible by resuspension of the hepatocytes in calcium-containing medium or addition of micromolar concentrations of vitamin E succinate to the calcium-deficient medium. Maintenance of vitamin E levels appears to be essential for limiting the effects of oxidative stress on

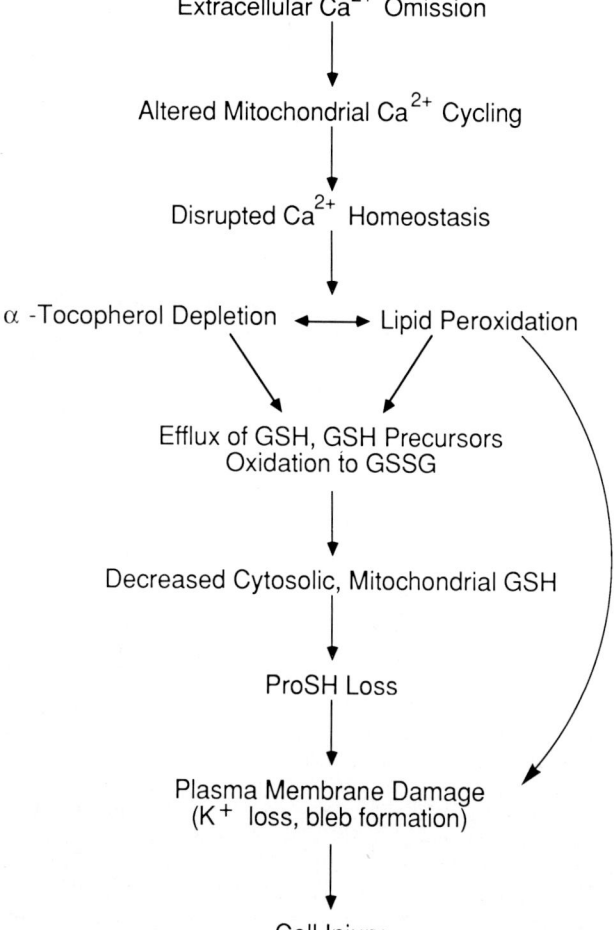

Figure 30–13. Calcium-omission model of oxidative stress to isolated hepatocytes: sequence of events leading to cellular injury.

Extracellular Ca²⁺ Omission

Altered Mitochondrial Ca²⁺ Cycling

Disrupted Ca²⁺ Homeostasis

α-Tocopherol Depletion ⟷ Lipid Peroxidation

Efflux of GSH, GSH Precursors
Oxidation to GSSG

Decreased Cytosolic, Mitochondrial GSH

ProSH Loss

Plasma Membrane Damage
(K⁺ loss, bleb formation)

Cell Injury

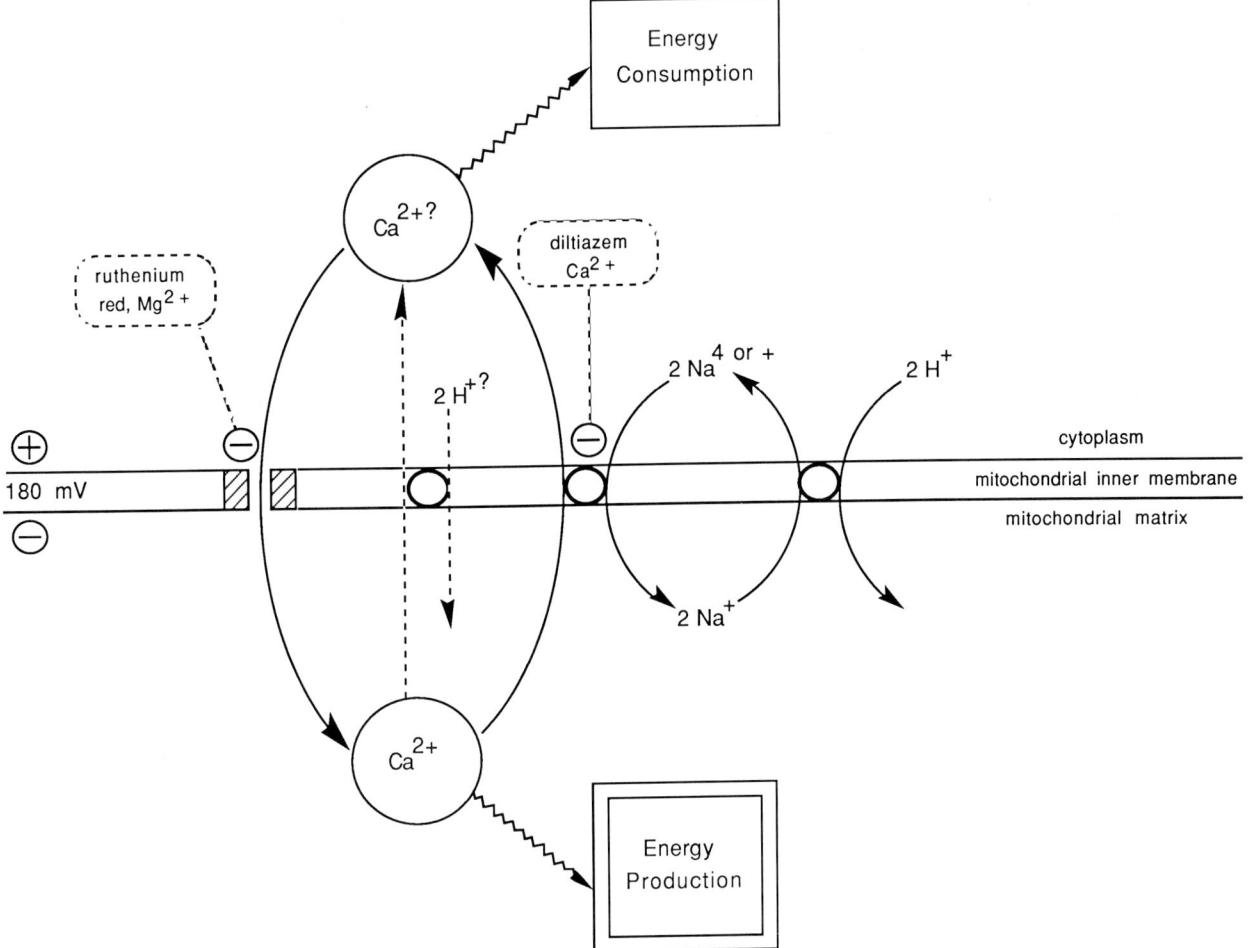

Figure 30–14. The Ca^{2+}-transport system of the inner membrane of vertebrate mitochondria and its effectors. (From McCormack JG, Denton RM. Trends Biochem Sci 11:258, 1986, with permission.)

membranes and thiols. Thus, changes in thiol redox status caused by efflux of GSH and the loss of vitamin E appear to predispose the plasma membrane to increasing permeability and massive blebbing.[155]

MORPHOLOGIC CHANGES DURING DRUG-INDUCED INJURY

Blebbing of the cell surface is an early consequence of hypoxic and toxic injury to cells.[142, 156–159] Since a rise in cytosolic free calcium has been suggested as the stimulus for bleb formation[135, 157, 159] and the final common pathway to irreversible cell injury,[83, 144, 159, 160] individual hepatocytes in culture have been monitored for "chemical hypoxia" induced by cyanide and iodoacetate.[161] During chemical hypoxia, free calcium in the cytosol did not change with bleb formation or before loss of cell viability. Cell death appears to be precipitated by a sudden breakdown of the permeability of the plasma membrane barrier, as would occur by rupture of a surface bleb.[161] The only change observed to accompany bleb formation was a fall of the mitochondrial membrane potential.[161] However, Andersson and Jones reported the persistence of the mitochondrial membrane potential in suspensions of isolated hepatocytes

during anoxia,[162] which may be essential for the maintenance of calcium homeostasis. An important question remaining is whether there is a trigger in calcium homeostasis that determines when the mitochondria begin to become actively involved in regulation of intracellular calcium. Calcium cycling resulting from low calcium levels created by omission of calcium from the media may be one of the best examples to date. Elucidation of the pathologic conditions that can initiate similar responses may be central to resolving the nature of the proximate mechanism of cell injury and death.

Changes in cell morphology and in the cytoskeleton occur during cell injury when that injury is related to oxidative stress. An example of such injury is that generated by stimulated polymorphonuclear leukocytes in areas of inflammation associated with tissue injury. These cells produce superoxide anion radicals and hydrogen peroxide as major oxidants and cause cell lysis within a few hours after exposure.[163–168] Oxidant production causes (1) oxidation of GSH; (2) loss of NAD,[169–172] concomitant with activation of poly-ADP ribose polymerase, and single-stranded breaks in DNA;[171] (3) loss of cellular ATP; and (4) elevation of intracellular free calcium. Cells that are injured and dying display morphologic changes that include swelling of the volume of cytoplasm and blebbing of the plasma membrane.[173] Membrane blebbing is associated with alteration in the redox state of GSH and intracellular homeostasis of calcium, which perturbs normal cytoskeletal organization. Since such alterations can be caused in hepatocytes as well as in other cell types by two well-known cytoskeletal toxins, cytochalasin B and phalloidin, considerable effort is being focused on determination of the mechanisms of such cell injury. A variety of drugs, including alkylating agents, induce the formation of blebbing in different cell types.[159, 174–176] One mechanism implicates redistribution of cellular filamentous (F-)actin in cells with blebs and changes in the globular (G-)actin:F-actin ratio.[73, 177, 178] These effects include considerable swelling of mitochondria and subcellular organelles within two hours of oxidant injury. Side-to-side aggregation of F-actin bundles (microfilaments) develop during this time. The injury also produces a marked increase in F-actin, associated rearrangement of the microfilaments, and simultaneous changes in the plasma membrane prior to cell death.[73, 177, 178] Thus, cytoskeletal changes during oxidant injury may have considerable importance for both the organization of subcellular organelles as well as the plasma membrane.

PREVENTION OF DRUG-INDUCED LIVER INJURY

When the mechanisms of bioactivation and detoxication of drugs are understood, it should be possible to devise several methods to prevent drug-induced liver injury. For example, modulation of the biochemical processes in bioactivation have been examined widely and include the co-administration of various protective agents (Table 30–3). These agents have effects ranging from inhibition of cytochrome P450–mediated bioactivation of drugs to reactive intermediates to stimulating the synthesis of GSH with precursor amino acids. In addition, antioxidants to protect against oxidative stress, including lipid peroxidation, have been shown to limit loss of hepatocyte viability in vitro. More recently, agents such as ruthenium red that modulate

calcium homeostasis have shown potential for protecting against liver injury.[134]

REFERENCES

1. Aldridge WN. Mechanisms of toxicity. New concepts are required in toxicology. Trends Pharmacol Sci 2:228, 1981.
2. Miller EC, Miller JA. Some historical perspectives on the metabolism of xenobiotic chemicals to reactive electrophiles. In: Anders MW, ed. Bioactivation of Foreign Compounds. Orlando, Fla.: Academic Press, 1985:3.
3. Anders MW, ed. Bioactivation of Foreign Compounds. Orlando, Academic Press, 1985.
4. Farmer PB. Metabolism and reactions of alkylating agents. Pharmacol Ther 35:301, 1987.
5. Guengerich FP, Liebler DC. Enzymatic activation of chemicals to toxic metabolites. CRC Crit Rev Toxicol 14:259, 1985.
6. Gillette JR. A perspective on the role of chemically reactive metabolites of foreign compounds in toxicity. II. Alterations in the kinetics of covalent binding. Biochem Pharmacol 23:2927, 1974.
7. Jollow DJ, Mitchell JR, Zampaglione N, et al. Bromobenzene-induced hepatic necrosis. Protective role of glutathione and endiene by 3,4-bromobenzene oxide as the hepatotoxic metabolite. Pharmacology 11:151, 1974.
8. van de Straat R, de Vries J, Debets AJJ, et al. The mechanism of prevention of paracetamol-induced hepatotoxicity by 3,5-dialkyl substitution. Biochem Pharmacol 36:2065, 1987.
9. van de Straat R. General introduction and objectives of this thesis; mechanism of paracetamol-induced cell injury. In: van de Straat R, ed. Paracetamol-Induced Hepatotoxicity and Prevention by Structural Modification. A Molecular Toxicological Study. Amsterdam, Free University Press, 1987.
10. Younes M, Siegers C-P. The role of iron in the paracetamol- and CCl$_4$-induced lipid peroxidation and hepatotoxicity. Chem Biol Interact 55:327, 1985.
11. van de Straat R, de Vries J, Groot EJ, et al. Paracetamol, 3-monoalkyl and 3,5-dialkyl derivates: comparison of their in vivo hepatotoxicity in mice. Toxicol Appl Pharmacol 89:183, 1987.
12. Needham WP, Shuster L, Kanel GC, et al. Liver damage from narcotics in mice. Toxicol Appl Pharmacol 58:157, 1981.
13. James RC, Goodman DR, Harbison RD. Hepatic glutathione and hepatotoxicity: changes induced by selective narcotics. J Pharmacol Exp Ther 221:708, 1982.
14. Correia MA, Krowich G, Caldera-Munoz P, et al. Morphine metabolism revisited. II. Isolation and chemical characterization of a glutathionyl morphine adduct from rat liver microsomal preparations. Chem Biol Interact 51:13, 1984.
15. Correia MA, Wong JS, Soliven E. Morphine metabolism revisited: I. Metabolic activation of morphine to a reactive species in rats. Chem Biol Interact 49:255, 1984.
16. Krowech G, Calder-Munoz PS, Straub K, et al. Morphine metabolism revisited. III. Confirmation of a novel metabolic pathway. Chem Biol Interact 58:29, 1986.
17. Mudge GH. Diuretics and other agents employed in the mobilization of edema fluid. In: Gilman AC, Goodman LS, Gilman A, eds. The Pharmacological Basis of Therapeutics, 6th ed. New York, Macmillan 1980:1843.
18. Weihe M, Potter WZ, Nelson WL, et al. Mechanism of dose threshold for furosemide hepatotoxicity. Toxicol Appl Pharmacol 29:90, 1974.
19. Uehleke H. The model system of microsomal drug activation and covalent binding to endoplasmic proteins. Proc Eur Soc Study Drug Toxicol 15:119, 1974.
20. Raha CR, Gallagher CH, Shubik P, et al. Covalent binding to protein of the K-region oxide of benzo[a]pyrene formed by microsome incubation. J Natl Cancer Inst (U.S.) 57:33, 1976.
21. Ketterer B. Interactions between carcinogens and proteins. Br Med Bull 36:71, 1980.
22. MacLeod MC, Kootstra A, Mansfield BK, et al. Specificity in interaction of benzo[a]pyrene with nuclear macromolecules: implication of derivatives of two dihydrodiols in protein binding. Proc Natl Acad Sci USA 77:6396, 1980.
23. Stout DL, Hemminki K, Becker FF. Covalent binding of 2-acetylaminofluorene, 2-amino-fluorene, and N-hydroxy-2-acetyl amino fluorene to rat liver nuclear DNA and protein in vivo and in vitro. Cancer Res 40:3579, 1980.
24. Jakoby WB, Keen JH. A triple-threat in detoxification: the glutathione S-transferase. Trends Biochem Sci 2:229, 1977.
25. Ohmi N, Bhargava M, Arias IM. Binding of 3'-methyl-N,N-dimethyl-4-aminoazobenzene metabolites to rat liver cytosol proteins and ligandin subunits. Cancer Res 41:3461, 1981.

TABLE 30–3. PREVENTION OF PARACETAMOL-INDUCED HEPATOTOXICITY BY CO-ADMINISTRATION OF PROTECTIVE AGENTS

Protective Agent	Mechanism of Prevention	References
Metyrapone	Inhibition of cytochrome P450	55
Cobaltous chloride		179
		180
N-acetylcysteine	Stimulation GSH resynthesis	181
Cysteamine	Inhibition cytochrome P450(?)	182
		183
Methionine		184
Ascorbic acid	Detoxication of reactive metabolite(?)	185
α-Tocopherol	Protection against oxidative stress(?)	186
Promethazine		187
		188
Acetylsalicylic acid	Stimulation glucose synthesis(?)	189
	Decrease of Ca^{2+} concentration	190
		191

Source: van de Straat R. In van de Straat R, ed. Paracetamol-Induced Hepatotoxicity and Prevention by Structural Modification. Amsterdam, Free University Press, 1987, with permission.

26. Reeve VE, Gallagher CH, Raha CR. The water-soluble and protein-bound metabolites of benzo[a]pyrene formed by rat liver. Biochem Pharmacol 30:749, 1981.

27. Lutz WK. In vivo covalent binding of organic chemicals to DNA as a quantitative indicator in the process of chemical carcinogenesis. Mutat Res 65:289, 1979.

28. Kosower NS, Kosower E. Glutathione status of cells. Int Rev Cytol 54:109, 1978.

29. Reed DJ, Beatty PW. Biosynthesis and regulation of glutathione. Toxicological implications. In: Hodgson E, Bend JR, Philpot RM, eds. Reviews in Biochemical Toxicology, Vol 2. New York, Elsevier Press, 1980:213.

30. Reed DJ. Regulation and function of glutathione in cells. In: Nygaard OF, Simic MG, eds. First Conference on Radioprotectors and Anticarcinogens. New York, Academic Press, 1983:153.

31. Boyd SC, Sesame HA, Boyd MR. High concentrations of glutathione in glandular stomach: possible implications for carcinogenesis. Science 205:1010, 1979.

32. Womack M, Kremmer KS, Rose WC. The relation of cysteine and methionine to growth. J Biol Chem 121:403, 1937.

33. White INH. Role of liver glutathione in acute toxicity of retroresine to rats. Chem Biol Interact 13:333, 1976.

34. Tateishi N, Higashi T, Naruse A, et al. Rat-liver glutathione. Possible role as a reservoir of cysteine. J Nutr 107:51, 1977.

35. Higashi T, Tateishi N, Naruse A, et al. Novel physiological role of liver glutathione as a reservoir of L-cysteine. J Biochem 82:117, 1977.

36. Cho ES, Sahyoun N, Stegink LD. Tissue glutathione as a cyst(e)ine reservoir during fasting and refeeding of rats. J Nutr 111:914, 1981.

37. Meredith MJ, Reed DJ. Status of the mitochondrial pool of glutathione in the isolated hepatocyte. J Biol Chem 257:3747, 1982.

38. Beck LV, Riecls VD, Duncan B. Diurnal variation in mouse and rat liver sulfhydryl. Proc Soc Exp Biol Med 97:229, 1958.

39. Calcutt G, Ting M. Diurnal variations in the rat tissue disulfide levels. Naturwissenschaften 56:419, 1969.

40. Jaeger RJ, Connolly RB, Murphy SD. Diurnal variation of hepatic glutathione concentration and its correlation with 1,1-dichloroethylene inhalation toxicity in rats. Res Commun Chem Pathol Pharmacol 6:465, 1973.

41. Lauterburg BH, Vaishnov Y, Stillwell WG, et al. The effects of age and glutathione depletion on hepatic glutathione turnover in vivo determined by acetaminophen probe analysis. J Pharmacol Exp Ther 213:54, 1980.

42. Reed DJ, Ellis WW. Influence of γ-glutamyl transpeptidase inactivation on the status of extracellular glutathione and glutathione conjugates. In: Snyder R, Parke CV, Kocsis JJ, et al, eds. Biological Reactive Intermediates IIA. New York, Plenum Press, 1982:75.

43. Davis N, Whipple C. The influence of fasting and various diets on the liver injury effected by chloroform anesthesia. Arch Intern Med 23:612, 1919.

44. Davis NC. The influence of diet upon liver injury produced by carbon tetrachloride. J Med Res 44:601, 1924.

45. Campbell R, Kosterlitz H. The effects of short-term changes in dietary protein in the response of the liver to carbon tetrachloride injury. Br J Exp Pathol 29:149, 1948.

46. Krishman N, Stenger RJ. Effects of starvation on the hepatotoxicity of carbon tetrachloride. Am J Pathol 49:239, 1966.

47. McLean AEM, McLean EK. Effect of diet and 1,1,1-tetra-chloro-2,2-bis-(p-chlorophenyl)ethane (DDT) on microsomal hydroxylating enzymes and on sensitivity of rats to carbon tetrachloride poisoning. Biochem J 100:564, 1966.

48. Highman B, Cyr WH, Streett RP Jr. Effect of x-irradiation and fasting on hepatotoxicity of carbon-tetrachloride in rats. Radiation Res 54:444, 1973.

49. Diaz Gomez MI, DeCastro CR, DeFerreyra EC, et al. Mechanistic studies on carbon tetrachloride hepatotoxicity in fasted and fed rats. Toxicol Appl Pharmacol 32:101, 1975.

50. Strubelt O, Dost-Kempf E, Siegers C-P, et al. The influence of fasting on the susceptibility of mice to hepatotoxic injury. Toxicol Appl Pharmacol 60:66, 1981.

51. Jaeger RJ, Connolly RB, Murphy SD. Effect of 18-hour fast and glutathione depletion on 1,1-dichloroethylene-induced hepatotoxicity and lethality in rats. Exp Mol Pathol 20:187, 1974.

52. Pessayre D, Dolder A, Artigou J-Y, et al. Effect of fasting on metabolite-mediated hepatotoxicity in the rat. Gastroenterology 77:264, 1979.

53. Pessayre D, Wanscheer J-C, Corbert B, et al. Additive effects of inducers and fasting on acetaminophen hepatotoxicity. Biochem Pharmacol 29:2219, 1980.

54. Maruyama E, Kojuma J, Higashi T, et al. Effect of diet on liver glutathione and glutathione reductase. J Biochem 63:398, 1968.

55. Mitchell JR, Jollow DJ, Potter WZ, et al. Acetaminophen-induced hepatic necrosis. 1. Role of drug-metabolism. J Pharmacol Exp Ther 187:185, 1973.

56. Siegers C-P, Schütt A, Strubelt O. Influence of some hepatotoxic agents on hepatic glutathione levels in mice. Proc Eur Soc Toxicol 18:160, 1977.

57. Vadi HV, Neal RA. Microsomal activation of thioacetamide-S-oxide to a metabolite(s) that covalently binds to calf thymus DNA and other polynucleotides. Chem Biol Int 35:25, 1981.

58. Welch RM. Toxicological implications of drug metabolism. Pharmacol Rev 30:457, 1979.

59. Kappus H, Sies H. Toxic drug effects associated with oxygen metabolism: redox cycling and lipid peroxidation. Experientia 37:1233, 1981.

60. Thor H, Moldéus P, Högberg J, et al. Toxicological aspects of food safety. Arch Toxicol Suppl 1:107, 1978.

61. Thor H, Moldéus P, Kristofersson A, et al. Metabolic activation and hepatotoxicity. Metabolism of bromobenzene in isolated hepatocytes. Arch Biochem Biophys 188:114, 1978.

62. Thor H, Moldéus P, Hermanson R, et al. Metabolic activation and hepatotoxicity. Toxicity of bromobenzene in hepatocytes isolated from phenobarbital-treated and diethylmaleate-treated rats. Arch Biochem Biophys 188:122, 1978.

63. Thor H, Moldéus P, Orrenius S. Metabolic activation and hepatotoxicity. Effect of cysteine, N-acetylcysteine, and methionine on glutathione biosynthesis and bromobenzene toxicity in isolated rat hepatocytes. Arch Biochem Biophys 192:405, 1979.

64. Högberg J, Orrenius S, Larson R. Lipid peroxidation in isolated hepatocytes. Eur J Biochem 50:595, 1975.

65. Högberg J, Kristofersson A. Correlation between glutathione levels and cellular damage in isolated hepatocytes. Eur J Biochem 74:77, 1977.

66. Babson JR, Abell NS, Reed DJ. Protective role of the glutathione redox cycle against adriamycin-mediated toxicity in isolated hepatocytes. Biochem Pharmacol 30:2299, 1981.

67. Meredith MJ, Reed DJ. Depletion in vitro of mitochondrial glutathione in rat hepatocytes and enhancement of lipid peroxidation by adriamycin and 1,3-bis(2-chloroethyl)-1-nitrosourea (BCNU). Biochem Pharmacol 32:1383, 1983.

68. Younes M, Siegers C-P. Mechanistic aspects of enhanced lipid peroxidation following glutathione depletion in vivo. Chem Biol Interact 34:257, 1981.

69. Lopez-Barea J, Lee C-Y. Mouse-liver glutathione reductase. Purification, kinetics, and regulation. Eur J Biochem 98:487, 1979.

70. Reed DJ. Regulation of reductive processes by glutathione. Biochem Pharmacol 35:7, 1986.

71. Thurman RG, Scholz R. Interaction of mixed-function oxidation with biosynthetic processes. 2. Inhibition of lipogenesis by aminopyrine in perfused rat liver. Eur J Biochem 38:73, 1973.

72. Weigl K, Sies H. Drug oxidations dependent on cytochrome P-450 in isolated hepatocytes. The role of the tricarboxylates and the aminotransferases in NADPH supply. Eur J Biochem 77:401, 1977.

73. Dang CV, Bell WR, Kaiser D, et al. Disorganization of cultured vascular endothelial cell monolayers by fibrinogen fragment D. Science 227:1487, 1985.

73a. Sies H, Wendel A, Bors W. Metabolism of organic hydroperoxides. In: Jakoby WB, Bend JR, Caldwell J, eds. Metabolic Basis of Detoxication, Metabolism of Functional Groups. New York, Academic Press, 1982:307.

74. Pinto RE, Bartley W. Changes in glutathione reductase and glutathione peroxidase activities in rat liver related to age and sex. Biochem J 109:34P, 1968.

75. Jones DP, Eklow L, Thor H, et al. Metabolism of hydrogen peroxide in isolated hepatocytes. Relative contributions of catalase and glutathione peroxidase in decomposition of endogenously generated H_2O_2. Arch Biochem Biophys 210:505, 1981.

76. Sies H, Moss KM. A role of mitochondrial glutathione peroxidase in modulating mitochondrial oxidations in liver. Eur J Biochem 84:377, 1978.

77. Sandy MS, Moldéus P, Ross D, et al. Cytotoxicity of the redox cycling compound diquat in isolated hepatocytes: involvement of hydrogen peroxide and transition metals. Arch Biochem Biophys 259:29, 1987.

78. Reed DJ. Cellular defense mechanisms against reactive metabolites. In: Anders MW, ed. Bioactivation of Foreign Compounds. Orlando, Fla.: Academic Press, 1985:71.

79. Muller A, Cadenas E, Graf P, et al. A novel biologically active seleno-organic compound—I. Glutathione peroxidase-like activity in vitro and antioxidant capacity of PZ 51 (Ebselen). Biochem Pharmacol 33:3235, 1984.

80. Keberle H. The biochemistry of desferrioxamine and its relation to iron metabolism. Ann NY Acad Sci 119:758, 1964.

81. Tribble DL, Aw TY, Jones DP. The pathophysiological significance of lipid peroxidation in oxidative cell injury. Hepatology 7:377, 1987.
82. Sies H, ed. Oxidative Stress. New York, Academic Press, 1985.
83. Bellomo G, Orrenius S. Altered thiol and calcium homeostasis in oxidative hepatocellular injury. Hepatology 5:876, 1985.
84. Zimmerman HJ. Experimental hepatotoxicity. In: Oskar Eichler, ed. Handbook of Experimental Pharmacology, Vol 16, Pt 5, Experimental Production of Diseases. Liver. New York, Springer-Verlag, 1976:1. Potential hazards of the pro-drug approach.
85. Gorrod JW. Potential hazards of the pro-drug approach. Chem Ind 7:457, 1980.
86. Sies H, Wefers H, Graf P, et al. Hepatic hydroperoxide metabolism: studies on redox cycling and generation of H_2O_2. In: Harris RA, Cornell NW, eds. Isolation, Characterization, and Use of Hepatocytes. New York, Elsevier Press, 1983:341.
87. Waydhas C, Weigl K, Sies H. The disposition of formaldehyde and formate arising from drug N-demethylations dependent on cytochrome P450 in hepatocytes and in perfused rat liver. Eur J Biochem 89:143, 1978.
88. Moore GA, O'Brien PJ, Orrenius S. Menadione (2-methyl-1,4-naphthoquinone)-induced Ca^{2+} release from rat-liver mitochondria is caused by NAD(P)H oxidation. Xenobiotica 16:873, 1986.
89. Smith PF, Alberts DW, Rush GF. Role of glutathione reductase during menadione-induced NADPH oxidation in isolated rat hepatocytes. Biochem Pharmacol 36:3879, 1987.
90. Albano E, Rundgren M, Harvison PJ, et al. Mechanism of N-acetyl-p-benzoquionone imine cytotoxicity. Mol Pharmacol 28:306, 1985.
91. Hewick DS. Reductive metabolism of nitrogen-containing functional groups. In: Jakoby WB, Bend JR, Caldwell J, eds. Metabolic Basis of Detoxication, Metabolism of Functional Groups. New York, Academic Press, 1982:151.
92. Mason RP, Josephy PD. In: Rickert DE, ed. Toxicity of Nitroaromatic Compounds. Washington, DC: Hemisphere, 1985:121.
93. Rosen GM, Rauchman EJ, Wilson RL Jr, et al. Production of superoxide during the metabolism of nitrazepam. Xenobiotica 14:785, 1984.
94. Bachur NR, Gordon SL, Gee MV. A general mechanism for microsomal activation of quinone anticancer agents to free radicals. Cancer Res 38:1745, 1978.
95. Christopherson BO. The inhibitory effect of reduced glutathione on the lipid peroxidation of the microsomal fraction and mitochondria. Biochem J 106:515, 1968.
96. McCay PB, Gibson DD, Fong K-L, et al. Effect of glutathione peroxidase activity on lipid peroxidation in biological membranes. Biochim Biophys Acta 431:459, 1976.
97. Yonaha M, Tampo Y. Bromosulfophthalein abolishes glutathione-dependent protection against lipid peroxidation in rat liver mitochondria. Biochem Pharmacol 36:2831, 1987.
98. Tirmenstein M, Reed DJ. Characterization of glutathione-dependent inhibition of lipid peroxidation of isolated rat liver nuclei. Arch Biochem Biophys 261:1, 1988.
99. Reddy CC, Sholz WW, Thomas CE, et al. Vitamin E–dependent reduced glutathione inhibition of rat liver microsomal lipid peroxidation. Life Sci 31:571, 1982.
100. Burk RF. Glutathione-dependent protection by rat liver microsomal protein against lipid peroxidation. Biochim Biophys Acta 757:21, 1983.
101. Burk RF, Trumble KR, Lawrence RA. Rat hepatic cystolic glutathione-dependent enzyme protection against lipid peroxidation in the NADPH-microsomal lipid peroxidation system. Biochim Biophys Acta 618:35, 1980.
102. Haenen GRMM, Bast A. Protection against lipid peroxidation by a microsomal glutathione-dependent latile factor. FEBS Lett 159:24, 1983.
103. Gibson DD, Hornbrook KR, McCay PB. Glutathione-dependent inhibition of lipid peroxidation by a soluble, heat-labile factor in animal tissues. Biochim Biophys Acta 620:572, 1980.
104. Gibson DD, Hawrylko J, McCay PB. GSH-dependent inhibition of lipid peroxidation: properties of a potent cytosolic system which protects cell membranes. Lipids 20:704, 1985.
105. Fairhurst A, Barber DJ, Clark B, et al. Development of the cytosolic defense system against microsomal lipid peroxidation in rat liver. Biochim Biophys Acta 752:491, 1983.
106. Takayanagi R, Takeshige K, Minakami S. NADH- and NADPH-dependent lipid peroxidation in bovine heart submitochondrial particles. Dependence on the rate of electron flow in the respiratory chain and an antioxidant role of ubiquinol. Biochem J 192:853, 1980.
107. Bindoli A, Cavallini L, Jocelyn P. Mitochondrial lipid peroxidation by cumene hydroperoxide and its prevention by succinate. Biochim Biophys Acta 681:496, 1982.
108. Mészaros L, Tihanyi K, Horvath I. Mitochondrial substrate oxidation-dependent protection against lipid peroxidation. Biochim Biophys Acta 713:675, 1982.
109. Flohé L, Zimmermann R. The role of GSH peroxidase in protecting the membrane of rat liver mitochondria. Biochim Biophys Acta 223:210, 1970.
110. McCay PB, Lai EK, Powell SR, et al. Vitamin E functions as an electron shuttle for glutathione-dependent "free radical reductase" activity in biological membrane. Fed Proc Fed Am Soc Exp Biol 45:1729, 1986.
111. Kraus P. Resolution, purification and some properties of three glutathione transferases from rat liver mitochondria. Hoppe-Seyler's Z Physiol Chem 361:9, 1980.
112. Morgenstern R, Lundqvist G, Andersson G, et al. The distribution of microsomal glutathione transferase among different organelles, different organs, and different organisms. Biochem Pharmacol 33:3609, 1984.
113. Wahlländer A, Soboll S, Sies H. Hepatic mitochondrial and cytosolic glutathione content and the subcellular distribution of GSH-S-transferases. FEBS Lett 97:138, 1979.
114. Green RC, O'Brien PJ. The cellular localization of glutathione peroxidase and its release from mitochondria during swelling. Biochim Biophys Acta 197:31, 1970.
115. Zakowski JJ, Tappel AL. Purification and properties of rat liver mitochondrial glutathione peroxidase. Biochim Biophys Acta 526:65, 1978.
116. Katki AP, Myers CE. Membrane-bound glutathione peroxidase-like activity in mitochondria. Biochem Biophys Res Commun 96:85, 1980.
117. Morgenstern R, Meijer J, DePierre JW, et al. Characterization of rat-liver microsomal glutathione S-transferase activity. Eur J Biochem 104:167, 1980.
118. Morgenstern R, Guthenberg C, DePierre JW. Microsomal glutathione S-transferase. Purification, initial characterization and demonstration that it is not identical to the cytosolic glutathione S-transferases A, B, and C. Eur J Biochem 128:243, 1982.
119. Morgenstern R, DePierre JW. Microsomal glutathione transferase. Purification in unactivated form and further characterization of the activation process, substrate specificity and amino acid composition. Eur J Biochem 134:591, 1983.
120. Reddy CC, Tu C-PD, Burgess JR, et al. Evidence for the occurrence of selenium-independent glutathione peroxidase activity in rat liver microsomes. Biochem Biophys Res Commun 101:970, 1981.
121. Morgenstern R, DePierre JW. In: Rydström J, Montelius J, Bengtsson M, eds. Extrahepatic Drug Metabolism and Chemical Carcinogenesis. New York, Elsevier Press, 1983:185.
122. Yonaha M, Tampo Y. Studies on protection by glutathione against lipid peroxidation in rat liver microsomes. Effect of bromosulfophthalein. Chem Pharm Bull (Tokyo) 34:4195, 1986.
123. Jakoby WB. The glutathione S-transferases: a group of multifunctional detoxification proteins. Adv Enzymol 46:383, 1978.
124. Ketterer B, Beale D, Taylor JB, et al. The genetic relationships and inducibility of soluble glutathione transferases of the rat liver. Biochem Soc Trans 11:466, 1983.
125. Ålin P, Jensson H, Guthenberg C, et al. Purification of major basic glutathione transferase isoenzymes from rat liver by use of affinity chromatography and fast protein liquid chromatofocusing. Anal Biochem 146:313, 1985.
126. Lawrence RA, Burk RF. Glutathione peroxidase activity in selenium-deficient rat liver. Biochem Biophys Res Commun 71:952, 1976.
127. Baars AJ, Jansen M, Arnoldussen S, et al. Inhibition of cytosolic rat hepatic glutathione S-transferase activities by bromosulfophthaleins. Experientia 38:426, 1982.
128. Lawrence RA, Parkhill LK, Burk RF. Hepatic cytosolic non–selenium-dependent glutathione peroxidase activity: its nature and the effect of selenium deficiency. J Nutr 108:981, 1978.
129. Lawrence RA, Burk RF. Species, tissue and subcellular distribution of non–Se dependent glutathione peroxidase activity. J Nutr 108:211, 1978.
130. Fiskum G. Mitochondrial respiration and calcium transport in tumor cells. In: Fiskum G, ed. Mitochondrial Physiology and Pathology. New York, Van Nostrand Reinhold Co, 1986:180.
131. Reed KC, Bygrave FL. The inhibition of mitochondrial calcium transport by lanthanides and ruthenium red. Biochem J 140:143, 1974.
132. Carafoli E. Intracellular calcium homeostasis. Annu Rev Biochem 56:395, 1987.
133. McCormack JG, Denton RM. Ca^{2+} as a second messenger within mitochondria. Trends Biochem Sci 11:258, 1986.
134. Thomas CE, Reed DJ. Effect of extracellular Ca^{2+} omission on isolated hepatocytes. II. Loss of mitochondrial membrane potential and protection by inhibitors of uniport Ca^{2+} transduction. J Pharmacol Exper Ther 245:501, 1988.
135. Moore M, Thor H, Moore G, et al. The toxicity of acetaminophen and N-acetyl-p-benzoquinone imine in isolated hepatocytes is associated with thiol depletion and increased cytosolic Ca^{2+}. J Biol Chem 260:13035, 1985.

136. DiMonte D, Bellomo G, Thor H, et al. Menadione-induced cytotoxicity is associated with protein thiol oxidation and alteration in intracellular Ca^{2+} homeostasis. Arch Biochem Biophys 235:343, 1984.

136a. Bellomo G, Thor H, Orrenius S. Increase in cytosolic Ca^{2+} concentration during t-cutyl hydroperoxide metabolism by isolated hepatocytes involves NADPH oxidation and mobilization of intracellular Ca^{2+} stores. FEBS Lett 168:38, 1984.

137. Webb JL. Sulfhydryl reagents (Chap. 4); Mercurials (Chap. 7). In: Webb JL, ed. Enzyme and Metabolic Inhibitors. Vol 2. New York, Academic Press, 1965.

138. Webb JL. Iodoacetate and iodoacetamide (Chap. 1); N-ethylmaleimide (Chap. 3); Arsenicals (Chap. 6); Comparison of SH reagents (Chap. 7). In: Webb JL, ed. Enzyme and Metabolic Inhibitors, Vol 3. New York, Academic Press, 1966.

139. Dean RT, Cheeseman KH. Vitamin E protects against free radical damage in lipid environments. Biochem Biophys Res Commun 148:1277, 1987.

140. Akerboom TPM, Bilzer M, Sies H. The relationship of biliary glutathione disulfide efflux and intracellular glutathione disulfide content in perfused rat liver. J Biol Chem 257:4248, 1982.

141. Pascoe GA, Reed DJ. Relationship between cellular calcium and vitamin E metabolism during protection against cell injury. Arch Biochem Biophys 253:287, 1987.

142. Trump BF, Pentilla A, Berezesky IK. Studies on cell surface conformation following injury. Virchows Arch [B] 29:281, 1979.

143. Farber JL. The role of calcium in cell death. Life Sci 29:1289, 1981.

144. Schanne FAX, Kane AB, Young EE, et al. Calcium dependence of toxic cell death: a final common pathway. Science 206:700, 1979.

145. Kane AB, Young EE, Schanne FAX, et al. Calcium dependence of phalloidin-induced liver cell death. Proc Natl Acad Sci USA 77:1177, 1980.

146. Smith MT, Thor H, Orrenius S. Toxic injury to hepatocytes is not dependent on extracellular calcium. Science 213:1257, 1981.

147. Stacey NH, Klaassen CD. Lack of protection against chemically induced cell injury to isolated hepatocytes by omission of calcium from the incubation medium. J Toxicol Environ Health 9:267, 1982.

148. Acosta D, Sorensen EMB. Role of calcium in cytotoxic injury of cultured hepatocytes. Ann NY Acad Sci 407:78, 1983.

149. Pascoe GA, Olafsdottir K, Reed DJ. Vitamin E protection against chemical-induced cell injury. I. Maintenance of cellular protein thiols as a cytoprotective mechanism. Arch Biochem Biophys 256:150, 1987.

150. Pascoe GA, Reed DJ. Vitamin E protection against chemical-induced cell injury. II. Evidence for a threshold effects of cellular α-tocopherol in prevention of adriamycin toxicity. Arch Biochem Biophys 256:159, 1987.

151. Pascoe GA, Farris MW, Olafsdottir K, et al. A role of vitamin E in protection against cell injury: maintenance of intracellular glutathione precursors and biosynthesis. Eur J Biochem 166:241, 1987.

152. Liebler DC, Kling DS, Reed DJ. Antioxidant protection of phospholipid bilayers by α-tocopherol. Control of α-tocopherol status and lipid peroxidation by ascorbic acid and glutathione. J Biol Chem 261:12114, 1986.

153. Fariss MW, Olafsdottir K, Reed DJ. Extracellular calcium protects isolated rat hepatocytes from injury. Biochem Biophys Res Commun 121:102, 1984.

154. Thomas CE, Reed DJ. Effect of extracellular Ca^{2+} omission on isolated hepatocytes. I. Induction of oxidative stress and cell injury. J Pharmacol Exper Therap 245:493, 1988.

155. Reed DJ, Pascoe GA, Olafsdottir K. Some aspects of cell defense mechanisms of glutathione and vitamin E during cell injury. Arch Toxicol [Suppl] 11:34, 1987.

156. Lemasters JJ, Ji S, Thurman RG. Centrilobular injury following hypoxia in isolated, perfused rat liver. Science 213:661, 1981.

157. Lemasters JJ, Stemkowski CJ, Ji S, et al. Cell surface changes and enzyme release during hypoxia and reoxygenation in the isolated, perfused rat liver. J Cell Biol 97:778, 1983.

158. Thor H, Hartzell P, Orrenius S. Potentiation of oxidative cell injury in hepatocytes which have accumulated Ca^{2+}. J Biol Chem 259:6612, 1985.

159. Jewell SA, Bellomo G, Thor H, et al. Bleb formation in hepatocytes during drug metabolism is caused by disturbances in thiol and calcium ion homeostasis. Science 217:1257, 1982.

160. Farber JL. Biology of disease: membrane injury and calcium homeostasis in the pathogenesis of coagulative necrosis. Lab Invest 47:114, 1982.

161. Lemasters JJ, DiGuiseppi J, Nieminen AL, et al. Blebbing, free Ca^{2+} and mitochondrial membrane potential preceding cell death in hepatocytes. Nature 325:78, 1987.

162. Andersson BS, Aw TY, Jones DP. Mitochondrial transmembrane potential and pH gradient during anoxia. Am J Physiol 252:C349, 1985.

163. Nathan CF, Silverstein SC, Breckner LH, et al. Extracellular cytolysis by activated macrophages and granulocytes. II. Hydrogen peroxide as a mediator of cytotoxicity. J Exp Med 149:100, 1979.

164. Simon RH, Scoggin CH, Patterson D. Hydrogen peroxide causes the fatal injury to human fibroblasts exposed to oxygen radicals. J Biol Chem 256:7181, 1981.

165. Weiss SJ, Young J, LoBuglio AF, et al. Role of hydrogen peroxide in neutrophil-mediated destruction of cultured endothelial cells. J Clin Invest 68:714, 1981.

166. Sacks T, Moldow CF, Craddock PR, et al. Oxygen radicals mediate endothelial cell damage by complement-stimulated granulocytes: an in vitro model of immune vascular damage. J Clin Invest 61:1161, 1978.

167. Martin WJ II. Neutrophils kill pulmonary endothelial cells by a hydrogen peroxide–dependent pathway. Am Rev Respir Dis 130:209, 1984.

168. Hinshaw DB, Sklar LA, Bohl B, et al. Cytoskeletal and morphologic impact of cellular oxidant injury. Am J Physiol 123:454, 1986.

169. Spragg RG, Hinshaw CB, Hyslop PA, et al. Alterations in adenosine triphosphate and energy change in cultured endothelial and P388D1 cells following oxidant injury. J Clin Invest 76:1471, 1985.

170. Schraufstatter IU, Hinshaw DB, Hyslop PA, et al. Glutathione cycle activity and pyridine nucleotide levels in oxidant-induced injury of cells. J Clin Invest 76:1131, 1985.

171. Schraufstatter IU, Hinshaw DB, Hyslop PA, et al. Oxidant injury of cells: DNA strand breaks activate polyadenosine diphosphateribose polymerase and lead to depletion of nicotinamide adenine dinucleotide. J Clin Invest 77:1312, 1986.

172. Bellomo G, Jewell SA, Thor H, et al. Regulation of intracellular calcium compartmentation: studies with isolated hepatocytes and t-butyl hydroperoxide. Proc Natl Acad Sci USA 79:6842, 1982.

173. Trump BF, Mergner WJ. The inflammatory process. In: Zweifach BW, et al, eds. Cell Injury, 2nd ed., Vol 1. New York, Academic Press, 1974:115.

174. Scott RE. Plasma membrane vesiculation: a new technique for isolation of plasma membranes. Science 194:743, 1976.

175. Scott RE, Perkins RG, Axchunke MA, et al. Plasma membrane vesiculation in 3T3 and SV 3T3 cells. I. Morphological and biochemical characterization. J Cell Sci 35:229, 1979.

176. Kinn SR, Allen TD. Conversion of blebs to microvilli: cell surface reorganization after trypsin. Differentiation 20:168, 1981.

177. Wu E, Tank DW, Webb WW. Unconstrained lateral diffusion of concanavalin A receptors on bulbous lymphocytes. Proc Natl Acad Sci USA 79:4962, 1982.

178. Tank DW, Wu E, Webb W. Enhanced molecular diffusibility in muscle membrane blebs: release of lateral constraints. J Cell Biol 92:207, 1982.

179. Jollow DJ, Mitchell JR, Potter WZ, et al. Acetaminophen-induced hepatic necrosis. II. Role of covalent binding in vivo. J Pharmacol Exp Ther 187:195 (1973).

180. Goldstein M, Nelson EB. Metyrapone as a treatment for acetaminophen (paracetamol) toxicity in mice. Res Commun Chem Pathol Pharmacol 23:203, 1979.

181. Labadarios N, Davis M, Portmann B, et al. Paracetamol-induced hepatic necrosis in the mouse—relationship between covalent binding, hepatic glutathione depletion and the protective effect of α-mercaptopropionylglycine. Biochem Pharmacol 26:31, 1977.

182. Gerber JG, MacDonald JS, Harbison RD, et al. Effect of N-acetylcysteine on hepatic covalent binding of paracetamol (acetaminophen) [letter]. Lancet 1:657, 1977.

183. Prescott LF. Paracetamol overdosage. Pharmacological considerations and clinical management. Drugs 25:290, 1983.

184. Prescott LF. The chief scientist report . . . prevention of hepatic necrosis following paracetamol overdosage. Health Bull 36:204, 1978.

185. McLean AEM, Nuttiall L. An in vitro model of liver injury using paracetamol treatment of liver slides and prevention of injury by some antioxidants. Biochem Pharmacol 27:425, 1978.

186. Devalia JL, Ogilvie RL, McLean AEM. Dissociation of cell death from covalent binding of paracetamol by flavones in a hepatocyte system. Biochem Pharmacol 31:3745, 1982.

187. Walker BE, Kelleher J, Dixon MF, et al. Vitamin E protection of the liver from paracetamol in the rat. Clin Sci Mol Med 47:449, 1974.

188. Raghuram TC, Krishnamurthi D, Kalamegham R. Effect of vitamin C on paracetamol hepatotoxicity. Toxicol Lett 2:175, 1978.

189. de Vries J, de Jong J, Lock FM, et al. Protection against paracetamol-induced hepatotoxicity by acetylsalicylic acid in rats. Toxicology 30:297, 1984.

190. Whitehouse LW, Paul CJ, Thomas BH. Effect of acetylsalicylic acid on a toxic dose of acetaminophen in the mouse. Toxicol Appl Pharmacol 38:571, 1976.

191. de Vries J. Induction and prevention of biochemical disturbances in hepatic necrosis. Trends Pharmacol Sci 4:393, 1983.

Drug-Induced Liver Disease

Nathan M. Bass, M.D., Ph.D. • Robert K. Ockner, M.D.

CLINICAL PERSPECTIVES

Recent advances in the understanding of infectious liver diseases (including viral, bacterial, rickettsial, fungal, and parasitic diseases) have led to important improvements in methods of diagnosis and treatment. Moreover, public health measures and, in the case of viral hepatitis, immunization procedures, offer the hope that the incidence and prevalence of these disorders may eventually decrease. In this context, it is perhaps paradoxical that the incidence of chemically induced liver disease may be increasing. That this should be the case undoubtedly reflects, at least in part, the same broad and fundamental changes that have proved so beneficial in the case of the infectious disorders. These changes include the expansion of science and technology and the widened accessibility of the fruits of that expansion to an increasing number of individuals. Thus, whereas viral hepatitis, schistosomiasis, yellow fever, and amebiasis may diminish in the wake of advancing technology, drug-induced liver disease, quite the opposite, is a direct and increasingly significant result of it.

To address this area in generalities is far easier than to deal in concrete facts. With a few notable exceptions, most statistical data concerning incidence and natural history are subject to several undoubtedly important errors. For example, drug-induced liver disease, like other forms of liver disease, may be clinically subtle or completely inapparent, so that estimates of incidence will be influenced critically by the method used to identify cases. Thus, although laboratory screening of all persons at risk will almost certainly detect liver injury more often than would reliance on clinical symptoms or signs, this approach may be overly sensitive, since in certain circumstances minor abnormalities of liver function may appear only transiently, may revert to normal despite continued administration of the agent, and may or may not be indicative of significant "hepatotoxicity." Conversely, even routine tests may not be sensitive enough to detect other forms of drug-induced liver disease (e.g., chronic methotrexate administration), which may appear only after many months or years. Since most available incidence figures are probably underestimates, and since case reports in the literature tend to be skewed toward more severe or fatal reactions, it is quite likely that estimates of case fatality rates tend to be high, and perceptions of natural history biased. Perhaps the most notable exception to these difficulties is the currently available body of data concerning the incidence and prognosis of clinical and subclinical liver injury associated with isoniazid administration, specifically as employed in the setting of single-drug "chemoprophylaxis" of tuberculosis.

Despite these general difficulties, the subject of drug-induced liver disease has been reviewed extensively,[1, 2] and some information is available that helps to place the broad problem of drug-induced liver disease in perspective. For example, 2 per cent of jaundiced patients admitted to general hospitals had drug-induced liver disease;[2, 3] this figure was substantially higher for elderly individuals.[2, 3] Drugs may account for approximately 25 per cent of instances of fulminant hepatitis,[4-6] and anywhere between a fourth and two thirds of patients with chronic active hepatitis.[7-9] Thus, among the more serious forms of liver disease (that is, those that have a chronic or fatal outcome), drugs are disproportionately represented.

Suspected drug-induced liver disease makes up between 4 and 7 per cent of all reports of adverse drug effects voluntarily reported to central registries.[10, 11] Although data available from these sources point to a relatively small group of frequently used drugs as producing the bulk of reported liver-related adverse effects, the variety of drugs that have been reported to induce liver disease is nevertheless substantial and ever increasing. Two recently published tabular compilations of drug-related liver pathology list over 150 therapeutic agents that have been implicated in the etiology of a broad spectrum of hepatic diseases.[12, 13]

CLINICAL SETTING—PROBLEMS IN DIAGNOSIS

Since drug-induced liver injury usually does not depend on pre-existing liver disease, its full range of severity may be expressed in any setting in which drugs are taken, from the relatively healthy ambulatory subject using an antibiotic or antidepressant to the more seriously ill or postoperative, hospitalized patient. Because of this, and because the presentation of drug-induced liver disease may be quite nonspecific (e.g., fever or a viral-like syndrome), it often is initially unclear whether a patient's deterioration represents progression or a complication of the underlying disorder, an unrelated event, or a drug reaction. Moreover, even if it becomes apparent (clinically or by laboratory testing) that liver function is impaired, a number of other diagnostic possibilities need to be considered, and these are not always easily distinguished from a drug-related problem. Among these are viral hepatitis (including posttransfusion), systemic bacterial infections, postoperative intrahepatic cholestasis, choledocholithiasis and/or acute pancreatitis, bile duct injury, congestive heart failure, and deterioration of pre-existing chronic liver disease that previously might have been well compensated or clinically inapparent. This broad differential diagnosis, together with the fact that the hepatotoxic potentials of most newly introduced agents are not known, makes it necessary for the clinician to remain constantly alert to the possibility that a seemingly nonspecific, unfavorable turn of events or change in liver function may represent drug-induced liver injury. Diagnosis is discussed in greater detail below; unfortunately, even when the diagnosis of drug-induced liver disease is considered, it may not be possible to confirm it with certainty. The exacerbation of liver disease upon reintroduction of a drug suspected of causing it in the first instance (rechallenge observation), although widely regarded as representing the most reliable "diagnostic test" for establishing a drug-related etiology, is potentially hazardous and rarely justifiable.

The prognosis of drug-induced liver disease is highly variable, and depends not only on the etiologic agent but also on the specific clinical circumstances. For some drugs, estimated case fatality rates may approach 50 per cent; such poor prognoses are for the most part limited to those agents that produce acute hepatic necrosis histologically similar to acute viral hepatitis. Other forms of drug-induced liver disease are virtually never fatal (e.g., estrogen-induced cholestasis), whereas still others may progress chronically and insidiously to cirrhosis (e.g., methotrexate-induced disease). Some are essentially benign in most respects, but uncertainties in their diagnosis may lead to unnecessarily expensive, invasive, or dangerous diagnostic or therapeutic interventions.

INDIVIDUAL SUSCEPTIBILITY AND MECHANISMS OF INJURY

It has long been recognized that most types of drug-induced liver injury can be classified as either predictable (usually dose-related), or unpredictable or "idiosyncratic" (usually unrelated to dose). Predictable forms often can be produced in experimental animals, and, if associated with liver cell necrosis, these characteristically affect predominantly a particular region of the hepatic lobule. Examples of agents causing lesions in this category include carbon tetrachloride and acetaminophen (centrilobular, or acinar zone 3), yellow phosphorus (mid-zonal, or acinar zone 2), and allyl alcohol (periportal, or acinar zone 1). Because of the predictability and dose-response relationships of the hepatic lesions they cause, these agents have been regarded as "direct hepatotoxins."

Most of the unpredictable or idiosyncratic forms of injury are more diffuse, consisting of necrosis and/or cholestasis, usually associated with a significant inflammatory reaction, but these processes, too, may be more localized. These reactions usually cannot be produced in experimental animals. Some agents (e.g., isoniazid, phenytoin) produce lesions histologically similar to viral hepatitis, which in some instances may be accompanied by systemic features such as fever, rash, arthralgias, or eosinophilia. Because of the unpredictability of these reactions with regard to both marked differences in individual susceptibilities and the apparent lack of dose-dependence, as well as the appearance, in some instances, of specific patterns of autoantibodies in the serum,[14] they had been assumed to represent forms of drug allergy in which the immune response is directed against the liver cell.

The validity of these earlier concepts increasingly has come into question because of important advances in the understanding of drug metabolism and the mechanism of hepatotoxicity. Thus, in several instances, so-called "direct" hepatotoxins actually do not injure the liver cell until after they have undergone biotransformation to toxic intermediates, which then interact with components of the cell.[15] Carbon tetrachloride and acetaminophen, among others, appear to act in this way. With regard to idiosyncratic hepatic drug reactions, not only has an immunologic mechanism not been established conclusively, but, at least in some instances, recent findings suggest an alternative mechanism in which the parent compound is converted to a toxic metabolite. For example, biotransformation of chlorpromazine converts it to a very large number of products, some of which are potentially toxic to the liver cell, whereas others are not, or are less so. It seems quite probable that idiosyncrasy (i.e., the apparent differences in individual susceptibilities to drug-induced liver injury) may represent corresponding and possibly genetically determined differences in either (1) the relative rates of several alternate pathways by which a drug may be converted to products of differing hepatotoxic potentials,[16] or (2) the efficiencies or completenesses with which a particular toxic product is "detoxified" via subsequent reactions.[17] An agent particularly well studied in regard to the multiplicity of potential influences on individual susceptibilities to hepatotoxicity is acetaminophen (discussed later in this chapter). The rate at which a toxic metabolite is formed from acetaminophen and the rate at which this metabolite is in turn "detoxified" may vary independently of each other and of the dose of the parent drug. Individual susceptibility, to the extent that it is related to rates of formation and disposition of the toxic products of drug metabolism, thus may be influenced by a variety of factors. It is important to keep in mind that a "toxic" product of drug metabolism could be immunogenic and lead to hepatic injury via immunologic mechanisms. Such mechanisms are not established, however. The factors influencing metabolism of drugs include genetic factors, age, sex, and other drugs or environmental agents that induce or otherwise influence the activity of metabolic pathways, or compete with the drug or its product for entry into a given pathway (Chap. 9).

Despite the significant advances that have led to the development of these concepts, it is important to recognize that the mechanism(s) by which various drugs and their metabolic products injure or kill the liver cell, or alter its function, is (are) largely unknown. Nonetheless, several concepts of drug hepatotoxicity have evolved that are useful and plausible in the formulation of an understanding of the area (Table 31-1).

Much recent research has focused on the final common pathway whereby drug-induced biochemical events such as covalent binding and lipid peroxidation ultimately lead to cell death. Disruption of cellular calcium homeostasis secondary to impairment of membrane calcium pump function has been intensively investigated in this regard. It is as yet unclear whether covalent binding or lipid peroxidation produced by direct hepatotoxins effect cell death specifically through disruption of calcium homeostasis, or if the observed alterations in cellular calcium flux are a terminal, nonspecific event in dying cells (see Chap. 30).[18, 19]

It should be noted that the examples shown are in many instances not unique expressions of hepatotoxicity for the indicated agent. Thus, although rifampin appears to block hepatic uptake of organic anions through an effect at the liver cell surface, it also may be associated with a viral hepatitis–like reaction. Similarly, although certain metabolites of chlorpromazine may cause cholestasis, in part through their effects on the cytoskeleton and on membranes (see Chap. 12), it is not clear whether or how this is related to the inflammation and liver cell necrosis that regularly accompany clinical chlorpromazine-induced cholestasis. Estrogen-induced cholestasis seems readily attributable to a direct effect on the physical properties of membranes, but the long-term and less frequent association between administration of estrogen and hepatocellular ad-

TABLE 31–1. POSTULATED MECHANISMS OF DRUG-INDUCED HEPATIC DISEASE

Effect	Example
Alteration of the physical properties of membranes	Estrogens
Inhibition of membrane enzymes (e.g., Na^+, K^+-ATPase)	Chlorpromazine metabolites
Interference with hepatic uptake processes	Rifampin
Impairment of cytoskeletal function	Chlorpromazine metabolites
Formation of insoluble complexes in bile	Chlorpromazine
Conversion to reactive intermediates:	
Electrophiles producing covalent modification of tissue macromolecules	Acetaminophen
Free radicals producing lipid peroxidation	Carbon tetrachloride
Redox-cycling with production of oxygen radicals	Nitrofurantoin

enoma and carcinoma seems to require invocation of a more complex pathogenesis. To the extent that information regarding the mechanism of hepatotoxicity is available, it is considered in the sections of this chapter that deal with specific agents. This topic is also discussed in Chapter 30.

HISTOLOGIC PATTERNS OF DRUG-INDUCED LIVER INJURY

GENERAL CONSIDERATIONS

The spectrum of drug-induced liver injury encompasses an extremely wide diversity of histologic changes. These range from an acute, reversible, clinically benign, and nearly inconsequential interference with bile flow, at the one extreme, to fatal massive necrosis, chronic hepatitis, or malignant tumor at the other. Because many agents are associated with relatively characteristic lesions, histology has provided one basis for the classification of drug-induced liver injury. Selected examples of each form are shown in Table 31–2. For some agents, the reactions are relatively stereotyped. For example, tetracycline-induced liver damage is manifested histologically by a characteristic (but nonspecific) form of fatty liver, and isoniazid-induced hepatitis comprises a spectrum of acute focal, submassive, or massive hepatocellular necrosis, all resembling the range of lesions seen with viral hepatitis. For other agents, a much broader range of responses may be elicited. For example, oral contraceptives may cause a bland, reversible cholestasis with little or no associated cellular necrosis or inflammation, an alteration in the composition of bile, and an increased propensity to cholesterol gallstone formation, or the development of a benign or malignant liver tumor. Similarly, isoniazid and methyldopa have been associated with both acute and chronic hepatitis, and phenylbutazone with an acute viral hepatitis–like lesion or granulomatous hepatitis.

As a corollary, the histologic features of drug-induced liver injury, while often relatively characteristic for a particular agent, are rarely, if ever, specific. Equally important, virtually all forms of drug-induced liver injury closely resemble other forms of liver disease not presently perceived as having chemical causes. In the context of these limitations, then, any classification of drug-induced liver

disease on the basis of histologic patterns must be based on the understanding that, whereas it is conceptually useful and may be diagnostically helpful, it often fails to provide specific or conclusive information regarding pathogenesis.

ZONAL NECROSIS

The hepatic injuries caused by many drugs and toxins appear to affect predominantly the cells in select regions of the hepatic lobule. Necrosis is either limited to the individual zones or at least is more prominent there, with apparent relative or absolute sparing of other zones. Agents that cause this type of injury are usually predictable direct or indirect hepatotoxins, the injurious effects of which are dose-dependent. Examples include acetaminophen and carbon tetrachloride, both of which cause predominantly centrilobular necrosis, and yellow phosphorus, which causes a mid-zonal lesion. Occasionally, halothane hepatitis may cause centrilobular necrosis, but often the lesion is indistinguishable from viral hepatitis. Often there is little or no inflammatory response or cellular infiltration, and damaged but not frankly necrotic cells may accumulate lipid (triglyceride). In addition to the morphologic changes, cellular injury is reflected by nonspecific clinical and laboratory evidence of liver dysfunction, which may range from asymptomatic abnormalities in the activity of liver enzymes in serum to fulminant liver failure. In most instances of acute injury of this kind, the process resolves completely or terminates fatally; there is no evidence that a chronic, self-sustaining form of liver injury is set in motion after a single acute exposure to the toxin. If exposure is chronic or recurring, however, the lesion may persist or progress, depending on the dose, the agent, and the patient's condition.

The basis for the relative selectivity of the lobular zone in which injury is most pronounced is not fully understood,

TABLE 31–2. HISTOLOGIC CLASSIFICATION OF DRUG-INDUCED LIVER DISEASE

Pattern	Examples
Zonal necrosis	Acetaminophen, carbon tetrachloride
Nonspecific hepatitis	Aspirin, oxacillin
Viral hepatitis-like lesion	Isoniazid, methyldopa
Granulomatous hepatitis	Quinidine, allopurinol
Chronic hepatitis	Methyldopa, nitrofurantoin
Fibrosis	Methotrexate
Cholestasis	
Inflammatory	Chlorpromazine, erythromycin estolate
Bland	Estrogens, anabolic steroids
Fatty liver	
Large globules	Ethanol, corticosteroids
Small droplets	Tetracycline, valproic acid
Vascular lesions	
Hepatic vein thrombosis	Oral contraceptives
Veno-occlusive disease	Certain antitumor agents
Non-cirrhotic portal hypertension	Vinyl chloride monomer
Peliosis hepatis	Anabolic steroids
Tumors	
Adenoma	Oral contraceptives, androgens
Focal nodular hyperplasia	Oral contraceptives
Carcinoma	Oral contraceptives, androgens
Angiosarcoma	Vinyl chloride monomer

but undoubtedly reflects to some extent intralobular differences in the determinants of the injurious process itself. For example, the abundance of the smooth endoplasmic reticulum and the activity of the cytochrome P450-dependent drug-metabolizing system are greatest in centrilobular hepatocytes. Those agents for which hepatotoxicity depends on the formation of a toxic metabolite via this system may be more likely to injure those cells in which the system is most active. This distribution, however, is undoubtedly influenced by the interaction of many other factors, including known or postulated lobular gradients in oxygen tension, drug concentration, rates of uptake, activity of alternative metabolic pathways (whose products may differ in toxicity), and cellular concentrations of potentially "protective" constituents, such as glutathione.

NONSPECIFIC HEPATITIS

This "pattern" of injury is characterized by a few scattered foci of hepatocellular necrosis, usually associated with a mononuclear cell infiltrate, and a variable portal inflammatory response. It lacks the characteristic features of viral hepatitis such as bile stasis, lobular disarray, and acidophil bodies, and, as its name implies, can be seen in a wide variety of clinical settings, including those in which the liver may not be primarily involved, such as sepsis or other systemic disorders. It is typical of many and diverse forms of drug-induced liver injury, including the clearly dose-dependent hepatotoxicity of aspirin and the lesions associated with certain semisynthetic analogs of penicillin. It virtually never is associated with serious or progressive hepatic decompensation or failure, and is fully reversible upon discontinuation of the responsible agent.

VIRAL HEPATITIS–LIKE REACTIONS

This form of injury is perhaps the most controversial and serious of all, and often poses especially difficult challenges to clinician, pharmacologist, and toxicologist alike. Because this lesion cannot be distinguished reliably from viral hepatitis, the resulting uncertainty of diagnosis may complicate management of the individual case. More broadly, over the years it has caused major confusion and controversy concerning the validity, incidence, significance, and natural history of such entities as halothane hepatitis and isoniazid-induced hepatitis, among others. Although in some instances, such as phenytoin-induced hepatitis, a prominent peripheral or tissue eosinophilia may suggest a nonviral etiology, this finding cannot be relied upon. Moreover, this group of reactions is characterized by a case fatality rate far in excess of that for acute viral hepatitis, and in the more severe cases, patterns of bridging, submassive, or massive necrosis may be seen. Indeed, of cases of acute bridging necrosis, a significant proportion may be accounted for by drug-induced hepatitis, but bridging necrosis per se does not necessarily indicate a chronic or fatal outcome.[20, 21] In addition to the above agents, this lesion has been associated with sulfonamides and inhibitors of monoamine oxidase.

As is true of most other forms of acute drug-induced liver disease, these lesions do not become self-perpetuating in the absence of continuing exposure to the injurious agent, although occasionally the course of disease may be prolonged, as in some patients with halothane hepatitis.[22]

If chronic hepatitis develops, it is almost always the result of continuing or repeated exposure.

GRANULOMATOUS HEPATITIS

Granulomatous lesions, typically consisting of circumscribed aggregates of epithelial histiocytes accompanied by variable numbers and types of inflammatory cells, represent part of the spectrum of hepatic inflammatory responses to medicinal agents. Several drugs may lead to granulomas with or without other manifestations of hepatic injury; typical examples include quinidine, allopurinol, phenylbutazone, sulfonamides, and sulfonylurea derivatives. However, many others also may produce this histopathologic lesion and, according to recent estimates, up to a third of cases of granulomatous hepatitis may result from therapeutic agents.[23] Granulomas resulting from drug-induced hepatic injury are invariably non-caseating and may contain abundant eosinophils. Their presence is generally taken as evidence of a hypersensitivity-based mechanism of injury.

CHRONIC HEPATITIS

That certain drugs may cause chronic hepatitis has been recognized only relatively recently.[7-9] However, the number of implicated agents continues to increase, and it seems likely that the apparent clinical incidence and importance of this type of reaction also will increase. Drug-induced chronic hepatitis is, in fact, a heterogeneous group of disorders that differ among themselves in pathogenesis and in histologic features (Table 31–3).

A drug-induced lesion indistinguishable from that of classic chronic active hepatitis was recognized initially as a complication of methyldopa or oxyphenisatin treatment, and since has been associated with isoniazid, sulfonamides, and nitrofurantoin therapy. A similar lesion has been found in a small number of chronic abusers of alcohol. Other forms of chronic hepatitis take the form of a focal nonspecific hepatic necrosis (e.g., that caused by aspirin) or centrilobular necrosis (e.g., that caused by acetaminophen).

Usually, the chronic forms of drug-induced liver injury depend on continued exposure to the agent and do not result from a self-perpetuating process set in motion by an acute insult. On the other hand, in very advanced cases of drug-induced chronic active hepatitis, resolution may be very slow despite discontinuation of the drug, or the lesion may progress to a fatal outcome over a period of weeks to months. In chronic aspirin- or acetaminophen-induced hep-

TABLE 31–3. DRUGS IMPLICATED IN THE ETIOLOGY OF CHRONIC HEPATITIS

Acetaminophen
Amiodarone
Aspirin
Dantrolene
Ethanol
Isoniazid
Methyldopa
Nitrofurantoin
Oxyphenisatin
Perhexilene maleate
Propylthiouracil
Sulfonamides

atotoxicity, prompt and complete resolution of the hepatic lesion after cessation of therapy is the rule. Rarely, chlorpromazine-induced cholestasis may be quite prolonged; although it may cause a clinical picture suggestive of primary biliary cirrhosis, this unusual complication would not ordinarily be regarded as a form of "chronic hepatitis."

Because these chronic forms of drug hepatotoxicity can be seen in patients taking readily available agents in doses regarded as therapeutic rather than toxic, the importance of the association may easily be overlooked in a given patient. For this reason, careful inquiry into use of both prescription and nonprescription drugs is essential in the evaluation of all patients with chronic liver disease.

CHOLESTASIS

Drugs can impair the formation of bile by interfering with any or all of the various hepatocellular mechanisms and structures involved in this process (Chap. 12). Two general histologic patterns are associated with drug-induced cholestasis. In one, cholestasis is accompanied by an inflammatory process that is especially prominent in the portal triads and, to a lesser extent, in the lobule itself, and is associated with variable hepatocellular necrosis. The inflammatory infiltrate is predominantly mononuclear, but may contain polymorphonuclear neutrophils or eosinophils. This type of reaction is often associated with systemic manifestations that include fever, rash, and arthralgias. It can be caused by a wide variety of drugs, including tranquilizers, antithyroid and hypoglycemic agents, and macrolide antibiotics such as erythromycin estolate. Chlorpromazine is the prototype of this class of agents.

In the second type of cholestatic drug reaction, the histologic features of inflammation and necrosis are minor or absent, and the lesion is characterized by a bland accumulation of bile in cells and canaliculi, principally centrilobular. This pattern characterizes the injury that can be caused by natural and synthetic estrogens, and by all 17α-substituted anabolic and androgenic steroids. Unlike the aforementioned inflammatory type of cholestatic reaction, the latter type of drug reaction usually results in only relatively mild systemic symptoms, except for pruritus, which can be quite severe.

In neither form does the process evolve to massive necrosis or a fatal outcome. Recovery after cessation of drug therapy is the rule. Recovery usually occurs within several weeks, although chlorpromazine reactions rarely may be quite prolonged.

FATTY LIVER

The lipid that accumulates in the liver in almost all forms of hepatotoxicity is predominantly triglyceride. The pathophysiologic abnormalities vary, depending on the agent, but in general they may be viewed as reflecting a rate of triglyceride formation that exceeds the rate of triglyceride disposition; *disposition* includes secretion into plasma in the form of triglyceride-rich lipoproteins, or hydrolysis to fatty acids and oxidation. There is no conclusive evidence that triglyceride in greater than normal amounts is injurious per se to the cell. Rather, accumulation of triglyceride in liver may be viewed as indicative of an abnormality in cellular metabolism that also may influence aspects of cellular function other than lipid metabolism, and thereby mediate toxicity.

There are two general histologic patterns of fatty liver. In the more common form, triglyceride is deposited in relatively large globules, which effectively fill the hepatocyte, displace the nucleus and other intracellular constituents to the periphery, and give the hepatocyte an adipocyte-like appearance. This large globular form of fat deposition characterizes the fatty liver associated with ethanol and corticosteroid administration, as well as with metabolic and nutritional disorders such as diabetes mellitus, obesity, hypertriglyceridemia, malnutrition, and the fatty liver seen after jejunoileal bypass surgery. Liver function may be relatively well preserved in the presence of fat deposition of this type, but can be altered to the extent that other processes such as alcoholic hepatitis are associated with it.

In a second histologic form of fatty liver, the fat is deposited in small droplets dispersed throughout the cytoplasm; the nucleus remains centrally located, and the cell itself retains its recognizability as a hepatocyte. This pattern is seen in only a few unusual circumstances, including tetracycline and valproic acid hepatotoxicity, Jamaican vomiting sickness, Reye's syndrome, fatty liver of pregnancy and certain rare inborn errors of metabolism. The pathogenesis is unknown except in the case of Jamaican vomiting sickness.[24] In this disorder, hypoglycin, a toxic principle from the unripened fruit of the ackee tree, causes impaired fatty acid oxidation and a more generalized disturbance in cellular metabolism that at least in part reflects its conversion to nonmetabolized derivatives of coenzyme A and carnitine, and thereby limits the availability of these critically important cofactors (Chap. 32). All the disorders leading to deposition of fat in small droplets are characterized by clinical and laboratory evidence of significantly disturbed hepatic function that, in its more severe forms, may include marked increases in serum transaminase activity, hypoglycemia, hyperammonemia, hepatic encephalopathy, and death in liver failure. Thus, the small droplet form of fat deposition reflects a potentially more serious disturbance of hepatocellular metabolism than does the large globular form of lipid accumulation.

Drug-induced lysosomal phospholipid storage (phospholipidosis) represents another type of hepatic lipid accumulation that may arise from the use of certain drugs, notably perhexilene maleate and amiodarone. The mechanism and significance of this distinctive morphologic entity are discussed further under the relevant drug headings.

VASCULAR LESIONS AND PORTAL HYPERTENSION

Apart from the fact that a number of drugs may cause chronic liver disease and thereby lead to the development of cirrhosis and portal hypertension, there are three drug- or toxin-associated disorders that cause portal hypertension, independent of primary liver disease. These are (1) hepatic vein thrombosis, which has been associated with, but not conclusively linked pathogenetically to, oral contraceptive use; (2) hepatic veno-occlusive disease, which has been observed in patients treated with 6-thioguanine as well as after the ingestion of pyrrolidizine alkaloids from plants of the genera *Senecio* and *Crotalaria* ("bush tea poisoning") (Chap. 32); (3) non-cirrhotic portal hypertension after chronic exposure to vinyl chloride monomer (Chap. 32). Peliosis hepatis, a dilation of sinusoids accompanied by replacement of zones of hepatocytes by blood-filled spaces, has been associated with chronic administration of androgenic and anabolic steroids, as well as with a variety of chronic wasting neoplastic and infectious diseases. Peliosis is not generally accompanied by portal hypertension.

TUMORS

Hepatic adenoma, focal nodular hyperplasia, and hepatocellular carcinoma have been associated with oral contraceptive use; less commonly, adenoma and carcinoma have been linked to anabolic steroid therapy. Angiosarcoma has been attributed to chronic exposure to vinyl chloride monomer (Chap. 45).

ANALGESIC, ANTI-INFLAMMATORY, AND MUSCLE RELAXANT DRUGS

ACETAMINOPHEN

Acetaminophen has enjoyed a long history as a relatively safe and well-tolerated analgesic agent. Beginning in about 1970, however, it became evident that, when taken in very large doses, the drug causes severe liver injury and death due to liver failure. It became popular, initially in Britain and increasingly in the United States, as an easily available method for committing suicide.[25-27] As the incidence of acetaminophen hepatotoxicity has increased, so has the appreciation of the broader clinical spectrum of the disorder, the experimental basis for an understanding of its pathogenesis, and approaches to treatment based on this understanding.

It is now recognized that acetaminophen hepatotoxicity occurs not only in persons who ingest massive amounts of the drug with suicidal intent but also in some individuals who ingest quantities within the therapeutic range.[28-30] Use of ethanol, or other inducers of hepatic drug metabolism, and nutritional state are among what may be many important determinants of significant individual differences in susceptibility.[28, 30-32] In addition to its clinical importance, therefore, acetaminophen hepatotoxicity stands virtually alone as a model of drug-induced liver disease in which fundamental concepts of drug metabolism and toxicity have proved directly translatable to pathogenesis and management.

Clinical and Laboratory Findings

After a massive acute ingestion, there is often a period of several hours in which the patient may experience diaphoresis, nausea, and vomiting. Typically, these subside and the patient enters a phase, lasting perhaps 24 hours, in which there may be no clinical or laboratory evidence of liver disease.[26, 27] During this period the patient may be judged erroneously to be out of danger, on the false premise that the ingested dose either was too small to be of concern or was not absorbed because of emesis or gastric aspiration. Presumably, this "latent" phase is the period during which there is progressive formation of toxic intermediates derived from acetaminophen metabolism, with progressive hepatic injury.

The latent phase ends with the onset of overt acute hepatocellular necrosis, including anorexia, nausea, vomiting, tender hepatomegaly, and, in the more severe cases, increasing jaundice and signs of liver failure and encephalopathy. Laboratory findings include variable increases in serum transaminase activity and bilirubin, and in prothrombin time. Transaminase levels of 20,000 IU/L are not unusual.[26] Although the degree of abnormality in those tests approximately reflects the extent of liver cell necrosis, the correspondence is imperfect. Thus, whereas in virtually all fatal cases serum transaminase activity exceeds 1000 IU/L at some point, most patients with transaminases in this range will survive,[33, 34] and even significant increases in prothrombin time and bilirubin do not necessarily indicate a fatal outcome. Conversely, patients whose liver tests are only mildly deranged generally have a favorable prognosis.[34] In non-fatal cases, recovery appears to be complete with restoration of normal liver function and structure on subsequent follow-up.[35]

Chronic acetaminophen hepatotoxicity has been associated with daily doses in the range of 3 to 8 g.[28-30] It may produce few or no symptoms, and may be clinically manifest only as a moderate increase in transaminase activity detected by routine screening. This mild disorder is completely reversible.

Histopathology

Very early changes in hepatocyte ultrastructure have been described in mice.[36] Clinically, the lesion of acute acetaminophen hepatotoxicity consists primarily of centrilobular or massive hepatic necrosis.[26, 27] Fat may be present, but the inflammatory response is relatively minor. As mentioned, available evidence suggests that histologically the liver returns to normal upon recovery.[35]

The chronic lesion is somewhat more variable and may consist of either centrilobular necrosis or a more nonspecific picture of focal or periportal hepatitis. Occasionally, it may resemble chronic active or chronic persistent hepatitis.[29, 37]

Diagnosis

Some patients will come to medical attention because of documented recent acetaminophen overdose. These patients may not have evident liver damage. Others may seek treatment for acute liver disease for which acute acetaminophen toxicity is one of several possible causes. Since active therapeutic intervention, if it is to be effective, must be initiated within 10 to 12 hours of ingestion (see below), it is important not only to document acetaminophen ingestion, but also to determine whether the dose was sufficient to cause life-threatening liver damage.

The latter question (i.e., the size and danger to life of the dose) has been particularly difficult to answer, for several reasons. First, although ingestion of 15 g or more is usually necessary to cause a severe or fatal case,[27] the history of the dose actually ingested, whether obtained from the patient or from others, is often unreliable.[38] Furthermore, the latent period between ingestion and the appearance of signs of liver damage may be quite misleading and may temporarily invalidate the clinical and laboratory findings customarily used for the assessment of liver disease. Finally, although acetaminophen hepatotoxicity is not immunologically mediated, there are important differences in individual susceptibilities such that serious toxicity may occur in one patient with a dose that in another would be relatively safe. For example, chronic ethanol use,[28, 31, 32] fasting,[39, 40] and prior induction of hepatic microsomal drug metabolism by other agents[41-45] all predispose to acetaminophen hepatotoxicity, and in such circumstances serious liver injury or death may occur with otherwise tolerable doses.

To help deal with these difficulties, determination of acetaminophen levels in blood has been employed with some success, on the basis of the empirical observation that serious liver injury usually occurs only in those patients in whom the plasma acetaminophen concentration at a given time after ingestion exceeds the line joining 200 mg/L at 4 hours with 30 mg/L at 15 hours on a semilogarithmic plot of plasma concentration as a function of time.[25, 26, 34] Although there is overlap, measurement of the blood acetaminophen level is quite helpful, both in confirming the ingestion and in providing an indication of the probability of serious toxicity.

Severe hepatocellular disease has developed in patients with chronic alcoholism who had taken acetaminophen in doses in or near the therapeutic range.[31, 32] In these patients, elevation of serum transaminases far in excess of values consistent with alcoholic hepatitis have been observed, although in keeping with underlying alcoholic liver disease, levels of aspartate aminotransferase have invariably exceeded those of alanine aminotransferase. When soliciting a history of acetaminophen use in patients with chronic alcoholism and evidence of acute severe liver injury, it is also important to inquire about acetaminophen-containing nonprescription drug combinations that may have been ingested for their alcohol content.[46]

The differential diagnosis of acute acetaminophen hepatotoxicity includes all other causes of acute hepatic necrosis, such as viral hepatitis and ethanol-induced and other forms of drug-induced liver injury, as well as acute deterioration of pre-existing chronic liver disease. Although it is important that these conditions be considered and, where possible, excluded, the importance of early institution of specific treatment of acetaminophen hepatotoxicity and its apparent safety necessitates that in the absence of definitive evidence to the contrary (e.g., very low blood acetaminophen levels), any patient with documented substantial acetaminophen ingestion should be considered at risk and managed accordingly.

Mechanism

An impressive body of evidence accumulated over the past decade indicates that acetaminophen hepatotoxicity is mediated by the formation of one or more toxic intermediates during the biotransformation of the parent compound.[41–44, 47] Thus, in animal studies, toxicity correlates not only with dose but with the activity of microsomal drug metabolizing enzymes. The current view of this interaction may be summarized as follows.

At low doses acetaminophen is principally conjugated with glucuronic acid or sulfate (Fig. 31–1), and these harmless conjugates are largely excreted in the urine. A minor fraction of the parent compound undergoes biotransformation via a specific isoenzyme of the microsomal cytochrome P450-dependent drug-metabolizing system.[48] This results in the formation of toxic intermediates, the best characterized of which is N-acetyl-p-benzoquinone imine (NAPQI), a highly reactive electrophile.[41, 49] NAPQI forms a conjugate with glutathione, which after further conversion to cysteine and N-acetylcysteine derivatives in the intestinal mucosa and renal tubules is excreted in the urine as a mercapturic acid.[50, 51] Detoxification via the glutathione

mechanism thus ordinarily provides the modest degree of protection needed at low doses of acetaminophen.[41–44]

Unfortunately, the glucuronide and sulfate conjugation pathways that predominate at low doses of acetaminophen are readily saturable.[52] As the dose of the drug increases, therefore, a correspondingly greater fraction becomes available for entry into the microsomal pathway, and subsequent conversion to toxic intermediates, the detoxification of which depends on conjugation with glutathione. As would be expected, as the ingested dose of acetaminophen is increased, cellular glutathione stores become progressively depleted.[44] If the formation of toxic intermediates is of sufficient magnitude, glutathione stores will fall below a critical level: that is, it no longer will be adequate to sustain this crucial detoxification reaction. At this point, the toxic intermediates react covalently with cellular constituents, especially proteins and other macromolecules essential for cellular homeostasis, and, presumably by this mechanism, effect their hepatotoxicity.[41–44, 53, 54]

The "threshold" phenomenon thus can be understood simply as the point at which the rate of formation of toxic intermediates exceeds the rate at which they can be detoxified by the glutathione mechanism. It is at once apparent that this threshold (which is, in effect, the determinant of individual susceptibility to acetaminophen toxicity) can vary up or down, depending on the rates of either or both of the two critical processes involved (microsomal production of toxic intermediates and their detoxification by glutathione), each of which is influenced in turn by several factors. For example, the rate of formation of toxic intermediates is not simply a function of drug dose or bioavailability, but also depends on the activity of the glucuronide and sulfate conjugating pathways, the availability of glucuronic acid and sulfate, and the activity of the cytochrome P450 pathway. Prior administration of drugs (e.g., phenobarbital and ethanol) that induce the microsomal cytochrome P450 pathway predisposes to acetaminophen hepatotoxicity,[27, 48] whereas inhibitors of the pathway,[41–44] including cimetidine,[55, 56] are protective. This undoubtedly accounts, at least in part, for the increased susceptibility to acetaminophen hepatotoxicity caused by prior use of ethanol, barbiturates, and other inducers. Indeed, there is evidence that ethanol induces the specific isoenzyme of cytochrome P450 responsible for the oxidation of both ethanol and acetaminophen.[48] This also provides an explanation, based on competitive inhibition, for the seemingly paradoxical protective effect of acute ethanol administration on acetaminophen-induced hepatotoxicity.[26, 48]

The threshold dose for hepatotoxicity will vary inversely with hepatocellular glutathione stores. For example, both fasting[39, 40] and ethanol[57] decrease hepatic glutathione concentrations and predispose to hepatotoxicity, whereas cysteine precursors, such as N-acetylcysteine and L-2-oxathiozolidine-4-carboxylate, increase hepatic glutathione stores by promoting glutathione synthesis and hence protect against acetaminophen toxicity.[58, 59] Although, to some extent, N-acetylcysteine also may increase the availability of sulfate,[60] the protective value of this is unclear.[61] Both propylthiouracil[62] and N-acetylcysteine[63] may also afford protection by acting as substitutes for glutathione, forming direct adducts with NAPQI, although in the case of N-acetylcysteine this probably represents a minor protective route.[59] Lipid peroxidation, possibly mediated via a free radical intermediate of acetaminophen metabolism,[64] also has been suggested as a mechanism for acetaminophen-induced liver injury.[40] Although the apparent protective

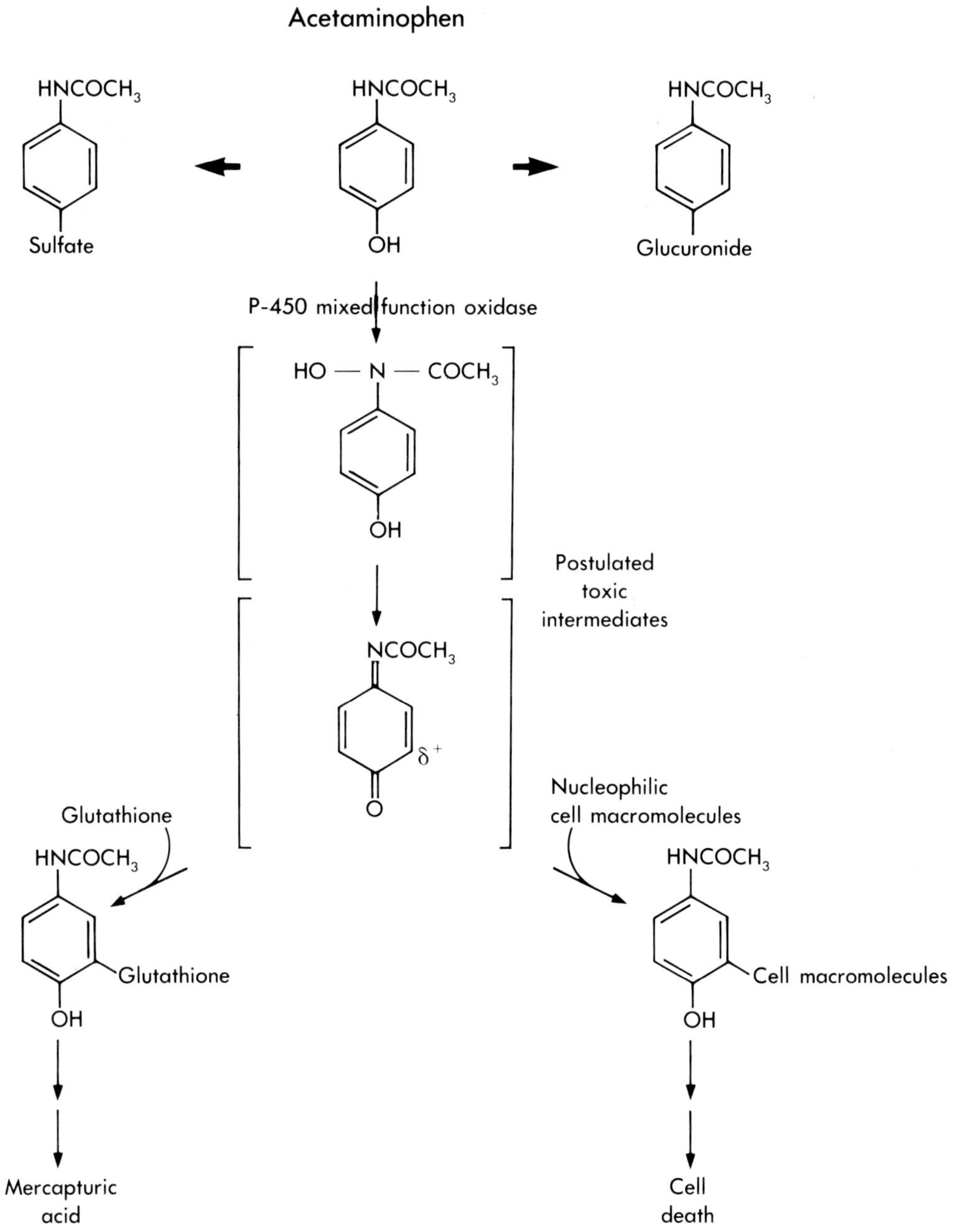

Figure 31–1. Pathways of acetaminophen metabolism. (From Mitchell JR, Jollow DJ. Gastroenterology 68:392, © by Williams & Wilkins, 1975.)

effect of vitamin E[65] as well as agents that increase glutathione[66] are explicable in relation to such a mechanism, available evidence does not support a causal role for lipid peroxidation in the injury but suggests, rather, that it may simply be a result of the injury.[67]

Although the evidence that cellular glutathione is protective against acetaminophen hepatotoxicity is compelling, there is less certainty that cellular injury is mediated primarily by the formation of covalent bonds between toxic intermediates of acetaminophen biotransformation (e.g., NAPQI) and cellular constituents. The covalent binding hypothesis has been challenged by reports that the protective effects of cimetidine,[68] N-acetylcysteine,[69] and α-mercapto-propionylglycine[70] are not associated with diminished overall formation of covalent adducts of acetaminophen to macromolecules. Subsequent work has criticized the methodology of these earlier studies and substantiated the inverse relationship between the protective effects of cimetidine[56] and N-acetylcysteine[71] and covalent modification of cellular macromolecules.

It is still disputed whether the primary pathway of acetaminophen-induced toxicity involves glutathione depletion via adduct formation with toxic intermediates and subsequent covalent binding of intermediates to cellular proteins, or whether toxic intermediates of the drug result in glutathione depletion via oxidation to glutathione disulfide with subsequent oxidation of cellular protein thiols.[62, 72–74] However, these two mechanisms are not necessarily mutually exclusive, although the predominance of one over the other may depend upon the experimental model investigated (e.g., isolated or cultured hepatocytes versus intact animals). Notwithstanding these uncertainties, available evidence suggests that either mechanism may result in impairment of proteins and/or cofactors involved in cellular calcium homeostasis,[75, 76] with accumulation of calcium in the cell cytosol leading to cell death. (See Chap. 30).

Treatment

On the basis of the available data, acetaminophen hepatotoxicity should be regarded as a potentially treatable disorder, not merely by discontinuation of the toxin and supportive care but by active pharmacologic intervention. As currently understood, the objective is to increase the stores of hepatocellular glutathione, thereby averting the toxicity of acetaminophen metabolites, which presumably have not yet reacted with critical cell constituents.

N-acetylcysteine is the drug of choice for patients with acetaminophen overdose. Thus, in the study by Prescott et al.,[34] only one of 62 patients treated with N-acetylcysteine within ten hours of taking acetaminophen developed severe liver damage (defined as a serum transaminase activity greater than 1000 IU/L), whereas 20 of 38 patients treated after ten hours and 33 of 57 given supportive care alone developed severe liver damage. Similarly, in the Rocky Mountain Poison Center multicenter study,[26] only four of 57 patients treated with N-acetylcysteine within ten hours of taking acetaminophen developed severe liver damage, whereas 15 of 52 patients treated between ten and 16 hours and 24 of 39 patients treated between 16 and 24 hours developed severe liver damage. Since the prognostic value of the serum transaminase activity could be questioned, it is significant that in the British trial[34] there were no deaths in the group treated early with N-acetylcysteine, but two and three deaths in the late treatment and untreated groups, respectively. N-acetylcysteine is both effective and rela-

tively innocuous. It may be administered orally or (in Britain) intravenously, but only if initiated within the first 10 to 12 hours after acetaminophen ingestion will it influence morbidity and mortality. As mentioned above, the decision to use the drug must often be made under circumstances in which information concerning the actual risk of severe acetaminophen hepatotoxicity (e.g., blood acetaminophen levels) is incomplete or inconclusive. Despite this, because of the importance of early institution of the drug, as well as the safety of N-acetylcysteine treatment, it should be employed in two clinical settings: (1) when acetaminophen blood levels and/or plasma disappearance $T_{1/2}$ indicate that the patient is at risk; (2) when blood acetaminophen levels are not rapidly available, but there is good reason to believe that a significant overdose has occurred. In these patients with documented or probable serious acetaminophen overdose, the threshold for institution of N-acetylcysteine treatment should be even lower when additional risk factors can be identified, such as chronic use of ethanol or drugs that induce microsomal drug metabolism, fasting, starvation, or protein malnutrition.

The treatment schedules currently employed involve administration of an initial dose of 140 mg/kg, p.o., followed by maintenance doses of 70 mg/kg q. 4 hr p.o. for a total of 72 hours.[26] The schedule employed by Prescott et al.[24] with a preparation appropriate for intravenous use was an initial dose of 150 mg/kg in 200 ml 5 per cent glucose over 15 minutes, followed by 50 mg/kg in 500 ml over 4 hours, and 100 mg/kg in 1 liter over the next 16 hours, for a total of 300 mg/kg over 20 hours. Unfortunately, the intravenous preparation is not generally available in the United States. In addition, other more standard approaches to drug overdose and acute hepatic injury are essential components of the care of these patients. They include initial gastric intubation and aspiration to recover any residual drug; the monitoring of vital signs; maintenance of fluid and electrolyte balance, oxygenation, and blood pressure; and customary management of severe liver injury and encephalopathy, if needed, as described in Chapter 17. Well over 90 per cent of patients may be expected to recover completely.

ASPIRIN

Like acetaminophen, aspirin is a well-documented cause of a dose-related, reversible form of hepatotoxicity. Unlike acetaminophen, neither its mechanism nor the basis for apparent differences in individual susceptibilities are understood.

The disorder is most commonly encountered in patients with chronic rheumatic diseases treated for several days or weeks with high-dose aspirin therapy and is manifest in most instances as an asymptomatic, subtle disturbance in liver function, as reflected by mild to moderate increases in serum transaminase activity and, much less commonly, subclinical hyperbilirubinemia.[77–81] Jaundice is quite uncommon, and severe clinical hepatitis rare, although nonfatal cases with hypoprothrombinemia and encephalopathy have been reported.[80, 82]

The histologic process associated with these functional abnormalities is a nonspecific focal hepatitis.[80] Massive or submassive necrosis has not been established as a consequence of high-dose aspirin therapy, and there is no apparent increase in hepatocellular fat. Thus, although the rare occurrence of acute encephalopathy and anicteric liver dysfunction in a child has suggested the possibility of a

Reye's-like syndrome,[83] hepatotoxicity in the setting of long-term high-dose aspirin therapy is associated with neither the characteristic histopathology nor the ominous prognosis of Reye's syndrome.[82, 83] Despite this, there is persisting concern regarding a possible association of aspirin use and Reye's syndrome.[84] Microvesicular hepatocellular fat, similar to that seen in Reye's syndrome, has been described in children with fatal salicylate intoxication,[85] but this is not a typical histologic feature of hepatotoxicity of high-dose aspirin therapy. In a patient with systemic lupus erythematosis, the biopsy picture resembled that of chronic active hepatitis,[78] but this is exceptional. Aspirin hepatotoxicity is rapidly and completely reversed when the drug is discontinued.

The dose dependency of the lesion is well established, but there are substantial differences in individual susceptibilities. Thus, whereas the injury usually is associated with serum salicylate levels in excess of 25 mg/dL (a daily dose of about 3 to 5 g in adults), there are numerous exceptions, and about 2 per cent of instances of toxicity occurred at levels of less than 10 mg/dL.[80] Certain groups of patients seem to be at greater risk, including those with juvenile rheumatoid arthritis, systemic lupus erythematosus, and rheumatoid arthritis. Indeed, it has been suggested that as many as 50 per cent of patients with juvenile rheumatoid arthritis taking therapeutic doses of aspirin will have increased serum transaminase activity.[81] It is not clear whether this apparent predisposition reflects only that these patients are more often exposed to potentially toxic doses of aspirin. It has been suggested that reduced serum albumin concentrations, by increasing the unbound fraction of aspirin, might predispose to injury.[86] Evidence in support of this concept has been obtained in studies of aspirin toxicity in monolayer cultures of hepatocytes,[87] but its significance with regard to clinical hepatotoxicity remains to be determined. It also has been suggested that alleviation of juvenile rheumatoid arthritis might in some way be promoted by hepatic dysfunction, regardless of cause.[81, 88] Hepatotoxicity also appears to occur with other salicylates, including sodium and choline salicylate,[77] but experience with these agents is limited.

An unusual reaction to aspirin was observed in a patient with adult onset of Still's disease.[89] This patient developed significant hepatotoxicity, microangiopathic hemolytic anemia, and disseminated intravascular coagulation while taking 3 to 6 g aspirin daily. This episode and a similar reaction occurring in response to aspirin rechallenge were treated with corticosteroids, and the patient's condition improved. It is not known whether this represented a distinctive form of aspirin hepatotoxicity or the superimposition of an aspirin-associated complication of the underlying disease process on otherwise ordinary aspirin hepatotoxicity.

OTHER AGENTS

Phenylbutazone. Phenylbutazone has been associated with overt hepatic injury in about 0.25 per cent of patients. The onset of the reaction usually occurs in the first six weeks of treatment but may be delayed by as much as one year. It is more common in adults than in children.[2, 90]

The reaction may take several forms. Most often the illness resembles viral hepatitis in its presentation, and in about 50 per cent of patients there may be antecedent fever, rash, or arthralgia. Clinical and laboratory findings are consistent with an acute hepatitis, and liver biopsy may show a typical viral hepatitis–like picture, submassive or massive necrosis. Fatal hepatitis may occur but is unusual. Less commonly, the appearance of the disorder may be cholestatic, with or without pruritus, and with little clinical or histologic evidence of significant hepatocellular necrosis. Non-caseating granulomas may accompany the hepatic reaction, usually in association with minor hepatocellular injury.[90] Histologic changes indistinguishable from those seen in primary biliary cirrhosis have been observed in one patient.[90]

The prognosis for all forms of phenylbutazone-associated hepatic injuries is good, although both the viral hepatitis–like and the granulomatous reaction have been associated with fatal outcomes. In the remainder, improvement accompanies discontinuation of the drug. There are anecdotal reports of the use of corticosteroids but their actual effect on the course of the disease is not defined.

The mechanism of the injury is unknown. Although certain clinical features suggest hypersensitivity to the drug, phenylbutazone is hepatotoxic in laboratory animals,[2] and overdoses with this drug have produced acute hepatic necrosis in humans.[90]

Allopurinol. Several case reports indicate that allopurinol may lead to liver cell injury, usually within a period of five weeks.[91, 92] Fever, skin rash, and eosinophilia are not uncommon, with moderate transaminase elevation and jaundice. Occasionally, there is a severe systemic reaction with vasculitis and renal failure.[93] Diuretic use and renal impairment may predispose toward the development of allopurinol hepatotoxicity.[91] The pathologic findings include centrilobular necrosis as well as features indistinguishable from viral hepatitis, with eosinophils being prominent. Massive hepatic necrosis also has been described,[94] but the disorder is rarely fatal. Granulomas, which may show a fibrin-ring structure similar to those seen in Q-fever,[95] are reported in about 50 per cent of liver biopsies and have also been described in bone marrow.[92]

Gold. Several case reports suggest that gold salts used in the treatment of rheumatoid arthritis occasionally cause a relatively noninflammatory, cholestatic form of liver injury.[96–98] The onset usually has occurred within a few weeks after the start of the course of drug administration, and has responded well to cessation of treatment. The prognosis has been uniformly good. The incidence and mechanism of toxicity are unknown.

Indomethacin, Ibuprofen, Naproxen. These and a number of other anti-inflammatory agents have been associated with variable hepatotoxicity.[2, 99, 100]

Sulindac. Several cases of painless jaundice with evidence of a mild hepatitis and variable cholestatic features have been attributed to sulindac.[101] Recovery upon withdrawal of the drug may take several months.

Benoxaprofen. This drug has been withdrawn following 31 deaths, mainly in elderly patients, from hepatorenal toxicity. The liver disease was typically cholestatic, with characteristic laminated concretions filling proliferated bile ductules, seen on histology.[102]

Dantrolene. This is an antispasmodic agent related to phenytoin. In a prospective study, prolonged (more than two months) use of the drug was associated with a 1.8 per cent incidence of liver function abnormalities; of the 19 affected patients, 6 were jaundiced and 3 died.[103] Additional experience indicates that significant liver injury caused by dantrolene occurs only after a month or more of use and is more likely to occur among patients 30 years old or older or when doses exceed 300 mg/day.[103] Clinically, the disease resembles acute or chronic viral hepatitis, and histologically it may be associated with bridging or submassive necrosis. A very high reported case fatality rate of 28 per cent may reflect a selection bias among the reported cases.[103] It has been recommended that liver tests be monitored in all patients treated with this agent.[103, 104] Experimental studies have shown that dantrolene is converted to an electrophilic metabolite by cytochrome P450 with covalent binding to hepatic proteins and inhibition of cytochrome P450.[105] This sequence of events, however, has not been shown to result in hepatic necrosis.

Chlorzoxazone. This centrally acting muscle relaxant has been implicated in several instances of acute hepatic injury, ranging in severity from a mild hepatitis to fatal massive hepatic necrosis.[106]

ANESTHETIC AGENTS

In contradistinction to the circumstances surrounding the use of most other categories of drugs and chemicals, the very use of anesthetic agents often implies a setting in which some changes in hepatic function, especially blood flow and oxygenation, are virtually inevitable.[107, 108] Although the anesthesia-associated decrease in splanchnic (thus, hepatic) blood flow and oxygenation is discussed in greater detail in Chapter 34, it deserves special emphasis, since it may be exaggerated under circumstances that cause systemic hypoxemia and hypotension and thereby may lead to overt anoxic liver injury. Moreover, recent studies indicate that the adequacy of oxygenation may exert a major influence on the hepatic metabolism of halogenated hydrocarbons such as halothane, and by this mechanism modulate their hepatotoxic potential. Clinically evident hepatotoxicity is a distinctly uncommon effect of the anesthetic agents currently in common use, and for practical purposes it occurs only in association with the administration of halothane and related haloalkanes such as methoxyflurane. Ethyl ether, nitrous oxide, and cyclopropane do not appear injurious to the liver directly.

HALOTHANE

Despite the numerous outstanding attributes of halothane as a general anesthetic agent, and despite early controversy and uncertainty as to its potential hepatotoxicity,[109, 110] it now seems clear that halothane can cause liver injury.[111–118] The earlier uncertainty stemmed in large part from the fact that halothane hepatotoxicity appears to be rare, that it can resemble severe acute viral hepatitis clinically and histologically, and that there are many other causes of postoperative (i.e., postanesthetic) jaundice and liver dysfunction.[119–122] Ultimately, however, the validity of halothane hepatotoxicity was unequivocally demonstrated in the report by Klatskin and Kimberg[123] of an anesthesiologist who, after repeated exposures to the agent, developed recurrent and progressive liver disease. In a controlled setting, administration of small amounts of halothane to this subject elicited a characteristic clinical, laboratory, and histologic response within hours.

Incidence and Epidemiology

Fortunately, the incidence of halothane hepatotoxicity is very low, approximating one case in 10,000 anesthesias.[111] The incidence is increased significantly, reaching perhaps

seven in 10,000, among patients undergoing repeated anesthesias.[115] This fact, together with the consistent finding that the majority of patients with clinically evident halothane hepatotoxicity have had prior experience with the agent, supports the concept that this lesion reflects a sensitization to the agent and is immunologically mediated. However, as is discussed below, there is increasing evidence that halothane hepatotoxicity reflects, at least in part, the injurious effects of one or more toxic products of halothane biotransformation. In addition to an increased risk among patients undergoing repeated exposures, it appears to be higher in female and obese subjects; its incidence is distinctly lower in children and young adults than in older adults.

Mechanism

As mentioned, the relative rarity of halothane hepatotoxicity, its increased frequency after prior exposure, and the fact that affected patients may have systemic features such as fever and eosinophilia, have suggested that this disorder is immunologically mediated. This concept is supported by the results of several studies,[124–129] including the recent demonstration in the sera of patients with fulminant hepatic failure after halothane anesthesia of an antibody that reacted with components of liver cell membranes from rabbits anesthetized with halothane.[130] Although compatible with immunologically mediated liver cell injury, these findings are subject to alternative interpretations.[131] Moreover, in studies of what is clearly a non-immunologically mediated carbon tetrachloride–induced hepatotoxicity in mice, a cellular immune response to liver cell antigens has been demonstrated, suggesting that the sensitization is the result of injury rather than the cause of it.[132]

An increasing body of evidence suggests that halothane hepatotoxicity is mediated by a toxic product of halothane biotransformation. Thus, halothane causes a variety of structural and functional changes in rat liver preparations.[133–139] In human subjects undergoing anesthesia, approximately 20 per cent of halothane is metabolized[140, 141] and morphologic changes not seen with other anesthetics are observed.[142] The principal products are trifluoracetic acid and bromide ion, neither of which appears to be hepatotoxic. However, in animal studies there was evidence of covalent binding of halothane to liver macromolecules, especially in animals pretreated with phenobarbital. Under aerobic conditions in which the inspired oxygen is high, this was not associated with hepatocellular necrosis. However, when rats were pretreated with inducers of microsomal drug-metabolizing enzymes and subjected to inhalation of 1 per cent halothane in a relatively oxygen-deficient atmosphere, centrilobular necrosis developed regularly, associated with increased serum transaminase activity, increased covalent binding of halothane metabolites to hepatic lipids, and inhibition of microsomal P450 activity.[141–151] These conditions favor metabolism of halothane via reductive pathways, and the formation of potentially toxic products (Fig. 31–2). Similar products (2-chloro-1,1,1-trifluoroethane and 2-chloro-1,1-difluoroethylene) are produced in a guinea pig model that does not require hypoxia or enzyme induction[152] and have been demonstrated in the expired air of human subjects undergoing halothane anesthesia, even at high oxygen tensions.[147, 148] Moreover, ethanolamine and cysteine conjugates of halothane metabolites have been demonstrated in the urines of some human subjects, adding further support to the concept that intermediates are

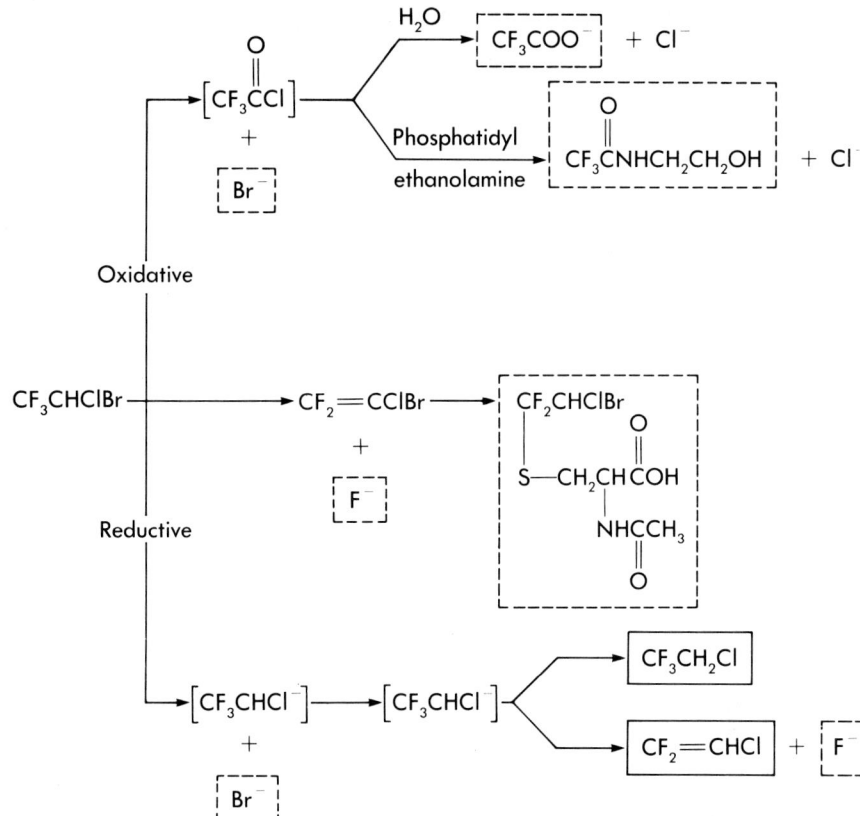

Figure 31–2. Schematic representation of hepatic microsomal biotransformation of halothane. [ ] = reactive intermediate; ⌐⌐⌐ = excreted in urine; ☐ = excreted in breath. (Modified from Cousins MJ, et al. Anesth Intensive Care 7:9, 1979, with permission.)

formed that may react with sulfhydryl groups of liver cell proteins and with lipids.[153] It is possible that the free radicals formed via reductive pathways[154–156] are the reactive intermediates of greatest significance under these conditions.

Individual differences in susceptibilities to the lesion may reflect differences in dose (e.g., obesity); intra- or postoperative systemic hypoxemia; impairment of splanchnic, hepatic or lobular blood flow; activity of reductive biotransformation pathways (possibly influenced by exposure to potential inducers); adequacy of cellular protective mechanisms; and genetic factors. Indeed, genetic differences in reductive metabolism of halothane have been identified in rats,[157] and the existence of a familial, probably genetic, susceptibility factor predisposing to halothane hepatitis in humans has been reported.[158] In view of the multiplicity of factors that influence the propensity to halothane hepatotoxicity, it may not be necessary to invoke an immunologic mechanism to account for the idiosyncratic nature of the reaction. As mentioned, however, this possibility is not excluded, either as the sole basis for the injury or in concert with the effect of a toxic intermediate.

Histopathology

In many instances the lesion associated with halothane hepatotoxicity has not been distinguishable from that of viral hepatitis, and this has caused considerable difficulty. It is especially a problem in massive hepatic necrosis, in which more specific histologic features often may be indistinguishable. Occasionally, there may be a significant eosinophilic infiltration and, less commonly, granuloma forma-

tion. In general, the spectrum of severity of lesions ranging from spotty necrosis to massive necrosis is related to repeated exposure to the agent.[159] In a significant number of cases, necrosis may be localized predominantly in the centrilobular zone, often associated with only a sparse inflammatory reaction. This pattern is similar to that caused by carbon tetrachloride and acetaminophen, which injure the liver via the formation of reactive intermediates. This finding, therefore, is of interest both because of its implications concerning the mechanism of halothane hepatotoxicity and because in some cases it permits differentiation from viral hepatitis. Unfortunately, this distinction is usually quite difficult on both clinical and histologic grounds.

Clinical Features

Symptoms and signs of halothane hepatotoxicity most often appear several days to two or at most three weeks after exposure.[117] This interval is characteristically reduced to a few days when there has been a previous exposure to halothane.[160] The clinical onset often begins with fever and in other respects is nonspecific, consisting of variable anorexia, nausea, myalgias, jaundice, and tender hepatomegaly.[111–113] In more severe cases, signs of liver failure develop, including ascites, encephalopathy, and coagulopathy. Skin and joint manifestations are uncommon.

There appears to be a relatively large group of up to 20 to 25 per cent of patients who develop mild, largely subclinical reactions to halothane.[116–118] In a subset of this group, hepatotoxicity may be manifested only by an elevated serum transaminase activity or postoperative fever. Because there are many causes other than halothane reaction for such phenomena in the postoperative patient, the true incidence of this mild form of the disease is unknown. Similarly, although most patients with clinically overt halothane hepatotoxicity in retrospect have had previous exposures to halothane, and many of these have had unexplained postoperative fevers, it is not known what proportion of the patients with mild or inapparent initial reactions would, if re-exposed, develop more overt liver injury. Despite this uncertainty, the generally accepted dictum that such patients, once identified, should not be exposed to halothane again is valid as a clinical guideline. It does seem clear that among patients with histories of recent halothane exposure, those who are re-exposed are more likely to have abnormal liver test results than is a control population.[161, 162] In neither of these reports were there serious reactions. In this respect, the situation may possibly be analogous to isoniazid hepatotoxicity, in which 10 to 20 per cent of patients develop mild and apparently self-limited reactions, whereas only 1 per cent have overt hepatitis; similar dichotomies are observed with other drugs. The relationship, if any, between these two patterns of hepatic dysfunction is unknown.

Laboratory findings are equally nonspecific and are chiefly characterized by prominent elevations in transaminase activity and, in more severe cases, prolonged prothrombin times.

On the basis of reported cases, the fatality rate among patients with halothane-associated fulminant hepatic failure approaches 80 per cent.[117] The overall mortality rate for all cases of halothane hepatotoxicity is undoubtedly lower. In some cases, especially those with more severe acute courses, resolution may be delayed considerably. Although it has been suggested that a chronic hepatitis may ensue,[163] more recent evidence suggests that even in the prolonged cases eventual resolution may be expected.[164]

Diagnosis and Differential Diagnosis

The nonspecificity of the clinical, laboratory, and histologic findings associated with halothane hepatotoxicity, and the multiplicity of causes of postoperative liver injury, make the diagnosis quite difficult. Indeed, it is likely that in most instances the diagnosis can only be inferred on the basis of a compatible history of exposure, post-exposure interval, and clinical and laboratory findings. Because of the potentially high case fatality rate, rechallenge with halothane is not recommended. If the findings are consistent and if other causes of postoperative jaundice, such as viral or drug-induced hepatitis, bile duct obstruction, postoperative cholestasis, sepsis, and hemolysis, can be excluded, it is best to assume that the patient has experienced a halothane reaction and to advise that this and related haloalkanes be avoided in the future. (See also Chap. 34.)

Prevention and Management

As noted, a careful history of prior anesthetic exposure is essential if halothane use is considered. For individuals in whom a series of anesthetic exposures is anticipated, another agent is preferred. Because halothane has been reported to contaminate vaporizer-equipped anesthesia machines and thereby cause a recurrence of hepatitis,[165] this potential should be dealt with in any patient with a history suggestive of halothane hepatitis.

The management of halothane hepatotoxicity is entirely supportive, including, if necessary in severe cases, measures directed against the complications of hepatic failure, such as encephalopathy, bleeding diathesis, hypoxia, and hypotension. Corticosteroids are of no proven value (see Chap. 17).

OTHER HALOALKANES

Methoxyflurane. This agent causes a hepatic injury very similar to that associated with halothane. Indeed, there is evidence for "cross-reactivity," in that some patients with a history of exposure to one agent may develop a reaction to the other.[117, 166] Methoxyflurane may also lead to hyperoxaluria and renal failure. Both methoxyflurane and halothane have caused hepatitis in individuals who have abused ("sniffed") these agents.[173–175]

Enflurane. Enflurane has been reported to cause liver injury.[167–169] The syndrome is similar to halothane hepatitis clinically and is associated with centrilobular necrosis. Prior exposure to either enflurane or halothane apparently is predisposing and shortens the latent period between exposure and clinical onset of illness.[168] It should be noted that the causal role of enflurane is disputed and that this issue remains unresolved.[170, 171] Both enflurane and methoxyflurane influence microsomal electron transport in vitro, but the possible relationship of this effect to hepatotoxicity is not known.[172]

Isoflurane. Isoflurane is the member of this class of agents that is least likely to cause hepatotoxicity, consistent with its extremely limited metabolism.[176] Its major disadvantage appears to be its greater cost.

ANTICONVULSANTS

PHENYTOIN

Chronic phenytoin use has been associated with a significant incidence of abnormal liver tests,[177] and structural abnormalities on liver biopsy.[178, 179] In addition, at least 45 cases of acute phenytoin-associated hepatic injury have been recorded. The acute cases have been remarkably similar to one another in clinical, laboratory, and histologic findings, and there is little doubt that the apparent causal relationship is valid.[180–183] The onset usually occurs after four to six weeks of drug administration, although it may be as early as one to two weeks, and is characterized by malaise, fever, lymphadenopathy, maculopapular rash, and vague abdominal complaints. Physical findings, in addition to rash and adenopathy, include variable hepatomegaly and jaundice, and, occasionally, splenomegaly. There is a moderate to marked leukocytosis; total leukocyte count occasionally may exceed 30,000/mm^3, with atypical lymphocytes and a relative and absolute eosinophilia. Liver function is significantly deranged, with moderate to marked increases in transaminase and alkaline phosphatase activity, bilirubin concentration, and prothrombin time. In the most severe cases, encephalopathy and other signs of progressive liver failure may ensue, and are poor prognostic signs. Histologically, the lesion resembles acute viral hepatitis, although there may be more than the usual number of eosinophils. In the most severe and fatal cases, there is massive hepatic necrosis, occasionally with a predominantly centrilobular localization. A granulomatous reaction also has been documented.[184] Treatment of the disorder is largely supportive.

Corticosteroids have been employed in a number of instances. They may improve the systemic, serum sickness–like features of the illness, but there is no evidence that they influence the course of the hepatic lesion or survival.[183] High dose (pulse) corticosteroids also have been employed with similar results.[185]

The pathogenesis of liver injury may involve both immunologic and toxic mechanisms. The apparent rarity of the disorder and its serum sickness and pseudolymphoma-like clinical features,[186] together with laboratory evidence suggestive of an immunologic response,[181, 187] are suggestive of drug hypersensitivity. That there may well be a component of this in the overall reaction is consistent with the fact that in several instances, rechallenge with the drug has led to a rapid reappearance of the systemic features.[188–192] It is of interest, however, that in only two of these cases[182, 192] was the response to rechallenge associated with abnormalities in liver tests. This would be consistent with the possibility that the liver injury is at least in part toxic, mediated by the formation of a reactive intermediate. In this connection, it is of interest that in its biotransformation, phenytoin is in part converted to a dihydrodiol derivative, possibly by way of an epoxide.[193] (Also see Chap. 9.) Epoxides are capable of reacting with sulfhydryl and other important reducing groups and may, in a manner analogous to that proposed for acetaminophen hepatotoxicity, cause liver cell injury via the formation of covalent bonds with critical cell constituents. If this is indeed the case, differences in individual susceptibilities could be explained by genetic or induced differences in rates and pathways of drug biotransformation. In fact, evidence has been presented that suggests that at least some of these patients are genetically predisposed to toxic liver injury related to a relative deficiency in their ability to detoxify arene oxides (e.g., via epoxide hydrolase).[17] On the other hand, such a mechanism would not appear to account for the prominent systemic features of the illness, for which an immunologic mechanism seems more plausible. Whereas it is conceivable that a toxic product of drug biotransformation might also elicit (as a hapten) an immune response, the relationship between the hepatic and systemic components of this drug-induced disorder remains speculative.

VALPROIC ACID (2-PROPYL-PENTANOIC ACID)

This newer agent is used principally in the treatment of petit mal epilepsy. It is a branched, medium-chain-length fatty acid, and is administered orally as the sodium salt. Although it is generally well tolerated, a number of side effects have been reported, including incidences as high as 44 per cent (average about 11 to 12 per cent) of mainly transient, asymptomatic, usually slight (< two fold) increases in serum transaminase activity.[194, 195] These usually occur after 10 to 12 weeks of drug therapy, and at least in some instances appear to be dose-dependent.[195]

Clinically overt liver damage is much less common, but its true incidence is unknown.[194–201] Whereas severe and sometimes fatal reactions are common among the available case reports, the full clinical, pathologic and prognostic spectra of the disease await definition. The clinical manifestations of overt valproic acid hepatotoxicity are similar to those of other forms of acute liver disease. There may be nonspecific systemic and digestive symptoms, such as fever, anorexia, and nausea, followed by the appearance of jaundice and, in severe cases, encephalopathy. Labora-

tory studies show variable increases in serum transaminase activity, bilirubin, alkaline phosphatase, and prothrombin time. Rash and eosinophilia are absent.[200]

Histologically, the disease is associated with centrilobular necrosis and the accumulation of fat in small droplets in the liver cells, similar to that observed in Reye's syndrome. Unlike Reye's syndrome, however, valproic acid hepatotoxicity also may be associated with evidence of bile ductular injury and submassive necrosis.[196] Indeed, it has been suggested that the bile secretory apparatus, canaliculi and ductules are the principal sites of injury, rather than the mitochondria. Perhaps reflecting this cholestatic component, the disorders also differ in that clinical jaundice is common in valproic acid toxicity, but distinctly uncommon in Reye's syndrome (Chapter 54). Nonetheless, at least three fatal cases have been reported in which elevated blood ammonia and transaminases, normal bilirubin, and microvesicular fat were reminiscent of Reye's syndrome.[200]

There has been considerable progress toward an understanding of the effects of valproic acid and its metabolites on intermediary metabolism and of their possible relationship to hepatotoxicity. Several studies, including some involving healthy human subjects, indicate that this agent significantly impairs mitochondrial oxidation of long-chain fatty acids, associated with a decrease in hepatocellular acetyl CoA and in serum levels of β-hydroxybutyrate and ketones and with impaired urea synthesis and gluconeogenesis.[202–208] Dicarboxylic aciduria may occur,[206, 209] but peroxisomal oxidation of fatty acids is not impaired.[210] Mice that are genetically deficient in ornithine transcarbamylase are far more sensitive to valproic acid than their normal counterparts,[211] consistent with the clinical impression that children with inborn errors in the urea cycle or other aspects of mitochondrial-dependent intermediary metabolism are most susceptible to valproate hepatotoxicity. The precise mechanism for the apparent valproate-induced aberration in mitochondrial function is not known, but accumulation of the coenzyme A derivatives of valproate and its major metabolites has been suggested,[203, 212] and is supported by the observation that phenobarbital enhances the ability of valproate to cause steatosis.[205, 213] Presumably, the accumulation of lipid as microvesicular steatosis is secondary to the impaired oxidation of fatty acids, analogous to other disorders associated with this picture, but this is not established.

Available evidence suggests that, unlike the hepatotoxic effects, valproic acid teratogenicity does not require its conversion to the coenzyme A derivative.[214] Over 90 per cent of the valproate excreted in bile is present as the glucuronide conjugate, and it causes an immediate bile acid-independent choleresis.[215] Valproic acid glucuronides, retained in plasma for prolonged periods because of hepatic and/or renal dysfunction, may undergo rearrangement, the biological consequences of which are unknown.[216]

There is no effective treatment for valproic acid hepatotoxicity, but spontaneous recovery after discontinuation of administration of the drug is the rule; fatalities appear to be rare. Rechallenge may elicit a recurrence,[202] although not invariably.[217] Routine monitoring of liver tests have been suggested, especially during the first six months of treatment when liver injury appears to be more common.[194, 199] However, as in other instances in which the incidence of asymptomatic and transient hepatic dysfunction greatly exceeds that of overt liver injury, the real usefulness of such monitoring is uncertain.

Carbamazepine. Hepatic injuries caused by this agent

have been well documented and, although the incidence is unknown, such injuries may be more common than has been appreciated.[218-223] The usual form of injury is a granulomatous reaction.[218, 219, 221, 223] The lesion, which may be associated with clinical and histologic evidence suggesting cholangitis,[220, 223] may be very slow to resolve, with residual abnormalities in alkaline phosphatase persisting for several months.[218] Occasionally, carbamazepine is associated with a predominant hepatocellular necrosis.[220] In one patient, carbamazepine induced a nonhereditary acute porphyria syndrome via direct inhibition of uroporphyrinogen I synthetase.[224] In another patient, this agent was believed to have predisposed to isoniazid hepatitis, secondary to induction of the latter's metabolism.[225] Management of carbamazepine hepatitis is supportive.

ANTIMICROBIALS

ANTIBACTERIAL AGENTS

Penicillins. Penicillin G has an excellent record of safety with regard to hepatotoxicity, and very few cases of penicillin G–induced liver damage have been recorded.[226] In contrast, a number of the semisynthetic penicillins apparently have been responsible for liver injury, and among these oxacillin is the best documented and characterized with respect to its hepatotoxic effects.

Oxacillin. Oxacillin hepatotoxicity has been the subject of several reports and in almost all instances has occurred in patients receiving large doses of the agent intravenously.[227-233] Although the serious infections for which this patient population is undergoing treatment also may adversely affect liver function, the causal relationship of the antibiotic itself to the liver dysfunction is well established. Thus, in some patients liver dysfunction appeared only after the infection was under control. Also, the reported clinical and laboratory features have been quite uniform in different patients, and generally there is rapid improvement after discontinuation of the drug.

The disorder, which usually first becomes manifest after a week or more of high-dose, intravenous oxacillin therapy, may be either asymptomatic or associated with low-grade fever; upper gastrointestinal symptoms such as anorexia, nausea, and vomiting; variable upper abdominal and right upper quadrant discomfort; and hepatomegaly. Laboratory findings include elevated serum transaminase (occasionally in excess of 1,000 units) and normal or slightly elevated alkaline phosphatase; bilirubin concentration is almost invariably normal. Rash, arthralgia, and eosinophilia are unusual. In the few cases in which biopsies have been performed, a nonspecific focal hepatitis has been present. The prognosis is uniformly excellent; in virtually all cases, rapid clinical and laboratory improvement has followed cessation of oxacillin therapy, and in most cases, liver tests have returned to normal within several weeks.

The mechanism of the injury is not known. Although an association of oxacillin hepatotoxicity with previous or subsequent evidence of penicillin allergy was reported in one series,[230] a convincing case cannot be made for an immunologic basis for the lesion. Rather, a toxic mechanism is suggested by the fact that almost all reported cases have followed high-dose administration of the drug for at least a week, and in many instances improvement has followed substitution of another penicillin analog, such as nafcillin,[227-230, 232, 233] for the oxacillin.

Although serious or lasting liver damage has not been attributed to oxacillin, it may be appropriate to monitor liver tests before, and at intervals during, prolonged parenteral high-dose administration of this agent. If significant abnormalities occur, substitution of an alternative drug should be considered.

Carbenicillin. This agent has been associated in four patients with a clinical, laboratory, and histologic syndrome similar to oxacillin hepatotoxicity. In all four, the disorder was elicited by subsequent rechallenge with the drug.[234] Liver tests in all patients improved when another penicillin analog was substituted, despite the fact that in one patient the hepatotoxicity had been associated with a serum sickness–like illness.

Cloxacillin. In a single, well-documented case report, cloxacillin has been associated with a hepatic injury quite unlike the nonspecific, anicteric focal hepatitis caused by oxacillin and carbenicillin.[235] In this case, proved by rechallenge, the patient developed marked cholestasis, with a serum bilirubin concentration of nearly 15 mg/dL, primarily direct-reacting, a fivefold elevation in alkaline phosphatase activity, and a normal to slightly increased transaminase activity. Recurrence of the syndrome within four days of rechallenge with oral cloxacillin and a positive macrophage migration-inhibition factor test were interpreted as suggesting a hypersensitivity reaction. *Flucloxacillin* has also been implicated in hepatic injury similar to that caused by cloxacillin, which was confirmed by rechallenge, in a single case.[236]

Erythromycin. A cholestatic reaction associated with significant portal inflammation and focal hepatic necrosis is a well-documented complication of erythromycin estolate administration,[226, 237-239] and more recently has been associated with erythromycin ethylsuccinate and erythromycin lactobionate.[238, 240, 241] Although the true incidence is unknown, it appears to occur more commonly in adults than in children. Among children, in fact, the incidence of liver test abnormalities caused by erythromycin estolate, erythromycin ethylsuccinate, and penicillin V are similar and occur with an incidence of generally less than 6 per cent.[242] Typically, the onset is one to four weeks after the agent is first administered, although it may occur earlier upon re-exposure. The symptoms are usually those of a nonspecific gastrointestinal upset, with or without fever, but upper abdominal or right upper quadrant pain is often prominent and may dominate the presentation. Hepatomegaly may or may not be present, and liver tests usually indicate both cholestasis and hepatocellular necrosis, with increased serum alkaline phosphatase and transaminase activities; serum bilirubin, if increased, is primarily direct-reacting. Liver biopsy demonstrates portal infiltrates, often with eosinophils, centrilobular cholestasis, and a few scattered foci of liver cell necrosis and acidophil bodies. The prognosis is excellent, with rapid and complete restoration of normal liver function and structure after withdrawal of the drug. Subsequent readministration of the drug usually elicits a similar clinical and laboratory response, often after only a day or two. This feature, together with the finding that eosinophils may be increased in the blood or the hepatic inflammatory infiltrate, suggests that the lesion has an allergic basis. However, erythromycin estolate causes a concentration-dependent impairment of bile flow in the isolated perfused rat liver and inhibition of canalicular membrane Mg- and NaK-ATPases,[243] and this and other in vitro studies suggest a direct hepatotoxic effect,[244-246] so that at the present time the pathogenesis remains undefined.

Two particularly important aspects of erythromycin hepatotoxicity deserve special emphasis. First, it was believed that only erythromycin estolate caused this lesion, but it is now evident that other preparations, including erythromycin ethylsuccinate and erythromycin lactobionate, may do the same, possibly with cross sensitization,[247] although their relative hepatotoxic potentials are unknown. Second, the clinical presentation of the lesion can resemble that of acute cholecystitis or ascending cholangitis so closely that it may not always be possible to distinguish erthyromycin hepatotoxicity from biliary tract disease on clinical grounds alone. Indeed, a false-positive ^{99m}Tc-DISIDA scan has been reported in this setting[248] and some patients with cholestasis secondary to erythromycin hepatotoxicity have been subjected to abdominal exploration.

Tetracyclines. This group of antibiotics rarely may cause an unusual and severe form of acute liver injury.[249–252] It has followed intravenous administration of the drug in high doses to patients with compromised renal function. The initial reports mostly involved women with acute pyelonephritis in the latter stages of pregnancy, but it later became apparent that nonpregnant patients were also at risk, and that oral tetracycline administration also could cause the syndrome.[250] Despite the latter variants, common features of the illness appear to be its occurrence in a setting in which blood levels of tetracycline are unusually high, and that for reasons as yet unknown, women, especially during pregnancy, appear to be at increased risk.

The clinical illness resembles viral hepatitis in its presentation, with nonspecific systemic and digestive complaints such as malaise, anorexia, nausea, vomiting, and upper abdominal discomfort. In pregnancy, premature labor may be precipitated. The course is often progressive, with deepening jaundice, encephalopathy, and hypoprothrombinemia, usually associated with azotemia and hyperamylasemia. Leukocytosis is often profound. Transaminase activities and bilirubin concentrations are moderately increased, and usually do not exceed 1,000 IU/L and 10 mg/dL, respectively. The advancing course of the illness may be complicated by hypoglycemia and its effects on mental status, as well as by hemorrhagic diathesis or gastrointestinal bleeding, and metabolic acidosis.

The histopathology of tetracycline hepatotoxicity consists of the accumulation of lipid, primarily triglyceride, in hepatocytes. The lipid is dispersed throughout the cell in small droplets, but the nucleus remains centrally located. Thus, this pattern differs strikingly from the fatty liver associated with ethanol ingestion, obesity, and diabetes mellitus, and superficially resembles that seen in only a few other disorders, including Reye's syndrome, fatty liver of pregnancy, Jamaica vomiting sickness, and valproic acid hepatotoxicity. Accordingly, this lesion, if found in a patient to whom tetracycline has recently been administered, strongly suggests the diagnosis of tetracycline hepatotoxicity, and in this respect it differs from the relatively nonspecific histologic abnormalities associated with most drug reactions.

The pathogenesis of the lesion has not been elucidated fully. The fact that high blood and tissue levels of the drug appear to be prerequisite suggests that hepatotoxicity represents a toxic effect of tetracycline or a metabolite rather than an immunologic phenomenon. Moreover, animal experiments clearly show that tetracycline interferes with the hepatic secretion of triglyceride-rich lipoproteins, both in vivo and in the isolated perfused rat liver.[253] Thus, although the precise mechanism for this secretory impairment is not known, the accumulation of fat seems understandable, at least in part, as the result of decreased lipid export from the cell. Not resolved by these animal experiments, however, is the basis for the more general and profound failure of hepatocyte function that characterizes the clinical syndrome. The presence of lipid in the hepatocyte per se does not satisfactorily explain these functional changes, and appears only to reflect the underlying metabolic disturbance, the nature and pathogenesis of which await elucidation. Since tetracycline is an inhibitor of protein synthesis, it conceivably could influence the availability of certain cell constituents that turn over rapidly, but this remains speculative.

Sulfonamides. Sulfonamides have been implicated in a form of hepatocellular necrosis, often associated with "allergic" features such as fever, arthralgia, rash, and eosinophilia.[226] The incidence is unknown. Agents for which the documentation is more or less adequate to support causality include sulfanilamide, sulfadimethoxine, azulfidine,[254–263] sulfamethoxazole,[264–266] sulfones,[267] sulfamethizole,[268] and sulfamethoxypyridizine.[268, 269] The latter two agents have been associated with a picture of chronic active hepatitis.[268, 269] Occasionally, a granulomatous reaction may be seen.[255, 260, 262]

The clinical onset of the reaction normally occurs within two weeks after the drug is started, but reactions may be delayed. As mentioned, the presentation is nonspecific, and is associated with laboratory evidence of liver cell necrosis, especially increased serum transaminase activity. Because of an expected bias toward more severe reactions among case reports, the case fatality rate is unknown, but it may exceed 10 per cent.[226] In the substantial majority of cases, however, complete recovery may be expected within several weeks to a few months after the medication is discontinued. If there is massive hepatic necrosis, death may occur early; late deaths may result from submassive necrosis. Although corticosteroids have been employed in the treatment of sulfonamide hepatitis, there is no clear evidence that they are beneficial.

Nitrofurantoins. These agents are now well established as an unusual cause of acute, usually cholestatic, and chronic forms[270–273] of liver injury. The incidence appears to be especially high in women, but this may reflect an increased exposure to the drug during treatment of urinary tract infections.

The acute syndrome is often associated with fever, rash, jaundice, and eosinophilia, and usually appears within a few weeks of the onset of drug administration. The clinical, laboratory, and histologic picture is predominantly cholestatic, although hepatocellular necrosis may be present. A granulomatous reaction has been documented.[274] The prognosis for complete recovery is good, and thus far none of the patients with overt acute disease has died of liver disease or has clearly progressed to chronic hepatitis.

Chronic active hepatitis with "lupoid" features has now been associated convincingly with chronic nitrofurantoin administration in several cases. The affected patients have been women who have taken the drug for at least four months, and often they are found to have hyperglobulinemia and positive tests for antinuclear and anti–smooth muscle antibodies. Cirrhosis developed in four patients. Two of 20 reported cases in one series died with massive necrosis, both having taken the drug for more than a year, and having continued to take it after the appearance of jaundice.[271] In the others, improvement followed discontinuation of the drug. Corticosteroids have been employed, but without clear benefit.

The mechanism of the injury is unknown.[273] Although many of the clinical and laboratory features suggest an immunologic process, some of these immunologic features also can be seen in chronic nitrofurantoin users who lack evidence of liver disease. Moreover, furan and related compounds such as furazolidone, furosemide, and the aflatoxins are hepatotoxic in vivo and in cell culture. It is quite possible that, as with a number of other agents, differences in individual susceptibility to agents may reflect metabolic rather than immunologic processes.

Other Antibacterial Agents. *Chloramphenicol* has been implicated in several cases of jaundice, reflecting hepatocellular necrosis and/or cholestasis. The mechanism is unclear, as is the possible relationship of the hepatic lesion to the bone marrow toxicity occasionally associated with it. *Clindamycin* administration has been associated with a 20 to 50 per cent incidence of elevated serum transaminase activity and, rarely, with jaundice.[226]

ANTIFUNGAL AND ANTIPARASITIC AGENTS

Griseofulvin may exacerbate acute intermittent porphyria (Chap. 14), and is hepatotoxic in rats and mice.[275] It may also cause transient hypertransaminasemia, and in two cases has been implicated as the cause of cholestatic jaundice.[276] *5-Fluorocytosine* also may cause transient transaminase elevations.[226] Hepatic injury caused by *amphotericin* is rare but has been documented.[277] *Ketoconazole* has been documented as a cause of significant liver damage,[278, 279] with an estimated incidence of approximately 1 in 15,000. The syndrome is rarely fatal. In 5 to 10 per cent of patients, a mild, transient, and reversible increase in serum transaminase activity may occur. About one third of patients experience nausea, emesis, or malaise, but rash and eosinophilia are lacking. Ketoconazole does exert a limited impairment of hepatic oxidative drug metabolism.[280] It has been suggested that consideration be given to routine monitoring of liver tests when ketoconazole is used, but opinions differ on this point.[278, 281] Miconazole, a related agent may influence cellular immune response and hepatic drug metabolism in mice.[282] Several of the agents used in the treatment of parasitic disease have been associated with liver injury. *Fansidar* (pyrimethamine plus sulfadoxine) has been linked to both a granulomatous reaction[283] and a fatal systemic toxic reaction associated with portal inflammatory infiltrates.[284] *Amodiaquine* has been associated with a syndrome of hepatic necrosis beginning 4 to 15 weeks after initiation of malaria prophylaxis.[285, 286] *Thiobendazole* may cause transient transaminase elevations. *Hycanthone* also may do the same and in addition may cause overt acute and occasionally fatal hepatic necrosis.[287]

ANTITUBERCULOUS AGENTS

ISONIAZID

Isoniazid has been important in the treatment of tuberculosis since the early 1950s. Despite a few case reports of associated liver injury, it was initially considered relatively safe and was not generally regarded as an important hepatotoxin. In the early 1970s, however, an outbreak of isoniazid-associated hepatitis triggered a reassessment of its hepatotoxic potential, and the clinical, epidemiologic, and biochemical investigations of the ensuing decade leave little

doubt that isoniazid can cause mild and occasionally fatal hepatic injury, although the possible mechanism or mechanisms involved remain in some doubt.

Incidence and Epidemiology

The hepatotoxicity of isoniazid has been documented most clearly in studies of populations undergoing single-drug chemoprophylaxis for positive tuberculin skin reactions. Two types of hepatic reaction can be identified, but the pathogenic and prognostic relationship between the two, if any, is unclear. The more common reaction, occurring in about 10 per cent or more of all recipients of isoniazid, consists of a mild, often entirely subclinical, nonspecific focal hepatitis that is apparently evanescent, occurs within the first few months of drug administration, and often subsides, even if the drug is continued.[288, 289] This mild, seemingly benign injury may occur somewhat less often in children than in adults,[290, 291] but it does occur in all age groups and has no clear relationship to sex, ethnic background, or the rate at which isoniazid is metabolized (acetylated) in the liver.[289]

The less common but far more severe and clinically important form of hepatic reaction to isoniazid is an overt hepatitis-like illness that occurs in approximately 1 per cent of all subjects.[292–297] Unlike the more usual less severe injury discussed above, this reaction shows a striking age dependency; it is very uncommon in children and teenagers[298, 299] and occurs with an incidence of 2 per cent or more in individuals 50 years old or older.[292, 293–296, 300] It has been suggested that more serious disease may occur predominantly in black women and Asian men,[294–296] but the effects of race and sex on incidence remain unclear because the number of cases has been relatively small and because in some of the more prominent earlier reports the subject populations themselves were skewed.[294, 296] Alcohol use may predispose to the lesion,[292, 296, 300] but the initial impression that rapid acetylators of the drug are at increased risk[293, 295] has not been supported by more recent evidence.[300–303]

Mild Isoniazid Hepatotoxicity

This common, seemingly benign lesion occurs in approximately 10 per cent of all subjects receiving single-drug isoniazid chemoprophylaxis.[288, 289, 291, 293, 295] It may be entirely asymptomatic, and is most often characterized by a mild increase in serum transaminase activity during the first few months of treatment.[289, 293] In virtually all, the lesion appears to be transient and self-limited, and liver tests revert to normal despite continued administration of the drug. Unfortunately, it can only be assumed that any associated histologic lesion also subsides, since results of follow-up liver biopsies in these patients have not been reported. By itself, the lesion appears to have no important short- or long-term adverse effect on liver function, morbidity, mortality, or successful completion of the intended course of drug treatment.[288, 289] It is of major importance, however, because its relative frequency and nonspecificity, and the timing of its onset have confounded the possible early detection and prevention of the much less common but potentially more severe overt isoniazid-induced hepatitis. For this reason, among others, serious doubt has been cast on the value of routine "prophylactic" monitoring of liver tests in patients taking isoniazid.[292]

Isoniazid-induced Hepatitis

The overall incidence of overt isoniazid-induced hepatitis is approximately 1 per cent, based on several studies of patients taking the drug for chemoprophylaxis of positive tuberculin reactions.[293-297, 302-305] It is rarely seen in patients less than 20 years old, and occurs in 2 per cent or more of those 50 years old or older.[292, 294-296, 300] The basis for the striking age dependency is not known, but is consistent with the more general perception that hepatic drug reactions are less common in children than in adults. In the case of the reaction to isoniazid, it has been suggested that the age dependency is only apparent, and in reality reflects a predisposition conferred by pre-existing liver disease.[306] The validity of this concept is unknown. The timing of the onset of hepatitis after drug treatment is begun is quite variable; about 50 per cent of cases occur within 2 months, whereas in a few cases onset may be delayed as long as 12 months.[294] Patients in whom the onset is delayed[294] or in whom isoniazid is continued after the onset of symptoms of hepatitis[297, 304] appear to be the most severely affected.

In virtually all aspects, including clinical, laboratory, and histologic findings, isoniazid-induced hepatitis is strikingly similar to viral hepatitis.[294, 295, 304, 307] It may present as a flu-like syndrome, with variable upper gastrointestinal symptoms and right upper quadrant discomfort, and may progress to jaundice and severe acute liver failure or may remain anicteric through a relatively brief illness. Any segment of the entire spectrum of the presentation and clinical course of viral hepatitis may be seen, from a mild acute hepatitis, to early death in liver failure, a more prolonged subacute course, or chronic active hepatitis. Physical findings are as would be expected, and include variable low-grade fever, jaundice, hepatomegaly, and signs of liver failure such as encephalopathy, bleeding tendency, and ascites. Notably infrequent are findings that might be regarded as evidence of drug "allergy" such as rash and arthritis. Routine laboratory studies reflect predominantly hepatocellular necrosis, with elevated serum transaminases and variable increases in alkaline phosphatase, bilirubin, and prothrombin time. The range of histologic findings also may encompass those seen in viral hepatitis, including the classic acute lesion, with or without bridging necrosis,[308] massive or submassive necrosis, chronic hepatitis.[309] The prognosis is distinctly worse than that associated with viral hepatitis, in that the case fatality rate approximates 10 per cent.[294, 295] Treatment is entirely supportive, as for acute viral hepatitis. There is no evidence that corticosteroids are beneficial in the treatment of the more severe acute or the chronic cases.

Prevention or early detection of significant isoniazid-induced hepatitis has proved elusive. Routine monitoring of liver tests, as mentioned, is of limited usefulness because apparently harmless transaminase elevations occur at least ten times more commonly than does the more serious lesion. Moreover, severe acute isoniazid-induced hepatitis may develop at any time. There is no interval that might be selected for monitoring of liver tests that reliably detects serious disease in its early stages. Reliance on symptoms alone has proved disappointing.[310] Perhaps the most practical approach is one that combines a conservative approach to the use of isoniazid chemoprophylaxis,[292, 296, 298] with careful instruction to the patient to report any symptoms suggesting intercurrent viral illness or liver disease, and testing of liver function as seems appropriate. In patients more than 35 years old, the risk-benefit ratio of routine isoniazid chemoprophylaxis becomes increasingly unfavorable,[292, 296, 311, 312] and in this group special care and a low threshold for discontinuing the drug are warranted.

Mechanism

Several features of isoniazid-induced hepatotoxicity suggest that it reflects the injurious effects of a chemical toxin. In support of this concept, mild liver injury is quite common, convincing evidence of drug allergy is lacking, and, as demonstrated in animal experiments, hepatic metabolism of isoniazid clearly leads to the formation of a potent hepatotoxin. Isoniazid is inactivated as an antituberculous agent by acetylation in the liver, which is the first reaction in its biotransformation sequence (Fig. 31–3). The product of this reaction, acetylisoniazid, appears harmless, per se, but it rapidly undergoes hydrolysis to monoacetylhydrazine. This intermediate is oxidized by the cytochrome P450-dependent drug metabolism pathway in the endoplasmic reticulum. The oxidized product of monoacetylhydrazine forms covalent bonds in vivo and in vitro with liver cell macromolecules,[295, 313] possibly accounting for its toxicity, although the mechanistic relationship between covalent binding of acetylhydrazine metabolites to macromolecules and the production of liver injury remains unclear.[314] An important aspect of the role of acetylation in the pathogenesis of isoniazid hepatotoxicity is that it implies that the generation of toxic intermediates may depend on the rates of formation of acetylisoniazid and monoacetylhydrazine, and hence that the acetylator phenotype may be an important determinant of individual susceptibility to isoniazid hepatotoxicity, with rapid acetylators of the drug being at greatest risk. However, although this view was supported by earlier studies of the acetylator phenotype in patients with isoniazid-induced hepatic dysfunction,[293-295] subsequent work has consistently failed to identify a greater risk of isoniazid-induced hepatitis among rapid acetylators than among slow acetylators[300-302] and has even suggested that the converse may be true—that is, that slow acetylators of isoniazid are in fact at greater risk.[303] Recent studies also indicate that rapid acetylators more rapidly acetylate not only the parent compound but also monoacetylhydrazine (the immediate percursor of the presumed toxic metabolite) to the relatively harmless diacetylhydrazine.[315, 316] The latter is excreted in the urine and thus precludes entry of the monoacetylhydrazine into the toxin-producing microsomal pathways. Thus, the rapid acetylator appears to be protected against excessive accumulation of toxic intermediates. On the other hand, this "protective" acetylation reaction that converts monoacetylhydrazine to diacetylhydrazine is inhibited by isoniazid itself,[317] whereas the half-life of elimination of monoacetylhydrazine is fivefold slower than that of isoniazid.[316] It might be expected, therefore, that slow acetylators, who at a given drug dose would have higher blood and tissue levels of isoniazid, would accumulate monoacetylhydrazine and be predisposed to hepatotoxicity.

Another potentially important route of toxic metabolite formation from isoniazid is the direct hydrolysis of the drug without prior acetylation (see Fig. 31–3). This reaction yields isonicotinic acid and hydrazine, the latter being a direct hepatotoxin.[318] Although this "direct pathway" of isoniazid metabolism accounts for only a minor fraction of the disposal of this drug, the proportion of isoniazid metabolized by this route is approximately tenfold greater in

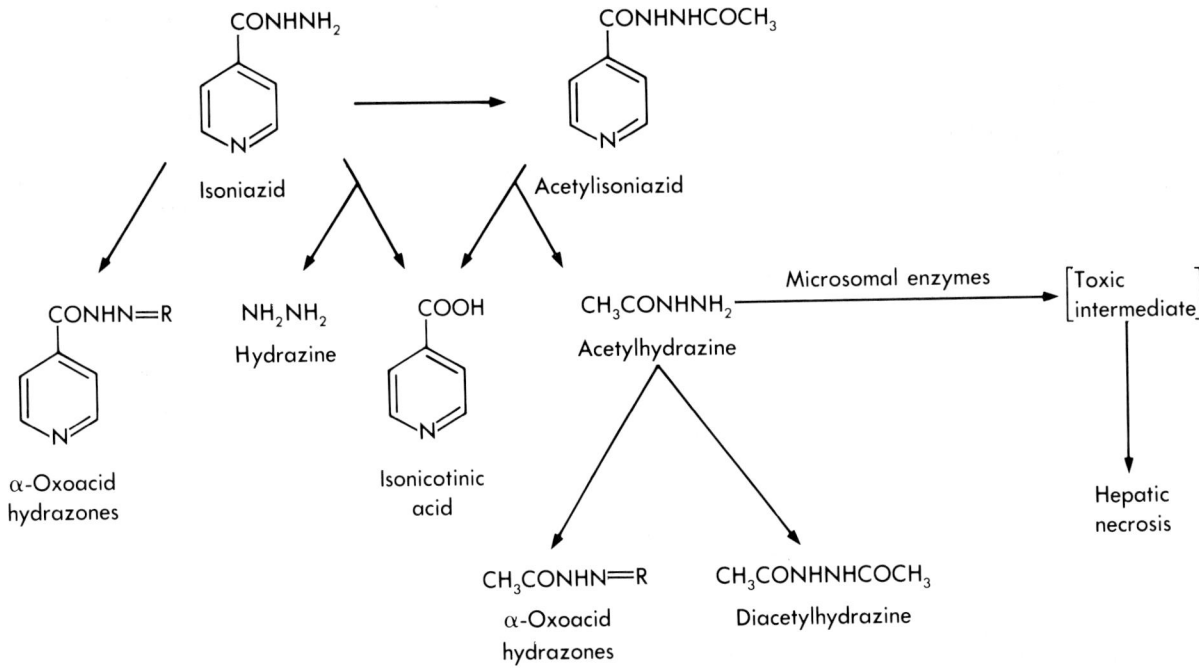

Figure 31–3. Pathways of isoniazid metabolism. (Adapted from Timbrell TA, et al. Clin Pharmacol Ther 22:602, 1977, with permission.)

slow acetylators than in rapid acetylators and is further increased by rifampicin administration.[319] This may have an important bearing upon the observation discussed below of a higher incidence of hepatotoxic sequelae among slow acetylators treated with isoniazid in combination with rifampicin.

RIFAMPIN

This more recently introduced agent has three distinct effects on the liver. First, rifampin produces predictable, dose-dependent impairment of the hepatic uptake of bilirubin, sulfobromophthalein (BSP), and bile acids.[320–322] The effect is reversible and its mechanism unknown, although available evidence suggests that it reflects an effect of rifampin at the hepatocyte surface. Second, rifampin is an inducer of drug metabolism in the endoplasmic reticulum,[323, 324] and thus may influence the biotransformation and, presumably, hepatotoxicity of other agents, including isoniazid.

Finally, rifampin has itself been associated with an acute viral hepatitis-like drug reaction not unlike that associated with isoniazid.[324, 325] The reported incidences of this reaction vary widely, however, and because the drug is almost always used in combination with other antituberculous agents, especially isoniazid, the actual incidence (indeed, the validity) of "rifampin hepatitis" remains unclear. It has been suggested that because rifampin induces microsomal drug metabolism, it may predispose to an especially severe and more rapidly appearing form of isoniazid-induced hepatitis,[324] but this interesting possibility, while compatible with the available evidence, is not conclusively established.

A recent study has also found a tenfold higher incidence of significant hepatotoxicity among slow acetylators than among rapid acetylators treated with isoniazid and rifampicin in combination.[326] Although the reason for this observed increase in the susceptibility of slow acetylators to the drug combination is unknown, it is compatible with the evidence discussed earlier that (1) slow acetylators are more likely to accumulate monoacetylhydrazine,[316] the substrate for (presumably rifampicin-inducible) cytochrome P450-generated toxic intermediate compounds; and (2) rifampicin increases hydrazine formation from the direct hydrolysis of isoniazid to a greater extent in slow acetylators than in rapid acetylators.[319] Children with tuberculous meningitis also have been noted to show a disproportionately high incidence of significant hepatotoxicity following treatment with isoniazid and rifampicin in combination,[326, 327] and this is likely to relate to a multitude of factors including higher dosages of isoniazid, nutritional factors, concomitant administration of cytochrome P450–inducing anticonvulsants, and closer monitoring of these critically ill patients.

OTHER ANTITUBERCULOUS AGENTS AND COMBINATION THERAPY

Para-aminosalicylic acid (PAS) has been implicated in a generalized serum sickness–like picture of drug allergy in as many as 5 per cent of patients, and in a hepatitis-like illness with features of cholestasis in about 1 per cent.[307] The case fatality rate of "PAS hepatitis" is probably about 10 per cent. Because of the frequency of adverse drug reactions and its relatively weak antimicrobial effect, this agent has fallen progressively into disuse. Whereas ethambutal and streptomycin are apparently free of hepatotoxicity, some of the secondary drugs, including ethionamide and pyrazinamide, have been associated with a hepatitis-like injury.[307] This may be a more frequent occurrence, comparable to the situation with isoniazid, when ethionamide is administered in combination with rifampicin.[328]

ANTINEOPLASTIC AND IMMUNOSUPPRESSIVE AGENTS

This diverse and rapidly growing group of drugs is associated with special problems in regard to hepatotoxicity. Whereas it is clear that several of these agents cause liver injury, assessment of the incidence, severity and, in some instances, even the validity of the association is much more difficult and uncertain than for most other groups of drugs. The reason for this is related to the nature of neoplastic disease itself and to the clinical circumstances that often surround the use of these agents. Thus, hepatic dysfunction in a patient with malignancy may be caused not only by a potentially hepatotoxic chemotherapeutic agent but also by metastases to the liver, opportunistic infections resulting from tumor- or drug-related immune suppression, post-transfusion hepatitis, shock, sepsis, other drugs used to treat infection or the symptoms of either the tumor itself or of its treatment. Because abnormalities of blood platelets and clotting function and other contraindications to liver biopsy are not infrequent in this setting, this procedure, which might otherwise clarify the basis for hepatic dysfunction, may not be feasible. The direct result of these uncertainties is that reports of abnormalities of liver function in patients receiving chemotherapy for neoplastic disease are numerous, but conclusively documented linkages of specific agents to pathologically defined liver injury is much less common. The effects on the liver of a wide variety of antineoplastic agents have been the subject of several recent reviews[329-332] and are summarized in Table 31-4.

ANTIMETABOLITES

Methotrexate. This agent has received major attention over the years as a potential hepatotoxin. Most of the current concepts of its long-term hepatotoxic potential have evolved from its use in a nonmalignant disease—namely, psoriasis. Initial judgments concerning long-term hepatotoxicity of methotrexate were complicated by the high incidence of pretreatment liver abnormalities in psoriatic patients, especially (but not exclusively) those who consumed alcohol excessively. However, a large body of evidence now points to the fact that chronic methotrexate therapy does indeed lead to fibrosis and cirrhosis.[333-339] It also seems clear that the risk of fibrosis and cirrhosis is reduced if the drug dose is minimized and is administered not more often than weekly.[333, 335, 336, 340] Total dose and duration of treatment also has been regarded as important. Although this is also not clearly established, most studies indicate that the incidence of cirrhosis is low with a total cumulative dose below 1.5 g.[338] In one series of patients treated with a single weekly oral dose of 25 mg for an average of 26 months, the incidence of cirrhosis was 6.8 per cent,[333] but the incidence was 25.6 per cent in patients receiving the same regimen for greater than 5 years.[337] On the other hand, a recent study of 30 patients receiving a single weekly dose of 15 mg for periods up to 10 years found progressive fibrosis in only two patients, both of whom had steatosis or fibrosis on pre-treatment liver biopsies and histories of alcohol abuse.[340] There remains a strong but as yet unproven impression that alcohol consumption increases the risk of fibrosis and cirrhosis in the setting of chronic methotrexate treatment.[337, 340] Other putative risk factors include diabetes, obesity, pre-existing hepatic abnormalities, previous arsenic treatment, impaired renal

TABLE 31-4. HEPATOTOXIC MANIFESTATIONS OF ANTINEOPLASTIC AGENTS

Veno-occlusive disease	Mitomycin C
	6-Thioguanine
	Azathioprine
	Cytabarine
	Dacarbazine
	Indicine-N-oxide
	Daunorubicin
	Combination chemotherapy
	Radiation therapy plus
	Cyclophosphamide
	Busulfan
	Carmustine
	Mitomycin C
	Other regimens
Hepatocellular necrosis	Frequent
	Mithramycin
	L-Aspariginase
	Streptozotocin
	Methotrexate (high dose)
	Rare
	Nitrosoureas
	6-Thioguanine
	Cytabarine
	Adriamycin
	5-Fluorouracil
	Cyclophosphamide
	Etoposide
Hepatic steatosis	L-Asparaginase
	Actinomycin-D
	Mitomycin C
	Bleomycin
	Methotrexate
Cholestasis	6-Mercaptopurine
	Azathioprine
	Busulfan
	Amsacrine
Fibrosis	Methotrexate
	Azathioprine
Sclerosing cholangitis	Floxuridine
Peliosis hepatis	Androgens
	Azathioprine
	Hydroxyurea
Hepatic neoplasms	Estrogens
	Androgens
	Methotrexate

function, and advanced age.[334, 335, 337-340] Cirrhosis attributable to methotrexate treatment may be complicated by portal hypertension and liver failure, but in the majority of patients the disease is subclinical and non-progressive. A single case report has raised the possibility that a methotrexate-associated hepatic fibrosis may evolve to hepatocellular carcinoma.[341]

A disturbing aspect of chronic methotrexate hepatotoxicity is that routine tests of liver function are not sensitive enough to serve alone as the basis for patient monitoring, since evolution to fibrosis has occurred despite normal test results. For this reason, it has become common practice to recommend liver biopsy prior to the institution of methotrexate treatment, and at regular intervals (after 1 to 1.5 g cumulative methotrexate doses) thereafter, for the duration of the treatment.[332, 338] The presence of significant liver disease at the initial evaluation, or its development during the course of treatment, is considered a relative contraindication to subsequent use of the drug.

As would be expected from the studies of patients with psoriasis, experience with higher-dose, chronic methotrexate treatment of malignancies also suggests that fibrosis may develop covertly.[329, 342] In addition, interval treatment is often associated with transient abnormalities of liver function, most of which normalize before the next treatment course.[343] Although the effect of methotrexate on folic acid metabolism is potentially injurious to all cell types, the mechanism of its hepatotoxicity is not known. Studies of hepatic ultrastructure indicate that hepatocyte damage is variable, and includes fat deposition, membrane whorls, and increased numbers of autophagic vacuoles; hyperplasia of Ito cells and increased numbers of residual bodies in Kupffer cells are also found.[344, 345] Significant changes also occur in biliary epithelium.[346] Since the liver cell population turns over very slowly, an important effect on DNA synthesis would seem unlikely. It is equally unclear whether toxicity is mediated by the parent compound or a metabolite. Evidence that choline-deficient fatty liver in rats is potentiated by methotrexate, and that this effect can be prevented by methionine and choline, has suggested that the injurious effects of the drug may reflect a general interference with hepatic methyl group metabolism.[347]

6-Mercaptopurine and Azathioprine. Although reliable incidence figures are not available, it appears that both of these agents (azathioprine is converted to 6-mercaptopurine in the liver) cause an apparently dose-dependent hepatotoxicity.[331, 332] The injury is primarily cholestatic, but also is associated with some hepatocellular necrosis. Abnormalities in liver tests appear one to two months after commencing therapy, but in most cases the lesion is reversible when the drug is discontinued. Whether recorded fatalities attributed to these agents were in fact caused by them is unclear. It is of interest that the hepatotoxicity of these agents has been demonstrated not only in patients with neoplastic disease but also in patients with chronic active hepatitis. In the latter condition, the dose dependency of the injurious effect was clearly demonstrated by the fact that a deteriorating clinical course associated with higher doses could be avoided with lower doses.[348] Azathioprine appears significantly less hepatotoxic than 6-mercaptopurine, and is used now in a low dose (50 mg) in the treatment of some patients with chronic active hepatitis.[349] The mechanism of the hepatotoxicity of either drug is not known, but it has been suggested that patients developing hepatotoxicity with azathioprine may convert this drug to 6-mercaptopurine at an unusually rapid rate.[329] Twelve cases of veno-occlusive disease have been reported in renal transplant patients treated with azathioprine and prednisone for periods between six months and nine years.[350, 351] The onset of the disease may be insidious, with progression to severe, often fatal liver failure and portal hypertension despite discontinuation of the drug. It has been suggested that concurrent infection with hepatotrophic viruses may be a factor in the development of veno-occlusive disease in renal transplant patients treated with azathioprine.[350]

6-Thioguanine. There have been several reports of veno-occlusive disease attributed to this agent in patients with acute leukemia.[332, 352, 353] In most instances, other drugs also have been used, but the temporal relationship of the onset of the hepatic disease to the institution of 6-thioguanine treatment strongly implicates this drug. The onset of veno-occlusive disease in this setting has been abrupt, with tender hepatomegaly and often minimal abnormalities in liver tests.[353] Clinical and, in some patients, histologic

resolution has occurred on stopping treatment with this agent (see Chap. 23).[352, 353]

5-Fluorouracil. Commonly used in treatment of malignancies of the digestive organs, 5-fluorouracil appears to produce little in the way of hepatotoxicity when given orally. However, the administration of the related drug floxuridine (FUDR) via constant-infusion pump into the hepatic artery for the treatment of hepatic metastases has resulted in abnormal liver function in almost all patients receiving this treatment.[354] Alkaline phosphatase elevations have been particularly marked, and jaundice common. Cholangiography and laparotomy in selected patients has revealed extensive fibrosis and stricturing of the biliary system (biliary sclerosis), particularly at the common hepatic duct bifurcation, as well as acalculous cholecystitis.[335] The pathogenesis appears to be a direct toxic effect of the drug delivered in high concentration to anatomic regions supplied mainly by the hepatic artery.

Cytosine arabinoside. Treatment with this drug has been accompanied by usually mild hepatic injury.[332]

NATURAL PRODUCTS

L-Asparaginase. Liver injury occurs in at least 50 per cent of patients treated with this indirect inhibitor of protein synthesis.[329, 330] The changes are usually mild, affect routine tests of liver function broadly, are associated with fatty liver, and revert rapidly to normal within two weeks after administration of the drug is discontinued. The mechanism of toxicity is not known with certainty, although it appears likely to result from impairment of hepatic protein synthesis secondary to depletion of asparagine stores. Impaired hepatic protein synthesis by L-asparaginase also is manifested by low serum levels of albumin, transferrin, and coagulation factors. Experimental evidence suggests that hepatotoxicity is more likely to follow treatment with microbial L-asparaginases, which contain significant glutaminase activity, than with varieties of the enzyme lacking this activity.[353]

Mithramycin. This drug produces a dose-related centrilobular hepatocellular necrosis that is thought to result from impaired protein synthesis secondary to inhibition of RNA transcription from DNA.[330–332] Almost all patients treated with this agent for embryonal carcinoma demonstrate hepatic injury, often with marked elevation of transaminases. Depression of coagulation factors, coupled with thrombocytopenia produced by the drug, may lead to a bleeding diathesis. The lower doses of mithramycin used to treat Paget's disease and hypercalcemia are better tolerated.[330, 332]

Adriamycin. This agent has been reported to produce a mild hepatitis in patients with acute leukemia.[357] Both adriamycin and *mitomycin C* have been implicated in instances of veno-occlusive disease,[332] and mitomycin C as well as *bleomycin* have also been associated with fatty liver.

Vinblastine and Vincristine. Vinblastine and vincristine, despite their general effects on microtubular function, have only rarely been linked to hepatotoxicity in man.

Cyclosporine. This immunosuppressant, widely used as an anti-rejection agent in organ transplantation, has been associated with hyperbilirubinemia and variable increases in transaminases in up to one third of patients receiving high doses of the drug.[358] The pathogenesis of this mild hepatic dysfunction is unknown, and it resolves completely at lower drug doses.

ALKYLATING AGENTS

Cyclophosphamide. Apart from a few instances of mild hepatic injury occurring in patients with collagen-vascular diseases,[359, 360] cyclophosphamide, as well as most related nitrogen mustards, appear to have low hepatotoxic potential. Similarly, *busulfan* appears not to cause liver injury. *Nitrosoureas* (BCNU, CCNU, methyl-CCNU) may cause mild and rapidly reversible elevations of serum liver enzyme activities and bilirubin concentrations in as many as 25 per cent of patients, associated with a variable hepatocellular necrosis.[329] *Streptozotocin* has been reported to cause mild and reversible liver dysfunction in 6 to 67 per cent of cases; the histologic features of this disorder are not defined.

Dacarbazine. This agent, used in the treatment of melanoma, has been reported to produce an aggressive form of veno-occlusive disease accompanied by massive hepatocellular necrosis in several patients.[361] Since the hepatic injury has usually manifested following the second cycle of treatment with dacarbazine and is often accompanied by eosinophilia, the pathogenesis may involve drug hypersensitivity.

DRUGS USED IN THE TREATMENT OF CARDIOVASCULAR DISEASE

ANTIHYPERTENSIVE AND DIURETIC AGENTS

Alpha-methyldopa. This agent has been clearly established as the cause of a wide spectrum of hepatic dysfunctions, ranging from asymptomatic and transient elevations of serum transaminase activity to acute and chronic active hepatitis, to fatal massive hepatic necrosis.[362–371] Asymptomatic increases in transaminase activity occur with reported frequencies ranging from 0 to 35 per cent, and averaging 6 per cent. In many instances, these abnormalities are discovered only as the result of routine laboratory screening and may disappear despite continued administration of the drug. In some, however, abnormalities may persist, necessitating discontinuation of the drug.

Overt acute hepatitis has been linked to methyldopa use in at least 100 cases. The clinical presentation, physical and laboratory findings, and histologic characteristics are, for practical purposes, indistinguishable from the spectrum of clinical and laboratory findings associated with acute viral hepatitis. The onset occurs within three months of starting the drug in more than 90 per cent of cases. In most, recovery is prompt and complete upon discontinuation of the drug, but bridging or submassive necrosis is not uncommon, and in approximately 10 per cent of reported cases fatal massive hepatic necrosis has ensued.

Methyldopa also has been reported to be a cause of chronic active hepatitis.[364, 367] Again, the clinical, laboratory, and histologic features of this syndrome do not distinguish it from chronic viral hepatitis or those forms of chronic hepatitis for which the causes are unknown. Although the hepatitis in these patients usually abates when the drug is discontinued, recovery may take many months.[366] In some cases, the disease appears to have passed the point of reversibility and progresses to a fatal outcome. In rare instances, cirrhosis has developed in patients following severe hepatic injury attributed to methyldopa.[372]

The pathogenesis of methyldopa-induced hepatitis has not been elucidated. An immunologically mediated form of "drug hypersensitivity" has been suggested because of the rather common occurrence of positive Coombs' tests,[363] and by more recent demonstration of positive tests for migration-inhibition factor and anti-nuclear and anti-smooth muscle antibodies in a case of methyldopa-induced hepatitis,[373] as well as evidence that methyldopa inhibits suppressor T-cell function and may thereby lead to unregulated antibody production.[374] Although consistent with a causal role for an immune response, these findings do not establish this concept conclusively, and clinical features suggestive of drug allergy (e.g., eosinophilia) are unusual. Furthermore, there is experimental evidence suggesting that the injury is mediated by a toxic drug metabolite. Thus, methyldopa is converted by human and rodent liver microsomes in the presence of NADPH and O_2 to a product that forms a covalent bond with proteins. That formation of this bond is inhibited by carbon monoxide, superoxide dismutase, ascorbic acid, ethylene diamine, and glutathione is taken as evidence that methyldopa is oxidized by cytochrome P450–generated superoxide anion (see Chap. 9 for details of this type of reaction) to a reactive semiquinone or quinone.[375, 376] A genetic predisposition to the adverse reaction has been suggested by the finding of presumed methyldopa hepatotoxicity in four members of a family.[370] If the proposed role for a toxic drug metabolite is correct, it is clear that nutritional and environmental factors also could influence individual susceptibility, and thus account for the relative scarcity of the overt hepatic reactions to the drug. A recent study has found that sera from patients with methyldopa-induced liver disease contain antibodies that bind to rabbit liver cell plasma membranes only after treatment with both methyldopa and a cytochrome P450–inducing agent.[377] These findings support the attractive hypothesis that antibody-mediated liver damage may occur with methyldopa after sensitization of the immune system to liver cell membranes immunologically altered by a metabolite of the drug, and thus both metabolic idiosyncracy and autoimmune mechanisms may be relevant in the pathogenesis of this disorder.

Because of the broad spectrum of liver disturbances that it may cause, methyldopa is probably best avoided in patients with liver disease. Although there is no evidence that such patients are at increased risk for methyldopa-induced hepatotoxicity, a deterioration in liver function occurring in this setting could be especially deleterious and at the least create diagnostic confusion. The possible value of monitoring liver tests is unclear, in view of the relatively high incidence of mild and apparently benign transaminase increases and the scarcity of overt liver disease. There is no evidence that corticosteroids favorably influence the course of acute or chronic methyldopa-induced hepatitis.

Hydralazine. Hydralazine rarely has been associated with a form of granulomatous hepatitis. In the reported cases, this has occurred in the setting of systemic lupus erythematosus–like hydralazine disease.[378, 379] The hepatic disorder is mild; reversibility is complete, including disappearance of granulomas, upon discontinuation of the drug. Hydralazine has also been reported to produce a clinical syndrome mimicking acute bacterial cholangitis.[380]

Captopril. Several documented cases of cholestatic hepatitis and at least one case of submassive hepatic necrosis have been attributed to this antihypertensive agent.[381] The onset of jaundice has followed the initiation of treatment by periods ranging from one week to ten months. Fever and eosinophilia have been prominent, suggesting a hypersensitivity mechanism of injury. Recovery following withdrawal of the drug has been the rule.

Other Agents. Scattered case reports have implicated *thiazides* and *furosemide* as causes of acute hepatic injury in man.[371] A dose-related furosemide-induced centrilobular necrosis in mice has been linked to the conversion of the parent compound to a toxic intermediate by the microsomal cytochrome P450 drug-metabolizing system.[382, 383]

Ticrynafen. This uricosuric diuretic, introduced in 1979, was withdrawn from use following the reporting of over 500 cases of hepatic injury attributable to the drug, with a mortality of about 7 per cent. Ticrynafen produced acute hepatocellular injury that in most cases was clinically indistinguishable from acute viral hepatitis, although it may also have resulted in chronic active hepatitis and cirrhosis in a few patients.[384]

ANTIARRHYTHMIC AGENTS

Quinidine. A few cases of mild, fully reversible, hepatic injury have been associated with quinidine administration.[385–387] In almost all, onset was characterized by fever within one to two weeks of starting the drug, and the injury was associated with variable systemic and upper gastrointestinal symptoms, transaminase and alkaline phosphatase elevations, and normal or only slightly elevated serum bilirubin concentrations. Liver biopsy findings have been variable, and may include a granulomatous reaction or hepatocellular necrosis and inflammation. In several cases the patients have been rechallenged with the drug after recovery, with the rapid recurrence of symptoms and abnormal liver tests. The pathogenesis is unknown, and both toxic and allergic mechanisms have been suggested. The prognosis has been uniformly good.

Amiodarone. This iodinated benzofuran derivative, when used in the treatment of refractory arrhythmias, produces an unusual form of hepatotoxicity similar to that previously documented for perhexilene maleate (see p. 777). Mild elevations of aminotransferase levels have been observed in between 15 and 40 per cent of patients recieving long-term therapy with amiodarone,[388, 389] although in some patients, values have returned to normal during continued treatment with this drug. Of major concern is the fact that in most instances in which serious hepatotoxicity from amiodarone has been described, the development of the liver disease has been insidious and asymptomatic, with mild to moderate elevations in transaminases and normal or mildly increased alkaline phosphatase levels.[390, 391] Jaundice is notably absent, and the commonest clinical finding is hepatomegaly. Liver biopsy has typically shown features similar to those found in alcoholic hepatitis, with steatosis, focal necrosis, focal (predominantly polymorphonuclear) leukocyte infiltrates, centrizonal fibrosis, and perinuclear (Mallory's) hyaline inclusions.[390, 391] The histologic appearances of cholangitis[390] may be present, and granulomas also have been observed.[392] In several cases, the liver lesion has progressed to a micronodular cirrhosis,[390] and death from liver failure has been reported.[393] In addition, evidence of hepatotoxicity may persist for several months after cessation of amiodarone treatment, an apparent consequence of the extremely slow elimination of this drug.[391] Liver biopsies from patients treated with amiodarone examined by electron microscopy consistently reveal a striking accumulation of concentric, whorled membranous arrays (myeloid figures) in lysosomes (Fig. 31–4) similar to those seen in

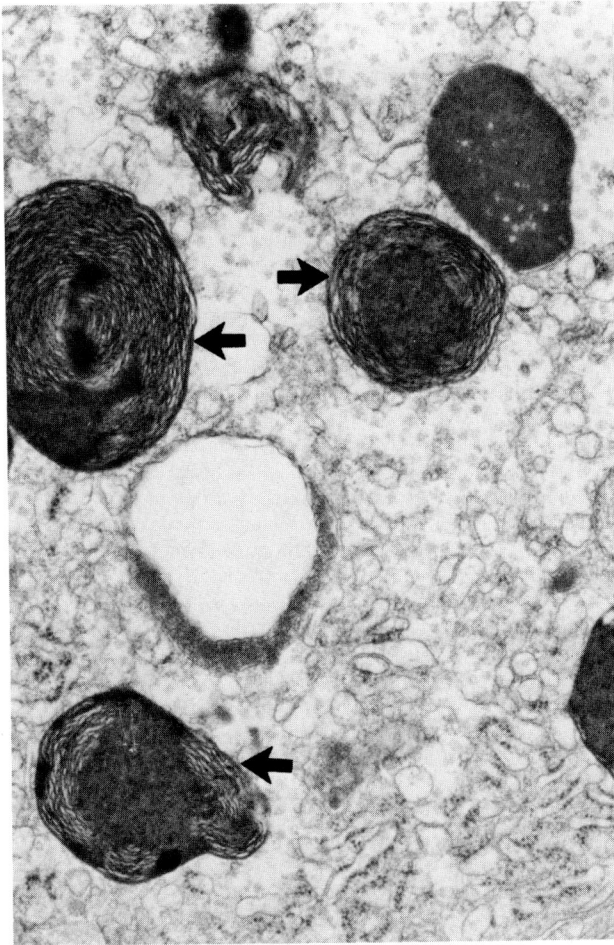

Figure 31–4. Electron micrograph of a hepatocyte from a patient treated with amiodarone. Lamellated bodies (arrows) are contained within lysosomes. These bodies are formed by the accumulation of phospholipids that normally are degraded within the lysosomes. × 31,000. (Courtesy of Dr. M. Barker.)

hereditary lipidoses such as Niemann-Pick and Tay-Sachs diseases.[390–392] These structures represent phospholipids stored in lysosomes and are found in extrahepatic tissues as well. The amphiphilic nature of amiodarone—a property it shares with other drugs such as perhexilene maleate, which also produce secondary phospholipid storage—leads to its entrapment in lysosomes, where it binds to phospholipids, protecting them from degradation by phospholipases and leading to their accumulation.[394] The accumulation of amiodarone in hepatic lysosomes also manifests as increased hepatic radiologic density on CT scanning.[395] It is unclear, however, whether the phospholipidosis produced by amiodarone treatment is of importance in the mechanism of clinically evident hepatotoxicity or merely an interesting but incidental phenomenon, since characteristic phospholipid inclusions also have been found in the livers of amiodarone-treated patients without any other histologic evidence of hepatic injury.[395]

Aprinidine. Another antiarrhythmic agent, aprinidine, has been linked to an acute hepatitis in a few cases.[396] The disorder is characterized by the onset of variable but mild systemic and digestive symptoms and mild to moderate increases in serum transaminase and alkaline phosphatase activities and bilirubin concentrations. Biopsy shows a mild, nonspecific hepatitis. Rechallenge has elicited the syndrome in at least one patient. The prognosis for complete recovery upon discontinuation of the drug is good. The mechanism is unknown.

Ajmaline. This antiarrhythmic drug is not currently available in the United States. Its use in Europe has been associated with a few cases of cholestatic jaundice developing one to three weeks after treatment is initiated.[397] Accompanying fever, chills, and abdominal pain may lead to a mistaken diagnosis of bacterial cholangitis. Eosinophilia is often prominent and liver biopsies have shown centrilobular cholestasis and portal inflammation. Liver function abnormalities may be slow to resolve following cessation of therapy.

Procainamide. This agent has been reported to cause a granulomatous hepatitis, documented by rechallenge, with eventual complete recovery.[398]

OTHER AGENTS

Perhexilene Maleate. Used in the treatment of angina pectoris, perhexilene maleate has been reported to cause liver dysfunction in several instances.[399–402] Most affected patients had taken the drug regularly for at least a year. Abnormalities in liver tests are variable, and patients may have clinical manifestations of liver disease such as jaundice, encephalopathy, and ascites. The liver injury produced by perhexilene maleate is similar to that encountered with amiodarone (see above). Liver biopsy shows a lesion similar to that of alcoholic hepatitis, and accumulation of phospholipid myeloid figures in lysosomes is seen on electron microscopy. The liver injury may progress to cirrhosis, and some patients have died in liver failure despite discontinuation of the drug. Perhexilene maleate belongs to the group of amphiphilic drugs including amiodarone (see above) that induce a secondary phospholipid storage disorder. In rats, short-term administration of perhexilene maleate increases total liver gangliosides and changes their composition.[403] However, the relationship of this drug-induced abnormality in glycolipid metabolism to the mechanism of hepatotoxicity remains to be established.

Papaverine. Papaverine may cause an acute hepatitis characterized by abnormal liver tests, hepatocellular necrosis, and cholestasis, with prominent eosinophilic portal infiltrates.[371, 404] The prognosis is good.

Verapamil. This papaverine derivative has been reported to rarely cause a mild hepatitis with variable cholestasis, recurring on rechallenge.[405–407]

Anticoagulants. Generalized hypersensitivity reactions are not uncommon with phenindione and have included hepatitis with both hepatocellular and cholestatic features.[408] *Warfarin*, on the other hand, appears to have little hepatotoxic potential. *Heparin* therapy has been found to result in minor to fivefold elevations in serum transaminase levels in up to 95 per cent of patients receiving this agent.[409] The mechanism of this transaminase increase is unknown, but values invariably return to normal during or after cessation of treatment.

Hypolipidemic Agents. *Cholestyramine, colestipol*, and *clofibrate*, and other such agents, have not been shown convincingly to cause liver disease. *Nicotinic acid*, however, occasionally appears to cause a dose-related cholestatic liver injury and, less commonly, hepatocellular necrosis. The mechanism is unknown, and complete recovery may be expected when the drug is reduced in dose or discontinued.[371]

HORMONES AND HORMONALLY ACTIVE DRUGS

ESTROGENIC STEROIDS

Both natural and synthetic estrogens influence liver structure and function in several important ways, including physiologic modulation of certain aspects of intermediary metabolism[410, 411] and a number of pathologic effects of clinical significance. Among these adverse effects are cholestasis, an apparent predisposition to cholesterol gallstone formation, the development of hepatic tumors, and the Budd-Chiari syndrome and other vascular lesions.

Estrogen-induced Cholestasis (*See also Chap. 54*)

Although it already had been recognized that estrogens could impair secretion of bile, the dramatic increase in the widespread use of contraceptive steroids in the late 1950s and early 1960s brought this fact to wider recognition.[412, 413] At about the same time, disorders of biliary secretion and clinical cholestasis associated with pregnancy were more clearly defined.[264] It soon became evident that the cholestasis associated with pregnancy and with oral contraceptive use could be viewed as variants of fundamentally the same pathophysiologic process, i.e., an adverse effect of estrogenic steroids on bile secretory function. It also was evident that there were marked differences in individual susceptibilities and responses to this particular impairment, despite the absence of any evidence that they were mediated immunologically.

Oral contraceptives uniformly cause subclinical impairment of sulfobromophthalein (BSP) transport maximum (T_{max}).[416] (See Chap. 25 for a discussion of this test.) This apparently is not related to any effect on hepatic conjugation or storage but represents a defect in the secretion of BSP into bile. Although it is demonstrable only by techniques that permit detection of subtle changes in BSP transport, minor, non-progressive, and reversible abnormalities in routine liver tests, such as serum alkaline phosphatase and transaminase activity, are not uncommon among users of oral contraceptives.[412] There appears to be no difference in effect on the liver between orally and vaginally administered estradiol of equivalent systemic potency.[413]

In contradistinction to these common and clinically subtle effects, a few patients develop overt cholestatic jaundice while taking oral contraceptives.[412] The incidence of this more exaggerated response is not known with certainty. It may occur less commonly as newer preparations contain less estrogen, but whether an apparent decrease in incidence simply reflects fewer case reports is not clear. In any case, it is evident that certain individuals are predisposed to the more exaggerated reaction, and incidences appear to be higher among Scandinavians[417] and Chileans.[418] The high incidence in Chile may reflect a genetically determined predisposition to estrogen-induced cholestasis among women of Auracanian Indian ancestry.[419] Women with histories of cholestasis of pregnancy[412] or with Dubin-Johnson syndrome[420] also are at increased risk.

Cholestasis Caused by Oral Contraceptives. This disorder usually appears within the first two months of treatment. It is manifested by pruritus and conjugated hyperbilirubinemia, associated with dark urine and light stools. There may be variable upper gastrointestinal symptoms or systemic symptoms such as fatigue and malaise, but as a rule these are minimal. Fever, arthralgia, rash, and other evidence of an inflammatory or allergic process are characteristically absent. There may or may not be minimal hepatomegaly, and there are no abnormal physical findings other than those attributable to the cholestasis itself. Laboratory studies add little; serum alkaline phosphatase and transaminase activities are slightly to moderately abnormal, whereas prothrombin time is usually normal. The histologic character of the lesion is that of a bland cholestatic process, most pronounced in the central areas where there is canalicular and hepatocellular bile stasis. Liver cell necrosis and inflammatory response are minimal or nonexistent. Upon discontinuation of the oral contraceptive, the syndrome rapidly and completely resolves, with return of liver function virtually to normal within two months in almost all cases. Occasionally, the use of oral contraceptives may serve to unmask clinically inapparent underlying chronic liver disease, such as early primary biliary cirrhosis. In such instances, liver tests may be unusually severely deranged during the cholestatic phase, or may fail to return completely to normal. Under such circumstances, the possibility of an underlying hepatobiliary disorder should be considered, and appropriate diagnostic studies performed as indicated.

The relationship of oral contraceptive use to acute viral hepatitis and other intercurrent liver disease has been examined. In one study[421] the incidence of viral hepatitis appeared to be increased in users as compared with nonusers, although this may have reflected other differences in lifestyles or exposure risks in the study population. After recovery from acute viral hepatitis, oral contraceptives appear to be well tolerated and do not seem to predispose to abnormal liver function.[422] Although there is no clear evidence that oral contraceptives aggravate the course of acute hepatitis, prudence dictates that these and other medications should be discontinued whenever possible during such an illness, if for no other reason than to simplify the clinical assessment of its course.

Intrahepatic Cholestasis of Pregnancy. This form of cholestasis has many similarities to that associated with oral contraceptives[414] and is discussed in detail in Chapter 54. It also is a bland, noninflammatory cholestatic process that in most women is subtle and usually manifests only pruritus, which commonly occurs in late pregnancy; in a few women, however, it may cause overt cholestatic jaundice. It almost always occurs late in pregnancy, when estrogen secretion rates are high, is not usually associated with significant systemic symptoms, and is rapidly and completely reversed after parturition. Contrary to earlier impressions, it now appears that this overt cholestatic syndrome is associated with a significantly increased risk of premature labor, fetal distress, and postpartum hemorrhage,[423, 424] but there is no evidence that it causes chronic or progressive liver disease; in this regard the prognosis is excellent. However, these patients are at increased risk for the development of jaundice if they subsequently use oral contraceptives.[412, 425]

Mechanism

That natural and synthetic estrogens are responsible for these two closely related cholestatic disorders is convincingly established on both clinical and experimental grounds.[412, 414, 426] Thus, estrogens alone can reproduce the clinical picture of cholestasis of pregnancy in susceptible subjects,[425] and in sufficient doses, increase the BSP T_{max} in

laboratory animals[427] and in both men and women.[428] Moreover, there is evidence for a direct effect of estrogenic steroids on several facets of liver function and structure thought to be important in the formation of bile. Estrogens decrease bile flow, biliary secretion of bile acids and other cholephilic anions, liver plasma membrane fluidity, and Na^+,K^+-ATPase activity in rats.[429–435] It has been suggested that estrogens increase biliary permeability.[429] However, recent evidence indicates that marker solutes used to assess junctional permeability also gain access to the canaliculus via transcytosis,[430] and that any permeability changes that do take place may be secondary to the cholestasis itself.[431] (These aspects of bile secretion are discussed in Chapter 12.) The choleretic effect of estrogens is not attributable to impaired bile acid uptake by the hepatocyte.[436] That the observed changes may reflect a fundamental alteration in the physical properties of membranes is suggested not only by direct evidence for such changes[433–435] but also by the observation that they are reversed in vivo by Triton WR-1339, a nonionic detergent.[437] In the case of the estrogens, however, the concept that this represents a direct effect of the native steroid does not account satisfactorily for the remarkable differences in individual susceptibilities to the effect, as demonstrated by the relative infrequency of overt cholestasis in pregnancy and among users of oral contraceptives. In this connection, it is of interest that ethinyl estradiol–induced cholestasis in rats is prevented by administration of S-adenosyl-L-methionine, and this effect is associated with increased excretion of methylated estrogen metabolites.[438] S-adenosyl-L-methionine also has been found to reverse cholestasis of pregnancy.[439] Possibly, genetic[440] or environmental factors influence the extent to which estrogenic steroids are converted to metabolic products of greater or lesser toxicity. The commonly recognized estrogen conjugates[441, 442] and bile acids[443, 444] are not believed to cause the syndrome, but D-ring glucuronides, present in urine during the third trimester, are clearly cholestatic.[445, 446] Tamoxifen, an estrogen antagonist, also has been associated with cholestasis.[447]

Oral Contraceptive–Associated Hepatic Tumors

These are discussed in detail in Chapter 45. In brief, the possible relationship between oral contraceptives and hepatic tumors was first pointed out in 1973.[448] Since then, several hundred cases have been reported, but the true incidence is unknown. Tumors associated with oral contraceptive use include hepatic adenomas, focal nodular hyperplasia, hepatocellular carcinoma, and, rarely, other malignancies,[449–463] although the data regarding hepatocellular carcinoma are conflicting,[458–461] as is the possible relationship with the fibrolamellar variant.[460, 462] An association with epithelioid hemangioendothelioma has been noted.[464] That these lesions also occur in persons who have not used oral contraceptives, including men, has complicated interpretation of the limited epidemiologic data available. That oral contraceptives are indeed responsible for at least some of these cases, however, is strongly suggested by the fact that lesions may regress after discontinuation of the drug.[465–467] However, the late development of hepatocellular carcinoma in one such patient has been interpreted as suggesting that long-term sonographic follow-up may be warranted.[468] Most of the reported patients are women who have taken oral contraceptives for more than five years.[451]

A particularly disturbing feature of these lesions, especially the adenomas, is their tendency to present suddenly and unexpectedly, with hemorrhage either into the tumor itself or into the peritoneal cavity, or as an abdominal mass. Focal nodular hyperplasia is more often asymptomatic, and found incidentally during investigations or operations conducted for other reasons. Unfortunately, adenoma and focal nodular hyperplasia most often are associated with little or no change in routine laboratory tests, so that their early detection by a screening program would require imaging techniques. Oral contraceptive-associated hepatocellular carcinoma does not appear to differ in any regard from similar lesions not associated with these agents.

Many of the estrogen-associated tumors are highly vascular and are more likely to bleed; this may reflect a direct estrogen effect on hepatic vascular and sinusoidal morphology. This concept is supported by clinical evidence that lesions are more vascular in users of oral contraceptives and during pregnancy,[453, 469] and that estrogens may alter hepatic sinusoidal structure in rats.[470] The mechanism(s) by which estrogens contribute to tumor formation is (are) unknown.[471]

Vascular Syndromes

Although an increased incidence of the Budd-Chiari syndrome in women taking oral contraceptives would be consistent with the general perception that thromboembolic disorders occur more often in this population, a definite causal relationship remains unproved. Instead, much of the relevant literature consists of case reports, rendering accurate estimation of incidence impossible.[472–474] Nonetheless, the association has been convincingly made, and it is therefore important that this diagnosis be considered in any patient taking oral contraceptives in whom there is rapid onset of hepatomegaly or hepatic dysfunction, or signs of portal hypertension. Although the mechanism of the effect remains unclear,[475] it has been suggested that oral contraceptives exacerbate an underlying thrombogenic condition, such as paroxysmal nocturnal hemoglobinuria, or an overt or forme fruste of a myeloproliferative disorder.[476, 477] Details of the clinical and diagnostic aspects of this syndrome and its management are discussed in Chapter 23. Peliosis hepatis,[478] unilobar hepatic vein obstruction,[479] and hepatic infarction[480] have been associated with oral contraceptive use.

Gallstones

There is convincing evidence that the incidence of gallstones is increased among users of oral contraceptives, reflecting an increase in the saturation of bile by cholesterol;[481–487] gallbladder contractility may also be impaired.[488] The estrogen effect on cholesterol saturation is ameliorated by S-adenosyl-L-methionine.[489] Accordingly, this additional potential cause of cholestasis should also be considered in the differential diagnosis of jaundice associated with oral contraceptive use. The pathogenesis of gallstones is discussed in Chapter 13.

ANDROGENS AND ANABOLIC STEROIDS

Cholestasis

A bland, reversible cholestatic reaction virtually identical to that seen in association with oral contraceptives or pregnancy may be caused by certain androgenic or anabolic steroids.[490] For the most part, these are agents in which the 17-carbon is α-substituted, such as methyltestosterone and norethandrolone; testosterone itself and its esters do not produce this response. The clinical and histologic picture also is the same as that of the reaction to oral contraceptives, and the lesion is entirely reversible. The similarities in the patterns of cholestasis produced by anabolic steroids and by estrogens suggest that they act by similar mechanisms. However, compared with the estrogen-induced lesion, anabolic steroid–induced cholestasis has been studied less extensively.

Peliosis Hepatis

This unusual condition is characterized by blood-filled spaces within the hepatic parenchyma that may or may not be lined with sinusoidal endothelium. It occurs in a variety of chronic, wasting diseases such as tuberculosis and malignancy, and in recipients of renal transplants, and it has been associated with chronic administration of androgenic-anabolic steroids.[491–496] It may be asymptomatic or may manifest clinically as hepatomegaly, liver failure, or intraperitoneal hemorrhage. It has been suggested that the lesion results from foci of liver cell necrosis, which then become hemorrhagic. More recently, it has been proposed that the lesion begins with hyperplasia of hepatocytes, associated with focal sinusoidal dilation, perhaps reflecting the anabolic steroid effect; sinusoidal occlusion or disruption is believed to result from the mechanical effect of subendothelial clusters of hepatocytes.[497] Since these steroids also are associated with the formation of hepatic tumors, this concept might provide a unifying hypothesis for the pathogenesis of both peliosis and neoplasm.

Tumors

Androgenic-anabolic steroids have been associated with the development of hepatic adenoma, hepatocellular carcinoma, and hepatic angiosarcoma.[498–500] Although long-term methyltestosterone in mice may cause dysplastic lesions,[501] such changes are not necessarily seen in human subjects receiving androgens.[502]

ORAL HYPOGLYCEMICS

Most of the commonly used agents in this category are innocuous with regard to the liver and only rarely have been associated with hepatic injury. The most common reaction is intrahepatic cholestasis, associated with variable but usually slight liver cell necrosis and seen in perhaps 0.5 per cent of patients who take chlorpropamide; it occurs much less often with tolbutamide and tolazamide.[503–505] The disorder usually becomes manifest in the first several weeks of treatment, is associated with clinical, laboratory, and biopsy evidence of cholestasis, and can be expected to resolve completely in virtually all cases, although the course of tolazamide hepatotoxicity may be quite prolonged.[505]

Less commonly, certain oral hypoglycemic agents, e.g., acetohexamide (and more recently glyburide[506]), cause a viral hepatitis–like picture of acute hepatocellular necrosis. Among these rare cases, fatalities have been recorded. Hepatic granulomas also have been described.

The mechanism of these hepatic drug reactions is unknown. It is of interest that, in an earlier review of the subject,[504] 8 of 25 reported instances of jaundice attributed to oral hypoglycemics occurred in patients who had other reasons for jaundice, and subsequent rechallenge with sulfonylureas of 6 of the remaining 17 patients in the series failed to reproduce the jaundice. Since features suggestive of "allergy" are inconstant, direct or indirect toxicity may account for the reaction in that small but uncertain number of patients who truly manifest sulfonylurea-induced hepatic injury. Biguanides do not appear to be associated with liver damage.

ANTITHYROID DRUGS

Clinically significant liver injury appears to be a distinctly uncommon side effect of this group of agents.[507] The available case reports suggest that it may take two different forms. The more common cholestatic form has been seen in association with *methimazole*. Its onset is usually two to four weeks after administration of the drug is started, but occasionally may be delayed. Symptoms are nonspecific, and occasionally include rash, fever, or adenopathy. Liver tests are primarily cholestatic, in that elevations of serum alkaline phosphatase are more striking than those of transaminases. Liver biopsy shows cholestasis, with relatively minor liver cell necrosis or inflammatory response. The prognosis appears to be good, in that no fatalities attributable to liver damage have been reported, but resolution of the process may take several months. *Carbimazole*, an agent related to methimazole, has been documented as a cause of a nonspecific hepatitis in which cholestatic features were absent.[508]

Propylthiouracil has been associated in several cases[509, 510] with a predominantly hepatocellular form of injury, which may be severe and even fatal, with massive hepatic necrosis. The mechanism of the hepatic reactions to antithyroid drugs is not known.

HISTAMINE-2 RECEPTOR ANTAGONISTS

Cimetidine has been reported to be a rare cause of jaundice associated with necrosis, which may be focal or confluent, and a polymorphonuclear and/or mononuclear infiltrate; it also has been associated with more subtle and presumably less significant changes in liver function in anicteric subjects.[511–514] Cimetidine also may influence the metabolism of other drugs, through its effect on drug-metabolizing enzymes (i.e., mixed function oxidases).[515] In vitro, this agent may damage DNA in hepatocyte cultures,[516] but the clinical relevance of this observation is not established.

Ranitidine also has been documented as hepatotoxic, associated histologically with focal necrosis, portal infiltrates, and mild cholestasis.[517–519]

PSYCHOACTIVE DRUGS

This broad class of agents includes a large number of compounds that differ in chemical structures, pharmacologic and physiologic effects, and hepatotoxic potentials.[520] The phenothiazines were among the earliest recognized causes of drug-induced cholestatic liver disease. *Iproniazid*, a hydrazine-containing monoamine oxidase inhibitor antidepressant, has largely fallen into disuse because of its

tendency to cause a frequently fatal acute hepatitis–like syndrome. Conversely, the tricyclic and tetracyclic antidepressants and the benzodiazepines appear much less hepatotoxic.

CHLORPROMAZINE

Soon after its introduction and widespread use approximately 30 years ago, it became apparent that chlorpromazine was a cause of liver damage and cholestatic jaundice. Because of its sporadic occurrence, certain clinical features, and the initial impression of a lack of clearly predictable hepatotoxicity in animals, chlorpromazine-induced cholestasis was assumed to reflect a form of drug hypersensitivity. However, there is now increasing evidence that chlorpromazine cholestasis is mediated directly by the parent compound or by the products of its hepatic biotransformation (see "Mechanism" below).

Incidence

The actual incidence of chlorpromazine-induced jaundice is unknown, but it is estimated as 0.5 to 1 per cent. As is true of hepatic injuries caused by many other agents, however, mild or subclinical hepatic dysfunction appears to be far more common than this, and may occur in as many as 50 per cent of chronic users. The incidence is lower in children and young adults. The relative infrequency of the overt acute lesion indicates substantial differences in individual susceptibilities, the possible basis of which is considered below.

Mechanism

Some patients with chlorpromazine-induced cholestasis have clinical and laboratory features suggestive of drug allergy, such as rash, eosinophilia, and the appearance in serum of antinuclear antibodies. These, together with the sporadic and unpredictable occurrence of the overt form of the reaction, have been taken as evidence that the injury is mediated immunologically, (i.e., that it represents a form of drug hypersensitivity). However, this concept is not convincingly supported, and seems less attractive in view of evidence that chlorpromazine and its metabolites may directly impair several aspects of liver cell function that appear important for secretion of bile. For example, in the isolated perfused rat liver, chlorpromazine and certain of its metabolites acutely inhibit bile and perfusate flow.[521–524] The effective dose, nature, and reversibility of this effect depend on the agent employed and on whether the animal had been treated previously with an inducer of microsomal drug metabolism.[524] In the rhesus monkey, chlorpromazine rapidly and reversibly inhibits bile acid and lipid secretion and bile acid-independent flow.[525] In vitro, chlorpromazine and its metabolites adversely affect the activities of plasma membrane Na^+, K^+-ATPase and Mg^{++}-ATPase,[526–528] solute transport,[528] membrane fluidity, and actin gelation and polymerization.[529] Although the precise roles of these variables in biliary secretion are not fully defined, their integrity appears necessary for the process to occur normally, as shown in a variety of experimental circumstances. Moreover, in each instance, the relative potencies of chlorpromazine and its metabolites in adversely affecting these variables are approximately the same (7,8-dihydroxychlor-promazine > 7-hydroxychlorpromazine > chlorpromazine > chlorpromazine sulfoxide), and the effective concentrations in vitro are similar to those present in serum during chlorpromazine administration. Chlorpromazine also forms insoluble 1:1 complexes with bile salts, and could inhibit bile secretion via this mechanism.[530] More recently, chlorpromazine has been shown to inhibit a number of secretory processes in other tissues, including intestine.[531, 532] This effect has been attributed to an interaction with calmodulin, an intracellular calcium-dependent regulator protein that, conceivably, could also be important in biliary secretion. Furthermore, it has been shown that chlorpromazine metabolites may be excreted in urine for many months after administration of the drug is discontinued, and this could account for the prolonged clinical cholestasis occasionally seen.

Taken together, the available evidence supports the concept that chlorpromazine-induced cholestasis is caused by a direct adverse effect of chlorpromazine and its metabolites on the cellular mechanism(s) involved in biliary secretion. As a corollary, it seems likely that individual differences in susceptibilities to this injury may reflect differences in the rates at which the parent compound is metabolized, the relative rates of its conversion to metabolites of differing hepatotoxic potencies, and the rates at which these toxic compounds are otherwise detoxified or excreted. Since all of these processes may be subject to modulation by a wide variety of poorly understood and potentially interacting pharmacologic, genetic, dietary, and environmental factors, one need not invoke an immunologic mechanism to account for the idiosyncratic nature of the reaction. Nonetheless, it remains a possibility that in some instances, chlorpromazine cholestasis may be partly or wholly mediated by an immunologic process. A recent study has shown that rats treated with chlorpromazine develop antibodies to the drug,[533] but the significance of this finding is unclear.

Histology

The lesion is the prototype of inflammatory drug-induced cholestasis. As in most other cholestatic conditions, cholestasis is most prominent in central zones. Inflammation is largely confined to the portal areas and consists primarily of mononuclear cells, with variable eosinophilia or neutrophilia. The smaller bile ducts are involved occasionally, and not infrequently there is hepatocellular necrosis in the lobule, associated with a predominantly lymphocytic inflammatory response and occasional acidophil bodies. Because of its nonspecificity, the reaction may not be distinguishable from that associated with biliary obstruction or ascending cholangitis.

Clinical Features

Chlorpromazine-induced jaundice almost always appears within three to five weeks after treatment is begun.[520] It may appear in the absence of other complaints or may be heralded by a variety of nonspecific gastrointestinal or systemic symptoms, including a flu-like syndrome, nausea, vomiting, and upper abdominal discomfort or frank pain. Pruritus may develop as the cholestasis becomes more prominent. Eosinophilia occurs in the majority of cases.

Alkaline phosphatase and cholesterol elevations in serum reflect the severity of the cholestasis; transaminase activity is slightly to moderately increased.

The prognosis is excellent. Nearly 75 per cent of reported patients recovered completely within three months of cessation of treatment with the drug. In a few patients, however, a significant cholestasis may persist for more than a year and may resemble primary biliary cirrhosis clinically and histologically. Unlike those who have primary biliary cirrhosis, however, patients with chronic chlorpromazine-induced jaundice usually recover within a few years. Only rarely does this chronic syndrome progress; it remains unclear whether this less favorable course in fact represents drug-induced primary biliary cirrhosis, the unmasking of previously unrecognized primary biliary cirrhosis, or the fortuitous association of two unusual diseases.

Diagnosis

An appropriate drug history, clinical and laboratory picture, and response to discontinuation of the drug would strongly suggest the diagnosis of chlorpromazine-induced cholestasis. As already mentioned, however, essentially all clinical and laboratory features, including histologic characteristics, are nonspecific. For this reason, the diagnosis can rarely be made unequivocally without rechallenge—a procedure which, while helpful in many patients, is not infallible, rarely is necessary for appropriate clinical management, and is not generally recommended. Rather, it is more important to exclude, by appropriate imaging techniques, other causes of transient cholestasis such as cholelithiasis and biliary duct obstruction. Liver biopsy may demonstrate histologic features that are consistent with the diagnosis but do not reliably exclude biliary duct obstruction.

Management

Discontinuation of the drug and symptomatic support, such as the use of colestipol or cholestyramine for itching, are appropriate. Since there is no evidence that corticosteroids are of significant benefit in reducing either the severity or the duration of the reaction, they should be avoided. In the more chronic cases, it may be necessary to provide fat-soluble vitamin supplements, especially when cholestyramine or colestipol treatment is employed. Other potentially correctable causes of cholestasis must be excluded.

Other Phenothiazines

Although cholestatic reactions similar to that caused by chlorpromazine have been associated with the use of other phenothiazines,[520] their incidence is unknown. Most agents in this group, however, appear to be no more hepatotoxic than chlorpromazine; with some agents, such as promazine and promethazine, cholestasis appears to be exceedingly rare or nonexistent.

OTHER PSYCHOACTIVE AGENTS

Antidepressants. Among the monoamine oxidase–inhibiting derivatives of hydrazine, iproniazid is the most widely recognized as a potential hepatotoxin. It produces an acute viral hepatitis–like injury, associated in fatal cases with massive or submassive necrosis. Iproniazid itself is no longer widely used, but other related compounds are available, the hepatotoxicities of which are documented but variable.[534] One of these agents, phenethylhydrazine, has produced hepatic angiosarcomas in mice, and this lesion has been found in one patient who had used the agent for at least six years.[535] Tranylcypromine, a monoamine oxidase inhibitor that does not contain hydrazine, has been reported to cause a viral hepatitis–like reaction. The tricyclic antidepressants, such as imipramine, desipramine, and amitriptylene, appear to be less frequently hepatotoxic, although there have been several recent reports of both cholestatic and hepatocellular types of liver injury following the use of these drugs, recurring on rechallenge.[520, 536] Cross-sensitization between drugs of this class also may occur.[537] The mechanism of hepatotoxicity is unknown, but experimental findings have involved both a direct toxic effect on the liver cell surface membrane dependent on the detergent properties of the tricyclic compounds,[538] and a mechanism dependent upon activation of these drugs to reactive, arylating intermediate compounds.[539] However, the clinical presentation of tricyclic antidepressant–induced hepatotoxicity is more compatible with a hypersensitivity mechanism.[536] Apart from a few isolated reports of mild hepatic reactions, the newer tetracyclic antidepressants have to date been relatively free of hepatotoxicity.

Benzodiazepines. These commonly used tranquilizers appear to have a very low hepatotoxic potential. Chlordiazepoxide, diazepam, and flurazepam have been associated with cholestasis in a few reported cases.[520, 540] There have been no reports of hepatotoxicity from midazolam.

Haloperidol. This agent may cause a cholestatic reaction, associated with portal infiltrates.[541] The incidence is uncertain, but appears to be less than 1 per cent.

MISCELLANEOUS DRUGS

Doxapram. A respiratory stimulant, doxapram has been reported to cause acute hepatotoxicity in at least two infants and one adult treated with this agent.[542, 543] It is of interest that in infants, the lesion was manifest clinically by hypoglycemia and increased serum transaminase activity, despite normal alkaline phosphatase and bilirubin values, and histologically by small-droplet fat deposition without significant inflammation or necrosis. While the mechanism is not known, the syndrome is reminiscent of Reye's syndrome and Jamaica vomiting sickness in many aspects. In the single adult case, hepatotoxicity manifested differently, as acute centrilobular hepatocellular necrosis.[543]

Disulfiram. An agent used in the aversion therapy of alcoholism, disulfiram has been reported to cause acute liver cell necrosis.[544–547] The clinical picture is quite similar to that of acute viral hepatitis, and at least one death has been reported due to fulminant hepatic failure.[546] The validity of the causal relationship has been well documented by recurrence of hepatitis on re-exposure to the drug in five patients. Most cases have occurred within two months of commencing treatment, and women appear to be more susceptible. The histologic findings are nonspecific, showing focal and zonal necrosis, with an inflammatory cell infiltrate often containing many eosinophils. Peripheral eosinophilia is, however, an uncommon feature.

Lergotrile Mesylate. This ergot derivative, used in the treatment of parkinsonism, caused increased serum trans-

aminase activities in 12 of 19 patients. It is associated with mild, nonspecific hepatocellular necrosis by light microscopy, but has unusual ultrastructural features, especially striking mitochondrial abnormalities.[548]

Retinoids. These agents (e.g., etretinate) are synthetic vitamin A analogs that have been used to treat a variety of dermatologic disorders including psoriasis and severe acne. Between 8 and 40 per cent of patients treated with etritinate have developed variable, usually minor increases in serum transaminases, which have usually returned to normal with continued treatment.[549, 550] Persistent transaminase abnormalities have been associated with nonspecific, usually mild histologic abnormalities. More serious histologic damage noted in some patients has been difficult to interpret in view of co-existent alcoholism, pre-existing liver disease, and previous treatment with methotrexate. Although related structurally to vitamin A, the synthetic retinoids are unlike the natural vitamin in that they do not appear to be stored in the liver over long periods of time and therefore would not be expected to produce liver damage via a mechanism analagous to vitamin A hepatotoxicity (see Chaps. 8 and 32). Indeed, a single report of hepatitis in a patient following one month of etretinate treatment, in whom striking eosinophilia was observed and in whom the hepatitis recurred upon rechallenge with the drug, suggests that hypersensitivity may be at least one mechanism whereby retinoids are capable of producing liver damage.[551]

REFERENCES

1. Zimmerman HJ, Maddrey WC. Toxic and drug-induced hepatitis. In: Schiff L, Schiff ER, eds. Diseases of the Liver. Philadelphia, JB Lippincott 1982:621.
2. Zimmerman HJ. Hepatotoxicity. New York, Appleton-Century-Crofts, 1978.
3. Koff RS, Gardiner R, Harinasuta V, et al. Profile of hyperbilirubinemia in three hospital populations. Clin Res 18:680, 1970.
4. Ritt DJ, Whelan G, Weiner DJ, et al. Acute hepatic necrosis with stupor or coma: an analysis of thirty-one patients. Medicine 48:151, 1969.
5. Caravati CM, Hooker TH. Acute massive hepatic necrosis with fatal liver failure. Am J Dig Dis 16:803, 1971.
6. Eastwood HOH. Causes of jaundice in the elderly: a survey of diagnosis and investigation. Gerontol Clin 13:69, 1971.
7. Maddrey WC, Boitnott JK. Drug-induced chronic liver disease. Gastroenterology 72:1348, 1977.
8. Maddrey WC, Boitnott JK. Drug-induced chronic hepatitis and cirrhosis. In: Popper H, Schaffner F, eds. Progress in Liver Diseases. Volume 6. New York, Grune and Stratton, 1979:595.
9. Zimmerman HJ. Drug-induced chronic hepatic disease. Med Clin North Am 63:567, 1979.
10. Jones JK. Suspected drug-induced hepatic reactions reported to the FDA's adverse reactions system: An overview. Semin Liver Dis 1:157, 1981.
11. Dossing M, Andreasen BP. Drug-induced liver disease in Denmark. An analysis of 572 cases of hepatoxicity reported to the Danish Board of adverse reactions to drugs. Scand J Gastroenterol 17:205, 1982.
12. Ludwig J, Axelsen R. Drug effects on the liver: an updated tabular compilation of drugs and drug-related hepatic diseases. Dig Dis Sci 28:651, 1983.
13. Tucker RA. Drugs and liver disease: a tabular compilation of drugs and the histopathological changes that can occur in the liver. Drug Intell Clin Pharmacol 16:569, 1982.
14. Homberg JC, Abuaf N, Helmy-Khalil S, et al. Drug-induced hepatitis associated with anticytoplasmic organelle autoantibodies. Hepatology 5:722, 1985.
15. Mitchell JR, Jollow DJ. Metabolic activation of drugs to toxic substances. Gastroenterology 68:392, 1975.
16. Jacqz E, Hall SD, Branch RA. Genetically determined polymorphisms in drug oxidation. Hepatology 6:1020, 1986.
17. Spielberg SP, Gordon GB, Blake DA, et al. Predisposition to phenytoin hepatotoxicity assessed in vitro. N Engl J Med 305:722, 1981.
18. Bellomo G, Orrenius S. Altered thiol and calcium homeostasis in oxidative hepatocellular injury. Hepatology 5:876, 1985.

19. Lemasters JJ, DiGuiseppi J, Nieminen A-L, et al. Blebbing, free Ca^{++} and mitochondrial membrane potential preceding cell death in hepatocytes. Nature 325:78, 1987.

20. Spitz RD, Keren DF, Boitnott JK, et al. Bridging hepatic necrosis. Etiology and prognosis. Am J Dig Dis 23:1076, 1978.

21. Ware AJ, Cuthbert JA, Shorey J, et al. A prospective trial of steroid therapy in severe viral hepatitis. The prognostic significance of bridging necrosis. Gastroenterology 80:219, 1981.

22. Miller DJ, Dwyer J, Klatskin G. Halothane hepatitis: benign resolution of a severe lesion. Ann Intern Med 89:212, 1978.

23. McMaster KR, Hennigar GR. Drug-induced granulomatous hepatitis. Lab Invest 44:61, 1981.

24. Kean EA, ed. Hypoglycin. New York, Academic Press 1975.

25. Prescott LF, Wright N, Roscoe P, et al. Plasma paracetamol half-life and hepatic necrosis in patients with paracetamol overdosage. Lancet 1:519, 1971.

26. Rumack BH. Acetaminophen overdose. Am J Med 75(suppl):104, 1983.

27. Black M. Acetaminophen hepatotoxicity. Ann Rev Med 35:577, 1984.

28. Barker JD, De-Carle DJ, Anuras S. Chronic excessive acetaminophen use and liver damage. Ann Intern Med 87:299, 1977.

29. Johnson GK, Tolman KG. Chronic liver disease and acetaminophen. Ann Intern Med 87:302, 1977.

30. Mitchell JR. Host susceptibility and acetaminophen liver injury. Ann Intern Med 87:377, 1977.

31. Leist MH, Gluskin LE, Payne JA. Enhanced toxicity of acetaminophen in alcoholics: report of three cases. J Clin Gastroenterol 7:55, 1985.

32. Seeff LB, Cuccherini BA, Zimmerman HJ, et al. Acetaminophen hepatotoxicity in alcoholics. A therapeutic misadventure. Ann Intern Med 104:399, 1986.

33. Ferguson DR, Snyder SK, Cameron AJ. Hepatotoxicity in acetaminophen poisoning. Mayo Clin Proc 52:246, 1977.

34. Prescott LF, Illingworth RN, Critchley JAJH, et al. Intravenous N-acetylcysteine: the treatment of choice for paracetamol poisoning. Br Med J 2:1097, 1979.

35. Hamlyn AN, Douglas AP, James OFW, et al. Liver function and structure in survivors of acetaminophen poisoning. Am J Dig Dis 22:605, 1977.

36. Walker RM, Racz WJ, McElligott TF. Scanning electron microscopic examination of acetaminophen-induced hepatotoxicity and congestion in mice. Am J Pathol 113:321, 1983.

37. Gerber MA, Kaufmann H, Klion F, et al. Acetaminophen associated hepatic injury. Report of two cases showing unusual portal tract reactions. Hum Pathol 11:37, 1980.

38. Ambre J, Alexander M. Liver toxicity after acetaminophen ingestion. Inadequacy of the dose estimate as an index of risk. JAMA 238:500, 1977.

39. Pessayre D, Dolder A, Artigou J-Y, et al. Effect of fasting on metabolite-mediated hepatotoxicity in the rat. Gastroenterology 77:264, 1979.

40. Wendel A, Feuerstein S, Konz K-H. Acute paracetamol intoxication of starved mice leads to lipid peroxidation in vivo. Biochem Pharmacol 28:2051, 1979.

41. Mitchell JR, Jollow DJ, Potter WZ, et al. Acetaminophen-induced hepatic necrosis. I. Role of drug metabolism. J Pharmacol Exp Ther 187:185, 1973.

42. Jollow DJ, Mitchell JR, Potter WZ, et al. Acetaminophen-induced hepatic necrosis. II. Role of covalent binding in vivo. J Pharmacol Exp Ther 187:195, 1973.

43. Potter WZ, Davis DC, Mitchell JR, et al. Acetaminophen-induced hepatic necrosis. III. Cytochrome P-450–mediated covalent binding in vitro. J Pharmacol Exp Ther 187:203, 1973.

44. Mitchell JR, Jollow DJ, Potter WZ, et al. Acetaminophen-induced hepatic necrosis. IV. Protective role of glutathione. J Pharmacol Exp Ther 187:211, 1973.

45. Pirotte JH. Apparent potentiation of hepatotoxicity from small doses of acetaminophen by phenobarbital. Ann Intern Med 101:403, 1984.

46. Johnson MW, Friedman PA, Mitch WE. Alcoholism, nonprescription drugs and hepatotoxicity. The risk from unknown acetaminophen ingestion. Am J Gastroenterol 76:530, 1981.

47. Rosen GM, Singletary WV, Rauckman EJ, et al. Acetaminophen hepatotoxicity: an alternative mechanism. Biochem Pharmacol 32:2053, 1983.

48. Black M, Raucy J. Acetaminophen, alcohol, and cytochrome P450. Ann Intern Med 104:427, 1986.

49. Holme JA, Dahlin DC, Nelson SD, et al. Cytotoxic effects of N-acetyl-p-benzoquinone imine, a common arylating intermediate of paracetamol and N-hydroxyparacetamol. Biochem Pharmacol 33:401, 1984.

50. Grafstrom R, Ormstad K, Moldeus P, et al. Paracetamol metabolism in the isolated perfused rat liver with further metabolism of a biliary paracetamol conjugate by the small intestine. Biochem Pharmacol 28:3573, 1979.

51. Inoue M, Okajima K, Morino Y. Metabolic coordination of liver and kidney in mercapturic acid biosynthesis in vivo. Hepatology 2:311, 1982.

52. Davis M, Simmons CJ, Harrison NG, et al. Paracetamol overdose in man: relationship between pattern of urinary metabolites and severity of liver damage. Q J Med 45:181, 1976.

53. Davis DC, Potter WZ, Jollow DJ, et al. Species differences in hepatic glutathione depletion, covalent binding and hepatic necrosis after acetaminophen. Life Sci 14:2099, 1974.

54. Rollins DE, von Bahr C, Glaumann H, et al. Acetaminophen: potentially toxic metabolite formed by human fetal and adult microsomes and isolated fetal liver cells. Science 205:1414, 1979.

55. Mitchell MC, Shenker S, Speeg KV. Selective inhibition of acetaminophen oxidation and toxicity by cimetidine and other histamine H$_2$-receptor antagonists in vivo and in vitro in the rat and in man. J Clin Invest 73:383, 1984.

56. Speeg KV, Mitchell MC, Maldonado AL. Additive protection of cimetidine and N-acetylcysteine treatment against acetaminophen-induced hepatic necrosis in the rat. J Pharmacol Exp Ther 234:550, 1985.

57. Lauterburg BH, Davies S, Mitchell JR. Ethanol suppresses hepatic glutathione synthesis in rats in vivo. J Pharmacol Exp Ther 230:7, 1984.

58. Hazelton GA, Hjelle JJ, Klaasen CD. Effects of cysteine pro-drugs on acetaminophen-induced hepatotoxicity. J Pharmacol Exp Ther 237:341, 1986.

59. Corcoran GB, Wong BK. Role of glutathione in prevention of acetaminophen-induced hepatotoxicity by N-acetyl-L-cysteine in vivo: studies with N-acetyl-D-cysteine in mice. J Pharmacol Exp Ther 238:54, 1986.

60. Lin JM, Levy G. Sulfate depletion after acetaminophen administration and replenishment by infusion of sodium sulfate or N-acetylcysteine in rats. Biochem Pharmacol 30:2723, 1981.

61. Hjelle JJ, Brzeznicka EA, Klaasen CD. Comparison of the effects of sodium sulfate and N-acetylcysteine on the hepatotoxicity of acetaminophen in mice. J Pharmacol Exp Ther 236:526, 1986.

62. Yamada T, Ludwig S, Kuhlenkamp J, et al. Direct protection against acetaminophen hepatotoxicity by propylthiouracil in vivo and in vitro in rats and mice. J Clin Invest 67:688, 1981.

63. Huggett A, Blair IA. The mechanism of paracetamol-induced hepatotoxicity: implications for therapy. Hum Toxicol 2:399, 1983.

64. Rosen GM, Singeltary WV, Rauckman EJ, et al. Acetaminophen hepatotoxicity: an alternative mechanism. Biochem Pharmacol 32:2053, 1983.

65. Walker BE, Kelleher J, Dixon MF, et al. Vitamin E protection of the liver from paracetamol in the rat. Clin Sci Molec Med 47:449, 1974.

66. Högberg J, Orrenius S, Larson RE. Lipid peroxidation in isolated hepatocytes. Eur J Biochem 50:595, 1975.

67. Mitchell JR, Smith CV, Hughes H, et al. Overview of alkylation and peroxidation mechanisms in acute lethal hepatocellular injury by chemically reactive metabolites. Semin Liv Dis 1:143, 1981.

68. Peterson FJ, Knodell RG, Lindemann NJ, et al. Prevention of acetaminophen and cocaine hepatotoxicity in mice by cimetidine treatment. Gastroenterology 85:122, 1983.

69. Gerber JG, MacDonald JS, Hartison RD, et al. Effect of N-acetylcysteine on hepatic covalent binding of paracetamol. Lancet 1:657, 1977.

70. Labradorios D, Davis M, Portmann B, et al. Paracetamol-induced hepatic necrosis in the mouse—relationship between covalent binding, hepatic glutathione depletion and the protective effect of α-mercapto-propionylglycine. Biochem Pharmacol 26:31, 1977.

71. Corcoran GB, Racz WJ, Smith CV, et al. Effects of N-acetylcysteine on acetaminophen covalent binding and hepatic necrosis in mice. J Pharmacol Exp Ther 232:864, 1985.

72. Gerson RJ, Casini A, Gilfor D, et al. Oxygen-mediated cell injury in the killing of cultured hepatocytes by acetaminophen. Biochem Biophys Res Commun 126:1129, 1985.

73. Smith CV, Mitchell JR. Acetaminophen hepatotoxicity in vivo is not accompanied by oxidant stress. Biochem Biophys Res Commun 133:329, 1985.

74. Tee LBG, Boobis AR, Huggett AC, et al. Reversal of acetaminophen toxicity in isolated hamster hepatocytes by dithiothreitol. Toxicol Appl Pharmacol 83:294, 1986.

75. Tsokos-Kuhn JO, Todd EL, McMillin-Wood JB, et al. ATP-dependent calcium uptake by rat liver plasma membrane vesicles. Effect of alkylating hepatotoxins in vivo. Molec Pharmacol 28:51, 1985.

76. Moore M, Thor H, Moore G, et al. The toxicity of acetaminophen and N-acetyl-p-benzoquinone imine in isolated hepatocytes is associated with thiol depletion and increased cytosolic Ca^{2+}. J Biol Chem 260:13035, 1985.

77. Rich RR, Johnson JS. Salicylate hepatotoxicity in patients with juvenile rheumatoid arthritis. Arthritis Rheum 16:1, 1973.

78. Seaman WE, Ishak KG, Plotz PH. Aspirin-induced hepatotoxicity in patients with systemic lupus erythematosus. Ann Intern Med 80:1, 1974.

79. Wolfe JD, Metzger AL, Goldstein RC. Aspirin hepatitis. Ann Intern Med 80:74, 1974.

80. Zimmerman HJ. Effects of aspirin and acetaminophen on the liver. Arch Intern Med 141:333, 1981.

81. Schaller JG. Chronic salicylate administration in juvenile rheumatoid arthritis: aspirin "hepatitis" and its clinical significance. Pediatrics 62(suppl.):916, 1978.

82. Ulshen MH, Grand RJ, Crain JD, et al. Hepatotoxicity with encephalopathy associated with aspirin therapy in rheumatoid arthritis. J Pediatr 93:1034, 1978.

83. Petty BG, Zahka KG, Bernstein MT. Aspirin hepatitis associated with encephalopathy. J Pediatr 93:881, 1978.

84. Hurwitz ES, Barrett MJ, Bregman D, et al. Public Health Service study on Reye's syndrome and medications. N Engl J Med 313:849, 1985.

85. Starko KM, Mullick FG. Hepatic and cerebral findings in children with fatal salicylate intoxication: further evidence for a causal relationship between salicylate and Reye's syndrome. Lancet 1:326, 1983.

86. Kanada SA, Kollig WM, Hindin BI. Aspirin hepatotoxicity. Am J Hosp Pharm 35:330, 1978.

87. Tolman KG, Peterson P, Gray P, et al. Hepatotoxicity of salicylates in monolayer cell cultures. Gastroenterology 74:205, 1978.

88. Bernstein BH, Singsen BH, King KK, et al. Aspirin-induced hepatotoxicity and its effect on juvenile rheumatoid arthritis. Am J Dis Child 131:659, 1977.

89. Sbarbaro JA, Bennett RM. Aspirin hepatotoxicity and disseminated intravascular coagulation. Ann Intern Med 86:183, 1977.

90. Benjamin SB, Ishak KG, Zimmerman HJ, et al. Phenylbutazone liver injury: a clinical-pathologic survey of 23 cases and review of the literature. Hepatology 1:255, 1981.

91. Al-Kawas FM, Seeff LB, Berendson RA, et al. Allopurinol hepatotoxicity. Report of two cases and review of the literature. Ann Intern Med 95:588, 1981.

92. Swank LA, Chejfec G, Nemchausky BA. Allopurinol-induced granulomatous hepatitis with cholangitis and a sarcoid-like reaction. Arch Intern Med 138:997, 1978.

93. Boyer TD, Sun N, Reynolds TB. Allopurinol hypersensitivity vasculitis and liver damage. West J Med 126:143, 1977.

94. Butler RC, Shah SM, Grunow WA, et al. Massive hepatic necrosis in a patient receiving allopurinol. JAMA 237:473, 1977.

95. Vanderstigel M, Zafrani ES, Lejonc JL, et al. Allopurinol hypersensitivity syndrome as a cause of hepatic fibrin-ring granulomas. Gastroenterology 90:188, 1986.

96. Schenker S, Olson KN, Dunn D, et al. Intrahepatic cholestasis due to therapy of rheumatoid arthritis. Gastroenterology 64:622, 1973.

97. Howrie DL, Gartner JC. Gold-induced hepatotoxocity: case report and review of the literature. J Rheumatol 9:727, 1982.

98. Lowthian PJ, Cleland LG, Vernon-Roberts B. Hepatotoxicity with aurothioglucose therapy. Arthr Rheum 27:230, 1984.

99. Bravo JF, Jacobson MP, Mertens BF. Fatty liver and pleural effusion with ibuprofen therapy. Ann Intern Med 87:200, 1977.

100. Stenpel DA, Miller JJ. Lymphopenia and hepatic toxicity with ibuprofen. J Pediatr 90:657, 1977.

101. Whittaker SJ, Amar JN, Wanless IR, et al. Sulindac hepatotoxicity. Gut 23:875, 1982.

102. Taggert M McA, Alderdice JM. Fatal cholestatic hepatitis in elderly patients taking benoxaprofen. Br Med J 284:1372, 1982.

103. Utili R, Boitnott JK, Zimmerman HJ. Dantrolene-associated hepatic injury. Gastroenterology 72:610, 1977.

104. Wilkinson SP, Portmann B, Williams R. Hepatitis from dantrolene sodium. Gut 20:33, 1979.

105. Arnold TH, Epps JM, Cook HR, et al. Dantrolene sodium. Urinary metabolites and hepatotoxicity. Res Commun Chem Pathol Pharmacol 39:381, 1983.

106. Powers BJ, Cattau EL, Zimmerman HJ. Chlorzoxazone hepatotoxic reactions. Arch Intern Med 146:1183, 1986.

107. Cooperman L-H, Wollman H, Marsh ML. Anesthesia and the liver. Surg Clin North Am 57:421, 1977.

108. Ngai SH. Effect of anesthetics on various organs. N Engl J Med 302:564, 1980.

109. Schaffner F. Hepatotoxicity of halothane. In: Ingelfinger FJ, ed. Controversy in Internal Medicine. Vol 2. Philadelphia, WB Saunders 1974:565.

110. Simpson BR, Strunin L, Walton B. Evidence for halothane hepatotoxicity is equivocal. In: Ingelfinger FJ, ed. Controversy in Internal Medicine. Vol 2. Philadelphia, WB Saunders 1974:580.

111. Carney FMT, Van Dyke RA. Halothane hepatitis: a critical review. Anesth Analg (Cleve.) 51:135, 1972.

112. Conn HO. Halothane-associated hepatitis. A disease of medical progress. Israel J Med Sci 10:404, 1974.

113. Moult PJA, Sherlock S. Halothane-related hepatitis. A clinical study of twenty-six cases. Q J Med 44:99, 1975.

114. Bottiger LE, Dalen E, Hallen B. Halothane-induced liver damage: an analysis of the material reported to the Swedish Adverse Drug Reaction Committee, 1966–1973. Acta Anesthesiol Scand 20:40, 1976.

115. Sherlock S. Halothane hepatitis. Lancet 2:364, 1978.

116. Pohl LR, Gillette JR. A perspective on halothane-induced hepatotoxicity. Anesth Analg 61:809, 1982.

117. Neuberger J, Williams R. Halothane anesthesia and liver damage. Br Med J 289:1136, 1984.

118. Halothane-associated liver damage (editorial). Lancet 1:1251, 1986.

119. Lindenbaum J, Leifer E. Hepatic necrosis associated with halothane anesthesia. N Engl J Med 268:525, 1963.

120. Mushin WW, Rosen M, Bowen DJ, et al. Halothane and liver dysfunction: a retrospective study. Br Med J 2:229, 1964.

121. Slater EM, Gibson JM, Dykes MHM, et al. Postoperative hepatic necrosis. Its incidence and diagnostic value in association with the administration of halothane. N Engl J Med 270:983, 1964.

122. Davidson CS, Babior B, Popper H. Concerning hepatotoxicity of halothane. N Engl J Med 275:1497, 1966.

123. Klatskin G, Kimberg DV. Recurrent hepatitis attributable to halothane sensitization in an anesthetist. N Engl J Med 280:515, 1969.

124. Paronetto F, Popper H. Lymphocyte stimulation induced by halothane in patients with hepatitis following exposure to halothane. N Engl J Med 283:277, 1970.

125. Williams BD, White N, Amlot PL, et al. Circulating immune complexes after repeated halothane anesthesia. Br Med J 2:159, 1977.

126. Price CD, Gibbs AR, Williams WJ. Halothane macrophage migration inhibition factor test in halothane-associated hepatitis. J Clin Pathol 30:312, 1977.

127. Vergani D, Tsantoulas D, Eddleston ALWF, et al. Sensitization of halothane-altered liver components in severe hepatic necrosis after halothane anesthesia. Lancet 2:801, 1978.

128. Satoh H, Fukuda Y, Anderson DK, et al. Immunological studies on the mechanism of halothane-induced hepatotoxicity: immunohistochemical evidence of trifluoroacetylated hepatocytes. J Pharmacol Exp Ther 233:857, 1985.

129. Neuberger J, Kenna JG. Halothane hepatitis: a model of immune mediated drug hepatotoxicity. Clin Sci 72:263, 1987.

130. Vergani D, Mieli-Vergani G, Alberti A, et al. Antibodies to the surface of halothane-altered rabbit hepatocytes in patients with severe halothane-associated hepatitis. N Engl J Med 303:66, 1980.

131. Dienstag JL. Halothane hepatitis. Allergy or idiosyncrasy. N Engl J Med 303:102, 1980.

132. Smith CI, Cooksley WGE, Powell LW. Cell-mediated immunity to liver antigen in toxic liver injury. I. Occurrence and specificity. II. Role in pathogenesis of liver damage. Clin Exp Immunol 39:607, 618, 1980.

133. Ross WT, Cardell RR, Jr. Effects of halothane on the ultrastructure of rat liver cells. Am J Anat 135:5, 1972.

134. Biebuyck JF, Lund P, Krebs HA. The effects of halothane on glycolysis and biosynthetic processes of the isolated perfused rat liver. Biochem J 128:711, 1972.

135. Biebuyck JF, Lund P, Krebs HA. The protective effect of oleate on metabolic changes produced by halothane in rat liver. Biochem J 128:721, 1972.

136. Berman MC, Ivanetich KM, Kench JE. The effects of halothane in hepatic microsomal electron transfer. Biochem J 148:179, 1975.

137. Mapes JP. Inhibition of lipogenesis by halothane in isolated rat liver cells. Biochem J 162:47, 1977.

138. Salhab AS, Nook NG, Dujovne CA. Hepatocyte responses to volatile anesthetics: changes in surface scanning and enzyme leakage. Anesth Analg (Cleve.) 57:605, 1978.

139. Aune H, Bessesen A, Olsen H, et al. Acute effects of halothane and enflurane on drug metabolism and protein synthesis in isolated rat hepatocytes. Acta Pharmacol Toxicol 53:363, 1983.

140. Rehder K, Forbes J, Alters H, et al. Halothane biotransformation in man: a quantitative study. Anesthesiology 28:711, 1967.

141. Brown B, Sipes IG. Biotransformation and hepatotoxicity of halothane. Biochem Pharmacol 26:2091, 1977.

142. Sindelar WF, Trulka TS, Gibbs PS. Evidence for acute cellular changes in human hepatocytes during anesthesia with halogenated agents. Surgery 92:520, 1982.

143. Sipes IG, Brown BR. An animal model of hepatotoxicity associated with halothane anesthesia. Anesthesiology 45:622, 1976.

144. Van Dyke RA, Gandolfi AJ. Anaerobic release of fluoride from halothane. Relationship to the binding of halothane metabolites to hepatic cellular constituents. Drug Metab Disposit 4:40, 1976.

145. Widger LA, Gandolfi AJ, Van Dyke RA. Hypoxia and halothane metabolism in vivo: release of inorganic fluoride and halothane

metabolite binding to cellular constituents. Anesthesiology 44:197, 1976.

146. Nastainczyk W, Ullrich V. Effect of oxygen concentration on the reaction of halothane with cytochrome P450 in liver microsomes and isolated perfused rat liver. Biochem Pharmacol 27:387, 1978.

147. Cousins MJ, Sharp JH, Gourlay GK, et al. Hepatotoxicity and halothane metabolism in an animal model with application for human toxicity. Anesth Intens Care 7:9, 1979.

148. Cousins MJ. Halothane and the liver: "firm ground" at last. Anesth Intens Care 7:5, 1979.

149. Gorsky BH, Cascorbi HF. Halothane hepatotoxicity and fluoride production in mice and rats. Anesthesiology 50:123, 1979.

150. McLain GE, Sipes IG, Brown BR. An animal model of halothane hepatotoxicity. Roles of enzyme induction and hypoxia. Anesthesiology 51:321, 1979.

151. Ross WT Jr, Daggy BP, Cardell RR Jr. Hepatic necrosis caused by halothane and hypoxia in phenobarbital-treated rats. Anesthesiology 51:327, 1979.

152. Lunam CA, Cousins MJ, Hall P de la M. Guinea-pig model of halothane-associated hepatotoxicity in the absence of enzyme induction and hypoxia. J Pharmacol Exp Ther 232:802, 1985.

153. Cohen EN, Trudell JR, Edmunds HN, et al. Urinary metabolites of halothane in man. Anesthesiology 43:392, 1975.

154. Plummer JL, Beckwith ALJ, Bastin FN, et al. Free radical formation in vivo and hepatotoxicity due to anesthesia with halothane. Anesthesiology 57:160, 1982.

155. De Groot H, Noll T. Halothane hepatotoxicity: relation between metabolic activation, hypoxia, covalent binding, lipid peroxidation and liver cell damage. Hepatology 3:601, 1983.

156. Lind RC, Gandolfe AJ, Sipes IG, et al. Oxygen concentrations required for reductive defluorination of halothane by rat hepatic microsomes. Anesth Analg 65:835, 1986.

157. Gourlay GK, Adams JF, Cousins MJ, et al. Genetic differences in reductive metabolism and hepatotoxicity of halothane in three rat strains. Anesthesiology 55:96, 1981.

158. Farrell G, Prendergast D, Murray M. Halothane hepatitis. Detection of a constitutional susceptibility factor. N Engl J Med 313:1310, 1985.

159. Benjamin SB, Goodman ZD, Ishak KG, et al. The morphologic spectrum of halothane-induced hepatic injury: analysis of 77 cases. Hepatology 5:1163, 1985.

160. Inman WHW, Mushin WW. Jaundice after repeated exposure to halothane: a further analysis of reports to the Committee on Safety of Medicines. Br Med J 2:1455, 1978.

161. Wright R, Eade OE, Chrisholm M, et al. Controlled prospective study of the effect of halothane on liver function of multiple exposures to halothane. Lancet 1:817, 1975.

162. Trowell J, Peto R, Smith AC. Controlled trial of repeated halothane anesthetics in patients with carcinoma of the uterine cervix treated with radium. Lancet 1:821, 1975.

163. Thomas FB. Chronic aggressive hepatitis induced by halothane. Ann Intern Med 81:487, 1974.

164. Miller DJ, Dwyer J, Klatskin G. Halothane hepatitis: benign resolution of a severe lesion. Ann Intern Med 89:212, 1978.

165. Varma RR, Whitesell RC, Iskandaremi MM. Halothane hepatitis without halothane, role of inapparent circuit contamination and its prevention. Hepatology 5:1159, 1985.

166. Joshi PH, Conn HO. The syndrome of methoxyflurane-associated hepatitis. Ann Intern Med 80:395, 1974.

167. Kline MM. Enflurane-associated hepatitis. Gastroenterology 79:126, 1980.

168. Lewis JH, Zimmerman HJ, Ishak KG, et al. Enflurane hepatotoxicity. A clinicopathologic study of 24 cases. Ann Intern Med 98:984, 1983.

169. White LB, DeTarnowsky GO, Mir JA, et al. Hepatotoxicity following enflurane anesthesia. Dig Dis Sci 26:466, 1981.

170. Eger EI, Smuckler EA, Ferrell LD, et al. Is enflurane hepatotoxic? Anesth Analg 65:21, 1986.

171. Seino H, Dohi S, Aiyoshi Y, et al. Postoperative hepatic dysfunction after halothane or enflurane anesthesia in patients with hyperthyroidism. Anesthesiology 64:123, 1986.

172. Ivanetich KM, Manca V, Harrison GG, et al. Enflurane and methoxyflurane: their interaction with hepatic microsomal stearate desaturase. Biochem Pharmacol 29:27, 1980.

173. Spencer JD, Raasch FO, Trefny FA. Halothane abuse in hospital personnel. JAMA 235:1034, 1976.

174. Min K-W, Cain GD, Sabel JS, et al. Methoxyflurane hepatitis. South Med J 70:1363, 1977.

175. Kaplan HG, Bakken J, Quadracci L, et al. Hepatitis caused by halothane sniffing. Ann Intern Med 90:797, 1979.

176. Isoflurane (editorial). Lancet 2:537, 1985.

177. Buch-Andreasen J, Lyngbye J, Trolle E. Abnormalities in liver function tests during long-term diphenylhydantoin therapy in epileptic outpatients. Acta Med Scand 194:261, 1973.

178. Pamperl H, Gradner W, Fridrich L, et al. Influence of long-term anticonvulsant treatment on liver ultrastructure in man. Liver 4:294, 1984.

179. Jezequel AM, Librari ML, Mosca P, et al. Changes induced in human liver by long-term anticonvulsant therapy. Liver 4:307, 1984.

180. Lee TJ, Carney CN, Lapis JL, et al. Diphenylhydantoin-induced hepatic necrosis. Gastroenterology 70:422, 1976.

181. Campbell CB, McGuffie C, Weedon AP, et al. Cholestatic liver disease associated with diphenylhydantoin therapy. Possible pathogenic importance of altered bile salt metabolism. Am J Dig Dis 22:255, 1977.

182. Brown M, Schubert T. Phenytoin hypersensitivity hepatitis and mononucleosis syndrome. J Clin Gastroenterol 8:469, 1986.

183. Powers NG, Carson SH. Idiosyncratic reactions to phenytoin. Clin Pediatr 26:120, 1987.

184. Cook IF, Shilkin KB, Reed WD. Phenytoin-induced granulomatous hepatitis. Aust NZ J Med 11:539, 1981.

185. Sherertz EF, Jegasdthy BV, Lazarus GS. Phenytoin hypersensitivity reaction presenting with toxic epidermal necrolysis and severe hepatitis. J Am Acad Derm 12:178, 1985.

186. Saltzstein SL, Ackerman LV. Lymphadenopathy induced by anticonvulsant drugs and mimicking clinically and pathologically malignant lymphomas. Cancer 12:164, 1959.

187. Kahn HD, Faquet GB, Agee JF, et al. Drug-induced liver injury. In vitro demonstration of hypersensitivity to both phenytoin and phenobarbital. Arch Int Med 144:1677, 1984.

188. Chaiken BH, Goldberg BI, Segal JP. Dilantin sensitivity. Report of a case of hepatitis with jaundice, pyrexia and exfoliative dermatitis. N Engl J Med 242:897, 1950.

189. Siegal S, Berkowitz J. Diphenylhydantoin hypersensitivity with infectious mononucleosis-like syndrome and jaundice. J Allerg 32:447, 1961.

190. Harinasuta U, Zimmerman HJ. Diphenylhydantoin sodium hepatitis. JAMA 203:1015, 1968.

191. Dhar GD, Pierach CA, Ahamed PN, et al. Diphenylhydantoin-induced hepatic necrosis. Postgrad Med 56:128, 1974.

192. Taylor JW, Stein MN, Murphy MJ, et al. Cholestatic liver dysfunction after long-term phenytoin therapy. Arch Neurol 41:500, 1984.

193. Chung T, Glazko AJ. Diphenylhydantoin biotransformation. In: Woodbury DM, Penry JK, Schmidt RP, eds. Antiepileptic Drugs. New York, Raven Press, 1972:149.

194. Browne TR. Valproic acid. N Engl J Med 302:661, 1980.

195. Coulter DL, Wu H, Allen RJ. Valproic acid therapy in childhood epilepsy. JAMA 244:785, 1980.

196. Suchy FJ, Balistreri WF, Buchino JJ, et al. Acute hepatic failure associated with the use of sodium valproate. N Engl J Med 300:962, 1979.

197. Gerber N, Dickinson RG, Harland, et al. Reye-like syndrome associated with valproic acid therapy. J Pediatr 95:142, 1979.

198. Ware S, Millward-Sadler GH. Acute liver disease associated with sodium valproate. Lancet 2:1110, 1980.

199. Sodium valproate and the liver (editorial). Lancet 2:1119, 1980.

200. Zimmerman HJ, Ishak KG. Valproate-induced hepatic injury: analyses of 23 fatal cases. Hepatology 2:291, 1982.

201. Powell-Jackson PR, Tredger JM, Williams R. Hepatotoxicity to sodium valproate: a review. Gut 25:673, 1984.

202. Itoh S, Yamada Y, Matsuo S, et al. Sodium valproate-induced liver injury. Am J Gastroenterol 77:875, 1982.

203. Turnbull DM, Bone AJ, Bartlett K, et al. The effects of valproate on intermediary metabolism in isolated rat hepatocytes and intact rats. Biochem Pharmacol 32:1887, 1983.

204. Coude FX, Grimber G, Pelet A, et al. Action of the antiepileptic drug, valproic acid, on fatty acid oxidation in isolated rat hepatocytes. Biochem Biophys Res Commun 115:730, 1983.

205. Kesterson JW, Grunneman GR, Machinist JM. The hepatotoxicity of valproic acid and its metabolites in rats. I. Toxicologic, biochemical and histopathologic studies. Hepatology 4:1143, 1984.

206. Grunneman G, Wang S-I, Kesterson JW, et al. The hepatotoxicity of valproic acid and its metabolites in rats. II. Intermediary and valproic acid metabolism. Hepatology 4:1153, 1984.

207. Turnbull OM, Dick DJ, Wilson L, et al. Valproate causes metabolic disturbances in normal man. J Neurol Neurosurg Psychiatr 49:405, 1986.

208. Hjelm M, Oberholzer V, Seakins J, et al. Valproate-induced inhibition of urea synthesis and hyperammonemia in healthy subjects. Lancet 2:859, 1986.

209. Mortensen PB, Gregersen N, Kolvraa S, et al. The occurrence of C6-C10-dicarboxylic acids in urine from patients and rats. Biochem Med 24:153, 1980.

210. Van den Branden C, Roels F. Peroxisomal β-oxidation and sodium valproate. Biochem Pharmacol 34:2147, 1985.

211. Qureshi IA, Letarte J, Tuchweber B, et al. Hepatotoxicity of sodium valproate in ornithine transcarbamylase-deficient mice. Toxicol Lett 25:297, 1985.

212. Acheampong A, Abbott FS. Synthesis and stereochemical determination of diunsaturated valproic acid analogs including its major diunsaturated metabolite. J Lip Res 26:1002, 1985.
213. Lewis JH, Zimmerman HJ, Garrett CT, et al. Valproate-induced hepatic steatogenesis in rats. Hepatology 2:870, 1982.
214. Brown NA, Farmer PB, Coakley M. Valproic acid teratogenicity: demonstration that the biochemical mechanism differs from that of valproate hepatotoxicity. Biochem Soc Trans 13:73, 1985.
215. Watkins JB, Klaassen CD. Choleretic effect of valproic acid in the rat. Hepatology 1:341, 1981.
216. Dickinson RG, Kluck RM, Hooper WD, et al. Rearrangement of valproate glucuronide in a patient with drug-associated hepatotoxicity and renal dysfunction. Epilepsia 26:589, 1985.
217. Ramsay RE. Safe readministration of valproate after an episode of hepatotoxicity. Ann Neurol 13:688, 1983.
218. Levy M, Goodman MW, Van Dyne BJ, et al. Granulomatous hepatitis secondary to carbamazepine. Ann Intern Med 95:64, 1981.
219. Mitchell MC, Boitnott JK, Arrequi A, et al. Granulomatous hepatitis associated with carbamazepine therapy. Am J Med 71:733, 1981.
220. Hopen G, Nesthus I, Laerum OD. Fatal carbamazepine-associated hepatitis. Acta Med Scand 210:333, 1981.
221. Soffer EE, Taylor RJ, Bertram PD, et al. Carbamazepine-induced liver injury. South Med J 76:681, 1983.
222. Ponte CD. Carbamazepine-induced thrombocytopenia, rash, and hepatic dysfunction. Drug Intell Clin Pharm 17:642, 1983.
223. Williams SJ, Ruppin DC, Grierson JM, et al. Carbamazepine hepatitis: the clinicopathological spectrum. J Gastroenterol Hepatol 1:159, 1986.
224. Laiwah AACY, Rapeport WG, Thompson GG, et al. Carbamazepine-induced non-hereditary acute porphyria. Lancet 1:790, 1983.
225. Wright JM, Stokes EF, Sweeney VP. Isoniazid-induced carbamazepine toxicity and vice versa. N Engl J Med 307:1325, 1982.
226. Zimmerman HJ. In: Hepatotoxicity. New York, Appleton-Century-Crofts 1978:468.
227. Dismukes WE. Oxacillin-induced hepatic dysfunction. JAMA 226:861, 1973.
228. Olans RN, Weiner LB. Reversible oxacillin hepatotoxicity. J Pediatr 89:835, 1976.
229. Bruckstein AH, Attia AA. Oxacillin hepatitis. Two patients with liver biopsy, and review of the literature. Am J Med 64:519, 1978.
230. Onorato IM, Axelrod JL. Hepatitis from intravenous high-dose oxacillin therapy. Findings in an adult population. Ann Intern Med 89:497, 1978.
231. Pollock AA, Berger SA, Simberkoff MS, et al. Hepatitis associated with high-dose oxacillin therapy. Arch Intern Med 138:915, 1978.
232. Olans RN. Antibiotic therapy for staphylococcal infections. Arch Intern Med 139:376, 1979.
233. Taylor C, Corrigan K, Steen S, et al. Oxacillin and hepatitis. Ann Intern Med 90:857, 1979.
234. Wilson FM, Belamaric J, Lauter CB, et al. Anicteric carbenicillin hepatitis. Eight episodes in four patients. JAMA 232:818, 1975.
235. Enat R, Pollack S, Ben-Arieh Y, et al. Cholestatic jaundice caused by cloxacillin: macrophage inhibition factor test in preventing rechallenge with hepatotoxic drugs. Br Med J 2:982, 1980.
236. Lobatto S, Dijkmans BAC, Maltie H, et al. Flucloxacillin-associated liver damage. Neth J Med 25:47, 1982.
237. Lunzer MR, Huang SN, Ward KM, et al. Jaundice due to erythromycin estolate. Gastroenterology 68:1284, 1975.
238. Zafrani ES, Ishak KG, Rudzki C. Cholestatic and hepatocellular injury associated with erythomycin esters. Report of nine cases. Am J Dig Dis 24:385, 1979.
239. Pessayre D, Larrey D, Funck-Brentano C, et al. Drug interactions and hepatitis produced by some macrolide antibiotics. J Antimicrob Chemother 16, suppl. A:181, 1985.
240. Viteri AL, Greene JF Jr, Dyck WP. Erythromycin ethylsuccinate-induced cholestasis. Gastroenterology 76:1007, 1979.
241. Diehl AM, Latham P, Boitnott JK, et al. Cholestatic hepatitis from erythromycin ethylsuccinate. Am J Med 76:931, 1984.
242. Ginsburg CM, and The Multicenter Pneumonia Study Group. A prospective study on the incidence of liver function abnormalities in children receiving erythromycin estolate, erythromycin ethylsuccinate or penicillin V for treatment of pneumonia. Pediatr Infect Dis 5:151, 1986.
243. Gaeta GB, Utili R, Adinolfi LE, et al. Characterization of the effects of erythromycin estolate and erythromycin base on the excretory function of the isolated rat liver. Toxicol Appl Pharmacol 80:185, 1985.
244. Sorenson EMB, Acosta D. Erythromycin estolate-induced toxicity in cultured rat hepatocytes. Toxicol Lett 27:73, 1985.
245. Richelmi P, Baldi C, Munzo L, et al. Erythromycin estolate impairs the mitochondrial and microsomal calcium homeostasis: correlation with hepatotoxicity. Arch Toxicol (suppl) 7:298, 1984.
246. Dujovne CA. Hepatotoxic and cellular uptake interactions among surface active components of erythromycin preparations. Biochem Pharmacol 27:1925, 1978.
247. Keeffe E, Reis TC, Berland JE. Hepatotoxicity to both erythromycin estolate and erythromycin ethylsuccinate. Dig Dis Sci 27:701, 1982.
248. Swayne LC, Kolc J. Erythromycin hepatotoxicity. A rare cause of a false-positive technetium-^{99}m DISIDA study. Clin Nucl Med 11:10, 1986.
249. Shultz JC, Adamson JS Jr, Workman WW, et al. Fetal liver disease after intravenous administration of tetracycline in high dosage. N Engl J Med 269:999, 1963.
250. Peters RL, Edmondson HA, Mikkelsen WP, et al. Tetracycline-induced fatty liver in nonpregnant patients. A report of six cases. Am J Surg 113:622, 1967.
251. Combes B, Whalley PJ, Adams RH. Tetracycline and the liver. In: Popper H, Schaffner F, eds. Progress in Liver Diseases, Volume 4. New York, Grune and Stratton 1972:589.
252. Burette A, Finet C, Prigogine T, et al. Acute hepatic injury associated with minocycline. Arch Intern Med 144:1491, 1984.
253. Breen KJ, Schenker S, Heimberg M. Fatty liver induced by tetracycline in the rat. Dose-response relationships and the effect of sex. Gastroenterology 69:714, 1975.
254. Jacobs E, Paulet P, Rahier J. Hypersensitivity reaction to sulfasalazine—another case. Gastroenterology 75:1193, 1975.
255. Callen JP, Soderstrom RM. Granulomatous hepatitis associated with salicylazosulfapyridine therapy. South Med J 71:1159, 1978.
256. Chester AC, Diamond LH, Schreiner GE. Hypersensitivity to salicylazosulfapyridine. Renal and hepatic toxic reactions. Arch Intern Med 138:1138, 1978.
257. Mihas AA, Goldenberg DJ, Slaughter RL. Sulfasalazine toxic reactions. Hepatitis, fever and skin rash with hypocomplementemia and immune complexes. JAMA 239:2590, 1978.
258. Sotolongo RP, Neefe LI, Rudzki C, et al. Hypersensitivity reaction to sulfasalazine with severe hepatotoxicity. Gastroenterology 75:95, 1978.
259. Gulley RM, Mirza A, Kelly CE. Hepatotoxicity of salicylazo-sulfapyridine. Am J Gastroenterol 72:561, 1979.
260. Namias A, Bhalotra R, Donowitz M. Reversible sulfasalazine-induced granulomatous hepatitis. J Clin Gastroenterol 3:193, 1981.
261. Lennard TWJ, Farndon JR. Sulphasalazine hepatotoxicity after 15 years' successful treatment for ulcerative colitis. Br Med J 287:96, 1983.
262. Fich A, Schwartz J, Braverman D, et al. Sulfasalazine hepatotoxicity. Am J Gastroenterol 79:401, 1984.
263. Ribe D, Benkov KJ, Thung S, et al. Fatal massive hepatic necrosis: a probable hypersensitivity reaction to sulfasalazine. Am J Gastroenterol 81:205, 1986.
264. Stevenson DK, Christie DL, Haas JE. Hepatic injury in a child caused by trimethoprin-sulfamethoxazole. Pediatrics 61:864, 1978.
265. Steinbrecher UP, Mishkin S. Sulfamethoxazole-induced hepatic injury. Dig Dis Sci 26:756, 1981.
266. Theis PW, Dull WL. Trimethoprim-sulfamethoxazole–induced cholestatic hepatitis. Inadvertent rechallenge. Arch Int Med 144:1691, 1984.
267. Johnson DA, Cattau EL Jr, Kuritsky JN, et al. Liver involvement in the sulfone syndrome. Arch Intern Med 146:875, 1986.
268. Ivarson I, Lundlin P. Multiple attacks of jaundice associated with repeated sulfonamide treatment. Acta Med Scand 206:219, 1979.
269. Tönder M, Nordöy A, Elgio G. Sulfonamide-induced chronic liver disease. Scand J Gastroenterol 9:93, 1974.
270. Hatoff DE, Cohen M, Schweigert BF, et al. Nitrofurantoin: another cause of drug-induced chronic active hepatitis? Am J Med 67:117, 1979.
271. Sharp JR, Ishak KG, Zimmerman HJ. Chronic active hepatitis and severe hepatic necrosis associated with nitrofurantoin. Ann Intern Med 92:14, 1980.
272. Black M, Rabin L, Schatz N. Nitrofurantoin-induced chronic hepatitis. Ann Intern Med 92:62, 1980.
273. Tolman KG. Nitrofurantoin and chronic active hepatitis. Ann Intern Med 92:119, 1980.
274. Sippel PJ, Agger WA. Nitrofurantoin-induced granulomatous hepatitis. Urology 18:177, 1981.
275. Denk H, Bernklau G, Kregler R. Effect of griseofulvin treatment and neoplastic transformation on transglutaminase activity in mouse liver. Liver 4:208, 1984.
276. Chiprut RO, Viteri A, Jamroz C, et al. Intrahepatic cholestasis after griseofulvin administration. Gastroenterology 70:1141, 1976.
277. Miller MA. Reversible hepatotoxicity related to amphotericin B. Can Med Assoc J 131:1245, 1984.
278. Lewis JH, Zimmerman HJ, Benson GD, et al. Hepatic injury associated with ketoconazole therapy. Analysis of 33 cases. Gastroenterology 86:503, 1984.

279. Rollman O, Loof L. Hepatic toxicity of ketoconazole. Br J Derm 108:376, 1983.

280. Brown MW, Maldonado AL, Meredith CG, et al. Effect of ketoconazole on hepatic oxidative drug metabolism. Clin Pharm Ther 37:290, 1985.

281. Boughton K. Ketoconazole and hepatic reactions. S Afr Med J 63:955, 1983.

282. Descotes J, Andre P, Tedne R, et al. Miconazole influence on both cellular immune response and hepatic drug metabolism in mice. J Immunopharmacol 7:171, 1985.

283. Lazar HP, Murphy RL, Phair VP. Fansidar and hepatic granulomas. Ann Intern Med 102:722, 1985.

284. Selby CD, Ladusans E, Smith PG. Fatal multisystemic toxicity associated with prophylaxis with pyramethine and sulfadoxine (Fansidar). Br Med J 290:113, 1985.

285. Larrey D, Castot A, Pessayre D, et al. Amodiaquine-induced hepatitis. A report of seven cases. Ann Intern Med 104:801, 1986.

286. Neftel KA, Woodtly W, Schmid M, et al. Amodiaquine induced agranulocytosis and liver damage. Br Med J 292:721, 1986.

287. Cohen C. Liver pathology in hycanthone hepatitis. Gastroenterology 75:103, 1978.

288. Bailey WC, Weill H, DeRouen TA, et al. The effect of isoniazid on transaminase levels. Ann Intern Med 81:200, 1974.

289. Mitchell JR, Long MW, Thorgeirsson UP, et al. Acetylation rates and monthly liver function tests during one year of isoniazid preventive therapy. Chest 68:181, 1975.

290. Beaudry PH, Brickman HF, Wise MB, et al. Liver enzyme disturbances during isoniazid chemoprophylaxis in children. Am Rev Resp Dis 110:581, 1974.

291. Litt IF, Cohen MI, McNamara H. Isoniazid hepatitis in adolescents. J Pediatr 89:133, 1976.

292. Tuberculosis Advisory Committee. Isoniazid-associated hepatitis: summary of the report of the tuberculosis advisory committee and special consultants to the Director, Center for Disease Control. Morbidity and Mortality 23:97, 1974.

293. Mitchell JR, Thorgeirsson UP, Black M, et al. Increased incidence of isoniazid hepatitis in rapid acetylators: possible relation to hydrazine metabolites. Clin Pharmacol Ther 18:70, 1975.

294. Black M, Mitchell JR, Zimmerman HJ, et al. Isoniazid-associated hepatitis in 114 patients. Gastroenterology 69:289, 1975.

295. Mitchell JR, Zimmerman HJ, Ishak KG, et al. Isoniazid liver injury: clinical spectrum, pathology and probable pathogenesis. Ann Intern Med 84:181, 1976.

296. Kopanoff DE, Snider DE Jr, Caras GJ. Isoniazid-related hepatitis. A U.S. Public Health Service Cooperative Surveillance Study. Am Rev Res Dis 117:991, 1978.

297. Comstock GW. New data on preventive treatment with isoniazid. Ann Intern Med 98:663, 1983.

298. Rapp RS, Campbell RW, Howell JC, et al. Isoniazid hepatotoxicity in children. Am Rev Res Dis 118:794, 1978.

299. Stein MT, Liang D. Clinical hepatotoxicity of isoniazid in children. Pediatrics 64:499, 1979.

300. Grönhagen-Riska C, Hellstrom PE, Froseth B. Predisposing factors in hepatitis induced by isoniazid-rifampin treatment of tuberculosis. Am Rev Res Dis 118:461, 1978.

301. Ellard GA, Mitchison DA, Girling DJ, et al. The hepatotoxicity of isoniazid among rapid and slow acetylators of the drug. Am Rev Resp Dis 118:628, 1978.

302. Gurumurthy P, Krishnamurthy MS, Nazareth O, et al. Lack of relationship between hepatic toxicity and acetylator phenotype in three thousand South Indian patients during treatment with isoniazid for tuberculosis. Am Rev Resp Dis 129:58, 1984.

303. Dickinson DS, Bailey WC, Hirschowitz BI, et al. Risk factors for isoniazid (INH)-induced liver dysfunction. J Clin Gastroenterol 3:271, 1981.

304. Maddrey WC, Boitnott JK. Isoniazid hepatitis. Ann Intern Med 79:1, 1973.

305. Israel HL. Isoniazid-associated hepatitis. Reconsideration of the indications for the administration of isoniazid. Gastroenterology 69:539, 1975.

306. Riska N. Hepatitis cases in isoniazid-treated groups and in a control group. Bull Int Union Against Tuberculosis 51:203, 1976.

307. Zimmerman HJ. In: Hepatotoxicity. New York, Appleton-Century-Crofts 1978:485.

308. Spitz RD, Keren DF, Boitnott JK, et al. Bridging hepatic necrosis. Etiology and prognosis. Dig Dis 23:1076, 1978.

309. Maddrey WC, Boitnott JK. Drug-induced chronic liver disease. Gastroenterology 72:1348, 1977.

310. Byrd RB, Horn BR, Griggs GA, et al. Isoniazid chemoprophylaxis. Association with detection and incidence of liver toxicity. JAMA 137:1130, 1977.

311. Comstock GW, Edwards PQ. The competing risks of tuberculosis and hepatitis for adult tuberculin reactors. Am Rev Res Dis 111:573, 1975.

312. Glassroth J, Robins AG, Snider DE Jr. Tuberculosis in the 1980's. N Engl J Med 302:1441, 1980.

313. Nelson SD, Mitchell JR, Timbrell JA, et al. Isoniazid and iproniazid: activation of metabolites to toxic intermediates in man and rat. Science 193:901, 1976.

314. Woodward KN, Timbrell JA. Acetylhydrazine hepatotoxicity: the role of covalent binding. Toxicology 30:65, 1984.

315. Timbrell TA, Wright JM, Baillie TA. Monoacetylhydrazine as a metabolite of isoniazid in man. Clin Pharmacol Ther 22:602, 1977.

316. Lauterburg BH, Smith CV, Todd EL, et al. Pharmacokinetics of the toxic hydrazine metabolites formed from isoniazid in humans. J Pharmacol Exp Ther 235:566, 1985.

317. Timbrell JA. Studies on the role of acetylhydrazine in isoniazid hepatotoxicity. Arch Toxicol Suppl 2:1, 1979.

318. Scales MD, Timbrell JA. Studies on hydrazine hepatotoxicity. 1. Pathological findings. J Toxicol Environ Health 10:941, 1982.

319. Ragupati Sarma G, Immanuel C, Kailasam S, et al. Rifampicin-induced release of hydrazine from isoniazid. A possible cause of hepatitis during treatment of tuberculosis with regimens containing isoniazid and rifampicin. Am Rev Resp Dis 133:1072, 1986.

320. Capelle P, Dhumeaux D, Mora M, et al. Effect of rifampicin on liver function in man. Gut 13:366, 1972.

321. Kenwright S, Levi AJ. Sites of competition in the selective hepatic uptake of rifamycin-SV, flavaspidic acid, bilirubin and bromosulphthalein. Gut 15:220, 1974.

322. Galeazzi R, Lorenzini I, Orlandi F. Rifampicin-induced elevation of serum bile acids in man. Dig Dis Sci 25:108, 1980.

323. Pessayre D, Mazel P. Induction and inhibition of hepatic drug metabolizing enzymes by rifampin. Biochem Pharmacol 25:943, 1976.

324. Pessayre V, Bentata M, Degott C, et al. Isoniazid-rifampin fulminant hepatitis. Gastroenterology 72:284, 1977.

325. Scheuer PJ, Summerfield JA, Lal S, et al. Rifampicin hepatitis. Clinical and histological study. Lancet 1:422, 1974.

326. Parthasarathy R, Ragupati Sarma G, Janardhanam B, et al. Hepatic toxicity in South Indian patients during treatment of tuberculosis with short-course regimens containing isoniazid, rifampicin and pyrazinamide. Tubercle 67:99, 1986.

327. O'Brien RJ, Long MW, Cross FS, et al. Hepatotoxicity from isoniazid and rifampicin among children treated for tuberculosis. Pediatrics 72:491, 1983.

328. Cartel JL, Naudillon Y, Artus JC, et al. Hepatotoxicity of the daily combination of 5 mg/kg prothionamide plus 10 mg/kg rifampin. Int J Lepr Mycobact Dis 53:15, 1985.

329. Menard DB, Gisselbrecht C, Marty M, et al. Antineoplastic agents and the liver. Gastroenterology 78:142, 1980.

330. Perry MC. Hepatotoxicity of chemotherapeutic agents. Semin Oncol 9:65, 1982.

331. McDonald GB, Tirumali N. Intestinal and liver toxicity of antineoplastic drugs. West J Med 140:250, 1984.

332. Zimmerman HJ. Hepatotoxic effects of oncotherapeutic agents. In: Popper H, Schaffner F, eds. Progress in Liver Diseases, Vol 8. Grune & Stratton, Orlando, 1986:621.

333. Dahl MGC, Gregory MM, Scheuer PJ. Methotrexate hepatotoxicity in psoriasis. Comparison of different dose regimens. Br Med J 1:654, 1972.

334. Nyfors A, Poulsen H. Liver biopsies from psoriatics related to methotrexate therapy. Acta Pathol Microbiol Scand (A) 84:253, 1976.

335. Weinstein G, Roenigk H, Maibach H, et al. Psoriasis-liver-methotrexate interactions. Arch Dermatol 108:36, 1973.

336. Podurgiel BJ, McGill DB, Ludwig J, et al. Liver injury associated with methotrexate therapy for psoriasis. Mayo Clin Proc 48:787, 1973.

337. Zachariae H, Kragballe K, Sogaard H. Methotrexate induced liver cirrhosis. Br J Dermatol 102:407, 1980.

338. Roenigk HH, Auerbach R, Maibach HI, et al. Methotrexate guidelines—revised. J Am Acad Dermatol 6:145, 1982.

339. Van de Kerkhoff PC, Hoefnagels WH, van Haelst UJ, et al. Methotrexate maintenance therapy and liver damage in psoriasis. Clin Exp Dermatol 10:194, 1985.

340. Lanse SB, Arnold GL, Gowans JD, et al. Low incidence of hepatotoxicity associated with long-term, low-dose oral methotrexate in treatment of refractory psoriasis, psoriatic arthritis, and rheumatoid arthritis. An acceptable risk/benefit ratio. Dig Dis Sci 30:104, 1985.

341. Ruymann FB, Mosijczuk AD, Sayers RJ. Hepatoma in child with methotrexate-induced hepatic fibrosis. JAMA 238:2631, 1977.

342. McIntosh S, Davidson DL, O'Brien RT, et al. Methotrexate hepatotoxicity in children with leukemia. J Pediat 90:1019, 1977.

343. Jaffe N, Traggis D. Toxicity of high-dose methotrexate (NSC-740) and citrovorum factor (NSC-3590) in osteogenic sarcoma. Cancer Chemother Rep 6:31, 1975.

344. Nyfors A, Hopwood D. Liver ultrastructure in psoriatics related to methotrexate therapy. 1. A prospective study of findings in hepatocytes from 24 patients before and after methotrexate treatment. Acta Pathol Microbiol Scand (A) 85:787, 1977.

345. Horvath E, Saibil FG, Kovacs K, et al. Fine structural changes in the liver of methotrexate treated psoriatics. Digestion 17:488, 1978.

346. Hopwood D, Nyfors A. Liver ultrastructure in psoriatics related to methotrexate therapy. 2. Findings in bile ducts from 11 methotrexate treated psoriatics and 2 controls. Acta Pathol Microbiol Scand (A) 85:801, 1977.

347. Tuma DJ, Barak AJ, Sorrell MF. Interaction of methotrexate with lipotropic factors in rat liver. Biochem Pharmacol 24:1327, 1975.

348. Mistilis SP, Blackburn CRB. The treatment of active chronic hepatitis with 6-mercaptopurine and azathioprine. Austral Ann Med 16:305, 1967.

349. Czaja AJ, Ludwig J, Beggenstoss AH, et al. Corticosteroid-treated chronic active hepatitis in remission. N Engl J Med 304:5, 1981.

350. Read AE, Wiesner RH, LaBreque DR, et al. Hepatic veno-occlusive disease associated with renal transplantation and azathioprine therapy. Ann Intern Med 104:651, 1986.

351. Katzka DA, Saul SH, Jorkasky D, et al. Azathioprine and hepatic veno-occlusive disease in renal transplant patients. Gastroenterology 90:446, 1986.

352. Krivoy N, Raz R, Carter A, et al. Reversible hepatic veno-occlusive disease with 6-thioguanine. Ann Intern Med 96:788, 1982.

353. D'Cruz CA, Wimmer RS, Harcke HT, et al. Veno-occlusive disease of the liver in children following chemotherapy for acute myelocytic leukemia. Cancer 52:1803, 1983.

354. Doria MI, Shepard KV, Levin B, et al. Liver pathology following hepatic arterial infusion chemotherapy. Hepatic toxicity with FUDR. Cancer 58:855, 1986.

355. Shea WJ, Demas BE, Goldberg HI, et al. Sclerosing cholangitis associated with hepatic arterial FUDR chemotherapy. Am J Radiol 146:717, 1986.

356. Durden DL, Salazar AM, Distasio JA. Kinetic analysis of hepatotoxicity associated with antineoplastic asparigenases. Cancer Res 43:1602, 1983.

357. Aviles A, Herrera J, Ramos E, et al. Hepatic injury during doxorubicin therapy. Arch Pathol Lab Med 108:912, 1984.

358. Starzl TE, Weil R, Iwatsuki S, et al. The use of cyclosporin A and prednisone in cadaver kidney transplantation. Surg Gynecol Obstet 151:17, 1980.

359. Bacon AM, Rosenberg SA. Cyclophosphamide hepatotoxicity in a patient with systemic lupus erythematosus. Ann Intern Med 97:62, 1982.

360. Goldberg JW, Lidsky MD. Cyclophosphamide-associated hepatotoxicity. South Med J 78:222, 1985.

361. Feaux de La Croix W, Runne U, Hauk H, et al. Acute liver dystrophy with thrombosis of hepatic veins: a fatal complication of dacarbazine treatment. Cancer Treat Rep 67:779, 1983.

362. Tysell JE Jr, Knauer CM. Hepatitis induced by methyldopa. Report of a case and a review of the literature. Dig Dis 16:849, 1971.

363. Rehman OU, Keith TA, Gall EA. Methyldopa-induced submassive hepatic necrosis. JAMA 224:1390, 1973.

364. Goldstein GB, Lam KC, Mistilis SP. Drug-induced active chronic hepatitis. Dig Dis 18:177, 1973.

365. Toghill PJ, Smith PG, Benton P, et al. Methyldopa liver damage. Br Med J 3:545, 1974.

366. Schweitzer IL, Peters RL. Acute submassive necrosis due to methyldopa. A case demonstrating possible initiation of chronic liver disease. Gastroenterology 66:1203, 1974.

367. Maddrey WC, Boitnott JK. Severe hepatitis from methyldopa. Gastroenterology 68:351, 1975.

368. Rodman JS, Deutsch DJ, Gutman SI. Methyldopa hepatitis. A report of six cases and review of the literature. Am J Med 60:941, 1976.

369. Thomas E, Rosenthal WS, Zapiach L, et al. Spectrum of methyldopa liver injury. Am J Gastroenterol 68:125, 1977.

370. Sotaniemi EA, Hokkanen OT, Ahokas JJ, et al. Hepatic injury and drug metabolism in patients with alpha-methyldopa-induced liver damage. Eur J Clin Pharmacol 12:429, 1977.

371. Zimmerman HJ. In: Hepatotoxicity. New York, Appleton-Century-Crofts 1978:510.

372. Arranto AJ, Sotaniemi EA. Histologic follow-up of alpha-methyldopa-induced liver injury. Scand J Gastroenterol 16:865, 1981.

373. Delpre G, Grinblat J, Kadish J, et al. Immunological studies in a case of hepatitis following methyldopa administration. Am J Med Sci 277:207, 1977.

374. Kirtland HH III, Mohler DN, Horwitz DA. Methyldopa inhibition of suppressor-lymphocyte function. A proposed cause of autoimmune hemolytic anemia. N Engl J Med 302:825, 1980.

375. Dybing E, Nelson SB, Mitchell JR, et al. Oxidation of α-methyldopa and other catechols by cytochrome P-450–generated superoxide anion: possible mechanism of methyldopa hepatitis. Molec Pharmacol 12:911, 1976.

376. Dybing E, Nelson SD. Metabolic activation of methyldopa and other catechols. Arch Toxicol (suppl) 1:117, 1978.

377. Neuberger J, Kenna JG, Nouri-Aria K, et al. Antibody mediated hepatocyte injury in methyldopa induced hepatotoxocity. Gut 261:1233, 1985.

378. Jori GP, Peschle C. Hydralazine disease associated with transient granulomas in the liver. Gastroenterology 64:1163, 1973.

379. Forster HS. Hepatitis from hydralazine. N Engl J Med 302:1362, 1980.

380. Myers JL, Augur NA. Hydralazine-induced cholangitis. Gastroenterology 87:1185, 1984.

381. Rahmat J, Gelfand RL, Gelfand MC, et al. Captopril-associated cholestatic jaundice. Ann Intern Med 102:56, 1985.

382. Mitchell JR, Potter WZ, Hinson JA, et al. Hepatic necrosis caused by furosemide. Nature 251:508, 1974.

383. Mitchell JR, Nelson WL, Potter WZ, et al. Metabolic activation of furosemide to a chemically reactive, hepatotoxic metabolite. J Pharmacol Exp Ther 199:41, 1976.

384. Zimmerman HJ, Lewis JH, Ishak KG. Ticrynafen-associated hepatic injury: analysis of 340 cases. Hepatology 4:315, 1984.

385. Chapek T, Lehrer B, Geltner D, et al. Quinidine-induced granulomatous hepatitis. Ann Intern Med 81:774, 1974.

386. Koch MJ, Seeff LB, Crumley CE, et al. Quinidine hepatotoxicity. A report of a case and review of the literature. Gastroenterology 70:1136, 1976.

387. Knobler H, Levij IS, Gavish D, et al. Quinidine-induced hepatitis: a common and reversible hypersensitivity reaction. Arch Intern Med 146:526, 1986.

388. Harris L, McKenna WJ, Rowland E, et al. Side effects of long-term amiodarone therapy. Circulation 67:45, 1983.

389. McGovern B, Garan H, Kelley E, et al. Adverse reactions during treatment with amiodarone hydrochloride. Br Med J 287:175, 1983.

390. Poucell S, Ireton J, Valencia-Mayoral P, et al. Amiodarone-associated phospholipidosis and fibrosis of the liver. Gastroenterology 86:926, 1984.

391. Simon JB, Manley PN, Brien JF, et al. Amiodarone hepatotoxicity simulating alcoholic liver disease. N Engl J Med 311:167, 1984.

392. Rigas B, Rosenfeld LE, Barwick KW, et al. Amiodarone hepatotoxocity. A clinicopathologic study of five patients. Ann Intern Med 104:348, 1986.

393. Rinder HM, Love JC, Wexler R. Amiodarone hepatotoxicity. N Engl J Med 314:318, 1986.

394. Lullman H, Lullman-Rauch R, Wasserman O. Drug-induced phospholipidosis. Crit Rev Toxicol 4:185, 1975.

395. Goldman IS, Winkler ML, Raper SE, et al. Increased hepatic density and phospholipidosis due to amiodarone. Am J Radiol 144:541, 1985.

396. Herlong HF, Reid PR, Boitnott JK, et al. Aprinidine hepatitis. Ann Intern Med 89:359, 1978.

397. Larrey D, Pessayre D, Duhamel G, et al. Prolonged cholestasis after ajmaline-induced acute hepatitis. J Hepatol 2:81, 1986.

398. Rotrensch HH, Yust I, Siegman-Igra Y, et al. Granulomatous hepatitis: a hypersensitivity response to procainamide. Ann Intern Med 89:646, 1978.

399. McDonald GSA. Liver damage after perhexilene maleate. Lancet 1:1056, 1977.

400. Paliard P, Vitrey D, Fournier G, et al. Perhexilene maleate-induced hepatitis. Digestion 17:419, 1978.

401. Pessayre D, Bichara M, Feldmann G, et al. Perhexilene maleate-induced cirrhosis. Gastroenterology 76:170, 1979.

402. Lewis D, Wainwright HC, Kew MC, et al. Liver damage associated with perhexilene maleate. Gut 20:186, 1979.

403. Hoenig V, Werner F. Effect of perhexilene maleate on lipid metabolism in the rat. III. Liver gangliosides after administration of high doses of perhexilene maleate. Pharmacol Res Commun 12:29, 1980.

404. Snider GB, Gogate SA. Clinical observations following papaverine therapy. Ohio State Med J 74:571, 1978.

405. Brodsky SJ, Cutler SS, Weiner DA. Hepatotoxicity due to treatment with verapamil. Ann Intern Med 94:490, 1981.

406. Guarascio P, D'Amato C, Sette P, et al. Liver damage from verapamil. Br Med J 288:362, 1984.

407. Hare DL, Horowitz JD. Verapamil hepatotoxicity: a hypersensitivity reaction. Am Heart J 11:610, 1986.

408. Gupta MC. Stomatitis, agranulocytosis and hepatitis due to phenindione sensitivity. J Ind Med Assoc 63:324, 1974.

409. Dukes GE, Sanders SW, Russo J, et al. Transaminase elevations in patients receiving bovine or porcine heparin. Ann Intern Med 100:646, 1984.

410. Mandour T, Kissebah A-H, Wynn V. Mechanism of oestrogen and progesterone effects on lipid and carbohydrate metabolism: alteration in the insulin:glucagon molar ratio and hepatic enzyme activity. Eur J Clin Invest 7:181, 1977.

411. Ockner R, Lysenko N, Manning JA, et al. Sex steroid modulation of fatty acid utilization and fatty acid binding protein concentration in rat liver. J Clin Invest 65:1013, 1980.

412. Ockner RK, Davidson CS. Hepatic effects of oral contraceptives. N Engl J Med 276:331, 1967.
413. Goegelsmann U, Mashchak A, Mishell DR. Comparison of hepatic impact of oral and vaginal administration of ethinyl estradiol. Am J Obstet Gynecol 151:568, 1985.
414. Kreek MJ. Female sex steroids and cholestasis. Semin Liver Dis 7:8, 1987.
415. Haemmerli UP. Jaundice during pregnancy, with special emphasis on recurrent jaundice during pregnancy and its differential diagnosis. Acta Med Scand (suppl) 444:1, 1966.
416. Kleiner GJ, Kresch L, Arias IM. Studies of hepatic excretory function. II. The effect of norethynodrel and mestranol on bromsulfalein sodium metabolism in women of childbearing age. N Engl J Med 273:420, 1965.
417. Larrson-Cohn U, Stenram U. Liver ultrastructure and function in icteric and non-icteric women using oral contraceptives. Acta Med Scand 181:257, 1967.
418. Orellana-Alcalde JM, Dominguez JP. Jaundice and oral contraceptive drugs. Lancet 2:1278, 1966.
419. Reyes H, et al. Prevalence of intrahepatic cholestasis of pregnancy in Chile. Ann Intern Med 88:487, 1978.
420. Cohen L, Lewis C, Anas IM. Pregnancy, oral contraceptives, and chronic familial jaundice with predominantly conjugated hyperbilirubinemia (Dubin-Johnson syndrome). Gastroenterology 62:1182, 1972.
421. Morrison AS, Jick H, Ory HW. Oral contraceptives and hepatitis. Lancet 1:1142, 1977.
422. Eisalo A, Konttinen A, Hietala O. Oral contraceptives after liver disease. Br Med J 3:561, 1971.
423. Johnston WG, Baskett TF. Obstetric cholestasis. A 14 year review. Am J Obstet Gynecol 133:299, 1979.
424. Wilson BRI, Haverkamp AD. Cholestatic jaundice of pregnancy: new perspectives. Obstet Gynecol 54:650, 1979.
425. Kreek MJ, Sleisenger MH, Jeffries GH. Recurrent cholestatic jaundice of pregnancy with demonstrated estrogen sensitivity. Am J Med 43:795, 1967.
426. Adlercreutz H, Tenhunen R. Some aspects of the interaction between natural and synthetic female sex hormones and the liver. Am J Med 49:630, 1970.
427. Gallagher TF, Mueller MN, Kappas A. Studies of the mechanism and structural specificity of estrogen effect on BSP metabolism. Trans Assoc Amer Physicians 78:187, 1965.
428. Mueller MN, Kappas A. Estrogen pharmacology. I. Influence of estradiol and estriol on hepatic disposal of sulfobromophthalein (BSP) in man. J Clin Invest 43:1905, 1964.
429. Forker EL. The effect of estrogen on bile formation in the rat. J Clin Invest 48:654, 1969.
430. Lake JR, Licko V, Van Dyke RW, Scharschmidt BF. Biliary secretion of fluid phase markers by the isolated perfused rat liver: The role of transcellular vesicular transport. J Clin Invest 76:676, 1985.
431. Jaeschke H, Trummer E, Krell H. Increases in biliary permeability subsequent to intrahepatic cholestasis by estradiol valerate in rats. Gastroenterology 93:533, 1987.
432. Davis RA, Kern F. Effects of ethinyl estradiol and phenobarbital on bile acid synthesis and biliary bile acid and cholesterol excretion. Gastroenterology 70:1130, 1976.
433. Davis RA, Kern F Jr, Showalter R, et al. Alterations of hepatic Na+, K+-ATPase and bile flow by estrogen: effects on liver surface membrane lipid structure and function. Proc Natl Acad Sci U.S.A. 75:4130, 1978.
434. Keeffe EB, Scharschmidt BF, Blankenship NM, et al. Studies of relationship among bile flow, liver plasma membrane NaK-ATPase and membrane microviscosity in the rat. J Clin Invest 64:1590, 1979.
435. Schreiber AJ, Simon FR. Estrogen-induced cholestasis: clues to pathogenesis and treatment. Hepatology 3:607, 1983.
436. Brock WJ, Durham S, Vore M. Characterization of the interaction between estrogen metabolites and taurocholate for uptake into hepatocytes. Lack of correlation between cholestasis and inhibition of taurocholate uptake. J Ster Biochem 20:1181, 1984.
437. Simon FR, Gonzales M, Sutherland E, et al. Reversal of ethinyl estradiol-induced bile secretory failure with Triton WR-1339. J Clin Invest 65:851, 1980.
438. Stramentinoli G, DiPadova C, Gualano M, et al. Ethinylestradiol-induced impairment of bile secretion in the rat: protective effects of S-adenosyl-L-methionine and its implication in estrogen metabolism. Gastroenterology 80:154, 1981.
439. Frezza M, Pozzato G, Chiesa L, et al. Reversal of intrahepatic cholestasis of pregnancy in women after high dose S-adenosyl-L-methionine administration. Hepatology 4:274, 1984.
440. Reyes H, Gonzales MC, Ribalta JR, et al. Prevalence of intrahepatic cholestasis of pregnancy in Chile. Ann Intern Med 88:487, 1978.
441. Tikkanen MJ, Adlercreutz H. Recurrent jaundice in pregnancy. III. Quantitative determination of urinary estriol conjugates, including studies in pruritus gravidarum. Am J Med 54:600, 1973.
442. Adlercreutz H, Tikkanen MJ, Wichmann K, et al. Recurrent jaundice in pregnancy. IV. Quantitative determination of urinary and biliary estrogens, including studies in pruritus gravidarum. J Clin Endocrinol Metab 38:51, 1974.
443. Thomassen PA. Urinary bile acids during development of recurrent cholestasis of pregnancy. Eur J Clin Invest 9:417, 1979.
444. Thomassen PA. Urinary bile acids in late pregnancy and in recurrent cholestasis of pregnancy. Eur J Clin Invest 9:425, 1979.
445. Adinolfi LE, Utili R, Gaeta GB, et al. Cholestasis induced by estradiol-17-beta-D-glucuronide: mechanisms and prevention by sodium taurocholate. Hepatology 4:30, 1984.
446. Vore M. Estrogen cholestasis. Membranes, metabolites or receptors? Gastroenterology 93:643, 1987.
447. Blackman AM, Amiel SA, Millis RR, Rubens RD. Tamoxifen and liver damage. Br Med J 289:288, 1984.
448. Baum JK, Holtz F, Bookstein JJ, et al. Possible association between benign hepatomas and oral contraceptives. Lancet 2:926, 1973.
449. Sherlock S. Hepatic adenomas and oral contraceptives. Gut 16:753, 1975.
450. Stauffer JQ, Lapinski MW, Honold DJ, et al. Focal nodular hyperplasia of the liver and intrahepatic hemorrhage in young women on oral contraceptives. Ann Intern Med 83:301, 1975.
451. Edmonson HA, Henderson B, Benton B. Liver-cell adenomas associated with use of oral contraceptives. N Engl J Med 294:470, 1976.
452. Mays ET, Christopherson WM, Mahr MM, et al. Hepatic changes in young women ingesting contraceptive steroids. Hepatic hemorrhage and primary hepatic tumors. JAMA 235:730, 1976.
453. Klatskin G. Hepatic tumors: possible relationship to use of oral contraceptives. Gastroenterology 73:386, 1977.
454. Christopherson WM, Mays ET, Barrows G. Hepatocellular carcinoma in young women on oral contraceptives. Lancet 2:38, 1978.
455. Neuberger J, Portman B, Nunnerly HB, et al. Oral-contraceptive-associated liver tumors; occurrence of malignancy and difficulties in diagnosis. Lancet 1:273, 1980.
456. Fitz JG. Oral contraceptives and benign tumors of the liver. West J Med 140:260, 1984.
457. Mays ET, Christoferson W. Hepatic tumors induced by sex steroids. Semin Liver Dis 4:147, 1984.
458. Goodman ZD, Ishak KG. Hepatocellular carcinomas in women: probable lack of etiologic association with oral contraceptives. Hepatology 2:440, 1982.
459. Henderson BE, Preston-Martin S, Edmondson HA, et al. Hepatocellular carcinoma and oral contraceptives. Br J Cancer 48:437, 1983.
460. Neuberger J, Forman D, Doll R, et al. Oral contraceptives and hepatocellular carcinoma. Br Med J 292:1355, 1986.
461. Forman D, Vincent TJ, Doll R. Cancer of the liver and the use of oral contraceptives. Br Med J 292:1357, 1986.
462. Francis IR, Agha FP, Thompson NW, et al. Fibrolamellar hepatocarcinoma: clinical, radiologic and pathologic features. Gastrointest Radiol 11:67, 1986.
463. Kerlin P, Davis GL, McGill DB, et al. Hepatic adenoma and focal nodular hyperplasia: clinical, pathologic, and radiologic features. Gastroenterology 84:994, 1983.
464. Dean PJ, Haggitt RC, O'Hara CJ. Malignant epithelial hemangioendothelioma of the liver in young women. Relationship to oral contraceptive use. Am J Surg Pathol 9:695, 1985.
465. Ross D, Pina J, Mirza M, et al. Regression of focal nodular hyperplasia after discontinuation of oral contraceptives. Ann Intern Med 85:203, 1976.
466. Edmonson HA, Reynolds TB, Henderson B, et al. Regression of liver cell adenomas associated with oral contraceptives. Ann Intern Med 86:180, 1977.
467. Ramseur WL, Cooper R. Asymptomatic liver cell adenomas. Another case of resolution after discontinuation of oral contraceptives. JAMA 239:1647, 1978.
468. Gordon SC, Reddy KR, Livingstone AS, et al. Resolution of a contraceptive-steroid–induced hepatic adenoma with subsequent evolution into hepatocellular carcinoma. Ann Intern Med 105:547, 1986.
469. Kent DR, Nissen ED, Nissen SE, et al. Effect of pregnancy on liver tumor associated with oral contraceptives. Obstet Gynecol 51:148, 1978.
470. Raufman J-P, Miller DL, Gumucio JJ. Estrogen-induced zonal changes in rat liver sinusoids. Gastroenterology 79:1174, 1980.
471. Porter LE, Van Thiel DH, Eagon PK. Estrogens and progestins as tumor inducers. Semin Liver Dis 7:24, 1987.
472. Hoyumpa AM, Schiff L, Helfman EL. Budd-Chiari syndrome in women taking oral contraceptives. Am J Med 50:137, 1971.
473. Wu S-M, Spurny OM, Klotz AP. Budd-Chiari syndrome after taking

oral contraceptives. A case report and review of 14 reported cases. Dig Dis 22:623, 1977.

474. Lewis JH, Tice HL, Zimmerman HJ. Budd-Chiari syndrome associated with oral contraceptive steroids. Review of treatment of 47 cases. Dig Dis Sci 28:673, 1983.

475. Maddrey WC. Hepatic vein thrombosis (Budd-Chiari syndrome): possible association with the rise of oral contraceptives. Semin Liver Dis 7:32, 1987.

476. Valla D, Le MG, Poynard T, et al. Risk of hepatic vein thrombosis in relation to recent use of oral contraceptives. A case control study. Gastroenterology 90:807, 1986.

477. Valla D, Casadevall N, Lacombe C, et al. Primary myeloproliferative disorder and hepatic vein thrombosis. A prospective study of euthyroid colony formation in vitro in 20 patients with Budd-Chiari syndrome. Ann Intern Med 103:329, 1985.

478. Schonberg LA. Peliosis hepatis and oral contraceptives. A case report. J Reprod Med 27:753, 1982.

479. Saint-Marc-Girardin MF, Zafrani ES, Prigent A, et al. Unilobular small hepatic vein obstruction: possible role of progestogen given as oral contraceptive. Gastroenterology 84:630, 1983.

480. Jacobs MB. Hepatic infarction related to oral contraceptive use. Arch Intern Med 144:642, 1984.

481. Pertsemlidis D, Panveliwalla D, Ahrens EH Jr. Effects of clofibrate and of an estrogen-progestin combination on fasting biliary lipids and cholic acid kinetics in man. Gastroenterology 66:565, 1974.

482. Bennion LJ, Ginsberg RL, Garnick MB, et al. Effects of oral contraceptives on the gallbladder bile of normal women. N Engl J Med 294:189, 1976.

483. The Coronary Drug Research Group. Gallbladder disease as a side effect of drugs influencing lipid metabolism. N Engl J Med 296:1185, 1977.

484. Anderson A, James OFW, MacDonald HS, et al. The effect of ethynyl oestradiol on biliary lipid composition in young men. Eur J Clin Invest 10:77, 1980.

485. Kern F. Epidemiology and natural history of gallstones. Semin Liver Dis 3:87, 1983.

486. Kern F, Everson GT, DeMark B, et al. Biliary lipids, bile acids, and gallbladder function in the human female: effects of contraceptive steroids. J Lab Clin Med 99:798, 1982.

487. Van Der Werf SD, Van Berge Henegouwen GP, Ruben AT, et al. Biliary lipids, bile acid metabolism, gallbladder motor function and small intestinal transit during ingestion of a sub-fifty oral contraceptive. J Hepatol 4:318, 1987.

488. Keane P, Colwell D, Baer HP, et al. Effects of age, gender, and female sex hormones upon contractility of the human gallbladder in vitro (strips). Surg Gynec Obstet 163:535, 1986.

489. Di Padova C, Tritappe R, Cammareri G, et al. S-adenosyl-L-methionine antagonizes ethynylestradiol-induced bile cholesterol supersaturation in humans without modifying the estrogen plasma kinetics. Gastroenterology 82:223, 1982.

490. Ishak KG. Hepatic lesions caused by anabolic and contraceptive steroids. Semin Liver Dis 1:116, 1981.

491. Bagheri SA, Boyer JL. Peliosis hepatis associated with androgenic-anabolic steroid therapy. Ann Intern Med 81:610, 1974.

492. Westaby D, Ogle SJ, Paradinas FJ, et al. Liver damage from long-term methyltestosterone. Lancet 2:261, 1977.

493. Nadell J, Kosek J. Peliosis hepatis. Twelve cases associated with oral androgen therapy. Arch Pathol Lab Med 101:405, 1977.

494. Chopra S, Edelstern A, Koff RS, et al. Peliosis hepatis in hematologic disease. JAMA 240:1153, 1978.

495. Degott C, Rueff B, Kreis H, et al. Peliosis hepatis in recipients of renal transplants. Gut 19:748, 1978.

496. Nuzzo JL, Manz HJ, Maxted WC. Peliosis hepatis after long-term androgen therapy. Urology 25:518, 1985.

497. Paradinas FJ, Bull TB, Westaby D, et al. Hyperplasia and prolapse of hepatocytes into hepatic veins during long-term methyl-testosterone therapy: possible relationships of these changes to the development of peliosis hepatis and liver tumors. Histopathology 1:225, 1977.

498. Johnson FL, Feagler JR, Lerner KG, et al. Association of androgenic-anabolic steroid therapy with development of hepatocellular carcinoma. Lancet 2:1273, 1972.

499. Falk H, Thomas LB, Popper H, et al. Hepatic angiosarcoma associated with androgenic-anabolic steroids. Lancet 2:1120, 1979.

500. Carrasco D, Prieto M, Pallardo L, et al. Multiple hepatic adenomas after long-term therapy with testosterone enanthate. J Hepatol 1:573, 1985.

501. Taylor W, Snowball S, Lesna M. The effects of long-term administration of methyltestosterone on the development of liver lesions in Balb/c mice. J Pathol 143:211, 1984.

502. Cicardi M, Bergamaschini L, Tucai A, et al. Morphologic evaluation of the liver in hereditary angioedema patients on long-term treatment with androgen derivatives. J Allerg Clin Immunol 72:294, 1983.

503. Schneider TL, Hornback KD, Knaiz JL, et al. Chlorpropamide hepatotoxicity: report of a case and review of the literature. Am J Gastroenterol 79:721, 1984.

504. Van Thiel DH, De Belle R, Mellow M, et al. Tolazamide hepatotoxicity. Gastroenterology 67:506, 1974.

505. Nakao NL, Gelb AM, Stenger RJ, et al. A case of chronic liver disease due to tolazamide. Gastroenterology 89:192, 1985.

506. Goodman RC, Dean PJ, Radparrar A, et al. Glyburide-induced hepatitis. Ann Intern Med 106:837, 1987.

507. Vitry AC, Goldman JM. Hepatotoxicity from antithyroid drugs. Hormone Res 21:229, 1985.

508. Lunzer M, Huang S-N, Ginsberg J, et al. Jaundice due to carbimazole. Gut 16:913, 1975.

509. Courty B-Z, Kauli R, Ben-Ari J, et al. Hepatitis associated with propylthiouracil treatment. Drug Intell Clin Pharmacol 19:740, 1985.

510. Parker WA. Propylthiouracil-induced hepatotoxicity. Clin Pharm 1:471, 1982.

511. Villeneuve JP, Warner HA. Cimetidine hepatitis. Gastroenterology 77:143, 1979.

512. McGuigan JE. A consideration of the adverse effects of cimetidine. Gastroenterology 80:181, 1981.

513. Van Steenbergen W, Vanstapel MJ, Desmet V, et al. Cimetidine-induced liver injury. J Hepatol 1:359, 1981.

514. Lorenzini I, Jezequel AM, Orlandi F. Cimetidine-induced hepatitis. Electron microscopic observations and clinical pattern of liver injury. Dig Dis Sci 26:275, 1981.

515. Nazario M. The hepatic and renal mechanisms of drug interactions with cimetidine. Drug Intell Clin Pharm 20:342, 1986.

516. Martelli A, Gavanna M, Gambino V, et al. Genotoxicity of cimetidine in primary cultures of rat hepatocytes. Mutat Res 120:133, 1983.

517. Souza Lima MA. Hepatitis associates with ranitidine. Ann Intern Med 101:207, 1984.

518. Black M, Scott WE, Kanter R. Possible ranitidine hepatotoxicity. Ann Intern Med 101:208, 1984.

519. Hiesse C, Cantarovich M, Santelli C, et al. Ranitidine hepatotoxicity in renal transplant patients. Lancet 1:1280, 1985.

520. Zimmerman HJ. In: Hepatotoxicity. New York, Appleton-Century-Crofts 1978:395.

521. Plaa GL, McGough EC, Blacker GJ, et al. Effect of thoridazine and chlorpromazine on rat liver hemodynamics. Am J Physiol 199:793, 1960.

522. Kendler J, Bowry S, Seeff LB, et al. Effect of chlorpromazine on the function of the perfused isolated liver. Biochem Pharmacol 20:2439, 1971.

523. Tavaloni N, Reed JS, Hruban Z, et al. Effect of chlorpromazine on hepatic perfusion and bile secretory function in the isolated perfused rat liver. J Lab Clin Med 94:726, 1979.

524. Tavaloni N, Boyer JL. Relationship between hepatic metabolism of chlorpromazine and cholestatic effects in the isolated perfused rat liver. J Pharmacol Exp Ther 214:269, 1980.

525. Ros E, Small DM, Carey MC. Effects of chlorpromazine hydrochloride on bile salt synthesis, bile formation and biliary lipid secretion in the Rhesus monkey: a model for chlorpromazine-induced cholestasis. Eur J Clin Invest 9:29, 1979.

526. Samuels AM, Carey MC. Effects of chlorpromazine hydrochloride and its metabolism on Mg^{2+}- and Na^+,K^+-ATPase activities of canalicular-enriched rat liver plasma membranes. Gastroenterology 74:1183, 1978.

527. Keeffe EB, Blankenship NM, Scharschmidt BF. Alteration of rat liver plasma membrane fluidity and ATPase activity by chlorpromazine hydrochloride and its metabolites. Gastroenterology 79:222, 1980.

528. Van Dyke RW, Scharschmidt BF. Effects of chlorpromazine on Na^+-K^+-ATPase pumping and solute transport in rat hepatocytes. Am J Physiol 253:G613, 1987.

529. Elias E, Boyer JL. Chlorpromazine and its metabolites alter polymerization and gelatin of actin. Science 206:1404, 1979.

530. Carey MC, Hirom PC, Small DM. A study of the physiochemical interactions between biliary lipids and chlorpromazine hydrochloride. Biochem J 153:519, 1976.

531. Smith PL, Field M. In vitro antisecretory effects of trifluoperazine and other neuroleptics in rabbit and human small intestine. Gastroenterology 78:1545, 1980.

532. Robins-Browne RM, Levine MM. Effect of chlorpromazine on intestinal secretion mediated by Escherichia coli heat-stable enterotoxin and 8-Br-cyclic GMP in infant mice. Gastroenterology 80:321, 1981.

533. Mullock BM, Hall DE, Shaw JL, et al. Immune responses to chlorpromazine in rats. Detection and relation to hepatotoxicity. Biochem Pharmacol 32:2733, 1983.

534. Pessayre D, De Saint-Louvent P, Degott C, et al. Iproclozide fulminant hepatitis. Possible role of enzyme induction. Gastroenterology 75:492, 1978.

535. Daneshmend TK, Scott GL, Bradfield JWB. Angiosarcoma of liver associated with phenelzine. Br Med J 1:1679, 1979.

536. Danan G, Bernuau J, Moullot X, et al. Amytriptyline-induced fulminant hepatitis. Digestion 30:179, 1984.

537. Larrey D, Rueff B, Pessayre D, et al. Cross hepatotoxicity between tricyclic antidepressants. Gut 27:726, 1986.

538. Yasuhara H, Dujovne CA, Veda I, et al. Hepatotoxicity and surface activity of tricyclic antidepressants. Toxicol Appl Pharmacol 47:47, 1979.

539. Kappus H, Remmer H. Irreversible protein binding of ^{14}C-imipramine with rat and human liver microsomes. Biochem Pharmacol 24:1079, 1975.

540. Fang MH, Ginsberg AL, Dobbins WO III: Cholestatic jaundice associated with flurazepam hydrochloride. Ann Intern Med 89:363, 1978.

541. Fuller CM, Yassinger S, Donlon P, et al. Haloperidol-induced liver disease. West J Med 127:515, 1977.

542. Hunt CE, Inwood RJ, Shannon DC. Respiratory and non-respiratory effects of doxapram in congenital central hypoventilation syndrome. Am Rev Resp Dis 119:263, 1979.

543. Fancourt GJ, Prendergast D, Murray M. Hepatic necrosis with doxapram hydrochloride. Postgrad Med J 61:833, 1985.

544. Keeffe EB, Smith FW. Disulfuram hypersensitivity hepatitis. JAMA 230:435, 1974.

545. Eisen HJ, Ginsberg AL. Disulfiram hepatotoxicity. Ann Intern Med 83:673, 1975.

546. Schade RR, Gray JA, Dekker A, et al. Fulminant hepatitis associated with disulfiram. Report of a case. Arch Intern Med 143:1271, 1983.

547. Bartle WR, Fisher MM, Kerenyi N. Disulfiram-induced hepatitis. Report of two cases and review of the literature. Dig Dis Sci 30:834, 1985.

548. Teychenne PF, Jones EA, Ishak KG, et al. Hepatocellular injury with distinctive mitochondrial changes induced by lergotrile mesylate: a dopaminergic ergot derivative. Gastroenterology 76:575, 1979.

549. Foged EK, Jacobsen FK. Side effects due to RO 10-9359 (Tigason). Dermatologica 164:395, 1982.

550. Glazer SD, Roenigk HH, Yokoo H, et al. A study of potential hepatotoxicity of etretinate used in the treatment of psoriasis. J Am Acad Dermatol 6:683, 1982.

551. Weiss VC, West DP, Ackerman R, et al. Hepatotoxic reactions in a patient treated with etretinate. Arch Dermatol 120:104, 1984.

32

Clinical Aspects of Liver Diseases Caused by Industrial and Environmental Toxins

Norman Gitlin, M.D.

The liver's potential for injury by ingested chemicals, toxins, or elements is very high because it is the first organ, after the gastrointestinal tract, that is exposed to these agents. Hepatic metabolism usually detoxifies these agents; however, hepatic metabolism of chemicals can result in metabolites that are considerably more hepatotoxic than the parent chemicals (see Chap. 9). The hepatotoxic effects in humans that result from accidental or intentional exposure to chemicals or toxins are protean and range from mild dysfunction to fulminant hepatic necrosis. The spectrum of hepatic responses to hepatotoxins includes abnormal liver function tests in asymptomatic patients, steatosis, hepatitis, acute necrosis, chronic active hepatitis, cirrhosis, veno-occlusive hepatic disease, and hepatic neoplasia. The realization that common and frequently used chemical compounds present carcinogenic hazards has stirred considerable apprehension and raised serious socioeconomic questions, not only for industrial workers exposed directly to these agents but also for the general public who unwittingly get exposed to these ubiquitous noxious agents in the environment, in the food they eat, or in their homes. The high frequency of liver exposure to environmental or occupational toxins and the similar clinical and biochemical presentations of toxic and nontoxic liver disease makes the differentiation between toxic and nontoxic hepatic disease difficult to recognize and prove. The response of the liver to a toxin is determined by a variety of factors such as dose, duration of exposure, route of exposure, age of the patient, simultaneous exposure to other drugs or toxins, the presence or lack of established liver disease, and an inherent sensitivity of the exposed individual to the noxious agent. Xenobiotics may react with nutrients and destroy them or make them unavailable because of altered absorption, competitive binding to proteins or changes in detoxification or metabolic rates. Nutritional deficiencies may enhance the toxic effects of chemicals. This is especially evident in impoverished societies, in which the socioeconomic burden of additional disease entities can be least afforded. In view of all these variables, the examining physician must have a high index of suspicion regarding toxins in the genesis of liver dysfunction. A history must include not only the drugs ingested but also whether there has been exposure to toxins in the environment—either accidentally or through occupation, work, or hobby. A list of some important chemicals and toxins, including their application and hepatotoxicity, is given in Table 32–1.

A variety of classifications has been used to group hepatotoxins according to the clinical picture they produce, for example, acute, subacute or chronic hepatitis, or according to the mechanism by which they produce their hepatotoxicity. Both methods are flawed because the clinical picture is often a spectrum of differing presentations

TABLE 32–1. SOME IMPORTANT CHEMICALS AND THEIR APPLICATION AND HEPATOTOXICITY*

CHEMICAL	USES	HEPATIC RESPONSES
Arsenic and inorganic salts	As pesticides and alloys; in production of dyes, ceramics, drugs, fireworks, paint, petroleum, ink, and semiconductors	Acute injury and death of parenchymal cells; cirrhosis; angiosarcoma
Beryllium	In alloys, cathode ray tubes, ceramics, electrical equipment, gas mantles, missiles, nuclear reactors, and refractory materials	Granulomata
Carbon tetrachloride	As degreasers, fat processors, fire extinguisher, fumigant, production of solvents: in fluorocarbons, ink, insecticides, lacquer, propellants, refrigerants, rubber and wax	Acute injury and death of parenchymal cells; ? cirrhosis; ? carcinoma
Dioxane	As solvent, degreaser, cement component; in production of adhesives, deodorants, detergents, emulsions, fats, glue, lacquer, oil, paint, polish, shoe cream, varnish remover, waxes; in histology laboratories	Subacute injury of parenchymal cells
Phosphorus (yellow)	In munitions, pyrotechnics, explosives, smoke bombs, fertilizers, rodenticides, bronze alloys, semiconductors, luminescent coatings, and chemical manufacture	Acute injury and death of parenchymal cells
Picric acid (2,4,6-trinitrophenol)	As copper etcher, forensic and biology laboratory chemical; in batteries, colored glass, disinfectants, drugs, dyes, explosives, matches, photography chemicals, and tanneries	Acute injury and death of parenchymal cells
Polychlorinated biphenyls	In cable insulation, dyes, electric equipment, herbicides, lacquers, paper treatment, plasticizers, resins, rubber textiles, flameproofer, transformers, and wood preservation	Subacute injury of parenchymal cells, proliferation of smooth endoplastic reticulum; ? cirrhosis; ? carcinoma
2,3,7,8-Tetrachloro-dibenzo-p-dioxin	Contaminant of commercial preparations of 2,4,5-trichlorophenoxyacetic acid, polychlorinated biphenyls, and other chlorinated compounds	Porphyria cutanea tarda; proliferation of small endoplasmic reticulum and some forms of associated monooxygenase enzymes
Tetrachloroethane	As dry-cleaning agent, fumigant, solvent, degreaser; in production of gaskets, lacquers, paints, phosphorus, resins, varnish, wax	Acute injury and death of parenchymal cells
Tetrachloroethylene	As solvent, degreaser, chemical intermediate, fumigant; in production of cellulose esters, gums, rubber, soap, vacuum tubes, wax, wool	Acute injury and death of parenchymal cells
2,4,5-Trinitrotoluene	As explosive	Acute and subacute injury and death of parenchymal cells
Vinyl chloride	As chemical intermediate and solvent; in production of polyvinyl chloride and resins	Fibrosis, noncirrhotic portal hypertension, cirrhosis, angiosarcoma, carcinoma

*Source: Modified from Pond SM, et al. West J Med 137:509, 1982.

depending on the dose, frequency, and duration of exposure to the hepatotoxic agent, and the mechanism of hepatotoxicity is often complex, multiple, and on many occasions speculative or unknown. In light of these limitations and the increasing number of hepatotoxic agents, this chapter will base its classification mostly on the clinical syndromes produced by the hepatotoxin and the origin of the hepatotoxin.

ACUTE LIVER DISEASE

CARBON TETRACHLORIDE

Carbon tetrachloride has had widespread use as a cleaning agent, solvent, fire extinguisher, grain fumigant, vermifuge (against hookworm), and intermediate in the synthesis of chlorofluorocarbons. The medical profession became aware of the menace of carbon tetrachloride as an industrial poison in the late nineteenth and early twentieth centuries. Yet approximately 710 million pounds of the chemical were manufactured in the United States in 1980.[1] Poisoning usually follows inhalation of the vapor in a poorly

ventilated environment, but it also occurs after the ingestion of contaminated food (especially grain) and ground water.[2,3] Absorption may occur through the skin.

Extrahepatic Manifestations

Acute poisoning with carbon tetrachloride becomes manifested as a multisystem disorder, involving especially the liver, kidneys, brain, lungs, adrenal glands, and myocardium.

Initially, carbon tetrachloride toxicity becomes manifested in the central nervous system. Confusion, dizziness, headaches, and visual impairment may evolve rapidly into coma and death as the anesthetic properties of carbon tetrachloride progress over a matter of minutes to hours. Renal failure accounts for the majority of deaths attributable to acute inhalational carbon tetrachloride toxicity.[4,5] On average, oliguria develops on the third day after exposure, although it may begin at any time during the first two weeks following exposure. Oliguria persists for 1 to 15 days, with an average of 8 days.[4] The renal failure is due to acute tubular necrosis, and it is both clinically and morphologically indistinguishable from tubular necrosis from other causes.[4]

Pulmonary changes, which are thought to reflect the underlying renal failure and hypervolemia, usually become manifested on the ninth day after exposure to carbon tetrachloride.[6] Patients become dyspneic and cyanotic. Fluffy hilar opacities are noted on radiographs, and on subsequent examinations they extend peripherally. Histologic findings consist of an exudate of fibrin with a pseudomembrane lining the alveolar walls.[6] The pulmonary changes are not considered to be a facet of the direct effects of carbon tetrachloride fumes, but rather a nonspecific systemic effect.

Other organs affected include the adrenal glands and the myocardium, in which there is cloudy swelling, fatty degeneration, and petechial hemorrhages that may be associated with dysrhythmias and reversible electrocardiographic changes.[7, 8] Congestive heart failure secondary to hypervolemia, and fluid retention consequent to renal failure, can occur. A hemorrhagic diathesis (subconjunctival hemorrhage, epistaxis, petechiae) subsequent to uremia and hepatic dysfunction may also occur. Experimental evidence indicates that carbon tetrachloride may be directly injurious to capillaries.[9] Hemolytic anemia may be present.[10]

Hepatic Manifestations

Carbon tetrachloride is a potent hepatotoxin, and a single exposure to it can rapidly lead to severe centrizonal necrosis and steatosis.[11–14] It is one of the most extensively studied of the hepatotoxins.[15] Apart from its acute hepatotoxic effects, chronic or intermittent exposure to it may cause cirrhosis and even lead to hepatic cancer in rats.[16–19] Evidence for cirrhosis and neoplasia in humans is less persuasive.[20, 21]

Factors Affecting Susceptibility

Carbon tetrachloride toxicity appears to be largely dependent on the metabolic transformation of the parent compound into a toxic metabolite.[11, 15, 22] This is accomplished by the mixed-function oxidase system of the liver (see Chap. 9). Factors that impair the capacity of the liver to metabolize carbon tetrachloride diminish its toxicity and vice versa. The observation in animals that an initial sublethal dose of carbon tetrachloride decreases or abolishes the hepatotoxicity of subsequent larger doses supports the concept that liver injury from nonlethal doses depresses the activity of the mixed-function oxidase system, preventing subsequent doses of carbon tetrachloride from being metabolized to its hepatotoxic metabolite.[11]

A wide variety of animals has been studied in experimental models. Recent studies have used mostly rats and mice and occasionally dogs or rabbits. Regardless of the mode of administration (oral, inhalation, subcutaneous, per rectum, or intraperitoneal) the hepatic lesions are similar. The toxicity is dose related, and as little as 0.176 ml/kg given orally caused hepatic necrosis in canines, and 0.02 ml/kg given orally or parenterally caused hepatic necrosis in rodents.[7, 14] Susceptibility varies according to the animal species. Chickens, birds, amphibians, and fish are very resistant to carbon tetrachloride hepatotoxicity.[11, 16, 23] Sex differences in rats indicate a greater male susceptibility, a difference consistent with a greater mixed-function oxidase

or mono-oxygenase activity in the male rat. Age and body weight have a profound influence on the toxicity of halocarbons. Newborn rats are resistant to carbon tetrachloride hepatotoxicity, whereas rats 4 to 21 days old are reported to be as sensitive as adults.[24, 25] Larger adult rats, 300- to 350-g animals, rarely exhibited hepatic necrosis and had lower serum enzyme levels than their 200- to 250-g counterparts.[17] The role of diet modifying susceptibility to carbon tetrachloride is not clear. Recent evidence favors a protective role afforded by short-term fasting or protein restriction.[26–28] This may be accounted for by a decrease in the functioning of the hepatic enzyme system that metabolizes and converts carbon tetrachloride to its toxic metabolite.[26, 28] A carbohydrate-deficient diet has a detrimental impact on carbon tetrachloride hepatotoxicity, possibly by virtue of a deficiency of protective liver glycogen stores or because of the concurrent high-fat diet, which causes a fatty liver, thereby concentrating carbon tetrachloride in the liver.[13, 26] Calcium may protect the liver from toxicity by stabilizing hepatic cell membranes.

Substances known to stimulate the hepatic microsomal enzyme system, such as dichlorodiphenyltrichloroethane (DDT) and barbiturates, potentiate the hepatotoxicity of carbon tetrachloride.[7, 29, 30] Likewise, the concomitant ingestion of alcohol enhances the hepatotoxicity of carbon tetrachloride, possibly because of enhanced microsomal activation and biotransformation of the carbon tetrachloride.[31]

Possible explanations for the effects of alcohol on carbon tetrachloride toxicity, other than that of inducing microsomal enzymes, include the cumulative effects of two known hepatotoxic agents, the additional storage of carbon tetrachloride in the fatty liver of alcoholics, and the alcohol-enhanced absorption of carbon tetrachloride in the gastrointestinal tract.[32–34] The induction of hepatic microsomal enzymes by alcohol and the consequent potentiation of carbon tetrachloride–induced hepatotoxicity is an attractive idea. A single dose of ethanol given many hours prior to the carbon tetrachloride also potentiates the hepatotoxicity of carbon tetrachloride when there is no steatosis or preexistent hepatic damage.[35–37] The maximum potentiation of carbon tetrachloride hepatotoxicity by alcohol occurs if the latter is administered 18 hours before the carbon tetrachloride.[36, 37] Mechanisms in addition to the induction of cytochrome P450 must be operative, however, for the ethanol-induced enhancement of carbon tetrachloride toxicity. An alternate explanation is that ethanol may provoke an output of catecholamines, which have been demonstrated to potentiate carbon tetrachloride hepatotoxicity.[38, 39] Increased fragility of liver mitochondria has been observed in rats fed ethanol chronically; it is possible that ethanol sensitizes the mitochondrial response to carbon tetrachloride.[40] In another study using rats, repetitive exposure to both ketones (acetone) and halogenated solvents (carbon tetrachloride) resulted in a potentiation of the severe chronic liver disease, with an accelerated appearance of cirrhosis.[41]

Several phenothiazines (chlorpromazine, promazine, and promethazine) and antihistamines have been shown to prevent hepatic necrosis induced by carbon tetrachloride.[42] This protection appears to be a manifestation of the membrane-stabilizing effects of these compounds.[42]

Mechanism of Hepatic Injury

The mechanism of hepatic injury produced by carbon tetrachloride is complex, multifactorial, and not completely understood. Considerable progress has been made in the

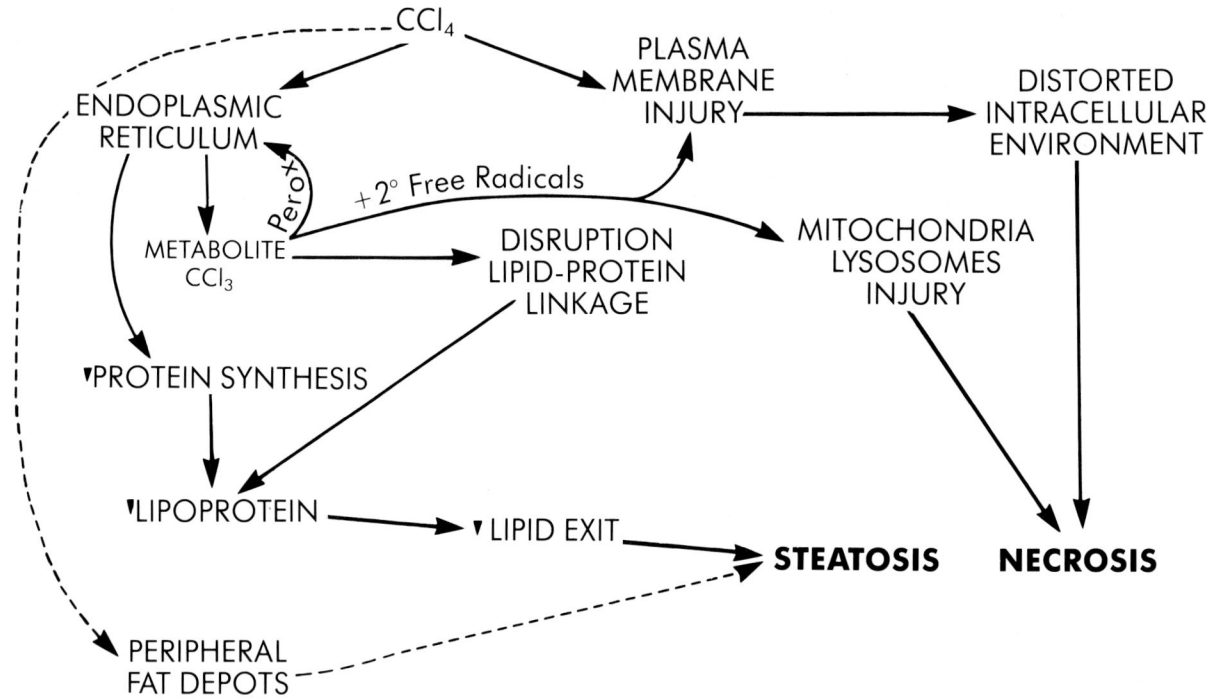

Figure 32–1. Carbon tetrachloride–induced hepatotoxicity. A suggested mechanism of production of the spectrum of liver manifestations. (Reproduced from Zimmerman HJ. Hepatotoxicity. New York, Appleton-Century-Crofts, 1978:208, with permission of the author and publisher.)

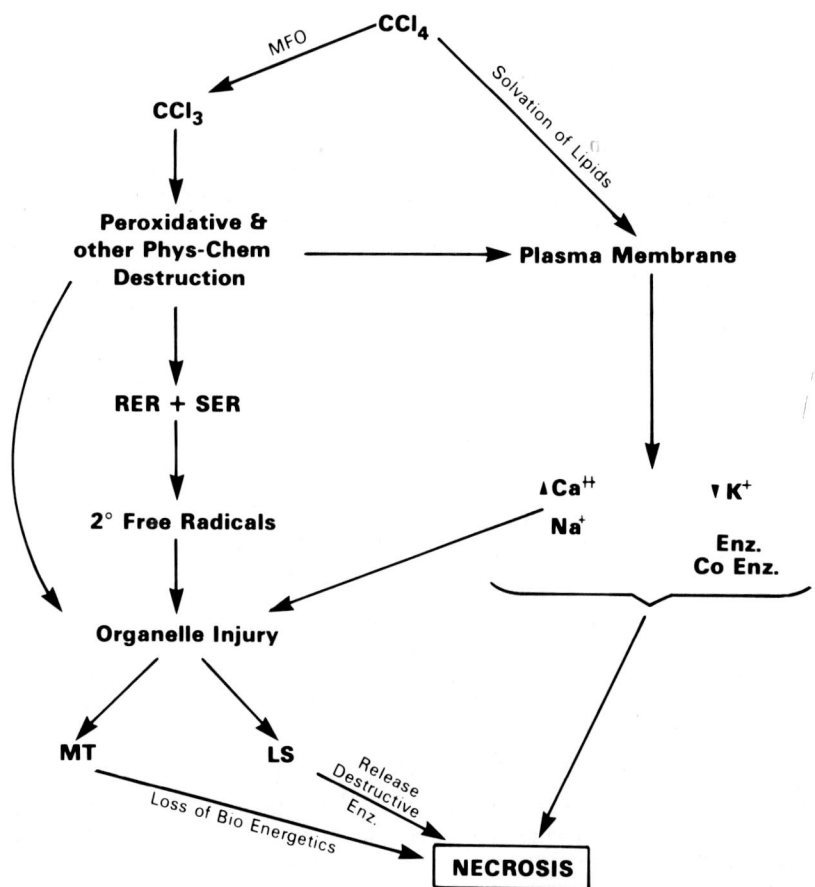

Figure 32–2. Carbon tetrachloride–induced hepatic necrosis. A suggested mechanism of its production. Plasma membranes, membranes of endoplasmic reticulum, and other organelles are injured by non-metabolized CCl_4, by free radicals (CCl_3), and by secondary free radicals formed from fatty acids of the membranes. This results in a cellular loss of potassium, enzymes, and coenzymes and a cellular gain of calcium and sodium. It also results in necrosis. (Reproduced from Zimmerman HJ. Hepatotoxicity. New York, Appleton-Century-Crofts, 1978:205, with permission of the author and publisher.)

elucidation of the mechanisms of hepatic damage since the original, and now debunked, concepts of centrizonal anoxia resulting from decreased sinusoidal blood flow and catecholamine induced steatosis.[15, 43] Carbon tetrachloride hepatotoxicity has two distinct, independent manifestations—fat accumulation and hepatic necrosis (Fig. 32–1).[15, 44] Fat accumulation is a rapid sequel to carbon tetrachloride hepatotoxicity, becoming manifested within one hour of exposure at the phase of peak hepatic concentrations of carbon tetrachloride. Hepatic necrosis becomes manifested after 3 to 12 hours and peaks at 24 to 36 hours after exposure to the hepatotoxin. Clear-cut evidence supports the idea that the two effects of carbon tetrachloride hepatotoxicity occur by partially independent mechanisms. Thus, certain agents protect selectively against either the steatosis or the necrosis.[44]

Steatosis. The steatosis in carbon tetrachloride toxicity is due to the impaired transport of triglycerides out of the hepatocyte, which results from a decrease in apolipoprotein synthesis, disruption of the binding of triglycerides to the apoprotein carrier, and impaired transport of lipoprotein across the cell membrane.[11, 15, 44, 45] Enhanced mobilization of triglyceride stores in peripheral tissues (adipocytes) contributes to the steatosis.[46, 47]

Hepatic Necrosis. The pathogenesis of the hepatonecrosis is complex and not fully understood. At least two separate mechanisms appear to be operative—an initial direct injury to the cell membrane and a subsequent toxicity induced by metabolites of carbon tetrachloride generated by a cytochrome P450–dependent step (Fig. 32–2).[48] There is experimental evidence that carbon tetrachloride–induced hepatic necrosis is in part a direct consequence of the solvent properties of carbon tetrachloride and that the necrosis is partially reversible.[48] It commences within minutes of exposure and manifests initially as a major injury to cell membranes and altered mitochondrial function.[48, 49] The damaged membranes become more permeable than normal. As a result, cellular loss of potassium and aspartate aminotransferase (AST) occurs. Subsequently there is damage to mitochondria (glutamate dehydrogenase release) and to lysosomes (acid phosphatase release).[48] Accumulation of intracellular calcium and water occurs. The damage to mitochondria disrupts oxidative phosphorylation, compounding the cellular necrosis.[45, 50] Likewise, the free lysomal enzymes aggravate the hepatic necrosis.[14] This chain of events produces hepatic necrosis that is partially reversible, depending on its extent. The initial phase of the hepatic necrosis is dose dependent and is a direct result of carbon tetrachloride. It cannot be prevented by inhibitors of cytochrome P450 nor by antioxidants.[48] Pretreatment with antihistamines and other substances known to stabilize membrane permeability prevent carbon tetrachloride–induced hepatic necrosis.[45] A second phase of damage, evident after three hours of exposure to carbon tetrachloride, is mediated through metabolites.[11, 28, 51–53] Free radicals generated by a cytochrome P450–dependent step are thought to induce injury by interacting with the unsaturated fatty acids of cell membranes. This causes lipid peroxidation and cross-linkage of the unsaturated fatty acids. In addition, free radicals bind covalently to macromolecules, including proteins, lipids, and nuclear and mitochondrial deoxyribonucleic acid (DNA).[11, 28, 51–53]

Carbon tetrachloride is metabolized in a series of reactions catalyzed by the cytochrome P450 system. The first product is the free radical $CCl_3 \cdot$, which is produced by homolytic cleavage of carbon tetrachloride. It causes hepatic damage by lipid peroxidation and reactions with proteins and DNA.[11, 28, 51–53] Reaction of $CCl_3 \cdot$ with unsaturated lipids generates secondary free radicals, producing further cellular and subcellular destruction. The localization of carbon tetrachloride–induced hepatonecrosis to the centrilobular area may be accounted for by the concentration in this area of the enzyme system that primarily metabolizes carbon tetrachloride.[54]

Susceptibility to carbon tetrachloride in animals is determined largely by the specific ability to metabolize it to the toxic radicals. The difference in susceptibility of newborn and 2-week-old rats, of animals on a protein-restricted diet, and of rats given agents that induce or inhibit cytochrome P450 supports the concept that hepatotoxicity depends on the metabolizing action of the endoplasmic reticulum and its production of a toxic radical.[11, 26, 29, 30, 55, 56] Certain animals that are unable to metabolize carbon tetrachloride manifest a minor degree of hepatotoxicity when exposed to it; this implies an additional mechanism of direct cellular damage by the parent metabolite or an unrecognized alternate metabolic pathway.[11] In humans, the hepatotoxicity is largely mediated by the metabolism of carbon tetrachloride to its toxic metabolite.[11, 22, 28, 51–53, 57] In summary, carbon tetrachloride instantly damages the plasma membrane, with a resultant loss of enzymes and a flux of ions out of the cell (Figs. 13–1 and 13–2). The carbon tetrachloride is then metabolized to a toxic free radical by cytochrome P450 in the endoplasmic reticulum. The toxic free radical, by peroxidation of lipids, disrupts membranes further and interferes with the synthesis and transport of lipoproteins, causing fat to accumulate in the hepatocyte. Peripheral fat, mobilized by the carbon tetrachloride, accumulates in the hepatocyte, compounding the steatosis.

Clinical Features

Accidental or intentional (suicidal) intoxication by carbon tetrachloride is relatively uncommon these days. Industrial or domestic accidents account for most cases. Industrial exposure usually occurs by inhalation of the fumes in a poorly ventilated environment. Domestic exposure occurs following the inhalation of the toxin in a confined unventilated area or more commonly following ingestion by alcoholics during a bout of alcoholic intoxication.[58–60] As previously mentioned, alcohol enhances hepatic susceptibility to carbon tetrachloride. As little as 5 ml of carbon tetrachloride has been sufficient to produce histologic evidence of necrosis.[61] The early theory that poisoning by ingestion produces mostly hepatic damage and that inhalation produces renal damage has been challenged.[34]

Within hours of inhalation or ingestion, dizziness and headache occur. Visual disturbances and confusion occur and reflect the anesthetic properties of carbon tetrachloride. Coma may occur rarely in carbon tetrachloride intoxication, resulting from profound neurologic inhibition. Gastrointestinal symptoms—nausea, vomiting, diarrhea, and abdominal pain—usually occur in the first 24 hours. Hemorrhagic gastritis can also occur. Features of liver disease become manifested usually after 24 to 48 hours, with a rapid increase in jaundice, an enlarged, tender liver; and a striking bleeding diathesis, with spontaneous hemorrhage. In severe cases, ascites and hepatic coma may ensue. Care must be taken to avoid attributing these signs and symptoms solely to the concurrent alcoholism that is frequently present. Evidence of liver disease may persist for three weeks before recovery occurs. Death, if caused by hepatic dysfunction, usually occurs within ten days of the onset of symptoms.

Renal failure reaches a peak especially during the second or third week after intoxication. Pulmonary edema occurs, with nonspecific clinical, histologic, and radiographic features similar in type to uremia.[6] Cardiac failure from hypervolemia—which is often iatrogenic because of over-zealous rehydration—renal failure, or sodium retention may occur and aggravate the pulmonary edema.

Laboratory Features

Within hours of experimentally induced histologic damage to the liver in animals, the serum transaminase levels rise. In humans, clinical evidence of liver disease manifests itself after 24 to 48 hours. The aminotransferases soar to extremely high levels, the AST level being somewhat higher than the alanine aminotransferase (ALT) level because of liberation of both mitochondrial and cytosolic enzymes.[62, 63] In survivors, the recovery is rapid, with enzyme values reverting to normal within two weeks. The alkaline phosphatase level is usually only mildly elevated. The bilirubin level rapidly rises, reflecting a variety of mechanisms—hepatocyte necrosis, hemolysis, destruction of cytochrome P450, and impaired renal excretion of bilirubin being the important ones. The serum albumin level often falls, reflecting the catabolic state and hemodilation.

Anemia occurs because of hemolysis and blood loss; it is usually mild, as is a neutrophilic leukocytosis of less than 20,000/mm³.[10] A profound impairment of coagulation is manifested early, and it accounts for the severe bleeding diathesis. A low prothrombin time as well as decreased levels of clotting factors produced by the liver occur within the first 24 hours. Other findings include protein, casts, erythrocytes, and epithelial cells in urine and an elevated blood urea nitrogen (BUN) level. Once azotemia occurs, the chemical derangements common to tubular necrosis develop.

Histologic Features

The major histologic abnormalities are found in the liver and kidney; changes are also present in the heart, lung, brain, adrenal glands, and pancreas.[5, 10, 58, 60, 64] The liver shows a centrilobular necrosis and varying amounts of fatty infiltration.

The location of the maximal hepatocyte damage is felt to correlate with the enzymic metabolic activities of the hepatocytes. Hepatocytes around the central vein have the greatest capacity to metabolize carbon tetrachloride to its free radical form. Prominent ballooning may precede the necrosis, and swollen granular cytoplasm with fading nuclei are seen. The renal changes are those of acute tubular necrosis.[10] The pulmonary changes include edema, fibrin exudates, a pseudomembrane lining the alveolar walls, and a thickening of the alveolar walls from a proliferation of fibroblasts and epithelium.[6] These changes probably reflect the renal failure rather than a specific pulmonary toxicity from carbon tetrachloride. A focal pancreatitis can occur, and the myocardium shows fatty changes and degeneration.[10]

Treatment and Prognosis

Awareness of the toxicity of carbon tetrachloride and the practice of appropriate prophylactic measures are universal in industry, but carelessness still accounts for domestic instances of toxicity. None of the agents used to prevent carbon tetrachloride hepatoxicity in animal research (antihistamines, antioxidants, and beta adrenergic blockers) is effective clinically. Depending on the severity of the hepatic pathologic condition and the subsequent renal dysfunction, a diet high in calories (mostly carbohydrates) is required. When there is no renal failure or encephalopathy, proteins may be supplied. There is no specific treatment; corticosteroids are ineffective, and the basic approach is mostly supportive treatment as in other forms of fulminant hepatic failure. The acute renal failure frequently requires hemodialysis. The correction of the bleeding state by the administration of fresh frozen plasma and other clotting factors is imperative. Meticulous attention to the patient's fluid and electrolyte status is important, not only to correct any dehydration but also to avoid hypervolemic complications that often accompany the subsequent renal failure. Radioimmunoassay of serum cholylglycine has been advocated in rat models as a sensitive and specific indicator of carbon tetrachloride–induced liver injury and its response to treatment.[65]

Anoxic conditions increase the ability of carbon tetrachloride to elevate ALT levels in male rats. The covalent binding of metabolites of carbon tetrachloride to cellular macromolecules may explain the potentiation of the toxicity of carbon tetrachloride by hypoxia.[66] Animal studies have shown that carbon dioxide–induced hyperventilation is effective in preventing carbon tetrachloride–induced hepatic toxicity by causing an increased pulmonary elimination of volatile halocarbons.[67] A hepatoprotective role against carbon tetrachloride–induced hepatotoxicity in rats has been attributed to prostacyclin (PGI₂), even when administered 24 hours after the initial intoxication by carbon tetrachloride.[68]

The prognosis after carbon tetrachloride intoxication varies, and a mortality rate between 10 and 25 per cent is reported.[59, 60, 69] Most of the deaths are from renal failure and occur during the second week after intoxication; hepatic causes of death account for about a quarter of all the fatalities and occur in the first week after intoxication. Patients surviving acute carbon tetrachloride toxic injury usually recover completely; rare cases of hepatic fibrosis and cirrhosis have been described.[21, 34] In animals, repeated exposure to combinations of carbon tetrachloride and other agents (acetone, phenobarbitone) may lead to cirrhosis and neoplasia.[18, 19, 30, 41]

HALOALKANES

Nitroaromatic Compounds

A variety of these compounds have been recognized as hepatotoxic in humans. *Dinitrophenol* has been associated with both hepatic necrosis and cholestasis after its ingestion.[70, 71] Its action is mediated by inhibiting oxidative phosphorylation. *Dinitrobenzene* has caused liver damage as has *nitrobenzene*.[72, 73] *Trinitrotoluene* (TNT) was responsible for a considerable amount of hepatotoxicity among munitions workers during the great World Wars. Since then, the incidence of TNT-induced hepatoxicity has decreased considerably, largely because of improved industrial techniques and methodology. The clinical picture of TNT toxicity was varied. Some patients developed fulminant hepatic necrosis and died rapidly. Others manifested subacute hepatic necrosis with ascites, portal hypertension, and liver failure.[74–76] Another group of patients survived, but macronodular cirrhosis developed.[77] The overall mortality rate for patients developing TNT hepatotoxicity was

25 per cent, and the incidence of hepatotoxicity from TNT ranged from 0.002 to 5 per cent.[78] TNT toxicity is the result of its absorption, which takes place mostly through the skin (enhanced by any grease on the skin); however, absorption through inhalation, ingestion, or via the mucous membranes can also occur.[79, 80] An individual difference in susceptibility exists. The mode of action of TNT toxicity is unknown. Formation of a toxic intermediate metabolites and interference with amino acid metabolism have been considered as possible mechanisms.

The clinical picture of intoxication with TNT was one of a latent period of two to four months during actual exposure, after which the onset of toxic symptoms occurred. These symptoms consisted of anorexia, asthenia, nausea, vomiting, abdominal pain with hepatomegaly, and jaundice. Thereafter some patients developed either fulminant hepatic failure or subacute hepatic failure (with ascites and portal hypertension). The extrahepatic manifestations of TNT intoxication included aplastic anemia, methemoglobinemia, and a rash. No specific treatment is available; prophylaxis and general nonspecific supportive measures are advocated.

Tetrachloroethane

This useful and effective solvent is no longer used in industry because of its hepatotoxic properties. It is considered to be less hepatotoxic than carbon tetrachloride or chloroform, and its hepatotoxicity reflects the effect of a sustained, intense industrial exposure rather than a primary intrinsic hepatotoxicity of the chemical.[81] It was used in both World Wars as a solvent with many applications, for example, to carry poison gas–neutralizing substances into cloth, in the manufacture of lacquers, and in the varnish of fabrics used as aircraft covers.

The portal of entry of tetrachloroethane into the systemic circulation was mostly by inhalation. Percutaneous routes and ingestion occasionally contributed to the hepatotoxicity. The effects on the liver depended on the dose and duration of toxic exposure. The mildest presentation was one of anorexia, nausea, vomiting, hepatomegaly, and the subsequent development of jaundice in the minority of instances.[82] Headache, asthenia, neurasthenia, and dizziness also occurred.[82] Terminating contact with the noxious agent usually resulted in a rapid and total resolution of the hepatic dysfunction. Continued exposure to tetrachloroethane would result in jaundice, tender and firm hepatomegaly, ascites and fulminant hepatic failure, and death in many but not all patients. The overall mortality rate has been reported to be 17 per cent.[82] The picture was one of a subacute hepatic necrosis rather than an acute necrosis.

The histologic findings were similar to those caused by carbon tetrachloride—zonal or massive hepatic necrosis, intact stroma, steatosis, and no hepatocyte regeneration.[82–84] Bile duct proliferation was evident.[85] In addition, evidence of subacute hepatic necrosis and postnecrotic fibrosis was noted in patients who died after a prolonged course. Fatty infiltration of the myocardium and the renal tubules also occurred, and a peripheral monocytosis has been stressed as being of diagnostic value.[86]

Trichloroethane

Various isomers exist; 1,1,2-trichloroethane is an established hepatotoxin and is no longer used. The isomer 1,1,1-trichloroethane (methylchloroform) has been regarded until recently as relatively nontoxic and has been used extensively as an industrial degreasing agent. It is estimated that 900,000 tons of the agent were used in 1979. The allowable concentration in the air is 350 parts/million (ppm). Experimental hepatotoxicity has been documented in mice. A single case report of hepatotoxicity in a human has been documented with ascites and hepatosplenomegaly. On histologic examination, fibrosis, perivenular sclerosis of the central vein, and subacute hepatic necrosis were evident.[87, 88]

Trichloroethylene

This solvent currently used in the dry cleaning industry was at one time also used as an anesthetic agent. Hepatotoxicity has been demonstrated in animal models. Human hepatotoxicity is rarely a sequel of occupational industrial exposure.[81] It is encountered more commonly in patients who have inhaled (sniffed) trichloroethylene as a form of drug abuse.[89] Such individuals manifest high transaminase levels, and acute hepatic and renal failure may follow. Apart for the extreme toxicities, recovery usually follows the withdrawal from exposure, but mild centrilobular fibrosis may complicate chronic drug abuse.[89, 90] An association between liver cancer and trichloroethylene exposure has not been proved.[91]

Tetrachloroethylene

This solvent appears to be as hepatotoxic as trichloroethylene.

Toluene

Toluene is a constituent of many commonly used products, for example, glue and paint. It has been suggested that it may be responsible for acute hepatocellular toxic effects and reversible renal failure in a "glue sniffer."[92] However, in a controlled study of car painters exposed to toluene, no significant hepatotoxic effect was detectable when compared with controls.[93] The difficulty in uncovering causal relationships in hepatic disorders when many chemicals are involved simultaneously has been evaluated and stressed.[94]

NITROPARAFFINS

The nitroparaffins (nitromethane, nitroethane, 1-nitropropane, and 2-nitropropane) are used extensively in industry as solvents for substances such as coating materials, inks, waxes, gums, dyes, and resins. They are considered to be less toxic than the aromatic nitrocompounds.

2-Nitropropane is used as a solvent in extractions and for protective coatings, adhesives, and printing inks. In 1977, 15 million pounds of nitroparaffins were used in the United States; 2-nitropropane accounted for about 80 per cent of this quantity.[95, 96] The National Institute for Occupational Safety and Health (NIOSH) estimates that 185,000 workers in the United States are potentially exposed to 2-nitropropane during its production and use.[95] No cases of oral ingestion of 2-nitropropane in humans have been reported. Inhalation of vapor is the only significant route of entry in humans, and it usually causes an initial headache and nausea. The substance cannot be recognized by odor until its concentration reaches about 160 ppm.[97] A report of four fatalities possibly attributed to 2-nitropropane has suggested that its toxic effects are underdiagnosed. Part of the problem is that it is rarely used alone as a solvent, and toxic effects are attributed to other chemicals used concurrently.[97] The clinical picture of hepatotoxicity resulting from 2-nitropropane includes acute fulminant hepatic failure with concurrent renal failure. The histologic findings include centrilobular necrosis of the liver, proliferation of bile ducts, cholestasis, steatosis, and mild inflammatory infiltrate in the periportal area. Recently, another report incriminated 2-nitropropane as a potent hepatotoxic agent.[98] Two construction workers applied an epoxy resin coating to a water main in an underground vault that was underventilated. No methods for protecting the respiratory tract or skin were employed. Analysis of sera from these individuals initially revealed 2-nitropropane concentrations of 13 μg/ml and 8.5 μg/ml, respectively, for each worker.[98] The former individual subsequently died of fulminant hepatic failure, whereas the latter individual survived.

Chlorinated nitroparaffins (1-chloro-1-nitroethane and 1-chloro-1-nitropropane) are known to produce steatosis in animals, and 1-1-dichloro-1-nitroethene has produced hemorrhagic centrizonal necrosis in animal models. No documented reports of human hepatotoxicity can be traced.

MUSHROOM POISONING

Mushroom poisoning occurs universally, especially in the fall season when people who are unfamiliar with the recognition of edible fungi harvest wild mushrooms and ingest them. About 90 per cent of the deaths due to mushroom poisoning in the United States and western Europe are attributed to the ingestion of *Amanita phalloides* (death cap). It is recognized by its olive green–brown cap, white gills, and white stem. The latter may have a greenish tinge and a broad volva or veil surrounding its base. Poisoning, at times fatal, can also occur following ingestion of mushrooms from the genera *Galerina, Russula,* and *Gyromitra.*[99, 100] The inhalation of the fumes produced from the genus *Gyromitra* can produce toxicity even without oral ingestion. The overall mortality rate following exposure to toxic mushrooms varies considerably. With recent advances in therapy, mortality rates range from 9.6 to 22.4 per cent for *Amanita.*[101, 102] Higher mortality rates of more than 50 per cent occur in children less than 10 years of age.[103] In the United States, *Amanita verna* (destroying angel) was the most common known cause of serious mushroom poisoning until 1970 when *Amanita phalloides* was identified for the first time.

Toxins and Pathophysiology

Wieland, and more recently, Faulstich in Wieland's laboratories in Heidelberg, Germany, have identified and established the structural formulae of the toxic cyclopeptides that cause poisoning by mushrooms.[103–108] Eight octapeptide amatoxins and seven hepapeptide phallotoxins and virotoxins have been isolated from mushrooms of the genus *Amanita* (Fig. 32–3). The amatoxins (of which the chief is α-amanitin) are cytotoxic, and five of them are among the most lethal toxins known. Usually the ingestion of one mushroom of *Amanita phalloides* results in severe poisoning, and three mushrooms (50 g) are usually a fatal dose, as they contain about 7 mg of amatoxins.[109] Wieland estimates that the lethal dose of amatoxins for humans is less than 0.1 mg/kg body weight.[109] The toxins bind to ribonucleic acid (RNA) polymerase B and inhibit the formation of messenger RNA thereby interfering with transcription of DNA.[110–115] This causes cellular necrosis, especially in cells that are exposed initially to the toxin and that have the most rapid rates of protein synthesis or turnover, or both—for example, cells in the gastrointestinal mucosa, hepatocytes, and the epithelial cells of the proximal convoluted tubule of the kidney. These effects are augmented because in the liver, the toxin is secreted into the bile and recycled via the enterohepatic circulation; in the kidney, the toxin is reabsorbed from the glomerular filtrate. The

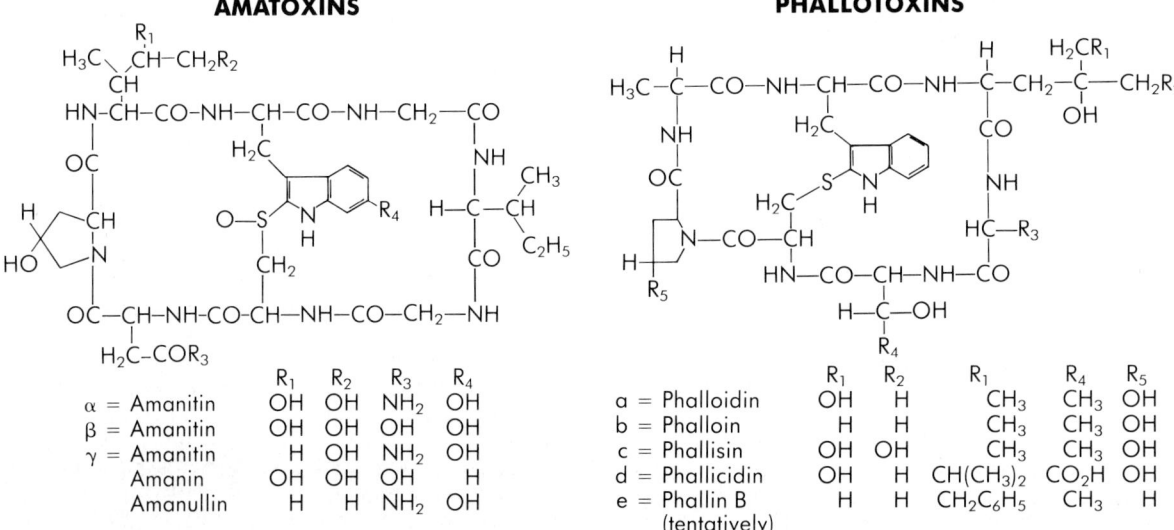

Figure 32–3. Structural formulae of (A) amatoxins and (B) phallotoxins. (Reproduced from Wieland T. Science 159:946, 1968, with permission. Copyright 1968 by the American Association for the Advancement of Science.)

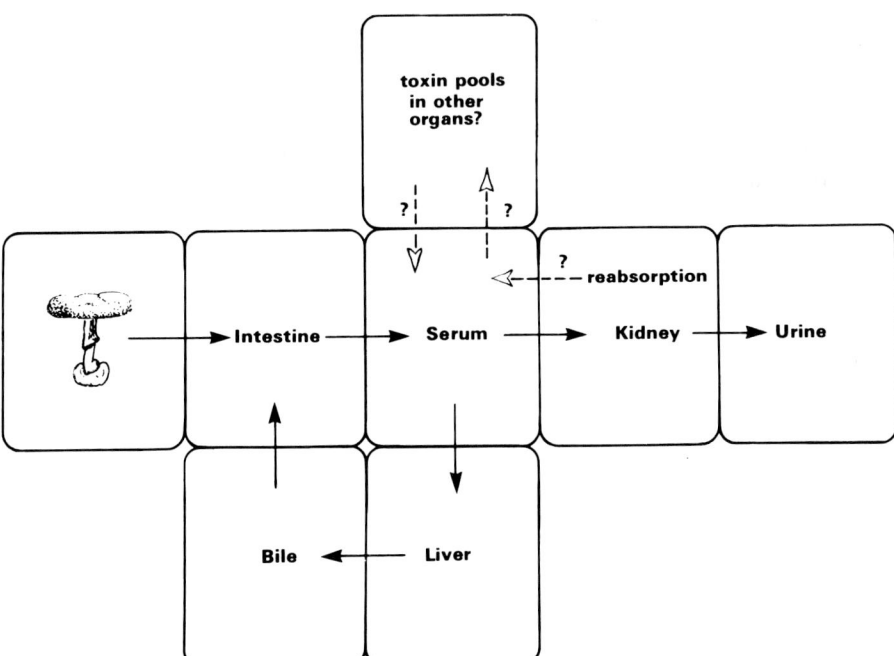

Figure 32–4. Pathways for metabolism of amatoxins during *Amanita* poisoning. (Reproduced from Faulstich H. Klin Wochenschr 57:1143, 1979, with permission.)

pathways for distribution of amatoxins during *Amanita* poisoning are shown in Figure 32–4. The concentration of amatoxin in the serum is dependent on several processes. Absorption from the gut and reabsorption through the enterohepatic circulation account for most of the concentration in serum. The kidney eliminates the major quantity of the toxin from the serum; it also may reabsorb some of the toxin. The molecular weight of α-amanitin is 900 kd. Preliminary evidence indicates that it does not cross the placenta even during the acute phase of intoxication.[116, 117]

The amatoxins are 10 to 20 times more toxic than the phallotoxins. The typical mechanism of the phallotoxins is shown by phalloidin, which acts on the polymerization-depolymerization cycle of actin, impairing the function of cell membranes.[118] Studies in vitro demonstrate that phalloidin increases the rate of polymerization of G-actin to F-actin and that it stabilizes polymerized actin. The actual contribution of each class of these two toxins to the clinical picture of poisoning by *Amanita phalloides* is still at issue. The phallotoxins probably are not absorbed from the gut, and according to Faulstich and Mitchel, the typical manifestations of *Amanita*-induced poisoning in humans are mainly (perhaps exclusively) caused by amatoxins.[110–119]

The virotoxins produce the same toxicologic symptoms as do the phallotoxins. They are not bicyclic peptides but monocyclic hepatopeptides.[108] The formulae and the variations of side chains leading to the six different virotoxins are shown in Figure 32–5. It is postulated that the virotoxins are derived from the phallotoxins or from a common precursor molecule. The toxicity of the virotoxins corresponds to that of the phallotoxins. They bind strongly to F-actin. Little is known about the mechanism of toxicity of the virotoxins.

Any eukaryotic cell can be damaged by amatoxin. However, the initial stage of the clinical picture is dominated by signs of damage to intestinal mucosa, and the later stages show mostly deterioration of hepatocyte function. Amatoxins enter hepatocytes more rapidly than other cell types. Since protein synthesis is active in hepatocytes,

these factors render them susceptible to the inhibitors of the transcription process.[119]

The hepatotoxicity attributed to *Gromitra esculenta* (false morel) is due to gyromitrin, which is hydrolyzed to monomethylhydrazine, which acts as a pyridoxine antagonist.[120]

Most of the toxins of poisonous mushrooms are thermostable, and many can persist for years after storage and desiccation.

Symptoms and Course

The characteristic course of poisoning by amatoxins has three stages. The first phase is delayed in onset, rarely commencing before 6 hours, and sometimes not until 24 hours, after ingestion of *Amanita*. Severe abdominal cramping, vomiting, and profuse cholera-like watery diarrhea occur for about 24 hours and may cause severe dehydration and hypotension. Next follows a phase of 24 to 36 hours, during which there is an apparent remission and abatement of the gastrointestinal symptoms. Abnormalities of liver enzymes become manifested during this phase. Finally, the third phase develops with its profound hepatic manifestations—jaundice, encephalopathy, hypoglycemia, hemorrhage, seizures, and coma. The mortality rate in patients in whom encephalopathy develops is very high.[120] Death usually occurs within a week and results from hepatic and renal failure with severe internal hemorrhagic manifestations and from the secondary effects on the cardiovascular and central nervous system. Studies of coagulation performed from the earliest phase of intoxication to the time of death or recovery in patients with *Amanita phalloides* poisoning have demonstrated a rapid, simultaneous fall in titers of all the clotting factors (except factor VIII), regardless of their individual biologic half-lives.[121] This unusual behavior was not due to increased fibrinolysis nor to disseminated intravascular coagulation. Its cause remains unexplained. A rise in fibrinogen and factor V levels and

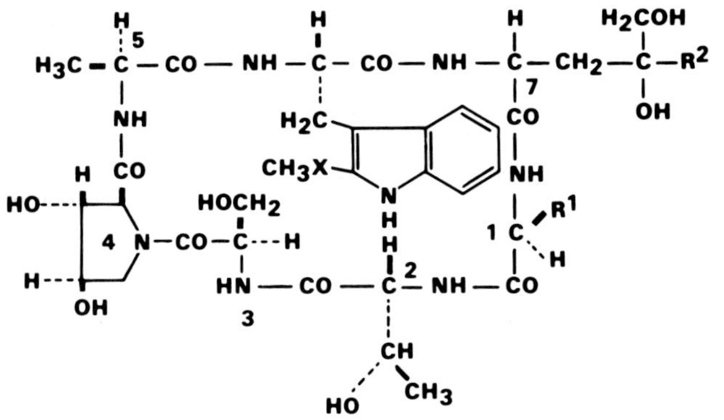

Name	X	R^1	R^2	Percent of total
Viroidin	SO$_2$	CH(CH$_3$)$_2$	CH$_3$	18
Desoxoviroidin	SO	CH(CH$_3$)$_2$	CH$_3$	4
Ala^1–viroidin	SO$_2$	CH$_3$	CH$_3$	
Ala^1–desoxoviroidin	SO	CH$_3$	CH$_3$	10
Viroisin	SO$_2$	CH(CH$_3$)$_2$	CH$_2$OH	49
Desoxoviroisin	SO	CH(CH$_3$)$_2$	CH$_2$OH	19

Figure 32–5. Structural formulae of the virotoxins. (Reprinted from Wieland T, Faulstich H. In: Keeler RF, Tu AT, eds. Handbook of Natural Toxins, Vol 1, 1983, by courtesy of Marcel Dekker, Inc.)

an increase in the prothrombin index are the earliest signs of recovery. If recovery occurs in the less serious cases, it may take as long as two to three weeks. However, recent evidence indicates that although poisoning by *Amanita phalloides* causes high mortality in the acute phase, it also ultimately causes chronic active hepatitis in some 20 per cent of survivors.[102, 122]

Hepatic Histologic Features

The histologic findings vary considerably, depending on the severity of the initial hepatic damage and the time interval following the ingestion of the hepatotoxic agent or agents. In mild liver damage, the histologic findings consist of vacuolated parenchymal degeneration and sporadic necrosis of hepatocytes.[102, 123, 124] Liver biopsies performed on the third day of illness in two patients who survived mushroom poisoning from *Amanita verna* revealed changes in both the periportal hepatocytes and the Kupffer cells. The hepatocytes contained fat droplets, karyolytic nuclei, and disrupted nucleoli. Electron microscopy of the latter showed paracrystalline inclusions. The cytoplasm showed mild fatty infiltration containing filamentous material. The sinusoids showed an increased prominence caused by swelling of the Kupffer cells (especially near the portal areas); occasional polymorphonuclear leukocytes were seen in the sinusoids. Another report of eight cases of nonfatal *Amanita phalloides* intoxication described a different histologic picture, with centrilobular necrosis, collapse, no initial significant inflammation, and no steatosis. Subsequently, mac-

rophages containing iron-positive ceroid pigment appeared in the necrotic area. The findings were fairly uniform and were typical but not specific.[125] In a recent large study of 64 patients with acute *Amanita* poisoning, biopsies were performed on the 15th day after the onset of symptoms in patients with mild or moderate hepatic dysfunction. Sinusoidal congestion was a major feature in the mild cases, and only sporadic necrotic cells were seen.[102]

The histologic findings in the severe, acute, and invariably fatal cases of *Amanita* hepatotoxicity show a fairly consistent morphologic picture, which contrasts distinctly with the preceding variable descriptions. The morphologic features are dominated by centrilobular necrosis, steatosis, sinusoidal congestion, and hemorrhagic necrosis.[102, 117] Experimental findings in animals given lethal doses of phalloidin by Agostini and co-workers have led these authors to consider the possibility that hepatic hemorrhage may be a crucial factor in precipating the hypovolemic shock encountered in these animals.[126–128]

The hepatic morphologic changes in patients surviving the acute phase of *Amanita* intoxication have been studied 6 to 12 months after apparent recovery from the acute phase.[102, 122] About 20 per cent of patients with initial acute *Amanita* intoxication and moderate or severe hepatic dysfunction (ALT levels > 1000 units and prolonged prothrombin activity levels) were subsequently found to have the histologic picture of chronic active hepatitis. A study of the serum transaminase levels in eight symptom-free patients was performed for 12 months after the original moderate or severe intoxication from *Amanita phalloides*. A fluctuating elevation of both AST and ALT levels was detected.

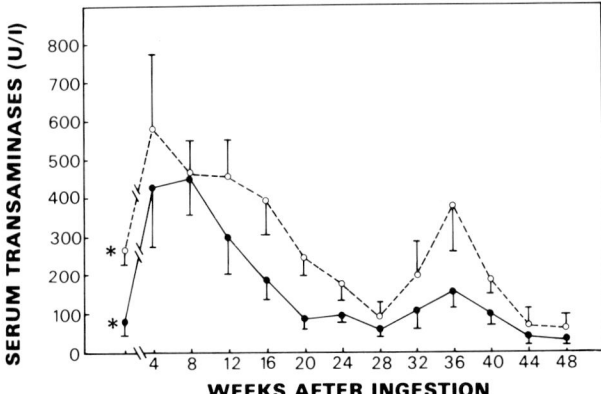

Figure 32–6. Twelve-month follow-up evaluation of serum transaminases in eight patients after *Amanita phalloides* poisoning. (Reproduced from Fantozzi R, et al. Klin Wochenschr 6:64, 1986, with permission.)

Means, SEM, * = transaminase values at time of discharge; open circles = ALT; closed circles = AST.

(Fig. 32–6)[122] Hepatic histologic features in these patients revealed a picture compatible with chronic active hepatitis at the six-month follow-up examination. A significant increase in plasma gamma globulin, as well as the presence of smooth muscle antibodies, cryoglobulins, and circulating immune complexes, characterized the group. The patients were free of serologic markers for hepatitis B virus. The authors postulated that severe but nonfatal *Amanita phalloides* poisoning eventually leads to chronic active hepatitis of the immunopathic variety in some of the survivors. The transaminase levels and prothrombin time appear to be the best indices of the initial severity of the liver disease and of the risk that asymptomatic chronic active hepatitis will eventually develop in survivors of the initial mushroom intoxication.[102, 122] *Amanita* poisoning presents a wide spectrum of hepatic histologic findings, ranging from massive hepatic necrosis to chronic active hepatitis. The results of a biopsy performed eight weeks after severe *Amanita* poisoning in a 5-year-old boy showed evidence suggestive of cirrhosis.[129]

Diagnosis

Apart from the obvious history of the ingestion of wild mushrooms and the possible identification of additional mushrooms by a qualified mycologist, the diagnosis requires an index of suspicion on the part of the physician. Definite confirmation of the diagnosis can be made by assaying gastric contents, blood, urine, and stool for α-amanitin by means of high-performance liquid chromatography (HPLC), thin-layer chromatography, or radioimmunoassay.[114, 116, 130, 131] As little as 10 ng is detectable by HPLC in serum samples from patients with *Amanita phalloides* poisoning.[131] The usual values for poisoning by α-amanitin are between 70 and 90 ng/ml.[131]

Management

Prevention of mushroom poisoning by avoiding the ingestion of wild, noncultivated mushrooms is a basic aim and goal. Widespread publicity about the need for extreme caution in identifying edible fungi is imperative. There are no visible signs on any mushroom that indicate with cer-

tainty whether it is toxic or not. A variety of instant home tests for determining the edibility of wild mushrooms has been offered. None is valid.

There is no specific antidote for the toxins of mushrooms. The major aim of therapy is to lower the serum concentration of the toxins as soon as possible and so shorten the period of exposure of highly susceptible cells (such as hepatocytes and renal tubular cells) to toxic levels. General measures should be initiated promptly regardless of the time interval following the ingestion of the toxins. The induction of vomiting (in the conscious patient with an intact gag reflex) or immediate gastric lavage is imperative. Thereafter the continuous aspiration of duodenal contents for 36 hours is advocated in order to remove any toxin recirculating via the enterohepatic circulation.[119, 132] Likewise the oral administration of activated charcoal in a dose of 60 to 100 g in adults and 30 to 60 g in children, repeated every 4 hours for 48 hours, is recommended in an endeavor to block the enterohepatic cycle of the toxins. If the patient is vomiting, the charcoal can be given through the distal port of a duodenal tube, and aspiration of the gastroduodenal fluid can be continued from the proximal port. Purgation with magnesium sulfate (adults, 30 g; children, 250 mg/kg) is also advisable. Intensive multisystem supportive measures may be required; they include correction of fluid and electrolyte imbalance, management of hepatic and renal failure, mechanical respiratory support, and administration of fresh frozen plasma to replace coagulation factors. Hemodialysis with activated charcoal hemoperfusion (to remove the mushroom toxin or toxins) is also advocated.[133] There were no deaths in eight patients who had ingested poisonous mushrooms (seven of whom had eaten a supposedly fatal dose) when this procedure was performed within 24 hours of ingestion. Hemodialysis and hemoperfusion have been advocated to enhance excretion of amatoxin.[119] Hemoperfusion may possibly prevent the cerebral edema associated with fulminant liver failure.[134, 135] Toxins of *Amanita* are easily dialyzed or adsorbed over charcoal or polymeric adsorbents.[136] However, plasma amanitin levels are very low in poisoning from *Amanita*, and they are not even near the experimental levels used to evaluate the kinetics of elimination. Often the amanitin levels are not measurable 14 hours after ingestion, suggesting that mushroom toxins have a high distribution volume, which would hamper any technique of blood purification.[137] Forced diuresis is effective in removing toxins from the blood, but there is a theoretic concern that it may increase renal toxicity.[114] However, patients with very high urinary levels of toxins measured by radioimmunoassay (as high as 57 ng/ml) showed no signs of renal impairment.[138] Large quantities of amatoxins (from 10,000 to 25,000 ng) were excreted in six patients treated with forced diuresis over a few hours.[138, 139] A high urinary flow rate achieves two goals: rapid reduction of the total body pool of amatoxins and a decrease in their urinary concentration, thus reducing the risk of renal toxicity.

Despite unimpressive clinical evidence of efficacy, various drugs have been and are being used in the treatment of intoxication by *Amanita phalloides*. Cytochrome *c* (its mechanism of protection is unknown), along with large doses of intravenous penicillin G (250 mg/kg/day), have been used.[102, 140, 141] The mechanism of action of penicillin is controversial. One hypothesis is that it displaces amatoxins from binding sites on plasma proteins, thus hastening renal excretion by glomerular filtration.[122, 141–143] This action is not supported by studies that fail to demonstrate significant binding of toxin to albumin.[144, 145] Other views are that penicillin inhibits the enterohepatic circulation of amatoxin and prevents the entry of toxin into hepatocytes or that sterilization of the bowel with resultant reduction of inhibitory neurotransmitters by enteric bacteria, underlies the utility of penicillin.[119] Silybin (20 to 50 mg/kg/day in divided doses), which is an active component of silymarin (a mixture of flavones found in the milk thistle *Silybum marianum*) is claimed to be antitoxic in animals and humans.[146, 147] Thioctic acid, vitamin C, bowel sterilization, and aggressive replacement of fluids and electrolytes are options favored by some. Thioctic acid (α-lipoic acid) a coenzyme for alpha-keto-dehydrogenases has been administered in the belief that it may be beneficial.[148–152] It has been credited in the United States and Europe with lowering the mortality rate. The dosage used is 50 to 150 mg administered intravenously every six hours. No well-controlled studies are available to prove or disprove the efficacy of therapy with thioctic acid. High doses of steroids (dexamethasone) are also advocated, but there are no experimental data to support their efficacy. In experimental intoxication with *Amanita phalloides*, ethanol has been shown to exert a favorable effect on the outcome.[153] Pretreatment of animals with antimicrobials and phenylbutazone afforded protection against amanitin hepatoxicity in mice.[154] Recently, orthotopic liver transplantation has been used successfully in the treatment of children with fulminant hepatic failure secondary to poisoning by *Amanita*.[129, 155]

A therapeutic protocol for *Amanita phalloides* poisoning, used extensively in Europe, follows the guidelines of Moroni and co-workers:

1. Correct fluid and electrolyte imbalance and acid-base status, and supply adequate glucose.

2. Administer activated charcoal orally and use continuous nasogastric aspiration.

3. Give intravenous dexamethasone, 20 to 40 mg daily, and intravenous thioctic acid, 500 mg daily.

4. Correct coagulation deficiencies with fresh frozen plasma and intravenous vitamin K₁, 40 mg daily.

5. Give penicillin G, 250 to 500 mg/kg daily, by continuous slow infusion.[141]

An American treatment protocol consists of (1) immediate dialysis; (2) electrolyte and fluid replacement; (3) administration of thioctic acid, 300 to 700 mg daily in intravenous glucose; (4) large doses of corticosteroids and cytochrome *c*; (5) emesis, catharsis, and activated charcoal therapy, especially if it is begun within six hours of the ingestion of toxin.[156]

HEPATOTOXIC METALS AND METALLOIDS IN HUMANS

Metals and metalloids rarely cause hepatotoxic effects in humans as a result of environmental or occupational contamination. Antimony, arsenic, beryllium, cadmium, chromium, copper, phosphorus, and thallium have on occasion proved to be hepatotoxic in humans. Iron, lead, mercury, and selenium may be responsible for human hepatotoxicity; however the evidence for this is not convincing. Hepatotoxicity by these agents in experimental models is more compelling.

Copper

Acute poisoning by copper is common in India, where it is ingested as a suicidal poison, or rarely it is ingested accidentally in amounts up to 100 g of copper sulfate.[157, 158]

In addition, hepatotoxic effects have been associated with the absorption of copper ions from the topical use of cupric sulfate, an astringent antiseptic.[159] Acute poisoning by copper becomes manifested as a metallic taste, nausea, repeated vomiting, and burning in the epigastrium in most patients. Diarrhea on the first day is common. Jaundice invariably occurred on the second or third day after ingestion in about a quarter of all patients reported in a study from India.[157] The authors also noted raised transaminase levels and hepatomegaly. Other findings of acute copper intoxication include shock, oliguria, anuria, hemoglobinuria, hematuria, melena, and coma (usually caused by renal failure). The jaundice is a combined result of the liver injury and its subsequent dysfunction together with the hemolysis of red blood cells, which is caused by the copper. Histologic findings include centrizonal hepatic necrosis, dilated central veins, cholestasis, bile thrombi in the liver, gastric mucosal erosions, and renal features of acute tubular necrosis with hemoglobin casts.[157, 160, 161] A significant relationship exists between the level of copper in blood and the severity of the disease process. The acute mortality rate was 14.6 per cent in one series.[157] Patients who died in the first 24 hours after poisoning exhibited shock. Later deaths were attributed to hepatic or renal complications. Management is largely supportive after attempts to remove the copper (gastric lavage) have been completed. There is no proof that corticosteroids or penicillamine are effective.

In view of the fact that absorbed copper is eventually excreted in the bile, it is not surprising that hepatic copper concentrations are high in chronic cholestatic conditions of the liver (see Chaps. 45 and 47).[162–169] The cause of the high hepatic copper concentration in Indian childhood cirrhosis is unknown. It may reflect high dietary intake of copper (from food stored or served in copper containers) in children with a genetic predisposition to excess copper retention.[166–168] The apparent familial pattern of Indian childhood cirrhosis (7 to 50 per cent of all cases) may only reflect a common familial pattern of exposure to copper.[167] Decreased hepatic levels of zinc and magnesium associated with high levels of copper have also been noted in Indian childhood cirrhosis. A secondary malabsorption of zinc and magnesium may account for these deficiencies. Supplementation with zinc has been suggested in the treatment of Wilson's disease, hepatic encephalopathy and, possibly, Indian childhood cirrhosis.[165]

Noncaseating hepatic granulomata containing copper inclusions have been reported in rural workers who used a copper solution to spray vineyards.[170] High amounts of copper have also been reported in the livers of patients with hepatocellular cancer.[171, 172]

Beryllium

Beryllium can cause multiple hepatic granulomata and a granulomatous disease resembling sarcoidosis.[173] Beryllium can be demonstrated in the granulomata by microemission spectrography.[174]

Iron

Acute accidental oral overdosage with iron in children has been associated with acute hepatic necrosis.[175] The patients manifest nausea, vomiting, gastrointestinal erosions, and bleeding. Shock ensues and may be fatal. In surviving patients, within three days jaundice, elevated transaminase levels, and a prolonged prothrombin time occur. Hepatic histologic characteristics show steatosis and periportal necrosis. The hepatic iron concentration is not strikingly increased.[176] Treatment is aimed at removal of the ingested iron by lavage and supportive measures. Desferrioxamine may be tried by the intravenous route to chelate and excrete excess iron; however, it may prove to be hazardous in its own right and induce shock in infants.[177] The administration of iron experimentally has not produced cirrhosis in animal models (see also Chap. 48).[178]

Phosphorus

The yellow form of phosphorus is extremely toxic, and as little as 60 mg may be fatal. Fortunately, poisoning by phosphorus is rare today. The course is often rapid, with death occurring within 24 hours of exposure. Occasionally it is less fulminant, with jaundice appearing on the fourth day; nevertheless, the overall mortality rate is 50 per cent. Diagnosis is suggested often by a garlic odor to the breath, the history, and phosphorescence of the stool and vomiting. There is no specific treatment. The histologic findings include a characteristic massive fatty infiltration (most evident in the periportal zone) and hepatic necrosis. Acute tubular necrosis and a fatty myocardium also occur.[179, 180] A long-term sequela in survivors includes periportal fibrosis.[181]

Antimony

Organic antimonials can cause steatosis in humans.[182] Whether or not they produce hepatic necrosis is debatable.[182] A newer antimony agent, stibocaptate, which is used in the treatment of schistosomiasis, leads to raised transaminase levels in two of three recipients. However, this appears to be reversible, and serious liver disease does not ensue.[183]

Thallium

Thallium can cause marked steatosis. However, the clinical picture is dominated by the neurologic manifestations of thallium intoxication.[184, 185] In rats, thallium chloride produced a dose-related loss of ribosomes from the endoplasmic reticulum, a proliferation of the rough endoplasmic reticulum, mitochondrial swelling, and an increase in the numbers of electron-dense autophagic lysosomes.[186] Thallium toxicity appears to arise from physical disruption of the membranes of subcellular organelles.

Lead

Lead intoxication is mostly a rare occupational hazard. It is encountered in children following the ingestion of lead from painted articles. Lead inhibits δ-aminolevulinic acid dehydratase (ALAD), causing a decrease in heme synthesis and an increase in δ-aminolevulinic acid synthetase (ALAS) activity. The net result is an increase in concentrations of δ-aminolevulinic acid (ALA) in blood and urine (see Chap. 14). ALA excretion in the urine is used as a screening test for lead poisoning, but it is relatively insensitive at low levels of lead intoxication.[187] Hepatotoxicity caused by inorganic lead was reported from Oviedo, Spain, where 85 patients were evaluated for lead toxicity.[188] The blood lead

threshold for hepatotoxicity was 75 to 80 μg/dl. Fifty per cent of patients with acute lead poisoning showed liver damage only when blood levels of lead exceeded 100 μg/dl. The histologic picture was that of a mild centrilobular hepatitis with fatty infiltration and deposition of hemosiderin. A rapid resolution of the liver disease occurred once the exposure to lead was terminated. Liver function tests did not correlate well with the extent of the hepatotoxicity; markers for lead (blood lead levels, urinary lead excretion, ALAD inhibition) were the best indices of hepatotoxicity.

Cadmium

There is abundant evidence that cadmium is hepatotoxic in experimental animals. Cadmium produces a wide spectrum of hepatotoxic effects, ranging from minor derangement of hepatic function to necrosis or cirrhosis.[189-194] In animals, cadmium-induced hepatotoxicity causes condensation of chromatin, with subsequent disturbance of ribosomal RNA synthesis.[195, 196] Increased hepatic levels of cadmium in Japanese subjects may be implicated in the genesis of cryptogenic liver disease.[191]

EPPING JAUNDICE (METHYLENEDIANILINE, MDA)

An epidemic of toxic hepatic damage was reported from Epping, England in 1965.[197, 198] Bread baked from flour contaminated with the aromatic amine methylenedianiline (an agent used in the manufacture of epoxy resin) was ingested, and it caused a cholestatic hepatitis in 84 people. Symptoms of the initial intoxication varied from abdominal pain, fever, rigors, and rash in 60 per cent of patients, to minimal or no symptoms in 33 per cent of affected patients. In 6 per cent of patients, jaundice was the initial complaint. Biochemical changes varied; most patients had moderately elevated serum bilirubin and alkaline phosphatase levels, but a number of patients had unexpectedly high transaminase levels. This unique mixed cholestatic-hepatocellular type of injury was also seen on histologic examination, in which bile stasis, variable hepatocyte necrosis, and a portal inflammatory infiltrate were commonly encountered.[198] Parenchymal inflammation was also evident, though to a lesser degree. The patients recovered usually after two or more weeks, although two patients had severe jaundice for three months. Two years after the exposure, a minority of patients had nonspecific symptoms of fatigue, irritability, depression, and fat intolerance. A slightly elevated level of aspartate transaminase was evident in six patients.[199]

A subsequent report of the hepatotoxicity that resulted from exposure to methylenedianiline revealed a similar acute clinical picture without detectable residual liver disease.[200] This was the first report of methylenedianiline causing a toxic hepatitis from an occupational exposure. Subsequently, there have been two reports of a reversible toxic hepatitis in workers handling an epoxy resin hardened by the addition of methylenedianiline powder.[201, 202] All the patients recovered without any apparent sequelae. Reexposure to methylenedianiline in two workers resulted in a recurrence of hepatitis.[201] The mechanism of hepatic injury associated with methylenedianiline is unknown. It is of unusual interest because it produces a predictable dosedependent direct hepatotoxicity that manifests as intrahepatic cholestasis and hepatocellular necrosis. The reports of hepatitis resulting from industrial exposure to methylenedianiline highlight the need for strict safety procedures in its use. Toxic manifestations follow its ingestion, inhalation, or absorption through the skin.

TOXIC RAPESEED OIL

A massive intoxication of tens of thousands of people occurred in Spain in 1981 following the consumption of adulterated rapeseed oil.[203] The syndrome was referred to as the toxic-epidemic syndrome. More than 350 people died. The causal agent was unidentified. The disease had a biphasic course. Initially, there was acute multisystem involvement with fever, arthralgia, rash, myalgia, conjuctivitis, digestive symptoms, and abdominal or chest pain, or both. Eosinophilia, raised levels of transaminases, alkaline phosphatase, γ-glutamyl transpeptidase, and IgE were commonly found. The majority of patients survived this phase. Three to 18 months after the attack episode, a third of the patients who survived the initial toxicity developed scleroderma, sicca (Sjögren's) syndrome, alopecia, pulmonary hypertension and respiratory failure.[204–206] Hepatic involvement occurred in 24.1 per cent of the victims, especially women in the fourth decade of life.[203] Most of the patients (91.6 per cent) with hepatic injury were asymptomatic. Elevation of γ-glutamyl transpeptidase was universal, and elevated alkaline phosphatase and transaminase levels were common. The bilirubin concentration was normal in the majority of patients. Histologic features included hepatocyte degeneration, cholestasis, a mixed cellular infiltration with a high eosinophil component, and acidophilic bodies—all similar to a drug-induced cholestatic hepatitis. Electron microscopy revealed lamellar inclusions, canalicular injury, giant mitochrondria, and hyperplastic smooth endoplasmic reticulum. Death from liver disease occurred in only one patient who had the Budd-Chiari syndrome and acute liver failure. Long-term histologic reassessment 30 months after the initial poisoning has shown that the eventual prognosis could be forecast according to the initial biochemical abnormalities.[204] Those patients with an initial transient elevation of transaminase levels recovered within two months. Those with initially raised transaminase and alkaline phosphatase levels mostly recovered or had evidence of a mild ongoing hepatitis. Of the patients who initially had jaundice, half continued to have an abnormal liver biochemistry profile at 30 months, and their histologic picture was suggestive of chronic biliary disease with cholestasis and a reduction in the septal biliary ducts. Many of these patients also had evidence of scleroderma, and there was an increased incidence of HLA-DR3 and HLA-DR4 among them.[207] This favors the hypothesis that the initial phase of toxicity was a direct toxic effect, whereas the secondary late phase was due to an autoimmune mechanism induced by the initial exposure to the toxin.

HEXACHLOROBENZENE

Hexachlorobenzene, a fungicide, contaminated grain and wheat in Turkey and caused a massive outbreak of porphyria cutanea tarda and liver disease with a significant mortality rate.[208, 209]

TANNIC ACID

Tannic acid was used in medicine for the treatment of burns and as a diagnostic material added to barium (it promoted barium to stick to the colonic mucosa, enhancing the diagnostic potential of the barium). Concentrations as high as 2 per cent tannic acid were used and resulted in hepatic necrosis, especially in patients with inflammatory bowel disease.[210] Tannic acid is no longer used for radiologic evaluation of the gut.

SUBACUTE LIVER DISEASE

COCAINE

Marks and Chapple first suggested that cocaine may be hepatotoxic in humans when they reported high transaminase levels and jaundice in chronic cocaine abusers.[211] Their observations did not conclusively incriminate cocaine as a hepatotoxic agent; but subsequent work in animals clearly implicated cocaine as a potent hepatotoxin when administered either acutely or chronically.[212]

Cocaine is a potent hepatotoxin in mice, causing fatty metamorphosis and necrosis with high serum transaminase levels.[212–216] It is converted in the liver by the hepatic microsomal enzymes cytochrome P450 and flavin adenine dinucleotide (FAD) containing mono-oxygenase to the active hepatotoxic metabolite norcocaine nitroxide.[217–220]

Cocaine is demethylated (or N-oxidized followed by demethylation) to produce norcocaine, which is rapidly oxidized to N-hydroxynorcocaine. This, in turn, is metabolized to norcocaine nitroxide (Fig. 32–7). This free radical is believed to be responsible for the hepatotoxicity of cocaine.

Cocaine → norcocaine → N-hydroxynorcocaine
$\qquad\qquad\qquad\qquad\qquad$ → norcocaine nitroxide

The mechanism of cocaine hepatotoxicity is due to the free radicals generated by this oxidative pathway (see Chap. 30).[221, 222] Ultrastructural changes noted in acute cocaine

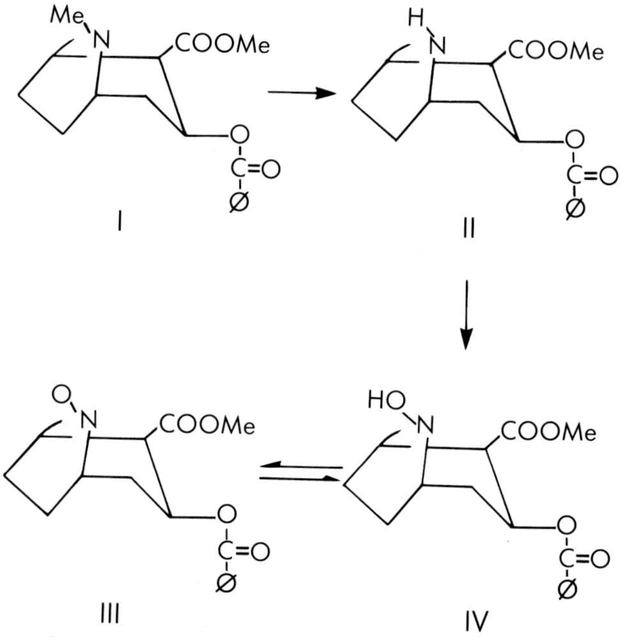

Figure 32–7. The structure of cocaine and its metabolites. (Reproduced from Rauckman EJ, et al. Mol Pharmacol 21:458, 1982, with permission.) I = cocaine; II = norcocaine; III = N-hydroxynorcocaine; IV = norcocaine nitroxide.

hepatotoxicity include dilation of rough endoplasmic reticulum, swelling of mitochondria, disruption of membranes, and changes in size, shape, and histochemical composition of peroxisomes.[213] In studies with mice, cimetidine effectively prevented cocaine-induced hepatic necrosis.[223] A plausible mechanism for this observed protection is that cimetidine interferes with cytochrome P450–mediated activation of the parent compound. Ethanol and barbiturates enhance cocaine-induced hepatotoxicity as has pretreatment of mice with diethyl maleate.[217, 224] The latter depletes intracellular glutathione.[221] The ethanol- and barbiturate-induced potentiation of cocaine-induced hepatotoxicity appears dependent on induction of hepatic cytochrome P450.

PYRROLIZIDINE (SENECIO)

Cattle in Nova Scotia were the first animals to be studied for the hepatic sequelae of veno-occlusive disease.[225, 226] The disease was recognized in humans in 1920 in South Africa. Since then it has been reported sporadically in widely scattered parts of the world.[227] It is endemic in the West Indies, and massive outbreaks have been reported from Ecuador, India, and Afghanistan. Isolated cases have occurred in the United States and in the United Kingdom.[228-233] Poisoning in humans has occurred by the contamination of cereals, barley, or bread and by the use of poisonous plants in traditional medicines or in bush tea. Most of the cases occurring in Jamaica were in children.[234-237]

The structure and ring numbering of pyrrolizidine is shown in Figure 32–8.[238] Two five-membered rings share a common nitrogen at position 4. All the toxic alkaloids are derivatives of 1-hydroxymethyl-1:2 dehydropyrrolizidine (see Fig. 32–8, II). The three essential requirements for hepatotoxicity are (1) the presence of a double bond at 1:2, (2) the presence of an ester group on the nucleus, and (3) at least one of the ester side chains must contain a branched carbon chain.[238] More than a hundred toxic pyrrolizidines have been identified. The mechanism of their hepatotoxic action is unknown, but they injure the hepatic microvessels. Hepatocyte RNA polymerase activity is decreased, which

is associated with a drop in the synthesis of RNA and DNA.[238] Single doses of pyrrolizidine alkaloids have a lasting effect in some tissues, especially in the liver. Affected cells accumulate nuclear chromatin and enlarge but fail to divide. The quantitative assay of pyrrolizidine alkaloids is by a colorimetric technique.[239]

Clinical Features of Pyrrolizidine Hepatotoxicity

The initial reports of poisoning from pyrrolizidine alkaloids in humans commented on its clinical similarity to the Budd-Chiari syndrome.[227, 240] The clinical syndrome associating hepatic damage secondary to pyrrolizidine alkaloid ingestion is that of veno-occlusive disease. Acute, subacute, and chronic hepatic injury in humans has been documented. *Acute veno-occlusive disease* is characterized by the rapid development of abdominal discomfort, often gross hepatomegaly, and ascites.[234, 237, 241] The liver is smooth, firm, and tender. Mild jaundice may be evident, and slight splenomegaly and edema of the legs may occur. Pleural effusions are not uncommon. The presence of collateral venous channels over the abdomen becomes manifested rapidly. There are no specific biochemical changes. Levels of transaminases are modestly elevated. Albumin levels are low (possibly reflecting previous underlying malnutrition). The levels of cholinesterase in sera tend to be low. The bilirubin is raised marginally.[237] The protein content of ascitic fluid is moderately increased (usually 2.0 to 2.5 g/dl). The duration of the acute phase varies from two to eight weeks, the average being four weeks.[237] The outcome is recovery, subacute or chronic disease, or fulminant hepatic failure. In the acute phase, the diagnosis is made from the history, the suggestive clinical picture, and the liver biopsy results.[237, 238] Rarely, pyrrolizidine intoxication in infants may appear to mimic Reye's syndrome.[242] The mean cumulative dose of alkaloids ingested prior to the development of acute hepatic veno-occlusive disease in three young Chinese women was estimated to be 18 mg/kg.[243]

Subacute veno-occlusive disease may develop imperceptibly from the acute phase or de novo from the onset.[237]

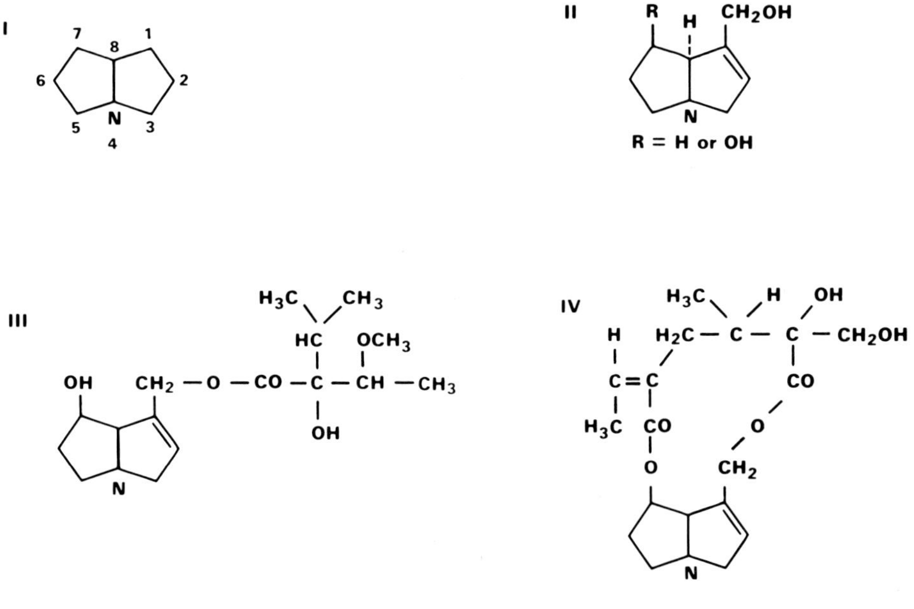

Figure 32–8. The structure and ring numbering of pyrrolizidine is shown in I. All toxic alkaloids are derivatives of the structure shown in II and are esters. Some are open esters, for example, heliotrine (III), and others are ring esters, for example, retrorsine (IV).

The patient is often asymptomatic, and the main findings are persistent hepatomegaly, varying quantities of ascitic fluid, and sometimes splenomegaly. The subacute phase may last months and may be punctuated by acute episodes similar to those described previously. Subacute disease may ultimately resolve, or more frequently it passes subclinically into the chronic stage of the disease.

Chronic veno-occlusive disease is characterized by cirrhosis that is often indistinguishable from that of other causes.[237] The cirrhosis can develop extremely rapidly; in one instance, marked cirrhosis was detected from a biopsy specimen three months after an initial biopsy was performed. The first biopsy specimen showed venous occlusion but no fibrosis.[237] In children, chronic veno-occlusive disease is associated frequently with an abdominal wall venous hum (Cruveilhier-Baumgarten syndrome).[237] Its occurrence and frequency may be an indication of the degree of venous obstruction and the ability of younger patients to form an extensive collateral circulation. Episodes of exacerbation with acute hepatic necrosis may occur in chronic disease. Chronic veno-occlusive disease is usually a sequel to the original acute intoxication; rarely, it is the result of chronic or repeated ingestion of the toxic alkaloid.[234, 237, 238, 244-246] A case report consistent with chronic pyrrolizidine intoxication causing veno-occlusive disease estimated that over a six-month period the patient consumed a minimum of 85 mg of pyrrolizidine alkaloids (15 µg/kg body weight/day).[246] The possible role of pyrrolizidine intoxication in the genesis of primary carcinoma of the liver in humans is debated.[238, 241, 245, 247]

Factors predisposing to the development of veno-occlusive disease are poorly understood and controversial. It is more common in children of all ages, except for those being breast fed.[237] This may be a reflection of an increased suspectibility in protein-malnourished children or of an increased risk of exposure in youth, or of an increased absolute dosage ingested by the young. Experimental attempts to clarify the role of nutrition in the genesis of the toxicity of alkaloids have produced conflicting and inconclusive results.[238, 245, 248] There is no evidence that protein deficiency causes a change in pyrrolizidine metabolism that leads to the production of toxic metabolites. In poorer socioeconomic societies, children may be exposed to larger absolute amounts of pyrrolizidine alkaloids because of the administration of bush tea or herbal medicine as a treatment for teething, gastroenteritis, or other illnesses or because their staple diet consists of mostly wheat or bread contaminated with pyrrolizidine alkaloids.[234, 237, 238, 241] Veno-occlusive disease has been reported less frequently in adults than in children.[227, 234, 237]

Histologic Features

In the acute stage of the disease, massive centrilobular sinusoidal congestion and necrosis are evident.[225, 238, 240, 249] The central hepatic veins show an endophlebitis obliterans hepatica, with uniform involvement throughout the liver (see Chap. 23). The main hepatic veins are normal. There is a concentric swelling of the subintimal tissues, consisting of edematous reticulated tissue containing fibrin and a few inflammatory cells. Also, there is congestion of the sinusoids, fatty infiltration, and variable necrosis of the centrilobular hepatocytes.[234, 238, 240] Necrosis varies in its intensity. In the later, chronic stages, reticular collagenous tissue is laid down. Ultimately fibrosis ensues. It is primarily non-

portal central fibrosis similar to that seen in the Budd-Chiari syndrome or in cardiac cirrhosis. As the fibrosis progresses, it produces ischemia of other hepatocytes, and the end result is the development of cirrhosis and a finely granular to nodular macroscopic appearance.[237] Megalocytosis (giant hepatocytes that are 10 to 20 times the normal size) is a striking feature of pyrrolizidine alkaloid hepatotoxicity.[250] They reflect the antimitotic action of the alkaloids on the hepatocytes, which permits growth but not cell division.[238, 250, 251] The cells contain a large nucleus, multiple centrioles, excess rough endoplasmic reticulum, and a disarray of organization of the cytoplasmic organelles.[250]

Treatment and Prognosis

There is no specific treatment available. Prophylaxis is a basic ground rule. Education of population groups regarding the hazards of alkaloids is an essential goal. In the acute phase of the illness, symptomatic treatment is the rule. The role of anticoagulants is not established. In an analysis of the prognosis following an acute attack of pyrrolizidine alkaloid–induced hepatotoxicity, Stuart and Bras noted that half their patients recovered completely from the acute attack, 20 per cent died of liver failure in the acute attack, and the remaining 30 per cent went on to a subacute form of veno-occlusive disease.[237] Two thirds of the patients who developed subacute illness ultimately had a complete resolution of their disease, and one third (10 per cent of the original group) had a progression to cirrhosis and died from bleeding varices. The overall total mortality rate for the acute illness was thus 30 per cent. Adult patients appear to have a worse prognosis than do children.[237] Death in the acute phase is caused most frequently by fulminant hepatic failure. In the chronic illness, death is caused mostly by the sequelae of portal hypertension.[237] Acute disease may evolve rapidly to chronic disease, with cirrhosis developing in as little as three months after initial exposure.[237]

CHRONIC LIVER DISEASE

AFLATOXINS

Since the recognition in England in 1960 that an epidemic of acute hemorrhagic hepatic necrosis (turkey X disease) in turkey poults, ducklings, and pheasants was caused by the contamination of their Brazilian peanut meal by metabolites of the fungus *Aspergillus flavus*, there has been extensive study of the hepatotoxic and hepatocarcinogenic effects of the aflatoxins.[252-254] The toxins produced by the fungus were designated *aflatoxins* from the contraction of *A. flavus* toxin. The aflatoxins are furanocoumarins. There are 12 naturally occurring parent forms and their metabolites. Some synthetic forms have been identified. Various thin-layer chromatography procedures for analysis of aflatoxins are available but are of limited usefulness, as they are semiquantitative and not automated. A reverse-phase HPLC analysis using post-column derivatization for enhancement of fluorescence appears promising.[255]

Aflatoxins have been classified into two major groups—aflatoxin B (AFB) and aflatoxin G (AFG) according to their chemical structure, fluorescence, and rate and position of migration on chromatography (Fig. 32–9).[256] AFB_1 is the most common aflatoxin contaminant found in

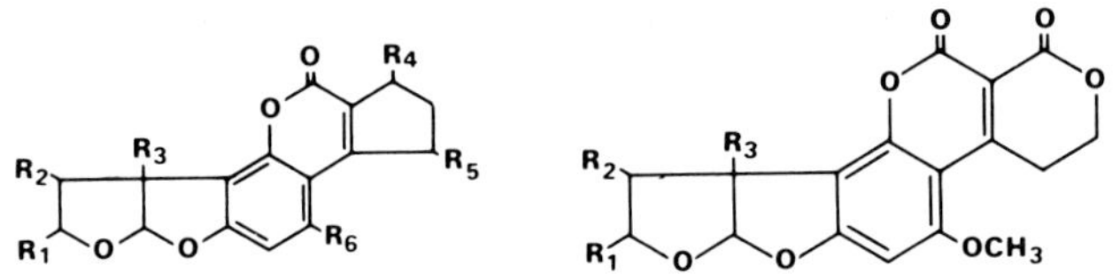

Figure 32–9. Structures of aflatoxins. A, AFB series of aflatoxins. B, the AFG series of aflatoxins. (Reproduced from Wogan GN. In: Okuda K, Peters RL, eds. Hepatocellular Carcinoma. New York, John Wiley & Sons, 1976:25, with permission.)

	R₁	R₂	R₃	R₄	R₅	R₆			R₁	R₂	R₃
B₁	H	H	H	=O	H	OCH₃		G₁	H	H	H
B₂	H₂	H₂	H	=O	H	OCH₃		G₂	H₂	H₂	H
B₂ₐ	HOH	H₂	H	=O	H	OCH₃		G₂ₐ	OH	H₂	H
M₁	H	H	OH	=O	H	OCH₃		GM₁	H	H	OH
M₂	H₂	H₂	OH	=O	H	OCH₃					
P₁	H	H	H	=O	H	OH					
Q₁	H	H	H	=O	OH	OCH₃					
R₀	H	H	H	OH	H	OCH₃					

food. It is also the most hepatotoxic and hepatocarcinogenic of the aflatoxins.²⁵⁷ The liver is the major organ affected most often by aflatoxins, and hepatocellular cancer is the most frequent neoplasm. Aflatoxin is estimated to be 1000-fold more carcinogenic than any other known agent.²⁵⁸ Occasionally malignancy associated with ingestion of aflatoxin may develop in the kidney and other organs.²⁵⁹ The *Aspergillus flavus* mould has been identified as a contaminant of a variety of nuts (especially peanuts and cashews), corn, wheat, barley, rice, cottonseed, and soy beans. It has been found in bread, milk, and cheese and in the soil. Circumstances favoring the production of the toxins include a warm and moist environment. Hence the greatest prevalence of contamination of foods by aflatoxin is in the tropics.²⁵⁶ Aflatoxin-induced acute hepatotoxicity in humans has followed the ingestion of contaminated maize, soybeans, and cassava.²⁶⁰ Minimal amounts of aflatoxin are commonly present in peanut butter and cows' milk, and many people regularly ingest aflatoxins in various concentrations.²⁶¹,²⁶² The metabolism of aflatoxins in mammals is in the liver. AFB₁ is metabolized by the microsomal mixed-function oxidase system to a variety of metabolites.²⁶³ The excretion of the parent molecule or metabolites is in the urine and milk. At present in the United States, the Food and Drug Administration permits a maximum aflatoxin level of 20 parts/billion (ppb) in peanut products ingested by the public. Stricter control has been advocated, and the risk of liver cancer at various aflatoxin exposures has been estimated (Table 32–2).²⁶⁴

Mechanism of Hepatotoxicity

Hepatic injury results from the rapid impairment of nucleic acid synthesis.²⁶⁵ In experimental models, there is a 90 per cent inhibition of the synthesis of RNA within 15 minutes of the administration of a lethal dose of AFB₁.²⁶⁵⁻²⁶⁷ This is associated with a marked inhibition of RNA polymerase, possibly because of the effect of aflatoxin on the chromatin template.²⁶⁵⁻²⁶⁷ The adverse effect of aflatoxin is thought to result from an interaction with nuclear chromatin rather than directly with RNA polymerase.²⁶⁵ The hepatic injury is mediated by active metabolites bearing hydroxyls at the R₁, R₃, R₄, and R₆ positions in AFB₁ and of AFG₁ (Fig. 32–9). Hepatotoxicity and carcinogenicity may be produced by different metabolites.²⁶⁵

Factors Influencing Susceptibility

Newborn and young animals are the most susceptible to toxicity. Considerable species differences in susceptibility exist, with ducklings, rabbit, and turkey poults being the most vulnerable and mice and sheep being the most resistant species.²⁵² Male animals are more susceptible to the hepatotoxic and carcinogenic effects of AFB₁.²⁵²,²⁶⁰ A reduced protein diet enhances the acute hepatotoxicity of AFB₁ in rats.²⁶⁸,²⁶⁹ Choline deficiency in rats reduces the hepatotoxicity of a single dose, but it enhances the toxicity and carcinogenicity of repeated doses.²⁷⁰ Malnutrition thus may be a factor in the genesis of cancer of the liver by virtue of enhancing the carcinogenic effects of aflatoxin. The effects of aflatoxins on animals are dose related. In

TABLE 32–2. RISK ESTIMATES OF LIVER CANCER AT VARIOUS AFLATOXIN EXPOSURES BASED ON A MODIFIED PEERS-LINSELL RELATIONSHIP*

Dietary Aflatoxin Level (ppb)	Crude Incidence Rate of Liver Cancer†	Predicted No. of Liver-Cancer Cases/Year
0.001	0.00265	5.8
0.005	0.01325	29.2
0.010	0.0265	58.3
0.050	0.1325	292
0.100	0.265	583
0.250	0.6625	1415
0.50	1.325	2915
1.0	2.65	5830

*Source: Reprinted with permission from Dichter CR, Risk estimates of liver cancer due to aflatoxin exposure from peanuts and peanut products. Copyright 1984, Pergamon Press plc. Food Chem Toxicol 22(6):431.
†Rate above background/100,000 persons/year. (Estimated United States, population = 220 million.)
A dietary aflatoxin level of 1.0 ppb is considered to be equivalent to 25 ng aflatoxin/kg body weight.

TABLE 32–3. AFLATOXIN INGESTION AND HEPATOMA INCIDENCE*

Country	Locale	Aflatoxin Intake (ng/kg/day)	Hepatoma Rate (per 10^5/year)
Kenya	High altitude	3.5	1.2
Thailand	Songkhla	5.0	2.0
Swaziland	Highveld	5.1	2.2
Kenya	Mid-altitude	5.9	2.5
Swaziland	Midveld	8.9	3.8
Kenya	Low altitude	10.0	4.0
Swaziland	Lebombo	15.4	4.3
Thailand	Ratburi	45.0	6.0
Swaziland	Lowveld	43.1	9.2
Mozambique	Inhambane	222.4	13.0

*Source: From Linsell CA, Peers FG. Trans R Soc Trop Med Hyg 71:471, 1977, with permission.

humans, the estimated aflatoxin intake from foods contaminated with the agent correlates with the frequency of primary liver cancer (Table 32–3).[271] A new role has been postulated for aflatoxin in the production of liver cancer. Rather than acting as a primary carcinogen, aflatoxins may act as cocarcinogens with hepatitis B virus. They may suppress the patient's cell-mediated immune response. This may increase the hepatitis B carrier rate, leading to chronic infection with hepatitis B virus, and the development of cirrhosis, and it may enhance the risk of eventually developing primary liver cancer.[272]

Hepatic Manifestations

Acute Hepatic Injury. Acute hepatotoxicity in animals secondary to aflatoxin exposure results in varying degrees of fatty infiltration, necrosis, bile duct duplication, inflammatory infiltrates, and congestion.[265] Histologic changes vary among species. The necrosis is mostly periportal in the turkey poult, rat, and cat. It is central in the pig, dog, and guinea pig and midzonal in the rabbit.[252, 273–276] Steatosis may be evident. In the monkey, the lesion simulates the histologic picture encountered in humans with Reye's syndrome.[277–278] Instances of Reye's syndrome in children have been associated with aflatoxin poisoning and aflatoxins have been detected in the livers of patients dying of Reye's syndrome.[277–281, 282, 283]

In humans, fulminant hepatic necrosis has complicated the ingestion of food contaminated with aflatoxins.[284] A mass intoxication of patients with aflatoxin-contaminated maize resulted in 106 fatalities among 397 exposed individuals in India.[260] The patients manifested fever, nausea, vomiting, and anorexia, followed by jaundice. They rapidly developed ascites, low serum albumin levels, edema of the legs, and portal hypertension. Males were affected more frequently than were females; infants were not affected. Death was usually from massive gastrointestinal bleeding. Hepatic coma was rare. Histologic examination of the liver revealed prominent proliferation of bile ducts, periductal fibrosis, and bile stasis. Hepatocytes usually were normal, apart from occasional multinuclear giant cells and hepatocytes with foamy cytoplasms. Acute aflatoxicosis thus appears to be a definite entity in humans.

Chronic Hepatic Injury. Cirrhosis has been induced in some animals after repeated exposure to aflatoxins.[275] In cattle, veno-occlusive lesions similar to those caused by

pyrrolidizone alkaloids may occur.[275, 285] Usually bile duct proliferation is the dominant morphologic change, and inflammation is usually sparse. Megalocytosis can develop in certain animal species. The evidence for chronic liver disease in humans resulting from repeated ingestion of aflatoxins is inconclusive. Unexplained cryptogenic cirrhosis and childhood cirrhosis in developing countries may be attributed in part to aflatoxin toxicity, but the evidence is not compelling. Further epidemiologic studies are necessary to clarify this vexing issue.[286]

The carcinogenic potential of aflatoxins and their metabolites is the most serious sequel to their effects on the human liver. Extensive studies in animals clearly indicate a high incidence of hepatic carcinoma.[287] Isolated reports have demonstrated levels of AFB_1 in the serum of patients with primary hepatic cancer.[288, 289] Epidemiologic studies point to an association between the quantity of ingested aflatoxin (from contaminated food) and the incidence of hepatocellular cancer in Africa (Fig. 32–10; Table 32–3).[271, 290–292] This epidemiologic evidence in humans and the conclusive evidence in animals indicating a hepatocarcinogenic role for aflatoxins support the hypothesis that aflatoxins, either alone or in combination with other oncogenic agents, are carcinogenic in humans.[293] Reports of hepatic cancer induced by aflatoxins in nonhuman primates further reinforces the concept of their carcinogenetic effects on the human liver.[256, 294]

It is ironic that aflatoxin is likely to contaminate the diet of humans in areas in which protein deficiency is rife and that its carcinogenic action is enhanced by the suppression of hepatic microsomal hydroxylation attendant upon protein deficiency.

PESTICIDES

Organochlorine Pesticides

The term *pesticide* includes herbicides, insecticides, and fungicides. They have different chemical structures and their toxicity varies. Millions of kilograms of pesticides

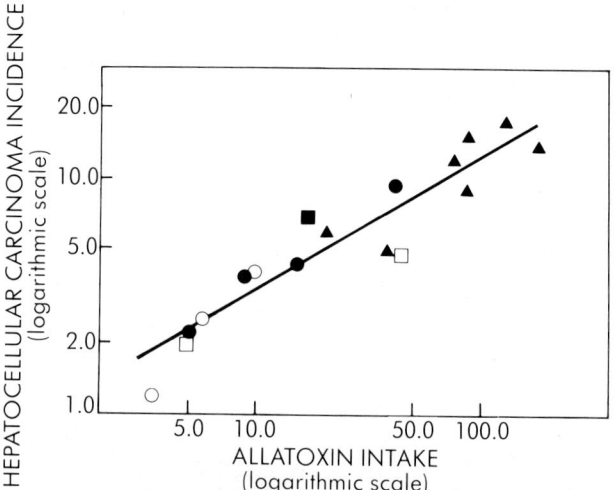

Figure 32–10. The relationship between dietary aflatoxin B exposure and the hepatocellular carcinoma rate (using a double logarithmic scale). (Reproduced from Van Rensberg SJ, et al. Br J Cancer 51:713, 1985, with permission.)
r = 0.95; P = <0.001; ○ = Kenya; □ = Thailand; ▲ = Mozambique; ● = Swaziland; ■ = Transkei.

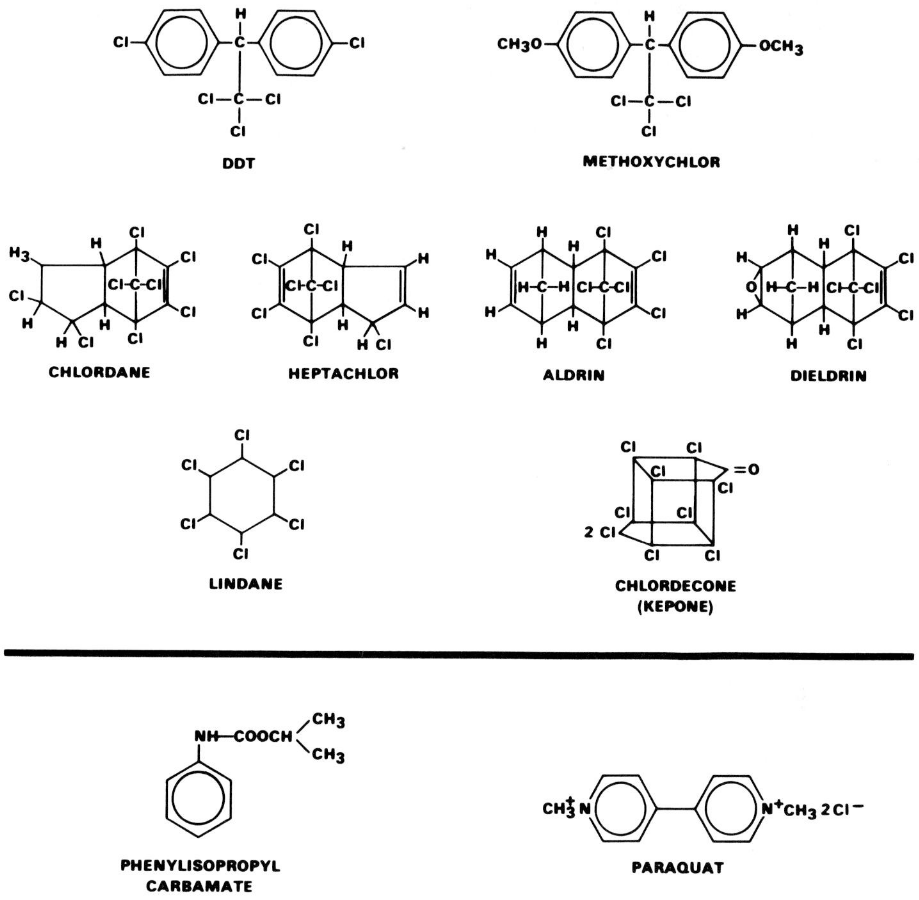

Figure 32-11. The structure of more commonly used pesticides. (Reproduced from Zimmerman HJ. Hepatotoxicity. New York, Appleton-Century-Crofts, 1978:313, with permission.)

have been produced and used, especially in agriculture. Consequently there has been considerable environmental pollution by these agents. Dichlorodiphenyltrichloroethane (DDT), the best known organochlorine compound, exhibits the properties of stability, nonvolatility, and slow biodegradability, which result in its persistence in the environment. Residual DDT has been detected in the environment a decade after a single application.[295, 296] The potential hepatotoxicity of the organochlorine pesticides has been a major concern. They are nonpolar and soluble in body fat, in which they are stored for considerable periods.[297, 298] They are also stored in the liver.[299, 300] The chemical structures of the more common pesticides—DDT, methoxychlor, chlordane, heptachlor, aldrin, dieldrin, lindane, and chlordecone—are shown in Figure 32-11. Exposure to the organochlorine pesticides may occur during their production, storage, delivery, or use. Environmental exposure may result directly or indirectly (secondary to ingested contaminated food or water). Accumulation of these products in the body follows their ingestion, inhalation, or percutaneous absorption.

The major concern regarding the organochlorine pesticides is whether they are hepatotoxic or hepatocarcinogenic in humans. Acute hepatotoxicity in humans has occurred following the rare accidental ingestion of large amounts of DDT.[301] Centrizonal necrosis and hepatic failure ensued after a single dose of nearly 6 g of DDT. Despite the massive production of DDT, there has been a striking lack of clinical or biochemical features suggestive of poisoning.[299] No disease entity has been documented despite

decades of industrial exposure, and only minor elevations of AST and sulfobromophthalein have been recorded.[298–300, 302, 303] Exposure to DDT dust may irritate the skin and eyes, but there has been no report of clear-cut liver injury following exposure to DDT in the United States. This is remarkable, since in some of the industrial workers, the exposure has continued for 20 years with absorption of quantities of DDT up to nearly 500 times the amount ingested daily by the average American adult. Hepatotoxicity of DDT has been documented in experimental animals, especially in mice and rats in whom steatosis and centrizonal hepatic necrosis occur.[304]

DDT is a potent inducer of mixed-function oxidase (see Chap. 9). This may result in an altered metabolism of avian sex hormones in the peregrine or hawk, with the production of thin egg shells.[305, 306] Another effect of the induction of mixed-function oxidase by DDT is the production of hepatotoxic and hepatocarcinogenic metabolites from parent chemicals or drugs already present in the environment or body.[307, 308] The enhancement of the hepatotoxic and hepatocarcinogenic effects of other unrelated chemicals is difficult to study in epidemiologic projects and more difficult to document conclusively. In rats fed DDT-contaminated food, hepatocellular enlargement, central cytoplasmic hyalinization, peripheral migration of ergastoplasm, and cytoplasmic inclusion bodies in the hepatocytes were seen under light microscopy.[309] Electron microscopy of these rat livers demonstrated a marked proliferation of agranular endoplasmic reticulum.

The question of the carcinogenicity of DDT in humans

has been deliberated for years. No study has provided evidence yet of a risk of cancer in humans exposed to DDT. Nevertheless, DDT is listed by the International Agency of Cancer (WHO) as a carcinogenic agent.[310] The Environmental Protection Agency banned the use of DDT in 1972, on the basis of potential carcinogenesis. Other pesticides—aldrin, dieldrin, and chlordane—have also been banned for similar reasons. The carcinogenic role of DDT is also disputed in experimental animals.[304, 311, 312] Hepatic cancer can be produced in mice, a species that is unusually susceptible to the induction of hepatic tumors. However, benign hepatic tumors develop in rats after chronic exposure to DDT.[312] Clearly, further epidemiologic studies are needed in order to resolve completely the hepatic carcinogenic potential of DDT in humans.

Chlordecone (Kepone)

This agent was responsible for neurologic and systemic abnormalities among workers at a manufacturing plant in Hopewell, Virginia.[313, 314] High concentrations of this chemical were detected in samples of blood, adipose tissues, and livers taken from the factory workers.[314, 315] In addition, contamination of the environment occurred, especially in a nearby river. Evidence of contamination by chlordecone of water and food products was still detectable a year after the factory closed. Animals exposed to chlordecone undergo liver cell injury and neoplastic changes.[316–319] Studies of exposed factory workers revealed neurologic and testicular changes as well as a high number of individuals with hepatomegaly and some with splenomegaly.[315] Liver function test results and sulfobromophthalein levels were generally normal. Liver biopsy results showed nonspecific findings, such as increased lipofuscin, steatosis, hyperglycogenation of nuclei, mild portal or lobular inflammatory infiltration, paracrystalline mitochrondrial inclusions, and marked proliferation of the smooth endoplasmic reticulum. The last finding suggests that chlordecone induces drug-metabolizing enzymes in the liver. Two to three years after exposure had ceased, the pesticide was no longer detectable in the tissues; the liver and spleen had reverted to normal size and the hepatic ultrastructure was normal.[315] The ultimate effects of exposure to chlordecone remain unknown.

Aldrin, Dieldrin

Exposure to these agents resulted in high concentrations of the agents in body fat of exposed workers, but no hepatic disease occurred. Adverse systemic effects, consisting of minor, nonspecific symptoms, rapidly resolved within weeks.[320]

Chlorophenoxy Herbicides

These agents produce minor evidence of hepatotoxicity in experimental animals.[321] The major effect on the liver appears to be the induction of the mixed-function oxidases of the hepatic microsomes. Hepatotoxic effects have been attributed to 2,4,5-trichlorophenoxy acetic acid (2,4,5-T). However, it is probable that the true hepatotoxic effect is due to contamination with 2,3,7,8-tetrachlorodibenzo-p-dioxin (TCDD), a potent hepatotoxic agent that causes centrizonal necrosis and porphyria.[322–324]

A major concern is whether the effects of exposure to two or more synthetic organic chemicals are likely to be more severe than those resulting from exposure to a single compound. Despite concurrent exposure to multiple organochlorine compounds, operators engaged in the manufacture or handling of mixtures of pesticides have not manifested hepatotoxic effects.[320]

Paraquat

Paraquat is the trade name of the dichloride salt of 1,1'-dimethyl-4,4'-dipyridylium, a powerful herbicide (Fig. 32–12). It is nonvolatile, nonflammable, and soluble in water. Accidental ingestion of 2 to 25 g of paraquat have resulted in shock, renal failure, jaundice, and pulmonary edema.[325, 326] Fatal and nonfatal cases of paraquat toxicity secondary to skin exposure and absorption in humans have been reported.[327, 328]

Histologic findings in livers of affected patients include congestion, centrilobular necrosis, acidophilic bodies, and fatty metamorphosis. Bile duct injury manifests as epithelial degeneration, necrosis, and cholestasis. Swollen bile epithelial cells, with partly vacuolated cytoplasm and destruction of the cell membrane, are seen. An infiltration with neutrophils and histiocytes in the intraductal and periductal tissues can occur. The severity of injury to the bile ducts increases as the size of the duct increases. It is felt that a direct corrosive effect of paraquat accounts for the ductal damage.[329] Cholestasis localized to the centrilobular area is often evident. It has been suggested that acute paraquat injury to the liver is biphasic; initially it is hepatocellular and after two days it becomes cholangiocellular.[326] Electron microscopy studies of livers from rats with paraquat poisoning revealed changes in the centrilobular hepatocytes, such as proliferation of the smooth endoplasmic reticulum together with mitochondrial swelling and transformation.[330] There is also thickening of the alveolar walls of the lung with edema and fibrin in the alveolar spaces, together with hemorrhage, an inflammatory infiltrate, and proximal tubular necrosis.[325] The acute pulmonary findings resemble those encountered in uremic pneumonitis. The pulmonary pathologic picture rapidly evolves into one of extensive fibrosis of the lung.[331]

Methyl Bromide

This chemical has widespread industrial use as a fumigant and insecticide despite its toxicity to humans and animals. A report of intoxication with methyl bromide stressed the protean neuropsychiatric manifestations and the apparent simulation of Reye's syndrome.[332] The hepatic histologic features, however, did not show the characteristic microvesicular fatty infiltration, and there was only moderate hepatocyte swelling and sinusoidal congestion.

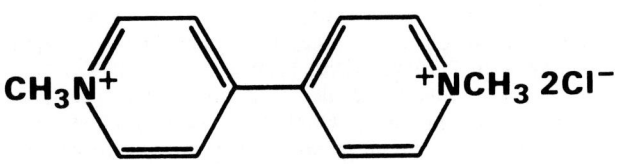

Figure 32–12. The structure of paraquat.

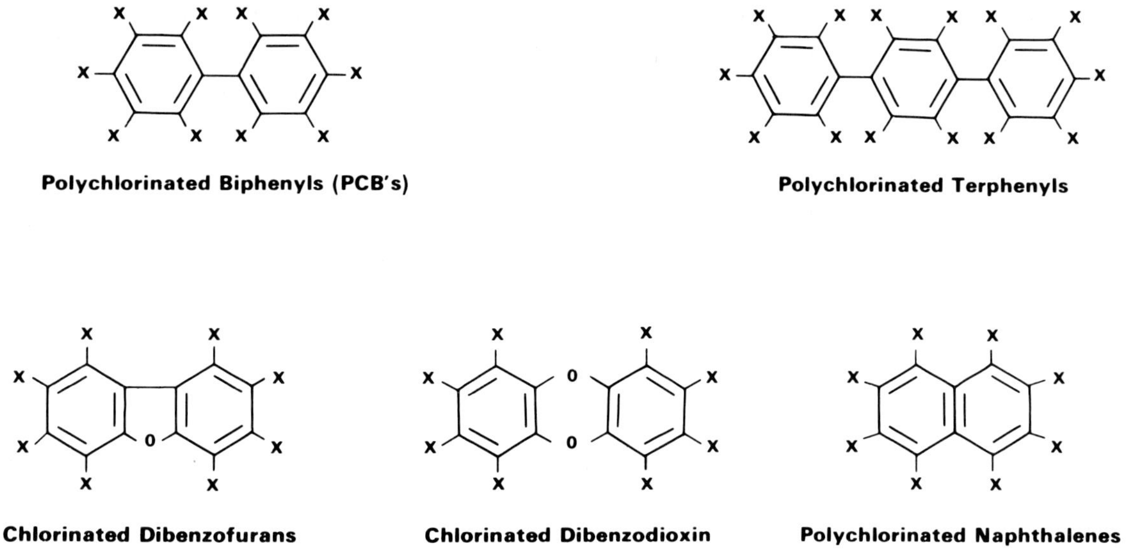

Figure 32–13. Structure of polychlorinated biphenyls (PCBs), terphenyls, dibenzofurans, dibenzodioxins, and naphthalenes. X represents possible chlorine substitution. (Reprinted with permission from Kimbrough RD. CRC Crit Rev Toxicol, 2:445, 1974. Copyright CRC Press Inc., Boca Raton, FL.)

POLYCHLORINATED BIPHENYLS

In the synthesis of chlorobiphenyls, isomeric mixtures are produced and are known as polychlorinated biphenyls (PCBs).[333] The biphenyl molecule, its numbering system, and examples of chlorobiphenyl compounds are shown in Figure 32–13.[334] Contaminants of PCBs, such as naphthalene, are themselves toxic and confound the precise evaluation and study of PCB toxicity. PCBs are used widely as insulating liquids in electrical capacitors, transformers, and nuclear reactors. Prior to 1971, PCBs were used widely in other fields. Since then, their application has been limited solely to closed electrical systems. NIOSH advocates an occupational environmental maximum of 1.0 μg of PCBs/m³ air.[335] PCBs have been detected in humans who do not work with it or are not directly exposed to it. PCBs are stored in the body in the fat and the liver. They are metabolized primarily in the liver by hydroxylation and subsequent conjugation with glucuronic acid.[334, 336] In animals and humans, chronic exposure results in induction of the cytochrome P450 system and induction of ALAS, producing porphyria.[333, 334, 337–341] PCBs can produce tumors, especially hepatocellular carcinomas in animals.[334, 337] The potential carcinogenic role of PCBs in humans is a major concern. The precise carcinogen is debatable. Some regard PCBs as direct carcinogens; others consider the metabolites (produced by cytochrome P450) carcinogenic. An alternative theory is that the carcinogenicity of unrelated chemicals is enhanced subsequent to metabolism by the PCB-induced cytochrome P450. PCBs appear to potentiate viral hepatitis in ducks, possibly because of an immunosuppressive action.[342]

Acute toxicity follows the accidental ingestion of PCBs. However, the major routes of absorption are through the skin and lungs. Acute intoxication of humans with PCBs, and also probably polychlorinated dibenzofurans, has been reported from Japan, where contaminated rice oil was ingested.[343, 344] The epidemic was known as Yusho (oil disease). It resulted in jaundice in 11 per cent of victims, as well as chloracne, conjunctivitis, neuropathy, edema of the eyelids, and congenital defects in infants born subse-

quently to women who were exposed to the rice oil. During the 1940's, cases of acute PCB toxicity were reported, manifesting as fatigue, anorexia, nausea, and edema of the face and hands. Jaundice was rare and when present often indicated poor prognosis in association with massive hepatic necrosis. Histologic features included mostly severe centrizonal necrosis with a rim of surviving periportal hepatocytes.[345, 346] In patients who survived the acute insult for only a few months, subacute hepatic necrosis or macronodular cirrhosis developed. Abnormal liver function test results have been recorded in workers exposed to PCBs; however, the reports have been poorly controlled and without histologic support.[347, 348] A significant increase of γ-glutamyl transpeptidase levels was noted in workers followed up to two years after handling PCBs. The raised enzyme levels correlated with the serum PCB levels.[349] Two cases of hepatocellular cancer have been reported in autopsy examinations of patients from the Yusho epidemic.[350] Epidemiologic studies evaluating the long-term effects of exposure to PCBs in humans have not as yet detected a significant increase in death from cirrhosis or carcinoma of the liver. However, it is prudent to keep human exposure to PCBs to a minimum until the long-term consequences of exposure are fully known. PCBs are stable and resist biodegradation, so despite the current limitations on its use, the widespread contamination of soil and water will pose risks for the community for a considerable time.

ARSENIC

A variety of acute and chronic hepatotoxic effects of arsenic and arsenical products has been recognized. Arsenic has been known to be a potent poison since antiquity. The association of liver disease and chronic arsenism was first reported in 1774.[351] Acute liver injury in humans is rare and it follows accidental, homicidal, or suicidal ingestion. Occupational and environmentally induced hepatic injury secondary to exposure to arsenic has been exclusively chronic. Chronic liver disease occurred among workers in vineyards (because of arsenic in insecticide sprays); it also occurred among patients with psoriasis given a 1% solution of arsenic trioxide (Fowler's solution) for sustained periods. Isolated episodes of poisoning occurred secondary to the ingestion of arsenic in well water, homemade alcoholic brews, or homemade drug formulae in India.[352-357] The WHO limit on the content of arsenic in water is less than 5 μg/dl. Wells in India and in areas of the United States have exceeded this limit considerably.[355-357]

Acute hepatotoxic manifestations of arsenic poisoning include an acute hepatic necrosis produced by large doses of arsenicals or a hypersensitivity reaction with fever, lymphadenopathy, rash, arthralgia, conjunctival suffusion, eosinophilia, and hepatitis. This is known as Milian's syndrome.[358] The histologic picture of the liver consists of severe steatosis and necrosis of varying degrees. There is a conflict of opinion as to whether the necrosis is in the peripheral or central zone.[359-361] The most important acute hepatotoxic lesion produced by arsenicals is intrahepatic obstructive jaundice associated with the administration of arsphenamine.[362] The patients manifest a cholestatic picture with elevated levels of bilirubin, alkaline phosphatase, and cholesterol. The histologic features show cholestasis with an eosinophil-rich portal infiltrate.[362] The cholestasis usually resolves, often after a period of months.[363] A syndrome similar to primary bilary cirrhosis may complicate cholestatic hepatitis caused by arsenic.[364, 365]

Chronic hepatotoxic manifestations of arsenic toxicity include steatosis, cirrhosis, presinusoidal intrahepatic portal hypertension (hepatoportal sclerosis), angiosarcoma, primary liver cell cancer, and possibly idiopathic portal hypertension.[353, 354, 359, 366-373] The angiosarcoma induced by arsenic may occur despite the lack of significant hepatic fibrosis. It resembles the hepatic lesions that complicate exposure to vinyl chloride and thorium dioxide (Thorotrast). The mechanism of hepatotoxicity of arsenic is thought to be its reaction with sulfydryl groups, which inhibit enzyme systems essential for cellular metabolism, and by the substitution of arsenate for the phosphate group of high-energy molecules.[374] Arsenic is a rare cause of liver disease today because its use in medicine, industry, and agriculture has dwindled.

SELENIUM

Selenium and its compounds are widely used in semiconductor technology, electrical engineering, glass, rubber, steel, and lubricants. Selenium is also used as a fungicide and in medications, and it is a by-product of the power industry that uses coal or petroleum. The annual world production of selenium is estimated to be 1100 to 1600 tons.[375] Selenium, like many other elements, has a bimodal effect. At lower concentrations it is an essential trace element for growth in humans and animals. The normal range of selenium in the blood is 10 to 37 μg/dl. Selenium deficiency in humans can result from the ingestion of a selenium-deficient diet in endemic areas where the soil is deficient in the element, or it may complicate chronic total parenteral nutrition. Selenium deficiency is reported to occur in alcoholics with cirrhosis.[376, 377] The biologic role of selenium is related to glutathione peroxidase, an enzyme that protects cellular membranes against lipid peroxidation, which may be an important mechanism in the pathogenesis of alcohol-induced liver damage (see Chap. 33).[376, 378, 379, 380-382] Low levels of selenium have been detected in blood from alcoholics with severe liver disease, there

being an inverse correlation in these patients between levels of selenium and bilirubin.[377] In higher concentrations selenium has toxic properties for humans and animals. Acute selenium poisoning from accidental ingestion or inhalation of selenium dioxide or hydrogen selenide has been reported.[383, 384] The liver histology revealed a diffuse microvacuolar steatosis in the hepatocytes.[383] The patient's breath and sweat had a garlic odor caused by the dimethyl selenide. There is no specific treatment for selenium intoxication; symptomatic measures are advocated. The hepatotoxicity of selenium probably is produced by the easy interchange of sulfur by selenium in the metabolism of certain amino acids, for example, methionine and cysteine, thus producing a deficiency of these amino acids. Selenium may also react with glutathione to form a selenotrisulfate derivative, which can inhibit protein synthesis.[385, 386] In large quantities and with chronic exposure, selenium can cause cirrhosis and possibly the development of hepatic neoplasia.[385] Selenium can have a severe ecologic impact on aquatic ecosystems, even when concentrations in water are low. Selenium affects fish, waterfowl, and marsh birds. Accumulation of selenium can be magnified in food chains in freshwater ecosystems. This biomagnification produces selenium toxicity in the animals inhabiting the water system.[387, 388] The current level of safety of selenium (52 μg/L in water catchments) has been challenged, and standards between 5 and 10 μg/L are suggested.[387, 388]

VINYL CHLORIDE

Polyvinyl chloride is manufactured by polymerization of vinyl chloride monomer. Vinyl chloride (CH_2=CHCl) is a halogenated aliphatic hydrocarbon structurally similar to trichloroethylene and other inhalational anesthetics. Its small molecular size allows easy absorption across all membranes. Polyvinyl chloride is used in the manufacture of a large variety of products, such as packaging material, clothing, toys, furniture, and building materials. Vinyl chloride has been used in aerosol hairsprays, disinfectants, deodorants, cleaning agents, and polishing material.

The manufacture of polyvinyl chloride has been growing steadily as the demand worldwide for plastics has increased over the past half century. Worldwide production of polyvinyl chloride was 18 billion pounds in 1972.[389] In 1973, attention was drawn to the first of two serious hepatic complications prevalent among workers in vinyl chloride plants.[390] Workers in Germany were found to have hepatic fibrosis, splenomegaly, and portal hypertension.[390] A year later, reports from Britain and the United States documented angiosarcoma of the liver in workers involved in the production of polyvinyl chloride.[391-393] Since then a number of cases of angiosarcoma of the liver, a previously rare tumor, have been detected in factory workers manufacturing polyvinyl chloride.[394-399] Systemic surveillance has led to the detection of noncirrhotic portal hypertension (hepatoportal sclerosis) in industrial workers exposed to vinyl chloride.[397, 400, 401] There has been considerable interest, therefore, in the toxicity of vinyl chloride.[402, 403] The hazards of vinyl chloride were considered initially to be occupational rather than environmental. Most patients with angiosarcoma had worked in polymer plants for periods of 12 to 28 years. However, the report of angiosarcoma in a patient living in the vicinity of a polyvinyl chloride manufacturing plant has raised the question of environmental pollution.[404] The manufacture of polyvinyl chloride from vinyl chloride causes the escape of 6 per cent of the monomer into the environment. It is uncertain what concentration of vinyl chloride in the atmosphere is hazardous.[405] In Britain, initial regulations set an upper limit for exposure of vinyl chloride in the environment to 50 ppm. In 1974, United States federal regulations reduced the exposure levels to 1 ppm. These levels have been followed almost universally.[406] Since then the occurrence of angiosarcoma has decreased rapidly. Monitoring of the atmosphere near a plant in the United States revealed concentrations of vinyl chloride as high as 40 parts/billion.[407] It is not known if factors other than the concentration and duration of exposure to vinyl chloride lead to hepatic sequelae. Alcohol, drugs, and undetermined agents (e.g., viruses) could be additional factors. At low levels of exposure to vinyl chloride, alcohol competes for the alcohol dehydrogenase system, leading to increased metabolism of vinyl chloride via the mixed-function oxidase system and increased production of chloro-oxirane compounds.[408–410] Recently, there have been two cases of angiosarcoma of the liver in workers extruding and manufacturing polyvinyl chloride. These patients raise the question as to whether contact with polyvinyl chloride, in addition to inhalation of the vapor released in polymerization of vinyl chloride, may be hazardous.[411]

Metabolism of Vinyl Chloride

Vinyl chloride enters the body mainly via the lungs, skin, and gastrointestinal tract. The neoplastic potential of the agent appears to depend on the conversion of vinyl chloride to an active metabolite, possibly an epoxide (see Chap. 9). The metabolism of vinyl chloride by different pathways depends on the dose.[389, 409] At concentrations less than 50 ppm, vinyl chloride is metabolized only by alcohol dehydrogenase. The products are chloroacetaldehyde and monochloroacetic acid. At levels greater than 50 ppm, oxidation by the peroxidase-catalase system becomes operative, producing chloroacetaldehyde. At concentrations greater than 250 ppm, metabolism by microsomal mixed-function oxidases occurs, forming chloroethylene oxide.[412] It appears that vinyl chloride or its reactive metabolites bind covalently to hepatic glutathione and are subsequently hydrolyzed and excreted in the urine as conjugates of cysteine.

Screening of Workers Exposed to Vinyl Chloride

To date, most cases of hepatic fibrosis and angiosarcomas in humans have been detected in workers exposed to vinyl chloride monomer gas during the production of polyvinyl chloride. Nevertheless, the possibility that food containers made of polyvinyl plastics may contain traces of the monomer and may contaminate food has been considered.[411, 413] Routine screening of plant employees, and rigid pollution restrictions are advocated.[389] A standard biochemical profile augmented by determinations of ALT and γ-glutamyl transpeptidase levels, and a routine liver-spleen scan are advocated every 6 to 12 months.[389] The best predictors of abnormal liver histologic changes are unknown. In a study of patients with abnormal findings on biopsy, 87 per cent had abnormal ALT levels, 80 per cent had abnormal AST levels, and 80 per cent had abnormal γ-glutamyl transpeptidase levels.[389] Every patient in whom all three test results were abnormal also had abnormal liver biopsies; however, normal values for each of these variables still may be associated with an abnormal histologic appearance. An abnormal plasma clearance of indocyanine green correlated with an abnormal hepatic histologic appearance. A low-dose indocyanine green clearance (0.5 mg/kg) gave the best single combination of sensitivity and specificity for detecting latent vinyl chloride–induced hepatic injury.[414, 415] Splenomegaly was not a useful predictor of hepatic histologic characteristics.[389] Original testing of prospective employees showed a 26 per cent abnormality rate for one or more tests. Alcoholism probably accounted for the high background rate of abnormal tests. A focal hepatocytic hyperplasia appears to be the earliest identifiable histologic change consistent with vinyl chloride exposure, and it is recommended as a screening test if liver biopsy is to be performed on chemical workers.[416] The use of fasting serum bile acids in the identification of vinyl chloride hepatotoxicity has been advocated.[417]

Hepatic Lesions Caused By Vinyl Chloride

Two different lesions in the liver can be attributed to the sequelae of vinyl chloride. One of the lesions, angiosarcoma of the liver, is frequently multicentric. The enlarged liver and spleen are tender, with easily audible bruits resulting from the intense vascularity. The angiosarcoma is often peripherally located in the liver and is associated with a terminal massive peritoneal hemorrhage. The other typical lesion is a variety of hepatic fibrosis, which is typical but not diagnostic. It is usually portal in distribution, often extending into the lobular parenchyma and even into the walls of the portal vein branches. Inflammatory cells may be seen around bile ducts. A form of capsular and subcapsular fibrosis is a most characteristic lesion.[390] Another variant of the fibrosis is a focal intralobular accumulation of connective tissue fibers, which is recognized under light microscopy only by special connective tissue stains. On electron microscopy, it is recognized by the presence of a dense, thin connective tissue coat surrounding the hepatocytes and associated with many fibroblasts and fat-containing mesenchymal Ito cells.[418]

Besides the fibrosis seen in all specimens, some patients have focal, irregular dilation of sinusoids. Vinyl chloride and its metabolites appear to induce hyperplasia of two types of cells: mesenchymal sinusoidal lining cells in the liver (and spleen) and the hepatocytes.[401] In the spleen this results in splenomegaly, and in the liver it results in fibrosis contributing to portal hypertension.[419] Substances related to vinyl chloride such as *vinyl bromide* or *vinylidine chloride* have produced similar lesions in experimental animals.[395]

Acute Hepatic and Extrahepatic Injury from Vinyl Chloride

Acute intoxication from vinyl chloride manifests essentially at the portal of entry into the body. Skin contact results in irritation and frostbite. The pharmacologic effects of vinyl chloride on the central nervous system cause dizziness, lightheadedness, and impaired vision. Gastrointestinal sequelae include nausea, vomiting (often coffee-ground), and abdominal pain. In severe, acute exposure (> 8000 ppm), hepatic necrosis can occur 24 to 48 hours after exposure. Raised levels of AST, ALT, and γ-glutamyl transpeptidase occur. Recovery usually is rapid, and long-term complications are rare. The histologic appearance of the liver in acute hepatic injury shows isolated necrosis of hepatocytes and occasional polymorphic infiltrates. Death is unusual in acute severe intoxication. If it occurs, it usually results from cardiac arrhythmia or respiratory arrest. Fulminant hepatic necrosis occurs rarely.

Other nonhepatic complications of vinyl chloride include *acro-osteolysis*—Raynaud's phenomenon accompanied by osteolysis of the terminal phalanges of the fingers and scleroderma-like skin changes.[420]

CYTOSTATIC AGENTS

Insidious hepatic injury associated with occupational exposure has been recognized. Personnel handling cytostatic agents during their daily duties in dealing with patients with cancer have developed increased mutagenicity in urine, enhanced frequency of chromosome gaps, and sister chromatid exchange.[421-423] Insidious liver injury after chronic handling of cytostatic drugs (bleomycin, vincristine, cyclophosphamide, ftorafur, doxorubicin, dacarbazine, chlormethehydrazine, 5-fluorouracil, and methotrexate) has been reported in three consecutive senior nurses in an oncologic department.[424] No single or specific hepatic lesion has been identified and the mechanism by which hepatotoxicity occurs is unknown. Inhalation or percutaneous absorption is the probable route of absorption. The need for precautions when handling large quantities of cytostatic agents over long periods has been addressed, and appropriate guidelines have been drafted.[425]

BENZYL CHLORIDE

Benzyl chloride is used mainly in the manufacture of dyes, perfumes, and pharmaceutical products. Ninety million pounds of benzyl chloride were manufactured in the United States in 1976. Abnormal liver function has been reported in workers exposed to 2 ppm.[426] Model studies in rats confirm the hepatotoxic potential of benzyl chloride. Rats exposed to the agent manifest a temporary elevation of hepatic enzymes, sulfobromophthalein retention, and decreased hepatic levels of glutathione, but no histologic changes.[427]

DIOXIN

Concerns regarding the health hazards caused by the chlorinated dibenzo-p-dioxins have been raised. Dioxins may arise as by-products of the manufacture of chlorinated phenols or as contaminants of herbicides and chemicals. The major focus has been on TCDD, a most potent porphyrinogenic agent.[428] Following an accident near Sevesco (Italy), a reversible secondary coproporphyrinuria developed in 22 per cent of exposed individuals.[429] Progression to porphyria cutanea tarda occurred only in individuals with a predisposition, that is, an inherited defect of uroporphyrinogen decarboxylase. Exposure of rats to TCDD resulted in increased liver weights. Most of the chemical was stored in the liver and fat tissues.[430]

PHTHALATE ESTERS

The term *phthalate esters* is reserved for the *ortho* form of benzenedicarboxylic acid, which is prepared by combining phthalic acid with a specific alcohol to form the desired ester.[431] These esters are produced industrially from phthalic anhydride rather than from the acid. The esters are colorless liquids that are poorly soluble in water but are soluble in solvents and oils. Phthalate esters have a wide spectrum of uses, by far the major application is as plasticizing agents for polyvinyl chloride.[431, 432] Dioctyl phthalate (DOP) and its isomer di-(2-ethylhexyl) phthalate (DEHP) are widely used plasticizers.

There are reports documenting that DEHP was present in tissues and organs of patients who previously had received blood that was stored in bags made of polyvinyl chloride plasticized with DEHP.[433-435] The leaching of the plasticizer DEHP from the polyvinyl chloride container appears to be dependent on the temperature and the lipid content of the fluid media contained in the tubing or container.[436, 437] Concerns regarding the safety of phthalate esters in humans have been raised, especially in the light of the current experience relating to the hepatotoxic and hepatocarcinogenic potential of these esters in animal models. Rodents fed DEHP sustained proliferation of peroxisomes in association with hepatomegaly and hypotriglyceridemia.[438, 439] Sustained proliferation of peroxisomes in the rodent liver has been associated with an increased incidence of hepatocellular carcinoma.[440, 441] DEHP has been implicated as a hepatocarcinogen in rats and mice in a long-term National Toxicology Program report.[442] Histologic examination of livers in rats given phthalate esters shows steatosis, congestion, dilation of smooth and rough endoplasmic reticulum, and swollen mitochondria.[443] A decreased concentration of glycogen in liver and blood glucose has been shown in rats fed DEHP. This suggests that DEHP affects both glycogenesis and glycogenolysis.[444] Despite the evidence for toxicity of DEHP in animals deliberately fed high doses of the agent on a chronic basis, there is no conclusive evidence for hepatotoxicity in humans secondary to the use in clinical medicine of polyvinyl chloride produced with DEHP. Phthalate esters have been detected in the urine of patients who have never received a transfusion, suggesting that environmental contamination may be a major source for their deposition in the body.[445] Further evaluation of this aspect of the problem and its implications, if any, is warranted.

REFERENCES

1. USITC (U.S. International Trade Commission). Preliminary report on U.S. Production of Selected Synthetic Organic Materials, Washington, DC, International Trade Commission, 1981.
2. Jagielski J, Scudamore KA, Heuser SG. Residues of carbon tetachloride and 1,2-dibromoethane in cereals and processed foods after liquid fumigant grain treatment for pest control. Pestic Sci 9:117, 1978.
3. United States of America and State of Louisiana v. Petro Processors of Louisiana Inc. U.S. District Court, Middle District of Louisiana, 1983:86, 171.
4. Guild WR, Young JV, Merrill JP. Anuria due to carbon tetrachloride intoxication. Ann Inter Med 48:1221, 1958.
5. Smetana H. Nephrosis due to carbon tetrachloride. Arch Intern Med 63:760, 1939.
6. Umiker W, Pearce J. Nature and genesis of pulmonary alterations in carbon tetrachloride poisoning. Arch Pathol 55:203, 1953.
7. Gardner GH, Grove RC, Gustafson RK, et al. Studies on the pathologic histology of experimental carbon tetrachloride poisoning. Bull Johns Hopkins Hosp 36:107, 1925.
8. Conway HB, Hoven F. Electrocardiographic changes in carbon tetrachloride poisoning: a report of a case. US Navy Med Bull 46:593, 1946.
9. Takasaka T. Ueber die lungenblutungen bei der akuten tetrachlormethanvergiftung. Deutsche Ztschr f d ges gerichtl Med 6:488, 1925.

10. Von Oettingen WF. The Halogenated Hydrocarbons of Industrial and Toxicological Importance. Amsterdam, Elsevier, 1964.

11. Recknagel RO, Glende EA Jr. Carbon tetrachloride hepatotoxicity: an example of lethal cleavage. CRC Crit Rev Toxicol 2:236, 1973.

12. Reynolds ES. Comparison of early injury to lower endoplasmic reticulum by halomethanes, hexachloroethane, benzene, toluene, bromobenzene, ethionine, thioacetamide and dimethylnitrosamine. Biochem Pharmacol 21:2255, 1972.

13. Drill VA. Hepatotoxic agents: mechanism of action and dietary relationship. Pharmacol Rev 4:1, 1952.

14. Rouiller Ch. Experimental toxic injury of the liver. In: Rouiller Ch, ed. The Liver, Vol II. New York, Academic Press, 1964:335.

15. Recknagel RO. Carbon tetrachloride hepatotoxicity. Pharmacol Rev 19:145, 1967.

16. Cameron GR, Karunaratne WAE. Carbon tetrachloride cirrhosis in relation to liver degeneration. J Pathol Bacteriol 42:1, 1936.

17. Bruckner JV, MacKenzie WF, Muralidhara S, et al. Oral toxicity of carbon tetrachloride: acute, subacute, and subchronic studies in rats. Fund Appl Toxicol 6:16, 1986.

18. Reuber MD, Glover EL. Hyperplastic and early neoplastic lesions of the liver in buffalo strain rats of various ages given subcutaneous carbon tetrachloride. J Natl Cancer Inst 38:891, 1967.

19. Hernberg S, Korkala M, Asikainen U, et al. Primary liver cancer and exposure to solvents. Int Arch Occup Environ Health 54:147, 1984.

20. Gitlin N. Carbon tetrachloride-induced cirrhosis? SA Med J 58:872, 1980.

21. Poindexter CA, Greene CH. Toxic cirrhosis of the liver. JAMA 102:2015, 1934.

22. Slater TF. Free radical mechanisms in tissue injury. Bristol, JW Arrowsmith, 1972:118.

23. Sastry KV, Agrawal VP. Effect of carbon tetrachloride on the hepatic alkaline and acid phosphatases in a teleost fish, *Heteropneustes fossilis*. Acta Anat 93:361, 1975.

24. Dawkins MJR. Carbon tetrachloride poisoning in the liver of the new born rat. J Pathol Bacteriol 85:189, 1963.

25. Cagen SZ, Klaassen CD. Hepatotoxicity of carbon tetrachloride in developing rats. Toxicol Appl Pharmacol 50:347, 1979.

26. Mclean AEM, Mclean EK. The effect of diet and DDT on microsomal hydroxylation and on sensitivity of rats to CCl_4 poisoning. Biochem J 105:1055, 1966.

27. Aterman K, Yuce R. Hepatoprotective substances: a partial assessment. In: Keppler D, ed. Pathogenesis and mechanism of liver cell necrosis. Lancaster, MTP Press, 1975:129.

28. Seawright AA, Mclean AGM. The effect of diet on carbon tetrachloride metabolism. Biochem J 105:1055, 1967.

29. Mahieu P, Geubel A, Rahier J, et al. Potentiation of carbon tetrachloride hepato-nephrotoxicity by phenobarbital in man, a case report. Int J Clin Pharmacol Res 3:427, 1983.

30. Garner RC, Mclean AEM. Increased susceptibility to carbon tetrachloride poisoning in the rat after pretreatment with oral phenobarbitone. Biochem Pharmacol 18:645, 1969.

31. Hasumura Y, Teschke R, Lieber CS. Increased carbon tetrachloride hepatotoxicity, and its mechanism, after chronic ethanol consumption. Gastroenterology 66:415, 1974.

32. Rosenthal SM. Some effects of alcohol upon the normal and damaged liver. J Pharmacol Exp Ther 38:291, 1930.

33. Schwarzmann V. Les hepatites toxiques experimentales. Rev Intern Hepatol 7:387, 1957.

34. Klatskin G. Toxic and drug induced hepatitis. In: Schiff L, ed. Diseases of the Liver, 4th ed. Philadelphia, JB Lippincott, 1975:604.

35. Cornish H, Adefuin J. Potentiation of carbon tetrachloride by aliphatic alcohols. Arch Environ Health 14:447, 1967.

36. Traiger GJ, Plaa GL. Relationship of alcohol metabolism to the potentiation of CCl_4 hepatotoxicity induced by aliphatic alcohols. J Pharmacol Exp Ther 183:481, 1972.

37. Traiger GJ, Plaa GL. Differences in the potentiation of carbon tetrachloride in rats by ethanol and isopropanol pretreatment. Toxicol Appl Pharmacol 20:105, 1971.

38. Wei E, Wong CK, Hine CH. Potentiation of carbon tetrachloride hepatotoxicity by ethanol and cold. Toxicol Appl Pharmacol 18:329, 1971.

39. Schwetz BA, Plaa GL. Catecholamine potentiation of carbon tetrachloride-induced hepatotoxicity in mice. Toxicol Appl Pharmacol 14:495, 1969.

40. Wei E, Wong LCK, Hine CH. Selective potentiation of carbon tetrachloride hepatotoxicity by ethanol. Arch Int Pharmacodyn 189:5, 1971.

41. Charbonneau M, Tuchweber B, Plaa GL. Acetone potentiation of chronic liver injury induced by repetitive administration of carbon tetrachloride. Hepatology 6:694, 1986.

42. Zimmerman HJ, Mao R, Israsena S. Phenothiazine inhibition of carbon tetrachloride cytotoxicity in vitro. Proc Soc Exp Biol Med 123:893, 1966.

43. Glynn LE, Himsworth HP. Intralobular circulation in acute liver injury by carbon tetrachloride. Clin Sci 19:63, 1948.

44. Farber E. Some fundamental aspects of liver injury. In: Kharina JM, Israel Y, Kalant H, eds. Alcoholic Liver Pathology. Toronto, Addiction Research Foundation of Ontario, 1975:289.

45. Judah JD, Mclean AEM, Mclean EK. Biochemical mechanisms of drug injury. Am J Med 49:609, 1970.

46. Schaffrir E, Khassis S. Role of enhanced fat mobilization in liver triglyceride accumulation in carbon tetrachloride-induced liver injury. Israel J Med Sci 5:975, 1969.

47. Kessler JI. The role of adipose tissue fatty acids in the pathogenesis of acute fatty liver. In: Paumgartner G, Presig R, eds. The Liver. Basel, Karger, 1973:278.

48. Berger ML, Bhatt H, Combes B, et al. CCl_4-induced toxicity in isolated hepatocytes: the importance of direct solvent injury. Hepatology 6:36, 1986.

49. Farber JL, El-Mofty SK. The biochemical pathology of liver cell necrosis. Am J Pathol 81:237, 1975.

50. Christie GS, Judah JD. Mechanism of action of carbon tetrachloride on liver cells. Proc Roy Soc Lond B 142:241, 1954.

51. Rao KS, Glende EA, Recknagel RO. Effect of drug pretreatment in carbon tetrachloride induced lipid peroxidation in rat liver microsomal lipids. Exp Mol Pathol 12:324, 1970.

52. Levy GN, Brabee MJ. Binding of carbon tetrachloride to rat hepatic mitochondrial DNA. Toxicol Lett 22:229, 1984.

53. Link B, Durk H, Thiel D, et al. Binding of trichloromethyl radicals to lipids of the hepatic endoplasmic reticulum during tetrachloromethane metabolism. Biochem J 223:577, 1984.

54. Slater TF. Necrogenic action of carbon tetrachloride in the rat: a speculative mechanism based on activation. Nature (Lond) 209:36, 1966.

55. Mclean AEM. Drugs, diet and liver injury. In: Gerok W, Sickinger K, eds. Drugs and the Liver. Stuttgart, F. K. Schattauer-Verlag, 1975:143.

56. Seawright AA, Steele DP, Mudie AW, et al. The effect of diet and drugs on hepatic microsomal amino pyrine *N*-demethylase activity in vitro and susceptibility to carbon tetrachloride in sheep. Res Vet Sci 13:245, 1972.

57. Wirtschafter ZT, Cronyn MW. Free radical mechanism for solvent toxicity. Arch Environ Health 9:186, 1964.

58. Moon HD. Pathology of fatal carbon tetrachloride poisoning with special reference to histogenesis of hepatic and renal lesions. Am J Pathol 26:1041, 1950.

59. Harden BL Jr. Carbon tetrachloride poisoning—a review. Industrial Med Surg 23:93, 1954.

60. Gennings RB. Fatal fulminant acute carbon tetrachloride poisoning. Arch Pathol 59:269, 1955.

61. Docherty JF, Burgess E. Action of carbon tetrachloride on the liver. Br Med J 2:907, 1922.

62. Wroblewski F. The clinical significance of transaminase activities of serum. Am J Med 27:911, 1959.

63. Wroblewski F. The clinical significance of alterations in transaminase activities of serum and other body fluids. Adv Clin Chem 1:313, 1958.

64. Kirkpatrick HJR, Sutherland JM. A fatal case of poisoning with carbon tetrachloride. J Clin Pathol 9:242, 1956.

65. Bolarin DM. Serum bile acid in the evaluation of colchicine treatment of carbon tetrachloride-induced liver injury. Exp Mol Pathol 41(3):331, 1984.

66. Shen ES, Garry VF, Anders MW. Effects of hypoxia on carbon tetrachloride hepatotoxicity. Biochem Pharmacol 31:3787, 1982.

67. Frenzl H, Heidenreich T, Gillert J, et al. Protective effect of CO_2-induced (hyperventilation) on the hepatotoxicity elicited by carbon tetrachloride. Liver 2:376, 1982.

68. Divald A, Ujhelyl E, Jeney A, et al. Hepatoprotective effects of prostacyclins on CCl_4-induced liver injury in rats. Exp Mol Pathol 42(2):163, 1985.

69. Dume T, Herms W, Schröder E, et al. Klinik und Therapie der tetrachlorkohlenstoff—vergiftung. Dtsch Med Wochenschr 94:1646, 1969.

70. Ottenberg R, Spiegel R. The present status of nonobstructive jaundice due to infectious and chemical agents. Causative agents, pathogenesis, interrelationships, clinical characteristics. Medicine 22:27, 1943.

71. Sidel M. Dinitrophenol poisoning causing jaundice. JAMA 103:254, 1934.

72. Browning E. Toxicology and Metabolism of Industrial Solvents. Amsterdam, Elsevier, 1965.

73. Spilsbury BH. Discussion on atrophy of the liver. Br Med J 2:583, 1920.

74. Livingstion-Learmouth A, Cunningham BM. Observations on the effects of trinitrotoluene on women workers. Lancet 2:261, 1916.
75. Martland HS. Trinitrotoluene poisoning. JAMA 68:835, 1917.
76. Pitton LA. The problem of the occupational environment. Chem Indust Sept. 20, 1975:768.
77. Davie TB. The pathology of T.N.T. poisoning. Proc Roy Soc Med (Lond) 35:553, 1942.
78. McConnell WJ, Flinn RH. Summary of twenty-two trinitrotoluene fatalities in World War II. J Med Hyg Toxicol 28:76, 1946.
79. Moore B. Toxic jaundice in munition workers and troops. Br Med J 1:155, 1917.
80. Barnes JAP. Toxic jaundice in munition workers and troops. Br Med J 1:155, 1917.
81. Von Oettingen WF. The Halogenated Hydrocarbons of Industrial and Toxicological Importance. Amsterdam, Elsevier, 1964.
82. Gurney R. Tetrachlorethane intoxication: early recognition of liver damage and means of prevention. Gastroenterology 1:1112, 1943.
83. Gurney R. Useful procedures in the early diagnosis of liver damage following exposure to the chlorinated hydrocarbons. NY State J Med 47:2566, 1947.
84. Wilcox WH. Toxic jaundice due to tetrachlorethane poisoning. A new type among aeroplane workers. Lancet 1:544, 1915.
85. Wilcox WW. Toxic jaundice. Lancet 2:57, 1931.
86. Minot GR, Smith LW. The blood in tetrachlorethane poisoning. Arch Intern Med 28:687, 1921.
87. McNutt NS, Amster RL, McConnell EE, et al. Hepatic lesions in mice after continuous inhalation exposure to 1,1,1-trichloroethane. Lab Invest 32:643, 1975.
88. Texter EC Jr, Grunow WA, Zimmerman HJ. Massive centrizonal necrosis of the liver due to inhalation of 1,1,1-trichloroethane. Gastroenterology 76(5):1260, 1979.
89. Baerg RD, Kimberg DV. Centrilobular hepatic necrosis and acute renal failure in "solvent sniffers." Ann Intern Med 73:713, 1970.
90. James WRL. Fatal addiction to trichloroethylene. Br J Ind Med 20:47, 1963.
91. Paddle GM. Incidence of liver cancer and trichloroethylene manufacture: joint study by industry and a cancer registry. Br Med J 286:846, 1983.
92. O'Brien ET, Yeoman WB, Hobby JAE. Hepatorenal damage from toluene in a glue sniffer. Br Med J 2:29, 1971.
93. Kurppa K, Husman K. Car painters' exposure to a mixture of organic solvents. Scand J Work Environ Health 8:137, 1982.
94. Dossing M, Ranek L. Isolated liver damage in chemical workers. Br J Ind Med 41:142, 1984.
95. Occupational Safety and Health Administration (OSHA) and National Institute for Occupational Safety and Health (NIOSH). Health hazard alert: 2-nitropropane. DHHS (NIOSH) Publication no. 80–142, 1980.
96. National Paint and Coatings Association (NPCA). Information released from NPCA's data bank, 1985.
97. Hine CH, Pasi A, Stephens BG. J Occup Med 20(5):333, 1978.
98. Acute hepatic failure after occupational exposure to 2-nitropropane. MMWR 34(43):659, 1985.
99. Rumack BH. Poisindex. Denver, Rocky Mountain Poison Center, 1982.
100. Mushroom poisoning among Laotian refugees—1981. Morbid Mortal Wk Rep 31:287, 1982.
101. Floersheim GL, Weber O, Tschumi P, et al. Die klinische Knollen-blatterpilzvergiftung (Amanita phalloides): Prognostische Faktoren und therapeutische Massnahmen: Eine Analyse anhand von 205 Fallen.
102. Bartoloni St Omer F, Giannini A, Botti P, et al. Amanita poisoning: A clinical-histopathological study of 64 cases of intoxication. Hepatogastroenterology 32:229, 1985.
103. Lynen F, Wieland U. Uber die giftstoffe des knollenblatter-pilzes. IV. Kristallisation von phalloidin. Justus Liebigs Ann Chem 533:93, 1937.
104. Wieland H, Hallermayer R. Uber die giftstoffe des knollen-blatter-pilzes. Justus Liebigs Ann Chem 548:1, 1941.
105. Wieland T, Wieland O. The toxic peptides of Amanita species. In: Kadis S, Ciegler A, Ajl SJ, eds. Microbial Toxins, Vol VIII, Fungal Toxins. New York, Academic Press 1972:249.
106. Wieland T, Faulstich H. Amatoxins, phallotoxins, phallolysin, and antamanide: the biologically active components of poisonous Amanita mushrooms. CRC Crit Rev Biochem 5(3):185, 1978.
107. Faulstich H. Structure of poisonous components of Amanita phalloides. Curr Probl Clin Biochem 71, 1977.
108. Wieland T, Faulstich H. Peptide toxins from Amanita. In: Keeler RF, and Tu AT, eds. Handbook of Natural Toxins, Vol 1. New York, Marcel Dekker, 1983:585.
109. Wieland T. Poisonous principles of mushrooms of the genus Amanita. Science 159:946, 1968.
110. Mitchel DH. Amanita mushroom poisoning. Ann Rev Med 31:51, 1980.
111. Lindell TJ, Weinberg F, Morris P, et al. Specific inhibition of nuclear RNA polymerase II by alpha-amanitin. Science 170:447, 1970.
112. Lindell TJ, Weinberg F, Morris PW, et al. Specific inhibition of nuclear RNA-polymerase-II by alpha-amanitin. Science 170:447, 1970.
113. Stirpe F, Fiume L. Studies on the pathogenesis of liver necrosis by a-amanitin. Biochem J 105:779, 1967.
114. Editorial. Mushroom poisoning. Lancet 2:351, 1980.
115. Wieland T. Poisonous principles of mushrooms of the genus Amanita. Science 159:946, 1968.
116. Belliardo F, Massano G, Accomo S. Amatoxins do not cross the placental barrier. Lancet 1:1381, 1983.
117. Slodkowska J, Szendzikowski S, Stetkiewicz J, et al. Obraz mikroskopowy zmian watroby I mechanizm ich rozwoju W Zatruciu muchomorem sromotnikowym. Pat Pol 1:55, 1980.
118. Wieland TH, Govindan VM. Phallotoxins bind to actin. FEBS Lett 46:351, 1974.
119. Faulstich H. New aspects of Amanita poisoning. Klin Wochenschr 57:1143, 1979.
120. Olson KR, Pond SM, Seward J, et al. Amanita phalloides-type poisoning. West J Med 137:282, 1982.
121. Meili EO, Frick PG, Straub PW. Coagulation changes during massive hepatic necrosis due to Amanita phalloides poisoning. Helv Med Acta 35:304, 1969.
122. Fantozzi R, Ledda F, Caramelli L, et al. Clinical findings and follow-up evaluation of an outbreak of mushroom poisoning—survey of Amanita phalloides poisoning. Klin Wochenschr 64:64, 1986.
123. Panner BJ, Hanss RJ. Hepatic injury in mushroom poisoning. Arch Pathol 87:35, 1969.
124. Slodkowska J, Szenozikowski S, Stetkiiewicz J, et al. Microscopical picture and mechanism of development of liver changes in mushroom poisoning. Patol Pol 31:55, 1980.
125. Wepler W, Opitz K. Histologic changes in the liver biopsy in Amanita phalloides intoxication. Hum Pathol 3:249, 1972.
126. Agostini B, Wieland TH, Lesh R. Decreased phalloidin toxicity in rats pretreated with D-galactosamine. Naturwissenschaften 64:649, 1977.
127. Agostini B, Wieland TH, Zimmerman R, et al. Hamorrhagische lebernekrose und schokerscheinungen bei phalloidinvergiftung. Verh Dtsch Ges Pathol 62:260, 1978.
128. Agostini B. Sistema reticolo-endoteliale (fagociti mononucleati) e intossicazione falloidinica. Da Atti del IV Congresso Nazionale della SIAP, 265-272 Messina 6.7.8. Novembre, 1981.
129. Pond SM, Olson KR, Woo OF, et al. Amatoxin poisoning in Northern California, 1982–1983. West J Med 145:204, 1986.
130. Fiume L, Busi C, Campadelli-Fiume G, et al. Production of antibodies to amanitins as the basis for their immunoassay. Experientia 31:1233, 1975.
131. Pastorello L, Tolentino D, D'Alterio M, et al. Determination of a-aminitin by high-performance liquid chromatography. J Chromatog 233:398, 1982.
132. Busi C, Fiume L, Costantino D, et al. Amanita toxins in gastroduodenal fluid of patients poisoned by the mushroom Amanita phalloides. N Engl J Med 300:800, 1979.
133. Wauters JP, Rossel C, Farquet JJ. Amanita phalloides poisoning treated by early charcoal haemoperfusion. Br Med J 2:1465, 1978.
134. Henry JA. Specific problems of drug intoxication. Br J Anaesth 58:223, 1986.
135. Canalese J, Gimson AES, Davis C, et al. Controlled trial of dexamethasone and mannitol for the cerebral oedema of fulminant hepatic failure. Gut 23:625, 1982.
136. Masini E, Blandina P, Mannaioni PF. Removal of alpha-amanitin from blood by hemoperfusion over uncoated charcoal. Experimental results. Contrib Nephrol 29:76, 1982.
137. Busi C, Fiume L, Costantino D, et al. Determination des amanitines dans le serum de patients intoxiques par l'Amanite phalloide. Nouv Presse Med 6:2855, 1977.
138. Vesconi S, Langer M, Costantino D. Mushroom poisoning and forced diuresis. Lancet 2:854, 1980.
139. Langer M, Vesconi S, Costantino D, et al. Pharmacodynamics amatoxins in human poisoning. In: Faulstich H, Kommerell B, Wieland T, eds. Amanita Toxins and Poisoning. New York, Witzstrock, 1979.
140. Floersheim GL. Curative potencies against a-Amanitin poisoning by cytochrome c. Science 177:808, 1972.
141. Moroni F, Fantozzi R, Masini E, et al. A trend in the therapy of Amanita phalloides poisoning. Arch Toxicol 36:111, 1976.
142. Floersheim GL. Antidotes to experimental a-amanitin poisoning. Nature (New Biol) 263:115, 1972.
143. Floersheim GL. Antagonistic effects against single lethal doses of Amanita phalloides. Naunyn-Schmiedelberg's Arch Pharmacol 293:171, 1976.
144. Fiume L, Sperti S, Montanaro L, et al. Amanitins do not bind to serum albumin. Lancet 1:1111, 1977.

145. Fiume L. Mechanism of action of amanitins. Curr Probl Clin Biochem 7:20, 1977.

146. Hruby K, Csomos G, Fuhrmann M, et al. Chemotherapy of *Amanita phalloides* poisoning with intravenous silibinin. Hum Toxicol 2:183, 1983.

147. Jahn W, Faulstich H, Wieland Th. Pharmacokinetics of (3H-) methyldehydroxy-methyl-a-amanitin in the isolated perfused rat liver, and the influence of several drugs. In: Faulstich H, Kommerell B, Wieland Th, eds. Amanita Toxins and Poisoning. Baden-Baden, Verlag Gerhard Witzstrock, 1980:79.

148. International Symposium on Thioctic Acid, Naples 1955: Thioctic acid, physics, chemistry and biology. Chem Abst 51:8153, 1957.

149. Schmidt U, Grafen P, Goedde HW. Chemistry and biochemistry of alpha lipoic acid. Angew Chem Int Ed Engl 4(10):845, 1965.

150. Kubicka J. Traitement des empoisonnements fongiques phalloidiniens en Tchecoslovaquie. Acta Mycol 4(2):373, 1968.

151. Finestone AJ, Berman R, Widmer B, et al. Thioctic acid treatment of acute mushroom poisoning. Pa Med 75(7):49, 1972.

152. Plotzker R, Jensen JM, Payne JA. *Amanita virosa* acute hepatic necrosis: treatment with thioctic acid. Am J Med Sci 283:79, 1982.

153. Floersheim GL, Bianchi L. Ethanol diminishes the toxicity of the mushroom *Amanita phalloides*. Experientia 40:1268, 1984.

154. Floersheim GL. Antidotes to experimental a-amanitin poisoning. Nature (New Biol) 236:115, 1972.

155. Woodle ES, Moody RR, Cox KL, et al. Orthotopic liver transplantation in a patient with *Amanita* poisoning. JAMA 253:69, 1985.

156. Rocky Mountain Poison Center. Poisindex, Micromedex, 1974.

157. Chuttani HK, Gupta PS, Gulati S, et al. Acute copper sulfate poisoning. Am J Med 39:849, 1965.

158. Ghosh S, Aggarwal VP. Accidental poisoning in childhood. J Indian Med Assoc 39:635, 1962.

159. Klatskin G. Drug-induced hepatic injury. In: Schaffner F, Sherlock S, Leevy CM, eds. The Liver and Its Diseases. New York, Intercontinental Medical Book, 1974:173.

160. Goldberg A, Willian CG, Jones RS, et al. Studies on copper metabolism. J Lab Clin Med 48:442, 1956.

161. Chuttani HK, Gupta PS, Gulati S, et al. Acute copper sulfate poisoning. Am J Med 39:849, 1965.

162. Tanner MS, Portmann B, Mowat AP, et al. Increased hepatic concentration in Indian childhood cirrhosis. Lancet 1:1203, 1979.

163. Sharda B, Bhandari B. Copper concentration in plasma, cells, liver, urine, hair and nails in hepatobiliary disorders in children. Indian Pediatr 21:167, 1984.

164. Sundaravalli N, Meena S, Baskar Raju B. Copper studies in liver disorders. Indian Pediatr 22:195, 1985.

165. Goksu N, Ozsoylu S. Hepatic and serum levels of zinc, copper, and magnesium in childhood cirrhosis. J Pediatr Gastroenterol Nutr 5:259, 1986.

166. Tanner MS, Kantajian AH, Bhave SH, et al. Early introduction of copper contaminated milk feeds as a possible cause of Indian childhood cirrhosis. Lancet 2:992, 1983.

167. Chaudhary SK. Environmental factors: extensive use of copper utensils and vegetarian diet in the causation of Indian childhood cirrhosis. Indian Pediatr 20:529, 1984.

168. Walshe JM. Copper: its role in the pathogenesis of liver disease. Semin Liver Dis 4(3):252, 1984.

169. Epstein O, Arborgh B, Sagiv M, et al. Is copper hepatotoxic in primary biliary cirrhosis? J Clin Pathol 34:1071, 1981.

170. Pimentel JC, Menezes AP. Liver granulomas containing copper vineyard sprayer's lung. Am Rev Resp Dis 111:189, 1975.

171. Lefkowitch JH, Muschel R, Price JB, et al. Copper and copper-binding protein in fibrolamellar liver cell carcinoma. Cancer 51:97, 1983.

172. Vecchio FM, Federico F. Copper and hepatocellular carcinoma. Digestion 35:109, 1986.

173. Sneddon IB. Berylliosis: a case report. Br Med J 1:1448, 1955.

174. Prine JR, Brokeshoulder SF, McVean DE, et al. Demonstration of the presence of beryllium in pulmonary granulomas. Am J Clin Pathol 45:448, 1966.

175. Luongo MA, Bjornson SS. The liver in ferrous sulfate poisoning. A report of three fatal cases in children and an experimental study. N Engl J Med 251:995, 1954.

176. Robotham JL, Troxler RF, Lietman PS. Iron poisoning: another energy crisis. Lancet 2:664, 1974.

177. Zimmerman HJ. Syndromes of environmental hepatotoxicity. In: Zimmerman HJ. Hepatotoxicity. New York, Appleton-Century-Crofts, 1978:290.

178. Bothwell TH, Charlton RW. Hemochromatosis. In: Schiff L, Schiff ER, eds. Diseases of the Liver, 5th ed. Philadelphia, JB Lippincott, 1982:1031.

179. Diaz-Rivera RS, Collazo PJ, Pons ER, et al. Acute phosphorous poisoning in man. A study of 56 cases. Medicine 29:269, 1950.

180. Salfelder K, Doehnert HR, Doehnert G, et al. Fatal phosphorous poisoning. A study of 45 autopsy cases. Beitr Pathol Bd 147:321, 1972.

181. Greenburger NJ, Robinson WL, Isselbacher KJ. Toxic hepatitis after the ingestion of phosphorus with subsequent recovery. Gastroenterology 47:179, 1964.

182. Klatskin G. Toxic and drug-induced hepatitis. In: Schiff L, ed. Diseases of the Liver, 4th ed. Philadelphia, JB Lippincott, 1975:604.

183. Manson-Bahr PEC. Antiprotozoal drugs. In: Meyler L, Herxheimer A, eds. Side Effects of Drugs, Vol. VII. Amsterdam, Excerpta Medica Foundation, 1972:409.

184. Editorial: Thallium. Lancet 2:564, 1974.

185. Fischl J. Aminoaciduria in thallium poisoning. Am J Med Sci 251:40, 1966.

186. Woods JS, Fowler BA. Alteration of hepatocellular structure and function by thallium chloride: ultrastructural, morphometric, and biochemical studies. Toxicol Appl Pharmacol 83:218, 1986.

187. Boeckx RL. Lead poisoning in children. Anal Chem 58:274A, 1986.

188. Sanchez JAC, de la Fuente JMCG, Castrillo JMA, et al. Hepatotoxicidad por plomo inorganico: resultados en 85 casos de saturnismo agudo. Gastroenterol Y Heapotol 8(1):24, 1985.

189. Webb M. Cadmium. Br Med Bull 31:246, 1975.

190. Singhal RL, Merali Z, Hrdina PD. Aspects of the biochemical toxicology of cadmium. Fed Proc 35:75, 1976.

191. Sumino D, Hayakawa D, Shibata T, et al. Heavy metals in normal Japanese tissues. Amounts of 15 heavy metals in 30 subjects. Arch Environ Health 30:487, 1975.

192. Santone KS, Acosta D. Cadmium toxicity in primary cultures of rat hepatocytes. J Toxicol Environ Health 10:169, 1982.

193. Sorensen EMB, Smith NKR, Boecker CS, et al. Calcium amelioration of cadmium-induced cytotoxicity in cultured rat hepatocytes. In Vitro 20(10):771, 1984.

194. Klimczak J, Wisniewska-Knypl JM, Kolakowski J. Stimulation of lipid peroxidation and heme oxygenase activity with inhibition of cytochrome P-450 mono-oxygenase in the liver of rats repeatedly exposed to cadmium. Toxicology 32:267, 1984.

195. Jongstra-Spaapen EJ, Morselt AFW, Copius Peereboom-Stegeman JHJ. Investigation of the mechanism of cadmium toxicity at cellular level. I. A light microscopical study. Arch Toxicol 52:91, 1983.

196. Morselt AFW, Copius Peereboom-Stegeman JHJ, Puvion E, et al. Investigation for the mechanism of cadmium toxicity at cellular level. II. An electron microscopical study. Arch Toxicol 52:99, 1983.

197. Kopelman H, Robertson MH, Saunders PG. The Epping jaundice. Br Med J 1:514, 1966.

198. Kopelman H, Scheuer P, Williams R. The liver lesion in Epping jaundice. Q J Med 35:553, 1966.

199. Kopelman H. The Epping jaundice after two years. Postgrad Med J 44:78, 1968.

200. McGill DB, Motto JD. An industrial outbreak of toxic hepatitis due to methylenedianiline. N Engl J Med 291(6):278, 1974.

201. Bastian PG. Occupational hepatitis caused by methylenedianiline. Med J Aust 141:553, 1984.

202. Williams SV, Bryan JA, Burk JR, et al. Toxic hepatitis and methylenedianiline. N Engl J Med 291:1256, 1974.

203. Solis-Herruzo JA, Castellano G, Colina F, et al. Hepatic injury in the toxic epidemic syndrome caused by ingestion of adulterated cooking oil (Spain, 1981). Hepatology 4(1):131, 1984.

204. Velicia R, Sanz C, Martinez-Barredo F, et al. Hepatic disease in the Spanish toxic oil syndrome. J Hepatol 3:59, 1986.

205. Toxic Epidemic Syndrome Study Group. Toxic epidemic syndrome—Spain 1981. Lancet 2:697, 1982.

206. Martinez-Tello FJ, Navas-Palacios JJ, Ricoy JR, et al. Pathology of new toxic syndrome caused by ingestion of adulterated oil in Spain. Virchows Arch 396:261, 1982.

207. Vicario TL, Serrano-Rios M, San Andres F, et al. HLA-DR3, DR4 increase in chronic stage of Spanish oil disease. Lancet 1:276, 1982.

208. Schmid R. Cutaneous porphyria in Turkey. N Engl J Med 263:397, 1960.

209. Peters HA. Hexachlorobenzene poisoning in Turkey. Fed Proc 35:2400, 1976.

210. Lucke HH, Hodge KE, Patt NL. Fatal liver damage after barium enemas containing tannic acid. Can Med Assoc J 89:111, 1963.

211. Marks V, Chapple PAL. Hepatic dysfunction in heroin and cocaine users. Br J Addict 62:189, 1967.

212. Shuster L, Quimby F, Bates A, et al. Liver damage from cocaine in mice. Life Sci 20:1035, 1977.

213. Gottfried MR, Kloss MW, Graham D, et al. Ultrastructure of experimental cocaine hepatotoxicity. Hepatology 6:299, 1986.

214. Evans MA, Harbison RD. Cocaine-induced hepatotoxicity in mice. Toxicol Appl Pharmacol 45:739, 1978.

215. Freeman RW, Harbison RD. Hepatic periportal necrosis induced by

chronic administration of cocaine. Biochem Pharmacol 30:777, 1981.

216. Kloss MW, Rosen GM, Rauckman EJ. Acute cocaine-induced hepatotoxicity in DBA/2a male mice. Toxicol Appl Pharmacol 65:75, 1982.

217. Evans MA, Dwivedi C, Harbison RD. Enhancement of cocaine-induced lethality of phenobarbitol. Adv Behav Biol 21:253, 1975.

218. Thompson ML, Shuster L, Shaw K. Cocaine-induced hepatic necrosis in mice: the role of cocaine metabolism. Biochem Pharmacol 28:2389, 1979.

219. Kloss MW, Cavagnaro J, Rosen GM, et al. Involvement of FAD-containing monooxygenase in cocaine-induced hepatotoxicity. Toxicol Appl Pharmacol 64:88, 1982.

220. Kloss MW, Rosen GM, Rauckman EJ. N-demethylation of cocaine to norcocaine: evidence for participation by cytochrome P-450 and FAD-containing monooxygenase. Mol Pharmacol 23:482, 1983.

221. Kloss MW, Rosen GM, Rauckman EJ. Cocaine-mediated hepatotoxicity. Biochem Pharmacol 33:169, 1984.

222. Rauckman EJ, Rosen GM, Cavagnaro J. Norcocaine nitroxide: a potential hepatotoxic metabolite of cocaine. Mol Pharmacol 21:458, 1982.

223. Peterson FJ, Knodell RG, Lindemann NJ, et al. Prevention of acetaminophen and cocaine hepatotoxicity in mice by cimetidine treatment. Gastroenterology 85:122, 1983.

224. Smith AC, Freeman RW, Harbison RD. Ethanol enhancement of cocaine-induced hepatotoxicity. Biochem Pharmacol 30:453, 1981.

225. Cushny AR. On the action of Senecio alkaloids and the causation of the hepatic cirrhosis of cattle. (Pictou, Molteno or Winton disease.) J Pharmacol Exp Ther 2:531, 1911.

226. Pethick WH. Special report on Pictou cattle disease. Health of Animals, Department of Agriculture of Canada, Ottawa, 1906.

227. Willmot FC, Robertson GW. Senecio disease or cirrhosis of the liver due to Senecio poisoning. Lancet 2:848, 1920.

228. Bras G, Hill KR. Veno-occlusive disease of the liver. Essential pathology. Lancet 2:161, 1956.

229. Lyford CL, Vergara GG, Moeller DD. Hepatic veno-occlusive disease originating in Ecuador. Gastroenterology 70:105, 1976.

230. Mohabbat O, Younos MS, Merzad AA, et al. An outbreak of hepatic veno-occlusive disease in North Western Afghanistan. Lancet 2:269, 1976.

231. Tandon BN, Tandon HD, Tandon RK, et al. An epidemic of veno-occlusive disease of liver in central India. Lancet 2:271, 1976.

232. Stillman AE, Huxtable R, Consroe P, et al. Hepatic veno-occlusive disease due to pyrrolizidine (Senecio) poisoning in Arizona. Gastroenterology 73:349, 1977.

233. McGee JO'D, Patrick RS, Wood CB, et al. A case of veno-occlusive disease of the liver in Britain associated with herbal tea consumption. J Clin Pathol 29:788, 1976.

234. Bras G, Jelliffe DB, Stuart KL. Veno-occlusive disease of liver with nonportal type of cirrhosis, occurring in Jamaica. Arch Pathol 57:285, 1954.

235. McFarlane AL, Branday WJ. Hepatic enlargement with ascites in children. Br Med J 1:838, 1945.

236. Royes K. Infantile hepatic cirrhosis in Jamaica. Caribbean Med J 10:16, 1948.

237. Stuart KL, Bras G. Veno-occlusive disease of the liver. Q J Med 26:291, 1957.

238. McLean EK. The toxic actions of pyrrolizidine (Senecio) alkaloids. Pharmacol Rev 22(4):429, 1970.

239. Mattocks AR. Spectrophotometric determination of unsaturated pyrrolizidine alkaloids. Anal Chem 39:443, 1967.

240. Selzer G, Parker RGF. Senecio poisoning exhibiting as Chiari's syndrome. Am J Pathol 27:885, 1951.

241. Schoental E. Liver disease and "natural" hepatotoxins. Bull WHO 29:823, 1963.

242. Fox DW, Hart MC, Bergeson PS, et al. Pyrrolizidine (Senecio) intoxication mimicking Reye syndrome. J Pediatr 93(6):980, 1978.

243. Kumana CR, Ng M, Lin HJ, et al. Herbal tea induced hepatic veno-occlusive disease: quantification of toxic alkaloid exposure in adults. Gut 26:101, 1985.

244. Srivastava RN. Veno-occlusive disease of the liver. Am Heart J 94(5):665, 1977.

245. Bull LB, Culvenor CCJ, Dick AT. The Pyrrolidizine Alkaloids. John Wiley & Sons, New York, 1968.

246. Ridker PM, Ohkuma S, McDermott WV, et al. Hepatic venocclusive disease associated with the consumption of pyrrolizidine-containing dietary supplements. Gastroenterology 88:1050, 1985.

247. Magee PN. Liver carcinogens in the human environment. In: Liver Cancer. IARC Scientific Publication No. 1. Lyon, WHO International Agency for Research on Cancer, 1971:110.

248. Jago MV. Factors affecting the chronic hepatotoxicity of pyrrolizidine alkaloids. J Pathol 105:1, 1971.

249. Davidson J. The action of retrorsine on rats liver. J Pathol Bacteriol 40:285, 1935.

250. Jago MV. The development of the hepatic megalobutosis of chronic pyrrolidizine poisoning. Am J Pathol 56:405, 1969.

251. Nolan JP, Scheig RL, Klatskin G. Delayed hepatitis and cirrhosis in weanling rats following a single dose of the Senecio alkaloid, lasiocarpine. Am J Pathol 49:129, 1966.

252. Butler WH. Liver injury induced by aflatoxin. In: Popper H, Schaffner F, eds. Progress in Liver Disease, Vol III. New York, Grune & Stratton, 1970:408.

253. Smith KM. Disease of turkey poults. Vet Rec 72:652, 1960.

254. Swarbrick O. Disease of turkey poults. Vet Rec 72:671, 1960.

255. Thiel PG, Stockenstrom S, Gathercole PS. Aflatoxin analysis by reverse phase HPLC using post-column derivatization for enhancement of fluorescence. J Liquid Chromatogr 9(1):103, 1986.

256. Wogan GN. Aflatoxins and their relationship to hepatocellular carcinoma. In: Okuda K, Peters RL, eds. Hepatocellular Carcinoma. New York, John Wiley & Sons, 1976:25.

257. Wogan GN. Structure-activity relationships in toxicity and carcinogenicity of aflatoxins and analogs. Cancer Res 31:1936, 1971.

258. Hutt MSR. Epidemiology of human primary liver cancer. In: Liver Cancer. IARC Scientific Publication No.1. WHO International Agency for Research on Cancer, Lyon, 1971:21.

259. Epstein SM, Bartus B, Farber E. Renal epithelium neoplasms induced in male Wistar rats by oral aflatoxin B1. Cancer Res 29:1045, 1969.

260. Krischnamarchari K, Nagarajan V, Bhat RV, et al. Hepatitis due to aflatoxins, an outbreak in Western India. Lancet 1:1061, 1975.

261. Wogan GN, Shank RC. Toxicity and carcinogenicity of aflatoxins. In: Pitts NN, Metcalfe RL, eds. Advances in Environmental Science and Technology, Vol II. New York, John Wiley & Sons, 1971:321.

262. Alpert ME, Hutt MSR, Wogan GN, et al. The association between aflatoxin in food and hepatoma frequency in Uganda. Cancer 28:253, 1971.

263. Enwonwu CO. The role of dietary aflatoxin in the genesis of hepatocellular cancer in developing countries. Lancet 2:956, 1984.

264. Dichter CR. Risk estimates of liver cancer due to aflatoxin exposure from peanuts and peanut products. Fd Chem Toxicol 22(6):431, 1984.

265. Wogan GN. Mycotoxins and liver injury. In: Gall EA, Mostofi FK, eds. The Liver. Baltimore, Williams & Wilkins, 1973:161.

266. Pong RS, Wogan GN. Time course and dose-response characteristics of aflatoxin B1 effects on rat liver RNA polymerase and ultrastructure. Cancer Res 30:299, 1970.

267. Petout MJ, McGee HA, Schabort JC. The effects of aflatoxin B1, aflatoxin B2 and steirgmatoxyotion on nuclear desoxyribonucleases from rat and mouse livers. Chem Biol Interact 3:353, 1971.

268. Rogers AE, Newberne PM. Diet and aflatoxin B1 toxicity in rats. Toxicol Appl Pharmacol 20:113, 1971.

269. Medhavan TV, Gopalan C. Effect of dietary protein on aflatoxin liver injury in weanling rats. Arch Pathol 80:123, 1968.

270. Rogers AE, Newberne PM. Aflatoxin B1 carcinogenesis in lipotrope deficient rats. Cancer Res 29:1965, 1969.

271. Linsell CA, Peers FG. Aflatoxin and liver cell cancer. Trans R Soc Trop Med Hyg 71:471, 1977.

272. Lutwick LI. Relation between aflatoxins and hepatitis-B virus and hepatocellular carcinoma. Lancet 1:755, 1979.

273. Armbrecht BH, Shalkop WT, Rollins LD, et al. Acute toxicity of aflatoxin B1 in Wethers. Nature (Lond) 225:1062, 1970.

274. Madhaven TV, Tulpule PG, Gopalan C. Aflatoxin-induced hepatic fibrosis in Rhesus monkeys. Arch Pathol 76:466, 1965.

275. Newberne PM, Butler WH. Acute and chronic effects of aflatoxin on the liver of domestic and laboratory animals; a review. Cancer Res 29:236, 1969.

276. Alpert E, Serck-Hanssen A, Rajagopolen B. Aflatoxin-induced hepatic injury in the African monkey. Arch Environ Health 20:723, 1970.

277. Bourgeois CH, Shank RC, Grossman RA, et al. Acute aflatoxin B1 toxicity in the macaque and its similarities to Reye's syndrome. Lab Invest 24:206, 1971.

278. Rogers AE. Toxicity and carcinogenicity of aflatoxins in experimental animals. In: Pollack JD, ed. Reye's Syndrome. New York, Grune & Stratton, 1974:135.

279. Chaves-Carballo E, Ellefson RD, Gomez MR. An aflatoxin in the liver of a patient with Reye-Johnson syndrome. Mayo Clin Proc 51:47, 1976.

280. Stora C, Dvorackova I, Ayraud N. Aflatoxin and Reye's syndrome. J Med 14(1):47, 1983.

281. Ryan NJ, Hogan GR, Hayes AW, et al. Aflatoxin B1: Its role in the etiology of Reye's syndrome. Pediatrics 64:71, 1979.

282. Becroft DMO, Webster DR. Aflatoxins and Reye's disease. Br Med J 2:117, 1972.

283. Dvorackova I, Zilkova J, Brodsky F, et al. Aflatoxin and liver damage with encephalopathy. Sb Ved Pr Lek Fak Univ Karlovy 15:521, 1972.

284. Serck-Hansen A. Aflatoxin-induced fatal hepatitis? Arch Environ Health 20:729, 1970.

285. Allcroft R. Aflatoxicosis in farm animals. In: Goldblatt LA, ed. Aflatoxin-Scientific. Background Control and Implications. New York, Academic Press, 1969:237.

286. Yadgiri B, Reddy V, Tulpule PG, et al. Aflatoxin in Indian childhood cirrhosis. Am J Clin Nutr 23:94, 1970.

287. Wogan GN, Newberne PM. Dose-response characteristics of aflatoxin B1 carcinogenesis in the rat. Cancer Res 27:2370, 1967.

288. Wray BB, Hayes AW. Aflatoxin B1 in the serum of a patient with primary hepatic carcinoma. Environ Res 22:400, 1980.

289. Phillips DL, Yourtree DM, Searles S. Presence of aflatoxin B1 in human liver in the United States. Toxicol Appl Pharmacol 36:403, 1976.

290. Peers FG, Linsell CA. Dietary aflatoxins and liver cancer—a population based study in Kenya. Br J Cancer 27:473, 1973.

291. Campbell TC, Stolloff L. Implications of mycotoxins for human health. J Agric Food Chem 22:1006, 1974.

292. Van Rensburg SJ, Cook-Mozaffari P, Van Schalkwyk DJ, et al. Hepatocellular carcinoma and dietary aflatoxin in Mozambique and Transkei. Br J Cancer 51:713, 1985.

293. Wogan GN. Aflatoxins and their relationship to hepatocellular carcinoma. In: Okuda K, Peters RL, eds. Hepatocellular Carcinoma. New York, John Wiley & Sons, 1976:25.

294. Adamson RH, Correa P, Dalgord DW. Occurrence of a primary liver carcinoma in Rhesus monkey fed aflatoxin B1. J Natl Cancer Inst 50:549, 1973.

295. Dimond JB, Kadunce RE, Getchell AS, et al. DDT residue persistence in red-backed salamanders in a natural environment. Bull Environ Contam Toxicol 3:194, 1968.

296. Dimond JB, Getchell AS, Blease JA. Accumulation and persistence of DDT in a lotic ecosystem. J Fish Res Bd Can 28:1877, 1971.

297. Council on Pharmacy and Chemistry. Pharmacologic and toxicologic aspects of DDT (Chlorophenothane U.S.P.). JAMA 145:728, 1951.

298. Editorial: Insecticide storage in adipose tissue. JAMA 145:735, 1951.

299. Laws ER, Willis CM, Curley A, et al. Long-term occupational exposure to DDT: Effect on the human liver. Arch Environ Health 27:318, 1973.

300. Morgan DP, Roan CC. Liver function in workers having high tissue stores of chlorinated hydrocarbon pesticides. Arch Environ Health 29:14, 1974.

301. Smith NJ. Death following accidental ingestion of DDT. JAMA 136:439, 1948.

302. Hayes WJ, Dale WE, Pirkle CI. Evidence of safety of long-term oral doses of DDT for man. Arch Environ Health 22:119, 1971.

303. Deichmann WB. The debate on DDT. Arch Toxikologie 29:1, 1972.

304. von Oettingen WF. The Halogenated Aliphatic, Olephinic, Cyclic, Aromatic and Aliphatic-Aromatic Hydrocarbons Including the Halogenated Insecticides. Their Toxicity and Potential Dangers. Washington, DC, US Dept HEW, US Government Printing Office, 1955.

305. Conney AH, Welch R, Kuntzman R, et al. Effects of environmental chemicals on the metabolism of drugs, carcinogens and body constituents in man. Ann NY Acad Sci 175:155, 1971.

306. Peakall DB. Pesticides and the reproduction of birds. Sci Am 222:72, 1970.

307. Fouts JR. Interactions of chemicals and drugs to produce effects on organ function. In: Lee DHK, Koten P, eds. Multiple Factors in the Causation of Environmentally Induced Disease. New York, Academic Press, 1972:109.

308. Mitchell JR, Gillette JR. Drug-chemical interactions as a factor in experimentally-induced disease. In: Lee DHK, Koten P, eds. Multiple Factors in the Causation of Environmentally Induced Disease. New York, Academic Press, 1972:119.

309. Ortega P. Light and electron microscopy of dichlorodiphenyltrichloroethane (DDT) poisoning in the rat liver. Lab Invest 15(4):657, 1966.

310. Tomatis L. The IARC program on the evaluation of the carcinogenic risk of chemicals to man. Ann NY Acad Sci 271:369, 1976.

311. Deichmann WB. Research, DDT and cancer. Indust Med 41:15, 1972.

312. Report of the Secretary's Commission on Pesticides and their Relationship to Environmental Health. Washington DC, US Dept of Health, Education and Welfare, December 1969:466.

313. Taylor JR, Selhorst JB, Houff SA, et al. Chlordencone intoxication in man. I. Clinical observations. Neurology (Minneapolis) 28:626, 1978.

314. Cohn WJ, Boylan JJ, Blanke RV, et al. Treatment of chlordecone (Kepone) toxicity with cholestyramine: results of a controlled clinical trial. N Engl J Med 298:243, 1978.

315. Guzelian PS, Vranian G, Boylan JJ, et al. Liver structure and function in patients poisoned with chlordecone (Kepone). Gastroenterology 78:206, 1980.

316. Atwal OS. Fatty changes and hepatic cell excretion in avian liver. An electron microscopical study of Kepone toxicity. J Comp Pathol 83:115, 1973.

317. Eroschenko VP, Wilson WO. Cellular changes in the gonads, livers and adrenal glands of Japanese quail as affected by the insecticide Kepone. Toxicol Appl Pharmacol 31:491, 1975.

318. Huber JJ. Some physiological effects of the insecticide Kepone in the laboratory mouse. Toxicol Appl Pharmacol 7:516, 1965.

319. Report on carcinogenesis bioassay of technical grade chlordecone (Kepone). Am Ind Hyg Assoc J 37:680, 1976.

320. Deichmann WB, MacDonald WE. Organochlorine pesticides and liver cancer deaths in the United States, 1930–1972. Ecotoxicol Environ Safety 1:89, 1977.

321. Rip JW, Cherry JH. Liver enlargement induced by the herbicide 2,4,5-trichlorophenoxyacetic acid (2,4,5-T). Agric Food Chem 24:245, 1976.

322. Poland AP, Smith D, Metter G, et al. A health survey of workers in a 2,4-D plant and 2,4,5-T plant. Arch Environ Health 22:316, 1971.

323. Fries GF, Marrow GS. Retention and excretion of 2,3,7,8-tetrachlorodibenzo-p-dioxin by rats. J Agric Food Chem 23:265, 1975.

324. Jones G, Butler WH. A morphological study of the liver lesion induced by 2,3,7,8-tetrachlorodibenzo-p-dioxin in rats. J Pathol 112:93, 1974.

325. Bullivant CM. Accidental poisoning by paraquat: report of two cases in man. Br Med J 1:1272, 1966.

326. Mullick FG, Ishak KG, Mahabir R, et al. Hepatic injury associated with paraquat toxicity in humans. Liver 1:209, 1981.

327. Jaros F. Acute percutaneous paraquat poisoning. Lancet 1:275, 1978.

328. Waight JJJ. Fatal percutaneous paraquat poisoning. JAMA 242:472, 1979.

329. Matsumoto T, Matsumori H, Kuwabara N, et al. A histopathological study of the liver in paraquat poisoning. An analysis of fourteen autopsy cases with emphasis on bile duct injury. Acta Pathol Jpn 30(6):859, 1980.

330. Matsumori H, Matsumoto T, Ishikawa H. Acute toxic effects of paraquat on ultrastructure of rat liver. Acta Pathol Jpn 34(3):507, 1984.

331. Parkinson C. The changing pattern of paraquat poisoning in man. Histopathology 4:171, 1980.

332. Shield LK, Coleman TL, Markesbery WR. Methyl bromide intoxication: neurologic features, including simulation of Reye syndrome. Neurology 27:959, 1977.

333. Pond SM. Effects on the liver of chemicals encountered in the workplace. West J Med 137(6):506, 1982.

334. Kimbrough RD. The toxicity of polychlorinated polycyclic compounds and related chemicals. CRC Crit Rev Toxicol 2:445, 1974.

335. National Institute for Occupational Safety and Health. A recommended standard of occupational exposure to . . . polychlorinated biphenyls. USDHEW (NIOSH) Publication No. 657012/337, 1979.

336. Peakall DB, Lincer JL. Polychlorinated biphenyls: Another long-life widespread chemical in the environment. Bioscience 20:958, 1970.

337. National Institute for Occupational Safety and Health. Criteria for a recommended standard—occupational exposure to polychlorinated biphenyls (PCBs). USDHEW (NIOSH) Publication No. 77–225, 1977.

338. Polychlorinated biphenyls and polybrominated biphenyls. IARC Monogr Eval Carcinog Risk Chem Hum 18:43, 1978.

339. Nicholson WJ, Moore JA, eds. Health effects of halogenated aromatic hydrocarbons. Ann NY Acad Sci 320:1, 1979.

340. Alvares AP, Kappas A. The inducing properties of polychlorinated biphenyls on hepatic monooxygenases. Clin Pharmacol Ther 22:809, 1977.

341. Alvares AP, Fischbein A, Anderson KE, et al. Alterations in drug metabolism in workers exposed to polychlorinated biphenyls. Clin Pharmacol Ther 22:140, 1977.

342. Friend M, Trainer DO. Polychlorinated biphenyls: interaction with duck hepatitis virus. Science 170:1314, 1970.

343. Kuratsune M, Yoshimura T, Matsuzaka J, et al. Epidemiologic study on Yusho, a poisoning caused by ingestion of rice oil contaminated with a commercial brand of polychlorinated biphenyls. Environ Health Perspect 1:119, 1972.

344. Kuratsune M. An epidemiological study on "Yusho" poisoning. Fubuoka Acta Medica 60:403, 1969.

345. Flinn FB, Jarvik NE. Actions of certain chlorinated naphthalenes on the liver. Proc Soc Exp Biol Med 35:118, 1936.

346. Flinn FB, Jarvik NE. Liver lesions caused by chlorinated naphthalene. Am J Hyg 27:19, 1938.

347. Maroni M, Colombi A, Cantoni S, et al. Occupational exposure to polychlorinated biphenyls in electrical workers—I. Environmental and blood polychlorinated biphenyls concentrations. Br J Ind Med 38:49, 1981.

348. Maroni M, Colombi A, Arbosti G, et al. Occupational exposure to

polychlorinated biphenyls in electrical workers—II. Health effects. Br J Ind Med 38:55, 1981.

349. Fischbein A. Liver function tests in workers with occupational exposure to polychlorinated biphenyls (PCBs): comparison with Yusho and Yu-Cheng. Environ Health Perspect 60:145, 1985.

350. Kikuchi M. Autopsy of patients with Yusho. Am J Ind Med 5:19, 1984.

351. Bang FL. De hydrope ex ingesto arsenico abservatio. Soc Med Havn Coll 1:307, 1774.

352. Roth F. Uber due Spatfolgen des chronishen Arsenismus der Mosel-winzer. Dtsch Med Wochneschr 82:211, 1957.

353. Morris JS, Schmid M, Newman S, et al. Arsenic and non-cirrhotic portal hypertension. Gastroenterology 66:86, 1974.

354. Viallet A, Guillaume E, Cote J, et al. Presinusoidal portal hypertension following chronic arsenic intoxication. Gastroenterology 62:177, 1972.

355. Dhawan D, Narang APS, Datta DV. Levels of arsenic in liver cirrhosis. Toxicol Lett 15:105, 1983.

356. Datta DV. Arsenic and non-cirrhotic portal hypertension. Lancet 1:433, 1976.

357. Feinglass EJ. Arsenic intoxication from well water in the United States. N Engl J Med 288:828, 1973.

358. Milian G. Arsenobenzol, erytheme et rubeole. Paris Med 23:131, 1917.

359. Von Glahn WC, Flinn FB, Keim WF Jr. Effect of certain arsenates on the liver. Arch Pathol 25:488, 1938.

360. Rouiller Ch. Experimental toxic injury of the liver. In: Rouiller Ch, ed. The Liver, Vol II. New York, Academic Press, 1964:335.

361. Foulerton AGR. On acute yellow atrophy of the liver and the fatty infiltration of the liver and kidney which results from the action of certain poisons on the liver. J Pathol 24:257, 1920.

362. Hanger FM Jr, Gutman AB. Post-arsphenamine jaundice apparently due to obstruction of intrahepatic biliary tract. JAMA 115:263, 1940.

363. Hartmann FL, Singer AG. Intrahepatic obstructive jaundice due to neoarsphenamine. Arch Derm Syph 53:620, 1946.

364. Haubrich WS, Sancetta SM. Spontaneous recovery from hepato-biliary disease with xanthomatosis. Gastroenterology 26:658, 1954.

365. Stolzer BL, Miller G, White WA, et al. Postarsenical obstructive jaundice complicated by xanthomatosis and diabetes mellitus. Am J Med 9:124, 1960.

366. Jhaveri SS. A case of cirrhosis and primary carcinoma of the liver in chronic industrial arsenical intoxication. Br J Indust Med 16:248, 1959.

367. Luchtrath H. Cirrhosis of the liver in chronic arsenical poisoning of vintners. Germ Med 2:127, 1972.

368. Kelynack TN, Kirby W, Delepine S, et al. Arsenical poisoning from beer-drinking. Lancet 2:1600, 1900.

369. Regelson W, Kim U, Ospina J, et al. Haemangioendothelial sarcoma of liver from chronic arsenic intoxication by Fowler's solution. Cancer 21:514, 1968.

370. Lander JJ, Stanley RJ, Sumner HW, et al. Angiosarcoma of the liver associated with Fowler's solution (potassium arsenite). Gastroenterology 68(6):1582, 1975.

371. Falk H, Caldwell GG, Ishak KG, et al. Arsenic-related hepatic angiosarcoma. Am J Indust Med 2:43, 1981.

372. Cowlishaw JL, Pollard EJ, Cowen AE, et al. Liver disease associated with chronic arsenic ingestion. Aust NZ J Med 9:310, 1979.

373. Chainuvati T, Viranuvatti V. Idiopathic portal hypertension and chronic arsenic poisoning. Digest Dis Sci 24(1):70, 1979.

374. Harvey SC. Heavy metals. In: Goodman LS, Gilman A, Gilman AG, et al., eds. The Pharmacological Basis of Therapeutics, 5th ed. New York, MacMillan Book Co, 1975:924.

375. Wiese U. Ullmanns Encyklopadie d. techn. Chemie, 4. Aufl., Verlag Chemie, Weinheim 21:227, 1982.

376. Korpela H, Kumpulainen J, Luoma PV, et al. Decreased serum selenium in alcoholics as related to liver structure and function. Am J Clin Nutr 42:147, 1985.

377. Dworkin B, Rosenthal WS, Jankowski RH, et al. Low blood selenium levels in alcoholics with and without advanced liver disease. Digest Dis Sci 30(9):838, 1985.

378. Rotruck JT, Pope AL, Ganther HE, et al. Biochemical roles as a component of glutathione peroxidase. Science 179:588, 1973.

379. Sunde RA, Hoekstra WG. Structure synthesis and function of glutathione peroxidase. Nutr Rev 38:265, 1980.

380. Suematsu T, Matsumura T, Sato N, et al. Lipid peroxidation in alcoholic liver disease in humans. Alcoholism 5:427, 1981.

381. Shaw S, Rubin KP, Lieber CS. Depressed hepatic glutathione and increased diene conjugate in alcoholic liver disease. Evidence of lipid peroxidation. Dig Dis Sci 28:585, 1983.

382. Lewis KO, Paton A. Could superoxide cause cirrhosis? Lancet 2:188, 1982.

383. Schellmann B, Raithel HJ, Schaller KH. Acute fatal selenium poisoning. Arch Toxicol 59:61, 1986.

384. Koppel C, Baudisch H, Koppel I. Fatal poisoning with selenium dioxide. Clin Toxicol 24(1):21, 1986.

385. Diplock AT. Metabolic aspects of selenium action and toxicity. CRC Crit Rev Toxicol 4:219, 1976.

386. Vernie LN, Bont WS, Emmelot P. Inhibition of in vitro amino acid incorporation by sodium selenite. Biochemistry 13:337, 1974.

387. Willett WC. Selenium and human cancer. Acta Pharmacol Toxicol 7:240, 1986.

388. Lemly AD. Ecological basis for regulating aquatic emmissions from the power industry: the case with selenium. Reg Toxicol Pharmacol 5:465, 1985.

389. Berk PD, Martin JF, Young RS, et al. Vinyl chloride-associated liver disease. Ann Intern Med 84:717, 1976.

390. Marsteller HJ, Lelbach WK, Muller R, et al. Chronischtoxische leber-schaden bei arbeitern in der PVC-produktion. Dtsch Med Wochenschr 98:2311, 1973.

391. Lee FI, Harry DS. Angiosarcoma of the liver in a vinyl chloride worker. Lancet 1:1316, 1974.

392. Creech J, Johnson MN, Block B. Angiosarcoma of the liver among polyvinyl chloride workers—Kentucky. Morbid Mortal Weekly Rep 23(6):49, 1974.

393. Creech JL Jr, Johnson MN. Angiosarcoma of the liver in the manufacture of polyvinyl chloride. J Occup Med 16:150, 1974.

394. Editorial: Vinyl chloride, P.V.C., and cancer. Lancet 1:1323, 1974.

395. Popper H, Selikoff IJ. Classical syndromes in occupational medicine. Pathological lessons from vinyl chloride angiosarcoma. Am J Indust Med 2:187, 1981.

396. Baxter PJ, Anthony PP, MacSween RNM, et al. Angiosarcoma of the liver in Great Britain, 1963–73. Br Med J 2:919, 1977.

397. Gedigk P, Muller R, Bechtelsheimer H. Morphology of liver damage among polyvinyl chloride production workers. A report on 51 cases. Ann NY Acad Sci 246:278, 1975.

398. Lee FI. Vinyl chloride-induced liver disease. J Roy Coll Phys Lond 16(4):226, 1982.

399. Heath CW Jr, Falk H. Characteristics of cases of angiosarcoma of the liver among vinyl chloride workers in the United States. Ann NY Acad Sci 246:231, 1975.

400. Smith PM, Williams DMJ, Crossley IP. Portal hypertension induced by vinyl chloride. Gut 16:402, 1975.

401. Popper H, Thomas LB. Alterations of liver and spleen among workers exposed to vinyl chloride. Ann NY Acad Sci 246:172, 1975.

402. Selikoff IJ, Hammond ED, eds. Toxicity of vinyl chloride-polyvinyl chloride. Ann NY Acad Sci 1:337, 1975.

403. Editorial: Vinyl chloride. The carcinogenic risk. Br Med J 2:134, 1976.

404. Schneider MJ. The fatal byproduct. Sciences 15:27, 1975.

405. Mancuso T. Comments for opening of discussion on "neoplastic effects." Ann NY Acad Sci 246:251, 1975.

406. Griciute L. The carcinogenicity of vinyl chloride. IARC Monogr 22:3, 1978.

407. Turshen M. Community health or company profits. Environ Action 8:11, 1976.

408. Radite MJ, Stemmer KL, Brown PG, et al. Effect of ethanol and vinyl chloride on the induction of liver tumours. Environ Health Perspect 21:153, 1977.

409. Tamburro CH. Relationship of vinyl monomers and liver cancers: angiosarcoma and hepatocellular carcinoma. Semin Liver Dis 4(2):158, 1984.

410. Radike MJ, Stemmer KL, Bingham E. Effect of ethanol on vinyl chloride carcinogenesis. Environ Health Perspect 41:59, 1981.

411. Maltoni C, Clini C, Vicini F, et al. Two cases of liver angiosarcoma among polyvinyl chloride (PVC) extruders of an Italian factory producing PVC bags and other containers. Am J Indust Med 5:297, 1984.

412. Hefner RE Jr, Watanabe PG, Gehring PG. Preliminary studies of the fate of inhaled vinyl chloride monomer in rats. Ann NY Acad Sci 246:135, 1975.

413. Van Esch FJ, Van Logten MJ. Vinyl chloride. A report of a European assessment. Food Cosmet Toxicol 13:121, 1975.

414. Tamburro CH, Creech JJ Jr, Davis A, et al. Indocyanine green clearance as the prospective indicator of hepatocellular chemical toxicity. Gastroenterology 75:989, 1978.

415. Tamburro CH, Greenberg RA. Effectiveness of federally required medical laboratory screening in the detection of chemical liver injury. Environ Health Perspect 41:117, 1981.

416. Tamburro CH, Makk L, Popper H. Early hepatic histological alterations among chemical (vinyl monomer) workers. Gastroenterology 77:A43, 1979.

417. Liss GM, Greenberg RA, Tamburro CH. Use of serum bile acids in the identification of vinyl chloride hepatotoxicity. Am J Med 78:68, 1985.

418. Triche T, Nanba K, Ishak K, et al. Hepatic ultrastructural changes in vinyl-chloride workers (Abstr). Clin Res 23:259, 1975.

419. Blendis LM, Smith PM, Lawrie BW, et al. Portal hypertension in vinyl chloride monomer workers. Gastroenterology 75:206, 1978.
420. Harris DK, Adams WGF. Acro-osteolysis occurring in men engaged in the polymerization of vinyl chloride. Br Med J 3:712, 1967.
421. Falck K, Grohn P, Sorsa M, et al. Mutagenicity in urine of nurses handling cytostatic drugs. Lancet 1:1250, 1979.
422. Norppa H, Sorsa M, Vainio H, et al. Increased sister chromatic exchange (SCE) frequencies in lymphocytes of nurses handling cytostatic drugs. Scand J Work Environ Health 6:299, 1980.
423. Waksvik H, Kiepp O, Brogger A. Chromosome analyses of nurses handling cytostatic agents. Cancer Treat Rep 65:607, 1981.
424. Sotaniemi EA, Sutinen S, Arranto AJ, et al. Liver damage in nurses handling cytostatic agents. Acta Med Scand 214:181, 1983.
425. Knowles RS, Virden JE. Handling of injectable antineoplastic agents. Br Med J 2:589, 1980.
426. Mihajlova TV. Benzyl chloride. In: Jenks W, ed. International Labor Office: Encyclopedia of Occupational Health and Safety, Vol 1. New York, McGraw-Hill Book Co, 1971:169.
427. Dahab GM, Gerges SE, Abdel-Rahman MS. Effect of benzyl chloride on rat liver functions. J Toxicol Environ Health 18:431, 1986.
428. Goldstein JA, Hickman P, Bergman H, et al. Hepatic porphyria induced by 2,3,7,8-tetrachlorodibenzo-p-dioxin in the mouse. Res Commun Chem Pathol Pharmacol 6:919, 1973.
429. Colombi AM. Subjective symptomatology prevalence as an additional criterion to define riskgroups exposed to TCDD in the Seveso area, Italy. In: Strik JJ TWA, Koeman JH, eds. Chemical Porphyria in Man. Amsterdam, North-Holland, 1979:83.
430. Fries GF, Marrow GS. Retention and excretion of 2,3,7,8-tetrachlorodibenzo-p-dioxin by rats. J Agr Food Chem 23(2):265, 1975.
431. Autian J. Toxicity and health threats of phthalate esters: review of the literature. Environ Health Perspect 4:3, 1973.
432. Gesler RM. Toxicology of di-2-ethylhexyl phthalate and other phthalic acid ester plasticizers. Environ Health Perspect 3:73, 1973.
433. Jaeger RJ, Rubin RJ. Plasticizers from plastic devices: extraction, metabolism, and accumulation by biological systems. Science 170:460, 1970.
434. Hillman LS, Goodwin SL, Sherman WR. Identification and measurement of plasticizer in neonatal tissues after umbilical catheters and blood products. N Engl J Med 292(8):381, 1975.
435. Mes J, Coffin DE, Campbell DS. Di-n-butyl- and di-2-ethylhexyl phthalate in human adipose tissue. Bull Environ Contamin Toxicol 12(6):721, 1974.
436. Kevy SV, Jacobson MS, Harmon WE. The need for a new plasticizer for polyvinyl chloride medical devices. Trans Am Soc Artif Intern Organs 27:386, 1981.
437. Kevy SV, Button LN, Jacobson MS. Toxicology of plastic devices having contact with blood. Comprehensive three year report. National Heart Lung Blood Institute, National Institutes of Health, Bethesda, MD, September 1975.
438. Reddy JK, Warren JR, Reddy MK, et al. Hepatic and renal effects of peroxisome proliferators: biological implications. Ann NY Acad Sci (In press.)
439. Moody DE, Reddy JK. Serum triglyceride and cholesterol contents in male rats receiving diets containing plasticizers and analogues of the ester 2-ethylhexanol. Toxicol Lett 10:379, 1982.
440. Warren JR, Lalwani ND, Reddy JK. Phthalate esters as peroxisome proliferator carcinogens. Environ Health Perspect 45:35, 1982.
441. Kluwe WM, Haseman JK, Douglas JF, et al. The carcinogenicity of dietary di (2-ethylhexyl) phthalate (DEHP) in Fischer 344 rats and B6C3F mice. J Toxicol Environ Health 10:797, 1982.
442. Albro PW, Corbett JT, Schroeder JL, et al. Pharmacokinetics, interactions with macromolecules and species differences in metabolism of DEHP. Environ Health Perspect 45:19, 1982.
443. Seth PK. Hepatic effects of phthalate esters. Environ Health Perspect 45:27, 1982.
444. Mushtag M, Srivastava SP, Seth PK. Effect of di-2-ethylhexyl phthalate (DEHP) on glycogen metabolism in rat liver. Toxicology 16:153, 1980.
445. Rubin RJ. Plasticizers in human tissues. N Engl J Med 278:1114, 1972.

33

Alcoholic Liver Disease

*David Zakim, M.D. • Thomas D. Boyer, M.D.
• Carolyn Montgomery, M.D.*

Alcohol abuse costs the U.S. more than $116 billion per year, of which about 12 per cent is for direct costs of medical care.[1, 2] Alcohol accounts for about 100,000 deaths per year in the United States.[3] A study of middle-aged men in Malmö, Sweden, over nearly six years in the early 1980s showed that premature deaths caused by alcoholism were as frequent as deaths resulting from cancer or coronary artery disease.[4] Nineteen per cent of the deaths due to alcoholism could be attributed to cirrhosis. The basic reason for this large epidemic of alcohol-related disease is that ethanol is an effective drug in relieving anxiety, depression, and the pressures of modern society. The easy availability of ethanol and the social acceptability of ethanol consumption are advertised widely and aggressively. About $1.2 billion is spent to advertise alcohol consumption as manly, facilitating sociability, leading to wealth and prestige, and enhancing romantic settings.[5] The industry promotes "responsible drinking" in its advertising. Yet it is known that the incidence of alcohol abuse increases rapidly as per

capita consumption increases and that the amount of alcohol drunk per event increases as frequency of drinking increases.[6, 7] The public seems unaware that chronic use of ethanol in the absence of addiction can lead to serious medical illness, the development of adverse social consequences of chronic use, or both.

Consumption of ethanol is widespread; about three quarters of the population of the United States use it. The incidence of alcoholism in the United States is approximately 7 per cent. In some states, such as California, it exceeds 10 per cent. We are therefore confronted with a social problem of enormous proportions—that is, a group of alcohol-related diseases that are completely preventable. The discussion in this chapter is limited to the impact of ethanol consumption on the incidence of hepatic disease, the possible causal relationship between ethanol use and liver disease, the clinical manifestations and course of ethanol-associated liver disease, and the management of these complications of ethanol abuse. Prevention (or treatment or both) of alcoholism is a problem for which we have no certain answers. Nor does there seem to be strong public resolve in this respect.[9] It is therefore clear that we will have to continue to manage the medical complications of alcoholism and to improve the usefulness of therapy. With regard to liver disease, we need to devise therapies that diminish the impact of ethanol on hepatic function. To do so depends on an understanding of the mechanisms by which ethanol ingestion leads to liver disease and whether ethanol per se is the cause of liver disease or whether ethanol abuse, environmental factors, and genetic predisposition act in concert to produce liver disease. Answers to these questions may be sought via experiments in animals aimed at elucidating the biochemical effects of ethanol metabolism and through studies of the natural history of ethanol-induced liver disease in patients. We hence devote a large portion of this chapter to a consideration of the biochemical basis for the hepatotoxicity of ethanol and to studies in experimental animals of ethanol-induced liver disease.

RELATIONSHIP BETWEEN ETHANOL CONSUMPTION AND THE INCIDENCE OF LIVER DISEASE

The concept of ethanol as a substance producing irreversible damage to the liver rests primarily on the clinicopathologic observation that cirrhosis with a fairly typical histologic appearance (see later) occurs in patients who consume large amounts of ethanol. Ethanol can be shown to have a variety of toxic effects on livers in otherwise normal animals, including normal men and women (Table 33–1), but whether any of these changes are cirrhogenic is debatable. Moreover, the animal models for ethanol-induced cirrhosis are not satisfactory (see later) and may indeed not apply to humans. Hence, it is important to keep in mind that epidemiologic evidence, not biochemical studies of the toxicity of ethanol, leads us to conclude that ethanol ingestion is an important factor in the genesis of

TABLE 33–1. SOME WAYS IN WHICH ETHANOL INGESTION CAN DIRECTLY OR INDIRECTLY STRESS LIVER CELL FUNCTION

Disorganizes the lipid portion of cell membranes, leading to adaptive changes in their composition
Increased fluidity and permeability of membranes
Impaired assembly of glycoproteins into membranes
Impaired secretion of glycoproteins
Impaired binding and internalization of large ligands
Formation of abnormal mitochondria
Impairment of transport of small ligands
Impairment of membrane-bound enzymes
Adaptive changes in lipid composition, leading to increased lipid peroxidation
Abnormal display of antigens on the plasma membrane
Alters the capacity of liver cells to cope with environmental toxins
Induces xenobiotic metabolizing enzymes
Directly inhibits xenobiotic metabolizing enzymes
Induces deficiency in mechanisms protecting against injury due to reactive metabolites
Enhances the toxicity of O_2
Oxidation of ethanol produces acetaldehyde, a toxic and reactive intermediate
Inhibits export of proteins from the liver
Modifies hepatic protein synthesis in fasted animals
Alters the metabolism of cofactors essential for enzymic activity—pyridoxine, folate, choline, Zn, vitamin E
Alters the oxidation—reduction potential of the liver cell
Induces malnutrition

cirrhosis; as for example, cirrhosis at autopsy is severalfold more frequent in alcoholics than in nonalcoholics.[10–12] Data on consumption reveal a positive correlation between average per capita ingestion of ethanol and the frequency of cirrhosis found post-mortem (Fig. 33–1) and show that decreases in the availability of ethanol-containing beverages are associated with declines in deaths due to cirrhosis (Fig. 33–2). These relationships are strengthened by the separate observation that the incidence of alcohol abuse increases with per capita consumption of alcohol.[6]

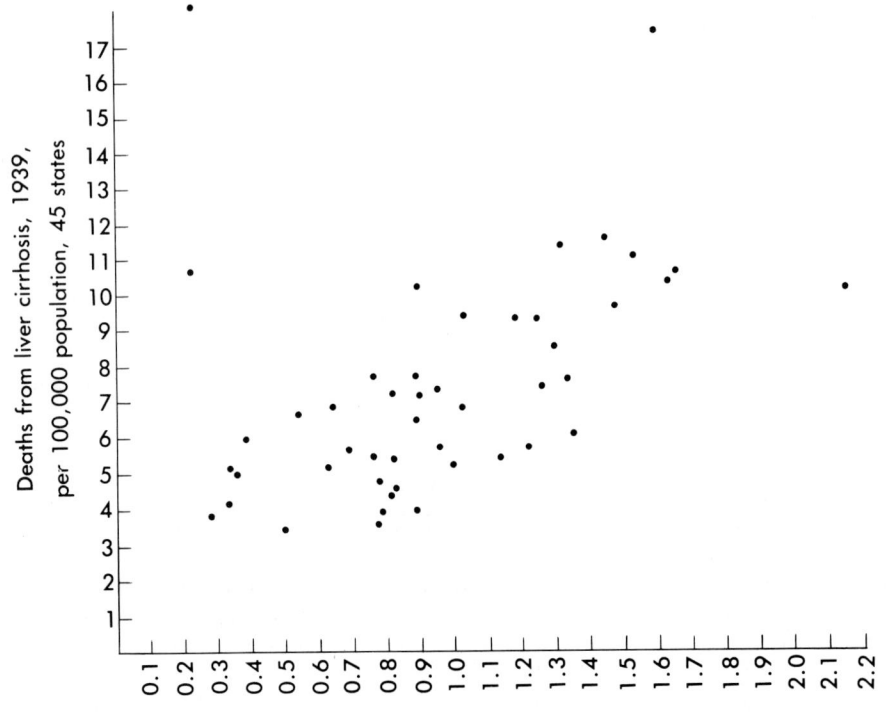

Figure 33–1. The relationship of death from cirrhosis of the liver per hundred thousand 1939 population of 45 states of the United States to the 1939 per capita consumption of absolute alcohol in the same states. (Reproduced from Jollife N, Jellinek EM. QJ Stud Alcohol 2:544, 1941, with permission.)

Deaths from liver cirrhosis, 1939, per 100,000 population, 45 states

Per capita consumption absolute alcohol (gallons), 1939

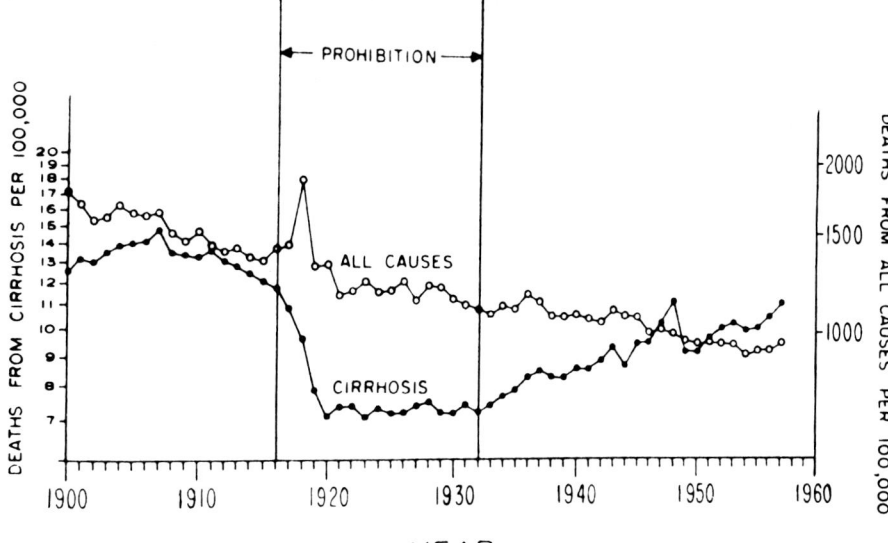

Figure 33–2. Cirrhosis mortality in the United States between 1900 and 1957 compared with death from all causes per 100,000. (From Martini GA, Bode CH. In: Engel A, Larsson T, eds. Alcoholic Cirrhosis and Other Toxic Hepatopathias. Stockholm, Nordiska Bokhandelns Förlag, 1970:315, with permission.)

Given the epidemiologic data indicating that ethanol causes liver disease (although the mechanism of its toxic effect[s] remains to be elucidated), the next logical question is, How much ethanol induces clinically significant liver disease? Lelbach, in Germany, studied in retrospect the relationship between consumption of ethanol and the incidence of liver disease by correlating consumption with histologic evidence of disease.[13,14] Not surprisingly, he found that the amount ingested and duration of intake were important factors in the induction of alcohol-associated liver disease. The incidence of biopsy-proven alcoholic hepatitis, cirrhosis, or both increased as consumption increased, and cirrhosis was most frequent in the subgroup of alcoholics who had drunk the most for the longest times (Fig. 33–3). On the other hand, no level or duration of consumption was associated uniformly with the appearance of clinically significant liver disease. Lelbach's patients had the highest incidence of cirrhosis of any group of alcoholic patients reported in the literature. Cirrhosis of the liver was present in 40 to 50 per cent of the alcoholic subgroup consuming the largest amount of ethanol for the longest time; but 60 per cent of patients consuming as much as 200 g/day of ethanol (for a 70-kg man or woman) for as long as ten years had normal liver biopsies or uncomplicated fatty livers. To put this level of ethanol intake into perspective we would point out that it is only slightly less than the maximum amount metabolized in 24 hours by a person weighing 70 kg.

Lelbach's data suggest that there is no threshold level of ethanol intake at which the risk of liver disease occurs abruptly, but that the relationship between risk and level of consumption is a smooth function. If there were a threshold level, in fact, this probably could not be discerned.[6] The dose-responsible curves (i.e., risk of liver disease as a function of intake) however are different for men and women. Risk increases faster for women for relatively low levels of consumption.[15] In addition, the course of liver disease appears to be accelerated in

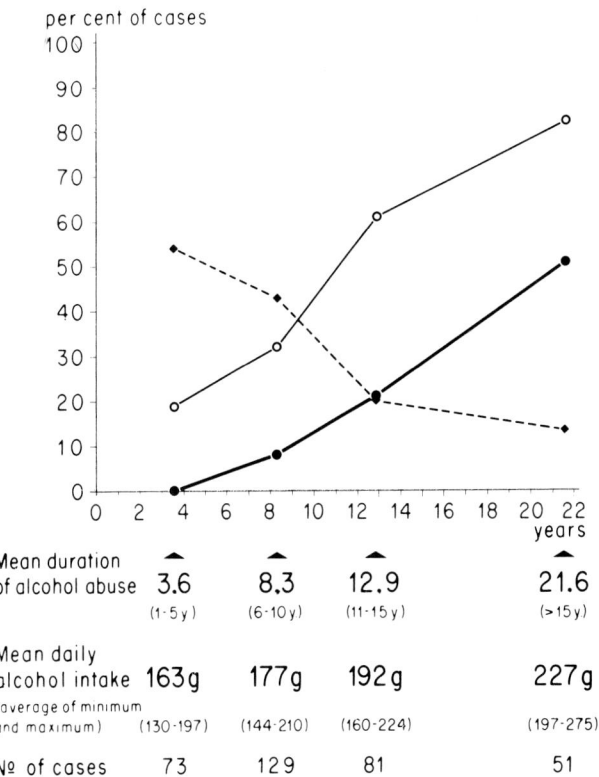

Figure 33–3. Relative frequency of cirrhosis and precirrhotic lesions and its relation to the volume of alcohol abuse among 334 drinkers. (Reproduced from Lelbach WK. Ann NY Acad Sci 252:85, 1975, with permission.)

women.[16-18] Fortunately, the incidence of alcoholism in women is about one sixth that in men.[19]

The incidence of cirrhosis in the hospitalized patients studied by Lelbach, was about 50 per cent for the group of patients drinking the largest amounts of ethanol for 20 years. Estimates of cirrhosis in the overall alcoholic population range from 8 to about 15 per cent.[20-25] There are several possible causes for this discrepancy. The populations in Lelbach's studies were self-selected, in that the patients admitted themselves to the hospital for detoxification. All studies of hospitalized patients may suffer from the same uncertainty: Do the patients in hospitals accurately reflect the larger group in the population using ethanol? On the other hand, the documentation of ethanol intake is far better in Lelbach's work than in other published surveys for the overall incidence of liver disease in abusers of alcohol. Recent surveys of the incidence of alcoholism and cirrhosis in several areas of the world can be found in Chapters 5 to 10 in reference 26. Whatever the exact incidence of liver disease in alcoholics, it is clear that some abusers of ethanol are resistant to its deleterious effects on the liver. Perhaps ethanol abuse that leads to cirrhosis requires malnutrition, a specific type of predisposed host, or the presence of factors not yet described. In order to give perspective to the complexity of this problem and to provide a basic level of background information for understanding of controversies in the literature, we review the metabolism of ethanol and the hepatotoxic effects of ethanol that are postulated.

OXIDATIVE METABOLISM OF ETHANOL

Ninety to ninety-five per cent of ingested ethanol is metabolized in the body to acetaldehyde and then to acetate.[27] The remainder is excreted intact via the lungs and kidneys and in sweat. Since oxidation in the liver accounts for nearly all ethanol metabolism (small amounts are oxidized in kidneys, muscles, intestines, and lungs), the study of ethanol metabolism has focused on oxidation by enzyme systems in this organ.

Ethanol oxidation is catalyzed by enzymes within the cytosolic compartment of the liver cell and by enzymes that are attached to the endoplasmic reticulum. The former system is quantitatively more significant compared with the latter.[28-31] Nevertheless, there is a great deal of interest in the oxidation of ethanol by membrane-bound enzymes.

OXIDATION OF ETHANOL BY THE COMBINED ACTIVITY OF ALCOHOL DEHYDROGENASES AND ALDEHYDE DEHYDROGENASES

Reactions [1] and [2] describe the predominant pathways for the oxidation of ethanol. Reaction [1], which is reversible, is catalyzed by alcohol dehydrogenases (ADH). Reaction [2] is catalyzed by aldehyde dehydrogenases.

$$C_2H_5OH + NAD^+ \leftrightharpoons C_2H_4O + NADH + H^+ \quad [1]$$
Ethanol   Acetaldehyde

$$C_2H_4O + NAD^+ \rightarrow C_2H_4O_2 + NADH + H^+ \quad [2]$$
Acetaldehyde   Acetate

Alcohol dehydrogenases (ADHs) are nonspecific enzymes. They catalyze the oxidations of a variety of alcohols to the corresponding aldehydes or ketones. ADHs catalyze

the oxidation of several physiologic intermediates, for example, glycerol to glyceraldehyde, retinol to retinal, and steroid alcohols to aldehydes. ADHs in humans comprise 20 isoenzyme forms, which are divided on the basis of molecular and catalytic properties into classes I, II, and III.[32-40] Class I consists of six basic isoforms composed of the peptide chains designated α, β, and γ in the combinations αα, αβ, αγ, ββ, βγ and γγ.[25] There is heterogeneity at the β and α gene loci.[39, 40] So there are more than six different possible isoforms in Class I in different people. The class II enzyme is referred to as π-alcohol dehydrogenase, and the class III enzyme as the χ-alcohol dehydrogenase.[39, 40] There is considerable homology between the α, β and γ peptides of the class I enzymes but not between subunits in different classes. Enzymes of different classes differ extensively in substrate specificities. For example, ethylene glycol and methanol are metabolized only by class I enzymes; ethanol is not metabolized by the class III enzyme.[39, 40] Ethanol is, in fact, a relatively poor substrate for all the isoforms of ADH, indicating that these enzymes have other biologic functions.[39-42]

The heterogeneity at the β locus affects the total ADH activity of affected individuals. The $\beta_2\beta_2$ variant (also known as ADH Bern or ADH oriental) has higher specific activity with ethanol as compared with the $\beta_1\beta_1$ enzyme.

The frequency of the β_2 variant depends on the population studied.[43, 44] It is present in 20 per cent of Swiss, 5 per cent of English, and 95 per cent of Japanese. The total hepatic activity of alcohol dehydrogenase in individuals with the atypical variety is four to five times greater than normal. Rates of metabolism of ethanol in vivo in those with the atypical enzyme are only slightly greater, however, than in the "normal" population.[45] The basis for this discordance between the activity of alcohol dehydrogenase and rates of utilization of ethanol in vivo is discussed later.

Mammalian tissues also contain several aldehyde dehydrogenases that catalyze Reaction [2]. In rat, there are two such enzymes in mitochondria, five in cytosol, and one in microsomes.[46-50] The individual enzymes have significantly different kinetic properties, such as different affinities for acetaldehyde. One of the two enzymes in mitochondria (located in the mitochondrial matrix) has a $K_m^{acetaldehyde}$ of 1 μM. Values for $K_m^{acetaldehyde}$ of the cytosolic isoforms range from 4.5 μM to as high as 13 mM. The concentrations of acetaldehyde in liver during active metabolism of ethanol are about 6 μM, which indicates that only the isoforms with small values for $K_m^{acetaldehyde}$ (i.e., high avidity for acetaldehyde) will contribute significantly to metabolism of acetaldehyde. The amounts of the different forms of aldehyde dehydrogenases in rat liver are unknown. This information would be helpful for deciding whether any acetaldehyde is metabolized by high K_m forms in the cytosol. Nevertheless, it is believed that in the rat, only the low K_m aldehyde dehydrogenase in mitochondria contributes significantly to the oxidation of acetaldehyde.

Human liver has at least four aldehyde dehydrogenases that oxidize acetaldehyde. One of these is similar to the low K_m mitochondrial enzyme in rat and generally is designated ALDH₂.[51-55] (The literature, however, also uses the designation ALDH I for this enzyme.) Its $K_m^{acetaldehyde}$ is 1 μM. None of the cytosolic aldehyde dehydrogenases in humans has an equally high affinity for acetaldehyde. Hence, as in the rat, metabolism of acetaldehyde, under normal conditions, is primarily due to the mitochondrial enzyme.

Polymorphism for ALDH₂ has been described in Chinese and Japanese patients, 50 per cent of whom lack an active form of ALDH$_2$.[51–55] Livers from these patients however contain a protein that reacts to an antibody against ALDH$_2$.[55] The rate of ethanol metabolism in individuals lacking an active ALDH$_2$ is not decreased,[52] but concentrations of acetaldehyde in blood are higher in these people as compared with groups possessing an active form of ALDH$_2$. Interestingly, the frequency of alcoholism is less in Japanese deficient in ALDH$_2$ compared with those with normal ALDH$_2$,[56] most likely because the former group experiences an unpleasant acetaldehyde-induced flushing reaction after ingesting alcohol.[57–62] Deficiency of ALDH$_2$ appears to occur only in Asians or in Native Americans, who are descendants of Asians.[63]

Investigators interested in alcoholism have suggested that the genetic basis for alcohol in humans may be linked to the diversity and the multiple allelic forms of the alcohol and aldehyde dehydrogenases.[40, 64] Ideas about the genetic basis for alcoholism remain controversial, however,[25, 65, 66] and the only direct evidence suggesting a genetic linkage between alcoholism and the enzymes of alcohol metabolism is the reported low incidence of alcoholism in Japanese with an abnormal ALDH$_2$.[56]

Deficiency of ALDH$_2$ can be detected with reasonable ease. The enzyme is normally present in hair roots, for example.[67] Moreover, individuals who lack ALDH$_2$ are sensitive (develop erythema) to patch-testing with ethanol because the enzyme is also absent from their skin.[68, 69] The sensitivity of these patients to patch-testing with ethanol can be blocked by prior treatment of the skin with inhibitors of alcohol dehydrogenase.[62] Thus, results from the patch test depend on the oxidation of ethanol to acetaldehyde, which then accumulates in and irritates the skin.

OXIDATION OF ETHANOL BY MICROSOMAL ENZYMES

It has been known for some time that microsomes derived from the hepatic endoplasmic reticulum catalyze the oxidation of ethanol. Interest was focused on this process in the 1960s by the work of Orme-Johnson and Ziegler[70] and Lieber and collaborators.[71–73] Lieber stressed that the microsomal oxidation of ethanol depended on the presence of microsomes, molecular oxygen, and the oxidized form of nicotinamide adenine dinucleotide phosphate (NADPH), the latter being a source of electrons. The stoichiometry of the oxidation of ethanol catalyzed by hepatic microsomes (Reaction [3]) is identical to reactions catalyzed by the microsomal cytochrome P450 (see Chapter 9). Since Reaction [3] was inhibited by carbon monoxide, a known inactivator of cytochrome P450, and since ethanol appeared to bind to cytochrome P450 and

CH$_3$CH$_2$OH + O$_2$ + NADPH + H$^+$ → CH$_3$CHO
Ethanol   Acetaldehyde
                          + NADP$^+$ + 2H$_2$O   [3]

was known to interfere with the metabolism of drugs via cytochrome P450,[28, 29, 31] it was proposed that one of the activities of cytochrome P450 of liver microsomes was to catalyze the oxidation of ethanol.[71–73] Lieber postulated that this was a specific system, which he named microsomal ethanol-oxidizing system (MEOS). The conclusion that cytochrome P450 could catalyze the oxidation of ethanol not only was compatible with several independent lines of evidence but was attractive because it provided a facile

explanation of metabolic adaptation to chronic ingestion of ethanol. Cytochrome P450 is an inducible enzyme system (see Chap. 9). Ingestion of ethanol, by acting as an inducer of cytochrome P450, would stimulate its own rate of oxidation.[74–76] Moreover, the affinity of MEOS for ethanol was low compared with the affinities for ethanol of the soluble forms of alcohol dehydrogenases described to that time. MEOS therefore was a useful concept for explaining why rates of ethanol metabolism increased as a function of chronic consumption and at concentrations of ethanol above those that saturated the soluble alcohol dehydrogenases. Questions were raised immediately, however, with regard to the validity of all these concepts and conclusions. These doubts could be divided into three major areas: (1) the quantitative importance of MEOS, (2) the role of MEOS in accounting for metabolism at high concentrations of ethanol, and (3) the identity of the enzyme referred to as MEOS—that is, was it cytochrome P450 or some other microsomal enzyme? Questions (1) and (2) were resolved easily in that most studies showed that MEOS, irrespective of its exact identity, accounted for the hepatic metabolism of small amounts of ethanol—perhaps as much as 10 per cent, but probably less.[28–31] Identification, purification, and characterization of the multiple isoforms of soluble alcohol dehydrogenase,[38–40] provided an explanation for the unexpectedly high rates of ethanol metabolism at concentrations far above those that saturate the high-affinity forms of alcohol dehydrogenase.[38]

Reaction [3] could describe the oxidation of ethanol by catalase, an enzyme bound to microsomes. Catalase catalyzes Reaction [4].[77]

$$H_2O_2 + C_2H_5OH \rightarrow CH_3CHO + 2H_2O \qquad [4]$$

H$_2$O$_2$ in this reaction is generated by flavoprotein oxidase enzymes (Reaction [5]), which are plentiful in microsomes.

$$NADPH + H^+ + O_2 \xrightarrow[\text{oxidase}]{\text{Flavoprotein}} H_2O_2 + NADP^+ \quad [5]$$

Addition of Reactions [4] and [5] yields the stoichiometry of Reaction [3]. The direct participation of cytochrome P450 in Reaction [3] cannot be inferred, therefore, on the basis of the stoichiometry of the oxidation of ethanol catalyzed by microsomes. The carbon monoxide-induced inhibition of microsomal-catalyzed oxidation of ethanol also is not a validation of the catalytic role of cytochrome P450 in the metabolism of ethanol because cytochrome P450 can generate H$_2$O$_2$, according to Reaction [5].

The oxidation of ethanol by microsomes is inhibited by specific inhibitors of catalase, or by removing catalase from microsomes,[78–83] but catalase does not account completely for all the oxidation of ethanol by microsomes.[84–85] NADPH-cytochrome c reductase produces OH (hydroxide radical) from H$_2$O$_2$.[86–88] Also, ·OH oxidizes alcohols nonenzymatically (Reaction [6]).

$$\cdot OH + \text{ethanol} \rightarrow \text{acetaldehyde} \qquad [6]$$

Oxidation of ethanol by catalase, by ·OH or by cytochrome P450-mediated reactions can be dissected out because each reaction can be inhibited selectively. When this is done, there is evidence for the involvement of P450 directly in the oxidation of ethanol.[76, 89–91] Note, however, that the stoichiometry of all three reactions for microsomal-catalyzed oxidation of ethanol are identical.

NON-OXIDATIVE PATHWAYS FOR THE METABOLISM OF ETHANOL

A nonoxidative pathway for ethanol metabolism was identified first in rabbit hearts. It was demonstrated that ethanol reacted with long-chain fatty acids to form ethyl esters.[92] This reaction has been documented in human hearts. The enzyme catalyzing the reaction has been purified.[93, 94] The esterification reaction is unusual in that there is a direct esterification of fatty acids with ethanol. By contrast, all esterification reactions of fatty acids with glycerol (but not cholesterol) require formation of the acyl coenzyme A (CoA) derivative, which depends on cleavage of adenosine triphosphate (ATP) to adenosine monophosphate (AMP) and inorganic pyrophosphate (PP_i). Esterification of fatty acids with ethanol occurs independently of CoA and ATP. Since ethyl esters accumulate in tissue, it was proposed that their formation accounted for the known deleterious effects of ethanol on myocardial metabolism and contractility.[95, 96]

In humans, the pancreas and liver have by far the largest enzymatic capacity for esterifying ethanol with long-chain fatty acids.[97] The esters are present in above normal amounts in a variety of tissues from alcoholics who have no ethanol in the blood at the time of death;[97] they are found in greater amounts in organs of patients dying while intoxicated. Although it has been proposed that the ethyl esters could have a deleterious effect on tissue and could account for the toxic effects of ethanol, there are no data as yet that connect the presence of the esters with pathogenic events in vivo.

Factors Determining the Rate of Oxidation of Ethanol by Alcohol Dehydrogenase

It is generally true that the rate of elimination of ethanol is zero order (constant) so long as the concentration of ethanol in vivo is higher than 50 mg/100 ml blood. The statement is not exactly correct, however, because the rate of metabolism of ethanol in humans increases at very high concentrations in blood. This is so because metabolism catalyzed by the class II type of ADH becomes increasingly larger at high concentrations of ethanol.[38] In fact, at high concentrations of ethanol (200 mg/100 ml) the elimination rate, due to metabolism, was nearly twice as great as at 50 mg/100 ml.[98] Moreover, this high rate was sustained until blood levels of ethanol fell to 25 mg/ml. The basis for this last effect is unclear. The high rates of ethanol metabolism at high concentrations of ethanol are observed in alcoholics and controls.[98, 99]

One can make a reasonable estimate of the rate of ethanol in an average, well-fed individual who is not a chronic user of large amounts of ethanol. This rate is about 100 mg ethanol/hour/kg body weight for as long as the plasma concentration of ethanol exceeds 50 mg/100 ml. There can be considerable variability, however, in the rate of oxidation of ethanol in intact humans. Nutritional state genetic polymorphism, alcohol dehydrogenases, and previous intake of ethanol influence rate of metabolism (see later).

The rate of oxidation of ethanol depends on the amount of alcohol dehydrogenase and the constraints under which it functions in the intact hepatocyte. It is uncertain whether the latter or former, limits metabolism in vivo. Reaction [1] is reversible, but levels of acetaldehyde in tissue and blood remain low as compared with those for ethanol during the metabolism of ethanol. In vivo, therefore, there is no tendency for Reaction [1] to come to equilibrium or to be reversed. On the other hand, the NADH produced in Reaction [1] is not as easily reoxidized to NAD^+ as the acetaldehyde is disposed of. Oxidation of ethanol hence alters the ratio of NAD^+ to NADH in the hepatocyte. The reduced form of the nucleotide (i.e., NADH) accumulates at the expense of the oxidized form. There is a considerable amount of evidence that the rate of reoxidation of NADH, not the amount, of alcohol dehydrogenase limits the metabolism of ethanol in an intact animal.[28, 29, 100–103] Direct observations in humans tend to confirm this idea. Thus, as previously mentioned, the rates of oxidation of ethanol in individuals with ADH_2 are only slightly faster than that in the "normal" population.[31] Since comprehension of some current views about the hepatotoxicity of ethanol (see the section on effects of ethanol on oxygen consumption) depends on an understanding of these events, we review briefly the reactions accounting for the reoxidation of NADH in hepatocytes.

Alcohol dehydrogenase is in the cytoplasm of the cell. NADH can be reoxidized to NAD^+ in this compartment according to the scheme in Reaction [7] (below). However, the amounts of substrates in these systems are limited as compared with the amount of ethanol usually ingested. These reactions hence cannot support the oxidation of ethanol. Instead, NADH produced by Reaction [1] must be transferred to the mitochondria to be oxidized by the electron-transport system. NADH and NAD^+ do not cross the inner membrane of the mitochondria, however (see Chap. 4). The hydrogen and electrons abstracted from ethanol and transferred to NAD^+ in Reaction [1] are shuttled across the inner mitochondrial membrane attached to carrier molecules, as depicted in Figure 33–4. The carrier systems for hydrogen and electrons, the malate-aspartate and α-glycerophosphate cycles, are the two most important such systems in liver.[104, 105]

Once inside the mitochondria, the reduced carriers are oxidized, thereby passing the hydrogen and electrons derived from ethanol to the components of the electron-transport chain. The energy of the oxidation-reduction reactions comprising the electron-transport system is conserved as ATP. Hence, ethanol oxidation is coupled to synthesis of ATP, and ethanol is a food. Its complete oxidation to CO_2 yields 7.1 calories/gm, a greater caloric yield than that derived from complete oxidation of carbohydrate or protein. The coupling of the oxidation of ethanol to the synthesis of ATP however limits the rate at which ethanol can be oxidized, because the rate of synthesis of ATP is regulated carefully: synthesis equals utilization. The rate of flow of electrons through the electron transport system and hence the rate of oxidation of NADH and glycerol-1-P is constrained in normal tissue by the rate at which the cell utilizes ATP. The rate of this last process may determine the maximal rate of ethanol oxidation in

$$\left.\begin{array}{l}\text{Pyruvate}\\\text{Dihydroxyacetone-P}\\\text{Glyceraldehyde}\\\text{Oxaloacetate}\end{array}\right\} + \text{NADH} + \text{H}^+ \longleftrightarrow \left\{\begin{array}{l}\text{lactate}\\\text{glycerol-1-P} + \text{NAD}^+\\\text{glycerol}\\\text{malate}\end{array}\right. \qquad [7]$$

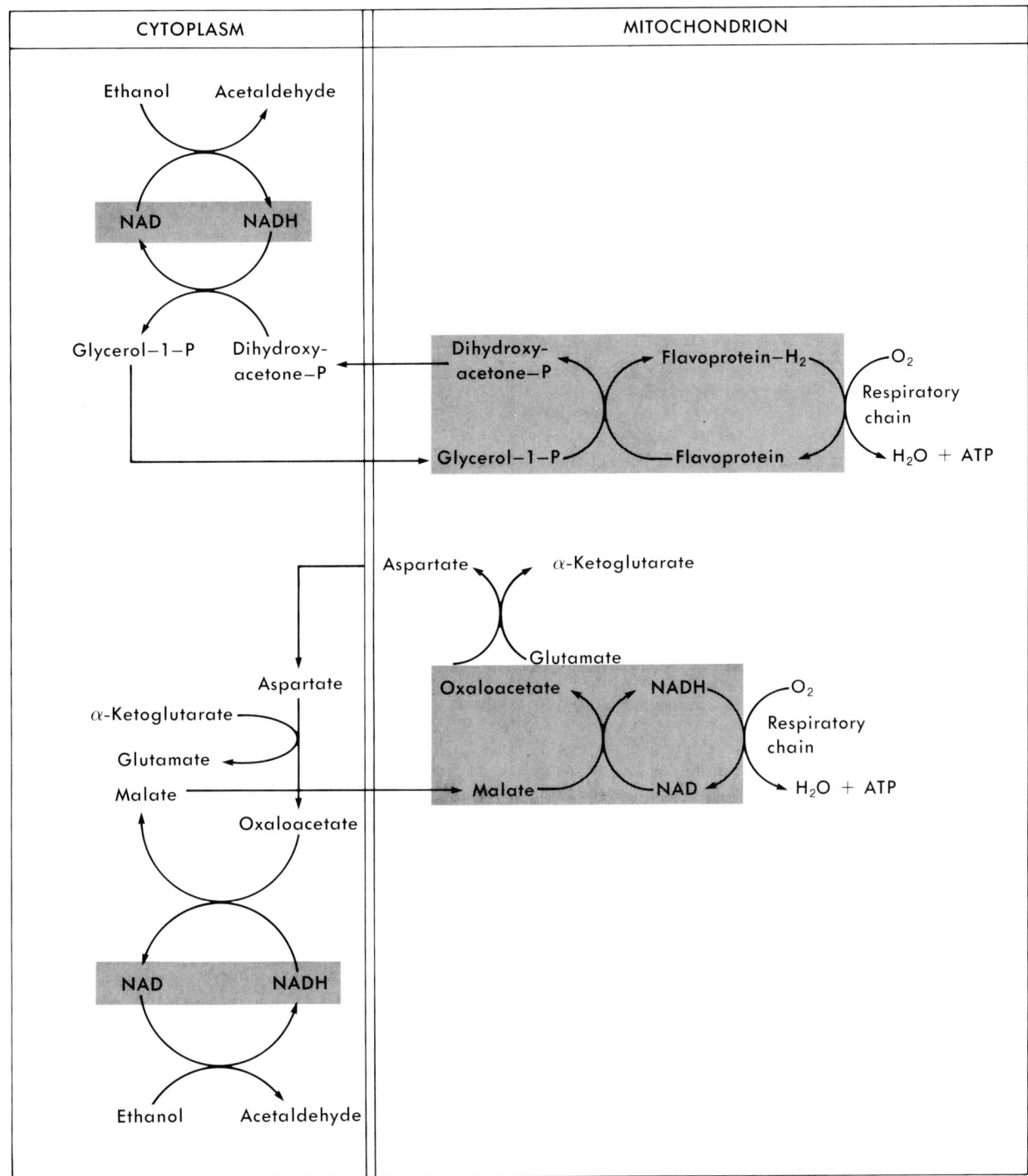

Figure 33–4. Shuttle systems for transporting electrons and hydrogen from cytoplasm to the mitochondrial respiratory chain.

fed animals. For example, uncouplers of oxidative phosphorylation, which allow the electron transport system to function independently of a supply of ADP, enhance the rate of metabolism of ethanol.[97, 98, 100] Fructose increases the rate of oxidation of ethanol by intact animals[105–107] because it increases the concentration of ADP in the cell (Reaction [8]).

$$\text{Fructose + ATP} \xrightarrow{\text{Fructokinase}} \text{fructose-1-P + ADP} \quad [8]$$

In addition, direct oxidation of NADH is coupled to reduction of fructose to sorbitol.

Calculations of the elimination rate for ethanol, based on the amounts and catalytic constants for alcohol dehydrogenases, predict with good accuracy, however, actual rates of elimination, both in humans and rats, whether fed or fasted.[64, 108–110] These data are posited to support the idea that the amounts of the dehydrogenases determine the elimination rate for ethanol. On the other hand, although the rate of oxidation of ethanol is thought to be increased in persons who use it on a chronic basis as compared with rates in those who consume it sporadically,[29, 101, 111-113] more recent studies suggest that the rate of oxidation does not increase with chronic consumption.[98]

Fasting diminishes the rate of oxidation of ethanol compared with the fed state.[102, 114] This is associated with a decrease in total alcohol dehydrogenase in the liver, but no change in the amount per gram liver.[107] The best evidence available is compatible with the idea that the rate of ethanol oxidation in fasted rats is limited by the activity of the shuttle systems for transporting reducing equivalents from the cytoplasm to the mitochondria. Treatment of fasted rats with agents that enhance the maximum capacity of either of the shuttle systems in Figure 33–4 increases the rate of oxidation of ethanol. The same treatments are without effect on the rate of oxidation of ethanol when administered to fed rats.[102, 114]

Diets deficient in protein, when fed to rats and alcoholic patients, decrease the alcohol and aldehyde dehydrogenases in liver.[114-119] The decrease in activity of the latter enzyme is no greater than for alcohol dehydrogenase in protein-restricted rats. Whether levels of alcohol dehydrogenase limit the metabolism of ethanol in vivo in protein-deficient animals or whether the activity of the shuttle systems does, as in fasting, is unstudied.

Metabolism of Acetaldehyde

Acetaldehyde levels in peripheral venous blood are at the level of detectability ($\sim 2\mu M$) after oral administration of ethanol to nonalcoholics.[120] Earlier data for levels of acetaldehyde in human blood, which reported higher values,[47-50, 119] were probably incorrect because of methodologic problems in quenching the production of acetaldehyde in blood.[120-122]

Only about 1 per cent of acetaldehyde produced in the liver from Reaction [2] leaves the liver.[46, 47] In addition, red blood cells (RBCs) oxidize acetaldehyde.[120, 123, 124] These two factors account for the low levels of acetaldehyde in peripheral blood in normal people. But levels of acetaldehyde in blood are higher in alcoholics with liver disease and alcoholics without evident liver disease than in nonalcoholic subjects given identical test doses of ethanol by any route (Fig. 33–5).[125-129] The basis for this difference in levels of acetaldehyde in the blood of alcoholics compared with nonalcoholics is probably reduced levels of aldehyde dehydrogenases in liver and RBCs of alcoholics.[125-129] Thus, rates of ethanol oxidation are equal in controls and alcoholics; so accumulation of acetaldehyde in alcoholics must reflect slower than normal rates of metabolism of acetaldehyde. Moreover, it has been found that the cytosolic isoform of aldehyde dehydrogenase in liver was reduced in alcoholics as compared with nonalcoholics.[127-129] Whether or not the mitochondrial form of the enzyme was reduced too was not clear.[126] The reduction of aldehyde dehydrogenase persists after abstention in some alcoholics,[128] but in others the abnormality disappears with abstention.[122] Whether these results are due to the presence and the extent of irreversible liver disease in some alcoholics has not been examined. Interestingly, the type of aldehyde dehydrogenase in RBCs is the same as the isoform that is reduced in cytosol from livers of alcoholics. The activity of this enzyme in RBCs also is decreased in alcoholics.[124] The activity of this same aldehyde dehydrogenase is decreased in liver in some patients with a variety of liver diseases that are not due to alcohol,[125] but levels of aldehyde dehydro-

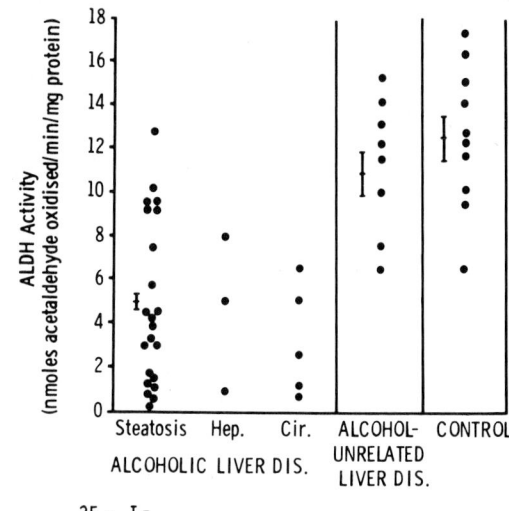

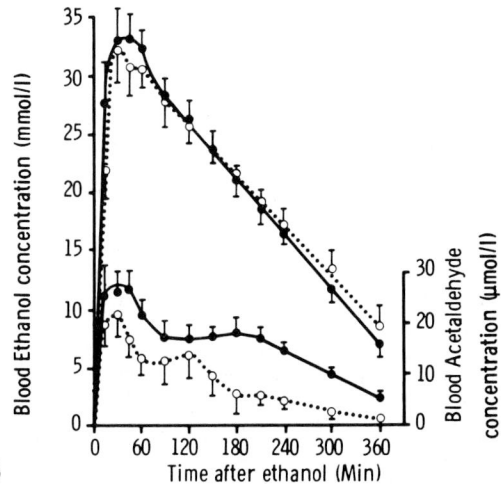

Figure 33–5. *A,* Activities of acetaldehyde dehydrogenase in liver biopsies from indicated groups of patients. B. Concentrations of ethanol and acetaldehyde (lower part of figure) in alcoholics (●) or controls (○) after a test dose of ethanol. (Reproduced from Palmer KR, Jenkins WJ. Gut 23:729, 1982, with permission.)

genase in RBCs have not been reported in this subset of patients. Patients with liver disease not due to alcohol have slightly greater concentrations of acetaldehyde in peripheral blood after administration of a test dose of ethanol as compared with controls.

As mentioned already, the mitochondrial form of aldehyde dehydrogenase is believed to be the only form of the enzyme in liver that catalyzes the oxidation of significant amounts of acetaldehyde. If, as claimed, alcoholic liver disease causes a selective reduction in a cytosolic aldehyde dehydrogenase and a decrease in rates of oxidation of acetaldehyde, then it is quite likely that cytosolic aldehyde dehydrogenase metabolizes significant amounts of acetaldehyde in normal liver.

The compromised metabolism of acetaldehyde in alcoholics may lead to its metabolism by a nonoxidative pathway. Evidence has been presented that 2,3-butanedione accumulates in serum after ingestion of ethanol and that levels are higher in alcoholics than in nonalcoholics.[130] The likely pathway for the synthesis of this compound is a condensation between hydroxyethylthiamine pyrophosphate (bound to the pyruvate dehydrogenase complex) and acetaldehyde to produce acetoin. The latter is reduced by NADH to 2,3-butanediol.

There is a positive correlation between the hepatic concentrations of ethanol and acetaldehyde. It is noteworthy, however, that the concentration of acetaldehyde is quite low compared with that of ethanol, even at high levels of the latter.[47, 48, 50, 121] The liver thus oxidizes acetaldehyde at a rate almost equal to its production. There are many uncertainties as to how this is accomplished. We say this because as mentioned already reoxidation of the NADH produced in Reaction [2] is effected by the enzymes of the mitochondrial electron-transport system, which may limit the rate of Reaction [1] in the fed state, by limiting the rate of reoxidation of the NADH. Yet oxidation of acetaldehyde keeps pace under almost all conditions with the rate of oxidation of ethanol. There appears to be a mechanism by which oxidation of acetaldehyde takes precedence over that of ethanol in order to ensure that acetaldehyde does not accumulate.

The rate of metabolism of acetaldehyde by liver mitochondria from rats fed ethanol on a chronic basis is slower than that by liver mitochondria from untreated rats,[131] suggesting that chronic exposure to ethanol may interfere with the oxidation of acetaldehyde in vivo. Measurement of aldehyde dehydrogenase activity in mitochondria from ethanol-treated rats demonstrates that their deficient metabolism of this intermediate is not due to a reduction in the amount of this enzyme but reflects a more complicated injury to mitochondrial function.[131]

Diet affects the metabolism of acetaldehyde. Levels of acetaldehyde are greater in rats fed diets containing low levels of protein,[117-119] but the relationship between levels of dietary protein and plasma levels of acetaldehyde after administration of a standard dose of ethanol is complex. The relationship is biphasic with regard to the amount of protein in the diet.[132] Also, after prolonged feeding of protein-deficient diets, levels of acetaldehyde in plasma are normal after administration of ethanol. After challenge of rats with ethanol, the concentration of acetaldehyde in liver is also affected by the amount of protein in the diet. As for the concentration of acetaldehyde in plasma, there is a biphasic response to levels of protein in the diet, but hepatic concentrations of acetaldehyde in response to ethanol administration do not become normal with persistent feeding of protein-deficient diets.[132] None of these effects of dietary protein can be explained on the basis of variable effects on the amounts of alcohol dehydrogenase and aldehyde dehydrogenase in liver.[117-119] Nor are there any data in this respect for humans. Nevertheless, any manipulation that alters the concentration of a potentially toxic agent deserves scrutiny. Of note for its potential application to humans is that starvation of rats markedly decreases plasma levels of acetaldehyde compared with rats fed normal or protein-restricted diets.[119] One should keep in mind, however, that starvation also decreases the elimination rate for ethanol. The effect of starvation on levels of acetaldehyde in liver is unknown.

METABOLIC CONSEQUENCES OF ETHANOL INGESTION

We need to know whether ethanol itself, independent of other factors, leads inexorably to liver disease. If this represents the true relationship between ethanol intake and liver disease, then from a strictly analytic view therapeutic efforts have to be directed toward persuading patients to cease abuse of ethanol, and toward altering the metabolism of ethanol or its metabolic consequences or both. If, on the other hand, the hepatotoxicity of ethanol depends on interactions with factors in the environment, the problem of ameliorating the deleterious effects of ethanol, at least with respect to hepatic function, might be easier to achieve.

Theories abound as to the manner in which ethanol ingestion directly produces liver disease. Most of these are based on observations of the effects of ethanol on the biochemistry and morphology of liver in experimental animals. These studies are important because they extend our opportunity to modify the effects of ethanol beyond what can be done in patients. Nevertheless, a great deal remains to be learned from observation of patients. As we try to emphasize in the following sections, for example, answers have not been sought to several direct, simple questions about the natural history of liver disease in the alcoholic.

PRODUCTION OF TOXINS VIA THE OXIDATION OF ETHANOL

ACETALDEHYDE

Acetaldehyde has several important pharmacologic and chemical effects; it is a vasoactive substance.[57, 58] Infusion in humans leads to a prompt flushing reaction on the trunk, especially the face. More serious symptoms are dyspnea and a sense of anxiety. A vascular reaction to acetaldehyde usually is not seen in individuals ingesting ethanol because the concentration of acetaldehyde in blood is too low to produce one.

The unpleasantness of the side-effects of acetaldehyde has been used therapeutically to encourage abusers of ethanol to abstain. The approach used is to administer an inhibitor of aldehyde dehydrogenase. Disulfiram (Antabuse) is the agent used for this purpose.[133, 134]

$$(C_2H_5)_2 - N - \overset{\overset{\textstyle S}{\|}}{C} - S - S - \overset{\overset{\textstyle S}{\|}}{C} - N\ (C_2H_5)_2$$
Disulfiram

The best evidence indicates that disulfiram forms a disulfide link with a thiol group of aldehyde dehydrogenase, thereby inhibiting it.[135] Maximum inhibition occurs between 16 and 40 hours after administration, and the effect of a single dose persists for several days, because the binding of disulfiram to aldehyde dehydrogenase is irreversible.[136] Also, the drug has a long half-life in the body.[137] Disulfiram-induced inhibition of aldehyde dehydrogenase is overcome only when new molecules of enzyme are synthesized. Experiments in vivo suggest that disulfiram does not have a uniform inhibitory effect on different isoenzymes of aldehyde dehydrogenase. The mitochondrial isoenzyme with a high affinity for acetaldehyde seems to be the form most sensitive to inhibition,[138] although the cytosolic forms in rat also are inhibited by disulfiram.[139] The symptoms experienced by a patient ingesting ethanol while under treatment with disulfiram are compatible with the idea that they are caused by acetaldehyde alone. In fact, acetaldehyde, when infused into patients who have previously experienced the ethanol-disulfiram reaction, evokes a response that is perceived by these patients as identical to it.

Disulfiram is not the only drug alleged to interfere with the metabolism of acetaldehyde. Pargyline and reserpine are inhibitors of aldehyde dehydrogenase.[140, 141] Disulfiram-ethanol–like reactions have been reported to occur after

ingestion of ethanol by patients being treated with sulfonylureas, phenylbutazone, metronidazole, and chemically
related compounds.[58, 141–147] However, the interactions between these drugs and ethanol have not been evaluated
carefully in patients in all instances. Metronidazole has no
demonstrable effect on the metabolism of acetaldehyde.
Sulfonylureas in combination with ethanol produce symptoms of acetaldehyde toxicity only at large doses of the
former. Recent studies of this last entity indicate that
naloxone prevents flushing in response to the combination
of ethanol and chlorpropamide.[147, 148] In addition, the flush
in these patients can be evoked by infusion of met-enceph-
alin. Ethanol-induced flushing in patients receiving chlorpropamide thus may have nothing to do with accumulation
of acetaldehyde and appears instead to be a dominantly
inherited trait in association with diabetes.[147, 148] Hence, the
clinical significance of the reported disulfiram-ethanol–like
interactions between ethanol and other drugs remains
clouded. By contrast, it is established that the edible
mushroom Coprinus atramentarius produces a disulfiram-
ethanol–like reaction when ingested with ethanol.

Acetaldehyde reacts readily with sulfhydryl and amino
groups, which are important functional groups in a large
number of enzymes. Acetaldehyde theoretically could inactivate many hepatocellular enzymes.[149–158] It reacts in
vitro with free amino groups on hemoglobin.[153–155] It also
probably reacts in vivo with hemoglobin, albumin, and
prothrombin[153, 156, 157] and with active site lysines in cytosolic
enzymes.[158] Acetaldehyde inhibits synthesis of proteins[149, 150]
and secretion of albumin and glycoproteins by liver.[151, 152]
Acetaldehyde also forms a covalent adduct with phosphatidylethanolamine,[159] which constitutes about 25 per cent of
the phospholipids in cellular membranes. All of these
reactions are nonenzymatic.

Whether or not reaction of acetaldehyde with proteins
is cytotoxic remains to be elucidated. The intracellular
proteins that react with acetaldehyde have not been identified, nor have the effects of acetaldehyde on their catalytic
functions been examined. It has been demonstrated, however, in intact animals and in perfused liver that the
metabolism of ethanol to acetaldehyde displaces pyridoxal
phosphate from hepatic proteins,[160, 161] including transaminases and glycogen phosphorylase. Displacement caused by
acetaldehyde would limit the rates of reactions catalyzed
by pyridoxal phosphate–requiring enzymes. Moreover, the
scheme accounts for the frequency of vitamin B_6 (pyridoxine) deficiency in alcoholics, in that displacement from
protein-binding sites facilitates degradation of pyridoxal
phosphate, the active form of vitamin B_6. Another mechanism by which acetaldehyde may alter cell function is by
competing with biogenic amines for metabolism by alde-
hydedehydrogenases.[162] A final possible mechanism by
which acetaldehyde may lead to liver disease is via a primary
effect on the synthesis of collagen.[163–165] This aspect of
alcoholic liver disease is described later on p. 842 (see also
Chap. 15).

EFFECTS OF ETHANOL ON THE STRUCTURE AND FUNCTION OF HEPATIC MITOCHONDRIA

Electron-microscopic examinations of liver biopsy
specimens from patients with alcohol-induced liver disease
often reveal striking abnormalities of the mitochondria such
as gross enlargement (Fig. 33–6) and swelling, a state that
alters mitochondrial function in vitro.[166, 167] Mitochondria in
livers from alcoholics also may contain granular deposits

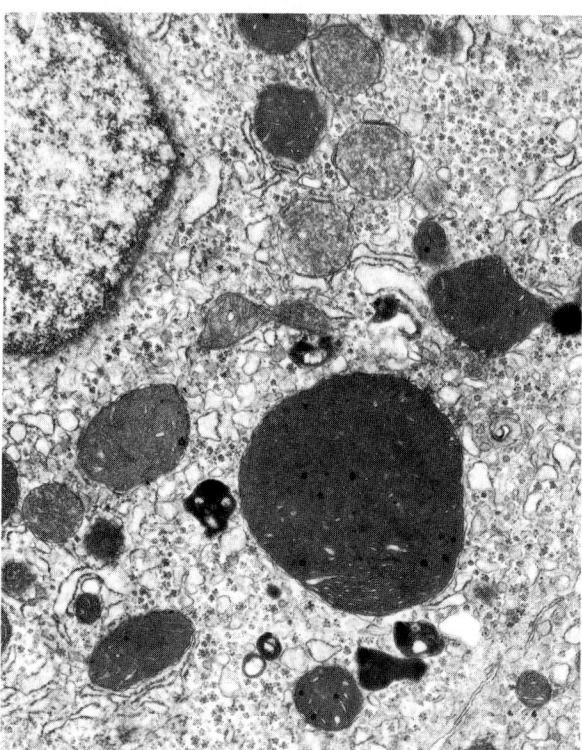

Figure 33–6. Electron micrograph of enlarged "megamitochondria" in
rat liver after administration of ethanol. A nucleus is in the upper left-hand
corner. Magnification × 32,300. (Courtesy of Dr. Sam French.)

and inclusions.[167] These morphologic abnormalities could
reflect an important mechanism through which ethanol
injures the hepatocyte.

Hepatic mitochondria isolated from animals fed
ethanol are more susceptible to induction of swelling in
vitro.[167, 168] Liver mitochondria from animals chronically
treated with ethanol compared with mitochondria from
control animals are abnormally permeable to several physiologic intermediates.[169, 170] Their content of respiratory
enzymes is also decreased, as is their capacity to oxidize a
variety of substrates.[167–179] There are blocks in the transfer
of electrons in the proximal portion of the electron transport
chain (the site I phosphorylation sequence). More recent
work suggests, too, that administration of ethanol inhibits
the flow of electrons through coupling sites II and III of
the electron transport complex.

Measurement of hepatic levels of acetaldehyde in
chronic alcoholics would be illuminating, because acetaldehyde in vitro inhibits mitochondrial respiration, especially
when respiration is coupled to oxidative phosphorylation—that is, acetaldehyde in vitro affects mitochondrial
function like ethanol in vivo.[173–176] The concentration of
acetaldehyde in vitro required to produce these effects is
greater than that known to occur in livers of experimental
animals, but the toxicity of acetaldehyde will depend on its
concentration and the duration of exposure.

THE PHYSICAL EFFECTS OF ETHANOL ON MEMBRANES

The effects of ethanol on mitochondrial function, and
indeed, its effects on other organelles of the hepatocytes
usually are considered to be consequences of the metabolism of ethanol. However, the best known effect of

ethanol—the capacity to induce narcosis—is related to its physical properties, not to metabolism. Thus, ethanol, like other lipid-soluble chemicals, is a membrane-active agent.

The functional properties of many proteins that are integral components of membranes are modulated by the chemical and physical properties of the membrane in which they are embedded.[180–183]

Many enzymes that are embedded within membranes of cells are sensitive to the chemical and physical properties of the lipid components of the membrane. The functions of these integral membrane-bound enzymes can be regulated to some extent by changes within the lipid portions of biologic membranes. This is not surprising, because the function of a protein depends on its conformation, which in turn depends on environmental conditions. The membrane lipids are a significant part of the proximate environment of membrane-bound proteins. So changes in the chemical and physical properties of these lipids can modify the function of proteins interacting with them.[184, 185] Whereas significant changes in the chemical composition and physical properties of the aqueous portion of the cell (e.g., ionic strength and pH) are not allowed, membranes normally tolerate significant changes in composition.[186] Although it has been shown for one membrane-protein from mammalian tissue (β-hydroxybutyrate dehydrogenase) that function depends on the presence of lipids with phosphocholine as the polar group,[187, 188] this type of dependence on a specific chemical group in a lipid is not characteristic for membrane-bound enzymes.[189] Instead, membrane-bound enzymes typically are sensitive to the physical state—specifically, the viscosity or fluidity—of the surrounding phospholipids.

Phospholipids are amphipathic molecules. They contain a polar region and a hydrophobic region. The former is the so-called head group of the phospholipid molecule and can be one of several different possible groups, for example, phosphocholine or phosphoethanolamine. The hydrophobic region of a phospholipid consists of the long hydrocarbon chains attached, usually via ester linkages to the 1 and 2 positions of the glycerol backbone of the molecule. These chains are at least 14 carbons long in humans. The hydrocarbon chains can be unsaturated to a variable extent. Typical of naturally occurring phospholipids is the presence of an unsaturated chain at position 2 and a saturated chain at position 1. Given the number of possible fatty acids (hydrocarbon region) that can be esterified with glycerol and the number of possible polar groups, there are hundreds of different species of phospholipids within the membranes of higher animals.

The phospholipids organize with each other so as to maximize the interaction of the hydrocarbon—or acyl tail—region of one molecule with the hydrocarbon regions of other. This arrangement excludes water from interacting with the nonpolar portions of the molecule and maximizes interactions between the polar regions and water. These thermodynamic requirements can be satisfied in a variety of ways, depending primarily on the structure of the polar region but also on the state of hydration of the polar groups and on the ionic strength and pH of the aqueous phase. Under conditions in vivo, including the natural abundance of phospholipids of different classes, the phospholipids organize as bilayers.

The manner in which phospholipids pack together seems to be their most important characteristic for modulating the function of enzymes embedded within phospholipid bilayers. The term *fluidity* has been used to describe and quantitate one important aspect of packing. The concept of fluidity is simple and can be understood in the

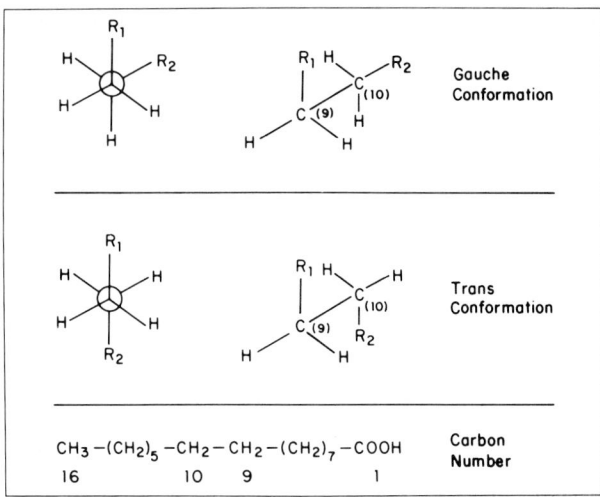

Figure 33–7. Effect of rotation about —C—C— bonds on conformation in fatty acids. The schematic is for rotation about the C-9–C-10 bond, but identical possibilities for conformation exist for all —C—C— bonds in the fatty acid. (Reproduced from Zakim D. Am J Med 80:645, 1986, with permission.)

following way. When the hydrocarbon chain of a phospholipid is fully saturated, there is free rotation around all of its carbon-carbon bonds. All positions of rotation are not equally probable, however, because of mutual repulsion between bulky groups when these are close to each other (Fig. 33–7). This familiar idea predicts that the most favorable conformation of the carbon-carbon bonds occurs when the bulky groups are trans. The least favorable position obviously is for the bulky groups—the proximal and distal regions of the hydrocarbon chain—to be cis or partially eclipsed. Thus, the most likely conformation of the acyl chains is with all carbon-carbon bonds as trans, as depicted in Figure 33–8. The acyl chains have maximal length in this configuration. More important, the cross-sectional area is minimal when all carbon-carbon bonds are trans. The energy barrier between trans and partially eclipsed, or gauche, conformations for each carbon-carbon bond is relatively low; the barrier is crossed easily at room temperature. Hence, there is a constant "wiggling" of the acyl chains of phospholipids as different carbon-carbon rotate from trans to gauche separately and together. Gauche configurations about a carbon-carbon bond have a kink in the chain. It can be seen in Figure 33–8 that acyl chains containing a kink have a larger cross-sectional area than chains in the all-trans state. This effect on cross-sectional

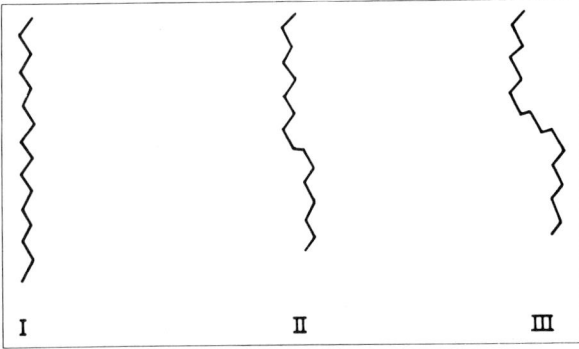

Figure 33–8. Extended views of conformational isomers of palmitate. (Reproduced from Zakim D. Am J Med 80:645, 1986, with permission.)

area is not important when we consider only a single molecule of phospholipid, but it is important in a bilayer in which there are thousands of phospholipid molecules. The packing together of many phospholipids makes it less likely that a carbon-carbon bond will rotate spontaneously from trans to gauche because introducing a kink in an otherwise all-trans chain increases the volume of the chain. The kink occurs only when the environment provides a sufficient volume to accommodate the kinked chain. So when phospholipids pack together, the creation of a kink in one acyl chain requires that surrounding chains be pushed aside. The extent to which trans-gauche changes occur therefore depends on the tightness of packing of the acyl chains, which in turn depends on van der Waals interactions. These interactions between two acyl chains are quite small, but the total energy of attraction becomes quite large when there are millions of chains limiting the wiggling of neighboring chains. The organization is cooperative, because close approximation of chains maximizes van der Waals energies. As these increase, wiggling is diminished. This in turn diminishes the volume occupied by a single chain, which increases van der Waals energies. Hence, the normal tendency for free rotation about the carbon-carbon bonds in a single acyl chain attached to an isolated molecule of phospholipid is constrained severely when there is an array of acyl chains. This constraint leads to high viscosities or low fluidities within the bilayer of a membrane. This tightness of packing can be disturbed in many ways: by unsaturated fatty acids, by introducing bulky detergent molecules, by substituting phosphocholine for phospho-ethanolamine, and so forth. Cholesterol has complex effects. It increases fluidity when added to a highly viscous (nonfluid) membrane but decreases fluidity when added to a highly fluid membrane.

Ethanol in vitro generally enhances the fluidity of biologic membranes.[190] Large amounts of ethanol (and other short-chain alcohols) can cause the basic bilayer structure to break down.[191, 192] These effects probably are not important in vivo. On the other hand, after chronic administration of ethanol, ethanol in vitro does not increase the "fluidity" of membranes from ethanol-treated animals to as great an extent as it increases fluidity of membranes from control animals.[193–198] Resistance to the membrane-active effects of ethanol, as defined by its effect on fluidity, can be attributed to an adaptive change in the lipid composition of the membrane.[195, 197, 199–203] The apparent adaptation of membranes is almost certainly not due to metabolism of ethanol but to its physical properties. The evidence for this idea is that exposure to ethanol leads to adaptive changes in the lipid compositions of membranes from *Escherichia coli* and Tetrahymena organisms, which do not oxidize ethanol.[204–206]

The physical interactions between ethanol and membranes in vitro are associated with acute changes in ATPase and several other enzymatic activities,[202, 203, 207, 208] decreased transport of amino acids[209, 210] and bile acids,[211] and an increased permeability of membranes to Na^+.[211] Chronic administration of ethanol is also associated with changes in the physical properties of membranes. For example, chronic administration of ethanol has been reported to enhance the solubility of halogenated anesthetics in liver membranes.[212] There appears to be an unusual limitation of glucose transport across hepatocyte plasma membranes during acute withdrawal after chronic administration of ethanol to rats.[213] In addition, administration of ethanol seems to interfere with the flow of glycoproteins from the Golgi to plasma membranes.[214] Interference by ethanol of secretion

of glycoproteins by liver could be one of the consequences of this effect, since mechanisms for the secretion of proteins and the assembly of proteins into membranes have many similarities.[214] The reported decrease in the number of glucagon receptors on hepatocyte plasma membranes[215] and reduced binding and internalization of asialoglycoproteins[216, 217] in rats fed alcohol on a chronic basis may be a reflection of an ethanol-induced abnormality in the "trafficking" of proteins to plasma membranes.[214] The effects of ethanol on membrane structure and function also may contribute to putative abnormalities of immune function in the alcoholic with liver disease (see later).

The most dramatic effects of chronic consumption of ethanol on membranes are on the morphology of mitochondria.[218–220] But, whether the "giant" mitochondria induced by ethanol (see Fig. 33–6) are unable to sustain the viability of hepatocytes is unclear. In addition, the morphologic changes of mitochondria in liver specimens from alcoholic patients are not specific. They are seen in specimens from obese patients and diabetics and increase as a function of the patient's age (see reference 167).

As mentioned above, studies with mitochondria in vitro indicate that ingestion of ethanol inhibits the respiration of intact hepatocytes secondary to decreased amounts of respiratory enzymes and inhibition of the coupled oxidation of several mitochondrial substrates. Various experiments with perfused liver, liver slices, and intact animals show, however, that chronic ingestion of ethanol increases mitochondrial respiration in intact hepatocytes.[111, 221–223] Oxygen consumption by liver is increased by chronic ingestion of ethanol in the preparations described, compared with controls. There is evidence, too, that hepatic synthesis and utilization of ATP are increased by ingestion of ethanol. (This evidence is discussed in the following section, Effects of Ethanol on Hepatic Consumption of Oxygen.) It therefore seems that the behavior of mitochondria in vitro does not correlate well with their function in intact cells. Nevertheless, it would be unwise to dismiss as biochemical curiosities the effects of ethanol on the function of hepatic mitochondria. First, careful scrutiny of the literature dealing with the toxic effects of ethanol on cells leads one to conclude that derangement of mitochondrial function is the only type of injury that is well established experimentally and that would diminish the viability of hepatocytes. Second, ethanol ingestion clearly has the capacity to alter the function of mitochondria in some environments. The biochemical functions of mitochondria deteriorate rapidly under the stress of isolation, for example.[203] Ethanol accelerates the rate of deterioration in vitro (Fig. 33–9).[203]

EFFECTS OF ETHANOL ON HEPATIC CONSUMPTION OF OXYGEN

There is a well-known lobular gradient of O_2 tension between portal and central vein cells (see Chap. 2). Hepatic levels of O_2 are low compared with those in other tissues, because 75 per cent of hepatic blood flow comes from the venous system rather than the arterial system. And the cells of the centrolobular regions of liver, which under normal conditions receive blood with the lowest concentration of O_2, are the cells principally affected in patients with alcoholic hepatitis (see the section Alcoholic Hepatitis). Therefore, it has been proposed that chronic ingestion of ethanol increases the consumption of O_2 by human liver to the point that centrolobular cells become anoxic. This leads to cell death, the morphologic constellation of central hyaline

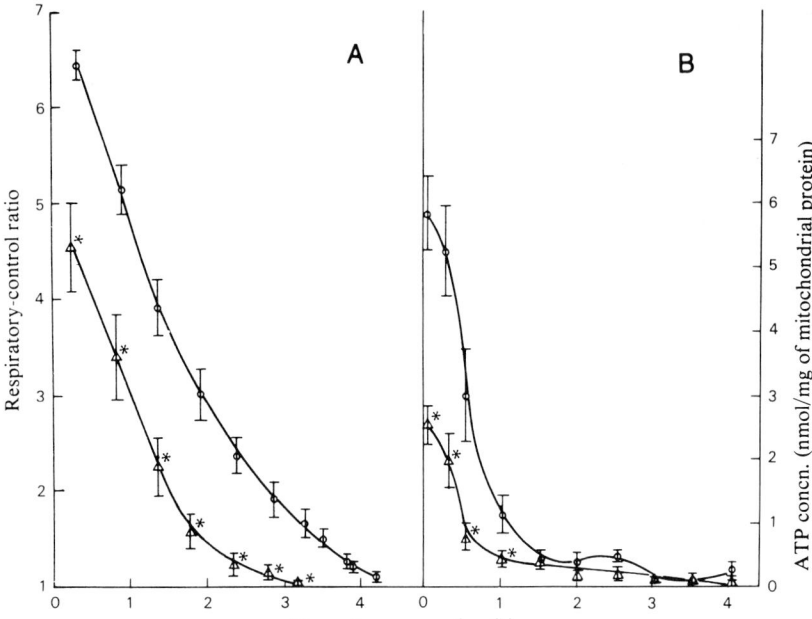

Figure 33–9. The effect of ethanol feeding on (*A*) respiratory control in hepatic mitochondria and (*B*) ATP. Control rats, $\bigcirc$; ethanol-fed rats, $\triangle$. There was a significant difference from liquid-diet controls ($P < 0.05$). Vertical bars represent $\pm$ SEM. (Reproduced from Spach PI, Parce JW, Cunningham CC. Biochem J 178:23, 1979, with permission.)

necrosis, and the clinical syndrome of alcoholic hepatitis. This hypothesis has been tested in rats by feeding ethanol chronically and then exposing the test animals to lower-than-normal O_2 tension in inspired air. Rats treated in this way develop extensive centrolobular necrosis.[224–228] Animals not exposed to ethanol prior to breathing air with a diminished content of O_2 do not develop hepatic necrosis. Clearly, ethanol can sensitize the liver to the noxious effects of low levels of inspired O_2. With these ideas and observations in mind we review the controversy about the effects of ethanol on O_2 consumption and consider whether ethanol induces a "hypermetabolic state" in the liver.

As previously mentioned, it has been believed for some time that chronic ingestion of ethanol induces a state in which ethanol oxidation is accelerated.[29, 101, 111–113] This concept began to change in the late 1970s when it was reported that a single prior dose of ethanol enhanced the elimination of a second dose given only a few hours later.[106, 229] This specific event, referred to as the swift increase in alcohol metabolism (SIAM), probably does not exist. It has not been reproduced in perfused livers with normal baseline levels of ethanol oxidation, for example.[230] Also, attempts to demonstrate it in intact animals yield equivocal data.[231–234] It is alleged to be present in a small percentage of normal individuals, but the data have not been published in a form that allows for complete evaluation.[232, 233] The proposal that the so-called SIAM is determined genetically in selected populations of men and women and experimental animals therefore seems premature.[232, 234–236] There is, however, a rapid adaptation in the metabolism of ethanol. Thus, as mentioned already, the zero order rate of metabolism in men and women with high concentrations of ethanol in blood (40–80 mM) is greater than for concentrations of 10 mM. The explanation offered for this phenomenon is that ethanol at the higher concentration begins to be metabolized by class II alcohol dehydrogenases, which have high K_ms for ethanol, in addition to metabolism by the low K_m form.[98] This explanation cannot be correct for at least two reasons. First, the best evidence, which has been reviewed already, is that the oxidation of ethanol is not regulated by the amounts of alcohol dehydrogenase but by the rate of reoxidation of NADH produced in Reactions [1] and [2].[28, 29, 100–103, 237] Second, once the high rate of ethanol metabolism was established by a dose that yielded a blood ethanol of 40 to 80 mM, this high rate persisted until the blood level fell below 5 mM. In other words, the rate of elimination was greater (by about 40 per cent) at equal concentrations of ethanol, depending on the recent past history of blood ethanol levels. Rates of elimination at 10 mM ethanol were increased in subjects in whom the blood alcohol levels were decreasing from an initial concentration of 40 to 80 mM. Perhaps this unexplained phenomenon of immediate and persistent adaptation of the oxidation of ethanol to high blood levels is what has been reported as the swift increase in alcohol metabolism. In any event, there is no adequate mechanism for this apparent, immediate adaptation in ethanol metabolism. That it occurs, however, reinforces the idea that ethanol metabolism is limited by the rate of reoxidation of NADH. It would seem, therefore, that any rapid adaptation would involve changes in this process. The possibilities are that high concentrations of ethanol uncouple oxidative phosphorylation, increase the concentrations of ADP in the cell, or somehow "capture" to a greater extent the coupled activity of the electron transport system in mitochondria. The first two possibilities would lead to an ethanol-induced increase in O_2 consumption by the liver. The last would not. It has been proposed that acute administration of ethanol increases the availability of adenosine diphosphate (ADP) because it increases ATPase activity in hepatocyte plasma membranes[222] or because it inhibits glycolysis.[229, 238] Both of these proposed mechanisms for increasing the concentration of ADP after ingestion of ethanol are located in the cytosol and thus should be expected to increase the concentration of ADP in this compartment. An abundance of NMR evidence shows that the concentration of ADP in cytosol of intact liver does not change significantly after an acute dose of ethanol.[239–242] The concentration of ADP in mitochondria is what directly controls the rate of electron transport, but this concentration cannot be measured by NMR techniques.

There are only limited data for the effects of ethanol

on O_2 consumption by liver. Hepatic O_2 consumption is decreased markedly in rats fed alcohol on a chronic basis (6 weeks) and then fasted for 12 hours prior to measurement of O_2 consumption.[243] This is not an unexpected finding given the changes in the composition, morphology, and function of liver mitochondria isolated from rats fed ethanol on a chronic basis.[167-179] In addition, hepatic O_2 consumption was decreased further when ethanol was given acutely to rats fed ethanol chronically.[244] When added to perfusate, ethanol stimulated O_2 consumption by rat livers from fed animals. Ethanol enhanced glucose-stimulated uptake of O_2 when added to perfusate of livers from fasted rats.[238] Baseline rates of O_2 uptake in this last work were low, however,[230] and the idea that ethanol acutely stimulated O_2 uptake in perfused livers with or without other oxidizable substrates has not been confirmed.[230]

Ethanol is also reported to increase portal blood flow to the liver (see reference 245 and references therein). The observed increases probably can be explained by mechanisms independent of any effects of ethanol.[246-248] Studies of hepatic blood flow and O_2 consumption in alcoholics or normal individuals given test doses of ethanol are limited. The rate of splanchnic O_2 consumption was reported to be increased in a group of poorly nourished alcoholics, and the O_2 saturation of hepatic vein blood in these patients was less than that in normal controls, a result compatible with the idea that centrolobular hepatocytes were close to a state of anoxia after chronic use of ethanol. Splanchnic consumption of O_2 in these patients returned to normal levels after prolonged abstention.[223] Hepatic lesions in the patients studied were limited to variable infiltrations of fat with or without small amounts of periportal fibrosis. In another single study, there was a positive correlation between rates of oxidation of ethanol and the histologic severity of liver disease in alcoholics.[249] On the other hand, moderate, acute doses of ethanol did not increase hepatic blood flow when given to normal individuals.[248]

Irrespective of whether ethanol induces hypoxia in centrolobular cells of the liver (by increasing consumption of O_2), it is important to point out the model of hepatic injury developed by Israel and coworkers depends on chronic administration of ethanol plus acute hypoxia.[224, 228, 250] Propylthiouracil protected against the injury induced by hypoxia, presumably because it induced a hypothyroid state. It has been demonstrated recently that inhibition of xanthine oxidase by allopurinol also protects the liver against damage caused by hypoxia,[251] which indicates the complexity of attributing causes to general types of effects. With regard to the applicability to men and women of the model of hypoxic liver damage, there is no evidence that ethanol directly induces a "hypermetabolic state" in humans. Perhaps, however, the narcotizing effect of large doses of ethanol and the relatively high incidences of pulmonary disease, anemia, or both among alcoholics are possible mechanisms for induction of anoxia in humans. Yet many, if not most, patients with alcoholic liver disease do not have an identifiable history of narcosis, acute lung disease, or acute severe anemia in close relationship to deterioration of liver function. If the model developed by Israel applies to human alcoholics, it would seem to be one of many factors that can contribute to cellular injury and would be limited to combined alcohol abuse and demonstrable anoxia.

Israel tried to alter the course of alcoholic liver disease by interdicting the putative hypermetabolic state induced by ethanol. The treatment plan was based on the observation that antithyroid agents protected ethanol-treated rats from development of centrolobular necrosis in response to anoxia. Israel and collaborators thus used propylthiouracil treatment for patients with alcoholic hepatitis. The data are interesting. The first reported clinical findings were that propylthiouracil might have enhanced slightly the rate of recovery from alcoholic hepatitis, as compared with no treatment. The study group, however, included a large number of patients with mild forms of this illness. In addition, propylthiouracil had no effect on the low mortality rate observed (8 deaths in 133 patients).[227, 228] No salutary effects of propylthiouracil were demonstrated in a second study of patients with more severe alcoholic hepatitis.[252] More recently, the results of long-term treatment of alcoholics with propylthiouracil have been reported.[253] Alcoholic patients with histologic abnormalities ranging from fatty liver to hepatitis with cirrhosis were treated for nearly two years with propylthiouracil. As compared with placebo, the treated group had a lower mortality, especially in patients who appeared to curb their intake of alcohol. This effect of propylthiouracil was independent of the change in alcohol intake, but the drug did not protect patients who appeared to maintain a high intake of alcohol. Levels of thyroxine decreased in treated patients but remained in the normal range. These data are potentially important and interesting. They do not, however, illuminate the mechanism of protection of propylthiouracil. They certainly do not constitute evidence for an ethanol-induced hypermetabolic state. More likely, propylthiouracil had effects on the liver independent of thyroid status or oxygenation of the organ or both.

THE EFFECTS OF ETHANOL ON THE METABOLISM OF FATTY ACIDS: ETHANOL-INDUCED FATTY LIVER

The central role of the liver in the metabolism of fatty acids and a pathogenetic discussion of fatty liver are presented in detail in Chapter 4. A general scheme of the circulation of fatty acids between peripheral tissues and liver is depicted in Figure 33–10. The amount of fatty acids in the liver depends on the balance between the processes of delivery and removal. The former are de novo synthesis in the liver and release from adipose tissue. The latter are oxidation of fatty acids and their resecretion as very low-density lipoproteins (VLDL). Ingestion of ethanol alters the rates of all these processes.[254]

Since the oxidation of ethanol is coupled to the synthesis of ATP, we would expect its metabolism to spare the utilization of other oxidizable fuels. Ingestion of ethanol appears to have a direct inhibitory effect on the Krebs cycle in hepatocytes.[176, 255-258]

Ethanol inhibits the oxidation of fatty acids to CO_2.[255] This can be explained, in part, by ethanol-induced enhancement of esterification of fatty acids.[257] The ethanol-induced shift in the ratio of NADH to NAD^+ in the cytoplasm of the hepatocyte drives the equilibrium of Reaction [9] to the right:[259]

$$\text{Dihydroxyacetone P} + \text{NADH} + \text{H}^+ \rightarrow \text{glycerol-1-P} + \text{NAD}^+ \qquad [9]$$

and as the concentration of glycerol-1-P increases, there is stimulation of the esterification of fatty acids.[259, 260] Ethanol, however, also inhibits the oxidation of medium-chain–length fatty acids that are not esterified efficiently in the liver. The block in oxidation of fatty acids is not at entry

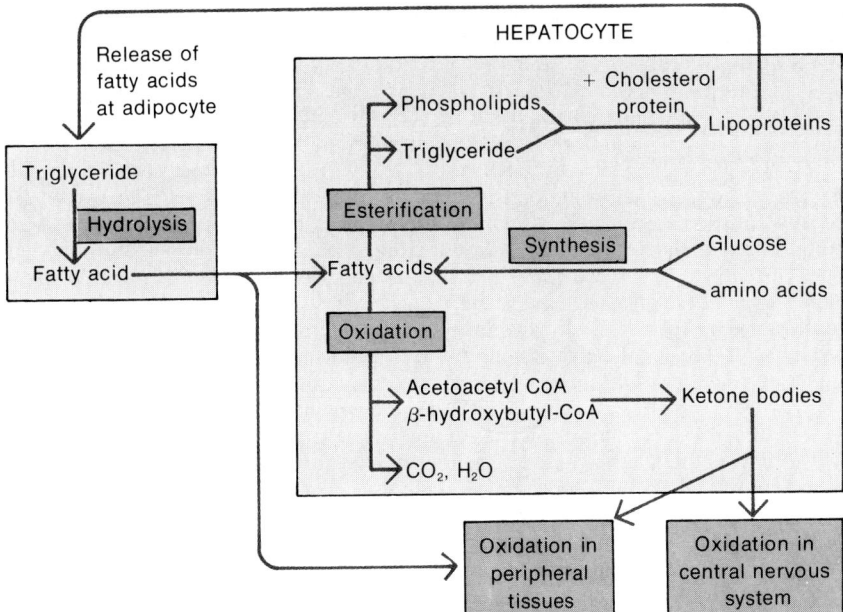

Figure 33–10. The flow of fatty acids between liver and adipose tissue. (Reproduced from Zakim D. In: Smith LH Jr, Thier SO, eds. International Textbook of Medicine, Vol 1. Pathophysiology, 2nd ed. WB Saunders, 1985:1267, with permission.)

to or within the β-oxidation cycle (see Chap. 4), but in the oxidation of the acetyl CoA produced by β-oxidation (Fig. 33–11).[257] It has been shown, too, that ethanol administration alters the capacity of liver mitochondria to oxidize acetyl CoA.[176, 256] The simplest explanation for these data is that ethanol increases the ratio of NADH to NAD$^+$, which, when elevated, inhibits several of the enzymes of the tricarboxylic acid cycle. The effect of ethanol on the activity of the tricarboxylic acid cycle is similar mechanistically to the suppression of these reactions in livers of fasted animals (see Chap. 4). On the other hand, the derangements of organization and function in liver mitochondria from ethanol-fed animals could underlie its effects on oxidation of acetyl CoA. In addition, recent data show that chronic consumption of ethanol decreases hepatic activity of carnitine palmitoyltransferase (see Chap. 4) and increases the sensitivity of this enzyme to inhibition by malonyl CoA.[261]

Since the activity of this enzyme determines, at least in part, the partitioning of fatty acids between oxidation and esterification,[262] its inhibition will tend to increase esterification of fatty acids.

Ethanol, via production of acetate, provides substantial amounts of 2-carbon substrate for the synthesis of fatty acids, a pathway that appears to be limited in the normal liver by the availability of substrate.[263, 264] Ingestion of ethanol hence is a good promoter of the synthesis of fatty acids,[258] adding further to fat in the livers of patients consuming ethanol.

Large doses of ethanol enhance the lipolytic rate in adipose tissue because of direct stimulatory effects on the adrenal[265, 266] and on the pituitary-adrenal axis.[266] Fatty acids released from adipose tissue after administration of large doses of ethanol are taken up by the liver.[267–270] Ethanol ingestion thus increases the rate of synthesis of triglycerides

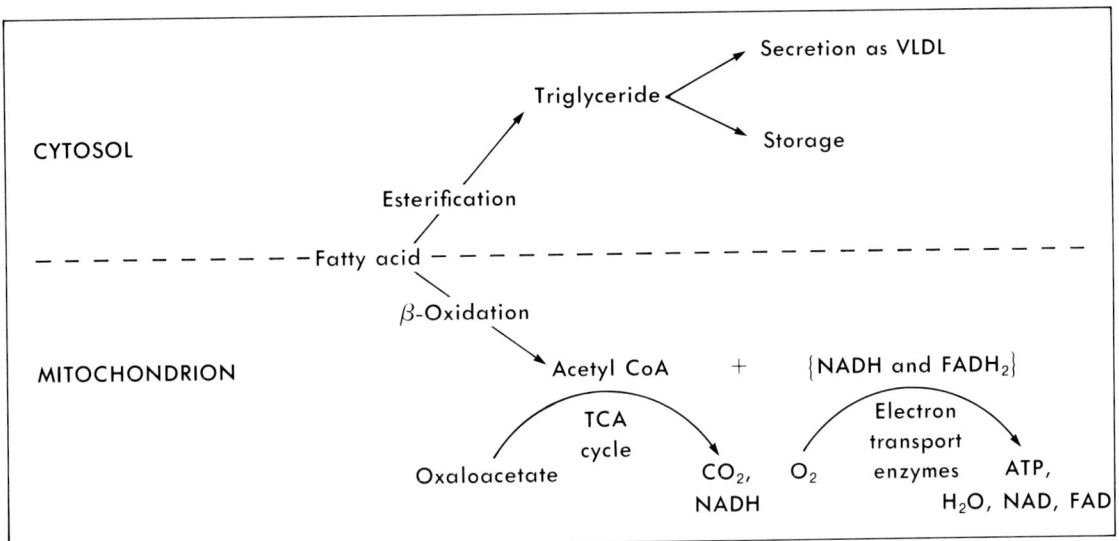

Figure 33–11. Disposition of fatty acids between esterification and oxidation. In ethanol-fed animals the block in oxidation of fatty acids is at the entry site into the TCA cycle, that is, the oxidation of acetyl CoA lost to CO_2. Ethanol also stimulates esterification of fatty acids.

in the liver by at least three separate mechanisms. And, not surprisingly, ingestion of ethanol leads to an accumulation of triglycerides in the liver.

The normal fate of hepatic triglycerides is incorporation into VLDL (Chap. 5), followed by secretion into the sinusoidal blood. Under normal conditions, the rates of the latter two processes are sufficient to keep triglycerides in the liver at low levels. When the triglyceride load increases because of increased synthesis of fatty acids or increased mobilization of fatty acids from adipose storage sites, the rates of synthesis and secretion of VLDL also increase. But increases in these rates depend acutely on increased concentrations of substrates for the synthetic and secretory enzymes. (Consider the relationship between velocity and substrate concentration for a single enzymatic reaction.) In other words, the normal liver cannot resecrete triglyceride as rapidly as it can make it. Hence, ethanol-induced fatty liver occurs in the absence of abnormalities of liver function (see Chaps. 4 and 5 for a more detailed discussion of fatty liver) and independent of nutritional state. Acute administration of ethanol does not appear to interfere with the synthesis or secretion of VLDL,[21, 271–273] unless the level in blood is sufficiently high to induce anesthesia. In humans, in fact, ethanol ingestion is a common cause of hyperlipidemia[274] (see also Chap. 5). The hyperlipidemia in these patients disappears during abstention.

Secretion of VLDL may be defective in patients with significant forms of ethanol-induced liver disease such as alcoholic hepatitis, cirrhosis, or both, because the synthesis and secretion of VLDL depend on synthesis of specific apoproteins and their incorporation into VLDL (see Chap. 5). It is reasonable to expect that some or all of these processes are functioning abnormally in patients with demonstrable abnormalities of liver cell function, as for example diminished synthesis of plasma proteins and less than normal capacity for detoxification of drugs and ammonia. Under these conditions, fatty liver in the alcoholic could reflect the result of increased synthesis of triglycerides plus inhibition of the synthesis and secretion of VLDL. There have been no experiments in alcoholics that specifically validate this assumption, but hyperlipidemia has been reported to be less common in alcoholics with cirrhosis as compared with alcoholics who do not have cirrhosis.[275]

The fatty liver in the ethanol abuser has been a well-known entity for many years. It has been stressed that ethanol-induced fatty liver is a toxic effect of ethanol per se that occurs independently of nutritional deficiency. Also, it has been suggested repeatedly that the fatty liver of the alcoholic is a harbinger of more serious liver disease and that the fatty liver is a natural event on the path to cirrhosis. No one today questions that fatty liver is a direct consequence of the biochemical and pharmacologic effects of ethanol. In this sense, fatty liver is a true toxic manifestation of the ingestion of ethanol, and it occurs in well-nourished alcoholics. In fact, careful attention to nutrition, even in a controlled setting, does not inhibit the development of ethanol-induced fatty liver. On the other hand, there is no evidence to indicate that fatty liver due to ethanol ingestion is the first step in the inexorable development of cirrhosis in the alcoholic or that it reflects a predisposition to this complication. In animals, for example, ethanol-induced fatty liver, which is produced easily in many species, is not a morbid condition. Animals with this lesion live a normal life span. Therefore, in and of itself, accumulation of fat does not appear to lead to irreversible changes in the function of liver cells, their normal morphologic organization, or both. Unfortunately, there are no adequate prospective studies in humans that deal with the natural history of alcohol-induced liver disease.

EFFECTS OF ETHANOL OXIDATION ON SYNTHESIS OF GLUCOSE

The most significant interaction between the metabolism of ethanol and glucose synthesis is that the former process inhibits the hepatic synthesis of glucose.[276–279] Ethanol does not alter the rate of hydrolysis of glycogen to glucose in a controlled setting, so inhibition of gluconeogenesis in response to ethanol is important clinically only in individuals who have no hepatic glycogen. A normal man or woman essentially is depleted of hepatic glycogen after about 48 hours of fasting. Normal subjects or alcoholics with and without liver disease may become hypoglycemic if they ingest ethanol at a time when they lack hepatic glycogen. This is a direct effect of ethanol on the liver and can be understood on the basis of the ethanol-induced shifts in the oxidation-reduction potential of the cytoplasmic compartment of the liver cell (Fig. 33–12). (Chap. 4 describes hepatic gluconeogenesis.) The increase in the ratio of NADH:NAD$^+$ during oxidation of ethanol shifts several oxidation-reduction couples to the reduced substrate: for example, oxaloacetate is reduced to malate, dihydroxyacetone-P is reduced to glycerol-1-P (Reaction [2]), and pyruvate is reduced to lactate. These intermediates are precursors of glucose. The ethanol-induced effect on levels of NADH thereby shunts intermediates of the gluconeogenic pathway away from the synthesis of glucose. A more important effect is that oxidation of ethanol interferes with the entry of carbon into the gluconeogenic pathway. This also is a consequence of the high NADH:NAD$^+$ ratio, which inhibits glutamate dehydrogenase (see the discussion of gluconeogenesis in Chap. 4).[280, 281] Glutamate dehydrogenase is an important enzyme in the synthesis of glucose, because it allows continued recycling of α-ketoglutarate in transaminase reactions, which provides for a continuous flow of carbon from amino acids to glucose. It has been found, too, that ethanol ingestion is associated with a reduction in the hepatic activity of two important gluconeogenic enzymes, pyruvate carboxylase and fructose-1,6-diphosphatase.[282] Measurement of the concentrations of gluconeogenic substrates in hepatocytes of fasted rats given ethanol suggests, however, that any changes in the activities of these two enzymes are less important than inhibition of the entry of substrates into the gluconeogenic pathway.[283]

The effects of ethanol on gluconeogenesis are self-limited. Inhibition of gluconeogenesis is present only so long as the NADH:NAD$^+$ ratio is elevated above normal. As soon as all administered ethanol is metabolized and NADH is reoxidized to NAD$^+$, the flow of substrate into and through the gluconeogenic pathway resumes. We want to stress, however, that ethanol-induced hypoglycemia can have serious clinical consequences requiring diagnosis and treatment with glucose. One should not delay administration of glucose while waiting for the ethanol to be metabolized completely. It also is important to appreciate that certain individuals are at high risk for development of ethanol-induced hypoglycemia: patients who are malnourished or thyrotoxic, those consuming high-protein diets with limited carbohydrates, and children.[284] Ethanol-induced hypoglycemia in children has a 25 per cent fatality rate.[284] The combination of ethanol and exogenous administration of insulin has produced severe hypoglycemia.[285]

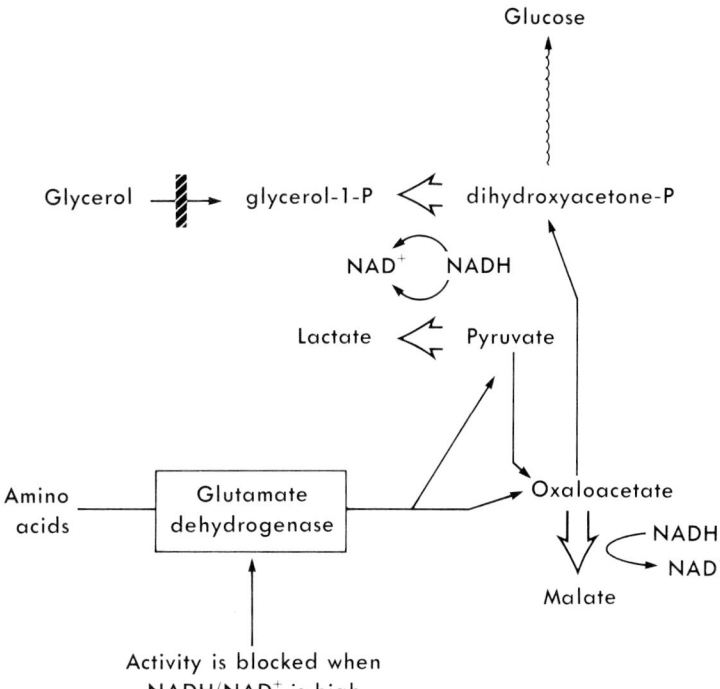

Figure 33–12. Effects of ethanol on synthesis of glucose. Ethanol blocks the flow of carbon to glucose by alteration in the ratios of lactate to pyruvate, dihydroxyacetone-P to glycerol-1-P, and oxaloacetate to malate secondary to increasing the ratio of NADH to NAD$^+$. Ethanol also leads to functional inhibition of glutamate dehydrogenase.

Obese patients and patients taking glucocorticoids are resistant to the hypoglycemic effects of ethanol.

Ethanol slightly decreases peripheral utilization of glucose.[286] In addition to direct interactions between the metabolism of ethanol and the synthesis of glucose, ethanol appears to influence the metabolism of glucose via effects on the endocrine system. Ethanol, when ingested by chronic users, interferes with the pituitary-adrenal axis, so that ethanol in this setting can limit the normal endocrine response to hypoglycemia,[287] potentiating the effects of ethanol on rates of gluconeogenesis and delaying recovery. Prior administration of ethanol enhances the response of the pancreatic cells to selected stimulators of insulin secretion. Ethanol, for example, potentiates arginine-induced but not glucagon-induced secretion of insulin by the pancreas.[288, 289]

Hypoglycemia presumed secondary to ingestion of ethanol has been reported to occur in well-fed individuals who were exercising vigorously in the cold.[288, 290] The mechanism of this phenomenon is unclear. Exercise, of course, potentiates utilization of glucose; but in the presence of hepatic glycogen, we would not expect hypoglycemia to ensue. It has been suggested, therefore, that ethanol ingestion may impede glycogenolysis. This point has not been documented and is difficult to accept in view of published studies of normal volunteers. It has also been reported that reactive hypoglycemia is potentiated by ethanol ingestion.[291, 292] Controlled studies in humans indicate that the combined intake of ethanol and a large sugar load may enhance insulin release.[277, 292] The timing of ethanol administration relative to glucose ingestion seems critical for duplicating this result.[292, 293]

ETHANOL INGESTION, LIPID PEROXIDATION, AND METABOLISM OF XENOBIOTICS

The phospholipids of cellular membranes contain a large proportion of polyunsaturated fatty acids, which are essential for maintaining the fluidity of the membrane and hence for the normal function of its constituent proteins. The carbon adjacent to the double bond, especially in a polyunsaturated fatty acid is highly susceptible to attack by free radicals (R·), which extract a proton, leaving behind a free-radical form of the acyl chain (Reaction [10]).[294–300]

$$\text{LIPID-H} + \text{R·} \rightarrow \text{LIPID·} + \text{RH} \qquad [10]$$

Oxygen can react with the lipid radical (Reaction [11]) to produce a peroxyradical that can react further with another unsaturated acyl chain (Reaction [12]) to produce

$$\text{LIPID·} + O_2 \rightarrow \text{LIPID-}O_2 \qquad [11]$$

$$\text{LIPID-}O_2\text{·} + \text{LIPID-H} \rightarrow \text{LIPID-OOH} + \text{LIPID·} \quad [12]$$

a lipid peroxide and a new lipid radical. The lipid peroxide can react further with Fe^{2+} and other transition metals to produce new free radicals (Reactions [13] and [14]).

$$\text{Lipid-OOH} + Fe^{2+} \rightarrow Fe^{3+} + OH^- + \text{Lipid-O·} \quad [13]$$

$$\text{Lipid-OOH} + Fe^{3+} \rightarrow \text{Lipid-}O_2 + H^+ + Fe^{2+} \quad [14]$$

This chain of radical formation obviously can cause extensive alterations in the lipid regions of membranes. In addition, the free radicals generated in the membrane can react with several functional groups in proteins, thereby altering the function of enzymes. The products of metabolism of the acyl peroxides—for example, reactive aldehyde—also will react with proteins and DNA, causing damage to the cell.[301–304]

The metabolism of many direct hepatotoxins is associated with generation of free radicals and peroxidation of membrane lipids (see Chaps. 30 and 32). Whether or not this kind of mechanism is critical for the initiation of hepatotoxicity is the subject of controversy,[301–304] but there is a fair amount of evidence to indicate that peroxidation of lipids at least contributes to the overall hepatotoxicity of many agents. Prior treatment with antioxidants diminishes the hepatotoxicity of carbon tetrachloride, for example.[305]

Normal metabolism within the liver cell gives rise constantly to toxic forms of oxygen.[296, 297, 306, 307] The superoxide anion of oxygen (O_2^-) is the most abundant of these. It is produced by a variety of flavin dehydrogenase enzymes and by cytochrome P450 (Fig. 33–13).[296, 297, 306, 307] (See also Chapter 9.) The O_2^- does not seem to be directly toxic, but it reacts with H_2O_2 to produce hydroxyl free radicals ($\cdot OH$) (Reaction [15]).

$$O_2^- + H_2O_2 \longrightarrow O_2 + OH^- + \cdot OH \quad [15]$$

Reaction [15] requires a catalyst in vivo, which probably is a form of Fe^{3+}.[86] The H_2O_2 for Reaction [15] can be produced by many flavoprotein oxidases (Reaction [5]). The hydroxyl radical ($\cdot OH$) is the proximate, toxic form of oxygen.

The superoxide anion is detoxified by the enzyme superoxide dismutase (Reaction [16]), which is distributed widely in tissues.[296–300]

$$2\ O_2^- + 2\ H^+ \longrightarrow H_2O_2 + O_2 \quad [16]$$

The H_2O_2 produced in Reaction [14] and the H_2O_2 produced in other reactions are detoxified by catalase and glutathione peroxidase (Reaction [17]).[308]

$$ROOH + 2\ GSH \longrightarrow ROH + GSSG + H_2O \quad [17]$$

The latter enzyme is abundant in the liver.[309] Reaction [17] is written to indicate that glutathione peroxidase reacts nonspecifically with a variety of peroxides, including those of fatty acids formed in Reaction [12]. Catalase, on the other hand, reacts only with H_2O_2. Thus, the activity of glutathione peroxidase is an important mechanism for protecting the cell against the toxicity of $\cdot OH$ and other free radicals. Oxidized glutathione (GSSG), one product of Reaction [17], is excreted into the bile.[310] This allows for monitoring the activity of Reaction [17] by collection of bile and measurement of the amount of GSSG present.

Liver contains two distinct forms of glutathione peroxidase, distinguished by the requirement of one of them for selenium.[311, 312] The non-selenium-requiring enzyme is glutathione-S-transferase B, which is known too as ligandin. Selenium deficiency in mice augments the toxicity of chemicals that are thought to produce excess superoxide anion.[313] In addition to the enzymatic mechanism for detoxifying activated forms of oxygen, the liver contains antioxidants, of which vitamin E, or α-tocopherol, is the best studied. Antioxidants detoxify free radicals, which abstract an elec-

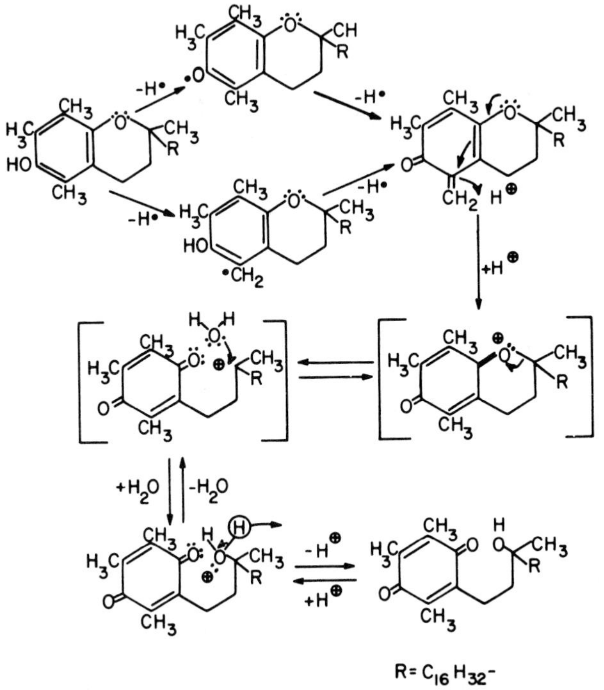

Figure 33–14. A mechanism for trapping of radicals by α-tocopherol. (Reprinted with permission from Tappel AL. Ann NY Acad Sci 203:12, 1973.)

tron from them (Fig. 33–14).[314] Deficiency of vitamin E is associated with enhanced rates of peroxidation of lipids.

There is a normal balance between production of toxic forms of O_2 and lipid peroxides on the one hand and mechanisms for detoxifying these intermediates on the other. Administration of ethanol or another toxic chemical can disturb this balance in a number of ways: by direct metabolism to a free radical, by increased production of toxic forms of O_2, and by destruction of normal, protective mechanisms for detoxifying free radicals (see also Chaps. 9 and 30). Ethanol is not metabolized to a free radical, but it can enhance mechanisms for the production of toxic forms of O_2 (Table 33–2) and at the same time modify mechanisms for detoxification of O_2^-. It appears in carefully controlled studies that ethanol increases peroxidation of lipids.[315–340] However, it is difficult to demonstrate consistently an effect of ethanol on peroxidation. This is not a surprising result, given the complexity and thus the difficulty in controlling the many variables in the system. The interrelations between different protective mechanisms (Table 33–2) indicate the many possible ways in which ethanol can modify the baseline effects of oxygen. Alcoholics with or without liver disease, for example, are deficient in α-tocopherol.[341] Tocopherols and glutathione protect against lipid peroxidation by independent pathways. Depletion of one will increase the stress on the other, but the status of tocopherol stores in liver influences the production of glutathione, because depletion of α-tocopherol leads to efflux from liver of precursors of glutathione (GSH).[342] Moreover, it appears that GSH, via a GSH-S-transferase–catalyzed reaction (Reaction [17]) converts radical forms of α-tocopherol to active forms.[343–345] Finally, whereas the glutathione concentration in liver cells is normal or only slightly depressed by chronic administration of ethanol, the concentration in mitochondria (about 15 per cent of the total in the liver) is decreased markedly in this setting, which could selectively lead to peroxidative change of mitochondria.[346] In spite of these data, one must keep in

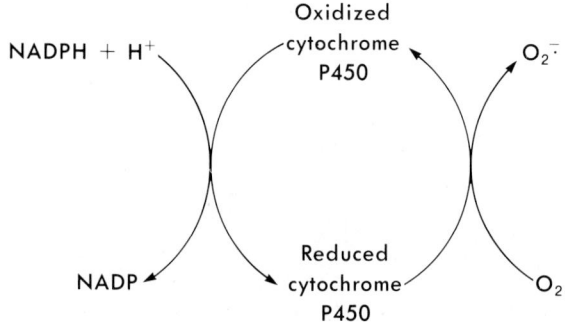

Figure 33–13. The generation of a toxic oxygen radical.

TABLE 33–2. MECHANISMS BY WHICH ETHANOL CAN ENHANCE PRODUCTION OF LIPID PEROXIDES

Enhanced Production of O_2^- and Other Toxic Forms of O_2
Induction of microsomal electron transport proteins
Increased production of NADPH (electron donor)
Increased amounts of unsaturated fatty acids in liver membranes
Oxidation of acetaldehyde by xanthine oxidase

Disorganization of Membranes Enhances the Attack of O_2^- on Unsaturated Lipids
Diminished Activity of Mechanisms for Detoxifying Free Radicals
Decreased total hepatic GSH in rats fed ethanol acutely but not chronically
Dietary deficiency of selenium (cofactor for glutathione peroxidase)
Deficiency of Zn (cofactor for superoxide dismutase)
Deficiency of vitamin E

mind that (1) there is no good evidence that ethanol-induced injury to the liver is due to lipid peroxidation; (2) there may be no correlation between production in vitro of lipid peroxides and their metabolic products by liver microsomes from alcohol-fed animals and lipid peroxidation in intact animals; and (3) finally, ethanol itself is a good quencher of free radicals.

EFFECTS OF ETHANOL ON SYNTHESIS AND SECRETION OF PROTEIN BY THE LIVER

The synthesis, glycosylation, sorting, and secretion of proteins are discussed in Chapter 6, which also includes a review of the known, specific effects of ethanol on hepatic metabolism of proteins. In addition to these effects, one must consider whether the synthesis of proteins becomes the limiting factor in the survival of liver cells under any set of experimental conditions. Some hepatotoxins are known to be inhibitors of hepatic protein synthesis, and a casual interpretation of this association suggests that the two phenomena are linked. They may be, but whether they are or not remains to be determined, because inhibiting the synthesis of a given protein will have an impact on the survival of a cell only when that protein is essential for the cell's life. We do not know which cellular proteins are essential for survival of liver cells, although we could make reasonable guesses. We do know, on the other hand, that the liver must have adaptive mechanisms for maintaining its critically important proteins. These mechanisms ensure survival of hepatocytes when conditions for maximal synthesis of proteins are not met—during severe malnutrition, for example. Data relating the toxicity of an agent to an effect on protein synthesis hence must be interpreted cautiously. Finally, although ethanol does inhibit the synthesis of some proteins, this effect is not general. Ethanol, for example, induces the synthesis of xenobiotic-metabolizing enzymes[347–349] (see the following section on drug metabolism).

EFFECTS OF ETHANOL ON HEPATIC DETOXIFICATION OF XENOBIOTICS

It is clear from the preceding discussion of lipid peroxidation that administration of ethanol will influence the toxicity of xenobiotics simply because ethanol will alter the

stress placed on systems that normally protect against liver damage caused by free radicals. In addition, ethanol will alter the metabolism of drugs directly (Table 33–3). Several lines of evidence indicate that this is an important problem for study and one that has more relevance to problems of disease in humans than many other lines of alcohol-related research.

Effects on P450 (see Chapter 9)

In humans and experimental animals, there is induction of a specific form of P450 that catalyzes, at relatively high rates, the oxidation of ethanol, isoniazid, aniline, acetaminophen, carbon tetrachloride, and several nitrosamines.[350–356] This specific form of P450 in humans is designated P450 HL$_j$.[354] Induction of P450s by ethanol is not limited to the liver,[355, 356] which is important medically because the likely connection between alcoholism and the increased incidence of cancer of the head, neck, and colorectal regions in alcoholics is induction by ethanol of cytochrome P450(s) that metabolize nitrosamines (and perhaps other agents) to proximate carcinogens.[357–360] Although it is clear that the P450 HL$_j$ form is increased in humans, in response to ethanol, other forms also may be induced.

Induction of P450 probably is the mechanism by which ethanol enhances the hepatotoxicity of CCl_4 and contributes to the toxicity of acetaminophen (see later) and cocaine.[361] In experimental animals, for example, prior treatment with a single dose of ethanol sensitizes the animal to the hepatotoxic effects of CCl_4. The interaction is greatest when the time between administrations of ethanol and CCl_4 is about 18 hours; it is independent of the metabolism of ethanol.[361–366] The ethanol-induced potentiation of toxicity is not limited to CCl_4 but extends to other halogenated hydrocarbons (including halothane), which are also metabolized by the P450 system.[361] The clinical correlate of enhanced toxicity caused by CCl_4 in ethanol-fed animals is that fatal CCl_4 poisoning in people occurs almost exclusively in alcoholics—that is, poisoning is almost never fatal in the nonalcoholic patient.[361] The significance of induction of P450 for acetaminophen-induced hepatotoxicity is more complex than for CCl_4 and is discussed at the end of this section.

Glucuronosyltransferase and Other Conjugating Reactions

Ethanol appears to be an inducer of this family of enzymes, which also are located in the endoplasmic reticulum of the liver and which represent the most important pathway for detoxification of xenobiotics by conjugation (Chap. 9). It is not proved, however, that prior administration of ethanol increases the amounts of any type of this enzyme. What is known is that glucuronidating activity, measured with many but not all substrates, is greater in liver microsomes from ethanol-fed rats than in microsomes

TABLE 33–3. MECHANISMS BY WHICH ETHANOL CAN MODIFY THE METABOLISM OF XENOBIOTICS

Selective induction of specific types of P450
Competitive inhibition of P450
Selective induction of glucuronosyltransferases
Decreased production of UDP-glucuronic acid
Stimulation of acetylation by increasing the hepatic concentration of acetyl-CoA

from controls.[367-370] However, if ethanol is being metabolized, it interferes with glucuronidation in intact animals by decreasing the hepatic concentration of uridine diphosphate (UDP)-glucuronic acid, probably as a result of the ethanol-induced increase in the ratio of NADH/NAD.[368, 371, 372]

Ethanol metabolism inhibits sulfation in association with decreases in the hepatic concentration of 3'phosphoadenosine-5'phosphosulfate (PAPS), which is the sulfo-donor in this detoxification reaction.[372] Chronic feeding of ethanol does not depress sulfotransferase activities. On an acute basis, ethanol would also be expected to decrease conjugation with glutathione because of its effects on the concentration of this intermediate (Table 33–3). The effects on conjugation with glutathione in chronically treated animals are uncertain because concentrations of glutathione are decreased in mitochondria but are normal in liver cytosol in these animals.[346] On the other hand, fasting per se leads to a decrease in total hepatic glutathione.[373] In the clinical setting, therefore, the effects of chronic intake of alcohol on conjugation with glutathione could be mediated by the influence of alcohol on nutrition.

Ethanol stimulates acetylation reactions because its metabolism increases concentrations of acetyl coenzyme A (acetyl-CoA) in liver (Reaction [2]).[361, 374, 375] Whether this effect has toxicologic significance—for example, whether increased rates of acetylation contribute to the increased hepatotoxicity of isoniazid in the alcoholic—is unstudied.

Alcohol and the Hepatotoxicity of Acetaminophen

Figure 33–15 depicts the major pathways for metabolism of acetaminophen (see also Chaps. 9 and 31). Ethanol should enhance the hepatotoxicity of acetaminophen, because it induces the type of P450 that metabolizes acetaminophen to reactive metabolites; it interferes with glucuronidation and sulfation; and at least acutely, it decreases the hepatic concentration of glutathione.

However ethanol and acetaminophen compete for the same P450, so in the presence of ethanol, metabolism of acetaminophen could be limited. Nevertheless, it is clear that ethanol augments the hepatotoxicity of acetaminophen in small laboratory animals.[361, 365, 376, 377] The important clinical question is whether ethanol enhances the hepatotoxicity of therapeutic doses of acetaminophen. The answer seems to be yes.[378-380] Several reports have shown that relatively large but therapeutic doses of acetaminophen cause acute hepatotoxicity and death in alcoholics.[378-380] But, in contrast to these data in people, chronic administration of ethanol did not augment the hepatotoxicity of therapeutic amounts of acetaminophen given to baboons.[381] Obviously, we cannot be certain of the significance of these discrepant results in humans and baboons. It is worthwhile to point out, nevertheless, that the environment of the baboons was controlled[39]—their dietary intake was controlled and constant, for example—whereas that for the patients was not.[378-380] The lesson from comparing the data in patients and experimental animals may be that the true hepatotoxicity of ethanol is much harder to demonstrate in the controlled experiment than in the world of clinical medicine because the hepatotoxicity of ethanol is determined to a considerable degree by undefined factors in a patient's environment and not simply by the intake of ethanol. We will return to this idea in the sections on animal models and ethanol-nutrient interactions.

Alcohol and the Hepatotoxicity of Vitamin A

Vitamin A is not a xenobiotic, but it is hepatotoxic, and its hepatotoxicity is potentiated by ethanol. In hypervitaminosis A in rats, there is a release of protease from liver lysosomes with swelling of rat liver mitochondria.[382] These phenomena reflect that excessive amounts of vitamin A decrease the stability of biologic membranes.[383, 384] Because of interactions between the hydroxyl of retinol and the phosphates in the polar region of the membrane, α-retinol, a biologically inactive analog of vitamin A, has lytic effects on membranes almost identical to those of retinol. Hence, the observed surface-active effects of retinol on membranes are not necessarily related to the physiologic action of this vitamin. It is possible also to produce the clinical manifestations of hypervitaminosis A in animals by administering large amounts of the all-trans-retinoic acid.[385, 386] The 13-cis-retinoic acid has no toxicity.[386]

The recommended daily intake of vitamin A by an adult is 5000 IU per day. Intakes severalfold (>40,000 IU/day) greater than this level, when prolonged for years, may lead to a chronic form of liver disease.[387-394] The amount of vitamin A ingested determines the interval between onset of excess intake and clinical manifestation of liver disease. Indeed, acute vitamin A intoxication occurs after massive intake. This has been reported to occur after ingestion of livers from animals whose livers contain enormous stores of vitamin A, such as fish and the polar bear. The more common cause of intoxication, however, is intake of vitamin A as a medication.

About half the patients with vitamin A intoxication have hepatomegaly and splenomegaly. Some of these patients have cirrhosis, with an elevated wedged hepatic vein pressure, and ascites may be present. The morphologic characteristics of the liver are variable in these patients.

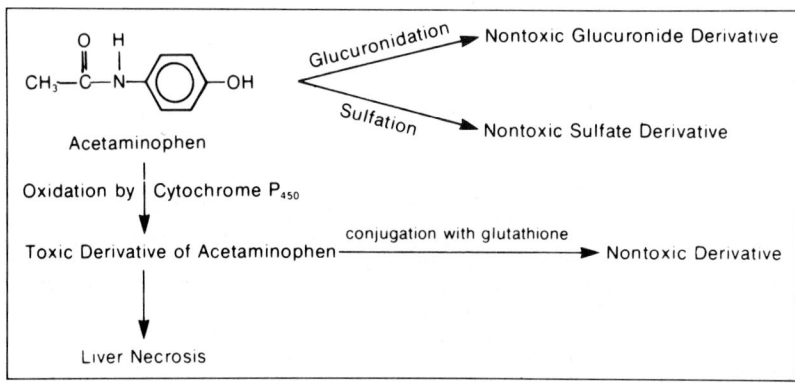

Figure 33–15. Metabolic pathways for the disposition of acetaminophen. Conjugation with glucuronic acid and sulfate are preferred to oxidation by P450; however, interference with the former pathways, and especially with glucuronidation, forces more substrate into the oxidative pathway, which produces toxic intermediates. (Reproduced from Zakim D. Am J Med 80:645, 1986, with permission.)

Changes range from nonspecific degeneration to fibrosis to cirrhosis. There may be sclerosis of portal and central veins as well as perisinusoidal fibrosis. The latter changes undoubtedly lead to the associated portal hypertension and ascites. In addition, storage of excess vitamin A in Kupffer cells leads to their swelling, and this may be an additional factor producing sinusoidal hypertension. Dilated vitamin A storage cells are seen typically in liver biopsy specimens from affected patients. Laboratory abnormalities in chronic vitamin A intoxication are not specific. Jaundice, when present, usually is mild.

It is important to appreciate that excess vitamin A causes liver disease that is potentially curable. Thus, discontinuation of exposure to excess vitamin A leads in many instances to complete recovery. This is not true, however, for patients in whom the disease has progressed to a cirrhotic stage; the manifestations of vitamin A–induced liver disease can persist in these patients. Nevertheless, it is reasonable to expect that removal of excess vitamin A from the diets of these patients will ameliorate some features of their disease. In addition to liver disease, vitamin A excess causes systemic signs and symptoms—for example, fever, night sweats, anemia, leukopenia, proteinuria, pruritus, loss of head and body hair, and bone pain and tenderness.

Hepatic storage capacity for vitamin A and serum levels of vitamin A–retinol-binding protein are decreased in cirrhotic as well as in many noncirrhotic forms of liver disease.[395] These changes can account for night blindness in patients with liver disease. In addition, zinc deficiency in cirrhosis can interfere with the metabolism of vitamin A in the retina (alcohol dehydrogenases contain zinc), which can cause night blindness even in the vitamin A–repleted patient.

Ethanol affects the metabolism of vitamin A in the absence of liver disease. Ethanol administration to rats and baboons depresses hepatic concentrations of vitamin A, probably because it enhances metabolism of vitamin A by P450 in the liver and promotes mobilization of vitamin A out of the liver.[396–400] These effects of ethanol clearly are independent of any extrahepatic effects of ethanol. Ethanol abuse in humans also decreases hepatic concentrations of vitamin A, the extent of the decrease from normal becoming larger as patients progress from fatty liver to alcoholic hepatitis to cirrhosis.[401] The presence of normal or deficient levels of zinc in experimental animals has an important impact on ethanol-induced changes in the metabolism of vitamin A. Deficiency of zinc diminishes the effect of ethanol on decreasing hepatic stores of vitamin A.[402] This is true as for ethanol-induced changes in the concentration of vitamin A in epithelial tissues as well.[402]

The problem of repleting the alcoholic with vitamin A is potentially difficult. Ethanol enhances the hepatotoxicity of vitamin A in experimental animals.[403] Nontoxic amounts of vitamin A (about 200 U/day, or about 5-fold greater than amounts usually fed to rats) fed in combination with ethanol, in a liquid diet, were associated with necrosis, inflammation, and fibrosis in rat liver.[403] These lesions did not occur in rats fed alcohol and lesser amounts of vitamin A, nor did they occur in rats fed 4000 U of vitamin A/day.[403] The basis of the toxic interaction between vitamin A and ethanol is unclear. Concentrations of vitamin A in livers from ethanol-fed animals were lower than in animals fed equal amounts of vitamin A (2000 U/day) and were in fact in the normal range.[403] It was concluded that a metabolic product of vitamin A, not vitamin A per se was the proximate toxin in the ethanol-fed rats.[404] But there are many equally plausible mechanisms, especially in view of

the multitude of effects ethanol has on membranes and the fact that vitamin A itself is a surface-active agent. The uncertainty about mechanism notwithstanding, the interaction between vitamin A (or acetaminophen) may provide an important *model* for the problem of alcoholic liver disease in humans. For, whereas vitamin A and ethanol can be nontoxic to the rat liver when administered separately, the combination becomes highly toxic. Interestingly, it has not been possible to connect any of the myriad toxic effects of alcohol *with liver disease in humans*, except for interactions between ethanol and toxins in the environment (e.g., acetaminophen).

MECHANISMS UNRELATED TO DIRECT LETHAL EFFECTS ON HEPATOCYTES

ALTERATIONS OF THE IMMUNE SYSTEM IN THE ALCOHOLIC

There has been speculation for a long time that alcohol-associated liver disease might be caused at least in part by immune attack on the liver.[405–415] The proposed mechanisms that could lead to liver disease on this basis and the evidence marshalled to support this idea (Table 33–4) range from observations of increased globulin levels in alcoholics with liver disease[406–409, 413] to observations that ethanol promotes expression of MHC class I antigens (see Chap. 42) on plasma membranes from a variety of nonhepatic cells in culture.[415] Omitted from Table 33–4 is the idea that people with HLA B8 and DR3 are at especially high risk for developing alcoholic liver disease. Observations to this effect have not been confirmed.[414] Also, despite the numerous observations that are compatible with an attack by the immune system on the liver in the alcoholic, there is no direct evidence for the idea that the immune system is a pathogenetic contributor to liver disease in these patients. In fact, the contrary is so. Numerous studies have failed to show a salutary effect of steroids (immune suppression) given to patients with alcoholic hepatitis (see later). In addition, although it is true that liver disease can progress from alcoholic hepatitis to cirrhosis in some alcoholics who purport to abstain from alcohol,[416, 417] there are no good data in these patients to support the notion that chronicity in them reflects an attack by the immune system on the liver. Other, unstudied pathogenetic mechanisms are more likely to account for progression of liver disease in these

TABLE 33–4. EVIDENCE FOR DERANGEMENT OF THE IMMUNE SYSTEM IN PATIENTS WITH ALCOHOLIC LIVER DISEASE

Humoral Factors
Increased levels of IgA and other immunoglobulins
Antinuclear antibodies or anti–smooth muscle antibodies in some patients
Antibodies to liver-specific protein
Antibodies to proteins changed by reaction with acetaldehyde ("neoantigens")
Antibodies to alcoholic hyalin

Cell-Mediated Factors
Alcoholic hyalin, acetaldehyde, or both transforms T lymphocytes, producing cytotoxic lymphocytes and humoral mediators of immunity
Patients with alcoholic hepatitis have circulating cells that are cytotoxic for liver cells
Alcohol increases reactivity of T and B cells
Alcohol promotes expression of MHC class I antigens (nonhepatic cells in culture)

patients—for example, progression as a natural consequence of vascular disarray in the diseased liver or perhaps infection with hepatitis B (see reference 418). Therefore, at present there really is no direct evidence that perturbation of the immune system contributes to liver disease in the alcoholic.

MACROPHAGE FUNCTION IN THE ALCOHOLIC

An interesting facet of the history of research on alcoholic liver disease was the idea first proposed by Rojkind that the effects of this disease could be ameliorated by preventing the fibrosis that accompanies it.[419–421] Work on this idea began prior to an appreciation of the full significance of the matrix of the liver for the function and development of liver cells as well as the importance of factors (cytokines) provoked by the inflammatory response in stimulating fibrogenesis. Recently, there has been an explosion of knowledge about cytokine-mediated inflammation and how, in addition to fibrogenesis, these mediators may be involved in pathogenetic mechanisms of liver diseases. These areas are reviewed in detail in Chapter 15. Although it is not clear as yet how this work will affect our ideas about the genesis of liver disease or the treatment of alcoholic liver disease, there is a reason to be hopeful. For example, a clinical trial of penicillamine, an inhibitor of fibrogenesis but not of the inflammatory response, was without effect on the progress of liver disease in alcoholics;[421] therapy in the future could be directed at the selective interdiction of inflammatory signals that incite cells in the liver to increase the synthesis of collagen, or it could be directed at preventing synthesis of collagen prior to its secretion from cells.[422, 423] Indeed, recent data show that a prostaglandin inhibited the generation of fibrous tissue in rats fed a cirrhogenic diet (deficient in choline and protein).[422] It must be admitted that treatment of these animals with prostaglandin may have altered the toxicity of the diet and inhibited synthesis of collagen in this manner. Nevertheless, it is clear that the course of dietary-induced cirrhosis can be altered dramatically with pharmacologic agents.

In addition to the inflammatory response within the parenchyma in alcoholic hepatitis, the metabolism of ethanol can have a direct effect on fibrogenesis. Acetaldehyde stimulates directly the production of collagen and noncollagen protein by fibroblasts grown in culture and within livers in intact animals.[163–165] Although as already mentioned little acetaldehyde leaves liver cells, there is more acetaldehyde in peripheral blood of alcoholics than normals, perhaps because they are deficient in aldehyde dehydrogenase (see p. 828). In addition, macrophages metabolize acetaldehyde via a P450-dependent pathway.[424, 425] The concentration of acetaldehyde in macrophages during oxidation of ethanol has not been measured. Nevertheless, there is an experimental basis for the idea that ethanol can modify macrophage function independently of effects on hepatocytes. There also may be a basis for ethanol-mediated effects on the direct liberation of cytotoxic substances from cells. Culture of macrophages in the presence of ethanol leads to production of a cytotoxic compound that is inactivated by heat.[426, 427] It also has been reported that a cytotoxic factor appears in serum of normal individuals given a test dose of ethanol.[428] These results are not convincing, but they are provocative. Obviously, this is an aspect of research in alcoholic liver disease that appears promising.

ANIMAL MODELS OF ALCOHOLIC LIVER DISEASE; INTERACTIONS BETWEEN ETHANOL AND NUTRITION

RATS

Table 33–1 presented a summary of the accepted toxic manifestations of ethanol in an experimental setting. Not all manifestations of ethanol's impact on liver function were listed, but the effects in Table 33–1 have been demonstrated to occur in rats. It is reasonable to ask for the evidence that any of these effects or all of them acting in concert, leads to cirrhosis in the rat. The answer is a clear-cut no.[429–434]

Rats fed large amounts of ethanol develop cirrhosis only when their diets are relatively low in choline.[429–434] For example, supplementation of the diet with choline allows the rat to adapt in some manner to the hepatotoxic consequences of ethanol. A diet that prevents the fibrosis and cirrhosis associated with feeding ethanol to rats does not alter the effects of ethanol on mitochondrial morphology and swelling and changes in the endoplasmic reticulum, nor does it prevent accumulation of fat in the liver and so forth; but all these toxic manifestations of ethanol administration appear to be self-limited events in the well-fed rat. The toxic effects of ethanol described to date establish conditions under which nutritional deficiency leads to cirrhosis and vice versa, but the toxic effects of ethanol per se (e.g., accumulation of fat, megamitochondria, lipid peroxidation) do not cause liver disease in the rat. Precisely what toxic effects of ethanol interact with dietary deficiency (or in fact with what dietary deficiency) to produce cirrhosis in the rat remain to be elucidated. All that really is known in this respect is that choline deficiency per se will cause cirrhosis in the rat when combined with protein deficiency[434] and that ethanol increases the choline requirement of the rat.[435–438]

The rat can synthesize choline-containing phosphatides (Fig. 33–16), but the rate of synthesis does not appear to be sufficient for meeting all the animal's needs. Choline hence is an essential dietary ingredient for the rat. Deficiency is associated almost immediately with an inability of the animal's liver to secrete VLDL. Fatty liver ensues. Fibrous tissue develops in the liver of the choline-deficient rat, and depending on the amount of dietary protein, the liver eventually becomes cirrhotic. There is no evidence of hepatitis during the development of cirrhosis, and the molecular events leading to cirrhosis in the choline-deficient rat are completely unknown. Nevertheless, given the importance of phosphatidylcholine for the structural and functional integrity of the plasma and intracellular membranes (in which it comprises two thirds of the phospholipids) of the hepatocyte and its role in maintaining the activities of some enzymes that are integral components of these membranes, it is not difficult to propose mechanisms by which choline deficiency can interfere with the viability of liver cells.

Choline deficiency per se is not sufficient for production of cirrhosis in the rat; the cirrhogenic potential of choline deficiency can be modulated. Cirrhosis is prevented by administration of nonabsorbable antibiotics to choline-deficient rats.[439] Fatty liver persists in these animals. Diets containing large amounts of protein also block the cirrhogenic effect of choline deficiency, so that choline deficiency leads to cirrhosis in the rat only when combined with a diet low in protein. Interestingly, the accumulation of fat in the livers of choline-deficient rats fed a high-protein diet is greater than that in animals fed a choline-deficient, low-

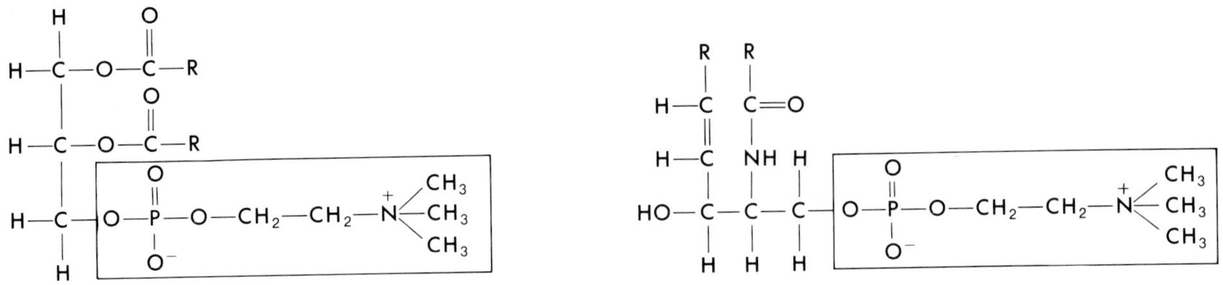

Figure 33–16. Choline-containing phosphatides.

protein diet. Thus, a high-protein diet does not correct choline deficiency but alters the hepatic response to it. Choline deficiency, therefore, is only one of the factors involved in the genesis of cirrhosis in the choline-deficient rat.

Secondary malnutrition occurs in rats fed ethanol on a chronic basis. Animals fed ethanol do not gain weight as rapidly as controls ingesting the same quantity of calories,[440] and these animals display evidence of multiple vitamin deficiencies despite a nutritionally adequate diet.[441, 442] What therefore is clear is that minimal daily requirements for nutrients determined for normal animals (humans probably included) do not apply to animals consuming large amounts of ethanol. One simple reason for this is the effect of ethanol on absorption of nutrients in the gut (Table 33–5).[443–447] Finally, the amounts of carbohydrate and fat fed along with ethanol have a profound effect on the genesis of cirrhosis and fibrosis in rat liver. Fibrosis does not occur if ethanol is substituted for fat instead of for sugar.[448, 449] The usual diets used to induce cirrhosis in the rat substitute ethanol for carbohydrates.

PRIMATES

The difficulties encountered in producing ethanol-induced cirrhosis in the rat independent of dietary manipulations led to the use of primates for this purpose. Lieber and coworkers reported in 1974 that chronic ingestion of ethanol by baboons led to fatty liver, alcoholic hepatitis, and cirrhosis.[450, 451] These effects were attributed to ethanol and were believed not to be dependent on prior induction of nutritional deficiencies. The basis for this interpretation of the data was that the animals were fed nutritionally adequate diets. The experiments appeared to be controlled, because one group of animals received the same amounts of protein, vitamins, and other nutrients fed to the experimental group, but the latter ingested ethanol in place of calories from carbohydrate. No abnormality of liver function occurred in the control group. It should be clear, however, that the design of nutritional experiments is exceedingly difficult because of the interactions between different nutrients and between drugs and nutrients. The proper control for experiments such as those reported,

given the state of knowledge about primate nutrition at that time and the demonstrated effects of alcohol on nutrition, would have been to test whether diets with varying amounts of essential nutrients (e.g., protein and choline) would ameliorate or exacerbate the effects of ethanol on liver function. This is especially important in primates because choline-deficient diets produce cirrhosis in them. The rate of progression of cirrhosis in such animals is dependent on the amount of fat in the diet, and depending on the animal's nutrition, can occur as early as two months after the onset of the experimental diet.[452–454] The conclusions drawn by Lieber and coworkers thus were open to question.[455] Rogers and colleagues found that the induction of cellular necrosis and extensive fibrosis in Rhesus monkeys in response to ethanol ingestion depended on the other components in the diet. The occurrence of these lesions in a small number of Rhesus monkeys fed large amounts of ethanol was prevented by increasing the amounts of protein and choline in their diets.[454, 455] These experiments, of course, do not provide information about the minimal daily requirements for these nutrients in a control population of Rhesus monkeys, but they provide an unequivocal indication that their levels in the diet are important for the genesis of ethanol-induced liver disease in primates. In considering the arguments in the literature on these issues the reader should keep in mind that choline supplements do not prevent many demonstrable toxic effects of ethanol in primates,[456] but they do prevent progressive disease as reflected by fibrosis.[454, 455, 455a]

There are many possible reasons why ethanol ingestion could alter the minimal daily requirements for choline as well as other nutrients. As mentioned already, ethanol ingestion increases the utilization of choline in the rat.[435–438] It also has important effects on the metabolism of folate, which can interact with the enzyme systems synthesizing choline. As shown in Figure 33–17, adequate stores of folate are important for synthesis of choline. Also, choline can serve as a source of $-CH_3$ groups for synthesis of methionine, thereby circumventing an ethanol-induced block of folate-mediated methyl transfer reactions (Chap. 21; reference 457). Sorting out the significant interactions between ethanol and the metabolism of nutrients obviously will be an enormously difficult task. These complexities probably explain why a fixed choline supplement that prevents ethanol-induced fibrosis in monkeys[454, 455a] does not do so in baboons.[456] The idea that ethanol per se is not toxic for baboons is underlined too by the observation that hepatic fibrosis develops in only one third of baboons fed ethanol. Two thirds of the animals fed ethanol plus a diet of questionable nutritional adequacy are able to compensate for the toxic effects of ethanol. This is not unlike the

TABLE 33–5. REVERSIBLE INTESTINAL ABNORMALITIES IN ALCOHOLICS WITHOUT LIVER DISEASE

Malabsorption of folic acid, thiamine, fat, nitrogen B_{12}, B_2
Decreased output of HCO_3 amylase, lipase, and chymotrypsin in response to secretin

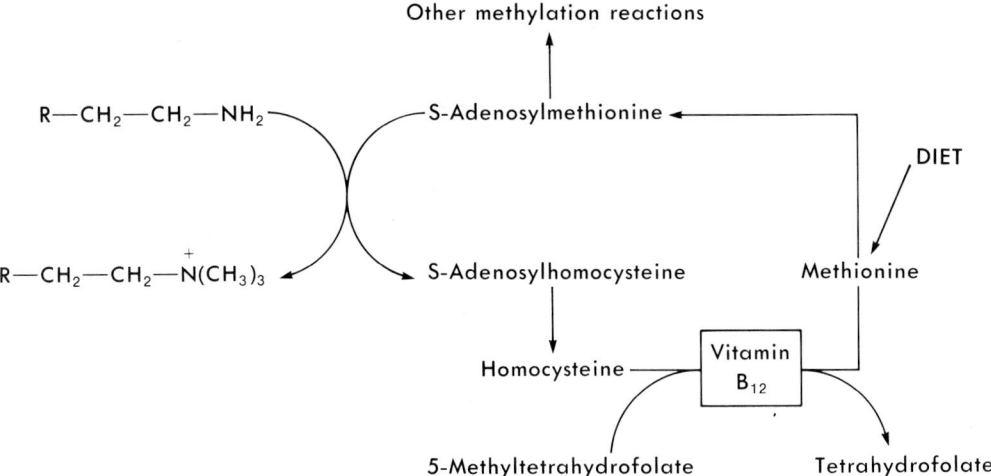

Figure 33–17. The synthesis of choline and its dependence on vitamin B_{12} and folate. $R\text{-}CH_2\text{-}CH_2\text{-}NH_2$ represents phosphatidyl ethanolamine, which is methylated three times to form phosphatidylcholine. Three moles of *S*-adenosylmethionine are required for synthesis of each mole of phosphatidylcholine. Regeneration of *S*-adenosylmethionine can be effected with dietary methionine or by synthesis of methionine from homocysteine. The latter conversion requires 5-methyltetrahydrofolate as a methyl group donor and vitamin B_{12} as cofactor. The scheme shows how choline- and methionine-deficient diets might induce folate deficiency by draining folate (the folate trap hypothesis) from DNA synthesis.

situation in humans. However, there is no good evidence that baboons ever develop alcoholic hepatitis.

HUMANS

There has been no long-term prospective study of the incidence of liver disease in alcoholic individuals. There are well-controlled studies of the effects of ethanol when administered to patients recovering from alcoholic hepatitis.[458–462] In one such study, the patients all had decompensated alcoholic cirrhosis.[458] After it was clear that the patients were able to eat, they were given large oral doses of ethanol. Patients consumed approximately 3000 calories each day, of which one third were derived from ethanol. The amount of ethanol ingested was sufficient in these patients to exceed their capacity to metabolize it completely within 24 hours. As liver function improved and the metabolic rate for ethanol increased, more ethanol was added to the diet. Liver function tests for the patients treated in this manner are shown in Figure 33–18. Data for a patient with acute sclerosing hyaline necrosis are shown in Figure 33–19. Clinical observations of the progress of the patients in this study indicated continued improvement over the course of the experiment. These results do not fit with the idea that ethanol is a direct hepatotoxin. Patients with decompensated, alcohol-induced liver disease recovered from their disease even while ingesting large amounts of ethanol so long as they also were consuming nutritionally adequate diets. The best available data from controlled investigations in humans indicate, therefore, that the response of humans to ethanol is similar to that of rats and primates. The data in humans imply that ethanol abuse is not the only factor essential for producing cirrhosis in the alcoholic, because, given an "adequate" diet, man adapts to the hepatotoxic effects of ethanol.

The idea that liver disease in the alcoholic is secondary to the malnutrition seen so frequently in this group, rather than to their alcohol intake per se, is an old one. This view has never been accepted as fact because malnutrition, defined as protein and calorie deprivation, does not cause irreversible liver disease in humans. During World War II, for example, the incidence of cirrhosis did not increase in

those areas in which starvation was present. Similarly, children who have kwashiorkor or marasmus do not develop cirrhosis. Since malnutrition cannot be shown to cause cirrhosis in humans (it does in rats and primates) it has been difficult to accept the concept that malnutrition in the alcoholic causes cirrhosis. Documentation that ethanol itself had deleterious effects on the function of the liver, causing, for example, fatty liver, abnormalities of endoplasmic reticulum, and swollen mitochondria, seemed to rationalize the idea that ethanol per se was the cause of cirrhosis in alcoholics and that diet was unimportant. However, the advances in biochemistry have taught us that most clinical diseases are the end-result of concerted effects, each of which may not cause clinical abnormality when

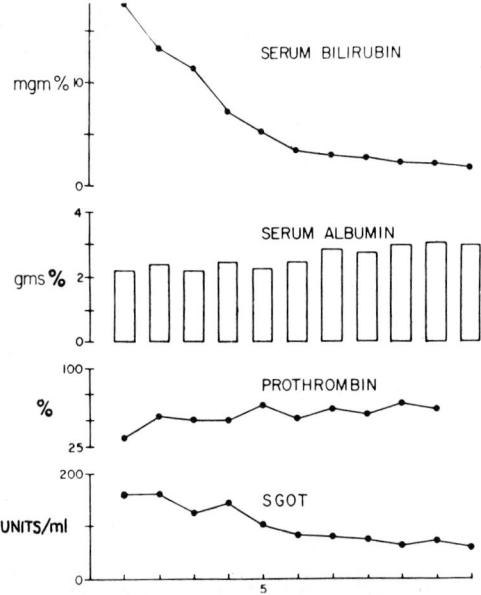

Figure 33–18. Composite results of laboratory tests performed on ten patients with alcoholic hepatitis who were given alcohol. Alcohol intake was increased to match an increasing alcohol metabolic rate. (Reproduced from Reynolds TB, et al. In: McIntyre NM, Sherlock S, eds. Therapeutic Agents and the Liver. Oxford, Blackwell Scientific Publications, 1965:131, with permission.)

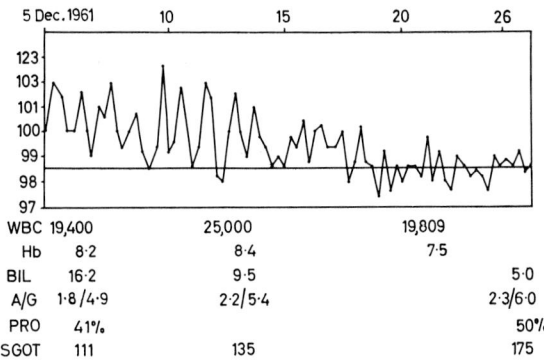

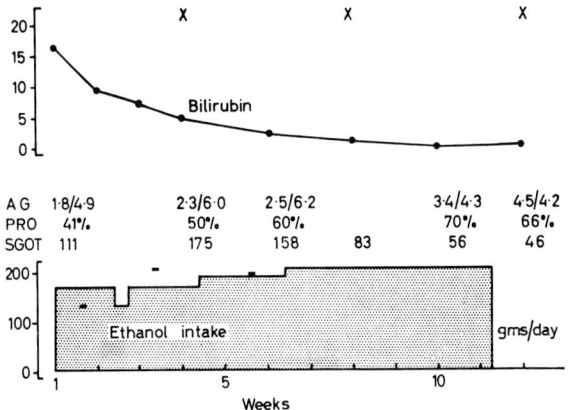

Figure 33–19. The top part of this figure reflects the clinical course of a patient with acute sclerosing hyaline necrosis. The two bottom sections are the results of laboratory tests of the patient. The small bars associated with the ethanol intake chart represent estimations of the alcohol metabolic rate. (Reproduced from Reynolds TB, et al. In: McIntyre NM, Sherlock S, eds. Therapeutic Agents and the Liver. Oxford, Blackwell Scientific Publications, 1965:131, with permission.)

acting alone. This is appreciated most easily in disease states secondary to inborn errors of metabolism. Patients lacking the hepatic form of fructose-1-P aldolase, for example, become ill after eating fructose, but are well so long as they avoid it.[463] Clinical disease, therefore, is not caused by either fructose or deficiency of fructose-1-P adolase, but by both acting in concert. Another example that is more relevant to disease in the alcoholic is the importance of ethanol and thiamine deficiency for producing Wernicke-Korsakoff syndrome. This disease is seen predominantly in malnourished alcoholics. Interestingly, however, those patients who develop Wernicke-Korsakoff psychosis, in addition to being alcoholics and thiamine deficient because of their alcoholism, have an apparently greater than normal requirement for thiamine because of a genetic abnormality. The affinity of transketolase from these patients for its cofactor thiamine-PP is abnormally low,[464, 465] which could explain why only a minority of malnourished alcoholics develop Wernicke-Korsakoff syndrome. With regard to the problem of ethanol-induced liver disease, some proponents seem to argue that malnutrition in the alcoholic is the causal factor; others argue that ethanol causes liver disease regardless of diet. Neither of these views is supported by experiments.

Nutritional Status of Alcoholics

Not all alcoholics are malnourished, nor do all alcoholics have liver disease. On the other hand, data in the

literature show that most alcoholics with liver disease are malnourished, on the basis of weight loss, specific evidence of malnutrition, or both.[466–480] This is true because ethanol interferes with intestinal absorption of nutrients and it diminishes appetite for nonethanolic calories, which can lead to further deficiencies in absorptive function (see Table 33–5). It is mentioned often that dietary histories of alcoholics fail to show diminished intake of protein in those with liver disease; yet objective studies of these same patients show repeatedly that abstention from alcohol and ingestion of a normal diet in a controlled setting corrects many abnormalities considered to reflect protein deficiency: weight gain, gain of muscle mass, correction of defective pancreatic secretion, and return of skin sensitivity to foreign antigens. Moreover, surveys of nutritional status in alcoholics consistently show that objective evidence of malnutrition is more prevalent in alcoholics with liver disease than in alcoholics without liver disease. Alcoholic patients with liver disease weigh less than they ideally should; alcoholics without liver disease are in excess of ideal body weight. Evidence of gross malnutrition is almost always present in patients with alcoholic liver disease and must be considered a significant and probably critical feature of their disease.

We should not assume that liver disease in the alcoholic patient, when it occurs, is continuously progressive. Clinical experience indicates that the intake of alcohol of a given patient with acute liver disease is not invariant. Instead, the history reveals quite frequently that admission to the hospital with acute decompensated liver disease was preceded by increasing intake of ethanol superimposed on a history of chronic alcoholism. Correlation of dietary intake with indices of liver function and without regard for the possible dynamic interactions between ethanol, diet, and hepatic function may give a skewed picture of the interrelations among these factors. Another problem that could confound studies of the relationship between ethanol, diet, and cirrhosis is that ethanol may interact not only with the diet but also with a genetic predisposition. That some malnourished alcoholics escape the problems of alcoholic hepatitis/cirrhosis is not evidence that malnutrition is not the critical pathogenic mechanism in those alcoholics that develop liver disease. Observations of the effects of ethanol in primates emphasize this idea.

Liver Disease in Patients Who Are Obese

An exceedingly interesting lesion is observed frequently (about 5 to 10 per cent of the time) in patients who are morbidly obese.[481–485] Liver biopsy specimens from these patients are strikingly similar to those from patients with alcohol-associated liver disease (see later). The frequency of the hepatic abnormalities increases to as much as 50 per cent in patients who have had jejunoileal bypass procedures for control of their obesity.[481–488] The jejunoileal bypass gives rise to several potential problems for the liver of the treated patient, who is deficient in essential nutrients, has a blind intestinal loop, and has abnormal hepatotoxic bile acids in serum.[487–490] The combination of these effects, especially the malnutrition, may account for the high incidence of severe hepatic lesions in patients who have had jejunoileal bypass procedures. In a few instances, the hepatic lesions found after bypass surgery have responded to intravenous hyperalimentation.[490–492] We do not know why this lesion is present in obese patients, but neither do we know very much about the nutrient balance in such patients.

CLINICAL FEATURES OF ALCOHOLIC LIVER DISEASE

DIAGNOSIS OF ALCOHOLIC LIVER DISEASE

Alcohol has replaced tuberculosis as the great imitator in modern medical practice. The major nonhepatic organs seriously affected by ethanol and the principal clinical manifestations of this involvement are listed in Table 33–6. It is important to remember that each of the illnesses listed in Table 33–6 can occur in concert with alcoholic liver disease. Thus, the patient who has alcoholic liver disease may be brought to medical attention initially because of a nonhepatic illness. The patient may lack symptoms referable to the liver. A slightly elevated serum AST or a palpable liver may be the only finding indicative of liver disease.

History

The initial step in determining whether liver disease is likely to be present is to assess the quantity of ethanol consumed by the patient. The average daily consumption of ethanol will indicate the probability that liver disease has developed. The form in which the ethanol is consumed has no effect on toxicity. Beer, for example, is as toxic as "hard" liquor for equal amounts of ethanol ingested. The grams of ethanol consumed based on intake of spirits, wine, or beer can be calculated by use of a suitable nomogram (Fig. 33–20).

The incidence of serious liver disease begins to rise with an average daily consumption of more than 40 to 60 g ethanol for a man and perhaps as little as 20 g for a woman.[493–495] These amounts of alcohol must be consumed

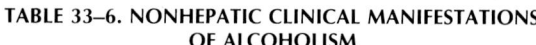

TABLE 33–6. NONHEPATIC CLINICAL MANIFESTATIONS OF ALCOHOLISM

Nervous System	Hematopoietic System
CNS	Leukopenia
Acute intoxication	Thrombocytopenia
Delirium tremens	Anemia
Wernicke-Korsakoff	Iron deficiency
encephalopathy	Folic acid deficiency
Cerebellar degeneration	Megaloblastic
Peripheral nervous system	Hemolytic
Peripheral neuropathy	**Musculoskeletal System**
Cardiovascular System	Acute rhabdomyolysis
Cardiomyopathy	Chronic proximal myopathy
Congestive heart failure	
Arrhythmias	

over a long period (many years) and should be thought of as general guidelines for risk, not absolutes.[12–14] Discovery that a patient drinks moderate to large amounts of ethanol is only one clue that can lead to the discovery of liver disease.

Symptoms

It is incorrect to think that patients with alcoholic liver disease always are symptomatic, with complaints such as jaundice, ascites, or gastrointestinal bleeding. Patients with alcoholic liver disease frequently have no symptoms referable to the liver. In one series of patients with biopsy-proven alcoholic liver disease, only 11 per cent had symptoms referable to the liver, whereas 35 per cent had complaints referable to the gastrointestinal tract.[496] Serious liver injury also may be present without any symptom.[497]

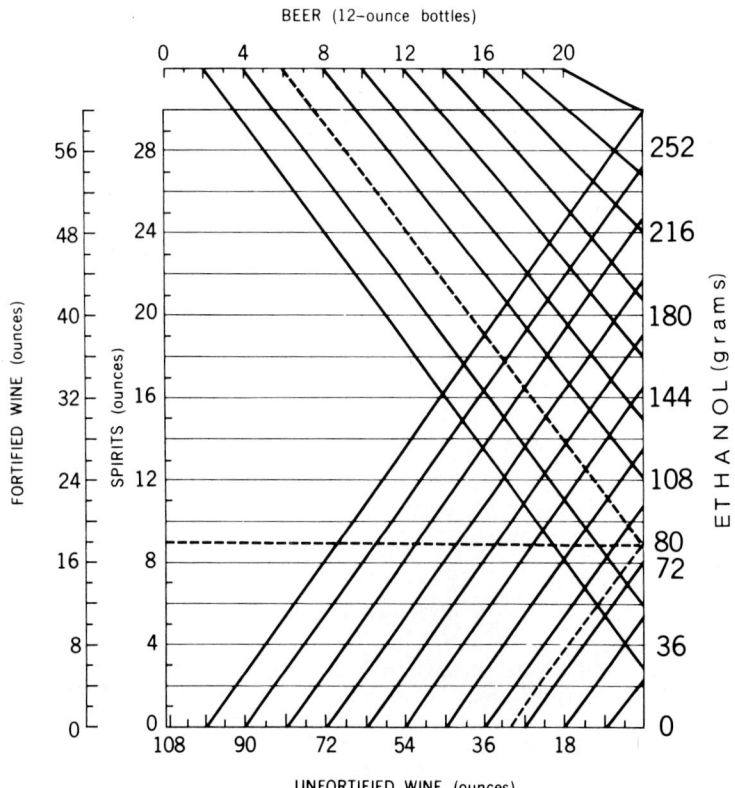

Figure 33–20. Alcoholic beverage conversion nomogram, calculated on the basis of beer, 5 per cent v/v; wine, 12.0 per cent v/v; fortified wine (e.g., sherry), 20 per cent v/v; and spirits, 40 per cent v/v ethanol. Specific gravity of ethanol, 0.78 g/ml; 1 ounce = 28.5 ml. Dashed lines indicate approximate levels of hazardous daily intake (30 ounces of wine, 9 ounces of spirits, 18 ounces of fortified wine, or six bottles of beer). (Reproduced from Rankin JG. In: Fisher MM, Rankin JG, eds. Alcohol and the Liver. Plenum Press, 1977:375, with permission.)

Physical Examination

The findings on physical examination will vary from entirely normal to the classic picture of hepatomegaly, jaundice, and ascites. In one series of asymptomatic patients, 50 per cent who had either cirrhosis or alcoholic hepatitis lacked hepatomegaly.[497]

Laboratory Tests

The ideal test for the diagnosis of any disorder is one that is sensitive (low incidence of false negatives) yet specific (few false positives). No test now available for the diagnosis of alcoholic liver injury fulfills either of these criteria. There are several tests, however, that at least warn that liver disease, type unspecified, may be present and that indicate the need for further evaluation.

Serum bilirubin and albumin are insensitive indices; when abnormal, they indicate significant hepatic injury.[498] Tests that are markers of cellular injury appear to be the most sensitive for detecting ethanol-induced hepatic injury. The tests of this type most commonly available are the determinations of serum AST and ALT. The AST is elevated in 43 to 100 per cent of patients with liver disease,[496–499] although the extent of elevation does not define the severity of the lesion.[500] Also, any disease of liver or muscle will elevate AST. The level of ALT in the blood is a poor marker of alcoholic hepatic injury. The serum levels of ALT are frequently normal or minimally elevated in severe ethanol-induced hepatic injury. The ALT level is almost always less than the AST level, and the AST:ALT ratio frequently exceeds 1.[499, 501] When ALT exceeds 300 Karmen units, ethanol is unlikely to be the cause of acute hepatic injury.

The reason for the depression of serum ALT in alcoholic liver disease is unclear. There are, however, data that support the idea that normal levels of ALT and elevated levels of AST in response to ethanol-induced hepatic necrosis reflect the effects of ethanol on the metabolism of pyridoxine and the concomitant induction of pyridoxine deficiency.[160, 161] Pyridoxal-5-phosphate is the cofactor for AST and ALT. Diet-induced pyridoxine deficiency had differential effects on the activities of AST and ALT.[502] Pyridoxine deficiency caused both serum and hepatic levels of AST and ALT to decline, but the decline in the activity of ALT was greater. Also, following the induction of hepatocellular necrosis, the AST:ALT ratio in serum was 1 in controls but approximately 5 in pyridoxine-deficient animals.[502] These data suggest that pyridoxine deficiency may account in part for the transaminase pattern seen in alcoholic liver injury. They probably also account for the observation that hepatic levels of ALT are lower in patients with alcoholic liver disease as compared with other forms of liver disease and with health, but that hepatic levels of AST are similarly depressed in alcoholic and non-alcoholic liver disease.[503] Further support for this hypothesis comes from observations that when pyridoxine was administered to pyridoxine-deficient patients with alcoholic hepatitis, liver ALT levels increased, whereas AST levels remained unchanged.[504] Partial correction of the pyridoxine deficiency therefore tended to lower the AST:ALT ratio.

Gamma-glutamyltranspeptidase (GGTP) is an enzyme located within cell membranes of several tissues. It is thought to be important for the cellular uptake of amino acids. The serum level of GGTP is believed to be a sensitive but nonspecific index of alcoholism and alcoholic hepatic

injury.[499] For example, in one study 16 per cent of a random sample of a male population had increased levels of GGTP, and in 75 per cent, the increase was due to excessive alcohol consumption.[499] It is believed that chronic ingestion of alcohol is necessary to increase serum activity of GGTP.[499, 505, 506] However, the plasma levels of GGTP correlate poorly with the total amount of alcohol consumed.[499] On the other hand, in one investigation, serum levels of GGTP were increased in only 67 per cent of patients with alcohol in their urine who were admitted to an alcoholism treatment unit.[507] In another series, 69 per cent of alcoholics had increased serum levels of GGTP, but patients with longer histories of drinking tended to have lower levels.[498] Some of the variability in these studies may reflect delays between admission to the hospital and measurement of GGTP activity, because the level of GGTP declines as the patient "dries out." On the other hand, the level of GGTP is so sensitive a test of liver injury that it is elevated in almost all forms of liver disease and hence is of little diagnostic usefulness in terms of suggesting a cause for the liver disease. In alcoholic hepatitis, GGTP may be increased far out of proportion to AST,[503] but the clinical utility of this difference has not been determined.

The increase in serum GGTP in alcoholics is felt to be due to an induction of the enzyme by ethanol.[508] The bases for this conclusion are (1) that chronic but not acute ingestion of ethanol elevates GGTP and (2) that known inducers of microsomal enzymes[509] also elevate serum GGTP. There are no data, however, on the actual levels of GGTP in the livers of alcoholics, and when ethanol was fed to rats, hepatic GGTP did not change.[510] Also, acute ingestion of ethanol has been found to increase serum GGTP.[511, 512] These last results suggest that hepatic injury, not induction of enzyme, causes increased serum GGTP in the alcoholic.

Measurement of the ratio in plasma of alpha amino-N-butyric acid to leucine has been proposed as a sensitive and specific marker for alcoholism. Shaw and co-workers measured this ratio in alcoholics, nonalcoholics, and ethanol-fed and control baboons. Those receiving ethanol had significantly higher ratios than did the controls.[513] Shaw and colleagues concluded that the elevation of the ratio was a direct result of ethanol ingestion not related to cellular injury. Two subsequent studies have failed to confirm this observation. Both studies found abnormalities in the ratio to be a nonspecific reflection of hepatocellular dysfunction.[514, 515] The differences in these studies have been reviewed.[516] Because of the requirement for an amino acid analyzer and the nonspecificity of the test, we do not feel that this ratio is of clinical use in the diagnosis of alcoholic liver disease.

Glutamate dehydrogenase is another enzyme that is proposed as a marker for alcohol-induced liver injury. This is a mitochondrial enzyme with greatest activity in zone 3 of Rappaport, which is the area of the liver lobule most severely involved in alcoholic liver disease. Van Waes and Lieber measured the levels of this enzyme in the blood of 100 alcoholics who had undergone liver biopsies. They then correlated the histologic findings with the serum levels of enzyme. The serum level of glutamate dehydrogenase correlated well with the amount of liver cell necrosis and was better in this respect than the AST. The incidences of false positives and false negatives were similar for AST and glutamate dehydrogenase.[500] The authors concluded that the serum level of glutamate dehydrogenase can effectively identify patients with active alcoholic hepatitis, including those who are asymptomatic. Two subsequent studies have failed to find serum glutamate dehydrogenase levels to correlate with the severity of hepatic injury.[517, 518] There is a mitochondrial form of AST, and its level in serum has also been used as a marker for alcoholism and alcoholic liver disease. In normals and patients with viral hepatitis, mitochondrial AST accounted for about 3 per cent of total serum AST activity, whereas in alcoholics it accounted for 11 to 13 per cent of total serum activity. Mitochondrial AST serum activity was a more sensitive test than was GGTP, glutamate dehydrogenase, or total AST for the diagnosis of alcoholism.[519]

Two rather simple tests appear to be useful in the diagnosis of alcoholism. One of these is the mean corpuscular volume of red cells (MCV). The MCV is higher in patients consuming more than four drinks daily than in those having one drink or less.[509] In addition, about one fourth of alcoholics will have elevated MCVs.[520] Also, elevations of serum uric acid are found in 10 per cent of alcoholics. The highest levels of uric acid are found in the heaviest drinkers.[509, 520] Each of these tests is nonspecific, but when combined with other observations, they all contribute to an accurate diagnosis of alcoholism and alcoholic liver disease. A number of authors have attempted to combine tests to increase sensitivity.[499] The value of this approach in diagnosing alcohol abuse on a case-by-case basis is unclear.

Liver Biopsy

Once the physician is confident that alcoholism is present and that hepatic injury is likely, it is important to establish the severity of the hepatic injury. This can be done only with liver biopsy. When or if one should biopsy the liver of a patient suspected to have alcoholic liver disease is a matter of philosophy. Patients who obviously have cirrhosis are usually subjected to biopsy without question, whereas when a patient has evidence of only minimal disease, biopsy is done with reluctance. Ironically, it is the patient with early injury who should be identified if one hopes to reduce the incidence of cirrhosis. It is the patient with early disease who would benefit most from a rehabilitation program. We believe, therefore, that biopsy should be performed whenever there is a reasonable suspicion of liver disease. One also should remember that alcoholics can have other types of liver disease. One study showed that 20 per cent of patients suspected to have alcoholic liver disease had other lesions on biopsy.[521] There were no clinical features or biochemical markers to differentiate between the alcoholic patients with alcoholic and those with nonalcoholic liver disease.

CLINICAL FORMS OF ALCOHOLIC LIVER DISEASE

Alcohol abuse is thought to lead to three forms of liver disease—fatty liver, alcoholic hepatitis, and cirrhosis. In the following discussion, each of these is discussed as a distinct clinical entity, although patients frequently have combinations of these three lesions, so that clinical features tend to overlap. The signs and symptoms of liver disease are generally a result of (1) hepatocellular necrosis including jaundice, nausea and vomiting, and tender hepatomegaly or (2) complications of portal hypertension including ascites, formation of portal-systemic collaterals, splenomegaly, and bleeding esophageal and gastric varices. Patients frequently have features of both hepatocellular necrosis

and portal hypertension. Other, less specific manifestations of liver disease that also may be present include gynecomastia, spider angiomas, parotid hypertrophy, and testicular atrophy.

Based on clinicopathologic considerations, several constellations of signs and symptoms can be identified in abusers of ethanol who have liver disease. The interrelationships between these conditions are depicted in Figure 33–21. Each entity cited is discussed here.

The signs and symptoms in alcoholic patients with liver disease vary with the stages of their illness. Many alcoholics with liver disease first come to medical attention because of the complications of cirrhosis, such as ascites, bleeding esophageal varices, or both. These patients often have no past history compatible with liver disease, despite long-term abuse of ethanol. Other patients may have long histories of hospitalizations because of symptomatic alcoholic hepatitis culminating eventually in cirrhosis. We do not know why alcoholism with liver disease follows such divergent courses. Presumably, however, some alcoholics have persistent subclinical alcoholic hepatitis, that is, they are well clinically but biopsy reveals the histologic lesion of alcoholic hepatitis. The destruction of liver cells may be sufficiently slow in these patients that they do not become symptomatic until cirrhosis is established. Liver disease may be discovered in such patients inadvertently or during evaluation for apparently unrelated disorders. Chemical tests of liver function are of no value in identifying alcoholics with asymptomatic alcoholic hepatitis, so we have no appreciation of the natural course of this entity.

Fatty Liver

Ethanol feeding induces fatty liver in both humans and animals. When ethanol was administered to normal volunteers for two to eight days, all developed fatty livers.[522] Fatty liver is the most common abnormality of hepatic morphology in the alcoholic population. In one series of alcoholics who lacked symptoms referable to the liver, biopsy showed that 33 per cent had fatty livers.[497] (The mechanism of ethanol induction of fatty liver is discussed earlier in this chapter.)

Clinical Presentation

Alcoholic fatty liver in the ambulatory population is largely asymptomatic. These patients frequently have no clinical or biochemical evidence of liver disease.[497] In studies of hospitalized patients, hepatomegaly is the most frequent finding (73 per cent). Jaundice, fluid retention, and splenomegaly are observed less frequently. Biochemical tests commonly are abnormal, with elevations of AST and bilirubin present in one third of patients.[523] Ascites, varices, and hepatic encephalopathy are indicative of a more ominous lesion than simple fatty liver.

Course and Prognosis

The long-term prognosis for patients with alcoholic fatty liver is unknown. There are no longitudinal studies that followed these patients over a number of years to determine which and how many will develop alcoholic hepatitis or cirrhosis, or both. In spite of this, the assumption has been that fatty liver is not a precirrhotic lesion. This conclusion is based on the fact that the fatty liver is reversible upon withdrawal of ethanol. In addition, nonal-

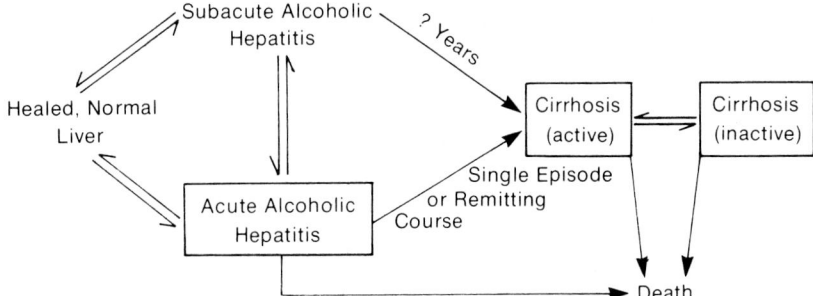

Figure 33–21. The clinical course of alcoholic liver disease. (Reproduced from Smith LH Jr, Thier S, eds. Pathophysiology of Disease. WB Saunders, 1981, with permission.)

coholic fatty liver does not lead to cirrhosis.[524–526, 528] In contradistinction to the finding of fat, perivenular sclerosis in the biopsy specimen from a patient with alcoholic steatosis is believed to be a marker for the subsequent development of cirrhosis.[524–526, 528] Although perivenular fibrosis may be a marker for an increased risk of developing cirrhosis, there is no evidence that the lesion progresses in the absence of ethanol abuse.

Fatty liver occurs in several conditions other than alcoholism (see Chap. 4). Most of these conditions are benign. However, as mentioned already, fatty liver in morbidly obese patients with or without jejunoileal bypass may be associated with other more serious lesions.[481–485] Similar findings in diabetics have now been reported.[529, 530]

Acute fatty liver may cause portal hypertension. Leevy measured wedged hepatic venous pressures in several patients with fatty livers and found them to be elevated.[523] The elevations were usually slight, but occasionally they were enough to produce visible varices. With resolution of the fatty livers, the varices disappeared and the wedged hepatic venous pressures returned to normal.[523] This increase followed by a fall in pressure is most likely due to corresponding changes in cell size (see Chap. 23).

The hospital course of a patient with fatty liver is usually benign. Occasionally, such a patient has a rapid downhill course and dies with liver failure. At autopsy, only severe alcoholic steatosis is found.[531] How this patient differs from the usual patient with fatty liver is unknown. Patients with fatty livers also may die suddenly. This uncommon event has been attributed to multiple cerebral and pulmonary fat emboli.[532]

Alcoholic Hepatitis

Alcoholic hepatitis is also referred to as acute sclerosing hyaline necrosis,[533] alcoholic steatonecrosis,[534] and florid cirrhosis.[535] The interest in this lesion stems from its relative specificity for alcoholic liver disease. Also, it is a precursor of cirrhosis and has associated high rates of morbidity and mortality.

Clinical Presentation

Alcoholic hepatitis is a histopathologic diagnosis. Thus, the patient may be asymptomatic or may be jaundiced and critically ill. The symptoms associated with alcoholic hepatitis are numerous but most commonly are anorexia, nausea, vomiting, abdominal pain, and weight loss.[533–537] Alcoholic hepatitis can be present, however, with a complete absence of symptoms. The most common physical finding is hepatomegaly, which occurs in 80 to 100 per cent of patients. Ascites, jaundice, fever, splenomegaly, and

encephalopathy are found in 10 to 70 per cent of patients, depending on the population studied.[533–537]

A biochemical diagnosis of alcoholic hepatitis is not possible, especially in the less severe forms of the disease. The AST is frequently elevated (70 to 80 per cent) but is usually less than 300 Karmen units and correlates poorly with the severity of the hepatic lesion. The ALT is minimally elevated or normal, and the AST:ALT ratio is almost always more than 1 and frequently greater than 2. However, this enzyme ratio is not specific for alcoholic hepatitis and may be present with other forms of chronic liver disease and fatty liver.[503] Again, the elevations of bilirubin and alkaline phosphatase are variable, with both normal and high values seen.[533–538] Leukocytosis, sometimes marked (80,000 to 100,000/mm³), is seen in 25 to 95 per cent of patients. The more severely ill patients are more likely to have marked leukocytosis.[533–537]

Diagnosis

The diagnosis of alcoholic hepatitis may be suspected on clinical grounds, but proof rests with liver biopsy. Patients who have fever, leukocytosis, jaundice, and tender hepatomegaly can be diagnosed as having alcoholic hepatitis with a fair degree of accuracy. However, the disease frequently is less obvious and can easily be confused with other illnesses. Patients who have alcoholic hepatitis can present perplexing problems of fevers of unknown origin or marked leukocytosis whose etiology is established only by liver biopsy. Also, hepatic abscesses, metastatic carcinoma, sepsis, and biliary tract disease can mimic alcoholic hepatitis, and vice versa. Errors in diagnosis can have disastrous consequences for the patient.[539]

Prognosis

The prognosis for patients who have acute alcoholic hepatitis is variable and depends upon the severity of the acute lesion and the presence or absence of underlying cirrhosis. Prognostic factors associated with significantly increased mortality include encephalopathy, spider angiomas, ascites, renal failure, and prolonged prothrombin time > 50 per cent of control.[536, 540–543] The variable clinical course is best exemplified by the study of Helman and associates.[541] Seven of 14 patients who had alcoholic hepatitis with encephalopathy in their group died, whereas none of the 22 patients without encephalopathy died. When alcoholic hepatitis is severe enough to prolong the prothrombin time to the extent that liver biopsy cannot be performed safely, the observed mortality is 42 per cent.[536] A serum bilirubin of greater than 20 mg/dl in concert with a prolonged prothrombin time also indicates a poor prognosis.[540] Thus, for patients who are asymptomatic or are outpatients, the acute prognosis is much better than for hospitalized patients. The prognosis is variable for the hospitalized patient.

The long-term prognosis for the patient who has alcoholic hepatitis is a function of several factors. The severity of the hepatic lesion and the presence or absence of cirrhosis appear to be most important.[536, 544] Alexander and coworkers followed for 5 years 164 patients with biopsy-proven acute alcoholic hepatitis.[545] The five-year survival rate in the patients with mild histologic lesions was approximately 70 per cent, and there was no increase in mortality after the third year. On the other hand, those who had severe lesions had a five-year survival rate of about 50 per cent, and mortality continued to increase throughout the period of observation. Fibrosis present on initial biopsy and ascites also were indicative of a poor prognosis. In a more recent study of patients with mild alcoholic hepatitis, the one-year mortality was 9 per cent, and by 30 months this had increased to 22 per cent. The initial presence of cirrhosis or ascites was associated with an increased mortality after two years of follow-up.[544] The effect of continued ethanol ingestion on survival is discussed in the next section, on cirrhosis.

The poor long-term prognosis of alcoholic hepatitis is in part caused by its progression to cirrhosis. In the series of Galambos,[536, 546] 61 patients who had alcoholic hepatitis without fibrosis had serial biopsies, and 38 per cent developed cirrhosis in less than five years. Interestingly, 52 per cent had persistent alcoholic hepatitis without developing cirrhosis. In only 10 per cent did the lesion of alcoholic hepatitis resolve without residual disease. Complete recovery was seen only in those patients who stopped drinking, although abstinence did not guarantee that cirrhosis would not develop. Similar observations have been made by others and suggest that alcoholic hepatitis can persist for years in a subclinical state with or without progression to cirrhosis.[547] It is unclear why cirrhosis develops in some but not all patients with the same histologic lesion.

Alcoholic hepatitis may lead to progressive hepatic fibrosis without the development of cirrhosis. In these patients, fibrosis is most severe in zone 3 of Rappaport, and there may be complete loss of terminal hepatic and sublobular veins. The major sequelae of this type of disease are the development of portal hypertension and ascites, because with the loss of the central veins, there is a marked increase in resistance to flow through the liver. The affected patients appear clinically to have cirrhosis, but there are no regenerative nodules, and the liver surface is smooth and appears grossly normal.[548] The reasons for the failure of regeneration in these patients are not understood.

Cirrhosis

Physicians equate cirrhosis with either a jaundiced patient or one who has ascites or bleeding varices. This, however, is not the case; only 60 per cent of patients with cirrhosis will have signs and symptoms of liver disease. The remaining 40 per cent of cases are discovered either accidentally or at autopsy.[549] One is left to question how the patients with quiescent disease arrive at cirrhosis from the earlier stages of fatty liver and alcoholic hepatitis. We know that some patients, when followed over relatively short intervals, have progressive fibrosis following alcoholic hepatitis.[546, 547] These patients, however, have overt liver disease. What about patients who had no knowledge of liver disease until they were found to have varices or ascites?

Did they also have recurrent bouts of subclinical alcoholic hepatitis, or is it possible to progress directly from alcoholic fatty liver to cirrhosis? This appears to be the case in nonhuman primates,[550] and small studies suggest that it may occur in humans,[526] but large prospective studies are needed to answer this question.

Clinical Features

Evidence of cirrhosis may be apparent or absent on physical examination. In addition, cirrhosis may coexist with fatty liver or alcoholic hepatitis. Liver biopsy is the only method by which the diagnosis can be established with certainty. Patients who have cirrhosis as well as acute hepatic injury generally seek medical advice because of symptoms referable to the acute hepatic injury. In patients with quiescent cirrhosis, symptoms due to portal hypertension—that is, ascites, encephalopathy, or bleeding varices—usually dominate the clinical picture.

The physical findings in a patient with cirrhosis may be numerous[551-554] or may be conspicuous by their absence (Table 33–7). Jaundice, when present, is usually indicative of coexistent alcoholic hepatitis or the development of a complication such as viral hepatitis, biliary obstruction, sepsis, or hemolysis. Spider angiomas, or arterial spiders, are frequently found in patients with alcoholic cirrhosis. Although poorly formed spiders may be seen in normal persons and may develop rapidly in patients with fulminant hepatic failure, in the author's experience large pulsating spiders are seen only in cirrhosis. Arterial spiders also have been found on the pleural surfaces.[551] The similarity of spiders to endometrial arteries suggests that hyperestrogenism is involved in their pathogenesis, but the exact mechanism of their formation has not been determined. Palmar erythema, although present in patients with cirrhosis, is a nonspecific finding. However, erythema extending onto the fingertips and periungual area suggests cirrhosis or another disease. Changes in the nails (Muehrcke's lines and white nails) are seen in all forms of cirrhosis.[552, 553] Dupuytren's contracture may be more common in alcoholics and in patients with alcoholic cirrhosis. On the other hand, the finding in an individual patient is not specific.[554] Asymptomatic enlargement of the parotid glands is seen with increased frequency in patients with alcoholic cirrhosis. The principal pathologic finding is fatty infiltration of the

TABLE 33–7. PHYSICAL FINDINGS IN CIRRHOSIS

	Percentage of Cases	
	Powell and Klatskin 283 Patients	Ratnoff and Patek 386 Patients
Palpable liver	95.8	75.4
Jaundice	67.5	65.3
Ascites	66.1	78.0
Spider angiomas	48.8	15.0
Dilated abdominal veins	47.0	23.6
Palpable spleen	45.6	44.0
Testicular atrophy	45.0	—
Palmar erythema	37.1	4.2
Fever not related to infection	21.6	24.5
Hepatic coma	17.7	—
Gynecomastia	15.0	—
Dupuytren's contractures	4.6	4.6

Source: Powell W, Klatskin G. Am J Med 44:406, 1968.
These are the major physical findings encountered during the period of observation of two large groups of patients with alcoholic cirrhosis.

gland.[555] Hepatomegaly is common in patients with alcoholic cirrhosis, but patients with advanced disease may have small livers. The liver, when palpable, is firm and may be tender if there is coexistent alcoholic hepatitis. Splenomegaly is common, but the size of the spleen correlates poorly with the severity of portal hypertension (see Chap. 23). Ascites and venous collaterals are indicative of portal hypertension.

The laboratory findings in alcoholic cirrhosis differ little from those in alcoholic hepatitis except that serum bilirubin and transaminases tend to be normal in quiescent cirrhosis. There may be hypoalbuminemia and hyperglobulinemia. However, all biochemical tests may be normal. Occasionally, the patient with alcoholic cirrhosis will have unconjugated hyperbilirubinemia. This is usually the result of hemolysis, and spur cells may be present in the blood (see Chap. 21).

Diagnosis

The diagnosis of alcoholic cirrhosis can be made with certainty only by liver biopsy. The findings of ascites, venous collaterals, and abnormal liver tests in an alcoholic are very suggestive of alcoholic cirrhosis. On the other hand, a similar clinical picture can be caused by any form of liver disease.

Prognosis

The prognosis for a patient with alcoholic cirrhosis is not determined by the presence of cirrhosis per se but by the presence or absence of complications of cirrhosis, for example, ascites or gastrointestinal bleeding. Powell and Klatskin[555a] studied the influences of certain clinical features and continued alcoholism on patient survival in 283 patients with histologically documented alcoholic cirrhosis. The five-year survival for patients without ascites, jaundice, or a history of hematemesis was 89 per cent in those who abstained from drinking. In contrast, it was 68 per cent in those who continued to drink (Fig. 33–22A). Following the onset of any of the complications mentioned, five-year survival was reduced to 60 per cent in the abstainers and 34 per cent in those who continued to abuse ethanol (Fig. 33–22B). Abstinence improved survival in those who developed jaundice or ascites (Fig. 33–23) but not in those with hematemesis (Fig. 33–24).[555a] A second study also showed that abstinence did not improve survival when varices were demonstrated.[556] In addition, when patients with alcoholic cirrhosis are stratified according to hepatitic function, clinical status and severity of cirrhosis (modified Child-Turcotte's criteria), those with the least severe disease (group A) had a two year probability of survival of > 90 per cent whereas those with severe disease (group C) the probability of survival was only 50 per cent after two years of follow-up.[557]

Pande and colleagues have studied this problem further by examining survival in a group of patients randomized for therapeutic portacaval shunts. They found no improvement in survival with abstinence.[558] The authors concluded that continued cell injury does not affect survival once the liver injury has advanced to the point of bleeding varices. Reynolds has taken exception to this belief and feels that continued alcoholism has a significant effect on the long-term prognosis of patients with portal hypertension.[559] In his experience, the only patients who have done well following randomization for portacaval shunts are those

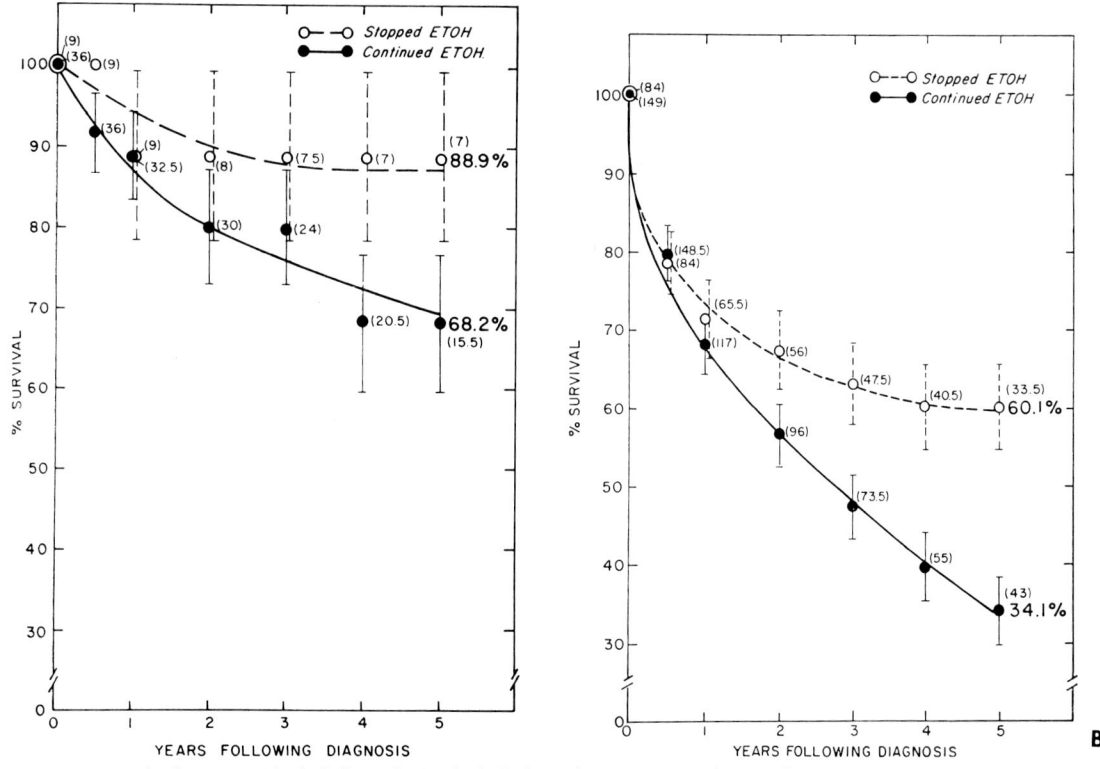

Figure 33–22. Survivals of patients with alcoholic cirrhosis who lacked jaundice, ascites, or a history of gastrointestinal bleeding (A) or had at least one of the three clinical features (B). (Reproduced from Powell W, Klatskin G, Am J Med 44, 406:1968, with permission.)

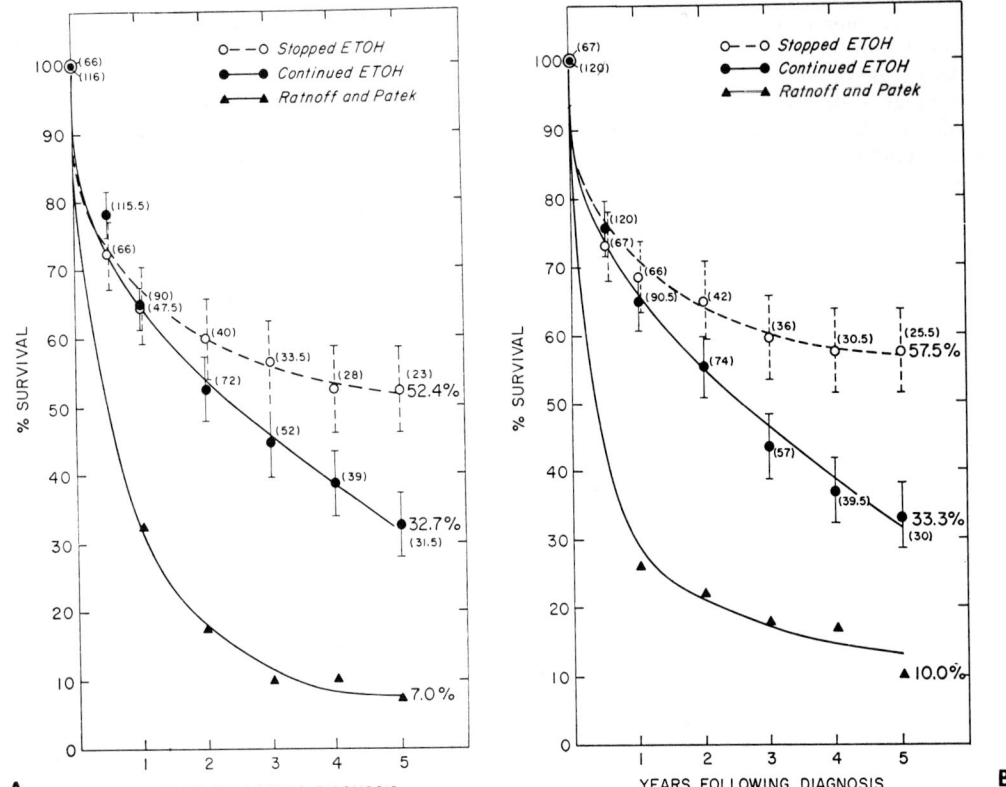

Figure 33–23. Influence of continued ethanol abuse on the survival of patients with alcoholic cirrhosis following onset of ascites (A) or jaundice (B). Results of the study by Ratnoff and Patek, published in 1942, are shown for comparison. (Reproduced from Powell W, Klatskin G. Am J Med 44:406, 1968, with permission.)

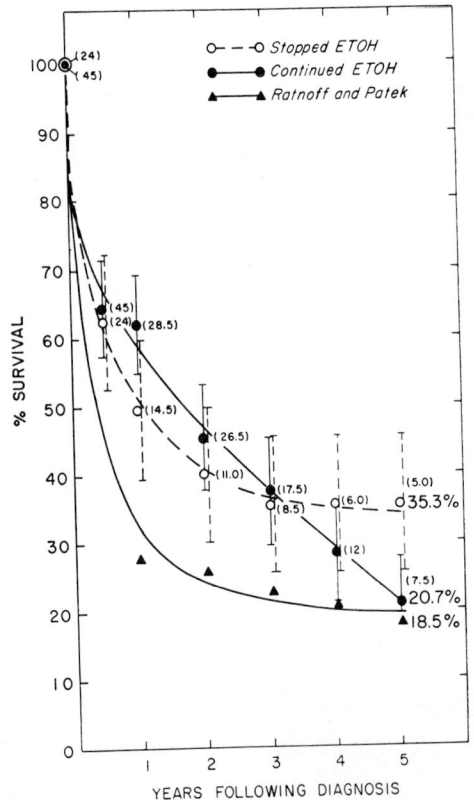

Figure 33–24. Influence of continued ethanol abuse on the survival of patients with alcoholic cirrhosis after the onset of hematemesis. (Reproduced from Powell W, Klatskin G. Am J Med 44:406, 1968, with permission.)

who stopped drinking. Although there are several patients who have survived portacaval shunts for four years or more despite continued drinking, these patients had severe medical problems.[559] In a recent study of the effect of propylthiouracil on alcohol liver disease, mortality in the placebo group was similar (25 to 26 per cent at two years) regardless of the amount of alcohol consumed (based on alcohol concentration in morning urine).[253] The uncertainty about the role of abstinence in survival is unlikely to be resolved because of the difficulties in obtaining accurate information from patients about their alcohol abuse.[561] However, the continued ingestion of ethanol is unlikely to be of any benefit to the patients, and every attempt should be made to help them to stop. The observations on the relationship of abstinence to survival underline the need to diagnose disease early when abstinence clearly will help.

THERAPY IN ALCOHOLIC LIVER DISEASE

Therapy in alcoholic liver disease has been directed at reducing the severity of alcoholic hepatitis or at trying to prevent hepatic fibrosis, or to reverse it. Agents used include corticosteroids, androgenic steroids, propylthiouracil, and colchicine. In addition, improvement in the nutritional state of the patient and stimulation of hepatic regeneration with insulin and glucagon have been used in an attempt to improve hepatic function.

CORTICOSTEROIDS

There are at least nine controlled trials of the efficacy of corticosteroids in alcoholic hepatitis.[540, 562–569] Most of the studies have come to the same conclusion. Steroids are of no benefit in the treatment of mild or moderately severe disease. The results differ, however, as to the efficacy of steroids in the treatment of severe disease (e.g., encephalopathy, marked icterus, prolonged prothrombin time, or ascites). Different investigators have come to different conclusions. The data from all of the studies that investigated the effect of steroids on the short-term (~30-day) survival of patients with acute alcoholic hepatitis and encephalopathy are summarized in Table 33–8. Most studies failed to show an effect on survival in these patients, although in two studies administration of steroids appeared to be beneficial. Two additional reports are worth mentioning, as the number of patients in both are unusually large. The patients investigated were considered to have severe alcoholic hepatitis based on a number of clinical criteria (e.g., encephalopathy, jaundice, and so forth). Maddrey and colleagues administered either prednisolone or a placebo to 55 patients with alcoholic hepatitis.[540] Fifteen patients had severe disease (high bilirubin and prolonged prothrombin time), and of this group, six of the eight placebo-treated patients died, whereas only one of the seven treated with prednisolone died. This study has been expanded into a multicentered trial in which prednisolone or a placebo was given to patients with severe alcoholic hepatitis. In a preliminary report of the first 67 patients, the short-term mortality in the placebo-treated group was 32 per cent, whereas it was only 6 per cent (P <0.01) in the group that received prednisolone.[567] The short-term efficacy of prednisolone in the treatment of severe alcoholic hepatitis also was investigated in a Veterans Administration (V.A.) cooperative study.[566] The short-term mortality in the severely ill patients was 29 per cent and was unaffected by the administration of prednisolone. Even in studies in which steroids appeared to be beneficial, there was no effect on the progression of hepatic fibrosis.[540] Additionally, the short-term administration of steroids appears to have no effect on long-term survival, regardless of the severity of the disease.[566] Given the uncertainty as to the efficacy of steroids in the treatment of alcoholic hepatitis and the possibility of serious side effects in these immunocompromised patients, we believe that corticosteroids should not be used in the management of patients with alcoholic hepatitis even as a measure of desperation.

ANABOLIC STEROIDS

Anabolic steroids have been used by a number of investigators in the treatment of alcoholic liver disease in hope of reversing the patient's catabolic state. Two recently

completed controlled trials have compared the efficacy of testosterone or oxandrolone to a placebo in the treatment of alcoholic liver disease. In a multicentered study from Copenhagen, testosterone (200 mg three times daily or a placebo) was administered to 221 men (134 treated and 87 controls) with alcoholic cirrhosis for an average of 28 months.[557] The mortality in the treated patients and controls, respectively, was 25 and 21 per cent. In addition, testosterone had no beneficial effect on liver tests or hepatic histology.[557, 570] In a V.A. cooperative study, oxandrolone or a placebo was administered to 173 (88 placebo and 85 oxandrolone) patients with alcoholic hepatitis for 30 days.[566] Oxandrolone had no effect on short-term (30-day) mortality of all classes of patients and also was without effect on the long-term survival of those with severe disease. However, of the patients with moderate alcoholic hepatitis who survived for one to two months, those who received oxandrolone appeared to have an improved long-term survival compared with the untreated controls or the patients who had received prednisolone for a similar period of time. Currently, it is clear that the use of testosterone in the treatment of alcoholic cirrhosis is not indicated. The use of oxandrolone in the severely ill patient with alcoholic hepatitis is also unwarranted. It is unclear whether it should be used in the less severely ill patient.

COLCHICINE

Colchicine interferes with assembly of microtubules and the transcellular movement of collagen and increases the production of collagenase in vitro.[419, 571] Colchicine has been found to reduce fibrosis in rats following CCl_4-induced injury[420] and has been applied in the treatment of primary biliary cirrhosis (see Chap. 44) and alcoholic liver disease. In a study in Mexico, cirrhotic patients (about 50 per cent with cirrhosis caused by ethanol) received either placebo or colchicine (1 mg five days a week) for as long as 48 months.[571] Survival may have been better in those receiving colchicine (75 per cent) compared with the placebo group (59 per cent), but this difference was not statistically significant. There appeared to be a decrease in fibrosis in three patients who received colchicine and a general clinical improvement in the colchicine but not the placebo group. This study has been continued, with some patients followed for up to 14 years. In a preliminary report, the cumulative five-year survival in the colchicine- and placebo-treated groups was 75 and 34 per cent, respectively (P <0.001).[572] In 18 per cent of the treated patients, histologic improvement was noted, whereas this was not observed in any of

TABLE 33–8. THE EFFICACY OF CORTICOSTEROIDS IN THE TREATMENT OF ALCOHOLIC HEPATITIS WITH ENCEPHALOPATHY IN SIX CONTROLLED TRIALS

Investigator	Control			Steroid Treatment			Significance of Difference
	No. in Study	Died		No. in Study	Died		
		NO.	%		NO.	%	
Helman[541]	6	6	100	9	1	11	P < 0.01
Porter[563]	8	7	88	8	6	75	ns
Campra[563]	10	8	80	8	4	50	ns
Blitzer[565]	2	1	50	3	2	67	ns
Lesesne[562]	7	7	100	7	2	29	P < 0.01
Depew[564]	13	7	54	15	8	53	ns
Theodassi[568]	14	10	71	20	19	95	ns

ns = not significant (P > 0.05).

the placebo-treated patients. Thirty months of therapy were required before any significant effect of colchicine could be seen. Clearly, if this therapy is to be of benefit then long-term compliance is required. It is unclear how effective colchicine is in alcoholic patients who continue to drink or in patients with active hepatocellular necrosis. The results with colchicine are encouraging; further studies are needed to clarify the role of this agent in the treatment of alcoholic liver disease. The data available so far do not warrant treatment with colchicine outside of controlled trials.

PROPYLTHIOURACIL

Work by Israel and colleagues suggests that a hypermetabolic state and hypoxia play major roles in the genesis of alcoholic liver disease (discussed earlier in this chapter). These investigators claimed that the putative hypermetabolic state induced by ethanol in animals could be abolished by propylthiouracil and that hypoxic liver damage could be prevented.[226] They studied the effect of propylthiouracil (300 mg/day for 30 days) on the rate of recovery of a group of patients with alcoholic liver disease. The administration of propylthiouracil was associated with an increase in the rate of clinical improvement but did not alter the survival of patients with alcoholic hepatitis.[227, 228] A study by a second group of investigators of the effect of propylthiouracil on the short-term survival of patients with alcoholic hepatitis failed to show any benefit of therapy.[574] Most recently, Orrego and colleagues have investigated the effect of long-term use of propylthiouracil on the clinical course of alcoholic liver disease.[253] They administered either 300 mg of propylthiouracil daily (N = 157) or a placebo (n = 153) to a group of patients with relative stable alcoholic liver disease for a maximum of two years. The cumulative mortality rate in the treated group (0.13) was significantly less than the placebo group (0.25). This positive effect was seen only in those with severe disease as the death rate in those with mild disease was so low as to prevent a meaningful comparison. The patients who benefited most from the propylthiouracil were those who had the lowest consumption of alcohol (based on the alcohol concentration in a morning urine), whereas the heavy drinkers were not protected by the drug. Although encouraging, the study is not without its faults, and serious side-effects may be associated with the use of propylthiouracil.[573] Therefore, caution is recommended in the use of this agent pending further studies and a better understanding of the genesis of alcoholic liver disease.

NUTRITIONAL SUPPORT

Malnutrition is a common feature of patients with alcoholic liver disease. The severity of protein-calorie malnutrition correlates with mortality and with the severity of liver disease.[575] If patients show improvement in their nutritional status during hospitalization, then their one-year survival is better than patients who fail to show similar improvement.[576] A number of studies have been performed that attempted to improve the nutritional state of patients with alcoholic liver disease in order to improve liver function and decrease mortality. A randomized controlled trial of supplemental amino acids given intravenously was performed in 35 patients with alcoholic hepatitis.[577] The controls and experimental subjects were offered a 3000-Kcal, 100-g protein diet with or without supplemental amino acids. Four of 18 patients in the control group died, whereas

none died in the treatment group. Hepatic function also improved in the supplemented group. Two subsequent studies have shown some improvement in hepatic function with supplemental intravenous amino acids; however, survival was unaffected.[578, 579] In addition, some patients receiving parenteral amino acids became septic from the indwelling catheters. Studies using oral supplements have also shown no clear benefit from this form of therapy.[580, 581] Although the results of the initial study were encouraging,[577] the lack of a clear beneficial effect in later studies and the risk of sepsis from indwelling catheters should limit intravenous supplementation to controlled trials. One of the most interesting results of these studies is that despite a high-protein intake there was not an increased incidence of encephalopathy compared with the control group. It seems reasonable, therefore, that patients receive oral supplements. This may improve both the patients' nutritional and immunologic states and therefore enhance recovery.

INSULIN AND GLUCAGON THERAPY

Hormones are known to stimulate hepatic regeneration, and it has been thought that the high mortality of alcoholic hepatitis may reflect in some patients a failure of hepatic regeneration. Two clinical trials that investigated the efficacy of insulin and glucagon in the treatment of alcoholic hepatitis have been published. In one study, 25 patients were randomized to receive a daily infusion of insulin and glucagon (given over 12 hours), and 25 patients served as controls.[582] Although there was some improvement over the three-week period of study in hepatic tests of those who received insulin and glucagon, there was no improvement in survival. Also, one patient died from hypoglycemia during the insulin and glucagon infusion. In a second study, 33 patients received daily infusions of insulin and glucagon and an equal number served as controls.[583] The mortality was 14 of 33 control patients and only 5 of 33 treated patients (P <0.02). In addition, hepatic tests improved more rapidly in those who received hormonal therapy. These two small studies of the use of insulin and glucagon to stimulate regeneration in patients with alcoholic hepatitis are encouraging. However, the use of insulin is dangerous, as these patients are already at risk for hypoglycemic episodes. The use of other hepatocyte growth factors, such as epidermal growth factor, would be safer and may now be possible with the successful cloning and preparation of the human forms of these agents.

THE HISTOPATHOLOGY OF ALCOHOLIC LIVER DISEASE*

FATTY LIVER

Fatty liver as mentioned already (Fig. 33–25) is the morphologic change most commonly observed in alcoholic liver disease. It may be present without inflammation or necrosis and can involve virtually every liver cell, doubling or tripling the organ's weight. On the other hand, relatively few liver cells may show this change; the actual numbers of involved hepatocytes generally vary, amounting to between 20 and 75 per cent. The triglyceride-bearing vacuoles are clearly defined, usually single, and occupy at least half of the hepatocyte's cytoplasm. Large vacuoles displace the nucleus peripherally in signet-ring fashion and may obscure

*This section was written by Dr. Carolyn Montgomery.

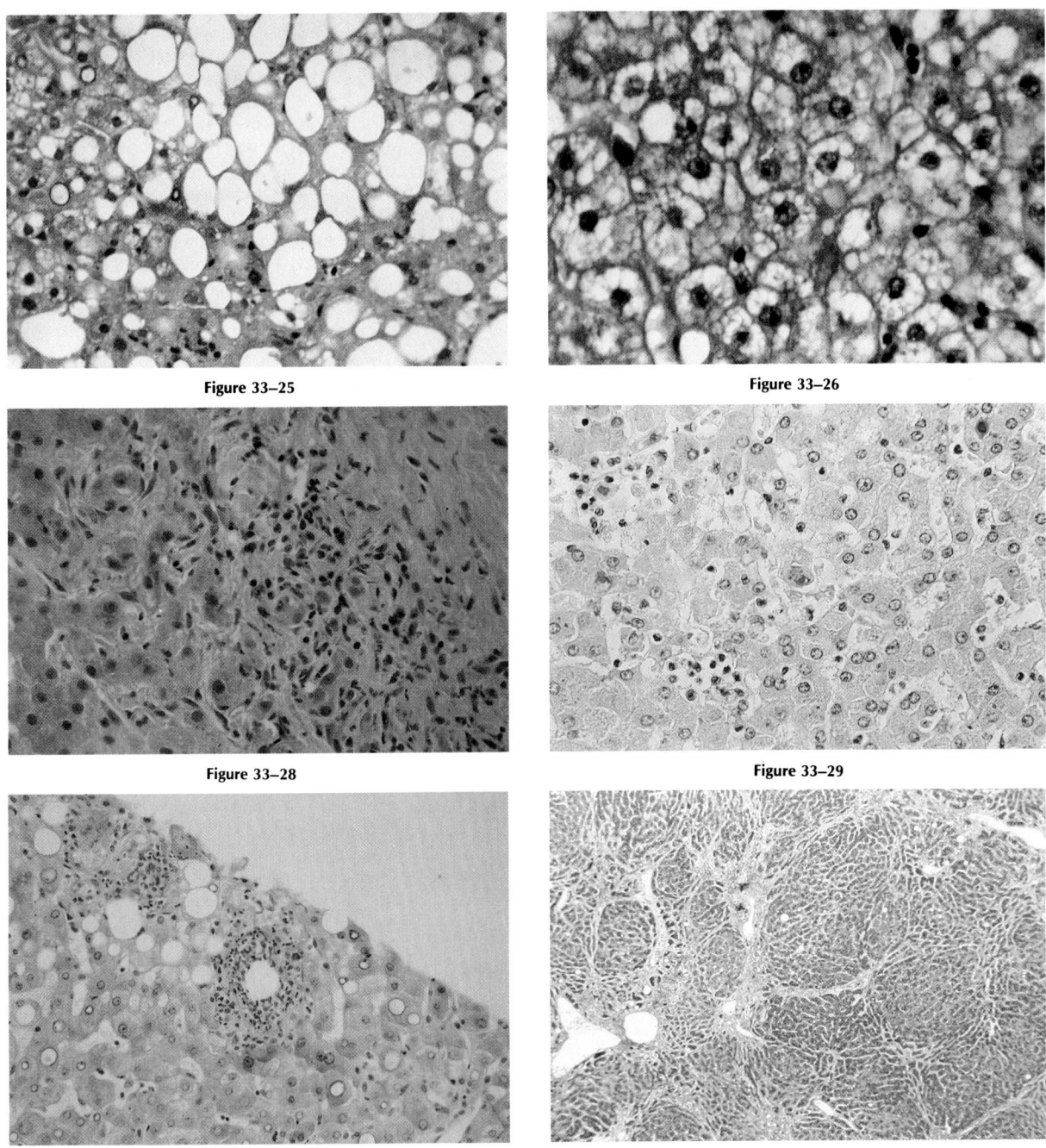

Figure 33–25

Figure 33–26

Figure 33–28

Figure 33–29

Figure 33–30

Figure 33–35

Figure 33–25. Nonspecific fatty change with typical large vacuoles. A few "diabetic" or glycogen nuclei are present in less involved cells. × 63.

Figure 33–26. Tetracycline toxicity with finely vacuolar fatty change in hepatocytes. × 160.

Figure 33–28. Chronic periportal inflammation and fibrosis with Mallory bodies in Wilson's disease. × 63.

Figure 33–29. Cytomegalic inclusion disease. Hepatitis with typical intranuclear and intracytoplasmic inclusions, mid-field. Notice also the numerous polymorphonuclear leukocytes. × 63.

Figure 33–30. "Lipogranuloma" of Q-fever encircled by eosinophils and neutrophils. × 63.

Figure 33–35. Cirrhosis of mixed nodularity. Regenerative nodules of sublobular size coexist with far larger, irregularly shaped regenerative pseudolobules. × 10.

it totally. Rupture of contiguous cells results in large aggregates or fatty "cysts." This evokes little, if any, reticuloendothelial or inflammatory response. There is no particularly consistent zonal distribution to the fatty change within hepatic lobules. The lesion is reversible within a few weeks to months, provided the patient consumes an adequate diet, avoids alcoholic beverages, and develops no intercurrent disease complication.

The same non-necrotic, noninflammatory fatty change, or steatosis, occurs in a wide variety of settings. Any systemically ill patient will have some vacuolated fatty liver cells. Severely protein-deficient as well as markedly obese individuals have significantly increased amounts of hepatic triglycerides with the same morphologic characteristics. Diabetes, juvenile or adult-onset, may be associated with fatty liver; the vacuoles in these patients are the most prominent in centrolobular cells. Numerous clear or "glycogen" nuclei in periportal hepatocytes may be helpful in arriving at this diagnosis. Diffuse fatty change with pericentral necrosis should suggest carbon tetrachloride poisoning; periportal fatty change with necrosis suggests phosphorus poisoning. Neither results in an appreciable inflammatory reaction, considering the amount of necrosis present.

Finely vacuolar or microvesicular fatty change without inflammation or necrosis is less common than the large vacuoles just discussed. It is seen in Reye's syndrome (Chap. 53) and in tetracycline toxicity (Fig. 33–26).[584, 585] Increased intracellular triglycerides are responsible for the pale, swollen, reticulated liver cells in which the vacuoles are very fine and difficult to delineate on routine stains. The hepatic nuclei are not displaced but remain central. Exactly the same picture but predominantly resulting from increased free fatty acids is seen with fatty liver of pregnancy.[586] In all three instances, virtually all liver cells are involved.

ACUTE ALCOHOLIC HEPATITIS

The histologic diagnosis of acute alcoholic hepatitis is classically based on a triad of fatty change, degeneration, and necrosis of hepatocytes, with or without Mallory bodies, and an inflammatory infiltrate of polymorphonuclear leukocytes, primarily within the lobule (Fig. 33–27). In addition, almost all patients with alcoholic hepatitis have increased amounts of intralobular connective tissue. None of the changes per se are pathognomonic of alcoholic injury, but the constellation of findings is generally accepted as diagnostic.

Mallory bodies, on staining with hematoxylin and eosin, consist of eosinophilic, intracellular aggregates of dense proteinaceous material, 2 to 3 μm in diameter. They are classically ropy or serpiginous in contour, and partially encircle, horseshoe fashion, the hepatocyte's nucleus. They are PAS-negative and Luxol fast blue–positive. Their characteristic electron microscopic appearance is one of randomly oriented filaments, often with parallel arrays at the periphery. Centrally, granular deposits of amorphous dense material may obscure the filamentous architecture. When measured as tubules across the outer walls, the filaments are 44 to 73 Å thick and appear to connect to plasma membranes, vesicles, and liver cell nuclei, as do normal intermediate filaments with various cell organelles.[587] The Mallory bodies gradually become less obvious and finally disappear within weeks to months following an acute episode of alcoholic hepatitis. Both fatty and less specific degenerative changes such as ballooning and inflammation subside earlier. First described in 1911, Mallory bodies came to be closely identified with alcoholic liver injury; they are indeed found in large proportions of hepatocytes in acute alcoholic hepatitis. They may be randomly dispersed, predominantly centrolobular, or, as the acute episode subsides, largely periportal. It is in this last location that the differential diagnosis of Wilson's disease and primary biliary cirrhosis should be considered, since Mallory bodies can be seen in both of these diseases.[588, 589] Neither fatty changes nor acute inflammatory cells are routinely encountered in Wilson's disease (Fig. 33–28) or primary biliary cirrhosis, whereas both are expected with alcoholic hepatitis.

Mallory bodies have been found in a variety of condi-

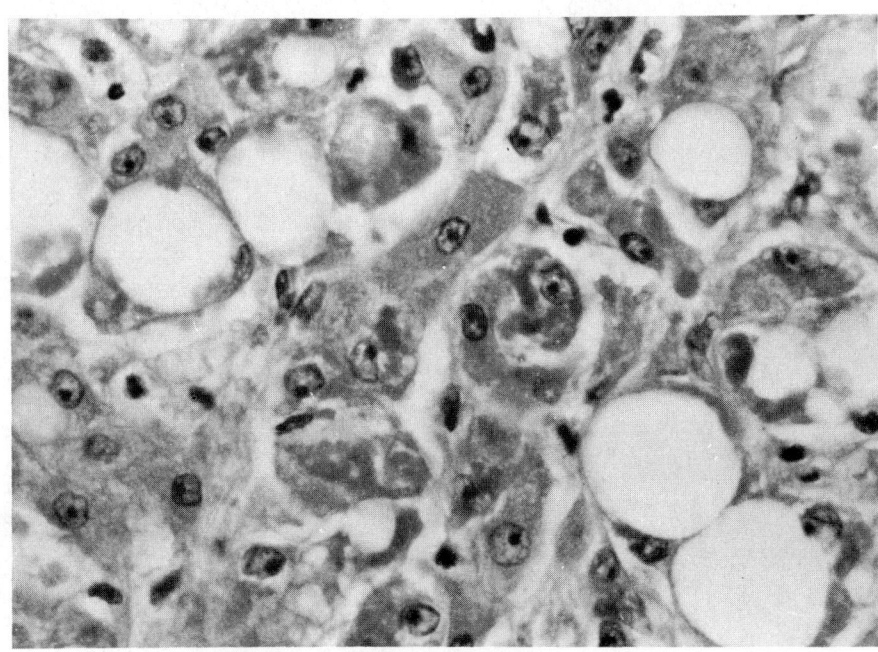

Figure 33–27. Mallory bodies and fatty changes in acute alcoholic hepatitis. × 480.

tions—for example, abetalipoproteinemia,[590] Indian childhood cirrhosis,[591] intestinal bypass surgery for morbid obesity,[592] perhexiline maleate hepatitis,[593] and hepatic injury due to amiodarone.[594] Mallory bodies have also been found in fatty livers of obese as well as diabetic patients.[485, 529] Indeed, they are not even confined to liver cells but have been described as occurring in alveolar epithelial cells following irradiation[595] and in patients with asbestosis.[596] Use of the appellation *alcoholic hyaline* should therefore be discontinued.

Neutrophilic leukocytes within the liver lobule should always suggest alcoholic hepatitis. They surround apparently healthy hepatocytes, hepatocytes with fatty change, hydropically swollen or overtly necrotic liver cells, or hepatocytes containing Mallory bodies. Neutrophils are distinctly unusual in the most common viral or toxic varieties of hepatitis. They are relatively rare in nonspecific reactive hepatitis. They can be seen in cytomegalovirus hepatitis (Fig. 33–29), but this condition also has the distinctive intranuclear and cytoplasmic viral inclusions within liver cells.[597] Neutrophils as well as eosinophils are found in conjunction with fatty liver in Q fever (Fig. 33–30). They show no zonal predilection within the lobule and tend often to surround characteristic lipogranulomas containing lipid vacuoles. True epithelioid granulomas may also be found.[598]

Cholestasis is usually minimal in alcoholic hepatitis. If it is pronounced, there may be an associated microscopic cholangitis that one can confuse with extrahepatic obstruction.[599] Acidophil bodies, mesenchymal reactions, bile duc-

tular proliferation, and increased iron stores may also be seen but are not particularly helpful diagnostically.

It is perhaps best to regard alcoholic hepatitis as an acute process that generally heals but usually with some residual scarring. The scarring takes place in the walls of central veins, in the space of Disse, and periportally (Fig. 33–31). Repeated episodes of acute injury have been seen to eventuate in significant amounts of cumulative fibrosis, which distort the lobular architecture sufficiently to mimic cirrhosis. Both reticulin and collagen obliterate sinusoids and encircle individual or small groups of hepatocytes.

Edmondson coined the term *sclerosing hyaline necrosis* to describe a form of noncirrhotic alcoholic liver injury in which central veins are preferentially involved by fibrosis, necrosis with Mallory bodies, and inflammation (Fig. 33–32).[600] The presence of considerable amounts of collagenous connective tissue can obscure the true central location of the lesion; at a superficial glance, one might suppose the area to be portal. The absence of ducts and the identification of true portal areas nearby will clarify matters. Central vein occlusion and actual obliteration by scarring may supervene in concert with progressive intralobular fibrosis. Fibrous septa can connect central and portal zones as well as encircle hepatocytes singly or in groups. We have seen this picture primarily in younger alcoholics and have observed in time progressive and diffuse lobular distortion by scarring. The process ultimately mimics micronodular cirrhosis, since lobules are converted into sublobular-sized aggregates of hepatocytes in association with impressive

Figure 33–31. Chronic alcoholic liver disease manifested by sclerosing hyaline necrosis. Portal-central and intralobular fibrosis are pronounced. × 75.

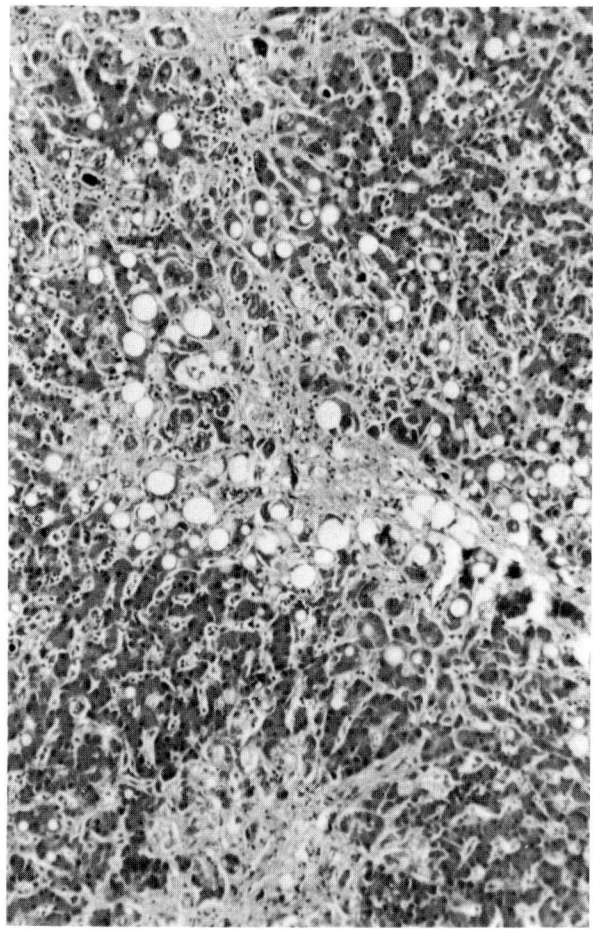

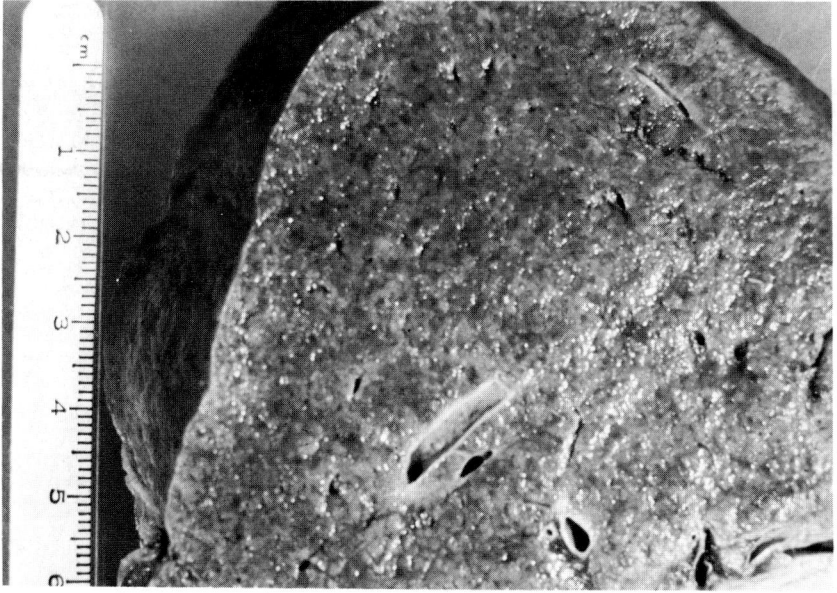

Figure 33–32. Chronic sclerosing hyaline necrosis. The distinction between this entity and true cirrhosis of the micronodular or monolobular type rests upon the absence or presence, respectively, of regeneration nodules.

amounts of fibrosis. Nonetheless, one should attempt to distinguish the diffuse fibrosis seen in chronic or healed sclerosing hyaline necrosis from true cirrhosis. Reticulin stains are sometimes helpful in distinguishing between distorted lobules of chronic alcoholic liver disease and regeneration nodules of cirrhosis.

CIRRHOSIS

The end-stage lesion of chronic alcoholic liver disease is cirrhosis (Figs. 33–33 to 33–35, p. 855). By definition, cirrhosis is a diffuse process of fibrosis and nodular parenchymal regeneration. Normal lobules measuring 1 mm are replaced by regenerative pseudolobules that are less than 1 cm (micronodular cirrhosis), larger than 1 cm (macronodular cirrhosis), or variably sized (mixed cirrhosis).[601] This classification system does not address pathogenesis. On the other hand, if one restricts micronodular cirrhosis to mean a unilobular, rather than multilobular, process, where each lobule is subdivided, the pseudolobules are truly quite fine. Several may lie within the width of a typical needle biopsy. This pattern of cirrhosis is relatively uncommon and suggests specific pathogenic mechanisms—for example, early chronic alcoholic liver disease, the effects of a few drugs and toxins, and some inherited childhood cirrhotic conditions.[602–604] The initial pattern of micronodular alcoholic cirrhosis is often altered in time by a number of insults—for example, additional episodes of hepatitis, gastrointestinal bleeding with hypotension and pseudolobular infarctions, and preferential blood flow. Patients develop mixed patterns of cirrhosis and may eventually have purely macronodular cirrhosis with pseudolobules as large as 5 cm. Since many diseases eventuate in macronodular cirrhosis, its pathogenesis in any given patient is often obscure.

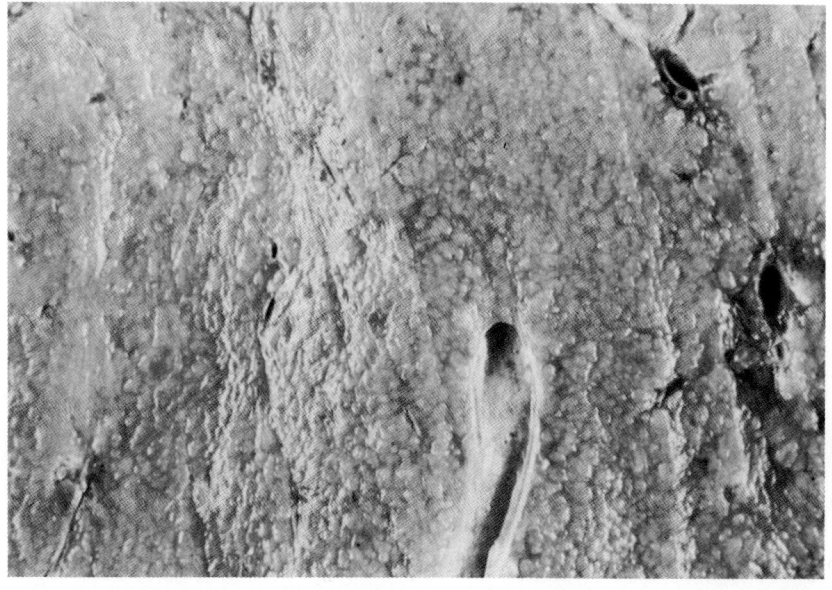

Figure 33–33. Micronodular cirrhosis. The regeneration nodules are small and uniform. The fibrosis that encircles them is delicate.

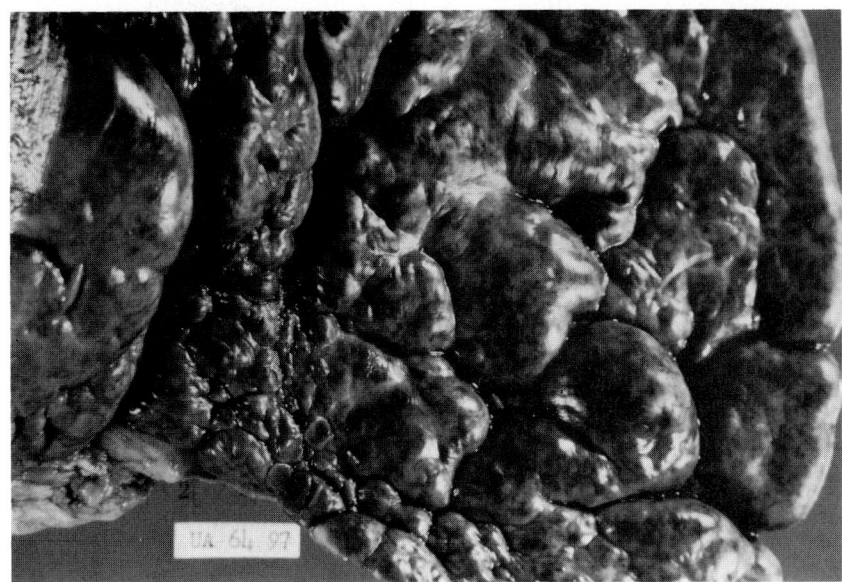

Figure 33–34. Macronodular or multilobular cirrhosis. Diameters of the regenerative nodules range from 0.5 to 5.0 cm.

CONCLUSION

In conclusion, the physician treating the alcoholic should keep in mind the variety of biologic, psychologic, and social causes and effects associated with chronic alcoholism. Treatment approaches should be flexible, supportive, and non-judgmental. The physician should expect that his patient will have occasional relapses, and should keep in mind that alcoholism is a disorder characterized by loss of control over drinking, chronicity, and a variety of biologic, psychologic, and social sequelae. The physician should see himself as the key figure in coordinating the treatment of his alcoholic patient. In some areas, he will want to refer the patient to appropriate medical, psychotherapeutic, and social service professionals. However, by conceptualizing himself as the central figure in treating the whole patient, he may have the greatest impact and best serve the needs of his patient.

REFERENCES

1. Harwood HJ, Napcitano DM, Kristiansen PL, et al. Economic costs to society of alcohol and drug abuse and mental illness: 1980. Research Triangle Institute: Report submitted to the Alcohol, Drug Abuse, and Mental Health Administration, Rockville, MD, 1984.
2. Board of Trustees Report. Alcohol. Advertising, counter advertising and depiction in the public media. JAMA 256:1485, 1986.
3. West LJ, ed. Alcoholism and Related Problems: Issues for the American Public. Prentice Hall, Englewood Cliffs, NJ: 1984.
4. Trell E, Kristenson H, Petersson B. A risk factor approach to alcohol related disease. Alcohol and Alcoholism 20:333, 1985.
5. Breed W, DeFoe JR. Themes in magazine alcohol advertisements: a critique. J Drug Issues 9:511, 1979.
6. Skog OJ. The wetness of drinking cultures: a key variable in the epidemiology of alcoholic liver disease. Acta Med Scand (Suppl) 703:157, 1985.
7. Cohalan D. Epidemiology: Alcohol use in American Society. In: Gomberg EL, White HR, Carpenter JD, eds. Alcohol Science and Society Revisited. University of Michigan Press, Ann Arbor, 1982:96–118.
8. Klaus A, Maxfield T. Social Problems of Alcoholism: The Present Need for Alcoholism Services in California. California Office of Alcoholism Publication, Sacramento, Calif., February 1977.
9. Kendell RE. Alcoholism: medical or political problem? Br Med J 1:367, 1979.
10. Gorwitz K, Bahn A, Warthen FJ, et al. Some epidemiological data on alcoholism in Maryland. Q J Stud Alcohol 31:423, 1970.
11. Schmidt W, DeLint J. Causes of death of alcoholics. Q J Stud Alcohol 33:171, 1972.
12. Lelbach WK. Quantitative aspects of drinking in alcoholic liver cirrhosis. In: Israel Y, Khanna J, Kalant H, eds. Alcoholic Liver Pathology. Addiction Research Foundation, Toronto, 1975.
13. Lelbach WK. Cirrhosis in the alcoholic and its relation to the volume of alcohol abuse. Ann NY Acad Sci 285:85, 1975.
14. Lelbach WK. Epidemiology of alcoholic liver disease. Prog Liver Dis 5:494, 1976.
15. Tuyns AJ, Pequignot G. Greater risk of ascitic cirrhosis in females in relation to alcohol consumption. Int J Epidem 13:53, 1984.
16. Spain DM. Portal cirrhosis of the liver: a review of 250 necropsies with reference to sex differences. Am J Clin Pathol 15:215, 1945.
17. Krasner N, Davis M, Portmann B, et al. Changing pattern of alcoholic liver disease in Great Britain: relation to sex and signs of autoimmunity. Br Med J 1:1487, 1977.
18. Morgan MY, Sherlock S. Sex-related differences among 100 patients with alcoholic liver disease. Br Med J 1:939, 1977.
19. Robins LN, Helzer JE, Weissman MM, et al. Lifetime prevalence of specific psychiatric disorders in three sites. Arch Gen Psychiatr 41:949, 1984.
20. Jolliffe N, Jellinek EM. Vitamin deficiencies and liver cirrhosis in alcoholism. VII. Cirrhosis of the liver. Q J Stud Alcohol 2:544, 1941.
21. Popham RE. The Jellinek alcoholism estimation formula and its application to Canadian data. Q J Stud Alcohol 17:559, 1956.
22. Klatskin G. Alcohol and its relation to liver damage. Gastroenterology 41:443, 1961.
23. Steiner PE. World problem in the cirrhotic diseases of the liver. Their incidence, frequency, types and etiology. Trop Geogr Med 16:175, 1964.
24. Bhathol PS, Wilkinson P, Clifton S, et al. The spectrum of liver disease in alcoholism. Aust NZ J Med 5:49, 1975.
25. Saunders JB, Williams R. The genetics of alcoholism: Is there an inherited susceptibility to alcohol-related problems? Alcohol Alcohol 3:189, 1983.
26. Hall PA, ed. Alcoholic Liver Disease Pathobiology, Epidemiology and Clinical Aspects. New York, John Wiley & Sons, 1985.
27. Lundquist F. The metabolism of ethanol. In: Israel Y, Mardonec J, eds. Biological Basis of Alcoholism. New York, John Wiley and Sons, 1971:1.
28. Williamson JR, Tischler M. Ethanol metabolism in perfused liver and isolated hepatocytes with associated methodologies. In: Majchrowicz E, Noble EP, eds. Biochemistry and Pharmacology of Ethanol. New York, Plenum, 1979:167.
29. Hawkins RD, Kalant H. The metabolism of ethanol and its metabolic effects. Pharmacol Rev 24:67, 1972.
30. Roach MD, Khan M, Knapp M, et al. Ethanol metabolism in vivo and the role of hepatic microsomal ethanol oxidation. Q J Stud Alcohol 33:751, 1972.
31. Lieber CS. Metabolism of ethanol. In: Lieber CS, ed. Metabolic Aspects of Alcoholism. Baltimore, University Park Press, 1977:1.
32. Branden CI, Jornvall H, Eklund H, et al. Alcohol dehydrogenases. In: Boyer PD, ed. The Enzymes. Volume XI. Third edition. New York, Academic Press, 1975:104.

33. Sytkowski AJ, Vallee BL. Metalloenzymes and ethanol metabolism liver alcoholic dehydrogenase. In: Majchrowicz E, Noble EP, eds. Biochemistry and Pharmacology of Ethanol. New York, Plenum, 1979:43.

34. Von Wartburg JP, Bethune JL, Vallee BL. Human liver—alcohol dehydrogenase: kinetic and physiochemical properties. Biochemistry 3:1775, 1964.

35. Blair AH, Vallee BL. Some catalytic properties of human liver alcohol dehydrogenase. Biochemistry 5:2026, 1966.

36. Smith H, Hopkinson DA, Harris H. Studies on the subunit structure and molecular size of the human alcohol dehydrogenase isoenzymes determined by the different loci ADH_1, ADH_2, and ADH_3. Ann Hum Gent 36:401, 1973.

37. Li TK, Magnes LJ. Identification of a distinct molecular form of alcohol dehydrogenase in human liver with high activity. Biochem Biophys Res Commun 63:202, 1975.

38. Li TK, Bosron WF, Dafeldecker WP, et al. Isolation of π-alcohol dehydrogenase of human liver: Is it a determinant of alcoholism? Proc Natl Acad Sci USA 74:4378, 1977.

39. Vallee BL, Bazzone TJ. Isoenzymes of human liver alcohol dehydrogenase. Curr Topics Biol Med Res 8:219, 1983.

40. Vallee BL. A novel approach to human ethanol metabolism: isoenzymes of alcohol dehydrogenases. Proc Cong Eur Brew Conv 20:65, 1985.

41. Wagner FW, Burger AR, Vallee BL. Kinetic properties of human liver alcohol dehydrogenase: oxidation of alcohols by class I isoenzymes. Biochemistry 22:1857, 1983.

42. Ditlow CD, Holmquist B, Morelock M, et al. Physical and enzymatic properties of a class II alcohol dehydrogenase isoenzyme of human liver: π ADH. Biochemistry 23:6363, 1984.

43. Von Wartburg JP, Papenberg J, Aebi H. An atypical human alcohol dehydrogenase. Can J Biochem 43:889, 1965.

44. Stamatoyannopoulos G, Chem SH, Fukul M. Liver alcohol dehydrogenase in Japanese. High population frequency of atypical form and its possible role in alcohol sensitivity. Am J Hum Genet 27:789, 1975.

45. Von Wartburg JP, Schürch PM. Atypical liver alcohol dehydrogenase. Ann NY Acad Sci 151:936, 1968.

46. Weiner H. Aldehyde dehydrogenase: mechanism of action and possible physiological roles. In: Majchrowicz E, Noble EP, eds. Biochemistry and Pharmacology of Ethanol. New York, Plenum, 1979:107.

47. Weiner H. Acetaldehyde metabolism. In: Majchrowicz F, Noble EP, eds. Biochemistry and Pharmacology of Ethanol. New York, Plenum, 1979:125.

48. Tank AW, Weiner H, Thurman JA. Enzymology and subcellular localization of aldehyde oxidation in rat liver. Oxidation of 3,4-dihydroxyphenylacetaldehyde derived from dopamine to 3,4-dihydroxyphenylacetic acid. Biochem Pharmacol 30:2365, 1981.

49. Corrall RJ, Havre P, Margolis J, et al. Subcellular site of acetaldehyde oxidation in rat liver. Biochem Pharmacol 25:17, 1976.

50. Eriksson CJP, Sippel HW. The distribution and metabolism of acetaldehyde in rats during ethanol oxidation. I. The distribution of acetaldehyde in liver, brain, blood and breath. Biochem Pharmacol 26:241, 1977.

51. Harada S, Agarval DP, Goedde HW. Electrophoretic and biochemical studies of human aldehyde dehydrogenase isoenzymes in various tissues. Life Sci 26:1773, 1980.

52. Mizoi Y, Tatsuno Y, Adachi J, et al. Alcohol sensitivity related to polymorphism of alcohol-metabolizing enzymes in Japanese. Pharmacol Biochem Behav 18:127, 1983.

53. Teng Y-S. Human liver aldehyde dehydrogenase in Chinese and Asiatic Indians: gene deletion and its possible implications in alcohol metabolism. Biochem Genet 19:107, 1981.

54. Yoshida A, Wang G, Dave V. Determination of genotypes of human aldehyde dehydrogenase $ALDH_2$ locus. Am J Human Genet 35:1107, 1983.

55. Impraim C, Wang G, Yoshida A. Structural mutation in a major human aldehyde dehydrogenase gene results in loss of enzyme activity. Am J Hum Genet 34:837, 1982.

56. Harada S, Agarawal DP, Goedde HW, et al. Aldehyde dehydrogenase isoenzyme variation and alcoholism in Japan. Pharmacol Biochem Behav 18. (Suppl)1:151, 1983.

57. Asmussen E, Hald J, Larsen V. The pharmacological action of acetaldehyde on the human organism. Acta Pharmacol Toxicol 4:311, 1948.

58. Truitt EJ Jr, Walsh MJ. The role of acetaldehyde in the actions of ethanol. In: Kissin B, Begleiter HB, eds. The Biology of Alcoholism. Volume 1. New York, Plenum, 1971:161.

59. Seto A, Tricomi S, Goodwin DW, et al. Biochemical correlates of ethanol-induced flushing in Orientals. J Stud Alcohol 39:1978.

60. Ewing JA, Rouse BA, Aderhold RM. Studies of the mechanism of Oriental hypersensitivity to alcohol. Currents in Alcoholism 5:45, 1979.

61. Harada S, Agarawal DP, Goedde HW. Aldehyde dehydrogenase deficiency as a cause of facial flushing reaction to alcohol in Japanese. Lancet ii:982, 1981.

62. Ikawa M, Impraim CC, Wang G, et al. Isolation and characterization of aldehyde dehydrogenase isoenzymes from usual and atypical human livers. J Biol Chem 258:6282, 1983.

63. Goedde HW, Agarwal DP, Harada S, et al. Aldehyde dehydrogenase polymorphism in North American, South American, and Mexican Indian populations. Am J Hum Genet 38:385, 1986.

64. Bosron WF, Li TK. Genetic polymorphism of human liver alcohol and aldehyde dehydrogenases, and their relationship to alcohol metabolism and alcoholism. Hepatology 6:502, 1986.

65. Saunders JB, Williams R. The genetics of alcoholism: Is there an inherited susceptibility to alcohol-related problems? Alcohol Alcohol 18:189, 1983.

66. Goodwin DW. Genetic influences in alcoholism. Adv Intern Med 32:283, 1987.

67. Harada S, Agarwal DP, Goedde HW. Isoenzyme variations in acetaldehyde dehydrogenase (EC 1.2.1.3) in human tissues. Hum Genet 44:181, 1978.

68. Wilhin JK, Fortner G. Cutaneous vascular sensitivity to lower alipathic alcohols and aldehydes in Orientals. Alcoholism 9:522, 1985.

69. Higuchi S, Muramatsu T, Saito M, et al. Ethanol patch test for low K_m aldehyde dehydrogenase deficiency. (Letter.) Lancet i:629, 1987.

70. Orme-Johnson WH, Ziegler DM. Alcohol mixed function oxidase activity of mammalian liver microsomes. Biochem Biophys Res Commun 21:78, 1965.

71. Lieber CS, DeCarli LM. Hepatic microsomal ethanol oxidizing system: in vitro characteristics and adaptive properties in vivo. J Biol Chem 245:2505, 1970.

72. Lieber CS, DeCarli LM. The role of hepatic microsomal ethanol oxidizing system (MEOS) for ethanol metabolism in vivo. J Pharmacol Exp Ther 181:279, 1972.

73. Cederbaum AI, Lieber CS, Rubin E. Effects of chronic ethanol treatment on mitochondrial functions damage to coupling site 1. Arch Biochem Biophys 165:560, 1975.

74. Koop DR, Morgan ET, Tarr GE, et al. Purification and characterization of a unique isozyme of cytochrome P-450 from liver microsomes of ethanol-treated rabbits. J Biol Chem 257:8472, 1982.

75. Morgan ET, Koop DR, Coon MJ. Catalytic activity of cytochrome P-450 isozyme 3a isolated from liver microsomes of ethanol-treated rabbits. J Biol Chem 257:13951, 1982.

76. Koop DR, Crump BL, Nordbloom GD, et al. Immunochemical evidence for induction of the alcohol-oxidizing cytochrome P_{450} of rabbit liver microsomes by diverse agents: ethanol, imidazole, trichlorethylene, acetone, pyrazole, and isoniazid. Proc Natl Acad Sci USA 82:4065, 1985.

77. Keilin D, Hartree ER. Properties of catalase. Catalysis of coupled oxidation of alcohol. Biochem J 39:293, 1945.

78. Isselbacher KJ, Carter EA. Ethanol oxidation by liver microsomes: evidence against a separate and distinct enzyme system. Biochem Biophys Res Commun 39:530, 1970.

79. Thurman RG, Ley HG, Scholz R. Hepatic microsomal ethanol oxidation: hydrogen peroxide formation and the role of catalase. Eur J Biochem 25:420, 1972.

80. Vatsis KP, Schulman MP. Absence of ethanol metabolism in acatalatic hepatic microsomes that oxidize drugs. Biochem Biophys Res Commun 52:588, 1973.

81. Oshino N, Oshino R, Chance B. The characteristics of 'peroxidatic' reaction of catalase in ethanol oxidation. Biochem J 131:555, 1973.

82. Ohnishi K, Lieber CS. Reconstitution of the microsomal ethanol-oxidizing system. J Biol Chem 252:7124, 1977.

83. Miwa GT, Levin W, Thomas PE, et al. The direct oxidation of ethanol by a catalase- and alcohol dehydrogenase-free reconstituted system containing cytochrome P-450. Arch Biochem Biophys 137:464, 1978.

84. Teschke R, Hasumura Y, Lieber CS. Hepatic microsomal ethanol-oxidizing system: solubilization; isolation, and characterization. Arch Biochem Biophys 163:404, 1974.

85. Teschke R, Hasamura Y, Lieber CS. Hepatic microsomal alcohol oxidizing system: affinity for methanol, ethanol, propanol and butanol. J Biol Chem 250:7397, 1975.

86. Fong KL, McCay PB, Poyer JL, et al. Evidence that peroxidation of lysosomal membranes is initiated by hydroxyl free radicals produced during flavin enzyme activity. J Biol Chem 248:7792, 1973.

87. Dorfman LM, Adams GE. Reactivity of the Hydroxyl Radical in Aqueous Solutions. NSRRS, p. 46. National Bureau of Standards, Washington, DC.

88. Cederbaum AI, Dicker E, Cohen G. Effect of hydroxyl radical scavengers on microsomal oxidation of alcohols and on associated microsomal reactions. Biochemistry 17:3058, 1978.

89. Krikun G, Lieber CS, Cederbaum AI. Increased microsomal oxidation

of ethanol by cytochrome P-450 and hydroxyl radical-dependent pathways after chronic ethanol consumption. Biochem Pharmacol 33:3309, 1984.

90. Krikun G, Cederbaum AI. Evaluation of microsomal pathways of oxidation of alcohols and hydroxyl radical scavenging agents with carbon monoxide and cobalt protoporphyrin IX. Biochem Pharmacol 34:2929, 1985.

91. Feierman DE, Cederbaum AI. Inhibition of microsomal oxidation of ethanol by pyrazole and 4-methylpyrazole in vitro. Biochem J 239:671, 1986.

92. Lange LG, Bergman SR, Sobel BE. Identification of fatty acid ethyl esters as products of rabbit myocardial ethanol metabolism. J Biol Chem 256:12968, 1981.

93. Lange LG, Sobel BE. Myocardial metabolites of ethanol. Circ Res 52:479, 1983.

94. Mogelson S, Lange LG. Non-oxidative ethanol metabolism in rabbit myocardium: purification to homogeneity of fatty acyl ethyl ester synthase. Biochemistry 23:4075, 1984.

95. Ryan TJ, Kororenidis G, Moschoz CB, et al. The acute metabolic and hemodynamic responses of the left ventricle to ethanol. J Clin Invest 45:270, 1966.

96. Lange LG, Sobel BE. Mitochondrial dysfunction induced by fatty acid ethyl esters, myocardial metabolites of ethanol. J Clin Invest 72:724, 1983.

97. Loposata EA, Lange LG. Presence of non-oxidative ethanol metabolism in human organs commonly damaged by ethanol abuse. Science 231:497, 1986.

98. Keiding S, Christian NJ, Damgaard SE, et al. Ethanol metabolism in heavy drinkers after massive and moderate alcohol intake. Biochem Pharm 32:3097, 1983.

99. Korsten MA, Matsuzaki S, Feinman L, et al. High blood acetaldehyde levels after ethanol administration. N Engl J Med 292:386, 1975.

100. Israel Y, Khanna JM, Lin J. Effect of 2,4 dinitrophenol on the rate of ethanol elimination in the rat in vivo. Biochem J 120:447, 1970.

101. Videla L, Israel Y. Factors that modify the metabolism of ethanol in rat liver and adaptive changes produced by its chronic administration. Biochem J 118:275, 1970.

102. Meijer AJ, Von Woerkon G, Williamson JR, et al. Rate limiting factors in the oxidation of ethanol by isolated rat liver cells. Biochem J 150:205, 1975.

103. Bucher T, Klingenberg M. Wege des Wasserstoffe in der Lebendigen Organisation. Angew Chem 70:552, 1958.

104. Klingenberg M, Bucher T. Glycerin 1-P und Flugmuskelmitochondrien. Biochem Z 334:1, 1961.

105. Grunnet N, Quistorff B, Thieden HID. Rate limiting factors in ethanol oxidation by isolated rat liver parenchymal cells. Effect of ethanol concentration on fructose, pyruvate, and pyrazole. Eur J Biochem 40:275, 1973.

106. Thurman RG, Ji S, Lemasters JJ. Lobular oxygen gradient: a possible role in alcohol-induced hepatotoxicity. In: Thurman RG, Kauffman FC, Jungerman K, eds. Regulation of Hepatic Metabolism. New York, Plenum, 1986:293.

107. Scholz R, Wohl H. Mechanism of the stimulatory effect of fructose on ethanol oxidation in perfused rat liver. Eur J Biochem 63:449, 1976.

108. Lumeng L, Bosron WF, Li TK. Quantitative correlation of ethanol elimination rates in vivo with liver alcohol dehydrogenase activities in fed, fasted and food restricted rats. Biochem Pharm 28:1547, 1979.

109. Wilson JS, Korsten MA, Lieber CS. The combined effects of protein deficiency and chronic ethanol administration on rat ethanol metabolism. Hepatology 6:823, 1986.

110. Crabb DW, Bosron WF, Li TK. Steady state kinetic properties of purified rat liver alcohol dehydrogenase: application to predicting alcohol elimination rates in vivo. Arch Biochem Biophys 224:299, 1983.

111. Videla L, Bernstein J, Israel Y. Metabolic alterations produced in the liver by chronic ethanol administration. Increased oxidative capacity. Biochem J 134:507, 1973.

112. Hawkins RD, Kalant H, Khanna JM. Effect of chronic intake of ethanol on rate of ethanol metabolism. Canad J Physiol Pharmacol 44:241, 1966.

113. Mendelson JH, Mello NK. Metabolism of ^{14}C ethanol and behavioral adaptation of alcoholics during experimentally induced intoxication. Trans Am Neurol Assoc 89:133, 1964.

114. Cederbaum AI, Dicker E, Rubin E. Transfer and reoxidation of reducing equivalents as the rate limiting steps in the oxidation of ethanol by liver cells isolated from fed and fasted rats. Arch Biochem Biophys 183:638, 1977.

115. Kerner E, Westerfeld WW. Effect of diet on rate of alcohol oxidation by the liver. Proc Soc Exp Biol Med 83:530, 1953.

116. Bode C. Factors influencing ethanol metabolism in man. In: Thurman RG, Yonetani T, Williamson JR, et al, eds. Alcohol and Aldehyde

Metabolizing Systems Vol. 1. New York, Academic Press, 1974:457.

117. Lindros KO, Pekkanen L, Kiovula T. Effect of low protein diet on acetaldehyde metabolism in rats. Acta Pharmacol Toxicol 40:134, 1977.

118. Lindros KO, Pekkanen L, Koivula T. Enzymatic and metabolic modification of hepatic ethanol and acetaldehyde oxidation by the dietary protein level. Biochem Pharmacol 28:2313, 1979.

119. Lindros KO. Regulatory factor in hepatic acetaldehyde metabolism during ethanol oxidation. In: Lindros KO, Eriksson CJP, eds. The Role of Acetaldehyde in the Actions of Ethanol. The Finnish Foundation for Alcohol Studies 23:67, 1975.

120. Nuutinen HU, Salaspuro MP, Valle M, et al. Blood acetaldehyde concentration gradient between hepatic and antecubital venous blood in ethanol-intoxicated alcoholics and controls. Eur J Clin Invest 14:306, 1984.

121. Eriksson CJP, Hilboni ME, Sovijarvi ARA. Difficulties in measuring human blood acetaldehyde concentration during ethanol intoxication. In: Begleiter H, ed. Biological Effects of Alcohol. New York, Plenum, 1979.

122. Truitt EB Jr. Blood acetaldehyde levels after alcohol consumption by alcoholic and non-alcoholic subjects. In: Biological Aspects of Alcohol, Advances in Mental Science. Volume 3. Austin, Tex, University of Texas Press, 1971:212.

123. Agarwal DP, Tobar-Rojas L, Meier-Taikman D, et al. Human erythrocyte aldehyde dehydrogenase: a biochemical marker of alcoholism? Alcohol Clin Exp Res 6:426, 1982.

124. Matthewson K, Record CO. Erythrocyte aldehyde dehydrogenase activity in alcoholic subjects and its value as a marker for hepatic aldehyde dehydrogenase in subjects with and without liver disease. Clin Sci 70:295, 1986.

125. Matthewson K, Al Mardini H, Bartlett K, et al. Impaired acetaldehyde metabolism in patients with nonalcoholic liver disorders. Gut 27:756, 1986.

126. Palmer KR, Jenkins WJ. Impaired acetaldehyde oxidation in alcoholics. Gut 23:729, 1982.

127. Jenkins WJ, Peter TJ. Selectively reduced hepatic acetaldehyde dehydrogenase in alcoholics. Lancet i:629, 1980.

128. Thomas M, Halsall S, Peters TJ. Role of hepatic acetaldehyde dehydrogenase in alcoholism: demonstration of a persisting reduction of cytosolic activity in abstaining patients. Lancet ii:1057, 1982.

129. Jenkins WJ, Cakebread K, Palmer KR. Effect of alcohol consumption on hepatic aldehyde dehydrogenase activity in alcoholic patients. Lancet i:1048, 1984.

130. Rutstein DD, Nickerson RJ, Vernon AA, et al. 2,3-butanediol: an unusual metabolite in the serum of seriously alcoholic men during acute intoxication. Lancet ii:534, 1983.

131. Hasumura Y, Teschke R, Lieber CS. Characteristics of acetaldehyde oxidation in rat liver mitochondria. J Biol Chem 251:4903, 1976.

132. Lindros KO, Pekkanen L, Koivula T. Biphasic influence of dietary protein levels on ethanol-derived acetaldehyde concentrations. Acta Pharmacol Toxicol 43:409, 1978.

133. Faiman M. Biochemical pharmacology of disulfuram. In: Majchrowicz E, Noble EP, eds. Biochemistry and Pharmacology of Ethanol. New York, Plenum, 1979.

134. Haley TJ. Disulfiram (tetraethylthioperoxydicarbonic diamide): a reappraisal of its toxicity and therapeutic applications. Drug Metab Rev 9:319, 1979.

135. Sanny CG, Weiner H. Inactivation of horse liver mitochondrial aldehyde dehydrogenase by disulfuram. Evidence that disulfiram is not an active-site–directed reagent. Biochem J 242:499, 1987.

136. Lundwall L, Baekeland F. Disulfiram treatment of alcoholism. J Nerv Ment Dis 153:381, 1971.

137. Ritchie JM. The aliphatic alcohols. In: Goodman LS, Gilman A, eds. The Pharmacological Basis of Therapeutics. Fourth ed. New York, MacMillan, 1970:135.

138. Berger D, Weiner J. In vivo interactions of chloral hydrate and disulfiram with the metabolism of catecholamines. In: Currents in Alcoholism 1:231, 1977.

139. Hellstrom-Lindahl E, Weiner H. Effects of disulfuram on oxidation of benzaldehyde and acetaldehyde in rat liver. Biochem Pharm 34:1529, 1985.

140. Cohen G, Heikkila RE, Allis B, et al. Destruction of sympathetic nerve terminals by 6-hydroxydopamine: protection by 1-phenyl-3-(2 thiazolyl)-2-thiourea, diethyl d-l-thiocarbamate, methimazole, cysteamine, ethanol and n-butanol. J Pharmacol Exp Ther 199:336, 1976.

141. Lebsack ME, Peterson DR, Collins AC, et al. Preferential inhibition of the low K_m aldehyde dehydrogenase activity by pargyline. Biochem Pharmacol 26:1151, 1977.

142. Kitson TM. The disulfiram-ethanol reaction. J Stud Alcohol 38:96, 1977.

143. Bonfiglio G, Donadio G. Results of the clinical testing of a new drug

"metronidazole" in the treatment of chronic alcoholism. Br J Addiction 62:249, 1967.

144. Truitt EB, Duritz G, Morgan AM, et al. Disulfiramlike actions produced by hypoglycemic sulfonylurea compounds. Q J Stud Alcohol 23:197, 1962.

145. Reeves DS, Davies AJ. Antabuse effect with cephalosporins. Lancet 2:540, 1980.

146. Kalant H, LeBlanc AE, Guttman M, et al. Metabolic and pharmacologic interaction of ethanol and metronidazole in the rat. Can J Physiol Pharmacol 50:476, 1972.

147. Leslie RDG, Pyke DA. Chlorpropamide-alcohol flushing: a dominantly inherited trait associated with diabetes. Br Med J 2:1519, 1978.

148. Leslie RDG, Pyke DA, Stubbs WA. Sensitivity to encephalin as a cause of non-insulin-dependent diabetes. Lancet 1:341, 1979.

149. Perin A, Scalabrino G, Sessa A, et al. In vitro inhibition of protein syntheses in rat liver as a consequence of ethanol metabolism. Biochim Biophys Acta 335:101, 1974.

150. Burke JP, Rubin E. The effects of ethanol and acetaldehyde on products of protein synthesis by liver mitochondria. Lab Invest 41:393, 1979.

151. Tuma DJ, Zetterman RK, Sorrel MK. Inhibition of glycoprotein secretion by ethanol and acetaldehyde in rat liver slices. Biochem Pharm 29:35, 1980.

152. Tuma DJ, Sorrel MF. Effect of ethanol on hepatic secretory protein. In: Galanter M, ed. Recent Developments in Alcoholism, Vol 2. New York, Plenum, 1984:159–180.

153. Stevens VJ, Fantl WJ, Newman CB, et al. Acetaldehyde adducts with hemoglobin. J Clin Invest 67:361, 1981.

154. Tsuboi KK, Thompson DJ, Rush EM, et al. Acetaldehyde-dependent changes in hemoglobin and oxygen affinity of human erythrocytes. Hemoglobin 5:241, 1981.

155. George RCS, Hoberman HD. Reaction of acetaldehyde with hemoglobin. J Biol Chem 261:6811, 1986.

156. Hoberman HD, Chiodo SM. Elevation of the hemoglobin A1 fraction in alcoholism. Alcohol Clin Exp Res 6:260, 1981.

157. Niemela O, Klajner F, Orrego H, et al. Antibodies against acetaldehyde-modified protein epitopes in human alcoholics. Hepatology 1:1210, 1987.

158. Mauch TJ, Donohue TM Jr, Zetterman RK, et al. Covalent binding of acetaldehyde selectively inhibits the catalytic activity of lysine-dependent enzymes. Hepatology 6:263, 1986.

159. Kenney WC. Interaction of acetaldehyde with phospholipids. Gastroenterology 79:1030, 1980.

160. Veitch RL, Lumeng L, Li TK. Vitamin B_6 metabolism in chronic alcohol abuse: the effect of ethanol oxidation on hepatic pyridoxal-5' phosphate metabolism. J Clin Invest 55:1026, 1975.

161. Lumeng L. The role of acetaldehyde in mediating the deleterious effect of ethanol on pyridoxal 5'-phosphate metabolism. J Clin Invest 62:286, 1978.

162. Helander A, Tottmar O. Effects of ethanol, acetaldehyde and disulfiram on the metabolism of biogenic aldehydes in isolated human blood cells and platelets. Biochem Pharm 36:3981, 1987.

163. Holt K, Bennett M, Chojkier M. Acetaldehyde stimulates collagen and non-collagen production by human fibroblasts. Hepatology 4:843, 1984.

164. Savolainen ER, Leo MA, Timpl R, et al. Acetaldehyde and lactate stimulate collagen synthesis of cultured baboon liver myofibroblasts. Gastroenterology 87:777, 1984.

165. Brenner DA, Chojkier M. Acetaldehyde increases collagen gene transcription in cultured human fibroblasts. J Biol Chem 262:17690, 1987.

166. Kiessling KH, Toke U. Degeneration of liver mitochondria in rats after prolonged alcohol consumption. Exp Cell Res 33:350, 1964.

167. French SW. Role of mitochondrial damage in alcoholic liver disease. In: Majchrowicz E, Noble EP, eds. Biochemistry and Pharmacology of Ethanol. New York, Plenum, 1979:409.

168. French SW. Fragility of liver mitochondria in ethanol-fed rats. Gastroenterology 54:1106, 1968.

169. Rubin E, Beattie DS, Lieber CS. Effects of ethanol on the biogenesis of mitochondrial membranes and associated mitochondrial functions. Lab Invest 23:620, 1970.

170. Christophersen BO. Effects of ethanol on mitochondrial oxidations. Biochim Biophys Acta 86:14, 1964.

171. Cederbaum AI, Lieber CS, Toth A, et al. Effects of ethanol and fat on the transport of reducing equivalents into rat liver mitochondria. J Biol Chem 248:4977, 1973.

172. Gordon ER. Mitochondrial functions in an ethanol-induced fatty liver. J Biol Chem 248:8271, 1973.

173. Cederbaum AI, Lieber CS, Rubin E. The effect of acetaldehyde on mitochondrial function. Arch Biochem Biophys 161:26, 1974.

174. Cederbaum AI, Rubin E. Molecular injury to mitochondria produced by ethanol and acetaldehyde. Fed Proc 34:2045, 1975.

175. Cederbaum AI, Lieber CS, Rubin E. Effect of acetaldehyde on fatty acid oxidation and ketogenesis by hepatic mitochondria. Arch Biochem Biophys 169:29, 1975.

176. Cederbaum AI, Lieber CS, Beattie DS, et al. Effect of chronic ingestion on fatty acid oxidation by hepatic mitochondria. J Biol Chem 250:5122, 1975.

177. Cederbaum AI, Lieber CS, Rubin E. Effect of chronic ethanol consumption and acetaldehyde on partial reactions of oxidative phosphorylation and CO_2 production from citric acid cycle intermediates. Arch Biochem Biophys 176:525, 1976.

178. Bernstein JD, Penniall R. Effects of chronic ethanol treatment upon rat liver mitochondria. Biochem Pharmacol 27:2337, 1978.

179. Schilling RJ, Reitz RC. A mechanism for ethanol induced damage to liver mitochondria structure and function. Biochim Biophys Acta 2:266, 1980.

180. Zakim D, Vessey DA. The effects of lipid-protein interactions on the kinetic parameter of microsomal UDP-glucuronyltransferase. In: Martonosi A, ed. The Enzymes of Biological Membranes. Volume 2. New York, Plenum, 1976:443.

181. Vessey DA, Zakim D. Membrane fluidity and the regulation of membrane-bound enzymes. Horizons Biochem Biophys 1:139, 1975.

182. Quinn PJ. The Molecular Biology of Cell Membranes. London, Macmillan, 1976.

183. Martonosi A, ed. The Enzymes of Biological Membranes. Volume 4. Electron Transport Systems and Receptors. New York, Plenum Press, 1976.

184. Zakim D. Interface between membrane biology and clinical medicine. Am J Med 80:645, 1986.

185. Sandermann H. Regulation of membrane enzymes by lipids. Biochim Biophys Acta 515:209, 1978.

186. Stubbs CD, Smith AD. The modification of mammalian membrane polyunsaturated fatty acid composition in relation to membrane fluidity and function. Biochim Biophys Acta 779:89, 1984.

187. Eibl HJ, Churchill P, McIntyre JO, et al. Optimal activation of D-β-hydroxybutyrate dehydrogenase with mitochondrial phospholipids can be mimicked with a ternary mixture of single molecular species of phospholipids. Biochem Int 4:551, 1982.

188. Churchill P, McIntyre JO, Eibl HJ, et al. Activation of D-β-hydroxybutyrate apodehydrogenase using molecular species of mixed fattyacyl phospholipids. J Biol Chem 258:208, 1983.

189. Devaux PF, Seigneuret M. Specificity of lipid-protein interactions as determined by spectroscopic techniques. Biochim Biophys Acta 822:63, 1987.

190. Chin JH, Goldstein DB. Effects of low concentrates of ethanol on the fluidity of spin-labeled erythrocyte and brain membranes. Mol Pharmacol 13:435, 1977.

191. Rowe ES. Lipid chain length and temperature dependence of ethanol-phosphatidylcholine interactions. Biochemistry 22:3299, 1983.

192. Herold LL, Rowe ES, Khalifah RG. ^{13}C-NMR and spectrophotometric studies of alcohol-lipid interactions. Chem Phys Lipids 43:215, 1987.

193. Chin JH, Goldstein DB. Drug tolerance in biomembranes: a spin-label study of the effects of ethanol. Science 196:684, 1977.

194. Johnson DA, Friedman HJ, Cooke R, et al. Adaptation of brain lipid bilayers to ethanol induced fluidization. Biochem Pharmacol 29:1673, 1980.

195. Johnson DA, Lee NM, Cooke R, et al. Ethanol-induced fluidization of brain lipid bilayers: required presence of cholesterol in membranes for expression of tolerance. Mol Pharmacol 15:739, 1979.

196. Goldstein DB. The effects of drugs on membrane fluidity. Ann Rev Pharmacol Toxicol 24:43, 1984.

197. Taraschi TF, Ellingson JS, Wu A, et al. Membrane tolerance to ethanol is rapidly lost after withdrawal: a model for studies of membrane adaptation. Proc Natl Acad Sci USA 83:3669, 1986.

198. Rottenberg H. Membrane solubility of ethanol in chronic alcoholism. The effect of ethanol feeding and its withdrawal on the protection by alcohol of rat red blood cells from hypotonic hemolysis. Biochim Biophys Acta 855:211, 1986.

199. French SW, Ihrig TJ, Morin RJ. Lipid composition of RBC ghosts, liver mitochondria and microsomes of ethanol-fed rats. Q J Stud Alcohol 31:801, 1970.

200. Thompson JA, Reitz RC. Studies on the acute and chronic effects of ethanol ingestion on choline oxidation. Ann NY Acad Sci 273:194, 1976.

201. Hosein EA, Hofmann I, Linder E. Ethanol and Mg^{2+}-stimulated ATPase. Arch Biochem Biophys 183:64, 1977.

202. Hosein EA, Lee H, Hofmann I. The influence of chronic ethanol feeding to rats on liver mitochondrial membrane structure and function. Can J Biochem 58:1147, 1980.

203. Spach PI, Parce JW, Cunningham CC. Effect of chronic ethanol administration on energy metabolism and phospholipase A_2 activity in rat liver. Biochem J 178:23, 1979.

204. Buthke TM, Ingram LO. Mechanism of ethanol-induced changes in

lipid composition of *Escherichia coli*: inhibition of saturated fatty acid synthesis in vivo. Biochemistry 17:637, 1978.

205. Berger B, Carty CE, Ingram LO. Alcohol-induced changes in the phospholipid molecular species of *Escherichia coli*. J Bacteriol 142:1040, 1980.

206. Nandini-Kishove SG, Mattox SM, Martin CE, et al. Membrane changes during growth of Tetrahymena in the presence of ethanol. Biochim Biophys Acta 551:315, 1979.

207. Swann AC. Free fatty acids and (Na$^+$,K$^+$)-ATPase: effects of cation regulation, enzyme conformation, and interactions with ethanol. Arch Biochem Biophys 233:354, 1984.

208. Dreiling CE, Schilling RJ, Reitz RC. Effects of chronic ethanol ingestion on the activity of rat liver mitochondrial 2′,3′-cyclic nucleotide 3′-phosphohydrolase. Biochim Biophys Acta 640:121, 1981.

209. Dorio RJ, Hock JB, Rubin E. Ethanol treatment selectively decreases neutral amino acid transport in cultured hepatocytes. J Biol Chem 259:11430, 1984.

210. O'Neill B, Weber F, Honig D, et al. Ethanol selectively affects Na$^+$ gradient-dependent intestinal transport systems. FEBS Lett 194:183, 1986.

211. Mills PR, Meier PJ, Smith DJ, et al. The effect of changes in the fluid state of rat liver plasma membrane on the transport of taurocholate. Hepatology 1:61, 1987.

212. Fassoulaki A, Eger EI II. Alcohol increases in solubility of anesthetics in the liver. Br J Anaesth 58:551, 1986.

213. Kosenko EA, Kaminsky YG. Limitation in glucose penetration from the liver into blood and other metabolic symptoms of ethanol withdrawal in rats. FEBS Lett 200:210, 1986.

214. Tuma DJ, Mailliard ME, Casey CA, et al. Ethanol-induced alterations of plasma membrane assembly in the liver. Biochim Biophys Acta 856:5171, 1986.

215. Lee H, Hosein EA. Chronic alcohol feeding and its withdrawal on the structure and function of the rat liver plasma membrane: a study with ^{125}I-labelled glucagon binding as a metabolic probe. Can J Physiol Pharmacol 60:1171, 1982.

216. Sharma RJ, Grant DA. A differential effect between the acute and chronic administration of ethanol on the endocytotic rate constant, k_e, for the internalization of asialoglycoproteins by hepatocytes. Biochim Biophys Acta 862:199, 1986.

217. Casey CA, Kragskow SL, Sorrell MF, et al. Chronic ethanol administration impairs the binding and endocytosis of asialo-orosomucoid in isolated hepatocytes. J Biol Chem 262:2704, 1987.

218. Kiessling K-H, Lindgren L, Strandberg B, et al. Electron microscopic study of liver mitochondria from human alcoholics. Acta Med Scand 85:413, 1964.

219. Uchida T, Kronborg I, Peters RL. Giant mitochondria in alcoholic liver disease—their identification, frequency and pathologic significance. Liver 4:29, 1984.

220. Stewart RV, Dincsoy HP. The significance of giant mitochondria in liver biopsies as observed by light microscopy. Am J Clin Pathol 78:293, 1982.

221. Israel Y, Videla L, Videla-Fernandez V, et al. Effects of chronic ethanol treatment and thyroxine administration on ethanol metabolism and liver oxidative capacity. J Pharmacol Exp Ther 192:565, 1975.

222. Thurman RG, McKenna WR, McCaffrey TB. Pathways responsible for the adaptive increase in ethanol utilization following chronic treatment with ethanol: inhibition studies with hemoglobin-free perfused rat liver. Mol Pharmacol 12:156, 1956.

223. Kessler BJ, Liebler JB, Bronfin GJ, et al. Hepatic blood flow and splanchnic oxygen consumption in alcoholic fatty liver. J Clin Invest 33:1338, 1954.

224. Videla L, Bernstein J, Israel Y. Metabolic alterations produced in the liver by chronic ethanol administration: changes related to energetic parameters of the cell. Biochem J 134:515, 1973.

225. Israel Y, Videla L, Bernstein J. Liver hypermetabolic state after chronic ethanol consumption. Hormonal inter-relations and pathogenic implications. Fed Proc 34:2052, 1975.

226. Israel Y, Kalant H, Orrego H, et al. Experimental alcohol induced hepatic necrosis: suppression by propylthiouracil. Proc Natl Acad Sci 72:1137, 1975.

227. Orrego H, Kalant H, Israel Y. Effect of short-term therapy with propylthiouracil in patients with alcoholic liver disease. Gastroenterology 76:105, 1979.

228. Israel Y, Walfish PG, Orrego H, et al. Thyroid hormones in alcoholic liver disease. Effect of treatment with 6-n-propylthiouracil. Gastroenterology 76:116, 1979.

229. Yuki T, Thurman RG. The swift increase in alcohol metabolism. Time course for the increase in hepatic oxygen uptake and the involvement of glycolysis. Biochem J 186:119, 1980.

230. Stowell KM, Crow KE. The effect of acute ethanol treatment on rates of oxygen uptake, ethanol oxidation and gluconeogenesis in isolated rat hepatocytes. Biochem J 262:595, 1985.

231. Braggins TJ, Crow KE. The effects of high ethanol doses on rates of ethanol oxidation in rats. A reassessment of factors controlling rates of ethanol oxidation in vivo. Eur J Biochem 119:633, 1981.

232. Cherin I, Thurman RG, Glassman E, et al. The swift increase in alcohol metabolism (SIAM) in humans: oral and intravenous studies. (Abstract.) Alcohol Clin Exp 7:366, 1983.

233. Cheren I, Glassman E, Thurman RG. The swift increase in alcohol metabolism in humans: dose response relations. (Abstract.) Alcohol 1:168, 1984.

234. Glassman EB, McLaughlin GA, Forman DT, et al. Role of alcohol dehydrogenase in the swift increase in alcohol metabolism (SIAM). Studies with deermice deficient in alcohol dehydrogenase. Biochem Pharmacol 34:3523, 1985.

235. Thurman RG. Ethanol elimination is inherited in rat. In: Thurman RG, ed. Alcohol and Aldehyde Metabolizing Systems, Vol 4. New York, Plenum, 1980:665.

236. Crownover BP, LaDine J, Bradford B, et al. Activation of ethanol metabolism in humans by fructose: importance of experimental design. J Pharmacol Exp Ther 236:574, 1986.

237. Hernandez-Munoz R, Diaz-Munoz M, Chagoya de Sanchez V. In vivo and in vitro adenosine stimulation of ethanol oxidation by hepatocytes and the role of the malate-aspartate shuttle. Biochim Biophys Acta 930:254, 1987.

238. Thurman RG, Scholz R. Interactions of glycolysis and respiration in perfused rat liver. Changes in oxygen uptake following addition of ethanol. Eur J Biochem 75:13, 1977.

239. Cunningham CC, Malloy CR, Radda GK. Effect of fasting and acute ethanol administration on the energy state of in vivo liver as measured by 31P-NMR spectroscopy. Biochim Biophys Acta 855:12, 1985.

240. Desmoulin F, Cossone PJ, Canioni P. Phosphorus-31 nuclear magnetic resonance study of phosphorylated metabolites compartmentation, intracellular pH and phosphorylation state during normoxia, hypoxia and ethanol perfusion, in the perfused rat liver. Eur J Biochem 162:151, 1987.

241. Helzberg JH, Brown MS, Smith DJ, et al. Metabolic state of the rat liver with ethanol: comparison of in vivo phosphorous nuclear magnetic resonance spectroscopy with freeze clamp assessment. Hepatology 7:83, 1987.

242. Desmoulin F, Canioni P, Crotte C, et al. Hepatic metabolism during acute ethanol administration: a phosphorus-31 nuclear magnetic resonance study on the perfused rat liver under normoxic or hypoxic conditions. Hepatology 7:315, 1987.

243. Kasahara A, Hayashi N, Kurosawa K, et al. Hepatic hemodynamics and oxygen consumption in alcoholic fatty liver assessed by organ-reflectance spectrophotometry and the hydrogen clearance method. Hepatology 6:87, 1986.

244. Sato N, Kamada T, Kawano S, et al. Effect of acute and chronic ethanol consumption on hepatic tissue oxygen tension in the rat. Pharmacol Biochem Behav (Suppl) 18:443, 1983.

245. McKaigney JP, Carmichael FJ, Saldivia V, et al. Role of ethanol metabolism in the ethanol-induced increase in splanchnic circulation. Am J Physiol 250:G518, 1986.

246. Svenson CK, Mauriello PM, Barde SH, et al. Effect of carbohydrates on estimated hepatic blood flow. Clin Pharmacol Ther 35:660, 1984.

247. Daneshmend TK, Jackson L, Roberts CJC. Physiological and pharmacological variability in hepatic blood flow in man. Br J Clin Pharmacol 11:491, 1981.

248. Edward DJ, Babiak LM, Beckman HB. The effect of a single oral dose of ethanol on hepatic blood flow in man. Eur J Clin Pharmacol 32:481, 1987.

249. Ugarte G, Iturriaga H, Pereda T. Possible relationship between the rate of ethanol metabolism and the severity of hepatic damage in chronic alcoholics. Am J Dig Dis 22:406, 1977.

250. Israel Y, Videla L, MacDonald A, et al. Metabolic alterations produced in the liver by chronic ethanol administration in comparison between the effects produced by ethanol and by thyroid hormones. Biochem J 134:523, 1973.

251. Younes M, Strubelt O. Enhancement of hypoxic liver damage by ethanol. Involvement of xanthine oxidase and the role of glycolysis. Biochem Pharmacol 36:2973, 1987.

252. Halle P, Pare P, Kaptein E, et al. Double-blinded controlled trial of propylthiouracil in patients with severe acute alcoholic hepatitis. Gastroenterology 82:925, 1982.

253. Orrego H, Blake JE, Blendis LM, et al. Long-term treatment of alcoholic liver disease with propylthiouracil. N Engl J Med 317:1421, 1987.

254. Baraona E, Lieber CS. Effects of ethanol on lipid metabolism. J Lipid Res 20:289, 1979.

255. Lieber CS, Schmid R. The effect of ethanol on fatty acid metabolism: stimulation of hepatic fatty acid synthesis in vitro. J Clin Invest 40:394, 1961.

256. Toth A, Lieber CS, Cederbaum AI, et al. Effects of ethanol and diet

on fatty acid oxidation by hepatic mitochondria. Gastroenterology 64:198, 1973.

257. Zakim D, Green J. Quantitative importance of reduced fatty acid oxidations in the pathogenesis of ethanol-fatty liver. Proc Soc Exp Biol Med 27:138, 1963.

258. Zakim D. Effect of ethanol on hepatic acyl-coenzyme A metabolism. Arch Biochem Biophys 111:253, 1965.

259. Nikkila EA, Ojala K. Role of hepatic l-d glycerophosphate and triglyceride synthesis in the production of fatty liver by ethanol. Proc Soc Exp Biol Med 113:814, 1963.

260. Ontko JA. Effects of ethanol on the metabolism of free fatty acids in isolated liver cells. J Lipid Res 14:78, 1973.

261. Guzman M, Castro J, Maquedano A. Ethanol feeding to rats reversibly decreases hepatic carnitine palmitoyltransferase activity and increases enzyme sensitivity to malonyl-CoA. Biochem Biophys Res Commun 149:443, 1987.

262. Zammit VA. Mechanisms of regulation of the partition of fatty acids between oxidation and esterification in the liver. Prog Lipid Res 23:39, 1984.

263. Zakim D, Pardini R, Herman RH, et al. Mechanism for the differential effects of high carbohydrate diets on lipogenesis in rat liver. Biochim Biophys Acta 144:242, 1967.

264. Zakim D, Herman RH. The regulation of fatty acid synthesis. Am J Clin Nutr 22:200, 1969.

265. Klingman GI, McGoodall C. Urinary epinephrine and levarterenol excretion during alcohol intoxication in dogs. J Pharmacol Exp Ther 121:313, 1957.

266. Forbes JC, Duncan GM. The effects of acute alcohol intoxication on the adrenal glands of rats and guinea pigs. Q J Stud Alcohol 12:355, 1951.

267. Schapiro RH, Scheig RL, Drummey GD, et al. Effect of prolonged ethanol ingestion on the transport and metabolism of lipids in man. N Engl J Med 272:610, 1965.

268. Brodie BB, Butler WM, Horning MG, et al. Alcohol-induced triglyceride deposition in liver through derangement of fat transport. Am J Clin Nutr 9:432, 1961.

269. Feigelson EG, Pfaff WW, Karmen A, et al. The role of plasma free fatty acids in the development of fatty liver. J Clin Invest 40:2171, 1961.

270. Kalant H, Khanna JM, Seymour F, et al. Acute alcoholic fatty liver. Metabolism or stress. Biochem Pharmacol 24:431, 1975.

271. Zakim D, Alexander D, Slesinger MH. The effect of ethanol on hepatic secretion of triglycerides into plasma. J Clin Invest 44:1115, 1965.

272. DiLuzio NR. An evaluation of plasma triglyceride formation as a factor in the development of ethanol-induced fatty liver. Life Sci 4:1373, 1965.

273. Hernell O, Johnson O. Effect of ethanol on plasma triglycerides in male and female rats. Lipids 8:503, 1973.

274. Chait A, Mancini M, February AW, et al. Clinical and metabolic study of alcoholic hyperlipemia. Lancet 2:62, 1972.

275. Marzo AP, Ghirardi D, Sardini D, et al. Serum lipids and total fatty acids in chronic alcoholic liver disease at different stages of cell damage. Klin Wochenschr 48:949, 1970.

276. Field JB, Williams HE, Mortimore GE, et al. Studies on the mechanism of ethanol-induced hypoglycemia. J Clin Invest 42:497, 1963.

277. Freinkel N, Singer DL, Arky RA, et al. Alcohol hypoglycemia. I. Carbohydrate metabolism of patients with clinical alcohol hypoglycemia and the experimental reproduction of the syndrome with pure ethanol. J Clin Invest 42:1112, 1963.

278. Forsander OA, Raiha N, Salasporo M, et al. Influence of ethanol on the liver metabolism of fed and starved rats. Biochem J 94:259, 1965.

279. Madison LL, Lochner A, Wolff J. Ethanol-induced hypoglycemia. Diabetes 16:252, 1967.

280. Frieden C. Glutamic dehydrogenase. III. The order of substrate addition in the enzymatic reaction. J Biol Chem 234:2891, 1959.

281. Ideo G, DeFranchis R, Del Ninno ED, et al. Decrease of rat liver glutamate dehydrogenase after chronic administration of ethanol. Enzymologia 43:245, 1972.

282. Stifel FB, Greene HL, Lufkin EG, et al. Acute effects of oral and intravenous ethanol on rat hepatic enzyme activities. Biochim Biophys Acta 428:633, 1976.

283. Zakim D. The effect of ethanol on the concentration of gluconeogenic intermediates in rat liver. Proc Soc Exp Biol Med 129:393, 1968.

284. Madison LL. Ethanol induced hypoglycemia. Adv Metab Dis 3:85, 1968.

285. Kreisberg RA, Siegal AM, Owen WC. Glucose-lactate interrelationships: effect of ethanol. J Clin Invest 50:175, 1971.

286. Arky RA, Veverbrants E, Abramson EA. Irreversible hypoglycemia: a complication of alcohol and insulin. JAMA 206:575, 1968.

287. Chalmers RJ, Bennie EH, Johnson RH, et al. The growth hormone response to insulin induced hypoglycemia in alcoholics. Psychol Med 7:607, 1977.

288. Kuhl C, Anderson O. Glucose- and tolbutamide-mediated insulin response after pure infusion with ethanol. Diabetes 23:821, 1974.

289. Cohen S. A review of hypoglycemia and alcoholism with and without liver disease. Ann NY Acad Sci 273:338, 1976.

290. Haight JSJ, Keatinge WR. Failure of thermoregulation in the cold during hypoglycemia induced by exercise and alcohol. J Physiol 229:87, 1973.

291. O'Keefe SJD, Marks V. Lunchtime gin and tonic: a cause of reactive hypoglycemia. Lancet 1:1286, 1977.

292. Metz R, Berger S, Mako M. Potentiation of the plasma insulin response to glucose by prior administration of alcohol. Diabetes 18:517, 1969.

293. Singh SP, Patel DG. Effects of ethanol on carbohydrate metabolism. I. Influence on oral glucose tolerance test. Metabolism 25:239, 1976.

293a. Bunyan J, Cawthorne MA, Diplock AT, et al. Vitamin E and hepatotoxic agents. Br J Nutr 23:309, 1969.

294. Demopoulus HB. The basis of free radical pathology. Fed Proc 32:1859, 1973.

295. Bus JS, Gibson JE. Lipid peroxidation and its role in toxicology. In: Hodgson E, Bend JR, Philpot RM, eds. Reviews in Biochemical Toxicology. I. New York, Elsevier-North Holland, 1979:125.

296. Fridovich I. Superoxide and evolution. Horizons Biochem Biophysics 1:1, 1974.

297. Chance B, Sies H, Baveris A. Hydroperoxide metabolism in mammalian organs. Physiol Rev 59:527, 1979.

298. Halliwell B, Gutteridge JMC. Oxygen toxicity, oxygen radicals, transition mutals and disease. Biochem J 219:1, 1984.

299. Halliwell B, Gutteridge JMC. The importance of free radicals and catalytic metal ions in human diseases. Mol Aspects Med 8:89, 1985.

300. Sevanian A, Hochstein P. Mechanisms and consequences of lipid peroxidation in biological systems. Ann Rev Nutr 5:365, 1985.

301. Younes M, Siegers C-P. Interrelation between lipid peroxidation and other hepatotoxic events. Biochem Pharmacol 33:2001, 1984.

302. Stacey NH, Kappus H. Comparison of methods of assessment of metal-induced lipid peroxidation in isolated rat hepatocytes. J Toxic Environ Health 9:277, 1982.

303. Poli G, Albano E, Dianzani HU. The role of lipid peroxidation in liver damage. Chem Phys Lipids 45:117, 1987.

304. Ungemach FR. Pathobiological mechanisms of hepatocellular damage following lipid peroxidation. Chem Phys Lipids 45:171, 1987.

305. Fallagher CH. The effect of antioxidants on poisoning by carbon tetrachloride. Aust J Exp Biol Med Sci 40:241, 1962.

306. Mason RP. Free radical metabolites of foreign compounds and their toxicological significance. In: Hodgson E, Bend JR, Philpot RM, eds. Review of Biochemical Toxicology. New York, Elsevier-North Holland, 1979:151.

307. McCoy PB, Poyer JL. Enzyme generated free radicals as initiators of lipid peroxidation in biological membranes. In: Martonosi A, ed. The Enzymes of Biological Membranes, Volume 4. New York, Plenum, 1976:239.

308. Mills GC. Hemoglobin catabolism. I. Glutathione peroxidase, an erythrocyte enzyme which protects hemoglobin from oxidative breakdown. J Biol Chem 229:189, 1957.

309. Mills GC. Glutathione peroxidase and the destruction of hydrogen peroxide in animal tissues. Arch Biochem Biophys 86:1, 1960.

310. Sies H, Wahllander A, Linke I, et al. Glutathione disulfide (GSSG) efflux from liver occurs via excretion into bile. Hoppe-Seyler's Z Physiol Chem 359:1151, 1979.

311. Flore L, Gunzler WA, Schock HH. Glutathione peroxidase: a selenoenzyme. FEBS Lett 32:132, 1973.

312. Lawrence RA, Burk RF. Species, tissue and subcellular distribution of non-SE-dependent glutathione peroxidase activity. J Nutr 108:211, 1978.

313. Bus JS, Aust SD, Gibson JE. Lipid peroxidation. A possible mechanism for paraquat toxicity. Res Commun Chem Pharmacol 11:31, 1975.

314. Tappel AL. Vitamin E and free radical peroxidation of lipids. Ann NY Acad Sci 203:12, 1973.

315. Diluzio NR. A mechanism on acute ethanol-induced fatty liver and the modification of liver injury by antioxidants. Lab Invest 15:50, 1966.

316. Comporti M, Hartman A, DiLuzio NR. Effect of in vivo and in vitro ethanol administration on liver lipid peroxidation. Lab Invest 16:616, 1967.

317. Hashimoto S, Recknagel RO. No chemical evidence of hepatic lipid peroxidation in acute ethanol toxicity. Exp Mol Pathol 8:225, 1968.

318. Reitz RC. A possible mechanism for the peroxidation of lipids due to chronic ethanol ingestion. Biochim Biophys Acta 380:145, 1975.

319. Kappus H, Koster U, Koster-Albrecht D, et al. Lipid peroxidation induced by ethanol and halogenated hydrocarbons in vivo or measured by ethane exhalation. In: Sies H, Wendel A, eds. Functions of Glutathione in Liver and Kidney. Berlin, Sprague-Verlag, 1978:176.

320. Koster U, Albrecht D, Kappus H. Evidence of carbon-tetrachloride- and ethanol-induced lipid peroxidation in vivo demonstrated by ethane production in mice and rats. Toxicol Appl Pharmacol 41:639, 1977.

321. Muller A, Sies H. Role of alcohol dehydrogenase activity and of acetaldehyde in ethanol-induced ethane and pentane production by isolate perfused rat liver. Biochem J 206:153, 1982.

322. Krikun G, Cederbaum AI. Effect of chronic ethanol consumption on microsomal lipid peroxidation. FEBS Lett 208:292, 1986.

323. Ishii H, Joly JG, Lieber CS. Effect of ethanol on the amount and enzyme activities of hepatic rough and smooth microsomal membranes. Biochim Biophys Acta 291:411, 1973.

324. Joly JG, Hetu C. Effects of chronic ethanol administration in the rat. Relative dependency on dietary lipids. I. Induction of hepatic drug-metabolizing enzyme in vitro. Biochem Pharmacol 24:1475, 1975.

325. Ioannides C, Lake BG, Parke DV. Enhancement of hepatic microsomal drug metabolism in vitro following ethanol administration. Xenobiotica 5:665, 1975.

326. Khanna JH, Kalant H, Yee Y, et al. Effect of chronic ethanol treatment on metabolism of drugs in vitro and in vivo. Biochem Pharmacol 25:329, 1976.

327. Personal communication.

328. McCoy GD. Differential effects of ethanol and other inducers of drug metabolism on the two forms of hamster liver microsomal aniline hydroxylase. Biochem Pharmacol 29:685, 1980.

329. Hammer CT, Wills ED. The role of lipid components of the diet in the regulation of the fatty acid composition of the rat liver endoplasmic reticulum and lipid peroxidation. Biochem J 174:585, 1978.

330. Kellogg EW, Fridovich I. Superoxide, hydrogen peroxide, and singlet oxygen in lipid peroxidation by a xanthine oxidase system. J Biol Chem 250:8812, 1975.

331. Shaw S, Jayatilleke E. Acetaldehyde-mediated hepatic lipid peroxidation: role of superoxide and ferritin. Biochem Biophys Res Com 143:984, 1987.

332. Sies H, Koch OR, Martino E, et al. Increased biliary glutathione disulfide release in chronically ethanol-treated rats. FEBS Lett 103:287, 1979.

333. MacDonald CM, Dow J, Moore MR. A possible protective role for sulphydryl compounds in acute alcoholic liver injury. Biochem Pharmacol 26:1529, 1977.

334. Fernandez V, Videla LA. Effect of acute and chronic ethanol ingestion on the content of reduced glutathion of various tissues of the rat. Experientia 37:392, 1981.

335. Morton S, Mitchell MC. Effects of chronic ethanol feeding on glutathione turnover in the rat. Biochem Pharmacol 34:1559, 1985.

336. Personal communication.

337. Vallee BL, Wacher WE, Bartholomay AF, et al. Zinc metabolism in hepatic dysfunction. I. Serum zinc concentrations in Laennec's cirrhosis and their validation by sequence analysis. N Engl J Med 135:403, 1956.

338. Helwig HL, Hoffer EM, Thulen WC, et al. Urinary and serum zinc levels in chronic alcoholism. Am J Clin Pathol 45:156, 1966.

339. Hannah JS, Soares JH. The effects of vitamin E on the ethanol metabolizing liver in the rat. Nutr Rep Int 19:733, 1979.

340. Benedetti A, Casini AF, Ferrali M, et al. Effects of diffusible products of peroxidation of rat liver microsomal lipid. Biochim J 180:303, 1979.

341. Tanner AR, Bantock I, Hinks L, et al. Depressed selenium and vitamin E levels in an alcoholic population. Possible relationship to hepatic injury through increased lipid peroxidation. Dig Dis Sci 31:1307, 1986.

342. Pascoe GA, Fariss MW, Olafsdottir K, et al. A role of vitamin E in protection against cell injury. Maintenance of intracellular glutathione precursors and biosynthesis. Eur J Biochem 166:241, 1987.

343. Yonaha M, Tampo Y. Bromosulfophthalein abolishes glutathione-dependent protection against lipid peroxidation in rat liver mitochondria. Biochem Pharmacol 36:2831, 1987.

344. Powell RS, McKay PB. Heat labile cytosolic factor mediates the effect of N-acetylcysteine (NAC) on adriamycin (ADR)-induced lipid peroxidation (LPO). Fed Proc 45:2626, 1986.

345. Jakoby WB. The glutathione S-transferases: a group of multifunctional detoxification proteins. Adv Enzymol 46:383, 1978.

346. Fernandez-Checa JC, Ookhtens M, Klapowitz N. Effect of chronic ethanol feeding on rat hepatocytic glutathione. Compartmentation, efflux, and response to incubation with ethanol. J Clin Invest 80:57, 1987.

347. Iseri OH, Lieber CS, Gottlieb LS. The ultrastructure of fatty liver induced by prolonged ethanol ingestion. Am J Pathol 48:535, 1966.

348. Rubin E, Hutterer F, Lieber CS. Ethanol increases hepatic smooth endoplasmic reticulum and drug metabolizing enzyme. Science 159:1469, 1968.

349. Joly J-G, Ishii H, Teschke R. Effect of chronic ethanol feeding on the activities and submicrosomal distribution of reduced nicotinamide adenine dinucleotide phosphate-cytochrome P-450 reductase and the demethylases for aminopyrine and ethylmorphine. Biochem Pharmacol 22:1532, 1983.

350. Koop DR, Nordblom GD, Coon MJ. Immunochemical evidence for a role of cytochrome P-450 in liver microsomal ethanol oxidation. Arch Biochem Biophys 235:228, 1984.

351. Koop DR, Crump BL, Nordblom GD, et al. Immunochemical evidence for induction of alcohol-oxidizing cytochrome P-450 of rabbit liver microsomes by diverse agents: ethanol, imidazole, trichloroethylene, acetone, pyrazole, and isoniazid. Proc Natl Acad Sci USA 82:4065, 1985.

352. Park SS, Ko IY, Patten C, et al. Monoclonal antibodies to ethanol-induced cytochrome P-450 that inhibit aniline and nitrosamine metabolism. Biochem Pharmacol 35:2855, 1986.

353. Fujii H, Ohmachi T, Sagami I, et al. Liver microsomal drug metabolism in ethanol-treated hamsters. Biochem Pharmacol 34:3881, 1985.

354. Wrighton SA, Thomas PE, Mulowa DT, et al. Characterization of ethanol-inducible human liver N-nitrosodimethylamine demethylase. Biochemistry 25:6731, 1986.

355. Ueng T-H, Friedman FK, Miller H, et al. Studies on ethanol-inducible cytochrome P-450 in rabbit liver, lungs and kidneys. Biochem Pharmacol 36:2689, 1987.

356. Rush GF, Adler VL, Hook JB. The effect of ethanol administration on renal and hepatic mixed-function oxidases in the Fischer 344 rat. Toxicol Lett 12:265, 1982.

357. McCoy GD, Wynder EL. Etiological and preventative implications in alcohol carcinogenesis. Can Res 39:2844, 1979.

358. Pollack ES, Nomura ANY, Heilbrun LK, et al. Prospective study of alcohol consumption and cancer. N Engl J Med 310:617, 1984.

359. Porta EA, Markell N, Dorado RD. Chronic alcoholism enhances hepatocarcinogenicity of dimethylnitrosamine in rats fed a marginally methyl-deficient diet. Hepatology 5:1120, 1985.

360. Sohn OS, Fiala ES, Puz C, et al. Enhancement of rat liver microsomal metabolism of azoxymethane to methylazoxymethanol by chronic ethanol administration: similarity to the microsomal metabolism of N-nitrosodimethylamine. Cancer Res 47:3123, 1987.

361. Zimmermann HJ. Effects of alcohol on other hepatotoxins. Alcoholism: Clin Exp Res 10:3, 1986.

362. Traiger GJ, Plaa GL. Relationship of alcohol metabolism to the potentiation of CCl4 hepatotoxicity induced by aliphatic alcohols. J Pharmacol Exp Ther 183:481, 1972.

363. Lamson PD, Gardner RK, Gustafson E, et al. The pharmacology and toxicology of carbon tetrachloride. J Pharmacol Exp Ther 22:215, 1923.

364. Klaasen CD, Plaa GL. Relative effects of various chlorinated hydrocarbons on liver and kidney functions in dogs. Toxicol Appl Pharmacol 10:119, 1975.

365. Strubelt U. Interactions between ethanol and other hepatotoxic agents. Biochem Pharmacol 29:1445, 1980.

366. Traiger GJ, Plaa GL. Relationship of alcohol metabolism to the potentiation of CCl4 hepatotoxicity induced by aliphatic alcohols. J Pharmacol Exp Ther 183:481, 1971.

367. Finley BL, Ashley PJ, Neptune AG, et al. Substrate-selective induction of rabbit hepatic UDP-glucuronosyltransferases by ethanol and other xenobiotics. Biochem Pharmacol 35:2875, 1986.

368. Bodd E, Gadebolt G, Christensson PI, et al. Mechanisms behind the inhibitory effect of ethanol on the conjugation of morphine in rat hepatocytes. J Pharmacol Exp Ther 239:887, 1986.

369. Sieg A, Seitz HK. Increased production, hepatic conjugation, and biliary secretion of bilirubin in the rat after chronic ethanol consumption. Gastroenterology 93:261, 1987.

370. Sweeny DJ, Reinke LA. Effect of ethanol feeding on hepatic microsomal UDP-glycuronyltransferase activity. Biochem Pharmacol 36:1381, 1987.

371. Moldeus P, Anderson B, Norling AI. Interaction of ethanol oxidation with glucuronidation in isolated hepatocytes. Biochem Pharmacol 27:2583, 1978.

372. Reinke LA, Moyer MJ, Notley KA. Diminished rates of glucuronidation and sulfation in perfused rat liver after chronic ethanol administration. Biochem Pharmacol 35:439, 1986.

373. Price VF, Miller MG, Jollow DJ. Mechanisms of fasting-induced potentiation of acetaminophen hepatotoxicity in the rat. Biochem Pharmacol 36:427, 1987.

374. Olsen H, Morland J. Ethanol-induced increase in drug acetylation in man and isolated rat liver cells. Br Med J 2:1260, 1978.

375. Olsen H. Interaction between drug acetylation and ethanol, acetate, pyruvate, citrate, and L-carnitine in isolated rat liver parenchymal cell. Acta Pharmacol Toxicol 50:67, 1982.

376. Moldeus P, Andersson B, Norling A, et al. Effect of chronic ethanol administration on drug metabolism in isolated hepatocytes with emphasis on paracetamol activation. Biochem Pharmacol 29:1741, 1980.

377. Sato C, Matsuda Y, Lieber CS. Increased hepatotoxicity of acetaminophen after chronic ethanol consumption in the rat. Gastroenterology 80:140, 1981.

378. Licht H, Seeff LB, Zimmermann HJ. Apparent potentiation of acetaminophen hepatotoxicity by alcohol. Ann Intern Med 92:511, 1980.

379. Leist MH, Gluskin LE, Payne JA. Enhanced toxicity of acetaminophen in alcoholics: report of three cases. J Clin Gastroenterol 7:55, 1985.

380. Seeff LB, Cuccherini BA, Zimmermann HJ, et al. Acetaminophen hepatotoxicity in alcoholics. Ann Intern Med 104:399, 1986.

381. Altomare E, Leo MA, Sato C, et al. Interaction of ethanol with acetaminophen metabolism in the baboon. Biochem Pharmacol 33:2207, 1984.

382. Dingle JT, Lucy JA. Vitamin A carotenoids and cell function. Biol Rev Cambridge Philosophic Soc 40:422, 1965.

383. Lucy JA. Some possible roles for vitamin A in membranes: micelle formation and electron transfer. Am J Clin Nutr 22:1033, 1969.

384. Roels OA, Anderson OR, Lui NST, et al. Vitamin A and membranes. Am J Clin Nutr 22:1020, 1969.

385. Thompson JN, Pitt GAJ. Vitamin A acid and hypervitaminosis A. Nature 188:672, 1960.

386. Nettesheim P, Williams MI. The influence of vitamin A on the susceptibility of the rat lung to 3-methylcholanthrene. Int J Cancer 17:351, 1976.

387. Josephs HW. Hypervitaminosis A. Am J Dis Child 67:33, 1944.

388. Stimson WH. Vitamin A intoxication in adults: report of case with a summary of the literature. N Engl J Med 265:369, 1961.

389. Soler-Bicheva J, Joscia JL. Chronic hypervitaminosis A: report of a case in an adult. Arch Intern Med 112:462, 1963.

390. Lane BP. Hepatic microanatomy in hypervitaminosis A in man and rat. Am J Pathol 53:591, 1968.

391. Rubin E, Floorman AF, Degnan T, et al. Hepatic injury in chronic hypervitaminosis A. Am J Dis Child 119:132, 1970.

392. Muenter MD, Perry HO, Ludwig J. Chronic vitamin A intoxication in adults. Hepatic, neurologic and dermatologic complications. Am J Med 50:129, 1971.

393. Personal Communication.

394. Russell RM, Boyer JL, Baghesi SA, et al. Hepatic injury from chronic hypervitaminosis A resulting in portal hypertension and ascites. N Engl J Med 291:435, 1974.

395. Popper H, Steigman F, Meyer KA, et al. Relation between hepatic and plasma concentrations of vitamin A in human beings. Arch Intern Med 72:439, 1943.

396. Roberts AB, Nichols MD, Newton DL, et al. In vitro metabolism of retinoic acid in hamster intestine and liver. J Biol Clin 254:6296, 1979.

397. Roberts AB, Frolik CA. Recent advances in the in vivo and in vitro metabolism of retinoic acid. Fed Proc 38:2524, 1979.

398. Sato M, Lieber CS. Increased metabolism of retinoic acid after chronic ethanol consumption in rat liver microsomes. Arch Biochem Biophys 213:551, 1982.

399. Sato M, Lieber CS. Hepatic vitamin A depletion after chronic ethanol consumption in baboons and rats. J Nutr 111:2015, 1981.

400. Sato M, Lieber CS. Changes in vitamin A status after acute ethanol administration in the rat. J Nutr 112:1188, 1982.

401. Leo MA, Lieber CS. Hepatic vitamin A depletion in alcoholic liver injury in man. N Engl J Med 137:597, 1982.

402. Mobarhan S, Layden TJ, Friedman H, et al. Depletion of liver and esophageal epithelium vitamin A after chronic moderate ethanol consumption in rats: inverse relation to zinc nutriture. Hepatology 6:615, 1986.

403. Leo MA, Arai M, Sato M, et al. Hepatotoxicity of vitamin A and ethanol in the rat. Gastroenterology 82:194, 1982.

404. Leo MA, Lieber CS. Interactions of ethanol with vitamin A. Alcohol Clin Exp Res 7:15, 1983.

405. Zetterman R, Luisada-Opper A, Leevy C. Alcoholic hepatitis. Cell-mediated immunological response to alcoholic hyaline. Gastroenterology 70:382, 1976.

406. MacSween RNA, Anthony RS, Farquharson M. Antibodies to alcohol altered hepatocytes in patients with alcoholic liver disease. Lancet ii:803, 1981.

407. Paronetto F. Immunologic factors in alcoholic liver diseases. Semin Liver Dis 1:232, 1981.

408. Kater L, Jobsis AC, Baart de la Faille-Kuyper EH, et al. Alcoholic hepatic disease: specificity of IgA deposits in liver. Am J Clin Pathol 71:51, 1970.

409. MacSween RNM, Anthony RS. Review: immune mechanisms in alcoholic liver disease. J Clin Lab Immunol 9:1, 1982.

410. Swerdlow MA, Chowdhury LN, Hoon T. Patterns of IgA deposition in liver tissues in alcoholic liver disease. Am J Clin Pathol 77:259, 1982.

411. McKay I. Genetic aspects of immunologically mediated liver disease. Semin Liver Dis 4:13, 1984.

412. Jovanovic R, Worner T, Lieber CS, et al. Lymphocyte subpopulations in patients with alcoholic liver disease. Dig Dis Sci 31:125, 1986.

413. Israel Y, Hurwitz E, Niemela O, et al. Monoclonal and polyclonal antibodies against acetaldehyde-containing epitopes and acetaldehyde-protein adducts. Proc Natl Acad Sci USA 83:7923, 1986.

414. Immunological abnormalities in alcoholic liver disease. (Editorial.) Lancet ii:605, 1983.

415. Parent LJ, Ehrlich R, Matis L, et al. Ethanol: an enhancer of major histocompatibility complex antigen expression. FASEB J 1:469, 1987.

416. Orrego H, Israel Y, Blendis LM. Alcoholic liver disease: information in search of knowledge. Hepatology 1:267, 1981.

417. Galambos J. Natural history of alcoholic hepatitis. III. Histological changes. Gastroenterology 63:1026, 1972.

418. Cuccurullo L, Rambaldi M, Iaquinto G, et al. Importance of showing HBsAg and HBcAg positivity in the liver for better etiological definition of chronic liver disease. J Clin Pathol 40:167, 1987.

419. Rojkind M, Dunn M. Hepatic fibrosis. Gastroenterology 76:849, 1979.

420. Rojkind M, Kershenobick D. Effect of colchicine on collagen, albumin and transferrin synthesis by cirrhotic rat liver slices. Biochim Biophys Acta 378:415, 1975.

421. Resnick R, Boitnolt J, Iber F, et al. Preliminary observations of d-penicillamine therapy in acute alcoholic liver disease. Digestion 11:257, 1974.

422. Ruwart MJ, Rush BD, Snyder KF, et al. 16,16-dimethyl prostaglandin E$_2$ delays collagen formation in nutritional injury in the rat liver. Hepatology 8:61, 1988.

423. Chojkier M, Brenner DA. Therapeutic strategies for hepatic fibrosis. Hepatology 8:176, 1988.

424. Wickramasinghe SN, Bond AN, Sloviter HA, et al. Metabolism of ethanol by human bone marrow cells. Acta Haematol 66:238, 1981.

425. Wickramasinghe SN. Observations on the biochemical basis of ethanol metabolism by human macrophages. Alcohol Alcohol 21:57, 1986.

426. Wickramasinghe SN. Supernatants from ethanol-containing macrophage cultures have cytotoxic activity. Alcohol Alcohol 21:263, 1986.

427. Wickramasinghe SN. Role of macrophages in the pathogenesis of alcohol-induced tissue damage. Br Med J [Clin Res] 294:1137, 1987.

428. Wickramasinghe SN, Gardner B, Barden G. Circulating cytotoxic protein generated after ethanol consumption: identification and mechanism of reaction with cells. Lancet ii:122, 1987.

429. Akira T, Porta EA, Hartroft WS. Regression of a dietary cirrhosis in rats fed alcohol and a "super diet." Evidence for the nonhepatotoxic nature of ethanol. Am J Clin Nutr 20:213, 1967.

430. Gomez-Dumm CLA, Porta EA, Hartroft WS, et al. A new experimental approach in the study of chronic alcoholism. II. Effects of high alcohol intake in rats fed diets of various adequacies. Lab Invest 18:365, 1968.

431. Koch OR, Porta EA, Hartroft WS. A new experimental approach in the study of chronic alcoholism. III. Role of alcohol versus sucrose- or fat-derived calories in hepatic damage. Lab Invest 18:379, 1968.

432. Koch OR, Porta EA, Hartroft WS. A new experimental approach in the study of chronic alcoholism. V. "Superdiet." Lab Invest 21:298, 1969.

433. Porta EA, Koch OR, Hartroft WS. Recovery from chronic hepatic lesions in rats fed alcohol and a solid superdiet. Am J Clin Nutr 25:881, 1972.

434. Hartroft WS. The liver—nutritional guardian of the body. In: Gall EA, Mostofi FK, eds. The Liver. Baltimore, Williams and Wilkins, 1973:131.

435. Klatskin G, Krehl WA, Conn HO. Effect of alcohol on choline requirement: changes in rat's liver following prolonged ingestion of alcohol. J Exp Med 100:605, 1954.

436. Fallon HJ, Gertman PM, Kemp ED. The effects of ethanol ingestion and choline deficiency on hepatic lecithin biosynthesis in the rat. Biochim Biophys Acta 187:94, 1969.

437. Tuma DJ, Keefer RC, Beckenhauer HC, et al. Effect of ethanol on uptake of choline by the isolated perfused rat liver. Biochim Biophys Acta 218:141, 1970.

438. Thompson JA, Reitz RC. Studies on the acute and chronic effects of ethanol ingestion on choline oxidation. Ann NY Acad Sci 273:194, 1976.

439. Rutenberg AM, Sonnenblick E, Koven E, et al. Role of intestinal

bacteria in the development of dietary cirrhosis in rats. J Exp Med 106:1, 1957.

440. Rao GA, Tsukamoto H, Larkin EC, et al. Nutritional inadequacy of diets for young growing rats used in models of chronic alcohol ingestion. Biochem Arch 1:97, 1985.

441. Frank O, Baker H. Vitamin profile in rats fed starch and liquid ethanolic diets. Am J Clin Nutr 33:221, 1980.

442. Rao GA, Larkin EC, Porta EA. Two decades of chronic alcoholism research with the misconception that liver damage occurred despite adequate nutrition. Biochem Arch 2:223, 1986.

443. Mezey E. Intestinal function in chronic alcoholism. Ann NY Acad Sci 252:215, 1975.

444. Pinto J, Huang YA, Rivlin RS. Mechanisms underlying the differential effects of ethanol on the bioavailability of riboflavin and flavin adenine dinucleotide. J Clin Invest 79:1343, 1984.

445. Mezey E, Potter JJ. Changes in exocrine pancreatic function produced by altered protein intake in drinking alcoholics. Johns Hopkins Med J 138:7, 1976.

446. Roggin GM, Iber FL, Kater RMH, Tobon F. Malabsorption in the chronic alcoholic. Johns Hopkins Med J 125:321, 1969.

447. Sarles H, Figarella C, Clemente F. The interaction of ethanol, dietary lipid and proteins on the pancreas. Digestion 4:13, 1971.

448. Tsukamoto H, French SW, Benson N, et al. Severe and progressive steatosis and focal necrosis in rat liver induced by continuous intragastric injustion of ethanol and low fat diet. Hepatology 5:224, 1985.

449. Tsukamoto H, Towner SJ, Ciofalo LM, et al. Ethanol-induced liver fibrosis in rats fed high fat diet. Hepatology 6:814, 1986.

450. Rubin E, Lieber CS. Fatty liver, alcoholic hepatitis and cirrhosis produced by alcohol in primates. N Engl J Med 290:128, 1974.

451. Lieber CS, DeCarli LM, Rubin E. Sequential production of fatty liver, hepatitis, and cirrhosis in subhuman primates fed ethanol with adequate diets. Proc Natl Acad Sci USA 72:437, 1975.

452. Wilgram GF. Experimental Laennec type of cirrhosis in monkeys. Ann Intern Med 51:1134, 1959.

453. Gaisford WD, Zuidema GD. Nutritional Laennec's cirrhosis in the Macaca mulatta monkey. J Surg Res 5:220, 1965.

454. Patek AJ Jr, Bowry S, Hayes KC. Cirrhosis of choline deficiency in rhesus monkey. Possible role of dietary cholesterol. Proc Soc Exp Biol Med 148:370, 1975.

455. Rogers AE, Fox JG, Whitney K, et al. Acute and chronic effects of ethanol in non human primates. In: Hayes KC, ed. Primates in Nutritional Research. New York, Academic Press, 1979:249.

455a. Mezey E, Potter JJ, French SW, et al. Effect of chronic ethanol feeding on hepatic collagen in the monkey. Hepatology 3:41, 1983.

456. Lieber CS, Leo MA, Mak KM, et al. Choline fails to prevent liver fibrosis in ethanol-fed baboons but causes toxicity. Hepatology 5:561, 1985.

457. Barak AJ, Beckewhauser HC, Tuma DJ, et al. Effects of prolonged ethanol feeding on methionine metabolism in rat liver. Biochem Cell Biol 65:230, 1987.

458. Reynolds TB, Redeker AG, Kuzma OT. Role of alcohol in pathogenesis of alcoholic cirrhosis. In: McIntyre NM, Sherlock S, eds. Therapeutic Agents and the Liver. Oxford, Blackwell, 1965:131.

459. Patek AJ, Post J. Treatment of cirrhosis of the liver by a nutritious diet and supplements rich in vitamins. J Clin Invest 20:481, 1941.

460. Volwiler W, Jones CM, Mallory TM. Criteria for the measurement of results of treatment in fatty cirrhosis. Gastroenterology 11:164, 1948.

461. Summerskill WHJ, Wolfe SJ, Davidson CS. Response to alcohol in chronic alcoholics with liver disease. Lancet 1:335, 1957.

462. Erenoglu E, Edreira JG, Patek AJ Jr. Observations on patients with Laennec's cirrhosis receiving alcohol while on controlled diets. Ann Intern Med 60:814, 1964.

463. Froesch ER. Essential fructosuria, hereditary fructose intolerance, and fructose-1,6-diphosphatase deficiency. In: Stanbury JB, Wyngaarden JB, Fredrickson DS, eds. The Metabolic Basis of Inherited Disease. Fourth edition. New York, McGraw-Hill, 1978:121.

464. Blass JP, Gibson GE. Abnormality of thiamine-requiring enzyme in patients with Wernicke-Korsakoff syndrome. N Engl J Med 297:1367, 1977.

465. Mukerjee AB, Svoronos S, Ghazanfari A, et al. An abnormality of transketolase in cultured fibroblasts from familial chronic alcoholic men and their male offspring. J Clin Invest 79:1039, 1987.

466. Mitchell MC, Herlong HF. Alcohol and nutrition: caloric value, bioenergetics, and relationship to liver damage. Ann Rev Nutr 6:457, 1986.

467. Mezey E. Liver disease and protein needs. Ann Rev Nutr 2:21, 1982.

468. World MJ, Ryle PR, Thomson AD. Alcoholic malnutrition and the small intestine. Alcohol Alcohol 20:89, 1985.

469. Mendenhall CL, Anderson S, Weesner RE, et al. Protein-calorie malnutrition associated with alcoholic hepatitis. Am J Med 76:211, 1984.

470. Mills PR, Shenkin A, Anthony RS, et al. Assessment of nutritional status and in vivo immune response in alcohol liver disease. Am J Clin Nutr 38:849, 1983.

471. Simko V, Connell AM, Banks B. Nutritional status in alcoholics with and without liver disease. Am J Clin Nutr 35:197, 1982.

472. Hurt RD, Higgins JA, Nelson RA, et al. Nutritional status of alcoholics before and after admission to an alcoholism treatment unit. Am J Clin Nutr 34:386, 1981.

473. Bunout D, Gattas V, Iturriaga H, et al. Nutritional status of alcoholic patients: its possible relationship to alcoholic liver disease. Am J Clin Nutr 38:469, 1983.

474. Patek AJ Jr, Toth IG, Sanders GA, et al. Alcohol and dietary factors in cirrhosis. An epidemiologic study of 304 alcoholic patients. Arch Intern Med 135:1053, 1975.

475. Small M, Longarini A, Zamcheck N. Disturbances of digestive physiology following acute drinking episodes in skid row alcoholics. Am J Med 27:575, 1959.

476. Leevy CM, Baker N, Ten-Hove W, et al. B-complex vitamins in liver disease of the alcoholic. Am J Clin Nutr 16:399, 1965.

477. Neville JN, Eagles JA, Samson G, et al. Nutritional status of alcoholics. Am J Clin Nutr 21:1329, 1968.

478. Pekkanen L, Forsander O. Nutritional implications of alcoholism. Nutr Bull 4:91, 1977.

479. Norton VP. Interrelationship of nutrition and voluntary alcohol consumption in experimental animals. Br J Addiction 72:205, 1977.

480. Korsten MA, Lieber CS. Nutrition in the alcoholic. Med Clin North Am 63:963, 1979.

481. Shibata HR, MacKenzie JR, Huary S-N. Morphological changes of the liver following small intestinal bypass for obesity. Arch Surg 103:229, 1971.

482. Kern WH, Payne JH, Dewind IT. Hepatic changes after small intestinal bypass for morbid obesity. Am J Clin Pathol 61:763, 1974.

483. Marrubbio AT, Buchwald H, Schwartz MZ, et al. Hepatic lesions of central pericellular fibrosis in morbid obesity, and after jejunoileal bypass. Am J Clin Pathol 66:684, 1976.

484. Galambos J, Willis C. Relationship between 505 paired liver tests and biopsies in 242 obese patients. Gastroenterology 74:11191, 1978.

485. Adler M, Schaffner F. Fatty liver, hepatitis and cirrhosis in obese patients. Am J Med 67:811, 1979.

486. Peters RL, Gay T, Reynolds TB. Post jejunoileal-bypass hepatic disease: its similarity to alcoholic hepatic disease. Am J Clin Pathol 63:318, 1975.

487. Galambos JT. Jejunoileal bypass and nutritional liver injury. Arch Pathol Med 100:229, 1976.

488. Iber FL, Cooper M. Jejunoileal bypass for the treatment of massive obesity. Prevalence, morbidity, and short- and long-term consequences. Am J Clin Nutr 30:4, 1977.

489. Moxley RT, Pozefsky T, Lockwood DH. Protein nutrition and liver disease after jejunoileal bypass for morbid obesity. N Engl J Med 290:921, 1974.

490. Campbell JM, Hunt TK, Karam JH, et al. Jejunoileal bypass as a treatment of morbid obesity. Arch Intern Med 135:602, 1977.

491. Sherr HP, Nair PP, White JJ, et al. Bile acid metabolism and hepatic disease following small bowel bypass for obesity. Am J Clin Nutr 27:1369, 1974.

492. Heimburger SL, Steiger E, Logerfo P, et al. Reversal of severe fatty hepatic infiltration after intestinal bypass for morbid obesity by calorie-free amino acid infusion. Am J Surg 129:1975.

493. Pequignot G, Tuyns AS, Berta JL. Ascitic cirrhosis in relation to alcohol consumption. Intl J Epidemiol 7:113, 1978.

494. Lieber CS. Ethanol and the liver: a decreasing "threshold" of toxicity. Am J Clin Nutr 32:1177, 1979.

495. Loft S, Olesen K-L, Dossing M. Increased susceptibility to liver disease in relation to alcohol consumption in women. Scand J Gastroenterol 22:1251, 1987.

496. Levi AJ, Chalmer DM. Recognition of alcoholic liver disease in a district general hospital. Gut 19:521, 1978.

497. Bruguera M, Bordas JM, Rodes J. Asymptomatic liver disease in alcoholics. Arch Pathol Lab Med 101:644, 1977.

498. Skude G. Amylase, hepatic enzymes and bilirubin in serum of chronic alcoholics. Acta Med Scand 201:53, 1977.

499. Salaspuro M. Use of enzymes for the diagnosis of alcohol-related organ damage. Enzyme 37:87, 1987.

500. VanWaes L, Lieber C. Glutamate dehydrogenase: a reliable marker of liver cell necrosis in the alcoholic. Br Med J 2:1508, 1977.

501. Cohen J, Kaplan M. The SGOT/SGPT ratio—an indicator of alcoholic liver injury. Dig Dis Sci 24:835, 1979.

502. Ludwig S, Kaplowitz N. Effect of pyridoxine deficiency on serum and liver transaminases in experimental liver injury in the rat. Gastroenterology 79:545, 1980.

503. Matloff D, Selinger M, Kaplan M. Hepatic transaminase activity in alcoholic liver disease. Gastroenterology 76:1195, 1979.

504. Diehl AM, Potter S, Boitnott J, et al. Relationship between pyridoxal

S¹-phosphate deficiency and aminotransferase levels in alcoholic hepatitis. Gastroenterology 86:632, 1984.

505. Rosalki S, Rau D, Lehmann D, et al. Determination of serum-glutamyltranspeptidase activity and its clinical applications. Annu Clin Biochem 7:143, 1970.

506. Rollason JG, Pincherle D, Robinson D. Serum gamma-glutamyltranspeptidase in relation to alcohol consumption. Clin Chim Acta 39:75, 1972.

507. Spencer-Peet J, Wood D, Glatt M. Screening test for alcoholism. Lancet 2:1089, 1973.

508. Fink R, Rosalki S. Clinical biochemistry of alcoholism. Clin Endocrinol Metab 7:297, 1978.

509. Whitfield J, Moss D, Neal G, et al. Changes in plasma-glutamyltranspeptidase activity associated with alterations in drug metabolism in man. Br Med J 1:316, 1973.

510. Morland J, Huseby NE, Sjoblum M, et al. Does chronic alcohol consumption really induce hepatic microsomal gamma-glutamyltransferase activity. Biochem Biophys Res Commun 77:1060, 1977.

511. Zein M, Discombe D. Serum gamma-glutamyltranspeptidase as a diagnostic aid. Lancet 2:748, 1970.

512. Freer DE. Effects of ethanol on the activity of selected enzymes in sera of healthy young adults. Clin Chem 23:2099, 1977.

513. Shaw S, Stimmel B, Lieber C. Plasma alpha amino-N-butyric acid to leucine ratio: an empirical biochemical marker of alcoholism. Science 194:1057, 1976.

514. Morgan M, Milsom J, Sherlock S. Ratio of plasma alpha-amino-N-butyric acid to leucine as an empirical marker of alcoholism: diagnostic value. Science 197:1183, 1977.

515. Dienstag J, Carter E, Wands J, et al. Plasma α-amino-N-butyric acid to leucine ratio: nonspecificity as a marker for alcoholism. Gastroenterology 75:561, 1978.

516. Mezey E. Ratio of plasma-α-amino-N-butyric acid to leucine in alcoholism. Gastroenterology 75:742, 1978.

517. Jenkins WJ, Rosalki SB, Foo Y, et al. Serum glutamate dehydrogenase is not a reliable marker of liver cell necrosis in alcoholics. J Clin Pathol 35:207, 1982.

518. Mills PR, Spooner RS, Russell RI, et al. Serum glutamate dehydrogenase as a marker of hepatocyte necrosis in alcoholic liver disease. Br Med J 23:754, 1981.

519. Nalpas B, Vassault A, Guillon AL, et al. Serum activity of mitochondrial aspartate aminotransferase: a sensitive marker of alcoholism with or without alcoholic hepatitis. Hepatology 4:893, 1984.

520. Morse R, Hurt R. Screening for alcoholism. JAMA 242:2688, 1979.

521. Levin DM, Baker AL, Rochman H, et al. Nonalcoholic liver disease: overlooked causes of liver injury in patients with heavy alcohol consumption. Am J Med 66:429, 1979.

522. Rubin E, Lieber C. Alcohol-induced hepatic injury in nonalcoholic volunteers. N Engl J Med 278:869, 1968.

523. Leevy C. Fatty liver: a study of 270 patients with biopsy proven fatty liver and a review of the literature. Medicine 41:249, 1962.

524. Creutzfeldt W, Frerichs H, Sickinger K. Liver diseases and diabetes mellitus. In: Popper H, Schaffner F, eds. Progress in Liver Diseases. III. New York, Grune and Stratton, 1970:371.

525. Massarrat S, Jordan G, Sahrhase G, et al. Follow-up study of patients with non-alcoholic and non-diabetic fatty liver. Acta Hepato-Gastroenterol 26:296, 1979.

526. Nakano M, Worner TM, Lieber CS. Perivenular fibrosis in alcoholic liver injury: ultrastructural and histologic progression. Gastroenterology 83:777, 1982.

527. VanWaes L, Lieber C. Early perivenular sclerosis in alcoholic fatty liver: an index of progressive liver injury. Gastroenterology 73:646, 1977.

528. Marbet UA, Bianchi L, Menry U, et al. Long-term histological evaluation of the natural history and prognostic factors of alcoholic liver disease. J Hepatol 4:364, 1987.

529. Falchuk K, Fiske S, Haggitt M, et al. Pericentral hepatic fibrosis and intracellular hyalin in diabetes mellitus. Gastroenterology 78:735, 1980.

530. Itoh S, Yougel T, Kawagoe K. Comparison between nonalcoholic steatohepatitis and alcoholic hepatitis. Am J Gastroenterol 82:650, 1987.

531. Morgan M, Sherlock S, Scheuer P. Acute cholestasis, hepatic failure and fatty liver in the alcoholic. Scand J Gastroenterol 13:299, 1978.

532. Lynch M, Raphael S, Dixon T. Fat embolism in chronic alcoholism. Arch Pathol 67:68, 1959.

533. Edmondson H, Peters R, Reynolds T, et al. Sclerosing hyaline necrosis of the liver in the chronic alcoholic. Ann Intern Med 59:646, 1963.

534. Birschback R, Harinasutau U, Zimmerman H. Alcoholic steatonecrosis. Gastroenterology 66:1195, 1974.

535. Popper H, Szanto P, Parthasarathy M. Florid cirrhosis, a review of 35 cases. Am J Clin Pathol 25:889, 1955.

536. Galambos J. Alcoholic hepatitis. In: Schaffner F, Sherlock S, Leevy

C, eds. The Liver and Its Diseases. New York, Intercontinental Medical Book Co, 1974:255.

537. French S, Burbige E. Alcoholic hepatitis: clinical, morphologic, pathogenic and therapeutic aspects. In: Popper H, Schaffner F, eds. Progress in Liver Diseases. VI. New York, Grune and Stratton, 1979:557.

538. Perrillo RP, Griffin P, Deschryver-Kecskemeti K, et al. Alcoholic liver disease presenting with marked elevation of serum alkaline phosphatase. A combined clinical and pathologic study. Am J Dig Dis 23:1061, 1978.

539. Mikkelson WP, Turrill F, Kern WH. Acute hyaline necrosis of the liver: a surgical trap. Am J Surg 116:266, 1968.

540. Maddrey W, Boitnott J, Bedine M, et al. Corticosteroid therapy of alcoholic hepatitis. Gastroenterology 75:193, 1978.

541. Helman R, Temko M, Nye S. Alcoholic hepatitis: natural history and evaluation of prednisolone therapy. Ann Intern Med 74:311, 1971.

542. Campra S, Hamlin E, Kirshbaum R, et al. Prednisone therapy of acute alcoholic hepatitis. Ann Intern Med 79:125, 1973.

543. Maddrey W. Alcoholic hepatitis: clinicopathologic features and therapy. Semin Liver Dis 8:91, 1988.

544. Goldberg S, Mendenhall C, Anderson S, et al. VA cooperative study on alcoholic hepatitis. IV. The significance of clinically mild alcoholic hepatitis—describing the population with minimal hyperbilirubinemia. Am J Gastroenterol 81:1029, 1986.

545. Alexander JF, Lischner W, Galambos J. Natural history of alcoholic hepatitis. II. The long term prognosis. Gastroenterology 56:515, 1971.

546. Galambos J. Natural history of alcoholic hepatitis. III. Histologic changes. Gastroenterology 63:1026, 1972.

547. Sorensen T, Orholm M, Bentsen K, et al. Prospective evaluation of alcohol abuse and alcoholic liver injury in men as predictors of development of cirrhosis. Lancet 2:241, 1984.

548. Reynolds T, Hidemura R, Michel H, et al. Portal hypertension without cirrhosis in alcoholic liver disease. Ann Intern Med 70:497, 1969.

549. Conn HL. Cirrhosis. In: Schiff L, ed. Diseases of the Liver. Philadelphia, JB Lippincott, 1975:833.

550. Popper H, Liever CS. Histogenesis of alcoholic fibrosis and cirrhosis in the baboon. Am J Pathol 98:695, 1980.

551. Bean WB. The cutaneous arterial spider. Medicine 24:243, 1945.

552. Muehrcke RC. The finger-nails in chronic hypoalbuminemia. A new physical sign. Br Med J 1:1327, 1956.

553. Terry R. White nails in hepatic cirrhosis. Lancet 1:757, 1964.

554. Wolfe J, Summerskill WH, Davidson CS. Thickening and contraction of the palmar fascia (Dupuytren's contracture) associated with alcoholism and hepatic cirrhosis. N Engl J Med 255:559, 1956.

555. Edmonson HA. Pathology of alcoholism. Am J Clin Pathol 74:725, 1980.

555a. Powell W, Klatskin G. Duration of survival in patients with Laennec's cirrhosis. Am J Med 44:406, 1956.

556. Soterakis J, Resnick R, Iber F. Effect of alcohol abstinence on survival in cirrhotic portal hypertension. Lancet 2:65, 1973.

557. Gluud C, et al. Testosterone treatment of men with alcoholic cirrhosis: a double-blind study. Hepatology 5:807, 1986.

558. Pande N, Resnick R, Yee W, et al. Cirrhotic portal hypertension: morbidity of continued alcoholism. Gastroenterology 74:64, 1978.

559. Reynolds TB. Good news for drinkers—or is it? Gastroenterology 74:153, 1978.

560. Personal communication.

561. Orrego H, Blendis L, Blake J, et al. Reliability of assessment of alcohol intake based on personal interviews in a liver clinic. Lancet 2:1354, 1979.

562. Lesesne HR, Bozymicki E, Fallon H. Treatment of alcoholic hepatitis with encephalopathy. Comparison of prednisolone with caloric supplements. Gastroenterology 79:169, 1978.

563. Porter HP, Simon F, Pope C, et al. Corticosteroid therapy in severe alcoholic hepatitis. N Engl J Med 284:1350, 1971.

564. Depew W, Boyer TB, Omata M, et al. Double-blind controlled trial of prednisolone therapy in patients with severe acute alcoholic hepatitis and spontaneous encephalopathy. Gastroenterology 78:524, 1980.

565. Blitzer B, Mutchnick M, Joshi P, et al. Adrenocorticosteroid therapy in alcoholic hepatitis. Am J Dig Dis 22:477, 1977.

566. Mendenhall CL, Anderson S, Garcia-Point P, et al. Short-term and long-term survival in patients with alcoholic hepatitis treated with oxandrolone and prednisolone. N Engl J Med 311:1464, 1984.

567. Maddrey W, Carithers R, Herlong H, et al. Prednisolone therapy in patients with severe alcoholic hepatitis: results of a multi-center trial. Hepatology 6:1202, 1986.

568. Theodossi A, Eddleston A, Williams R. Controlled trial of methyl prednisolone therapy in severe acute alcoholic hepatitis. Gut 23:75, 1982.

569. Shumaker J, Resnick R, Galambos J, et al. A controlled trial of 6-

methylprednisolone in acute alcoholic hepatitis. Am J Gastroenterol 69:443, 1978.

570. Gluud C, Christoffersen P, Eriksen J, et al. No effect of long-term oral testosterone treatment on liver morphology in men with alcoholic cirrhosis. Am J Gastroenterol 82:660, 1987.

571. Kershenobick D, Uribe M, Suarez O, et al. Treatment of cirrhosis with colchicine. A double-blind randomized trial. Gastroenterology 77:532, 1979.

572. Kershenobich D, Vargas F, Garcia-Tsau G, et al. Colchicine in the treatment of cirrhosis of the liver. N Eng J Med 318:1709, 1988.

573. Halle P, Pare P, Kaptein E, et al. Propylthiouracil therapy in severe acute alcoholic hepatitis. (Abstract.) Gastroenterology 79:1024, 1980.

574. Propylthiouracil and alcoholic liver disease. (Editorial.) Lancet 1:450, 1988.

575. Achord J. Malnutrition and the role of nutritional support in alcoholic liver disease. Am J Gastroenterol 82:1, 1987.

576. Mendenhall C, Tosch T, Weesner R, et al. VA cooperative study on alcoholic hepatitis. II. Prognostic significance of protein-calorie malnutrition. Am J Clin Nutr 43:213, 1986.

577. Nasrallah S, Galambos JT. Aminoacid therapy of alcoholic hepatitis. Lancet 2:1276, 1980.

578. Diehl A, Boitnott J, Herlong G, et al. Effect of parenteral amino acid supplementation in alcoholic hepatitis. Hepatology 5:57, 1985.

579. Naveau S, Pelletier G, Poynard T, et al. A randomized clinical trial of supplementary pareneral nutrition in jaundiced alcoholic cirrhotic patients. Hepatology 6:270, 1986.

580. Calvey H, Davis M, Williams R. Controlled trial of nutritional supplementation with or without branched-chain amino acid enrichment in the treatment of acute alcoholic hepatitis. J Hepatol 1:141, 1985.

581. Mendenhall C, Bongiovanni G, Goldberg S, et al. VA cooperative study on alcoholic hepatitis III: Changes in protein-calorie malnutrition associated with 30 days of hospitalization with and without enteral nutritional therapy. 9:590, 1985.

582. Baker A, Jaspan J, Haines N, et al. A randomized clinical trial of insulin and glucagon infusion for treatment of alcoholic hepatitis: progress report in 50 patients. Gastroenterology 84:1410, 1981.

583. Feher J, Cornides A, Romony A, et al. A prospective multicenter study of insulin and glucagon infusion therapy.

584. Bove KE, McAdams KJ, Partin JC, et al. The hepatic lesion in Reye's syndrome. Gastroenterology 69:685, 1975.

585. Combes B. Tetracycline in man. In: Gerok W, Sickinger K, eds. Proceedings III International Symposium: Drugs and Liver. Stuttgart, Schattaner, 1973:263.

586. Kunelis CT, Peters RL, Edmondson HA. Fatty liver of pregnancy and its relationship to tetracycline therapy. Am J Med 38:359, 1965.

587. French SW. The Mallory body: structure, composition, and pathogenesis. Hepatology 1:76, 1981.

588. Sternlieb I. Evolution of the hepatic lesion in Wilson's disease (hepatolenticular degeneration). In: Popper H, Schaffner F, eds. Progress in Liver Diseases. IV. New York, Grune and Stratton, 1973:511.

589. Monroe S, French SW, Zamboni L. Mallory bodies in a case of primary biliary cirrhosis: an ultrastructural and morphogenetic study. Am J Clin Pathol 59:254, 1973.

590. Partin JS, Partin JC, Schubert WK, et al. Liver ultrastructure in abetalipoproteinemia: evolution of micronodular cirrhosis. Gastroenterology 67:107, 1974.

591. Roy S, Ramalingaswami V, Nayak NC. An ultrastructural study of the liver in Indian childhood cirrhosis with particular reference to the structure of cytoplasmic hyaline. Gut 12:693, 1971.

592. Peters RL. Patterns of hepatic morphology in jejunoileal bypass patients. Am J Clin Nutr 30:53, 1977.

593. Paliard P, Vitrey D, Fournier G, et al. Perihexiline maleate-induced hepatitis. Digestion 17:419, 1978.

594. Parcell S, Ireton J, Valencia-Mayoral P, et al. Amiodarone-associated phospholipidosis and fibrosis of the liver: light, immunohistochemical and electron microscopic studies. Gastroenterology 86:926, 1984.

595. Warnock ML, Press M, Churg A. Further observations on cytoplasmic hyaline in the lung. Hum Pathol 11:59, 1980.

596. Kuhn C III, Kuo T-T. Cytoplasmic hyalin in asbestosis. A reaction of injured alvcolar epithelium. Arch Pathol 95:190, 1973.

597. Wong T, Warner NE. Cytomegalic inclusion disease in adults: report of 14 cases with review of literature. Arch Pathol 74:403.

598. Bernstein M, Edmundson HA, Barbour BH. The liver lesion in Q-fever. Arch Intern Med 116:491, 1965.

599. Afshani P, Littenberg GD, Wollman J, et al. Significance of microscopic cholangitis in alcoholic liver disease. Gastroenterology 75:1045, 1978.

600. Edmondson HA, Peters RL, Reynolds HB, et al. Sclerosing hyaline necrosis of the liver in the chronic alcoholic. Ann Intern Med 59:646, 1963.

601. Leevy CM, Tygstrup N. Standardization of nomenclature diagnostic criteria and diagnostic methodology for diseases of the liver and biliary tract. S. Karger, Basel. In: Fogarty International Proceedings, No 22, DHEW Publication No. (NIH) 76-725, 1976, Washington, DC US Government Printing Office.

602. Rubin E, Popper H. The evolution of human cirrhosis deduced from observations in experimental animals. Medicine 46:163, 1967.

603. Millward-Sadler GH, Ryan TJ. Methotrexate-induced liver disease in psoriasis. Br J Dermatol 90:661, 1974.

604. Nayak NC, Ramalingaswami V. Indian childhood cirrhosis. Clin Gastroenterol 4:333, 1975.

34

Postoperative Hepatic Dysfunction

Geoffrey C. Farrell, M.D., F.R.A.C.P.

ABBREVIATIONS
ALT = alanine aminotransferase
AST = aspartate aminotransferase
CDF = 2-chloro-1,1-difluoroethylene
CTF = 2-chloro-1,1,1-trifluoroethane
FI_{O_2} = fraction of inspired gas that is oxygen
Pa_{O_2} = arterial partial pressure of oxygen
TFA = trifluoroacetic acid

When confronted with a problem of hepatic dysfunction in the postoperative period, the clinician needs to consider the pharmacologic effects of anesthesia on hepatic function in the normal and the diseased liver, as well as the potential of anesthetic agents to produce hepatotoxicity. It should also be borne in mind that hepatic necrosis, viral hepatitis, biliary obstruction, and other disorders of the hepatobiliary system may be present coincidentally or in response to factors such as intraoperative hypotension and hypoxia, blood transfusion, surgical trauma, other drugs,

TABLE 34–1. CAUSES OF POSTOPERATIVE HEPATIC
DYSFUNCTION

Exacerbation of pre-existent liver disease
  Viral hepatitis
  Chronic liver disease
Hepatic drug reactions
  Anesthetic agents
    Halothane hepatitis
    Methoxyflurane hepatitis
    Enflurane hepatitis
    Other anesthetic agents
  Other drugs
Post-transfusion hepatitis
Ischemic liver injury
Extrahepatic biliary obstruction
  Bile duct injury
  Choledocholithiasis
  Postoperative pancreatitis
  Acalculous cholecystitis
Poorly explained postoperative jaundice
  Increased pigment load
  Benign postoperative cholestasis
  Bacterial infection
  Multifactorial jaundice in the critically ill patient

and bacterial infection. In this chapter, each of these problems is considered as the basis for a discussion of the diagnosis (Table 34–1) and management of hepatobiliary disease in the postoperative period.

EFFECTS OF ANESTHESIA AND SURGERY ON THE NORMAL LIVER

The effects of general anesthetic agents on the liver include reduced hepatic blood flow, altered tissue oxygen content, changes in intermediary metabolism, and effects on hepatic drug metabolism. The process of surgery itself produces similar changes that add to and may often be quantitatively more important than the pharmacologic effects of anesthetic agents.

HEPATIC BLOOD FLOW

General anesthesia may produce profound reductions in hepatic blood flow.[1-5] This has been studied most extensively for halothane,[3-5] but diethyl ether, methoxyflurane,[6] cyclopropane, enflurane, fluroxene, and isoflurane all produce similar effects.[7-9] In individual cases, almost complete cessation of hepatic arterial flow has been demonstrated by arteriograms performed during halothane anesthesia.[3, 4] A proportion of the reduction in hepatic blood flow that occurs during halothane anesthesia is due to arterial hypotension, which results from the depressant effect of halothane on cardiac output and a fall in total peripheral resistance.[8, 10] However, a specific increase in hepatic vasomotor tone at the arterial, sinusoidal, or venous level has also been suggested.[3] The combination of arterial hypotension and hepatic artery vasoconstriction probably accounts for the reduction in hepatic blood flow. In one study, ether and halothane anesthesia produced a 12 and a 16 per cent reduction in hepatic blood flow, respectively.[9] However, the estimated hepatic blood flow fell an extra 6 to 10 per cent during extra-abdominal procedures such as herniorrhaphy, and it was reduced by more than 50 per cent during upper abdominal operations. In another study, methoxyflu-

rane reduced splanchnic blood flow by 50 per cent and hepatic venous oxygen tension by 30 per cent.[6]

The result of reduced hepatic blood flow, especially via the hepatic artery, which supplies about 50 per cent of the hepatic requirement for oxygen, is to reduce the hepatic supply of oxygen and hence to produce the potential for tissue hypoxia, especially in centrizonal regions.[11, 12] Also during anesthesia, hepatic extraction of oxygen may be increased relative to hepatic blood flow, thus increasing the likelihood of centrilobular hypoxia. These factors may be relevant to the exacerbation of hepatic dysfunction following surgery in patients with underlying liver disease (see later). It is also a possible explanation for tissue hypoxia, which could be important in facilitating halothane-induced hepatotoxicity (see later).

INTERMEDIARY METABOLISM

Anesthetic agents promote glycogenolysis in the isolated perfused rat liver,[13] intact rats,[14] and humans.[5] Some agents, in particular halothane, also inhibit gluconeogenesis and ureagenesis.[13, 14] Halothane probably alters intermediary metabolism by a direct mechanism, since identical changes can be produced when halothane is added to mitochondria in vitro.[15, 16] The changes appear to result from interruption of the mitochondrial electron transport chain at the stage of reduced nicotinamide adenine dinucleotide (NADH) dehydrogenase. The resultant effect is a substantially decreased tissue content of ATP.[13] All these metabolic changes reverse rapidly upon withdrawal of halothane; hence their relevance to clinically apparent hepatic dysfunction after surgery remains unclear.

HEPATIC DRUG METABOLISM

Several volatile anesthetic agents, including diethyl ether, chloroform, halothane, methoxyflurane, fluroxene, and enflurane, interact with the cytochrome P450–dependent hepatic mixed function oxidase system.[17-23] During this interaction, inhibition of drug metabolism may occur.[19, 20, 22] In some circumstances, cytochrome P450 may be destroyed by fluroxene, methoxyflurane,[20] or halothane;[22, 24–26] the potential relevance of this observation to anesthetic-induced liver injury is considered later. Anesthetic concentrations of halothane or enflurane also inhibit conjugation of sulfobromophthalein sodium by glutathione transferase[27–30] and conjugation of paracetamol by glucuronosyl transferase or sulfotransferase.[31]

Drug metabolism appears to be enhanced in the postoperative period, and general anesthetic agents are partly responsible for this effect.[32–34] Four days after minor surgery, for which halothane had been administered, antipyrine clearance was increased by 26 per cent, but in patients who had received ketamine, no change was observed.[34] In another study, antipyrine clearance appeared to be stimulated in patients given either halothane or neurolept anesthesia.[33] Antipyrine clearance was stimulated three days after a halothane anesthetic in patients who had been subjected to a short procedure (less than two hours), whereas it was impaired in those who had been subjected to a prolonged operation (more than four hours).[3, 4] It is thus difficult to separate the effects of drugs used for premedication and anesthesia and the metabolic effects of surgery itself. The stimulating effect of halothane on antipyrine metabolism, which is seen after shorter surgery, lasts for between one and four weeks.[35] It seems likely that only trace concentrations of halothane are required for induction of drug metabolism, since occupational exposure to halothane in unscavenged operating rooms increased antipyrine clearance in exposed personnel by 29 per cent.[33] It is not known whether the effects of surgery and anesthesia on drug metabolism are clinically important, but a possible effect of halothane in stimulating its own biotransformation could be relevant to halothane-induced hepatotoxicity. In contrast to halothane, enflurane anesthesia does not appear to affect antipyrine metabolism.[36]

EFFECTS OF ANESTHESIA AND SURGERY ON HEPATIC FUNCTION IN PATIENTS WITH LIVER DISEASE

ACUTE HEPATITIS

The effects of surgery and anesthesia on hepatic function in patients with hepatitis appear to depend on the etiology and chronicity of the liver disease and the type of operative procedure. These factors relate to the severity of the preoperative liver disease, to the combined effects of reduced hepatic blood flow and diminished oxygenation, and to the deleterious effects of anesthesia and surgery on intermediary metabolism in the liver. In one early series of 42 patients with viral hepatitis submitted to laparotomy,[37] there was a 10 per cent mortality and an additional 12 per cent incidence of major, nonfatal complications. Postoperative hepatic decompensation was more likely when a more extensive procedure had been performed.[37] Among 16 patients with drug-induced hepatitis, however, anesthesia was uncomplicated.[37] In another survey, 5 deaths and 4 severe exacerbations were observed among 12 patients with apparent viral hepatitis who underwent surgery.[38] As a result of these observations, several authorities have counseled against performing surgery in the presence of viral hepatitis.[39]

Among 46,923 patients submitted to surgery at the Massachusetts General Hospital, 73 patients developed clinical features of hepatic dysfunction between 12 hours and 6 weeks after general anesthesia.[40] Of these 73 patients, 30 were found to have preoperative hepatic dysfunction. The perioperative mortality among the patients with preoperative hepatic dysfunction was over 90 per cent, but it is unclear whether this represented death from fulminant hepatitis or from decompensated chronic liver disease in that the study did not distinguish between acute viral hepatitis and chronic active hepatitis. In an Australian study, Hardy and Hughes in 1968 reviewed 30 patients with presumed viral hepatitis who underwent laparotomy.[39] No adverse sequelae were observed among 14 patients with acute viral hepatitis, but 2 of 16 patients with chronic hepatitis died in the immediate postoperative period. It cannot be concluded with certainty that anesthesia and surgery cause deterioration of uncomplicated acute viral hepatitis; this is an important consideration in light of the suggestion that postoperative fulminant hepatic failure may be attributed to occult viral hepatitis.[41-44]

CHRONIC LIVER DISEASE

There is no doubt that anesthesia and surgery in patients with cirrhosis and other forms of chronic active liver disease are hazardous. Among 11,808 patients operated on for nonmalignant disease of the biliary tract over a 46-year period at Cornell Medical Center, liver disease, usually cirrhosis, was a major factor associated with postoperative mortality.[45] In another review of 33 patients with cirrhosis who had been subjected to cholecystectomy, other biliary procedures, or both, 8 deaths and 10 instances of excessive bleeding were observed.[46] The perioperative mortality was 100 per cent in five patients in whom a bile duct procedure was performed. Aranha and colleagues noted a similar experience.[47] In this study, the operative mortality for cholecystectomy in patients with cirrhosis and a normal prothrombin time was 9.3 per cent, and in those with a prolonged prothrombin time, it was 83 per cent. Dobernech and coworkers reported an increased mortality for many operative procedures in patients with cirrhosis[48] and a 35 per cent mortality for intraperitoneal operations on the alimentary tract. Jaundice and a prolonged prothrombin time were predictors of a poor outcome. These studies suggest that hepatic function is the key factor in predicting outcome of surgery in patients with chronic liver disease. This has been confirmed in a study of 38 patients with known or suspected liver disease.[49] Thirty of the 31 patients with normal preoperative aminopyrine breath tests survived; 6 of 7 patients with abnormal breath tests died. Clearly, patients with cirrhosis should be submitted to elective operative procedures only after the most careful consideration. In particular, intra-abdominal procedures or surgery on a patient with poor hepatic function should be avoided if possible.

The relative contributions of general anesthesia and surgery in causing the deterioration of liver function are difficult to assess. General anesthesia in patients with cirrhosis may exacerbate systemic hypoxemia or produce hypoxemia for the first time.[50] This circumstance may be due to suppression of cardiac output and vasodilation, resulting in pulmonary arteriovenous shunting.[50] Halothane, with its more potent vasodilatory properties, appears to be particularly liable to produce this effect, and recommendations about preoxygenation and use of other agents have been made.[50, 51] However, halothane anesthesia (without surgery) did not exacerbate hepatic dysfunction in rats with experimental cirrhosis.[52] Moreover, the varying outcomes of different types of surgery suggest that the operative procedure itself is of prime importance. Several authors have suggested that halothane is a highly satisfactory anesthetic agent for portacaval shunt surgery,[48, 53] and it may be the best agent for hepatobiliary surgery.[28, 54-57]

HALOTHANE-INDUCED HEPATIC INJURY

In this chapter, the term *halothane hepatitis* will be used synonymously with the more precise term *halothane-induced hepatic injury*. Halothane hepatitis is a rare disorder characterized by the development of clinical and biochemical features resembling acute viral hepatitis within 21 days of a halothane anesthetic.[51, 58-60] As yet, there is no generally accepted diagnostic test to prove conclusively that halothane is the cause of such a reaction.[44, 61] It is essential, therefore, that the diagnosis be made only after excluding viral hepatitis and other causes of liver disease in the postoperative period (Table 34-1).[44, 58-62] The likelihood that halothane hepatitis is the correct diagnosis is increased by a past history of unexplained postoperative fever or jaundice that was delayed in appearance after a halothane anesthetic, by the presence of eosinophilia, and by hepatic morphology suggestive of drug-induced liver injury. The problem of defining the cause has bedeviled the recognition and study of the clinical entity of halothane-induced liver injury, and some authors still prefer the term *unexplained hepatitis following halothane anesthesia.*[44] An additional problem is whether the biochemical abnormalities that occur in the absence of clinical features of liver injury are related in any way to the clinical entity of halothane hepatitis.[60, 61, 63–66]

HISTORY OF THE HALOTHANE CONTROVERSY

The introduction of halothane (2-chloro-2-bromo-1,1,1-trifluoroethane) was hailed as a major development in general anesthesia, given the numerous desirable attributes of halothane.[67] It is nonflammable and nonexplosive and can be administered in accurately metered doses by calibrated vaporizers. It has a pharmacokinetic profile that results in smooth induction and rapid recovery from anesthesia, and it causes few postoperative side effects such as vomiting. It is not an irritant to the respiratory tract. Halothane is regarded by most anesthetists as close to the ideal anesthetic. After extensive testing of its safety, halothane was introduced into Great Britain in 1956 and into the United States in 1958. By 1962 it was the most popular general anesthetic agent, accounting for 48.5 per cent of anesthetic administrations in the United States. It supplanted agents such as diethyl ether, trichlorethylene, and cyclopropane.

Many anesthetists have been reluctant to accept halothane-induced hepatitis as a distinct entity.[41, 43, 44, 57, 68] The reasons for this attitude include the popularity and overall safety of halothane, the excessive rarity of unequivocal halothane-induced hepatitis, the historic difficulties in excluding viral hepatitis, and the perception of some anesthetists that internists and pathologists were inappropriate parties to comment on an anesthetic problem.[43, 69–74] Even now that the entity halothane hepatitis is widely recognized,[60, 61, 75] some authorities are still unconvinced of the etiologic role of halothane.[44] It should be noted that the highest estimate of the frequency of halothane hepatitis is one case for every 6000 instances of repeated halothane administration within four weeks. On this basis, it is estimated that no more than one in three anesthetists will see a single case of halothane jaundice in their entire professional lifetime.[76]

Hepatic injury occurring after exposure to haloalkane anesthetic agents other than halothane (e.g., carbon tetrachloride and chloroform) has been recognized since the mid-nineteenth century.[77, 78] Acute and delayed chloroform-induced hepatotoxicity were hazards of anesthesia until the late 1950s, and rare instances of chloroform-induced hepatotoxicity still occur after "recreational" use of chloroform.[79] There have never been any extensive surveys of the prevalence of chloroform hepatitis, however. In fact, the unequivocal identification of chloroform as the cause of postoperative jaundice would have posed even greater difficulties than have been experienced for halothane because of the greater chance of intraoperative hypoxia, hypercarbia, and hypotension in the era when chloroform was used as an anesthetic.

Only sporadic case reports of jaundice or fatal hepatic necrosis appeared in the first three years after the release of halothane,[80–82] but by 1963 there were in excess of 40 published reports,[54, 83–86] and by 1968 the number exceded 400.[77, 87] Assessment of these reports by present criteria suggests that halothane itself cannot be incriminated as the sole responsible factor in all cases and that halothane-induced hepatitis was overdiagnosed (e.g., the sex ratio of 67 per cent males[77] is the opposite of later series; Table 34–2). Moreover, the animal studies conducted until 1963 failed to show a dose-dependent, direct toxic effect of halothane on the liver,[67, 77, 78] and in patients halothane appeared to be no more likely to alter liver function tests[53, 54, 77, 88, 89] or hepatic histology than did ethyl ether or cyclopropane.[55, 77]

Retrospective surveys of 350,000 halothane anesthetics indicated that postoperative jaundice and hepatic failure were uncommon complications.[28, 54, 55, 77, 88, 90–94] The incidence of massive hepatic necrosis after operations for which halothane was administered was 0.88 per 100,000 anes-

TABLE 34–2. CLINICAL DATA IN REPORTED SERIES OF PATIENTS WITH HALOTHANE HEPATITIS

Study	No. of cases	Mean Age (yrs)	Sex (% female)	Obesity (%)	Multiple Halothane Exposure (%)	Last 2 exposures <28 days apart* (%)	Eosinophilia (%)	Mortality (%)	Comments
Trey[99]	13	53	69	NR	100	100	NR	77	Fulminant hepatic failure study
Peters[97]	49	50	65	77	69	85	NR	76	Includes autopsy series
Klion[105]	42	21–77	52	NR	71	NR	47	67	Biased by referral of autopsy material
Hughes[114]	6	58	100	NR	100	100	NR	33	Selected, carcinoma of cervix
Inman[103]	130	57	67	NR	82	80	few	51	Reports to U.K. Committee on Safety of Medicine
Moult[116]	26	59	69	Common	92	83	8	42	Majority referred because of liver failure
Böttiger[107]	94	50	65	NR	82	NR	NR	14	Reports to Swedish Adverse Drug Reactions Committee
Walton[117]	76	53	70	38	95	56	32	20	Prospective survey; allergic history 21%
Neuberger[65]	48	57	65	68	94	60	NR	79	Liver failure unit, other drug allergies 33%
Farrell[118]	11	53	73	73	91	60	9	9	Selected for recovered patients
Otsuka[66]	38	40	63	32	42	38	67	0	Selected for recovered patients
Nomura[143]	8	41	100	NR	38	67	62	25	7 patients taking phenobarbital
All Studies	541	53	66	51	81	70	<36	52	

*Percentage of cases exposed to two or more halothane anesthetics.
NR = not recorded.

thetics, whereas for other agents it was 0.73 per 100,000 anesthetics.[56] Despite these data, the number of case reports incriminating halothane led the manufacturer to issue a warning in May 1963, "The administration of halothane to patients with known liver or biliary tract disease is not recommended." Some institutions had come by then to restricting the use of halothane to a few specific instances.

With this background, the National Halothane Study was undertaken by a multidisciplinary group of investigators.[56, 57] It embraced a multicenter retrospective review of necropsy reports of deaths within six weeks of surgery.[56, 57, 95] In all 10,171 reports were surveyed from 34 participating institutions, out of an estimated 856,515 anesthetics, of which 254,898 were halothane. The principal findings of the National Halothane Study were[56, 57]

1. Vindication of the overall safety of halothane, which was associated with a perioperative mortality of 1.87 per cent. This figure compared favorably with the mortality for other agents (1.93 per cent). Outcome was no worse among patients with biliary tract disease, when halothane was administered, compared with other agents.

2. Confirmation of the rarity of fatal, massive hepatic necrosis after surgery and anesthesia. The overall incidence appeared to be about one case in 10,000 operations and was not more common after halothane anesthesia.

3. About 90 per cent of cases of fatal hepatic necrosis after general anesthesia could be explained by factors such as shock, hypoxia, surgical trauma, sepsis, and preexistent liver disease; thus, only 10 per cent of cases remained unexplained.

Although all these findings have been universally accepted, there have been differing interpretations and opinions about the rare cases of hepatic necrosis occurring after halothane anesthesia that could not be attributed to other causes.[57, 95–97] Criticisms of the National Halothane Study have included concerns about the adequacy of case collection and identification; an autopsy rate of 60 per cent; incomplete autopsies; autolysis of specimens; retrospective collation of clinical, operative, and laboratory data; and doubt about whether previously reported cases of possible halothane hepatitis should have been included or excluded.[43, 59, 62, 73, 97] Among the 10,171 autopsy reports (many gleaned from a second round of searching and reviewing), 197 cases of fatal hepatic necrosis were identified, 82 with massive hepatic necrosis and 115 with intermediate hepatic necrosis. When the six pathologists on the panel were asked to interpret the likely cause of liver injury from histologic appearances alone, "opinions were greatly individualized and showed little uniformity."[95] Members of the committee then were given a summary of the clinical courses, operative procedures, laboratory data, and other necropsy findings. With this information in addition to their assessment of hepatic histology, they were asked again to indicate their impressions of the causative basis for hepatic necrosis. Certain histologic features such as zonal necrosis, hemorrhagic lesions, and a collapsed central reticulin framework were regarded as indicative of shock, anoxia, and sepsis.

The majority of the committee identified 19 cases in which there was not a readily explicable cause, 9 of massive hepatic necrosis and 10 of intermediate hepatic necrosis. Halothane was the anesthetic used in 14 (74 per cent) of these cases, whereas it was used in only 30 per cent of all anesthetic administrations. Most reviewers have discussed only the nine cases of massive hepatic necrosis; in these halothane was the anesthetic used on seven occasions, cyclopropane once, and ethylene once. The small numbers mean that apparent differences between agents could have

occurred by chance.[56] These data have been used to derive an incidence of massive hepatic necrosis induced by halothane of 1 in 35,000 administrations. However, this is a minimum figure, since there was disagreement amongst pathologists as to the correct number of cases of unexplained massive hepatic necrosis. Estimates ranged from 7 to 15.[96] In a separate review of the clinical records and pathologic specimens available from 71 cases of massive hepatic necrosis that had been considered previously in the National Halothane Study, Babior and Davidson considered that the histologic and clinical assessment was in good agreement with a "vascular" cause, usually shock or cardiac failure, in 56 cases.[98] The remaining 15 cases were designated as a "hepatitis"; 3 of the patients had been noted to be jaundiced before surgery. Eleven of the 15 patients had been administered halothane, but the 4 who had been given another agent included all 3 cases of preexistent hepatitis. Hence halothane anesthesia was used in 11 of the 12 cases of unexplained postoperative hepatitis, compared with 18 of 56 in the "vascular" group and 30 per cent overall. Moreover, in 5 of the 9 cases of unexplained massive hepatic necrosis (or 11 of 13, according to Trey)[99], more than one anesthetic had been administered in the month before death, and in 4 instances both anesthetics contained halothane. Only 9 per cent of all patients given halothane anesthetics received this agent on multiple occasions.[56] The risk for massive hepatic necrosis (of any cause) after multiple halothane anesthetics was thus 7.1/10,000 for halothane and 2.1/10,000 for other agents.[56, 77, 99] These data are more indicative of an etiologic role for halothane than might be suggested by the official report of the National Halothane Study, which states, "The study has not entirely ruled out a rare relationship between halothane and massive hepatic necrosis."[56, 57]

RECOGNITION OF HALOTHANE HEPATITIS AS AN ENTITY

Controversy followed the release of the report of the National Halothane Study,[41–43, 53, 70–73] and it was another decade before there was widespread acceptance of halothane-induced hepatitis as a separate entity.[58, 73, 74, 100, 101] The most conclusive evidence that this was a form of drug-induced liver injury was the clear propensity for halothane-induced hepatitis to occur after multiple halothane administrations and the description of cases in which exacerbations of hepatitis occurred after reexposure (Table 34–2).[53, 73, 83, 99, 100, 102, 103] In addition, it was recognized increasingly that halothane hepatitis occurred with rather predictable clinical features. Morphologic features of drug-induced liver injury were sometimes present. Risk factors for individual susceptibility could be identified, and eventually, from the mid 1970s, most cases of viral hepatitis could be excluded by serologic tests for hepatitis B and hepatitis A.

Recurrence of liver disease after reexposure to the inciting agent remains the "gold standard" for diagnosis of drug-induced liver disease. There are now many well-documented cases in which hepatocellular necrosis has occurred after inadvertent reexposure to halothane anesthesia.[83, 102, 103] Moreover, there are several reports of anesthetists,[66, 83, 104–107] surgeons,[65] nurses,[108, 109] one laboratory technician,[110] and one factory worker,[105] who developed unexplained hepatitis-like illnesses that recurred following occupational reexposure to halothane.[111] Hepatitis has also been described in three individuals who sniffed halothane repeatedly in order to obtain a drug "high."[112] In two anesthetists suspected of having halothane-induced hepatitis, a deliberate challenge test was performed by reexposure to small amounts of halothane.[104, 106]

Reexposure to halothane has generally been associated with an accelerated onset of symptoms (Table 34–3).[58, 59, 103] The case described by Klatskin and Kimberg is particularly convincing.[106] The patient, an anesthetist, had a history of recurrent hepatitis, which led to the development of cirrhosis. Multiple relapses were coincident with the patient's return to work and reexposure to halothane. Challenge with a small dose of halothane resulted in chills, fever, and myalgia within 6 hours and was associated with biochemical and histologic evidence of hepatitis within 24 hours.[106]

The importance of multiple exposures in the pathogenesis of halothane-induced liver injury is now established (Table 34–2).[65, 66, 77, 84, 97, 103, 105, 107, 113–118] In one early report, Lindenbaum and Leifer noted recurrences of fever and jaundice in three patients after repeated halothane anesthesia.[84] Trey and coauthors found that 27 of 35 patients with fulminant hepatic failure following recent exposure to halothane had received multiple halothane anesthetics.[113] Hughes and Powell reported six patients with recurrent hepatitis following multiple halothane anesthetics for insertion of radium implants for carcinoma of the uterine cervix.[114] Episodes of hepatitis disappeared when a policy against giving multiple halothane anesthetics for this procedure was implemented. Inman and Mushin analyzed data from 130 doctor-reported instances of jaundice following anesthesia and noted that 82 per cent of patients had been exposed to halothane on more than one occasion, and in 80 per cent of these patients, repeat exposure was within 28 days.[76, 103] Moreover, there was a significant relationship between the number of exposures and the rapidity with which jaundice developed (Fig. 34–1). Sharpstone and colleagues reported on 11 patients with halothane hepatitis, 6 of whom died from massive hepatic necrosis. In nine patients, unexplained fever had occurred after a previous halothane anesthetic.[119] In three patients, jaundice had occurred after an earlier exposure (in one case, without fever). These data are more convincing than two earlier reports of smaller numbers of patients with a history of postoperative jaundice who were reexposed to halothane without recurrence of jaundice.[92, 117] The characteristic clinical picture of halothane hepatitis is of some value in distinguishing this disorder from other causes of postoperative jaundice and also from viral hepatitis.[58, 59]

By the late 1970s, the accumulated epidemiologic data, the special clinical and morphologic features, the availability of hepatitis B and hepatitis A serologies, and most persuasively, the evidence of rechallenge studies had led

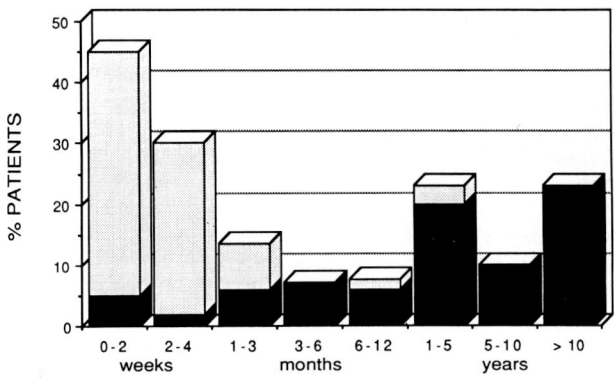

Figure 34–1. The interval between anesthetics among patients with unexplained jaundice after halothane anesthesia (hatched bars) and controls (solid bars). (Modified from Inman HW, Moshin WW. Br Med J 1:5, 1974, with permission.)

most authorities to recognize the existence of halothane-induced hepatitis as a real entity.[58, 73, 74, 100, 101] However, controversy and uncertainty continue to surround many aspects of halothane hepatitis, especially the following: (1) whether the mechanism producing the disorder is an immunologic or a chemical one; (2) the relevance of animal models, in particular the role of hypoxia; and (3) the ethical and medicolegal issues surrounding the present but diminishing use of this otherwise safe and useful anesthetic agent.

INCIDENCE OF HALOTHANE-INDUCED HEPATIC INJURY

The frequency with which halothane-induced hepatitis progresses to fatal fulminant hepatic failure was estimated in the National Halothane Study to be 1:35,000 anesthetic administrations. This is almost certainly a gross underestimate of the incidence of clinically overt halothane hepatitis, since it seems unlikely that more than 50 per cent of cases are fatal (see Table 34–2).[59, 107, 120] An incidence of between 1:6,000 and 1:22,000 administrations of halothane appears to be a more realistic figure.[59, 76, 107] Among patients treated for fulminant hepatic failure, halothane hepatitis remains an important cause;[59, 65, 99] halothane is probably the most common cause of a fatal hepatic drug reaction.[120]

It has been suggested that clinically overt cases of halothane hepatitis represent the most extreme end of a spectrum of hepatotoxicity. In early prospective studies, biochemical tests of liver disease were no more common after single halothane administrations than after other agents.[28, 54, 55, 77, 88, 89] However, more recent studies have observed elevations of serum aminotransferases from five days to three weeks after repeated halothane anesthetics.[121–125] Among 152 patients who had received a halothane anesthetic within one year and then required a second operative procedure, Wright and coworkers randomly allocated one half to be given halothane and the other half a different anesthetic.[121] Serum aspartate aminotransferase (AST) levels were significantly higher in the halothane group, and were outside the normal range in 20 per cent of halothane recipients compared with 5 per cent of controls. In one patient in the halothane group, serum AST rose tenfold, and hepatocellular necrosis was present on liver biopsy. Two other patients in the halothane group whose ALT level had risen at least twofold showed a similar

TABLE 34–3. AVERAGE TIME (DAYS) BETWEEN LAST HALOTHANE EXPOSURE AND ONSET OF FEVER AND JAUNDICE

Study	Single Exposure Fever	Single Exposure Jaundice	Multiple Exposures Fever	Multiple Exposures Jaundice
Klion[105]	—	11	—	8
Trey[99]	—	—	—	7*
Moult[116]	—	—	8	5
Inman[103]	—	12	—	6
Walton[117]	—	—	—	6*
Böttiger[107]	7	8	4	7
Neuberger[65]	—	—	—	5*

*In these studies, the time was calculated from all patients, although small numbers exposed only once were included.

reaction to a third exposure to halothane, although they had not shown a reaction to an intervening control anesthetic. In another study of repeated anesthesia, patients were given either a halothane or a nonhalothane anesthetic (not methoxyflurane) for implantation of radon rods.[122] In 4 of the 18 patients given repeated halothane administrations, serum alanine aminotransferase (ALT) levels rose above 100 U/l (normal, less than 35 U/l); such a rise did not occur in any of the 21 patients given a different anesthetic. A third prospective study of liver enzymes following repeat administrations of halothane or enflurane, this time in patients undergoing minor urological procedures, demonstrated that disordered liver function tests were more frequent following halothane anesthesia.[123] This tendency was more pronounced as the number of anesthetic administrations increased and was increased by the presence of obesity and short intervals between reexposures.[124, 125] By contrast, it is noteworthy that in none of the studies demonstrating elevations of aminotransferase after repeat administration of halothane did patients develop jaundice or symptoms of hepatitis. Also, in other studies, increases in serum levels of aminotransferase following repeated halothane anesthesia (not always within 28 days) were no more common than after enflurane or other agents;[126, 127] however in one of these studies, sampling was confined to the first three postoperative days.[127]

RISK FACTORS FOR HALOTHANE HEPATITIS

Halothane-induced hepatitis is not dose dependent. Massive overdose of halothane does not cause hepatocellular necrosis.[128, 129] The duration of halothane anesthesia and the amount given do not appear related to unexplained postoperative hepatic necrosis (see Table 34–2 and references 65, 103, 107, 114, 116). Individuals who suffer from this rare disorder do so because of one or more factors that render them unusually susceptible to liver damage after exposure to halothane.[51, 53, 59, 61, 65, 130] The importance of repeated administrations of halothane has been outlined (see Table 34–2). Some possible ways in which this may be related to chemical or immunologic mechanisms are discussed later, but reexposure in a patient with previous, unexplained hepatitis following halothane administration does not always result in another episode of hepatitis.[92, 117]

Age and gender are both risk factors for halothane hepatitis (see Table 34–2). Most large series indicate that about two thirds of cases occur in women. This sex ratio is similar to most other idiosyncratic hepatic drug reactions.[131] Adults appear to be at greater risk (see Table 34–2). However, the magnitude of heightened risk with increasing age is not known. Cases occurring in childhood are infrequent,[75, 132–135] but patients as young as 11 months have been described.[136, 137]

Another consistent observation is that obese patients are at increased risk for halothane-induced hepatitis (see Table 34–2).[65, 97, 116–118] Obesity is also associated with abnormal serum aminotransferase levels after repeated halothane anesthetics.[125] The stereotypic patient with halothane-induced hepatitis is an obese, postmenopausal female who has had multiple halothane anesthetics within 28 days. The frequency with which this description fits patients with halothane hepatitis most likely accounts for the apparent predilection of this disorder for patients being treated with radon implants for carcinoma of the cervix.[63] Why obesity predisposes to hepatic necrosis after halothane anesthesia is unclear, but obesity increases bodily and perhaps hepatic

stores of halothane[101] and is associated with an increased production of both oxidative[137] and reductive metabolites,[138, 139] indicating enhanced biotransformation of halothane. Obesity also may increase the risk of postoperative hypoxia.[101]

Several studies have noted the presence of allergic tendencies, including rhinitis, asthma, and penicillin and other drug allergy, in patients with halothane-induced hepatitis.[53, 65, 86, 94, 116, 117] However, there are insufficient data to know whether the incidence of these common problems in patients with halothane hepatitis is greater than would be expected in carefully matched groups of patients. Hoft and colleagues observed apparent halothane hepatitis in two closely related members of three separate families.[140] Farrell and co-workers found a defect in the resistance of lymphocytes to cell damage mediated by reactive metabolites in 10 of 11 patients who appeared to have halothane hepatitis.[118] The same defect was present in about 50 per cent of nonaffected family members. The abnormality was present in individuals of both sexes and in more than one generation, thus suggesting that it was inherited.[118]

Among the animal models of halothane-induced hepatotoxicity (see later), one requires a particular genetic strain of rat, induction of hepatic drug metabolizing enzymes by pretreatment with phenobarbital, and administration of halothane under slightly hypoxic conditions.[44, 51, 61, 141] Most studies have not noted a particular association between treatment with microsomal enzyme-inducing agents and halothane-induced hepatitis in patients (see Table 34–2). Greene reviewed 393 patients given single halothane anesthetics at the time they were being treated with anticonvulsants, which in 294 instances included phenobarbital.[142] Only two patients developed hepatitis after surgery. In neither instance did the clinical features suggest that halothane could be incriminated. More recently, Nomura and colleagues reported a different experience among Japanese patients undergoing brain surgery under halothane anesthesia.[143] The incidence of symptomatic halothane-induced liver injury in the patients receiving phenobarbital was 7 per 100, compared with 1 per 179 among those who were not. Only three of the seven phenobarbital-treated patients with apparent halothane-induced hepatitis had previously received halothane.[143]

CLINICAL AND LABORATORY FEATURES OF HALOTHANE HEPATITIS

Fever is the first symptom in at least 75 per cent of patients. There is in many patients a previous history of unexplained, postoperative fever that was delayed in onset (see Table 34–2). In the infrequent cases of halothane-induced hepatitis occurring after a single exposure to halothane, fever was noted 6 to 14 days after operation (Table 34–3).[58, 59, 105, 107] After more than one exposure, the median time to fever is six days; but onset as early as the first postoperative day has been reported.[65, 103, 116–118, 143] Early onset often has been associated with a fatal outcome. Fever in halothane hepatitis, unlike that in viral hepatitis, is often hectic with chills and sweats. About 10 per cent of patients may exhibit a rash during the febrile phase. After a further two to five days of fever (depending on previous exposure), symptoms of hepatitis occur, such as anorexia, malaise, nausea, and right upper quadrant abdominal pain. Dark urine and jaundice are then evident in most patients, but anicteric cases occur. Early on, the liver may be enlarged and tender, but later in severe cases it may shrink. In such cases, drowsiness, confusion, coagulation disorder, and, eventually, coma ensue, often with death occurring within ten days of onset. The established phase of the illness is indistinguishable from viral hepatitis and fulminant hepatic failure of other causes.

Biochemical tests of liver disease are those expected for acute hepatocellular necrosis. The serum bilirubin concentration is usually raised. Serum aminotransferase levels are elevated at least tenfold but may fall toward the terminal phase of the illness, presumably because of failure of hepatic protein synthesis. Levels of serum alkaline phosphatase and γ-glutamyl transpeptidase usually are increased, but not strikingly so. The prothrombin time is one of the best prognostic indicators; a prothrombin time of more than 20 seconds indicates a high likelihood of a fatal outcome.[105, 116]

The frequency of eosinophilia, with or without neutropenia, varies in different reports between 11 and 40 per cent (see Table 34–2). The lower figure seems to represent the more common experience. Aplastic anemia has been described as an extremely rare complication.[144] Renal failure is thought to occur most often in the late stages as a complication of terminal hepatic failure (see Chap. 18).[116] However, at least six cases have been reported in which the authors considered that nephrotoxicity was directly due to halothane.[118, 145, 146] Gelman has drawn attention to some similarities with methoxyflurane nephrotoxicity and suggested a similar mechanism.[146]

HISTOLOGIC ASSESSMENT

Liver biopsy need not be performed in every case but should be considered when other diagnoses cannot be excluded satisfactorily, especially when further anesthesia is contemplated. It is unclear how often the morphologic features on liver biopsy indicate clearly that a drug hepatitis is the likely diagnosis in an individual case.[43, 44, 73] Many biopsies show spotty parenchymal necrosis with infiltrates in portal areas and thus cannot be distinguished from viral hepatitis.[59, 95, 147, 148] However, necrosis that is disproportionately severe for the clinical picture, and especially sharply demarcated centrizonal necrosis,[97] steatosis, and plentiful eosinophils in the inflammatory infiltrate,[105] are features in favor of a drug etiology.[149] Hepatic granulomas or, more often, poorly formed aggregates of mononuclear cells (pseudogranulomas) have been reported rarely in halothane hepatitis.[105, 150, 151] But, like eosinophils, they are a common feature in any series of liver biopsies.[152] The electronmicrographic features of halothane-induced hepatitis include expansion and swelling of the smooth endoplasmic reticulum but with preservation of the rough endoplasmic reticulum.[53, 105, 147, 148] Occasional herniations of the plasma membrane into the sinusoid may be seen, but this feature also occurs in viral hepatitis.[53] The predominant feature is damage to mitochondria with breaks in the outer membrane, infolding of the inner membrane, and crystalline inclusions.[53, 105, 147] The mitochondrial lesions are regarded by some workers as helpful in distinguishing halothane hepatitis from viral hepatitis.[53, 105, 147] However, one is left with the impression that electronmicroscopic changes are likely to be of limited value in individual cases.[147]

COURSE AND PROGNOSIS

An important unanswered question is whether asymptomatic elevations of serum transaminases, as seen in prospective studies of repeat halothane anesthesia, are a separate, self-limited type of hepatotoxicity[60, 61, 65, 66] or whether they are part of a spectrum of disease severity. In most reported series of halothane hepatitis, there is a bias toward more severe cases, but recent studies have suggested that less severe cases could be more common (see Table 34–2). Hence, whereas the reported mortality ranges from 10 to 80 per cent, the higher figures are undoubtedly due to referral bias (see Table 34–2). A more realistic figure for the overall mortality is probably 10 to 30 per cent.[107, 117] Adverse prognostic factors (Table 34–4) include age of more than 60 years, obesity, a number of halothane exposures with short intervals between them, previous episodes of postoperative jaundice, a short time between anesthesia and the onset of jaundice, serum bilirubin concentration exceeding 200 μmol/L, and prothrombin time of more than 20 seconds.[65, 97, 103, 107, 116, 117]

In patients who survive, defervescence, return of appetite, and improved well-being occur after five to ten days. Complete clinical recovery is then usual. Follow-up studies of liver histology show restitution of normal hepatic architecture. There are only three well-documented cases of chronicity. In one case, the patient was an anesthetist subjected to repeated exposure to halothane. This man developed cirrhosis.[106] In the other two patients, a lesion resembling chronic active hepatitis was found on liver biopsy four months after the postoperative event.[153, 154] These patients are unusual. It is arguable whether halothane is a bona fide cause of chronic liver disease in these or other patients.[131] Further doubt on this matter arises from the possibility that halothane exposure may exacerbate autoimmune chronic active hepatitis.[155, 156] This would provide an alternative explanation for rare patients with chronic liver disease that seemingly was precipitated by halothane and was responsive to treatment with corticosteroids.[157]

MANAGEMENT

Management is supportive. There are no reports of the use of potential hepatoprotective agents for this disorder. Severe cases are best cared for in a unit experienced in the management of acute liver failure, since optimal conservative management still offers the best chance of a favorable outcome (see Chap. 17). Liver transplantation may be considered in individual cases,[75] but optimal timing is unclear.[158] Resolution of halothane hepatitis may be prolonged.[159] In one such case, a prompt improvement was noted after introduction of corticosteroids.[157] Patients who have survived an episode of halothane-induced hepatitis should be cautioned against further exposure to halothane and should be encouraged to wear a medic-alert bracelet or similar identification.

TABLE 34–4. ADVERSE PROGNOSTIC FACTORS IN PATIENTS WITH HALOTHANE-INDUCED HEPATITIS

Over 60 years of age
Obesity
Multiple exposures to halothane
Short interval between exposures
Previous episodes of jaundice after exposure to halothane
Short interval between anesthesia and onset of jaundice
Serum bilirubin concentration greater than 200 μmol/L
Prothrombin time greater than 20 seconds

PREVENTION

Halothane-induced hepatitis could be avoided if the use of this anesthetic agent was discontinued. In view of the overall safety of halothane compared with other anesthetic agents and the rarity of halothane-induced hepatitis, this course of action has never seemed appropriate.[44, 77, 101] Despite these considerations, the use of halothane in North America and to a lesser extent in the United Kingdom has decreased considerably in recent years because of concern about litigation.[44, 75] If the following guidelines are adhered to, 80 to 90 per cent of cases of halothane-induced hepatitis could be avoided.[44, 75, 76, 126] The previous anesthetic history should always be considered. Halothane is contraindicated when there has been unexplained jaundice, nausea, or unexplained late-onset fever occurring after an earlier procedure for which halothane was or could have been given. Halothane should be avoided if there is a family history of halothane hepatitis.[44, 61, 75, 140] When considering use of multiple anesthetics within 28 days, the risk of halothane hepatitis is unacceptable in obese, postmenopausal women now that equally satisfactory (albeit much more expensive) alternatives are available.[160–162] In other groups, including children, the risk of unexplained hepatitis is less, and the advantages of halothane over other agents need to be balanced against this rare side effect. It is recommended that administration of halothane should not be repeated within a short period,[163] but whether there is a safe period after three months or six months is unclear.[44, 75, 164] When electing to avoid halothane, the possibility of cross reactivity with methoxyflurane and enflurane should be considered (see later). It seems likely that isoflurane is the haloalkane anesthetic of choice.[75] A halothane-free circuit and operating room should also be used, because halothane hepatotoxicity appears at least in part to be *dose-independent*, and halothane can be leached out of the rubber tubing and carbon dioxide–absorbent and other equipment used in anesthetic machines. Halothane is present in easily detectable amounts even in scavenged operating suites.[111, 165]

MECHANISMS OF HALOTHANE-INDUCED LIVER INJURY

Initial concern about the potential hepatotoxicity of halothane was based on the knowledge that other haloalkanes, including carbon tetrachloride and chloroform, produced dose-dependent liver injury.[77, 78] However, the early animal studies together with a vast clinical experience indicate that halothane is not a potent, direct hepatotoxin,[66, 77, 78, 94, 166] although minor ultrastructural changes are present in the liver after chronic exposure to halothane.[167, 168] It was initially believed that halothane was chemically inert and was not metabolized by mammals. This concept is incorrect.[44, 77, 101, 169, 170] About 20 per cent of the dose of halothane absorbed during an inhalational anesthetic is metabolized, predominantly in the liver, by cytochrome P450–dependent microsomal enzymes.[77, 101, 169, 170] Metabolism is slow and capacity limited,[171, 172] but because of prolonged storage of halothane in the body, it continues for several days after anesthesia.[101]

Three principal hypotheses have been advanced to explain halothane-induced hepatitis. One view is that it is a form of chemical hepatotoxicity, which is initiated by the metabolism of halothane to reactive metabolites.[44, 51, 59–62, 170] In rat models, a critical feature is the presence of a mild degree of tissue hypoxia.[44, 59, 146, 170, 172–175] It has now become evident, however, that severe tissue hypoxia itself may cause a form of liver injury that appears to be similar to halothane-induced hepatitis.[44, 176–178] A second proposal is that halothane could produce hepatic necrosis purely on the basis of hepatic ischemia.[44, 176–178] The third idea is that halothane-induced hepatitis is a form of hypersensitivity, or drug allergy, resulting from an immunologic response to halothane or more likely to metabolites of halothane that have reacted with constituents of the liver cell.[53, 65, 130] The immune and chemotoxicity hypotheses are not mutually exclusive.[59, 64, 130]

HALOTHANE METABOLISM

The structures of halothane and other haloalkane anesthetic agents are presented in Figure 34–2. During inhalational anesthesia, 6 to 11 g of halothane are absorbed and distributed into body fat, liver, and brain.[179, 180] Following recovery from anesthesia, halothane is excreted slowly and may be detected in breath for at least six days.[101, 180–182] Metabolites of halothane, including bromide ion and trifluoroacetic acid (TFA), can be detected in urine for up to three weeks.[183, 184] The rate of halothane metabolism appears to be determined genetically[185] but also may be influenced by environmental factors such as occupational exposure to halothane[52, 181] and treatment with inducers of microsomal enzymes.[146, 170, 176, 186]

Halothane is metabolized by two major pathways (Fig. 34–3), both of which are catalyzed by hepatic cytochrome P450–dependent microsomal enzymes.[170, 176, 187–189] The first pathway requires molecular oxygen and so is termed the *oxidative pathway*. The second pathway is independent of and partially inhibited by oxygen.[19, 190, 191] This is usually called the *reductive pathway*, although *anaerobic metabolism* is a more precise term.[62] Although oxygen inhibits the anaerobic metabolism of halothane in vitro, when halothane is administered in air (or 100 per cent O_2) to human subjects, a proportion of metabolism will proceed via the reductive pathway.[192, 193]

Admininistration of inducers of cytochrome P450, such as phenobarbital,[186, 194] polychlorinated biphenyl (Araclor

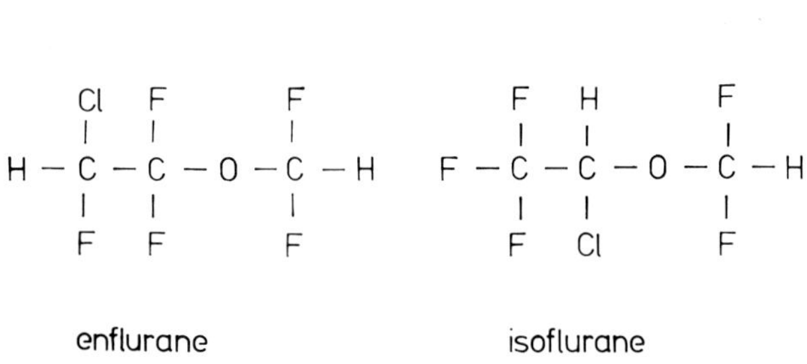

Figure 34–2. Structures of halothane (2-bromo-2-chloro-1,1,1-trifluoroethane), methoxyflurane (2,2-dichloro-1,1-difluoroethyl methyl ether), enflurane (2-chloro-1-[difluoromethoxy]-1,1,2-trifluoroethane), and isoflurane (1-chloro-1-[fluoromethoxy]-2,2,2-trifluoroethane).

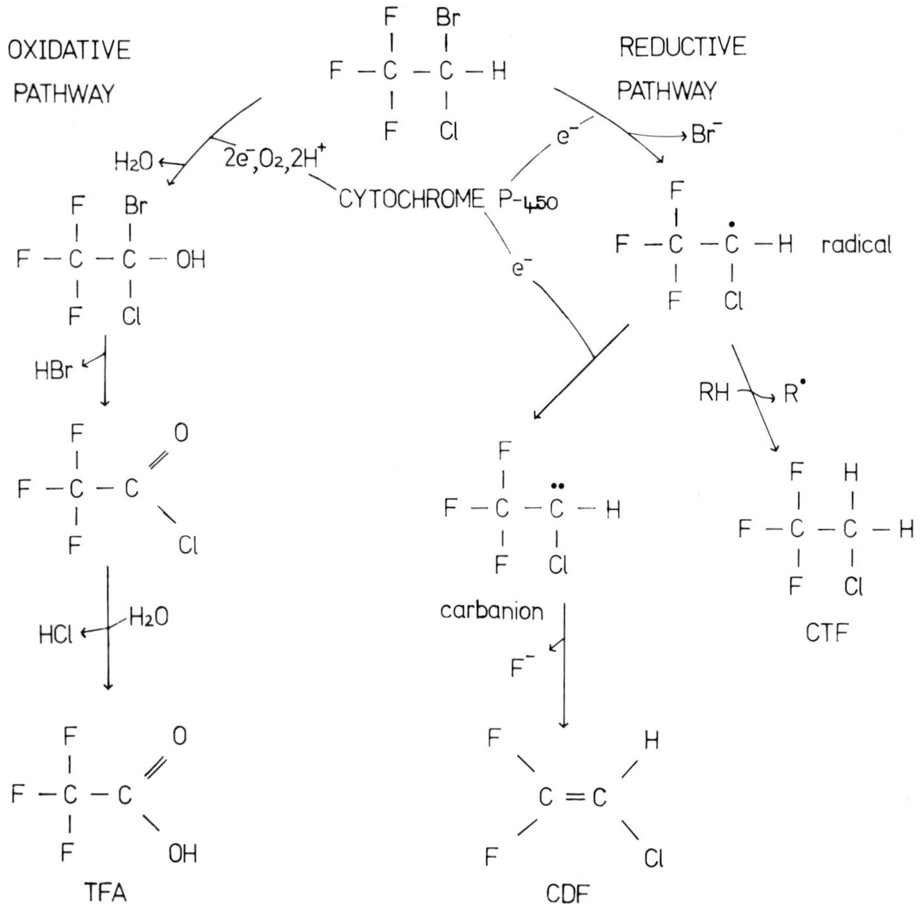

Figure 34–3. Pathways of halothane metabolism. TFA, trifluoroacetic acid; CTF, 2-chloro-1,1,1-trifluoroethane. CDF, 2-chloro-1,1-difluorethylene.

1254),[173, 195] and ethyl alcohol,[196] but not 3-methylcholanthrene,[22, 25, 26, 174, 197] increases halothane metabolism in experimental animals.[169] Halothane induces its own metabolism in mice,[179, 198] but not in rats.[44, 169] In humans, it has been suggested that chronic exposure to halothane in operating theaters increases the rate of halothane metabolism among anesthetists.[185] In patients, obesity appears to be associated with higher fluoride levels after halothane anesthesia, thereby suggesting a greater extent of anaerobic metabolism.[138, 139] This could be because obesity increases the risk of intraoperative or postoperative hypoxia, thereby favoring the reductive pathway of halothane metabolism.[101]

Oxidative metabolism of halothane results in formation of a trifluoroacylhalide (CF_3-COX) and liberation of inorganic bromide and chloride (Fig. 34–3). Trifluoroacylhalide is a chemically reactive species. It combines with water to yield the stable and inert TFA. Alternatively, it may bind to macromolecules in the vicinity of its production, particularly to the fatty acyl side chains of phospholipids. In rats, TFA adducts can be detected in hepatic microsomes and plasma membranes four hours after exposure to halothane.[199] Binding to plasma membrane in the intact liver can be demonstrated by immunofluorescence and is most evident in hepatocytes in centrolobular zones.[199, 200] Despite this, there is no evidence that the oxidative pathway of halothane metabolism results directly in cytotoxicity.[44, 51, 170, 176]

The principal products of the reductive pathway of halothane metabolism are fluoride and bromide ions (excreted in urine) and the volatile metabolites 2-chloro-1,1,1-trifluoroethane (CTF) and 2-chloro-1,1-difluoroethylene (CDF) (excreted in the breath).[51, 141, 169, 176, 201–210] Reductive metabolism can be stimulated by systemic and regional hypoxia produced by ligation of the hepatic artery in vivo or by reduction of hepatic perfusion in the isolated perfused rat liver.[101, 204, 211, 212] Reductive metabolism of halothane can proceed only via the formation of unstable and reactive intermediates (Fig. 34–3).[19, 202, 205, 213–216] CTF, an end-product of reductive halothane metabolism, may itself be hepatotoxic, since it causes liver necrosis when injected into the portal vein of rats.[217]

Metabolites of halothane produced by oxidative metabolism can bind to membrane phospholipids.[183, 199] Those produced by anaerobic metabolism bind to both phospholipids[174, 206, 207] and microsomal proteins.[24] In the case of cytochrome P450, such binding results in the destruction of the hemoprotein.[22, 24–26] The adducts formed from reactions between metabolites of halothane and phospholipids probably are excised within 12 hours and excreted in urine.[205] Anaerobic metabolites have been found in urine as conjugates with cysteine,[183] but there is little evidence that these metabolites are conjugated with glutathione.[218–220]

EXPERIMENTAL MODELS OF HALOTHANE-INDUCED LIVER INJURY

Whether or not animal models have relevance to the mechanism of halothane hepatitis in patients, the study of these models has provided strong evidence that the reactive metabolites produced during reductive halothane metabolism can initiate hepatotoxicity. A review of the relevant data is beyond the scope of this chapter. However, to summarize, halothane-induced hepatotoxicity in the rat has three critical components—enzyme induction of cytochrome P450, genetic strain, and hypoxia.[44, 51, 59, 170, 218] Liver injury occurs only when cytochrome P450 levels are increased and it is abolished by inhibition of halothane metabolism. The selectivity of phenobarbital, polychlorinated biphenyl, and ethanol but not 3-methylcholanthrene as appropriate inducing agents indicates the relevance of particular pathways of halothane metabolism. Male rats may be more susceptible than females because of their higher activity of hepatic drug metabolizing enzymes. Also, the strain of rat is important for demonstrating the hepatotoxicity of halothane. This may reflect genetic control of metabolic pathways, but nonmetabolic determinants of individual susceptibility have been suggested. The third requirement for halothane-induced hepatotoxicity in rats is the presence of mild hypoxia, which as already mentioned promotes reductive metabolism of halothane. The use of hypoxia has caused misgivings about the relevance to humans of observations made in the hypoxic rat.[176, 178, 220]

In the initial studies with the phenobarbital-treated hypoxic rat, controls consisted of animals exposed to the same mildly hypoxic atmosphere.[141, 173–175, 203] An important problem with this model is that systemic and hepatic concentrations of oxygen may be lower in the halothane-anesthetized animals owing to the respiratory and circulatory effects of halothane;[3–5, 44, 178, 221–223] it is known, for example, that halothane disturbs hepatic circulation to a greater extent than enflurane or isoflurane when used in equipotent doses.[177, 178] Hence, liver necrosis in the hypoxic rat could be the direct result of tissue ischemia rather than the indirect effect of enhanced anaerobic metabolism of halothane. Ischemic necrosis results from an imbalance between oxygen supply and the tissue demands for oxygen utilization. It seems likely that phenobarbital treatment, hyperthyroidism, feeding, and increased body temperature all increase the oxygen needs of the liver.[44, 176–178] However, phenobarbital pretreatment is also associated with an increase in fluoride production and with enhanced covalent binding of halothane metabolites to tissue components, whereas liver injury is prevented by inhibition of halothane metabolism.[141, 170, 173, 174, 197, 205, 211] These findings are more indicative of a crucial role for halothane biotransformation in the production of liver injury. Controversy about the role of hypoxia in the rat models has led to the search for a more acceptable animal model of halothane hepatitis.[176, 178, 220]

Hepatic necrosis can be produced in guinea pigs by administration of halothane in the absence of enzyme induction or hypoxia.[224–226] Earlier workers were interested in determining whether repeated halothane exposure would produce the accelerated onset of hepatic necrosis that is seen in humans. They found instead that the incidence of lesions is equal after single or multiple administrations of halothane.[224] Lunam and her coworkers have characterized the guinea pig model of halothane-associated hepatotoxicity.[226] Following 4 hours of exposure to 1 per cent halothane in air, about 65 per cent of animals have lesions consisting of either confluent centrizonal necrosis or scattered foci of necrosis throughout the hepatic lobule. Hepatocellular necrosis is evident on the second day after anesthesia, and recovery is complete by the seventh day.[226] Administration of the cytochrome P450 inhibitor SKF-525A decreases the incidence and severity of hepatic injury and decreases exhalation of the volatile metabolites CTF and CDF. Isoflurane anesthesia produces similar reductions in mean arterial pressure and in Pa_{O_2}, as does halothane, but it is not associated with hepatotoxicity in the guinea pig.[226] Hence, it seems that halothane-induced liver necrosis in the guinea pig is not caused by the effects of anesthesia on hepatic oxygenation but rather by the production of hepatotoxic metabolites of halothane.

POSSIBLE MECHANISMS LEADING TO CELL DEATH

Although metabolic activation of halothane to reactive metabolites seems likely as the initial step in hepatotoxicity, the mechanism by which such metabolites produce cell death has yet to be defined.[170] In the case of carbon tetrachloride, there is no direct evidence that covalent binding of radicals to cellular macromolecules is decisive for cell death.[170] There has been considerable interest, however, in lipid peroxidation as a propagating mechanism of liver cell injury caused by carbon tetrachloride and halothane.[173, 219, 227–230] Data for halothane have been inconsistent, but De Groot and Noll have provided an explanation for this discordance.[231] Under anaerobic conditions or at a Pa_{O_2} above 10 mmHg, no halothane-induced formation of malondialdehyde (reflecting lipid peroxidation) was detected. Between these extremes significant malondialdehyde was formed. Thus, for halothane-induced peroxidation of lipids to occur, the Pa_{O_2} should be low enough to permit reductive metabolism of halothane to form CF_3CHCl radicals but high enough to promote formation of lipid peroxides.[170, 230] The median hepatic concentration of oxygen in vivo is about 22 mmHg. The range is from 1 to 56 mmHg.[232]

In the case of hepatotoxicity caused by carbon tetrachloride, there are altered fluxes of cell calcium. These may be important in mediating cell damage, because sustained elevations of cytosolic calcium impair the function of microfilaments and activate phospholipases, proteases, and endonucleases.[233–236] Among the several homeostatic mechanisms that constrain rises in the cytosolic concentration of calcium in liver cells, cellular extrusion of calcium by a calcium pump in plasma membranes, and uptake of calcium by the endoplasmic reticulum, which is catalyzed by a calcium pump, appear to be most important.[234, 235] Preincubation of microsomes with halothane inactivates irreversibly ATP-dependent calcium transport.[237] This, too, appears to occur in intact liver 24 hours after exposure of guinea pigs to 1 per cent halothane in air.[238] These preliminary indications of disordered calcium homeostasis in halothane-induced hepatic injury are of considerable interest, especially because malignant hyperpyrexia, a rare complication of halothane, is mediated by inappropriate release of calcium from within skeletal muscle cells and lymphocytes.[239, 240]

EVIDENCE FOR AN IMMUNE MECHANISM

Several of the clinicopathologic features of halothane-induced hepatitis could be explained by some kind of immune hypersensitivity.[53, 58, 59, 65, 105, 130] The importance of repeated exposures, the accelerated response with increasing numbers of exposures, and occasional hepatotoxicity after reexposure to small amounts of halothane are consistent with prior "sensitization."[106, 241] More direct evidence for an immunologic disturbance is the presence of organelle-specific antibodies in serum. Doniach and co-workers[242] and Rodriguez and colleagues[243] detected antimitochondrial antibodies in serum from a total of 11 of 13 patients. Since then, however, antimitochrondrial antibodies have been found in a minority of patients and usually only in low titer.[53, 116, 117, 244, 245] The evidence for antiliver/kidney microsomal antibodies is more impressive. These have been detected in 20 to 50 per cent of patients with halothane-induced hepatitis,[65, 117, 244] but they are also found in patients with other causes of acute hepatocellular necrosis.[199, 245] Furthermore, the organelle-specific auto-antibodies remain detectable in patients with halothane-induced hepatitis for variable intervals.[242, 244] These observations diminish the likelihood that the antiliver/kidney microsomal antibodies are of pathogenetic importance. Circulating immune complexes were reported in six patients with fulminant hepatic failure related to halothane[246] and in one patient in whom a serum-sickness–like illness was a prominent feature of hepatitis following repeated exposures to halothane.[247] It has been proposed that such findings are consistent with a role for circulating immune complexes in contributing to liver injury,[246] but direct evidence is lacking.

It has been suggested that halothane-induced hepatitis occurs in perimenopausal females who are predisposed to organ-specific autoimmune disease.[117] In one study of English patients, however, the frequency of human leukocyte antigen (HLA) A and B locus antigens was unremarkable.[248] Similarly, there was no overall difference in the frequency of histocompatibility antigens among 38 Japanese patients compared with controls.[66] In the latter study, however, when patients were considered according to the presence (24 patients) or absence (14 patients) of jaundice, it was noted that DR2 was significantly more common in the jaundiced patients and Bw44 in those who were not jaundiced. In addition, the frequency of haplotype Aw24-Bw52-DR2 was higher in the jaundiced group (haplotype frequency = 0.2362) than in patients without jaundice (haplotype frequency = 0). The authors suggest that there may be two groups of patients with halothane-induced hepatitis, that these would have different genetic backgrounds, and that the gene determining susceptibility to jaundice after halothane anesthesia is in the HLA region of the sixth chromosome. It is noteworthy in this context that the Bw52-DR2-MT haplotype is strongly associated with primary biliary cirrhosis in Japanese patients.[66]

Evidence that cell-mediated immunity is involved in the mediation of halothane-induced hepatic necrosis has been sought by studies of lymphocyte stimulation in vitro.[249–252] Using ^{3}H-thymidine incorporation as an index of blast transformation, Paronetto and Popper found positive tests in 10 of 15 patients during an episode of halothane-induced hepatitis.[249] After recovery, two patients were retested and found to have negative tests. Inhibition of leukocyte migration was also demonstrated in the presence of halothane in the majority of patients with halothane-induced hepatitis.[251, 252] On the other hand, the results of other studies using blast transformation or inhibition of leukocyte migration in the presence of halothane have been negative;[250, 253–256] cross-reactivity with other agents and false-positive results also have been described.[252, 257] Walton and his colleagues were unable to demonstrate cellular hypersensitivity to trifluoroacetylated human liver–specific protein in patients with halothane-induced hepatitis.[256]

Studies from the Kings College Hospital in London have provided firmer evidence for a possible immune mechanism in halothane-induced hepatitis.[130] Leukocytes of patients recovering from halothane hepatitis were exposed to homogenized hepatocytes from halothane-exposed rabbits. In 9 of 11 patients, leukocyte migration was either increased or decreased compared with individuals exposed to halothane without ill-effect.[258] Antibodies were detected in 9 of 14 sera from 11 patients with halothane-induced hepatitis.[259] These antibodies bound in a granular pattern to "halothane-altered" rabbit hepatocytes but not to untreated cells or hepatocytes exposed to diethyl ether. The antibodies stimulated mononuclear cells from normal individuals to be cytotoxic to halothane-altered (but not to ether-treated) hepatocytes from rabbit. Lymphocytes from three of four patients with severe unexplained hepatitis following halothane anesthesia were demonstrably cytotoxic towards halothane-exposed rabbit hepatocytes.[260] Thus, antibodies and antibody-dependent cytotoxicity were present in 9 of 11 patients with halothane hepatitis.[249, 250] However, in four of these nine patients, antibodies were not detectable until eight weeks after the onset of liver injury. Although it has been suggested that this may be due to initial absorption of antibodies onto liver or to their concealment within circulating immune complexes,[246] the possibility remains that the antibodies were secondary to liver damage.[130] More recently, an enzyme-linked immunosorbent assay has been developed to recognize antibodies directed at the cell surface membrane of halothane-exposed rabbit hepatocytes.[261] This test identified antibodies in 16 of 24 patients with halothane-induced hepatitis and was negative in 26 healthy individuals, 17 people exposed to halothane without ill-effect, and 32 patients with other forms of liver disease.[261]

The hypotheses for immune or chemical mediation of halothane-induced hepatitis are not mutually exclusive.[59, 61, 101, 112] In theory, for example, there may be two (or three) types of halothane-induced liver injury.[60, 64–66, 75, 262] It is proposed, in fact, that one type consists of a mild, self-limited lesion resembling that seen in prospective studies of patients exposed repeatedly to halothane (see the preceding, p. 874)[63, 121–125] and possibly the nonjaundiced group of patients described by Otsuka and associates.[66] This type is considered to result from chemical toxicity.[60, 64, 75] The second, more severe, type may result from an accelerated immune response to cell constituents that have been altered by reacting with metabolites of halothane.[64, 65, 199, 200] Thus, Neuberger and coauthors have suggested that antibody-dependent cytotoxicity in patients with halothane-induced hepatitis is directed at determinants in the plasma membrane that are formed after the oxidative metabolism of halothane.[263] Support for this concept is that trifluoroacetyl adducts are present in the plasma membrane after exposing rat hepatocytes to halothane.[199, 200] Attempts to demonstrate an enhancement of halothane-induced liver injury in guinea pigs[256, 264] or in mice or rats[265] by sensitizing animals to trifluoroacetylated serum proteins have failed.

HEPATOTOXICITY OF OTHER ANESTHETIC AGENTS

METHOXYFLURANE

Methoxyflurane (Penthrane; see Fig. 34–1) was introduced in 1960 and became a commonly used general anesthetic agent, especially for eye surgery. Sporadic reports of hepatotoxicity,[266–268] nephrotoxicity, or both have appeared.[269–271] Two reviews of methoxyflurane hepatitis have been published.[270, 271] Although some cases of hepatic necrosis occurring after methoxyflurane anesthesia may have been caused by other factors, the similarity to halothane-associated hepatotoxicity together with metabolic pathways for biotransformation of methoxyflurane that predispose to hepatotoxicity support the conclusion that methoxyflurane-induced hepatitis is a real entity.[272-274] Among 24 patients with suspected methoxyflurane hepatitis, the underlying risk factors and clinical features were similar to those for halothane-induced hepatitis.[271] Two thirds of the patients were women and about one half were obese. Prior exposure to methoxyflurane was common (40 per cent of cases) but less than that among patients with halothane hepatitis. A few cases have been reported in which hepatic necrosis occurred after administration of methoxyflurane to patients with previous exposure to halothane only.[84, 271, 275] These reports raise the possibility of cross-sensitivity between halothane and methoxyflurane.

Fever was the presenting symptom in one half the patients with methoxyflurane-induced hepatitis. It appeared from as early as a few hours until 14 days (mean, 4 days) after surgery. There was a shorter latent period in patients who had received this agent previously.[271] Clinical and biochemical features of hepatitis were evident about two days after the onset of fever. The incidence of eosinophilia was about 20 per cent;[269, 271] less than 10 per cent of patients develop a rash.[271] A history of other allergic disorders was volunteered in 20 per cent of patients. The histologic features of methoxyflurane-induced hepatotoxicity appear to be indistinguishable from viral hepatitis. Among reported cases, the mortality of methoxyflurane-induced hepatitis has been about 60 per cent.[270, 271] Approximately 57 per cent of inhaled methoxyflurane undergoes metabolism,[276] and pretreatment with phenobarbital increases metabolism further.[272, 273] Production of large amounts of fluoride ion by cytochrome P450–catalyzed oxidation in hepatic endoplasmic reticulum is thought to cause the renal injury.[277]

Unlike patients with a suspected reaction to halothane, none with a suspected reaction to methoxyflurane has been challenged deliberately. The high mortality is a clear contraindication to such a study. Moreover, the evidence for cross-sensitization between halothane and methoxyflurane is sufficient to recommend that both agents be avoided in a patient who has exhibited unexplained postoperative fever of delayed onset, hepatitis after either agent, or both.[101, 271]

A proportion of individuals (about 20 per cent) who develop methoxyflurane-induced hepatotoxicity also develop methoxyflurane-induced nephrotoxicity.[270, 271] The exact relationship between the hepatitis and nephrotoxicity is unclear. Methoxyflurane-induced nephrotoxicity is characterized by a renal tubular defect resulting in failure to concentrate urine and unresponsiveness to vasopressin.[271, 277] This impairment of renal function usually is manifest immediately after surgery and lasts for as long as three weeks. Rarely, it may persist and may be associated with interstitial fibrosis and chronic renal failure.[271, 277] The mechanism is thought to be a direct renal tubular toxicity of fluoride ion produced by metabolism of the drug.[277] However, oxalate is another potentially nephrotoxic metabolite of methoxyflurane, and calcium oxalate crystals have been observed in the kidneys of patients with methoxyflurane-induced renal failure.[277] Although methoxyflurane possesses a number of desirable properties, including a potent analgesic effect, its use has declined markedly in the last decade because of nephrotoxicity.

FLUROXENE

A few case reports of severe hepatic necrosis after anesthesia have been attributed to fluroxene (2,2,2-trifluoroethyl vinyl ether).[97, 278, 279] This agent is metabolized by hepatic microsomal enzymes, and its biotransformation is enhanced by phenobarbital.[280] It is thus of interest that fluroxene has been reported to cause fatal hepatic necrosis in rats pretreated with phenobarbital.[281] Fluroxene is no longer used because of flammability and a tendency to produce postoperative nausea and vomiting.

ENFLURANE

Enflurane (see Fig. 34–1) was introduced in 1963. By 1983 it was estimated to have been administered to over 20 million patients.[282] Despite this widespread use, only 10 cases of hepatic injury were ascribed to enflurane during this time.[44, 282-289] In many of the reported cases, other causes of postoperative hepatic injury had not been discounted.[282, 290] In considering 58 suspected cases of enflurane-induced hepatitis, including the 10 previously published cases, Lewis and colleagues accepted only 24 in which viral hepatitis, other drugs, or other liver diseases could not be incriminated.[291] Moreover, it is not clear whether contamination of the anesthetic apparatus with halothane was possible in any of these patients.[111, 165] This could be relevant because seven patients had previously been administered halothane, and two of these had experienced postoperative fever and eosinophilia on the earlier occasion.[291] The possibility remains that some cases attributed to enflurane were actually cases of halothane-induced hepatitis. Nevertheless, in the only patient deliberately rechallenged with enflurane, recurrence of hepatotoxicity was documented.[286]

Among the 24 patients regarded as having enflurane-induced hepatotoxicity, the clinical, biochemical, and histologic features were similar to those of halothane-induced hepatitis.[291] Postoperative fever, usually beginning within 72 hours of anesthesia, was a presenting feature in 19 patients. Surgery had been relatively minor in two thirds of the patients and was unlikely to have produced shock or hypoxia. However, in some of the eight patients who had been subjected to laparotomy, the occurrence of transient shock or hypotension had been recorded. Only three patients were obese, and the sex incidence was equal. Jaundice appeared in 19 patients between 3 and 19 days (mean, 8 days) after anesthesia, and symptoms of hepatitis were reported in 40 per cent of cases. In five patients, a progressive course, with hepatic encephalopathy, acute renal failure, and death, occurred. Biochemical abnormalities were typical of hepatocellular necrosis, with serum aminotransferase levels being greater than 500 U/L in most cases. Histologic evidence of liver cell degeneration and necrosis always was apparent. Centrizonal necrosis or ballooning degeneration in acinar zone 3 was the predominant lesion in at least half the cases.[291] Two thirds of the patients had been exposed previously to either enflurane (nine instances) or halothane (seven instances). The latent period from the time of exposure to the onset of symptoms was shorter in these patients than in those without previous exposure. The possibility of hypersensitivity to enflurane with cross-reactivity to halothane has been raised on the basis of these observations, although Lewis and coauthors considered that "metabolic idiosyncrasy" was more likely.[291]

The criteria for recognizing enflurane-induced hepatitis as an entity were exclusion of other potential causes of postoperative hepatic dysfunction and the presence of "a consistent set of clinical features and a histologic pattern of injury suggesting a hepatic drug reaction."[291] It has been argued that these are "soft" criteria.[282, 290] The problems inherent in interpreting such limited data are exemplified by the fact that other experts who reviewed essentially the same material reached a different conclusion.[290] Among 88 cases of liver injury attributed to enflurane, the data were insufficient in 30 instances to assess the role of other variables. Other factors known to produce hepatic necrosis were present in 43 ("unlikely" group); and in only 15 patients ("possible enflurane hepatitis") were no other factors evident.[290] The authors were unable to find consistent morphologic features from either the "possible" or "unlikely" groups of cases. Female gender, a history of allergy, prior anesthesia with a halogenated anesthetic, onset of symptoms within five days, nausea, chills, and a serum AST more than ten times the normal value were more common in the "possible enflurane hepatitis" group. The issue of the existence of enflurane-induced hepatitis is thus not settled.[44, 282] Measurements of aminotransferases in serum after multiple exposures have given conflicting results.[123, 125, 127, 291, 292] Elevations of ALT were observed in 25 per cent of patients receiving enflurane on two or more occasions, but hepatotoxicity appeared to be minimal.[125] Apart from the occasional nonspecific allergic features of eosinophilia and rash, there are no data that provide insight into a possible mechanism for enflurane-induced hepatitis in patients. The Gastroenterology Drug Advisory Committee of the FDA did conclude in 1984 that there was a link between exposure to enflurane and liver damage.[44] If such a link exists, enflurane-induced hepatitis is rarer than halothane hepatitis, but the potential for cross-reactivity with halothane seems possible.

The mechanism by which enflurane could produce liver injury is unclear. The potential for hepatotoxicity of halothane, methoxyflurane, enflurane, and isoflurane appears to be roughly in proportion to the extent to which they undergo biotransformation. Enflurane, being less lipid-soluble than halothane, is stored in the body for a shorter time and only about 2.4 per cent of enflurane is metabolized.[293, 294] Metabolism is catalyzed by the cytochrome P450 system, but only oxidative mechanisms are involved.[20, 293–295] It seems unlikely, therefore, that radicals or other reactive metabolites are generated.[295] The form of cytochrome P450 that catalyzes enflurane metabolism is induced by phenobarbital and isoniazid.[20, 295] The initial step in enflurane metabolism is oxidation of the chlorofluoromethyl group (Fig. 34–4) to yield alcohol intermediates. These undergo spontaneous dehydrohalogenation to form acylhalides, which in turn form ionic halide and a carboxylic acid derivative. The relatively inert nature of enflurane would seem to indicate little potential for the proposed mechanism of metabolic idiosyncrasy.[291]

Hepatic necrosis can be produced in animals anesthetized with enflurane but only with a much lower oxygen supply:demand ratio than for halothane-induced liver injury.[177] Enflurane (and isoflurane) produced a mild degree of hepatocellular necrosis in about 25 per cent of rats pretreated with 3,3',5-triiodothyronine (T3), compared with more severe injury in 75 per cent of such animals exposed to halothane.[296] In other studies, enflurane was administered to rats, using moderately hypoxic conditions ($FI_{O_2} = 10$ per cent) and heating to prevent the hypothermia that otherwise occurs during haloalkane anesthesia. Hepatic necrosis after enflurane occurred only in animals kept at 37°C, in contrast to halothane, in which liver injury was present also in hypothermic rats.[210, 221, 297] Unlike halothane-associated hepatotoxicity, phenobarbital pretreatment had no effect on the incidence or severity of necrotic lesions caused by enflurane. These factors, together with the temporal pattern of enzyme release, which is not delayed, suggest that liver injury in the enflurane animal models is due to hepatic ischemia. There is no evidence that metabolism of enflurane is related to liver injury. Since enflurane anesthesia produces hepatic necrosis in animals only under extreme conditions, it seems unlikely that these observations have any relevance to possible rare episodes of idiosyncratic hepatic necrosis in humans.

ISOFLURANE

Isoflurane is a structural isomer of enflurane (see Fig. 34–1). It was produced in 1965 but was not released for clinical use until 1980. It is less soluble in blood and lipid compared with halothane, and the minimum alveolar concentration required for anesthesia is thus 1.5 times less than for halothane.[160, 161, 176] Only 0.17 per cent of the isoflurane taken up during anesthesia appears as urinary metabolites.[161] This lack of biotransformation of isoflurane may explain why no convincing cases of postoperative hepatotoxicity have been ascribed to it.[75, 161, 298, 299] In animals, isoflurane appears to resemble enflurane in being associated with hypoxic liver injury when unfavorable conditions of hepatic oxygen supply and demand exist.[82, 210, 296, 297] It seems safe to administer isoflurane to patients with a previous history of hepatotoxicity associated with halothane, methoxyflurane, or enflurane.[44, 75, 178]

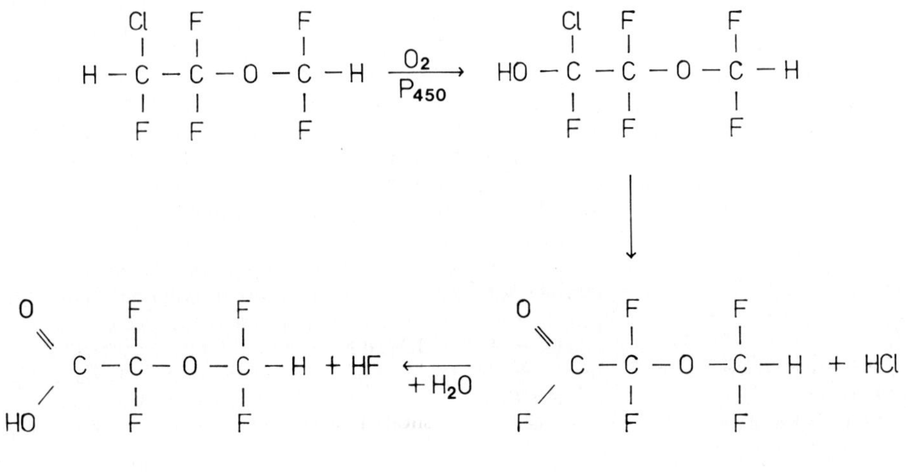

Figure 34–4. Pathway of enflurane metabolism. (Modified from Burke TR, et al. Drug Metab Dispos 9:19, 1981, © by Am. Soc. for Pharm. & Exp. Therapeutics.)

OTHER AGENTS

There is no evidence that nitrous oxide, thiopental, or narcotics (such as fentanyl) are hepatotoxic per se in the doses used in anesthesia. In phenobarbital-pretreated rats exposed to halothane under mildly hypoxic conditions (FI_{O_2} = 14 per cent), nitrous oxide appeared to potentiate marginally liver injury.[300] When phenobarbital-pretreated rats were exposed to severe hypoxia (FI_{O_2} = 7.5 per cent), hepatic injury occurred after exposure to 92.5 per cent nitrous oxide but not after enflurane, isoflurane, or thiopental. Fentanyl (but not nitrous oxide) was associated with centrolobular hepatic injury after exposure of rats to 9 per cent oxygen.[300] It has been concluded that all anesthetics can potentiate hypoxic liver injury in rats.[290] However, these observations are of dubious relevance to unexplained hepatic injury after anesthesia in humans.

UNEXPLAINED POSTOPERATIVE JAUNDICE

The overall incidence of jaundice following anesthesia and major surgery is probably less than 1 per cent.[301, 302] It is more common in critically ill patients and after trauma.[303] Exclusion of patients with underlying liver disease, posttransfusion hepatitis, extrahepatic biliary obstruction, or hepatic drug reactions leaves a large proportion of patients who have jaundice that is not readily explained. It seems likely that postoperative jaundice in such patients results from the interaction of a number of factors on the hepatic mechanism for excretion of bilirubin.[301, 302] In contrast to halothane hepatitis, this type of jaundice is more common after abdominal or cardiac surgery, after multiple traumas, and after prolonged operations.[303–306] The major contributing factors appear to be multiple blood transfusions, bacterial infection, shock, and hypoxia.

PATHOPHYSIOLOGY OF UNEXPLAINED POSTOPERATIVE JAUNDICE

Increased Pigment Load

About 10 per cent of erythrocytes in a 500-ml unit of stored blood undergoes hemolysis within 24 hours of transfusion. This liberates 7.5 g of hemoglobin, from which 250 mg of bilirubin is produced.[302] The normal liver should handle this increased load of pigment without elevation of the serum bilirubin concentration, but in the multitransfused, seriously ill postoperative patient, the bilirubin load from transfused blood may exceed the hepatic excretory capacity. Absorption of blood from large hematomas or hemolysis caused by factors such as prosthetic heart valves or glucose-6 phosphatase deficiency has the same effect. It appears that the excretory function of the liver is most affected by the nonspecific effects of surgery and anesthesia, because the resultant hyperbilirubinemia is composed of increased levels of conjugated bilirubin as well as unconjugated bilirubin (see Chap. 11).

Impaired Secretion of Bile

The term *benign postoperative intrahepatic cholestasis* was coined by Schmid and colleagues for a condition in which jaundice occurred early after surgery in the absence of other clinical and pathological features of hepatobiliary

disease.[304] A similar condition had been recognized earlier by French and German physicians.[307, 308] In most such patients, jaundice occurs within two to four days after surgery, reaches maximum intensity between 3 and 10 days, and then fades rapidly.[304, 306] Whereas pale stools and dark urine occur, fever, pruritus, symptoms of hepatitis, and evidence of hepatocellular failure are absent. The liver and spleen are not enlarged, and peripheral stigmata of liver disease are not present. Liver tests show a predominant elevation of total bilirubin in serum, which is composed of both conjugated and unconjugated bilirubin. Serum aminotransferases are characteristically normal or marginally elevated, with AST levels usually higher than those of ALT.[304, 306] Serum alkaline phosphatase is either normal or mild to moderately elevated. The prothrombin time, serum albumin, and levels of ammonia are minimally abnormal. The principal histologic findings in this disorder are preservation of the hepatic architecture and no evidence of hepatocellular necrosis, even at autopsy.[301, 304–306] Morphologic features of cholestasis are predominant, with canalicular bile plugs and staining of bile pigment in centrolobular liver cells but no evidence of extrahepatic biliary obstruction. A similar histologic "cholestasis" is seen in some other hyperbilirubinemic states, such as the Crigler-Najjar type I syndrome.[309, 310] There may be some swelling of centrolobular hepatocytes and fatty change in severe cases. The term *cholestasis* is probably not a good description of this entity, which is better regarded as an acquired disorder of hepatic bilirubin transport. Subclinical degrees of impaired excretory function, as detected by impaired sulfobromophthalein excretion, have been reported in about 50 per cent of patients following general anesthesia and surgery.[27–29, 77, 86, 311]

Most patients have received blood transfusions, but the blood has not always been old, and frank hemolysis usually is not present. The severity of the associated illness is such that postoperative mortality is high, 50 per cent in the series of Schmid and co-workers.[304] However, failure of hepatic synthetic functions and hepatic encephalopathy do not occur, thus supporting the concept that this is primarily a disorder of hepatobiliary excretion. The term *benign* pertains to the fact that jaundice itself, in this situation, is a postoperative complication of little consequence. It does not influence the outcome.

Bacterial Infection

Jaundice may complicate pneumococcal pneumonia, although this once common finding is now rare with prompt institution of antibiotic treatment.[312] Localized or systemic infection with gram-negative or gram-positive organisms may also be associated with a raised serum concentration of bilirubin.[313–315] The mechanism is unclear, but may be related to impaired bile secretion and to shortened red cell life span, resulting in increased production of bilirubin.[312, 316] In children, the presence of an infection such as an abdominal abscess or bacteremia may result in jaundice.[312] In adults, sepsis often is important in the multifactorial postoperative jaundice that occurs in critically ill patients.[312, 317]

Shock and Hypoxia

Prolonged hypotension and hypoxia may result in centrolobular hepatic necrosis. Ischemic hepatitis is best recognized as a complication of cardiac failure,[318, 319] but it may result from shock and hypoxia during surgery. This is most frequent after cardiac surgery, particularly for multiple valve replacement.[305] Ischemic hepatitis may be associated with very high serum levels of aminotransferase occurring within hours of surgery.[318, 319]

Among patients admitted with shock secondary to trauma, postoperative jaundice is uncommon, in one series occurring in about 2 per cent of cases.[303] Hyperbilirubinemia may be associated with up to tenfold elevations of serum AST. Centrolobular congestion with or without associated hepatocellular necrosis may be evident on histologic examination.[303] More often, multiple trauma, shock, and hypoxia together with blood transfusion, sepsis, and anesthesia are contributory factors to jaundice in critically ill patients, as alluded to earlier. In such cases, the prognosis is that of the underlying condition. Liver failure does not occur, and recovery is associated with complete resolution of hepatic morphology and excretory function.

OTHER CAUSES OF HEPATIC DYSFUNCTION IN THE POSTOPERATIVE PERIOD

Hepatobiliary disorders that occur for the first time in the postoperative period are listed in Table 34–1. A more detailed discussion of these conditions is outlined in the appropriate chapters. The following is a brief account of how such disorders are distinguished from halothane-induced hepatitis, ischemic hepatitis, and postoperative cholestasis (Table 34–5).

POST-TRANSFUSION HEPATITIS

Post-transfusion hepatitis differs from the previously discussed disorders because of its delayed onset. Hepatitis B is now rare after blood transfusion, and the incubation period is rarely shorter than six weeks. Non-A, non-B post-transfusion hepatitis usually has an incubation period of at least three weeks and on this basis can usually be distinguished from halothane-induced hepatitis.[320] Other viruses, such as cytomegalovirus and Epstein-Barr virus, are rare causes of post-transfusion hepatitis and are diagnosed by appropriate serologic tests. Post-transfusion hepatitis may cause clinical and laboratory features that are identical to those found with halothane-induced hepatitis, except that a very high fever and chills or eosinophilia are rare in viral hepatitis but common with halothane-induced hepatitis.

BILIARY OBSTRUCTION

Biliary obstruction may cause jaundice in the postoperative period when caused by surgical trauma to a major bile duct, retained gallstone in the common bile duct, or postoperative pancreatitis. These disorders are suggested by the clinical context and result in cholestasis of later onset than benign postoperative cholestasis (Table 34–5). Abdominal ultrasound will demonstrate dilation of the common bile duct when a low obstruction is present. Cholangiography, via a T-tube if one is present, is the definitive investigation and should be performed to define the site and nature of biliary obstruction. Acalculous cholecystitis may present in the postoperative period and is occasionally associated with jaundice.[321, 322] It is discussed elsewhere (Chap. 58).

OTHER HEPATIC DRUG REACTIONS

Other drug reactions may occur in the postoperative period. These should be suspected in any patient with unexplained cholestasis or hepatitis, especially when drugs have recently been commenced. Commonly incriminated agents are antibiotics such as cotrimoxazole, nitrofurantoin, and cloxacillin and anticonvulsants such as carbamazepine, sex steroids, and phenothiazines when used as tranquilizers or antiemetic agents. The clinicopathologic spectrum of reactions produced by such agents is discussed elsewhere (Chap. 31). In some cases, it may be impossible to distinguish between a reaction to, for example, isoniazid started two weeks before surgery and halothane-induced hepatitis. Unless one of the agents is uniquely valuable for that patient, an appropriate course of action is to withdraw all possible offending drugs and to caution against further use of halothane.

APPROACH TO THE PATIENT WITH JAUNDICE OR HEPATITIS IN THE POSTOPERATIVE PERIOD

The clinical features remain the most helpful factors leading to a correct diagnosis and appropriate course of action. Such features as antecedent symptoms of liver disease, a history of heavy alcohol ingestion, risk factors for hepatitis B or non-A, non-B infection, and recent

TABLE 34–5. CONTRASTING FEATURES OF DISORDERS CAUSING POSTOPERATIVE HEPATIC DYSFUNCTION

Disorder	Type of Surgery	Blood Transfusion	Previous Halothane Anesthetic	Fever	Onset Jaundice	Major Clinical Features	ALT U/L	BR	SAP
Halothane hepatitis	Often minor, usually repeated procedures	No	Yes	Usual, delayed onset	2–15 days	Fever, anorexia, nausea, jaundice	>500	↑	± ↑
Post-transfusion hepatitis	Required blood, especially cardiovascular	Yes	No	Minimal, late	3–10 weeks	Anorexia, nausea, fatigue	>100	± ↑	± ↑
Benign postoperative cholestasis	Complicated, abdominal, trauma	Yes	±	Common, due to bacterial sepsis	0–4 days	Critically ill patient	<100	↑ ↑	± ↑
Extrahepatic biliary obstruction	Biliary	No	No	±	Variable, often late	Pain, pruritus, jaundice	<100	↑	↑

± indicates variable responses; ± ↑, ↑, ↑ ↑ are arbitrary grades of abnormality.
BR = bilirubin.
SAP = serum alkaline phosphatase.

medication exposure may all suggest a possible cause. It should be remembered that asymptomatic liver disease may have been present before surgery.[61, 323] The time and mode of onset of symptoms will assist in distinguishing benign postoperative cholestasis, halothane hepatitis, extrahepatic biliary obstruction, and post-transfusion hepatitis (Table 34–5). High fever with chills commencing two to ten days after a halothane anesthetic and followed a few days later by symptoms of hepatitis and jaundice suggest halothane hepatitis if other etiologies are unlikely. Halothane hepatitis is much more likely if there is history of previous untoward reaction to halothane (delayed-onset of fever, nausea, or jaundice) and when repeated administrations have been given within 28 days. Post-transfusion hepatitis has a much later onset and fever is less prominent. Extrahepatic biliary obstruction should be suspected following biliary tract surgery or when epigastric pain and vomiting could be due to postoperative pancreatitis. Benign postoperative cholestasis is more likely when jaundice occurs within a few days of major surgery, when multiple blood transfusions have been given, and if shock, hypoxia, and sepsis have been part of the clinical picture.

In general, simple investigations will help strengthen the clinical suspicion of one of the above disorders (Table 34–5). A tenfold or more elevation of serum levels of aminotransferase is indicative of hepatocellular necrosis such as would be caused by viral hepatitis, ischemic hepatitis, or reaction to a drug, including halothane hepatitis. Serology for hepatitis viruses should be performed. Predominant elevation of serum alkaline phosphatase and other biliary enzymes occurs with extrahepatic biliary obstruction and less so with benign postoperative cholestasis. Abdominal ultrasound should be performed to help exclude extrahepatic biliary obstruction, and serum amylase estimations will aid the diagnosis of postoperative pancreatitis. Only in exceptional cases will further investigations, such as cholangiography, be required. Liver biopsy should be reserved for situations in which the diagnosis is not evident, and especially when the illness is severe and protracted. Histologic appearances will help distinguish hepatonecrotic lesions from cholestasis and may provide further evidence to support the possible diagnosis of halothane hepatitis.

REFERENCES

1. Price HL, Deutsch S, Davidson IA. Can general anesthetics produce splanchnic visceral hypoxia by reducing regional blood flow? Anesthesiology 27:24, 1966.
2. Epstein RM, Deutsch S, Cooperman LH. Splanchnic circulation during halothane anesthesia and hypercapnia in normal man. Anesthesiology 27:654, 1966.
3. Berger PE, Culham JAG, Fitz CR, et al. Slowing of hepatic blood flow by halothane: angiographic manifestations. Radiology 118:303, 1976.
4. Benumof JL, Bookstein JJ, Saidman LJ, et al. Diminished hepatic arterial flow during halothane administration. Anesthesiology 45:545, 1976.
5. Andreen M, Brandt R, Strandell T, et al. Hepatic gluconeogenesis during halothane anaesthesia in man. Acta Anaesthiol Scand 25:453, 1981.
6. Libonati M, Malsch E, Price HL, et al. Splanchnic circulation in man during methoxyflurane anesthesia. Anesthesiology 38:466, 1973.
7. Galindo A. Hepatic circulation and hepatic function during anesthesia and surgery. II. Effect of various anesthetic agents. Can Anaesth Soc J 12:337, 1965.
8. Larson CP, Mazze RI, Cooperman LH, et al. Effects of anesthesia on cerebral, renal and splanchnic circulations: recent developments. Anesthesiology 41:169, 1974.
9. Gelman SI. Disturbances in hepatic blood flow during anesthesia and surgery. Arch Surg 111:881, 1976.
10. Eger EI II, Smith NT, Stoelting RK, et al. Cardiovascular effects of halothane in man. Anesthesiology 32:396, 1970.
11. Lemasters JJ, Ji S, Thurman RG. Centrilobular injury following hypoxia in isolated, perfused rat liver. Science 213:661, 1981.
12. Shoemaker WC, Szanto PB, Fitch LB, et al. Hepatic physiologic and morphologic alterations in hemorrhagic shock. Surg Gynecol Obstet 118:828, 1964.
13. Biebuyck JF, Lund P, Krels HA. The effects of halothane (2-bromo-2-chloro-1,1,1-trifluoroethane) on glycolysis and biosynthetic processes of the isolated perfused rat liver. Biochem J 128:711, 1972.
14. Biebuyck JF, Lund P. Effects of halothane and other anesthetic agents on the concentrations of rat liver metabolites in vivo. Mol Pharmacol 10:474, 1974.
15. Hoech GP Jr, Matteo RS, Fink BR. Effect of halothane on oxygen consumption of rat brain, liver and heart and anaerobic glycolysis of rat brain. Anesthesiology 27:770, 1966.
16. Miller RN, Hunter FE Jr. The effect of halothane on electron transport, oxidative phosphorylation and swelling in rat liver mitochondria. Mol Pharmacol 6:67, 1970.
17. Reitbrock I, Lazarus G, Otterbein A. Effect of halothane on the hepatic drug metabolizing system. Arch Pharmacol 273:422, 1972.
18. Brown BR Jr, Sagalyn AM. Hepatic microsomal enzyme induction by inhalation anesthetics: mechanism in the rat. Anesthesiology 40:152, 1974.
19. Nastainczyk W, Ullrich V, Sies H. Effect of oxygen concentration on the reaction of halothane with cytochrome P450 in liver microsomes and isolated perfused rat liver. Biochem Pharmacol 27:387, 1978.
20. Ivanetich KM, Lucas SA, Marsh JA. Enflurane and methoxyflurane. Their interaction with hepatic cytochrome P-450 in vitro. Biochem Pharmacol 28:785, 1979.
21. Poppers PJ. Hepatic drug metabolism and anesthesia. Anaesthetist 29:55, 1980.
22. Krieter PA, Van Dyke RA. Cytochrome P-450 and halothane metabolism. Decrease in rat liver microsomal P-450 in vitro. Chem Biol Interact 44:219, 1983.
23. Enosawa SI, Nakazawa Y. Changes in cytochrome P-450 molecular species in rat liver in chloroform intoxication. Biochem Pharmacol 35:1555, 1986.
24. Uehleke H, Hellmer KH, Tabarelli-Poplawski S. Metabolic activation of halothane and its covalent binding to liver endoplasmic proteins in vitro. Arch Pharmacol 279:39, 1973.
25. Ross WT, Cardell RR Jr. Proliferation of smooth endoplasmic reticulum and induction of microsomal drug-metabolizing enzymes after ether or halothane. Anesthesiology 48:325, 1978.
26. de Groot H, Harnisch U, Noll T. Suicidal inactivation of microsomal cytochrome P-450 by halothane under hypoxic conditions. Biochem Biophys Res Commun 107:885, 1982.
27. Geller W, Tagnon HJ. Liver dysfunction following abdominal operations. The significance of postoperative hyperbilirubinemia. Arch Intern Med 86:908, 1950.
28. Keeri-Szanto M, Lafleur F. Postanaesthetic complications in a general hospital: a statistical study. Can Anaesth Soc J 10:531, 1963.
29. Beibuyck JF, Saunders SJ, Harrison GG, et al. Multiple halothane exposure and hepatic bromsulphthalein clearance. Br Med J 1:668, 1970.
30. Dale O, Nilsen OG. Glutathione and glutathione S-tranferases in rat liver after inhalation of halothane and enflurane. Toxicol Lett 23:61, 1984.
31. Aune H, Bessesen A, Olsen H, et al. Acute effects of halothane and enflurane on drug metabolism and protein synthesis in isolated rat hepatocytes. Acta Pharmacol Toxicol 55:363, 1983.
32. Pessayre D, Allemand H, Benoist C, et al. Effect of surgery under general anaesthesia on antipyrine clearance. Br J Clin Pharmacol 6:505, 1978.
33. Duvaldestin P, Mazze RI, Nivoche Y, et al. Enzyme induction following surgery with halothane and neurolept anesthesia. Anesth Analg 60:319, 1981.
34. St. Haxholdt O, Loft S, Clemmensen A, et al. Increased hepatic microsomal activity after halothane anaesthesia in children. Anaesthesia 41:579, 1986.
35. Nimmo WS, Thompson PG, Prescott LF. Microsomal enzyme induction after halothane anaesthesia. Br J Clin Pharmacol 12:433, 1981.
36. Duvaldestin P, Mauge F, Desmonts J-M. Enflurane anesthesia and antipyrine metabolism. Clin Pharmacol Ther 29:61, 1981.
37. Harville DH, Summerskill WHJ. Surgery in acute hepatitis. JAMA 184:257, 1963.
38. Turner MD, Sherlock S. In: Smith R, Sherlock S, eds. Surgery of the gallbladder and bile ducts. London, Butterworth and Co., 1964.
39. Hardy KJ, Hughes ESR. Laparotomy in viral hepatitis. Med J Aust 1:710, 1968.
40. Dykes MHM, Walzer SG. Preoperative and postoperative hepatic dysfunction. Surg Gynecol Obstet 124:747, 1967.

41. Simpson BR, Strunin L, Walton B. The halothane dilemma: a case for the defence. Br Med J 4:96, 1971.
42. Dykes MHM, Gilbert JP, McPeek B. Halothane in the United States. An appraisal of the literature on "Halothane Hepatitis" and the American reaction to it. Br J Anaesth 44:925, 1972.
43. Simpson BR, Strunin L, Walton B. Evidence for halothane hepatotoxicity is equivocal. In: Ingelfinger FJ, Ebert RV, Finland M, et al, eds. Controversy in Internal Medicine 2. Philadelphia, WB Saunders, 1972:580–594.
44. Stock JG, Strunin L. Unexplained hepatitis following halothane. Anesthesiology 63:424, 1985.
45. McSherry CK, Glenn F. The incidence and causes of death following surgery for nonmalignant biliary tract disease. Ann Surg 191:271, 1980.
46. Schwartz SI. Biliary tract surgery and cirrhosis: a critical combination. Surgery 90:577, 1981.
47. Aranha GV, Sontag SJ, Greenlee HB. Cholecystectomy in cirrhotic patients: a formidable operation. Am J Surg 143:55, 1982.
48. Doberneck RC, Sterling WA, Allison DC. Morbidity and mortality after operation in nonbleeding cirrhotic patients. Am J Surg 146:306, 1983.
49. Gill RA, Goodman MW, Golfus GR, et al. Aminopyrine breath test predicts surgical risk for patients with liver disease. Ann Surg 198:701, 1983.
50. Kaplan JA, Bitner RL, Dripps RD. Hypoxia, hyperdynamic circulation, and the hazards of general anesthesia in patients with hepatic cirrhosis. Anesthesiology 35:427, 1971.
51. Cousins MJ. Halothane hepatitis: What's new? Drugs 19:1, 1980.
52. Maze M, Smith CM, Baden JM. Halothane anesthesia does not exacerbate hepatic dysfunction in cirrhotic rats. Anesthesiology 62:1, 1985.
53. Schaffner F. Halothane hepatitis. In: Ingelfinger FJ, Ebert RV, Finland M, et al, eds. Controversy in Internal Medicine, vol 2. Philadelphia, WB Saunders, 1974:565–579.
54. Mushin WW, Rosen M, Bowen DJ, et al. Halothane and liver dysfunction: a retrospective study. Br Med J 2:329, 1964.
55. Dawson B, Adson MA, Dockerty MB, et al. Hepatic function tests: postoperative changes with halothane or diethyl ether anesthesia. Mayo Clin Proc 41:599, 1966.
56. Subcommittee on the National Halothane Study of Committee on Anesthesia, National Academy of Sciences—National Research Council. Summary of the national halothane study: possible association between halothane anesthesia and post-operative hepatic necrosis. JAMA 197:775, 1966.
57. Bunker JP. Final report of the national halothane study. Anesthesiology 29:231, 1968.
58. Sherlock S. Halothane hepatitis. Lancet 2:364, 1978.
59. Touloukian J, Kaplowitz N. Halothane-induced hepatic disease. Semin Liver Dis 1:134, 1981.
60. Halothane-associated liver damage. (Editorial.) Lancet 1:1251, 1986.
61. Brown BR Jr. Halothane hepatitis revisited. N Engl J Med 313:1347, 1985.
62. Brown BR Jr. Drugs, their complications and some new agents. Halogenated analgesics and hepatotoxicity. S Afr Med J 59:422, 1981.
63. Halothane. (Editorial.) Lancet 1:841, 1975.
64. Pohl LR, Gillette JR. A perspective on halothane-induced hepatotoxicity. Anesth Analg 61:809, 1982.
65. Neuberger J, Williams R. Halothane anaesthesia and liver damage. Br Med J 289:1136, 1984.
66. Otsuka S, Yamamoto M, Kasuya S, et al. HLA antigens in patients with unexplained hepatitis following halothane anaesthesia. Acta Anaesthesiol Scand 29:497, 1985.
67. v. Dardel O, Holmdahl MH, Norlander OP. A new modular system for anaesthesia and resuscitation. Acta Anaesthesiol Scand [Suppl] 26:5, 1966.
68. Strunin L. Hepatitis and halothane. Br J Anaesth 48:1035, 1976.
69. Stephen CR. Halothane and liver damage. N Engl J Med 280:561, 1969.
70. Strunin L, Simpson BR. Halothane in Britain today. Br J Anaesth 44:919, 1972.
71. Bunker JP. The Hepatotoxicity of Halothane. In: Ingelfinger FS, Ebert RV, Finland M, et al, eds. Controversy in Internal Medicine 2. Philadelphia, WB Saunders, 1974:595.
72. Cascorbi HF, Gravenstein JS. Silent death. Anesthesiology 40:319, 1974.
73. Conn HO. Halothane-associated hepatitis. A disease of medical progress. Israel J Med Sci 10:404, 1974.
74. Johnstone M. Halothane hepatitis. Lancet 2:526, 1978.
75. Blogg CE. Halothane and the liver: the problem revisited and made obsolete. Br Med J 292:1691, 1986.
76. Mushin WW, Rosen M, Jones EV. Post-halothane jaundice in relation to previous administration of halothane. Br Med J 3:18, 1971.
77. Little DM. Effects of halothane on hepatic function. In: Greene NM, ed. Clinical Anesthesia. 1. Halothane. Oxford, Blackwell Scientific Publications, 1968:85.
78. Johnstone M. Halothane: the first five years. Anesthesiology 22:591, 1961.
79. Hutchens KS, Kung M. "Experimentation" with chloroform. Am J Med 78:715, 1985.
80. Virtue RW, Payne KW. Postoperative death after fluorothane. Anesthesiology 19:562, 1958.
81. Barton JDM. Jaundice and halothane. Lancet 1:1097, 1959.
82. Temple RL, Cote RA, Gorens SW. Massive hepatic necrosis following general anesthesia. Anesth Analg 41:586, 1962.
83. Tygstrup N. Halothane hepatitis. Lancet 2:466, 1963.
84. Lindenbaum J, Leifer E. Hepatic necrosis associated with halothane anesthesia. N Engl J Med 268:525, 1963.
85. Bunker JP, Blumenfeld CM. Liver necrosis after halothane anesthesia. Cause or coincidence? N Engl J Med 268:531, 1963.
86. Blackburn WR, Ngai SH, Lindenbaum J. Morphologic changes in hepatic necrosis following halothane anesthesia in man. Anesthesiology 25:270, 1964.
87. Belcher HV, Remsberg JRS. Halothane anesthesia, hepatic necrosis, and death: report of a case. Surv Anesth 12:406, 1968.
88. DeBacker LJ, Longnecker DS. Prospective and retrospective searches for liver necrosis following halothane anesthesia. JAMA 195:157, 1966.
89. Beckman V, Brohult J, Reichard H. Elevations of liver enzyme activities in serum after halothane, ether and spinal anaesthesias. Acta Anaesth Scand 10:55, 1966.
90. Samrah ME. Liver damage after halothane. Br Med J 1:1736, 1963.
91. Slater EM, Gibson JM, Dykes MHM, et al. Postoperative hepatic necrosis. Its incidence and diagnostic value in association with the administration of halothane. N Engl J Med 270:983, 1964.
92. Dykes MHM, Walzer SG, Slater EM, et al. Acute parenchymatous hepatic disease following general anesthesia. Clinical appraisal of hepatotoxicity following administration of halothane. JAMA 193:339, 1965.
93. Dodson ME. The proof of guilt. A study of case reports of postoperative jaundice. Br J Anaesth 44:207, 1972.
94. Carney FMT, Van Dyke RA. Halothane hepatitis: a critical review. Anesth Analg 51:135, 1972.
95. Gall EA. Report of the pathology panel. National Halothane Study. Anesthesiology 29:233, 1968.
96. Davidson CS, Babior B, Popper H. Concerning hepatotoxicity of halothane. N Engl J Med 275:1497, 1966.
97. Peters RL, Edmondson HA, Reynolds TB, et al. Hepatic necrosis associated with halothane anesthesia. Am J Med 47:748, 1969.
98. Babior BM, Davidson CS. Postoperative massive liver necrosis. A clinical and pathological study. N Engl J Med 276:645, 1967.
99. Trey C, Lipworth L, Davidson CS. The clinical syndrome of halothane hepatitis. Anesth Analg 48:1033, 1969.
100. Coombes B. Halothane-induced liver damage—an entity. N Engl J Med 280:558, 1969.
101. Cousins MJ. Halothane and the liver: "firm ground" at last? Anaesth Intensive Care, 7:5, 1979.
102. Winkler K, Sejersen P, Rask H. Halothane. Lancet 2:902, 1965.
103. Inman WHW, Mushin WW. Jaundice after repeated exposure to halothane: an analysis of reports to the Committee on Safety of Medicines. Br Med J 1:5, 1974.
104. Belfrage S, Ahlgren I, Axelson S. Halothane hepatitis in an anaesthetist. Lancet 2:1466, 1966.
105. Klion FM, Schaffner F, Popper H. Hepatitis after exposure to halothane. Ann Intern Med 71:467, 1969.
106. Klatskin G, Kimberg DV. Recurrent hepatitis attributable to halothane sensitization in an anesthetist. N Engl J Med 280:515, 1969.
107. Böttiger LE, Dalén E, Hallén B. Halothane-induced liver damage: an analysis of the material reported to the Swedish Adverse Drug Reaction Committee, 1966–1973. Acta Anaesth Scand 20:40, 1976.
108. Keiding S, Døssing M, Hardt F. A nurse with liver injury associated with occupational exposure to halothane in a recovery unit. Dan Med Bull 31:255, 1984.
109. Lund I, Skulberg A, Helle I. Occupational hazard of halothane. Lancet 2:528, 1974.
110. Johnston CI, Mendelsohn F. Halothane hepatitis in a laboratory technician. Aust NZ J Med 2:171, 1971.
111. Marier JR. Halogenated hydrocarbon environmental pollution: the special case of halogenated anesthetics. Environ Res 28:212, 1982.
112. Kaplan HG, Bakken J, Quadracci L, et al. Hepatitis caused by halothane sniffing. Ann Intern Med 90:797, 1979.
113. Trey C, Lipworth L, Chalmers TC, et al. Fulminant hepatic failure. Presumable contribution of halothane. N Engl J Med 279:798, 1968.
114. Hughes M, Powell LW. Recurrent hepatitis in patients receiving

multiple halothane anaesthetics for radium treatment of carcinoma of the cervix uteri. Gastroenterology 58:790, 1970.

115. Paull A, Kerr Grant A. Halothane hepatitis. A report of five cases. Med J Aust 1:954, 1974.

116. Moult PJA, Sherlock S. Halothane-related hepatitis. A clinical study of twenty-six cases. Q J Med 44:99, 1975.

117. Walton B, Simpson BR, Strunin L, et al. Unexplained hepatitis following halothane. Br Med J 1:1171, 1976.

118. Farrell G, Prendergast D, Murray M. Halothane hepatitis. Detection of a constitutional susceptibility factor. N Engl J Med 313:1310, 1985.

119. Sharpstone P, Medley DRK, Williams R. Halothane hepatitis—a preventable disease? Br Med J 1:448, 1971.

120. Døssing M, Andreasen PB. Drug-induced liver disease in Denmark. Scand J Gastroenterol 17:205, 1982.

121. Trowell J, Peto R, Crampton-Smith A. Controlled trial of repeated halothane anaesthetics in patients with carcinoma of the uterine cervix treated with radium. Lancet 1:821, 1975.

122. Wright R, Eade OE, Chisholm M, et al. Controlled prospective study of the effect on liver function of multiple exposures to halothane. Lancet 1:817, 1975.

123. Fee JPH, Black GW, Dundee JW, et al. A prospective study of liver enzyme and other changes following repeat administration of halothane and enflurane. Br J Anaesth 51:1133, 1979.

124. Dundee JW, McIlroy PDA, Fee JPH, et al. Prospective study of liver function following repeat halothane and enflurane. J R Soc Med 74:286, 1981.

125. Dundee JW. Problems of multiple inhalation anaesthetics. Br J Anaesth 53:63S, 1981.

126. McEwan J. Liver function tests following anesthesia. Br J Anaesth 48:1065, 1976.

127. Allen PJ, Downing JW. A prospective study of hepatocellular function after repeated exposures to halothane or enflurane in women undergoing radium therapy for cervical cancer. Br J Anaesth 49:1035, 1977.

128. Curelaru I, St Stanciu V, Nicolau V, et al. A case of recovery from coma produced by the ingestion of 250 ml of halothane. Br J Anaesth 40:283, 1968.

129. Kopriva CJ, Lowenstein E. An anesthetic accident: cardiovascular collapse from liquid halothane delivery. Anesthesiology 30:246, 1969.

130. Dienstag JL. Halothane hepatitis. Allergy or idiosyncrasy? N Engl J Med 303:102, 1980.

131. Seef LB. Drug-induced chronic liver disease, with emphasis on chronic active hepatitis. Semin Liver Dis 1:104, 1981.

132. Campbell RL, Small EW, Lesesne HR, et al. Fatal hepatic necrosis after halothane anesthesia in a boy with juvenile rheumatoid arthritis: a case report. Anesth Analg 56:589, 1977.

133. Wark HJ. Postoperative jaundice in children. The influence of halothane. Anaesthesia 38:237, 1983.

134. Warner LO, Beach TP, Garvin JP, et al. Halothane and children: the first quarter century. Anesth Analg 63:838, 1984.

135. Walton B. Halothane hepatitis in children. Anaesthesia 41:575, 1986.

136. Lewis RB, Blair M. Halothane hepatitis in a young child. Br J Anaesth 54:349, 1982.

137. Whitburn RH, Sumner E. Halothane hepatitis in an 11-month-old child. Anaesthesia 41:611, 1986.

138. Bentley JB, Vaughan RW, Gandolfi J, et al. Halothane biotransformation in obese and nonobese patients. Anesthesiology 57:94, 1982.

139. Young SR, Stoelting RK, Peterson C, et al. Anesthetic biotransformation and renal function in obese patients during and after methoxyflurane or halothane anesthesia. Anesthesiology 42:451, 1975.

140. Hoft RH, Bunker JP, Goodman HI. Halothane hepatitis in three pairs of closely related women. N Engl J Med 304:1023, 1981.

141. Gourlay GK, Adams JF, Cousins MJ, et al. Genetic differences in reductive metabolism and hepatotoxicity of halothane in three rat strains. Anesthesiology 55:96, 1981.

142. Greene NM. Halothane anesthesia and hepatitis in a high-risk population. N Engl J Med 289:304, 1973.

143. Nomura F, Hatano H, Ohnishi K, et al. Effects of anticonvulsant agents on halothane-induced liver injury in human subjects and experimental animals. Hepatology 6:952, 1986.

144. Jurgensen JC, Abraham JP, Hardy WW. Erythroid aplasia after halothane hepatitis. Report of a case. Am J Dig Dis 15:577, 1970.

145. Murisasco A, Saingra S, Auffray JP, et al. A case of acute reversible renal failure associated with halothane-induced liver disease. Clin Nephrol 15:44, 1981.

146. Gelman ML, Lichtenstein NS. Halothane-induced nephrotoxicity. Urology 17:323, 1981.

147. Uzunalimoglu B, Yardley JH, Boitnott JK. The liver in mild halothane hepatitis. Light and electron microscopic findings with special reference to the mononuclear cell infiltrate. Am J Pathol 61:457, 1970.

148. Wills EJ, Walton B. A morphologic study of unexplained hepatitis following halothane anesthesia. Am J Pathol 91:11, 1978.

149. Review by an International Group: Guidelines for diagnosis of therapeutic drug-induced liver injury in liver biopsies. Lancet 1:854, 1974.

150. Shah IA, Brandt H. Halothane-associated granulomatous hepatitis. Digestion 28:245, 1983.

151. Dordal E, Glagov S, Orlando RA, et al. Fatal halothane hepatitis with transient granulomas. N Engl J Med 283:357, 1970.

152. Neville E, Piyasena KHG, James DG. Granulomas of the liver. Postgrad Med J 51:361, 1975.

153. Thomas FB. Chronic aggressive hepatitis induced by halothane. Ann Intern Med 81:487, 1974.

154. Kronborg IJ, Evans DTP, Mackay IR, et al. Chronic hepatitis after successive halothane anesthetics. Digestion 27:123, 1983.

155. Camilleri M, Victorino RMM, Hodgson HJF. Halothane aggravation of chronic liver disease. Acta Med Port 5:194, 1984.

156. Dykes MHM. Is halothane hepatitis chronic active hepatitis? There may be a need to control the challenge test. Anesthesiology 46:233, 1977.

157. Moore DH, Benson GD. Prolonged halothane hepatitis: prompt resolution of severe lesion with corticosteroid therapy. Dig Dis Sci 31:1269, 1986.

158. Peleman RR, Gavaler JS, Van Thiel DH, et al. Orthotopic liver transplantation for acute and subacute hepatic failure in adults. Hepatology 7:484, 1987.

159. Miller DJ, Dwyer J, Klatskin G. Halothane hepatitis: benign resolution of a severe lesion. Ann Intern Med 89:212, 1978.

160. Corall IM. Isoflurane: the need for new volatile agents. Anaesthesia 38:1035, 1983.

161. Eger FI II. The pharmacology of isoflurane. Br J Anaesth 56:71S, 1984.

162. Crawford JS. Halothane and the liver. Br Med J 293:334, 1986.

163. Inman WHW, Mushin WW. Jaundice after repeated exposure to halothane: a further analysis of reports to the Committee on Safety of Medicines. Br Med J 2:1455, 1978.

164. Bruce DL. What is a "safe" interval between halothane exposures? JAMA 221:1140, 1972.

165. Dykes MHM, Laasberg LH. Clinical implications of halothane contamination of the anesthetic circle. Anesthesiology 35:648, 1971.

166. Jones WM, Margolis G, Stephen CR. Hepatotoxicity of inhalation anesthetic drugs. Anesthesiology 19:715, 1958.

167. Chang LW, Dudley AW Jr, Lee YK, et al. Ultrastructural studies of the hepatocytes after chronic exposure to low levels of halothane. Exp Mol Pathol 23:35, 1975.

168. Plummer JL, Hall P de la M, Cousins MJ, et al. Hepatic injury in rats due to prolonged sub-anaesthetic halothane exposure. Acta Pharmacol Toxicol 53:16, 1983.

169. Brown BR, Sipes IG. Biotransformation and hepatotoxicity of halothane. Biochem Pharmacol 26:2091, 1977.

170. de Groot H, Noll T. Halothane hepatotoxicity: relation between metabolic activation, hypoxia, covalent binding, lipid peroxidation and liver cell damage. Hepatology 3:601, 1983.

171. Sawyer DC, Eger EI II, Bahlman SH, et al. Concentration dependence of hepatic halothane metabolism. Anesthesiology 34:230, 1971.

172. Fiserova-Bergerova V, Kawiecki RW. Effects of exposure concentrations on distribution of halothane metabolites in the body. Drug Metab Dispos 12:98, 1984.

173. Sipes IG, Brown BR Jr. An animal model of hepatotoxicity associated with halothane anaesthesia. Anesthesiology 15:622, 1976.

174. McLain GE, Sipes IG, Brown BR Jr. An animal model of halothane hepatotoxicity: role of enzyme induction and hypoxia. Anesthesiology 51:321, 1979.

175. Jee RC, Sipes IG, Gandolfi AJ, et al. Factors influencing halothane hepatotoxicity in the rat hypoxic model. Toxicol Appl Pharmacol 52:267, 1980.

176. Van Dyke RA. Hepatic centrilobular necrosis in rats after exposure to halothane, enflurane or isoflurane. Anesth Analg 61:812, 1982.

177. Gelman S. Are the requirements of hepatic injury with halothane and enflurane in rats really different? Anesth Analg 65:539, 1986.

178. Gelman S. Halothane hepatotoxicity—again? Anesth Analg 65:831, 1986.

179. Cohen EN, Hood N. Application of low-temperature autoradiography to studies of the uptake and metabolism of volatile anesthetics in the mouse. III. Halothane. Anesthesiology 31:553, 1969.

180. Cohen EN. Metabolism of halothane-2 ^{14}C in the mouse. Anesthesiology 31:560, 1969.

181. Cascorbi HF, Blake DA, Helrich M. Differences in the biotransformation of halothane in man. Anesthesiology 32:119, 1970.

182. Tinker JH, Gandolfi AJ, Van Dyke RA. Elevation of plasma bromide levels in patients following halothane anesthesia: time correlation with total halothane dosage. Anesthesiology 44:194, 1976.

183. Cohen EN, Trudell JR, Edmunds HN. Urinary metabolites of halothane in man. Anesthesiology 43:392, 1975.
184. Stier A, Alter H, Hessler O, et al. Urinary excretion of bromide in halothane anesthesia. Anesth Analg 43:723, 1964.
185. Cascorbi HF, Vesell ES, Blake DA, et al. Halothane biotransformation in man. Ann NY Acad Sci 179:244, 1971.
186. Van Dyke RA. Metabolism of volatile anesthetics. III. Induction of microsomal dechlorinating and ether-cleaving enzymes. J Pharmacol Exp Ther 154:364, 1966.
187. Van Dyke RA, Chenoweth MB, Larsen ER. Synthesis and metabolism of halothane-1-^{14}C. Nature 204:470, 1964.
188. Van Dyke RA, Chenoweth MB, Van Poznak A. Metabolism of volatile anesthetics. I. Conversion in vivo of several anesthetics to $^{14}CO_2$ and chloride. Biochem Pharmacol 13:1239, 1964.
189. Van Dyke RA, Chenoweth MB. The metabolism of volatile anesthetics. II. In vitro metabolism of methoxyflurane and halothane in rat liver slices and cell fractions. Biochem Pharmacol 14:603, 1965.
190. Fujii K, Miki N, Sugiyama T, et al. Anaerobic dehalogenation of halothane by reconstituted liver microsomal cytochrome P-450 enzyme system. Biochem Biophys Res Commun 102:507, 1981.
191. Lind RC, Gandolfi AJ, Sipes IG, et al. Oxygen concentrations required for reductive defluorination of halothane by rat hepatic microsomes. Anesth Analg 65:835, 1986.
192. Plummer JL, Van der Walt JH, Cousins MJ. Reductive metabolism of halothane in children. Anaesth Intensive Care 12:293, 1984.
193. Cousins MJ, Sharp H, Gourlay GK, et al. Hepatotoxicity and halothane metabolism in an animal model with application for human toxicity. Anaesth Intensive Care 7:9, 1979.
194. Stenger RJ, Johnson EA, Rosenthal WS. Effects of phenobarbital pretreatment on the response of rat liver to halothane administration. Proc Soc Exp Biol Med 140:1319, 1972.
195. Reynolds ES, Moslen MT. Halothane hepatotoxicity: enhancement by polychlorinated biphenyl pretreatment. Anaesthesiology 47:19, 1977.
196. Takagi T, Ishii H, Takahashi H, et al. Potentiation of halothane hepatotoxicity by chronic ethanol administration in rat: an animal model of halothane hepatitis. Pharmacol Biochem Behav 18:461, 1983.
197. Rao GS. A study of the mechanism of halothane-induced liver necrosis. Role of covalent binding of halothane metabolites to liver proteins in the rat. J Med Chem 20:262, 1977.
198. Cohen EN. Metabolism of the volatile anesthetics. Anesthesiology 85:193, 1971.
199. Satoh H, Fukuda Y, Anderson DK, et al. Immunological studies on the mechanism of halothane-induced hepatotoxicity: immunohistochemical evidence of trifluoroacetylated hepatocytes. J Pharmacol Exp Ther 233:857, 1985.
200. Satoh H, Gillette JR, Davies HW, et al. Immunochemical evidence of trifluoroacetylated cytochrome P-450 in the liver of halothane-treated rats. Mol Pharmacol 28:468, 1985.
201. Mukai S, Morio M, Fujii K, et al. Volatile metabolites of halothane in the rabbit. Anesthesiology 47:248, 1977.
202. Sharp JH, Trudell JR, Cohen EN. Volatile metabolites and decomposition products of halothane in man. Anesthesiology 50:2, 1979.
203. Sipes IG, Gandolfi AJ, Pohl LR, et al. Comparison of the biotransformation and hepatotoxicity of halothane and deuterated halothane. J Pharmacol Exp Ther 214:716, 1980.
204. Van Dyke RA, Wood CL. Binding of radioactivity from ^{14}C-labeled halothane in isolated perfused rat livers. Anesthesiology 38:328, 1973.
205. Van Dyke RA, Gandolfi AJ. Studies on irreversible binding of radioactivity from [^{14}C]halothane to rat hepatic microsomal lipids and protein. Drug Metab Dispos 2:469, 1974.
206. Baker MT, Van Dyke RA. Reductive halothane metabolite formation and halothane binding in rat hepatic microsomes. Chem Biol Interact 49:121, 1984.
207. Trudell JR, Bosterling B, Trevor AJ. Reductive metabolism of halothane by human and rabbit cytochrome P-450. Binding of 1-chloro-2,2,2-trifluoroethyl radical to phospholipids. Mol Pharmacol 21:710, 1982.
208. Gandolfi AJ, White RD, Sipes IG, et al. Bioactivation and covalent binding of halothane. Studies with [^{3}H]$^-$ and [^{14}C]halothane. J Pharmacol Exp Ther 214:721, 1980.
209. Plummer JL, Wanwimolruk S, Jenner MA, et al. Effects of cimetidine and ranitidine on halothane metabolism and hepatotoxicity in an animal model. Drug Metab Dispos 12:106, 1984.
210. Lind RC, Gandolfi AJ, Sipes IG, et al. Comparison of the requirements for hepatic injury with halothane and enflurane in rats. Anesth Analg 64:955, 1985.
211. Widger LA, Gandolfi AJ, Van Dyke RA. Hypoxia and halothane metabolism in vivo: release of inorganic fluoride and halothane metabolite binding to cellular constituents. Anesthesiology 44:197, 1976.
212. Harper MH, Collins P, Johnson BH, et al. Postanesthetic hepatic injury in rats: influence of alterations in hepatic blood flow, surgery, and anesthesia time. Anesth Analg 61:79, 1982.
213. Goldblum A, Loew GH. Quantum chemical studies of anaerobic reductive metabolism of halothane by cytochrome P-450. Chem Biol Interact 32:83, 1980.
214. Siegers C-P, Fruhling A, Younes M. Influence of dithiocarb, (+)-catechin and silybine on halothane hepatotoxicity in the hypoxic rat model. Acta Pharmacol Toxicol 53:125, 1983.
215. Poyer JL, McCay PB. In vivo spin-trapping of radicals formed during halothane metabolism. Biochem Pharmacol 30:1517, 1981.
216. Plummer JL, Beckwith ALJ, Bastin FN, et al. Free radical formation in vivo and hepatotoxicity due to anesthesia with halothane. Anesthesiology 57:160, 1982.
217. Brown BR, Sipes IG, Baker RK. Halothane hepatotoxicity and the reduced derivative 1,1,1-trifluoro-2-chloroethane. Environ Health Perspect 21:185, 1977.
218. Van Dyke RA. Metabolism of anesthetic agents: toxic implications. Acta Anaesth Scand (Suppl) 75:7, 1982.
219. Tribble DL, Aw TY, Jones DP. The pathophysiological significance of lipid peroxidation in oxidative cell injury. Hepatology 7:377, 1987.
220. Strunin L, Harrison LJ, Davies JM. Etiology of halothane hepatotoxicity. Anesthesiology 58:391, 1983.
221. Shingu K, Eger EI II, Johnson BH, et al. Hepatic injury induced by anesthetic agents in rats. Anesth Analg 62:140, 1983.
222. Shingu K, Eger EI II, Johnson BH. Hypoxia may be more important than reductive metabolism in halothane-induced hepatic injury. Anesth Analg 61:824, 1982.
223. Shingu K, Eger EI II, Johnson BH. Hypoxia per se can produce hepatic damage without death in rats. Anesth Analg 61:820, 1982.
224. Hughes HC, Lang CM. Hepatic necrosis produced by repeated administration of halothane to guinea pigs. Anesthesiology 36:466, 1972.
225. Reves JG, McCracken LE. Failure to induce hepatic pathology in animals sensitized to a halothane metabolite and subsequently challenged with halothane. Anesth Analg 55:235, 1976.
226. Lunam CA, Cousins MJ, Hall P de la M. Guinea-pig model of halothane-associated hepatotoxicity in the absence of enzyme induction and hypoxia. J Pharmacol Exp Ther 232:802, 1985.
227. Brown BR Jr, Sipes IG, Sagalyn AM. Mechanisms of acute hepatic toxicity: chloroform, halothane, and glutathione. Anesthesiology 41:554, 1974.
228. Harrison GG, Manca V. The effect of exposure to halogenated anesthetics on liver glutathione levels in rats. S Afr Med J 55:555, 1979.
229. Brown BR Jr. Hepatic microsomal lipoperoxidation and inhalation anesthetics: a biochemical and morphologic study in the rat. Anesthesiology 36:458, 1972.
230. Wood CL, Gandolfi AJ, Van Dyke RA. Lipid binding of a halothane metabolite. Relationship to lipid peroxidation in vitro. Drug Metab Dispos 4:305, 1976.
231. de Groot H, Noll T. The crucial role of hypoxia in halothane-induced lipid peroxidation. Biochem Biophys Res Commun 119:139, 1984.
232. Kessler M. Normal and critical O_2 supply of the liver. In: Lubbers DW, Luft UC, Thews G, et al, eds. Oxygen transport in blood and tissue. Stuttgart, Georg Thieme Verlag, 1968:242.
233. Recknagel RO. A new direction in the study of CCl_4 hepatotoxicity. Life Sci 33:401, 1983.
234. Long RM, Moore L. Elevated cytosolic calcium in rat hepatocytes exposed to carbon tetrachloride. J Pharmacol Exp Ther 238:186, 1986.
235. Bellomo G, Orrenius S. Altered thiol and calcium homeostasis in oxidative hepatocellular injury. Hepatology 5:876, 1985.
236. Moore M, Thor H, Moore G, et al. The toxicity of acetaminophen and N-acetyl-P-benzoquinone imine in isolated hepatocytes is associated with thiol depletion and increased cytosolic Ca^{2+}. J Biol Chem 260:13035, 1985.
237. Zucker JR, Diamond EM, Berman MC. Effect of halothane on calcium transport in isolated hepatic endoplasmic reticulum. Br J Anaesth 54:981, 1982.
238. Farrell GC, Mahoney J, Bilous M, et al. Altered hepatic calcium homeostasis in guinea pigs with halothane-induced hepatotoxicity. J Pharmacol Exp Ther 247:751, 1988.
239. Nelson TE, Flewellen EH. The malignant hyperthermia syndrome. N Engl J Med 309:416, 1983.
240. Klip A, Britt BA, Elliott ME, et al. Anesthetic-induced increase in ionised calcium in blood mononuclear cells from malignant hyperthermia patients. Lancet 1:463, 1987.
241. Chapman BA, Laurenson VG, Cook HB. Halothane hepatitis: toxicity or hypersensitivity? NZ Med J 98:793, 1985.
242. Doniach D, Roitt IM, Walker JG, et al. Tissue antibodies in primary biliary cirrhosis, active chronic (lupoid) hepatitis, cryptogenic cirrhosis and other liver diseases and their clinical implications. Clin Exp Immunol 1:237, 1966.
243. Rodriguez M, Paronetto F, Schaffner F, et al. Antimitochondrial

antibodies in jaundice following drug administration. JAMA 208:148, 1969.

244. Homberg J-C, Abuf N, Helmy-Khalil S, et al. Drug-induced hepatitis associated with anticytoplasmic organelle autoantibodies. Hepatology 5:722, 1985.

245. Mackay IR. Induction by drugs of hepatitis and autoantibodies to cell organelles: significance and interpretation. Hepatology 5:904, 1985.

246. Canalese J, Wyke RJ, Vergani D, et al. Circulating immune complexes in patients with fulminant hepatic failure. Gut 22:845, 1981.

247. Williams BD, White N, Amlot PL, et al. Circulating immune complexes after repeated halothane anesthesia. Br Med J 2:159, 1977.

248. Eade OE, Grice D, Krawitt EL, et al. HLA A and B locus antigens in patients with unexplained hepatitis following halothane anaesthesia. Tissues Antigens 17:428, 1981.

249. Paronetto F, Popper H. Lymphocyte stimulation induced by halothane in patients with hepatitis following exposure to halothane. N Engl J Med 283:277, 1970.

250. Moult PJA, Adjukiewicz AB, Gaylarde PM, et al. Lymphocyte transformation in halothane-related hepatitis. Br Med J 2:69, 1975.

251. Price CD, Gibbs AR, Williams WJ. Evaluation of the macrophage migration inhibition test in halothane-induced hepatitis (halothane MIF test). J Clin Pathol 30:96, 1977.

252. Nunez-Gornes JF, Marx JJ Jr, Motszko C. Leukocyte migration inhibition in halothane-induced hepatitis. Clin Immunol Immunopathol 14:30, 1979.

253. Davies GE, Holmes JE. Drug-induced immunological effects on the liver. Br J Anaesth 44:941, 1972.

254. Walton B, Dumonde DC, Williams C, et al. Failure to demonstrate increased lymphocyte transformation in patients with postoperative jaundice and physicians with alleged halothane sensitivity. Br J Anaesth 44:904, 1972.

255. Walton B, Hamblin A, Dumonde DC, et al. Further immunological investigations in patients with possible halothane hepatitis. Br J Anaesth 47:908, 1975.

256. Walton B, Hamblin A, Dumonde DC, et al. Absence of cellular hypersensitivity in patients with unexplained hepatitis following halothane. Anesthesiology 44:391, 1976.

257. Lecky JH, Cohen PJ. Hepatic dysfunction without jaundice following administration of halothane. Anaesthesiology 33:371, 1970.

258. Vergani D, Tsantoulas D, Eddleston ALWF, et al. Sensitisation to halothane-altered liver components in severe hepatic necrosis after halothane anaesthesia. Lancet 2:801, 1978.

259. Vergani D, Mieli-Vergani G, Alberti A, et al. Antibodies to the surface of halothane-altered rabbit hepatocytes in patients with severe halothane-associated hepatitis. N Engl J Med 303:66, 1980.

260. Mieli-Vergani G, Vergani D, Tredger JM, et al. Lymphocyte cytotoxicity to halothane-altered hepatocytes in patients with severe hepatic necrosis following halothane anaesthesia. J Clin Lab Immunol 4:49, 1980.

261. Kenna JG, Neuberger J, Williams R. An enzyme-linked immunosorbent assay for detection of antibodies against halothane-altered hepatocyte antigens. J Immunol Methods 75:3, 1984.

262. Davis M, Eddleston ALWF, Neuberger JM, et al. Halothane hepatitis. N Engl J Med 303:1123, 1980.

263. Neuberger J, Mieli-Vergani G, Tredger JM, et al. Oxidative metabolism of halothane in the production of altered hepatocyte membrane antigens in acute halothane-induced hepatic necrosis. Gut 22:669, 1981.

264. Reves JG, McCracken LE Jr. Hepatic pathology and skin test reactions to trifluoro-acetylated autologous protein after repeated halothane anaesthesia in the guineapig. Br J Anaesth 48:419, 1976.

265. Ford DJ, Coyle DE, Harrington JF. Effects of hypersensitivity to a halothane metabolite on halothane-induced liver damage. Anesthesiology 60:141, 1984.

266. Stefanini M, Herland A, Kosyak EP. Fatal massive necrosis of the liver after repeated exposure to methoxyflurane. Anesthesiology 32:374, 1970.

267. Katz S. Hepatic coma associated with methoxyflurane anesthesia. Report of a case. Am J Dig Dis 15:733, 1970.

268. Brenner AI, Kaplan MM. Recurrent hepatitis due to methoxyflurane anesthesia. N Engl J Med 284:961, 1971.

269. Elkington SG, Goffinet JA, Conn HO. Renal and hepatic injury associated with methoxyflurane anesthesia. Ann Intern Med 69:1229, 1968.

270. Litwiller RW, DiFazio CA, Carron H. Postmethoxyflurane hepatitis: a clinical entity. South Med J 67:351, 1974.

271. Joshi PH, Conn HO. The syndrome of methoxyflurane-associated hepatitis. Ann Intern Med 80:395, 1974.

272. Murray WJ, Fleming PJ. Defluorination of methoxyflurane during anesthesia. Anesthesiology 37:620, 1972.

273. Mazze RI, Hitt BA, Cousins MJ. Effect of enzyme induction with phenobarbital on the in vivo and in vitro defluorination of isoflurane and methoxyflurane. J Pharmacol Exp Ther 190:523, 1974.

274. Holaday DA, Fiserova-Bergerova V. Fate of fluorinated metabolites of inhalation anesthetics in man. Drug Metab Rev 9:61, 1979.

275. Judson JA, de Jough HJ, Walmsley JBW. Possible cross-sensitivity between halothane and methoxyflurane: report of a case. Anesthesiology 35:527, 1971.

276. Plummer JL, Hall P de la M, Jenner MA, et al. Hepatic and renal effects of prolonged exposure of rats to 50 ppm methoxyflurane. Acta Pharmacol Toxicol 57:176, 1985.

277. Cousins MJ, Mazze RI, Kosek JC, et al. The etiology of methoxyflurane nephrotoxicity. J Pharmacol Exp Ther 190:530, 1974.

278. Harris JA, Cromwell TH. Jaundice following fluroxene anesthesia. Anesthesiology 37:462, 1972.

279. Reynolds ES, Brown BR Jr, Vandam LD. Massive hepatic necrosis after fluroxene anesthesia—a case of drug interaction? N Engl J Med 286:530, 1972.

280. Blake DA, Rozman RS, Cascorbi HF, et al. Anaesthesia. LXXIV. Biotransformation of fluroxene-I. Metabolism in mice and dogs in vivo. Biochem Pharmacol 16:1237, 1967.

281. Smith JS, Harrison GG. The effects of multiple anaesthetics on the livers of rats subjected to microsomal enzyme induction. S Afr Med J 47:797, 1973.

282. Dykes MHM. Is enflurane hepatotoxic? Anesthesiology 61:235, 1984.

283. Van Der Reis L, Askin SJ, Frecker GN, et al. Hepatic necrosis after enflurane anesthesia. JAMA 227:76, 1974.

284. Ona FV, Patanella H, Ayub A. Hepatitis associated with enflurane anesthesia. Anesth Analg 59:146, 1980.

285. Vacanti CJ, Lynch TG. Hepatitis following enflurane. Anesth Analg 59:890, 1980.

286. Kline MM. Enflurane-associated hepatitis. Gastroenterology 79:126, 1980.

287. White LB, DeTarnowsky GO, Mir JA, et al. Hepatotoxicity following enflurane anesthesia. Dig Dis Sci 26:466, 1981.

288. Masone RJ, Goldfarb JP, Manzione NC, et al. Enflurane hepatitis. J Clin Gastroenterol 4:541, 1982.

289. Sigurdsson J, Hreidarsson AB, Thjodleifsson B. Enflurane hepatitis: a report of a case with a previous history of halothane hepatitis. Acta Anaesth Scand 29:495, 1985.

290. Eger EI II, Smuckler EA, Ferrell LD, et al. Is enflurane hepatotoxic? Anesth Analg 65:21, 1986.

291. Lewis JH, Zimmerman HJ, Ishak KG, et al. Enflurane hepatotoxicity. Ann Intern Med 98:984, 1983.

292. Plummer JL, Hall P de la M, Jenner MA, et al. Effects of chronic inhalation of halothane, enflurane or isoflurane in rats. Br J Anaesth 58:517, 1986.

293. Chase RE, Holaday DA, Fiserova-Bergerova V, et al. The biotransformation of ethrane in man. Anesthesiology 35:262, 1972.

294. Hitt BA, Mazze RI, Beppu WJ, et al. Enflurane metabolism in rats and man. J Pharmacol Exp Ther 203:193, 1977.

295. Burke TR, Branchflower RV, Lees DE, et al. Mechanism of defluorination of enflurane. Drug Metab Dispos 9:19, 1981.

296. Berman ML, Kuhnert L, Phythyon JM, et al. Isoflurane and enflurane-induced hepatic necrosis in triiodothyronine-pretreated rats. Anesthesiology 58:1, 1983.

297. Harper MH, Collins P, Johnson B, et al. Hepatic injury following halothane, enflurane, and isoflurane anesthesia in rats. Anesthesiology 56:14, 1982.

298. Allan LG, Hussey JA, Howie J, et al. Hepatic glutathione S-transferase release after halothane anaesthesia: open randomised comparison with isoflurane. Lancet 1:771, 1987.

299. Lambert DH. Isoflurane and hepatic dysfunction. Anesth Analg 64:456, 1985.

300. Ross JAS, Monk SJ, Duffy SW. Effect of nitrous oxide on halothane-induced hepatotoxicity in hypoxic, enzyme-induced rats. Br J Anaesth 56:527, 1984.

301. LaMont JT, Isselbacher KJ. Postoperative jaundice. N Engl J Med 288:305, 1973.

302. LaMont JT. Postoperative jaundice. Surg Clin North Am 54:637, 1974.

303. Nunes G, Blaisdell FW, Margaretten W. Mechanism of hepatic dysfunction following shock and trauma. Arch Surg 100:546, 1970.

304. Schmid M, Hefti ML, Gattiker R, et al. Benign postoperative intrahepatic cholestasis. N Engl J Med 272:546, 1965.

305. Sanderson RG, Ellison JH, Benson JA, et al. Jaundice following open-heart surgery. Ann Surg 165:217, 1967.

306. Kantrowitz PA, Jones WA, Greenberger NJ, et al. Severe postoperative hyperbilirubinemia simulating obstructive jaundice. N Engl J Med 276:591, 1967.

307. Caroli J, Paraf A, Champeau J, et al. La icteres de la gastrectomie. Arch mal app digest 39:1057, 1950.

308. Pichlmayr I, Stich W. Der bilirubinostatische Ikterus—eine neue Ikterusform beim Zusammentreffen von Operation, Narkose und Bluttransfusion. Klin Wochenschr 40:665, 1962.

309. Wolkoff AW, Chowdhury JR, Gartner LA, et al. Crigler-Najjar syndrome (type 1) in an adult male. Gastroenterology 76:840, 1979.

310. Farrell GC, Gollan JL, Stevens SMB, et al. Crigler-Najjar type 1 syndrome: absence of hepatic bilirubin UDP-glucuronyl transferase activity and therapeutic response to light. Aust NZ J Med 12:280, 1982.
311. Tagnon HJ, Robbins GF, Nichols MP. The effect of surgical operations on the Bromsulfalein-retention test. N Engl J Med 238:556, 1958.
312. Zimmerman HJ, Fang M, Utili R, et al. Jaundice due to bacterial infection. Gastroenterology 77:362, 1979.
313. Fahrländer H, Huber F, Gloor F. Intraheptic retention of bile in severe bacterial infections. Gastroenterology 47:590, 1964.
314. Eley A, Hargreaves T, Lambert HP. Jaundice in severe infections. Br Med J 2:75, 1965.
315. Vermillion SE, Gregg JA, Bagenstoss AH, et al. Jaundice associated with bacteremia. Arch Intern Med 124:611, 1969.
316. Miller DJ, Keeton GR, Webber BL, et al. Jaundice in severe bacterial infection. Gastroenterology 71:94, 1976.

317. Norton L, Moore G, Eiseman B. Liver failure in the post-operative patient: the role of sepsis and immunological deficiency. Surgery 78:6, 1975.
318. Gibson PR, Dudley FJ. Ischemic hepatitis: clinical features, diagnosis and prognosis. Aust NZ J Med 14:822, 1984.
319. Ischaemic hepatitis. (Editorial.) Lancet 1:1019, 1985.
320. Dienstag JL. Non-A, non-B hepatitis. 1. Recognition, epidemiology, and clinical features. Gastroenterology 85:439, 1983.
321. Howard RJ, Delaney JP. Postoperative cholecystitis. Am J Dig Dis 17:213, 1972.
322. Glenn F, Becker CG. Acute acalculous cholecystitis. An increasing entity. Ann Surg 195:131, 1982.
323. Marx GF, Nagayoshi M, Shoukas JA, et al. Unsuspected infectious hepatitis in surgical patients. JAMA 205:793, 1968.

IV B.   Infectious Agents and Liver Disease

35

Biology of Human Hepatitis Viruses

William S. Robinson, M.D.

THE RECOGNITION OF HEPATITIS VIRUSES IN HUMANS

Hippocrates described infectious icterus, which may have been viral hepatitis, more than 2000 years ago, and epidemic jaundice has been recognized since the middle ages. Hepatitis has occurred frequently in military and civilian populations during wars, and its importance sometimes approached that of plague and cholera as a cause of pandemics in Europe in past centuries. Although leptospirosis, yellow fever, and malaria probably were not distinguished from viral hepatitis in early times, most of the disease recognized as infectious or epidemic icterus was undoubtedly what we know today as infectious hepatitis or hepatitis A. Studies in the early part of this century defined the epidemiologic features of infectious hepatitis. For example, Pickles studied a rural English population in the 1930s and concluded that infectious icterus could be transmitted by personal contact and that the incubation period was several weeks.[1]

Hepatitis transmitted by inoculation with serum was recognized much later than was infectious hepatitis. In retrospect, the first report of long incubation or serum hepatitis was probably that of Lurman in 1855,[2] who reported jaundice in 15 per cent of 1285 shipyard workers up to six months after vaccination with smallpox vaccine containing human lymph. Early in this century, with the widespread use of venipuncture, arsenotherapy, and vaccines and the observation of associated cases of hepatitis, blood-borne hepatitis was recognized. In 1926, Flaum and associates suggested that patients acquiring hepatitis in a diabetic clinic in Sweden were infected with contaminated needles and syringes.[3] Inadequately sterilized syringes were also probably responsible for transmission of serum hepatitis in venereal disease clinics administering arsenotherapy.[4, 5] The use of plasma from convalescents for prophylaxis of measles and mumps was observed to be followed in up to six months by hepatitis.[6-8] Similarly, the administration of yellow fever vaccine containing human serum was noted to be followed by hepatitis after a long incubation period.[9] In 1942 more than 28,000 American soldiers developed jaundice, and 62 of them died following inoculation with yellow fever vaccine containing filtered pooled human serum and apparently serum hepatitis virus.[10] With this background, it was inevitable that hepatitis following blood transfusion and pooled plasma administration would be recognized.[11, 12] Eventually it was recognized that there were healthy carriers of the serum hepatitis virus and that it was unwise to use these individuals as blood donors.

Although these observations on natural and accidental infections suggested the existence of more than one hepatitis agent in humans, studies of human transmission carried out in the 1940s and 1950s provided much more complete evidence for this.[14-23] At least two agents, designated infectious hepatitis virus (IHV) and serum hepatitis virus (SHV), were distinguished by differences demonstrated in cross-protection transmission studies, by the regular presence of IHV and never SHV in feces of infected patients, by the common occurrence of persistent infection in chronic carriers of SHV in the blood (never observed with IHV), and by the ability to prevent infectious hepatitis but not serum hepatitis with immune serum globulin. Fecal-oral or contact transmission was associated with the sporadic and epidemic patterns of IHV infection, and SHV appeared to be transmitted percutaneously by blood and blood products, resulting in different epidemiologic features. These hepatitis agents were shown by Sietz filtration to have sizes consistent with those of viruses.[14, 24, 25] Further progress in understanding hepatitis viruses, as compared with other viruses that are pathogenic for humans, has come only in the last two decades. In large part this was because investigators failed to infect convenient experimental animals or tissue culture cells with hepatitis viruses.

The finding of a viral antigen (now called hepatitis B surface antigen [HBsAg]) in the blood of patients with serum hepatitis in the 1960s and the transmission of a virus from such patients to chimpanzees were the first steps in identification of a specific virus, now designated hepatitis B virus (HBV).[26–29] The successful infection of marmosets with a virus from the feces of patients with infectious hepatitis and the finding of a viral antigen in the feces of such patients led to the identification of the infectious hepatitis virus now called hepatitis A virus (HAV).[30–32] These discoveries led to methods for detecting the infectious viruses, viral antigens, and viral antibodies so that further characterization of both HAV and HBV and a much more complete understanding of the course of infection and the epidemiology of both viruses have recently been possible. Although they both infect liver cells primarily, it is now clear that HAV (a picornavirus) and HBV (a small deoxyribonucleic acid [DNA] virus) are completely unrelated. They have different structural and biologic properties.

In the past decade, at least three additional human hepatitis viruses have been recognized. The use of specific serologic tests to identify infections with HAV and HBV led to the recognition of hepatitis that followed blood transfusions and was not caused by HAV or HBV or by other recognized viruses that can cause post-transfusion hepatitis in humans, such as cytomegalovirus (CMV) and Epstein-Barr virus (EBV).[33–35] Thus there exists at least one additional agent (currently referred to as post-transfusion non-A, non-B hepatitis or PT-NANB hepatitis agents) that causes serum hepatitis in humans. This and possibly other agents have been transmitted serially in chimpanzees and have been shown to cause persistent infection in humans with virus continuously in the blood. It is known too that the epidemiologic features of these agents are like those for HBV. However, these agents have not yet been identified with certainty as antigenic, ultrastructural, and chemical entities.

More recently, epidemics of acute hepatitis have been caused in various parts of the world by a water-borne agent that does not cross-react serologically with any previously known hepatitis virus.[36] This disease has been called epidemic or enterically transmitted non-A, non-B hepatitis (ET-NANB hepatitis). It has epidemiologic features like those of hepatitis A. It appears to be caused by an agent that is different from the one associated with PT-NANB. Virus-like particles have been observed in the feces of patients with ET-NANB, and the agent of ET-NANB hepatitis has been transmitted to *Cynomolgus* monkeys and marmosets.

Finally, a defective virus containing a circular ribonucleic acid (RNA) called hepatitis delta virus or HDV appears to replicate only in liver infected with HBV (or other hepadnaviruses). It acquires a viral envelope containing HBsAg.[37] HDV is a significant cause of severe acute and chronic hepatitis in patients with acute or chronic HBV infection.

THE SPECTRUM OF VIRUSES THAT INVOLVE THE LIVER IN HUMANS AND OTHER VERTEBRATES

Although most cases of viral hepatitis in humans appear to be caused by infection with only a few viruses (Table 35–1) and, as described previously, these infections were recognized long before specific knowledge of viruses existed, it has become clear in the era of modern virology that many viruses with widely different characteristics and from many of the recognized virus groups may be associated with acute and chronic hepatitis in humans and in a wide variety of other vertebrates. Many of these viruses are listed in Table 35–2. A discussion of the viruses of subhuman species listed in Table 35–1 is beyond the scope of this chapter, but they are listed to illustrate the spectrum of viruses that may infect and lead to injury of hepatocytes, and because some provide useful models for studying the mechanism of viral-induced hepatic injury. The references listed in Table 35–1 for each virus review evidence for their association with hepatitis. By far the most interesting hepatitis viruses of nonhuman species are the viruses recently discovered in Eastern woodchucks,[40] Beechey ground squirrels,[41] and Pekin ducks in China and the United States.[42]

TABLE 35–1. VIRUSES THAT MAY INVOLVE THE LIVERS OF VERTEBRATES

I. RNA Viruses
  A. Picornaviruses (enteroviruses)
    1. Duck hepatitis virus[36, 37]
    2. Hepatitis A virus (humans)
    3. Coxsackie viruses (humans)
    4. Echo viruses (humans)
  B. Corona viruses
    1. Murine hepatitis viruses[36, 37]
  C. Togaviruses
    Flavivirus subgroup
    1. Yellow fever virus (humans)
    Alphavirus subgroup
    2. Rubella virus (humans)
  D. Arenaviruses
    1. Junin virus (humans)
    2. Machupo virus (humans)
    3. Lassa virus (humans)
    4. Rift Valley fever virus (humans)

  E. Rhabdoviruses
    1. Marburg virus (humans)
    2. Ebola virus (humans)
  F. Reoviruses
    1. Cause hepatitis in suckling mice[36, 37]
  G. Paramyxoviruses
    1. Measles virus (humans)
II. DNA Viruses
  A. Parvoviruses
    1. Kilham rat virus[36, 37]
  B. Adenoviruses
    1. Infectious canine hepatitis virus[36, 37]
    2. Human adenoviruses?
  C. Hepadnaviruses
    1. Hepatitis B virus (humans)
    2. Woodchuck hepatitis virus[38]
    3. Ground squirrel hepatitis[39]
    4. Pekin duck hepatitis virus[40]

  D. Herpesviruses
    1. Cytomegalovirus (humans)
    2. Epstein-Barr virus (humans)
    3. Herpes simplex virus (humans)
    4. Varicella zoster virus (humans)
  E. Poxviruses
    1. Ectromelia (mousepox) virus[36, 37]

III. Agents Causing Infectious Hepatitis Thought to Be Viral (Viruses Unclassified)
  A. Non-A, non-B hepatitis viruses (humans)
  B. Agent causing hepatitis in horses[36]
  C. Agent causing hepatitis in goslings[36]
  D. Agent causing hepatitis in turkeys[36]
  E. Agent causing hepatitis in pheasants[36]

TABLE 35–2. VIRUSES COMMON IN THE UNITED STATES ASSOCIATED WITH THE ACUTE VIRAL HEPATITIS (AVH) SYNDROME (1981)

Agent	Approximate Contribution to AVH Cases (%)		
	Epidemic Disease	*Endemic Disease*	*Post-transfusion*
Hepatitis A virus (HAV)	90	25–50	<1
Hepatitis B virus (HBV)	5	25–50	10
Non-A, non-B hepatitis viruses	5	25	90
Cytomegalovirus (CMV)	—	<1	<1
Epstein-Barr virus (EBV)	—	<1	<1
Herpes simplex virus (HSV)	—	<1	—
Varicella zoster virus (VZV)	—	<1	—
Measles virus	—	<1	—
Rubella virus	—	<1	—
Coxsackie viruses	—	<1	—

They are listed in Table 35–1 under the virus family name Hepadnaviruses.[43] These viruses are closely related to HBV. They share unique antigenic, molecular, and ultrastructural features of HBV (to be described later in the section on HBV), and they cause a similar persistent infection, which is associated with chronic hepatitis, hepatocellular carcinoma (HCC), and in some cases extrahepatic immune complex disease. The hepadnaviruses and their infections are so similar to HBV in humans that they provide ideal models for studying disease pathogenesis, treatment, and control of viruses of this class. These viruses are much more closely related and biologically similar to HBV, for example, than the coxsackievirus, the polio virus, and the echovirus are to HAV. The polio virus, coxsackievirus, echovirus, and HAV are all small RNA viruses of the Picornavirus group and have similar structures and mechanisms of replication, but these viruses are not serologically related, and there are major differences in their biologic behavior.

This chapter will describe in detail only the common hepatitis viruses of humans (HAV, HBV, HDV, PT-NANB hepatitis viruses, and ET-NANB hepatitis viruses). The other human viruses that may involve the liver (Tables 35–2 and 35–3) will be discussed only briefly. All the human herpesviruses are known to involve the liver under some circumstances. Although most primary CMV infections are not clinically apparent, some degree of liver involvement is usually a feature of almost all forms of clinically apparent primary infection, including congenital infection,[44, 45] post-perfusion and post–blood transfusion syndromes,[46–49] disseminated disease in an immunocompromised host,[50] and heterophile-negative mononucleosis in previously healthy adults.[51–53] Icteric or anicteric hepatitis may be the principal manifestation of CMV infection.[52–56] Similarly, most primary EBV infections are not clinically apparent, but when they

are, such as infectious mononucleosis, some liver function abnormality is almost always present.[57] In some cases, however, hepatitis may be both severe and the predominant clinical feature.[58] Infrequent cases of hepatitis following blood transfusion appear to be due to EBV infection.[33–34] Herpes simplex virus (HSV) infections rarely involve the liver in adults, although liver involvement is common in generalized HSV infection in newborns.[59–61] Hepatic involvement is also described in generalized HSV infections in severely malnourished children.[62, 63] In adults, HSV hepatitis, although rare, has been seen most often in patients undergoing immunosuppressive therapy or in pregnancy and is accompanied almost always by oral, labial, esophageal, genital, or other cutaneous or mucous membrane vesicular lesions, often with dissemination to other viscera.[64–66] Very rarely HSV hepatitis has been reported in an apparently immunologically normal host without a cutaneous or mucous membrane lesion.[67] Overt hepatitis associated with varicella zoster virus (VZV) infection is also unusual.[68] When it occurs, it is almost always part of widely disseminated disease.[68, 69] It rarely appears in previously healthy individuals,[70] and it appears more commonly in immunocompromised hosts.[71] Conversely, mild or subclinical hepatitis appears to be common during uncomplicated childhood chickenpox.[72]

Hepatitis has also been reported in measles virus infection in adults and in severely immunosuppressed children.[73–75] Hepatomegaly and hepatitis can be a feature of congenital rubella virus infection,[76] but liver disease has not been reported with rubella in older children and adults.

Coxsackieviruses, usually of group B, have been associated with hepatitis as part of severe multisystem disease, usually in neonates and rarely in adults.[77–79] Similar syndromes with echoviruses have been reported.[80, 81]

Finally, whether adenoviruses ever cause hepatitis in humans is not clear, although several different human adenovirus types have been isolated from feces and plasma of a few patients with acute hepatitis.[82–84] Since adenoviruses may commonly persist in the gastrointestinal tract of asymptomatic individuals, with fecal shedding, more direct evidence of hepatic involvement with these viruses during hepatitis is needed before a causal relationship can be assumed.

The viruses listed in Table 35–3 and designated exotic viruses most often involve the liver during the course of severe generalized disease, with widespread clinical manifestations such as rash and hemorrhagic diathesis, and cardiac, renal, and other organ involvement. These viruses do not occur in the United States, but infections could be acquired by travelers to tropical South or Central America

TABLE 35–3. EXOTIC VIRAL INFECTIONS OF THE LIVER NOT SEEN IN THE UNITED STATES

Togaviruses
  Yellow fever virus

Arenaviruses
  Junin virus (causes Argentinian hemorrhagic fever)
  Machupo virus (causes Bolivian hemorrhagic fever)
  Lassa virus (causes Lassa fever)
  Rift Valley fever virus

Rhabdoviruses?
  Marburg virus (causes Marburg disease)
  Ebola virus

(yellow fever virus, Junin virus, and Machupo virus) or Africa (yellow fever virus, Lassa virus, Rift Valley fever virus, and Marburgh and Ebola viruses), or from biologic materials transported to the United States from endemic areas.[85, 86] Although the viruses listed in Tables 35–2 and 35–3 are known to involve the liver, the list should not be considered to include all viruses that potentially can infect the human liver. In fact, it is possible that any virus to which humans are susceptible could, under the right circumstances, involve the liver. This possibility would be expected to be increased for many viruses in the immunocompromised host.

One clinically relevant distinction between the common hepatitis viruses of humans (HAV, HBV, HDV, and NANB hepatitis viruses) and the other human viruses listed in Tables 35–2 and 35–3 (which are sometimes associated with hepatitis) appears to be their tissue tropism. The viruses in Tables 35–2 and 35–3—except for HAV, HBV, HDV, and probably NANB hepatitis viruses—infect a wide variety of tissues in addition to hepatic tissue. Infection with these viruses involves the liver infrequently when compared with involvement of other tissues. When hepatitis occurs during infection with these viruses, it is usually only one feature of a more widespread disease. Only rarely is hepatitis the predominant feature of the illness, as for example infrequently in EBV or CMV infections. HAV and HBV clearly have a much more narrow tissue tropism and may infect hepatocytes exclusively. Whether such exclusive liver tropism is also a feature of the other common hepatitis viruses of humans (NANB hepatitis viruses) remains to be finally established, but injury to organs other than the liver has not yet been associated with infection with these agents. Thus it seems appropriate to include "hepatitis" in the names of these viruses and not in the names of the viruses causing more widespread infection.

HEPATITIS B VIRUS AND OTHER HEPADNAVIRUSES

The hepadnavirus family includes HBV,[43, 87, 88] woodchuck hepatitis virus (WHV),[40] ground squirrel hepatitis virus (GSHV),[40] and duck hepatitis B virus (DHBV).[42] These very similar viruses share unique features, which define the virus family. In high-prevalence geographic regions, the liver disease associated with chronic HBV infection is more important numerically than is acute hepatitis B. Chronic HBV infection may be the single most common cause of chronic liver disease and liver cancer in humans.[89, 90] All hepadnaviruses share the propensity for silent infection in early life, leading to persistent infection. HCC clearly is associated with longstanding, persistent infection in humans,[89, 90] woodchucks,[40, 91, 92] and ground squirrels.[93] Hepadnaviruses have an interesting molecular structure and mechanism of replication, and they appear to share certain important features with retroviruses, indicating that they are phylogenetically related to retroviruses. A characteristic feature of almost all active hepadnavirus infections is the continuous presence in the blood of noninfectious and sometimes infectious viral forms, usually in high concentrations.

VIRAL FORMS IN THE BLOOD

Particulate hepatitis B viral forms in the blood of HBV-infected patients were identified and characterized following the discovery of the antigen on the surfaces of these viral forms. HBsAg was discovered in 1965 by Blumberg and co-workers while they were investigating human sera for protein polymorphism.[94] The antigen was first found in the serum of an Australian aborigine when a precipitin line formed in agar gel diffusion between that serum and a serum from a patient with hemophilia who had received multiple transfusions. Thus the antigen was first named Australia antigen.[95] It was not recognized immediately to be a viral antigen. Several years of investigation led to its eventual association with acute hepatitis B.[26–28] It was first renamed hepatitis-associated antigen (HAA) and then given its current name, hepatitis B surface antigen. HBsAg in the blood remains the most useful marker of active HBV infection. HBsAg appears in the blood exclusively as a component of the virion and incomplete viral forms. No soluble or low molecular weight forms have been detected.[96, 97] The serum of infected patients has been the principal source of viral material for physical characterization of HBV, since this virus has not been grown in tissue culture.

Small spherical particles that are heterogeneous in size and appearance (diameters from approximately 16 to 25 nm and called 22-nm particles) and filamentous or rod-shaped particles (approximately 22 nm wide and up to several hundred nanometers in length) (Fig. 35–1) were the HBsAg particulate forms first observed in electron micrographs by Bayer and co-workers in 1968.[97] These are the most numerous HBsAg-bearing particles in the sera of most HBV-infected patients. They consist of protein, carbohydrate, and lipid. No nucleic acid is found in them. They are considered to be incomplete viral coat particles. In 1970 a larger and more complex HBsAg-bearing particle (Figs. 35–1 through 35–3) was described by Dane and co-workers.[98] Strong evidence now indicates that this so-called Dane particle is the complete hepatitis B virion. The virion has a diameter of approximately 42 nm, with a lipid-containing outer layer or envelope, which is approximately 7 nm in width, and an electron-dense spherical internal core or nucleocapsid, which is 28 nm in diameter.[98, 99] The surface of the virion shares antigenic determinants (HBsAg) with the incomplete viral forms (22-nm spherical and filamentous particles).[98, 99] The outer envelope of the virion with HBsAg can be removed by treatment with nonionic detergents such as Nonidet P-40 (NP-40), leaving free core particles (Figs. 35–2 and 35–3) containing the virus-specified hepatitis B core antigen (HBcAg), which is antigenically distinct from HBsAg.[99] The viral core (Figs. 35–2 and 35–3) also contains the viral DNA,[100] with a covalently attached polypeptide,[101] DNA polymerase activity,[102, 103] protein kinase activity,[104] and apparently the third antigen associated with HBV infection—hepatitis B e antigen (HBeAg)—in a cryptic form.[105] In addition to virions with electron-dense centers, virions with empty cores (Fig. 35–1) are found in almost all preparations.

The size of the hepatitis B virion, estimated by electron microscopy to be 42 nm in diameter, is consistent with ultrafiltration studies showing that the infectious agent passes through Seitz filters with an average pore diameter of 52 nm.[25] The concentrations of physical virions in serum measured by electron microscopy (undetectable in some sera to between 10^5 and 10^9 particles/ml) are consistent with directly measured concentrations of infectious HBV.[106–111] Inoculation of 1 ml of some undiluted HBsAg-reactive sera has failed to infect chimpanzees,[107] suggesting that such patients circulate HBsAg only in the form of incomplete particles and not complete virions. Sera from other patients,

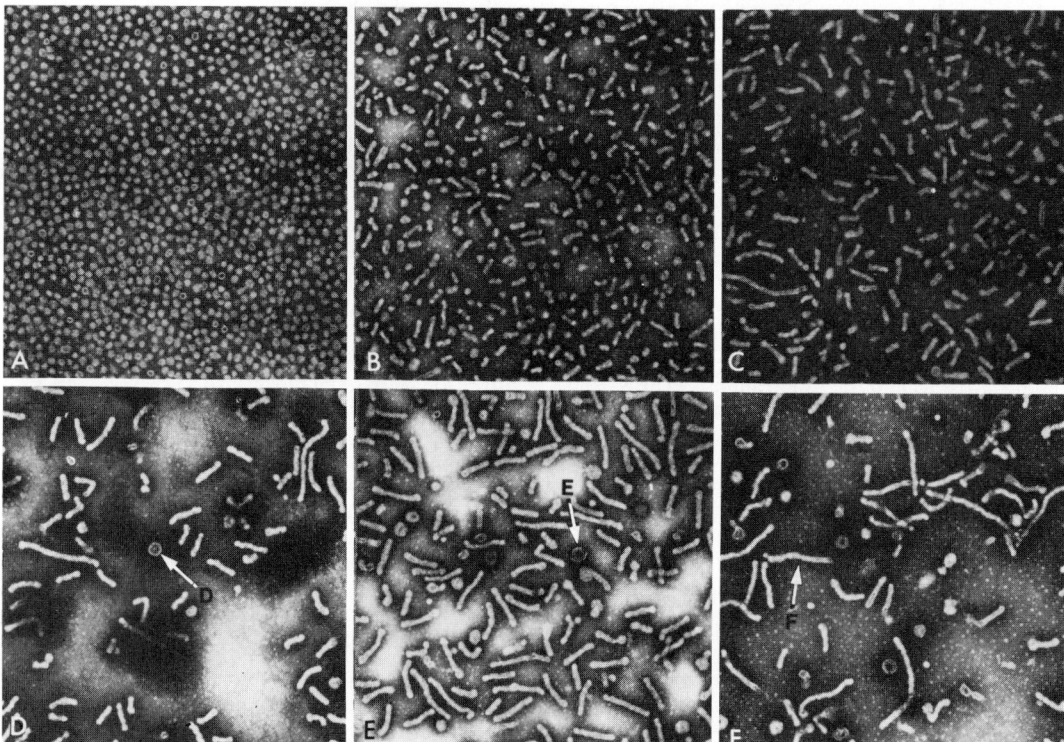

Figure 35–1. Electron micrograph of hepatitis B viral forms in the blood of an infected patient. *A* to *F* represent sucrose density gradient fractions after rate zonal sedimentation of particles. *D* indicates a virion with electron-dense core. *E* shows an empty virion, and *F* indicates a filamentous form. (Modified from Gerin JL. Fractions 1:1, 1976.)

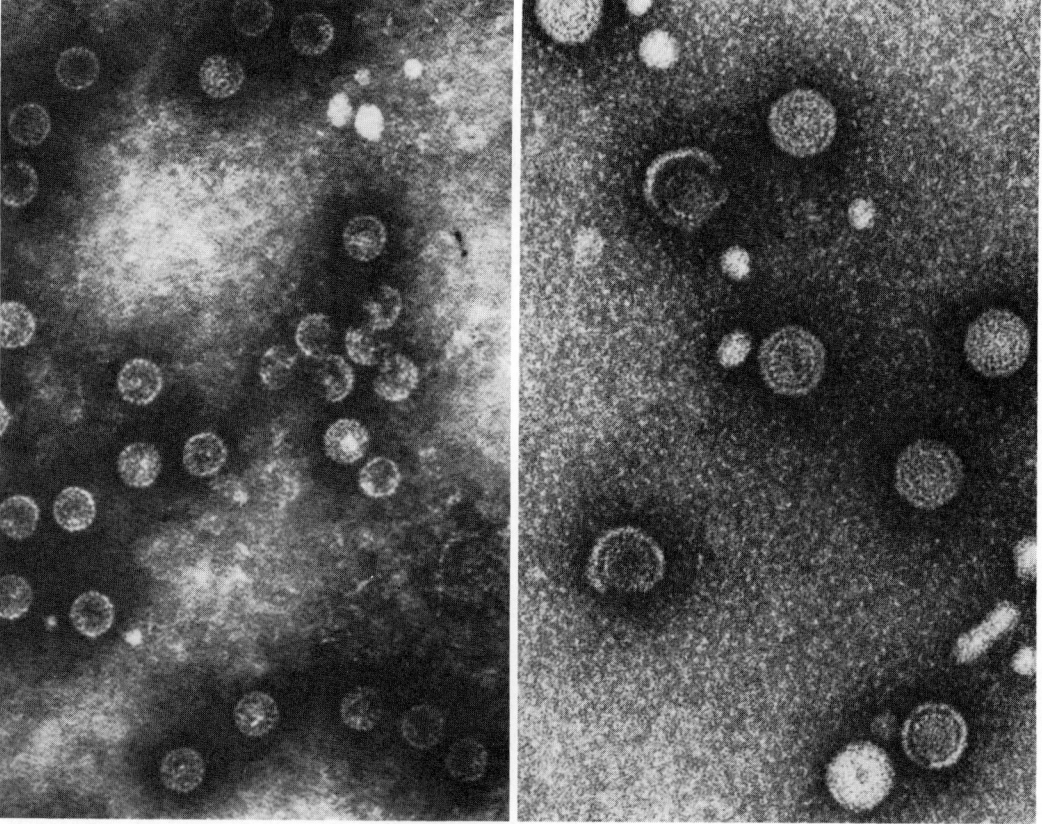

Figure 35–2. Electron micrograph of virions (*right*) and virion cores after detergent (NP 40) treatment of virions (*left*). (Experiment by June Ameida.)

1. *HBsAg* (a, d/y, w/r) bearing particles in blood.

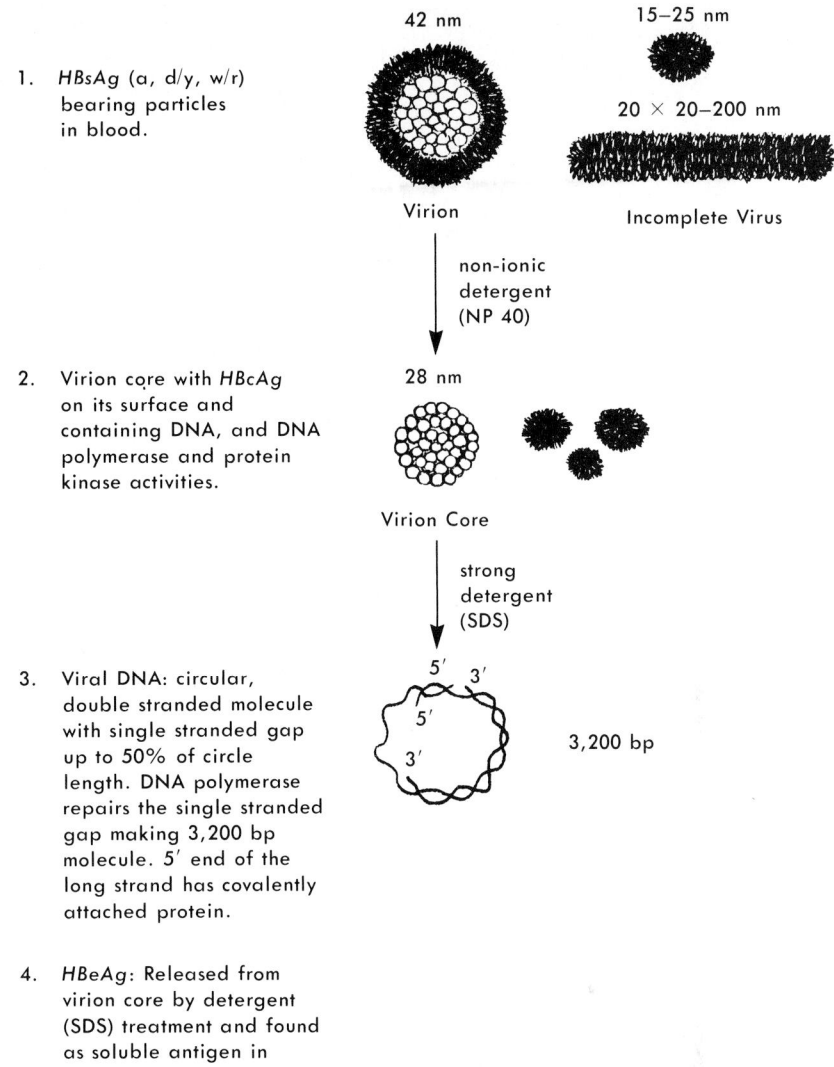

42 nm

15–25 nm

20 × 20–200 nm

Virion

Incomplete Virus

non-ionic detergent (NP 40)

2. Virion core with *HBcAg* on its surface and containing DNA, and DNA polymerase and protein kinase activities.

28 nm

Virion Core

strong detergent (SDS)

3. Viral DNA: circular, double stranded molecule with single stranded gap up to 50% of circle length. DNA polymerase repairs the single stranded gap making 3,200 bp molecule. 5′ end of the long strand has covalently attached protein.

5′   3′

5′

3′

3,200 bp

4. *HBeAg*: Released from virion core by detergent (SDS) treatment and found as soluble antigen in serum.

Figure 35–3. Schematic representation of hepatitis B viral forms found in the blood of infected patients.

in contrast, have infected humans or chimpanzees in dilutions up to 10^{-7} or 10^{-8},[107–110] indicating the presence of high concentrations of infectious virions. However, there has been no reported direct comparison between carefully measured concentrations of virion particles and quantitative titers of infectious HBV in the same sera. It has been shown that physical concentration and partial purification of virions results in preparations that are infectious at a higher dilution (10^{10}) than that reported for unconcentrated serum.[111] The concentrations of incomplete viral forms in serum usually greatly exceed the concentrations of complete virions. Concentrations of 22-nm spherical particles of 10^{14}/ml or higher have been found in some sera,[111–113] indicating that these particles outnumber virions by 10^4 or more in most sera.

HBV has been shown to retain infectivity for humans when stored in serum at 30 to 32°C for 15 years.[114] Infectivity for human volunteers is not lost at 60°C for up to four hours,[115] but it is lost at 60°C for 10 hours when in albumin solution,[116] although it is not completely lost in whole serum.[117, 118] Infectivity in serum was destroyed at 98°C for 1 minute or 20 minutes.[119, 120] Infectivity has also been destroyed by dry heat at 160°C for one hour.[121]

The same spectrum of viral forms has been found in

the blood of animals infected with WHV, GSHV, and DHBV. The complete virions of WHV and GSHV appear, however, to be slightly larger (47-nm diameter) than hepatitis B virions.[40, 41]

HEPADNAVIRUS GENOME STRUCTURE

The genomes of hepadnaviruses are among the smallest of all known viruses. The form of the hepadnavirus genome in virions from the blood of infected individuals is a small circular DNA molecule that is partially single-stranded (shown schematically in Fig. 35–4).[100, 122–124] The DNA of the three mammalian viruses contains single-stranded regions that vary in length from approximately 15 to 60 per cent of the circle length in different molecules.[40, 41, 122–124] The single-stranded region of DHBV is apparently much smaller, and many full-length double-stranded molecules are packaged in virions.[42] The DNA in hepadnaviruses consists, therefore, of a long strand (this is the minus DNA strand, since its sequence is complementary to that of viral messenger RNA) of constant length (between 3000 and 3300 bases in different hepadnaviruses) in all molecules and a short (or plus) strand that varies in length between 1700

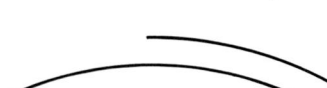

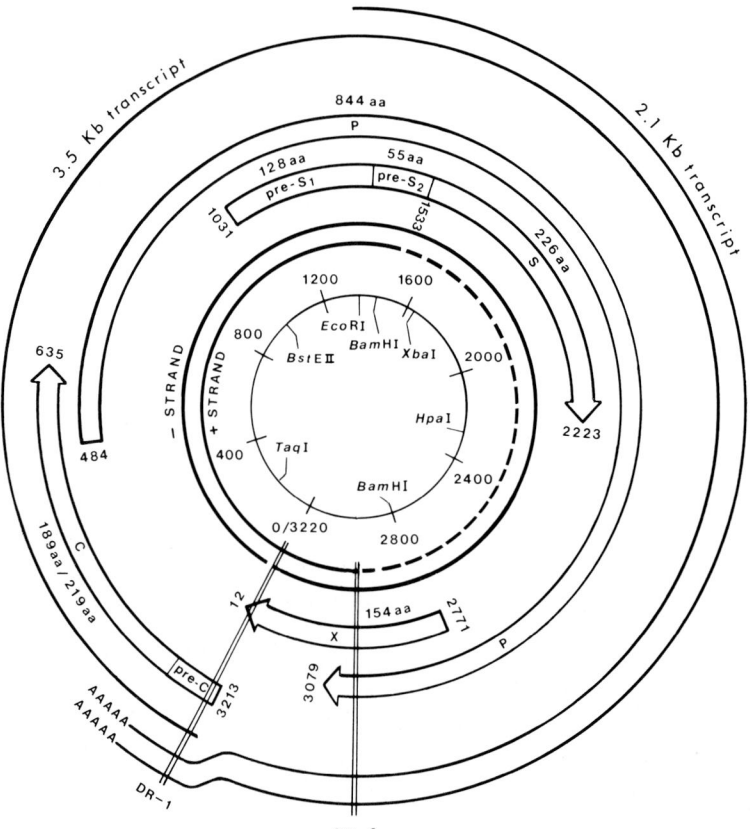

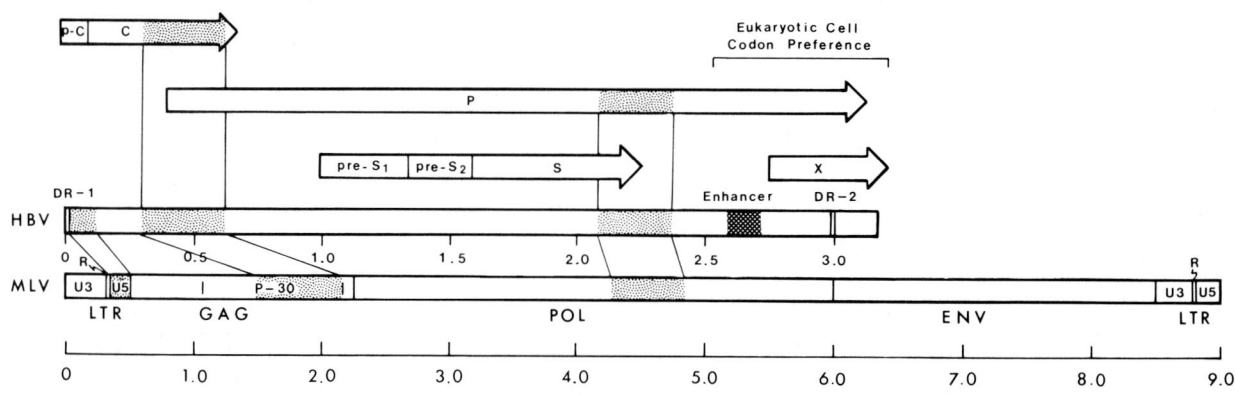

Figure 35–4. Physical and genetic map of HBV DNA and murine leukemia virus (MLV). In the circular map of HBV DNA, the *broken line* in the short (+) DNA strand represents the region within which the 3' end of the + strand may occur in different molecules, and the corresponding region of the long strand is that which may be single-stranded in different molecules. The restriction sites and locations of the nick in the − strand, the 5' end of the + strand, and the location of the single-stranded region have been reported by Siddiqui and colleagues,[128] and the open reading frames (*large arrows*) and 11 bp direct repeat sequences (*DR-1 and DR-2*) are found in the nucleotide sequence published by Valenzuela and co-workers.[138] The RNA transcripts are as mapped by Moroy and associates and Enders and co-workers.[151, 152] In the HBV genome represented as a linear sequence, the transcriptional enhancer location is that reported by Shaul and colleagues and Tognoni and associates.[153, 154] The murine leukemia virus proviral DNA structure is as reviewed by Coffin.[812] The regions of shared nucleotide sequence homology (*stippled regions*) are those described by Miller and Robinson and Toh and co-workers.[156, 813]

and 2800 bases in different molecules. DNA polymerase activity in the virion repairs the single-stranded region in the viral DNA to make fully double-stranded molecules.[40–42, 125, 126] DNA synthesis is initiated for this reaction at the 3' end of the short strand, which occurs at different sites within a specific region (50 per cent) of the DNA in different molecules. DNA synthesis is terminated when the uniquely located 5' end of the short strand is reached. The virus strand is not a closed circle; a nick exists at a unique site approximately 225 base pairs (bp) from the 5' end of the plus strand in mammalian viruses and 69 bp in DHBV DNA.[127–130] An approximately nine-nucleotide terminal rep-

etition (r) has been shown in the minus DNA strand of DHBV and GSHV,[129, 131] which may be important in circularizing the DNA and in template switching during synthesis of the plus DNA strand (see Genome Replication and Fig. 35–5). The circular DNA of the mammalian viruses can be converted to a linear form with single-stranded cohesive ends by selectively denaturing the 225-bp region between the 5' ends of the short and long strands using heat under appropriate conditions.[127] The resulting linear form can be recircularized by reassociation of the complementary single-stranded ends.

The 5' ends of both the long and short strands of HBV

Figure 35–5. Scheme of proposed mechanism of hepadnavirus DNA replication.

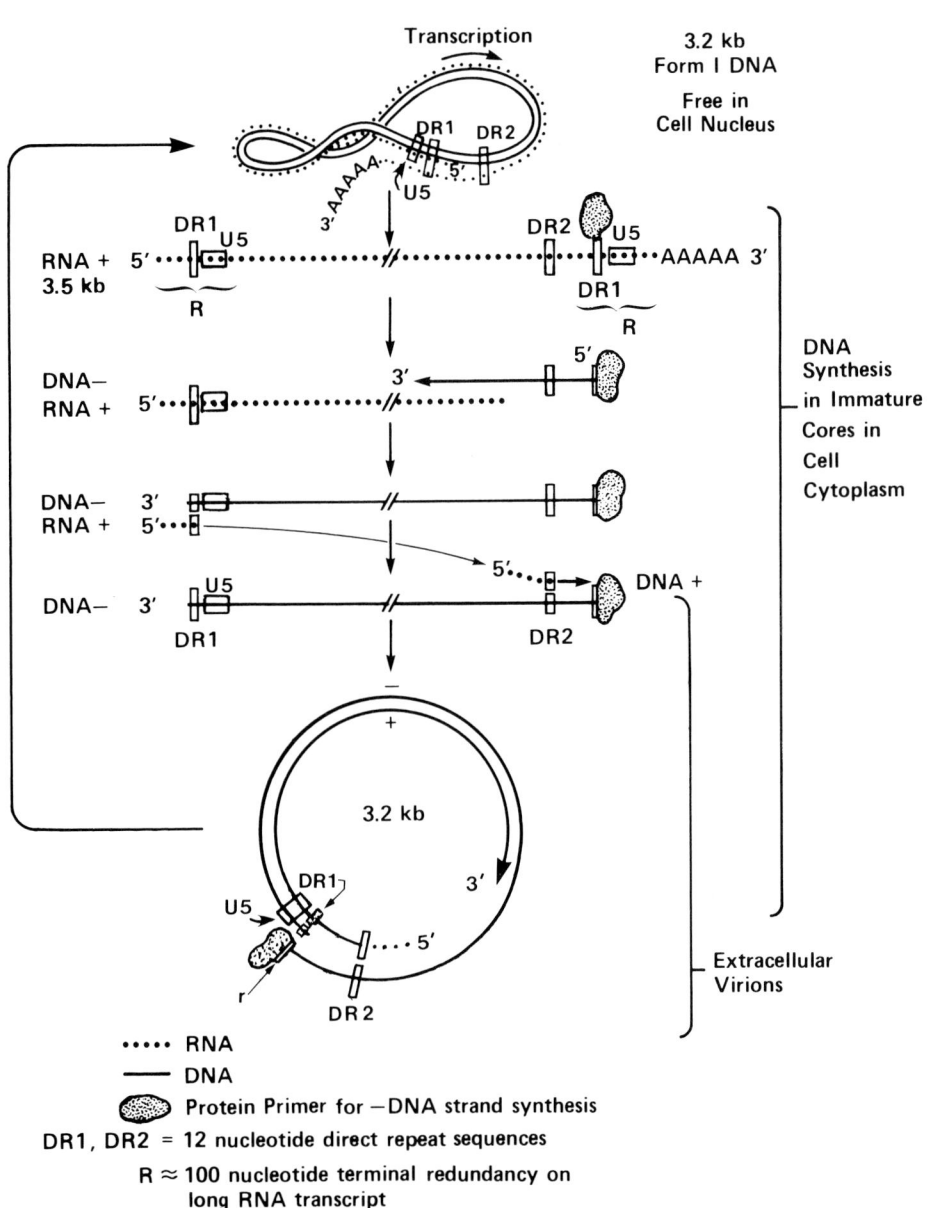

HEPADNAVIRUS GENOME REPLICATION

····· RNA
—— DNA
● Protein Primer for –DNA strand synthesis
DR1, DR2 = 12 nucleotide direct repeat sequences
R ≈ 100 nucleotide terminal redundancy on long RNA transcript
U5 = U5–homologous sequence
r = nine–nucleotide direct terminal repeat in the –DNA strand

DNA appear to be blocked in a manner that prevents phosphorylation with polynucleotide kinase.[101] A polypeptide appears to be attached covalently to the 5' end of the long strand of HBV,[101] DHBV,[132] and GSHV[133] DNA isolated from virions.[133] This undoubtedly prevents phosphorylation of this strand. Evidence with DHBV and GSHV suggests that this protein functions as a primer for synthesis of the viral minus DNA strand.[132, 133] Recently a 19-nucleotide, capped oligoribonucleotide covalently attached to the 5' end of the plus DNA strand of DHBV and GSHV,[11, 129] which appears to function as a primer for synthesis of this DNA strand, has been described. This capped oligoribonucleotide undoubtedly accounts for the inability to phosphorylate the 5' end of the plus DNA strand. The unusual virion DNA structure of hepadnaviruses results from packaging into the virions, which are released from cells, incompletely replicated viral DNA molecules consisting of complete minus strands (the first strand to be synthesized) and variably completed plus strands, with the primer for each strand remaining covalently attached to the 5' ends (see Virus Replication and Fig. 35–5).

The complete nucleotide sequences of the cloned DNA of nine HBV isolates,[134–141] two DHBV isolates,[142, 143] and one each of WHV and GSHV have been reported.[144, 145] The genomes of the three mammalian viruses have four long open reading frames in the complete or long (minus) DNA strand. They have similar locations in each virus with respect to the cohesive ends of the DNA (Fig. 35–4). The genes for the major virion polypeptides have been identified. The C gene specifies the major viral core or nucleocapsid polypeptide of 22,000 daltons and the 16,000-dalton polypeptide with HBeAg specificity described further on, and this open reading frame sometimes includes a short pre-C (precore) sequence. The S gene, including pre-S_1, pre-S_2, and S regions, specifies the viral surface antigen–reactive polypeptides in the virion (Dane particle) envelope and in incomplete viral forms (surface antigen particles) found in serum and liver of infected individuals. They consist of the glycosylated and nonglycosylated forms of three polypeptides of 24,000, 31,000, and 38,000 daltons coded respectively by S alone, pre-S_2, and S, and by pre-S_1, pre-S_2 and S regions of the S open reading frame described in detail further on. The P gene appears to specify the virion-associated DNA polymerase (or reverse transcriptase). The small X gene appears to specify a polypeptide that may activate viral transcription and has been detected in the livers of some infected patients.[147, 148] The C, P, pre-S_2, and S open reading frames are approximately the same size and occupy the same relative genomic positions in all mammalian hepadnaviruses. The pre-S_1 region varies somewhat in size in different viruses, suggesting that the polypeptide sequence specified by this DNA sequence is less functionally critical than that specified by the pre-S_2 and S regions. The pre-C sequence similarly varies in size in differently sequenced HBV genomes. The size of the X gene varies by up to 50 per cent among nine different HBV isolates, and the X open reading frame has been nearly deleted in DHBV.

Several other functionally important elements have been identified in hepadnavirus genomes. They include 11-bp direct repeat sequences (5'TTCACCTCTGC3') designated DR1 and DR2, which are approximately 225 bp apart in the mammalian viruses (Fig. 35–4). They appear to be critical for viral DNA replication (Fig. 35–5). The 5' end of the minus DNA strand occurs within DR1 and the 5' end of the plus DNA strand occurs at the 3' boundary of DR2.[129, 149] Transcriptional control elements that have been

identified include two promoter sequences. One in the pre-S_1 region appears to direct synthesis of a 2.1-kilobase (kb) RNA transcript that probably functions as messenger for pre-S_2 and S gene–specified polypeptides.[150] Another, upstream from the start of the C gene,[151, 152] appears to direct synthesis of a greater than genome length (3.5-kb) RNA transcript that may function as messenger for synthesis of C– and P gene–specified polypeptides and appears to serve as a template for synthesis of the virus minus DNA strand by reverse transcription. These are the major viral transcripts that appear to be unspliced and to have different 5' ends but colinear, polyadenylated 3' ends. A transcriptional enhancer element has been localized to a region approximately 450 bp upstream from the C gene promoter and occurs either immediately upstream from the start of the X gene in viruses with a short (typical) X gene or within the 5' end of that open reading frame in viruses with a long X gene (e.g., in HBV subtype *adr*).[153, 154] Glucocorticoids increase levels of HBsAg expression in HBV-infected patients in vivo and in HCC cell lines expressing HBsAg in culture. Recently, dexamethasone has been shown to stimulate expression of chloramphenicol aminotransferase (CAT) driven by the promoter when a region of HBV DNA was inserted into plasmid pA$_{10}$CAT.[154a] The glucocorticoid-responsive region of HBV DNA was localized to the S region of the S open reading frame, and a 15-nucleotide sequence (5' NCAANNTGTYCT 3') similar to other known glucocorticoid-responsive DNA elements was identified in that region (approximately 2097 to 2112 on the map in Fig. 35–4). This glucocorticoid-responsive, enhancer-like sequence is distinct from the enhancer sequence described earlier. A polyadenylation signal that appears to be used by both major transcripts described previously lies within the beginning of the C gene and approximately 20 bp upstream from the 3' end of the minus DNA strand.[150, 155] Finally, a highly conserved 60- to 70-bp sequence with a high degree of homology with the U-5 sequence of the retrovirus long terminal repeat (LTR) is present just downstream from DR1 and within the pre-C region of the genome (Fig. 35–4).[156]

Figure 35–4 also shows the linear arrangement of the four genes of a typical murine leukemia virus for comparison with the hepadnavirus genome. The *gag, pol,* and *env* gene products are functionally analogous to the C, P, and S genes, respectively, of hepadnaviruses. The terminal regions of retrovirus RNA are duplicated at the ends of the proviral DNA synthesized in infected cells by reverse transcription of the virion RNA. This LTR sequence contains a short sequence, U-5, derived from the 5' end of genomic RNA and a U-3 region derived from the 3' end of genomic RNA. U-3 appears to contain transcriptional and other viral control sequences.

There are three regions of the hepadnavirus genome with nucleotide sequence homology with specific regions of retroviral genomes.[156] They are shown in Figure 35–4. The most highly conserved sequence is the U-5 region of the LTR of retroviruses and a 111-nucleotide sequence just upstream from the C gene of hepadnaviruses. Regions of significant sequence homology are also present in the retroviral and hepadnaviral *gag* and *core* genes respectively, and in the *pol* genes of the two virus families (and of cauliflower mosaic virus).

The presence of significant homology in genes with comparable functions (e.g., nucleocapsid and polymerase) and control regions (e.g., U-5), suggests that hepadnaviruses and retroviruses (and cauliflower mosaic virus) are phylogenetically related. No such homology is found between hepadnaviruses and viruses of other families. The preservation of sequences in a major portion of the P-30 region of the *gag* gene and a middle region of the *pol* gene of retroviruses with functionally and structurally analogous genes of hepadnaviruses (and the *pol* gene of cauliflower mosaic virus) suggests that the conserved sequences specify functionally important peptide regions within the protein gene products that have little tolerance for change. Similarly the highly conserved U-5 sequence in retroviruses and the U-5 homologous sequence in hepadnaviruses must be essential sequences with important functions for viruses in these two families. Among retroviruses, the murine type C retroviruses and endogenous retroviral sequences found in human and other primate genomes share the greatest homology with mammalian hepadnaviruses,[156] suggesting that they have diverged most recently from a common ancestor.

Analysis of the codon preferences of hepadnavirus genes has shown that the hepadnavirus S, C, and P genes are like typical eukaryotic viral genes in this respect and the X gene, in contrast, has a codon preference that is more similar to eukaryotic cell genes, suggesting that the X gene sequence may have been derived from cellular DNA,[150] as are retroviral oncogenes and some other retroviral sequences.

HEPADNAVIRUS GENOME REPLICATION

Recent studies of hepadnaviral RNA and DNA forms in infected hepatic tissue and synthesis of viral DNA strands indicate that hepadnavirus DNA replicates by a reverse transcriptase mechanism first shown for DHBV replication.[157] Hepatic tissue of infected animals has been used to date because no infected cell culture system has been available. The most detailed findings have been made with DHBV,[131, 132, 149, 157, 158] and more recently with GSHV,[129] and have been substantiated in some respects for HBV-infected human liver.[159–161] The model shown in Figure 35–5 for replication of hepadnaviruses is based on that proposed by Summers and Mason and Lien and colleagues for DHBV replication and by Seeger and colleagues for GSHV.[129, 131, 157] Following entry of virus into liver cells, the infecting viral genome is converted to 3200-bp closed circular (cc) viral DNA, which is found in abundance in the cell nucleus. This conversion requires removal of the oligoribonucleotide from the 5' end of the plus strand, removal of the protein and one nine-nucleotide terminal redundancy (r) from the minus strand of virion DNA, and ligation of the ends of both strands to form cc viral DNA molecules. This ccDNA found in the cell nucleus probably functions as a template for transcription and formation of viral messenger RNA, including a longer than genome length transcript with the DR2 sequence near the polyadenylated 3' end, and the DR1 sequence and U-5 homologous sequence at both ends within the 200 to 300 nucleotide terminal redundancy. This transcript then serves as a template for viral minus-strand DNA synthesis. This long RNA transcript, newly synthesized viral DNA polymerase (reverse transcriptase), and a protein of unknown origin, which functions as a primer for minus DNA strand synthesis, are assembled with the major structural polypeptide of the viral core into core particles or viral nucleocapsids. Viral minus-strand DNA synthesis by reverse transcriptase within the core particles in the cell cytoplasm is initiated within the DR1 sequence (probably near the 3' end of the RNA template), using the protein primer. If the DR1 sequence

at the same end (e.g., 3') of the RNA template is always the site for initiation of DNA minus-strand synthesis, the protein primer or reverse transcriptase, or both, not only must recognize the DR1 or some neighboring sequence such as the U-5 homologous sequence but also must distinguish the two ends of the RNA template, perhaps by recognizing a sequence unique to one end of the RNA (i.e., a sequence not within R). The RNA template appears to be degraded by RNase H-like activity as DNA synthesis proceeds. The primer for synthesis of the viral DNA plus-strand synthesis is a 19- or 20-oligoribonucleotide with a sequence corresponding to that of a 5' terminal fragment of the RNA template containing the DR1 sequence. DNA plus-strand synthesis is initiated at the last nucleotide of DR2 near the 5' end of the minus DNA strand template. This suggests that the oligoribonucleotide primer is generated from the 5' end of the RNA template by ribonuclease action and that the RNA fragment is then dissociated from the completed 3' end of the newly synthesized minus DNA strand and translocated by an unknown mechanism to the 5' end of the minus DNA strand, at which point it base pairs with the DR2 sequence in the minus strand for initiation of DNA plus-strand synthesis at the boundary of the DR2 sequence. When the 3' end of the elongating DNA plus strand reaches the 5' end of the DNA minus strand template, it must switch templates to the 3' end of the DNA minus strand, forming a circular molecule. The 3' end of the new plus strand dissociated from the 5' end of the minus strand would contain a sequence complimentary to the short terminal redundancy (r) of the minus strand. This complementary sequence in the plus strand could then base pair with r at the 3' end of the minus DNA strand, resulting in circularization of the DNA and positioning the 3' end of the minus strand for use as a template for continued elongation of the DNA plus strand. This mechanism of replication shares many features with the reverse transcriptase mechanism of retroviruses and is an unusual mechanism for DNA viruses (observed only for hepadnaviruses and cauliflower mosaic virus).

Hepadnavirus core particles are assembled into complete virions with HBsAg and cell membrane lipid-containing envelopes. In the case of HBV, virus formation and release from the cell apparently can take place at almost any step after intracellular assembly of the core particle, since virions (Dane particles) found in the blood may contain DNA-RNA hybrid molecules as well as partially single-stranded, circular DNA molecules. Endogenous DNA polymerase activity in the virions catalyzes the incorporation of nucleotides into minus DNA strands of the former and plus DNA strands of the latter.[160]

In addition to the episomal viral DNA forms involved in virus replication described earlier, other episomal forms and integrated viral DNA have been found in infected cells. Nonintegrated oligomeric forms of viral DNA have recently been demonstrated in lymphocytes from the blood of chronic HBV carrier humans and chimpanzees and WHV-infected woodchucks.[162, 163] The origin and function of these episomal DNA forms are unknown.

Evidence of integrated HBV DNA sequences in at least some infected livers and most cases of HCC has been obtained by restriction endonuclease digestion of tissue DNA and Southern blot analysis. Evidence for viral integration in some studies of chronically HBV-infected human liver has consisted of finding one or more DNA fragments containing viral DNA sequences that are larger than unit-length viral DNA (3200 bp) after, but not before, digestion of cell DNA with a restriction enzyme (e.g., Hind III), for which no recognition sites exist in the viral DNA.[164, 165] The specific high molecular weight Hind III DNA fragments containing viral sequences have been found to be different in the liver of each individual chronically infected patient. The ability to detect such DNA fragments by Southern blot analysis has been interpreted to mean that viral DNA is integrated in the same site in many different cells of the liver of each chronically infected patient, but the site is different in individual patients. Other viruses, such as retroviruses, that readily integrate into cellular DNA appear to do so at many and possibly random sites in the cellular DNA. Specific sites of integration are not detected in DNA of infected tissue by the experimental strategy just described for HBV unless the cells are of clonal origin (e.g., as are cells in most viral-induced tumors).[166]

Other studies of HBV-infected livers have obtained evidence for random integration by detecting subgenomic-sized DNA fragments with HBV DNA sequence after digestion of infected liver DNA with a restriction enzyme that cleaves HBV DNA at more than one site and detecting no fragments of any specific size after Hind III digestion and Southern blot analysis.[167, 168] Southern blot analysis of DNA from livers of many infected humans, woodchucks, ground squirrels, and ducks has failed to demonstrate high molecular weight viral DNA forms suggestive of integration. This would suggest that integration of hepadnaviruses probably does not occur in all infected cells, and under some conditions of infection integration may be present in few, if any, cells.

The state of viral DNA in HCC has been examined by Southern blot analysis. Replicating forms of viral DNA and evidence for integrated viral DNA have been detected in some but not all human HCC,[167–176] woodchuck HCC,[177–179] and ground squirrel HCC,[93] and in human cell lines isolated from HCC.[169, 180–184] Restriction endonuclease Hind III (an enzyme that cleaves cellular DNA at specific sites but does not cleave most HBV DNA), digestion of tumor DNA, and Southern blot analysis have revealed DNA fragments (usually one to four) apparently containing viral DNA sequences that are larger than unit length (3200 bp) viral DNA and are similar to those described earlier for nontumorous infected liver. This suggests that viral DNA may be integrated at a few specific cellular DNA sites in such HCC tissue, but always at different sites in different tumors. The presence of unique integration sites and the rough correspondence of the viral genome copy number/cell and the number of integration sites in tumors without replicating viral DNA suggest that the cells of these tumors are of clonal origin, and when multiple sites of integration exist, they probably arise through DNA rearrangements of an original single integration.[168]

Cloning and sequence analysis of integrated viral DNA with flanking cellular DNA sequences has proved that viral sequences are integrated into host DNA of HCC. In almost all cases of woodchuck and human tumors and human HCC cell lines studied to date, the integrated viral DNA contains extensive deletions and rearrangements, which are different for each HBV integration.[178, 185–189] The site in viral DNA that joins cellular DNA among 30 or more cloned HBV integrations that have been analyzed is near the 5' end of the minus DNA strand in approximately 50 per cent of instances, near the 5' end of the plus DNA strand in a few instances, and at other (possibly random) viral genome sites in the others.[187] The apparently more frequent integration near the ends of the DNA strands (particularly the end of the minus strand) suggests that the ends of virion DNA strands (and particularly the minus strand) or a nucleotide sequence in that region plays a role in many hepadnavirus integrations. The evidence to date indicates that the cloned flanking cellular sequences are not the same for any two integrations and that these sequences do not correspond to known proto-oncogene sequences.[185, 186] At this time, there is no demonstrated difference between the state of integrated viral DNA in HCC and that in infected nontumorous liver.

The evidence suggests that hepadnavirus integrations are sporadic and may occur more commonly with longer duration of infection, and possibly with liver injury and regeneration. Also, rearrangements and deletions (at least in HCC) appear to be the rule in the integrated viral genomes. Thus, hepadnavirus integrations are more similar to those of DNA viruses such as SV 40 than to retroviruses, which undergo precise and orderly integration in all infected cells. Some HCC cell lines in culture, containing HBV only as integrated viral DNA, have been found to express the S gene and no other viral genes. Similarly, livers of chronically infected patients, in which integrated viral DNA and no episomal or replicating viral DNA forms can be detected by Southern blot analysis, have been shown to contain HBsAg in some cells (detected by immunofluorescence) but no HBcAg. The blood of such patients contains HBsAg particles but no particles with HBcAg, viral DNA, or DNA polymerase activity and, at least sometimes, no infectious HBV. Thus HBsAg appears to be expressed without virus replication. The expression of the S gene and not other viral genes in cells with only integrated virus may occur because the intact S gene, its promoter, and the viral enhancer are preserved in many integrations (e.g., when the ends of the integrated viral DNA are near the 5' end of the minus DNA strand (see Fig. 35–4), but integrated viral sequences necessary for synthesis of the long transcript, which appears to function as messenger for core and *pol* gene products and serves as template for viral DNA synthesis and thus is essential for viral replication (i.e., an integrated DNA sequence consisting of more than one intact viral genome is necessary to generate a greater than genome length transcript with terminal repeats) are probably never formed during natural HBV infection.

ANTIGENIC AND MOLECULAR STRUCTURE OF HEPATITIS B SURFACE ANTIGEN

The surface of the HBsAg-bearing particles is antigenically complex. At least five antigenic specificities may be found on HBsAg particles. A group-specific determinant (*a*) is shared by all HBsAg preparations, and two pairs of subtype determinants (*d,y* and *w,r*), which are for the most part mutually exclusive and thus usually behave as alleles, have been demonstrated.[190–192] Antigenic heterogeneity of the *w* determinants and additional determinants such as q and x or g have also been described.[193] The eight HBsAg subtypes *ayw*, *ayw₂*, *ayw₃*, *ayw₄*, *ayr*, *adw₂*, *adw₄*, and *adr* have been identified.[193] Isolated and usually single cases from the Far East with unusual combinations of HBsAg subtype determinants, such as *awr*, *adwr*, *adyw*, *adyr*, and *adywr*, have been reported.[193] The subtype determinants in these cases are found on the same particles, suggesting that phenotypic mixing or unusual genetic recombinants have formed during mixed infections.

Immunization with highly purified HBsAg particles results in protection against HBV infection,[194] as does administration of immunoglobulin preparations with a high titer of antibody against HBsAg (anti-HBs),[195, 196] indicating that the immune response to this antigen during infection provides protection against reinfection. The viral protein containing HBsAg specificity is coded by the viral S gene. As expected, the antigenic subtype found in secondary cases of HBV infection is always the same as the subtype of the index case or the original source used in experimental infections.[197, 198] HBsAg subtypes have provided very useful markers for epidemiologic studies of the spread of virus in populations and in individual cases of transmission.

For chemical characterization of HBsAg, 22-nm spherical and filamentous particles can be purified by gel filtration, rate zonal sedimentation, and equilibrium centrifugation in CsCl density gradients.[199] The buoyant density of 22-nm specific and filamentous particles in CsCl is approximately 1.18 g/ml,[200] reflecting a significant lipid content (approximately 30 per cent by weight). The higher buoyant density of virions (approximately 1.28 g/ml for virions with DNA-containing cores and 1.24 g/ml for those with empty cores) reflects the contribution of their high buoyant-density nucleocapsids.[201] Lipid analysis of highly purified preparations of 22-nm HBsAg particles has revealed a mixture of lipids similar to that found in enveloped viruses and suggesting a host cell origin for the lipid.[202, 203]

Several polypeptides with apparent molecular weights between 24,000 and 42,000 daltons have been isolated from purified preparations of HBsAg 22-nm particles of subtypes *adw*, *ays*, and *adr* by sodium dodecyl sulfate–containing polyacrylamide gel electrophoresis (SDS-PAGE), all of which contain HBsAg specificity as described previously. The isolated major polypeptides (24,000 and 27,000 daltons) were shown to contain the group and type-specific determinants of HBsAg and to induce anti-HBs when used to immunize animals.[204–208] Higher molecular weight minor polypeptides were shown to contain the same group and type-specific HBsAg determinants,[204, 208] suggesting that the polypeptides were not unique but shared at least some amino acid sequences with the smaller major polypeptides.

Chemical reduction and alkylation were shown to greatly reduce the HBsAg reactivity of HBsAg particles,[209, 210] indicating that disulfide bonds in the polypeptide were necessary for this reactivity. When polypeptides are isolated after chemical reduction and SDS-PAGE, they must be reoxidized to obtain maximum HBsAg reactivity.

More recently it has been shown that the two smallest polypeptides (24,000 and 27,000 daltons) that are present in greatest amount in HBsAg preparations represent, respectively, the 226–amino acid polypeptide and the glycosylated form of the same polypeptide coded by the S region of the S open reading frame (designated P-24^s and GP-27^s, respectively).[146] Two sets of larger polypeptides are minor components found in HBsAg preparations containing virions. They are a 30,000-dalton (281–amino acid) polypeptide consisting of 55 amino acids coded by pre-S$_2$ plus the 226 amino acid coded by the S region of the S open reading frame and the glycosylated form of the same polypeptide (33,000 daltons) designated P-31^s and GP-33^s, respectively, and a 39,000-dalton (389– to 400–amino acid) polypeptide consisting of 108 to 119 amino acids coded by the pre-S$_1$ region plus sequences coded by the pre-S$_2$ and S regions of the S gene and a glycosylated form of the same polypeptide (42,000 daltons) designated P-39^s and GP-42^s, respectively. Antigenic specificities of polypeptide sequences coded by pre-S$_1$, pre-S$_2$, and S regions of the S open reading frame have all been found on the surface of virions (Dane particles).[211] HBsAg preparations containing no virions and only small spherical and filamentous HBsAg forms (without core or viral DNA) appear to contain the S-coded polypep-

tides (P-24^s and GP-27^s) with little or no pre-S$_1$– or pre-S$_2$– containing polypeptides (P-31^s, GP-33^s, P-39^s, or GP-42^s).[212] Thus virions appear to have antigenic specificities on their surfaces (pre-S$_1$ and pre-S$_2$) that are not present on other HBsAg particles. Following primary HBV infection, patients develop anti-pre-S$_1$, anti-pre-S$_2$, and anti-S, indicating all of these antigenic specificities are expressed during primary infection.[212] Pepsin digestion of HBsAg preparations destroys pre-S$_1$ and pre-S$_2$ determinants but not S.[212] Thus the HBV vaccine produced from HBsAg from plasma and treated with pepsin in its manufacture contains no pre-S$_1$ or pre-S$_2$ determinants,[212] yet it provides protection against HBV infection,[213, 214] indicating that an immune response to S determinants alone can be protective.

Synthetic peptides with amino acid sequences corresponding to specific regions of pre-S$_1$–, pre-S$_2$–, and S-coded polypeptides and predicted to be surface regions of protein because of their hydrophobic nature have been used to better localize different antigenic specificities and investigate their functional importance. A synthetic peptide with an amino acid sequence corresponding to residues 110–137 of the 226–amino acid polypeptide specified by the S region induced antibody in rabbits with subtype reactivity to d/y specificities and some reactivity with the group determinant *a*.[215] Immunization of chimpanzees with this peptide provided partial protection against infection following challenge with HBV. Peptide 138–149 appeared to have strong *a* specificity and reacted strongly with antiserum following immunization with the plasma-derived vaccine.[216, 217] Peptide 139–147 similarly was shown to have *a* specificity.[218] S immunogenicity and antigenicity are known to be destroyed by chemical reduction of HBsAg and are restored by re-formation of disulfide bonds,[219] and the same properties can be shown for peptide 122–137 cyclized through a disulfide bond between cysteine residues. This peptide manifested *a* and *y* specificities, and as an immunogen it protected chimpanzees against infection by an HBV challenge.[219] Peptide 122–137 was also shown by Gerin and co-workers to have d/y specificity.[220] These studies localize to some degree group *a* and subtype specificities of the S antigen and confirm that S determinants alone (without pre-S$_1$ and pre-S$_2$) can induce protective immunity.

Synthetic peptides corresponding to amino acid sequences of the pre-S region have also been studied. Specifically, residues 12–32 (pre-S$_1$) and 120–145 (the N-terminal 26 amino acids of pre-S$_2$) have been shown to contain antigenic specificities that correspond to those on the surface of virions.[212] Peptide 12–32 (pre-S$_1$) and antibody to this peptide appeared to block binding of virions to human HCC cell line Hep G2 and peptide 120–140 (pre-S$_2$) did not,[221] suggesting that pre-S$_1$ on the surface of virions may mediate virus attachment to cells. Peptide 120–140 (pre-S$_2$) was more immunogenic in mice than were peptides containing S determinants alone, and mice with genetically determined inability to respond to S were responsive to pre-S$_2$.[222] Peptide 120–140 is also said to induce neutralizing antibody.[223] Because the pre-S$_2$ determinant appears to be protective and more immunogenic than S, it has been advocated as an important determinant to be included in an HBV vaccine, particularly for individuals who respond poorly or not at all to the vaccine containing only S.

Although HBsAg determinants clearly reside in polypeptide chains, the isolated polypeptides react significantly less strongly with anti-HBs and are less immunogenic than are intact HBsAg particles. Treatment of intact HBsAg particles with periodate or glycosidases and neuraminidase results in significant loss of HBsAg reactivity,[224] suggesting that carbohydrate is on the particle surface and permits purification of the particles, for example, by affinity chromatography on concanavalin A columns.[225] The binding of HBsAg particles to a sialic acid–specific lectin before neuraminidase digestion and to a β-galactosidase–specific peanut lectin after suggests that these two sugars may be the terminal and subterminal residues of the surface carbohydrate.[226, 227] Protease treatment does not destroy the HBsAg reactivity of intact HBsAg particles as it does that of free polypeptides,[224] suggesting that critical parts of the HBsAg-reactive polypeptides are unavailable to proteases in assembled particles, although pre-S determinants are destroyed.[212]

Preparations of 22-nm particles consistently appear to contain small amounts of serum protein components that have not been removed by extensive purification.[228–230] Whether these are minor intrinsic constituents of the particles, are only avidly bound to the particle surface, or are just contaminating the preparation and copurifying with HBsAg is in some cases not yet clear. The only serum component present in large enough amounts in purified HBsAg preparations to be detected by Coomassie blue staining on SDS gels apparently is human serum albumin (HSA), which comigrates as a separate polypeptide with one of the viral specific polypeptides.[231] In this regard it is of interest that several laboratories have reported that HBsAg particles contain receptors for polymerized HSA,[232–234] and avid binding of HSA to such sites might account for the finding of significant amounts of this protein in purified HBsAg preparations. It has been speculated that polymerized HSA is involved in attachment of HBV to cells,[235] but the fact that only glutaraldehyde-polymerized HSA and not naturally occurring polymerized HSA binds HBsAg and evidence that pre-S$_1$ determinants of the virus may bind directly to cells raise doubts about the role of polymerized HSA in this regard.[221, 234]

It has been claimed that virions may have surface antigenic determinants (e.g., HBeAg) other than pre-S determinants that are not present on the other particulate HBsAg forms,[237] but others have failed to confirm this finding.[238, 239]

The surface antigens of WHV and GSHV demonstrate significant, although minimal, specific cross-reaction with HBsAg.[240, 241] The two major polypeptides of the GSHV surface antigen are similar, although distinctly smaller, than those of HBsAg, and only one third of the tryptic peptides of the polypeptides of GSHV surface antigen and HBsAg are identical and two thirds are distinct.[241] These results indicate that although GSHV and WHV are closely related to HBV, they are not the same virus, and the two probably diverged from a common ancestor in the distant past.

THE HEPATITIS B VIRION CORE AND HEPATITIS B e ANTIGEN

The virion core bears HBcAg, and this antigen is found in the blood only as an internal component of virions. No free HBcAg has been detected in serum. The virion core is illustrated in Figures 35–2 and 35–3. HBcAg-bearing particles, with the electron microscopic appearance of virion cores, have also been isolated from homogenates of HBV-infected liver.[242] A significant fraction of HBcAg particles isolated from virions and a smaller fraction of those isolated from infected liver have been shown to have a high buoyant density in CsCl (1.38 g/ml) and to contain DNA and DNA polymerase activity.[201, 243] However, most HBcAg particles from infected liver tissue,[201, 243] and many from virions,[200, 201]

appear to have lower buoyant densities (1.33 g/ml) and to be empty particles with little or no DNA, and they manifest no DNA polymerase activity.

Although the antigenic specificities of HBcAg from different sources have not been carefully compared, no antigenic heterogeneity or variation has been described. The core antigens of WHV and GSHV cross-react to a small extent with HBcAg.[40, 41]

The e antigen was discovered in 1972 and was shown to be physically and antigenically distinct from HBsAg and HBcAg.[244] It was found to be a soluble antigen in serum with a size estimated to be 300,000 daltons by gel filtration chromatography.[245] More recent evidence indicated that HBeAg is a complex of antigens. Up to three precipitin lines, designated e$_1$, e$_2$, and e$_3$, may be detected by agar gel diffusion in sera from individual patients.[246–249] Different investigators have given different numeric designations to the three components,[250] so a standard nomenclature is not yet agreed upon.

Highly purified Dane particle cores and liver-derived HBcAg particles contain a single predominant polypeptide with an apparent size of approximately 22,000 daltons (P-22^c).[201, 251] P-22^c is a 183– to 185–amino acid polypeptide coded by the C open reading frame. Thirty-four to 36 amino acids at the carboxy terminus of P-22^c are rich in arginine and thus highly basic, a property that would promote binding to viral DNA. A pre-C sequence in the open reading frame, which is variable in length but on average could be expected to code for approximately 29 amino acids, is not known to be expressed during natural infection. It has been suggested that it might function as a signal peptide and be cleaved from P-22^c during secretion and processing.[252] HBcAg specificity is lost when core particles are disrupted with detergent or urea and HBeAg specificity appears.[105, 253–255] The free isolated P-22^c does not react with anti-HBc but does react with anti-HBe.[105] P-22^c has been expressed in bacterial cells containing the C gene in a plasmid expression vector,[252, 256] and it appears to self-assemble in bacteria into 22-nm particles with HBcAg specificity. P-25 (P-22^c + pre-C) expressed in bacteria will not assemble into core particles and does not manifest HBcAg specificity but reacts as HBeAg.[252]

Recent evidence indicates that the originally discovered high molecular weight HBeAg form (300,000 daltons) in serum was a complex of HBeAg with immunoglobulin IgG.[257, 258] A 16,000 dalton polypeptide (P-16^e), with an amino acid sequence identical to the amino terminal end of P-22^c, is the naturally occurring polypeptide with HBeAg specificity in serum.[259] This suggests that cleavage of P-22^c in a manner that removes the DNA binding carboxy terminal sequence may be the mechanism for formation of P-16^e. Recently, an amino acid sequence in the amino terminal region of P-22^c has been found to correspond to the active site of proteases such as trypsin.[260] This suggests that P-22^c may have protease activity.

Protein kinase activity has been found in virion cores and HBcAg particles from HBV-infected hepatic tissue.[104] The major 22,000-dalton polypeptide of core particles is heavily phosphorylated by this activity. Under some conditions, P-22^c is cleaved to a protein of 16,000 daltons.[104] Whether this cleavage represents formation of HBeAg (P-16^e) by self-cleavage of P-22^c after phosphorylation is not yet clear. Some other enveloped viruses also contain protein kinase activity that phosphorylates virion polypeptides closely associated with the viral nucleic acid. The role of this activity in HBV infection and replication is not yet clear.

An important clinical feature of HBeAg is the high correlation of its occurrence in sera of HBV-infected patients with high concentrations of virions and infectious HBV,[107, 109, 261-264] indicating that HBeAg and virions are produced together during the infection. This suggests that in HBV-infected patients with active virus replication in the liver, C gene expression yields P-22^c, which is assembled into core particles with HBcAg specificity within hepatocytes (some of which are then assembled into virions that leave the cell). In addition, the cleavage product of P-22^c (i.e., P-16^c) leaves the cell in a soluble form and is found in serum as HBeAg. Without virus replication—for example, when only HBsAg is expressed—HBeAg is probably never formed, since the C gene is not expressed. Serum HBeAg remains a useful clinical marker for active HBV replication.

HEPATITIS B VIRUS INFECTION

Host Range

HBV has a narrow host range that is probably restricted to humans and some other primates. Tests for HBsAg in sera of captive nonhuman primates has revealed infection in chimpanzees,[265-269] gibbons,[266, 270] orangutans,[266, 271] African green monkeys,[272] and squirrel monkeys.[271, 273] Testing for anti-HBs has revealed evidence of past infection in the same species as well as baboons, Celebes apes, macaques and some other Old World monkeys, and some New World monkeys.[266, 271] Only negative test results have been found in numerous other primate species. It is not clear in these studies whether HBV infection occurred in any of the nonhuman primates in their natural habitat in the wild or whether the virus was always acquired in captivity by exposure to humans. It seems possible that natural infection with HBV or a cross-reacting hepadnavirus may occur at least in some of these species.

HBV has been transmitted experimentally to chimpanzees,[29, 268, 269] which are highly susceptible and demonstrate patterns of infection like those in humans (see Course of Infection) except for less severe liver disease. Experimental infection has also been reported in gibbons,[270] African green monkeys,[272] rhesus monkeys,[273] and wooly monkeys.[202] The latter three species appear much more resistant to infection than chimpanzees and humans because much higher doses of virus are required and infection is irregular. Infection, when it occurs, is transient and little or no liver disease is seen. Because of this, these monkeys are unsuitable as animal models for HBV infection and for infectivity titrations. No successful infection of subprimate species has been reported.

Tissue and Cell Tropism

The balance of evidence at this time suggests that HBV infects and replicates readily only in hepatocytes and less well in a few other cell types in humans and chimpanzees. Although HBsAg can be detected by immunofluorescence in tissues other than liver,[274-276] the clumped pattern of staining in blood vessels, glomeruli, and phagocytic cells is different from the diffuse cytoplasmic and cell surface patterns of staining observed in hepatocytes replicating HBV and suggests intravascular antigen rather than replicating virus in the nonhepatic sites. Deposition of HBsAg without HBV infection in nonhepatic sites is not unexpected, since this antigen circulates in high concentrations in the blood and appears in most body fluids and secretions. The fact that HBV infection may be confined to hepatocytes in persistently infected chimpanzees was suggested by the finding of nuclear HBcAg detected by immunofluorescent antibody staining only in hepatocytes and not in other cell types.[276] A report of permanent eradication of HBV in a persistently infected patient after orthotopic liver transplantation indicates that virus replication existed in no site other than the liver in that patient. Conversely, the finding of HBsAg in pancreatic juice,[278] and HBsAg and HBcAg detected by immunofluorescent antibody staining in occasional cells in the pancreas of HBsAg-positive patients,[279] suggests that the pancreas is at least sometimes a site of limited HBV infection. The pancreas of Pekin ducks appears to be the site of more regular and extensive infection with DHBV as revealed by a more increased hybridization of a DHBV DNA probe with pancreatic tissue DNA than occurred with DNA of other nonhepatic tissues (although much less than with hepatic DNA).[42] HBV DNA has also been found in small numbers of peripheral blood cells in chronically infected humans and chimpanzees.[163, 280, 281] WHV DNA has been found in blood cells of infected woodchucks.[163] Lymphocytes appear to be the predominant cell type containing virus.

A final observation suggesting a possible nonhepatic site of HBV infection is the finding of anti-HBs of the IgA class in feces of infected and convalescent subjects.[282] Viral IgA antibody in the gastrointestinal tract is usually considered to be the result of active mucosal infection. There is, however, no more direct evidence of HBV infection of the gastrointestinal tract mucosa at this time. HBsAg has been found irregularly and in very low titer in feces, and no evidence for infectious virus in feces has been found in transmission studies (see Epidemiology).

Although highly infectious for susceptible intact hosts, HBV has not been shown to reproducibly infect cells in culture. It is not yet clear if a special cell type (e.g., hepatocyte) that is not available in culture is needed or if some other factor is responsible for the failure so far to infect cells in culture. Recently DHBV has been shown to infect and replicate in primary duck hepatocyte cultures when the cells are exposed to virus within a few hours of the time they are transplanted from liver.[283]

Immunofluorescence antibody staining for HBcAg has revealed diffuse staining, mostly of hepatocyte nuclei and less commonly of cell cytoplasm.[29, 284, 285] Electron microscopic examination has revealed particles with the appearance of both full and empty Dane particle cores, mostly in nuclei of infected hepatocytes.[286-288] HBcAg-reactive particles have been purified from infected liver.[242, 243] Most appear to have a low buoyant density, do not contain viral DNA, and do not manifest DNA polymerase activity.[201, 243] Only a fraction of HBcAg particles from some livers contain DNA and demonstrate DNA polymerase activity.[200, 201]

In contrast, HBsAg has been located exclusively in hepatocyte cytoplasm and at the cell surface and not in nuclei.[29, 284, 285] Electron microscopic examination of infected cells has not revealed abundant HBsAg forms in cytoplasm or cell surface. The exact mode and site of formation of these particles is thus uncertain. No budding viral forms have been detected as can be observed with other enveloped viruses. It is presumed, however, that HBsAg particles are released from cells in a manner that does not require cell disruption. The virion envelope containing cellular lipid and possibly host proteins, as well as the virus-specified polypeptides, is formed around the virion nucleocapsid.

During the acute phase of HBV infection, almost all hepatocytes appear to be infected.[29] A variable number of hepatocytes contain detectable viral antigen at any given time during persistent infection. Liver tissue from persistently infected humans and chimpanzees has revealed different patterns of viral antigen synthesis in different cells. Immunofluorescent antibody staining of liver sections containing HBsAg and HBcAg has shown that most infected cells stain only for HBsAg (in the cytoplasm), fewer have only detectable HBcAg (in the nucleus), and even fewer cells appear to contain both HBsAg and HBcAg.[29, 284, 285] The number of infected cells detected by immunofluorescent antibody staining during persistent infection can vary from less than 1 per cent to virtually 100 per cent of hepatocytes. The relative number of cells with detectable HBsAg only, detectable HBcAg only, or both antigens varies widely in individual patients.[29, 285] In the livers of some chronic carriers, only cells synthesizing HBsAg exclusively can be found.[29, 285] In all chronic carriers producing relatively high concentrations of Dane particles, significant numbers of cells synthesizing HBcAg can be found in the liver.[289] The observation that the number of cells synthesizing HBsAg almost always exceeds the number synthesizing HBcAg in most infected livers correlates with the fact that 22-nm spherical and filamentous HBsAg forms greatly outnumber Dane particles in the sera of most infected patients. The different patterns of viral antigen synthesis in individual cells of chronically infected liver detected by immunofluorescent antibody staining indicates that individual viral genes are expressed differently in different cells. This may account for the widely different relative numbers of the viral forms found in the blood of different patients. It is possible, but not proved, that cells with only HBsAg detected by immunofluorescent antibody staining contain only integrated viral DNA, since some cells with only integrated virus appear to express the S gene and not other viral genes (see Genome Replication).

THE COURSE OF THE VIRUS INFECTION

Studies of natural HBV infections in humans and experimental infections in humans and chimpanzees have defined several patterns of infection with this virus. Most primary infections in adults are self-limited and resolve completely within six months of onset. Most infections also appear to be subclinical and are detected only by serologic testing and other methods. Some infections fail to resolve, become persistent, and may continue for many years. A unique feature of infection with HBV is the continuous presence of viral forms in the blood during active infection in almost all patients. These forms are detected most commonly by their antigenicity (e.g., HBsAg). Tests for HBsAg essentially detect the incomplete viral forms described previously (22-nm particles and filaments), which greatly outnumber complete virions in most patients. Although most persistently infected patients appear to have complete infectious virus in the blood, as well as incomplete viral forms, some such patients appear to have no infectious virus. The presence of viral forms in the blood that can be detected by serologic testing and other methods, and the immune response to the viral antigens offers markers that can be used to follow the course of HBV infections. Several patterns of infection that define the spectrum of responses to this virus will be described here in detail.

Self-limited Hepatitis B Surface Antigen–Positive Primary Infection

This pattern of self-limited HBsAg-positive infection is one in which HBsAg can be detected transiently in the blood. It is the most common pattern of primary HBV infection in adults. HBsAg is usually the first viral marker to appear in the blood after HBV infection (Fig. 35–6). The presence of this antigen is considered to be synonymous

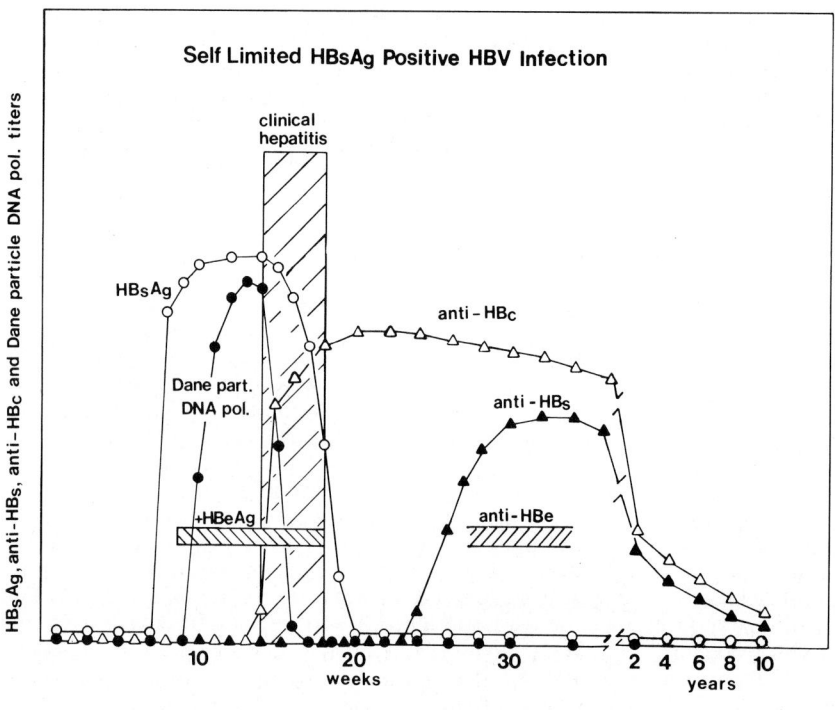

Figure 35–6. Schematic representation of viral markers in the blood throughout the course of self-limited HBsAg-positive primary HBV infection.

with active infection. HBsAg can be detected as early as 1 or 2 weeks and as late as 11 or 12 weeks after exposure to HBV when very sensitive assays are used.[290, 291] Evidence of hepatitis was found to follow the appearance of HBsAg by an average of four weeks (usual range, one to seven weeks) and after at least three to six weeks in different studies.[291, 292] In self-limited infections, HBsAg was found to remain detectable by complement fixation in the blood for 1 to 6 weeks in most patients,[292] although it may persist for up to 20 weeks.[291] Patients who remain HBsAg-positive for less than seven weeks appear to develop symptomatic hepatitis rarely.[291] The severity of hepatitis as measured by bilirubin elevations has been roughly correlated with the duration of HBsAg positivity in patients with self-limited experimental infections.[291] As symptoms and jaundice clear, the HBsAg titer usually falls, and HBsAg becomes undetectable in most symptomatic patients several weeks after the resolution of hepatitis. However, in experimental transmission studies, 9 per cent of patients became HBsAg-negative even before the onset of symptoms, and 28 per cent were HBsAg-negative by the time symptoms had resolved.[291]

HBeAg is another regular and early marker of HBV infection, as depicted in Figure 35–6. Highly sensitive assays, such as passive hemagglutination and radioimmunoassay,[293–298] have demonstrated that HBeAg appears simultaneously or within a few days of the appearance of HBsAg in all or almost all primary infections. Its titer peaks and then declines in parallel with HBsAg. The prevalence of HBeAg declines constantly over the first ten weeks after the onset of symptoms.[298] HBeAg usually disappears just before the disappearance of HBsAg in self-limited infections. Patients who remain HBeAg-positive for ten weeks or longer appear likely to become persistently infected.[297] Anti-HBe appears in most patients at the time HBeAg becomes undetectable or shortly thereafter. Anti-HBe persists for one to two years after resolution of HBV infection.[290]

The third viral marker in order of appearance is DNA and DNA polymerase–containing virions. These particles, detected by their DNA polymerase activity or by hybridization for viral DNA, appear in the blood of most patients soon after the appearance of HBsAg. They rise to high concentrations during the late incubation period of hepatitis B and fall with the onset of hepatic disease,[299, 300] as shown in Figure 35–6.

A fourth marker of infection, which appears in virtually all patients and before the onset of hepatic injury in most, is anti-HBc, which is the antibody directed against the internal antigen of virions. Anti-HBc usually can be detected three to five weeks after the appearance of HBsAg in the blood and before the onset of clinically apparent hepatitis,[290, 291, 300] as shown in Figure 35–6. Anti-HBc titers usually rise during the period of HBsAg positivity, level off, and eventually fall after HBsAg becomes undetectable. The highest titers of anti-HBc appear in patients with the longest period of HBsAg positivity.[300] Anti-HBc titers fall three- to fourfold in the first year following acute infection and then drop more slowly.[301] Anti-HBc can still be detected by immunoelectro-osmophoresis five to six years after acute infection in most patients.[290, 301] The high correlation between the prevalence of anti-HBc detected by immunoelectro-osmophoresis or radioimmunoassay and anti-HBs detected by radioimmunoassay indicates that the two antibodies persist for a similar time after acute self-limited infections.

Although most of the anti-HBc activity is of the IgG class, IgM anti-HBc has been found in almost all patients

with acute hepatitis B.[303–306] Using a sensitive enzyme-linked immunosolvent assay (ELISA), the anti-HBc IgM titer was found to decline rapidly after disappearance of HBsAg in 40 per cent of cases with self-limited acute hepatitis B. The decline was slow in the remainder of patients, with 20 per cent still showing positivity after two years.[306]

Antibody to HBsAg (anti-HBs) has been shown to appear during antigenemia and before the onset of clinically apparent hepatitis in the 10 to 20 per cent of patients who develop arthritis and rash associated with immune complex formation.[307] Complexes between HBsAg and anti-HBs have also been detected in a significant fraction of acute hepatitis B cases without well-recognized immune complex disease.[308–310] In most patients with self-limited HBV infection, however, anti-HBs can be detected only after HBsAg disappears from the blood,[23, 290–292, 300, 311] as illustrated in Figure 35–6. Anti-HBs cannot be detected even by the most sensitive tests in many patients immediately after HBsAg disappears. There is a time interval of up to several months between the disappearance of detectable HBsAg and the appearance of anti-HBs in approximately one half of patients with self-limited infections.[291, 300] In approximately 10 per cent of patients with transient antigenemia, anti-HBs never appears when tested for by the most sensitive assays.[291] In patients with measurable anti-HBs responses, the antibody titer rises slowly during recovery and may still be rising 6 to 12 months after the disappearance of HBsAg.[291, 300] In contrast to the anti-HBc response, the highest titers of anti-HBs appear in those patients with the shortest period of antigenemia.[291] This antibody may persist for years after HBV infection and is associated with protection against reinfection.[23, 312–314]

In contrast to the extensive studies of viral markers in the blood early in the course of primary HBV infection, only a few investigators have examined the state of virus in the cells of the liver at this early time. During the late incubation period and early during the acute disease almost all hepatocytes have been reported to test positive for HBsAg and HBcAg by immunofluorescent staining.[29, 284, 285] During acute hepatitis B, the state of viral DNA in liver has not been adequately studied, although evidence for integrated viral DNA has been reported in two patients.[315] However, the forms of virus in blood and antigen expression in liver suggest that almost all hepatocytes are replicating complete virions during the early stages of primary infection.

Self-limited Primary Infections Without Detectable Serum Hepatis B Surface Antigen

A significant fraction of patients with evidence of acute self-limited primary HBV infection apparently never have detectable HBsAg in the blood. Anti-HBs usually appears 4 to 12 weeks after exposure to HBV (at about the time HBsAg appears in patients with detectable antigen), and the titer typically rises rapidly to high levels and is sustained,[291] as depicted in Figure 35–7. An anti-HBc response is also detected, but the antibody usually appears only in low titer and may not persist for as long as in patients manifesting antigenemia.[291] IgM anti-HBc is probably found regularly in these patients, since it was detected in each of 31 patients with apparent acute hepatitis B who tested HBsAg-negative from the time of their admission to the hospital.[306] Although some of the patients in this study may have been HBsAg-positive before testing began, some undoubtedly had HBsAg-negative primary infections. In-

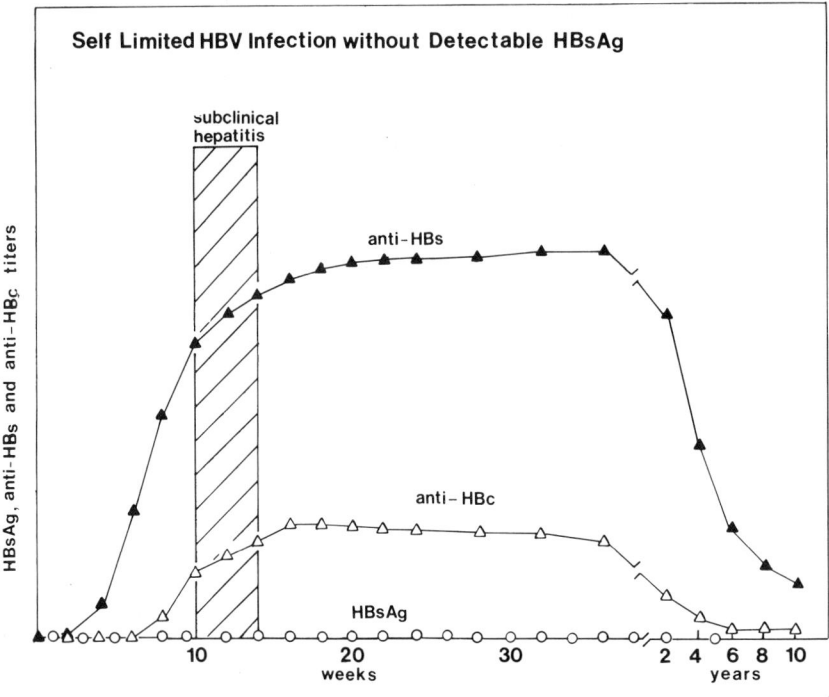

Figure 35–7. Schematic representation of the serologic response throughout the course of HBsAg-negative primary HBV infection.

fections associated with a primary antibody response without detectable HBsAg in the blood are usually accompanied by asymptomatic disease, with only minor elevations in serum transaminase activity.[300, 312, 316] Although the patterns of anti-HBs and anti-HBc response differ in order and relative magnitude compared with the responses of patients with detectable antigenemia, the fact that both the antibodies (including IgM anti-HBc) and liver function abnormalities appear after a length of time that is consistent with the incubation period of HBV infection indicates that actual infection with HBV has taken place. DNA polymerase–containing virions and HBeAg have not been studied in such cases. No studies have been done to assess the state of virus in liver cells during infection of this kind.

In a large series of adult patients experimentally infected with HBV, 70 per cent had self-limited infection with transient HBsAg positivity, and 23 per cent had no detectable antigenemia but had a primary anti-HBs and anti-HBc response.[291] The frequency of each response after natural infection would probably depend on the infecting dose of virus and other factors that might differ for different populations.

Hepatitis B Surface Antigen–Positive Persistent Hepatitis B Virus Infection

Patients who remain HBsAg-positive for 20 weeks or longer after primary infection are very likely to remain positive indefinitely and are designated chronic HBsAg carriers (Fig. 35–8). Virions (Dane particles) can be detected by electron microscopy,[317–319] DNA polymerase activity,[289, 318] HBcAg,[319] or virion DNA in the blood of a significant percentage of persistently infected patients who test positive for HBsAg.[320] Approximately 50 per cent of persistently infected patients tested positive by a sensitive assay for virion DNA polymerase, and 5 to 10 per cent had very high levels.[318] All patients with detectable virion DNA

polymerase in the blood have HBcAg detected by immunofluorescence in liver biopsies,[289] and when a highly sensitive assay for virions is used, all patients with HBcAg in liver have been found to have detectable virions in serum.[321]

Almost all persistently infected patients have high titers of anti-HBc in the blood,[291] as shown in Figure 35–8. The titers of this antibody are significantly higher during persistent infection than during most self-limited infections or in convalescence.[291] Although most of the anti-HBc is undoubtedly in the IgG fraction, interestingly IgM anti-HBc continues to be made and can be detected indefinitely in the serum of most persistently infected patients.[306, 321]

As described earlier, HBeAg can be detected in the serum of almost all patients early in primary HBV infection, and anti-HBe appears in almost all patients during resolution of the infection. Conversely, in persistent infection sensitive assays, such as radioimmunoassay or passive hemagglutination, have detected HBeAg in one fourth to one half of patients, and anti-HBe was detected in almost all the remainder.[293, 322] When less sensitive assays are used, neither marker may be detected in 50 per cent or more of persistently infected patients.[323–326] The observation that the high molecular weight form of HBeAg in serum represents a complex between HBeAg and immunoglobulin suggests that the anti-HBe may be produced by many or all HBeAg-positive patients, but is present exclusively as a complex with HBeAg so that no free antibody can be detected.[257, 258] There is a very high correlation between the presence of HBeAg in serum and virions detected by electron microscopy or by their DNA polymerase activity.[261–264, 327]

There is a wide range of HBsAg titers in persistently infected patients. In general, those with the highest titers of infectious virus and detectable virion DNA polymerase activity or HBeAg, or both, have the highest titers of HBsAg.[312, 316, 328, 329]

The most sensitive assay for complete virions is infectivity titrations by inoculation into susceptible hosts such as humans or chimpanzees, because as described previously,

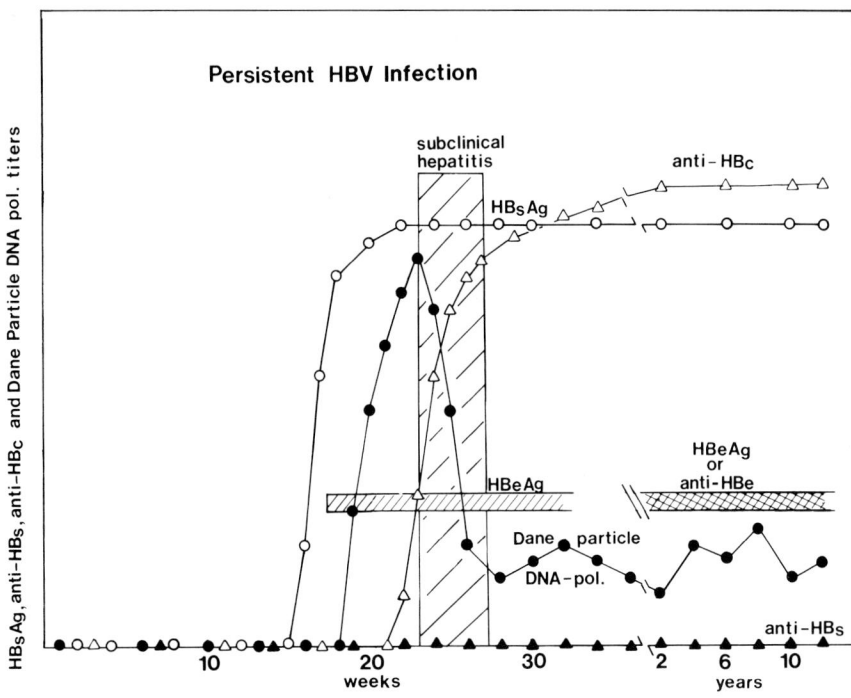

Figure 35–8. Schematic representation of viral markers in the blood throughout the course of HBV infection that becomes persistent.

infectious HBV can be demonstrated in some sera after dilution by as much as 10^8.[107, 108] Although most HBsAg carriers have high titers of infectious HBV in serum, some carriers appear to have no detectable infectious virus. The highest titers of virus are found in patients with detectable HBeAg or virion DNA polymerase activity, or both, in serum.[107, 108] Patients without these markers or with anti-HBe have much lower titers of virus.[108] Recently, undiluted sera from six HBsAg carriers without detectable virion DNA polymerase or HBeAg failed to infect chimpanzees.[107] This was a direct demonstration that some persistently infected patients who continue to produce HBsAg do not produce detectable amounts of infectious HBV. These patients appear to be HBsAg carriers without detectable virion DNA polymerase or HBeAg. The percentage of HBsAg carriers who have no detectable infectious virus is not known. Patients with detectable virion DNA polymerase and HBeAg in sera, but not those without these markers, appear to be highly contagious,[262, 330, 331] which is in agreement with the data on titers of infectious HBV in the blood. A few HBsAg carriers with HBeAg and DNA and DNA polymerase–containing virions in the blood have free replicating forms of viral DNA (closed and relaxed circular, and linear double-stranded, single-stranded, and DNA-RNA hybrids) and probably integrated viral DNA in the liver,[159, 165, 315, 332] providing biochemical evidence that complete virus replication is proceeding in at least some cells. A variable number of liver cells in such patients appear to contain HBsAg or HBcAg, or both, as detected by immunofluorescent staining. These patients frequently, but not always, have chronic persistent or chronic active hepatitis (CAH).[327, 333, 334]

Investigation of a few HBsAg carriers with no detectable DNA and DNA polymerase–containing virions or HBeAg in the blood has revealed evidence of integrated sequences of viral DNA but no detectable free viral DNA forms or HBcAg in liver cells.[159, 165, 315, 332] As already described, not all cells (and frequently only a fraction of cells) are HBsAg-positive by immunofluorescent staining. These findings and the infectivity studies cited previously indicate that these patients are replicating complete virus at a very low level or not at all, and the only viral gene expressed appears to be the HBsAg gene in an integrated state. Many but not all of these patients appear to have little or no liver disease and are considered to be "healthy carriers."[284, 327, 333]

Anti-HBs has been regularly detected as a complex with HBsAg in the serum of patients with certain extrahepatic disease syndromes such as HBV-associated polyarteritis nodosa and membranous glomerulonephritis.[307] In addition, there is evidence for HBsAg–anti-HBs complexes in the serum of a significant percentage of persistently infected patients with chronic liver disease and in some so-called healthy carriers,[308–310] indicating that in at least some patients anti-HBs is made in the face of ongoing persistent infection and without significant associated disease. Standard assays for anti-HBs rarely detect this antibody in persistently infected subjects because of the great antigen excess in their sera. It is not known whether the anti-HBs response in these patients is quantitatively diminished; however, the frequent presence of this antibody, anti-HBc, and anti-HBe during persistent HBV infection suggests that complete immunologic tolerance to these viral antigens does not account for the persistence of infection.

The long-term natural history of persistent HBV infection is not completely defined. Prolonged infection (e.g., for many years) appears to be the rule for most chronic carriers. HBsAg positivity lasting as long as 20 years has been documented.[334] The titers of HBsAg and levels of virion DNA polymerase have been shown to be relatively stable over a period of weeks or a few months,[289] but increasing evidence suggests that persistent HBV infections tend to wind down spontaneously over a period of many months to years, with HBsAg titers slowly falling and virion DNA polymerase and HBeAg titers falling below the level of detection with time. In one prospective study of persistently infected patients with significant levels of virion DNA polymerase activity in their sera, levels of virion DNA polymerase spontaneously fell to undetectable levels in approximately 10 per cent of patients/year. A similar rate of disappearance was observed for serum HBeAg.[289] In a different group of patients with HBeAg, this antigen disappeared from serum in 45 per cent of patients over a two- to seven-year period.[335] Similar spontaneous disappearance of HBeAg or virion DNA polymerase activity, or both, has been shown in many other cases.[264, 333, 335–338] Anti-HBe eventually can be detected in most patients after they become HBeAg-negative. In HBsAg carriers without virion DNA polymerase activity or HBeAg in serum, these markers have been observed infrequently to reappear spontaneously.[339, 340] The interval between onset of infection and the time when HBeAg and virion levels become undetectable varies greatly in different individuals. These markers may remain detectable in persistently infected patients for years; clearly, the duration of infection correlates strongly with the presence of detectable HBeAg and virions. Spontaneous clearance of all viral markers of active HBV infection, although unusual, can occur at any time. Combined data from three different studies showed that HBsAg became undetectable at a rate of approximately 2 per cent/year. This group of patients included a total of 800 HBsAg-positive blood donors, most of whom were undoubtedly chronic carriers. Individual follow-ups ranged from 2 to 44 months.[341–343] In another study of persistently infected patients, most of whom had chronic hepatitis, HBsAg became undetectable in 1.5 per cent of cases over a ten-month period.[289] Spontaneous disappearance of HBsAg in persistently infected patients has been observed in numerous other cases.[264, 333, 344] A number of factors that appear to influence the incidence of persistent infection—such as age, sex, immunologic status, and possibly race—also may influence rates of spontaneous remission, but preliminary data suggesting that persistent infections resolve in females at a faster rate than in males are the only evidence bearing on these factors.[345]

Hepatitis Surface Antigen–Negative Persistent Hepatitis B Virus Infection

There is good evidence that some patients with persistent HBV infection do not have detectable HBsAg in their serum. Hoofnagle and co-workers described a patient with persistent HBV infection, a high anti-HBc titer, and a titer of HBsAg that fluctuated just above and below the level of detection by radioimmunoassay.[291] At certain times, the patient's serum was HBsAg-negative by the most sensitive tests, although active infection apparently continued. A small but significant percentage of blood donors whose sera test HBsAg-negative by the most sensitive assays transmit HBV infection to recipients of their blood.[346–348] Some of these donors could be in the incubation period of hepatitis B before the appearance of detectable HBsAg. Most probably they are persistently infected but have HBsAg levels below the level of detection. Finally, cases of chronic hepatitis without detectable HBsAg have been ascribed to active HBV infection because of persistent high titers of anti-HBc.[349]

Exogenous Factors That May Alter the Course of Persistent Hepatitis B Virus Infection

Corticosteroid therapy appears to alter the course of persistent HBV infection. Initiation of approximately 20 to 30 mg of prednisone/day is followed rapidly and regularly by a rise in virion DNA polymerase activity and HBsAg titers in blood.[350] Occasionally HBsAg-negative patients with anti-HBc or anti-HBs will become HBsAg-positive during immunosuppressive therapy.[351, 352] This suggests that HBV may be present in a latent state in some patients and that virus replication can be activated in such patients by immunosuppression. Withdrawal of corticosteroids is usually associated with a fall in HBsAg titers and virion DNA polymerase levels, the latter sometimes to undetectable levels.[350] The mechanism of the effects observed with corticosteroids is not understood, but suppression of the immune response may be involved or activation of the steroid-responsive element in the HBV genome (154a), as corticosteroids appear to have a direct stimulatory effect on the replication of some other viruses, independent of effects on the immune system.[353]

Antiviral agents α-interferon and adenine arabinoside inhibit replication of HBV in all persistently infected patients.[289, 319, 354, 355] Experimental treatment with either antiviral agent or with the two together is accompanied by a rapid reduction in the level of virions in the serum of all patients and a much more gradual reduction of HBsAg titers in some patients. These antivirals thus may act primarily on a step involved in virion production and not production of incomplete HBsAg particles. Permanent disappearance of only virions and HBeAg in some patients and disappearance of those markers as well as HBsAg in a few patients have been observed (see Management of Hepatitis B). Although these responses to antiviral treatment have been well documented, the frequency with which each response occurs can be determined only in carefully designed trials including placebo-treated controls.

Finally, several cases have been observed in which HBeAg and virion DNA polymerase have fallen to undetectable levels and HBsAg titers have fallen significantly in persistently infected patients during intercurrent infection with other agents such as HAV (W. S. Robinson, unpublished results) and HDV (see Hepatitis D Virus). More evidence is needed to establish the frequency of such effects and elucidate a mechanism.

Secondary Immune Response After Exposure to Hepatitis B Virus

Patients with anti-HBs at the time of exposure to HBV (and HBsAg) may have a secondary anti-HBs response with a rapid and marked rise in titer of this antibody.[291] Although anti-HBc can be detected in the serum of most of these patients, no change in the titer of this antibody has been observed.[291] The speed of the anti-HBs response and the lack of liver function abnormalities suggest that these patients are not reinfected by the HBV challenge but experience a secondary anti-HBs response after re-exposure to HBsAg.

PROTECTIVE IMMUNITY

Anti-HBs in the serum of convalescent patients appears to confer almost complete resistance to reinfection. The anti-HBs produced after primary HBV infection is primarily of anti-a specificity, although anti-d, anti-y, or other type of specific antibody appropriate to the subtype of the infecting virus may also appear.[356] Protection against reinfection with HBV of either the same or a different subtype has been shown,[312] suggesting that immunity is probably conferred on the most part by anti-a. In exceptional cases, however, second infections with HBV have been reported in patients with anti-HBs,[357–359] and in some cases HBV of a different subtype has infected individuals with antibody of restricted (e.g., only subtype) specificity.[357] It has also been shown that chimpanzees can be reinfected when challenge doses are sufficiently large, even when the identical strain of HBV is used for both the initial and the challenge exposures.[312, 360] Second infection with HBV, overcoming immunity by either mechanism, must be unusual because individuals having multiple episodes of acute viral hepatitis have not been found to develop hepatitis B more than once.[361–363]

Although evidence from primary immunization with purified HBsAg (following which anti-HBs appears and anti-HBc does not) and passive immunization with high-titer anti-HBs indicates that anti-HBs protects against reinfection,[313, 314] patients with anti-HBc and no detectable anti-HBs have also been shown to resist reinfection.[291] More recently, immunization of chimpanzees with HBcAg purified from infected liver and HBcAg produced in bacterial cells transformed with a plasmid expression vector containing the HBcAg gene led to protection of the animals against challenge with HBV.[364, 365] Anti-HBe also appears to be protective.[366] These results suggest that the immune response to HBcAg and HBeAg plays a role in protecting against HBV infection, and the question whether HBcAg as well as HBsAg could be used as a vaccine is raised. Since anti-HBc appears to be directed against an internal virion antigen, it is unlikely that this antibody directly neutralizes viral infectivity. Cellular immune mechanisms may make such patients resistant to reinfection, although the role of cellular immunity in resistance to reinfection and in resolution of ongoing infection is unclear.

DISEASES ASSOCIATED WITH HEPATITIS B VIRUS INFECTION

Acute and Chronic Hepatitis B

The syndromes of acute and chronic hepatitis B are associated with hepatocellular necrosis and inflammatory responses in HBV-infected liver. Primary HBV infection may be associated with little or no liver disease or with acute hepatitis of severity that varies from mild to fulminant.[367] Persistent HBV infection is sometimes associated with a histologically normal or nearly normal liver and normal liver function and sometimes with syndromes designated chronic persistent hepatitis (CPH) or chronic active hepatitis (CAH).[367] CPH is considered not to be progressive and CAH may be more severe and progress to cirrhosis. The mechanism of liver cell injury in hepatitis B has not been established, but there has been much conjecture about the role of the immune response.[368, 369] Several factors have been identified that appear to correlate with the severity of acute or chronic hepatitis B and that may provide clues about pathogenesis. Among them is the infecting dose of virus. High doses of HBV usually result in shorter incubation periods and more severe acute hepatitis than do low infecting doses.[107] A second factor appears to be age. An HBV infection at a very young age is usually associated with mild (almost always subclinical) initial hepatitis.[370, 371] Anecdotal cases suggest that HBV infections are associated with milder initial disease in immunologically impaired hosts than in immunologically normal individuals.[372, 373]

These observations raise the possibility that the immune response may influence the severity of acute hepatitis B.

During acute and chronic HBV infection there is almost always a humoral immune response to HBcAg and frequently to HBsAg.[291, 308–310] During chronic infection there is a humoral immune response to HBeAg.[293, 322, 331] There is also evidence that humoral immunity to hepatic (host) antigens occurs in chronic hepatitis B.[268] However, a role for the humoral immune response in hepatic injury would appear to be excluded by the observation that severe acute and chronic viral hepatitis can occur without an intact humoral immune response, such as in patients with agammaglobulinemia.[374]

Cellular immune responses directed against HBsAg, HBcAg, and liver cell antigens in acute and chronic HBV infection have also been detected by numerous investigators.[368, 369] Specific cellular immune reactivity to HBsAg has been detected by leukocyte migration inhibition and lymphocyte transformation assays during acute hepatitis B. It has been detected variably during chronic hepatitis B and most strongly and regularly during recovery and early convalescence. Cellular sensitization to HBsAg measured by these assays is frequently undetectable or weak in HBsAg carriers without liver disease. The localization of HBsAg on the cell surface in patients with CAH (in contrast to its cytoplasmic location in those with little or no liver disease) is considered to be an appropriate state for immune attack directed at HBsAg.[284, 285] Conversely, circulating cytotoxic effector T cells directed against HBsAg-bearing target cells have not been demonstrated clearly. Claims for the cytotoxicity of lymphocytes from patients with hepatitis B against artificial or nonphysiologic target cells, such as avian erythrocytes bearing chemically coupled HBsAg, have been made, but antigen-specific cytotoxic effector cell activity against human HCC cell lines producing HBsAg has not been detected.[368, 369] In these studies, target cells were not HLA-matched with the lymphocyte donors, a condition that probably is necessary for optimum detection of antigen-specific cytotoxicity.[375] Thus, no convincing evidence of lymphocyte cytotoxicity directed against cells bearing HBsAg has been reported, although optimum testing for such cytotoxic effector cell activity may not have been carried out. Evidence has been presented for the cytotoxicity of peripheral blood cells for autologous hepatocytes in chronic hepatitis B. This effect is blocked by anti-HBc, suggesting that HBcAg may be the target antigen for the cytotoxic cell.[376, 377] This is currently considered a likely mechanism that may contribute to liver injury in hepatitis B.

Cellular sensitization to host antigens in viral hepatitis has been demonstrated by several investigators.[369] Sensitization to a liver-specific hepatocyte surface membrane lipoprotein (liver-specific protein, or LSP) has been detected in approximately one half of patients with acute hepatitis B, but it is transient and has not been demonstrated following recovery.[378, 379] Reactivity to the same antigen has also been detected in most patients with CAH (whether they are HBsAg-positive or not). Suppressor T-cell activity is also depressed in the blood of patients with acute and chronic hepatitis B and returns to normal with recovery.[380]

The findings described here have led some to conclude that cellular reactivity to HBsAg and hepatocyte antigens (e.g., LSP) is significant for liver injury in acute and chronic hepatitis B, but this mechanism is not yet proved. The failure so far to demonstrate clear cytotoxic effector T cells directed against HBsAg-bearing target cells in patients with hepatitis B, in fact, leaves in doubt whether HBsAg is an important target antigen.

Certain viral markers in the serum and liver of persistently infected patients appear to be present more often when significant chronic hepatitis is present. HBeAg and virion DNA polymerase activity in serum,[323-327, 381, 382] and HBcAg as well as HBsAg in the liver detected by immunofluorescent staining,[284, 285, 327] are often found in patients with CAH or CPH. There is little difference between the prevalence of these markers, however, in CAH and CPH.[323-325, 327] In contrast, healthy carriers,[381-383] including those with little or no abnormality documented by liver biopsy,[327, 384] appear most often to be HBeAg-negative, virion DNA polymerase–negative,[327] and frequently anti-HBe positive.[325, 327, 382-384] Liver biopsy results from these patients reveal only HBsAg and no HBcAg, as determined by immunofluorescent staining.[284, 285, 327] These findings suggest that complete virus replication proceeds more often in liver cells of patients with chronic hepatitis B as compared with livers of carriers. Little or no hepatitis is present in the latter, and most often expression of HBsAg is the only viral gene product detected. These findings support the possibility that it is the cellular immune response directed at HBcAg or HBeAg (or some as yet undescribed viral antigen) rather than at HBsAg that is responsible for hepatic injury during HBV infection.

A prominent reason often given to support the hypothesis that liver cell injury in hepatitis B is caused by immune attack is the belief that HBV is not a cytopathic virus. The evidence for this idea is that hepatoma cell lines in culture containing the entire HBV genome but expressing only HBsAg, that is, not replicating complete virus, have no apparent impairment in growth or function.[385, 386] Also, healthy carriers producing only HBsAg may have little or no liver injury.[327] These observations do not exclude the possibility, however, that the infection is cytopathic when HBV-infected cells express HBcAg, HBeAg, and other viral gene products in addition to HBsAg and are replicating viral DNA. For example, expression of HBsAg by an HCC cell line in culture resulted in no impairment in cell function or growth, but when the same cells were made to express HBcAg, a cytopathic effect was observed.[387] In addition, the association of hepatitis with HBeAg in serum and HBcAg in liver, as described earlier, is consistent with such a mechanism. Thus a direct cytotoxic effect of the virus must still be considered a possible mechanism for hepatic injury by HBV.

A final mechanism for liver cell injury in some cases during HBV infection appears to be coinfection with a second cytopathic virus—HDV. This mechanism is described in Hepatitis D Virus.

Hepatocellular Carcinoma

Within the limits of the data available, there appears to be a good correlation between the worldwide geographic distribution of HCC and active HBV infection, with the highest frequency of both occurring in sub-Saharan Africa and Southeast Asia).[89] In addition, active HBV infection occurs significantly more frequently in patients with HCC than in controls in both high- and low-incidence geographic areas of HCC.[89] A recent prospective study of HBsAg-positive and HBsAg-negative middle-aged men in Taiwan revealed an incidence of HCC that was more than 300 times higher in the HBsAg-positive group than in the

HBsAg-negative group.[90] Similar results have been obtained in Japan.[388]

The high incidence of persistent HBV infection in mothers of HCC patients, in contrast to that in fathers,[389] suggests that transmission from mothers to newborn or infant children may be a frequent mode and time of HBV infection in HCC patients. The finding of low serum HBsAg titers and no HBeAg, together with the rare occurrence of hepatic HBcAg in most HCC patients,[89, 390] also suggests that the persistent infections in HCC patients are of long duration. If HBV infection does occur frequently at very early ages in HCC patients in areas of high HCC incidence, the age distribution of patients with clinically recognized tumors would suggest that these tumors appear after a mean duration of approximately 35 years of HBV infection.[391] Very few cases of HCC occur in children.[391] Between 60 and 90 per cent of HCC patients have coexisting cirrhosis,[90, 391-394] suggesting that this lesion in association with persistent HBV infection may predispose a person to HCC, although clearly cirrhosis need not be present.

HBV infection in humans is not the only hepadnavirus infection associated with HCC. In fact, a much higher incidence of HCC formation occurs in WHV-infected woodchucks and in GSHV-infected ground squirrels than is observed in humans infected with HBV.[40, 92, 395] HCC develops in approximately one third of infected animals in captivity each year; no tumors have been observed in uninfected animals.

Several studies have evaluated the state of virus in HCC tissue from humans and woodchucks and in tissue culture lines from human HCC. Immunofluorescent antibody staining and immunoperoxidase staining usually do not detect HBsAg in tumor tissue from patients with HBsAg in blood and HBsAg or HBcAg, or both, in nontumorous liver cells. Some studies have reported small numbers of HBsAg-positive cells in tumors.[394] HBcAg has been detected even more rarely. Thus few tumor cells appear to express either viral gene product in amounts that can be detected by immunofluorescent antibody staining.

Viral DNA has been found in approximately 75 per cent of tumors but not in the remaining 25 per cent.[396] In addition to free episomal genome-length (3200 bp) viral DNA forms, integrated viral DNA can be detected in many, although not all, cases of HCC).[167, 171, 172, 180, 181, 183, 315, 397] Integration occurs at a few (usually one to four) specific cellular DNA sites in tumors, but always at different sites in different tumors. The integrated viral DNA contains extensive deletions and rearrangements, which are different for each integrated viral sequence. No known cellular oncogene sequences have been detected in the cellular DNA flanking viral inserts.[185] Thus although there is a strong association between longstanding hepadnavirus infection and HCC formation in humans, woodchucks, and ground squirrels and viral DNA is found integrated in the cellular DNA of many tumors, exactly how these viruses are involved in HCC formation is not clear.

Additional Syndromes Associated with Hepatitis B Virus Infection

Syndromes with extrahepatic manifestations have been associated with HBV infection, and for some there is evidence that HBsAg–anti-HBs complexes play a role in pathogenesis.[307, 398] The serum sickness–like syndrome—consisting of fever, rash, urticaria, arthralgias, and sometimes acute arthritis—which occurs in 10 to 20 per cent of patients during the incubation period of acute hepatitis B, is accompanied by HBsAg-antibody complexes and low levels of complement components in serum, synovial fluid, and synovial membranes from involved joints.[299, 400]

In several series, one third to one half of patients with biopsy proven polyarteritis nodosa have had persistent HBV infection.[298, 307] Among all HBsAg carriers, however, this syndrome occurs infrequently (1 of 43 in one series).[291a] Such patients have low serum complement levels and circulating HBsAg–anti-HBs complexes. Immune complexes and complement components have also been regularly detected in diseased vessels by immunofluorescent staining.[401, 402]

A significant number of cases of membranous glomerulonephritis have been associated with CAH and persistent HBV infection.[307, 398] Immune complex deposits can be found along the subepithelial surfaces of glomerular basement membranes by electron microscopy, and nodular deposits of HBsAg, immune globulin, and C_3 in glomeruli have been observed by immunofluorescent staining in these cases.[403-407]

Several additional syndromes with unknown pathogenesis have also been associated with HBV infection. Infantile papular acrodermatitis appears to be associated frequently with persistent HBV infection in Mediterranean countries and Japan.[408, 409] In a series of 19 patients with essential mixed cryoglobulinemia, cryoprecipitates were shown to contain HBsAg in 6 cases and anti-HBs in 11 cases,[410] suggesting that some cases of cryoglobulinemia may be related to HBV infection. This association, however, could not be confirmed in a subsequent study.[411] A significant number of cases of aplastic anemia have been observed following acute viral hepatitis.[412] Although in most cases the specific hepatitis virus has not been identified, in a few cases acute hepatitis B has been documented.[413, 414] The basis of this apparent association is not yet clear. Further work is needed to clarify the pathogenesis of these syndromes and to determine whether HBsAg-antibody complexes or HBV infection in some other way plays an important role.

Clearly, infections with HBV and other hepadnaviruses have protean manifestations, and different, distinct pathogenetic mechanisms appear to be responsible for a number of different disease syndromes.

DIAGNOSTIC TESTING FOR HEPATITIS B VIRUS INFECTION

A diagnosis of acute viral hepatitis can usually be made from clinical findings, and the responsible viral agent is often suspected from the epidemiologic setting and features such as the incubation period; however, only virus-specific tests can conclusively identify the infecting virus. Highly sensitive and specific tests for HBsAg, anti-HBs, anti-HBc, anti-HBc IgM, HBeAg, and anti-HBe are specific for HBV. They are diagnostically useful and commercially available. Tests specific for Dane particles or viral DNA and DNA polymerase–containing virions are available only in research laboratories. Table 35–4 shows typical serologic test findings at different stages of HBV infection and in convalescence. This table does not include all variations and does not convey the dynamic nature of infection during which individual markers appear and disappear (not always in the same order in different patients) during the evolution of infection, as indicated in Figures 35–6 through 35–7.

Tests for serum HBsAg, anti-HBs, anti-HBc, and anti-HBc IgM are important when clinically evaluating patients for active and past HBV infection.[415, 416] HBsAg is the most important and commonly used marker for active infection, because its presence in serum indicates active infection with HBV in almost all cases, the rare exception being after passive transfer of HBsAg (e.g., by blood transfusion). Sera or other body fluids or secretions should be considered infectious when HBsAg is present.

When serum tests positive for HBsAg in patients with apparent acute hepatitis, acute hepatitis B is suggested, although superimposed hepatitis caused by another agent or acute exacerbations of CAH may give similar findings in a patient with persistent HBV infection. Falling titers of HBsAg or rising anti-HBc titers and positive anti-HBc IgM, or both, in such patients suggest acute hepatitis B (see Fig. 35–6). As described in Course of Infection, HBsAg can never be detected in some patients with acute HBV infection (see Fig. 35–7); in some, HBsAg becomes undetectable before the end of clinical disease, and in a few, it becomes undetectable even before the onset of disease. In such patients with acute hepatitis, the diagnosis of HBV infection may be established only by the presence of anti-HBc IgM, a rising titer of anti-HBc, or the subsequent appearance of anti-HBs, or all of these.

Without detectable anti-HBc, the presence of HBsAg suggests early infection (i.e., during the first few weeks after the patient becomes HBsAg-positive and before the appearance of anti-HBc (see Fig. 35–6). HBsAg would also occur alone in any infected patient unable to mount an antibody response (e.g., as in agammaglobulinemia). HBsAg in the presence of anti-HBc IgM suggests primary infection sometime after the early period (see Fig. 35–6), and a high titer of anti-HBc without anti-HBc IgM suggests persistent infection (see Fig. 35–8). Anti-HBc titers are usually significantly higher during persistent infection than during or following self-limited infection.[291, 415, 416]

TABLE 35–4. TITERS OF SEVERAL HBV MARKERS IN HIGH-HBsAg–TITER SERUM

Serum Dilution	HBsAg				Virions/ml†	Virion DNA Polymerase Activity† (cpm/ml)	HBeAg (RIA)†	Infectivity for Chimpanzees†
	Protein*	Particles/ml*	CEP*	RIA*				
Undiluted	100 μg/ml	10^{13}	+	+	10^9	10^5	+	+
10^{-1}	10 μg/ml	10^{12}	+	+	10^8	10^4	+	+
10^{-2}	1 μg/ml	10^{11}	+	+	10^7	10^3	+	+
10^{-3}	100 ng/ml	10^{10}	−	+	10^6	10^2	+	+
10^{-4}	10 ng/ml	10^9	−	+	10^5	10	−	+
10^{-5}	1 ng/ml	10^8	−	+	10^4	−	−	+
10^{-6}	100 pg/ml	10^7	−	−	10^3	−	−	+
10^{-7}	10 pg/ml	10^6	−	−	10^2	−	−	+
10^{-8}	1 pg/ml	10^5	−	−	10	−	−	−

*Data of Hoofnagle[104] for single high-HBsAg-titer serum.

†Data of Robinson (unpublished results) for a different serum with HBsAg and infectivity titers similar to those of the serum examined by Hoofnagle.

The presence of anti-HBs and anti-HBc without HBsAg and anti-HBc IgM indicates past infection with HBV and immunity.[291, 415, 416] In general, the more recent the infection, the higher the titers of these antibodies. The presence of either anti-HBs or anti-HBc alone in low titers most commonly occurs after infection in the distant past in individuals who have since lost the second antibody. Anti-HBc alone may be present in relatively high titer after the disappearance of HBsAg and before the appearance of anti-HBs (see Fig. 35–6), thus indicating recent infection. Anti-HBc is the only antibody detected after self-limited infection in 10 per cent of patients in whom detectable anti-HBs never develops.

Infrequently, blood containing high titers of anti-HBc but no detectable HBsAg has been shown to transmit HBV infection to recipients.[291] Such blood probably comes from persistently infected patients or those with self-limited infection who have HBsAg titers that are too low for detection by even the most sensitive assays. Thus blood containing anti-HBc alone, particularly when in high titer, should be considered potentially infectious.

The presence of anti-HBs without anti-HBc and HBsAg indicates past HBV infection or past vaccination for HBV.[291, 415, 416] Low titers of anti-HBs in patients without past HBV vaccination suggest infection in the distant past in patients in whom anti-HBc had fallen to undetectable levels. High titers of anti-HBs alone may occur after a secondary anti-HBs response following exposure to HBV and HBsAg (e.g., by receiving HBsAg-containing blood products or immunization with HBV vaccine) without reinfection, which would result in a rise in anti-HBc as well as anti-HBs levels. Blood containing detectable anti-HBs appears to transmit HBV infection rarely if ever.[417, 418] Passive transfer of HBsAg, anti-HBs or anti-HBc, or all of these, after transfusion with blood containing the appropriate serologic activity, can produce any of the patterns described.

Although analysis of a single blood sample may provide an accurate diagnosis in some cases, a second sample one month or more after the first, or serial samples, may be required to fully establish HBV infection and the stage of infection or convalescence in some patients. For example, falling HBsAg titers in serial blood samples suggests resolving acute infection (see Fig. 35–6). A fourfold or greater rise in the anti-HBc titer and anti-HBc IgM suggests ongoing infection (see Figs. 35–6 and 35–7). Such a rise in anti-HBs suggests recent infection (see Figs. 35–6 and 35–7) or a secondary response after exposure to HBsAg without infection. Persistent infection (i.e., the chronic carrier state) usually cannot be established until HBsAg has been shown to be present for at least six months.

Assays for Dane particles, HBeAg, and anti-HBe in serum are also clinically useful for assessing patients with HBV infection. Dane particles (detected by DNA polymerase activity) or viral DNA content (detected by nucleic acid hybridization) and HBeAg are not found in serum without detectable HBsAg.[318, 320] High levels of DNA polymerase activity in Dane particles, and HBeAg, appear regularly in the late incubation period of hepatitis B, and their presence with HBsAg in sera of patients without anti-HBc suggests an early stage of infection (see Fig. 35–6). The presence of Dane particles and HBeAg during acute or persistent infection may be used to identify patients who are more likely to transmit infection to others. Infected patients without these markers are less likely to infect others. As described in the next section (Epidemiology), the presence of these activities correlates well with trans-

mission of HBV infection from carriers via a percutaneous route,[362, 419] from pregnant carriers to their newborn infants,[329, 330, 371, 420] from medical care personnel—such as dentists—to their patients,[421] and from individuals with persistent infection to their sexual contacts.[422] HBsAg carriers with anti-HBe in their serum appear to transmit infection by these routes much less frequently. These correlations are not absolute, however.[423] Some blood containing HBsAg and anti-HBe has been shown to contain infectious HBV,[107, 424] although in much lower titer than in blood containing HBeAg.[107] Thus, whereas these viral markers clearly can distinguish between infected patients who readily transmit infection and those unlikely to infect others (at least by certain routes of transmission), the outcome of contacts with infected patients in individual cases cannot be predicted with certainty from knowledge of these viral markers because the correlations are not absolute.

EPIDEMIOLOGY

Incidence of Primary Hepatitis B Virus Infection

It has been estimated by the Centers for Disease Control that there are approximately 200,000 primary HBV infections/year in the United States.[425] Most are in young adults, and approximately one fourth are associated with acute icteric disease. More than 10,000 individuals are hospitalized with hepatitis B each year, and 250 die with fulminant hepatitis B. The infection fails to resolve in between 6 and 10 per cent and these patients become persistently infected (chronic HBsAg carriers). The lifetime risk of HBV infection is estimated to be 5 per cent for the whole population of the United States, but for certain high-risk groups it may reach nearly 100 per cent.

Most cases of acute hepatitis B in the United States are in young adults, unlike the younger age distribution of hepatitis A.[345] The age distribution is related to the circumstances leading to transmission (see further on). More cases occur in males than in females,[345] again unlike hepatitis A, for which there is no apparent sex difference in incidence. The incidence of acute hepatitis B differs in different populations within the United States (Table 35–5).[425] Percutaneous drug users; patients receiving blood transfusions or some other blood products and those requiring hemodialysis; laboratory personnel who work with human blood, serum, and blood products; homosexuals and others with frequent and different sexual contacts; and medical and dental personnel who have frequent contact with blood are at greatest risk. Blood donor screening for HBsAg by the most sensitive tests, and a shift away from paid blood donors to the use of volunteer donors, greatly reduced but did not completely eliminate post-transfusion hepatitis B during the 1970s.[34, 346–348, 426] Recent studies of post-transfusion hepatitis indicate that 5 to 10 per cent of cases are still hepatitis B. Most of them occur after transfusion of blood that tests negative for HBsAg by the most sensitive tests available, indicating that this test does not detect every individual with infectious HBV in the blood.

The prevalence of serum antibody to HBsAg (anti-HBs), indicating past HBV infection or vaccination (as seen in results from the most sensitive techniques) increases with age in the general population in the United States, up to a maximum at around ages 30 to 45 years. Approximately 5 to 20 per cent of people older than this group test positive in most studies.[345, 427] The prevalence of anti-HBs in serum

TABLE 35–5. PREVALENCE OF SEROLOGIC MARKERS OF HBV INFECTION IN DIFFERENT POPULATION GROUPS IN UNITED STATES GROUPED ACCORDING TO RISK OF INFECTION*

	Prevalence of Serologic Markers of HBV Infection	
	HBsAg (%)	All Markers† (%)
High Risk		
Immigrants and refugees from areas of high HBV endemism	13	70–85
Clients in institutions for the mentally retarded	10–20	35–80
Users of illicit parenteral drugs	7	60–80
Homosexually active males	6	35–80
Household contacts of HBV carriers	3–6	30–60
Patients of hemodialysis units	3–10	20–80
Intermediate Risk		
Prisoners (male)	1–8	10–80
Staff of institutions for the mentally retarded	1	10–25
Health-care workers frequent blood contact	1–2	15–30
Low Risk		
Health-care workers no or infrequent blood contact	0.3	3–10
Healthy adults (first-time volunteer blood donors)	0.3	3–5

*Data from the CDC.[276]

†All markers include HBsAg, anti-HBs, and anti-HBc.

also differs significantly in different populations within the United States. The groups described as at increased risk of acute hepatitis B have the highest prevalence of serum anti-HBs (Table 35–5). Different socioeconomic groups also have different risks for infection. Cherubin and associates found the frequency of anti-HBs to be 44, 18, and 10 per cent for people older than 30 years of age in sections of Harlem, Staten Island, and Park Avenue in New York City, respectively.[428]

Primary HBV infections occur at much higher frequencies and at much earlier ages in geographic areas of the world with high prevalence, such as in parts of Asia and Africa.[345] This undoubtedly reflects the fact that the important routes of transmission (see Routes of Transmission) are different from those in the United States and most often appear to involve transmission from infected mothers to their children. In countries such as Senegal, Thailand, and Taiwan, infection rates are very high in infants and continue through early childhood, at which time the prevalence of HBsAg in serum may exceed 25 per cent.[345] In Panama, New Guinea, the Solomon Islands, and Greenland, and in Indians in Alaska, infant infection rates are relatively low and increase rapidly during early childhood.[345] In all these populations, the prevalence of serum anti-HBs reaches a plateau, which is usually greater than 50 per cent between ages 10 and 19 years.[345]

Although clinically apparent acute viral hepatitis, which is often severe, was the first manifestation of primary HBV infection to be recognized, it is now clear that this is probably not the most common response to infection, except possibly when infection involves iatrogenic routes of transmission to susceptible adults such as by blood transfusion or other direct percutaneous transfer of virus-containing serum. In geographic areas of the world where infection rates are very high and take place at early ages, and the routes of transmission do not involve overt percutaneous transfer, primary infections appear most often to be clinically silent or mild, as is the persistent infection that appears to be a common outcome of primary infection in

that setting. Similarly, the natural infections of woodchucks, ground squirrels, and ducks by the respective hepadnaviruses that are related to HBV appear to be silent until late manifestations of disease (e.g., hepatoma) appear in some animals. Thus much of the severe acute viral hepatitis that was first associated with primary HBV infection appears to be a manifestation of medical procedures and other practices (e.g., blood transfusions and illicit parenteral drug abuse) peculiar to technologically advanced cultures.

Persistent Infection with Hepatitis B Virus

Persistent or chronic HBV infection (usually designated the HBsAg carrier state) is one of the most common persistent viral infections in humans. It has been estimated that more than 170 million people in the world today are persistently infected with HBV.[89] A large percentage of these cases are in eastern Asia and sub-Saharan Africa, where the prevalence of chronic infection is very high, and associated chronic liver disease and liver cancer are among the most important health problems. It is estimated that there are between 400,000 and 800,000 chronic carriers in the United States. As many as 25 per cent of them may have chronic active hepatitis.[425] As many as 4000 patients may die each year of hepatitis B–induced cirrhosis, and 800 patients may die from liver cancer. Although infection apparently terminates in a small number of long-established chronic carriers who then become HBsAg-negative (approximately 2 per cent/year),[289, 341–343] most chronic carriers remain infected for many years,[334] and infection for life appears to be common.

The HBsAg carrier rate varies from 0.1 to 20 per cent in different populations.[89] The incidence of the HBsAg carrier state is related most importantly to the incidence and the age of onset of primary infection. There are other host and viral factors that appear to increase the risk for developing persistent infection. They may be important in establishing carrier rates for some epidemiologic groups. A genetic predisposition for persistent infection has been suggested by family studies in which the chronic carrier state appeared to cluster in families, with a distribution consistent with segregation as an autosomal recessive trait.[429, 430] An association between persistent infection and certain HLA types has been reported,[431] but these findings have not been confirmed.[432, 433] Some evidence suggests that following primary HBV infection, New York residents of Chinese origin are more likely to become carriers than are white residents.[434] Whether this represents a genetic predisposition for persistent HBV infection remains to be determined.

Very young age appears to be one of the most important factors predisposing to persistent HBV infection. Approximately 5 to 10 per cent of adults with acute hepatitis B in the United States become chronically infected,[291, 291a] but persistent infection almost invariably follows acute neonatal hepatitis B, which most commonly is anicteric.[370, 371] The HBsAg carrier state appears to be most common in young adults in the United States, and the frequency in men is several times that in women in this age group.[345] The higher proportion of men to women carriers observed in many populations is due at least in part to the greater probability that men will become persistently infected after primary infection as well as to the apparently more rapid rate at which the carrier state is terminated in women.[345, 435–437]

Ancedotal cases suggest that immunosuppression may be associated with milder initial disease and more frequent persistent infection than occurs in immunologically normal individuals. For example, HBV infection in renal dialysis patients frequently becomes persistent.[438] Finally, the HBsAg carrier state appears to be more common in patients with certain diseases—such as Down's syndrome, lepromatous leprosy, and chronic lymphocytic leukemia—than in the general population.[436, 437] Although the mechanism by which each of these conditions leads to persistent infection is not clear, a common mechanism could be a modified or inadequate immune response so that the virus is not eliminated as it is after most acute infections.

The infecting dose of virus and the severity of initial disease also appear to correlate with the probability for developing persistent infection. Persistent infection occurs more frequently after initial anicteric hepatitis than it does with initial icteric disease.[107, 439] Survivors of fulminant hepatitis rarely become persistently infected, and HBsAg carriers frequently give no history of recognized acute hepatitis.[291a] Experimental infections with different dilutions of infectious serum suggest that lower doses of virus result more often in long incubation periods, mild initial disease, and subsequent chronic infection when compared with larger virus doses.[107] This relationship has been so regular that the infecting dose can usually be estimated from the incubation period in experimental transmission studies.[107, 109, 312] There is no evidence that hepatitis B virus strains (e.g., HBsAg subtypes) have different virulence or propensity for persistent infection.

Striking differences occur in HBsAg carrier rates in different populations in the United States and different geographic areas of the world. In most areas of the United States, less than 0.1 per cent of volunteer blood donors have been found to be HBsAg-positive,[89] and almost all are chronic HBsAg carriers, whereas the carrier rate in paid donors is usually closer to 1 per cent. Among certain populations—such as percutaneous drug abusers, patients in some hemodialysis centers, and certain homosexual populations—the carrier rate may be 1 to 5 per cent.[440] These high rates appear to reflect the frequent exposure to virus experienced by members of these groups. The carrier rates in most western European countries are similar to those in the United States,[89] but in other endemic areas of the world, such as many countries in Africa, Asia, and Oceania, the rate may be as high as 20 per cent. Almost all HBsAg-negative adults test positive for anti-HBs or anti-HBc, or both, indicating past infection.[89, 345, 436] The increased carrier rates in some developing countries may be related not only to poor sanitary conditions and increased exposure at very early ages but also to differences in predisposition for chronic infection on a genetic, nutritional, or other basis in different populations. Transmission of virus from persistently infected mothers to newborn or young infants, who then usually develop persistent infection, has been estimated to account for 40 per cent of carriers in Taiwan.[420, 441]

There is an uneven geographic distribution of HBsAg subtypes among HBsAg carriers in the world. As described earlier, almost all antigens contain either determinants *d* or *y* and either *w* or *r*. The *d* determinant is common in the United States, northern Europe, Asia, and Oceania. The *y* determinant is found at a lower frequency in these regions.[442, 443] The *d* determinant, to the near exclusion of *y*, is found in Japan. The *y* determinant (and rarely *d*) is found in Africa and in Australian aborigines; *y* also is found frequently in India and around the Mediterranean. The *w* determinant predominates in Europe, the United States, Africa, India, Australia, and Oceania. The *r* determinant

predominates in Japan, China, and Southeast Asia. Subtypes *adw*, *ady*, and *adr* are each found in extensive geographic regions of the world. Subtype *ayr* is more rare in the world, although it is found commonly in small populations in Oceania. The geographic distributions of subtypes probably reflect the locations of their origins—that is, diversion from a common HBsAg ancestor—and the migrations of infected human populations.

Routes of Transmission of Hepatitis B Virus

The only important source or reservoir of virus for human infections is humans themselves. No important animal reservoir is known. Although some higher primates other than humans may be infected in nature (see Virus Host Range), there is no evidence that they are important sources for human infection. If nonhuman primates are infected in nature, it is unlikely they would infect humans, because transmission from infected individuals requires specific patterns of intimate contact (to be described further on). Some environmental surfaces such as toothbrushes, razors, needles, toys, and so on may mediate person to person transmission in some cases, but there are no important environmental reservoirs such as water or food as are sometimes involved in the transmission of HAV to large numbers of individuals. HBV does not appear to be present very often in feces. There is no evidence for fecal-oral transmisison, as there is for HAV. These features of HBV, and the particular kinds of close contact required for transmission, probably account for the infrequent epidemic pattern of spread, in contrast to many agents that are spread by enteric (e.g., HAV) or respiratory routes. Persistent infections in which infectious HBV may be present continuously in the blood and certain other body fluids represent a stable human reservoir of virus, so HBV can be maintained indefinitely, even in small isolated populations (e.g., some island populations).

Although blood and blood products are the best-documented sources of infectious virus, HBsAg has also been found in feces, urine, bile, sweat, tears, saliva, semen, breast milk, vaginal secretions, cerebrospinal fluid, synovial fluid, and cord blood. Only serum,[107] saliva,[270, 444] and semen have actually been shown to contain infectious HBV in experimental transmission studies.[444] The report of transmission through the bite of an infected patient is consistent with the presence of HBV in saliva.[445] During the 1940s, more than 50 attempts to transmit serum hepatitis to human volunteers using feces from persons after experimental infection were unsuccessful,[18, 19] suggesting that infectious HBV probably enters feces infrequently when no gastrointestinal bleeding is present. Thus feces must not be a common source of virus for HBV infections acquired in the community.[446] Other body fluids have not been tested for infectious virus. Often the concentrations of HBsAg in fluids other than the serum of infected patients are low or are not detectable at all. When present, antigen sometimes can be demonstrated only after concentration. When infectious virus is also present in such fluids, its concentration is undoubtedly lower than that in serum. As mentioned already, infectious HBV has been shown to be present in blood without detectable HBsAg,[34, 346–348, 426] so the failure to detect antigen does not exclude the presence of infectious virus.

Several specific routes of transmission appear to be well established. The most important routes of transmission in the United States are undoubtedly by percutaneous transfer and probably mucous membrane contact with blood and possibly other body fluids (e.g., saliva) and by heterosexual and homosexual contacts. Direct percutaneous inoculation of virus by needles can occur with contaminated blood or blood products, hemodialysis, tattooing, ear piercing, acupuncture, sharing needles during illicit drug use, or accidental needle sticks by hospital personnel. Clearly HBV is commonly transmitted by routes other than these overt parenteral ones.[440] Infectious material contacting open skin breaks or mucous membranes such as the eye can be expected to result in infection. Because HBV is quite stable, transmission by means of environmental surfaces that may contact mucous membranes or open skin breaks—such as toothbrushes, baby bottles, toys, eating utensils, and razors—[447, 448] or hospital equipment—such as respirators, endoscopes,[449, 450] or laboratory glassware and instruments—[451]can be expected. In households, transmission is more common from HBV-infected patients to sexual partners than to other kinds of household contacts.[331, 452–454] HBV infection rates are unusually high among female prostitutes and male homosexuals,[455–457] who are commonly exposed to many different sexual partners. Cases of apparent direct transmission from HBV-infected persons to susceptible individuals following sexual intercourse have been reported.[422] The exact route of transmission in these cases is not yet proved, but it seems likely that sexual contact would be among the most common circumstances leading to HBV transmission in populations with high carrier rates. The demonstration of infectious virus in semen and saliva of infected patients supports the possibility of venereal transmission.[444]

Health care personnel have been shown to be at greater risk for HBV infection than is the general public,[458–460] and this is undoubtedly caused by their more frequent exposure to infected patients. The specific routes of transmission from patients to medical and dental workers are not known, although it appears that the greater the direct exposure to blood and serum—for example, as for surgeons and workers in renal dialysis units[460, 461]—the greater the frequency of HBV infection.

A few persistently infected physicians,[462] dentists,[421] and oral surgeons,[463, 464] as well as acutely infected health care personnel,[465, 466] have been implicated in the transmission of HBV infection to multiple patient contacts, but most health care personnel who are carriers,[467] as well as those with acute infection,[467, 468] appear to represent little risk to their patients. Transmission of infection from only certain chronic HBsAg carrier women and not others to their newborn infants has been observed.[329, 420] Transmission of virus from chronic carriers via administration of their blood products or via accidental needle puncture in a medical setting has been observed frequently. Although these are the best-documented instances of the spread of HBV infection from chronic carriers, transmission also appears to occur commonly from chronic carriers to sexual contacts, and those taking illicit drugs by self-injection using shared needles,[422, 454, 456] and by other routes described earlier. However, proof of transmission from patients during the persistent phase of infection rather than during the acute phase has not been demonstrated as clearly for the latter routes of transmission.

Infection after oral intake of infectious material has been demonstrated. The dose of virus needed for successful infection by the oral route appears to be higher than that needed for parenteral infection.[23] Also, oral infection does not occur via the intestinal tract, but through small breaks postulated to regularly exist in the oral mucosa. Experi-

mental transmission showed, for example, that two susceptible chimpanzees failed to become infected by infectious material placed directly in their stomachs but were infected by an oral spray of infectious material after their gums were brushed lightly with a toothbrush.[469] It is not clear how important an oral portal of entry is in community-acquired infections. There is no evidence that the fecal-oral route plays a significant role in HBV transmission.

Evidence consistent with an intestinal phase of HBV infection is lacking. In fact, HBsAg and HBcAg have not been detected by immunofluorescence in the cells of any tissue except liver.[470] Further investigation will be required to establish whether intestinal or other mucosal surfaces actually contain cells susceptible to infection by HBV. Although it appears that food and water are almost never sources of virus for HBV infections, HBsAg has been detected in clams from coastal waters into which untreated sewage has been drained.[471] Despite this finding, published outbreaks of shellfish-associated hepatitis have not been of type B.

Persistent viremia would appear to be a favorable condition for transmission by blood-feeding insects such as mosquitoes. Some populations of wild mosquitoes and bedbugs caught in Africa and the United States contain HBsAg.[472–475] Nevertheless, there has been no direct demonstration of transmission to humans by insect vectors. Unlike arboviruses, HBV probably will not infect insects, so passive transfer would be required.

In areas of the world where HBV infection rates are much higher than in the United States, there would appear to be less opportunity for virus transmission by overt parenteral routes. Other routes of transmission appear to be much more important. In this setting, transmission from infected mothers to newborn infants or young children appears to account for a very large percentage of HBV infections. Transmission to neonates from chronic carrier mothers and mothers with acute hepatitis B in the third trimester or first two months postpartum has been documented in the United States,[370, 371] as well as in highly endemic populations.[329, 420] In Taiwan it has been estimated that 40 to 50 per cent of HBsAg carriers acquired their infection in the perinatal period.[329] Only 5 to 10 per cent of these cases appear to have been infected in utero. The others appear to have been infected at the time of delivery by exposure to maternal blood.[476] Many infants not infected perinatally are infected in the first few months or years of life, probably by contact with their infected mothers or siblings, although the exact routes of transmission are not known. Clustering of carriers in families in which mothers are infected is consistent with this pattern of spread.[389, 477] The presence of HBsAg in maternal milk suggests that breast feeding might be an important route, although one study suggests that this may not be the case.[478] Mastication of food by mothers before feeding to infants is common in some cultures, and this might be expected to lead to infection of infants in those populations. Other kinds of intimate contact between mothers and children, as well as between siblings, are undoubtedly important.

The presence of significant concentrations of Dane particles or HBeAg, or both, in the blood correlates with the transmission of infection from carrier mothers to neonates,[329, 330, 371, 388] from carriers to normal health care personnel accidentally inoculated with contaminated needles,[345, 419] from carrier health care personnel to patient contacts,[421, 461–464] and among sexual partners in households.[331] The regular appearance of Dane particles in high concentrations and of HBeAg in the serum of patients during the late incubation period of acute hepatitis B suggests that this is a time when patients are probably highly contagious,[299, 300] as the few chronic HBsAg carriers with high Dane particle concentrations or HBeAg, or both, in their blood appear to be. The very frequent transmission of infection from mothers with acute hepatitis B during the third trimester of pregnancy or the first two months postpartum is consistent with this finding.[370, 371]

HEPATITIS DELTA VIRUS

HDV is among the most recently discovered and characterized human hepatitis viruses. It is a particularly interesting human virus. First, it appears to be a virus with a small circular RNA. It is defective and requires HBV or a similar hepadnavirus for its replication. Thus HDV has been found only in patients with simultaneous acute or chronic HBV infection. Second, HDV infections can become chronic in chronic HBsAg carriers. As in chronic HBV infections, HDV can persist in liver and blood for many months or years. Third, HDV appears frequently to inhibit or suppress replication of HBV. Fourth, it is a pathogenic agent. Patients with acute or chronic HDV infection appear to commonly (or possibly always) have active liver disease. The mechanisms for variation in the severity of liver disease associated with acute and chronic HBV infections are not well understood. The discovery of HDV and recognition of its pathogenic nature, and its apparent dependence on HBV, have raised the question of how often concomitant HDV and HBV infection accounts for severe acute or chronic hepatitis B. Most interest has focused on three syndromes: severe acute hepatitis B (and particularly fulminant hepatitis B), episodes of acute hepatitis in chronic HBV carriers, and severe chronic hepatitis B.

VIROLOGY

HDV is a transmissible RNA virus whose genome is unrelated to (i.e., does not share demonstrable nucleotide sequence homology with) those of HBV, HAV, or other viruses whose nucleotide sequences are known.[479–481] However, HDV does appear to be dependent on HBV for its replication, because it has not been found in patients without evidence of active HBV infection. Delta antigen was discovered by immunofluorescent staining in 1977 in Italy. It was found to be a nuclear antigen distinct from HBsAg, HBcAg, and HBeAg in hepatocytes of some HBV carriers. There is a high prevalence of HDV in Italy.[482] Hepatitis delta antigen (HDAg), purified from hepatic tissue, is a protein with a molecular weight of approximately 68,000 daltons. In serum it appears as an internal component of a discrete subpopulation of approximately 36-nm HBsAg particles or virions containing RNA.[483–485] The 36-nm virions were found in concentrations between 10^9 and 10^{10} particles/ml of serum. They had a buoyant density of 1.25 g/ml in CsCl density gradients and contained surface HBsAg polypeptides similar to those in HBV Dane particles (ie., 95 per cent P-24/GP-27, 5 per cent GP-33/GP-36, and 1 per cent P-39/GP-42) as well as two polypeptides of 27 and 29 kilodaltons (P-27 and P-29) that reacted specifically with anti-HDAg, suggesting that they may be coded by the HDV genome.[486] The RNA (approximately 1750 bases) is smaller than that of other known RNA viruses.[479–481] It is circular, single-stranded, and highly base-paired.[487, 488, 488a] This structure is reminiscent of the RNA of plant viroids,

which exist extracellularly without a protein coat. A cDNA clone of the RNA has been sequenced, and the presence of open reading frames suggests that the virion RNA is a plus strand (i.e., contains the sequence of messenger RNA).[480, 481, 489]

Inoculation of sera containing delta antigen into delta antigen–negative HBsAg-carrier chimpanzees results in the appearance of delta antigen in hepatocyte nuclei of these animals. HBsAg-bearing particles with internal delta antigen and RNA appear in the blood. HBcAg disappears from liver, the titer of HBsAg falls in serum, and serum alanine aminotransferase (ALT) levels rise.[490] These findings have led to the interesting concept that delta antigen is an antigen of an infectious RNA virus (HDV) that is defective in that its replication requires coinfection with HBV (a helper virus). Phenotypic mixing results in delta antigen and RNA-containing particles within HBsAg-containing virion envelopes. Infection with the delta agent results in hepatic injury and suppression of HBV replication. This apparent relationship of HDV and HBV is similar in many ways to that of other defective viruses, such as Bryan Rous sarcoma virus, which acquires its viral envelope antigen by phenotypic mixing with an avian leukosis (helper) virus.[491] HDV has recently been shown to infect woodchucks infected with WHV, which is closely related to HBV.[492] This indicates that hepadnaviruses other than HBV can function as helper viruses for HDV, and the host range of HDV (unlike that of HBV) extends beyond humans and chimpanzees to at least these rodents. Despite this, HDV has not yet been found to occur in nonhuman species under natural conditions, although apparently there is potential for this possibility.

The titer of infectious HDV can be very high and can exceed that of HBV in at least some human sera. In virus titration studies in chimpanzees, one specimen of human serum containing HBV and HDV no longer transmitted HBV to uninfected animals after a 10^{-7} dilution, but still transmitted HDV to an HBsAg-carrier animal when diluted 10^{-11}.[493] Infectious HDV (and HBV) can be present in blood without detectable HBsAg (by the most sensitive tests) as shown by post-transfusion hepatitis studies in which HBV and HDV coinfection was observed after transfusion with HBsAg-negative blood.[494]

HEPATITIS DELTA VIRUS INFECTION AND ASSOCIATED DISEASE

Infection with HDV can occur at the time of primary HBV infection (simultaneous primary infection), or primary HDV infection can occur any time during chronic HBV infection.

Simultaneous Primary Infection with Hepatitis B Virus and Hepatitis Delta Virus

Many simultaneous primary HBV-HDV infections are associated with little evidence of extensive HDV replication (HDAg detected only transiently in liver and not in serum).[490, 495, 496] In such cases there is usually minimal liver disease and HBsAg is often detected only transiently in serum. In these cases, HDV replication is thought to be limited by minimal HBV infection. The only serum marker of HDV infection in such cases may be an anti-HDAg IgM response (Fig. 35–9A).

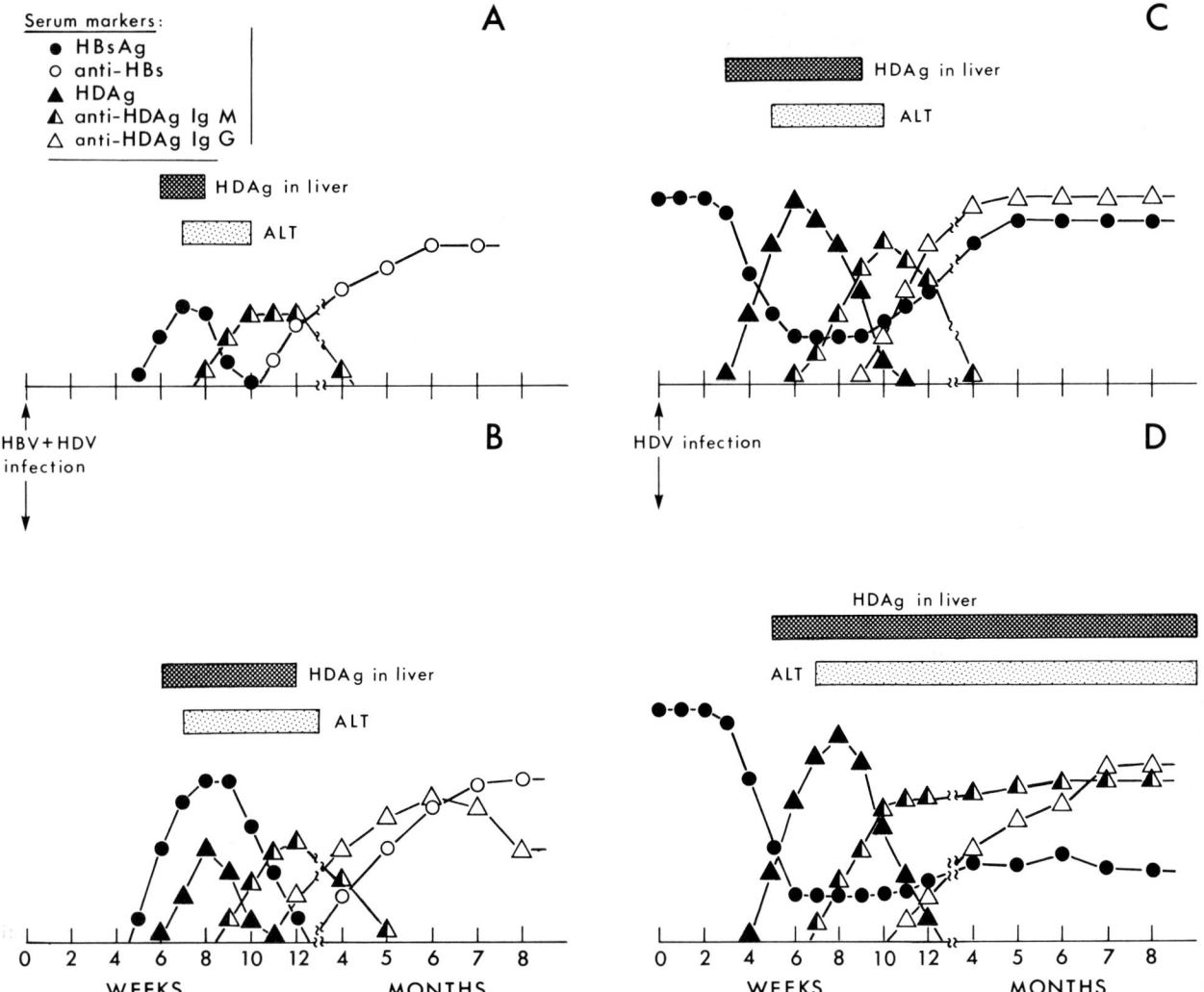

Figure 35–9. Typical patterns of serologic markers during hepatitis D virus (HDV) infection. Simultaneous primary infection with HDB and HBV is usually self-limited and resolves (i.e., does not become chronic), and HDAg may (*B*) or may not (*A*) be detected in serum. Following such HDV infections without detectable HD-antigenemia, an anti-HDAg IgG response may not be detected (*A*). HDV superinfection of HBsAg carriers may be self-limited and resolve (*C*) or become chronic (*D*) with persisting HDAg in liver and anti-HDAg IgM in serum. (Modified from Rizetto M, Verme G. J Hepatol 1:187, 1985.)

In some simultaneous primary HBV-HDV infections, HDV replication is more extensive, as evidenced by HDAg detected in the blood and in the liver for a more prolonged period (Fig. 35–9*B*). This is thought to be the consequence of more extensive HBV replication. Such patients often have severe or fulminant hepatitis.[495] In general, HD antigenemia appears to correlate with the degree of liver injury, and thus its presence suggests the potential for severe hepatitis.[495] In patients who survive simultaneous primary HBV-HDV infection, almost all have hepatitis that resolves and does not become chronic.[496] The acute hepatitis that results from simultaneous primary HDV-HBV infection cannot be distinguished on clinical grounds from primary infection with HBV alone, but such simultaneous infections have been observed on occasion to follow a biphasic course (possibly because of sequential expression of HBV and HDV.[489, 497, 498] Simultaneous infections are associated with a higher incidence of fulminant hepatitis than is observed in primary HBV infection alone.[498–501] There is no evidence that simultaneous primary infection with HDV and HBV affects the risk of becoming an HBV carrier. The incubation period or time from exposure to onset of acute hepatitis

following simultaneous HDV-HBV infection of chimpanzees has been between 4 and 20 weeks.

Primary Hepatitis Delta Virus Infection of Hepatitis B Virus Carriers

Primary HDV infections appear to occur more frequently as superinfections of chronic HBV carriers than as simultaneous primary HBV-HDV infection. Although HDV superinfections of HBV carriers can be asymptomatic, more often there is extensive HDV replication, which is thought to occur because HBV infection is already established. In general, more severe liver disease occurs in this setting than after simultaneous primary HBV-HDV infection. Symptomatic hepatitis (incubation period three to six weeks in chimpanzees) and on occasion fulminant hepatitis lead to chronic HDV infection, with significant chronic hepatitis in patients who survive the acute disease.[21, 22, 499, 500] HDV superinfection of chronic HBV carriers leads to HDAg in serum and liver and anti-HDAg IgM and IgG responses (Fig. 35–9*B* and *C*).[490, 495] HDV superinfection of

TABLE 35–6. HEPATITIS DELTA VIRUS AND HEPATITIS B VIRUS MARKERS DURING STAGES OF HEPATITIS DELTA VIRUS INFECTION

	HBsAg	Anti-HBc		Anti-HdAg		HDAg		HDV RNA	
		IgM	IgG	IgM	IgG	Serum	Liver	Serum	Liver
Acute HDV infection	+	±	+	±	±	±	+	+	+
Chronic HDV infection	+	±	+	+	+ (high titer)	−	+	+	+
Past HDV infection	±	±	+	−	±	−	−	−	−

asymptomatic HBV carriers can be confused with acute hepatitis B when the HBV carrier state is not previously suspected,[502] unless appropriate testing is done to demonstrate primary HDV infection (anti-HDAg IgM and IgG seroconversions) and to suggest that HBV infection is chronic (e.g., negative anti-HBc IgM and positive [high-titer] anti-HBc IgG in an HBsAg-positive patient suggests chronic HBV infection) (Table 35–6). HDV superinfection of an HBV carrier can be mistaken for a flare-up of chronic hepatitis B unless testing is done to demonstrate primary HDV infection. How often primary HDV infection accounts for apparent exacerbations of hepatitis in HBV carriers in the United States is not clear, since testing for HDV has not been widely used.

Hepatitis Delta Virus and Fulminant Hepatitis B

The exact proportion of acute fulminant hepatitis B cases that are associated with HDV infection (either HDV superinfection of HBsAg carriers or simultaneous primary HBV-HDV infection) and the proportion with primary HBV infection alone appears to depend on the geographic region and other factors that influence the prevalence of HDV infection in the patient population in question. In populations with a high prevalence of HDV, simultaneous infection with HDV has been reported to occur in a high percentage of cases of fulminant hepatitis B (e.g., 25 of 82 [30 per cent] cases reported in Italy and 14 of 34 [41 per cent] cases of intravenous drug users in Los Angeles).[500] Conversely, in geographic regions of low prevalence, such as certain populations in the United States and Ireland,[503, 504] HDV appears to be present in only a small percentage of fulminant hepatitis B cases, and thus it probably plays no role in most cases in these populations.

Chronic Hepatitis Delta Virus Infection

HDV infection of HBV carriers can be self-limited and can resolve (Fig. 35–9C). More often it becomes chronic and is accompanied by chronic hepatitis (Fig. 35–9D). Chronic HDV infections probably result almost exclusively from primary HDV infection of chronic HBV carriers, since simultaneous primary HBV-HDV infection has been found rarely if ever to lead to chronic HDV infection.[498, 502] The fact that chronic HDV infection is a common outcome of HDV superinfection of HBV carriers is also suggested by evidence that chronic hepatitis is at least fivefold more common than normal liver function in anti-HDAg–positive HBV carriers. For example, in a study in Italy, 20 of 24 HBsAg carriers developed CAH after superinfection with HDV.[499] More extensive studies using methods more critical than anti-HDAg testing alone are needed to document the frequency of chronic HDV infection in the United States.

In both self-limited HDV infection of HBsAg carriers and HDV infections that become persistent, HDAg has been detected by radioimmunoassay in serum during the late incubation period and early after the onset of disease,[490, 495, 505] but not in serum during chronic HDV infection.[495, 506] A recent study has detected HDAg in the serum of five patients with chronic HDV infection using the immunoblotting technique, which is a procedure that is not affected by the presence of anti-HDAg in the serum.[507] It was postulated that HDAg was not detected in serum of chronic HDV carriers in prior studies using radioimmunoassay because the antigen in such sera is in complex with anti-HDAg. If HDAg can be shown to be present regularly in serum during chronic HDV infections, and a clinically useful assay for its detection can be developed, it will provide a simple direct test for chronic HDV infection.[507] HDV RNA can be detected in serum by hybridization with a HDV cDNA probe. HDAg and HDV RNA can be detected in liver in almost all patients throughout chronic HDV infection.[480, 489] The only readily available serologic markers for distinguishing chronic or persisting HDV infection from past HDV infection that did not persist in chronic HBV carriers are anti-HDAg IgM and anti-HDAg IgG. Assays for these markers are commercially available. In some studies, anti-HDAg IgG has been detected in serum of patients with either chronic or past HDV infection, and in patients with chronic HDV infection the titer has been reported to be high.[507, 508] Anti-HDAg IgM appears to persist in serum throughout chronic HDV infection but does not persist in patients with past or resolved HDV infection (Fig. 35–9C and D).[495, 509, 510] Thus, a positive test result for anti-HDAg IgM in an HBV carrier, or anti-HDAg IgG in high titer, or both, is evidence for ongoing chronic HDV infection and the likelihood that infectious HDV is in the blood.[495] Chronic HDV infections appear to represent the most important reservoir of HDV. Infected humans are the only known source of HDV for transmission to other humans.

Hepatitis Delta Virus and Chronic Liver Disease

Many or all patients with chronic HDV infection appear to have active liver disease, and chronic HDV infection appears to be present in a high percentage of HBsAg carriers with chronic liver disease in some patient populations. For example, in a geographic area in Italy where HDV prevalence is high, 32 per cent of HBsAg carriers with CAH and 52 per cent with cirrhosis had intrahepatic HDAg (direct evidence of ongoing HDV infection). None of a group of HBsAg carriers without liver disease had detectable HDAg.[511] Other studies have shown similar correlations.[512] Another study in Italy found that almost all HBsAg-positive children with CAH or cirrhosis, or both, had coexisting chronic HDV infection, suggesting a greater importance for HDV than for other factors in the development of chronic liver disease in HBsAg-positive children in that country.[513] The prevalence of chronic HDV infection in HBsAg carriers with liver disease is lower in populations in the United States than in Italy, although some subpopulations in the United States have a high prevalence of HDV, for example, intravenous drug users. As in Italy, in the United States chronic HDV infection is common in HBV carriers with significant liver disease.[514] Many patients with chronic HDV infection and liver disease have symptoms,[512, 514, 515] but significant and serious liver disease with the potential for progression (CAH or cirrhosis, or both) can occur in asymptomatic carriers. In a large study in Italy of apparently healthy and asymptomatic prospective blood donors who tested HBsAg-positive, 38 per cent of those who tested positive for anti-HDAg but only 9 per cent of those without anti-HDAg had abnormal liver function test results. Liver biopsy of the asymptomatic HBsAg carriers with abnormal liver function revealed that 61 per cent of those who tested positive for anti-HDAg had CAH or cirrhosis, or both, and only 19 per cent of those without anti-HDAg had such abnormalities.[516] These results are consistent with previous liver biopsy studies showing that only 1 to 5 per cent of all asymptomatic, apparently healthy HBsAg carriers have CAH or cirrhosis, or both,[517-526] and this indicates that the presence of serum anti-HDAg greatly increases the risk of occult, serious liver disease.[516] It has been recommended that the presence of serum anti-HDAg in asymptomatic HBsAg carriers be an indication for liver biopsy.[516] The overall impact of HDV on chronic hepatitis B in the United States, which is a low-prevalence area for both HBV and HDV, remains to be determined when testing for HDV becomes more widely available. The mechanism of liver cell injury associated with HDV infection has not been studied. Two studies have failed to find evidence for an association of HDV infection and HCC in HBV carriers.[527, 528]

Hepatitis Delta Virus Infection Suppresses Hepatitis B Virus Replication

HDV infection of HBV carriers frequently appears to alter the course of HBV infection. HBcAg in livers of HBV carrier chimpanzees disappears, and HBsAg titers fall following HDV infection.[490] In some human carriers, HBeAg and Dane particles in the blood disappear, and occasionally even serum HBsAg has been observed to disappear following primary HDV superinfection of an HBV carrier.[529] There is also evidence that replication of HBV may be suppressed during chronic HDV infection. Several studies have demonstrated that most HBsAg carriers with evidence of chronic HDV infection test anti-HBe-positive and HBeAg and HBV DNA polymerase–negative,[512, 515] which is a serologic pattern consistent with little or no HBV replication. In a recent study,[530] very few patients with chronic HDV infection and chronic hepatitis had evidence of HBV replication. Only 2 of 13 HBsAg-positive patients with HDAg in liver biopsy specimens had detectable HBV DNA and HBcAg in liver, only 4 of 21 patients had weakly detectable HBV DNA in serum, and only 2 of 21 patients had serum HBeAg, which are all markers of HBV replication.[530] The evidence for limited or undetectable replication of HBV in most HBsAg carriers with chronic HDV infection suggests that HDV persists most often when it infects HBsAg carriers with little or no HBV replication, or that chronic HDV infection itself inhibits HBV replica-

tion, as occurs during primary HDV infection.[531] Patients with chronic hepatitis B and no evidence of HDV infection frequently have evidence of active HBV replication, for example, HBV DNA in serum and HBcAg in liver.[532] These differences suggest that markers for HBV replication may help determine which patients with chronic hepatitis B are coinfected with HDV. The mechanism of the effects of HDV on HBV replication is unknown.

EPIDEMIOLOGY OF HEPATITIS DELTA VIRUS

Serologic studies have shown a high prevalence of anti-delta among HBsAg carriers in southern Italy,[533, 534] other Mediterranean populations,[535] North Africa,[536] and the Middle East, which are all areas that are moderately endemic for HBV. In developing countries with high HBV endemism, anti-delta has been found in parts of West Africa, the South Pacific, and South America.[537, 538] In parts of the Amazon Basin, HDV infection is highly endemic and may have been present in these populations for many years. In highly endemic areas, transmission of HDV is thought to occur through intimate contacts and routes of transmission known for HBV in populations highly endemic for that virus. In some areas of the world that are highly endemic for HBV there is little evidence of HDV infection, including China, Taiwan, Japan, Burma, and other areas of Asia where testing has been done.[536, 538] Although the prevalence of anti-HDAg in HBsAg carriers is low in most of the western Pacific, there are isolated foci with very high prevalence, such as the islands of Hauru and Hiue and western Samoa.[538] In geographic regions with low endemism for HBV (i.e., HBsAg carrier rates are less than 1 per cent), such as the United States, northern Europe and Australia, anti-delta prevalence is between 1 and 10 per cent in HBsAg carriers.[517] In these regions, anti-HDAg is found mostly among parenteral drug users, hemophiliacs, and polytransfused patients who are HBV carriers.[517, 533] Thus the transmission of HDV in these populations must be predominantly by parenteral routes involving blood and blood products. HDV is found rarely among HBV carrier homosexual men in the United States, but this may be changing because sporadic cases of HDV infection are now occurring outside the high-risk groups in the United States. Delta antigen has not been found in HBsAg-negative patients. However, low titers of anti-delta have been observed occasionally in polytransfused HBsAg-negative patients. These patients have anti-HBs or other evidence of past HBV infection. Immune serum globulin prepared from plasma collected in the United States 40 years ago contains anti-HDAg, indicating that HDV has been in the population of the United States for at least that long.[539]

HDV may spread into populations with a low prevalence of HDV, and a high prevalence of HBV when introduced by infected individuals and transmitted by intimate contact or parenteral routes to HBV carriers.[540] For example, anti-HDAg was not present in Swedish drug addicts before 1973. Over the next decade, the prevalence of anti-HDAg increased from 0 to 75 per cent of HBsAg-carrier addicts.[541] HDV is similarly thought to have spread from southern to northern Italy through population migrations over several years.[542] HDV also appears to cause dramatic and explosive epidemics of severe acute, often fulminant, and chronic hepatitis, presumably when newly introduced into populations with a high prevalence of HBV but no HDV. In an epidemic in Yucpa Indians in Venezuela (a small population with a high prevalence of HBV carriers), there were 149 cases of hepatitis over three years with 34 deaths. More than 22 patients developed chronic hepatitis.[501] Eighty-six per cent of HBsAg-positive patients had anti-HDAg, and HDAg was detected in liver at autopsy in seven of nine cases. Most cases appeared to represent HDV superinfection of HBV carriers among children and young adults. The most likely route of transmission in children was considered to be close contact with individuals having open skin breaks (almost all children in that population had one of several skin diseases) and living in poverty under crowded conditions. Acupuncture and sexual contacts were considered possible factors in transmission among adults. Severe hepatitis, termed *Labrea fever* in the Amazon valley in Brazil and *hepatitis of Sierra Nevada de Santa Marta* in small villages in northern Colombia,[543, 544] which is thought to have been recurrent in those populations over many decades, has been associated recently with HDV infection. In Worcester, Massachusetts, more than 200 drug addicts have been involved in an outbreak of HDV since 1983; nine deaths have occurred.[545]

There is a risk of HDV infection from therapeutic use of blood and blood products. The prevalence of anti-HDAg in prospective United States blood donors with serum HBsAg is reported to be 3 to 12 per cent.[546] Thus the risk of transfusion-acquired HBV plus HDV, compared with HBV alone, is probably less than 1 to 30. Although most blood containing HBV is eliminated by screening donors for HBsAg, HBV transmission still occurs from infrequent HBsAg-negative donor blood (in significantly less than 1 to 100 recipients of HBsAg-negative blood).[547] Thus the risk of HDV transmission is undoubtedly less than 1 in 3000 transfusions, a small but not negligible risk. The risk may vary with the donor population. The same demographic factors that increase the likelihood of HBV and NANB hepatitis viruses in commercial donors can be expected to increase the risk of HDV, strengthening the need for a shift from paid to volunteer blood donors.

Although the risk of HDV infection from a single blood transfusion is very low, the risk from repeated use of some blood products (e.g., factor VIII) prepared from large plasma pools is very high. In some studies,[494, 548] 27 to 100 per cent of HBsAg-positive hemophilia patients in Europe and the United States were found to have serum anti-HDAg in high titers, suggesting chronic HDV infection at a very high frequency. Although there are no reports of HDV transmission from immune serum globulin, anti-HDAg was found in 75 per cent or more of immune serum globulin lots prepared before 1970 (and as early as 1944), in 45 per cent of those prepared in 1971 and 1972, and in none prepared since 1973.[539] Anti-HDAg was found in 38 per cent of immune serum globulin lots prepared in the United States in 1981 and 1982.[549] The apparent decline with time in the prevalence of anti-HDAg in lots of immune serum globulin undoubtedly represents the impact of screening of blood donors for HBsAg, which was introduced in the 1970s. Screening for HBsAg can be expected to eliminate almost all HDV-containing plasma. Although immune serum globulin has a good record of safety, HBsAg has been found in some lots (at least in lots prepared before HBsAg screening),[550] and transmission of both HBV and NANB hepatitis by immune serum globulin has been reported,[551–553] suggesting the potential for HDV transmission. The evidence that infectious titers of HDV may exceed the titer of infectious HBV in some sera and that HDV infection has been transmitted by HBsAg-negative blood suggests that infectious HDV could be present in immune serum globulin without detectable HBsAg and even without in-

fectious HBV.[493, 494] Conversely, the presence of anti-HDAg in immune serum globulin does not indicate certain infectivity for HDV.

DIAGNOSIS OF HEPATITIS DELTA VIRUS INFECTION

The diagnosis of acute or chronic HDV infection cannot be made on clinical grounds alone, because the associated clinical syndromes are not distinctive enough. Severe or fulminant hepatitis B, acute hepatitis B with a biphasic course, CAH B (especially without evidence of HBV replication), episodes of acute hepatitis in HBsAg carriers in which hepatitis A has been excluded, and hepatitis B in individuals in groups at high risk for HDV are some clinical and demographic features suggesting the possibility of HDV coinfection. Specific testing for HDV is indicated in such cases. Figure 35–9 demonstrates schematically the evolution of serologic and other HDV and HBV markers during acute and chronic HDV infection. These changes were discussed earlier in Infection and Disease. Table 35–6 lists the test results considered most common or typical in different stages of HDV infection. The only commercially available tests for HDV markers at this time are the ELISA for anti-HDAg IgG and anti-HDAg IgM. Diagnosis of acute or primary HDV infection in an HBsAg-positive patient with clinical or laboratory evidence of acute hepatitis, or both, can be made by demonstrating an anti-HDAg IgM or antiHDAg IgG seroconversion, or both.[490, 495, 510] Anti-HDAg IgG may appear late during the acute illness or may even remain undetectable in acute self-limited cases.[554] Tests for this antibody hence have limited usefulness for diagnosis of acute HDV infection. Some workers have claimed that anti-HDAg IgM is the best marker for acute infection with HDV and that it may be the only marker, in patients with transient, mild, and limited HBV infection.[510] Others find, however, that anti-HDAg IgM is present infrequently in acute infection and is never the only marker.[505] Instead the latter study found the most sensitive test of primary HDV infection to be serum HDAg by ELISA in the first two weeks of illness.[505] Whether these discrepancies represent differences in test performance, different patient popultions, or other differences remains to be seen. Clearly, detection of HDAg or HDV RNA, or both, in serum and liver gives the most direct evidence of active HDV infection and may be the most sensitive indicator of primary infection. However, tests for these markers are not available commercially and can be done at this time only in a few research laboratories. Primary HDV infection can accompany primary HBV infection or can occur as superinfection of chronic HBV carriers. The presence or lack of anti-HBc IgM in HBsAg-positive patients has been used commonly to distinguish, respectively, primary or acute HBV infection from chronic HBV carriers in many studies of HDV infection.[494, 498, 500, 508]

Distinguishing chronic HDV infection from resolved or past HDV infection in an HBsAg carrier using only anti-HDAg IgG and IgM testing is not definitive in many cases. The persistence of anti-HDAg IgM or very high titers of anti-HDAg IgG, or both,[495, 507–510] is suggestive of persisting HDV infection, but exactly how often either marker is present without persisting HDV infection or is not present when virus continues to replicate in liver is not clear for all populations. More work is needed to establish the diagnostic power of these markers. Again more direct and probably more sensitive evidence for ongoing chronic HDV infection is provided by detection of HDV RNA alone or in combination with HDAg in serum,[480, 489, 507] and HDAg or HDV RNA in liver.[480, 490, 506, 508, 511, 512]

CONTROL OF HEPATITIS DELTA VIRUS INFECTIONS

Prevention of HBV infection by vaccination or other measures will prevent HDV infections, since HDV appears to depend upon HBV for its replication. Perinatal, sexual, or percutaneous exposure of HBV-susceptible individuals to sera or other body fluids of patients known to carry HDV should be treated as for any other exposure to HBV.[496] HBV carriers are also at risk for HDV infection, particularly if they are in one of the high-risk groups for HBV infection, for example, parenteral drug users, homosexuals, and so on. In such cases, there are no specific measures that can prevent HDV infection other than avoiding exposure to the virus. As described in Epidemiology, there is a small risk of HDV transmission by blood transfusion. Use of volunteer blood donors in preference to paid donors should reduce the risk of HDV as it does transmission of HBV and NANB hepatitis virus. The potential for HDV infection and serious disease would seem to be greatest for transfusion of HBsAg carriers. It has been suggested that HBsAg carriers receive only HBsAg-negative (by third-generation testing) and anti-HDAg–negative blood, with normal transaminase levels, from volunteer donors.[494]

The risk of transmission of HDV by some blood products prepared from pooled plasma (e.g., factor VIII) is much greater than from single-unit blood transfusion, and pooled plasma products should be used (particularly in HBsAg carriers) only for strong clinical indications. No cases of HDV transmission by immune serum globulin have been documented, but the potential for this (as described in Epidemiology) exists. Immune serum globulin should not be given to HBsAg carriers without a firm indication because of the potential that small amounts of HDV could produce significant disease in these patients. Without ongoing HBV infection, HDV would only infect individuals that were simultaneously and newly infected with HBV. In such cases there would be much less potential for serious disease. Exclusion of not only HBsAg-positive but also anti-HDAg–positive plasma, plasma with elevated aminotransferase levels, and use of plasma from populations with a low risk for hepatitis are measures that would provide blood products made from pooled plasma with a lower chance of contamination with HDV or other known hepatitis viruses.

HEPATITIS A VIRUS

The transmission of HAV to experimental animals (first to marmosets in 1969 and then to chimpanzees in 1975),[30, 31, 555, 556] the identification of viral antigen in feces in 1973,[32] and the propagation of HAV in tissue culture more recently, in 1979,[557] have permitted progress in the characterization of the virion and its replication, and in the investigation of the course of infection and the epidemiology of HAV.

THE INFECTIOUS VIRUS AND HOST RANGE

The host range of HAV is restricted to humans, chimpanzees, and several species of South American *San-*

quinus marmoset (Tamaran) monkeys. Humans appear to be the only host in nature. Experimental infection of *S. fuscicollis*, *S. nigricollis* (white-lipped marmoset), and *S. oedipus* (cotton-topped marmoset) was first shown clearly by Deinhardt and co-workers in studies using control and virus-containing specimens under code.[30, 31] Lorenze and associates, Mascoli and co-workers, and Provost and colleagues confirmed infection of marmosets using the highly susceptible *S. mystax* (white-mustached marmoset).[558–560] Provost and colleagues and Holmes and co-workers showed that human convalescent serum would neutralize the infectivity for marmosets. *S. labiatus*, also known as *Jacchus rufiventer* or *Markina labiata*, and *S. mystax* are the species most susceptible to HAV infection. *S. nigricollis* and *S. fuscicollis* are intermediate, and *S. oedipus* is among the most resistant species.[560, 561] Serial passage in rubiventer marmosets results in adaptation of the virus so that 100 per cent of the animals can be infected with an incubation period of only seven days.[562] Marmoset infection results in disease with histologic and biochemical changes similar to those in humans.

A hepatitis A–like illness in animal caretakers after close exposure to chimpanzees was first described in 1961.[563, 564] Later it was documented serologically to be due to hepatitis A.[565] Following the development of assays for hepatitis A antigen (HAAg) and antibody to HAAg (anti-HA), experimental transmission of HAV to chimpanzees by oral and parenteral routes was demonstrated by Maynard and co-workers and Deinstag and co-workers.[555, 556] The hepatitis following HAV infection of chimpanzees is extremely mild. Attempts to infect other primates as well as lower animal species have not been clearly successful to date.[566]

Propagation of HAV in tissue culture was first reported in 1979.[557] Virus passed 31 times through marmosets was used to infect fetal rhesus monkey kidney cells. Since then, several investigators have infected different cell types, including human hepatoma cell lines and primary African green monkey cells,[567–569] with HAV directly from feces of naturally infected humans. HAV appears to be mostly cell-associated and produces little or no cytopathic effect in cell culture.[557, 568] In some studies,[567, 569] a long (e.g., four week) eclipse period between inoculation of the culture and appearance of viral antigen in the cells has been observed,[570, 571] whereas in other studies, HAAg has appeared more rapidly (e.g., four days).

The agent causing infectious hepatitis in human volunteers was shown to pass through a Seitz filter, which retains bacteria,[19, 24] indicating that the agent is smaller than bacteria. No more precise sizing of the infectious agent of hepatitis A has been reported.

Little information is available on the stability of HAV to chemical and physical agents. HAV infectivity for human volunteers was destroyed by 100° C for 20 minutes or 1 minute and 160° C dry heat for 60 minutes,[572–574] but survived 60° C heat for 1 hour.[560] Infectivity of HAV in water was destroyed by chlorination, and the concentration required depended on the organic content of the water.[575] HAV has been inactivated by ultraviolet irradiation and 1:4000 formalin but not by ether or acid (pH 3 for three hours).[560] The virus is also quite stable during storage at 4° C and −20° C.

HEPATITIS A ANTIGEN FORMS IN FECES AND LIVER

Feinstone and colleagues first described virus-like particles in the feces of patients experimentally infected with

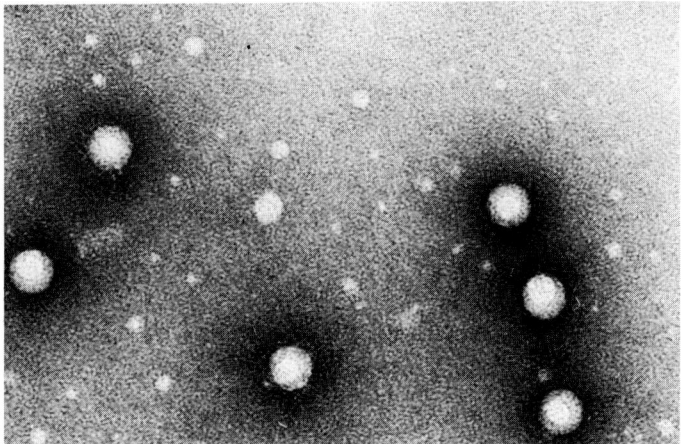

Figure 35–10. Electron micrograph of HAAg particles purified from feces of an HAV-infected patient. (Experiment by Dr. John Gerin.)

HAV.[32] The particles were immunoprecipitated by serum from patients in the convalescent phase of infection, but not those in the acute phase. The particles thus were considered to be HAV antigen forms. Similar particles were observed during natural infections. Their presence in feces was temporally associated with the illness. The particles were uniform in size and appearance, being spherical structures 27 nm in diameter (Fig. 35–10). Both full and empty particles were observed. Similar particles were observed in liver extracts, bile, and serum of HAV-infected *S. mystax*.[576] The major component of HAAg particles purified from infected human and chimpanzee feces and from marmoset liver had a buoyant density in CsCl of approximately 1.34 g/ml.[576–580] Empty particles appeared at density 1.29 to 1.30 g/ml.[578, 580–582] Another less well defined component of HAAg was found in the density range of 1.38 to 1.44 g/ml in variable amounts in different preparations.[577, 582] The sedimentation coefficient of full particles was 160 S.[578] The size and appearance in electron micrographs and the buoyant density and sedimentation coefficient are nearly identical with those for poliovirus. There is no clearly documented antigenic variation in HAAg from patients in different geographic areas of the world. Protection of individuals by passive immunization with immune serum globulin collected in other areas of the world supports the concept that HAV is antigenically similar in different parts of the world.[583, 584]

Chemical characterization of HAAg particles has been limited by the relatively small amount of material available from any source. Analysis of the polypeptides of 27-nm HAAg particles purified from the feces of HAV-infected patients reveals four polypeptides with approximate molecular weights of 32,000, 26,000, 22,000, and 10,000 daltons.[585–588] These polypeptides are near the size of polypeptides VP1, VP2, VP3, and VP4 of poliovirus.[589] A 59,000- or 66,000-dalton polypeptide has also been observed in some studies.[586, 587] This is somewhat larger than polio VP0, which is an uncleaved precursor of VP2 and VP4 in immature polio virions.[590]

Virus-like HAAg particles purified from feces of HAV-infected patients contain single-stranded RNA molecules that contain a polyA sequence.[587, 591, 592] This suggests that HAV is a positive-stranded virus (i.e., virions contain the messenger RNA strand) with RNA similar to that of poliovirus.

c-DNA made from RNA extracted from HAAg particles from feces or marmoset liver and infected monkey kidney cells in culture has been cloned and sequenced, and the results are consistent with a genome organization and size similar to that of other picornaviruses.[593–595]

HAAg has been detected by direct immunofluorescence in liver tissue of experimentally infected chimpanzees and marmosets.[596, 597] Specific staining was in a finely granular pattern in the cytoplasm and not in the nucleus of hepatocytes distributed diffusely throughout the liver. Localization of HAAg by immunofluorescence in hepatocyte cytoplasm is consistent with the finding of 27-nm particles that are indistinguishable by electron microscopy from those in feces in vesicles within hepatocyte cytoplasm of experimentally infected chimpanzees.[580] The cytoplasmic location of HAAg is consistent with the cellular site of synthesis of other small RNA viruses, such as polio.[598–600]

Tissue sites at which HAV replicates have been investigated by immunofluorescent staining with anti-HAAg using tissues of chimpanzees and marmosets after parenteral and oral infection.[592, 596, 597, 601] HAAg is synthesized in hepatocytes of all infected animals. There is no evidence that viral antigen is synthesized in other tissues. It seems likely, however, that some cells in the gastrointestinal tract are susceptible to HAV infection, since infections in humans occur so readily by the oral route. HAV is similar in many important ways to poliovirus, suggesting that it should be classified as an enterovirus along with poliovirus, coxsackievirus, and echovirus. The viruses have similar sizes, ultrastructures, and polypeptide compositions, as well as RNA size, structure, and polyA content. HAV, like enteroviruses, is resistant to acid, replicates in the cell cytoplasm, is transmitted almost exclusively by the fecal-oral route, and causes epidemic disease.

THE COURSE OF HEPATITIS A VIRUS INFECTION

HAV infection can be associated with anicteric or icteric hepatitis, and in general the illness in children is milder and has a shorter course than it does in adults. Estimates of the ratio of anicteric to icteric cases in several studies have ranged from 12:1 in experimentally infected young children,[686] 9:1 in young adults and children in Alaska,[602] 2:1 in Holy Cross College football players and patients aged 13 to 31 years in a New England mental institution,[687, 688] 1.1:1 in institutionalized handicapped children in Los Angeles,[689] 1:1.7 in a community outbreak,[690] 1:2 in an institution for the mentally retarded in Virginia,[691] to 1:3.5 in U.S. Navy recruits.[608] Age appears to influence the severity of hepatitis A in that young children appear to have a higher proportion of anicteric, mild disease than adults. The infecting dose of virus and other factors may also be important.

The incubation period after experimental infection was between 14 and 49 days in human volunteer studies in the 1940s.[692, 693] The incubation period in epidemic, serologically verified hepatitis A resulting from common-vehicle exposure during brief defined periods is between 20 and 45 days, with a mean around 28 days in several studies.[657, 674, 676, 681, 694]

Relapse seven to ten weeks after rapid recovery from the initial disease appears to be an unusual, but well-documented course for hepatitis A.[631a, 696] No documented HAV infections have been reported to be followed by chronic hepatitis, and no evidence of HAV infection has been found in cases of CAH.[697] Most infections are associated with acute, self-limited icteric or anicteric illness. Infrequent cases are associated with hepatic encephalopathy or fulminant hepatitis.[697-699]

Serologic markers of HAV infection can be detected well before the onset of symptoms or evidence of liver disease (Fig. 35–11). The first evidence of viral infection in chimpanzees is the appearance of HAAg detected by immunofluorescent antibody staining in liver one or two weeks after infection (Fig. 35–11).[596] At the same time, 27-nm virus-like particles are detected by electron microscopy in vesicles within hepatocyte cytoplasm.[580] Antigen has been observed in marmoset liver as early as one week after infection.[562] Within a few days, HAAg can be detected in feces and bile by immune electron microscopy and radioimmunoassay in these animals.[580, 596, 700] HAAg has been detected in feces several days before and usually reaches a maximum concentration about the time of the first aspartate aminotransferase (AST) elevation in experimentally infected human subjects.[625, 628, 629] Fecal HAAg detected by radioimmunoassay, which appears to be more sensitive than immune electron microscopy, was found up to 7 days after the onset of bilirubinuria in 67 per cent of patients and 8

to 16 days after in 33 per cent of patients in one study,[631] and was found 5 to 10 days after onset of jaundice in another study.[626, 627] The period over which HAAg is detectable in feces is similar to the period of fecal infectivity described in Epidemiology. Bile may be the source of fecal HAAg, since antigen has not been detected in bowel mucosa after infection of chimpanzees by parenteral or oral routes.[596, 597, 601] There appears to be a rough correlation between the severity of hepatitis A and the concentration of fecal HAAg. Many patients with anicteric hepatitis A apparently have no HAAg detectable by serologic assays.[608, 626] Antigen has been detected in the blood before the onset of disease,[597] but the time of its appearance and duration in the blood are not well defined.

HAAg usually can be detected by staining with immunofluorescent antibody for a longer period than by radioimmunoassay in blood or feces. HAAg has been detected in chimpanzee liver for a period of four to five weeks. Low levels regularly persist after alanine aminotransferase (ALT) levels have returned to normal.[596] Titers of anti-HAAg detected by immune adherence hemagglutination (IAHA), following acute hepatitis A, rise to a maximum in about 10 to 16 weeks.[701, 702] Antibody can be detected earlier in the course of infection by more sensitive tests. Anti-HAAg was found by radioimmunoassay at the time of onset of jaundice and by immune electron microscopy before the peak AST levels.[702]

The immunoglobulin class containing most of the anti-HA in acute-phase sera (between onset of symptoms and peak of icterus) is IgM, and in convalescent sera it is IgG.[703] Anti-HAAg can be detected for many years following most infections.

IMMUNE RESPONSE, IMMUNITY, AND DISEASE PATHOGENESIS

The presence of anti-HAAg in serum indicates immunity and resistance to reinfection. Recently anti-HAAg IgA

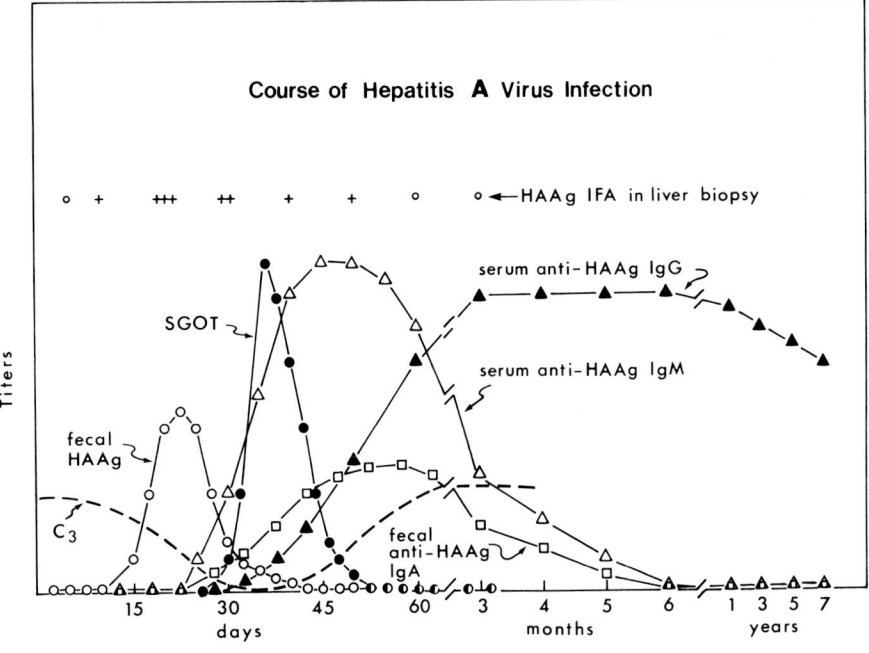

Figure 35–11. Schematic representation of viral markers in the blood, liver, and feces throughout the course of primary HAV infection.

was found in feces of patients with acute hepatitis A (Fig. 35–11). It disappeared within several months.[704] This suggests that intestinal epithelium may be infected by HAV at some time during the course of infection although, as described earlier, there is no direct evidence for HAAg synthesis in the bowel of chimpanzees or marmosets after parenteral or oral infection. The importance of local antibody in resistance or reinfection has not been proved, but it may be important by analogy with immunity against other viruses that infect by the enteric route. Thus an oral vaccine that stimulates local immunity might be effective, as it is with viruses such as polio. HAV infection appears to result in solid immunity. Reinfections, if they occur, must be rare. Experimental transmission to human volunteers of clinical hepatitis or serologically documented HAV and subsequent rechallenge has shown resistance to reinfection by the same virus,[19, 705, 706] but no resistance to serum hepatitis virus or serologically documented HBV was found.[19, 705, 706] Studies of multiple episodes of apparent viral hepatitis by natural routes of transmission have not found individuals with more than a single episode of HAV infection, although HAV infection can follow HBV and vice versa.[707–709] These studies indicate that homologous immunity develops on first infection with HAV.

The histopathologic changes in liver during acute hepatitis A are indistinguishable from those described for hepatitis B, and the mechanisms of hepatic injury are unknown. Because limited amounts of HAAg are available, investigation of the specific cellular immune response during HAV infection and its role in hepatic injury are not well studied.[608]

Although transient arthralgias, and occasionally arthritis and rash, occur during the incubation period of hepatitis A,[608] they are apparently less frequent than in hepatitis B. The pathogenesis of the joint and skin involvement associated with HAV infection has not been studied as extensively as with HBV. However, HAAg and anti-HAAg have been detected in the same serum;[597] anticomplementary activity occurs during the incubation period of hepatitis A,[710] and low C3 levels are found during acute hepatitis A.[711] All are consistent with immune complex formation, but the importance of these changes for HAV-associated disease has not been proved.

VIRAL DIAGNOSIS

Several methods have been used for making a specific diagnosis of HAV infection. Two specific serologic assays are readily available for clinical use, since there are commercial versions of each.

The most useful approach for making a serologic diagnosis of acute hepatitis A is testing for anti-HAAg IgM in serum.[703, 712–715] With an optimally designed test, virtually all patients are anti-HAAg IgM–positive by the time of onset of symptoms and test negative by three to six months after onset of symptoms (Fig. 35–11).[716] A sensitive and specific radioimmunoassay is produced commercially, making this test generally available for clinical use. It should permit an accurate diagnosis to be made in 90 to 100 per cent of cases of hepatitis A in a clinical setting. Because of its relatively short half-life after HAV infection, anti-HAAg IgM is much less likely to be acquired passively (e.g., by blood transfusion) than is anti-HAAg IgG.

A specific diagnosis can sometimes be made by demonstrating a significant total anti-HAAg (IgM + IgG) response. Anti-HAAg titers have been determined by complement fixation (CF),[701, 710] IAHA,[577, 701, 717] immune electron microscopy,[32] and radioimmunoassay.[718, 720] The latter two methods appear to be more sensitive than the former. A highly sensitive and specific radioimmunoassay for total anti-HAAg is available commercially. A fourfold or greater rise in titer between sera collected during the acute illness and that collected two or three weeks later suggests acute infection (Fig. 35–11). An exception would be a rise caused by passive acquisition of anti-HA (e.g., by blood transfusion or immune serum globulin administration). In clinical settings, however, a specific diagnosis probably can be made only about half the time with this approach because many patients already have detectable anti-HAAg at the time the first sample of serum is obtained, and a fourfold rise in titer cannot be shown. In addition, a diagnosis cannot be made during the acute illness, since testing of convalescent serum is required. Several features of the response can be used to attempt to distinguish active infection from passive acquisition of anti-HAAg. The antibody titers following HAV infection are usually much higher than expected by passive transfer,[596] the presence of anti-HAAg as IgM would suggest recent infection,[703] and the titer of passively acquired anti-HAAg can be expected to have fallen below the level of detection before six months, unlike the anti-HAAg resulting from active infection, which would last longer.

At this time, tests for total anti-HAAg are most useful to determine the immune status of individuals as evidence of past infection and thus resistance to reinfection. Knowledge of the anti-HAAg status of individual patients is useful in determining the need for passive immunization before or after exposure.

Other diagnostic approaches are currently available in only a few research laboratories. One method tests fecal specimens for HAAg by immune electron microscopy,[32, 608, 625, 628–630] ELISA,[721] or radioimmunoassay.[721, 722] However, as described previously, fecal HAAg reaches a maximum concentration about the time the AST determination first becomes abnormal (Fig. 35–11).[625, 628, 630] HAAg can be detected infrequently after this time. In one study, HAAg particles were found by immune electron microscopy in fecal specimens of only 17 of 44 patients during the first week of hospitalization with icteric hepatitis A. No specimens tested positive more than two days after the peak of jaundice.[608] No positive results were found in 13 anicteric cases. Testing of feces by radioimmunoassay and ELISA appears to be technically simpler than using immune electron microscopy.[608, 721] However, examination of feces, even early in the course of the acute icteric hepatitis A, does not ensure finding HAAg particles. A negative result late in the illness (e.g., after AST levels peak) in icteric cases, or at any time after the onset of symptoms in anicteric cases, has little diagnostic significance. In a clinical setting, probably little more than a fourth of hepatitis A cases can be identified by examining feces for HAAg.

Immunofluorescent staining of liver biopsy specimens from HAV-infected chimpanzees indicates that HAAg can be detected in liver for around two weeks after the ALT level peaks (Fig. 35–11).[596] If the same were true in humans, a specific diagnosis might be made by liver biopsy later in the course of the illness than is possible by testing for fecal HAAg. The opportunity to make a diagnosis in this way does not arise frequently, however, since liver biopsy usually is not indicated clinically during acute viral hepatitis.

Recently, testing for fecal anti-HAAg IgA has been used to diagnose acute hepatitis A.[704] Since these antibodies appear to become undetectable within a few months of the acute illness (Fig. 35–11), their presence during acute hepatitis suggests recent HAV infection. These findings must be repeated and extended before their usefulness for clinical diagnosis will be certain.

EPIDEMIOLOGY

The epidemiology of HAV differs from that of HBV because of several significant differences in the biologic behavior of the two viruses. Persistent infection with continuous viremia does not occur with HAV as it does with HBV. Hence, transmission via parenteral routes almost never occurs with HAV. No form of persistent infection has been documented for HAV and no animal or other reservoir is known, so this virus must be maintained in a population by serial transmission from patients with acute disease to susceptible individuals. In isolated populations of limited size, HAV disappears after epidemics that follow its introduction from outside. The virus can reappear years later, again when brought in from outside.[601–604] This behavior in small isolated populations is similar to that of measles, mumps, rubella, and poliomyelitis viruses,[605] which do not commonly cause persistent infection in humans and for which no reservoir outside of humans is known.

The Incidence of Infection

The number of cases of hepatitis A in the United States is not known precisely because hepatitis A is not a reportable disease, and not all cases of viral hepatitis are evaluated by specific HAV serologic properties. Approximately 60,000 cases of acute viral hepatitis are identified each year by the Centers for Disease Control, and approximately one half are considered to be hepatitis A.[606] The actual number of HAV infections in the United States is probably severalfold higher, since most primary infections are subclinical, and clinically apparent infections are under-reported. Thirty to 50 per cent of the adult population of the United States has serologic evidence of past HAV infection; only 3 to 5 per cent recall an illness suggesting or documented to be viral hepatitis.[607] The ratio of anicteric to icteric cases has been reported to be as high as 12:1 and as low as 1:3 in different outbreaks and experimental transmission studies.[608] The highest incidence of reported cases of hepatitis A is in adolescents and young adults.[606] Males and females appear to be equally susceptible,[606, 607] and the highest incidence in the United States in past years has occurred during autumn and winter.

The prevalence of antibody to HAAg (anti-HAAg) as evidence of past infection varies among different populations in the United States and has been used to estimate the contribution of HAV to adult hepatitis cases in several urban populations. For example, of all hepatitis cases presenting to one Los Angeles Hospital, 50 to 60 per cent were associated with HBV, 20 per cent were associated with HAV, and 20 to 30 per cent were neither type A nor type B hepatitis.[609] The prevalence of anti-HAAg is higher in populations of low socioeconomic status than in those of upper socioeconomic status.[610] HAV infection rates are high in circumstances of poor sanitation or crowded living conditions, or both, such as in schools, military facilities, prisons, and so on.[607] High-risk groups in the United States include homosexual men and children and staff in day care centers,[611–613] groups in which close physical contact appears to promote spread of enterically transmitted infections.

Secondary attack rates are high in members of households (particularly children) with an index case. The risk of hepatitis A in day care centers is greatest when large numbers of diapered children under the age of 2 years are cared for. Infection in the children is usually asymptomatic, and spread from infected children to household contacts provides the majority of recognized cases.[613]

Seroepidemiologic studies reveal striking differences in incidence of anti-HAAg in the populations of different areas of the world.[607, 614] In general, the highest rates of HAV infection are in economically developing countries, in which housing and sanitation are poor. In such areas, antibody appears at very early ages, and most infections at these ages appears to be subclinical and anicteric.[614] In a representative study, by adulthood more than 90 per cent of the population in a developing country was found to have antibody, compared with around 20 per cent in the United States.[615] In the population of some countries, such as the United States and Switzerland, serologic evidence of past infection with both HAV and HBV is relatively low. In others, such as Senegal and Taiwan, the incidence of both is relatively high, and in countries such as Belgium, Israel, and Yugoslavia, HAV infection rates appear to be relatively high and HBV infection appears to be relatively low.[607] Thus, although HAV infection is worldwide, it is not evenly distributed. In addition, the relative differences in infection rates for HAV and HBV in different populations support the conclusion that the factors enhancing infection are not the same for both viruses.

Routes of Hepatitis A Virus Transmission

Fecal Shedding of Virus Contact Transmission

The most common manner of HAV transmission is through close person to person contact, probably by the fecal-oral route. Table 35–7 summarizes the results of several studies, which show that infectious HAV has been detected in feces from two to three weeks before to eight days after the onset of jaundice. No infectivity has been found 4 weeks or more before, or 19 days or more after the onset of jaundice. These results probably define the time of virus shedding for most infected patients, although the number of cases in which infectivity has been studied is relatively small and some patients undoubtedly fall outside these limits.

No case of chronic HAV shedding (beyond 90 days) has been documented either after experimental infection of human subjects or in more recent studies of HAAg excretion during experimental and natural infections. Epidemiologic evidence also suggests that persistent HAV excretion must occur infrequently if at all. The disappearance of hepatitis A in small isolated populations after an epidemic is consistent with the view that persistent HAV shedding does not occur at a high enough frequency to maintain HAV in these populations.[602–604, 640–643] Nevertheless, although chronic fecal shedding of HAV has not been documented, many more cases of infection must be studied by methods that specifically identify HAV to finally establish whether or not persistent infection ever occurs.

Involvement of Nonfecal Sources of Hepatitis A Virus Contact Transmission

There is little evidence for important sources of virus other than feces to account for contact transmission. Infectivity for human volunteers was reported with nasophar-

TABLE 35–7. DETECTION OF INFECTIOUS HEPATITIS A VIRUS IN FECES OF INFECTED PATIENTS

Number of Infected Fecal Donors	Time of Fecal Collection			Tests for Infectivity			
	Days after Experimental Infection	Days after Onset of Symptoms	Days before (−) or after (+) Onset of Jaundice	Test System	No. Infected No. Inoculated	Outcome	Reference
1*	7		−34	Marmoset	0/6	−	Deinhardt et al.[655]
3†	11		−28 to −35 days pooled	Human	0/8	−	Krugman et al.[656]
3†	25		−14 to −21 days pooled	Human	4/11	+	Krugman et al.[656]
1*	33		−8	Marmoset	2/6	+	Deinhardt et al.[655]
1*	38		−3	Marmoset	66	+	Deinhardt et al.[655]
			1	Human			Havens et al.[546]
			3	Human		+	Havens et al.[546]
7		3–10 days pooled		Chimpanzee		+	Maynard et al.[657]
1*	47		6	Marmoset	4/5	+	Deinhardt et al.[655]
3†			1–8 days pooled	Human	16/37	+	Krugman et al.[656]
			8	Human		+	Havens et al.[546]
1			19	Human		−	Havens[583]
			20	Human		−	Havens[583]
5		29–26 days pooled		Human		−	Havens[583]
3			19–33 days pooled	Human		−	Krugman et al.[506]
1			32	Human		−	Krugman et al.[506]
1			33	Human		−	Neefe et al.[658]
1			43	Human		−	Neefe et al.[658]

*Samples from the same patient
†Samples from the same three patients.

angeal washings from two to seven patients with hepatitis considered (although not established) to be type A.[644] However, in other studies experimental transmission was not successful in 15 subjects challenged with specimens taken from the late incubation period and preicteric and icteric phases of hepatitis.[623, 645] These results suggest that respiratory secretions contain infectious HAV infrequently, if at all, and transmission by contact or aerosol via such secretions would be an unlikely event. Consistent with this is the regular observation that transmission is limited to close contacts rather than by the more casual contact associated with transmission of some respiratory viruses.

Urine collected just before or at the time of onset of jaundice appears to contain low levels of infectious HAV in some patients. Three of 6 subjects in one study and 1 of 12 in another were infected by urine samples.[618, 620] In contrast, three other studies reported a failure to infect a total of 29 subjects with urine of patients with clinically diagnosed hepatitis A and one patient with serologically proven HAV infection.[601, 623, 644, 645] Although urine has been implicated in non-experimental transmission in rare instances,[646] it seems unlikely that urine is commonly involved in infections in the community.

There is little evidence bearing on the risk of HAV transmission during heterosexual contact. Conversely, a high prevalence of anti-HAAg in homosexual males indicates high infection rates in this population.[611, 612] Specific routes of transmission are not proved. The well-documented presence of infectious HAV in feces (Table 35–7) and more limited studies indicating infectivity in saliva suggest these could be sources of virus for transmission during homosexual contact.[601] No cases of intrauterine infection with HAV have been reported, and in six cases of acute hepatitis A followed prospectively in pregnant women (three occurring at the time of delivery), there was no evidence of infection in the newborn infants.[647]

Viremia and Percutaneous Transmission

Although transient viremia has been documented after HAV infection, percutaneous transfer of blood or serum appears to be an infrequent route of transmission. Data on the period when infectious virus is present in the blood are less complete than for fecal virus. Virus has been found in blood during the later half of the incubation period. The time when viremia is terminated in most patients is not well established. Negative test results for susceptibility to infection in human subjects must be interpreted, however. The susceptibility of the subjects used for testing was unknown. The period of antigenemia in experimentally infected chimpanzees is brief and occurs exclusively during the late incubation period of hepatitis A. These results suggest that viremia is present for a limited period and probably most often during the late incubation period of hepatitis A. Because the data on infectivity in blood and on antigenemia are quite limited, more investigation with improved methods will be needed to establish conclusively the frequency, duration, and precise time limits of viremia in HAV infection in humans.

Because the incubation period of hepatitis A and the period of viremia are much shorter than they are for hepatitis B, and because persistent infection does not occur, the period for potential percutaneous transmission of HAV from asymptomatic patients is clearly less than it is for HBV. Epidemiologic evidence supports this view. Although multiply-transfused children have been found to have a much higher frequency of anti-HBs than do nontransfused populations, the frequency of anti-HAAg has been found to be the same.[651] Similarly, patients and staff of hemodialysis centers have not been found to have a higher incidence of anti-HAAg (unlike anti-HBs) than that expected for groups of similar demographic characteristics.[652] Studies of post-transfusion hepatitis have failed to reveal cases of hepatitis A by specific serologic testing.[653-656] Thus, percutaneous transmission of HAV is possible theoretically, but except for experimental transmission, it has not been demonstrated unequivocally. It is insignificant for infections in the community.

Food and Water

Besides the spread of HAV by close personal contact, water and food are documented vehicles for transmission.[657-662] Numerous examples of epidemic and endemic hepatitis A have been associated with ingestion of shellfish.[663-670] Sewage contaminating raw clams has been implicated most often in causing disease, but contaminated oysters,[664, 668, 670] mussels,[669] and steamed clams have also been reported.[667] Milk-borne hepatitis A has been described and is thought to follow the use of contaminated water to wash milk containers and equipment.[671, 672] Transmission via other food and drink has been reported on numerous occasions.[648, 664, 673-681] In some instances, a food handler with hepatitis A has been implicated as the source.[648, 673, 675-678]

Nonhuman Primate Exposure

Many cases of infectious hepatitis, which is indistinguishable clinically from hepatitis A, have followed contact with chimpanzees and a few other nonhuman primates.[563-565, 682-683a] Such cases have been confirmed serologically to be type A hepatitis.[684] In all cases, animals in captivity with previous contact with humans were involved. It is most likely that the animals in these cases were first infected by contact with humans rather than being infected before they were captured. The infection causes subclinical illness in nonhuman primates. Much of the epidemiologic experimental transmission and serologic evidence concerning HAV transmission has recently been reviewed by Mosley.[685]

POST-TRANSFUSION NON-A, NON-B HEPATITIS

PT-NANB hepatitis was clearly recognized in the mid-1970s after blood donor screening by sensitive assays for HBsAg. Elimination of the use of many paid donors and the greater use of volunteer donors led to a significant reduction in post-transfusion hepatitis B.[33, 34, 723-726] The overall incidence of post-transfusion hepatitis remained unexpectedly high, and newly developed assays for HAV and tests for CMV and EBV revealed that these agents were infrequently involved.[33, 34, 726, 727] Thus, most cases of post-transfusion hepatitis since that time meet criteria (i.e., exclusion of known viruses or other identifiable causative factors) for NANB hepatitis. Transmission of the disease to chimpanzees and marmosets indicates that many cases of PT-NANB hepatitis are caused by infectious agents,[728-733] although no virus or other infectious agent proved to be responsible for this disease has been identified with certainty as an antigenic, ultrastructural, or molecular entity at this time.

CAUSATIVE AGENT

The causative agent of PT-NANB hepatitis has not been defined physically. The most important experimental advance in defining the agent has been the transmission of an infectious agent to chimpanzees and more recently to marmosets.[10-13, 17, 18, 723-733, 735, 736] The direct demonstration of a transmissible agent provided an assay for the agent and an animal model of the disease. An agent has been transmitted to chimpanzees with serum from several human cases and has been serially transmitted in chimpanzees using serum or plasma from animals at the time of acute or chronic hepatitis.[728-731, 735, 736] The agent has recently been identified and an assay has been developed that detects antibodies to this agent.[814, 815]

It is not clear how many different agents may be associated with PT-NANB hepatitis, but several findings suggest that there may be more than one. First, two or more episodes of NANB hepatitis have been described in hemophiliacs given multiple doses of factor VIII,[738, 739] as well as in others with biopsy diagnosed viral hepatitis.[740] Second, an unusually wide range of incubation periods has been observed for PT-NANB hepatitis.[723, 741-745] Third, infectious serum from several different patients with NANB hepatitis was consistently found to produce either nuclear or cytoplasmic ultrastructural changes in hepatocytes of experimentally infected chimpanzees.[747] The ultrastructural patterns were consistent during serial passage in chimpanzees. The different changes could reflect different infectious agents. Fourth, three different studies have shown apparent sequential infection in individual chimpanzees with PT-NANB hepatitis–inducing inocula from two different sources.[748-750] If PT-NANB hepatitis leads to solid immunity against the infecting agent, these results would indicate that at least two antigenically different PT-NANB hepatitis agents exist. Other cross-challenge experiments suggest, however, that not all agents in sera of patients with PT-NANB hepatitis are different, since cross-challenge in chimpanzees has shown apparent cross-protection when serum from patients from different parts of the United States was used.[751] Formalin inactivates the infectivity of the NANB hepatitis–inducing agent in the sera of patients with chronic NANB hepatitis.[752, 753] This result is of interest because it suggests that the formalin treatment used in the preparation of HBV vaccines made from viral antigen purified from patient plasma may eliminate the risk of NANB agents in the vaccine.

There have been numerous reports of the detection of apparently unique antigen-antibody systems in the sera of patients and chimpanzees with NANB hepatitis when human convalescent sera or sera from polytransfused patients was used as the source of antibody.[753-758] Each result has been difficult to confirm in other laboratories, and only one of these tests has successfully identified sera known to contain NANB agents within a panel of sera sent to several laboratories to evaluate the test methods.[759, 815] Immunofluorescent staining of liver tissue with convalescent-phase sera has also been described.[755] The relationship that these antigens and the antibodies used for their detection may have to infectious agents of NANB hepatitis and whether they will be useful diagnostically is not yet clear. Some may represent autoantigen-antibody or other reactions that are not virus-specific. The difficulty encountered in detecting an agent-specific antigen in sera that clearly do contain infectious NANB hepatitis agents suggests that the concentration of specific antigen must be significantly lower than the concentration of HBsAg in sera of most HBV-infected patients, although the titers of infectious NANB hepatitis agents in at least some sera appear to be comparable to the titers of HBV in the serum of HBV-infected patients.[733, 760-762]

In addition to antigen, virus-like particulate structures have been observed in serum and plasma of humans and chimpanzees with NANB hepatitis. Bradley and co-workers have observed 27-nm spherical particles (CsCl buoyant density 1.30 g/ml) in serum and hepatocyte cytoplasm of infected chimpanzees,[735, 750] and Yoshizawa and colleagues have seen similar particles in human serum containing a NANB hepatitis agent and in hepatocyte cytoplasm of chimpanzees with NANB hepatitis.[750, 763] The properties of these particles are similar to those of small RNA viruses (picornaviruses). Other reports of hepatocyte intranuclear particles and HBV-like particles in serum have been less consistent. Whether any of these particulate structures or antigen-antibody systems represent causative agents of NANB hepatitis remains to be proved. Thus, it seems likely that one or more viruses are responsible for most cases of NANB hepatitis. However, it is not clear how many infectious agents exist, whether they are all viruses or other types of infectious agents, and even whether some cases now clinically diagnosed as NANB hepatitis are caused by factors other than infectious agents.

EPIDEMIOLOGY

Clinical Setting and Incidence of Infection

There has been a tenfold or more reduction in the incidence and a fivefold reduction in the mortality rate of post-transfusion hepatitis B since the mid-1970s.[764] The recognition that there is a very high risk from the use of blood from commercial donors, which led to the exclusion of paid donors and greater use of volunteer donors,[725, 726, 765] and the screening of all donors for HBsAg by sensitive assays,[766] accounts for the reduction in hepatitis B. Despite the reduction, the overall incidence of post-transfusion hepatitis remains high and almost all cases today meet the criteria for NANB hepatitis. Approximately 5 to 10 per cent of patients who develop hepatitis following transfusion with radioimmunoassay blood tested from volunteer donors are infected with HBV or rarely with CMV, EBV, or HAV.[33, 34] Thus, approximately 90 per cent of cases can be designated NANB hepatitis. Most cases are mild, and 70 to 80 per cent are anicteric.[74, 743] The source of transfused blood clearly influences the incidence of post-transfusion NANB hepatitis, since it was found to develop in 6 to 7 per cent of recipients of blood from volunteer donors, compared with 17 to 35 per cent in those receiving blood from paid donors.[742, 743] If infectious NANB agents are involved in most or all cases, it would indicate a remarkably high incidence of carriers of these agents in the healthy blood donor population. The apparent high incidence in donor blood suggests that there could be multiple causes for these cases.

Many viral hepatitis cases not related to blood transfusion also meet the criteria for NANB hepatitis. In Costa Rica, 12 per cent of cases of endemic hepatitis were found to be NANB hepatitis.[767] In a study of hepatitis patients admitted to referral hospitals in the United States, 50 per cent were hepatitis B, 25 per cent were hepatitis A, and 25 per cent were NANB hepatitis.[768] A study of patients in the United States, many of whom were intravenous drug users with two or more episodes of hepatitis, demonstrated 7 per cent to have hepatitis A, 40 per cent to have hepatitis B, and 53 per cent to have NANB hepatitis.[738] In an outbreak of viral hepatitis in an oncology unit, all 15 cases proved to be NANB hepatitis, rather than hepatitis A as suspected clinically. Another nosocomial outbreak of mild NANB hepatitis involved 34 healthy young persons who underwent plasmaphoresis at a single center in Europe.[769] Thus, it appears that 25 to 50 per cent of sporadic hepatitis cases in

some settings in the United States and abroad are due to NANB hepatitis agents. In some instances, NANB hepatitis demonstrates the epidemiologic behavior of classic blood-borne serum hepatitis, and in other cases it behaves like infectious hepatitis and may be related to the epidemic form of NANB hepatitis described in the next chapter, which is undoubtedly caused by a different agent or agents than PT-NANB hepatitis. Identification of the agents and development of diagnostic tests will be necessary to distinguish the different viruses with certainty.

Routes of Transmission

Probably not all routes of transmission of the blood-borne NANB hepatitis are known at this time. The best established route is by parenteral transfer of blood and other blood products including platelets and factor VIII and factor IX concentrates. This is consistent with persistent infection and continuous viremia in the donor population, as occurs with HBV. Thus NANB hepatitis may also be transmitted by other mechanisms involving transfer of blood or serum percutaneously—such as accidental needlesticks by medical personnel, percutaneous drug abuse, tattooing, and so on—as is hepatitis B. The common occurrence of NANB hepatitis in illicit parenteral drug users is consistent with this route of transmission.[770] Increasing evidence suggests that NANB hepatitis may be spread in the community by nonpercutaneous routes, although such routes have not been precisely defined and the relationship of the agents in such cases to that of more typical PT-NANB hepatitis is not established. NANB hepatitis is apparently no more common in homosexual populations than in the general population, suggesting that homosexual contacts do not promote transmission as they apparently do for HBV and HAV.[54-57]

In a recent study,[371] six of nine newborns of mothers with acute NANB hepatitis in the third trimester developed very mild liver function abnormalities, suggesting the possibility that the agent was transmitted from mother to infant. None of three infants born to mothers who had NANB in the second trimester had any liver function abnormality. Further investigation will be required to determine more clearly whether the abnormalities found in the infants were due to infection with NANB hepatitis agents.

THE COURSE OF POST-TRANSFUSION NON-A, NON-B HEPATITIS AND CLINICAL MANIFESTATIONS

The incubation period or time between exposure and onset of symptoms or first abnormal liver function has been studied best for PT-NANB hepatitis. The mean time between transfusion and the first abnormal liver function (usually elevated serum ALT levels) was approximately seven to eight weeks in three different studies,[741-744] and there was a significant peak frequency near that time.[743] This incubation period is between those for hepatitis A and hepatitis B. As mentioned already, however, the range of incubation periods has been unusually wide. Ninety-two per cent of cases were between five and ten weeks,[741, 744] but cases with incubation periods as short as 2 weeks and as long as 26 weeks have been reported.[742] A peak or clustering of cases around 12 or 13 weeks was found in one study.[743] Others have also reported long (three to four months) incubation periods for PT-NANB hepatitis.[723] Other studies have consistently observed short (<30 days) incubation periods.[745] An incubation period around 20 days for NANB following administration of factor VIII concentrates has been described.[735] Although the differences in incubation periods for PT-NANB hepatitis in different studies and within individual studies could reflect different infecting agents, different incubation periods could also result from different infecting doses of virus or other unknown factors.

Acute NANB hepatitis is not distinguishable clinically from hepatitis A or hepatitis B in individual cases. PT-NANB hepatitis tends to be mild during the acute phase,[741, 744, 771, 772] although approximately one third of cases following blood transfusion were found to have peak serum ALT values greater than 800 IU, less than 10 per cent had ALT levels greater than 2000 IU,[741, 746] and 20 to 30 per cent were icteric.[741, 744] NANB hepatitis can be fulminant. Redeker found nearly equal proportions of HBV and NANB hepatitis in a series of cases of fulminant hepatitis in Los Angeles.[773]

Chronic hepatitis is a frequent sequel to PT-NANB hepatitis. Abnormal liver functioning has been reported to persist for more than one year in 10 to 60 per cent of cases.[741–744, 771] Similar results have been found in the follow-up of NANB hepatitis in a hemodialysis unit and hemophiliacs receiving factor VIII and factor IX concentrates in different studies.[772, 774] CAH has been found in 30 to 90 per cent of biopsied cases of chronic hepatitis following PT-NANB hepatitis.[744, 771, 772–777] Cirrhosis has developed in occasional cases.[741, 744, 771, 776] How long the chronic hepatitis persists in these patients is not clear, but abnormal liver functioning has been found to resolve after one to three years in a few patients.[741, 744, 771] Thus, potentially serious long-term liver disease appears to develop in a significant percentage of patients with PT-NANB hepatitis. However, the prognosis may be better than that for CAH of other causes. Resolution appears to occur in time in some patients.

The risk of developing chronic hepatitis appears to correlate with the severity of acute PT-NANB hepatitis. Among 12 patients who developed chronic hepatitis in one study, 3 had icteric hepatitis initially and 9 were anicteric.[741, 744] Eight of nine patients with serum ALT levels greater than 300 IU recovered, and one patient developed CAH. CAH developed in eight of nine anicteric patients with serum ALT levels less than 300 IU, and only one patient recovered.[741, 744] The differences are highly significant.

The common development of CAH following PT-NANB hepatitis and the apparent frequent occurrence of infectious NANB agents in the population suggests that many cases of CAH that are not associated with HBV infection may be related to infection with NANB hepatitis agents.

In addition to the chronic liver disease that commonly develops following acute PT-NANB, persistence of virus in the blood has been documented. The studies are limited because detection of virus is difficult and requires inoculation of chimpanzees or marmosets. One patient was shown to have a NANB hepatitis agent in the blood over a six-year interval,[778] and several others showed the agent in the blood for eight to ten months.[749] Transmissible NANB hepatitis agent has been shown to persist in the serum of infected chimpanzees for at least 16 months.[779] The high incidence of NANB hepatitis following blood transfusion, as described earlier, is also consistent with frequent persistence of the infectious agents in the blood of apparently healthy blood donors.

NANB hepatitis not associated with blood transfusion may have a different outcome than that occurring after transfusion. No cases of chronic hepatitis appeared to follow 70 cases of NANB hepatitis unrelated to blood transfusion.[777] Whether the different outcome reflects different infectious agents, differences in the infecting dose of virus and severity of initial disease, or other factors remains to be determined.

CLINICAL DIAGNOSIS

Without a virus-specific test for PT-NANB hepatitis, a diagnosis in a clinical setting can only be tentative and depends on excluding identifiable hepatitis viruses (e.g., HAV, HBV, EBV, CMV, and so on). Exposure to hepatotoxic chemicals, drugs, and other noninfectious factors also must be excluded. The most definitive diagnosis can be made by inoculation of chimpanzees or marmosets.

Blood donors with elevated serum ALT levels transmit NANB hepatitis more frequently than do donors with normal values, although many donors with elevated serum ALT levels appear not to transmit hepatitis.[741, 780] The incidence of post-transfusion hepatitis is proportional to the level of ALT in donor blood.[781, 782] In one study,[781] hepatitis developed in 10 of 11 recipients of blood with ALT values greater than 45 IU. Eliminating donors with ALT levels greater than 45 IU would have excluded 3 per cent of the donors and 45 per cent of those transmitting NANB hepatitis. In another study, an exclusion level of 2.25 standard deviations (SD) above the normal mean ALT value would have excluded 33 per cent of blood units that transmitted NANB hepatitis, but only 1.6 per cent of the noninfectious blood donors.[782] These findings suggest that an ALT exclusion level can be chosen to eliminate high-risk donors without excluding an unacceptable percentage of noninfectious donors. In lieu of a specific test for NANB hepatitis in blood donors, ALT screening of donors should be considered. Since ALT levels vary with age, sex, alcohol use, and geographic region, more work will be required to define ALT exclusion levels that may be cost-effective for different donor populations.

PREVENTION OF POST-TRANSFUSION NON-A, NON-B HEPATITIS

Prevention of PT-NANB hepatitis can be best accomplished by measures of environmental control, which are effective for control of HBV and are described earlier.

Several double-blind, randomized, controlled trials to evaluate the effect of immune serum globulin for prevention of PT-NANB hepatitis have been reported.[783–786] In two studies,[783, 784] there was no evidence of protection, and in two other studies significant protection was shown.[785, 786] The greatest effect appeared to be a reduction in the incidence of icteric cases, but prevention of infection and progression to chronic hepatitis may also have resulted. Although passive immunization for prevention of PT-NANB hepatitis transmitted by other routes has not been investigated, the fact that immune serum globulin may on occasion provide some protection against PT-NANB hepatitis suggests that it might be effective in other settings. Thus immune serum globulin could be administered to individuals with direct percutaneous, open skin break, or mucous membrane exposure to serum or blood of infected patients—the same indications recommended for passive prophylaxis after exposure to HBV (see Chap. 37).

Whether immune serum globulin should be used for prevention of PT-NANB hepatitis is not agreed upon. Although it appears that immune serum globulin can provide some protection, its expense and the limited supply would preclude its use with all transfusions. Some have recommended that immune serum globulin might be given to recipients of three units or more of blood for whom the risk of PT-NANB hepatitis is high.[787]

EPIDEMIC ENTERICALLY TRANSMITTED NON-A, NON-B HEPATITIS

Large epidemics of viral hepatitis have been observed in various parts of southern Asia over the past 30 years. The acute hepatitis in these outbreaks has been indistinguishable from hepatitis A or B. No chronic disease developed, young adults were primarily affected (it is infrequent in children), there was a high mortality rate in pregnant women, and often the source of the infection appeared to be water contaminated with sewage. One such outbreak in New Delhi, India, involving 29,000 cases exposed to water contaminated with raw sewage, was described in 1957.[788] Such outbreaks were considered to be hepatitis A, since they were similar epidemiologically and clinically to outbreaks of infectious hepatitis in Europe and the United States. When HAV was identified and specific serologic tests were developed for its detection, analysis in 1980 of stored sera from the large New Delhi epidemic of the 1950s and study of a similar water-borne epidemic in Kashmir, India, involving 275 cases in 1978 to 1979 revealed no evidence of HAV or HBV.[789, 790] The disease in these outbreaks was designated NANB hepatitis. Many similar outbreaks, as well as sporadic cases of NANB hepatitis not associated with exposure to parenteral blood, have since been reported in many developing countries of Asia and outside Asia.

CAUSATIVE AGENT

Electron microscopic examination of stool samples from patients early in the course of epidemic NANB hepatitis by investigators from the Soviet Union,[791] India,[792] and the United States have revealed 27- to 30-nm viruslike particles.[792, 793] These particles are aggregated by convalescent sera and not by sera from the acute stage of disease or by antibody to HAV, suggesting that they contain antigens of the causative agent, which is distinct from HAV. Such particles from patients in Pakistan have been aggregated by sera from Nepalese,[793] Burmese,[794] and East African patients,[794] suggesting that antigenically identical or cross-reacting agents cause this epidemic disease in different parts of the world. The fecal particles from patients in these countries and from the Soviet Union were similar morphologically.[791] The causative agent in the epidemics in other geographic regions has not been similarly characterized.

Acute hepatitis, confirmed by histologic appearance and serum ALT elevations, developed in marmosets inoculated with stool samples from patients with epidemic NANB hepatitis from Nepal. Their stools contained particles that were morphologically identical to those in human cases, and they developed antibodies that agglutinated the particles in stools of the same animal, the human patient

from Nepal providing the inoculum for the animal and human patients from a different geographic region (Pakistan).[793] The agent has also been transmitted to *Cynomolgus* monkeys but not to chimpanzees.[795]

These studies suggest that an antigen (possibly the virion) of the causative agent of epidemic NANB hepatitis has been found in stool of infected patients. It has the appearance of a small non-enveloped virus, and it can be transmitted to marmosets and *Cynomolgus* monkeys. The agent is clearly antigenically distinct from HAV, and work is in progress to develop a more convenient diagnostic test for this agent.

EPIDEMIOLOGY

Epidemics of apparent water-borne NANB hepatitis have been described in India,[796-798] Nepal,[792] Burma,[799, 800] the central Asian part of the Soviet Union,[791] Algeria and other parts of North Africa,[801] China (C. B. Liu, personal communication), Afghanistan and Pakistan,[793, 802] Japan,[803] Mexico (G. Ornelas, personal communication), and in refugee camps in East Africa (Somalia and Sudan).[794] Epidemics have occurred as discrete common-source outbreaks related to exposure to contaminated water, or outbreaks may be prolonged over one to two years, with increased attack rates during the monsoon rains. Similar epidemics of hepatitis A do not occur in adults in these geographic regions, since almost all individuals in these populations are infected with HAV in childhood, and almost all adults are immune. This difference in age distribution of hepatitis A and epidemic NANB hepatitis in these Asian countries appears to be a significant epidemiologic difference, possibly related to a difference in the intensity of exposure to the two agents in childhood or to a failure of infection with the agent of NANB hepatitis to produce long-lasting protective immunity as does infection with HAV. Epidemics of similar NANB hepatitis have not been documented in the United States or western Europe.

The observation that preimmune and other control human sera do not aggregate particles suggests that the agent of epidemic NANB hepatitis is not a widespread enteric agent, as is HAV, or that antibody to it is not long-lasting in these Asian populations.[793] The observation that immune serum globulin preparations from the United States do not protect against epidemic NANB hepatitis suggests that infections with the agent are rare and that the prevalence of antibody is very low in the United States or that if antibody to the agent is present in the immune serum globulin manufactured in the United States, it is not protective.[792]

More than one half of sporadic cases of acute viral hepatitis in adults not related to epidemics in these Asian countries have also been shown to be NANB hepatitis.[796] These cases have an age distribution that is similar to that of the epidemic disease. They are more common during the monsoon season, show no history of parenteral exposure, and apparently do not lead to chronic disease. It is presumed, but not proved, that they are caused by the same agent or agents that cause epidemic NANB hepatitis.[804] The name enterically transmitted non-A, non-B (ET-NANB) hepatitis has been suggested for both the epidemic and sporadic forms of this disease.[804] A significant percentage of cases of sporadic, community acquired hepatitis unrelated to blood transfusions has also been reported to be NANB hepatitis in other parts of the world, including Costa Rica,[767] the United States,[768] England,[805] and Australia.[806] In addition, NANB hepatitis following raw shellfish consumption has been reported in the United States and Great Britain.[752, 807] Whether these sporadic cases represent infections with the agents of PT-NANB hepatitis, ET-NANB hepatitis, or other agents is not yet clear, but it seems likely that some could be caused by agents of ET-NANB hepatitis.

Recently, three cases of NANB hepatitis were reported in Los Angeles over a ten-month period in Pakistani men who had recently lived in or traveled to Pakistan and who had no history of parenteral exposure.[793] Virologic and pathologic features were like those found in cases of epidemic NANB hepatitis, suggesting that these cases were caused by the agent of epidemic, enterically transmitted NANB hepatitis. Water-borne NANB hepatitis has also been documented in Americans visiting Nepal during epidemics.[792] Thus, it is clear that this disease may occur in overseas travelers, and more cases can be expected to occur in the United States in individuals who have recently traveled from epidemic or highly endemic geographic areas.

An average incubation period of 35 to 40 days was observed in the epidemic disease reported in Delhi and Kashmir, India,[789, 790, 791] Nepal,[792] and Burma,[799] and in experimental human infections.[791]

Not all possible routes of transmission of this agent have been carefully investigated, but clearly the enteric route of infection and a source of drinking water contaminated with human sewage has been the rule for the well-studied epidemics of this disease. Cases among household contacts raise the question of person to person spread.[789, 790]

COURSE OF DISEASE AND PATHOLOGIC FEATURES

Enterically transmitted NANB hepatitis cannot be distinguished from other forms of viral hepatitis on clinical grounds alone in individual cases. However, certain features may occur more or less frequently in disease associated with different agents. More than 50 per cent of patients with ET-NANB hepatitis have fever,[790, 792, 797, 808] compared with those with PT-NANB hepatitis in which fever is uncommon. Up to one third of patients with ET-NANB in one study have been reported to have arthralgias,[792] and arthralgias are less common in other viral hepatitides. Although the disease is usually mild among individuals who survive, severe hepatitis with a high mortality rate can occur. A mortality rate of 12 per cent was observed in one study,[797] but it was similar to that in PT-NANB hepatitis and hepatitis A (<1 per cent) in another study.[789, 809] The most severe disease has been consistently observed in pregnant women,[790, 792, 794] with mortality rates reported to be 20 to 39 per cent, unlike PT-NANB hepatitis in which the mortality rate in pregnant women is no different from that in other groups. Fetal wastage has been reported to be common.[790] Symptoms and liver function abnormalities have been observed to resolve within six weeks in most surviving patients.[790, 797] Unlike PT-NANB hepatitis, in which chronic hepatitis develops in more than 50 per cent of patients,[735, 744] chronic hepatitis has not been observed after ET-NANB hepatitis.

Marked cholestasis, gland-like acinar formation, and preserved lobular structure have been observed in several reported cases of ET-NANB hepatitis,[790, 793, 810] and this is in contrast to the usual findings of parenchymal injury and inflammation observed in hepatitis associated with other

agents.[811] Clinical features frequently correlate with this histologic picture. Marked jaundice and other features of a predominantly cholestatic clinical picture have been reported in cases of ET-NANB hepatitis, although a clinical picture of severe parenchymal injury can also occur.[793]

Clinical Diagnosis

Without diagnostic testing specific for the agent of ET-NANB hepatitis, a presumptive diagnosis can be made by excluding other hepatitis agents for which specific diagnostic testing is available and by ruling out parenteral exposure such as illicit intravenous drug use, recent blood transfusion, or parenteral exposure to other blood products. In addition, history of exposure to water or shellfish potentially contaminated with sewage, association with epidemic disease, and clinical findings of a cholestatic picture might support the presumption of ET-NANB hepatitis. Immune electron microscopy on fecal specimens from the early phase of the disease using convalescent sera of proven cases might provide more specific diagnostic information, but such testing is available only in a few research laboratories.

Prevention

During epidemics of ET-NANB hepatitis, efforts should be made to prevent transmission. Water sources should be examined for sources of fecal contamination that can be eliminated, and water should be boiled or chlorinated before consumption. Improved sanitation and other efforts such as education to prevent person to person spread should be emphasized. Although immune serum globulin manufactured from American donors does not appear to protect against disease,[792] the efficacy of immune serum globulin from endemic populations is untested. The best protection for travelers from low endemic areas, such as the United States, to highly endemic or epidemic areas is the same as for preventing all enteric diseases, namely avoiding potentially contaminated water and uncooked food.

REFERENCES

1. Pickles WN. Epidemiology in Country Practice. Bristol, John Wright and Sons, 1939:110.
2. Lurman A. Eine icterus epidemic. Berl Klin Wochenscher 22:20, 1855.
3. Flaum A, Malmros H, Persson E. Eine nosocomiale icterus epidemic. Acta Med Scand (Suppl)16:544, 1926.
4. Bigger JW, Dubi SD. Jaundice in syphilitics under treatment. Lancet 1:457, 1943.
5. MacCallum FO. Transmission of arsenotherapy jaundice by blood: failure with feces and nasopharyngeal washing. Lancet 1:342, 1945.
6. McNatty AS. Great Britain Ministry Health Report of Chief Medical Officer, Annual Report, London, 1937.
7. Propert SA. Hepatitis after prophylactic serum. Br Med J 2:677, 1938.
8. Beeson PB, Chesney G, McFarlan AM. Hepatitis following injection of mumps convalescent plasma. Lancet 1(24):814, 1944.
9. Findlay GM, MacCallum FO. Note on acute hepatitis and yellow fever immunization. Trans Soc Trop Med Gyg 31:297, 1937.
10. Anonymous. Jaundice following yellow fever vaccine. JAMA 119:1110, 1942.
11. Beeson PB. Jaundice occurring one to four months after transfusion of blood or plasma. JAMA 121:1332, 1943.
12. Morgan HW, Williamson DAJ. Jaundice following administration of human blood products. Br Med J 1:750, 1943.
13. Stokes J, Berk JE, Malamut LL. The carrier state of viral hepatitis. JAMA 154:1059, 1954.
14. Voegt H. Zur Aetiologie der Hepatitis Epidemica. Muchen Med Wochenschr 89:76, 1942.
15. Havens WP, Ward R, Drill VA, et al. Experimental production of hepatitis by feeding icterogenic materials. Proc Soc Exp Biol Med 57:206, 1944.

16. MacCallum FO, Bradley WH. Transmission of infective hepatitis to human volunteers. Lancet 2:228, 1944.
17. Havens WP. Experiment in cross immunity between infectious and homologous serum jaundice. Proc Soc Exp Biol Med 59:148, 1945.
18. Neefe JR, Stokes J Jr, Reinhold JG. Oral administration to volunteers of feces from patients with homologous serum hepatitis and infectious (epidemic) hepatitis. Am J Med Sci 210:29, 1945.
19. Neefe JR, Gellis SS, Stokes J Jr. Homologous serum hepatitis and infectious (epidemic) hepatitis: studies in volunteers bearing on immunological and other characteristics of the etiological agents. Am J Med 1:3, 1946.
20. Ward R, Krugman S, Giles JP, et al. Infectious hepatitis: studies of its natural history and prevention. N Engl J Med 258:407, 1958.
21. Krugman S, Ward R, Giles JP. The natural history of infectious hepatitis. Am J Med 32:717, 1962.
22. Krugman S, Giles JP, Hammon J. Infectious hepatitis: evidence for two distinctive clinical, epidemiological and immunological types of infection. JAMA 200:365, 1967.
23. Krugman S, Giles JP. Viral hepatitis: new light on an old disease. JAMA 212:1019, 1970.
24. Havens WP. Properties of the etiologic in infectious hepatitis. Proc Soc Exp Biol Med 58:203, 1945.
25. McCollum RW. The size of serum hepatitis virus. Proc Soc Exp Biol Med 81:157, 1952.
26. Blumberg BS, Gerstley JS, Hungerford DA, et al. A serum antigen (Australia antigen) in Down's syndrome leukemia and hepatitis. Ann Intern Med 66:924, 1967.
27. Okachi K, Murakami S. Observations on Australia antigen in Japanese. Vox Sang 15:374, 1968.
28. Prince AM. An antigen detected in the blood during the incubation period of serum hepatitis. Proc Nat Acad Sci USA 60:814, 1968.
29. Barker LF, Chisari F, McGrath PP, et al. Transmission of type B viral hepatitis to chimpanzees. J Infect Dis 127:648, 1973.
30. Homes AW, Wolfe L, Rosenblate H, et al. Hepatitis in marmosets: induction of disease with coded specimens from a human volunteer study. Science 165:816, 1969.
31. Holmes AW, Wolfe L, Deinhardt F, et al. Transmission of human hepatitis to marmosets: further coded studies. J Infect Dis 124:520, 1971.
32. Feinstone SM, Kapikian AZ, Purcell RW. Hepatitis A: detection by immune electron microscopy of a virus-like antigen associated with acute illness. Science 182:1026, 1973.
33. Feinstone SM, Kapikian AZ, Purcell RH, et al. Transfusion associated hepatitis not due to viral hepatitis type A or B. N Engl J Med 282:767, 1975.
34. Knodell RG, Conrad ME, Dienstag JL, et al. Etiological spectrum of post-transfusion hepatitis. Gastroenterology 69:1278, 1975.
35. Alter HL, Purcell RH, Feinstone SM, et al. NonA/nonB hepatitis: a review and interim report of an ongoing prospective study. In: Vyas GN, Cohen SN, Schmid R, eds: Viral Hepatitis: A Contemporary Assessment of Etiology, Epidemiology, Pathogenesis and Prevention. Philadelphia, Franklin Institute Press, 1978:359.
36. Centers for Disease Control. Enterically transmitted nonA, nonB hepatitis. MMWR 36:241, 1987.
37. Rizzeto M, Caulse MG, Gerin JL, et al. Transmission of hepatitis B virus-associated delta antigen to chimpanzees. J Infect Dis 141:590, 1980.
38. Andrewes C, Pereira HG. Viruses of Vertebrates. Baltimore, Williams & Wilkins, 1974:451.
39. Sabesin SM, Koff RS: Pathogenesis of experimental viral hepatitis. N Engl J Med 290:944, 996, 1974.
40. Summers J, Smolec JM, Snyder R. A virus similar to human hepatitis B virus associated with hepatitis and hepatoma in woodchucks. Proc Natl Acad Sci USA 75:4533, 1978.
41. Marion PL, Oshiro L, Regnery DC, et al. A virus in Beechey ground squirrels that is related to hepatitis B virus of man. Proc Natl Acad Sci USA 77:2941, 1980.
42. Mason W, Seal G, Summers J. A virus of Pekin ducks with structural relatedness to human hepatitis B virus. J Virol 36:829, 1980.
43. Robinson WS. Genetic variation among hepatitis B and related viruses. Ann NY Acad Sci 354:371, 1980.
44. Weller TH. The cytomegalovirus. Ubiquitous agents with protein clinical manifestations. N Engl J Med 285:203, 267, 1971.
45. Weller TH, Hanshaw JB. Virologic and clinical observations on cytomegalic inclusion disease. N Engl J Med 266:1233, 1962.
46. Lang DJ, Hanshaw JB. Cytomegalovirus infection and the postperfusion syndrome: recognition of primary infections in four patients. N Engl J Med 280:1145, 1969.
47. Foster KM, Jack I. A prospective study of the role of cytomegalovirus in post-transfusion mononucleosis. N Engl J Med 280:1311, 1969.
48. Kantor GL, Goldberg LS, Johnson BL, et al. Immunologic abnormalities induced by postperfusion cytomegalovirus infection. Ann Intern Med 73:553, 1970.
49. Prince AM, Szmuness W, Millian SJ, et al. A serologic study of cytomegalovirus infections associated with blood transfusions. N Engl J Med 284:1125, 1971.
50. Wong TW, Warner NE. Cytomegalic inclusion disease in adults. Arch Pathol 74:403, 1962.
51. Klemola E, Kaarianinen L. Cytomegalovirus as a possible cause of a disease resembling infectious mononucleosis. Br Med J 2:1099, 1965.
52. Klemola E, von Essen R, Wager O, et al. Cytomegalovirus mononucleosis in previously healthy individuals: five new cases and followup of 13 previously published cases. Ann Intern Med 71:11, 1969.
53. Carlstrom G, Alden J, Belfrage S, et al. Acquired cytomegalovirus infection. Br Med J 2:521, 1968.
54. Lamb SG, Stern H. Cytomegalovirus mononucleosis with jaundice as the presenting sign. Lancet 2:1003, 1966.
55. Toghill PL, Bailey ME, Williams R, et al. Cytomegalovirus hepatitis in the adult. Lancet 1:1351, 1967.
56. Carter AR. Cytomegalovirus disease presenting as hepatitis. Br Med J 3:786, 1968.
57. Kilpatrick ZM. Structural and functional abnormalities of liver in infectious mononucleosis. Arch Intern Med 117:47, 1966.
58. Jain S, Sherlock S. Infectious mononucleosis with jaundice anemia and encephalopathy. Br Med J 2:54, 1975.
59. Hass GM. Hepato-adrenal necrosis with intranuclear inclusion bodies. Am J Pathol 11:127, 1935.
60. Quilligan JJ, Wilson JL. Fatal herpes simplex infection in newborn infant. J Lab Clin Med 38:742, 1951.
61. Zueler WW, Stulberg CS. Herpes simplex virus as the cause of fulminating visceral disease and hepatitis in infancy. Am J Dis Child 83:421, 1952.
62. Becker W, Naude W du T, Kipps A, et al. Virus studies in disseminated herpes simplex infections: associated with malnutrition in children. S Afr Med J 37:74, 1963.
63. Kipps A, Becker W, Wainright J, et al. Fatal disseminated primary herpes virus infection in children: epidemiology based on 93 non-neonatal cases. S Afr Med J 41:647, 1967.
64. Keane JT, Malkinson FD, Bryant J, et al. Herpes hominis hepatitis and disseminated intravascular coagulation: occurrence in an adult with pemphigus vulgaris. Arch Intern Med 136:1312, 1976.
65. Flewett TH, Parker RGF, Philip AM. Acute hepatitis due to herpes simplex virus in an adult. J Clin Pathol 22:60, 1969.
66. Goyette RE, Conowho EM, Heiger LR. Fulminant herpes virus hominis hepatitis during pregnancy. Obstet Gynecol 43:191, 1974.
67. Eron L, Kosinski K, Hirsch MS. Hepatitis in an adult caused by herpes simplex virus type I. Gastroenterology 71:500, 1976.
68. Krugman S, Ward R. Infectious Diseases of Children, 4th ed. St. Louis, CV Mosley, 1973:412.
69. Cheatham WJ, Weller TH, Polan TF, et al. Varicella: report of two fetal cases with necropsy, virus isolation and serologic studies. Am J Pathol 32:1015, 1956.
70. Blair AW, Jamieson WM, Smith GH. Complications and death in chicken-pox. Br Med J 2:981, 1965.
71. Scheinman JI, Stamler FW. Cyclophosphamide and fatal varicella. J Pediatr 74:117, 1969.
72. Pitel PA, McCormick KL, Fitzberald E, et al. Subclinical hepatic changes in varicella infection. Pediatrics 64:631, 1980.
73. Siegel D, Hirschman SZ. Hepatic dysfunction in acute measles infection of adults. Arch Intern Med 137:1178, 1977.
74. Nickell MD, Cannady PB, Schwitzer GA. Subclinical hepatitis in rubeola infections in young adults. Ann Intern Med 90:354, 1979.
75. Mawhinney H, Allen IV, Beare JM, et al. Dysgammaglobulinemia complicated by disseminated measles. Br Med J 2:380, 1971.
76. Esterly JR, Shusser RJ, Reubner BH. Hepatic lesions in the congenital rubella syndrome. J Pediatr 71:676, 1967.
77. O'Shaughnessey WJ, Beuchner HA. Hepatitis associated with a coxsackie B5 virus infection during late pregnancy. JAMA 179:71, 1962.
78. Morris JA, Elisberg BL, Pond WL, et al. Hepatitis associated with coxsackie virus group A, type 4. N Engl J Med 267:1230, 1962.
79. Sun NC, Smith VM. Hepatitis associated with mycocarditis: unusual manifestation of infection with coxsackie virus group B, type 3. N Engl J Med 274:190, 1966.
80. Schleissner LA, Portnoy B. Hepatitis and pneumonia associated with ECHO virus, type 9, infection in two adult siblings. Ann Intern Med 68:1315, 1968.
81. Hughes JR, Wilfert CM, Moore M, et al. ECHO virus 14 infection associated with fatal neonatal hepatic necrosis. Am J Dis Child 123:61, 1972.
82. Davis EV. Isolation of virus from children with infectious hepatitis. Science 133:1059, 1961.
83. Hartwell WV, Love GJ, Eidenbock MP. Adenovirus in blood clots from cases of infectious hepatitis. Science 152:1390, 1966.

84. Strong WB. Adenovirus isolation from patients with infectious hepatitis. CDC Hepatitis Surveillance Report 22. Atlanta, GA, 1965:17.

85. Johnson KM. Ebola virus and hemorrhagic fever: Andromeda strain or localized pathogen. Ann Intern Med 91:117, 1979.

86. Center for Disease Control: Recommendations for initial management of suspected or confirmed cases of Lassa fever. Morbid Mortal Weekly Rep 28:35, 1979.

87. Robinson WS, Marion PL, Feitelson M, et al. The hepadnavirus group: hepatitis B and related viruses. In: Szmuness W, Alter HJ, Maynard JE, eds. Viral Hepatitis. Philadelphia, Franklin Institute Press, 1982:57.

88. Gust ID, Coulepis AG, et al. Taxonomic classification of hepatitis B virus. Intervirology 25:14, 1986.

89. Szmuness W. Hepatocellular carcinoma and the hepatitis B virus: evidence for a causal association. Prog Med Virol 24:40, 1978.

90. Beasley RP, Lin CC, Hwang LY, et al. Hepatocellular carcinoma and hepatitis B virus: a prospective study of 22,707 men in Taiwan. Lancet 2:1129, 1981.

91. Snyder RL, Summers J. In: Viruses in Naturally Occurring Cancers, Cold Spring Harbor Conferences on Cell Proliferation, Vol 7. Cold Spring Harbor, New York, 1980:447.

92. Popper H, Shih JWK, Gerin JL, et al. Woodchuck hepatitis and hepatocellular carcinoma: correlation of histologic with virologic observations. Hepatology 1:91, 1981.

93. Marion PL, Robinson WS. Unpublished results.

94. Blumberg BS, Alter HJ, Visnich S. A "new" antigen in leukemia sera. JAMA 191:541, 1965.

95. Alter HJ, Blumberg BS. Further studies on a "new" human isoprecipitin system (Australia antigen). Blood 27:297, 1966.

96. LeBouvier GL, McCollum RW. Australia (hepatitis associated) antigen: Physicochemical and immunological characteristics. Adv Virus Res 16:357, 1970.

97. Bayer ME, Blumberg BS, Werner B. Particles associated with Australia antigen in the sera of patients with leukemia, Down's syndrome and hepatitis. Nature (London) 218:1057, 1968.

98. Dane DS, Cameron CH, Briggs M. Virus-like particles in serum of patients with Australia antigen associated hepatitis. Lancet 2:695, 1970.

99. Almeida JD, Rubenstein D, Stott EJ. New antigen antibody system in Australia antigen positive hepatitis. Lancet 2:1225, 1971.

100. Robinson WS, Clayton DA, Greenman RL. DNA of a human hepatitis B virus candidate. J Virol 14:384, 1974.

101. Gerlich W, Robinson WS. Hepatitis B virus contains protein attached to the 5' terminus of its complete DNA strand. Cell 21:801, 1980.

102. Kaplan PM, Greenman RL, Gerin JL, et al. DNA polymerase associated with human hepatitis B antigen. J Virol 12:995, 1973.

103. Robinson WS, Greenman RL. DNA polymerase in the core of the human hepatitis B virus candidate. J Virol 13:1231, 1974.

104. Albin C, Robinson WS. Protein kinase activity in hepatitis B virus. J Virol 34:297, 1980.

105. Takahashi K, Akahane Y, Gotanda T, et al. Demonstration of hepatitis e antigen in the core of Dane particles. J Immunol 122:275, 1979.

106. Almeida JD. Individual morphological variation seen in Australia antigen positive sera. Am J Dis Child 123:303, 1972.

107. Barker LF, Murray R. Relationship of virus dose of incubation time of clinical hepatitis and time of appearance of hepatitis-associated antigen. Am J Med Sci 263:27, 1972.

108. Scullard G, Greenberg HB, Smith JL, et al. Antiviral treatment of chronic hepatitis B virus infection: infectious virus cannot be detected in patient serum after permanent responses to treatment. Hepatology 2:39, 1982.

109. Shikata T, Karasawa T, Abe K, et al. Hepatitis B e antigens and infectivity of hepatitis B virus. J Infect Dis 136:571, 1977.

110. Barker LF, Murray R, Purcell RH. Hepatitis B virus infection in chimpanzee titration of subtypes. J Infect Dis 132:451, 1975.

111. Thomssen R, Gerlich W, Stamm B, et al. Infectivity of purified hepatitis virus particles. N Engl J Med 296:396, 1977.

112. Hoofnagle JH. Hepatitis B surface antigen (HBsAg) and antibody (anti-HBs). In: Bianchi L, Gerok W, Stickinger K, et al, eds. Virus and the Liver. Lancaster, England, MIP Press Ltd, 1980:27.

113. Kim CY, Tilles JG. Purification and biophysical characterization of hepatitis B antigen. J Clin Invest 52:1176, 1970.

114. Redeker AG, Hopkins CE, Jackson B, et al. A controlled study of the safety of pooled plasma stored in the liquid state at 30–32°C for 6 months. Transfusion 8:60, 1968.

115. Murray R, DieFenbach WC. Effect of heat on the agent of homolgous serum hepatitis. Proc Soc Exp Biol Med 84:230, 1953.

116. Gellis SS, Neefe JR, Stokes J Jr, et al. Chemical, clinical and immunological studies on the products of human plasma fractionation. XXXVI. Inactivation of the virus of homologous serum hepatitis in solution of normal serum albumin by means of heat. J Clin Invest 27:239, 1948.

117. Soulier JP, Blatix C, Courouce AM, et al. Prevention of virus B hepatitis (SH virus). Am J Dis Child 123:429, 1972.

118. Shikata T, Karasawa T, Abe K, et al. Incomplete inactivation of hepatitis B virus after heat treatment at 60°C for 10 hours. J Infect Dis 138:242, 1978.

119. Krugman S, Giles JP, Hammond J. Hepatitis virus: effect of heat infectivity and antigenicity of MS-1 and MS-2 strains. J Infect Dis 122:432, 1970.

120. Wewalka F. Zur Epidemiologie des Ikterus bei der antisyphlitischen Behandlung. Schweiz Z Allg Pathol 16:307, 1953.

121. Salaman MH, Williams DI, King AJ, et al. Prevention of jaundice resulting from antisyphilitic treatment. Lancet 2:7, 1944.

122. Summers JA, O'Connell A, Millman I. Genome of hepatitis B virus: restriction enzyme cleavage and structure of DNA extracted from Dane particles. Proc Natl Acad Sci USA 72:4597, 1975.

123. Landers TA, Greenberg HB, Robinson WS. Structure of hepatitis B Dane particle DNA and nature of the endogenous DNA polymerase reaction. J Virol 23:368, 1977.

124. Hruska JF, Clayton DA, Rubenstein JLR, et al. Structure of hepatitis B Dane particle DNA before and after the Dane particle DNA polymerase reaction. J Virol 21:666, 1977.

125. Kaplan PM, Greenman RL, Gerin JL, et al. DNA polymerase associated with human hepatitis B antigen. J Virol 12:995, 1973.

126. Robinson WS, Greenman RL. DNA polymerase in the core of the human hepatitis B virus candidate. J Virol 13:1231, 1974.

127. Sattler F, Robinson WS. Hepatitis B viral DNA molecules have cohesive ends. J Virol 32:226, 1979.

128. Siddiqui A, Sattler FR, Robinson WS. Restriction endonuclease cleavage map and location of unique features of the DNA of hepatitis B virus, subtype adw₂. Proc Natl Acad Sci USA 76:4664, 1979.

129. Seeger C, Ganem D, Varmus HE. Biochemical and genetic evidence for the hepatitis B virus replication strategy. Science 232:477, 1986.

130. Molnar-Kimber KL, Summers JW, Mason WS. Abstracts: initiation sites of DNA synthesis of duck hepatitis B virus. The 1984 International Symposium on Viral Hepatitis, San Francisco, 1984:86.

131. Lien J-M, Aldrich CE, Mason WS. Evidence that a capped oligoribonucleotide is the primer for duck hepatitis B virus plus-strand DNA synthesis. J Virol 57:229, 1986.

132. Molnar-Kimber K, Summers J, Taylor J, et al. Protein covalently bound to minus-strand DNA intermediates of duck hepatitis B virus. J Virol 45:165, 1983.

133. Ganem D, Greenbaum L, Varmus HE. Virion DNA of ground squirrel hepatitis virus: structural analysis and molecular cloning. J Virol 44:374, 1982.

134. Fujiyama A, Miyanohara A, Nozaki C, et al. Cloning and structural analyses of hepatitis B virus DNAs, subtype adr. Nucleic Acids Res 11:4601, 1983.

135. Ono Y, Onda H, Sasada R, et al. The complete nucleotide sequences of the cloned hepatitis B virus DNA; subtype adr and adw. Nucleic Acids Res 11:1747, 1983.

136. Kobayshi M, Koike K. Complete nucleotide sequence of hepatitis B virus DNA of subtype adr and its conserved gene organization. Gene 30:227, 1984.

137. Gan R-B, Chu M-J, Shen L-P, et al. The complete nucleotide sequence of the adr subtype hepatitis B virus DNA pADR-1. Acta Biochimica Biophys Sinica 16:316, 1984.

138. Valenzuela P, Quiroga M, Zaldivar J, et al. The nucleotide sequence of the hepatitis B genome and the identification of the major viral genes. In: Fields B, Jaenisch R, Fox CF, eds. Animal Virus Genetics. New York, Academic Press, 1980:57.

139. Galibert F, Mandart E, Fitoussi F, et al. Nucleotide sequence of hepatitis B virus genome (subtype ayw) cloned in E. coli. Nature (London) 281:646, 1979.

140. Bichko V, Pushko P, Dreilina D, et al. Subtype ayw variant of hepatitis B virus. DNA primary structure analysis. FEBS Lett 185:208, 1985.

141. Pasek M, Goto T, Gilbert W, et al. Hepatitis B virus genes and their expression in E. coli. Nature 282:575–579, 1979.

142. Mandart E, Kay A, Galibert F. Nucleotide sequence of a cloned duck hepatitis B virus genome: comparison with woodchuck and human hepatitis B virus sequences. J Virol 49:782, 1984.

143. Sprengel R, Kuhn C, Will H, et al. Cloned duck hepatitis B virus DNA is infectious in Pekin ducks. J Med Virol 15:323, 1985.

144. Galibert F, Chen TN, Mandart E. Nucleotide sequence of a cloned woodchuck hepatitis virus genome: comparison with the hepatitis B virus sequence. J Virol 41:51, 1982.

145. Seeger C, Ganem D, Varmus HE. The nucleotide sequence of an infectious molecularly cloned genome of the ground squirrel hepatitis B virus. J Virol 51:367, 1984.

146. Tiollais P, Pourcel C, Dejean A. The hepatitis B virus. Nature 317:489, 1985.

147. Moriarty AM, Alexander H, Lerner RA. Antibodies to peptides detect

new hepatitis B antigen: serological correlation with hepatocellular carcinoma. Science 227:429, 1985.

148. Kay A, Mandart E, Trepo C, et al. The HBV HBX gene expressed in *E. coli* is recognised by sera from hepatitis patients. EMBO J 4:1287, 1985.

149. Molnar-Kimber KL, Summers J, Mason WS. Mapping of the cohesive overlap of duck hepatitis B virus DNA and of the site of initiation of reverse transcription. J Virol 51:181, 1984.

150. Cattaneo R, Will H, Hernandez N, et al. Signals regulating hepatitis B surface antigen transcription. Nature 305:336, 1983.

151. Moroy T, Etiemble J, Trepo C, et al. Transcription of woodchuck hepatitis virus in the chronically infected liver. EMBO J 4:1507, 1985.

152. Enders GH, Ganem D, Varmus H. Mapping the major transcripts of ground squirrel hepatitis virus: the presumptive template for reverse transcriptase is terminally redundant. Cell 42:297, 1985.

153. Shaul Y, Rutter WJ, Laub O. A human hepatitis B viral enhancer element. EMBO J 4:427, 1985.

154. Tognoni A, Cattaneo R, Sertling E, et al. A novel expression selection approach allows precise mapping of the hepatitis B virus enhancer. Nucleic Acids Res 13:7457, 1985.

154a. Tur-Kaspa R, Burk R, Shaul Y, et al. Hepatitis B virus DNA contains a glucocorticoid-responsive element. Proc Natl Acad Sci USA 83:1627–1631, 1986.

155. Cattaneo R, Will H, Schaller H. Hepatitis B virus transcription in the infected liver. EMBO J 3:2192, 1984.

156. Miller RH, Robinson WS. Common evolutionary origin of hepatitis B virus and retroviruses. Proc Natl Acad Sci 83:2531, 1986.

157. Summers J, Mason WS. Replication of the genome of a hepatitis B-like virus by reverse transcription of an RNA intermediate. Cell 29:403, 1982.

158. Mason WS, Aldrich C, Summers J, et al. A symmetric replication of duck hepatitis B virus DNA in liver cells (free minus-strand DNA). Proc Natl Acad Sci USA 79:3997, 1982.

159. Miller RH, Robinson WS. Hepatitis B viral forms in infected liver. Virology 139:53, 1984.

160. Miller RH, Tran C-T, Robinson WS. Hepatitis B virus particles of plasma and liver contain viral DNA-RNA hybrid molecules. Virology 139:53, 1984.

161. Miller RH, Marion PL, Robinson WS. Hepatitis B viral DNA-RNA hybrid molecules in particles from infected liver are converted to viral DNA molecules during an endogenous DNA polymerase reaction. Virology 139:64, 1984.

162. Yoffe B, Noonan CA, Melnick JL, et al. Hepatitis B virus DNA in mononuclear cells and analysis of cell subsets for presence of replicative intermediates of viral DNA. J Infect Dis 153:471, 1985.

163. Korba BD, Wells F, Tennant BC, et al. Hepadnavirus infection of peripheral blood lymphocytes *in vivo*: woodchuck and chimpanzee models of viral hepatitis. J Virol 58:1, 1986.

164. Brechot C, Hadchouel M, Scotto J, et al. State of hepatitis B virus DNA in hepatocytes of patients with hepatitis B surface antigen-positive and -negative liver disease. Proc Natl Acad Sci 78:3906, 1981.

165. Kam W, Rall L, Smuckler E, et al. Hepatitis B viral DNA in liver and serum of asymptomatic carriers. Proc Natl Acad Sci USA 79:7522, 1982.

166. Varmus H, Swanstrom R. Replication of retroviruses. In: Weiss R, Teich N, Varmus H, et al., eds. RNA Tumor Viruses. New York, Cold Spring Harbor Press, 1982:369.

167. Koshy R, Maupas P, Muller R, et al. Detection of hepatitis B virus-specific DNA in the genomes of human hepatocellular carcinoma and liver cirrhosis tissues. J Gen Virol 57:95, 1981.

168. Miller RH, Lee SC, Liaw YF, et al. Hepatitis B viral DNA in infected human liver and in hepatocellular carcinoma. J Infect Dis 151:1081, 1985.

169. Brechot C, Pourcel C, Louise A, et al. Presence of integrated hepatitis B virus DNA sequences in cellular DNA of human hepatocellular carcinoma. Nature (London) 286:533, 1980.

170. Brechot C, Pourcel C, Louise A, et al. Detection of hepatitis B virus DNA sequences in human hepatocellular carcinoma in an integrated form. Prog Med Virol 27:99, 1981.

171. Brechot C, Pourcel C, Hadchouel M, et al. State of hepatitis B virus DNA in liver diseases. Hepatology 2:27S, 1982.

172. Shafritz DA, Shouval D, Sherman H, et al. Integration of hepatitis B virus DNA into the genome of liver cells in chronic liver disease and hepatocellular carcinoma. N Engl Med J 305:1067, 1981.

173. Shafritz D, Kew M. Indentification of integrated hepatitis B virus DNA sequences in human hepatocellular carcinoma. Hepatology 1:1, 1981.

174. Shafritz DA. Hepatitis B virus DNA molecules in the liver of HBsAg carriers: mechanistic considerations in the pathogenesis of hepatocellular carcinoma. Hepatology 2:35S, 1982.

175. Chen DS, Hoyer BH, Nelson J, et al. Detection and properties of

hepatitis B virus DNA in liver tissue from patients with hepatocellular carcinoma. Hepatology 2:425, 1982.

176. Hino O, Kitagawa T, Koike K, et al. Detection of hepatitis B virus DNA in hepatocellular carcinoma in Japan. Hepatology 4:90, 1984.

177. Summers J, Smolec JM, Werner BG, et al. Hepatitis B virus and woodchuck hepatitis virus are members of a novel class of DNA viruses. In: Viruses in Naturally Occurring Tumors. Cold Spring Harbor Conference on Cell proliferation VII. New York, Cold Spring Harbor Press, 1980:459.

178. Ogston CW, Jonak GJ, Rogler CE, et al. Cloning and structural analysis of integrated woodchuck hepatitis virus sequences from hepatocellular carcinomas of woodchucks. Cell 29:385, 1982.

179. Mitamura K, Hoyer B, Ponzetto A, et al. Woodchuck hepatitis virus DNA in woodchuck liver tissue. Hepatology 2:47A, 1982.

180. Marion PL, Salazar FH, Alexander JJ, et al. The state of hepatitis B viral DNA in a human hepatoma cell line. J Virol 33:795, 1980.

181. Chakroborty P, Ruiz-Opzao N, Shouval D, et al. Identification of integrated hepatitis B virus DNA and expression of viral DNA in an HBsAg producing human hepatocellular carcinoma cell line. Nature 286:531, 1980.

182. Edman J, Gray P, Valenzuela P, et al. Integration of pattern of hepatitis B virus DNA sequences in human hepatoma cell lines. Nature (London) 286:535, 1980.

183. Twist EM, Clark HF, Aden AP, et al. Integration pattern of hepatitis B virus DNA sequences in human hepatoma cell lines. J Virol 37:239, 1981.

184. Miller RH, Robinson WS. Integrated hepatitis B virus DNA sequences specifying the major viral core polypeptide are methylated in PLC/PRF/5 cells. Proc Natl Acad Sci USA 80:2534, 1983.

185. Fung Y-KT, Lai CL, Todd D, et al. An amplified domain of cellular DNA containing a subgenomic insert of hepatitis B virus DNA in a human hepatoma. In: Vyas G, Alter H, Hoofnagle J, eds. The 1984 International Symposium on Viral Hepatitis.

186. Fung Y-KT, Lai CL, Lok A, et al. Analysis of HBV-associated human hepatocellular carcinoma for oncogene expression and structure rearrangement. In: Molecular Biology of Hepatitis B Viruses. Cold Spring Harbor, New York, Cold Spring Harbor Press 1985:80.

187. Matsubara K, Nagaya A, Fukushige T, et al. Studies with junctions between integrated HBV-DNA and host chromosomal DNA. In: Molecular Biology of Hepatitis B Viruses. Cold Spring Harbor, New York, Cold Spring Harbor Press 1985:82.

188. Standring D, Rall L, Laub O, et al. Hepatitis B virus encodes a DNA polymerase III transcript. Molec Cell Biol 3:1774, 1983.

189. Dejean A, Brechot C, Tiollais P, et al. Characterization of integrated hepatitis B viral DNA cloned from a human hepatoma and the hepatoma-derived cell line PLC/PRF/5. Proc Natl Acad Sci USA 80:2505, 1983; 81:5350, 1984.

190. LeBouvier GL. The heterogenicity of Australia antigen. J Infect Dis 123:671, 1971.

191. Bancroft WH, Mundo FK, Russel PK. Detection of additional determinants of hepatitis B antigen. J Immunol 109:842, 1972.

192. Courouce-Pauty AM, Soulier JP. Further data on HBs antigen subtypes—geographical distribution. Vox Sang 27:533, 1974.

193. Courouce AM, Holland PV, Muller JY, et al. HBsAg antigen subtypes. Proceedings of the International Workshop on HBs antigen subtypes. Bibli Haematologica 42:1, 1976.

194. Purcell RH, Gerin JL. Hepatitis B subunit vaccine: a preliminary report of safety and efficacy tests in chimpanzees. Am J Med Sci 270:395, 1975.

195. Seef LB, Zimmerman HJ, Wright EC, et al. Efficacy of hepatitis B immune serum globulin after accidental exposure: preliminary report of the Veterans Administration Cooperative Study. Lancet 2:938, 1975.

196. Redeker AG, Mosley JW, Gocke DJ, et al. Hepatitis B immune globulin as a prophylactic measure for spouses exposed in acute type B hepatitis. N Engl J Med 293:1055, 1975.

197. Le Bouvier GL. Seroanalysis by immunodiffusion: the subtypes of type B hepatitis virus. In: Vyas GN, Perkins A, Schmid R, eds. Hepatitis and Blood Transfusions. New York, Grune & Stratton, 1972:97.

198. Mosley JW, Edwards VM, Meihaus JE, et al. Subdeterminants d and y of hepatitis B antigen as epidemiologic markers. Am J Epidemiol 95:529, 1972.

199. Gerin JL, Holland PV, Purcell RH. Australia antigen: large scale purification from human serum and biochemical studies of its proteins. J Virol 17:569, 1971.

200. Kaplan PM, Ford EC, Purcell RH, et al. Demonstration of subpopulations of Dane particles. J Virol 17:885, 1976.

201. Hruska JF, Robinson WS. The proteins of hepatitis B Dane particle cores. J Med Virol 1:119, 1977.

202. Kim CY, Bissell DM. Stability of the lipid and protein of hepatitis-associated (Australia) antigen. J Infect Dis 123:470, 1971.

203. Steiner S, Huebner MT, Dreesman GR. Major polar lipids of hepatitis B antigen preparations: evidence for the presence of glycosphingolipid. J Virol 14:572, 1974.

204. Gerin GL. Structure of hepatitis B antigen (HBeAg). In: Robinson WS, Fox CF, eds. Mechanisms of Virus Diseases. Menlo Park, CA, WA Benjamin, 1974:215.

205. Dreesman GR, Chairez R, Suarez M, et al. Production of antibody to individual polypeptides derived from purified hepatitis B antigen. J Virol 16:508, 1975.

206. Shish JW, Gerin JL. Immunochemistry of hepatitis antibodies to the constituent polypeptides. J Immunol 115:634, 1975.

207. Gold JWM, Shih JW, Purcell RH, et al. Characterization of antibodies to the structural polypeptides of HBsAg: evidence for subtype-specific determinants. J Immunol 117:1404, 1976.

208. Shih JW, Gerin JL. Proteins of hepatitis B surface antigen. J Virol 21:347, 1976.

209. Vyas GN, Rao K, Ibrahim AB. Australia antigen (hepatitis B antigen): a conformational antigen dependent on disulfide bonds. Science 178:1300, 1972.

210. Dreesman GR, Hollinger FB, McCombs RM, et al. Alteration of hepatitis B antigen (HB Ag) determinants by reduction and alkylation. J Gen Virol 19:129, 1973.

211. Hermann KH, Goldman U, Schwarz W, et al. Large surface proteins of hepatitis B virus containing preS square. J Virol 52:396, 1984.

212. Neurath AR, Kent SBH, Strick N, et al. HBV contains preS gene coded domains. Nature 315:154, 1985.

213. Szmuness W, Stevens CE, Harley EJ, et al. Hepatitis B vaccine: demonstration of efficacy in a controlled clinical trial in a high-risk population in the United States. N Engl J Med 303:835, 1980.

214. Beasley RP, Hwang LY, Lee CY, et al. Prevention of perinatally transmitted hepatitis B virus infection with hepatitis B immune globulin and hepatitis B vaccine. Lancet 2:1099, 1983.

215. Gerin JL, Alexander H, Shih JW, et al. Chemically synthesized peptides of hepatitis B surface antigen duplicate the d/y specificities and induce subtype-specific antibodies in chimpanzees. Proc Natl Acad Sci USA 80:236, 1983.

216. Prince AM, Ikram H, Hopp TP. Hepatitis B virus vaccine: identification of HBsAg/a and HBsAg/d but not HBsAg/y subtype antigenic determinants on synthetic immunogenic peptide. Immunology 79:579, 1982.

217. Brown SE, Howard CE, Zuckerman AJ, et al. Affinity of ab response in man to hepatitis B vaccine determined by synthetic peptide. Lancet 2:184, 1984.

218. Bhatnager PK, Papas E, Blum HE, et al. Immune response to synthetic peptide analogues of hepatitis B surface antigen-specific for the a determinant. Proc Natl Acad Sci USA 79:4400, 1982.

219. Kennedy RC, Dreesman GR, Sparrow JT, et al. Inhibition of a common human anti-hepatitis B surface antigen idiotype by cyclic synthetic peptide. J Virol 46:653, 1983.

220. Gerin JL, Alexander H, Shi JW, et al. Chemical synthesis of peptides of HBsAg duplicate the d/4 specificities and induce subtype specific ab in chimpanzees. Proc Natl Assoc Sci 80:2365, 1983.

221. Neurath AR, Strick N, Kent SB, et al. Identification and chemical synthesis of a host cell receptor binding site on hepatitis B virus. Cell 45:429, 1986.

222. Milich DR, Thornton GB, Neurath AR, et al. Enhanced immunogenicity of the preS region of HBsAg. Science 228:1195, 1986.

223. Kent S. Unpublished results.

224. Burrell CJ, Leadbetter G, MacKay P, et al. Tryptic cleavage of antibody binding sites from hepatitis B surface antigen particles. J Gen Virol 33:41, 1976.

225. Neurath AR, Prince AM, Giacalone J. Large scale purification of hepatitis B surface antigen using affinity chromatography. Experimentia 34:414, 1978.

226. Neurath AR, Hashimoto N, Prince AM. Sialyl residues in determining the life span of the antigen in serum and in eliciting an immunological response. J Gen Virol 27:81, 1975.

227. Neurath AR, Strick N, Huang CY. Properties of delipidated hepatitis B surface antigen (HBsAg) and preparation of its proteolytic cleavage fragments carrying HBsAg antigenic determinants. Intervirology 10:265, 1978.

228. Millman I, Hutanen H, Merino F, et al. Australia antigen: physical and chemical properties. Res Commun Chem Pathol Pharmacol 2:667, 1971.

229. Neurath AR, Prince AM, Lippin A. Hepatitis B antigen: Antigenic site related to human serum proteins revealed by affinity chromatography. Proc Natl Acad Sci USA 71:2663, 1974.

229a. Redeker AC. Viral hepatitis—clinical aspects. Am J Med Sci 270:9, 1975.

230. Burrell CJ. Host components in hepatitis B antigen. J Gen Virol 27:117, 1975.

231. Shih JWK, Tan PL, Gerin JL. Relationship of large hepatitis B surface antigen polypeptide to human serum albumin. Infect Immun 28:459, 1980.

232. Hollinger FB, Dreesman GR. Hepatitis B virus antigen and albumin receptors. Gastroenterology 76:641, 1979.

233. Imai M, Yanase Y, Nojiri T, et al. A receptor for polymerized human and chimpanzee albumins on hepatitis B virus particles occurring with HBeAg. Gastroenterology 76:242, 1979.

234. Neurath AR, Strick N. Radioimmunoassay of albumin-binding sites associated with HBsAg: correlation of results with the presence of e-antigen in serum. Intervirology 11:128, 1979.

235. Machida A, Kishimoto S, Ohnuma H, et al. A polypeptide containing 55 amino acid residues coded by the pre-S region of hepatitis B virus deoxyribonucleic acid bears the receptor for polymerized human as well as chimpanzee albumins. Gastroenterology 86:910, 1984.

236. Yu MW, Finlayson JS, Shih JW. Interaction between various polymerized human albumins and hepatitis B surface antigen. J Virol 55:736, 1985.

237. Neurath AR, Trepo C, Chen M, et al. Identification of additional antigenic sites on Dane particles and tubular forms of hepatitis B surface antigen. J Gen Virol 30:277, 1976.

238. Takahashi K, Yamashita S, Imai M, et al. Failure of antibody to e antigen to precipitate DNe particles containing DNA polymerase activity and hepatitis B core antigen. J Gen Virol 38:431, 1978.

239. Gerin JL, Shih JWK, McCuliffe VJ, et al. Antigens of the hepatitis B virus: failure to detect HBeAg on the surfaces of HBsAg forms. J Gen Virol 38:561, 1978.

240. Werner BG, Smolec JM, Snyder RM, et al. Serologic relationship of woodchuck hepatitis virus and human hepatitis B virus. J Virol 32:314, 1979.

241. Gerlich W, Feitelson M, Marion PL, et al. Structural relationships between the surface antigens of ground squirrel hepatitis virus and human hepatitis B virus. J Virol 36:787, 1980.

242. Hoofnagle JH, Gerety RJ, Barker LS. Antibody to hepatitis B virus core in man. Lancet 2:869, 1973.

243. Robinson WS, Lutwick LI. Hepatitis B virus: a cause of persistent virus infection in man. In: Baltimore D, Huang A, Fox CF, eds: Animal Virology. New York, Academic Press, 1976:787.

244. Magnius LO, Espmark JA. New specificities in Australia antigen-positive sera distinct from Le Bouvier determinants. J Immunol 109:1017, 1972.

245. Magnius LO. Characterization of a new antigen-antibody system associated with hepatitis B. Clin Exp Immunol 20:209, 1975.

246. Williams A, LeBouvier G. Heterogeneity and thermolability of "e." Bibl Haematologica 42:71, 1976.

247. Tabor E, Gerety RJ, Barker LF. Detection of e antigen during acute and chronic hepatitis B virus infections in chimpanzees. J Infect Dis 136:541, 1977.

248. Miller DJ, Williams AE, LeBouvier GL, et al. Hepatitis B in hemodialysis patients: significance of HBeAg. Gastroenterology 74:1208, 1978.

249. Courouce-Pauty AM, Plancon A. e Antigen and anti-e in two categories of chronic carriers of hepatitis B surface antigen. Vox Sang 34:231, 1978.

250. Murphy B, Tabor E, McAuliffe V, et al. Third component HBeAg/3, of hepatitis Be antigen system identified by three different double diffusion techniques. J Clin Microbiol 8:349, 1978.

251. Budkowska A, Shih JWK, Gerin JL. Immunochemistry and polypeptide composition of hepatitis B core antigen (HBcAg). J Immunol 118:1300, 1977.

252. Uy A, Bruss V, Gerlich WH, et al. Pre-core sequence of hepatitis B virus inducing e antigen and membrane association of the viral core protein. Virology 155:89, 1986.

253. Neurath AR, Strick N. Association of hepatitis B e-antigen (HBeAg) determinants with the core of Dane particles. J Gen Virol 42:645, 1979.

254. Budkowska A, Kalinowska B, Nowoslowski A. Identification of two HBeAg subspecificities revealed by chemical treatment and enzymatic digestion of liver-derived HBcAg. J Immunol 123:1415, 1979.

255. Ohori H, Onodera S, Ishida N. Demonstration of hepatitis B e antigen (HBeAg) in association with intact Dane particles. J Gen Virol 43:423, 1979.

256. Stahl S, MacKay P, Magazin M, et al. Hepatitis B virus core antigen: synthesis in Escherichia coli and application in diagnosis. Proc Natl Acad Sci USA 79:1606, 1982.

257. Takahashi K, Imai M, Miyakawa Y, et al. Duality of hepatitis B e antigen in serum of persons infected with hepatitis B virus: Evidence for non-identity of e antigen and immunoglobulin. Proc Natl Acad Sci USA 75:1952, 1978.

258. Takahashi K, Miyakawa Y, Gotanda T, et al. Shift from free "small" hepatitis B e antigen to IgG-bound "large" form in the circulation

of human beings and a chimpanzee acutely infected with hepatitis B virus. Gastroenterology 77:1193, 1979.

259. Neurath AR, Szmuness W, Stevens CE, et al. Radioimmunoassay and some properties of human antibodies to hepatitis B core antigen. J Gen Virol 38:549, 1978.

260. Miller RH. Proteolytic self cleavage of hepatitis B virus core may generate serum e antigen. Science (In press.)

261. Hindman SH, Gravelle CR, Murphy BL, et al. "e" Antigen, Dane particles, and serum DNA polymerase activity in HBsAg carriers. Ann Intern Med 85:458, 1976.

262. Alter HJ, Seeff LB, Kaplan PM, et al. Type B hepatitis: the infectivity of blood positive for e antigen and DNA polymerase after accidental needlestick exposure. N Engl J Med 295:909, 1976.

263. Takahashi K, Imai M, Tsuda F, et al. Association of Dane particles with e antigen in the serum of asymptomatic carriers of hepatitis B surface antigen. J Immunol 117:102, 1976.

264. Nordenfeldt E, Andren-Sandberg M. Dane particle associated DNA polymerase and e antigen: relation to chronic hepatitis among carriers of hepatitis B surface antigen. J Infect Dis 134:85, 1976.

265. Maynard JE, Hartwell WV, Berquist KR. Hepatitis associated antigen in chimpanzees. J Infect Dis 126:660, 1971.

266. World Health Organization. Viral hepatitis: Report of a scientific group. WHO Tech Rep Ser 512, 1973.

267. Lichter EA. Chimpanzee antibodies to Australia antigen. Nature 224:810, 1969.

268. Prince AM. Infection of chimpanzees with hepatitis B virus. In Vyas GN, Perkins HA, Schmid R, eds.: Hepatitis and Blood Transfusions. New York, Grune & Stratton, 1972:403.

269. Markenson JH, Gerety RJ, Hoofnagle JH. Effects of cyclophosphamide on hepatitis B virus infection and challenge in chimpanzees. J Infect Dis 131:79, 1975.

270. Bancroft WH, Snitbhan R, Scott RM, et al. Transmission of hepatitis B virus to gibbons by exposure to human saliva containing hepatitis B surface antigen. J Infect Dis 135:79, 1977.

271. Barker LF, Maynard JE, Purcell RH, et al. Viral hepatitis, type B, in experimental animals. Am J Med Sci 270:189, 1975.

272. London TW, Milman I, Sutnick AI. Transmission, replication and passage of Australia antigen in African green monkeys (vervets). Clin Res 18:636, 1970.

273. London WT, Alter HJ, Lander J. Serial transmission in rhesus monkeys of an agent related to hepatitis-associated antigen. J Infect Dis 125:382, 1972.

274. Nowoslawski A, Krawczyuski K, Brzosko WJ. Tissue localization of Australia antigen immune complexes in acute and chronic hepatitis and liver cirrhosis. Am J Pathol 68:31, 1972.

275. Shikata T. Australia antigen in liver tissue. Jpn J Exp Med 43:231, 1973.

276. Murphy BL, Peterson JM, Ebert JW. Immunofluorescent localization of hepatitis B antigens in chimpanzee tissues. Intervirology 6:207, 1975.

277. Johnson PJ, Wansbrough-Jones MH, Portmann B. Familial HBsAg positive hepatoma: treatment with orthotopic liver transplantation and specific immunoglobulin. Br Med J 1:216, 1978.

278. Hoefs JC, Renner IG, Ashcavai M, et al. Hepatitis B surface antigen in pancreatic and biliary secretion. Gastroenterology 79:191, 1980.

279. Karasawa T, Tsukagoshi S, Yoshimura M, et al. Light microscopic localization of hepatitis B virus antigens in the human pancreas: possibility of multiplication of hepatitis B virus in the human pancreas. Gastroenterology 81:998, 1981.

280. Romet-Lemonne JL, McLane MF, Elfassi E, et al. Hepatitis B virus infection in cultured human lymphoblastoid cells. Science 221:667, 1983.

281. Lie-Injo LE, Balasegaram M, Lopez CG, et al. Hepatitis B virus DNA in liver and white blood cells of patients with hepatoma. DNA 2:301, 1983.

282. Ogra PL. Immunologic aspects of hepatitis associated antigens and antibody in body fluids. J Immunol 11:1197, 1973.

283. Tuttleman JS, Pugh JC, Summers JW. In vitro experimental infection of primary duck hepatocyte cultures with DHBV. J Virol 58:17, 1986.

284. Gudat F, Bianchi O, Sonnabend W. Pattern of core and surface expression in liver tissue reflects state of specific immune response in hepatitis B. Lab Invest 32:1, 1975.

285. Ray MB, Desmet VI, Bradburne AF. Distribution patterns of hepatitis B surface antigen (HBsAg in liver of hepatitis patients). Gastroenterology 71:462, 1976.

286. Almeida JD, Watterson AP, Trowel JM, et al. The finding of virus-like particles in two Australia-antigen-positive human livers. Microbios 2:145, 1970.

287. Huang SA. Hepatitis associated antigen hepatitis: an electronmicroscopic study of virus-like particles in liver cells. Am J Pathol 64:783, 1971.

288. Camamia F, DeBac C, Ricci G. Virus-like particles within hepatocytes of Australia antigen carriers. Am J Dis Child 123:309, 1972.

289. Scullard GH, Pollard RB, Smith JL, et al. Antiviral treatment of chronic hepatitis B virus infection. I. Changes in viral markers with interferon combined with adenine arabinoside. J Infect Dis 143:772, 1981.

290. Krugman S, Overby LR, Mushahwar IK, et al. Viral hepatitis, type B: studies on natural history and prevention reexamined. N Engl Med J 300:101, 1979.

291. Hoofnagle JH, Seeff LB, Bales ZB, et al. Serologic responses in hepatitis B. In: Vyas GN, Cohen SN, Schmid R, eds. Viral Hepatitis: A Contemporary Assessment of Etiology, Epidemiology, Pathogenesis and Prevention. Philadelphia, Franklin Institute Press, 1978:219.

291a. Redeker AG. Viral hepatitis: clinical aspects. Am J Med Sci 270:9–16, 1975.

292. Shulman RN. Hepatitis-associated antigen. Am J Med 49:669, 1971.

293. Takahashi K, Fukuda M, Baba K, et al. Determination of e antigen and antibody to e by means of passive hemagglutination method. J Immunol 119:1556, 1977.

294. Aikawa T, Sairenji H, Furuta S, et al. Seroconversion from hepatitis B e antigen to anti-HBe in acute hepatitis B virus infection. N Engl J Med 298:439, 1978.

295. Fields HA, Bradley DW, Davis C, et al. Radioimmunoassay for the detection of hepatitis B e antigen (HBeAg) and its antibody (anti-HBe). J Immunol 121:273, 1978.

296. Myakawa Y, Akahane Y, Gotand T. Application of microtiter solid phase radioimmunoassay to the determination of hepatitis B "e" antigen. J Immunol 122:273, 1979.

297. Ling C, Mushahwar IK, Overby LR, et al. Hepatitis B e antigen and its correlation with other serologic markers in chimpanzees. Infect Immun 24:352, 1979.

298. Aldershvile J, Frosner GG, Nielsen JO, et al. Hepatitis B e antigen and antibody radioimmunoassay in acute hepatitis B surface antigen-positive hepatitis. J Infect Dis 141:293, 1980.

299. Kaplan PM, Gerin JL, Alter HJ. Hepatitis B-specific DNA polymerase activity during post-transfusion hepatitis. Nature 249:762, 1974.

300. Krugman S, Hoofnagle JH, Gerety RJ, et al. Viral hepatitis type B: DNA polymerase activity and antibody to hepatitis B core antigen. N Engl J Med 290:1331, 1974.

301. Hansson BG. Age and sex-related distribution of antibodies to hepatitis B surface and core antigens in Swedish population. Acta Pathol Microbiol Scand Sect B 84:342, 1976.

302. Hansson BG. Persistence of antibody to hepatitis B core antigen. J Clin Microbiol 6:209, 1977.

303. Brzosko WJ, Mikulska B, Cianciara J, et al. Immunoglobulin classes of antibody to hepatitis B core antigen. J Infect Dis 132:1, 1975.

304. Cohen BJ. The IgM antibody responses to the core antigen of hepatitis B virus. J Med Virol 3:141, 1978.

305. Neimeijer P, Gips CH. Antibodies and the infectivity of serum in hepatitis B. N Engl J Med 299:958, 1978.

306. Gerlich WH, Luer W, Thomssen R. Diagnosis of acute and inapparent hepatitis B virus infections by measurement of IgM antibody to hepatitis B core antigen. J Infect Dis 142:95, 1980.

307. Gocke DJ. Extrahepatic manifestations of viral hepatitis. A J Med Sci 270:49, 1975.

308. Almeida JD, Waterson AP. Immune complexes in hepatitis. Lancet 2:983, 1969.

309. Madalinski L, Bragiel I. HBsAg immune complexes in the course of infection with hepatitis B virus. Clin Exp Immunol 36:371, 1979.

310. Lambert PH, Tribollet E, Celada A, et al. Quantitation of immunoglobulin associated HBs antigen in patients with acute and chronic hepatitis, in healthy carriers, and in polyarteritis nodosa. J Clin Lab Immunol 3:1, 1980.

311. Lander JJ, Giles JP, Purcell RH. Viral hepatitis type B (MS-2 strain): detection of antibody after primary infection. N Engl J Med 283:303, 1970.

312. Barker LF, Maynard JE, Purcell RH, et al. Hepatitis B virus infection in chimpanzees: titration of subtypes. J Infect Dis 132:451, 1975.

313. Purcell RH, Gerin JL. Hepatitis B subunit vaccine: a preliminary report of safety and efficacy tests in chimpanzees. Am J Med Sci 270:395, 1975.

314. Seef LB, Wright EC, Zimmerman HJ, et al. Type B hepatitis after needle-stick exposure: prevention with hepatitis B immune globulin. A final report of the Veterans Administration Cooperative Study. Ann Intern Med 88:285, 1978.

315. Brechot C, Hadchouel M, Scotto J, et al. State of hepatitis B virus DNA in hepatocytes of patients with hepatitis B surface antigen-positive and -negative liver disease. Proc Natl Acad Sci 78:3906, 1981.

316. Hoofnagle JH. Hepatitis B surface antigen (HBsAg) and antibody (anti-HBs). In: Bianchi L, Gerok W, Sickinger K, et al., eds. Virus and the Liver. Lancaster, MTP Press, 1980:27.

317. Nielsen JO, Nielsen MH, Elling P. Differential distribution of Australia-antigen-associated particles in patients with liver disease and normal carriers. N Engl J Med 288:484, 1973.

318. Robinson WS. DNA and DNA polymerase in the core of Dane particles. Am J Med Sci 270:151, 1975.
319. Greenberg HB, Pollard RB, Lutwixk LI, et al. Effect of human leukocyte interferon on hepatitis B virus infection in patients with chronic active hepatitis. N Engl J Med 295:517, 1976.
320. Kryger P, Mathiesen LR, Aldershvile J, et al. Presence and meaning of anti-HBc IgM as determined by ELISA in patients with acute type B hepatitis and healthy HBsAg carriers. Hepatology 1:233, 1981.
321. Bonino F, Hoyer B, Moriarty A, et al. Hepatitis B virus DNA in the sera of HBsAg carriers: a marker of active HBV replication in the liver. Gastroenterology 79:1009, 1980.
322. Aldershvile J, Skinhoj P, Frosner GG, et al. The expression pattern of hepatitis B e antigen and antibody in different ethnic and clinical groups of hepatitis B surface antigen carriers. J Infect Dis 142:18, 1980.
323. Eleftheriou N, Heathcoate J, Thomas HC, et al. Incidence and clinical significance of e antigen and antibody in acute and chronic liver diseases. Lancet 2:1171, 1975.
324. Smith JL, Murphy BL, Auslander MO, et al. Studies of the "e" antigen in acute and chronic hepatitis. Gastroenterology 71:208, 1976.
325. Nielsen JO, Dietrichson O, Juhl E. Incidence and meaning of the "e" determinant among hepatitis-B-antigen positive patients with acute and chronic liver diseases. Lancet 2:913, 1974.
326. Fay O, Tanno H, Ronocoroni M, et al. Prognostic implications of the e antigen of hepatitis B virus. JAMA 238:2501, 1977.
327. Hess G, Arnold W, Shih JWK, et al. Expression of hepatitis B virus-specific markers in asymptomatic hepatitis B surface antigen carriers. Infect Immun 17:550, 1977.
328. Andres LL, Sawhney VK, Scullard GH, et al. Dane particle DNA polymerase and HBeAg: impact on clinical, laboratory, and histologic findings in hepatitis B-associated chronic liver disease. Hepatology 1:583, 1981.
329. Beasley RP, Trepo C, Stevens CE, et al. The e antigen and vertical transmission of hepatitis B surface antigen. Am J Epidemiol 105:94, 1977.
330. Okada K, Kainiyama I, Inometa M, et al. e Antigen and anti-e in the serum of asymptomatic carrier mothers as indicators of positive and negative transmission of hepatitis B virus in their infants. N Engl J Med 294:746, 1976.
331. Perrillo RP, Gelb L, Campbell C, et al. Hepatitis B e antigen, DNA polymerase activity, and infection of household contacts with hepatitis B virus. Gastroenterology 76:1319, 1979.
332. Koshy R, Maupas P, Muller R, et al. Detection of hepatitis B virus-specific DNA in the genomes of human hepatocellular carcinoma and liver cirrhosis tissue. J Gen Virol 57:95, 1981.
333. Norkrans G, Nordenfeldt E, Hermodsson ES, et al. Long-term follow-up of chronic hepatitis patients with HBsAg, HBeAg and Dane particle associated DNA polymerase. Scand J Infect Dis 12:159, 1980.
334. Zuckerman AJ, Taylor PE. Persistence of the serum hepatitis (SH-Australia) antigen for many years. Nature 223:81, 1969.
335. Realdi G, Alberti A, Rugge M, et al. Seroconversion from hepatitis B e antigen to anti-HBe in chronic hepatitis B virus infection. Gastroenterology 79:195, 1980.
336. Aikawa T, Seirenji S, Furuta S, et al. Seroconversion from hepatitis B e antigen to anti-HBe in acute hepatitis B virus infection. N Engl J Med 298:439, 1978.
337. Alberti A, Diana S, Scullard GM, et al. Full and empty Dane particles in chronic hepatitis virus infection: relationship to hepatitis B e antigen and presence of liver damage. Gastroenterology 75:869, 1978.
338. Hoofnagle JH, Seef LB, Dusheiko GM, et al. Seroconversion from hepatitis B e antigen to antibody during chronic type B hepatitis. Gastroenterology 79:1026, 1980.
339. Perrillo RP, Campbell CR, Saunders GE, et al. Spontaneous clearance and reactivation of HBV infection among male homosexuals with chronic type B hepatitis. Ann Intern Med 100:43, 1984.
340. Davis GL, Hoofnagle JH, Waggoner JG. Spontaneous reactivation of chronic hepatitis B virus infection. Gastroenterology 86:230, 1984.
341. Szmuness W, Prince AM, Brotman B. Hepatitis B antigen and antibody in blood donors: an epidemiologic study. J Infect Dis 127:17, 1973.
342. Helske T. Carriers of hepatitis B antigen and transfusion hepatitis in Finland. Scand J Haematol (Suppl) 22:1, 1974.
343. Sampliner RE, Hamilton FA, Iseri OA. The liver histology and frequency of clearance of the hepatitis B surface antigen in chronic carriers. Am J Med Sci 277:17, 1979.
344. Feinman SV, Cooter N, Sinclair JC, et al. Clinical and epidemiological significance of the HBsAg (Australia antigen): carrier state. Gastroenterology 68:113, 1975.
345. Szmuness W, Harley EJ, Ikran H, et al. Sociodemographic aspects of the epidemiology of hepatitis B. In: Vyas GN, Cohen SN, Schmid R, eds. Viral Hepatitis. Philadelphia, Franklin Institute Press, 1978:297.
346. Hollinger FB, Werch J, Melnick JL. A prospective study indicating
347. Alter HJ, Holland PV, Purcell RH. The emerging patterns of post-transfusion hepatitis. Am J Med Sci 270:329, 1975.
348. Hoofnagle JH, Seeff LB, Bales ZB, et al. The Veterans Administration Hepatitis Cooperative Study Group. Type B hepatitis after transfusion with blood containing antibody to hepatitis B core antigen. N Engl J Med 298:1379, 1978.
349. Bories P, Coursaget P, Degott C, et al. Antibody to hepatitis B core antigen in chronic active hepatitis. Br Med J 1:396, 1978.
350. Scullard GH, Smith CI, Merigan TC, et al. Effect of immunosuppressive therapy on viral markers in chronic active hepatitis B. Gastroenterology 81:978, 1981.
351. Nagington J, Cossart YE, Cohen BJ. Reactivation of hepatitis B after transplantation operations. Lancet 1:558, 1977.
352. Wands JR, Chura CM, Roll FJ, et al. Serial studies of hepatitis associated antigen and antibody in patients receiving anti-tumor chemotherapy for myeloproliferative and lymphoproliferative disorders. Gastroenterology 68:105, 1975.
353. Ringold G, Yamamoto KR, Thompkins GM, et al. Dexamethasone-mediated induction of mouse mammary tumor virus RNA: A system for studying glucocorticoid action. Cell 6:299, 1975.
354. Pollard RB, Smith JL, Beal A, et al. Effect of vidarabine on chronic hepatitis B virus infection. JAMA 239:1648, 1978.
355. Scullard GH, Andres LL, Greenberg HB, et al. Antiviral treatment of chronic hepatitis B virus infection: improvement in liver disease with interferon and adenine arabinoside. Hepatology 1:228, 1981.
356. Gold JWM, Alter HJ, Holland PV. Passive hemagglutination assay for antibody to subtypes of hepatitis B antigen. J Immunol 117:2260, 1976.
357. Koziol DE, Alter HJ, Dirchner JP. Development of HBsAg positive hepatitis despite previous existence of antibody to HBsAg. J Immunol 117:2260, 1976.
358. Sherertz RJ, Spindel E, Hoofnagle JH. Antibody to hepatitis B surface antigen may not always indicate immunity to hepatitis B virus infection. N Engl J Med 309:1519, 1983.
359. Linnemann CC, Askey PA. Susceptibility to hepatitis B despite high titer anti-HBs antibody. Lancet 1:346, 1984.
360. Trepo CG, Prince AM. Absence of complete homologous immunity to hepatitis B infection after massive exposure. Ann Intern Med 85:427, 1976.
361. Karvountzis GG, Mosley JW, Redecker AG. Serologic characterization of patients with two episodes of acute viral hepatitis. Am J Med 58:815, 1975.
362. Mosley JW. Hepatitis types B and non-B: epidemiologic background. JAMA 233:967, 1975.
363. Mosley JW, Redecker AG, Feinstone SM. Multiple hepatitis viruses in multiple attacks of acute viral hepatitis. N Engl J Med 296:75, 1977.
364. Tabor E, Gerety RJ. Possible role of immune response to hepatitis B core antigen in protection against hepatitis B infection. Lancet 1:172, 1984.
365. Murray K, Bruce SA, Hinnen A, et al. Hepatitis B virus antigens made in microbial cells immunise against viral infection. EMBO J 3:645, 1984.
366. Prince AM. Mechanism of protection against hepatitis B infection by immunization with hepatitis B virus cores. Lancet 1:512, 1984.
367. Peters RL. Viral hepatitis: a pathologic spectrum. Am J Med Sci 270:17, 1975.
368. Edgington TS, Chisari FV. Immunological aspects of hepatitis B infection. Am J Med Sci 270:213, 1975.
369. Dienstag JL, Khan AK, Klingenstein RJ, et al. Immunopathogenesis of liver disease associated with hepatitis B. In: Szmuness W, Alter HJ, Maynards JE, eds. Viral Hepatitis. Philadelphia, Franklin Institute Press, 1982:231.
370. Schweitzer IL, Dunn AEF, Peters RL, et al. Viral hepatitis in neonates and infants. Am J Med 55:762, 1973.
371. Tong MJ, Thursby M, Rakela J, et al. Studies of the maternal-infant transmission of the viruses which cause acute hepatitis. Gastroenterology 80:999, 1981.
372. London WT, DiFiglia M, Sutnick AI, et al. An epidemic of hepatitis in a chronic hemodialysis unit. N Engl J Med 281:571, 1969.
373. Nordenfeldt E, Lindholm T, Dailquist E. A hepatitis epidemic in a dialysis unit: occurrence of persistence of Australia-antigen among patients and staff. Acta Pathol Microbiol Scand (B) 78:692, 1970.
374. Good RA, Page AR. Fatal complications of virus hepatitis in two patients with agammaglobulinemia. Am J Med 29:804, 1960.
375. Dienstag JL, Bhan AK. Enhanced in vitro cell-mediated cytotoxicity in chronic hepatitis B virus infection: absence of specificity for virus-expressed antigen on target cell membranes. J Immunol 125:2269, 1980.
376. Eddleston ALWF, Mondelle M, Mieli-Vergani G, et al. Lymphocyte cytotoxicity to autologous hepatocytes in chronic hepatitis B virus infection. Hepatology 2:122s, 1982.
377. Naumov NW, Mondelli M, Alexander GJM, et al. Relationship be-

tween expression of hepatitis B virus antigens in isolated hepatocytes and autologous lymphocyte cytotoxicity in patients with chronic hepatitis B virus infection. Hepatology 4:13, 1984.

378. Lee WM, Reed WD, Osman CG, et al. Immune responses to the hepatitis B surface antigen and liver-specific lipoprotein in acute type B hepatitis. Gut 18:250, 1977.

379. Moussouros A, Cochrane AMG, Thomson AD. Transient lymphocyte mediated hepatotoxicity in acute viral hepatitis. Gut 16:835, 1975.

380. Chisari FW, Castle KL, Xavier C, et al. Functional properties of lymphocyte subpopulations in hepatitis B virus infection: I. Suppressor cell control of T-lymphocyte responsiveness. J Immunol 126:38, 1981.

381. Trepo CG, Magnius LO, Schaefer RA, et al. Detection of e antigen and antibody: correlations with hepatitis B surface and hepatitis B core antigen, liver disease, and outcome in hepatitis B infections. Gastroenterology 71:804, 1976.

382. Aldershvile J, Nielsen JO, Dietrichson O, et al. Long-term followup of e antigen (HBeAg) positive acute viral hepatitis. Scand J Gastroenterol 14:845, 1979.

383. Magnius LO, Lindholm A, Lundin P, et al. A new antigen-antibody system. Clinical significance in long term carriers of hepatitis B surface antigen. JAMA 231:356, 1975.

384. Reinicke V, Dybkjaer E, Poulsen H, et al. A study of Australia-antigen-positive blood donors and their recipients, with special reference to liver histology. N Engl J Med 286:867, 1972.

385. Macnab GM, Alexander JJ, Lecatsas G, et al. Hepatitis B surface antigen produced by a human hepatoma cell line. Br J Cancer 34:509, 1976.

386. Marion PL, Salazar FH, Alexander JJ, et al. Polypeptides of hepatitis B virus surface antigen produced by a human cell line. J Virol 32:796, 1979.

387. Yoakum GH, Korba BE, Lechner JR, et al. High-frequency transfection and cytopathology of hepatitis B virus core antigen gene in human cells. Science 222:385, 1983.

388. Obata H, Hayashi N, Motoike Y. A prospective study of development of hepatocellular carcinoma from liver cirrhosis with persistent hepatitis B virus infection. Int J Cancer 25:741, 1980.

389. Larouze B, London WT, Saimot G, et al. Host responses to hepatitis-B infection in patients with primary hepatic carcinoma and their families: a case-control study in Senegal, West Africa. Lancet 2:534, 1976.

390. Nishioka K, Hirayama T, Sekine T, et al. Australia antigen and hepatocellular carcinoma. Gann Monogr Can Res 14:167, 1973.

391. Steiner PE. Cancer of the liver and cirrhosis in trans-Saharan Africa and the United States of America. Cancer 13:1085, 1960.

392. Trichopoulos D, Violaki M, Sparros L, et al. Epidemiology of hepatitis B and primary hepatic carcinoma. Lancet 2:1038, 1975.

393. Peters RL. Pathology of hepatocellular carcinoma. In: Okuda K, Peters RL, eds. Hepatocellular Carcinoma, New York, John Wiley & Sons, 1976:107.

394. Kew MD. Hepatoma and HBV. In: Vyas GM, Cohen SN, Schmid R, eds. Viral Hepatitis: A Contemporary Assessment of Etiology, Epidemiology, Pathogenesis and Prevention. Philadelphia, Franklin Institute Press, 1978:439.

395. Marion PL, VanDavelaar MJ, Knight SS, et al. Hepatocellular carcinoma in ground squirrels persistently infected with ground squirrel hepatitis virus. Proc Natl Acad Sci USA 83:4543, 1986.

396. Robinson WS, Miller RH, Klote L, et al. Hepatitis B virus and hepatocellular carcinoma. In: Vyas GN, ed. Viral Hepatitis and Liver Disease. Orlando, Florida: Grune & Stratton, Inc., 1984:245.

397. Edman JC, Gray P, Valenzuela P, et al. Integration pattern of hepatitis B virus DNA sequences in human hepatoma cell lines. J Virol 37:238, 1981.

398. Gocke JD. Immune complex phenomena associated with hepatitis. In: Vyas GN, Cohen SN, Schmidt R, eds. Viral Hepatitis: A Contemporary Assessment. Philadelphia, Franklin Institute Press, 1978:277.

399. Schumacher HR, Gall EP. Arthritis in acute hepatitis and chronic active hepatitis: pathology of the synovial membrane with evidence for the presence of Australia antigen in synovial membranes. Am J Med 57:655, 1974.

400. Wands JR, Mann EA, Isselbacher KJ. The pathogenesis of arthritis associated with acute hepatitis B surface antigen positive hepatitis. Complement activation and characterization of circulating immune complexes. J Clin Invest 55:930, 1975.

401. Gocke DJ, Hsu K, Morgan C, et al. Vasculitis in association with Australia antigen. J Exp Med 134:330s, 1971.

402. Fye KH, Becker MJ, Theofilopoulos AN, et al. Immune complexes in hepatitis B antigen associated polyarteritis nodosa: detection by antibody dependent cell mediate cytotoxicity in Raji cell assay. Am J Med 62:783, 1977.

403. Combes B, Stastny P, Shorey J, et al. Glomerulonephritis with deposition of Australia antigen-antibody complexes in glomerular basement membrane. Lancet 2:234, 1971.

404. Kohler PF, Croniln RE, Hammond WS. Chronic membranous glomerulonephritis caused by hepatitis B antigen-antibody immune complexes. Ann Intern Med 81:488, 1974.

405. Knieser WR, Jens EH, Howenthal DT, et al. Pathogenesis of renal disease associated with viral hepatitis. Arch Pathol 97:193, 1974.

406. Ozawa T, Levisohn P, Orsini E, McIntosh RH. Acute immune complex disease associated with hepatitis. Arch Pathol Lab Med 100:484, 1976.

407. McIntosh RH, Koss MN, Gocke DJ. The nature and incidence of cryoproteins in hepatitis B antigen (HBsAg) positive patients. J Med 45:23, 1976.

408. Gianotti F. Papular acrodermatitis of childhood: an Australia antigen disease. Arch Dis Child 48:794, 1973.

409. Ishimaru Y, Ishimaru H, Toda G, et al. An epidemic infantile papular acrodermatitis in Japan associated with hepatitis B surface antigen subtype ayw. Lancet 1:707, 1976.

410. Levo Y, Gorevic PD, Kassab HJ, et al. Association between hepatitis B virus and essential mixed cryoglobulinemia. N Engl J Med 296:1501, 1977.

411. Popp JW, Dienstag JL, Wands JR, et al. Essential mixed cryoglobulinemia without evidence for hepatitis B virus infection. Ann Intern Med 92:383, 1980.

412. Hagler L, Pastore RN, Bergin JJ. Aplastic anemia following viral hepatitis. Medicine 54:139, 1975.

413. Nakamura S, Sato T, Maeda T, et al. Viral hepatitis B and aplastic anemia. Tohoku J Exp Med 116:101, 1975.

414. Casciato DA, Klein CA, Kaplowitz N, et al. Aplastic anemia associated with type B viral hepatitis. Arch Intern Med 138:1557, 1978.

415. Hoofnagle JH. Type B viral hepatitis: virology, serology and clinical course. Semin Liver Dis 1:7, 1981.

416. Overby LR, Ling CM, Decker RH, et al. Serodiagnostic profiles of viral hepatitis. In: Szmuness W, Alter HJ, Maynard JE, eds. Viral Hepatitis: 1981 International Symposium. Philadelphia, Franklin Institute Press, 1982:169.

417. Aach RD, Alter HJ, Hollinger FB, et al. Risk of transfusing blood containing antibody to hepatitis B surface antigen. Lancet 2:190, 1974.

418. Renton PH, Wadsworth LD. Infectivity of blood containing hepatitis B antibody. Lancet 1:736, 1975.

419. Grady GF, Gitnick FL, Prince AM. Relation of e antigen to infectivity of HBsAg-positive inoculation among medical personnel. Lancet 2:492, 1976.

420. Stevens CE, Beasley RP, Tsui V, et al. Vertical transmission of hepatitis B antigen in Taiwan. N Engl J Med 292:771, 1975.

421. Levin ML, Maddrey CW, Wands JR. Hepatitis B transmission by dentists. JAMA 228:1139, 1974.

422. Wright RA. Hepatitis B and the HBsAg carrier: an outbreak related to sexual contact. JAMA 232:717, 1975.

423. Schweitzer IL, Edwards VM, Brezina M. E antigen in HBsAg-carrier mothers. N Engl J Med 293:940, 1975.

424. Berquist KR, Maynard JE, Murphy BL. Infectivity of serum containing HBsAg and antibody to e antigen. Lancet 1:1026, 1976.

425. Centers for Disease Control. Inactivated hepatitis B virus vaccine. Morbid Mortal Weekly Rep 31:318, 1982.

426. Holland PV. Available methods to further reduce post-transfusion hepatitis. In: Szmuness W, Alter HJ, Maynard JE, eds. Viral Hepatitis. Philadelphia, Franklin Institute Press, 1982:563.

427. Lander JJ, Holland PV, Alter HJ, et al. Antibody to hepatitis-associated antigen. Frequency and pattern of response as detected by radioimmunoprecipitation. JAMA 220:1079–1081, 1972.

428. Cherubin CE, Purcell RH, Landers JJ, et al. Acquisition of antibody to hepatitis B antigen in three socioeconomically different medical populations. Lancet 2:149, 1972.

429. Blumberg BS, Friedlander JS, Woodside A, et al. Hepatitis and Australia antigen: autosomal recessive inheritance of susceptibility to infection in humans. Proc Natl Acad Sci 62:1108, 1969.

430. Grossman RA, Benenson MW, Scott RM, et al. An epidemiologic study of hepatitis B virus in Bangkok, Thailand. Am J Epidemiol 101:144, 1975.

431. Hillis WD, Hillis A, Bias WB, et al. Association of hepatitis B surface antigenemia with HLA locus B specificities. N Engl J Med 296:1310, 1977.

432. Stevens EC, Beasley RP. Lack of an autosomal recessive genetic influence in the vertical transmission of hepatitis B antigen. Nature 260:715, 1976.

433. Patterson MJ, Hourani MR, Mayor GH, et al. HLA antigens and hepatitis B virus. N Engl J Med 297:1124, 1977.

434. Szmuness W, Stevens CE, Ikram H, et al. Prevalence of hepatitis B virus infection and hepatocellular carcinoma in Chinese-Americans. J Infect Dis 137:822, 1978.

435. Mosley JW. Epidemiologic implications of changing trends in type A and type B hepatitis. In: Vyas GN, Perkins HA, Schmid R, eds. Hepatitis and Blood Transfusion. New York, Grune & Stratton, 1972:349.

436. Blumberg BS. Australia antigen: the history of its discovery with comments on genetic and family aspects. In: Vyas GN, Perkins HA, Schmid R, eds. Hepatitis and Blood Transfusion. New York, Grune & Stratton, 1972:63.

437. Blumberg BS, Sutnick AI, London WT, et al. Sex distribution of Australia antigen. Arch Intern Med 130:231, 1972.

438. London WT, Drew JS, Lustbader DE, et al. Host response to hepatitis B infection in patients in a chronic hemodialysis unit. Kidney Int 12:51, 1977.

439. Krugman S. Hepatitis B immune globulin. In: Vyas GN, Perkins HA, Schmid R, eds. Hepatitis and Blood Transfusion. New York, Grune & Stratton, 1972:349.

440. Szmuness W, Much WM, Prince AM, et al. On the role of sexual behavior in the spread of hepatitis B infection. Ann Intern Med 83:489, 1975.

441. Beasley RP, Hwang LY, Lin CC, et al. Incidence of hepatitis B virus infections in preschool children in Taiwan. J Infect Dis 147:185, 1982.

442. Mazzur S, Burget S, Blumberg BS. Geographical distribution of Australia antigen determinants d, y and w. Nature 247:38, 1974.

443. Bancroft WH, Holland PV, Mazzur S, et al. The geographical distribution of HBsAg subtypes. Bibl Haematol 42:42, 1976.

444. Alter JH, Purcell RH, Gerin JL. Transmission of hepatitis B to chimpanzees by hepatitis B surface antigen-positive saliva and semen. Infect Immun 16:928, 1977.

445. Center for Disease Control. Hepatitis transmitted by a human bite. Morbid Mortal Week Rep 23:24, 1974.

446. Prince AM, Hargrove RI, Szmuness W. Immunologic distinction between infectious and serum hepatitis. N Engl J Med 282:987, 1970.

447. Gocke DJ. Type B hepatitis—good news and bad news. N Engl J Med 291:1409, 1974.

448. Pattison CP, Boyer KM, Maynard JE. Epidemic hepatitis in a clinical laboratory: possible association with computer card handling. JAMA 230:854, 1974.

449. Morris IM, Cattle DS, Smits BJ. Endoscopy and transmission of hepatitis B. Lancet 2:1152, 1975.

450. McDonald GB, Silverstein FE. Can gastrointestinal endoscopy transmit hepatitis B to patients? Gastrointest Endosc 22:168, 1975.

451. Lauer JL, Van Drunen NA, Washburn JW, et al. Transmission of hepatitis B virus in clinical laboratory areas. J Infect Dis 140:513, 1979.

452. Mirick GS, Shank RE. An epidemic of serum hepatitis studied under controlled conditions. Trans Am Climatol Assoc 71:176, 1959.

453. Hersh T, Melnick JL, Goyal RK, et al. Nonparenteral transmission of viral hepatitis type B (Australia antigen-associated serum hepatitis). N Engl J Med 285:1363, 1971.

454. Heathcote J, Gateau P, Sherlock S. Role of hepatitis B antigen carriers in non-parenteral transmission of hepatitis B virus. Lancet 2:370, 1974.

455. Papaevangllon D, Trichopoulos D, Kemagtinon, et al. Prevalence of hepatitis B antigen and antibody in prostitutes. Br Med J 2:256, 1975.

456. Szmuness W, Much WM, Prince AM. On the role of sexual behavior in the spread of hepatitis B infection. Ann Intern Med 83:489, 1975.

457. Dietzman DE, Harmisch JP, Ray CG, et al. Hepatitis B surface antigen (HBsAg) and antibody to HBsAg: prevalence in homosexual and heterosexual men. JAMA 238:2625, 1977.

458. Lewis TL, Alter HJ, Chalmers TC. A comparison of the frequency of hepatitis B antigen and antibody in hospital and non-hospital personnel. N Engl J Med 289:647, 1973.

459. Mosley JW, Edwards VM, Casey BS. Hepatitis virus infection in dentists. N Engl J Med 293:730, 1975.

460. Maynard JE. Viral hepatitis as an occupational hazard in the health care professional. In: Vyas GN, Cohen SN, Schmid R, eds. Viral Hepatitis. A Contemporary Assessment of Etiology, Epidemiology, Pathogenesis and Prevention. Philadelphia, Franklin Institute Press, 1978:321.

461. Rosenberg JL, Jones DP, Lipitz LR. Viral hepatitis: an occupational hazard to surgeons. JAMA 223:395, 1973.

462. Graf JP, Moeschlin P. Risk to contacts of a medical practitioner carrying HBsAg. N Engl J Med 293:197, 1975.

463. Goodwin D, Fannin SL, McCracker BB. An oral surgeon related hepatitis B outbreak. In: California Morbidity (California State Department of Health), April 16, 1976.

464. **Rimland D, Parkin WE, Miller GB. Hepatitis B outbreak traced to an oral surgeon. N Engl J Med 296:153, 1977.**

465. Syndmen DR, Hindman SH, Wineland MD. Nosocomial viral hepatitis B: a cluster among staff with subsequent transmission to patients. Ann Intern Med 85:573, 1976.

466. Garibaldi RA, Rasmussen CM, Holmes AW. Hospital acquired serum hepatitis: report of an outbreak. JAMA 219:1577, 1972.

467. Alter HJ, Chalmer TC, Freeman BM. Health-care workers positive for hepatitis B surface antigen: are their contacts at risk? N Engl J Med 292:454, 1975.

468. Williams SV, Pattison CP, Berquist KR. Dental infection with hepatitis B. JAMA 232:1231, 1975.

469. Centers for Disease Control. Hepatitis Surveillance Report, No. 41, September, 1977.

470. Ogra PL. Immunologic aspects of hepatitis associated antigen and antibody in body fluids. J Immunol 110:1197, 1974.

471. Mohoney P, Gleischner G, Millman I. Australia antigen: detection and transmission in shellfish. Science 183:80, 1974.

472. Prince AM, Metselaar D, Kapuko GW. Hepatitis B antigen in wild caught mosquitoes in Africa. Lancet 2:247, 1972.

473. Brotman B, Prince AM, Godfrey HK. Role of arthropods in transmission of hepatitis B virus in the tropics. Lancet 1:1305, 1973.

474. Wills W, Laroiuze B, London WT. Hepatitis B in bedbugs from Senegal. Lancet 2:217, 1977.

475. Dick SJ, Tamborro CH, Leevy CM. Hepatitis B antigen in urban caught mosquitoes. JAMA 229:1627, 1974.

476. Beasley RP, Hwang LY, Lee GC, et al. Prevention of perinatally transmitted hepatitis B virus infections with hepatitis B immuneglobulin and hepatitis B vaccine. Lancet 2:1099, 1983.

477. Ohbayashi A, Okochi K, Mayumi M, et al. Familial clustering of asymptomatic carriers of Australia antigen and patients with primary liver disease and primary liver cancer. Gastroenterology 62:618, 1972.

478. Beasley RP, Stevens CE, Shiao IS, et al. Evidence against breast feeding as a mechanism for vertical transmission of hepatitis B. Lancet 2:740, 1975.

479. Hoyer W, Bonino F, Ponzetta A. Properties of delta associated ribonucleic acid. In: Verme G, Bonino F, Rizzetto M, eds. Viral Hepatitis and Delta Infection (Progress in Clinical and Biological Research, Vol. 143). New York, Alan R. Liss, 1983:91.

480. Gerin JL. Personal communication.

481. Denniston KJ, Hoyer BH, Smedile A, et al. Cloned fragment of the hepatitis delta virus RNA genome: sequence and diagnostic application. Science 232:873, 1986.

482. Rizzetto M, Canese MG, Arico S. Immunofluorescence detection of a new antigen system (delta/anti-delta) associated to the hepatitis B virus in the liver and the serum of HBsAg carriers. Gut 18:997, 1977.

483. Rizzetto M, Hoyer B, Canese MG, et al. Delta agent: the association of delta antigen with hepatitis B surface antigen and ribonucleic acid in the serum of delta-infected chimpanzees. Proc Natl Acad Sci USA 77:6124, 1980.

484. Bonino F, Hoyer B, Shih JWK, et al. Delta hepatitis agent—structural and antigenic properties of the delta-associated particle. Infect Immun 43:1000, 1984.

485. Rizzetto M, Shih JWK, Gerin JL. The hepatitis B virus associated delta antigen: isolation from liver, development of solid phase radioimmunoassay for delta antigen, and anti-delta antigen and partial characteristics of delta antigen. J Immunol 125:318, 1980.

486. Bonino F, Heermann KH, Rizzetto M, et al. Hepatitis delta virus: protein composition of delta antigen and its hepatitis B virus derived envelope. J Virol 58:945, 1986.

487. Wang KS, Choo QL, Weiner AJ, et al. Structure, sequence and expression of the hepatitis delta viral genome. Nature 323:508, 1987.

488. Kos A, Dijkema R, Arnberg AC, et al. The hepatitis delta virus possesses a circular RNA. Nature 323:558, 1987.

488a. Makino S, Chang MF, Shieh CK, et al. Molecular cloning and sequencing of human hepatitis delta virus RNA. Nature 329:343, 1987.

489. Smedile A, Rizzetto M, Bonino F, et al. Serum delta-associated RNA (DAR) in chronic HBV carriers infected with the delta agent (Abstr 3A9). In: International Symposium on Viral Hepatitis, March 8–10, 1984, San Francisco.

490. Rizzetto M, Canese MG, Gerin JL, et al. Transmission of the hepatitis B virus-associated delta antigen to chimpanzees. J Infect Dis 141:590, 1980.

491. Weiss RA. Experimental biology and assay of RNA tumor viruses. In: Weiss RA, Teich N, Varmus H, et al., eds. RNA Tumor Viruses. New York, Cold Spring Harbor Laboratory, 1982:209.

492. Rizzetto M. The delta agent. Hepatology 3:729, 1983.

493. Purcell RH, Gerin JL, Rizzetto M, et al. Experimental transmission of delta agent to chimpanzees. Prog Clin Biol Res 143:79, 1983.

494. Rosina F, Saracco G, Rizzetto M. Risk of post-transfusion infection with delta virus. A multicenter study. N Engl J Med 312:1488, 1985.

495. Rizzetto M, Verme G. Delta hepatitis—present status. J Hepatol 1:187, 1985.

496. Smedile A, Dentico P, Zanethi A, et al. Infection with delta agent in chronic HBsAg carriers. Gastroenterology 81:992, 1981.

497. Moestrup T, Hansson BG, Widell A, et al. Clinical aspects of delta infection. Br Med J 286:87, 1983.
498. Caredda F, Rossi E, Monforte A, et al. Hepatitis B virus associated coinfection and superinfection with delta. J Infect Dis 151:925, 1985.
499. Smedile A, Farci P, Verme G. Influence of delta infection on severity of hepatitis B. Lancet 2:945, 1982.
500. Govindarajan S, Chin KP, Redeker AG, et al. Fulminant B viral hepatitis: role of delta agent. Gastroenterology 86:1417, 1984.
501. Hadler S, Monzon M, Ponzetto A, et al. Delta virus infection and serum hepatitis: an epidemic in the Yucpa Indians of Venezuela. Ann Intern Med 100:339, 1984.
502. Farci P, Smedile A, Lavarini C, et al. Delta hepatitis in inapparent carriers of hepatitis B surface antigen. Gastroenterology 85:665, 1983.
503. Tabor E, Ponzetto A, Gerin JL, et al. Does delta agent contribute to fulminant hepatitis? Lancet 1:765, 1983.
504. Shattock A, Morgan B, Peutherer J, et al. High incidence of delta antigen in serum. Lancet 2:104, 1983.
505. Buti M, Esteban R, Jardi R, et al. Serologic diagnosis of acute delta hepatitis. J Med Virol 18:81, 1986.
506. Rizzetto M, Shiuh JWK, Gocke DJ, et al. Incidence and significance of antibodies to delta antigen in hepatitis B virus infection. Lancet 2:986, 1979.
507. Bergmann KF, Gerin JL. Antigen of hepatitis delta virus in the liver and serum of humans and animals. J Infect Dis 154:702, 1986.
508. Farci P, Smedile A, Lavarani C, et al. Delta infection: a factor of transition to chronicity of acute HBsAg hepatitis. J Med Virol (In press.)
509. Farci P, Lindsay I, Aragona M. IgM anti-delta: a marker of active delta hepatitis. Hepatology 4:1096, 1984.
510. Smedile A, Lavarini C, Crivelli O, et al. Radioimmunoassay detection of IgM antibodies to HBV associated delta antigen: clinical significance in delta infection. J Med Virol 9:131, 1982.
511. Columbo M, Cambieri R, Rumi M, et al. Long-term delta superinfection in hepatitis B surface antigen carriers and its relationship to the course of chronic hepatitis. Gastroenterology 85:235, 1983.
512. Rizzetto M, Verme G, Recchia S. Chronic hepatitis in carriers of hepatitis B surface antigen, with intrahepatic expression of delta antigen: an active and progressing disease unresponsive to immunosuppressive treatment. Ann Intern Med 98:437, 1983.
513. Farci P, Barbera C, Navone C, et al. Infection with the delta agent in children. Gut 1:4, 1985.
514. Govindarajan S, Kanel GC, Peters RL. Prevalence of delta antibody among chronic hepatitis B virus infected patients in Los Angeles area: its correlation with liver biopsy diagnosis. Gastroenterology 85:160, 1983.
515. Hadziyannis SJ. Delta antigen positive chronic liver disease in Greece: clinical aspects and natural course. In: Verme G, Bonino F, Rizzetto M, eds. Viral Hepatitis and Delta Infection. New York, Alan R Liss, 1983:207.
516. Arico S, Aragona M, Rizzetto M, et al. Clinical significance of antibody to the hepatitis delta virus in symptomless HBsAg carriers. Lancet 2:356, 1985.
517. Reinecke V, Dybkjaer E, Poulsen H, et al. A study of Australia antigen-positive blood donors and their recipients, with special references to liver histology. N Engl J Med 286:867, 1972.
518. Ricci G, De Bac C, Caramia F. Hepatitis B antigen: an epidemiologic and histologic study. J Infect Dis 128:125, 1973.
519. Woolf IL, Boyes BE, Jones DM, et al. Asymptomatic liver disease in hepatitis B antigen carriers. J Clin Pathol 27:348, 1974.
520. Lesnicar J, Zaversnik H, Ferluga D, et al. The significance of HB antigenemia in apparently healthy persons in the clinic for liver diseases. Acta Hepato-Gastroenterol 22:297, 1975.
521. Feinman SV, Cooter N, Sinclair JC, et al. Clinical and epidemiological significance of the HBsAg (Australian antigen) carrier state. Gastroenterology 68:113, 1975.
522. Piccinino F, Sagnelli F, Manzillo G, et al. Liver histology in 34 HBsAg long-term healthy carriers. Acta Hepato-Gastroenterol 23:148, 1977.
523. Shrago SS, Auslander MO, Gitnick GL. Hepatic pathologic condition in asymptomatic Australia antigen carriers. Arch Pathol Lab Med 101:648, 1977.
524. Valasco M, Gonzalez-Ceron M, De la Fuenta C, et al. Clinical and pathological study of asymptomatic HBsAg carriers in Chile. Gut 19:569, 1978.
525. Koretz RI, Lewin KJ, Rebhun DJ, et al. Hepatitis B surface antigen carriers—to biopsy or not to biopsy. Gastroenterology 75:860, 1978.
526. DeFranchis R, D'Arminio A, Vecchi M, et al. Chronic asymptomatic HBsAg carriers: histologic abnormalities and diagnostic and prognostic value of serologic markers of the HBV. Gastroenterology 79:521, 1980.
527. Govindarjan S, Hevia FJ, Peters RL. Prevalence of delta antigen/antibody in B-viral associated hepatocellular carcinoma. Cancer 53:1692, 1984.
528. Jew MC, Dusheiko GM, Hadziyannis S, et al. Does delta infection play a part in the pathogenesis of hepatitis B virus related hepatocellular carcinoma? Br Med J 288:1727, 1984.
529. Garcia G, Merigan TC, Robinson WS. Unpublished results.
530. Hadziyannis SJ, Sherman M, Lieberman HM, et al. Liver disease activity and HBV replication in chronic delta antigen positive hepatitis B virus carriers. Hepatology 4:544, 1985.
531. Caredda F, D'Arminio Monforte A, Rossi E, et al. Prospective study of epidemic delta infection in drug addicts. In Verme G, Bonino F, Rizzetto M, eds. Viral Hepatitis and Delta Infection. Progress in Clinical and Biological Research, Vol 143. New York, Alan R Liss, 1983:91.
532. Hadziyannis SJ, Lieberman HM, Karvountzis GG, et al. Analysis of liver disease, nuclear HBcAg, viral replication and hepatitis B virus DNA in liver and serum of HBeAg vs. anti-HBe positive carriers of hepatitis B virus. Hepatology 3:656, 1983.
533. Rizzetto M, Purcell RH, Gerin JL. Epidemiology of HBV-associated data agent: geographical distribution of anti-delta and prevalence of polytransfused HBsAg carriers. Lancet 1:1215, 1980.
534. Smedile A, Lavarini C, Farci P, et al. Epidemiologic patterns of infection with the hepatitis B virus associated delta agent in Italy. Am J Epidemiol 117:223, 1983.
535. Hadziyannis S, Hatzakis A, Karamanos B. Clinical features of chronic delta infection. In: Vyas GN, Dienstag JL, Hoofnagle JH, eds. Viral Hepatitis. New York, Grune & Stratton, 1984:701.
536. Ponzetta A, Forzani E, Shafi MS. Delta agent infection in Saudi Arabia: a general population study. In: Vyas GN, Dienstag JL, Hoofnagle JH, eds. Viral Hepatitis. New York, Grune & Stratton, 1984:634.
537. CDC Hepatitis Surveillance Report 49:7, 1985.
538. Dimitrakakis M, Crowe S, Gust I. Prevalence of delta infection in the Western Pacific Region. J Med Virol 18:335, 1986.
539. Ponzetto A, Hoofnagle JH, Seeff LB. Antibody to the hepatitis B virus-associated delta-agent in immune serum globulins. Gastroenterology 87:1212, 1984.
540. Bonino F, Caporaso N, Denico P, et al. Familial clustering and spreading of hepatitis delta virus infection. J Hepatol 1:221, 1985.
541. Hansson BG, Moestrup T, Widell A, et al. Infection with delta agent in Sweden: introduction of a new hepatitis agent. J Infect Dis 146:472, 1982.
542. Smedile A, Lavarini C, Farci P, et al. Epidemiologic patterns of infection with the hepatitis B virus-associated delta agent in Italy. Am J Epidemiol 117:223, 1983.
543. Purcell RH, Gerin JL. Epidemiology of delta agent: an introduction. In: Verme G, Bonino F, Rizzetto M, eds. Viral Hepatitis and Delta Infection. New York, Alan Liss, 1983:113.
544. Ljunggren KE, Patarroyo ME, Engle R, et al. Viral hepatitis in Colombia: a study of the Sierra Nevada de Santa Marta. Hepatology 5:299, 1984.
545. Ukena T, Morse LJ, Gurwitz A, et al. Delta hepatitis—Massachusetts. Morbid Mortal Week Rep 33:483, 1984.
546. Nath N, Fang CT, Berberian H, et al. Antibodies to delta antigen in asymptomatic HBsAg reactive blood donors in the United States and its association with other markers of hepatitis B virus. Am J Epidemiol 122:218, 1985.
547. Aach RD, Kahn RA. Post-transfusion hepatitis: current perspectives. Ann Intern Med 92:539, 1980.
548. Rizzetto M, Morello C, Mannucci PM, et al. Delta infection and liver disease in hemophilic carriers of hepatitis B surface antigen. J Infect Dis 145:18, 1982.
549. Ponzetto A, Forzani B, Hele C, et al. Infection with hepatitis delta virus. N Engl J Med 314:517, 1986.
550. Hoofnagle JH, Waggoner JG. Hepatitis A and B virus markers in immune serum globulin. Gastroenterology 78:259, 1980.
551. Tabor E, Gerety RJ. Transmission of hepatitis B by immune serum globulin. Lancet 2:1293, 1979.
552. Petrilli FL, Crovari P, De Flora S. Hepatitis B in subjects treated with a drug containing immunoglobulins. J Infect Dis 135:252, 1977.
553. Lane RS. Non-A, non-B hepatitis from intravenous immunoglobulin. Lancet 2:974, 1983.
554. Thomas HC. The delta agent comes of age. Gut 26:1, 1985.
555. Maynard JE, Bradley DW, Gravelle CR, et al. Preliminary studies of hepatitis A in chimpanzees. J Infect Dis 131:194, 1975.
556. Dienstag JL, Feinstone SM, Purcell RH. Experimental infection of chimpanzees with hepatitis A virus. J Infect Dis 132:532, 1975.
557. Provost PJ, Hilleman MR. Propagation of human hepatitis A virus in cell culture in vitro. Proc Soc Exp Biol Med 160:213, 1979.
558. Lorenz D, Barker L, Stevens D, et al. Hepatitis in the marmoset, Sanguinus mystax. Proc Soc Biol Med 135:348, 1970.
559. Mascoli CC, Ittensohn OL, Villarejos VM, et al. Recovery of hepatitis

agents in the marmoset from human cases occurring in Costa Rica. Proc Soc Exp Biol Med 142:276, 1973.

560. Provost PJ, Ittensohn OL, Villarejos VM, et al. Etiologic relationship of marmoset-propagated CR 326 hepatitis A virus to hepatitis in man. Proc Soc Exp Biol Med 142:1257, 1973.

561. Holmes AW, Deinhardt F, Wolfe G, et al. Specific neutralization of human hepatitis A in marmoset monkeys. Nature 243:419, 1973.

562. Provost PJ, Villarejos VM, Hilleman MR. Suitability of the rufiventer marmoset as a host animal for human hepatitis A virus. Proc Soc Exp Biol Med 155:283, 1977.

563. Hillis W. An outbreak of infectious hepatitis among chimpanzee handlers at a U.S. Air Force Base. Am J Hyg 73:316, 1961.

564. Hillis W. Viral hepatitis associated with sub-human primates. Transfusion 3:445, 1963.

565. Mosley JW, Reinhardt HP, Hassler FR. Chimpanzee-associated hepatitis: an outbreak in Oklahoma. JAMA 199:695, 1967.

566. Dienstag JL, Mathiesen JR, Purcell RH. Test methods and animal models for hepatitis A virus infection. In: Vyas GN, Cohen SN, Schmidt R, eds. Viral Hepatitis: A Contemporary Assessment of Etiology, Epidemiology, Pathogenesis and Prevention. Philadelphia, Franklin Institute Press, 1978:13.

567. Frosner GG, Deinhardt F, Scheid R, et al. Infection 7:303, 1979.

568. Alexander JJ, Macnab G, Saunders R. Perspect Virol 10:103, 1978.

569. Daemer RJ, Feinstone SM, Gust ID, et al. Propagation of human hepatitis A virus in African green monkey kidney cell culture: primary isolation and serial passage. Infect Immun 32:388, 1981.

570. Balayan MS, Andzhaprize AG, Tol'skaia EA, et al. Viprosy Virus Logii 6:675, 1979.

571. Locarnini SA, Coulepis AG, Westaway EG, et al. Restricted replication of human hepatitis A virus in cell culture: intracellular biochemical study. J Virol 37:216, 1981.

572. Wewalka F. Zur Epidemiologie des Ikterus bei der antisyphilitischen Behandlung. Schweiz Z Allg Path 16:307, 1953.

573. Krugman S, Giles JP, Hammond J. Hepatitis virus: effect of heat on infectivity and antigenicity of MS-1 and MS-2 strains. J Infect Dis 122:432, 1970.

574. Salaman MH, Williams DL, King AJ, et al. Prevention of jaundice resulting from antisyphilitic treatment. Lancet 2:7, 1944.

575. Neefe JR, Baty JB, Reinhold JL, et al. Inactivation of the virus of infectious hepatitis in drinking water. Am J Public Health 37:365, 1947.

576. Provost PJ, Wolanski BS, Miller WJ, et al. Physical, chemical, and morphologic dimensions of human hepatitis A virus strain CR 326 (38578). Proc Soc Exp Biol Med 148:532, 1975.

577. Moritsugu Y, Dienstag JL, Valdesnso J, et al. Purification of hepatitis A antigen from feces and detection of antigen and antibody by immune adherence hemagglutination. Infect Immun 13:898, 1976.

578. Siegl G, Frosner GG. Characterization and classification of virus particles associated with hepatitis A: 1. Size, density and sedimentation. J Virol 26:40, 1978.

579. Bradley DW, Hornbeck CL, Gravelle CR, et al. CsCl banding of hepatitis A-associated virus-like particles. J Infect Dis 131:304, 1975.

580. Schulman AN, Dienstag JL, Jackson DR, et al. Hepatitis A antigen particles in liver, bile, and stool of chimpanzees. J Infect Dis 134:80, 1976.

581. Feinstone SM, Kapikian AZ, Gerin JL, et al. Buoyant density of the hepatitis A virus-like particle in cesium chloride. J Virol 13:1412, 1972.

582. Bradley DW, Gravelle CR, Cook EH, et al. Cyclic excretion of hepatitis A virus in experimentally infected chimpanzees. J Med Virol 1:113, 1977.

583. Woodson RD, Clinton JJ. Hepatitis prophylaxis abroad: effectiveness of immune serum globulin in protecting Peace Corps volunteers. JAMA 209:1053, 1969.

584. Anonymous. Prophylactic gamma globulin for prevention of endemic hepatitis. Effects of U.S. gamma globulin upon incidence of viral hepatitis and other infectious diseases in U.S. soldiers abroad. Arch Intern Med 128:723, 1971.

585. Coulepis AG, Locarnini SA, Ferris AA, et al. The polypeptides of hepatitis A virus. Intervirology 10:24, 1978.

586. Coulepis AG, Locarnini SA, Gust ID. Iodination of hepatitis A virus reveals a fourth structural polypeptide. J Virol 35:572, 1980.

587. Feinstone SM, Moritsugu Y, Shih JWK, et al. Characterization of hepatitis A virus. In: Vyas GN, Cohen SN, Schmidt R, eds. Viral Hepatitis: A Contemporary Assessment of Etiology, Epidemiology, Pathogenesis and Prevention. Philadelphia, Franklin Institute Press, 1978:41.

588. Tratschin JD, Siegl G, Frosner GG, et al. Characterization and classification of virus particles associated with hepatitis A. III. Structural proteins. J Virol 38:151, 1981.

589. Maizel JW, Phillips BA, Summers DF. Composition of artificially produced and naturally occurring empty capsids of polio virus type 1. Virology 32:692, 1967.

590. Maizel JW, Summers DF. Evidence for large precursor proteins in poliovirus synthesis. Proc Natl Acad Sci USA 59:966, 1968.

591. Siegl G, Frosner GG. Characterization and classification of virus particles associated with hepatitis A: II. Type and configuration of nucleic acid. J Virol 26:48, 1978.

592. Coulepis AG, Tannock GA, Locarnini SA, et al. Evidence that the genome of hepatitis A virus consists of single stranded RNA. J Virol 37:473, 1981.

593. Von der Holm K, Winneacker EL, Deinhardt F, et al. J Virol Methods 2:37, 1981.

594. Gust ID, Locarnini SA, Coulepis AG, et al. The Biology of Hepatitis A Virus. In: Deinhardt F, Deinhardt J, eds. Viral Hepatitis: Laboratory and Clinical Science. New York, Marcel Dekker, 1983:35.

595. Ticehurst JR, Racainello VR, Baroudy BM, et al. Molecular cloning and characterization of hepatitis A virus cDNA. Proc Natl Acad Sci 80:5885, 1983.

596. Mathiesen LR, Feinstone SM, Purcell RH, et al. Detection of hepatitis A antigen by immunofluorescence. Infect Immun 18:524, 1977.

597. Mathiesen LR, Drucker J, Lorenz D, et al. Localization of hepatitis A antigen in marmoset organs during acute infection with hepatitis A virus. J Infect Dis 138:369, 1978.

598. Franklin RM, Rosner J. Localization of RNA synthesis in meningovirus infected L. cells. Biochem Biophys Acta 55:240, 1961.

599. Franklin RM, Baltimore D. Patterns of macromolecular synthesis in normal and virus-infected mammalian cells. Cold Spring Harbor Symposia on Quant Biol 27:175, 1962.

600. Dales S, Eggers HJ, Tamm I, et al. Electron microscopic study of the formation of poliovirus. Virology 26:379, 1965.

601. Feinstone SM, Purcell RH. New methods for the serodiagnosis of hepatitis A. Gastroenterology 78:1092, 1980.

602. Maynard JE. Infectious hepatitis at Fort Yukon, Alaska—report of an outbreak, 1960–61. Am J Public Health 53:31, 1963.

603. Skinhoj P, McNair A, Anderson ST. Hepatitis and hepatitis B antigen in Greenland. Am J Epidemiol 99:50, 1974.

604. Skinhoj P, Mikkelsen F, Hollinger B. Hepatitis A in Greenland: importance of specific antibody testing in epidemiologic surveillance. Am J Epidemiol 105:140, 1977.

605. Black FL, Hierholzer WJ, Pinheire F, et al. Evidence for persistence of infectious agents in isolated human populations. Am J Epidemiol 100:230, 1974.

606. Centers for Disease Control: Hepatitis Surveillance Report Number 48, 1982.

607. Dienstag JL, Szmuness W, Stevens CE, et al. Hepatitis A virus infection: new insights from seroepidemiologic studies. J Infect Dis 137:328, 1978.

608. Routenberg JA, Dienstag JL, Harrison WO, et al. A food-borne outbreak of hepatitis A: clinical and laboratory features of acute and protracted illness. Am J Med Sci 278:123, 1979.

609. Dienstag JL, Alaama A, Mosley JW, et al. Etiology of sporadic hepatitis B surface antigen negative hepatitis. Ann Intern Med 87:1, 1977.

610. Szmuness W, Dienstag JL, Purcell RH, et al. Distribution of antibody to hepatitis A antigen in urban adult populations. N Engl J Med 295:755, 1976.

611. Corey L, Holmes KK. Sexual transmission of hepatitis A in homosexual men: incidence and mechanism. N Engl J Med 302:435, 1980.

612. Fawaz KA, Watloff DS. Viral hepatitis in homosexual men. Gastroenterology 81:537, 1981.

613. Centers for Disease Control. Morbidity and Mortality Weekly Report. 29:565, 1980.

614. Szmuness W, Dienstag JL, Purcell RH, et al. The prevalence of antibody to hepatitis A antigen in various parts of the world. Am J Epidemiol 106:392, 1977.

615. Villarejos VM, Provost PJ, Ittensohn OL, et al. Seroepidemiologic investigations of human hepatitis caused by A, B, and a possible third virus. Proc Soc Exp Biol Med 152:525, 1976.

616. Krugman S, Ward R, Giles JP. The natural history of infectious hepatitis. Am J Med 32:717, 1962.

617. Havens WP, Ward R, Drill VA, et al. Experimental production of hepatitis by feeding icterogenic materials. Proc Soc Exp Biol Med 57:206, 1944.

618. Giles JP, Liebhaber H, Drugman S, et al. Early viremia and viruria in infectious hepatitis. Virology 24:107, 1964.

619. Boggs JD, Melnick JL, Conrad ME, et al. Viral hepatitis—clinical and tissue culture studies. JAMA 214:1041, 1970.

620. Findlay GM, Willcox RR. Transmission of infective hepatitis by feces and virus. Lancet 1:212, 1945.

621. Deinhardt F, Peterson D, Cross G, et al. Hepatitis in marmosets. Am J Med Sci 270:73, 1975.

622. Drugman S, Ward R, Giles JP, et al. Infectious hepatitis: detection of virus during incubation and in clinically inapparent infection. N Engl J Med 261:729, 1959.

623. Havens WP. Period of infectivity of patients with experimentally induced infectious hepatitis. J Exp Med 83:251, 1946.

624. Neffe JR, Stokes J Jr, Reinhold JG. Oral administration to volunteers

of feces from patients with homologous serum hepatitis and infection (epidemic) hepatitis. Am J Med Sci 210:29, 1945.

625. Dienstag JL, Feinstone SM, Kapikian AZ, et al. Faecal shedding of hepatitis-A antigen. Lancet 1:765, 1975.

626. Frosner GG, Overby LR, Flehmig B, et al. Seroepidemiological investigation of patients and family contacts in an epidemic of hepatitis A. J Med Virol 1:163, 1977.

627. Dienstag JL, Routenberg JA, Purcell RH, et al. Foodhandler-associated outbreak of hepatitis A. Ann Intern Med 83:647, 1975.

628. Rakela J, Mosley JW. Fecal excretion of hepatitis A virus in humans. J Infect Dis 135:933, 1977.

629. Flehmig B, Frank H, Frosner GG, et al. Hepatitis A virus particles in stools of patients from a natural hepatitis outbreak in Germany. Med Microbiol Immunol 163:209, 1977.

630. Hopkins R, Scott TG. Hepatitis A antigen in Edinburgh. Lancet 2:206, 1976.

631. Locarnini SA, Gust ID, Ferris AA, et al. Prospective study of acute viral hepatitis with particular reference to hepatitis A. Bull WHO 54:199, 1976.

631a. Sjogren MH, Tanno H, Fay O, et al. Hepatitis A virus in stool during clinical relapse. Ann Intern Med 106:221, 1987.

632. Mao JS, Yu PH, Ding ZS, et al. Patterns of shedding of hepatitis A virus antigen in feces and of antibody responses in patients with naturally acquired type A hepatitis. J Infect Dis 142:654, 1980.

633. Ward R, Krugman S, Giles JP, et al. Infectious hepatitis: studies of its natural history and prevention. N Engl J Med 258:407, 1958.

634. Knight V, Drake ME, Belden EA, et al. Characteristics of spread of infectious hepatitis in schools and households in an epidemic in a rural area. Am J Hyg 59:1, 1954.

635. Batten PL, Runte VE, Skinner HG. Infectious hepatitis: infectiousness during the presymptomatic phase of the disease. Am J Gyg 77;129, 1963.

636. Mosley JW, Smithers WW. Infectious hepatitis: report of an outbreak probably caused by drinking water. N Engl J Med 257:590, 1957.

637. Leger RT, Boyer KM, Pattison CP, et al. Hepatitis A: report of the common-source outbreak with recovery of a possible etiologic agent. I. Epidemiologic studies. J Infect Dis 131:163, 1975.

638. Dull HB, Doege TC, Mosley JW. An outbreak of infectious hepatitis associated with a school cafeteria. South Med J 56:475, 1963.

639. Denes AE, Smith JL, Hindman SH, et al. Food borne hepatitis A infection: a report of two urban restaurant-associated outbreaks. Am J Epidemiol 105:1059, 1977.

640. Ashley A. Use of gamma globulin for control of infectious hepatitis in an institution for the mentally retarded. N Engl J Med 252:88, 1955.

641. Drake ME, Ming C. Gamma globulin in epidemic hepatitis. JAMA 155:1302, 1954.

642. Mathew EB, Dietzman DE, Madden DL, et al. A major epidemic of infectious hepatitis in an institution for the mentally retarded. Am J Epidemiol 98:199, 1973.

643. Horstman DM, Havens WP, Deutsch J. Infectious hepatitis in childhood: report of 2 institutional outbreaks and comparison of disease in adults and children. J Pediatr 30:381, 1947.

644. MacCallum FO, Bradley WH. Transmission of infective hepatitis to human volunteers. Lancet 2:228, 1944.

645. Neefe JR, Stokes J. An epidemic of infectious hepatitis apparently due to a water-borne agent. JAMA 128:1063, 1945.

646. Joseph PR, Miller JD, Henderson DA. An outbreak of hepatitis traced to food contamination. N Engl J Med 273:188, 1965.

647. Tong MJ, Thursby M, Rakela J, et al. Studies of the maternal-infant transmission of the viruses which cause acute hepatitis. Gastroenterology 80:999, 1981.

648. Barker JF, Dienstag JL, Lorenz DE, et al. Serologic and animal inoculation studies of a communal outbreak of viral hepatitis, type A. Am J Med Sci 274:247, 1977.

649. Harden AG, Barondess JA, Parker B. Transmission of infectious hepatitis by transfusion of whole blood. N Engl J Med 253:923, 1955.

650. Francis T Jr, Frisch AW, Quilligan JJ Jr. Demonstration of infectious hepatitis virus in presymptomatic period after transfer by transfusion. Proc Soc Exp Biol Med 61:276, 1946.

651. Stevens CE, Silbert JA, Miller DR, et al. Serologic evidence of hepatitis A and B virus infections in thalassemia patients: a retrospective study. Transfusion 18:94, 1978.

652. Szmuness W, Dienstag JL, Purcell RH, et al. Type A hepatitis and hemodialysis: a seroepidemiologic study in 15 U.S. centers. Ann Intern Med 87:8, 1977.

653. Feinstone SM, Kapikian AZ, Purcell RH, et al. Transfusion associated hepatitis not due to viral hepatitis type A or B. N Engl J Med 292:767, 1975.

654. Knodell RG, Conrad ME, Dienstag JL, et al. Etiologic spectrum of post-transfusion-associated hepatitis. Gastroenterology 69:1278, 1975.

655. Alter HJ, Purcell RH, Holland PV, et al. Clinical and serological analysis of transfusion-associated hepatitis. Lancet 2:838, 1975.

656. Dienstag JL, Feinstone SM, Purcell RH. Clinical and serological analysis of transfusion-associated hepatitis. Lancet 1:56, 1977.

657. Tucker CB, Owen WH, Farrell MS. Outbreak of infectious hepatitis apparently transmitted through water. South Med J 47:732, 1954.

658. Bryan JA, Lehmann JD, Stetiady IF, et al. An outbreak of hepatitis A associated with recreational lake water. Am J Epidemiol 99:145, 1974.

659. Rindge ME, Mason JO, Elsea WR. Infectious hepatitis: report of an outbreak in a small Connecticut school due to water-borne transmission. JAMA 180:33, 1962.

660. Mosley JW, Schrack WD Jr, Densham TW, et al. Infectious hepatitis in Clearwater County, Pennsylvania. I. A probable water-borne epidemic. Am J Med 26:555, 1959.

661. Poskanzer DC, Beadenkoph WG. Water-borne infectious hepatitis epidemic from a chlorinated municipal supply. Public Health Rep 76:745, 1961.

662. Morse LJ, Bryan JA, Hurley JP, et al. The Holy Cross football team hepatitis outbreak. JAMA 219:706, 1972.

663. Roos B. Hepatitis epidemic conveyed by oysters. Svenska Tkar 53:989, 1956.

664. Mason JO, McLean WR. Infectious hepatitis traced to the consumption of raw oysters. Am J Hyg 75:90, 1962.

665. Dougherty WJ, Altman R. Viral hepatitis in New Jersey 1960–61. Am J Med 32:704, 1962.

666. Ruddy SJ, Johnson RF, Mosley JW, et al. An epidemic of clam-associated hepatitis. JAMA 208:649, 1969.

667. Koff RS, Sear HS. Internal temperature of steamed clams: viral hepatitis in a group of Boston hospitals. III. Importance of exposure to shellfish in a non-epidemic period. N Engl J Med 276:737, 1967.

668. Portnoy BL, Mackowiak PA, Caraway CT, et al. Oyster-associated hepatitis—failure of shellfish certification program to prevent outbreaks. JAMA 233:1065, 1975.

669. Dienstag JL, Gust ID, Lucas CR, et al. Mussel-associated viral hepatitis type A: serological confirmation. Lancet 1:561, 1976.

670. Mackowiak PA, Caraway CT, Portnoy BL. Oyster-associated hepatitis: lessons from the Louisiana experience. Am J Epidemiol 103:181, 1976.

671. Murphy WJ, Petrie LM, Work SD. Outbreak of infectious hepatitis, apparently milk-borne. Am J Public Health 36:169, 1946.

672. Raska K, Heich J, Jezek A, et al. A milk-borne infectious hepatitis epidemic. J Hyg Epidemiol Microbiol Immunol 10:413, 1966.

673. Read MR, Bancroft H, Doull JA, et al. Infectious hepatitis—presumably food-borne outbreak. Am J Public Health 36:367, 1946.

674. Ballance GA. Epidemic of infective hepatitis in an Oxford college. Br Med J 1:1071, 1954.

675. Joseph PR, Miller JD, Henderson DA. An outbreak of hepatitis traced to food contamination. N Engl J Med 173:188, 1965.

676. Philip JN, Hamilton TP, Albert TJ, et al. Infectious hepatitis outbreak with mai tai as the vehicle of transmission. Am J Epidemiol 97:50, 1973.

677. Levy BS, Fontaine RE, Smith CA, et al. A large food borne outbreak of hepatitis A possible transmission by oropharyageal secretions. JAMA 234:289, 1975.

678. Meyers JD, Rom JF, Tihen WS, et al. Food-borne hepatitis A in a general hospital—epidemiologic study of an outbreak attributed to sandwiches. JAMA 231:1049, 1975.

679. Dienstag JL, Routenberg JA, Purcell RH, et al. Food-handler-associated outbreak of hepatitis type A—an immune electron microscopic study. Ann Infect Med 83:647, 1975.

680. Schoenbaum SC, Baker O, Jezek Z. Common-source epidemic hepatitis due to glazed and iced pastries. Am J Epidemiol 104:74, 1976.

681. Eisenstein AB, Aach RD, Jacobsohn W, et al. An epidemic of infectious hepatitis in a general hospital: probable transmission by contaminated orange juice. JAMA 185:171, 1963.

682. Ruddy SJ, Mosley JW, Held JR. Chimpanzee-associated viral hepatitis in 1963. Am J Epidemiol 86:634, 1967.

683. Friedmann CTH, Dinnes MR, Bernstein JF, et al. Chimpanzee-associated infectious hepatitis among personnel at an animal hospital. J Am Vet Med Assoc 159:541, 1971.

683a. Davenport FM, Hennessy AV, Christopher N, et al. A common source multihousehold outbreak of chimpanzee-associated hepatitis in humans. Am J Epidemiol 83:146, 1966.

684. Dienstag JL, Davenport FM, McCollum RW, et al. Non-human primate associated viral hepatitis type A: serologic evidence of hepatitis A virus infection. JAMA 236:462, 1976.

685. Mosley JW. Epidemiology of HAV Infection. In: Vyas GN, Cohen SN, Schmidt R, eds. Viral Hepatitis: A Contemporary Assessment of Etiology, Epidemiology, Pathogenesis and Prevention. Philadelphia, The Franklin Institute Press, 1978:85.

686. Krugman S, Ward R, Giles JP, et al. Infectious hepatitis: studies on the effect of gamma globulin on the incidence of inapparent infection. JAMA 174:823, 1960.
687. Wacker WEC, Riodan JF, Snodgrass PJ, et al. The Holy Cross hepatitis outbreak: clinical and chemical abnormalities. Arch Intern Med 130:357, 1972.
688. Hindman SH, Maynard JE, Bradley DW, et al. Simultaneous infection with type A and B hepatitis viruses. Am J Epidemiol 105:135, 1977.
689. Rakela J, Nugent E, Mosley JW. Viral hepatitis: enzyme assays and serologic procedures in the study of an epidemic. Am J Epidemiol 106:493, 1977.
690. Schneider AJ, Mosley JW. Studies of variations of glutamic-oxalacetic transaminase in serum in infectious hepatitis. Pediatrics 24:367, 1959.
691. Matthew EB, Dietzman DE, Madden DL, et al. A major epidemic of infectious hepatitis in an institution for the mentally retarded. Am J Epidemiol 98:199, 1973.
692. Havens WP. Infectious hepatitis. Medicine 27:279, 1948.
693. MacCallus FO. Infective hepatitis: studies in East Anglia during the period 1943–47. London, Medical Res Council Special Rep Series, No. 273, HMS Office, 1951.
694. Wallace EC. Infectious hepatitis: report of an outbreak, apparently water-borne. Med J Aust 1:101, 1958.
695. Bromberg K, Newhall PN, Peter G. Hepatitis A and meningoencephalitis. JAMA 247:815, 1982.
696. Gruer LD, McKenrick MW, Beeching NJ, et al. Relapsing hepatitis associated with hepatitis A virus. Lancet 2:163, 1982.
697. Rakela J, Redeker AG, Edwards VM, et al. Hepatitis A virus infection in fulminant hepatitis and chronic active hepatitis. Gastroenterology 74:879, 1979.
698. Dienstag JL, Alaama A, Mosley JW, et al. Etiology of sporadic hepatitis B surface antigen-negative hepatitis. Ann Intern Med 87:1, 1977.
699. Rakela J, Mosley JW, Redeker AG, et al. The role of hepatitis A virus in fulminant hepatitis. Gastroenterology 69:854, 1975.
700. Bradley DW, Hollinger FB, Hornbeck CL, et al. Isolation and characterization of hepatitis A virus. Am J Clin Pathol 65:876, 1976.
701. Krugman S, Friedman H, Lattimer C. Viral hepatitis type A: identification by specific complement fixation and immune adherence tests. N Engl J Med 292:1141, 1975.
702. Rakela J, Stevenson D, Edwards V, et al. Antibodies to hepatitis A virus: patterns by two procedures. J Clin Microbiol 5:110, 1977.
703. Bradley DW, Maynard JE, Kindman SH, et al. Serodiagnosis of viral hepatitis A: detection of acute-phase immunoglobulin M antihepatitis A virus by radioimmunoassay. J Clin Microbiol 5:521, 1977.
704. Yoshizawa H, Itah Y, Iwakim S, et al. Diagnosis of type a hepatitis by fecal IgA antibody against hepatitis A antigen. Gastroenterology 78:114, 1980.
705. Havens WP. Experiment in cross immunity between infectious and homologous serum jaundice. Proc Soc Exp Biol Med 59:148, 1945.
706. Krugman S, Giles JP, Hammond J. Infectious hepatitis: evidence for two distinctive clinical, epidemiological and immunological types of infection. JAMA 200:365, 1967.
707. Karvountzis GG, Mosley JW, Redeker AG. Serologic characteristics of patients with two episodes of acute viral hepatitis. Am J Med 58:815, 1975.
708. Mosley JW. Hepatitis types B and non-B: epidemiologic background. JAMA 233:967, 1975.
709. Mosley JW, Redeker AG, Feinstone SM, et al. Multiple hepatitis viruses in multiple attacks of acute viral hepatitis. N Engl J Med 296:75, 1977.
710. Provost PJ, Ittensohn OL, Villarejos VM, et al. A specific complement fixation test for human hepatitis A employing CR 326 virus antigen: diagnosis and epidemiology. Proc Soc Exp Biol Med 148:962, 1975.
711. Baer GM, Walker JA, Yager PA. Studies of an outbreak of acute hepatitis A: I. Complement level fluctuation. J Med Virol 1:1, 1977.
712. Locarnini SA, Coulepis AG, Stratton AM, et al. Solid-phase enzyme-linked immunoabsorbent assay for detection of hepatitis A-specific immunoglobulin M. J Clin Microbiol 9:459, 1979.
713. Frosner GG, Scheid R, Wolf H, et al. Immunoglobulin M anti-hepatitis A virus determination by reorienting gradient centrifugation for diagnosis of acute hepatitis A. J Clin Microbiol 9:476, 1979.
714. Flehmig B, Ranke M, Berthold H, et al. A solid-phase radioimmunoassay for detection of IgM antibodies to hepatitis A virus. J Infect Dis 140:169, 1979.
715. Duermeyer W, Wielaard F, Van der Veen J. A new principle for the detection of specific IgM antibodies applied in an ELISA for hepatitis A. J Med Virol 4:25, 1979.
716. Roggendorf M, Frosner GG, Deinhardt F, et al. Comparison of solid

717. Miller WJ, Provost PJ, McAleer WJ, et al. Specific immune adherence assay for human hepatitis A antibody. Application to diagnostic and epidemiologic investigations. Proc Soc Exp Biol Med 149:254, 1975.
718. Hollinger FB, Bradley DW, Maynard JE, et al. Detection of hepatitis A viral antigen by radioimmunoassay. J Immunol 115:1464, 1975.
719. Purcell RH, Wong DC, Moritsugu Y, et al. A microtiter solid-phase radioimmunoassay for hepatitis A antigen and antibody. J Immunol 116:349, 1976.
720. Hollinger FB, Bradley DW, Dressman GR, et al. Detection of viral hepatitis type A. Am J Clin Pathol 65:854, 1976.
721. Locarnini SA, Garland SM, Lehmann NI, et al. Solid phase enzyme-linked immunoabsorbant assay for detection of hepatitis A virus. J Clin Microbiol 8:277, 1978.
722. Coursaget P, Maupas P, Hibon P, et al. Hepatitis A diagnosis in man: radioimmunoassay for hepatitis A antigen detection in feces. J Med Virol 6:53, 1980.
723. Prince AM, Brotman B, Grady GF, et al. Long-incubation post-transfusion hepatitis without serological evidence of exposure to hepatitis B virus. Lancet 2:241, 1974.
724. Hollinger FB, Werch J, Melnick JL. A prospective study indicating that double-antibody radioimmunoassay reduces the incidence of post-transfusion hepatitis.
725. Alter HJ, Holland PV, Purcell RH. The emerging pattern of post-transfusion hepatitis. Am J Med Sci 270:329, 1975.
726. Alter HJ, Purcell RH, Holland PV, et al. Clinical and serological analysis of transfusion-associated hepatitis. Lancet 2:838, 1975.
727. Deinstag JL, Feinstone SM, Purcell RH, et al. Clinical and serological analysis of transfusion-associated hepatitis. Lancet 1:560, 1977.
728. Alter HJ, Purcell RH, Holland PV, et al. Transmissible agent in non-A, non-B hepatitis. Lancet 1:459, 1978.
729. Tabor E, Gerety BJ, Drucker JA, et al. Transmission of non-A, non-B hepatitis from man to chimpanzee. Lancet 1:463, 1978.
730. Hollinger FB, Gitnick GL, Aach RD, et al. Non-A, non-B hepatitis transmission in chimpanzees: a project of the transfusion-transmitted viruses study group. Intervirology 10:60, 1978.
731. Prince AM, Brotman B, van der Ende MC, et al. In: Vyas GN, Cohen SN, Schmid R, eds. Viral Hepatitis: A Contemporary Assessment of Etiology, Epidemiology, Pathogenesis and Prevention. Philadelphia, Franklin Institute Press, 1978:633.
732. Feinstone SM, Deines H, Alter HJ, et al. Studies on non-A, non-B hepatitis in chimpanzees and marmosets. Gastroenterology 79:1072, 1980.
733. Feinstone SM, Alter HJ, Dienes HR, et al. Non-A, non-B hepatitis in chimpanzees and marmosets. J Infect Dis 144:588, 1981.
734. Gerety RJ. Non A, Non B Hepatitis. New York, Academic Press, 1981.
735. Bradley DW, Cook EH, Maynard JE, et al. Experimental infection of chimpanzees with antihemophilic (factor VIII) materials: recovery of virus-like particles associated with non A, non B hepatitis. J Med Virol 3:253, 1979.
736. Wyke RJ, Tsiquaye KN, Thornton A, et al. Transfusion of non-A non-B hepatitis to chimpanzees by factor-IX concentrates after fatal complications in patients with chronic liver disease. Lancet 1:520, 1979.
737. Tabor E, April M, Seeff LB, et al. Acute non-A non-B hepatitis. Gastroenterology 76:680, 1979.
738. Craske J, Spooner RJD, Vandervelds EM. Evidence for existence of at least two types of factor VIII associated non-A, non-B transfusion hepatitis. Lancet 2:1051, 1978.
739. Hruby MA, Schauf W. Transfusion-related short-incubation hepatitis in hemophilic patients. JAMA 240:1355, 1978.
740. Mosley JW, Redeker AG, Feinstone SM, et al. Multiple hepatitis viruses in multiple attacks of acute viral hepatitis. N Engl J Med 296:75, 1977.
741. Alter HJ, Purcell RH, Feinstone SM, et al. Non A, non B hepatitis: a review and interim report of an ongoing prospective study. In: Vyas GN, Cohen SN, Schmid R, eds. Viral Hepatitis: A Contemporary Assessment of Etiology, Epidemiology, Pathogenesis and Prevention. Philadelphia, Franklin Institute Press, 1978:359.
742. Seeff LB, Wright EC, Zimmerman HJ, et al. Post-transfusion hepatitis, 1973–1975: A Veterans Administration cooperative study. In: Vyas GN, Cohen SN, Schmid R, eds. Viral Hepatitis: A Contemporary Assessment of Etiology, Epidemiology, Pathogenesis and Prevention. Philadelphia, Franklin Institute Press, 1978:383.
743. Aach RD, Lander JL, Sherman LA, et al. Transfusion-transmitted viruses: interim analysis of hepatitis among transfused and non-transfused patients. In: Vyas GN, Cohen SN, Schmid R, eds. Viral Hepatitis: A Contemporary Assessment of Etiology, Epidemiology, Pathogenesis and Prevention. Philadelphia, Franklin Institute Press, 1978:383.

744. Berman M, Alter HJ, Ishak KG, et al. Chronic sequelae of non A, non B hepatitis. Ann Intern Med 91:1, 1979.

745. Meyers JD, Dienstag JL, Purcell RH, et al. Parenterally transmitted non-A, non-B hepatitis: an epidemic reassessed. Ann Intern Med 87:57, 1977.

746. Myers JD, Dienstag JL, Purcell RH, et al. Parenterally transmitted non A, non B hepatitis: an epidemic reassessed. Ann Intern Med 87:57, 1977.

747. Shimizu YK, Feinstone SM, Purcell RH, et al. Non-A, non-B hepatitis: ultrastructural evidence for two agents in experimentally infected chimpanzees. Science 205:197 1979.

748. Tsiquaye KN, Zuckerman AJ. New human hepatitis virus (letter). Lancet 1:1135, 1979.

749. Bradley DW, Maynard JE, Cook EH, et al. Non A, non B hepatitis in experimentally infected chimpanzees: cross-challenge and electron microscopic studies. J Med Virol 6:202, 1980.

750. Hollinger FB, Mosley JW, Szmuness W, et al. Transfusion-transmitted viruses study: experimental evidence for two non A, non B hepatitis agents. J Infect Dis 142:400, 1980.

751. Tabor E, Aprim M, Seeff LB, et al. Acquired immunity to human non-A, non-B hepatitis: cross-challenge of chimpanzees with three infectious human sera. J Infect Dis 140:789, 1979.

752. Tabor E, Gerety RJ. Inactivation of an agent of non A, non B hepatitis by formalin. J Infect Dis 142:767, 1980.

753. Shirachi R, Shiraishi H, Tateda A, et al. Hepatitis "c" antigen in non-A, non-B post-transfusion hepatitis. Lancet 2:853, 1978.

754. Vitvitski L, Prince AM, Trepo C, et al. Detection of virus-associated antigen in serum and liver of patients with non A, non B hepatitis. Lancet 2:1263, 1979.

755. Kabiri M, Tabor E, Gerety RJ. Antigen-antibody system associated with non-A, non-B hepatitis detected by indirect immunofluorescence. Lancet 2:221, 1979.

756. Tabor E, Mitchell FO, Goudeau AM, et al. Detection of an antigen-antibody system in serum associated with human non-A, non-B hepatitis. J Med Virol 4:161, 1979.

757. Chircu LV, Pezzella M, Lacava V, et al. Post-transfusion hepatitis: antigen/antibody system correlated with non A, non B hepatitis. J Med Virol 6:147, 1980.

758. Prince AM, Brotman B, Van den Ende MC, et al. Non A-non B hepatitis identification of virus-specific antigen and antibody: a preliminary report. In Vyas GN, Cohen SN, Schmid R, eds. Viral Hepatitis: A Contemporary Assessment of Etiology, Epidemiology, Pathogenesis and Prevention. Philadelphia, Franklin Institute Press, 1978:633.

759. Alter HJ, Purcell RH, Feinstone SM, et al. Non-A, non-B hepatitis: its relationship to cytomegalovirus, to chronic hepatitis, and to direct and indirect test methods. In: Szmuness W, Alter HJ, Maynard JE, eds. Viral Hepatitis. 1981 International Symposium. New York, The Franklin Institute Press, 1981:279.

760. Barker LF, Murray R. Relationship of virus dose to incubation time of clinical hepatitis and time of appearance of hepatitis-associated antigen. Am J Med Sci 263:27, 1972.

761. Shikata T, Karasawa T, Abe K, et al. Hepatitis B e antigens and infectivity of hepatitis B virus. J Infect Dis 136:571, 1977.

762. Scullard G, Greenberg HB, Smith JL, et al. Antiviral treatment of chronic hepatitis B virus infection: infectious virus cannot be detected in patient serum after permanent responses to treatment. Hepatology 2:39, 1982.

763. Yoshizawa H, Akahane Y, Itoh Y, et al. Virus-like particles in a plasma fraction (fibrinogen) and in the circulation of apparently healthy blood donors capable of inducing non A, non B hepatitis in chimpanzees and humans. Gastroenterology 79:512, 1980.

764. Goldfield M, Black HC, Bill J. The consequences of administering blood pretested for HBsAg by third generation techniques: A progress report. Am J Med Sci 270:335, 1975.

765. Alter HJ, Holland PV, Purcell RH, et al. Post-transfusion hepatitis after exclusion of commercial and hepatitis-B antigen-positive donors. Ann Intern Med 77:691, 1972.

766. Hollinger FB, Dreesman GR, Fields H, et al. HBcAg, anti-HBc and DNA polymerase activity in transfused recipients followed prospectively. Am J Med Sci 270:343, 1975.

767. Villarejos VM, Visona KA, Eduarte CA, et al. Evidence for viral hepatitis other than type A or type B among persons in Costa Rica. N Engl J Med 293:1350, 1975.

768. Dienstag JL, Alaama A, Mosley JW, et al. Etiology of sporadic hepatitis B surface antigen negative hepatitis. Ann Intern Med 87:1, 1977.

769. Martini GA, Reiter HJ, Kalbfleisch H. Acute and chronic non A, non B Hepatitis. Abstracts of the International Symposium on Viral Hepatitis. Munich, Germany, 1979:22.

770. Hollinger FB, Alter JH. Summary of workshop B-6: non A non B hepatitis. In: Vyas GN, Cohen SN, Schmid R, eds. Viral Hepatitis: A Contemporary Assessment of Etiology, Epidemiology, Pathogenesis and Prevention. Philadelphia, Franklin Institute Press, 1978:697.

771. Koretz RL, Stone O, Gitnick GL. The long-term course of non-A, non-B hepatitis. Gastroenterology 79:893, 1980.

772. Kim HC, Saidi P, Ackley AM, et al. Prevalence of type B and non-A, non-B hepatitis in hemophilia: relationship to chronic liver disease. Gastroenterology 79:1159, 1980.

773. Redeker AG. Advances in clinical aspects of acute and chronic liver disease of viral origin. In: Vyas GN, Cohen SN, Schmid R, eds. Viral Hepatitis: A Contemporary Assessment of Etiology, Epidemiology, Pathogenesis and Prevention. Philadelphia, Franklin Institute Press, 1978:425.

774. Galbraith RM, Deinstag JL, Purcell RH, et al. Non-A, non-B hepatitis associated with chronic liver disease in a haemodialysis unit. Lancet 1:951, 1979.

775. Koretz RL, Suffin SC, Gitnick GL. Post-transfusion chronic liver disease. Gastroenterology 71:797, 1976.

776. Knodell RG, Conrad ME, Ishak KG. Development of liver disease after acute non-A, non-B post-transfusion hepatitis: role of α-globulin prophylaxis in its prevention. Gastroenterology 72:902, 1977.

777. Rakela J, Redeker AG. Long term follow-up after HBsAg negative hepatitis. Gastroenterology 73:1241, 1977.

778. Tabor E, Seeff LB, Gerety RJ. Chronic non-A, non-B hepatitis carrier state. N Engl J Med 303:140, 1980.

779. Bradley DW, Maynard JE, Popper H, et al. Persistent non-A, non-B hepatitis in experimentally infected chimpanzees. J Infect Dis 143:210, 1981.

780. Goldfield M, Bill J, Colosimo F. The control of transfusion associated hepatitis. In: Vyas GN, Cohen SN, Schmid R, eds. Viral Hepatitis: A Contemporary Assessment of Etiology, Epidemiology, Pathogenesis and Prevention, Philadelphia, Franklin Institute Press, 1978:405.

781. Aach RD, Szmuness W, Mosley JW, et al. Serum alanine aminotransferase of donors in relation to the risk of non A, non B hepatitis. N Engl J Med 304:989, 1981.

782. Alter HJ, Purcell RH, Holland PV, et al. Donor transaminase and recipient hepatitis: impact on blood transfusion service. JAMA 246:630, 1981.

783. Knodell RG, Conrad ME, Ginsberg AL, et al. Efficacy of prophylactic gamma-globulin in preventing non A, non B post-transfusion hepatitis. Lancet 1:557, 1976.

784. Kuhns WJ, Prince AM, Brotman B, et al. A clinical and laboratory evaluation of immune serum globulin from donors with a history of hepatitis: attempted prevention of post-transfusion hepatitis. Am J Med Sci 272:255, 1976.

785. Seeff LB, Zimmerman HJ, Wright EC, et al. A randomized double blind controlled trial of the efficacy of immune serum globulin for the prevention of post-transfusion hepatitis. Gastroenterology 72:111, 1977.

786. Kikuchi K, Tateda A, The Venoglobulin Research Group. J Jpn Soc Blood Transfus 24:2, 1980.

787. Seeff LB, Hoofnagle JH. Immunoprophylaxis of viral hepatitis. Gastroenterology 77:161, 1979.

788. Viswanathan E. Infectious hepatitis in Delhi (1955–56): a critical study—observations in pregnant women. Indian J Med Res (Suppl) 45:1, 1957.

789. Wong DC, Purcell RH, Screenivasan MA, et al. Epidemic and endemic hepatitis in India: evidence for non A/non-B hepatitis virus etiology. Lancet 2:876, 1980.

790. Khuroo MS. Study of an epidemic of non-A, non-B hepatitis: possibility of another human hepatitis virus distinct from post-transfusion non-A, non-B type. Am J Med 68:818, 1980.

791. Balayan MS, Andjaparidze AG, Savinskaya SS, et al. Evidence for a virus in non-A, non-B hepatitis transmitted via the fecal-oral route. Intervirology 20:34, 1983.

792. Kane MA, Bradley DW, Shrestha SM, et al. Epidemic non-A, non-B hepatitis in Nepal: recovery of a possible etiologic agent and transmission studies in marmosets. JAMA 252:3140, 1984.

793. De Cock KM, Bradley DW, Sanford NL, et al. Epidemic non-A, non-B hepatitis in patients from Pakistan. Ann Intern Med 106:227, 1987.

794. Enterically transmitted non-A, non-B hepatitis—East Africa. MMWR 36:24, 1987.

795. Bradley DW, Krawczynski K, Cook EH, et al. Enterically transmitted (epidemic) non-A, non-B hepatitis (ET-NANB). Serial passage of the disease in Cynomolgus monkeys and recovery of disease-associated 27–29 nm virus-like particles from case and primate stools. Abstracts of the 1987 International Symposium on Viral Hepatitis and Liver Disease. London, 1987:31A.

796. Khuroo MS, Duemeyer W, Zargar SA, et al. Acute sporadic non-A, non-B hepatitis in India. Am J Epidemiol 118:360, 1983.

797. Tandon BN, Boshi YK, Jain SK, et al. An epidemic of non-A, non-B hepatitis in north India. Indian J Med Res 75:739, 1982.

798. Screenivasan MA, Banerjee K, Pandya PG, et al. Epidemiological investigations of an outbreak of infectious hepatitis in Ahmedabad city during 1975–76. Indian J Med Res 67:197, 1978.

799. Myint H, Soe MM, Khin T, et al. A clinical and epidemiological study of an epidemic of non-A, non-B hepatitis in Rangoon. Am J Trop Med Hyg 34:1183, 1985.

800. Shew S, Soe MM. Epidemiological criteria as indication of non-A, non-B hepatitis in a community (letter). Lancet 2:828, 1985.

801. Belabbes H, Benatallah A, Bouguermouh A. Non-A, non-B epidemic viral hepatitis in Algeria: strong evidence for its water spread. In: Vyas GN, Dienstag JL, Hoofnagle JH, eds. Viral Hepatitis and Liver Disease. Orlando, Florida: Grune & Stratton, Inc., 1984:637.

802. Maynard JE. Epidemic non-A, non-B hepatitis. Semin Liver Dis, 4(4):336, 1984.

803. Yamauchi M, Nakajima H, Kimura K, et al. An epidemic of non-A, non-B hepatitis in Japan. Am J Gastroenterol 78:652, 1983.

804. Centers for Disease Control. New horizons. Enterically transmitted non-A, non-B hepatitis. Hepatitis Surveillance, Report 50, 1986:10.

805. Farrow LJ, Stewart JS, Stern H, et al. Non-A, non-B hepatitis in west London. Lancet 1:982, 1981.

806. Gust ID. A comparison of the epidemiology of hepatitis type A and B. In: Szmuness W, Alter HJ, Maynard JE, eds. Viral Hepatitis. Philadelphia, Franklin Institute Press. 1982:129.

807. Bamber M, Thomas HC, Bannister B, et al. Acute type A, B, and non-A, non-B hepatitis in a hospital population in London: clinical and epidemiological features. Gut 24:561, 1983.

808. Chakraborty S, Datta M, Pasha ST, et al. Non-A, non-B viral hepatitis: a common-source outbreak traced to sewage contamination of drinking water. J Commun Dis 14:41, 1982.

809. Rekela J, Redeker AG, Edwards VM, et al. Hepatitis A virus infection in fulminant hepatitis and chronic active hepatitis. Gasterenterology 74:879, 1978.

810. Gupta DN, Smetana HF. The histopathology of viral hepatitis seen in the Delhi epidemic (1955–1956). Indian J Med Res (Suppl)45:101, 1957.

811. Edmondson HA, Peters RL. Liver. In: Anderson WAD, Kissane IM, eds. Pathology, 8th ed. St. Louis, CV Mosby Co, 1985:1096.

812. Coffin JC. Structure of the retroviral genome. In: Weiss R, Teich N, Varmus H, et al., eds. RNA tumor viruses. New York, Cold Spring Harbor Press, 1982:261.

813. Toh H, Hayashida H, Miyata T. Sequence homology between retroviral reverse transcriptase and putative polymerases of hepatitis B virus and cauliflower mosaic virus. Nature 305:827, 1983.

814. Choo Q-L, Kuo G, Weiner AJ, et al. Isolation of a cDNA clone derived from a blood born non-A, non-B hepatitis genome. Science 244:359, 1989.

815. Kuo G, Choo Q-L, Alter HJ, et al. An assay for circulating antibodies to a major etiologic virus of human non-A, non-B hepatitis. Science 244:362, 1989.

36

Hepatitis B Virus Persistence, Chronic Liver Disease, and Primary Liver Cancer

David A. Shafritz, M.D. • Morris Sherman, M.B., B.Ch., Ph.D. • Ran Tur-Kaspa, M.D.

ABBREVIATIONS

HBcAg = hepatitis B core antigen
HBeAg = hepatitis B e (early) antigen
HBsAg = hepatitis B surface antigen
HBV = hepatitis B virus
HCC = hepatocellular carcinoma

The question as to whether hepatitis B virus (HBV) causes hepatocellular carcinoma (HCC) has to date been answered best by epidemiologic studies. Precisely how HBV causes HCC remains unclear, however. A general theme emerging from molecular studies is that HBV has the capacity to integrate into the host genome, perhaps related to its basic structure and/or mechanism of replication, both of which show strong analogies to retroviruses (see Chap. 35). At or subsequent to the initial integration event, there are modifications of both viral and cellular sequences leading to mutagenesis of both the viral and cellular genome. Multiple steps involving both host and viral factors may then lead to cellular transformation and selection of hepatocytes with oncogenic potential.

EPIDEMIOLOGIC AND CLINICAL STUDIES

WORLD-WIDE INCIDENCE OF HEPATOCELLULAR CARCINOMA (See also Chap. 45)

HCC is reported to be the eighth most frequent cancer in the world, accounting for approximately 260,000 new cases each year.[1] This conclusion is based on estimates gleaned from 75 cancer registries, worldwide, and synthesized by the WHO International Agency for Research on Cancer (IARC) and the Union International Contra Cancrum (UICC).[2] These data, however, must be regarded as incomplete, since reliable estimates of the incidence of HCC are not available from many areas of the world where HCC is common. In these areas, cancer registries do not exist or are only poorly kept. Furthermore, many estimates of the incidence of HCC are based on autopsy data, which of necessity are biased.

According to these data, the incidence of HCC varies greatly in different parts of the world. The highest incidence is found in the black population of Zimbabwe (formerly Rhodesia) and Maputo (formerly Mozambique), where the age-standardized incidence has been recorded as high as

106.9/100,000/year.[1–4] HCC accounts for 65.5 per cent of all male cancer deaths and 31 per cent of deaths in females in these areas.[5,6] Elsewhere in Africa and in Southeast Asia, for example, China, Taiwan, Vietnam, and Korea, the incidence of HCC varies from 20 to 100/100,000/year. HCC is the third most common cause of cancer death in Chinese and Japanese men and is the fourth and fifth most frequent cause in Chinese and Japanese females, respectively.[7,8]

Areas of intermediate incidence of HCC include Japan, Switzerland, and Bulgaria (10 to 20/100,000/year) and Poland, Rumania, Western Europe, and Yugoslavia (5 to 9/100,000/year). Areas of lowest incidence include the United States, United Kingdom, Canada, Scandinavia, and South Africa (whites)—<5/100,000 population/year.

HEPATOCELLULAR CARCINOMA AND HEPATITIS B VIRUS INFECTION

There is now clear epidemiologic evidence that chronic hepatitic B virus infection is causally related to HCC. Some estimates suggest that HBV may be responsible for 80 per cent of all HCC worldwide. Evidence for this association

has been obtained from several different lines of epidemiologic investigation.

1. There is a strong geographic concordance between endemic HBV infection and a high incidence of HCC (Fig. 36–1). For instance, in China, Southeast Asia, and South Africa (blacks), as much as 10 to 15 per cent of the population may be HBV carriers. These areas also have the highest incidence of HCC.[9,10] Areas of somewhat lower incidence of HCC, such as Greece, Italy, and the Mediterranean basin,[1–4] have correspondingly lower rates of HBV infection (3 to 5 per cent of the population may be carriers).[9] Conversely, those areas of the world where HBV is uncommon (that is, North America and Western Europe, where 0.1 to 0.5 per cent of the population are carriers)[9] have a low incidence of HCC.[1–4] Yet within areas of low incidence of HCC, pockets of high HBV endemicity exist.[11,12] Many Southeast Asian communities in North American cities have a higher prevalence of chronic HBV infection than the rest of the population.[9,13] Similarly, these populations have a higher incidence of HCC than their neighbors with low HBV incidence. By contrast, in an area with a high prevalence of HBV, such as South Africa, the white community, which has a level of HBV endemicity approaching that seen in North America, has a low incidence of HCC.[4]

Figure 36–1. A, Worldwide distribution of hepatitis B virus. B, Worldwide distribution of primary hepatocellular carcinoma. (Modified from Maupas P, Melnick JL. Prog Med Virol 27:1, 1981, with permission of S. Karger AG, Basel.)

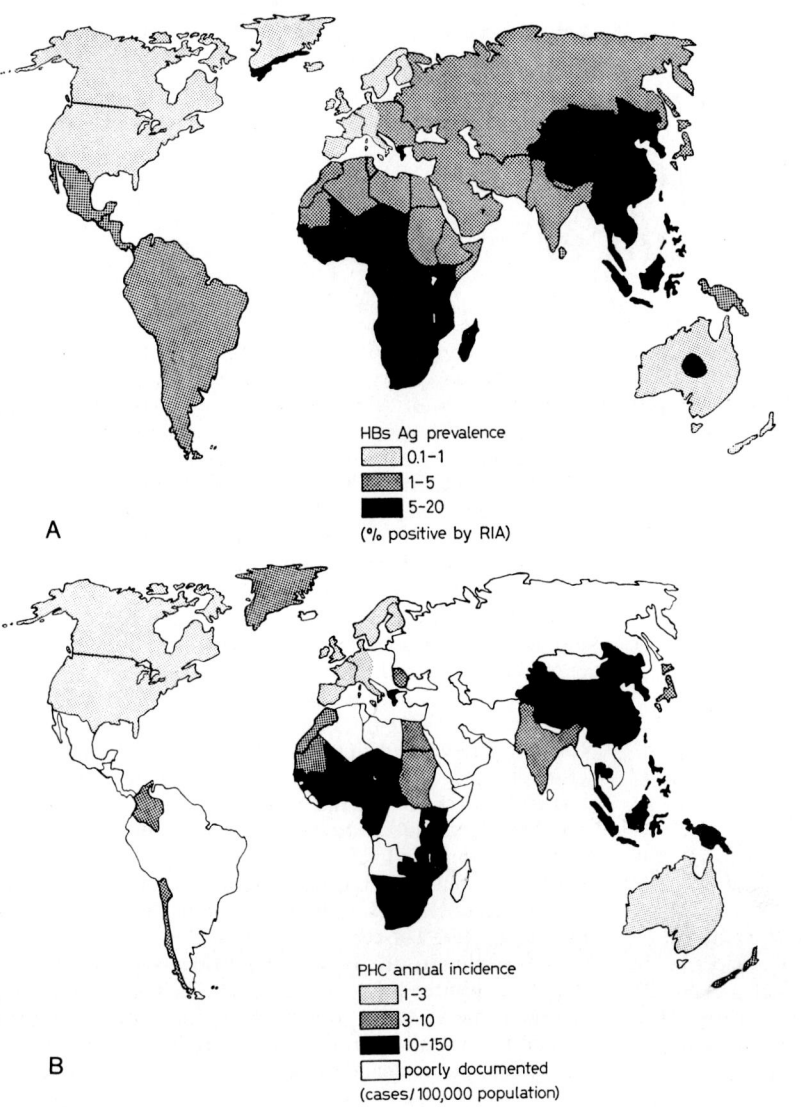

A

HBs Ag prevalence
- ▨ 0.1–1
- ▨ 1–5
- ■ 5–20

(% positive by RIA)

B

PHC annual incidence
- ▨ 1–3
- ▨ 3–10
- ■ 10–150
- ☐ poorly documented

(cases/100,000 population)

2. Patients who have HCC, whether in areas with high or low incidence of HCC, frequently have evidence of current or previous HBV infection (Table 36–1). Prospective and retrospective studies have shown that in areas of high incidence of HCC, more than 90 per cent of HCC arises in patients with markers of HBV infection, that is, either hepatitis B surface antigen (HBsAg)–positive or anti–hepatitis B core (HBc)–positive.[9, 14–20] Even in those parts of the world where HBV is less prevalent and other diseases such as hemochromatosis and alcoholic cirrhosis contribute to the incidence of HCC, evidence of HBV infection is still present in more than 40 per cent of patients with HCC.[9]

3. Prospective studies have yielded the most complete and convincing evidence that HBV is causally linked to HCC. The largest of these studies was that performed in Taiwan by Beasley and his associates.[14] The most recent report of this ongoing study showed that of an initial population of 22,707 men of whom 3454 were HBsAg-positive (15.2 per cent), 116 individuals developed HCC.[21] Of these, 113 were HBsAg-positive, one was anti-HBs and anti-HBc positive, and two were anti-HBs positive only. The annual incidence of HCC in these Chinese male HBsAg carriers was 527/100,000 (Table 36–2). The relative risk of an HBsAg carrier developing HCC in this study was 217. As Table 36–2 shows, in HBsAg carriers the incidence of and relative risk for HCC increases dramatically in the presence of cirrhosis. Other additional risk factors in these patients were a previous history of hepatitis, the presence of IgM anti-HBc, and increasing age. It has been estimated that the lifetime risk of death from cirrhosis, HCC, or both in these HBsAg carriers will be 40 to 50 per cent.

In a prospective study of 3130 Japanese male railway workers, a similar annual incidence of HCC was found in HBsAg-positive individuals.[15]

TABLE 36–1. HEPATITIS B VIRUS MARKERS IN PATIENTS WITH HEPATOCELLULAR CARCINOMA (HCC) IN VARIOUS COUNTRIES

	Patients with HCC (%)	Control Populations (%)
HBsAg		
Greece	55	4.7
Spain	19.3	2.0
United States	14.7	1
Senegal	51.9	12.0
Mozambique	62.1	14.3
Uganda	47.0	6.0
Zambia	63.0	7.5
South Africa	59.5	9.0
Taiwan	54.8	12.2
Singapore	35.8	4.1
Japan	37.3	2.6
Vietnam	80.3	24.5
Anti-HBc		
Greece	70.0	31.9
Spain	87.0	14.8
United States	48.5	1
Senegal	87.3	26.0
South Africa	86.0	31.7
Hong Kong	70.3	36.2

Source: Blumberg B, London WT, Curr Probl Cancer 6(12):1, 1982, with permission.

Anti-HBc = anti–hepatitis B core antigen.

TABLE 36–2. RISK AND INCIDENCE OF HEPATOCELLULAR CARCINOMA IN TAIWAN

Recruitment status	Risk of HCC 100,000/year	Relative risk
All HBsAg-positive subjects	528	217
Ages		
20–29	0	
30–39	122	
40–49	274	
50–59	854	
60–69	1331	
With cirrhosis	2419	961
Without cirrhosis	505	201
All HBsAg-negative subjects	2.6	
Anti-HBs–positive	2.1	
Anti-HBs, anti-HBc–positive	7.1	

Source: Modified from Beasley RP, et al. Lancet 2:1124, 1981.

THE INFLUENCE OF AGE, RACE, AND SEX

The prospective studies previously described included only male subjects. Equivalent figures for females do not exist. However, it is known that HCC occurs more frequently in males than females by at least four to eightfold in African and Asian populations[22–25] and about twofold in Caucasian populations.[26] The reason for this difference is unknown.

Race per se does not appear to be a factor in the development of HCC. Rather, the different incidence in different racial groups reflects the endemicity of HBV infection, not racial factors. South African blacks have a high incidence of HCC, but North American blacks, in whom the incidence of HBV infection is low, have a correspondingly low incidence of HCC.[27]

The age at which HCC develops differs in Southeast Asians and in South African blacks. In Southeast Asian populations, the incidence of HCC increases with age,[21, 22, 23] whereas in South African blacks, the incidence is highest in the 25 to 40 age group.[28, 29] In both areas, HCC is uncommon in patients younger than 20 years of age, although the incidence in this age group in these high prevalence areas is still significantly higher than in areas of low prevalence.[29] Rural African blacks with HCC tend to be younger than their urban counterparts. Again, the cause for this difference is not known, but it has been suggested that some of these differences may be due in part to the presence or absence of co-carcinogens acting in concert with HBV.

CO-CARCINOGENS

In the Taiwan study,[14] the high incidence of HCC in HBV carriers combined with the absence of HCC in HBV marker–negative patients made it unnecessary to invoke additional carcinogenic factors. Nonetheless, evidence from other sources strongly suggests that co-carcinogenic factors may be important in the pathogenesis of HCC. As discussed before, male gender is itself an important pathogenetic factor. In addition, there are several observations of differing HCC incidence in neighboring populations that have similar prevalences of HBV. Rural South African blacks who are HBsAg-positive have a higher incidence of HCC than do urban HBsAg-positive blacks, who also tend to get their tumors about ten years later.[30, 31]

The main chemical co-carcinogen that has been implicated in the pathogenesis of HCC is aflatoxin B1 (see Chap. 45).[32-36] Several studies of rural populations in central Africa and Southeast Asia have demonstrated a high daily intake of aflatoxin B1 and have correlated the incidence of HCC in these populations with the amount of aflatoxin ingested daily.[34-37] However, whereas aflatoxin ingestion may be a factor in rural areas of Africa and Southeast Asia, it is unlikely to be an important co-carcinogen in large cities and in North America or Western Europe.

Cirrhosis as a Co-carcinogen

The question has been raised whether HBV is of itself carcinogenic or whether the risk of HCC is related to the presence of cirrhosis. It is well known that cirrhosis from any cause may be associated with the development of HCC. Such a relationship has been demonstrated in patients with hemochromatosis (Chap. 48), alpha$_1$-antitrypsin deficiency (Chap. 50), or hereditary tyrosinemia (Chap. 49).[38-40] In Europe and North America, alcoholic cirrhosis is the form of non-HBV–related cirrhosis that may be associated with HCC (Chap. 45).[41] In cirrhosis other than that associated with HBV, the relative risk of HCC is not known; but the risk of malignant transformation, although greater than in noncirrhotics, is generally considered to be low.

In Asia, 80 to 90 per cent of HCCs develop in cirrhotic livers. In Africa, the prevalence of cirrhosis in patients with HCC is less (~60 per cent). In most instances, the cirrhosis is of a macronodular variety and has been shown to precede the onset of HCC.

The Taiwan prospective study of HBsAg carriers showed that the presence of cirrhosis in an HBsAg carrier greatly increased the risk of HCC (Table 36–2). No tumors developed in 30 patients who were HBsAg-negative with cirrhosis. In contrast, Zaman and colleagues,[42] in a study of 613 HBsAg carriers, were unable to show that HBV infection was an independent risk factor for HCC over and above the risk conferred by the presence of cirrhosis. In this study, few patients were of Asian origin. Therefore, the differences between this study and previous studies performed in Asia may relate to the age at which the HBV infection was acquired. In Southeast Asians, horizontal transmission in the neonatal period occurs frequently, whereas in Caucasians this is a less common form of transmission.

Thus, the question of whether chronic HBV infection is an independent risk factor for HCC or if HBV causes HCC by causing cirrhosis is not entirely settled. However, since the incidence of HCC in HBsAg-positive patients with no liver disease and with chronic active hepatitis in the absence of cirrhosis is also increased,[21, 43] it is likely that HBV is indeed a carcinogenic agent, but whether it is an initiator or promoter of tumor is not clear.

SCREENING PROGRAMS FOR EARLY DETECTION OF HEPATOCELLULAR CARCINOMA

Because therapy of HCC is so dismal, aside from surgical removal of small tumors, it seems logical to try to devise a regimen whereby HCC can be detected early, at a stage where less radical surgery, less severe cirrhosis, and smaller tumor size might make resection feasible. Indeed, such programs have been devised, most notably in China, Taiwan, and Japan.[44-47] Tang and co-workers have described large-scale screening of asymptomatic high-risk populations by using alpha fetoprotein (AFP) as a tumor marker. Such screening programs have a low yield of HCC (5 to 15 tumors/100,000 population screened). On the other hand, screening of HBsAg carriers should have a much higher yield. Projections from the Taiwan study suggest that 0.5 per cent of male carriers will develop HCC per year. Under these circumstances, a screening program that has a high sensitivity and specificity becomes a much more cost-effective endeavor.

A Suitable Marker for HCC

Elevation of serum alpha fetoprotein (AFP) has long been recognized as a marker for HCC.[48, 49] An AFP of 0.5 ng/ml in the correct clinical setting is diagnostic of HCC. Lesser elevations of AFP, however, cannot differentiate between HCC and chronic liver disease. It has been shown that AFP measurements may be elevated in 66 to 77 per cent of patients with small HCCs (<3 cm), although only 26 to 53 per cent of measurements were diagnostically elevated.[44, 45, 49-51] Several observers have noted, however, that even when AFP is not diagnostically elevated, a sudden sharp rise in AFP is often evidence of HCC.[44, 46]

Because the false-negative and false-positive rate of AFP is rather high,[40] other tests have also been used for screening. Tang and associates compared AFP levels with aspartate aminotransferase (AST) levels.[46, 52] In patients with active liver disease—mainly chronic active hepatitis or active cirrhosis—both AST and AFP may be elevated. In inactive cirrhosis, both are usually low. With small HCCs, AFP may rise, but AST usually remains low. The sensitivity of this method of screening has not been assessed. Other serologic tests that have been used to predict the presence of HCC include carcinoembryonic antigen,[53] acid isoferritins,[54] placental D-alkaline phosphatase,[55] γ-glutamyltranspeptidase,[56] and several hepatoma-specific antigens. None of these tests have proved to be as reliable as AFP, but their role in AFP-negative tumors has not been evaluated systematically.

Real-time ultrasonography is frequently used in Japan and Taiwan to complement AFP measurements. Various investigators have shown that ultrasound can detect up to 92 per cent of all tumors less than 5 cm and 91 per cent of all lesions less than 3 cm.[50, 51] Other investigators have not shown such impressive results. A single report has objectively assessed the sensitivity and specificity of ultrasound in diagnosing liver tumors and in particular, HCC.[57] Ultrasound has a sensitivity of 94.4 per cent, a specificity of 98.7 per cent, and an overall accuracy of 98.8 per cent in diagnosing liver tumors. In this study, sensitivity in diagnosing masses as HCC was 58.9 per cent, although once diagnosed, specificity was 99.9 per cent. Invasive radiologic modalities, such as various forms of angiography, may be more accurate than sonography but cannot be recommended as screening tests.

PROLONGED SUBCLINICAL GROWTH

Sheu and co-workers, using ultrasound, showed that small HCCs may remain subclinical for prolonged periods.[58] They estimated tumor doubling times to be between 29 and

398 days. The median subclinical growth period was 3.2 years, with a range of 9.6 months to 10.9 years. If ultrasonography is to be used for screening, a suitable screening period would be every four to five months. This is based on the least time which a 1-cm tumor would take to grow to 3 cm, that is, four to six months. These figures however refer only to the growth of tumors after initial detection. They give no information about the interval of screening necessary to pick up tumors growing from undetectable to minimum detectable size. The validity of these estimates also needs to be confirmed in areas of the world where HCC sometimes seems to have a different biologic behavior.

A SUITABLE INTERVENTION

Tang and colleagues and others have shown that resection of small hepatomas detected by screening is feasible even in cirrhotic patients.[46, 52] In China, up to 49 per cent of clinically detectable tumors may be resectable. The resectability rate rises to 65 per cent for subclinical HCCs detected by population screening. These workers gave an operative mortality in clinical tumors of 12.4 per cent, but in subclinical tumors operative mortality was less than 3 per cent. In Japan, 9 per cent of HCCs were resectable in 1980,[59] whereas in 1984, 24 per cent of a similar series of patients were resectable.[60] This increase is attributed to earlier diagnosis.

Tang and colleagues report that early resection is feasible because the extent of the resection is more limited, so that cirrhosis presents less of a problem.[52] Tumors can be removed by simple excision, wedge resection, or segmentectomy, all less drastic than hepatic lobectomy. The amount of liver tissue remaining after a more limited resection than hemihepatectomy is apparently sufficient to allow adequate liver function in the postoperative period.

Furthermore, it has been suggested that cirrhosis progresses over the period of subclinical growth of the tumor.[61] Therefore, resection of small tumors may result in improved mortality rates because the liver disease is less severe at this time.

Ebara and associates have shown that the three-year survival of untreated small (<3 cm) tumors is 12.8 per cent, while the one-year survival is 90.7 per cent.[62] Based on these figures, if surgery offers less than 10 per cent operative mortality and better than 15 to 20 per cent three-year survival, then surgery is better than no treatment. There are no published studies on chemotherapy of small HCCs. Dr. Tang's group reports a 33.3 per cent five-year survival following surgery.[46] However, since the figures quoted above are culled from several reports, the studies described therein probably are not strictly comparable. Furthermore, as discussed previously, these estimates of survival do not take lead-time bias into account.

SCREENING: THE JAPANESE EXPERIENCE

Although screening programs are well established in Japan, the success reported by Tang and colleagues in China has not been duplicated.[61] In Japan, many tumors detected by screening (nearly 50 per cent) were already unresectable. Of concern in setting up a screening program based upon the presence of HBsAg in serum is the finding that although the incidence of HCC has doubled in Japan over 15 years, the frequency of HBV-related HCC has diminished, thus reducing the value of HBsAg as a pre-screening test.[63] Up to 40 per cent of HBsAg-negative patients with HCC in Japan have a prior history of blood transfusion, raising the specter of non-A, non-B hepatitis as a cause of HCC.[61] In Japan, because of these factors, all high-risk patients, that is, HBsAg-positive patients as well as HBsAg-negative patients with liver disease, patients with a past history of liver disease or transfusion, and those with a family history of liver disease all are candidates for regular screening by ultrasonography. This kind of program however is of value only in populations in which HCC is common and may not be applicable in North America or Europe. Even less is known about the potential benefit of screening patients with HBsAg-negative cirrhosis.

SCREENING FOR HCC AS A MEDICAL POLICY

Other questions concerning screening of HBV carriers still remain to be addressed. Should all HBsAg-positive carriers be screened or only those over a certain age? Should noncirrhotic HBsAg-positive patients be screened? If not, with how much certainty can the diagnosis of cirrhosis be excluded (short of liver biopsy)? How frequently should screening be performed? Furthermore, there is no indication of whether screening is cost effective. It may be difficult to justify screening a 20-year-old patient who develops a tumor at age 70-plus years. On the other hand, if this patient develops a tumor at age 40 to 50 years, cost-benefit analysis would probably show that screening was cost efficient.

Because of these unanswered questions and the uncertain benefits of screening of HBsAg carriers (or other patients with cirrhosis), routine screening of such patients cannot be recommended as public policy at this time. Despite this limitation, it is likely that many practitioners will screen their patients who are HBsAg-positive or who have cirrhosis. Furthermore, patients are likely to demand screening more frequently as they become better educated about the risks of the HBV-carrier state.

MOLECULAR STUDIES OF HBV-RELATED CHRONIC LIVER DISEASE AND HCC

USE OF RECOMBINANT HBV DNA PROBES

The advent of molecular cloning has permitted detailed analysis of the structure and nucleotide sequence of the HBV genome and preparation of highly sensitive and specific cloned HBV DNA probes for detecting HBV DNA sequences in infected tissue specimens. The procedure is known as molecular hybridization, or Southern blot analysis. In essence, cellular DNA is extracted from the tissue of interest and is subjected to digestion with restriction endonucleases. These enzymes recognize specific hexanucleotide sequences and cleave high molecular weight DNA into fragments ranging in size from ~2000 to 10,000 nucleotides. The "digested" DNA can be spread out in manageable pieces, which can be separated by size by gel electrophoresis. Following electrophoresis, the DNA is transferred to a nitrocellulose filter or other solid support matrix to which the DNA can be bound irreversibly. The filter is incubated with a specific radiolabeled probe prepared from cloned repurified DNA (hybridization). The labeled DNA probe will bind to complementary DNA sequences attached to the filter, and the hybrid molecules can be detected by autoradiography.

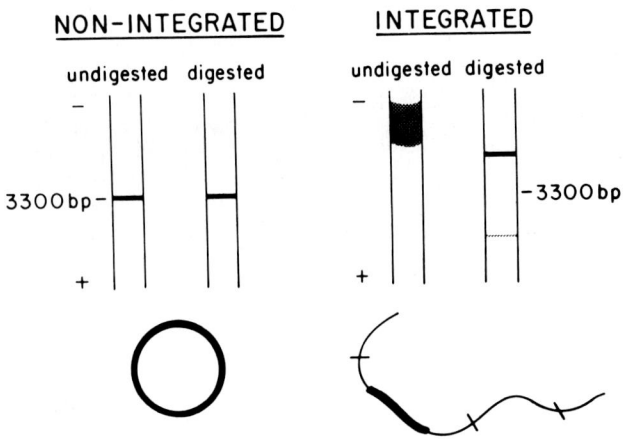

Figure 36–2. Use of restriction enzyme digestion. Southern blot transfer and molecular hybridization with a cloned HBV DNA probe to identify and show the molecular forms of hepatitis B virus DNA in extracts from human liver or tumor tissue. (See text and references 83 and 85 for explanation.)

This technique has been used to study the relationship between HBV infection and HCC. The strategy for these experiments is outlined in Figure 36–2. Free HBV virions can be differentiated from HBV DNA integrated into the patient's genome by using a restriction enzyme that does not cleave within the HBV genome. Full length, double-stranded HBV DNA migrates on gel electrophoresis as a single band at ~3200 to 3300 base pairs. If HBV DNA is integrated into the cellular genome, HBV sequences in a DNA extract that has not been digested with a restriction enzyme will appear as a diffuse band of high molecular weight at the top of the gel. If HBV DNA is randomly integrated into numerous different sites in the genome of different cells, digestion with restriction enzyme will produce HBV DNA sequences in larger pieces of DNA of various sizes. The fragments reacting with a probe for HBV DNA will then spread throughout the gel. These molecules may be detectable as a diffuse smear on hybridization analysis or may not be detectable if present in too low an amount. However, if HBV DNA is integrated into a specific site(s) in cellular DNA, then restriction enzyme digestion will produce specific, discrete hybridization bands representing these integrations. If the restriction enzyme used does not recognize any sequence in HBV DNA, all integrated viral sequences should remain in molecules larger than 3200 to 3300 base pairs, except for *fragments* of integrated viral DNA that could migrate in molecules of smaller size. Use of a series of restriction enzymes with either no cleavage site in HBV DNA or different specific cleavage sites within the HBV genome can unambiguously establish the presence or absence of integrated sequences of HBV.

HYBRIDIZATION STUDIES IN HUMAN HCC CELL LINES

Initial molecular studies demonstrating integration of HBV into the genome of a liver tumor were performed in the PLC/PRF/5 cell line (Fig. 36–3),[64–67] originally established by J. Alexander and colleagues. The HCC tumor was from a young Mozambican male who was a chronic HBV carrier.[68] This cell line produces HBsAg[68] and under some conditions, low levels of HBcAg[69, 70] but no other known HBV gene products. There are no replicating or free virus molecules in PLC/PRF/5 cells (Fig. 36–3). Analysis of integrated HBV DNA sequences has shown that there is no intact full-length copy of the viral genome in this cell line. Instead, fragments of HBV DNA are integrated into at least seven distinct cellular sites.[71] All of these integrations have been cloned and mapped by restriction enzyme analysis. DNA sequencing has revealed a duplication and inversion of viral sequences in one case

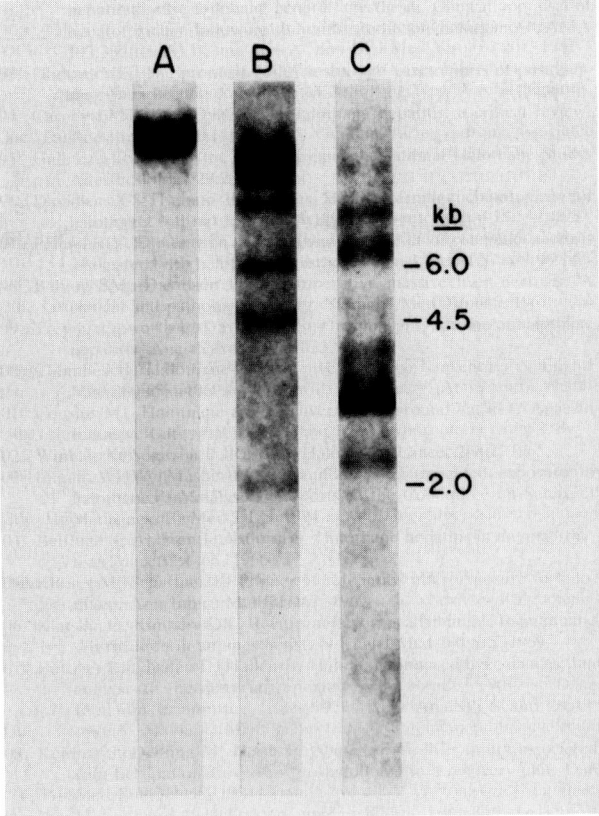

Figure 36–3. Hybridization pattern of hepatitis B virus DNA sequences in human hepatocellular carcinoma cell line PLC/PRF/5. *Lane A,* undigested DNA, showing that all HBV DNA sequences are present in high–molecular weight DNA and that there is neither free virus nor replicative forms in this cell line. *Lane B,* DNA digested with restriction enzyme Hind III, which recognizes no site in HBV DNA. Each band represents a separate restriction fragment containing integrated HBV DNA sequences. *Lane C,* DNA digested with restriction enzyme EcoR1, which recognizes one site in HBV DNA. This enzyme produces a greater number of bands hybridizing with the HBV DNA probe because some of the integrated viral sequences contain internal sites for EcoR1.

and deletion of viral sequences in another. Rearrangements of host cellular sequences flanking integrated HBV DNA have also been found,[71-73] as well as amplification and transposition of viral and cellular flanking sequences subsequent to the initial integration event.[74-77] These changes suggest that HBV DNA can have a strong mutagenic effect on cellular DNA once it has become integrated into the cellular genome. This property has been previously recognized in several viruses that are oncogenic in animal model systems, such as SV40 and adenoviruses, and may represent a general feature of oncogenic DNA viruses.[78, 79] Other cell lines derived from HCCs in viral carriers or in patients previously infected with HBV and showing antibodies to viral proteins in the serum at the time of tumor development also contain integrated HBV genomes.[80-82]

HBV DNA INTEGRATIONS IN PRIMARY HCCS

Shortly after the discovery of integrated HBV DNA in the PLC/PRF/5 cell line, studies by several investigators showed that the vast majority of primary HCCs from viral carriers also contained HBV DNA integrated into unique sites within the host genome.[66, 83-86] Banding patterns of integrated HBV DNA varied in different tumors, and individual tumors often contained multiple viral DNA integrations (Fig. 36–4). This suggested that individual hepatocytes can accumulate multiple integrations during chronic infection or that several integrations could occur simultaneously during transformation. The fact that viral DNA integrations were also present in "normal" liver tissue

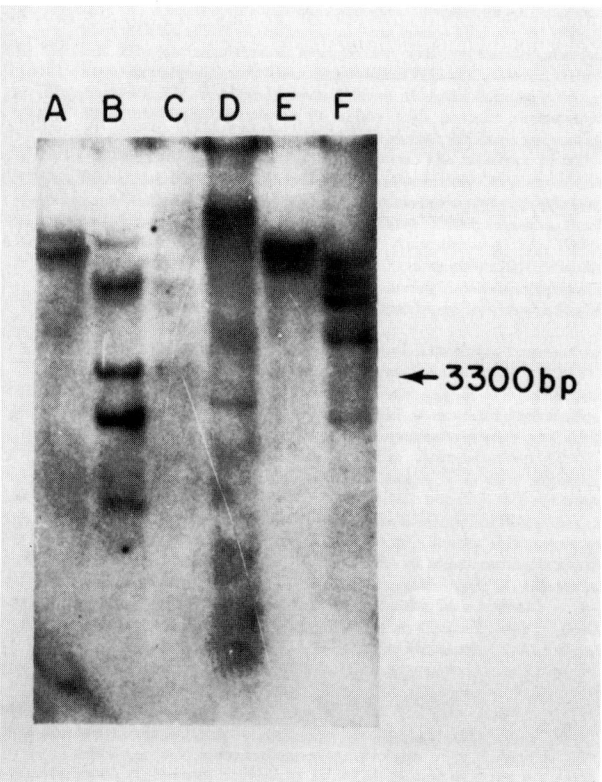

Figure 36–4. Molecular hybridization analysis showing integration of HBV-DNA into unique sites in the host genome of hepatocellular carcinoma tissue. Each band of hybridization represents a separate integration of HBV sequences. The arrow at 3300 bp indicates the migration position of full-length free HBV genomes.

in HCC patients raised the possibility that these integrations may play a role in the transformation process.[85-87] In addition, HBV DNA integration was also found in the liver cell genome of patients with no evidence of HCC.[85, 86, 88-90]

HBV integrations from HCCs often contain multiple arrangements, including deletions, inversions, and direct and inverted duplications.[74, 75, 81, 91, 92] However, some HBV integrations in HCCs contain a greater than unit length HBV DNA sequence with an apparently intact copy of the genome.[73, 76] Extrachromosomal, high molecular weight "novel" forms of viral DNA have also been found in livers from woodchuck and ground squirrel carriers of hepatitis virus.[93, 94] These molecules are comprised of oligomeric, greater than unit length viral DNAs with deletions, duplications, and rearrangements of viral sequences. These structural rearrangements are similar to those observed in woodchuck hepatitis virus (WHV) integrations in woodchuck HCCs.[95] It has been suggested that novel forms may represent a by-product of defective genome replication during viral persistence and could represent a precursor of integrations involved in hepatic oncogenesis.[93] Although novel forms have not been identified in humans, several integrations have recently been cloned, mapped, and partially sequenced from the liver of HBV carriers without HCC.[96] These integrated HBV sequences show modified structures similar to those found in HCC tissue.

In 30 to 50 per cent of HBV DNA integrations, in which the junctions between normal cellular DNA have been mapped and sequenced, a short, repeated sequence of 11 nucleotides, referred to as DR1 (see Chap. 35), has been found at one junction.[72, 73, 92, 97] This suggests that DR1 may be involved in a specific recombination event with an analogous sequence in the host cell. However, the precise mechanism for this process has not yet been established.

In different tumors, HBV DNA integrations have been found on chromosomes 6, 9, and 11 with, also, a translocation between chromosomes 17 and 18.[91, 92] These integrations are usually associated with deletions of cellular genes. Other HBV integrations in HCC or HCC cell lines have been identified on chromosomes 2, 3, 4, 7, 12, 15, and 18. Therefore, many chromosomes are involved in HBV integrations associated with HCC, and it remains to be determined whether these integrations are located at random sites or in chromosomal regions specifically associated with oncogenesis. Interestingly, an HBV integration isolated from a primary HCC and located on chromosome 11p is in the same region that contains the locus of the oncogene for Wilms's tumor.[98]

The ability of HBV to integrate into cellular DNA during chronic infection is consistent with its potential function as a tumor initiator. For retroviruses, this has been shown to occur either by direct transfer of oncogenes carried by the virus[99, 100] or by activation of cellular proto-oncogenes through insertion of viral gene regulatory signals (promoters or enhancers) into the cellular genome.[101] To date, however, hepadna viruses have not been shown to contain a viral oncogene, although three HBV gene promoters, an HBV enhancer, and a glucocorticoid responsive element (GRE) have been identified.[102-105] Dejean and co-workers have also identified an HBV integration at the 5' boundary of a gene having partial homology with the erb A oncogene and the glucocorticoid receptor, which are structurally related.[106, 107] This HBV integration is located on chromosome 3. They suggest that the erb A/steroid receptor–related gene (referred to as hap) regulates the transcription of a crucial target gene. In the specific tumor in which this integration has been found, the erb A oncogene-like sequence is truncated and is perhaps inappro-priately expressed as a consequence of HBV integration, thus contributing to cell transformation.[108] Apart from this report, no HBV DNA integration has been shown to occur immediately adjacent to any known cellular proto-onco-gene.[73, 75, 81] However, several studies in woodchucks and humans suggest enhanced expression of c-myc or N-ras on-cogenes in HCC tissues as compared to normal liver.[109, 110]

HBV DNA INTEGRATION IN NONMALIGNANT LIVER TISSUE

In regions of liver adjacent to tumor tissue, HBV DNA integration into the host genome has been found with the same pattern, a partially related pattern, or a totally differ-ent one, compared with tumor.[84-87] This suggests that inte-gration of HBV sequences into host DNA precedes hepatic oncogenesis. As indicated previously, HBV DNA integra-tion into the liver genome of HBV carriers without HCC has also been reported.[84-86, 88-90] The additional finding in some cases of integrated HBV DNA in discrete bands after restriction enzyme digestion of total liver DNA suggests that these integrations are present in precisely the same genomic location in many cells. These cells are most likely derived from single hepatocytes that have already under-gone clonal expansion and are therefore transformed but do not have the morphologic appearance of a malignancy (see later).

EVOLUTION OF HCC IN HBV CARRIERS

Generally, HBV carriers with HCC show lower levels of viremia than HBV carriers without HCC,[111, 112] and the viral DNA integration process is thought to precede hepatic oncogenesis by months or years.[84-86, 89, 113] In areas where HBV carrier rates and HCC incidence are high (such as Africa and Asia), initial infection occurs during infancy or early childhood, and most HBV carriers have converted to anti–hepatitis B early antigen (anti-HBe) status long before malignancy develops.[112, 114] During the course of persistent HBV infection, the level of viremia gradually decreases over time, and a significant portion of carriers convert spontaneously from hepatitis B early antigen (HBeAg) to anti-HBe status associated with cessation of virus produc-tion.[115-119] The molecular forms of HBV DNA present in hepatic tissues of patients who are viremic (HBsAg- and HBeAg-positive—HBsAg+/HBeAg+) are full-length, free HBV genomes and lower molecular weight viral DNA replicative intermediates (Fig. 36–5). However, in carriers who are no longer viremic (usually anti-HBe+), only high molecular weight, integrated HBV DNA or integrated forms plus free genomes are present in the liver. In a well-studied group of HBsAg carriers from South Africa who developed HCC, markedly reduced levels of viremia were observed, even when such patients remained HBeAg-pos-itive.[111, 112]

REPLICATING VERSUS NONREPLICATING STATES OF PERSISTENT HBV INFECTION

At present, the most sensitive and definitive test for viremia is the detection of HBV DNA in the serum by molecular hybridization. This test can be performed by directly applying a small amount of serum (5 to 10 μl) to a filter[111] or by extracting DNA from the serum and applying

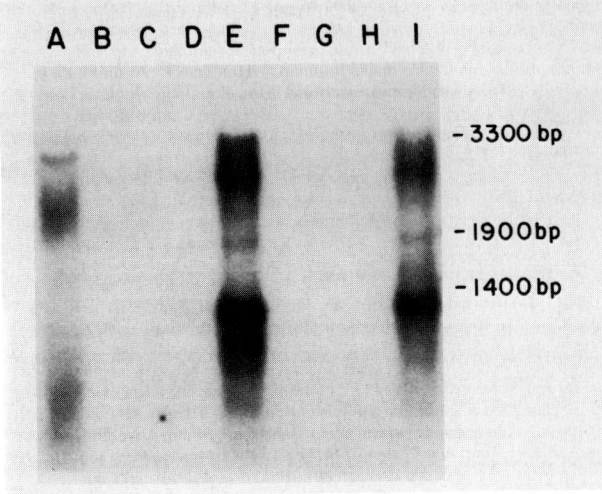

Figure 36–5. Identification of full-length free HBV genomes and lower molecular weight replicative forms of HBV DNA in liver tissue of an HBV carrier actively secreting virus. *Lanes A, E,* and *I* are from short-term HBV carriers (from six months to two years) who were serologically HBsAg+/HBeAg+, and *lanes B, C, D, F, G* and *H* were from noncarriers. The band present at ~3300 base pairs represents the full-length double-stranded HBV genome. Lower molecular weight, partially double-stranded HBV DNA molecules are present between 2200 and 3000 base pairs, and partial single-stranded HBV DNA molecules are seen below 1400 base pairs. A band seen at ~1900 base pairs represents either full-length single-stranded HBV DNA or supercoiled molecules of full-length double-stranded HBV DNA, which migrate more rapidly in the gel than relaxed circular or linear forms of the complete genome because of their supercoiled configuration.

it to the filter[88, 89, 120-122] and then hybridizing the filter with a purified HBV DNA probe (Fig. 36–6). As few as 5000 to 10,000 molecules of HBV DNA (~ 0.05 pgm) can be detected by this method. This test can be positive indepen-dent of the HBeAg/anti-HBe status.[111, 122-126] Nearly all

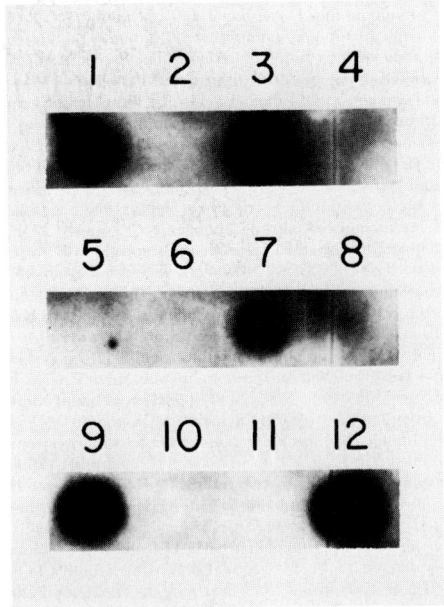

Figure 36–6. Spot hybridization test to detect HBV DNA sequences in human serum. In this test, 5 to 10 μl of serum is applied directly to a nitrocellulose filter and hybridized with a cloned repurified HBV DNA probe. Alternatively, total DNA can be first extracted from an aliquot of serum (200 μl to 1.0 ml) and then applied to the filter. Spots 1, 3, and 7 are from HBsAg+/HBeAg+ carriers; spot 9 is from a patient with acute HBV infection, and spot 12 is from an HBsAg+/anti-HBe+ carrier. Spots 2, 4, 5, 6, 8, 10, and 11 are from noninfected control sera or patients who spontaneously cleared a previous HBV infection (anti-HBs+/anti-HBc+).

HBeAg[+] patients show HBV DNA in serum. A significant proportion of anti-HBe[+] patients also show HBV DNA in serum (Table 36–3). This was unexpected in view of the generally accepted notion that most HBsAg carriers who are anti-HBe[+] no longer actively replicate virus. The percentage of HBsAg[+]/anti-HBe[+] patients who are also HBV DNA–positive can vary considerably, depending on the population studied.[111, 120–127] In the general pool of HBsAg[+]/anti-HBe[+] carriers, only a small percentage will be serologically HBV DNA–positive. However, among HBsAg[+]/anti-HBe[+] carriers being evaluated or followed for active liver disease, a large proportion (up to 50 per cent or more) may be HBV DNA–seropositive.[90, 123–127] These patients also demonstrate other evidence of active virus replication in liver tissue, such as the presence of viral core antigen.[90, 127] Such patients often show virulent, chronic active hepatitis progressing to cirrhosis within a few years.[125–127] Therefore, under certain circumstances, detection of HBV DNA in the serum by hybridization represents a prognostically useful test in HBsAg carriers who are HBeAg-negative (HBeAg), anti-HBe[+], or both. Hopefully, simplified, nonradioactive versions of this test will become available for routine use within the next few years.

In many fewer cases, patients can be anti-HBs[+] and anti-HBe[+] and still show hybridization of serum with HBV DNA probes.[122, 128–130] In these patients, it would seem that HBV infection is continuing even though antibodies to specific viral proteins have been produced. In other cases, patients have been completely negative for HBV by routinely used immunologic tests but still show positive hybridization of serum with HBV DNA probes.[122, 128–130] The precise interpretation of these findings requires further study.

The preceding studies have led to the identification of permissive and nonpermissive states of HBV replication in the livers of long-term carriers of HBsAg.[89, 90, 120, 125, 127, 131–133] During the permissive stage, cells continue to replicate virus, and the patients show continued activity of liver disease. During the nonpermissive state, which generally occurs later during the course of persistent infection, hepatocytes do not replicate the virus, and the patients show little or no activity of the liver disease. In permissive infection, the bulk of HBV DNA in hepatocytes is in free virions or replicating forms, and integration into the host genome is not observed. However, during this period, HBV DNA integration is probably occurring at many sites throughout the host genome. This may not be detected readily by the usual method of Southern blot analysis because of its diffuse nature and a high level of free virions and lower molecular weight of replicative forms.[85, 88–90] In nonpermissive infection, it is often possible to observe the multiple integrations as a smear of hybridization in the high–molecular weight region of the gel (Fig. 36–7). In some nonpermissive infections, unique bands of HBV DNA

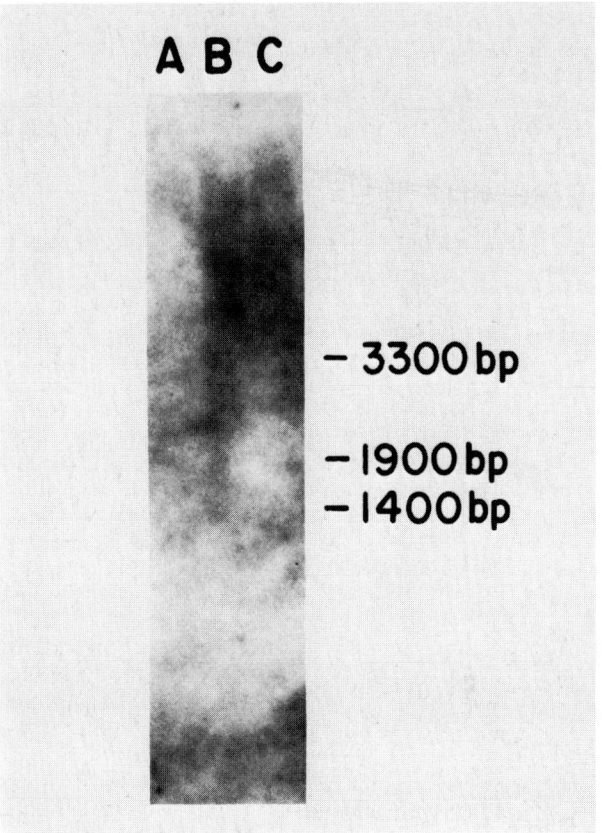

Figure 36–7. Molecular hybridization analysis for HBV-DNA sequences in liver tissue from long-term viral carriers without HCC. *Lanes B* and *C*, from individuals who have been HBsAg carriers for at least 8 to 10 years, show a diffuse pattern of integrated HBV-DNA. *Lane A* is a control from a non-HBV carrier with primary biliary cirrhosis and shows no hybridization with the HBV-DNA probe.

integration have been observed (Fig. 36–8).[88, 90] In these patients, Hadziyannis and colleagues[90] and Shafritz and Hadziyannis[131] have noted clusters or nodular accumulations of cells, all producing HBsAg (Fig. 36–9). Histologically, these clusters of cells appear as small regenerative nodules, but their uniform expression of HBsAg and the presence of integrated HBV DNA in unique banding patterns suggests that they represent clonally expanded foci of transformed hepatocytes. A mixed type of persistent infection may also occur in which features of replicating and nonreplicating infection are found in different regions of the same liver.

POSSIBLE ASSOCIATED ROLE OF CHEMICAL CARCINOGENS

Since many HCCs, especially those observed in Western countries, occur in non–HBV-infected individuals (e.g., those associated with alcoholic cirrhosis, hemochromatosis, α_1-antitrypsin deficiency, mycotoxins, and chemical carcinogens), other pathologic states can lead to hepatic oncogenesis. Factors that stimulate chromosomal aberrations have been associated with increased risk of neoplasia,[134] and agents such as benzpyrene, acetaminofluorine, aflatoxin, and so forth, which damage DNA, clearly cause HCC. A similar process may be occurring with HBV, since HBV integrations are often associated with deletion of ad-

TABLE 36–3. DETECTION OF HBV DNA IN SERUM COMPARED WITH HBeAg/ANTI-BHe STATUS IN HBsAg CARRIERS

HBeAg[+]		Anti-HBe[+]		Reference
HBV DNA positive/total patients studied				
9/9	(100%)	9/16	(56%)	Bonino et al.[120]
72/81	(89%)	7/16	(44%)	Scotto et al.[122]
28/28	(100%)	16/32	(50%)	Lieberman et al.[111]
—	—	28/106	(26%)	Negro et al.[123]
52/54	(96%)	14/22	(64%)	Chu et al.[124]
368/446	(83%)	131/551	(24%)	Matsuyama[126]

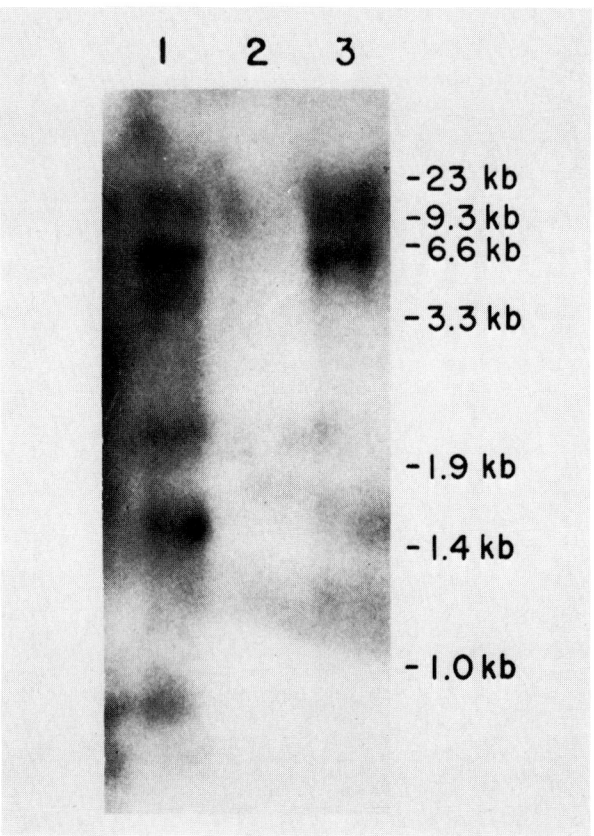

Figure 36–8. Integrated HBV-DNA in a unique banding pattern from long-term HBV carriers. *Lanes 1* and *3* are from two long-term HBsAg⁺/anti-HBe⁺ carriers and show discrete bands of integrated HBV-DNA but little or no free replicating virus. *Lane 2* is from a control biopsy from a non-HBV carrier and shows no hybridization with the HBV-DNA probe.

jacent cellular sequences at the site of integration.[72–74, 91, 97] However, it should be noted that HCC developed in eight of eight woodchuck carriers infected experimentally with WHV and maintained on diets free of all known carcinogens.[135] Therefore, like other oncogenic viruses, hepadna viruses can induce oncogenesis in the apparent absence of co-carcinogens. However, co-carcinogens could hasten the oncogenic process in a synergistic fashion by increasing the total number of mutagenic events in the liver cell DNA pool. This is consistent with the notion that oncogenesis occurs in a multistage process[136] and that mutation or altered expression of multiple genes or different combinations of genes may be involved.[137]

MODEL OF PERSISTENT HBV INFECTION AND DEVELOPMENT OF HCC

Evidence cited above indicates that integration of HBV DNA occurs before or during the oncogenic process, but this does not prove that HBV itself is oncogenic. If neoplasia arises frequently in HBV-bearing livers and if random integration of HBV DNA occurs frequently (that is, in many cells in such livers), then tumors arising in those livers will often contain integrated HBV DNA, whether or not the integrated viral DNA itself is wholly or partly responsible for the oncogenic change. This does not exclude HBV from a role in oncogenicity but merely implies that neoplastic change may occur by an epigenetic mechanism.

From information currently available, one can generate the following hypothesis (illustrated schematically in Fig. 36–10). At some stage during the progression of the carrier state, or perhaps as early as the initial acute infection, HBV DNA integration occurs (stage I). Hepatocytes expressing all, or at least some, specific viral proteins are

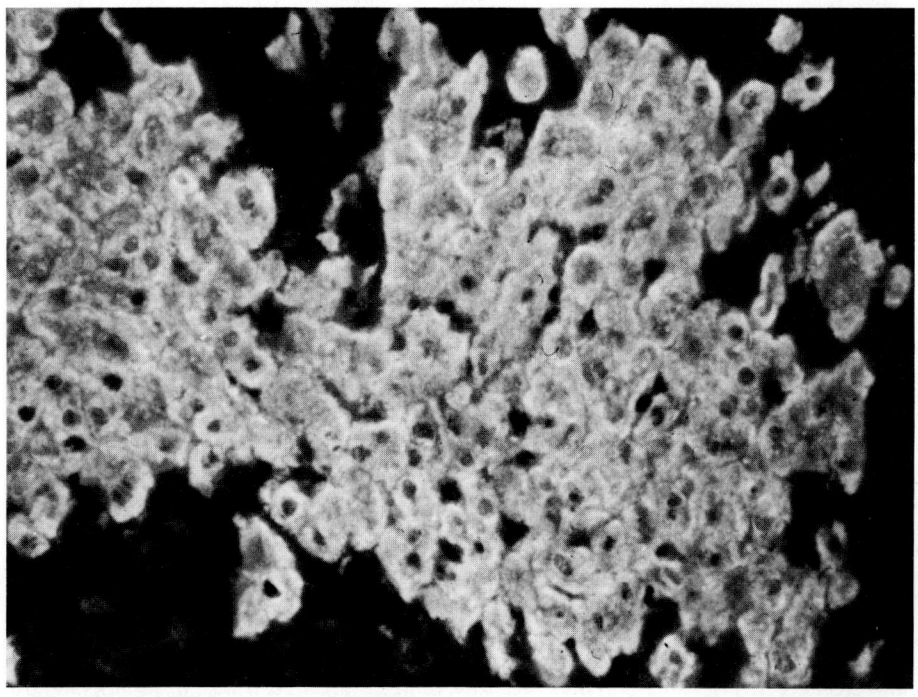

Figure 36–9. Nodular distribution of hepatocytes expressing HBsAg in a long-term carrier without evidence of hepatocellular carcinoma. Large clusters of hepatocytes show HBsAg in the cytoplasm by immunofluorescence. In conjunction with discrete bands of integrated HBV-DNA on hybridization analysis, these results suggest that focal accumulations of HBsAg-producing cells may represent clonal expansions of single hepatocytes containing integrated HBV-DNA.

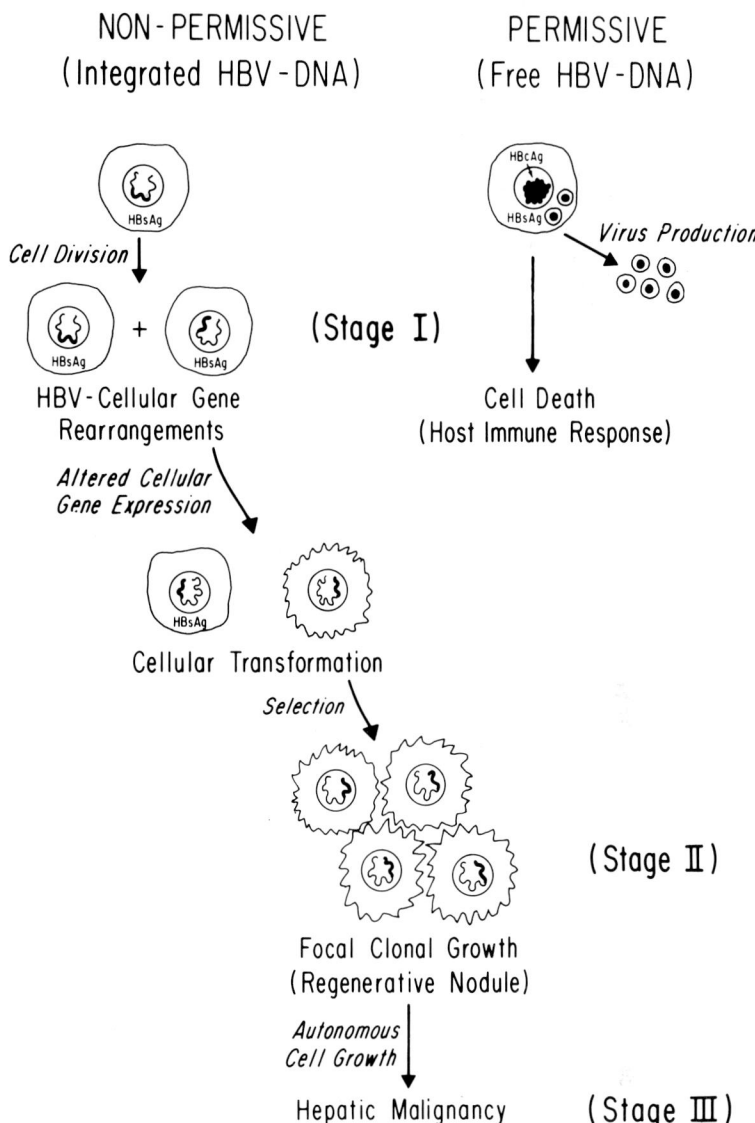

Figure 36–10. Hypothetic states or events during persistent hepatitis B virus infection that might ultimately lead to development of hepatocellular carcinoma.

efficiently removed by host immunologic defense mechanisms. However, integration of HBV DNA, which is probably a random event or can occur at many sites in the host genome, may result in altered expression of viral antigens. Under these circumstances, the specific recognition factor or factors for host immune surveillance may not be expressed or may be expressed to a reduced degree in cells containing integrated, as opposed to free, virion HBV DNA. Therefore, cells containing integrated HBV DNA might be preferentially retained within the liver parenchyma in contrast to cells actively replicating virus. With time, the normal process of cell division would therefore accelerate the accumulation of cells containing integrated HBV DNA. At this stage, HBV DNA would be integrated into multiple sites within the host genome and would appear as a diffuse smear on Southern blot hybridization, reflecting this dispersed distribution. Cell division is essential to this stage, so that factors stimulating cycles of hepatocyte necrosis and regeneration (such as ethanol, hepatotoxins, chemical carcinogens, super infection with other viruses, and the like) may potentiate early selection events.[113, 131, 138, 139] Disruption of the nuclear-cytoplasmic boundary during cell division, destabilization of the cellular genome during mitosis, or

both may also augment integration of viral genomes and cause rearrangement, deletion, or modification of integrated HBV DNA and/or adjacent cellular sequences.[138–140] This process would be accentuated further during repeated cycles of liver regeneration.

Subsequently, a clone or several clones of hepatocytes containing integrated HBV DNA may become selected for preferential survival, or multiplication or both by factors at present unknown (stage II). This selection may be dependent upon the functional state or the chromosomal location of integrated HBV DNA. On restriction analysis and Southern blotting, these selected cells would show discrete bands of integrated HBV DNA. Under the influence of still other factors (such as host immune surveillance, nutritional state, hormones, environmental toxins, or carcinogens), one or more of the selected clones may give rise eventually to a malignant tumor (stage III).

The above model predicts that multiple, independent, primary HCCs, with different HBV DNA integration patterns, could occur in the same liver and that development of a second primary after resection of a solitary lesion would occur with increased frequency in such patients. Both of these phenomena have been observed.

REFERENCES

1. Parkin DM, Stjernsward J, Muir CS. Cancer Control. Estimates of the world-wide frequency of 12 major cancers. WHO Bull 62:163, 1984.
2. Waterhouse J, Muir C, Correa P, et al. Cancer incidence in five continents. Lyon, World Health Organization, 1977.
3. Higginson J. The geographical pathology of primary liver cancer. Cancer Res 23:1624, 1963.
4. Dunham LJ, Bailar JC. World maps of cancer mortality rates and frequency rates. J Natl Cancer Inst 41:155, 1968.
5. Kew MC, Geddes EW. Hepatocellular carcinoma in rural South African blacks. Medicine 61:98, 1961.
6. Prates MD, Torres FO. A cancer survey in Lourenco Marques, Portuguese East Africa. J Natl Cancer Inst 35:729, 1965.
7. Yu SZ. Epidemiology of primary liver cancer. In: Tang ZY, ed. Subclinical Hepatocellular Carcinoma. Beijing, China Academic Publishers, 1985:198.
8. Annual Report of Demographic Statistics in Japan, 1985. Tokyo, Health and Welfare Statistics Association 1986:54. Quoted in Okuda K. Early recognition of hepatocellular carcinoma. Hepatology 6:729, 1986.
9. Szmuness W. Hepatocellular carcinoma and the hepatitis B virus: evidence for a causal relationship. Prog Med Virol 24, 40, 1978.
10. Okuda K, Beasley RP. In: Okuda K, Mackay I, eds. Hepatocellular Carcinoma. Union Internationale Contra Cancrum Report 17:9, 1982.
11. Munoz N, Linsell A. Epidemiology of primary liver cancer. In: Correa P, Haenszel W, eds. Epidemiology of Cancer of the Digestive Tract. Martinus Nijhoff Publishers, 1982:161.
12. Linsell DA, Higginson J. The geographic pathology of liver cell cancer. In: Cameron HM, Linsell DA, Warwick GP, eds. Liver Cell Cancer. Amsterdam, Elsevier, 1976:1.
13. King H, Henszel W. Cancer mortality among foreign and native born Chinese in the United States. J Chronic Dis 26:623, 1973.
14. Beasley RP, Hwang LY, Lin CC, et al. Hepatocellular carcinoma and HBV: a prospective study of 22,707 men in Taiwan. Lancet 2:1124, 1981.
15. Obata H, Hayashi N, Motoike Y, et al. A prospective study on the development of hepatocellular carcinoma from liver cirrhosis with persistent hepatitis B virus infection. Int J Cancer 25:741, 1979.
16. Prince AM, Szmuness W, Michau V, et al. A case control/study of the association between primary liver cancer and hepatitis B infection in Senegal. Int J Cancer 16:376, 1975.
17. Tong MJ, Sun SCM, Schaefer BT, et al. Hepatitis-associated antigen and hepatocellular carcinoma in Taiwan. Ann Intern Med 75:687, 1971.
18. Yarrish RL, Werner BJ, Blumberg BS. Association of hepatitis B virus infection with hepatocellular carcinoma in American patients. Int J Cancer 26:711, 1980.
19. MacNab GM, Urbanowicz JM, Geddes EW, et al. Hepatitis B surface antigen and antibody in Bantu patients with primary hepatocellular carcinoma. Br J Cancer 33:544, 1976.
20. Trichopoulos D, Gerety RJ, Sparros L, et al. Hepatitis B and primary hepatocellular carcinoma. J Natl Cancer Inst 58:1147, 1977.
21. Beasley RP, Hwang LY. Epidemiology of hepatocellular carcinoma. In: Vyas GN, Dienstag JL, Hoofnagle JH, eds. Viral Hepatitis and Liver Disease. Grune & Stratton, Orlando, Fla. 1984:209.
22. Okuda K. Clinical aspects of hepatocellular carcinoma—analysis of 134 cases. In: Okuda K, Peters RL, eds. Hepatocellular Carcinoma. New York, John Wiley & Sons, 1976:387.
23. Bagshaw A, Cameron HM. The clinical problem of liver cell cancer in a high-incidence area. In: Cameron HM, Linsell DA, Warwick UP, eds. Liver Cell Cancer. Amsterdam, Elsevier, 1976:45.
24. Sung J-L, Wang TH, Yu J-Y. A clinical study in primary carcinoma of the liver in Taiwan. Am J Dig Dis 12:1036, 1967.
25. Hutt MSR. Epidemiology of human primary liver cancer. In: Liver Cancer. Lyon, World Health Organization, Scientific Publications, 1970:1.
26. Ihde DC, Sherlock P, Winawer SJ, et al. Clinical manifestations of hepatoma. Am J Med 56:83, 1974.
27. Young JL Jr, Percy CL, Asire AJ, eds. Surveillance epidemiology and end results incidence and mortality data 1973–1977. Natl Cancer Inst Monograph 57. Washington, DC, NIH Publication 1981:1.
28. Prates MD. Cancer and cirrhosis of the liver in the Portuguese East African. Acta Univ Int Contra Cancrum 17:718, 1961.
29. Kew MC, Marcus R, Geddes EW. Some characteristics of Mozambican Shangaans with primary hepatocellular cancer. S Afr Med J 51:306, 1977.
30. Lin T-Y. Tumors of the liver: primary malignant tumors. In: Bockus HL, ed. Gastroenterology, 3rd ed. Philadelphia, WB Saunders, 1976:522.
31. Kew MC, Rossouw E, Hodkinson J, et al. Hepatitis B virus status of South African blacks with hepatocellular carcinoma: comparison between rural and urban patients. Hepatology 3:65, 1983.
32. Keen P, Martin P. Is aflatoxin carcinogenic in man? The evidence in Switzerland. Trop Geogr Med 23:44, 1971.
33. Alpert ME, Hutt MSR, Wogan GW, et al. The association between aflatoxin content of food and hepatoma frequency in Uganda. Cancer 28:253, 1971.
34. Peers FG, Gilman JA, Linsell DA. Dietary aflatoxins and human liver cancer. A study in Switzerland. Int J Cancer 17:167, 1976.
35. Peers FG, Linsell DA. Dietary aflatoxins and liver cancer—a population-based study in Kenya. Br J Cancer 27:473, 1973.
36. Shank RC, Gordon JE, Wogan FW, et al. Dietary aflatoxins and human liver cancer. III. Field survey of rural Thai families for ingested aflatoxins. Food Chem Toxicol 10:71, 1972.
37. van Resnburg SJ, van der Watt JJ, Purchase IFH, et al. Primary liver cancer rate and aflatoxin intake in a high cancer area. S Afr Med J 48:2508a–2508d, 1974.
38. Bomford A, Williams R. Long-term effects of venesection therapy in idiopathic haemochromotosis. O J Med 80:611, 1976.
39. MacSween RNM. A clinicopathological review of 100 cases of primary malignant tumors of the liver. J Clin Pathol 27:669, 1974.
40. Omata M, Ashcavai M, Liew C-T, et al. Hepatocellular carcinoma in the USA: etiologic considerations. Gastroenterology 76:279, 1979.
41. Lee FI. Cirrhosis and hepatoma in alcoholics. Gut 7:77, 1966.
42. Zaman SN, Melia WM, Johnson RD, et al. Risk factors in the development of hepatocellular carcinoma in cirrhosis. A prospective study of 613 patients. Lancet i:1356–1359, 1985.
43. Anthony PP. Cancer of the liver: pathogenesis and recent etiological factors. Trans R Soc Trop Med Hyg 72:466, 1977.
44. Kubo Y, Okuda K, Musha H, et al. Detection of hepatocellular carcinoma during a clinical follow-up of chronic liver disease. Observations in 31 patients. Gastroenterology 74:578, 1978.
45. Chen DS, Sung JL, Shen JL, et al. Serum alpha fetoprotein in the early stage of hepatocellular carcinoma. Gastroenterology 86:1404, 1984.
46. Tang ZY, Ying YY, Gu TJ. Hepatocellular carcinoma: changing concepts in recent years. In: Popper H, Schaffner F, eds. Progress in Liver Diseases, Vol 7. New York, Grune & Stratton, 1982:637.
47. Chen DS, Sheu JC, Sung JL, et al. Small hepatocellular carcinoma—a clinicopathological study in thirteen patients. Gastroenterology 83:1109, 1983.
48. O'Conor GT, Tatarinov YS, Abelev GI, et al. A collaborative study for the evaluation of a serologic test for primary liver cancer. Cancer 25:1091, 1970.
49. Chen DS, Sung JL. Serum alpha-fetoprotein in hepatocellular carcinoma. Cancer 40:779, 1977.
50. Shinegawa T, Ohto M, Kimura K, et al. Diagnosis and features of small hepatocellular carcinoma with emphasis on the utility of real-time ultrasonography. A study in 51 patients. Gastroenterology 86:495, 1984.
51. Liaw YF, Tai DI, Chu CM, et al. Early detection of hepatocellular carcinoma in patients with chronic type B hepatitis. A prospective study. Gastroenterology 90:263, 1986.
52. Tang ZY, Yu YQ, Lin ZY, et al. Clinical research of primary liver cancer. Chinese Med J 96:247, 1983.
53. Macnab GM, Urbanowicz JM, Kew MC. Carcinoembryonic antigen in hepatocellular carcinoma. Br J Cancer 38:51, 1978.
54. Kew MC, Torrance DJ, Derman D, et al. Serum and tumor ferritins in primary liver cancer. Gut 19:294, 1978.
55. Warnock ML, Reisman R. Variant alkaline phosphatase in hepatocellular carcinoma. Clin Chem Acta 25:5, 1969.
56. Fujisawa K, Kurihara N, Kojima N, et al. In: Leevy CM, ed. Diseases of the liver and biliary tract. Fifth Quadrennial Meeting of International Association for the Study of Liver (IASL). Basel, S. Karger, 1976.
57. Tanaka S, Kitamura T, Oshina A, et al. Diagnostic accuracy of ultrasonography for hepatocellular carcinoma. Cancer 58:344, 1986.
58. Sheu JC, Sung JL, Chen DS, et al. Growth rate of asymptomatic hepatocellular carcinoma and its clinical implications. Gastroenterology 89:259, 1985.
59. Okuda K. The Liver Cancer Study Group of Japan. Primary liver cancers in Japan. Cancer 45:2663, 1980.
60. The Liver Cancer Study Group of Japan. Primary liver cancer in Japan. Cancer 54:1757, 1984.
61. Ebara M, Ohto M, Shinegawa T, et al. Natural history of minute hepatocellular carcinoma smaller than three centimeters complicating cirrhosis. A study in 22 patients. Gastroenterology 90:289, 1986.
62. Okuda K. Early recognition of hepatocellular carcinoma. Hepatology 6:729, 1986.
63. Okuda K, Fujimoto I, Hanai A, et al. Changing incidence of hepatocellular carcinoma in Japan. Cancer Res 47:4967, 1987.

64. Marion PL, Salazar FH, Alexander JJ, et al. State of hepatitis B viral DNA in a human hepatoma cell line. J Virol 33:795, 1980.
65. Chakraborty PR, Ruiz-Opazo N, Shouval D, et al. Identification of integrated hepatitis B virus DNA and expression of viral RNA in an HBsAg-producing human hepatocellular carcinoma cell line. Nature 286:531, 1980.
66. Brechot C, Pourcel C, Louise A, et al. Presence of integrated hepatitis B virus DNA sequences in cellular DNA of human hepatocellular carcinoma. Nature 286:533, 1980.
67. Edman JC, Gray P, Valenzuela P, et al. Integration of hepatitis B virus sequences and their expression in a human hepatoma cell. Nature 286:535, 1980.
68. Macnab GM, Alexander JJ, Lacatsas G, et al. Hepatitis B surface antigen produced by a human hepatoma cell line. Br J Cancer 34:505, 1976.
69. Yoakum GH, Korba BE, Lechner JF, et al. High frequency transfection and cytopathology of the hepatitis B virus core antigen gene in human cells. Science 22:385, 1983.
70. Marquardt O, Freytag von Loringhoven A, Frosner GG. Expression of hepatitis B virus core antigen gene is induced in human hepatoma cells by their growth in nude mice. J Gen Virol 65:1443, 1984.
71. Shaul Y, Ziemer M, Garcia P, et al. Cloning and analysis of integrated hepatitis virus sequences from a human hepatoma cell line. J Virol 51:776, 1984.
72. Koshy R, Koch S, Freytag von Loringhoven A, et al. Integration of hepatitis B virus DNA: evidence for integration in the single-stranded gap. Cell 34:215, 1983.
73. Dejean A, Brechot C, Tiollais P, et al. Characterization of integrated hepatitis B viral DNA cloned from a human hepatoma and the hepatoma derived cell line PLC/PRF/5. Proc Natl Acad Sci USA 80:2505, 1983.
74. Ziemer M, Garcia P, Shaul Y, et al. Sequence of hepatitis B virus DNA incorporated into the genome of a human hepatoma cell line. J Virol 53:885, 1985.
75. Koch S, Freytag von Loringhoven A, Hofschneider H, et al. Amplification and rearrangement in hepatoma cell DNA associated with integrated hepatitis B virus DNA. EMBO J 3:2185, 1984.
76. Koch S, Freytag von Loringhoven A, Kahmanu R, et al. The genetic organization of integrated hepatitis B virus DNA in the human hepatoma cell line PLC/PRF/5. Nucleic Acids Res 12:6871, 1984.
77. Ou HH, Rutter WJ. Hybrid hepatitis B virus host transcripts in a human hepatoma cell. Proc Natl Acad Sci USA 82:83, 1985.
78. Botchan M, Stringer J, Mitchison T, Sambrook J. Integration and excision of SV40 DNA from the chromosome of a transformed cell. Cell 20:143, 1980.
79. Sambrook J, Green R, Stringer J, et al. Analysis of the site of integration of viral DNA sequences in rat cells transformed by adenovirus or SV40. Cold Spring Harbor Symp Quant Biol 44:569, 1980.
80. Twist EM, Clark HF, Aden DP, et al. Integration pattern of hepatitis B virus DNA sequences in human hepatoma cell lines. J Virol 37:239, 1981.
81. Koike K, Koyabashi M, Mizusawa H, et al. Rearrangement of the surface antigen gene of hepatitis B virus integrated in the human hepatoma cell lines. Nucleic Acids Res 11:5391, 1983.
82. He L, Shih C, Isselbacher KJ, et al. Integration of HBV into genome of a new hepatocellular carcinoma cell line (CUSPF). Gastroenterology 84:1184, 1983.
83. Shafritz DA, Kew MC. Identification of integrated hepatitis B virus DNA sequences in human hepatocellular carcinomas. Hepatology 1:1, 1981.
84. Brechot C, Hadchouel M, Scotto J, et al. State of hepatitis B virus DNA in hepatocytes of patients with hepatitis B surface antigen positive and negative liver disease. Proc Natl Acad Sci USA 78:3906, 1981.
85. Shafritz DA, Shouval D, Sherman HI, et al. Integration of hepatitis B virus DNA into the genome of liver cells in chronic liver disease and hepatocellular carcinoma. N Engl J Med 395:1067, 1981.
86. Koshy R, Maupas P, Muller K, Hofschneider PH: Detection of hepatitis B virus specific DNA in the genomes of human hepatocellular carcinoma and liver cirrhosis tissues. J Gen Virol 57:95, 1981.
87. Chen DS, Hoyer BH, Nelson J, et al. Detection and properties of hepatitis B viral DNA in liver tissues from patients with hepatocellular carcinoma. Hepatology 2:42S, 1982.
88. Brechot C, Hadchouel M, Scotto J, et al. Detection of hepatitis B virus DNA in liver and serum: a direct appraisal of the carrier state. Lancet 2:765, 1981.
89. Kam W, Rall LB, Smuckler EA, et al. Hepatitis B viral DNA in liver and serum of asymptomatic carriers. Proc Natl Acad Sci USA 79:7522, 1982.
90. Hadziyannis SJ, Lieberman HM, Karvountzis GG, et al. Analysis of liver disease, nuclear HBeAg, viral replication and hepatitis B virus DNA in liver and serum of HBeAg vs. anti-HBe positive carriers of hepatitis B virus. Hepatology 31:656, 1983.
91. Rogler CE, Sherman M, Su CY, et al. Deletion in chromosome 11p associated with a hepatitis B integration site in hepatocellular carcinoma. Science 230:319, 1985.
92. Hino O, Shows B, Rogler CE. Hepatitis B virus integration site in hepatocellular carcinoma at chromosome 17:18 translocation. Proc Natl Acad Sci USA 83:8338, 1986.
93. Rogler CE, Summers J. Novel forms of woodchuck hepatitis virus DNA isolated from chronically infected woodchuck liver nuclei. J Virol 44:852, 1982.
94. Marion PL, Robinson WS, Rogler CE, et al. High molecular weight GSHV-specific DNA in chronically infected ground squirrel liver. J Cell Biochem, 19(Suppl 5):203, 1982.
95. Ogston CW, Jonak GJ, Rogler CE, et al. Cloning and structural analysis of integrated woodchuck hepatitis virus sequences from hepatocellular carcinomas of woodchucks. Cell 29:385, 1982.
96. Yaginuma K, Kobayashi H, Kobayashi M, et al. Multiple integration sites of hepatitis B virus in hepatocellular carcinoma and chronic active hepatitis tissues from children. J Virol 61:1808, 1987.
97. Dejean A, Sonigo P, Wain-Hobson S, et al. Specific hepatitis B virus integration in hepatocellular carcinoma DNA through a viral 11–base-pair direct repeat. Proc Natl Acad Sci USA 81:5350, 1984.
98. Koufos A, Hansen MF, Lampkin BC, et al. Loss of alleles at loci on human chromosome 11 during genesis of Wilms's tumor. Nature 309:170, 1984.
99. Land H, Parada LF, Weinberg RA. Cellular oncogenes and multistep oncogenesis. Science 222:771, 1984.
100. Bishop JM. Viral oncogenes. Cell 42:23, 1985.
101. Payne GS, Bishop JM, Varmus HE. Multiple arrangements of viral DNA and activated host oncogenes in bursal lymphomas. Nature 295:209, 1982.
102. Tiollais P, Pourcel C, DeJean A. The hepatitis B virus. Nature 317:489, 1985.
103. Shaul Y, Rutter WJ, Laub O. A human hepatitis B viral enhancer element. EMBO J 4:427, 1985.
104. Tognoni A, Cattaneo R, Serfling E, et al. A novel expression-selection approach allows precise mapping of the hepatitis B virus enhancer. Nucleic Acids Res 13:7457, 1985.
105. Tur-Kaspa R, Burk RD, Shaul Y, et al. Hepatitis B virus DNA contains a glucocorticoid-responsive enhancer element. Proc Natl Acad Sci USA 83:1627, 1986.
106. Dejean A, Bouguelenet L, Grzeschik KH, et al. Hepatitis B virus DNA integration in a sequence homologous to v-erb-A and steroid receptor genes in a hepatocellular carcinoma. Nature 322:70, 1986.
107. Weinberger C, Hallenberg SM, Rosenfeld MG, et al. Domain structure of human glucocorticoid receptor and its relationship to the v-erb-A oncogene product. Nature 318:670, 1985.
108. Mösöy T, Marchio A, Etiemble J, et al. Two different mechanisms for hepatitis B virus-induced hepatocellular carcinoma. In: Zuckerman AJ, ed. Viral Hepatitis and Liver Disease. Alan R. Liss, New York, 1988:737.
109. Moroy T, Marchio A, Etiemble J, et al. Rearrangement and enhanced expression of c-myc in hepatocellular carcinoma of hepatitis virus–infected woodchucks. Nature 324:276, 1986.
110. Gu J-R, Hu L-F, Cheng Y-C, et al. Oncogenes in human primary hepatic cancer. J Cell Physiol (Suppl) 4:13, 1986.
111. Lieberman HM, LaBrecque DR, Kew MC, et al. Detection of hepatitis B virus directly in human serum by a simplified molecular hybridization test. Comparison to HBeAg/anti-HBe status in HBsAg carriers. Hepatology 3:286, 1983.
112. Song E, Dusheiko GM, Bowyer S, et al. Hepatitis B virus replication in South African blacks with HBsAg-positive hepatocellular carcinoma. Hepatology 4:608, 1984.
113. Lieberman HM, Shafritz DA. Persistent hepatitis B virus infection and hepatocellular carcinoma. In: Popper H, Schaffner F, eds. Progress in Liver Diseases, Vol 8. Grune & Stratton, Orlando, Fla. 1986:395.
114. Chung WK, Sun HS, Park DH, et al. Primary hepatocellular carcinoma and hepatitis B virus infection in Korea. J Med Virol 11:99, 1983.
115. Realdi G, Alberti A, Rugge M, et al. Seroconversion from hepatitis Be antigen to anti-HBe in chronic hepatitis B virus infection. Gastroenterology 79:195, 1980.
116. Hoofnagle JH, Dusheiko CM, Seef LB, et al. Seroconversion from hepatitis Be antigen to antibody in chronic type B hepatitis. Ann Intern Med 94:744, 1981.
117. Liaw Y, Chu C, Su I, et al. Clinical and histological events preceding hepatitis Be antigen seroconversion in chronic type B hepatitis. Gastroenterology 84:216, 1983.
118. Dusheiko GM, Bowyer SM, Sjögren MH, et al. Replication of hepatitis

B virus in adult carriers in an endemic area. J Infect Dis 152:566, 1985.

119. Fattovich G, Rugge M, Brollo L, et al. Clinical, virologic and histologic outcome following seroconversion from HBeAg to anti-HBe in chronic hepatitis type B. Hepatology 6:167, 1986.

120. Bonino F, Hoyer B, Nelson J, et al. Hepatitis B virus DNA in the sera of HBsAg carriers: a marker of active hepatitis B virus replication in the liver. Hepatology 1:386, 1981.

121. Berninger M, Hammer M, Hoyer B, et al. An assay for the detection of the DNA genome of hepatitis B virus in serum. J Med Virol 9:57, 1982.

122. Scotto J, Hadchouel M, Henry C, et al. Detection of hepatitis B virus DNA in serum by a simple spot hybridization technique: comparison with results for other viral markers. Hepatology 3:279, 1983.

123. Negro F, Chiaberge E, Oliviero S, et al. Hepatitis B virus DNA (HBV-DNA) in anti-HBe positive sera. Liver 4:177, 1984.

124. Chu CM, Karayiannis P, Fowler MJF, et al. Natural history of chronic hepatitis B virus infection in Taiwan: studies of hepatitis B virus DNA in serum. Hepatology 5:431, 1985.

125. Yokosuka O, Omata M, Imazeki F, et al. Active and inactive replication of hepatitis B virus deoxyribonucleic acid in chronic liver disease. Gastroenterology 89:610, 1985.

126. Matsuyama Y, Omata M, Yokosuka O, et al. Discordance of hepatitis Be antigen/antibody and hepatitis B virus deoxyribonucleic acid in serum. Analysis of 1063 specimens. Gastroenterology 89:1104, 1985.

127. Bonino F, Rosina F, Rizzetto M, et al. Chronic hepatitis in HBsAg carriers with serum HBV-DNA and anti-HBe. Gastroenterology 90:1268, 1986.

128. Shafritz DA, Lieberman HM, Isselbacher KJ, et al. Monoclonal radioimmunoassays for hepatitis B surface antigen: demonstration of hepatitis B virus DNA or related sequences in serum and viral epitopes in immune complexes. Proc Natl Acad Sci USA 79:5675, 1982.

129. Lieberman HM, Young EM, Wydro RM, et al. Analysis of hepatitis B virus DNA in human serum by a simplified molecular hybridi-

zation test: studies in relation to HBeAg/anti-HBe status. Clin Res 31:476A, 1983.

130. Brechot C, Degas F, Lugassy C, et al. Hepatitis B virus DNA in patients with chronic liver disease and negative tests for hepatitis B surface antigen. N Engl J Med 312:270, 1985.

131. Shafritz DA, Hadziyannis SJ. Hepatitis B virus DNA in liver and serum, viral antigens and antibodies, virus replication, and liver disease activity in patients with persistent hepatitis B virus infection. In: Chisari FV, ed. Advances in Hepatitis Research. New York, Masson Press, 1984:80.

132. Fowler MJF, Monjardino J, Weller IVD, et al. An analysis of the liver and serum of patients with chronic hepatitis or primary liver carcinoma and the effect of therapy with adenine arabinoside monophosphate. Gut 25:611, 1984.

133. Miller RH, Lee S-C, Lioro Y-F, et al. Hepatitis B viral DNA in infected human liver and in hepatocellular carcinoma. J Infect Dis 151:1081, 1985.

134. Klein G. The role of gene dosage and genetic transpositions in carcinogenesis. Nature 294:313, 1981.

135. Popper H, Roth L, Purcell RH, et al. Hepatocarcinogenecity of the woodchuck hepatitis virus. Proc Natl Acad Sci USA 84:866, 1987.

136. Geissler E, Theile M. Virus-induced gene mutations of eukaryotic cells. Hum Genet 63:1, 1983.

137. Sinn E, Muller W, Pattengale P, et al. Coexpression of MMTV/v-Ha-ras and MMTV/c-myc genes in transgenic mice: synergistic action on oncogenes in vivo. Cell 49:465, 1987.

138. Popper H, Gerber MA, Thung SN. The relation of hepatocellular carcinoma to infection with hepatitis B and related viruses in man and animals. Hepatology (Suppl) 2:10S, 1982.

139. Shafritz DA. Hepatitis B virus DNA molecules in the liver of HBsAg carriers: mechanistic considerations in the pathogenesis of hepatocellular carcinoma. Hepatology (Suppl) 2:35S, 1982.

140. Popper H, Shafritz DA, Hoofnagle JH. Relation of the hepatitis B virus carrier state to hepatocellular carcinoma. Hepatology 7:764, 1987.

37

Diagnosis, Therapy, and Prognosis of Viral Hepatitis

Leonard B. Seeff, M.D.

ABBREVIATIONS

AFP = alpha-fetoprotein
ALT = alanine aminotransferase
anti-HAV = antibody to hepatitis A virus
anti-HBc = antibody to HBcAg
anti-HBe = antibody to HBeAg
anti-HBs = antibody to HBsAg
AST = aspartate aminotransferase
CH50 = total serum hemolytic complement activity
HAV = hepatitis A virus
HBcAg = hepatitis B core antigen
HBeAg = hepatitis B e antigen
HBIG = hepatitis B immune globulin
HBsAg = hepatitis B surface antigen
HBV = hepatitis B virus
IG = immune serum globulin
LCAT = lecithin:cholesterol acyltransferase
PHA = passive hemagglutination
HDV = hepatitis delta virus

HISTORY

Viral hepatitis is believed to date back to antiquity.[1] Reference to it can be found in the Babylonian Talmud (fifth century B.C.), and Hippocrates is thought to have been aware of the entity, referring to it as the "fourth kind of jaundice." In the eighth century A.D., Pope Zacharias informed St. Boniface, Archbishop of Mainz, that jaundice was contagious.[2] There was little further mention of the disease until 1791, when Herlitz, in Göttingen, reported an epidemic of jaundice among civilians and introduced the term *icterus epidemicus*. In the intervening period to the beginning of the present century, hepatitis was referred to only occasionally, usually as occurring in outbreaks, particularly during times of war. Indeed, the French referred to the disease as jaundisse des camp and the Germans as Soldatengelbsucht.

Even though hepatitis was recognized to be an epidemic illness, Bamberger, in 1858, suggested that it was caused by inflammation and obstruction of the ostium of the common bile duct and hence that it was an obstructive and not, as was later realized, a parenchymal form of jaundice.[3] A decade later, Virchow came to the same conclusion when he found, in an autopsy performed on a person who had died of hepatitis, that the common bile duct was plugged by mucus.[4] Thus was born the term *catarrhal* jaundice.

It was first considered likely that hepatitis could be the result of infection of the hepatic parenchyma toward the end of the nineteenth century,[5, 6] but the possibility that the infectious agent might be a virus was suggested only as recently as 1918.[7] A clear description of the illness and its differentiation from Weil's disease was reported by Blumer in 1923, when he detailed 63 epidemics of infectious hepatitis in the United States occurring between 1812 and 1920.[8] He clearly defined the disease as affecting children and young adults, as having an incubation period as long as 28 days, as being spread mainly through person to person contact, and as having its greatest incidence in fall and winter. Similar findings were recorded in other epidemiologic surveys undertaken before World War II in the United States and in England.[9, 10] However, proof of the infectious nature of the disease was fully established only by a series of studies conducted during and just after World War II, which involved feeding contaminated material to human volunteers.[11–14]

To facilitate study of the disease, it was necessary to develop tests capable of defining the presence of hepatic injury and of distinguishing between obstructive and hepatocellular jaundice. The earlier tests found to be useful included the van den Bergh test and determinations of urinary urobilinogen, sulfobromophthalein excretion, cephalin flocculation, thymol turbidity, and serum alkaline phosphatase. However, precision of diagnosis became possible only in 1939 when percutaneous needle aspiration biopsy of the liver was introduced by Roholm and Iversen,[15] and particularly after aminotransferase (transaminase) assays were developed and reported by Karmen and colleagues in 1955.[16, 17] These latter tests permitted recognition of hepatitis when no accompanying symptoms were present.

The first description of percutaneously transmitted hepatitis is attributed to a report by Lurman in 1885.[18] He noticed that jaundice developed in 191 of 1339 workers at a shipyard in Bremen, Germany two to eight months after they were vaccinated against smallpox with glycerinated human lymph. Most authorities have regarded this as an outbreak of hepatitis B, although it has recently been suggested that it might instead have represented an outbreak of non-A, non-B hepatitis.[19] Numerous other reports of percutaneously transmitted hepatitis followed, the earlier ones involving, in particular, persons who attended clinics at which injections were given for the treatment of diabetes and syphilis.[20–24] It was later realized that many instances of jaundice in these clinics, originally believed to be the result of drug hepatotoxicity, were probably the result of transmission of viral hepatitis.[25] The largest outbreak of percutaneously transmitted hepatitis occurred in 1942 when it developed in almost 50,000 American soldiers who were inoculated with a yellow fever vaccine; 62 of them died.[26] Previous studies of the yellow fever vaccine identified a filterable hepatitis agent in the human serum used to culture yellow fever virus.[27] The responsible hepatitis virus has been determined to be hepatitis B. The actual number of infected soldiers exceeded 330,000, the majority of whom had no symptoms of jaundice.[27a] In 1943, Beeson in the United States and Morgan and Williamson in Great Britain reported for the first time an association between the transfusion of blood or plasma and the development of hepatitis.[28, 29]

The features that distinguish infectious hepatitis (IH) from serum hepatitis (SH) became more apparent as a result of the numerous experiments with human volunteers conducted in the 1940s.[11–14, 30, 31] These studies defined two immunologically distinct diseases that were characterized by different incubation periods and differed in modes of transmission, each being associated with homologous, but not heterologous, immunity. The virus of each of these diseases was present in the blood during the incubation period, but only the hepatitis A virus (HAV) was found in the stools. Investigators also established during the 1940s that immune serum globulin, now called immune globulin (IG), provided effective prophylaxis against hepatitis A.[32–34] The existence of a prolonged carrier state presumed to be for hepatitis B was recognized in the following decade.[35, 36]

For many years, the two types of hepatitis were described by a variety of different names. One of them, known in England as infective hepatitis and in Russia as Botkin's disease, was variously referred to in the United States as epidemic jaundice, epidemic hepatitis, acute catarrhal jaundice, IH, and short-incubation hepatitis. The terms applied to the other form included homologous serum hepatitis, postinoculation jaundice, post-transfusion hepatitis, SH, and long-incubation hepatitis. In 1947, MacCallum proposed the names hepatitis A and hepatitis B,[37] which rapidly received worldwide acceptance.

In 1958, Ward and associates reported the first of what was to become a series of human studies involving mentally retarded inmates of the Willowbrook State School in New York.[38] Guided primarily by Dr. Saul Krugman, these studies added information about the epidemiology and the natural history of the disease and confirmed the existence of the two distinct types of hepatitis, MS-1 hepatitis (equivalent to hepatitis A), and MS-2 hepatitis (equivalent to hepatitis B).[39–42] The studies also demonstrated that hepatitis B could be transmitted by both percutaneous and oral routes, and eventually that the Australia antigen was a specific marker for hepatitis B. Further, they helped to confirm the efficacy and mode of action of IG and hepatitis B immune globulin (HBIG), developed evidence that active immunization against hepatitis B could be induced, and clearly detailed the serologic and immunologic responses in hepatitis A and hepatitis B.[43–51]

For many years, all attempts to isolate and propagate the hepatitis viruses in tissue culture met with failure.[52] Indeed, the hepatitis B virus (HBV) has not yet been grown in tissue culture. However, Provost and Hilleman reported in 1979 the reliable and repeated propagation of human HAV in primary explant cell cultures of marmoset (a small South American monkey) livers and in the normal fetal rhesus monkey kidney cell line.[53] In part, their success can be attributed to the availability of an inoculum highly characterized for infectivity, as well as sensitive and specific biochemical and serologic tests with which to identify infection. Indeed, all of the original attempts to define a susceptible animal for study failed simply because these indices of infection were not then in existence. In view of the earlier failures, interest in animal models lagged until the early 1960s, when Hillis reported an epidemic of hepatitis A among animal handlers of newly imported chimpanzees at a United States Air Force base.[54] Spurred by this report, investigators once again turned to the study of nonhuman primates. The first encouraging report came from Deinhardt and co-workers, who chose for evaluation various species of marmoset on the assumption that this relatively vicious animal with rare human contact would be unlikely to have immunity against viral hepatitis.[55] They found that after inoculating the marmoset with acute-phase sera from humans with viral hepatitis, biochemical and histologic changes compatible with hepatitis developed. These findings were subsequently confirmed by the same investigators and others, demonstrating specifically the susceptibility of the marmoset species.[56–59] Later, other investigators showed that the chimpanzee could also serve as an animal model for hepatitis A transmission.[60, 61] Success in the transmission of hepatitis B to animals was not achieved until several years after the discovery of the putative viral agent, although early studies had demonstrated the presence of the viral antigen in naturally infected chimpanzees.[62–64] In a series of studies, chimpanzees, gibbons, orangutans and, to a lesser extent, rhesus monkeys were found to be susceptible to HBV infection.[65–68] The recent discovery of a disease much like hepatitis B affecting woodchucks, ground squirrels, and Pekin ducks represents an exciting development with important research potential.[69–69b]

An extensive and initially frustrating search for specific tests to diagnose hepatitis A and hepatitis B was begun in the 1940s. Several agglutination tests were devised, all appearing at the outset to be promising, but all finally proving to be nonspecific.[70–74] The search for the viral agents themselves was even more diligent and protracted,[75] and the reported isolations were even more ubiquitous.[75–82] Indeed, in a review published in 1968, Hersey and Shaw noted that 23 classified and 6 or more unclassified viral agents had been implicated at one time or another as the cause of viral hepatitis.[83] One abortive discovery that initially excited much attention was the finding reported in 1970 of an antigen believed to be related to HAV.[84] Referred to as the epidemic hepatitis–associated antigen or the Milan antigen, it was identified originally in 90 per cent of individuals involved in three separate epidemics of short-incubation hepatitis during the first two weeks of their illness. It was later determined to be an abnormal serum lipoprotein that was associated with liver disease but not directly related to viral hepatitis.[85]

The long, arid period in the search for a virus was finally broken in the mid-1960s with the discovery by Dr. Baruch Blumberg of the hepatitis B surface antigen (HBsAg, Australia antigen) and its antibody (anti-HBs).[86] This initiated a series of events that led to the description of the morphologic and immunochemical features of HBV, the development of specific passive and active hepatitis B immunoprophylaxis, the etiologic association of HBV with primary hepatocellular carcinoma, the identification and description of HAV by Feinstone and colleagues,[87] and finally, the recognition of another common form of hepatitis that was not caused by either the A or B virus and hence was designated non-A, non-B hepatitis. For his discovery, which set these events in motion, Dr. Blumberg was awarded a Nobel Prize in 1977.[88] Most recent is the report of an antibody test for the post-transfusion type of non-A, non-B hepatitis.[989]

Since Blumberg's discovery, many investigators from various parts of the world have helped to fill in the pieces of the fascinating jigsaw puzzle constituting the features of the various types of viral hepatitis.[69–127w] Some of the highlights are shown in Tables 37–1, 37–2, 37–3, and 37–4. Individual achievements are discussed in this and other chapters of this book.

CLINICAL FEATURES

The present discussion of the clinical features of hepatitis excludes all but the most pertinent of epidemiologic associations, the serologic and immunologic events (for these, see Chap. 35), fulminant hepatitis (see Chap. 17), and chronic hepatitis (see Chap. 38).

At the outset, it must be stressed that there are no pathognomonic clinical, physical, or biochemical features of viral hepatitis. Indeed, the diagnosis depends on the accumulation of a constellation of findings that taken together suggest the presence of hepatocellular necrosis. The illness may develop without any clinical sign or symptom, nonspecific symptoms may be present for a short time only, or symptoms may occur, with or without jaundice, and persist for a protracted period. There are no features that unequivocally distinguish the individual types of hepatitis, even though there are components that seem more characteristic for one form than for the others. One factor previously considered to have diagnostic relevance is the incubation period. However, although the incubation periods of the various hepatitis viruses differ, they can overlap sufficiently to obscure this diagnostic characteristic. Even the modes of transmission may not serve to differentiate them from one another. Contrary to early concepts, it is now established that, like HBV, HAV can also be transmitted through oral and percutaneous routes, albeit with differing degrees of ease.[42, 127x, 127y] Accordingly, it is not surprising that the traditionally accepted epidemiologic approach to distinguishing hepatitis A from hepatitis B was frequently in error. For example, Bryan and Gregg, using HBsAg testing, analyzed the cases of viral hepatitis reported to the Centers for Disease Control (CDC) between 1970 and 1973 and found that physicians had misdiagnosed as many as 24 per cent of cases of hepatitis B.[128] Another confounding factor is that the conditions that favor the transmission of HBV seem to be the same as those that promote transmission of the previously unrecognized non-A, non-B, and delta hepatitis viruses.[129–129c]

Although certain epidemiologic patterns can provide some help in defining the different hepatitis viruses, definitive distinction necessitates specific serologic identification. The following sections present a summary of general clinical features that may occur in viral hepatitis of any type. Characteristics other than serologic features that appear to differentiate the viral illnesses are also discussed.

GENERAL SYMPTOMATOLOGY

Early Prodromal Phase

In approximately a fourth of patients, principally, but not exclusively, those incubating hepatitis B, the illness is heralded by a serum sickness–like syndrome, consisting variably of fever, arthralgia, arthritis, rash, and angioneurotic edema. These symptoms, when they occur, usually begin two to three weeks before jaundice develops. Generally they disappear before jaundice emerges, sometimes concomitant with its onset. Less frequently, they may persist for variable periods during the course of the acute illness. Rarely, arthritis may remain even beyond recovery from the acute illness. A more detailed description of these syndromes appears later.

TABLE 37–1. HISTORICAL PERSPECTIVES IN HEPATITIS B RESEARCH SINCE THE DISCOVERY OF THE AUSTRALIA ANTIGEN

Item	Year	Reference	Item	Year	Reference
Discovery of the Australia antigen (hepatitis B surface antigen, antibody; HBsAg, antiHBs)	1965	Blumberg et al.[86]	Refinement of radioimmunoassay test for HBsAg	1972	Ling and Overby[103]
			Transmission of HBV infection to chimpanzees	1972	Maynard et al.[65]
Association of Australia antigen with viral hepatitis	1967	Blumberg et al.[89]	Identification of hepatitis B e antigen and antibody (HBeAg, anti-HBe)	1972	Magnius and Espmark[104]
Association of Australia antigen with serum hepatitis	1968	Prince[90]	Association of DNA-polymerase with Dane particle cores	1973	Kaplan et al.[105]
Identification of 20-nm spherical and filamentous viral particles in plasma	1968	Bayer et al.[91]	Demonstration of double-stranded Dane particle–associated DNA	1974	Robinson and Greenman[106]
Proof of specific association of HBsAg and hepatitis B	1969	Giles et al.[92]	Refinement of hepatitis B vaccine	1975	Purcell and Gerin[107]
Recognition of different HBsAg specificities, i.e., subtypes	1969	Levene and Blumberg[93]	Demonstration of synthesis of HBsAg by hepatoma cell line (PLC/PRF/5)	1976	Macnab et al.[107a]
Identification of 42-nm double-shelled viral particles (Dane particles, presumptive HBV*)	1970	Dane et al.[94]	Characterization of polypeptides and amino acid sequences of HBsAg	1977	Peterson et al.[107b]
Development of heat-inactivated vaccine from HBsAg-containing serum	1970	Krugman et al.[45]	Identification of woodchuck hepatitis virus	1978	Summers et al.[69]
Association found between chronic HBV infection and primary hepatocellular carcinoma	1970	Sherlock et al.[95]	Cloning of HBV DNA	1979	Burrell et al.[108]
			Demonstration of receptors on HBV for polymerized albumin	1979	Imai et al.[107c]
Development of radioimmunoassay test for HBsAg	1970	Walsh et al.[96]	Establishment of efficacy of HBV vaccine in humans	1980	Szmuness et al.[107d]
Recognition of HBsAg, anti-HBs immune-complex extrahepatic disease	1970	Gocke et al.[97]	Identification of HBV-like virus in Beechey ground squirrels	1980	Marion et al.[69a]
Purification of Australia antigen	1971	Gerin et al.[98]	Description of structure of HBV DNA	1981	Tiollais et al.[107e]
Disruption of Dane particle with release of core; establishment of hepatitis B core antigen, antibody system (HBcAg, anti-HBc) distinct from HBsAg, anti-HBs	1971	Almeida et al.[99]	Demonstration of HBV DNA in serum	1981	Brechot et al.[107f]
			Categorization of HBV as hepadnavirus, type 1	1982	Melnick et al.[107g]
			Delineation of genetic characteristics of HBV genome	1983	Delius et al.[107h]
Discovery of DNA polymerase in preparations of particulate antigen isolated from serum	1971	Hirschman et al.[100]	Development of recombinant HBV vaccine	1984	McAleer et al.[107i]
Characterization of antigen subtypes of HBsAg	1971	Le Bouvier[101]	Characterization of pre-S domain of HBV	1985	Neurath et al.[107j]
Development of hepatitis B immune globulin	1971	Prince et al.[102]	Propagation of HBV by transfection of human hepatoma cell line with cloned HBV DNA	1986	Sureau et al.[107k]

*HBV = hepatitis B virus.

TABLE 37–2. HISTORIC PERSPECTIVES IN HEPATITIS A RESEARCH SINCE THE IDENTIFICATION OF THE SPECIFIC VIRUS

Item	Year	Reference
Identification of the hepatitis A virus, antigen and antibody (HAV, anti-HAV) following experimental inoculation	1973	Feinstone et al.[87]
Transmission of HAV infection to marmosets	1973	Mascoli et al.[110]
Identification of HAV particles in a naturally occurring epidemic	1975	Gravelle et al.[111]
Establishment of HAV as an RNA virus	1975	Provost et al.[112]
Development of a complement fixation test for hepatitis A	1975	Provost et al.[112a]
Development of an immune adherence assay test specific for hepatitis A	1975	Miller et al.[113]
Development of a radioimmunoassay specific for hepatitis A	1975	Hollinger et al.[114]
Experimental infection of chimpanzees with HAV	1975	Dienstag et al.[61]
Establishment of anti-HAV prevalence by age and socioeconomic status in the United States	1976	Szmuness et al.[116]
Development of radioimmunoassay-IgM blocking test for diagnosis during the acute phase	1977	Bradley et al.[117]
Development of enzyme-linked immunoadsorbent assay for anti-HAV	1978	Mathiesen et al.[117a]
Development of inactivated HAV vaccine effective after experimental infection of marmosets	1978	Provost and Hilleman[118]
Propagation of human HAV in cell cultures of marmoset livers and rhesus kidney	1979	Provost and Hilleman[53]
Transmission of HAV to macaque monkey	1981	Mao et al.[118a]
Categorization of HAV as enterovirus, type 72, within the picornavirus group	1982	Melnick[107g]
Transmission of HAV to owl monkeys	1983	LeDuc et al.[118b]
Molecular cloning of HAV cDNA	1983	Ticehurst et al.[118c]
Detection of HAV RNA by hybridization	1985	Jansen et al.[118d]

TABLE 37–3. HISTORIC PERSPECTIVES IN NON-A, NON-B HEPATITIS RESEARCH SINCE RECOGNITION OF ITS EXISTENCE

Item	Year	Reference
Recognition of entity of non-A, non-B hepatitis by epidemiologic analysis	1974	Prince et al.[119]
Evidence that non-A, non-B hepatitis is transmitted by blood products	1975	Feinstone et al.[115]
Evidence for the existence of sporadic non-A, non-B hepatitis	1975	Villarejos et al.[120]
Identification of ultra-short incubation period non-A, non-B hepatitis in recipients of coagulation factors	1975	Craske et al.[120a]
Evidence from epidemiologic analysis of existence of at least three viruses	1977	Mosley et al.[121]
Experimental transmission of non-A, non-B hepatitis to humans and establishment of carrier state	1977	Hoofnagle et al.[122]
Transmission of non-A, non-B hepatitis to chimpanzees	1978	Alter et al.[123] Tabor et al.[124]
Development of an immunodiffusion assay for the detection of a non-A, non-B antigen and antibody	1978	Shirachi et al.[125]
Development of indirect immunofluorescence and counterelectrophoresis tests believed to detect an antigen-antibody system associated with non-A, non-B hepatitis	1979	Kabiri et al.[126] Tabor[127]
Demonstration of ultrastructural changes in livers of chimpanzees, suggesting two distinct agents	1979	Shimizu et al.[127a]
Recovery of putative virus-like particles associated with non-A, non-B hepatitis	1979	Bradley et al.[127b]
Evidence that the non-A, non-B hepatitis is inactivated by formalin	1980	Tabor et al.[127c]
Evidence for two non-A, non-B hepatitis agents based on chimpanzee cross-challenge experiments	1980	Hollinger et al.[127d]
Experimental proof of carrier state for non-A, non-B hepatitis	1980	Tabor et al.[127e]
Separation of two distinct non-A, non-B hepatitis viruses on physicochemical grounds	1983	Bradley et al.[127f]
Suggested relationship of non-A, non-B hepatitis to retroviruses	1984	Seto et al.[127g] Prince et al.[127h]
Questioning of etiologic relationship of retrovirus	1986	Bradley et al.[127i]
First report of epidemic non-A, non-B hepatitis (unrecognized)	1957	Viswanathan[127j]
Demonstration of lack of association of epidemic non-A, non-B hepatitis with hepatitis A and B viruses	1980	Wong et al.[127k]
Confirmation of epidemic non-A, non-B hepatitis	1982	Tandon et al.[127l]
Identification of fecal virus-like particles in persons with epidemic non-A, non-B hepatitis	1983	Balayan et al.[127m]
Development of specific test for non-A, non-B hepatitis	1989	Kuo et al.[989]

TABLE 37–4. HISTORIC PERSPECTIVES IN HEPATITIS D (DELTA) RESEARCH SINCE RECOGNITION OF ITS EXISTENCE

Item	Year	Reference
Identification of delta antigen and antibody	1977	Rizzetto et al.[127n]
Development of sensitive radioimmunoassay for detection of delta antigen and antibody	1980	Rizzetto et al.[127o]
Transmission of delta antigen to chimpanzees	1980	Rizzetto et al.[127p]
Definition of the RNA genome of the delta agent	1980	Rizzetto et al.[127q]
Effect of acute delta infection on severity of acute hepatitis B	1982	Smedile et al.[127r]
Association of delta infection with progressive chronic liver disease	1983	Rizzetto et al.[127s]
Transmission of delta antigen to woodchucks	1984	Ponzetto et al.[127t]
Identification of delta agent in early United States immune globulins	1984	Ponzetto et al.[127u]
Association of delta antigen infection with fulminant hepatitis	1984	Govindarajan et al.[127v]
Cloning of cDNA fragment of delta RNA genome	1986	Denniston et al.[127w]

Preicteric Phase

Nonspecific constitutional symptoms, as well as symptoms referable to the respiratory and gastrointestinal tracts, may develop, appearing insidiously or abruptly. These symptoms include malaise, unusual fatigue, myalgia, anorexia, nausea, and occasionally vomiting. Associated with these symptoms is a change in taste and smell, with concomitant aversion to food and often to cigarettes. As a result, slight to moderate weight loss may ensue. Coryza, headache, photophobia, fever and, less commonly, pharyngitis and cough may also occur, particularly in association with hepatitis A. Often, but not invariably, patients complain of mild to moderate midepigastric or right upper quadrant pain and, on occasion, diarrhea. An early view held that the diarrhea resulted from intestinal involvement by the hepatitis virus,[130] but this has been questioned,[131, 132] as is discussed later.

Physical examination may be quite unrevealing, or it may identify lymphadenopathy (involving particularly the posterior cervical region), hepatomegaly, and splenomegaly (5 to 10 per cent). The hepatic enlargement is generally only slight; a markedly enlarged liver is uncommon. The liver edge is usually rounded, soft to moderately firm, and only slightly tender to palpation or to percussion over the lower ribs. Spider nevi may be found rarely in self-limited acute viral hepatitis.

There are no pathognomonic laboratory abnormalities associated with viral hepatitis. The most sensitive tests for identifying the development or presence of hepatocellular disease are aminotransferase determinations—aspartate aminotransferase (AST) and alanine aminotransferase (ALT). Also characteristic of the preicteric phase is the development of dark urine, resulting from the excretion of bilirubin into the urine. Bilirubinuria usually precedes the onset of overt hyperbilirubinemia. The color of the stool may be light because of reduced excretion of bilirubin into the gastrointestinal tract.

In a variable proportion of individuals, particularly the young, the disease may subside slowly without jaundice developing. This anicteric form of hepatitis may occur following infection by any of the hepatitis viruses, but it appears to be more common among children with hepatitis A and those with non-A, non-B hepatitis. The duration of the preicteric phases varies considerably, ranging from two to three days to as much as two to three weeks. The development of jaundice signals the beginning of the icteric phase.

Icteric Phase

The frequencies of the various symptoms and signs noted in three collected series of acute, predominantly icteric cases, are shown in Table 37–5. The first is an instance of serologically defined hepatitis A that occurred as a food-borne outbreak;[133] the second represents an analysis of a large number of cases, presumed to be hepatitis A in origin, in patients admitted to a United States field hospital in France during World War II;[134] the third is a careful assessment of a subgroup of 4083 United States soldiers, admitted to Camp Polk, Louisiana between May and September 1942, in whom hepatitis developed after they received yellow fever vaccine that was stabilized with pooled human serum.[134a] The latter outbreak has recently been identified as the result of hepatitis B infection.[27a] The variable frequencies of the recorded manifestations are apparent, as no marked discrepancy is noted between the cases of hepatitis A and hepatitis B.

With the onset of jaundice, the fever declines and general constitutional symptoms begin to subside. Sometimes, however, there may be a transient worsening of anorexia, nausea, and vomiting, followed by clinical improvement. The physical findings at this time are similar to those described for the preicteric phase, but with the obvious addition of scleral icterus and yellowish-tinged skin. Pruritus may lead to scratching and excoriations of the skin.

Convalescent Phase

Jaundice usually begins to wane within a few days to a week (particularly in children), but it may persist for as long as four to six weeks. At this time, weakness, headache, anorexia, and the olfactory and gustatory abnormalities generally disappear. In addition, the enlarged liver and spleen begin to shrink, pruritus abates, and a sense of well-being returns. In the majority of patients (85 to 100 per cent, depending on the specific virus), full recovery is achieved by six months after the onset of disease.

LABORATORY FINDINGS

A large number of hematologic and biochemical abnormalities occur during the incubation period and course of viral hepatitis. Some represent changes that strongly suggest the presence of acute necroinflammatory disease and therefore have important diagnostic relevance. Others are abnormalities that occur concomitant with acute viral hepatitis, but they are not diagnostic.

TABLE 37–5. INITIAL SYMPTOMS AND SIGNS IN THREE CAREFULLY ANALYZED HEPATITIS OUTBREAKS, TWO OF THEM SEROLOGICALLY DEFINED

Author (Ref.) Responsible Virus No. Patients	Rootenberg et al[123] Hepatitis A 130	Zimmerman et al[134] Probable Hepatitis A 260	Turner et al[134a] Hepatitis B 196
Symptoms (%)			
Malaise	76	94	Common
Anorexia	71	96	70
Dark urine	65	94	77
Nausea	61	81	58
Vomiting	NS	37	20
Scleral icterus	48	NS	NS
Abdominal pain	26	68	32
Respiratory symptoms	24	20	NS
Headache	19	57	Common
Fever	18	52	Rare
Myalgia	14	NS	Common
Rash	14	NS	NS
Arthralgias	10	NS	NS
Itching	NS	26	Common
No. symptoms	14	NS	Common
Signs (%)			
Jaundice	70	90	Almost all
Hepatomegaly	14	69	39–50
Tender liver	39	86	20
Splenomegaly	3	21	NS
Fever	NS	72	NS
Rash	8	1	NS
Bradycardia	NS	40	NS

NS = not stated.

Tests with Diagnostic Relevance

Serum Enzymes

Enzymes increase in the blood as a result of their release from necrotic tissues, because their production is increased or because their disposition is impaired by biliary obstruction or renal failure.[135] Clearly, the first of these mechanisms is the one responsible for the increases that occur during acute viral hepatitis.

Several enzymes are helpful in diagnosing viral hepatitis. Among them are ornithine carbamyltransferase, sorbitol dehydrogenase, glutamate dehydrogenase, isocitrate dehydrogenase, malate dehydrogenase, and guanase. However, none of them is superior to the aminotransferases AST and ALT as an indicator of the disease. These two enzymes are the most sensitive of those evaluated in routine biochemical tests for establishing the diagnosis of acute viral hepatitis. Indeed, they are the first determinations to become abnormal as the disease develops and frequently the last to return to normal as it subsides. Normal values of these enzymes should exclude a diagnosis of acute (though not necessarily chronic) viral hepatitis.

Aminotransferases may reach levels greater than 100 times the upper limit of normal.[136–143] Enzyme elevations always precede jaundice; ALT determinations are usually more abnormal than AST determinations in both the early and late stages of acute hepatitis; in general, abnormal values are greater in icteric than in anicteric hepatitis.

The development of the first abnormal aminotransferase values is currently regarded as signaling the beginning of the illness and hence defines the incubation period. Studies of the aminotransferases have shown differences between hepatitis viruses regarding the timing of enzyme abnormalities (incubation period), the rapidity of enzyme elevations, and the pattern and duration of the abnormalities during the course of the illness. Krugman and colleagues found under experimental circumstances that disease developed in children exposed to hepatitis A after incubation periods of 30 to 38 days, with the enzymes remaining abnormal for 3 to 19 days.[42] Exposure to hepatitis B led to disease with incubation periods of 41 to 108 days, a more gradual rise in enzyme values, and persistence of abnormal activity for 35 to 200 days. Another finding of this study was that the incubation period after exposure to hepatitis B varied with the route of infection: after parenteral inoculation, the incubation period was 41 to 91 days, whereas with oral administration, using viral concentrations that were 50 times greater than those used for parenteral inoculation, the incubation period was 88 to 108 days. Barker and Murray have demonstrated that the incubation period of hepatitis B is a function not only of the route of viral entry but also of the dose of virus.[144] They found that the incubation time of clinical hepatitis and the appearance of HBsAg varied inversely with the dose of virus inoculated, as defined by a series of dilutions of an icterogenic pool of HBsAg-positive human plasma. More recently, HBsAg was detected in the blood as early as six days after exposure.[51] Thus, hepatitis A and hepatitis B can have overlapping incubation periods. The incubation period of non-A, non-B hepatitis has been defined best in a series of large-scale prospective studies of post-transfusion hepatitis.[144a] These findings indicate that the incubation period ranges from 2 to 26 weeks but that the vast majority of cases occurs 5 to 12 weeks after transfusion, the mean interval being 7.8 weeks. In one study, post-transfusion non-A, non-B hepatitis could be subdivided into two groups.[125] In the first group, characterized by a monophasic elevation of ALT, the incubation period was 5.7 weeks. The elevation of ALT persisted for five to eight weeks. In the second group, characterized by biphasic elevations of ALT, the average incubation period was 7.2 weeks, and abnormal enzyme levels persisted for 17.5 weeks. Conceivably, this could represent two separate transfusion-transmitted non-A, non-B hepatitis viruses, a supposition supported by experimental evidence derived from chimpanzee cross-challenge studies and from physicochemical studies that suggest the existence of two agents.[144b-144d] There may be a third parenteral non-A, non-B hepatitis agent that induces illness after an even shorter incubation period (four weeks or less), which is identified following transfusion of clotting factor concentrates.[144e, 144f] Whether this represents an entirely separate viral agent or a shortened incubation period as a consequence of high concentrations of virus in the pooled concentrate is not known. Finally, there is another non-A, non-B viral agent, unrelated to the parenterally transmitted form or forms, that is referred to as epidemic (or enteric) non-A, non-B hepatitis because it is transmitted via the oral-fecal route.[144g, 144h, 144i] The incubation period for this disease, like that of hepatitis A, ranges between 15 and 40 days. Biphasic disease has also been noted in hepatitis delta infection.[129c] In the circumstance of acute coinfection with hepatitis B, the first peak of illness can generally be attributed to the hepatitis B infection and the second peak, which is detected after a mean interval from the first of approximately 17 days, is attributed to infection by the hepatitis delta virus (HDV).

The rate of regression of abnormal aminotransferase values has also been examined. In one study, the levels of AST and ALT declined by 11.7 per cent and 10.5 per cent, respectively, of the peak values/day, but with slower rates of subsidence late in the disease.[145] This study also showed that results of liver tests were more severely deranged for patients with hepatitis B, that the duration of aminotransferase elevations exceeded that of hyperbilirubinemia, and that ALT values remained abnormal longer than did those of AST. No significant difference between the rates of improvement of the aminotransferase levels was found in this study of hepatitis A and hepatitis B, as defined clinically. In other studies, the durations of illness have been found to be longer for hepatitis B and non-A, non-B hepatitis than for hepatitis A.[146, 147] One characteristic finding, but not an invariable one, in patients with non-A, non-B hepatitis, is the fluctuating pattern of enzyme activity.[144a] This phenomenon tends to obscure the termination point of the disease, since it may be observed for several months.

The degree of elevation of the aminotransferases and the AST to ALT ratio have also been reported to be useful in the diagnosis of acute viral hepatitis. Values for the aminotransferases, particularly ALT, that are greater than 300 IU/L (eight times the upper limit of normal) strongly support a diagnosis of acute hepatocellular necrosis. The uppermost abnormal value uncommonly exceeds 3000 to 4000 IU/L; indeed, values in excess of these levels almost always indicate toxic or vascular rather than viral injury.[147a] Although there is a tendency for aminotransferase activity to be higher in patients with icteric or symptomatic disease when compared with those with asymptomatic disease, extremely high values can be seen in the latter circumstance. There appears to be little correlation between the degree of enzyme activity and prognosis. With regard to the AST to ALT ratio, a value of less than 1 is characteristic of acute viral hepatitis,[143, 148-150] but it is rarely found in alcoholic liver disease.[149, 151, 152] Only occasionally is the ratio greater than 2 in viral hepatitis,[149, 152] and it is an occurrence that is more likely when the serum enzymes are markedly elevated

or when the hepatitis develops in the presence of pre-existing alcoholic cirrhosis.[153]

Other enzymes, none of which is important in diagnosis, have also been studied in the course of viral hepatitis. Among them are the lysosomal enzymes, β-glucuronidase, and α-1,4-glucosidase,[154-157] an isoenzyme of 5'nucleotide phosphodiesterase,[158, 159] and a urinary metabolite of the microsomal enzyme, cytochrome P450.[160, 161] However, enzymes that are measured more commonly are alkaline phosphatase and lactate dehydrogenase (LDH) as part of a panel consisting of the AST, ALT, alkaline phosphatase, and LDH determinations. With certain exceptions, neither of the latter two enzymes is markedly elevated during acute viral hepatitis. Although the level of serum alkaline phosphatase is almost always abnormal, it rarely exceeds four times the upper limit of normal in the uncomplicated case. The exception is the sometimes unusual increase in alkaline phosphatase that may occur in the cholestatic variant of acute viral hepatitis (see further on). Although LDH values are almost always elevated during acute viral hepatitis, the increase is only modest in comparison with the elevations of the aminotransferases.

Because of the central role of the liver in drug metabolism (Chap. 10), it can be expected that drug disposition will be severely impaired in acute hepatocellular disease. Numerous studies of drug metabolism rates in patients with acute hepatitis have revealed impairment,[162-167] no change,[168, 169] or acceleration of drug metabolism.[170]

Flocculation Tests

These tests, said to measure serum colloid stability, depend on the depression of albumin and $α_1$-globulin levels, changes in the albumin complex, an increase in the gamma globulin level, and other changes in serum proteins.[171, 172] Among the many flocculation tests that have been devised, only the cephalin flocculation test, thymol turbidity test, and occasionally, the thymol flocculation test have been used in the United States with any regularity. Results of both the thymol turbidity test and the cephalin flocculation test are usually abnormal in hepatitis A and less frequently in hepatitis B.[42, 173] The tests are not specific and, accordingly, are rarely used now that serum enzyme determinations are available.

Serum Bilirubin

By convention, it is generally accepted that a bilirubin value of 2.5 to 3.0 mg/dl (the level at which jaundice becomes clinically detectable) or greater establishes the presence of icteric hepatitis. Both conjugated and unconjugated bilirubin levels are elevated in hepatocellular forms of jaundice. The precise mechanism responsible for the elevations is unknown. One theory is that they result from a reversal of the normal polarity of the hepatocyte, which permits conjugated bilirubin to be regurgitated back into the blood.[174] Total bilirubin levels rarely exceed 20 mg/dl. After reaching its peak, bilirubin begins to decline by slightly more than 50 per cent/week, usually reaching normal levels in two to four weeks.[145] Bilirubin values in excess of 30 mg/dl always signify an additional bilirubin load coming from overproduction (hemolysis) or failure of excretion (renal failure). Such marked hyperbilirubinemia may be seen when viral hepatitis occurs in individuals who have glucose-6-phosphate dehydrogenase deficiency or sickle cell anemia.[175-178]

Abnormal but Nonspecific Tests

Hematologic Changes

Hematologic changes in acute viral hepatitis include mild anemia, a low reticulocyte count, reduction of the red blood cell survival time, macrocytosis, leukopenia, atypical lymphocytosis, megaloblastic changes, and mild to moderate thrombocytopenia.

Leukopenia, which develops in the preicteric phase of hepatitis, is the hematologic change most commonly observed.[134, 179-182] In 10 per cent of cases, the leukocyte count is less than 5000/mm[3]. This is accompanied by a reversal of the neutrophil to lymphocyte ratio, which is characterized by granulocytopenia and a relative lymphocytosis, frequently with atypical lymphocytes. The cause of the leukopenia has not been established, although it is believed to result from direct bone marrow depression. In addition to the reduction in the number of neutrophils, their functional capacity may be depressed in some patients with acute viral hepatitis,[183] as well as in children who are HBsAg carriers.[184] An inhibitory factor appears to reside in the serum, but it has not been defined. A leukocyte count of more than 12,000 cells/mm[3] in uncomplicated viral hepatitis is sufficiently rare that it warrants a search for an alternative explanation. Severe leukocytosis is, however, frequently associated with fulminant viral hepatitis.

Anemia is a far less frequent occurrence, even though shortened red blood cell survival appears to be common in acute viral hepatitis.[184a-184c] When present, it is usually mild.[179] Its cause has not been clearly established. One suggestion is that, like leukopenia, it might be the result of temporary bone marrow depression in the early stages of hepatitis.[130] However, hemolysis has also been seen in acute viral hepatitis.[130] In one study, hemolysis was found to persist for as long as three years after recovery from hepatitis.[185]

Asymptomatic or slightly symptomatic *thrombocytopenia* has been described as occurring during hepatitis, but its frequency has not been determined.[186]

The overtly pathologic effects of viral hepatitis on the hematologic system are discussed later.

Changes Related to Protein Metabolism

Serum albumin, because of its relatively extended half-life of two to three weeks, is depressed only minimally or is not decreased at all in acute viral hepatitis. Other serum proteins that may be depressed in acute viral hepatitis include the mucoproteins,[187] the haptoglobins,[188-190] prealbumin,[150, 189] and α-lipoprotein.[150, 191] An increase in *acute-phase reactants* (α$_1$-antitrypsin, orosomucoid, haptoglobin, C-reactive protein, fibrinogen, antichymotrypsin) does not occur in viral hepatitis.[189]

Immunoglobulin levels have been found to be increased during acute viral hepatitis by many,[192, 193] but not all,[189, 194] investigators. Furthermore, it has been suggested that the specific immunoglobulin fractions that increase vary according to the type of hepatitis virus involved in the infection.[195-198] Wollheim reported a moderate, sustained increase in IgG levels during both hepatitis A and hepatitis B; in contrast, IgM values were found to be increased markedly in hepatitis A only.[195] The exclusivity of IgM elevations for hepatitis A has been validated by Mosley and co-workers and others.[195a-198] Andersen and Ladefoged have suggested that smooth muscle antibody of the IgM class may account for part of the increase in serum IgM

levels.[199] In one study, IgE levels were found to be elevated in 50 per cent of patients with hepatitis caused by any virus.[150] In another study, IgE elevation was found in patients with HBsAg-positive but not HBsAg-negative hepatitis.[198] The durations of immunoglobulin elevations following acute viral hepatitis are variable.[196, 200]

Changes in *serum complement levels* in acute viral hepatitis have been described. High, low, and normal values have been reported. Fox and associates, in a study of single serum samples, observed that C3 levels remained normal during self-limited acute viral hepatitis but were markedly reduced if massive necrosis of the liver occurred.[201] They could not determine whether this represented decreased synthesis or increased consumption of complement. In a later study, Kosmidis and Leader-Williams found that in 94 per cent of patients with either HBsAg-positive or HBsAg-negative acute hepatitis, C3 levels declined initially and then rose gradually to normal.[202] Because the hypocomplementemia occurred long before hepatocellular disease had been fully established, and because it developed abruptly, it was suggested that it was due to the formation of immune complexes rather than to the effects of acute hepatocellular necrosis. Similar findings by Alpert and colleagues of reductions in total serum hemolytic complement activity (CH50), C3, and C4 concomitant with the highest serum HBsAg titers and with severe joint symptoms seemed to confirm this hypothesis.[203] Interestingly, similar changes have been found in acute hepatitis A, but without the same temporal relationships.[204] Nevertheless, both hepatitis A and hepatitis B were accompanied early in the clinical phase of the illness by reductions of C1q, C5, C4, C3, and even C7, with C3d present in the initial but not subsequent blood samples.[205] This pattern is compatible with activation of the classic pathway, again suggesting the presence of immune complexes.

The presence in adult serum of *alpha fetoprotein* (AFP), which is synthesized normally by fetal liver cells, yolk sac cells, and the fetal gastrointestinal tract,[206] was considered originally to be diagnostic for primary hepatocellular carcinoma or teratoblastoma, or both.[207] As the sensitivity of the test procedure improved, it was possible to show small amounts of AFP in normal serum and somewhat larger concentrations in the presence of other malignant tumors and in other forms of liver disease, as well as in acute viral hepatitis.[208-218] Although AFP was reported initially to be present in those patients who had HBsAg-positive hepatitis only,[210] a subsequent study has shown that it is present in 97 per cent of all patients with acute hepatitis, regardless of antigenic status.[212] In the latter study, AFP concentrations in a fourth of the cases increased as aminotransferase values declined, suggesting that this change reflected enhanced synthesis of AFP during hepatocellular regeneration. Subsequently, Karvountsis and Redeker suggested that the detection of AFP during acute hepatitis represented a sign of good prognosis.[214] They found AFP in 57 per cent of patients with fulminant hepatitis, the prevalence being significantly greater for those who survived (85 per cent) than for those who died (39 per cent). They also detected AFP in 30 per cent of nonfatal cases of acute hepatitis, the frequency rising with increasing severity of disease. Thus, 78 per cent of patients whose prothrombin concentrations were less than 20 per cent had sera that were AFP-positive, as opposed to only 4.3 per cent of those whose prothrombin levels never fell to less than 60 per cent. They therefore concluded that the presence of AFP heralded active hepatocyte regeneration. Furthermore, they suggested that failure to detect AFP in serum of a patient with severe hepatitis should be considered an ominous sign. Bloomer and colleagues also found a relationship between AFP and the severity and duration of hepatitis,[215] and they agreed that its presence probably indicated hepatic regeneration, since the levels rose concomitant with the decline in aminotransferase values. Moreover, they proposed that the very high AFP levels found in patients with severe necroinflammatory disease could be accounted for by a greater stimulus to regeneration. They did not agree, however, that the ability to detect AFP in a patient with massive hepatic necrosis necessarily represented a good prognostic indicator.[216] Rather, they found that the increase in AFP, reflecting active regeneration, did not occur until the second week of illness, regardless of the outcome, so its presence merely related to the duration of survival after onset of the illness. Most recently, Alpert and Feller concluded that AFP synthesis following massive hepatic necrosis does not represent hepatocellular regeneration.[217] Although they found elevated AFP concentrations in acute and chronic active hepatitis, and particularly in hepatic necrosis, they could not demonstrate increased levels during the regenerative phase following resection of as much as 75 per cent of the liver. Whether there is a relationship between the presence or persistence of AFP in persons with HBsAg-positive hepatitis and the subsequent development of HBsAg-associated hepatocellular carcinoma is still to be determined. In one study, no special relationship was found between AFP and the healthy HBsAg carrier state.[218]

Deoxyribonuclease (DNA)-*binding antibodies*, which are present in low titer in normal serum, increase commensurate with the severity of cellular necrosis and persist at an elevated level until cellular destruction abates. Villarejos and co-workers have suggested that the measurement of antibodies to single-stranded DNA represents a remarkably accurate test for the early diagnosis of icteric and anicteric hepatitis.[219] They found that in both hepatitis A and hepatitis B, anti-DNA titers increased rapidly one to two weeks before clinical or biochemical evidence of hepatic disease appeared and that they fell together with the return of normal aminotransferase levels.

The anticipation that viral hepatitis induces detectable *interferon* activity was not borne out by several early studies.[219a, 219b] More recent studies have shown that mononuclear cells in peripheral blood from patients with acute hepatitis can produce interferon.[219c, 219d] This phenomenon could not be documented in an in vitro experiment.[219e]

Changes Related to Lipid Metabolism

Abnormalities of *cholesterol* and *cholesterol esters* may be found in patients with liver disease (see Chap. 5). From a purely diagnostic viewpoint, the measurement of cholesterol has its greatest value in the identification of obstructive jaundice. Nevertheless, in acute parenchymal disease, the ratio of esterified to free serum cholesterol decreases. This was originally ascribed to a decrease in ester synthesis because of hepatocellular dysfunction. The mechanism (see Chap. 5) seems to be an impairment in the hepatic synthesis and release of the enzyme lecithin:cholesterol acyltransferase (LCAT) because of the liver damage.[220-226] The extent of LCAT impairment parallels the severity of hepatic damage, and the enzyme returns to normal when clinical improvement occurs.[227]

Serum triglycerides may be increased during the course of acute viral hepatitis.[227] Suggested mechanisms have included a reduction in hepatic triglyceride lipase activity or

a decrease in extrahepatic lipoprotein lipase activity, or both.[150, 228] Skrede and co-workers observed that the concentrations, lipid compositions, and electron microscopic appearances of the lipoproteins are often abnormal in acute hepatitis.[150] They reported finding a faint or even invisible α-lipoprotein band and the disappearance of the pre-beta band on electrophoresis.

Numerous studies beginning in the mid-1950s demonstrated that the concentrations of *bile acids* in serum are markedly increased during the icteric phase of acute viral hepatitis.[229-233] Tests devised since then have included studies of bile acid metabolism following intravenous injection,[234, 235] measurement of total bile acids in the fasting state and two hours postprandially,[233, 236, 237] and the measurement of individual bile salts using sensitive radioimmunoassay procedures.[238, 239] In an early study of the metabolism of intravenously injected isotopic cholic acid, Theodor and associates found a prolongation of the cholic acid half-life during acute viral hepatitis.[234] Cronholm and colleagues studied the sequential changes of bile acids during viral hepatitis and found that in the icteric phase, the concentration of deoxycholic acid was almost negligible, whereas cholic acid and chenodeoxycholic acid concentrations were increased 50 to 100 times.[240] The bile acid levels subsequently declined, returning to normal at about the same time as did the serum bilirubin.

The assay of serum bile acids appears to be a sensitive measure of the presence of liver disease. However, it is unclear whether measurement of the levels or types of bile acids in the serum is in any way superior to other tests.[233, 238, 239, 241-243] In this reviewer's opinion, measurements of serum bile acids do not provide enough clinical information to warrant their routine use. Preliminary reports suggest that measurement of the sulfate conjugates of lithocholate may differentiate between hepatitis A and hepatitis B,[239] and that elevated levels of bile acids may identify carriers of hepatitis;[244] however, these reports need confirmation.

Other Tests

Trace Metal and Vitamin Measurements

Serum iron levels in patients with acute viral hepatitis are generally elevated. The levels usually reach maximum about two to three weeks after the onset of jaundice.[245-247] It is believed that the excess serum iron comes from necrotic hepatocytes, a view supported by the observation of a decrease in stainable iron in liver biopsy specimens during the acute phase of the illness and its reappearance in increased amounts in Kupffer cells and hepatocytes during convalescence.[248] However, Felton and colleagues have reported that elevated serum iron levels occur not only when there is hepatocellular necrosis but also in persons who are HBsAg carriers.[249] The explanation of the latter finding is unclear.[250, 251] A test believed to have diagnostic significance is the measurement of iron levels in urine following the intramuscular injection of deferoxamine.[252, 253] Iron levels are reportedly markedly elevated during acute hepatitis.

Other metals that have been found in increased amounts in serum in acute hepatitis are *manganese, copper*, and *zinc*.[254-256] Also, *serum vitamin B_{12}* is greatly increased,[257] presumably as a result of the hepatocellular necrosis.[258] Alternatively, it may be the result of the excessive binding of vitamin B_{12} to transcobalamins I and II that has been demonstrated to occur during acute hepatitis.[259]

Glucose Metabolism

Hypoglycemia is an uncommon manifestation of uncomplicated viral hepatitis despite the fact that acute hepatocellular necrosis can potentially impair carbohydrate metabolism.[260] However, blood sugar abnormalities may be found if actively sought. Felig and co-workers have reported that more than half of patients with acute viral hepatitis whom they studied had fasting hypoglycemia, which they attributed to impaired gluconeogenesis.[261] This finding has been disputed.[262, 263] Several investigators have reported glucose intolerance to oral and intravenous glucose loads.[261, 263–266] In one extensive study of glucose tolerance in viral hepatitis, increased fasting blood levels of insulin, growth hormone, lactate, 2-oxoglutarate, glutamate, glutamine, and triglycerides were found.[263] Fasting levels of ketones, glycerol, and free fatty acids were normal. From these data it appears that viral hepatitis can be associated with glucose intolerance and insulin resistance. The mechanism for insulin resistance in acute viral hepatitis is unclear (see also Chap. 4).

Hypoglycemia is reported to develop in as many as 10 per cent of patients with fulminant hepatic failure,[267] as well as in other forms of liver disease.[268] The low blood sugar level may be extremely difficult to treat. It may recur despite treatment, and it may cause the deaths of many patients with fulminant hepatitis (see Chap. 17).

Sulfobromophthalein Excretion Test

Kinetics of sulfobromophthalein during acute viral hepatitis have been evaluated carefully by Preisig and co-workers.[269] They studied 22 patients who had acute viral hepatitis, on admission to the hospital and again during convalescence, by measuring the rate of maximal sulfobromophthalein transport (T_{max}) and the relative sulfobromophthalein storage capacity (S). Initially, both T_{max} and S were reduced, T_{max} being more markedly affected than S. During convalescence, S returned to normal more rapidly than did T_{max}. The investigators concluded that rates of healing of the parenchyma and the portal tracts differ, with parenchymal function returning to normal more promptly than biliary function. Although these findings are interesting, they have no practical significance, as sulfobromophthalein clearance is not used in the diagnosis of viral hepatitis. Similar information is derived by performing the *indocyanine green clearance test*.[270]

Equally nonspecific for the diagnosis of acute viral hepatitis is the measurement of the *erythrocyte sedimentation rate* (ESR). In one study, an elevated ESR was found only in patients with HBsAg-negative hepatitis.[271] This result needs confirmation.

COMPARATIVE FEATURES OF HEPATITIS A, HEPATITIS B, AND NON-A, NON-B HEPATITIS

Some of the features that characterize and distinguish the illnesses caused by the different hepatitis viruses are shown in Table 37–6. Hepatitis A most closely resembles epidemic non-A, non-B hepatitis, both of which differ from the three parenterally transmitted forms—namely, hepatitis B, parenteral non-A, non-B hepatitis, and delta hepatitis or hepatitis D. The mildest form of illness is that caused by HAV, particularly among children and young adolescents, the vast majority (>80 per cent) of whom are

asymptomatic and anicteric.[271a, 271b] It is therefore not surprising that the population of the United States shows a progressive increase in the prevalence of antibody to hepatitis A with advancing age without historic evidence of preceding overt illness.[116] In contrast, jaundice almost always develops in adults.[271c] The disease is characterized by its short period of viremia, its oral-fecal mode of transmission, its abridged incubation period, its high frequency of fever and occasional association with diarrhea,[271d] and its lack of a carrier state and progression to chronic hepatitis. Although the majority of patients with hepatitis A recover within four to six weeks, some may have sustained illness for up to a year;[271e] others may appear to recover and then clinical relapse develops 30 to 90 days after the primary episode.[271f] Rarely, the disease may manifest itself as intrahepatic cholestasis with prolonged jaundice and pruritus.[271g] Because of the short viremic phase of hepatitis A, parenteral transmission is exceedingly rare, but it has been reported.[127x, 127y] Epidemic non-A, non-B hepatitis has similar characteristics, being transmitted by the fecal-oral route and resolving without the development of chronic hepatitis.[127k, 148h] The majority of outbreaks have followed flooding conditions in the face of poor sanitation facilities. The disease has been reported from India, Nepal, Burma, Pakistan, and the Soviet Union and, most recently, Mexico.[271h] A small number of cases have been seen in the United States, imported from Pakistan.[271i] The clinical manifestations differ from hepatitis A in that there is a longer incubation period and a higher mortality rate,[271h] particularly among pregnant women.[127j, 127k] The three parenterally transmitted viruses produce disease that is characterized by a longer incubation period, insidious onset, lack of fever, a carrier state, and the potential for culmination in chronic hepatitis. Hepatitis B is frequently an asymptomatic disease, particularly in neonates, young children, and immunosuppressed persons, all of whom are at high risk for the development of chronic hepatitis and primary hepatocellular carcinoma. Parenteral non-A, non-B hepatitis, which is defined most clearly as a transfusion-related disease, is even more insidious than hepatitis B, presenting less frequently with either symptoms or jaundice.[144a] Peak aminotransferase values also tend to be lower than in hepatitis B. A characteristic feature is the fluctuating pattern of aminotransferase activity, thus hindering the ability to accurately define termination of the illness. Determining this end point is particularly important, since progression to chronic hepatitis seems to evolve more frequently than it does following acute hepatitis B. Despite several reports of the development of liver cancer in persons presumed to have had non-A, non-B hepatitis,[271k, 271l, 271m] a direct causal relationship cannot be confirmed without a definitive serologic test. Undoubtedly the most serious of these viral illnesses is that caused by HDV. This defective agent, dependent for its survival and replication in humans on HBV, induces disease only in the presence of HBV, either in coinfecting with HBV, or as superinfection in individuals who are already carriers of HBV.[271n] The disease appears to be endemic to certain geographic areas of the world (southern Italy, the Middle East, southern Europe, and parts of South America). In other areas (such as the United States), it is confined at present to high-risk groups such as drug addicts and hemophiliacs. Surprisingly, its prevalence among homosexual men and Asian populations, among whom hepatitis B is widely disseminated, is relatively low. Coinfection may become manifested in one of three ways. The first is a pattern indistinguishable from typical acute hepatitis B, including complete resolution. The second is that of bi-

TABLE 37–6. COMPARISON OF HEPATITIS TYPES A, B, NON-A, NON-B (PARENTERAL AND EPIDEMIC), AND D

Feature	Hepatitis				
	A	B	PNANB	ENANB	D
Clinical Presentation					
Age group	Primarily young	All ages	All ages	Mostly adults	All ages
Onset	Abrupt	Insidious	Insidious	Abrupt	Insidious
Incubation period					
Range (days)	15–50	28–160	14–160		
Mean (days)	± 30	± 8	± 50	± 40	
Symptoms					
Arthralgia, rash	Uncommon	Common	Uncommon	Common	Uncommon
Fever	Common	Uncommon	Uncommon	Common	Common
Nausea, Vomiting	Common	Common	Common	Common	Common
Jaundice	Uncommon in children	More common in hepatitis A	Uncommon	Common	Common
Laboratory Data					
Duration of enzyme	Short	Prolonged	Like hepatitis B		Like hepatitis B
Increase (days)	3–49	35–200	?	?	?
IgM elevation			?	?	?
Virus	RNA	DNA	?	?	RNA
Location of virus					
Blood	Transient	Prolonged	Prolonged	?Transient	Prolonged
Stool	Yes	No	No	Yes	No
Elsewhere	?	Yes	?	?	?
Outcome					
Severity of acute disease	Mild	Moderate	Mild	High in frequency	Moderate to high
Mortality	Low, 1%	Low 1–3%	Low, 2%	Moderate, ± 3%	High, 5%
Chronic hepatitis	No	Yes	Yes	No	Yes
Chronic carrier	No	Yes	Yes	No	Yes
Liver carrier	No	Yes	Possible	No	?
Relapse	Yes	Yes	?	?	?
Transmission					
Oral	+	±	?No	+	?No
Percutaneous	Rare	+	+	−	+
Sexual	+	+	−	?	+
Perinatal	−	+	±	?	−
Animal models					
Marmosets	+	−	−	?	
Chimpanzees	+	+	+	+	+

PNANB = parenteral non-A, non-B; ENANB = epidemic non-A, non-B.

phasic disease, the first peak representing the HBV infection and the second representing the HDV infection.[129c] The third pattern is the development of fulminant hepatitis, associated with a high mortality rate.[127r, 127v] Fulminant hepatitis is especially frequent in the setting of superinfection. This illness, which is almost invariably fatal, has been identified in several past epidemics in South America,[271o, 271p] as well as among drug addicts in the United States.[129a] Chronic HDV infection also may ensue in the setting of superinfection, greatly enhancing the likelihood of progression to serious chronic hepatitis.[271q, 271r] Indeed, this sequel is far more common when there is dual infection with HBV and HDV than when chronic HBV infection exists alone.

CLINICAL FORMS OF EXPRESSION AND OUTCOMES OF VIRAL HEPATITIS

ANICTERIC HEPATITIS

Anicteric hepatitis is the predominant form of expression of the diseases caused by all of the hepatitis viruses.

Because anicteric hepatitis is often asymptomatic, the determination of its relative frequency had to await the advent of prospective biochemical monitoring and the development of serologic tests. One of the several large-scale prospective studies that permitted this determination was the Veterans Administration cooperative study of post-transfusion hepatitis, in which all individuals who received blood transfusions were monitored by aminotransferase determinations and serologic testing every two weeks for six months.[272] Anicteric hepatitis, as determined biochemically, was found to develop five times more frequently than icteric hepatitis. Moreover, when the disease was defined by both biochemical and serologic parameters, the ratio of anicteric to icteric hepatitis was 15:1. Similar results have come from other prospective studies using frequent biochemical monitoring, most of which show a lower frequency of icterus in individuals with non-A, non-B hepatitis than in those with hepatitis B.[273–276a] In hepatitis A, the ratio of anicteric to icteric hepatitis is high as well, particularly in children.[42] Even in adults, anicteric hepatitis A can exceed icteric disease in frequency, although icteric hepatitis is a more common finding.[271c] For example, among 97 football players, managers, and coaches at a school in Massachusetts who were exposed to an HAV-contaminated drinking fountain, hepatitis developed in 90 individuals, but only a third had icteric disease.[277, 278] Finally, high rates of anicteric hepatitis A and hepatitis B can be inferred from serologic surveys showing prevalences of antibodies to these two viruses in excess of historic evidence of overt hepatic illness.[116, 279–282]

When anicteric hepatitis is asymptomatic, its clinical manifestations are similar to those of icteric hepatitis.[283] Indeed, it is not yet understood why icteric hepatitis develops in some patients, whereas anicteric disease develops in others. In general, anicteric hepatitis is milder than icteric disease, as judged by the lower frequency of symptoms, the lesser elevations of the aminotransferase levels,[272] the lower mortality rate, and the lesser histologic abnormalities.[284] Sometimes, biochemical and histologic abnormalities are identical to those of icteric hepatitis, with the obvious exception of hyperbilirubinemia. Furthermore, even histologic evidence of bridging and multilobular necrosis may be found in anicteric hepatitis and may result in progression to chronic liver disease without the appearance of clinical icterus at any time.[285] It has been suggested that subclinical disease is more likely to advance to chronic hepatitis than is overt icteric disease.[286–287a] Certainly, chronic hepatitis B without preceding overt hepatitis is a common finding in immunocompromised hosts, such as patients treated with dialysis and renal transplantation;[288–291] individuals with blood dyscrasias;[292, 293] and those with Down's syndrome.[294] This can be compared with the disease that affects medical personnel working with these individuals, which is generally icteric and self-limited.[295, 296]

ICTERIC HEPATITIS

The clinical and laboratory findings associated with icteric hepatitis have been described; the serologic changes are discussed in Chapter 35. Self-limited disease is the outcome in 99 per cent or more of cases of acute hepatitis A,[41, 297] in 1 to 90 per cent of cases of acute hepatitis B,[27a, 298] and in 60 per cent or more of cases of acute non-A, non-B hepatitis.[144a, 147, 299] Self-limited implies that symptoms disappear and bilirubin and aminotransferase values return to normal by the end of four months. However, approximately 10 per cent of patients have persistently abnormal aminotransferase levels for periods in excess of 100 days, usually without clinical symptoms or abnormal physical findings. Liver biopsy specimens of such patients reveal occasional focal areas of parenchymal degeneration and necrosis, sometimes with acidophilic bodies and usually with inflammatory cells, but more commonly with portal lymphocytic infiltration without fibrosis. This entity, referred to as prolonged hepatitis,[300] protracted hepatitis,[298] transaminitis,[301] or asymptomatic chronic hepatitis,[302] is believed to have a benign outcome. It may be difficult to distinguish from the even more extended entity of unresolved or chronic persistent hepatitis, which is also benign.[298, 303, 304] Even more confusing is the entity of *chronic lobular hepatitis*. As defined by Popper and Schaffner, it consists of viral hepatitis of more than three months' duration, but with histologic changes identical to those of acute viral hepatitis.[305] Wilkinson and co-workers have described the clinical courses of five such cases.[306] All patients were males with apparent HBsAg-negative acute viral hepatitis; their aminotransferase levels were elevated to between 500 and 3000 IU/L, and they tested positive for autoantibodies (antinuclear, antimitochondrial, or anti–smooth muscle)

and hyperglobulinemia. Their subsequent courses, after periods ranging at the time of the report from eight months to eight and a half years, were characterized by numerous remissions and relapses, each associated with striking elevations of aminotransferase levels. Three patients were treated with corticosteroids, and two of them had remissions while treatment was maintained. The histologic appearance of the liver during each relapse was characteristic of acute viral hepatitis, and cirrhosis did not develop in any patient, even after eight and a half years. The disease in these patients was believed to be the result of a single viral infection, rather than an autoimmune form of chronic hepatitis, or of two or more viral infections, each of which it superficially resembled. Similar observations come from a more recent study.[306a]

In some patients, the acute illness appears to resolve completely and then undergoes "re-exacerbation" or relapse, as defined by the reappearance of symptoms and recurrence of biochemical abnormalities suggestive of acute necroinflammatory disease. As already noted, this has been clearly documented in patients with acute hepatitis A and is a common manifestation of parenteral non-A, non-B hepatitis,[276a] a disease in which widely fluctuating enzyme activity (from abnormal to normal and back again to abnormal values) is regularly observed. Re-exacerbation has not been demonstrated in acute hepatitis B, except when delta hepatitis coinfection has occurred, at which time the second enzyme peak, representing the delta virus–induced injury, may be mistaken for a relapse. Individuals with chronic hepatitis B, in whom disease has evolved into a quiescent, nonreplicative phase, may experience reactivation following treatment with chemotherapeutic agents, immunosuppressive drugs, or corticosteroids, especially if these agents are rapidly withdrawn.[306b] Carriers, principally those in high-risk categories (e.g., drug addicts, hemophiliacs) may also appear to have an episode of reactivation in the rare instance of superinfection with HAV, non-A, non-B hepatitis, and HDV. In an even smaller group (< 3 per cent), the disease persists and even worsens over a period of one to three months. This is manifested by continuing or increasing jaundice, a gradual deterioration of the coagulation factors, the persistence of markedly abnormal aminotransferase levels, and the development of asterixis and spider nevi and of features suggestive of portal hypertension, such as splenomegaly, ascites, peripheral edema, and occasionally varices and hepatic encephalopathy. This entity has been referred to variously as subacute hepatic necrosis,[307] submassive hepatic necrosis,[308] subacute or subchronic atrophy of the liver,[309, 310] and subacute hepatitis.[311] Features that have appeared to correlate with the appearance of this complication have included the development of hepatitis in persons older than 40 years of age,[307] drug addiction,[312] the insidious onset of anicteric disease,[287, 307] the development of HBsAg-positive hepatitis with persistence of the antigen,[307, 313] the presence of complicating disease,[307] the presence of antibodies such as antinuclear, anti–smooth muscle, and antimitochondrial antibodies,[314] and the development of hypoprothrombinemia and hypoalbuminemia associated with hypergammaglobulinemia.[307, 312] However, the finding that has received the most attention and has been most controversial is the histologic correlate of *bridging necrosis*, which represents zones of necrosis bridging adjacent portal triads or central veins, or both. Klatskin reported in 1958 that this morphologic feature represented a poor prognostic indicator in anicteric hepatitis,[285] and together with Boyer in 1970, he again showed it was an equally important indicator of a poor outcome for patients with overt icteric hepatitis.[307] Thus, they found in a retrospective analysis that 52 per cent of 170 patients with biopsy proven acute viral hepatitis had features of bridging necrosis; in 19 per cent of these patients the disease advanced to cirrhosis. This was in contradistinction to the outcome among the remaining 118 patients without bridging necrosis, all of whom recovered completely. It was concluded, therefore, that the finding of intralobular bridging necrosis of portal triads or central veins during the acute phase of hepatitis is associated with a poor prognosis. The view that the presence of bridging necrosis during acute hepatitis has serious consequences seemed to be affirmed by the results of another retrospective analysis. Ware and associates, in an evaluation of 57 patients with bridging necrosis, reported that one of them died, and chronic liver disease developed in eight others.[315] Fourteen other subjects were lost to follow-up. Two thirds of these patients were HBsAg-positive. Thus, the results of these two studies suggest that a third to two thirds of patients who have bridging necrosis during acute viral hepatitis suffer serious complications. It is of note that in a third study of 42 patients with bridging necrosis, drugs were believed to be responsible for almost half of the cases.[316] The outcome, once the drugs were discontinued, was significantly better than the outcome when the lesion had not been caused by a drug.

The least common complication is *fulminant hepatitis*.[298] This term is applied when hepatic failure occurs abruptly during the first four weeks of the acute illness. Fulminant hepatitis is discussed in Chapter 17 and therefore is not described here. However, it should be noted that, unlike survivors of subacute hepatic necrosis, the disease in survivors of fulminant hepatitis does not appear to progress to chronic liver disease. Karvountzis and co-workers reported that all of 22 patients who had survived acute viral hepatitis with coma and who were subjected to long-term follow-up evaluation showed complete clinical and biochemical resolution within 45 to 75 days of the acute onset.[321] Furthermore, none of 13 patients who later had liver biopsies were found to have disease that could be related to the fulminant hepatitis.

Chronic hepatitis as a sequel to the acute disease is more common than the other complications already described. The frequency of this complication relates, in part, to the virus causing the acute disease. Redeker, in a study of 429 patients with acute hepatitis B who were followed for one to five years, found that nearly 90 per cent recovered entirely without residua, less than 1 per cent died with fulminant hepatitis, and almost 10 per cent advanced to chronic liver disease.[298] In a third of the patients in whom chronic hepatitis developed, there were histologic features of chronic active hepatitis, and in two thirds of the patients, there were histologic features of chronic persistent hepatitis. Similar results were observed in another prospective study involving 500 patients with acute viral hepatitis, conducted by the Copenhagen Hepatitis Study Group.[322] In this study, the persistence of HBsAg beyond 13 weeks after the onset of disease correlated closely with progression to chronic hepatitis B, an outcome that occurred in 4 per cent of the cases.[313] The rate of progression to chronic hepatitis B was similar in yet another study from Scandinavia involving 440 patients.[323] In contrast, the carrier rate was less than 1 per cent (40-year follow-up) among patients with acute hepatitis B caused by contaminated yellow fever vaccine.[27a] Factors that increase the likelihood of chronicity include infection in the neonatal period,[324] infection in immunosuppressed individuals,[293] infection in renal dialysis and kidney transplant patients,[288–291] the use of corticosteroids during acute hepatitis,[287] the high frequency of exposure of certain groups such as drug addicts and persons with hemophilia,[281, 325, 326] the development of subclinical disease,[286–287a] and the persistence of HBsAg for periods exceeding 13 weeks,[313] of HBeAg for periods of 10 weeks or more,[327] and of HBsAg complexes with immunoglobulin (IgM; antibody directed against polymerized human serum albumin bound to HBsAg) beyond 5 weeks.[327a] Perhaps the most important determinant is the age at which the initial infection occurs; chronicity evolves in 90 to 95 per cent of neonates and in approximately 20 per cent of children,[327b–327e] but in only 1 to 10 per cent of adults.[27a, 298, 327f]

The progression of acute non-A, non-B hepatitis to chronic liver disease has been documented. Indeed, the frequency of this occurrence seems to be higher following acute non-A, non-B hepatitis than following acute hepatitis B. Chronic hepatitis, as defined by the persistence of enzyme abnormalities for a period of six months or more, has been reported in 10 to 70 per cent of patients evaluated in numerous prospective studies of post-transfusion hepatitis. The majority of investigators report a frequency in excess of 50 per cent.[144a, 327g] Sporadic non-A, non-B hepatitis also culminates in chronic hepatitis, although the frequency has tended to be somewhat lower.[144a] A group at particular risk for the development of chronic non-A, non-B hepatitis are individuals with hemophilia.[327h] Liver biopsy specimens have revealed chronic liver disease (chronic active hepatitis or cirrhosis, or both) in more than 50 per cent of such individuals.[328–330] A small number of such patients progress rapidly to liver failure and death, but the vast majority have an insidious course that is usually free of symptoms. In one major study, the disease process was noted to subside, as indicated by the gradual return of enzyme levels to normal in association with liver biopsy results indicating a change from chronic active to chronic persistent disease.[147] Further long-term studies are needed to determine with greater precision the outcome of this important disease.

Hepatitis A does not progress to chronic liver disease. Krarup and Roholm, in early histologic studies, described the presence of cirrhosis following acute hepatitis,[331] but this was viewed by Chalmers as a coincidental finding.[332] His belief that cirrhosis was not a sequel to acute hepatitis was supported by two long-term follow-up studies, one conducted 10 years and the other 20 years after the acute illness.[333, 334] No increased incidence of chronic hepatitis was found. In retrospect, it is likely that the first of Chalmer's studies probably represented an outbreak of acute hepatitis A. The second has now proved to be the result of HBV infection that led to a negligible HBsAg carrier rate.[27a] Two recent studies of established hepatitis A—one involving children at the Willowbrook School infected with the MS-1 strain of HAV and the other an outbreak among naval recruits[41, 133]—also failed to demonstrate progression to chronic hepatitis.[297] Additional evidence comes from studies of patients with established chronic hepatitis, in whom the prevalence of anti-HAV is no greater than that in matched controls without chronic hepatitis.[335, 336]

CHOLESTATIC VIRAL HEPATITIS

The third and least common clinical variant is cholestatic viral hepatitis. First described in the mid-1930s by Eppinger as a "cholangitic" form of hepatitis,[337] and referred to by Watson and Hoffbauer in 1946 as "cholangiolitic hepatitis,"[338] this entity has been reported on at least a half dozen occasions.[271g, 339–344] It is characterized by fever, marked pruritus, unusual elevations of serum alkaline phosphatase and serum bilirubin levels (usually in excess of 15 mg/dl), prolongation of the prothrombin time, elevation of serum cholesterol levels, an increased ESR, no urobilinogenuria, clay-colored stools, and a prolonged course. Early investigators believed it to be a precursor of "cholangiolitic" or primary biliary cirrhosis,[338] but in later studies it was found to be followed by complete recovery. Three regional epidemics have been reported from an Army hospital in San Antonio, Texas,[342] from Delhi, India,[343] following a waterborne epidemic (now known to be caused by epidemic non-A, non-B hepatitis), and from Accra, Ghana.[344] In the latter two reports, hepatitis was associated with a higher complication rate in pregnant than in nonpregnant women, as well as a high fetal death rate. The most recent report implicated hepatitis A.[271g] The cause of this variant of acute hepatitis is unknown; an early suggestion that it results because of obstruction or damage to the intrahepatic bile channels has been rejected.[338, 339, 341, 342] The outcome of cholestatic viral hepatitis is good, although jaundice may be protracted, lasting as long as eight months. There are no obvious sequelae of this disease.

HISTOPATHOLOGIC FEATURES OF VIRAL HEPATITIS

The wide array of histologic abnormalities of the liver occurring in viral hepatitis serves to differentiate acute from chronic disease. Ishak has classified the histopathologic changes of viral hepatitis as follows:[248, 345]
A. Acute infection
    1. Acute classic viral hepatitis
    2. Acute viral hepatitis with submassive necrosis
    3. Acute viral hepatitis with massive necrosis
    4. Acute cholestatic viral hepatitis
    5. Persistent (unresolved) hepatitis

B. Chronic infection
    1. The chronic hepatitis B antigen carrier
    2. Chronic persistent viral hepatitis
    3. Chronic active viral hepatitis
    4. Chronic cholestatic viral hepatitis
    5. Posthepatic cirrhosis
C. Viral hepatitis and hepatocellular carcinoma

The present discussion is confined to a description of the histologic changes in acute viral hepatitis and in the HBsAg carrier state. The pathologic findings in chronic hepatitis are described in Chapter 38. At the outset, it should be noted that the view held until recently was that the viruses of hepatitis A and hepatitis B caused identical morphologic changes in the liver. Data from a study of liver tissue from chimpanzees inoculated with specific hepatitis strains now suggest that subtle differences exist.[346] Furthermore, careful study of large numbers of liver biopsy specimens from patients with serologically well-defined viral hepatitis reveals morphologic clues to etiology. One should also note that icteric hepatitis and anicteric hepatitis produce similar histologic changes, with quantitative differences seen only occasionally.

LIGHT-MICROSCOPIC FEATURES OF ACUTE VIRAL HEPATITIS

ACUTE CLASSIC VIRAL HEPATITIS

During the acute phase of the illness, the histologic changes, which occur in varying degrees and combinations, include lobular disarray, smudging of cellular outlines, ballooning and acidophilic degeneration, acidophilic (free hyaline, Councilman-like) bodies, areas of focal necrosis, lymphocytic parenchymal and portal inflammation, cholestasis, Kupffer cell and macrophage hypertrophy and hyperplasia, and the deposition of lipofuscin within these reticuloendothelial cells (Fig. 37–1). Lobular disarray is the

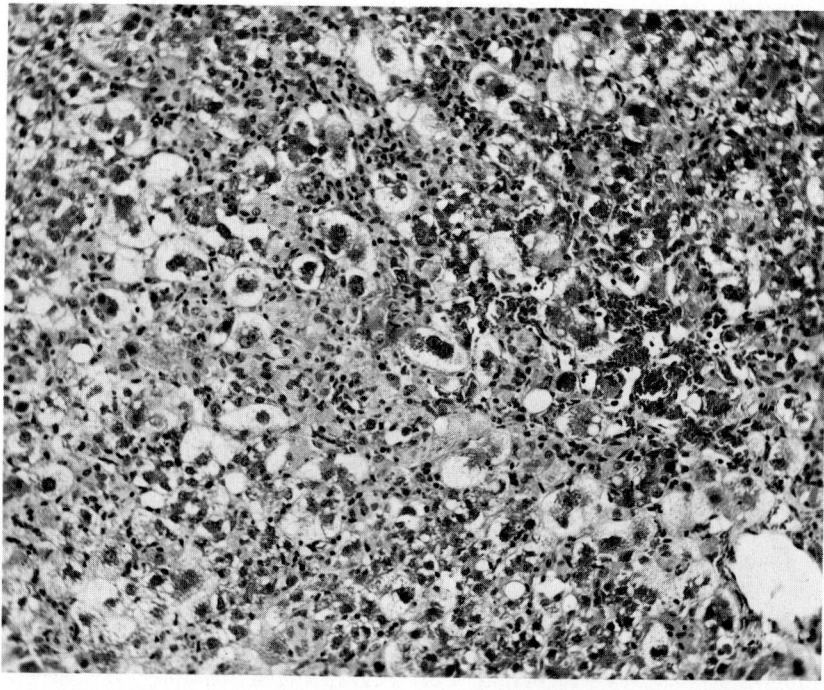

Figure 37–1. Acute viral hepatitis, showing lobular disarray, ballooning degeneration, mild hepatocellular necrosis with an acidophilic body, and slight inflammation. Cellular outlines are smudged, and anisocytosis and anisonucleosis can be seen (hematoxylin and eosin, × 145; AFIP Neg. No. 71–1394. Courtesy of K. Ishak).

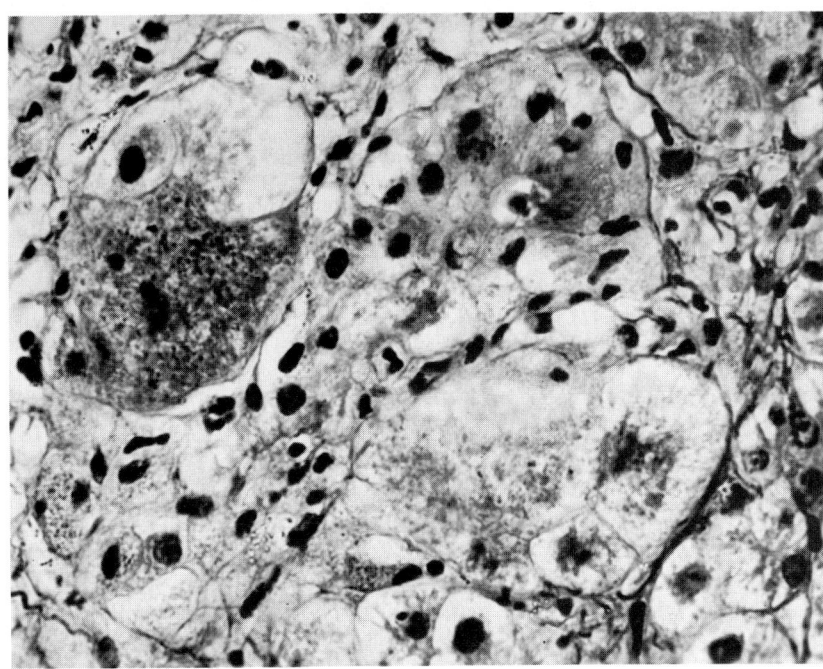

Figure 37–2. Acute viral hepatitis, showing markedly ballooned hepatocytes with lysed cell membranes and empty cytoplasm (hematoxylin and eosin, × 530; AFIP Neg. No. 70–10577. Courtesy of K. Ishak).

result of a combination of anisocytosis, anisonucleosis, binucleation, smudging of cell outlines, focal necrosis, and reticuloendothelial cell activation. Cells showing ballooning degeneration, as the name implies, are markedly swollen, with smudged cell membranes and rarefied cytoplasm (Fig. 37–2). In contrast, cells undergoing acidophilic degeneration are shrunken, angulated, and deeply eosinophilic in color (Fig. 37–3). Ultimately, the latter cells round up, usually lose their nuclei, free themselves from the surrounding hepatocytes by entering the space of Disse, and there await destruction and removal through engulfment by Kupffer cells. Although lymphocytes are the predominant inflammatory cells present, occasional eosinophils and neu-

trophils may also be found. Plasma cells are rarely seen. In drug abusers in whom hepatitis develops, the inflammatory response is characterized by an unusual predominance of eosinophilic leukocytes in portal areas and in foci of necrosis.[345, 347] Also, birefringent material, believed to be talc or other extraneous material that has been added to the narcotic drug, is often deposited in Kupffer cells and portal macrophages.[348] These particles may also be responsible for the small granuloma-like lesions sometimes seen in the livers of narcotic drug abusers. The presence of fat, which was believed by earlier investigators to be rare or nonexistent in acute hepatitis, can be seen (sometimes in large quantities) in persons with non-A, non-B hepatitis or hep-

Figure 37–3. Acute viral hepatitis, showing a focus of acute necrosis with an acidophilic body and lymphocytic infiltration (hematoxylin and eosin, × 680; AFIP Neg. No. 70–1880. Courtesy of K. Ishak).

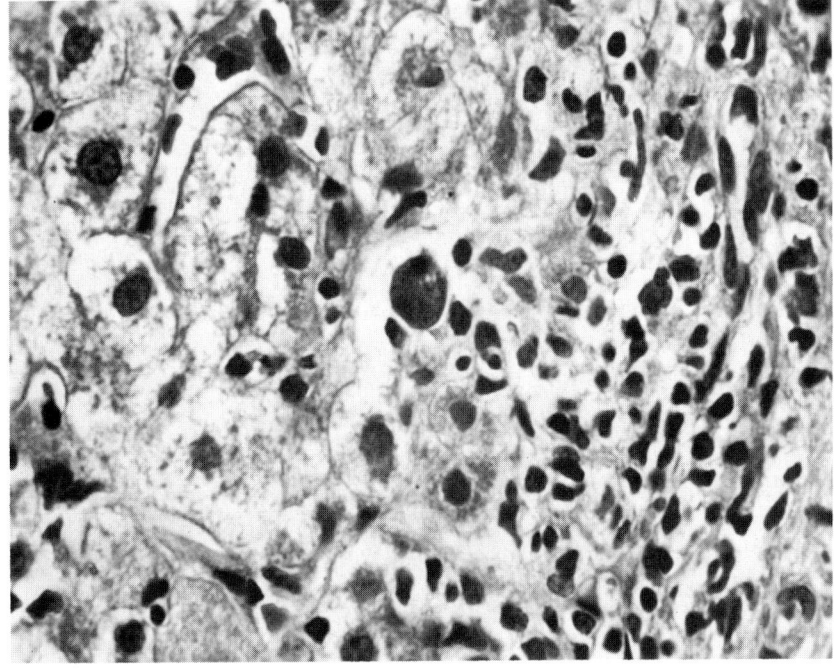

atitis D. Both macro- and microvesicular droplets may be identified.

As the disease subsides, evidence of regeneration, characterized by binucleation and mitoses, becomes prominent. The reticuloendothelial cells remain hypertrophied and can be seen to contain lipofuscin and hemosiderin. Centrilobular cholestasis may become apparent during this phase. Finally, the changes that have occurred all begin to recede.

ACUTE VIRAL HEPATITIS WITH SUBMASSIVE NECROSIS

In some instances, the areas of necrosis may be more extensive, involving the entire central or mid-zone, or both, but sparing the remaining one third to two thirds of the lobule (Fig. 37–4). The liver cells in the necrotic areas drop out, the reticulum framework becomes condensed, and the sinusoids are dilated and filled with inflammatory cells. Necrotic zones that are adjacent may become linked together to form bridging necrosis, a feature believed to be a forerunner of hepatic failure or cirrhosis.[307] The bridges seem to develop on the border of the acini of Rappaport farthest from the origin of the oxygen-rich blood entering from the portal tracts.[349] The central veins may be involved by endophlebitis, and in the rest of the parenchyma, combinations of ballooning degeneration, acidophilic bodies, cholestasis, and regeneration of surviving tissue that produces a nodular appearance may be present.

ACUTE VIRAL HEPATITIS WITH MASSIVE NECROSIS

In this even less common situation, the necrosis is widespread, affecting all zones of the lobule, and it is accompanied by prominent cholangiolar proliferation (Fig. 37–5). Massive necrosis may involve only part of the liver or the entire organ. When all lobules are simultaneously involved, death is inevitable. Usually, the necrosis develops in episodes, and death will occur only when a critical amount of hepatic parenchyma has become involved. Data from a study using stereologic estimation of hepatocyte volume suggest that death is the invariable outcome when the hepatocyte volume falls to less than 35 to 45 per cent.[350] Another finding is inflammation, with mononuclear cells still predominating, although neutrophils may be seen infiltrating the cholangioles. Surprisingly, cirrhosis appears to be an uncommon sequel of fulminant hepatitis despite the extensive necrosis.[321, 351]

ACUTE CHOLESTATIC VIRAL HEPATITIS

The cholestatic variant of viral hepatitis is characterized histologically by prominent cholestasis, dilated canaliculi forming pseudoglands, and periportal proliferation of cholangioles. Hepatocyte degeneration may be variably present, but ballooning degeneration is common. The hypertrophied Kupffer cells are usually found to contain bile as well as lipofuscin. There is a sparsity of acidophilic bodies.[345]

PERSISTENT (UNRESOLVED) VIRAL HEPATITIS

The morphologic features suggesting that acute disease has not resolved include mild to moderate hepatocellular unrest, occasional acidophilic bodies, rare and small foci of necrosis, minimal focal Kupffer cell hypertrophy, minimal and patchy parenchymal and portal inflammation with plasma cells, insignificant periportal fibrosis, and no evidence of piecemeal necrosis (Fig. 37–6). Furthermore, beyond six months after infection, the Kupffer cells should not contain either lipofuscin or hemosiderin. If the patient has a relapse following development of persistent hepatitis, the liver biopsy specimen will show the reappearance of centrilobular ballooning and cholestasis.

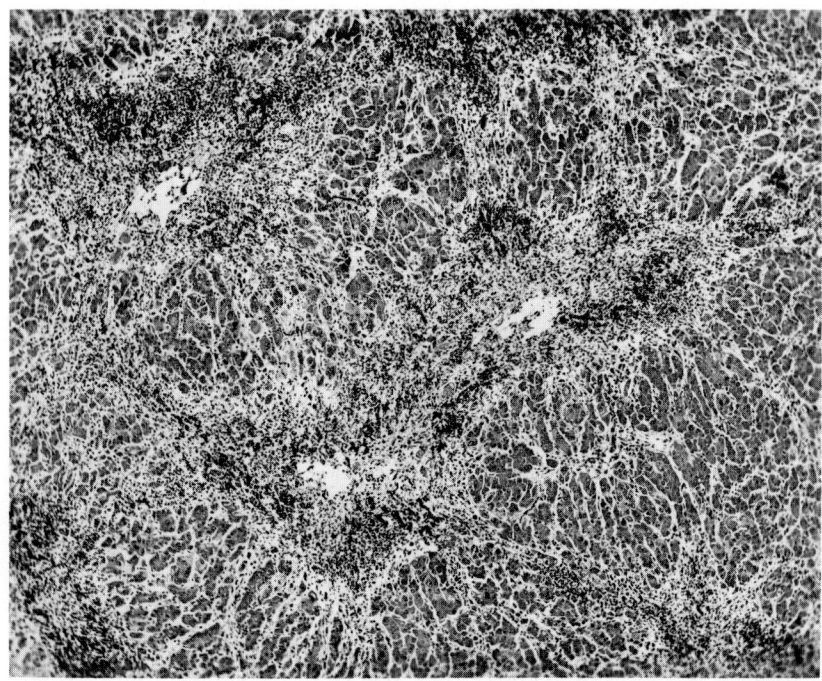

Figure 37–4. Acute viral hepatitis with submassive necrosis. Centrilobular zones of necrosis are linked together by bridges of necrosis (bridging necrosis) (hematoxylin and eosin, × 50; AFIP Neg. No. 74–4232. Courtesy of K. Ishak).

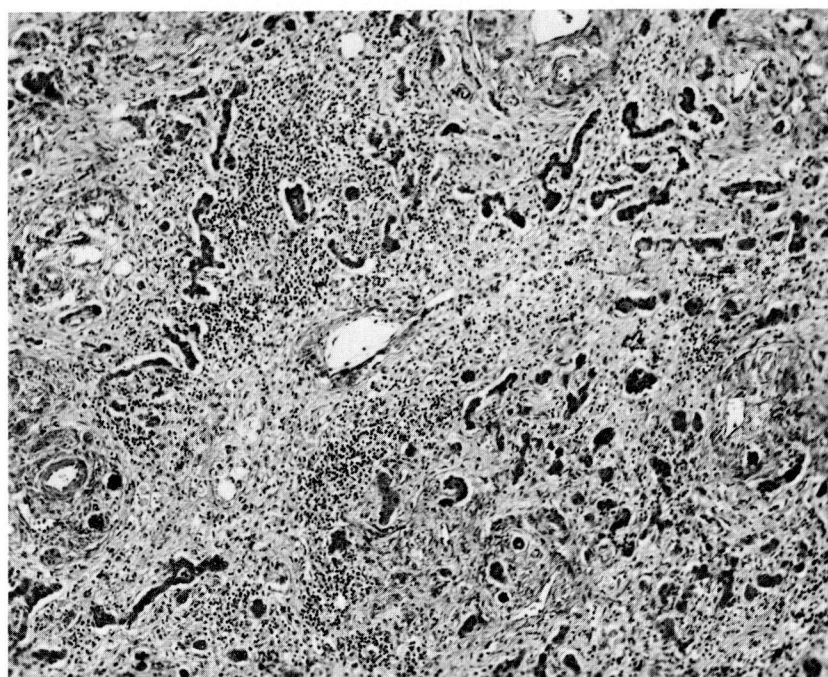

Figure 37–5. Acute viral hepatitis with massive necrosis, all of the hepatocytes having dropped out, leaving behind proliferating periportal cholangioles and inflamed portal areas (hematoxylin and eosin, × 55; AFIP Neg. No. 71–1231. Courtesy of K. Ishak).

There will be an increase in acidophilic degeneration and acidophilic bodies, lipofuscin will reaccumulate in Kupffer cells, and portal inflammation will increase. The typical findings in acute, subsiding, and persistent (unresolved) hepatitis are shown in Table 37–7.

Much effort has been expended to define morphologic features that predict the ultimate outcome of the hepatic disease. Unfortunately, no completely reliable feature has yet been determined. Piecemeal necrosis during the acute attack does not necessarily imply a poor outcome. Popper has suggested that the following factors should be considered disturbing: (1) alteration of bile ducts in portal tracts,

(2) the presence of central to central or central to portal bridging necrosis, and (3) the early admixture of plasma cells with portal and lobular inflammatory exudates.[352] The study of chimpanzees infected with defined hepatitis inocula has provided support for some of these criteria.[346]

ULTRASTRUCTURAL CHANGES IN ACUTE VIRAL HEPATITIS

Cells showing ballooning degeneration on light microscopy are seen by electron microscopy as light cells with

Figure 37–6. Persistent (unresolved) hepatitis, showing mild hepatocellular unrest, an acidophilic body, and Kupffer cell hypertrophy (hematoxylin and eosin, × 440; AFIP Neg. No. 75–2481. Courtesy of K. Ishak).

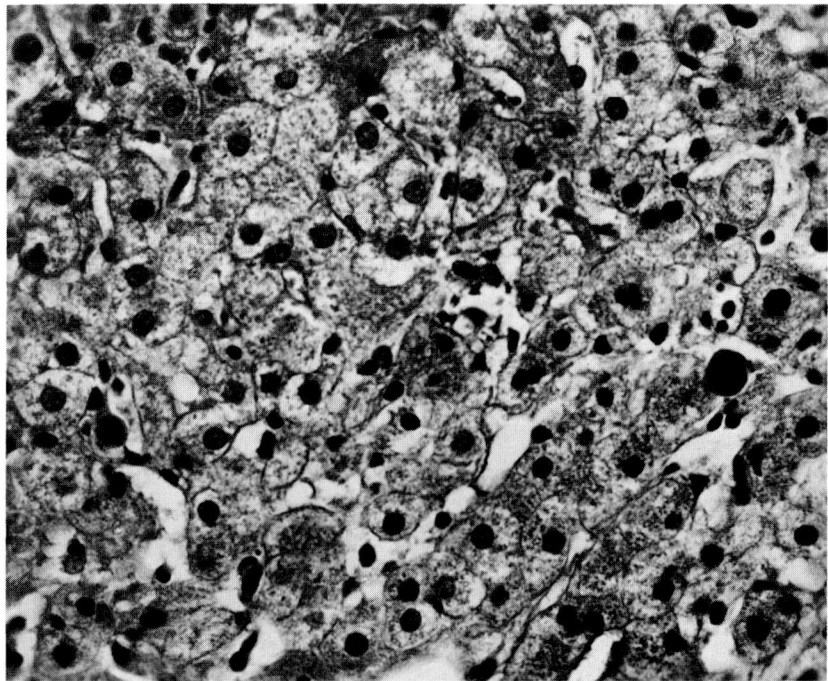

TABLE 37–7. MORPHOLOGIC FEATURES OF ACUTE, SUBSIDING, AND PERSISTENT VIRAL HEPATITIS*

Morphologic Change	Acute	Subsiding	Persistent
Ballooning degeneration	+ + +	+	+ to + + (relapse)
Focal necrosis	+ +	+	+ to + + +
Focal inflammation	L	L	P
Acidophilic degeneration and acidophilic bodies	+ + +	+	+ to + +
Cholestasis	0 to +	+ +	0 to + +
Unicellular regeneration	+	+ +	+ +
Fat	0	0 to +	0 to +
Kupffer cell hypertrophy and hyperplasia	+ + +	+ + +	0 to + +
Lipofuscin in Kupffer cells	+ +	+ + +	0 to + +
Hemosiderin in Kupffer cells	0	+	0 to + +
Portal inflammation	L (diffuse)	L (patchy)	P (patchy)

*Data courtesy of K. G. Ishak (personal communication).

0 = absent; + = unusual; + + = moderate; + + + = marked; L = lymphocyte; P = plasma cell.

dilated cisternae of rough endoplasmic reticulum.[350, 353] Polyribosomes are dilated and reduced in number. Hyaloplasm appears floccular with reduced electron density, and there is loss of glycogen. Mitochondria are swollen, and degenerating cells have swollen villi. Cells undergoing acidophilic degeneration, appearing as markedly electron-dense (dense cells), are shrunken and angulated and show loss of organelles and microvilli. Eventually, they become rounded and pass into the space of Disse and the sinusoids. Here they become surrounded by interdigitating processes of markedly hypertrophied Kupffer cells, which ultimately digest them. The Kupffer cells are also found to contain multilobed lipofuscin. In the subsiding phase of hepatitis, the lysosomes contain both lipofuscin and fine hemosiderin granules. In the cholestatic form of acute viral hepatitis, cholestasis can be seen in association with markedly dilated canaliculi containing fibrillar and granular material.

LIGHT-MICROSCOPIC AND ELECTRON MICROSCOPIC FEATURES OF THE CHRONIC HEPATITIS B ANTIGEN CARRIER

Persons who are HBsAg carriers may have no clinical, biochemical, or histologic evidence of liver disease, or they may have associated chronic liver disease manifesting as chronic persistent hepatitis, chronic active hepatitis, cirrhosis, or hepatocellular carcinoma. The present discussion is confined to a description of the morphologic features of the liver in the carrier state only. Descriptions of the histologic changes of chronic hepatitis and of hepatocellular carcinoma appear in other chapters.

The characteristic finding in the liver of the HBsAg carrier is the presence of ground-glass hepatocytes (Fig. 37–7). This association was first made in 1972 by Hadziyannis and co-workers,[354] although similar cells had previously

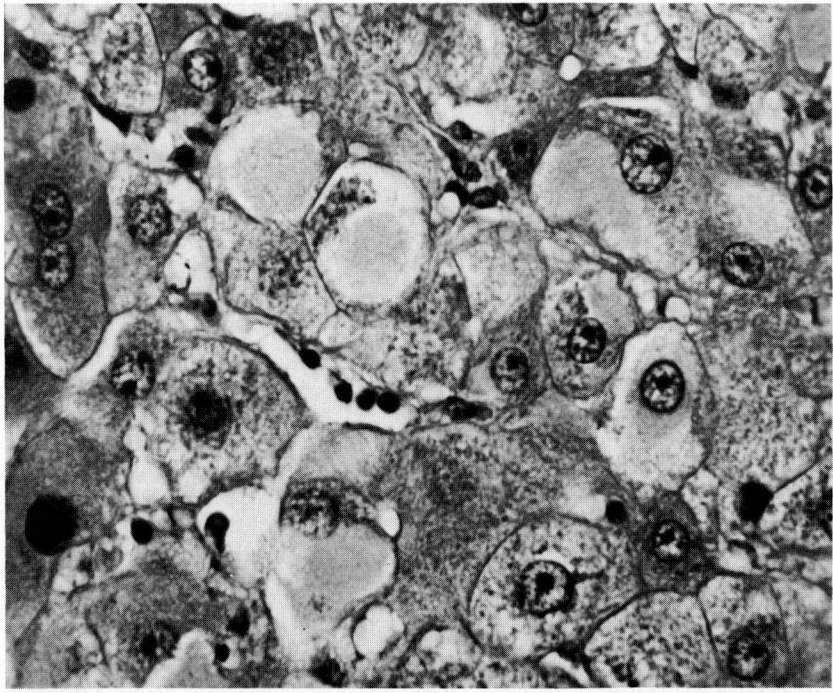

Figure 37–7. Ground-glass cells in the liver of an HBsAg carrier, showing also enlarged hyperchromatic nuclei with prominent nucleoli (hematoxylin and eosin, × 530; AFIP Neg. No. 74–9138. Courtesy of K. Ishak).

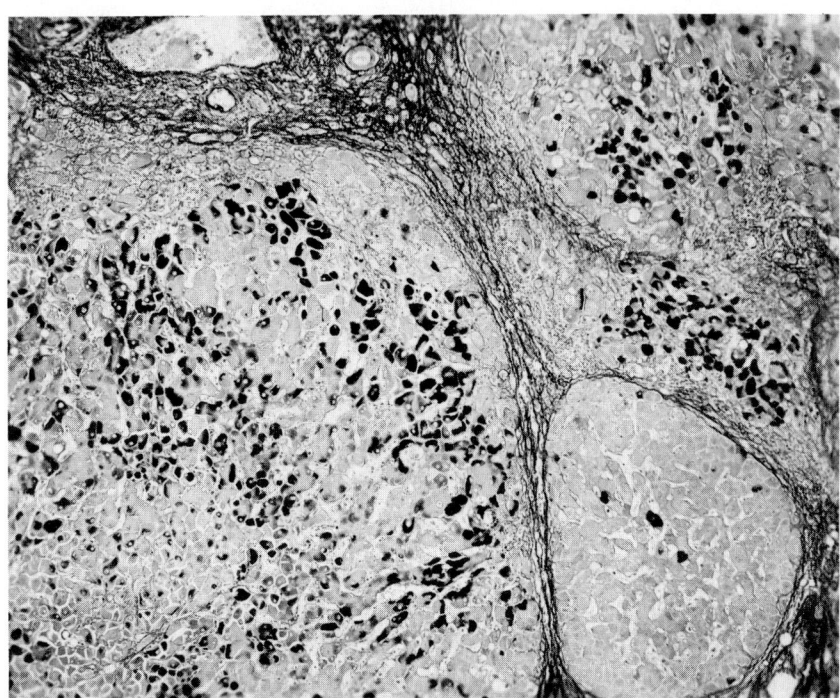

Figure 37–8. HBsAg carrier patient with multilobular necrosis and heavy deposition of HBsAg in hepatocytes, visible as dark black angulated cells (aldehyde fuchsin, × 60; AFIP Neg. No. 78–3093. Courtesy of K. Ishak).

been described by Klinge and Bannasch in 1968 as occurring in the livers of persons who had received drugs capable of stimulating the microsomal biotransformation system.[355] Indeed, these investigators were able to demonstrate an increase in the smooth endoplasmic reticulum of the affected cells. Later, Klinge and co-workers also reported the presence of ground-glass cells in the livers of asymptomatic HBsAg carriers.[356] Shortly thereafter, Shikata and colleagues described several methods for staining HBsAg in formalin-fixed paraffin-embedded sections.[357] They suggested that HBsAg had an affinity to certain dyes because of the presence of disulfide bonds, HBsAg having been shown to have high levels of cystine. Subsequent studies using the aldehyde fuchsin and the orcein methods showed that they both stained ground-glass cells in liver specimens from HBsAg-positive patients with and without chronic hepatitis (Fig. 37–8) but that they did not stain HBsAg-positive cells in acute hepatitis.[358, 359] The positively stained cells appeared to be more numerous in the livers of carriers, in which they were often arranged in groups or cords, than in livers of patients with chronic hepatitis or cirrhosis, in which they tended to be scattered throughout the hepatic lobule, present sometimes singly and sometimes in clusters. Ultrastructural studies have demonstrated that the stains identify tubular and circular structures 20 to 30 nm in size that are present in the dilated cisternae of excess endoplasmic reticulum. These structures, found only in the cytoplasm of hepatocytes, are believed to represent the coat material (HBsAg) of the hepatitis B virus.[358] Furthermore, it is these viral particles that appear to take up the stain, and not the hypertrophied endoplasmic reticulum, since ground-glass cells secondary to drug therapy are not stained by the methods tested by Shikata and associates. It is of practical importance that these stains have been found to provide positive results even when the liver biopsy material has been stored for many years. Finally, it should be noted that these stains are not specific for HBsAg. They have been found to identify lipofuscin pigment, bile, and

copper.[360, 361] Immunofluorescent and electron microscopic studies have shown the presence of HBsAg in the cytoplasm of hepatocytes (tubular structures 20 to 30 nm in size, located in cisternae of proliferated smooth endoplasmic reticulum, giving a ground-glass appearance), and the presence of hepatitis B core antigen (HBcAg) in the hepatocyte nuclei (noncoated viral particles, 20 to 25 nm in diameter).[362–365] Immunohistochemical procedures capable of tissue localization of HBcAg and HBsAg in formalin-fixed paraffin sections have also been developed.[365] Gudat and co-workers correlated the pattern of HBcAg and HBsAg expression with clinical and light-microscopic characteristics and proposed that there are four reaction types, with diagnostic and prognostic implications.[366, 367] They suggest that immune responsiveness determines the reaction pattern, the key mechanism being immune elimination of affected cells. According to this concept, between efficient elimination (type I) and effective immunosuppression (type II), there is graded elimination insufficiency found in chronic forms (types III and IV), which explains the persistence and perhaps also the aggressiveness of HBV infection.

PATHOLOGIC EFFECTS OF VIRAL HEPATITIS ON ORGANS OTHER THAN THE LIVER

Even before the discovery of HBsAg, it was recognized that abnormalities in other organ systems sometimes developed in persons with viral hepatitis. When specific hepatitis-related serologic tests became available, interest in the extrahepatic manifestations of viral hepatitis grew, for a number of reasons. First, the serologic tests made it possible to define several disease entities not formerly regarded as being associated with viral hepatitis. Second, certain of the nonhepatic manifestations could be clearly linked to the prodromal stages of viral hepatitis, thus permitting early recognition of the viral infection with or without manifested hepatic disease. Third, the use of sophisticated immunologic procedures to study the pathogenesis of these entities also expanded knowledge regarding the pathogenesis of the hepatic disease itself.

At present, the numerous extrahepatic manifestations of viral hepatitis may be viewed as consisting of two broad categories—those for which the pathogenesis has not been fully defined and those believed, on the basis of developing data, to be mediated by circulating immune complexes containing HBsAg and anti-HBs. The two categories are discussed separately. It is highly likely, however, that the categoric distinctions will change as more is learned about the immunologic bases for their development.

NONHEPATIC DISORDERS ASSOCIATED WITH VIRAL HEPATITIS NOT KNOWN TO BE MEDIATED BY CIRCULATING IMMUNE COMPLEXES

Cardiac Manifestations

Several reports in the past 30 years have described cardiac abnormalities in viral hepatitis.[368-375] Most have been derived from retrospective studies involving analysis of pathologic findings in the hearts of patients who have died with fulminant hepatic disease.[368-371] Because no effort has been made to evaluate the cardiovascular system prospectively in routine cases of viral hepatitis, the frequency of cardiac involvement is not known. However, based on the sparsity of reports, it appears that patients with complicated hepatitis rarely manifest important cardiac disease, whereas in fulminant hepatitis, cardiac disease may contribute to the cause of death.

In 1944 Lucke, reporting the pathologic findings in fulminant viral hepatitis, noted cloudy swelling and vacuolization of myocardial fibers, as well as hemorrhage into the intraventricular septum.[368] Subsequent postmortem studies confirmed and extended these observations.[369-371] Thus, the features of myocarditis include foci of necrosis of isolated muscle bundles surrounded by an inflammatory response, the necrosis frequently involving the left branch of the bundle of His. There are also widespread petechial hemorrhages, fatty degeneration of the myocardium, and edema of the subendocardial connective tissue, resulting in flabby dilated ventricles. Pericardial effusion, frequently hemorrhagic, has also been reported.[372] In one instance, bloody fluid from the pericardial sac was shown to be HBsAg-positive.[373]

The pathogenesis of the myocarditis and pericarditis is not established. It may result from a direct effect of the hepatitis virus—analogous to the myocarditis that occurs in other viral infections such as viral influenza, coxsackievirus B infection, poliomyelitis, measles, and chickenpox—or from the formation of immune complexes.[373] However, immunologic studies to define the presence of immune complexes have not been reported. Hemorrhagic pericarditis, occurring most frequently in fulminant hepatitis, presumably results from the accompanying severe coagulation disturbances.

The clinical findings in affected patients include electrocardiographic abnormalities, prolonged hypotension, progressive cardiomegaly, pulmonary edema, and sudden death.[374, 375] The electrocardiogram has been reported to show low-voltage left axis deviation, T-wave changes, prolonged P-R and Q-T intervals, and a variety of arrhythmias, including atrial fibrillation, ventricular premature contractions, atrial flutter, tachycardias, and sinus bradycardia.

The original view that sinus bradycardia results from depression of the sinoatrial node by high levels of circulating bilirubin seems not to be borne out by clinical facts. Bradycardia is found when jaundice is not present, and most jaundiced patients do not have bradycardia. The bradycardia, when present, may reflect inflammation of the myocardial conduction system.[375]

Pulmonary Manifestations

Pleural effusion is the only pulmonary abnormality that has been attributed to viral hepatitis.[376-382] Its frequency is uncertain, but effusions are rare.

The fluid, when described, has had the characteristics of an exudate. In addition, HBsAg, antibody to HBcAg (anti-HBc), hepatitis B e antigen (HBeAg), and 42- and 22-nm viral particles have been identified in the effusion.[381, 382] Most instances of pleural effusion have occurred in patients with overt hepatitis B, but it has also been found in HBsAg-positive anicteric hepatitis.[382] It has been suggested that the effusion represents an element of the serum sickness syndrome,[380] although this remains to be proved. The effusion usually disappears spontaneously as the hepatic disease abates. Hence, rare though it is, HBV infection should be a diagnostic consideration whenever there is a cryptogenic pleural effusion. The finding of HBV markers in pleural fluid indicates that this is another body fluid capable of transmitting the disease to the unwary.

Gastrointestinal Tract Manifestations

Endoscopic examinations during the early years of this procedure,[383-385] radiology,[385] and gastric acid secretion studies[386] all revealed only minimal abnormalities in the stomach. However, in one study, mild hypertrophic gastritis was commonly observed in patients with acute viral hepatitis.[384]

Greater attention has been given to an examination of the intestinal tract because of the report from Lucke in 1944 of the finding of phlegmonous inflammation of the gastrointestinal tract in 15 per cent of 125 cases of fatal epidemic hepatitis.[368] However, in a more recent report, the development of acute diffuse hemorrhagic necrosis of the bowel (enteritis gravis) in a patient with viral hepatitis was considered a chance association.[387] Investigators in Italy, who obtained tissue by peroral biopsy of the small bowel, found subtotal and total villous atrophy and abnormal epithelium in jejunal biopsy specimens.[388] They also observed increased numbers of mucus-filled goblet cells and intestinal inflammation of the villous stroma. Repeat jejunal biopsies that were obtained following recovery from the hepatic disease demonstrated marked improvement. Similar abnormalities were found in a study involving United States soldiers who had acquired hepatitis in Korea.[130] However, opposing results were found in a more recent study, conducted among servicemen stationed in the United States.[131] In this study, jejunal biopsy specimens were obtained from 18 patients with hepatitis and compared in a blinded fashion with specimens from patients without hepatitis. Slight abnormalities were found, but the changes were seen in all biopsy specimens. There were no distinguishing features to separate the two groups of patients. The authors concluded that intestinal abnormalities in hepatitis were uncommon, and they attributed the previously reported abnormal findings to intestinal changes resulting from residence in tropical areas of the world.

A similarly negative report has come from a Canadian study of patients with liver disease and steatorrhea.[132] Jejunal biopsies showed no evidence of histologic abnormality in any of five patients with viral hepatitis and steatorrhea, nor was there any instance of impaired absorption of nutrients by the small bowel (normal D-xylose absorption and Schilling test). The authors proposed that the malabsorption of fat in their patients was due to a micellar phase effect secondary to reduced concentrations of conjugated bile salts within the intestine. Indeed, low concentrations of conjugated bile acid have been demonstrated in intestinal contents of patients with acute viral hepatitis following a fatty meal.[389]

Uncommonly, severe diarrhea associated with abdominal cramping may predate the development of acute hepatitis A. This may be the result of two separate illnesses—gastroenteritis and hepatitis A—acquired simultaneously from the same source; at least two such outbreaks have been reported following the ingestion of contaminated raw clams.[271d, 390] There is little evidence to support a direct effect of HAV on the intestinal mucosa. In a study using highly sophisticated procedures, the virus could not be demonstrated in the gastrointestinal tract of marmosets or chimpanzees infected with this agent through the intravenous route.[391, 392]

The availability of sensitive serologic tests has provided the opportunity to track the path of HBV through the gastrointestinal tract. Beginning in the mouth, HBsAg has been found in gingival crevicular fluid,[392a] as well as in nasopharyngeal secretions and saliva.[392b–392f] Salivary HBsAg is potentially an important source for viral transmission,[392g, 392h] as was recognized in early human volunteer studies.[392i] HBsAg has been sought but not found in gastric juice and duodenal aspirates,[392j, 392k, 392l] but it has been identified in bile and pancreatic juice.[392k, 392l, 392m] Early reports of the detection of HBsAg in stool conflicted with the observations in the mid-1940s that feces was not a source of transmission of hepatitis B.[392d, 392n–392r] Additional studies failed to confirm these earlier findings.[392e, 392s–392u] These suggest that intestinal contents, such as carboxypeptidase A, might denature HBsAg.[392l, 392v, 392w, 393, 394]

Pancreatic Involvement

It has been known for more than 40 years that viral hepatitis and acute pancreatitis can coexist.[395–401] Most instances of overt pancreatitis have occurred in association with fulminant hepatitis, and hence the most reliable figures come from autopsy examinations. Necropsy studies have defined pancreatic involvement in 12 to 40 per cent of patients with fatal hepatitis, with pathologic changes ranging from slight pancreatic edema to severe hemorrhagic pancreatitis. It has been suggested that the pancreatic necrosis may be triggered by disseminated intravascular coagulation.[402]

The frequency of pancreatic involvement in uncomplicated viral hepatitis is uncertain. In one study, elevated amylase levels in serum and urine were found in 30 per cent of nonfatal cases of viral hepatitis.[399] However, isoenzyme studies to distinguish pancreatic from hepatic amylase have yielded conflicting results.[403] Nevertheless, the demonstration of pancreatic isoenzymes in the blood of some patients,[397] the report of radiographic evidence of pancreatitis,[397] and the pathologic changes already cited all suggest that pancreatitis does complicate viral hepatitis, albeit with uncertain frequency.

Of note is the accumulating evidence that the pancreas might represent an important nonhepatic site of HBV replication. In one compelling report, HBsAg could be demonstrated by immunofluorescent techniques in the pancreas of 18 of 30 HBsAg-infected persons, and HBcAg was detected in six of these individuals.[403a]

A disturbance in pancreatic endocrine function in patients with hepatitis has also been reported. One group of investigators observed abnormal glucose tolerance in 50 per cent of patients with viral hepatitis.[404] In another report involving viral hepatitis, 4 of 100 patients seen by a single physician developed frank, although ultimately reversible, diabetes mellitus.[405] The diabetes was attributed to direct invasion of the pancreas by the hepatitis virus. However, it is possible that hyperglycemia might have developed for other reasons, such as widespread severe malnutrition and enforced massive glucose intake.

Hematologic Manifestations

Viral hepatitis can be associated with two forms of hematologic alterations. The first, already described, is a normal, common manifestation of acute viral hepatitis, is usually slight, and almost always reverts to normal as the hepatic disease abates. The other develops as a rare, usually severe, unexpected complication that frequently causes death.

Aplastic anemia in association with viral hepatitis was first reported in 1955 by Lorenz and Quaiser.[406] Since then more than 200 additional cases have been described as a complication of most, if not all, the different hepatitis types.[406–411b] A comprehensive picture of this entity has emerged from a careful review of the literature by Hagler and co-workers.[407] Pancytopenia develops more frequently in males than in females. The average age at onset is approximately 20 years. Occasionally, only some of the blood elements are affected.[410] The hematologic abnormalities are usually present within a year of the hepatic disease, but in a few instances they have developed later. The average interval between the onset of hepatitis and the onset of the pancytopenia is 9.3 weeks. The associated hepatic disease usually is mild to moderate, and the patient frequently is in the recovery phase when the aplasia develops. Liver biopsies, when done, have shown the features of subsiding hepatitis. Bone marrow examination shows hypoplasia or aplasia. Treatment with adrenal corticosteroids alone or with androgenic agents, splenectomy, and bone marrow transplantation has not been particularly successful. The latter modality, however, appears to be promising in selected cases.[409] Only 15 per cent of patients survive the illness, with death occurring an average of 20 weeks after the onset of hepatitis and 11 weeks after the onset of pancytopenia. The survival rate has been lower in females than in males. Many theories have been offered for the pathogenesis of this complication, but none has received universal acceptance. The one with the widest appeal is that the virus directly invades the marrow, causing chromosomal changes that interfere with cell replication and viability.

An extremely uncommon complication is isolated *agranulocytosis*.[412, 413] Fewer than ten patients with this complication have been reported. In such cases, total leukocyte counts may be normal, but neutrophilic cells usually amount to less than 5 per cent. Bone marrow examination shows hypercellularity and granulocytic hyperplasia, with maturation arrest at the myelocyte stage. In some of the reported cases, an associated hypogammaglob-ulinemia has been found, which may enhance the suscep-tibility of the patient to the adverse effects of the hepatitis virus. Death from this complication has been reported.

Severe *hemolytic anemia*, accompanied by reticulocy-tosis and leukocytosis, occasionally may complicate the course of acute viral hepatitis.[175–178, 344, 414–416] The hematocrit and hemoglobin values of these patients decline dramati-cally in association with marked elevations in serum bili-rubin that are inconsistent with the apparent severity of the liver disease. The cause of hemolysis is undefined in most cases, but in some, glucose-6-phosphate dehydrogenase deficiency has been implicated.[175–178, 344, 415, 416] The postulated mechanism of hemolysis in glucose-6-phosphate dehydro-genase deficiency in patients with hepatitis is that impaired liver function permits the accumulation of metabolites that oxidize red blood cell sulfhydryl groups. These agents cause oxidative destruction of glucose-6-phosphate dehydrogen-ase-deficient erythrocytes, but not of normal erythro-cytes.[175, 176] It must be remembered that a diagnosis of glucose-6-phosphate dehydrogenase deficiency is difficult to confirm during the hemolytic crisis, because the older red blood cells are destroyed selectively during hemolysis. The younger cells that remain have normal glucose-6-phosphate dehydrogenase activity. Tests to establish the enzymatic deficiency should be carried out after recovery from the hemolytic crisis.

Marked hyperbilirubinemia occurs in patients with *sickle cell anemia* in whom viral hepatitis develops.[178] Values of bilirubin between 43 mg/dl and 103 mg/dl have been reported. The very high values are presumably the result of the additive effects of enhanced hemolysis resulting from the infectious process and the inability of the damaged liver to excrete the increased pigment load. Also of interest is the fact that persons with nonlymphocytic leukemia who develop acute viral hepatitis appear to undergo transient improvement of their leukemic state.[413a, 413b]

Depression of coagulation factors synthesized by the liver with the development of *disseminated intravascular coagulation* is a common finding in fulminant hepatitis.[402, 417, 418] This is discussed in Chapter 17.

Profoundly important is the discovery in recent years that, like the pancreas, white blood cells appear to be another nonhepatic site of hepatitis B viral replication. Using molecular biologic techniques, HBV DNA sequences have been found in peripheral blood mononuclear cells or leukocytes of persons with acquired immunodeficiency syn-drome and in the bone marrow of children with leuke-mia.[418a–418f]

Neurologic Manifestations

Neurologic manifestations, which are intrinsic to ful-minant hepatitis, may take many forms. However, in the uncomplicated case of acute viral hepatitis, neurologic alterations are relatively uncommon.[419] There have been isolated reports of aseptic meningitis,[420, 421] encephalitis,[422, 423, 423a] myelitis,[421–424] seizures,[421, 425–427] and status epilepticus during the course of viral hepatitis.[428]

The development of encephalomyeloradiculitis (Guil-lain-Barré syndrome) has also been noted as a complication of hepatitis.[429, 430] As has been meticulously detailed recently by Tabor,[430a] seven cases have been attributed to hepatitis A and eight cases to hepatitis B.[430b–432] All patients recovered

with little deficit. A study of cerebrospinal fluid in some of the patients has revealed the presence of HBsAg and, in at least one instance, HBsAg–anti-HBs immune com-plexes.[430j, 430m]

A somewhat more frequent neurologic manifestation is polyneuritis,[433, 440a] usually manifesting as peripheral neu-ropathy but also found affecting cranial nerves. Even among patients with viral hepatitis who do not have overt neuro-logic symptoms, impairment of nerve conduction velocities can be demonstrated, abating as the disease subsides.[435, 436] Possible pathogenetic mechanisms are viral damage of nerve cell bodies directly, as occurs in poliomyelitis, or induction by the virus of an abnormal immune response detrimental to neural tissue. Support for the latter sugges-tion comes from a study of a patient with chronic active hepatitis and peripheral neuropathy, in whom there were serum cryoprotein complexes composed of IgM, IgG, HBsAg, and Dane particles.[437]

In regard to cranial nerve involvement, there is a report of trigeminal sensory neuropathy occurring in a 26-year-old man in whom viral hepatitis developed.[438] Also, in view of the frequent loss of appetite and alteration in food preferences, it is not surprising that impairment of gustatory and olfactory acuity can be demonstrated by objective measurements.[439, 440] Both show measurable improvement as the illness subsides. A suggested mechanism for the disturbed olfaction derives from the finding that retinal binding protein, the specific transport protein for vitamin A (see Chap. 8), is decreased during acute viral hepatitis.[440] Vitamin A is believed to be important for olfaction.[440]

Mononeuritis multiplex, an asymmetric sensorimotor neuropathy, is commonly found in patients with HBsAg-positive periarteritis nodosa and is a consequence of nec-rotizing vasculitis of the vasa vasorum.[440b–440d] It is not clear whether immune complexes are responsible for this disor-der.

Some patients who have acute viral hepatitis have psychologic disturbances.[441] On occasion, symptoms of poor concentration, fatigability, right upper quadrant tenderness, and exaggerated concern regarding the presence of liver disease may persist for many months after all evidence of acute hepatitis disappears. This so-called posthepatitis syn-drome occurs more commonly in soldiers than in civilians and in medical than in nonmedical personnel.[442, 443]

Genital Tract Manifestations

Studies of the uterine cervices of female patients with viral hepatitis show a high incidence of cytologic abnor-malities.[444, 445] In one study, a third of women with the disease had abnormal cytologic findings, and half of them had the changes of carcinoma in situ.[444] In another study, 8.5 per cent of 93 women admitted to a hospital with hepatitis had cytologic abnormalities (of these, 12.5 per cent had invasive cancer).[445] This figure can be compared with the prevalence rate of cytologic abnormalities of 2.15 per cent among female patients admitted to that hospital for diseases other than hepatitis. From this it was concluded that women with hepatitis represent a high-risk group for the development of cytologic changes consistent with neo-plasia of the cervical epithelium. The authors did not indicate what effect resolution of the hepatic disease had on the abnormal cytologic findings, but they nevertheless urged that a Papanicolaou smear be included during the physical examination of every female patient with hepatitis.

NONHEPATIC DISORDERS IN VIRAL HEPATITIS BELIEVED TO BE MEDIATED BY CIRCULATING IMMUNE COMPLEXES

Serum Sickness–like Syndrome

Acute viral hepatitis is sometimes heralded by a serum sickness–like complex consisting of fever, arthralgia, arthritis, rash, angioneurotic edema, and occasionally, hematuria and proteinuria.[446–456] Sir Robert Graves is credited with having recognized, in 1843, that arthralgias and arthritis may develop during the prodromal phase of hepatitis.[455] The first detailed investigation and report of the arthritis of hepatitis in the United States came from Alpert and colleagues in 1971.[446] More than 100 cases of rheumatologic abnormalities in viral hepatitis have been reported. A number of them have come from the United States.[452]

Joint manifestations are common in patients with viral hepatitis, with reported incidences as high as 50 per cent. Most investigators identify these manifestations in 5 to 25 per cent of patients. The frequency of arthritic complaints depends on the manner in which the information is obtained. Unless it is specifically sought, the patient may not relate the occurrence of joint symptoms. They sometimes disappear as early as two to three weeks before the onset of hepatitis-related symptoms, and arthritis may occur in association with anicteric hepatitis.[451]

Arthralgias occur with the same frequency in both sexes; arthritis is more common in females. The ages affected are spread widely. Hepatitis with joint problems has been reported to appear as late as the eighth decade of life and as early as adolescence. However, it is a rare event in preadolescence, perhaps because of the relative infrequency of hepatitis B in younger people. Early reports suggested that joint symptoms occurred in both hepatitis A and hepatitis B.[447, 448] It now appears that they are a manifestation of hepatitis B almost exclusively, and perhaps of non-A, non-B hepatitis. There have been instances in which hepatitis B preceded by severe arthritis has developed in several individuals after exposure to the same source. This has led to the view that a specific arthritogenic strain of HBV may exist.[453]

The average duration of joint symptoms is estimated to be approximately 20 days. Symptoms usually disappear with the onset of jaundice. Sometimes, however, they persist into the beginning of overt hepatitis, and occasionally they remain after the hepatic disease subsides. Ultimately, the symptoms disappear, leaving no residual deformity. Joint involvement may be localized or generalized. It is usually symmetric, with swelling, tenderness, and inflammation. The areas most frequently involved, in approximate decreasing order of frequency, are the proximal interphalangeal joints, knees, ankles, shoulders, wrists, small joints of the feet, elbows, cervical spine, hips, and lumbar spine. Rarely, subcutaneous nodules are present on extensor surfaces.[447, 450] Morning stiffness is common. The presence of HBsAg in synovial membranes has been reported.[454] Synovial fluid, originally described as a noninflammatory exudate (leukocyte count < 5000/mm³, predominantly mononuclear cells), frequently shows evidence of inflammation, similar to the synovial fluid changes in rheumatoid arthritis.[449, 453] The fluid is usually HBsAg-positive (occasionally even before the appearance of HBsAg in serum) and is low in total CH50.[449]

Serial studies of patients with arthritis and viral hepatitis strongly support the involvement of circulating immune complexes in the pathogenesis of the arthritis. The complexes activate the classic and alternative complement pathways.[203, 456] During the period of acute joint symptoms, HBsAg titers in the blood and joint fluid are high, and serum and joint fluid complement levels are low. Cryoprotein–immune complexes have been identified in the majority of patients with hepatitis with or without arthritis. However, C3, C4, C5, IgA, and specific IgG complement-fixing subtypes (IgG 1; IgG 3) can be detected in the complexes of those with arthritis only. The cryoprotein complexes in patients with arthritis contain anti-HBs, which is often present in higher concentrations in joint fluid than in plasma. Occasionally anti-HBs is found in joint fluid before it appears in serum. Finally, C3 activator fragments of the properdin complex, which activate the alternative pathway, have been demonstrated in serum of persons with arthritis but not in those without arthritis. After the disappearance of joint symptoms, complement levels normalize, and HBsAg titers in serum begin to decline. The differential diagnosis includes rheumatoid arthritis and gonococcal arthritis. A comparison of rheumatoid arthritis with HBV-related arthritis is shown in Table 37–8.

Skin rashes commonly accompany the joint manifestations.[457–461] They may be urticarial,[459, 459a] macular, maculopapular,[449] erythematous, purpural,[454, 461] petechial, nodular,[450] or scarlatiniform,[457] or circinate and annular erythematous plaques may appear. Sometimes, the rash may be present without joint manifestations. In either case, it usually disappears with the onset of jaundice. The designation of the rash as an immune complex phenomenon is based on the finding in serum of complement changes similar to those described for arthritis, the identification of necrotizing vasculitis and venulitis on light-microscopic examination of the skin, and the identification by immunofluorescence of fibrin, C3, IgM, and HBsAg in cutaneous vessel walls.[459]

The joint and skin changes ultimately disappear as hepatic disease subsides. Less commonly, a severe multisystem disease may develop, with various combinations of fever and renal, heart, gastrointestinal tract, and nervous system disease, in addition to the arthritis and dermatitis.[462]

TABLE 37–8. COMPARISON BETWEEN RHEUMATOID AND HBsAg-POSITIVE ARTHRITIDES*

	Rheumatoid Arthritis	HBsAg-positive Arthritis
Symmetric, polyarticular arthritis	+	+
Morning stiffness	+	+
Nonmigratory arthritis	+	+
Sharply localized tenderness	−	+
Red, warm overlying skin	+	−
Synovial thickening	+	−
Rash	−	+
Fever, anemia, ↑ ESR	+	−
Serum HBsAg	−	+
Rheumatoid factor	+	−
Total serum hemolytic complement activity	± ↓	+ + ↓ ↓
Joint fluid leukocyte count	> 5000 cells/mm³	< 5000 cells/mm³
Joint fluid differential	Predominantly polymorphonuclear	Predominantly mononuclear
Joint deformity and destruction	+	−

Source: Adapted from McCarty DS, Ormiste V. Arch Intern Med 132:264, copyright 1973, American Medical Association.

The course of this form of the disease is prolonged, and it may terminate in death. Presumably, multisystem involvement stems from a widespread vasculitis.

Polyarteritis Nodosa

The presence of arteritis in persons dying of serum sickness was first observed in 1937 by Clarke and Kaplan.[463] Ten years later, Paull suggested a relationship between viral hepatitis and polyarteritis nodosa when he reported that three of four Army officers who developed vasculitis following yellow fever vaccination had had evidence of viral hepatitis prior to death.[464] The link to HBsAg came in 1970 when Trepo and associates in France and Gocke and associates in the United States independently described the presence of HBsAg in serum or in the vascular lesions of patients with biopsy proven polyarteritis nodosa. This association has been found in more than 50 patients.[97, 465–474] Furthermore, recent studies show that 36 to 69 per cent of patients with established polyarteritis nodosa are HBsAg-positive.[474]

Persons of all ages and of both sexes may be affected. The manifestations of vasculitis usually precede the development of acute hepatitis B, but occasionally they follow it. An acute Raynaud's disease–like syndrome with digital vasospasm and infarction has been reported.[471] Necrotizing vasculitis may be found in persons with chronic HBV infection and in drug abusers, particularly those who abuse methamphetamines.[469] Whether the vasculitis in the latter group is due to a direct toxic effect of methamphetamines or to other unidentified chemical agents, or whether it is related to associated HBV infection, is not yet established. In all instances, persistence of the vascular disease and of HBsAg parallel one another.

Symptoms include arthralgias, mononeuritis, fever, abdominal pain, renal disease, hypertension, central nervous system abnormalities, and rashes. HBsAg-positive and negative patients with polyarteritis nodosa have similar frequencies of each of these manifestations, but there are slightly higher frequencies of renal disease, rash, and central nervous system abnormalities in those who are HBsAg-negative.[473] Also, episcleritis seems to be confined to patients with polyarteritis nodosa who are HBsAg-negative. As might be expected, the frequency and extent of the abnormalities disclosed by biochemical tests of liver function are greater in those who are HBsAg-positive. There is, however, no apparent relationship between the severity of the vascular complications and the severity of the hepatic disease. Accordingly, it is apparent that all persons in whom multisystem disease suggestive of polyarteritis nodosa develops, even when overt evidence of hepatic disease is not present should be tested for HBsAg.

Diagnosis requires first that the entity be considered when a patient seeks treatment for seemingly unrelated manifestations involving numerous organs. On tissue biopsy specimens, small arteries show fibrinoid necrosis and perivascular infiltration containing mononuclear and polymorphonuclear leukocytes. Acute lesions are found mainly in small arteries, and older lesions, consisting of focal or diffuse fibrous replacement of the media and obliteration of the lumen, predominate in medium-sized and larger arteries. Sometimes, confirmation by tissue biopsy may be difficult because of the patchy nature of the disease. Angiography is a potentially useful diagnostic tool.[475] The most common findings are microaneurysms, stenosis, and occlusion of vessels in multiple organs, particularly in the kidneys and liver.

The pathogenesis is unclear. Certainly, HBsAg is present in the serum throughout the course of the disease. Furthermore, HBsAg, immunoglobulins (IgG and IgM), and complement have been demonstrated by immunofluorescence in recent exudative hyaline and fibrinoid lesions in the walls of the blood vessels. However, there have been varying results concerning the presence of immune complexes in the serum. Some investigators have found immune complexes,[465, 470, 472, 474] and others have not.[468, 469] During the acute phase of the disease, HBsAg is present and CH50 and C3 titers are low. As the disease subsides, HBsAg may disappear and anti-HBs may appear. The course of the disease is variable, but there is a mortality rate of about 40 per cent within three years, a rate no different from that found for HBsAg-negative polyarteritis nodosa.

Glomerulonephritis

In contrast to the other nonhepatic disorders, renal disease in association with viral hepatitis was recognized long before the discovery of HBsAg.[130, 476] Renal disease may manifest itself at the same time as acute viral hepatitis, overt disease of the two organ systems may not occur simultaneously, or renal disease may develop in patients with inapparent or no liver disease.[477–484] Combes and associates, in 1971, were the first to demonstrate the presence of HBV complexes in the kidney of a person with glomerulonephritis.[477] The patient, with known chronic hepatitis as a sequel to acute post-transfusion hepatitis B, developed severe proteinuria, hypoalbuminemia, and peripheral edema. Renal biopsy specimens revealed membranous glomerulonephritis. Immunofluorescence showed deposits throughout glomerular capillary loops containing IgG, C3, and HBsAg. The liver biopsy specimen also contained HBsAg, demonstrated by immunofluorescence, and the serum was HBsAg-positive. Circulating immune complexes could not be detected. Although this was the first human case in which viral immune complexes appeared responsible for renal disease, viral immune complexes had already been established as a cause for renal disease in animals, for example, Aleutian disease of minks and lymphocytic choriomeningitis in mice.[485, 486]

There have now been almost 50 reports of HBV-related renal disease. In the majority, the renal lesions are membranous and membranoproliferative glomerulonephritis, but there are rare instances of epimembranous glomerulonephritis and focal glomerulosclerosis. More than half of the reported patients have had no apparent accompanying liver disease. In most cases, immunofluorescence has shown IgG, IgM, C3, and HBsAg in granular deposits along the glomerular basement membrane and within the mesangium. Cryoprecipitates containing HBsAg, anti-HBs, IgG, IgM, C3, and occasionally C4 have also been detected, suggesting their involvement in the pathogenesis of renal disease. With rare exceptions, glomerulonephritis has been reported to occur only in patients with HBV infection. However, Ecknoyan and co-workers observed renal morphologic changes in seven patients with acute viral hepatitis, only four of whom had HBsAg-positive sera.[479] Either the serologic test used in this study (counterelectrophoresis) was too insensitive to identify HBsAg in all seven patients, or other viruses, most likely those associated with non-A, non-B hepatitis, are also capable of inducing immune complex–related renal disease.

The frequency with which immune complex–mediated glomerulonephritis is initiated with HBV infection is not fully established. In one study from Japan, 163 children subjected to renal biopsy because of proteinuria and hematuria were tested for HBsAg, and 18 (11 per cent) were found to be positive.[482] This included all 11 children whose renal biopsy specimens showed membranous nephropathy and 7 of the 152 children with other renal lesions. The ages of these children ranged from 4 to 15 years. Other studies of large numbers of persons with glomerulonephritis report a frequency of 31 per cent and 16.8 per cent, respectively.[486a, 486b] Even more startling figures were reported from Poland. Of 52 unselected kidney biopsy specimens from children with the clinical diagnosis of nephrosis or glomerulonephritis, or both, 32 had features of an immune complex–related disease (variable amounts of IgG, IgM, IgA, and β1C).[484] Of these 32 children, 18 (56.2 per cent) had immune deposits of HBsAg–anti-HBs complexes present in renal glomeruli, including almost all those with the features of membranous or membranoproliferative glomerulonephritis. All 18 of these children had either HBsAg or anti-HBc in their sera. The circumstances of HBV exposure for most of the children of this study could not be determined. In the study from Japan, it was suggested that transmission had occurred from mother to child at the time of birth. The mothers of 6 of the 11 children with HBsAg-associated membranous glomerulonephritis had HBsAg-positive sera; an additional serum sample was positive for anti-HBs.

The widely held view is that the immune complexes responsible for causing renal disease contain HBsAg–anti-HBs. However, an interesting alternative explanation has been offered by Takekoshi and colleagues.[483] They indicate that only complexes with molecular weights of one million daltons or less are precipitated into the glomerular basement membrane to induce glomerulonephritis. Since HBsAg has a molecular weight of three million daltons, whereas that of HBeAg, even when associated with IgG, is no greater than 300,000 daltons, they suggest that the implicated immune complexes consist of HBeAg–anti-HBe. Support for this view comes from a more recent report from Japan.[486c]

It is apparent from these data that HBV is responsible for a major portion of the definable immune complex–related renal diseases in children. Immunoprophylaxis against hepatitis may afford the unique opportunity of preventing a considerable proportion of the glomerulonephritides of childhood.

A report of some interest documents recovery from HBsAg-associated glomerulonephritis following spontaneous clearance of HBsAg.[486d] Unfortunately, permanent loss of HBsAg is a rare phenomenon; it remains to be determined whether clearance of HBsAg induced by antiviral agents might represent a useful form of treatment for this condition.

Mixed Cryoglobulinemia

It has been suggested recently that mixed cryoglobulinemia may be initiated by HBV infection.[487, 488] The diagnosis of this condition has required the finding of mixed (IgM-IgG) cryoprotein not obviously associated with infection or with collagen-vascular or lymphoproliferative diseases. The disease presents as the clinical triad of weakness, purpura, and arthralgias. A systemic vasculitis, involving the kidneys in particular, causes most of the deaths. This entity can be distinguished from polyarteritis nodosa by the lack of eosinophilia, by the paucity of neurologic and abdominal symptoms, and by the involvement of small vessels only. Also, aneurysmal formations are not found in patients with mixed cryoglobulinemia.

The precipitating cause of this entity has been elusive, and hence the term *essential mixed cryoglobulinemia* has been applied. However, in a recent study, Levo and associates found HBsAg or anti-HBs, or both in the sera of more than half of patients with mixed cryoglobulinemia. Three fourths had cryoprecipitates in their sera.[488] The prevalence of anti-HBs exceeded that of HBsAg in sera and cryoprecipitates. Electron microscopic studies of four cryoprecipitates revealed HBV-like particles. Clinical and biochemical evaluations demonstrated overt liver disease in only a few instances (<15 per cent), although the majority of patients had hepatomegaly or abnormal results of biochemical tests of liver functions.[487] Liver biopsy results from some of the patients demonstrated a spectrum of histologic changes from slight, nonspecific inflammation to chronic active hepatitis with cirrhosis. However, liver disease was clinically negligible in most of the patients even after prolonged follow-up. Death from hepatic failure was a rare event.

The association between HBV infection and mixed cryoglobulinemia has, however, been questioned.[489] Investigators at the Massachusetts General Hospital were unable to detect HBsAg in sera or cryoprecipitates from any of 12 patients with essential mixed cryoprecipitates. Markers for HBV were detectable in sera of almost a fourth of patients with secondary cryoglobulinemia. Furthermore, there was little definable liver disease in the former group of patients, leading to the conclusion that in most instances essential cryoglobulinemia remains a disease of unknown cause.

Mixed cryoglobulins have been sought in various forms of liver disease and have been found commonly even without the presence of the clinical syndrome of mixed cryoglobulinemia.[490] The liver diseases involved include acute and chronic HBsAg-positive hepatitis, as well as the HBsAg carrier state, with the highest quantities of cryoprecipitates found in acute hepatitis. When mixed cryoglobulins are detected in patients who are HBsAg-positive, they have the biologic properties of immune complexes and are associated with acute or chronic serum sickness. Cryoprecipitates have also been found in HBsAg-negative patients with liver disease, but in these circumstances they do not contain HBsAg or anti-HBs and do not have the biologic properties of immune complexes.[490]

Papular Acrodermatitis of Childhood (Gianotti's Disease)

This skin disease of childhood is viewed generally as an immune complex–related disorder, but this has not been proved. First recognized in 1955 by Gianotti,[491] and known to be associated with HBsAg since 1970, it is characterized by skin eruptions, lymphadenopathy and lymphadenitis, and mild, usually anicteric, acute viral hepatitis. It primarily affects young children.[491–496] The children affected range in age from several months to 10 years. In an epidemic of the disease in Matsuyama City, Japan, 153 cases occurred in a period of two and a half years, and 91.7 per cent of the patients were younger than 4 years of age.[492, 494] In that series, boys and girls were approximately equally affected. Also of note is that 14 adults developed acute hepatitis with jaundice 3 to 14 months after their offspring had been found to have acrodermatitis.[494]

The disease begins with the onset of skin eruptions, which are usually flat, erythematopapular, and do not itch. They appear symmetrically on the face, buttocks and limbs, usually, but not always, sparing the trunk, and not involving the mucous membranes. Infants tend to have large (5 to 10 mm) papules, whereas older children develop smaller (1 to 2 mm) papules. The eruption takes several days to evolve and lasts approximately 15 to 20 days. Lymph node enlargement, involving mainly the inguinal and axillary areas, may last two to three months. Early in the course of the disease, it is possible to detect HBsAg and HBeAg in the serum. Ultimately, anti-HBs and anti-HBe are found in those children who are HBsAg-negative. An early view was that the HBsAg in this disease is virtually always of the *ayw* subtype (see Chap. 35). It appears now, however, that no single subtype is responsible for the skin disorder.[496a, 496b]

The sera of approximately two thirds to three fourths of the affected children ultimately became HBsAg-negative. The chance that this would occur increased with the age at onset of disease. In contrast, more than 40 per cent of infants who acquired the disease when they were less than a year old had HBsAg-positive sera a year later.[494]

Evidence of acute hepatitis may coincide with the onset of the skin eruption or, more commonly, will begin as the dermatitis starts to wane. Aminotransferase levels are often high (1000 to 2000 IU/L). Serum bilirubin levels are almost always normal in affected children, but the occasional adult who acquires the disease from a child is likely to have jaundice. In the few instances in which a liver biopsy has been performed in those with persisting HBsAg, chronic active hepatitis has been found.[493]

The pathogenesis of the skin disease is unclear at present. Immunocytochemical studies fail to identify HBsAg or HBcAg in skin biopsy samples. Furthermore, the clinical features of an immune complex–related vasculitis have not been identified. Gianotti has postulated that papular acrodermatitis of childhood is the clinical manifestation of primary natural infection with HBV that is acquired via mucous membranes or the skin.[495]

Polymyalgia Rheumatica

Polymyalgia rheumatica, a disease of unknown cause related to giant-cell arteritis, is characterized by generalized aching, particularly of the shoulder girdle, severe morning stiffness, and an elevated ESR without features of rheumatoid arthritis, neoplasia, or intercurrent disease. Because it is thought to be an immunologic disorder, perhaps triggered by a viral infection, several studies have been undertaken to determine whether HBV infection might be implicated. Bacon and associates studied 13 consecutive patients with the disorder to determine whether any of a large number of viral organisms they measured could be responsible for initiating the illness.[497] Their only positive finding was the presence of anti-HBs in 75 per cent of untreated cases; HBsAg was not found. Although they were unable to demonstrate circulating immune complexes, they suggested, in light of the remarkably high prevalence of anti-HBs, that this viral antibody could be an important component of a presumptive complex and urged further studies in this direction. In another study, HBsAg was demonstrated in the serum and temporal artery of a patient with polymyalgia rheumatica. Two recent studies have failed to demonstrate this association.[498–500] In one of these studies, HBV markers were not found significantly more frequently in 36 patients with polymyalgia rheumatica

alone, in 8 patients with giant cell arteritis and polymyalgia, and in 14 patients with giant cell arteritis alone than in 100 selected controls.[500]

VIRAL HEPATITIS OCCURRING IN SPECIFIC CIRCUMSTANCES

VIRAL HEPATITIS AND PREGNANCY

Two considerations of obvious concern when viral hepatitis occurs in pregnancy are (1) does viral hepatitis have an unusual effect on the pregnant woman? and (2) does viral hepatitis have an adverse effect on the fetus or newborn baby? (See also Chap. 54.)

Early reports from the Middle East,[501–504] India,[271j, 505–508a] and Africa,[344, 509–509b] described viral hepatitis in pregnancy, particularly in the third trimester, as manifesting with unusual severity, often progressing to fulminant hepatitis. However, in other studies, mostly from Western countries,[510–515] hepatitis was not found to be unusually severe in pregnant women. It has been inferred, therefore, that the factors responsible for a poor prognosis are a suboptimal nutritional status of the pregnant mother, and perhaps, inadequate prenatal care. Further support comes from a recent study from Israel showing a similar severity of hepatitis in pregnant and nonpregnant women during 1967 to 1977, a period of rising socioeconomic status in that country,[515a] in contrast to the higher mortality rate found in pregnant women in earlier studies when socioeconomic conditions were poor.[501, 515b] Thus, viral hepatitis appears to be no more dangerous to the well-nourished pregnant woman than it is to the nonpregnant woman.

The effects on the fetus of hepatitis in the mother are reported to include increased frequencies of abortion, stillbirth, prematurity, and congenital anomalies.[501, 505, 506, 516–518, 522–524b] Other reports have not confirmed all of these complications,[512, 514, 519, 520] but Hieber and co-workers recently reaffirmed the increased incidence of premature deliveries in pregnant women with viral hepatitis.[515] A particular concern is that viral hepatitis in pregnancy might cause intrauterine death or congenital malformations. Siegel and associates found increased fetal mortality when viral hepatitis developed in the third trimester.[517] However, subsequent studies suggest that there is no relationship between viral hepatitis in pregnancy and congenital malformations of the fetus.[521, 525–531]

The most obvious risk to the neonate of a mother with viral hepatitis is the possible transmission of disease. In 1951, Stokes and colleagues suggested that mothers who were hepatitis carriers could transmit the disease to their newborn infants at birth.[532] These investigators were able to produce viral hepatitis in volunteers by inoculating them with sera obtained both from a two-month-old baby with hepatitis and from its asymptomatic mother. Almost 20 years later, Gillespie and co-workers reported for the first time the detection of HBsAg in a mother as well as in her infant in whom hepatitis had developed.[533] This finding was confirmed by numerous subsequent surveys, and studies were soon undertaken to determine the factors responsible for HBV transmission in these circumstances. Other early data that suggested the likelihood of vertical transmission of HBV were the reports of familial HBV-related chronic liver disease and hepatocellular carcinoma clustering around an HBsAg-positive mother.[534–536] Indeed, in one such study, a remarkably high proportion of mothers of patients with hepatocellular carcinoma were found to be

HBsAg-positive, in contradistinction to an HBsAg frequency among the fathers that was no different from that of the general population.[537]

Factors that appear to determine the frequency of vertical transmission include the manifestation of the disease in the pregnant woman (acute versus chronic), the period in the pregnancy during which the acute illness develops, the mother's infectivity (as measured by the presence or lack of HBeAg), and her racial and geographic origins. Acute hepatitis during pregnancy is clearly associated with transmission of disease to the infant. Schweitzer and associates reported in 1972 that HBsAg developed in 10 of 26 babies born to 26 mothers who had acute hepatitis B during pregnancy.[538] The frequency of transmission appeared to be related to the timing of the acute illness in the mother: HBsAg was present in 33 per cent of babies born to mothers in whom acute hepatitis developed between conception and the eighth month of gestation. It was found in 47 per cent of babies of mothers in whom the disease occurred between the sixth month of gestation and the second postpartum month. None of the babies whose mothers developed hepatitis during the second to sixth months postpartum tested HBsAg-positive. In a separate study, HBsAg was not found in any of 6 infants whose mothers became ill during the first trimester of pregnancy, but it was present in 1 of the 4 infants whose mothers' disease developed in the second trimester, in 7 of 11 infants whose mothers experienced onset of disease in the third trimester, and in 5 of 6 infants whose mothers contracted acute hepatitis during the first two postpartum months.[539] Data from yet another study from California showed remarkably similar results; no transmission resulted if the hepatitis occurred in the first trimester, but it rose progressively to 6 per cent when acute hepatitis developed in the second trimester, to 67 per cent if it occurred in the third trimester, and to 100 per cent if the disease began shortly after delivery.[540] The outcome is different when the mother is a hepatitis carrier. Evidence of HBV infection was present in only 1 of 21 babies born to asymptomatic carrier mothers, but in 13 of 27 infants whose mothers had had acute hepatitis.[539] Gerety and Schweitzer found that HBV infection developed in 67 per cent of infants born to mothers with acute hepatitis, compared with 36 per cent whose mothers were asymptomatic carriers.[540a]

Other studies, both in the United States and elsewhere,[541-543] have confirmed the high transmission rate when acute hepatitis occurs in pregnancy, particularly during the last trimester. However, the rates of transmission by asymptomatic carrier pregnant mothers to their infants have varied considerably,[544-560a] as shown in Table 37-8. With few exceptions, the rates of transmission from carrier mothers are low in the United States and in most of western Europe, but they are considerably higher in Asian countries. In the one United States study showing a high transmission rate,[540] a large proportion of mothers were found to have HBeAg-positive sera, a factor known to carry a high risk. The explanation offered by Dupuy and co-workers for the unexpectedly high rates found in France is that the frequent blood sampling in their study simply increased the opportunity for finding a transiently positive result.[552]

The strikingly higher frequency of transmission that occurs in carrier mothers who are Asian may result, in part, from the high carrier rate of the general population in that area of the world. However, there may also be differences in racial susceptibilities, best exemplified by the data of Derso and colleagues and Woo and associates.[551, 551a] In a survey to detect asymptomatic pregnant carriers in West Midlands, England, a firm relationship was found between the frequency of HBV transmission and the ethnic origin of the mother. Thus, none of the babies born to 39 European mothers developed HBV infection, whereas the incidences were 8 per cent for Asian babies, 30 per cent for Afro-Caribbean babies, and 64 per cent for Chinese babies. HBV infection was found in 5 per cent of 92 non-Chinese and 44 per cent of Chinese babies born to carrier mothers in a second study.[551a] One explanation for the variability in rates of transmission relates to differences in inherited susceptibilities. Blumberg and co-workers expressed strong views,[561] later supported by Carbonara and colleagues,[561, 562] that the antigen was inherited as a simple mendelian recessive trait. Petrakis and Lederberg subsequently outlined the difficulties entailed in substantiating this theory.[563] A later report by Peters and associates of disparate responses of monozygotic twins to HBV infection seemed to refute this theory.[564]

Numerous investigators have attempted to define the degree of infectivity of the mother and to determine the route or routes by which the infection of the infant takes place. Stevens and associates, in a study conducted in Taiwan, found that the risk of neonatal antigenemia was increased when the mother's serum HBsAg titer was high, when HBeAg was present in the baby's cord blood, or when HBsAg positivity was present in the baby's older siblings.[555] Not all of these risk factors have been confirmed by others. One item about which there is general agreement is the extreme risk associated with the presence of HBeAg in the mother's blood at the time of delivery. More than 80 per cent of HBeAg-positive mothers transmit HBV to their offspring, whereas transmission occurs in fewer than a fourth of instances when the mother is anti-HBe–positive (Table 37–9). It was believed originally that the presence of anti-HBe in the mother denoted complete lack of infectivity and that anti-HBe–positive plasma might even be useful for immunoprophylaxis.[557] The first-mentioned view is not entirely correct, as demonstrated in Table 37–10 by the data of Derso and co-workers and Stevens and colleagues,[551, 560] and is indicated also by several reports demonstrating transmission of hepatitis B from HBsAg- and anti-HBe–positive mothers to their newborn infants.[540, 564-564c] Nevertheless, it is apparent that the presence of anti-HBe defines far lesser infectivity than does the presence of HBeAg.

An understanding of the route of HBV transmission is important for many reasons, but particularly for purposes of immunoprophylaxis. If transmission occurs in utero, immunoprophylaxis at birth probably would be of little benefit. To study this, samples of cord blood have been examined for the presence of HBsAg and for other HBV markers. Early studies, using only moderately sensitive tests, failed to detect HBsAg in cord blood,[546, 565-570] but in later studies, HBsAg was often found.[538-540a, 547, 549, 551, 553, 555, 556, 558, 559, 571, 572] Also, both anti-HBc and Dane particles have been identified in cord blood of babies born to carrier mothers,[547, 573, 574] sometimes without detectable HBsAg. These findings suggest transplacental transmission. However, it is probable that anti-HBc found in the infants' blood shortly after birth is simply a consequence of passive transfer, since it has been shown to lack IgM specificity and to disappear rapidly.[574a] Furthermore, circumstantial evidence indicates that infection probably occurs during the perinatal period; certainly, the birth process offers ample opportunity for transmission to occur. During delivery, the infant is in direct contact with the mother's blood, fre-

TABLE 37–9. PREVALENCE OF HBsAg IN PREGNANT WOMEN AND FREQUENCY OF TRANSMISSION OF HEPATITIS B VIRUS FROM ASYMPTOMATIC CARRIER MOTHERS TO INFANTS

Reference	Country	HBsAg-positive Mothers		HBsAg-positive Babies	
		% of Pregnancies	*No. Carriers*	*No.*	*%*
Skinhoj et al. (1972)[544]	Denmark	0.1	81	0/36	0
Schweitzer et al. (1973)[539]	United States	NR	21	1/21	4.8
Aziz et al. (1973)[546]	Pakistan	1.5	16	1/14	7.1
Papaevangelou et al. (1974)[547]	Greece	NR	12	1/15	6.7
Schweitzer (1975)[548]	United States	NR	36	6/36	16.7
Kew et al. (1975)[549]	S. Africa	0.16	7	1/7	14.3
Gerety and Schweitzer (1977)[540]	United States	NR	12	5/14	35.7
Waterson et al. (1977)[550]	England	0.5	36	2/36	5.6
Derso et al. (1978)[551]	England	0.1	122	17/122	13.9
Dupuy et al. (1978)[552]	France	0.6	17	8/12	67.0
Moroni et al. (1978)[553]	Italy	1.8	98	0/37	0
Mollica et al. (1979)[572]	Italy	2.8	18	4/18	22.2
Okada et al. (1975)[554]	Japan	2.3	139	8/11	72.7
Stevens et al. (1975)[555]	Taiwan	15.2	158	63/158	29.9
Anderson et al. (1975)[556]	Taiwan	7.5	41	27/43	62.8
Okada et al. (1976)[557]	Japan	NR	17	10/17	58.8
Shiraki et al. (1977)[558]	Japan	NR	23	10/19	52.6
Miyakawa and Mayumi (1978)[908]	Japan	NR	84	25/84	29.8
Lee et al. (1978)[559]	Hong Kong	6.6	125	26/37	70.2
Stevens et al. (1979)[560]	Taiwan	NR	65	48/65	73.8

NR = not reported.

quently suffers minor cuts and superficial abrasions, and often swallows blood or amniotic fluid. Indeed, amniotic fluid in carrier mothers can be HBsAg-positive.[549, 559] Lee and associates found that gastric aspirates from neonates born to HBsAg-positive mothers were HBsAg-positive.[559] Another suggested mode of oral transmission is through breast-feeding. Breast milk of infected mothers frequently is HBsAg-positive, usually in low titer.[575, 576] However, the data of Beasley and Stevens do not support this mechanism; they did not find a difference in outcomes between breast-fed and non–breast-fed babies of HBsAg-positive mothers.[577] Taking all of these findings into account, it is currently believed that transplacental transmission is probably extremely uncommon and that the likeliest period for HBV transmission is the time of delivery. This conclusion is supported by the poor correlation between the presence of HBsAg in cord blood and in amniotic fluid and the hepatitis outcome in the baby. Furthermore, hepatitis in the baby generally develops with an incubation period most consistent with infection occurring at delivery; antigenemia usually develops after an initial period of HBsAg negativity, and anti-HBc in cord blood usually disappears rapidly from the blood of the infant, suggesting passive transfer from the mother. Particularly compelling is the fact that combined passive-active immunoprophylaxis administered shortly after delivery prevents nearly 95 per cent of cases

of hepatitis B in the neonate, an outcome that could not be anticipated if transplacental transmission were the rule rather than the exception.[560a]

It should be noted that HBV infection in the very young is not always the consequence of perinatal transmission. The results of surveys of young children and their mothers in Ovambaland suggest that in this area, horizontal transmission is the more likely route of transfer.[577a]

The most frequent outcome of infection in the neonate is chronic antigenemia.[539, 540a, 544, 555, 556, 560, 560a] Sometimes this is associated with chronic liver disease,[552, 577b, 578, 579] and by inference, the development of hepatocellular carcinoma later in life. The high carrier rate that develops in neonates is believed to be the result of either the immunologic tolerance that exists in the immature infant or genetic susceptibility.[561, 562, 578] Although genetic susceptibility had been considered likely because of the different rates of transmission by asymptomatic carrier Oriental and white mothers, this theory became less attractive when it was found that Oriental and white babies are equally susceptible if their mothers contract acute viral hepatitis late in pregnancy. The concept of reduced immunologic tolerance in neonates also has been recently questioned. Whatever the mechanism, the result is the development of persistent antigenemia, with or without low-grade enzyme abnormalities, often with histologic evidence of established chronic

TABLE 37–10. RELATIONSHIP BETWEEN HBeAg–ANTI-HBe IN THE MOTHER AND THE DEVELOPMENT OF HBsAg IN THE INFANT

Reference	Test Procedure	Mother HBeAg +		Mother Anti-HBe–Positive		Mother Anti-HBe–Negative	
		No.	*% Infected Infants*	*No.*	*% Infected Infants*	*No.*	*% Infected Infants*
Okada et al. (1976)[557]	ID	10	100	7	0	6	33
Miyakawa and Mayumi (1978)[908]	PHA	25	100	59	0	0	—
Lee et al. (1978)[559]	RH	22	95	0	—	15	33
Derso et al. (1978)[551]	ID	7	86	13	23	11	36
Stevens et al. (1979)[560]	RIA	47	96	14	21	4	0

ID = immunodiffusion; PHA = passive hemagglutination; RH = rheophoresis; RIA = radioimmunoassay.

liver disease ranging from chronic persistent hepatitis to cirrhosis.[578, 579] Indeed, Dunn and co-workers, in an examination of the ultrastructure of liver explants from neonates in whom acute hepatitis B developed, identified virus-like particles in nuclei, which were thought to represent the mature intracellular form of the hepatitis virus.[580]

Occasionally, neonates contract acute viral hepatitis that may progress to fulminant hepatic failure.[581–584] Dupuy and colleagues reported the deaths of 8 of 14 infants less than six months of age in whom acute hepatitis developed.[582] A disturbing feature is that HBV carrier mothers may transmit the virus to each succeeding child,[583, 584] and the disease may prove fatal to more than one child. Mollica and co-workers reported an instance in which a carrier mother appeared to infect each of her six children, four of whom died between 38 and 75 days of age.[584] Similarly, Fawaz and colleagues reported two successive cases of maternal-fetal transmission of fatal hepatitis B from the same mother.[583] If transmission of the disease occurs at birth, it is reasonable to assume that the process might be interrupted by delivering the infant by cesarean section. However, Grady found that a cesarean section performed on a chimpanzee failed to prevent transmission to the baby chimpanzee.[585] Also, Beasley and Stevens, in Taiwan, found no difference between outcomes in human infants born naturally and by cesarean section.[577] This finding has been taken to support the concept of transplacental transmission, a conclusion not accepted by all.

Data similar to those just described with respect to the viruses of hepatitis A and non-A, non-B hepatitis are meager, so it is not certain how frequently these agents are transmitted by the maternal-fetal route. Because of the short viremic phase of HAV, transplacental transmission seems unlikely unless delivery occurs during the incubation period of hepatitis A. During this time, transmission can conceivably result from contact with either infectious blood or stools. In one attempt to study this entity, Tong and associates found no evidence of disease in five infants born to mothers who had acute hepatitis A in the third trimester.[586] They detected anti-HAV in the cord blood of two infants, but in declining titers in a sequence consistent with passive immunization. With regard to non-A, non-B hepatitis, it seems likely that perinatal transmission does occur, but confirmation must await the development of specific test procedures. In the same study, Tong and colleagues found that six of nine infants whose mothers appeared to have had acute non-A, non-B hepatitis in the third trimester developed transient aminotransferase abnormalities.[586] Gupta and co-workers also reported a single instance of what was considered to be maternal-fetal transmission of HBsAg-negative hepatitis from a mother who had fulminant antigen-negative hepatitis during labor.[587] The validity of this case is uncertain, since pertinent sophisticated serologic testing was not performed. Perinatal transmission of the delta virus is extremely rare.[587a, 587b] Because it is dependent on HBV for its replication, delta infection in the newborn can occur only if HBV is also transferred from mother to infant. HBV carriers who are superinfected with HDV are usually anti-HBe–positive and therefore are far less likely to transmit HBV to the newborn. Clearly, further studies are needed. At the present time, the only available means of interrupting perinatal transmission is through the use of immunoprophylaxis. The available data on this topic are discussed later.

Other causes of jaundice in pregnancy include intrahepatic cholestasis of pregnancy and acute fatty metamorphosis of pregnancy.[588–592] They are discussed in Chapter 54.

ORAL CONTRACEPTIVES IN ACUTE VIRAL HEPATITIS

In light of the interrelationship between pregnancy and viral hepatitis, a question that must be considered is whether oral contraceptives adversely affect the patient with acute viral hepatitis. The question is pertinent also because oral contraceptives have been recognized to be associated with hepatic dysfunction and with a number of lesions in women who do not have hepatitis.[593–595] Members of the Boston Collaborative Drug Surveillance Program found that hepatitis appeared to occur more frequently in women who used oral contraceptives than in those who did not.[596] However, Jenny and Markoff found that the use of oral contraceptives by women with chronic liver disease was not associated with unusual hepatic dysfunction.[597] Similarly, Schweitzer and co-workers, in a retrospective analysis, could find no difference in the severity of acute hepatitis and its sequelae between 34 women who had used oral contraceptives through major portions or the entire courses of their acute illness and a matched group of 34 women who had never used oral contraceptives.[598] These data suggest that oral contraceptives can be used in an unrestricted manner during the course of acute viral hepatitis. However, sexual contacts during the acute illness should be discouraged because of the possibility of transmission of the viral disease.

VIRAL HEPATITIS AND THE DUBIN-JOHNSON SYNDROME

In the Dubin-Johnson syndrome, which is a benign congenital disorder inherited as an autosomal recessive trait, chronic nonconjugated hyperbilirubinemia is associated with a secondary rise in sulfobromophthalein during the course of an extended sulfobromophthalein test (see Chap. 25); typical changes in urinary coproporphyrins with a normal total value but with more than 80 per cent excreted as coproporphyrin 1; poor radiologic visualization of the biliary tree; and, most characteristically, a black coloration of the liver, resulting from the accumulation of a dense melanin-like large granular pigment, most pronounced in the centrilobular zones (see also Chaps. 11 and 12).[599] An interesting observation is that the pigment typically disappears from the liver during the course of acute hepatitis and then reaccumulates over several years following recovery from the disease.[600–602] The precise reason for the loss of pigment is not known, but it may be the result of its extrusion from damaged parenchymal cells followed by uptake and disposition by the reticuloendothelial system.[603]

VIRAL HEPATITIS AND MONOCLONAL GAMMOPATHIES

There are several reports of cases in which various monoclonal gammopathies have undergone apparent total remission following the development of acute viral hepatitis. Complete clinical and hematologic remission of multiple myeloma that occurred in a woman with the disease and lasted two years after acute viral hepatitis developed has been reported.[604] Another patient, who had a plasma cell dyscrasia, was reported to have had a remission lasting at least five years following an episode of acute hepatitis.[605] Finally, there are two reports of cases in which patients with Waldenström's macroglobulinemia had either partial or complete remissions following episodes of acute hepatitis.[606, 607] The remission in the latter case lasted at least three and a half years. The mechanism of this response is unknown, but it may relate to the production of interferon or to a direct effect of the virus, causing cellular destruction or chromosomal changes.

TREATMENT OF ACUTE HEPATITIS

In contradistinction to the serologic and epidemiologic aspects of acute viral hepatitis, there have been no significant advances in treatment. Indeed, any changes that have taken place have been in the direction of removing items that once represented standard treatment rather than adding specific therapeutic modalities. This section is devoted to a review of the treatment of acute viral hepatitis only. The treatments of fulminant and chronic hepatitis are discussed in Chapters 17 and 38, respectively.

The treatment of acute hepatitis continues to depend on supportive care, the avoidance of liver-damaging circumstances, and the institution of uncertainly effective heroic measures if the disease begins an inexorably downhill course. Provided there is adequate family and medical support, the majority of patients with uncomplicated acute viral hepatitis can be treated in their homes. Hospitalization for isolation purposes is not warranted. In the first place, the most infectious period of hepatitis A, and perhaps also of the other forms of hepatitis, precedes the onset of symptoms. If transmission of the disease were to occur, it would probably have done so by the time the patient is first seen. Second, provided that appropriate hygienic measures and proper use of immunoprophylaxis are maintained (discussed in detail later), the likelihood of subsequent transmission is small.

Adequate home care requires that proper medical attention be available. The patient should probably be seen by appropriate health care personnel, on two or three occasions during the first week of illness then at lesser intervals as necessary provided that there is no worsening of the illness. Biochemical tests should be performed at least twice a week while enzyme values are rising, weekly after they have plateaued, and at one- to two-week intervals during the subsiding phase. It is appropriate to follow these values to the point at which they normalize. Hospitalization is warranted if severe symptoms of anorexia or vomiting, or both, persist, or if mentation changes or results of biochemical tests worsen. The biochemical abnormalities that should lead to the consideration of hospitalization are a rising bilirubin value (>15 to 20 mg/dl), the persistence of hyperbilirubinemia at a plateau for two to three weeks, an increasing prothrombin time, rapidly falling aminotransferase activity despite a rising bilirubin level, evidence of hepatic encephalopathy, the development of other evidence of hepatic failure (falling albumin levels, ascites, and so on), and a persistence or plateau of elevation of aminotransferase levels (>200 IU/L) for more than six weeks. Otherwise, supportive care should be provided as described in the following sections.

EVALUATION

A presumptive etiologic diagnosis can usually be made from the detailed historic interview, careful questioning about the use of all drugs (prescription and over the counter), and a physical examination. Appropriate biochemical and serologic tests and, if necessary, additional immunologic tests and imaging procedures, will almost always yield a definitive diagnosis.

A general physical examination should include determination of liver and spleen sizes. Disturbing findings include the presence of an unusually large and firm liver, together with splenomegaly and spider nevi, all of which should lead to consideration of the diagnosis of chronic liver disease. Also of concern is sudden, rapid shrinking of the liver. This occurs in fulminant hepatitis as the liver stroma collapses.

Minimal biochemical and serologic testing requires evaluation of serum bilirubin, aminotransferases, alkaline phosphatase, serum protein levels, the prothrombin time, and for the presence of HBsAg and anti-HAV. Additional serologic tests, such as IgM anti-HAV, IgM anti-HBc, and IgM anti-HDV, can be performed as needed. Of the biochemical tests, the prothrombin time represents the most important prognostic indicator.[418, 608] Prolongation of the prothrombin time by more than 3 seconds may forbode the development of progressive disease.

A routine liver biopsy is unnecessary. However, it should be performed, provided that coagulation indices permit, when there is reason to suspect that the diagnosis might be an exacerbation of chronic liver disease rather than an episode of acute hepatitis, or when the disease runs an atypical, protracted course (persisting symptoms or severe biochemical abnormalities for more than four weeks). Liver biopsy should be considered also if the low-grade aminotransferase abnormalities together with HBsAg persist for more than 16 weeks. This combination suggests a possible transition to chronic hepatitis. If the initial test for HBsAg is positive, it is imperative to repeat the procedure to establish a return to a negative result.

BED REST

The requirement that patients with acute viral hepatitis be treated with bed rest and a high protein intake came from studies of servicemen conducted shortly after World War II.[609] The approach seemed justified by observations indicating that hepatic blood flow is decreased by erect posture during exercise.[609a, 610, 610a] This view remained unchallenged until Swift and co-workers, in 1950 and Chalmers and colleagues, in 1955 demonstrated that strict bed rest appeared to confer no benefit.[611, 112] It was found that ad libitum ward activity together with a one-hour rest period after each meal did not prolong the disease; also, physical reconditioning following the return of biochemical test results to normal did not produce relapse.[612] When the same patients were re-evaluated ten years later, none of them showed evidence of serious chronic liver disease, nor had there been increased mortality among them when compared with a selected group of nonhospitalized controls.[333] Similar results were obtained in another study in which children with acute hepatitis were treated either with strict bed rest or with ad libitum diets and activity.[613] These studies did not, however, examine the effect of exercise. Krikler and Zilberg reported the development of fulminant hepatitis in five patients who unwittingly participated in strenuous competitive activity just prior to hospitalization for acute hepatitis; three of these patients died.[614] Since this was a retrospective observation, and an earlier report had indicated that physical exercise did not compromise recovery from acute hepatitis,[614a] a controlled study that involved 199 United States servicemen in Vietnam with acute hepatitis was undertaken. The individuals were urged to perform strenuous exercise (calisthenics, a one-mile run, filling sand bags, painting buildings) for three hours a day, and their course was compared with that of an equal number assigned to a rest ward (a short walk to the mess hall three times a day and bed rest at the patient's discretion).[615] No adverse effect of this strenuous activity was found in these previously healthy young men. Similar results were observed in a later study in which patients with viral hepatitis were stressed by moderately heavy bicycle exercise.[616] Although other investigators found that hepatic blood flow was increased when measured at bed rest with the patient in the supine position, no negative effect of exercise was found in eight patients with hepatitis whose bilirubin values were less than 4 mg/dl. In two children who had bilirubin values of 9.6 and 5.8 mg/dl, respectively, exercise appeared to provoke a relapse in one and a slight delay in the recovery of the other.[617]

Taken together, these data suggest that little harm is likely to result if patients with acute hepatitis are not treated with strict bed rest. Conversely, strenuous activity may not be advisable, particularly when the patient is an older person who is not physically fit. The following program seems to be a reasonable approach. Bed rest with bathroom privileges should be advised while the bilirubin level is rising, if the prothrombin time is prolonged by more than 3 seconds, if the patient is severely symptomatic, or if the patient is more than 40 years of age.[618] With alleviation of symptoms and improvement in biochemical values, ambulation within the bounds of fatigability can be permitted. If symptoms recur or biochemical deterioration occurs in this setting, activity should be restricted until improvement again ensues. There would seem to be little purpose in restricting activity when there is continued low-grade elevation of aminotransferase levels (less than 100 IU/L) without symptoms, jaundice, or serologic evidence of persistent disease.

DIET

The anorexia common during early acute hepatitis is due, in part, to disordered gustatory acuity.[439] It therefore becomes a challenge to induce the patient to eat. In one study, the use of a high-protein diet appeared to be associated with a 20 per cent reduction in the duration of the acute illness,[612] although no obvious long-term benefit was found in this study,[333] nor in another one in which a high-calorie, high-protein, low-fat diet was evaluated.[618a] Nevertheless, provided there is no evidence of hepatic encephalopathy and the patient can tolerate it, a high-protein diet may be encouraged. Generally, nausea and anorexia are least severe in the morning. To capitalize on this, the major proportion of calories can be offered at breakfast. Sometimes it may be necessary to provide many small feedings of a high-caloric liquid formula, taking care not to employ high-glucose concentrations because these patients may have impaired ability to excrete a normal water load. Severe, continued vomiting will obviously necessitate fluid and electrolyte replacement. Fatty foods need not be restricted unless they produce nausea; dairy fats seem to be better tolerated in the anorectic patient than do animal fats. Vitamin supplementation is unnecessary unless a specific deficiency already exists.

DRUGS

All drugs, particularly narcotics, analgesics, and tranquilizers, should be avoided during the course of acute hepatic disease. If nausea and vomiting persist, and drug treatment is believed to be essential, judicious use of small doses of metoclopramide or phenothiazines may be considered. Sedatives should almost never be given, since their elimination is impaired in patients with hepatic disease. It has been shown that oxazepam is excreted at a normal rate by patients with hepatitis,[619] but clinical safety during the course of hepatitis has yet to be clearly established. No purpose is served in administering vitamin K_1, although it may improve abnormal prothrombin times in patients who have cholestatic liver disease. Oral contraceptives are usually proscribed. However, as already mentioned, no deleterious effect was found in a retrospective comparison of women with hepatitis who were users and those who were nonusers.[598] Drinking alcohol is also prohibited, based on early studies suggesting that its use predisposes to relapse or progression to fulminant hepatitis.[620] This proscription should remain even though an early study showed no important effect on serum enzymes in persons with acute viral hepatitis who were infused with 80 mg of ethanol,[620a] and a later study in chimpanzees of the effect of ethanol infusion during HBV infection did not demonstrate an alteration in the course of the disease.[621]

Early studies suggested that the use of corticosteroids could hasten recovery from acute viral hepatitis.[622, 623, 623a] Their administration rapidly reduced the serum bilirubin values in the majority of patients with acute hepatitis.[623b] Later studies comparing corticosteroids with placebos failed to substantiate the findings of a beneficial effect.[624] Furthermore, it has been suggested that corticosteroid treatment may predispose to a higher rate of relapse,[625] and also that it interferes with the normal immune response and hence may promote development of chronic hepatitis.[626] Accordingly, the use of corticosteroids for uncomplicated viral hepatitis is neither justified nor helpful.

There has also been uncertainty regarding the role of corticosteroids in the treatment of severe acute viral hepatitis or subacute hepatic necrosis as manifested by bridging hepatic necrosis. Because early studies suggested that corticosteroids were beneficial for the treatment of acute and chronic hepatitis,[317, 318] Gregory and associates undertook a controlled trial among patients defined as having severe hepatitis (at least one of the following: total bilirubin >25 mg/dl; prothrombin time <50 per cent of normal; serum albumin <2.5 mg/dl; ascites, encephalopathy, edema, or bridging necrosis on liver biopsy) provided that the duration of the illness had not exceeded three months.[319] The patients were assigned randomly to receive methylprednisolone or a placebo. The results suggested that corticosteroids not only were not helpful but also were possibly even harmful. Ware and colleagues, in another controlled trial of patients with severe viral hepatitis of less than one month's duration, also found no benefit from treatment with corticosteroids.[320] An unexpected finding in the latter study was that bridging necrosis did not have prognostic significance. Accordingly, these investigators concluded that routine early liver biopsies are unnecessary for prognostic purposes, and indeed, that they could be misleading. Thus, current data suggest that corticosteroids confer no benefit in the treatment of acute fulminant hepatitis,[626a–626c] subacute hepatic necrosis, and probably even virus-related chronic active hepatitis,[626d, 626e] and, in fact, may be harmful because of their ability to promote replication of the hepatitis B virus.

Elective surgery is precluded during acute viral hepatitis. Unequivocal objective evidence of the dangers of surgery is scanty. It was suggested during the period when surgical exploration was the only means of distinguishing medical from surgical jaundice that abdominal exploration might be hazardous.[341, 627] In the only major effort to examine the effects of surgery during acute hepatitis, Harville and Summerskill found that patients with acute drug-related hepatitis were not adversely affected when subjected to laparotomy, whereas those with acute viral hepatitis suffered severe consequences.[628] Of the 42 patients with acute viral hepatitis who were subjected to surgery, 5 died within three weeks of surgery and nonfatal major complications developed in 5 other patients.

NEW FORMS OF TREATMENT

A variety of new treatment modalities have emerged recently. Their effects are aimed directly at inhibition of viral synthesis or at alteration of the immune response. These therapies have had their primary evaluation in patients with chronic viral liver disease. A few have been examined in patients with acute hepatic disease. Among these therapies are two antiviral agents, ribavirin and isoprinosine; a flavonoid, (+)-cyanidanol-3; an immunostimulant, levamisole; and an immunotherapeutic agent, high-titer anti-HBs.

Ribavirin, a synthetic triazole nucleoside, has antiviral activity against DNA and RNA viruses in vitro and in vivo. The drug inhibits synthesis of viral nucleic acid.[629] It appeared in one study to be moderately effective in reducing mortality among mice infected with a strain of murine hepatitis, an RNA virus, but only marginally effective in hamsters infected with equine abortion virus, a DNA virus.[630] In a small double-blind study involving human hepatitis conducted in Brazil, ribavirin was found to be associated with significant decreases in serum bilirubin and aminotransferase values between the fifth and tenth days of illness.[631] No other clinical data were made available.

Isoprinosine, which inhibits viral RNA and DNA from transmitting their own genetic codes to the host, and which has been claimed to be of benefit in treating herpes zoster and herpes simplex, measles, varicella, influenza, and subacute sclerosing panencephalitis, has also been reported to be effective in the treatment of viral hepatitis.[632] However, in a prospective, double-blind, controlled trial conducted among 81 patients with clinical acute viral hepatitis, no positive effect of the drug was found.[633]

The flavonoid, (+)-cyanidanol-3, a powerful free-radical scavenger, has also been tested in a double-blind, controlled trial.[634] Although the drug was reported to accelerate the disappearance of HBsAg, to reduce serum bilirubin, and to relieve symptoms of anorexia, nausea, and pruritus without detectable side effects, the differences were not sufficient to warrant its use at this time. Further studies are necessary.

Levamisole, a nonspecific immunostimulant that acts by restoring defective macrophage activity or disturbed T-cell function, has been examined in a trial in which 50 consecutive patients received either the drug or a placebo.[635] The levamisole-treated patients lost HBsAg earlier and recovered from the acute disease sooner than did those given the placebo. The conclusion by the investigators was that levamisole may be used in some cases, but they cautioned against the harmful effects of possible enhanced cellular immune destruction with potential massive necrosis.

A double-blind, placebo-controlled, randomized study to evaluate transfer factor for acute hepatitis B has been performed.[635a] No significant beneficial effect was noted.

Finally, the use of anti-HBs infusions has been evaluated in patients with fulminant hepatitis B and in those with HBsAg-positive chronic active hepatitis.[636, 637] In neither was the course of the disease altered by these infusions.

All of these studies are of interest, but none of the drugs tested can be recommended as routine treatment. There are several reasons for this. First, most instances of viral hepatitis are self-limited and hence do not require treatment. Second, many of the studies of the efficacy of drugs have been small and poorly organized. Third, data available regarding toxicity are insufficient. They seem better suited for evaluation in patients with chronic virus-induced liver disease.

PREVENTION OF VIRAL HEPATITIS

Two major components are necessary in order to contain the spread of viral hepatitis. The first, and one that is often forgotten or neglected in the haste to initiate immunoprophylaxis, is the development and institution of general measures that help to check transmission of the virus. For this approach to be effective, it is essential to have a thorough knowledge of the epidemiology and natural history of the viral disease. The second component is the appropriate use of passive and active immunoprophylaxis that can be applied either in anticipation of exposure (pre-exposure prophylaxis) or following definitive exposure to the disease (postexposure prophylaxis). Once again, it is essential that the natural history and seroepidemiology of each of the various types of hepatitis be fully understood to facilitate rational decisions in regard to appropriateness, form, type, dose, and frequency of administration of the globulin and vaccine products.

GENERAL MEASURES TO AVERT TRANSMISSION OF HEPATITIS

A detailed knowledge of the modes of spread of hepatitis is a prerequisite for the design of effective preventive public health measures. These measures must take into account that humans and, to a lesser extent, nonhuman primates, are the only recognized reservoirs of the hepatitis viruses. It appears, however, that certain insects may on occasion act as vectors for the transmission of hepatitis B. Accordingly, the basic principle in preventing spread of the disease is to restrict or avoid direct contact with human body fluids and secretions that may harbor the viruses.

Hepatitis A

Early studies of hepatitis A demonstrated evidence of infectivity of both blood and feces starting about two to three weeks before the onset of jaundice and lasting about three days beyond disease onset in blood and eight days beyond in feces.[14, 41, 638-640a] Efforts to transmit the disease to volunteers with blood and feces obtained beyond these time periods were unsuccessful.[41, 640a, 640b] These data, derived from experimental transmission studies, have since been confirmed. Immune electron microscopy demonstrates HAV particles in the stools during this period. The number of viral particles rapidly diminishes after serum aminotransferase levels reach their peak;[640c, 641] although they have been detected in stool as long as two to two and a half weeks after peak enzyme values have been reached.[642] On the basis of this information, the contagious period for hepatitis A is now considered to be from the latter half of the incubation period to shortly after the onset of overt illness. Careful analysis of a household outbreak in one study suggested that transmission probably occurs most often close to the time that symptoms develop.[641]

Contaminated stools represent the primary source of transmission of hepatitis A. Unlike hepatitis B and non-A, non-B hepatitis, there is no carrier state for hepatitis A and hence transmission by blood, as might occur following transfusion, is exceedingly rare, although it has been reported.[127x, 127y, 643] Thus, the principal mode of transmission of this viral disease from person to person is through direct fecal-oral contact and, less frequently, it is transmitted through ingestion of fecally contaminated water or foodstuffs.[277, 278, 297, 644–651] In the former instance, spread of the disease is enhanced when there is close and prolonged contact with an individual incubating the disease. Accordingly, those at risk include all susceptible household contacts, as well as other persons living together in close proximity, as occurs in Army camps, during Army maneuvers, in prisons, in day care centers,[271b, 651a] and in institutions for the mentally retarded. Homosexual men, particularly those who have oral-anal contact, are particularly susceptible.[651b, 651c] Poor personal hygiene and substandard sanitation will, of course, greatly increase the chance of spread.

In the United States, spread of the disease through contaminated water and foodstuffs has been relatively uncommon, but waterborne transmission has occurred, primarily from urinary or fecal contamination of underground wells or contamination of drinking water through imperfect plumbing lines.[277–279, 647, 648–649a, 652–655] Many foodstuffs have been implicated in hepatitis transmission.[297, 650, 651, 656–660] With the exception of shellfish-associated hepatitis, which represents a specific and well-defined epidemiologic entity,[271d, 390, 661–663] most food-related outbreaks have occurred merely as isolated incidents.

Americans are far more likely to acquire waterborne or food-borne HAV when they visit or reside in areas of the world where the disease is endemic. The prevalence of anti-HAV in United States–born and –raised populations, even taking into account the modifying factors of age and socioeconomic status, is comparatively low, making them vulnerable when transposed to areas of high risk. These areas include North Africa, parts of the Middle East, India and Pakistan, and parts of Asia and Central and South America. As shown in several studies involving American missionaries and Peace Corps workers living abroad, the risk of acquiring hepatitis appears to remain constant during the first ten years of residence in these countries.[664–668]

Another high-risk situation is close, prolonged contact with newly imported nonhuman primates. There have been numerous instances of hepatitis developing in veterinarians, zookeepers, scientists, and other handlers of these animals.[54, 669–672] Most have occurred when the individuals were working with chimpanzees, but gorillas, orangutans, gibbons, the woolly monkey, and Celebes apes have also been responsible for some outbreaks.

General measures to contain hepatitis A depend upon defined public health procedures aimed at preventing contamination of water and food. They include proper handling of raw sewage, filtration and chlorination of water, and the maintenance of adequate separation between sewage disposal and drinking-water facilities through appropriate sanitary engineering. Special attention is paid to shellfish harvesting areas, since the danger from these mollusks rests on their ability to accumulate from the water, retain, and concentrate viral contaminants, which are then transmitted to humans who eat them raw or partially cooked. However, even bacteriologic monitoring and certification of the safety of these harvesting areas does not ensure complete safety, as evidenced by a large outbreak of hepatitis A that occurred two months after flooding of the Mississippi River. This epidemic was traced to contamination of a certified commercial Louisiana oyster bed fed by the river.[663, 673]

Maintenance of safe food requires that exemplary hygiene and sanitary precautions be practiced by all food handlers. Ideally, they should behave as if they are always in the asymptomatic, incubation phase of hepatitis A, constantly excreting HAV in their stools. Thus, regular hand-washing, particularly after bowel evacuation, is mandatory for all such workers. Also, insects that may contaminate food and water through fecal soilage should be eliminated from all areas in which food is handled or sold.

Once hepatitis develops, it becomes necessary to curtail its spread. In the past it was required that the hospitalized patients be isolated in a private room, that there be use of separate toilet facilities, and that every staff member wear gown and gloves when entering the room. On the basis of the serologic pattern of hepatitis A as now defined, the rarity of nosocomial hepatitis A infection,[674, 675] and the lack of a higher prevalence of anti-HAV among health care professionals than among nonmedical persons of similar socioeconomic status, it has been suggested by authoritative public health officials that such measures are no longer necessary.[676] The current recommendation is that precautions in the use of needles be continued, but that otherwise the same care be taken in disposing of the urine and feces of hepatitis patients as is applied to handling such materials from all other hospitalized patients, that is, that gloves be worn when handling bedpans, fecal material, or instruments that come in contact with the intestinal tract. The following general measures are considered appropriate for the individual patient with hepatitis. Separate thermometers should be used and retained in the patient's room in a disinfectant (e.g., 0.2 per cent iodine in 70 to 90 per cent alcohol) and then washed with soap and water, rinsed, and dried when the patient leaves. If bedpans are needed, the same one should always be assigned to the patient, and it should be disinfected and sterilized when no longer needed. Urine and feces collected in the bedpan should be flushed directly down the toilet. Separate toilet facilities are not needed for the ambulatory patient. The patient should always carefully wash his hands after the use of toilet facilities.

Medical personnel without skin disease need to wear gloves only when there is direct contact with blood or feces. In these circumstances, careful subsequent washing of the hands also is required. Masks and gowns are not needed unless it is expected that there is likely to be splattering of the patient's blood. Disposable needles and syringes should always be used and should be discarded in an impervious bag for ultimate incineration or autoclaving. Instruments that come in contact with blood or feces should be thoroughly washed and sterilized or disinfected. Visitors need not be restricted, but food should not be shared. These precautions apply to patients cared for in the home or the hospital. Utensils and crockery can be sterilized adequately by cleaning in a hot-water dishwasher.

Little can be done to stem a waterborne outbreak other than to recognize its origin and prohibit drinking of the water. Krugman and associates have shown that boiling contaminated water at 98° C for 1 minute inactivates HAV.[44] Persons working with newly imported primates should be advised to wear gloves at all times when there is expectation of potential exposure to the blood or feces of these animals. Such persons should have regular tests performed for anti-HAV, and if necessary, should receive immunoprophylaxis, as is discussed later.

Hepatitis B

From an epidemiologic and preventive viewpoint, hepatitis B differs in important ways from hepatitis A. First, the virus is usually present in the blood longer in acute hepatitis B than in acute hepatitis A, averaging approximately six weeks. Second, a carrier state exists for hepatitis B only, and HBV may persist in the blood indefinitely. Third, HBsAg can be detected in virtually all body fluids, secretions, and excretions, with the exception of feces.[382, 392a-m, 392t, 392w, 393, 394, 449, 453, 575, 677-686] Added to this is the fact that HBV is an extremely hardy agent, capable of withstanding wide extremes of temperature and humidity, as well as the effects of numerous chemical agents. The virus remains stable after storage for 15 years at −20° C;[687] for 24 months at −80° C;[688] for six months at room temperature;[689] for three to four weeks on a dried glass surface maintained at ambient temperature;[689] for at least seven days at 44° C, depending on the diluent and pH;[689] and for four hours at 60° C.[690] It also remains viable after repeated cycles of freezing and thawing over a period of six months.[689] Antigenicity, but not infectivity, is retained after heating for 1 minute at 98° C,[44] but it is lost after heating for an hour at 85° C or for 5 minutes at 100° C. It had been widely accepted that heat treatment at 60° C for ten hours inactivates HBV, but results of recent studies have cast doubt on this view.[691-693] With regard to chemical agents, HBV has been shown to withstand exposure to ultraviolet irradiation and extraction with ether, benzalkonium chloride, and alcohol.[694-698] Conversely, it is inactivated by β-propiolactone,[699] glutaraldehyde,[700] chloroform,[701] formalin (1:4000), pepsin, and urea (8 M).[702]

It is thus apparent that the modes of transmission of the two viral diseases are likely to be different, as are the strategies required to interrupt their transmission. For many years, it was believed that hepatitis A could be transmitted via both blood and stool, whereas blood was the only vehicle for transmission of hepatitis B. The present view is that blood and all body fluids identified as being HBsAg-positive are potential sources for transmission. In support of this are the reports of the identification of HBV particles in saliva, semen, and various body effusions, and the circumstantial and experimental evidence that these secretions are capable of effecting virus transfer.[382, 392a-392i, 449, 453, 575, 703, 704] Indeed, hepatitis B is clearly identified as a sexually transmitted virus, with a high rate of infection occurring among prostitutes and promiscuous homosexual men.[705-707, 707b] Thus, hepatitis B is now recognized to be transmissible by both percutaneous and nonpercutaneous routes.

Of these modes of transmission, the percutaneous route, involving direct blood to blood contact across an interrupted barrier of skin or mucous membrane, is the more easily envisioned and definable. The most flagrant example of this is the exposure to large volumes of blood that occurs as a result of transfusion of blood or blood products,[28, 273-275, 708-712] although the frequency of type B post-transfusion hepatitis has declined to negligible levels since the introduction of routine screening of blood donors

for HBsAg.[712a, 712b] Other easily identifiable forms of percutaneous exposure, but to smaller volumes of blood, include accidental puncture of the skin with a blood-contaminated needle,[713, 714] a splash of blood in the eyes,[715] injection with unsterilized needles shared with others,[281, 716-721a] and exposure to instruments used to perform procedures such as tattooing,[722-725] ear piercing,[726] acupuncture,[727, 728] or neurologic sensory examination.[729] Less obvious are instances in which blood or other contaminated body fluids enter the circulatory system through inapparent abrasions or cuts in the skin or mucous membranes as, for example, the sharing of razors or toothbrushes,[729a] or through skin made permeable by dermatologic abnormalities.[730] Insects can act as vectors to transfer infection by biting or perhaps by contaminating foods.[731-735]

Persons susceptible to percutaneous hepatitis transmission are obviously those whose occupations or ways of life bring them into direct and regular contact with blood or blood products. These individuals include blood recipients, particularly those who need frequent or massive transfusions;[736-740, 740a] medical and paramedical personnel,[741-747] particularly those working in hemodialysis units,[288, 289, 295, 748-750] oncology units,[751] clinical laboratories,[752-756] and morgues;[757] dental personnel,[758-763] especially oral surgeons who work in a bloody field; drug abusers who share needles indiscriminately with other potentially infected persons;[281, 716-721a] patients in hemodialysis units;[749, 750, 763a] and those who undergo renal transplantation.[763b] A special risk group comprises neonates born to HBsAg-positive mothers, the presumed route of exposure being percutaneous entry through skin abrasions or perhaps ingestion of HBV-contaminated blood at the time of delivery.[538-560a]

The precise mechanisms and circumstances of the nonpercutaneous forms of exposure are not so well established. It is assumed that in the majority of instances, the virus is ingested.[42, 382a-i, 382u, 677, 764-767] Another route of entry that has been considered is the respiratory tract.[392e, 768, 769] The most apparent form of oral exposure is the circumstance in which a laboratory worker accidentally pipettes HBsAg-positive blood or blood-derived reagents into the mouth. Less certain is the view that transmission of hepatitis B during intimate hetero- or homosexual contact is the result of the ingestion of HBsAg-positive saliva or semen.[392c, 392e, 703, 705-707, 707a, 707b, 770-773] The evidence indicating that environmental surface contamination with HBsAg occurs in areas of high blood concentration and usage suggests the possibility that hand-oral transmission might be another mechanism for viral transfer.[697, 774, 775] Airborne transmission with inhalation of the virus is suggested because HBsAg has been found in sneeze and cough specimens and saliva.[392e] There is evidence, too, that aerosolization of blood develops in the immediate vicinity of blood centrifuges and dental drills.[776, 777] Circumstantial evidence from several outbreaks suggests that airborne transmission is the best explanation for spread of the disease.[768, 769] Suffice it to say, it is often impossible to establish the mode of transmission in the individual sporadic case of hepatitis B.

The prevention or containment of this ubiquitous virus requires detailed attention to the many circumstances surrounding its transmission. Thus, efforts to deal with post-transfusion hepatitis include a more critical assessment of the need for blood transfusions, elimination or reduction of the use of blood products established to be unusually infectious (e.g., pooled plasma, fibrinogen, prothrombin complex concentrates),[740a, 778-781a] the introduction of testing of blood donors for HBsAg, with interdiction of those found to be positive, the reduction in reliance on paid-donor blood (a most important step),[712a-712c] and the continued search for other blood markers, such as anti-HBc,[782] that might be capable of further reducing the incidence of post-transfusion hepatitis B.

Other approaches have included efforts to reduce infectivity by attempting to inactivate HBV and the non-A, non-B hepatitis virus. These attempts have included heating procedures,[782a-782c] the addition of high-titer anti-HBs in the form of HBIG with the aim of neutralizing HBV,[782d] the addition of formalin,[782e, 782f] and the use of frozen deglycerolized red blood cells.[782g] The latter approach has proved to be inneffective.[782h, 782i]

Non-A, non-B post-transfusion hepatitis continues to be the major concern because of the lack of a specific viral marker that would identify potentially harmful blood. Accordingly, surrogate tests have been sought. Despite early discouraging results regarding the potential infectivity of donor blood found to have increased aminotransferase activity,[782j, 782k] interest in the technique was renewed,[782l] with data suggesting efficacy of this approach from two large studies.[782m, 782n] Retrospective analysis of the collected information prompted the conclusion that if donor blood with increased levels of ALT had been eliminated, the frequency of non-A, non-B post-transfusion hepatitis could have been reduced by about one-third to one-half. Even though the majority of donor blood units with increased ALT activity do not appear to be infectious,[782m, 782n] and despite the evidence that most instances of ALT elevations in the donor blood appear ascribable to events other than hepatitis, for example, obesity, alcoholism, and drugs,[782o-782r] the blood-banking community in the United States has elected to introduce routine ALT testing of all donor blood and to interdict that blood showing increased activity. A similar correlation has been found between donor blood with detectable anti-HBc and the development of non-A, non-B post-transfusion hepatitis.[782s, 782t] Accordingly, testing for this antibody has also become a routine screening procedure for all blood donors.

Other mechanical modes of transmission are dealt with by reducing the chances of environmental contamination, by attempting to inactivate the virus if contamination does occur through the use of appropriate disinfection and sterilization procedures,[697, 783, 784] by eliminating cross-transfer of blood through the use of disposable needles and other equipment, and by the maintenance of meticulous hygienic procedures.

Critically important components of the prevention program in the hospital setting are the institution of hospital-wide surveillance with the aid of a designated safety officer and the introduction of continuing education for hospital personnel regarding modes of spread of the hepatitis viruses.[676] Surveillance should include serologic analyses of all hospitalized patients with viral hepatitis, as well as regular serologic screening of patients and personnel in certain high-risk areas, such as the hemodialysis unit. For their own protection, hospital personnel should be aware of all patients known to be HBsAg-positive and whether or not they have acute hepatic damage, and all blood and other specimens obtained from them should be clearly labeled as being potentially infectious to ensure special precautions in their handling. This should not lead to complacency with the handling of non-labeled vials, since they may nevertheless harbor the hepatitis virus. Hospital personnel likely to come into contact with HBsAg-positive blood should wear gloves. If splashing of blood or other fluids can be anticipated, gown and mask should be worn. Persons who have dermatitis should be urged to wear gloves

at all times until the skin disease has healed. Regular instructions should be given regarding the best methods to discard needles and syringes. Used needles should never be recapped, forcibly bent, or broken, because these procedures increase the chances for an accidental puncture. Instead, they should be discarded into a prominently labeled puncture-resistant and impervious container for incineration or autoclaving. They should never be thrown into open garbage containers, in which they represent a hazard to cleaning and janitorial staff members. Syringes should be cleansed thoroughly of all blood under a running tap. All personnel should wash their hands thoroughly after each contact with a patient with hepatitis, using a foot- or elbow-operated faucet.

Special precautions are required for certain high-risk areas of the hospital, the most important of which are the hemodialysis and hematology-oncology units.[785] The following procedures have been recommended for containing the hepatitis problem in the hemodialysis unit. Whenever possible, anti-HBs–positive personnel should be selected to work in the unit, since they are immune to reinfection with hepatitis B. Personnel who are anti-HBs–negative should receive the hepatitis B vaccine, as will be described later. They should not be permitted to eat or smoke on the unit. They should be instructed to wear gloves and gowns when performing functions such as handling shunts, drawing blood, dismantling dialysis equipment, or changing bedpans. They should be made aware of which patients are HBsAg-positive and should practice scrupulous personal hygiene and aseptic techniques when dealing with them. All accidental needle punctures should be reported immediately. The patients should be screened for HBsAg prior to admission to the dialysis unit, and HBsAg screening of personnel and patients should be continued at regular three- to six-month intervals after acceptance onto the unit. Patients who are HBsAg-positive should be segregated from those who are HBsAg-negative and, whenever possible, sharing of equipment by these two groups should be avoided. All patients should be prohibited from eating or smoking while the dialysis procedure is in progress, and they should refrain from sharing personal items with other patients at any time.

All nondisposable instruments and medical equipment for reuse, whether on or off the dialysis unit, should be carefully dismantled, thoroughly washed with soap and water, and then sterilized or disinfected as appropriate. Sterilization by heating is the treatment of choice for all instruments and objects that can be so handled. It is accomplished through applying steam under pressure (autoclaving) at 121° C (250° F) for 15 minutes, by boiling for 20 minutes, or by exposure to dry heat at 170° C (340° F) for 60 minutes.[697, 785] Sterilization by gas is also feasible, using ethylene oxide for 3.5 to 16 hours, depending on the object and the manufacturer's recommendations.[786] Chemical disinfection, presumed although not proved conclusively to be effective, includes the use of sodium hypochlorite, 5000 to 10,000 ppm available chlorine (0.5 to 1.0 per cent) for 30 minutes (for pipettes, slides, glassware, and other nonmetallic objects, since hypochlorite corrodes metal, or to wipe surfaces contaminated with blood); 40 per cent aqueous formalin (16 per cent aqueous formaldehyde) for 12 hours; formalin, 20 per cent in 70 per cent alcohol, for 18 hours; and 2 per cent alkalinized glutaraldehyde for 10 hours. Glutaraldehyde has proved to be particularly useful in the disinfection of fragile instruments, such as endoscopes.[700, 787]

Persons working in clinical pathology laboratories,

morgues, dental clinics, and other high-risk areas should be made aware of all patients and specimens known to be HBsAg-positive. Gloves and other protective clothing should be worn as appropriate. However, caution should be practiced in the handling of all specimens, even when they are not explicitly labeled as being derived from HBsAg-positive patients.

Hospitalized patients with hepatitis B always represent a potential hazard to medical personnel, as hepatitis B is a major nosocomial illness. Efforts to reduce transmission of the disease are aimed primarily at reducing percutaneous transmission by instituting the precautions outlined previously. Since HBsAg is not found in feces, precautions in handling feces are not required. There is also concern regarding the reverse problem, namely, that hospital staff may represent a threat to patients. Indeed, because of the high rate of nosocomial infection, health care workers represent a group with a distinct likelihood of becoming HBV carriers. It is not surprising, therefore, that there have been instances of hepatitis B in patients traced back to exposure to medical personnel who tested positive for HBsAg.[788, 789] Nevertheless, prospective studies of nurses and physicians who are carriers of HBsAg show that transmission of hepatitis B to their patients during the course of normal working activities is uncommon unless a break in technique occurs in the course of routine hospital activities.[790, 791] Accordingly, restriction of normal activities simply on the basis of HBsAg positivity would seem at present to be unwarranted. Instead, the health care carrier should be made acutely aware of the modes of hepatitis transmission and should apply rigorous measures to reduce the chances of their occurring. These measures should include regular hand washing, scrupulous aseptic techniques, and the use of gloves when any break in the skin can be identified. Serologic testing of HBsAg-positive persons should be performed regularly, since it is now apparent that some individuals convert to HBsAg negativity even after six months.[792, 793] Testing for HBeAg should also be undertaken. Its presence identifies a person who is more likely to transmit the disease than is a person who is HBeAg-negative or anti-HBe–positive.[794–795b] However, the lack of HBeAg in the HBV carrier does not necessarily denote lack of infectivity. Several investigators have observed HBV DNA or IgM anti-HBc in serum without detectable HBeAg,[795c–795f] and transmission of hepatitis B by anti-HBe–positive persons has been noted, even though it is evident that such individuals are clearly less infectious. These carriers should be especially careful to avoid circumstances that might promote disease transmission. Also, their activities should be regularly monitored, and if any evidence of disease transmission is found, they might require transfer to areas involving less intimate patient contact.

Patients with hepatitis who are not hospitalized should be treated with the same precautions. Since hepatitis B in the household is transmitted most commonly to spouses or to others having intimate sexual contact with the patient, such contact should be minimized during the acute illness.[771–773, 796–798] All members of the household should be educated with regard to the modes of spread of the disease. In particular, they should be warned against the sharing of items such as toothbrushes, razors, washcloths, and other personal effects.

Because of the high frequency of maternal-neonatal transmission of HBV, particularly when acute illness develops during the third trimester, pregnant women should be warned against working in high-risk areas. Carriers of HBsAg who work as food handlers do not appear to pose a direct threat to others. Nevertheless, it is prudent to suggest that they alter their occupation to one in which direct contact with food is not required. If this cannot be accomplished, they must be instructed to take particular care to avoid all situations that might favor viral transmission.

Non-A, Non-B Hepatitis

Because there is no serologic marker for non-A, non-B hepatitis, the exact mechanisms and routes of transmission have not been clearly established. However, in view of the many epidemiologic similarities between hepatitis B and non-A, non-B hepatitis, it is reasonable to assume that the modes of transmission of the two diseases are also similar. Epidemiologic and primate transmission studies indicate that the viral agent is present in blood and that there exists a prolonged carrier state even without biochemical evidence of liver disease. In light of the accumulating data suggesting that non-A, non-B hepatitis is transmitted via both percutaneous and nonpercutaneous routes, it is conceivable that saliva and other body fluids might harbor the agent as they do the virus of hepatitis B.

Currently identified circumstances of percutaneous transmission are those of transfusion of blood and blood products and of indiscriminate sharing of needles by narcotic drug abusers.[115, 121, 643, 799–804] Confirmation of the infectivity of blood during acute disease, and even for a prolonged period thereafter, comes from experimental studies that have shown that humans and chimpanzees respond to inoculation with blood believed to harbor the agent by developing non-A, non-B hepatitis.[121–124, 323, 803, 805] Nonpercutaneous transmission is assumed from the various reports from around the world of sporadic instances of this viral disease unassociated with a history of percutaneous exposure.[120, 324, 806, 807]

General preventive measures are presumably the same as those outlined for hepatitis B. Worthy of comment are data that show that blood obtained from commercial donors is far more likely to be associated with post-transfusion non-A, non-B hepatitis than is blood derived from volunteer donors.[272] Lacking specific serologic tests, efforts are in progress to identify other markers of potentially infectious donor blood. Some correlation has been found between donor blood with elevated levels of aminotransferases or carcinoembryonic antigen, or the presence in donor blood of anti-HBc and the ultimate development of hepatitis.[244, 782m, 782n, 782s, 782t, 808] Accordingly, until a specific test for non-A, non-B hepatitis becomes available (one may be imminent), the best means of preventing this disease is to eliminate the routine use of donor blood from paid donors.

PASSIVE IMMUNOPROPHYLAXIS

A second line of defense, once those of the general preventive measures have been breeched, is to resort to immunoprophylaxis. The concept of immunotherapy was devised before the turn of the last century, when von Behring and Kitasoto developed an antitoxin against diphtheria using rabbit serum.[809] Globulin extracts from humans were produced in the early 1930s, and studies with them soon showed that they were capable of preventing measles.[810, 811] However, general use of gamma globulin became practical only after Cohn and associates, in 1944, developed an effective, safe method of plasma fractionation.[812] In this procedure, gamma globulin is precipitated as fraction II at a specific ionic strength, temperature, and ethanol concentration, in the process of which antibody is concentrated to nearly 25 times the concentration in the original plasma.[813] Early clinical evaluation of gamma globulin produced by the Cohn fractionation method showed that even when derived from infectious material, it did not transmit hepatitis.[814] More recent studies of gamma globulin made from starting material known to be HBsAg-positive have demonstrated that the HBsAg and other HBV-related indices (HBeAg, DNA polymerase, Dane particles) do not appear in fraction II, but instead migrate to later fractions, primarily fraction III.[815–817] In keeping with this is the fact that despite the millions of doses of gamma globulin that have been administered since its introduction as an agent of immunoprophylaxis, there have been only a handful of reported instances of transmission of hepatitis B attributed to this product.[818–823] The best characterized of these was an outbreak that occurred in Italy in 1974 following the use of an antiallergy drug that contained gamma globulin.[818] The implicated globulin had been prepared in the United States by the Cohn method from a plasma pool that was HBsAg-negative by counterelectrophoresis, but that was later found by the more sensitive radioimmunoassay procedure to contain both HBsAg and anti-HBc.[819] Despite this occurrence, HBsAg-positive lots are extremely rare, a fact evident even before the advent of mandatory screening of all blood donors for HBsAg in 1972. Less than 1 per cent of more than 1000 lots of IG submitted to the Bureau of Biologics prior to 1973 were found to test positive, and since then no positive lot has been identified by routine serologic testing.[824] It is reasonable to assume that gamma globulin produced from appropriately screened donor pools (as is now the requirement in the United States and in many other parts of the world) will not transmit hepatitis B.

The product used in the United States is IG, and as already stated was known in the past as immune serum globulin (ISG). It is licensed by the Bureau of Biologics, Food and Drug Administration. It is produced from pools consisting of a minimum of 1000 donors, the source material being outdated blood, deliberately plasmapheresed paid donors, or placental material. It is a 16.5 per cent solution, stabilized by glycine and preserved with thimerosal, a mercury derivative. Because anti-HAV could not be measured in the past, it was required that IG contain specific titers of antibody against diphtheria, measles, and poliovirus, type I to meet standardization criteria. Studies in the United States and elsewhere have since shown that all lots of IG do contain anti-HAV, as might have been expected, but with varying titers as measured by immune adherence hemagglutination (IAHA), ranging from 1:220 to 1:16,000, although usually in excess of 1:1000.[113, 825] In the United States, the prevalence and the titer of anti-HAV have been shown to correlate directly with both low socioeconomic status and age.[117, 826] A concern expressed that anti-HAV titers in IG prepared in the United States might decline to negligible levels because of ever-improving public health protective measures and sanitation is not supported by results of a recent study. Hoofnagle and Waggoner examined 62 lots of IG prepared between 1962 and 1977 and found no change during this period in the anti-HAV titers, which ranged from 1:500 to 1:4000 and averaged 1:1000.[827] This was in direct contradistinction to the HBV indices. Prior to 1972, HBsAg could be demonstrated frequently (78 per cent of lots studied, but only after the IG had been subjected to ultracentrifugation), anti-HBc was demonstrable in high titers (mean 1:8000), and anti-HBs was present

infrequently in low titers. After that year, coincident with and presumably as a result of the requirement that all blood donors be screened by sensitive tests, HBsAg could not be identified, anti-HBc titers declined tenfold, and anti-HBs prevalence and titers increased. Clearly, the findings prior to 1972 were the result of a complex of HBsAg and anti-HBs.

The half-life of IG is important in determining the frequency of its administration. Half-lives have been found to range from 13.1 to 37 days, depending on the method of study. Recent sophisticated studies have shown that IgG has a half-life of about 21 days.[828–831]

Adverse reactions are, fortunately, uncommon when IG is given via the intramuscular route. The incidence of the mild allergic reactions of arthralgia, rash, and fever is approximately 1 per cent.[272, 275, 832] Rarely, the IG additives may cause the allergic reaction.[833] The chance that an adverse reaction will occur is higher, however, in IgA-deficient children who have received frequent IG injections.[834] Severe anaphylactic reactions are rare unless the IG is administered intravenously.[833–838]

Because IG and HBIG are derived from pooled human plasma, the most important potential adverse reaction is the transmission of the human immunodeficiency virus (HIV). Currently, there are three lines of evidence to indicate that this concern seems unwarranted. First, investigators have shown that after spiking pooled serum with HIV, ethanol fractionation removes the virus by a factor exceeding 1×10^{15} in vitro infectious units (IVIU)/ml.[838a] Second, efforts to culture HIV from IG and HBIG lots that are positive for anti-HIV have been unsuccessful. Third, recipients of IG or HSIG that were known to be positive for anti-HIV showed no serologic evidence or signs or symptoms related to the acquired immunodeficiency syndrome.[838b] Even though anti-HIV can be detected in these recipients after administration, the antibody disappears within six months, indicating that its initial appearance is a consequence of passive transfer from the globulin.[838c]

There are two broad categories of use of IG for immunoprophylaxis. It can be given after exposure has already occurred, and this is known as postexposure prophylaxis. Alternatively, IG may be given in anticipation of exposure, and this is referred to as pre-exposure prophylaxis.

Prophylaxis of Hepatitis A

Evaluation of the efficacy of IG during the early years of its use was handicapped because specific serologic tests were lacking. As is now known, differentiation of hepatitis A from hepatitis B on purely epidemiologic grounds was far from accurate. Furthermore, antibody responses and titers in IG could not be determined and, as has been pointed out, HBV-related antibodies have been in a state of flux. Nevertheless, in numerous studies conducted over the years in several countries, IG has proved to be highly effective in prophylaxis of hepatitis A when administered appropriately.

The efficacy of IG in preventing hepatitis A was established in 1944 in three separate studies, one involving summer campers in the United States exposed to contaminated well water,[32] one involving United States soldiers stationed in the Mediterranean littoral,[33] and the third involving institutionalized children.[34] Many studies have been conducted in various parts of the world since then, and they not only have confirmed the original results but also in the process have attempted to define the circumstances of need, optimal dose, effectiveness, and mechanism of action of IG.

The circumstances of need for immunoprophylaxis against hepatitis A, based on the transmission characteristics of the disease and on epidemiologic studies, have been described. To recapitulate, because maximal viral excretion in stools predates the development of acute disease, populations at risk are those who are in regular, close contact with persons incubating hepatitis A, particularly when personal hygiene and sanitary conditions are substandard. Thus, when used for postexposure prophylaxis, prime candidates in the United States are all contacts who live in the same household or in the same institution,[640, 839–840a] such as in those for the mentally retarded,[38, 40, 841, 842] prisons, or army camps. The more casual contacts that occur in schools, hospitals, offices, and factories appear to represent no great risk. Other potential candidates for immunoprophylaxis are persons who drink contaminated water or eat contaminated food.[277, 297, 390, 647, 648, 650–653, 656–663] However, in practical terms, by the time the epidemic is recognized and the vehicle of transmission is identified, so much time has usually elapsed that little benefit is thought to be gained from IG administration.[651] Pre-exposure prophylaxis is warranted for susceptible (anti-HAV–negative) international travelers to certain parts of the world (discussed earlier), particularly if they deviate from the usual tourist paths,[664–668] as well as for susceptible persons who work continuously with newly imported primates.[669–672]

Attempts to define an optimum dose were mandated in part by the high cost and limited supply of IG in the 1950s and 1960s. The dose used in the original study by Stokes and Neefe, 0.15 ml/kg (equivalent to 0.3 ml/kg), was determined to be 90 per cent effective in reducing the incidence of hepatitis. In other studies, progressively lower doses were found to be effective. For example, in yet another study by Stokes and colleagues, involving an epidemic in a training school for children,[843] and in a study conducted by Hsia and co-workers among household contacts,[839] 0.02 ml/kg appeared effective. An even lower dose, 0.01 ml/kg, was found to be effective in several other pre- and postexposure studies,[844–846] although in one, 0.02 ml/kg appeared to be more effective than did 0.01 ml/kg.[844] To ensure efficacy, the former dose of 0.02 ml/kg has been chosen, and it has been proved by field experience to provide adequate postexposure prophylaxis. A practical and convenient formulation has been to administer 0.5 ml of IG to children weighing less than 50 pounds, 1.0 ml to persons weighing 50 to 100 pounds, and 2.0 ml to persons weighing more than 100 pounds.[840a] Pre-exposure prophylaxis for travelers requires a slightly different immunization regimen, particularly if there is a likelihood of prolonged exposure. For a visit of short duration (<2 months) to areas of the world in which hepatitis A is endemic, a single injection of 0.02 ml/kg body weight will generally suffice.[840a] If the visit is more prolonged, and especially if rural areas of poor sanitation are included, a dose of 0.06 ml/kg body weight every five months is considered necessary. The need for immunoprophylaxis may be averted, however, if serologic testing identifies the presence of anti-HAV. Indeed, prescreening is particularly important if repetitive doses are contemplated.

Levels of anti-HAV achieved after IG administration are relatively low when compared with those that follow natural infection. Indeed, anti-HAV cannot be detected by the readily available immunoassay methods, but specific anti-HAV neutralizing antibody can be defined by a radioimmunofocus inhibition assay.[847]

As a prelude to a discussion of efficacy, it should be remembered that the purpose of immunoprophylaxis is to administer specific antibody in sufficient quantity and at an optimal time to be able to counteract the effect of an alien antigen. In the case of IG, anti-HAV specificity has been established through biologic and serologic studies. Furthermore, the specificity of anti-HAV is the same throughout the world; studies have demonstrated that IG prepared from donors in one part of the world effectively protects against hepatitis A in another part of the world.[848] The quantity of anti-HAV in the final IG preparation is dependent, of course, on the amounts present in the blood of individual donors to the pool. As mentioned earlier these vary; some of the reasons for the variation have been defined. There is also evidence to suggest that the method of preparation influences efficacy. Mosley and co-workers found that one lot of IG prepared by the Cohn fractionation method had high levels of certain measurable viral antibodies and was 87 per cent effective in protecting against hepatitis A; another lot, derived by ammonium sulfate preparation, was found to have lower levels of the same antibodies and to be only 47 per cent protective.[849] It is apparent that the timing of IG administration also influences efficacy, being greater the closer in time IG is given to the moment of exposure. Unfortunately, a protection rate of 100 per cent is almost impossible to achieve. Because of the time lag between actual viral transmission and the development of overt illness, different contacts will have had variable time intervals from their exposure to the receipt of IG, and hence hepatitis might be too advanced in the incubation period for them to derive benefit from the IG. Cases of hepatitis that develop within seven to ten days of inoculation probably fall into this category.[850] It is generally accepted that IG can profitably be administered as long as two weeks after exposure. Mosley and Galambos have suggested that the interval can be extended to six weeks.[851] Suffice it to say that field trials in the United States and other countries have demonstrated remarkable efficacy when IG is used to prevent hepatitis A outbreaks. In the United States, the efficacy rate is reported to be 80 to 90 per cent;[852] in New Zealand, 80 per cent;[853] and in Britain, it is 84 to 87 per cent.[854]

The mechanism of action of IG has both theoretic and practical importance. It is believed that there are three different means whereby immunization can be achieved.[843] *Passive immunization* occurs as the result of transmission of sufficient quantities of neutralizing antibody to inhibit both clinical disease and subclinical infection. The result is that long-lasting immunity does not develop. *Active immunization* requires administration of inactivated antigen that induces development of specific antibody. This form of immunization does produce long-lasting immunity. A third type has been called *passive-active immunization*. For this to occur, there must be sufficient antibody transferred to attenuate but not to entirely prevent the disease. This must be accompanied also by an infecting exposure that produces a specific subclinical infection, followed by the development of endogenous long-lasting antibody. With regard to IG, evidence against active immunization as its mechanism of action in preventing hepatitis A has been derived from several studies. In one such study, Stokes and associates were able to induce hepatitis with infectious material in mentally retarded persons previously exposed to hepatitis and given IG.[843] In another study, Werhle and Hammon found equal incidences of hepatitis among persons who had been given IG and those who had been given gelatin several years earlier during a field trial of prophylaxis against poliomyelitis.[855] The argument against passive immunization has centered around the fact that IG evaluated in early studies appeared to be protective for as long as nine months—far exceeding the half-life of IG—and that rechallenging these individuals with infectious inocula induced hepatitis in a relatively small number.[843] Support for the concept of passive-active immunization has come from several studies. In these studies, exposed persons were selected to receive IG or to remain untreated and were then followed by aminotransferase testing to assess the frequency of development of hepatitis.[40] Although the incidences of hepatitis in the two groups were the same, the majority of cases of hepatitis in the IG recipients were subclinical. These observations have come mostly from experimental, and hence artificial, studies and therefore may not be entirely applicable to naturally acquired infection. Since anti-HAV titers in IG differ, as do the timings of administration schedules, it can be predicted that there will be different mechanisms of effect. Indeed, reanalysis of stored serum samples from a study conducted earlier by Krugman and colleagues seemed to confirm that there is variability in the mechanism of action of IG in preventing hepatitis A.[48] They found that clinical hepatitis developed in all 14 susceptible inmates of a home for the mentally retarded and that anti-HAV subsequently developed after they were given 0.1 ml of a 1:2 dilution of acute-phase serum from a child with hepatitis A. In contrast, clinical hepatitis did not develop in eight susceptible inmates given the acute-phase serum plus 0.2 ml/kg IG. However, two of these patients developed anti-HAV. Thus, two of the eight individuals (25 per cent) experienced only subclinical infection, the form of protection that occurs as a result of passive-active immunization, whereas six of eight patients (75 per cent) had neither clinical nor subclinical disease, findings compatible with the mechanism of passive immunization.

Prophylaxis of Hepatitis B

Confusion regarding the efficacy of immunoprophylaxis for hepatitis B began with the first studies. This was obviously a result of the inability to identify the presence of HBV, so the designation of cases as hepatitis B was often in error, and specific anti-HBs–containing globulin could not be chosen for use. Indeed, the earliest studies of hepatitis B prophylaxis were aimed at preventing post-transfusion hepatitis, in the mistaken belief that all such cases were hepatitis B,[856, 857] and it is therefore not surprising that the results were in conflict. The first controlled trial in recent times demonstrating an apparent efficacy of IG in preventing hepatitis B, which was conducted among United States soldiers stationed in Korea, was reported in 1971.[858] Participants in that trial were divided into four groups and selected to receive two injections of IG, five to seven months apart, in doses of 10 ml, 5 ml, or 2 ml, or to receive a placebo. The IG was later shown to contain modest titers of anti-HBs (1:1256 by radioimmunoassay).[859] HBsAg-positive and HBsAg-negative hepatitis developed significantly less frequently in recipients of the 10-ml and 5-ml doses than in subjects in the other two groups.[859a] In the same year, Prince and co-workers reported the development of a globulin product from a single donor with hemophilia that contained anti-HBs in a titer of 1:256,000 by passive hemagglutination.[860] This came to be known as HBIG. Krugman and associates, using this globulin preparation, showed that it was 60 to 70 per cent effective in preventing hepatitis B in children experimentally infected with HBV, whereas conventional IG provided 40 per cent protection.[46] The infection rate was 100 per cent in those given neither preparation. Other effects were that HBIG recipients who contracted hepatitis had prolonged incubation periods and a lower frequency of HBsAg carriage. In that study, HBIG appeared to be effective through the mechanism of passive-active immunization. The same HBIG preparation was again evaluated in another study, this time for the circumstance of endemically acquired hepatitis B, specifically that occurring in institutions for the mentally retarded.[861] In this double-blind study, HBIG was compared with conventional IG (prepared prior to 1972 and containing anti-HBs in a titer of 1:16), and a group of subjects who refused either injection was also studied. The conclusions reached were that the two globulin products were equally effective, that neither promoted the HBV carrier state, and that IG permitted passive-active immunization, whereas HBIG inhibited such immunization. On the basis of these provocative results, it was apparent that appropriately designed controlled trials were needed. During the decade of the 1970s, four pre-exposure and four postexposure prophylaxis studies were performed.[713, 714, 797, 862–866] Numerous other uncontrolled studies have also been performed.

Pertinent data from the four pre-exposure prophylaxis studies of HBIG for hepatitis B are shown in Table 37–11. All these studies involved patients and medical staff members in high-risk areas of the hospital, primarily the hemodialysis unit. In the study of Desmyter and colleagues,

TABLE 37–11. EFFICACIES OF IMMUNE GLOBULIN (IG) AND HEPATITIS B IMMUNE GLOBULIN (HBIG) IN PREVENTION OF HEPATITIS B PRE-EXPOSURE PROPHYLAXIS

Reference	Group Studied	No. Patients	Months Followed	Amount and No. of Injections	Incidence of Hepatitis B (Incidence of HBsAg) (%)		
					HBIG	IG	NIL
Desmyter et al.[862]	Dialysis patients	29	16	5 ml × 2	13.3 (13.3)	42.9* (71.4)	—
Iwarson et al.[863]	High-risk medical staff	235	28	3 ml × 2	1.7 (6.9)	3.8 (7.8)	10.4 —
Kleinknecht et al.[864]	Dialysis patients	28	14–30	3–5 ml × 9–17	0.0 (0.0)	—	77 (77)
Prince et al.[865]	Dialysis patients	284	12	3 ml × 2	12.1 (18.7)	14.1 (21.7)	—
	Dialysis staff	282	12	3 ml × 2	4.5 (5.6)	10.3 (11.3)	—

*IG with no detectable anti-HBs.

the HBIG used contained an anti-HBs titer of 1:25,000 as measured by passive hemagglutination (PHA), whereas the IG had no detectable anti-HBs.[862] Current IG with moderate titers and a true placebo were not tested. The investigators concluded that the HBIG had both modified and prevented hepatitis B. The HBIG in the study by Iwarson and co-workers contained anti-HBs titers of 1:355,000 by PHA and the titer in the IG was 1:100.[863] An untreated control group consisting of persons unwilling to receive either injection also participated. There was no significant difference between the two globulin products, both appearing effective when compared with the untreated but not randomly selected control group. Kleinknecht and associates randomly selected subjects to receive HBIG with a titer of 1:64,000 by PHA, leaving the control group untreated.[864] The HBIG was reported to be remarkably effective. In the study of Prince and colleagues, patients and medical staff members received one of three globulin preparations—one with a titer of 1:500,000 by PHA, one with a titer of 1:5000 by PHA, and one with a titer of 1:50 by PHA.[865] A true placebo was not used. Among the patients, the high-titered globulin was significantly more effective than were the other two globulins 8 months after randomization, but this changed to a nonsignificant difference at 12 months. Results for staff members were similar, but in this group the incidence of hepatitis at the end of the 12-month period was considerably lower in the recipients of the high-titered material when compared with the recipients of the low-titered material (4.5 versus 10.3 per cent), even though this difference also was not significant. They concluded that HBIG was not superior to IG in preventing the acquisition of hepatitis B by dialysis patients. The considerably lower incidence found in staff members treated with HBIG, coupled with the apparently prolonged incubation of the disease when it did occur, suggested to them that greater efficacy could probably be achieved by the use of multiple injections. By that time, it was already apparent that general preventive measures alone were useful in reducing the incidence of hemodialysis-associated hepatitis.[867]

The data from the four postexposure studies are shown in Table 37–12. Redeker and co-workers studied the sexual contacts of persons with acute hepatitis B, such contact having taken place within two to four weeks of onset of the illness.[797] Either HBIG (with anti-HBs titers of 1:200,000 by PHA) or IG (prepared from anti-HBs–negative plasma units) was administered by random selection within 7 to 30 days of the recognition of hepatitis in the partner. The data demonstrated a remarkably beneficial effect of HBIG. There were some misgivings about this study, however.[868] The particular concern that follow-up was too brief has since been addressed by Mosley, who reported unchanged results after the study patients had

undergone more prolonged evaluation.[869] The two studies evaluating the efficacy of HBIG in preventing hepatitis B following accidental needle-stick exposure have shown conflicting results. In the study by Grady and Lee, the globulin products tested were the same as those used by Prince and co-workers in their study in hemodialysis units.[713] The conclusion reached was that HBIG seemed only to extend the incubation period of hepatitis B and not to prevent it. In the Veterans Administration cooperative study, the HBIG used contained an anti-HBs titer of 1:100,000 by PHA, whereas the IG had no detectable anti-HBs.[714] Currently available IG and a true placebo were not included in the evaluation. The IG had been prepared in 1944 and kept in a lyophilized form until the initiation of the Veterans Administration cooperative study. The conclusion reached in this study was that the HBIG reduced the incidence of icteric hepatitis B significantly and that it also extended the incubation period. Of importance is that in these two needle-stick studies, the chance of transmission of hepatitis was significantly greater when the donor blood was both HBeAg- and HBsAg-positive.[794, 795] Also, in both studies, persons exposed by accidental needle-stick appeared to be protected against hepatitis if they were already anti-HBs– positive at the time of the accident. In the study of hepatitis transmitted from mothers to infants, conducted by Beasley and co-workers, a small dose of HBIG (PHA titer of 1:200,000) given within seven days of birth was compared with a larger dose of IG (with no detectable anti-HBs) and an albumin placebo.[866] No significant reduction in the incidence of hepatitis B was found in the infants, although the onset of hepatitis in HBIG recipients was markedly delayed. Also found was a reduction in the HBV carrier rate when HBIG was given within 48 hours of birth. As in the needle-stick studies, the most important determinant for transmission was the presence of HBeAg in the mother. Although HBIG was not significantly more effective than the other two products, the investigators were sufficiently impressed with the evidence of a reduction in the carrier rate following early inoculation that they were prompted to initiate a second trial.[869a] This one, a randomized, double-blind, placebo-controlled study, involved the administration of HBIG within hours of birth and again at three and six months of age. The results did not demonstrate a reduction in the overall infection rate, but it did confirm the decrease in the HBsAg carrier rate with a calculated efficacy of 71 per cent.

Several other uncontrolled but noteworthy trials deserve mention. In a study conducted in Britain under the auspices of a Combined Medical Research Council, all persons exposed by accidental needle-stick to HBsAg-positive material were given 500 mg HBIG within 14 days of the accident.[870] Acute hepatitis B developed in 3 per cent of the subjects, and anti-HBs developed in an additional 2

TABLE 37–12. EFFICACIES OF IMMUNE GLOBULIN (IG) AND HEPATITIS B IMMUNE GLOBULIN (HBIG) IN PREVENTION OF HEPATITIS B POSTEXPOSURE PROPHYLAXIS

Reference	Group Studied	No. Patients	Months Followed	Amount and No. of Injections	Incidence of Hepatitis B (Incidence of HBsAg) (%)		
					HBIG	IG	NIL
Redeker et al[797]	Sexual contacts	58	>5	5 ml × 1	4	27	—
Grady and Lee[713]	Accidental needle-stick	435	>9	3 ml × 2	9.8	12.3	—
Seeff et al.[714]	Accidental needle-stick	419	>9	5 ml × 2	1.4	5.9*	—
					(3.2)	(5.9)	
Beasley and Stevens[866]	Neonates	109	12	0.2 ml × 1	(55.9)	(75.0)*	(64.1)

*IG with no detectable anti-HBs.

per cent. The conclusion reached was that the results resembled those of the Veterans Administration needle-stick study, supporting the view that HBIG is protective. Six uncontrolled studies of immunoprophylaxis aimed at interrupting mother to infant transmission of HBV have also been reported. In four of them, HBIG appeared to be protective,[871-874] in the fifth a large dose of conventional IG appeared protective,[875] and in the sixth study, conventional IG provided no benefit.[876] Of the four studies that showed benefits from HBIG, one was a trial in which repeated doses of HBIG were administered.[874] The recipients first were given HBIG within 48 hours of birth in a dose of 0.5 ml/kg, followed by monthly doses of 0.16 ml/kg for a period of six months. This regimen afforded complete protection, even when the mother was HBeAg-positive. In this study, neonates of HBsAg-positive, HBeAg-positive mothers were randomized into one of three treatment groups. The first group received 1.0 ml of saline at birth and at three and six months; 94 per cent became infected and 91 per cent remained carriers. The second group was given 1.0 ml of HBIG within hours of birth and 1.0 ml of saline at three and six months; 79 per cent became infected and 50 per cent remained HBsAg-positive. The third group received 0.5 ml of HBIG diluted in 0.5 ml IG immediately after birth and again at three and six months; nevertheless, 75 per cent became infected, although only 23 per cent remained carriers, for an efficacy rate of 75 per cent. Thus, the study demonstrated unequivocally that HBIG in this setting prevented HBsAg rather than HBV infection, the response of passive-active immunization.

The positive studies have been analyzed carefully to determine the mechanism of action of HBIG. In one of these studies, conducted by Krugman and colleagues, HBIG was shown to attenuate but not entirely prevent hepatitis B, suggesting that passive-active immunization had resulted.[46, 47] In the Veterans Administration cooperative needle-stick study, it was believed originally that HBIG had acted by producing passive immunization, whereas IG was thought to have induced passive-active immunization against hepatitis B.[877] Earlier investigations by others had also suggested that IG was capable of preventing hepatitis B by the mechanism of passive-active immunization.[858, 861, 863] However, after additional testing of stored sera from the Veterans Administration study was undertaken and the data were reanalyzed, these conclusions were reversed.[878] With the addition of anti-HBc testing, it became apparent that the total incidence of HBV infection in the Veterans Administration study was the same regardless of whether the patients received IG or HBIG; only the incidence of overt hepatitis was significantly reduced by the HBIG. These new data suggested that HBIG had been effective through passive-active immunization. In contrast, the IG, which had been manufactured in 1944, was found by ultracentrifugation analysis to contain small amounts of HBsAg and could have behaved as an immunizing vaccine. Accordingly, it was suggested that the conclusion reached in the earlier two studies that IG had acted through passive-active immunization was probably incorrect, for the same reasons.[858, 861] The IG used in these studies had been prepared prior to 1972 and could therefore also have behaved as a modified vaccine. Indeed, this effect has since been demonstrated for one of these two IG preparations. Lemon and associates have reported that in re-evaluating the original IG used in the Korean study using new and sophisticated techniques, they were unable to detect anti-HBs as originally reported, but instead found small quantities of HBsAg and anti-HBc.[879] This supports the hypothesis that it probably did confer immunity by active rather than passive-active immunization.

Like IG, HBIG is licensed by the Bureau of Biologics, Food and Drug Administration. The current United States standard preparation has an anti-HBs titer of approximately 1:100,000. Recipients of this product are subject to the same adverse effects as those listed for IG. In addition, it has been suggested that HBIG given to HBsAg-positive persons has the potential for inducing an immune complex disorder.[636, 637, 880] Although no such complication has been reported, it is believed prudent to check the HBsAg status of all prospective HBIG recipients.[881] Another concern that had been expressed earlier was that HBIG might favor the development of the HBV carrier state. This has proved to be unfounded.

Prophylaxis of Post-transfusion and Non-A, Non-B Hepatitis

As mentioned earlier, studies of immunoprophylaxis of post-transfusion hepatitis conducted in the 1940s produced conflicting results. This prompted additional investigations in several countries, each group of investigators hoping to clarify the prevailing uncertainties. Since these studies, the data of which are summarized in Table 37–13, spanned a period of approximately 30 years, it is not surprising that uniformity of results was not achieved.[272, 275, 882-891] During this time there were many important advances, including improvements in medical technology, greater sophistication in the conduct of large-scale trials, the development of specific serologic tests, and the production of specific immunoglobulins. Other important pertinent items recognized during this 30-year period were that post-transfusion hepatitis and hepatitis B are not the same entity; that hepatitis A rarely causes post-transfusion hepatitis; and that another virus (or viruses) exists, which, following the introduction of HBsAg testing of donor blood and the consequent decline in hepatitis B, is now responsible for the majority of cases of post-transfusion hepatitis. A change in the anti-HBs levels of IG was also found during the course of the various studies. Since many of these facts were derived as a result of the studies, they could not be taken into account when designing the trials. Accordingly, none of the trials can now be considered to have been ideally designed. Only four of them were developed in fact as randomized, double-blind, controlled trials, and in these trials, different forms, doses, and schedules of immunoprophylaxis were tested.[272, 887, 891, 892]

Furthermore, only three studies (including two of the four just referred to) were conducted at times when it was possible to identify the existence of non-A, non-B hepatitis.[887, 891, 892] These three studies were the only ones in which HBIG was evaluated, but the majority of cases of post-transfusion hepatitis that developed in them were caused by the virus or viruses of non-A, non-B hepatitis.

The efficacy of the immunoglobulins in preventing the specific types of post-transfusion viral hepatitis can be determined from these four large studies.[272, 887, 891, 892] As shown in Table 37–14, none of them demonstrated any beneficial effect of IG in preventing the development of post-transfusion hepatitis B. The effects of HBIG could not be determined, since the studies in which they were evaluated began after post-transfusion hepatitis B had virtually disappeared as a result of routine HBsAg screening of all blood donors.

Three studies permit evaluation of the effects of im-

TABLE 37–13. EFFICACY OF IMMUNE GLOBULIN (IG) IN THE PREVENTION OF POST-TRANSFUSION HEPATITIS

Reference*	Study Design	No. Patients	Amount and No. of Injections	Mean No. of Transfusions	Incidence of Hepatitis (%)			
					Total		Icteric	
					NO TREATMENT	IG	NO TREATMENT	ISG
Grossman et al.[882]	—	768	10 ml × 2	NA	8.9	1.3†	—	—
Csapo et al.[883]	—	387	8 mg/kg × 1	5.5	7.3	0.6†	—	—
Mirick et al.[884]	I	1311	10 ml × 2–3	5.5	9.5	7.1	4.0	1.6†
Creutzfeldt et al.[885]	I	251	10 ml × 2	1.5	10.6	4.0†	2.0	0.0†
Katz et al.[886]	I	3989	10 ml × 1	2.1	1.7	1.4	0.9	0.3†
Knodell et al.[887]	R,D	279	10 ml × 1	12.0	13.8	6.0	8.5	1.1†
Seeff et al.[272]	I,R,D	2204	10 ml × 2	3.3	12.1	9.8	2.5	1.3†
Duncan et al.[888]	—	5780	10 ml × 1	NA	0.9	1.2	—	—
Holland et al.[889]	R	167	10 ml × 2	24.0	13.3	16.6	7.1	13.0
Spellberg and Berman[890]	I,R	100	10 ml × 2	3.8	19.1	22.6	8.5	5.6
Grady et al.[275]	R,D	5189	10 ml × 3	7.7	3.3	3.2	—	—
Kuhns et al.[891]	I,R,D	195	10 ml × 2	10.0	25.0	26.0	12.0	10.0

*In order of year of study and efficacy of IG.
†Significant difference.
I = intensive follow-up; R = randomized; D = double-blind; NA = not available.

munoprophylaxis of post-transfusion non-A, non-B hepatitis (Table 37–15).[272, 887, 891] In the study of Kuhns and colleagues, IG did not prevent the development of either anicteric or icteric hepatitis.[891] In the other two studies, one from the Walter Reed Army Institute of Research,[887] and the other from the Veterans Administration cooperative study,[272] IG did produce significant reductions, but only in icteric post-transfusion non-A, non-B hepatitis. In the first of these two studies,[887] IG was also found to significantly reduce the chances of progression from acute to chronic hepatitis.[299] In the Veterans Administration study, a striking association was found between the use of paid blood donors and the development of non-A, non-B hepatitis. Indeed, it was estimated that a greater reduction in icteric non-A, non-B hepatitis would have been achieved by eliminating paid blood donors than was actually achieved by the use of IG.[272]

On the basis of these collected data, it appears that IG confers no benefit in the prevention of post-transfusion hepatitis B; the data are insufficient to permit assessment of the use of HBIG for this purpose. However, the accrued information does suggest that IG, acting perhaps through passive-active immunization, has a partially beneficial effect (50 to 80 per cent) in preventing post-transfusion non-A, non-B hepatitis. Nevertheless, because of the uncertain nature of these data, the evidence that interdicting paid donor blood clearly reduces the frequency of non-A, non-B hepatitis and the promise of beneficial effects from the elimination of donor blood with raised ALT activity or detectable anti-HBc, there seems little enthusiasm for recommending IG as a routine pretransfusion procedure. There is, however, more support for its use in the setting of percutaneous exposure to potential viral-containing

serum, the Immunization Practices Advisory Committee suggesting the use of a single injection of IG (0.06 ml/kg body weight) in this circumstance.[840a] Additional support for this posture is derived from a recent reanalysis of the immunoprophylaxis study conducted in Korea between 1967 and 1970.[858] This recasting suggested that the pre-exposure administration of 5 or 10 ml of IG significantly reduced the frequency of acquisition of endemic non-A, non-B hepatitis.[859a] Resort to routine immunoprophylaxis might be considered in the future when tests for non-A, non-B hepatitis become available, since this will permit the development of a globulin product with specific antibodies directed against this type of hepatitis.

ACTIVE IMMUNOPROPHYLAXIS

HEPATITIS A

Both inactivated and attenuated vaccines have been developed. The first vaccine was prepared from marmoset livers that had been infected with the CR326 strain of HAV.[118, 118c] Partially purified HAV, extracted from the livers, was inactivated with formalin and then injected subcutaneously into marmosets at biweekly intervals for eight doses, producing protective antibody as demonstrated by challenge of the marmosets with live HAV. The same strain has been used to develop an immunogenic and protective vaccine in fetal rhesus kidney cells (FRhK6).[893, 894] More recently, a formalin-inactivated HAV vaccine, prepared in green monkey kidney cells, has been shown to be immunogenic as well as protective in owl monkeys.[895] A similar vaccine made from MRC-5 cells infected with the

TABLE 37–14. EFFICACIES OF IMMUNE GLOBULIN (IG) AND HEPATITIS B IMMUNE GLOBULIN (HBIG) IN PREVENTION OF POST-TRANSFUSION HEPATITIS B

Reference	No. of Patients	HBsAg Screening Radioimmunoassay	Incidence of Post-transfusion Hepatitis B (%)		
			Placebo	IG	HBIG
Kuhns et al.[891]	195	No	7.8	7.5	—
Knodell et al.[887]	279	No	1.1	1.1	0.0
Seeff et al.[272]	2204	No	2.6	2.1	—
Seeff et al.[892]	969	Yes	—	0.4	0.4

TABLE 37–15. EFFICACY OF IMMUNE GLOBULIN (IG) IN THE PREVENTION OF POST-TRANSFUSION NON-A, NON-B, HEPATITIS

Reference	No. Patients	Incidence of Non-A, Non-B Hepatitis (%)			
		Anicteric		Icteric	
		PLACEBO	IG	PLACEBO	IG
Kuhns et al.[891]	195	8.8	11.8	7.8	6.4
Knodell et al.[887]	279	5.3	4.9	7.4	1.1*
Seeff et al.[272]	2204	7.7	6.9	1.8	0.8*

*Significant difference, P < 0.05.

HM-175 strain of HAV has been found to be safe and immunogenic in studies of human volunteers.[896, 897] Nevertheless, for a number of reasons, including cost, attention is being directed toward the development of attenuated vaccines.[895] Several efforts are in progress toward the development of such a vaccine.[898–903] The first was made possible by the success in generating numerous variants of HAV from the CR326 and CR326F strains through passage in FRhK6 and MRC-5 cell cultures.[898–900] Selected variants, particularly the more highly passaged ones, when inoculated into marmosets and chimpanzees, exhibited reduced virulence and protected the animals against challenge with virulent HAV. Efforts continue in the search for ideal replicating variants that do not produce liver cell necrosis and that stimulate protective antibody, but the work is handicapped by the lack of a specific marker for attenuation. It can be anticipated that recombinant gene technology will permit the development of genetically engineered hepatitis A vaccines. The genome of HAV has been cloned, and work on nucleotide sequencing is in progress.[904–907] A number of novel approaches are being considered, aided considerably by new techniques that can produce larger amounts of HAV than have been generated by current systems for cell culture.[908, 909]

HEPATITIS B

The studies that pioneered the development of the hepatitis B vaccine were those undertaken in the early 1970s by Krugman and colleagues.[44, 45, 47, 51] These investigators administered to susceptible subjects serum known to be infectious for hepatitis B, which was diluted 1:10 and boiled at 98° C for 1 minute, and they found that it induced production of anti-HBs. Approximately 70 per cent of the individuals inoculated were either completely or partially protected against subsequent challenge with live HBV. Thus, despite the fact that HBV could not be cultured at that time, the evidence that the immunizing antigen appeared to be the 22-nm HBsAg particle permitted the development of a vaccine by extracting and purifying HBsAg from carriers.

PRODUCTION OF CURRENTLY AVAILABLE VACCINES IN THE UNITED STATES

The first commercially available hepatitis B vaccine was produced by Merck, Sharp & Dohme by plasmapheresing HBV carriers and then subjecting the pooled plasma to a number of biophysical procedures.[910, 911] The technique employed then and still applied to the plasma-derived vaccine used currently in the United States is as follows: the serum pool is defibrinated with calcium and is concentrated with ammonium sulfate precipitation, following which it is subjected to isopyknic banding with sodium bromide and rate zonal sedimentation through a sucrose gradient. The latter two steps remove 10^4 chimpanzee infectious doses (CID) of HBV/ml. Three virus-inactivating steps are then applied—(1) pepsin digestion at pH 2.1 and a temperature of 37° C, (2) treatment with 8M urea, and (3) treatment with formalin 1:4000. These three procedures each inactivate 10^5 or more CID of HBV/ml as well as all known groups of animal viruses,[912, 913] including HIV.[914] Finally, aluminum hydroxide is added as an adjuvant, together with thimerosal, 1:20,000, a preservative. Many other plasma-derived vaccines have since been developed in other countries by differing techniques and have been found to be equally, and in some instances even more, immunogenic.[913–918]

Production of the recombinant vaccine begins with the isolation of the gene that codes for HBsAg (the S gene) from an HBV DNA fragment. A plasmid is then constructed that contains the S gene, which can be cloned in either *Escherichia coli* or common bakers' yeast (*Saccharomyces cerevisiae*).[919, 920] The commercially produced vaccine employs yeast for this purpose because of its superior gene expression.[921] The inserted HBsAg (subtype *adw*) undergoes continuous replication, at which time it is harvested by yeast cell disruption after which it is purified through two chromatography steps (hydrophobic adsorption and size exclusion). The product is then subjected to sterile filtration and is inactivated with formaldehyde. Finally, like the plasma vaccine, aluminum hydroxide is added as an adjuvant, and the preservative thimerosal is also added. The recombinant vaccine differs from the plasma vaccine in that it contains slightly smaller particles (17 to 25 nm) and it is not glycosylated (25 per cent of the plasma vaccine is glycosylated). Up to 4 per cent yeast protein may be detected, but there is no yeast DNA.

Immunogenicity

Early studies with the vaccine were directed toward determining safety and immunogenicity in both chimpanzees and humans.[913, 914, 922–924] The measure of immunogenicity is the development of anti-HBs alone, since vaccine production excludes the actual HBV, leaving only the noninfectious HBsAg particles as the immunizing agent. (The development of anti-HBc indicates actual infection.)

Although a number of small trials were first undertaken among health care workers, the studies that clearly established immunogenicity and efficacy of the plasma vaccine were two trials conducted in the United States that involved homosexual men and hemodialysis staff members.[925–927] In the first study, which was a classic double-blind, controlled trial, 549 homosexual men received three injections of hepatitis B vaccine, and 534 homosexual men received a placebo, in doses of 40 μg each at zero, one, and six months.

Subjects were evaluated for a period of one year.[925] Anti-HBs was detected in 76.2 per cent of the subjects at the end of one month, in 78 per cent of the subjects at the end of two months, and in 95.4 per cent at the end of six months. Among this latter group, the degree of response was good (>20 ratio units [RU]) in 90.5 per cent of subjects, fair (10 to 20 RU) in 2.9 per cent of subjects, and poor (2.2 to 10 RU) in 2 per cent of subjects. Ratio units are calculated by comparing net counts/minute of the ^{125}I–anti-HBs that remains attached to HBsAg at the end of the radioimmunoassay procedure in the test sample (test sample counts/minute minus background counts/minute) with the counts/minute of the negative mean control. A positive result requires the counts/minute of the test sample to exceed the counts/minute of the negative sample by a factor of 2.1. Similar results were noted in the second trial involving homosexual men, except that the seroconversion rate following the third injection was only 85 per cent.[926] This lower rate of immunogenicity was attributed later to decreased potency of the vaccine secondary to storage in the frozen state, which induces granular precipitation and an enhanced rate of settling.[928] Accordingly, it is now required that the vaccine be stored at 2° to 6° C and not frozen. The trial among staff members of hemodialysis units, in whom a seroconversion rate of 96 per cent was found, confirmed the results of the first two studies.

A series of investigations followed to determine the degree of immunogenicity of the plasma vaccine in a variety of populations.[929] Emerging from these investigations were several conclusions. First, immunogenicity was high (>95 per cent) in all immunocompetent adult populations. Second, an excellent response was noted in infants and neonates given as little as 10 μg of vaccine, the rates ranging between 95 and 100 per cent,[930–932] which was an unusual response in neonates given other vaccines. Third, immunodeficient populations, such as hemodialysis and transplant patients, showed a poor rate of seroconversion (<65 per cent), even when given vaccine in doses twice those used in otherwise normal persons.[933–937] Fourth, women appeared more likely than men to mount an immune response, also achieving higher anti-HBs titers.[934, 938] These last conclusions have been disputed.[939] Finally, receipt of the injection in the buttock appeared to be associated with a lesser frequency of seroconversion than after injection into the deltoid muscle (in the adult) or lateral part of the thigh (in the infant), presumably because the large volume of fat in the buttock impedes mobilization of the vaccine.[940]

The immunogenicity of the recombinant vaccine, with respect both to frequency of immune response and the titer of anti-HBs achieved, has been reported to be only a little less or quite similar to that of the plasma vaccine.[941–946] Furthermore, the biologic quality of the anti-HBs induced by both vaccines seems identical.[921, 947] Thus the two vaccines appear to be interchangeable.

Duration of Antibody Persistence

Information regarding the duration of antibody persistence is sparse at present. In the one major study bearing on this question, homosexual men who participated in one of the early trials were re-evaluated five years after completion of the vaccination process.[926, 948] Among the subjects whose maximal response exceeds 9.9 RU, 15 per cent no longer had detectable anti-HBs by five years; an additional 27 per cent had levels that had fallen to less than 10 RU. If the peak level had been between 10 and 49 RU, the

antibody retention rate would have been only 30 per cent; if it had risen to about 100 RU, 93 per cent would still test positive at five years. These data attest to the importance of the third (booster) dose of vaccine, which is especially responsible for the increase in antibody titer.

Vaccine Efficacy

The high immunogenicity rate of the vaccine in non-immunocompromised individuals is paralleled by its remarkable protective efficacy in them. In one study involving homosexual men who received three doses of vaccine of 40 μg each, the second dose was given one month after the first and the third dose was given six months after the first.[925] The calculated efficacy rate for all HBV events was 81.4 per cent, whereas for clinical hepatitis B it was 92.1 per cent. When these calculations were applied only to individuals who had received all three doses and in whom a good antibody response (>10 RU) had developed, the rates increased to 94.9 and 100 per cent, respectively. Indeed, the development of HBV events in recipients of all three doses was confined in all but one instance to persons who were either nonresponders or weak responders. The HBV event in the single individual with a good response consisted of the development of anti-HBc only. Also noteworthy in this study was the evidence that the vaccine appeared to modify the illness that was already incubating when the first dose was administered, suggesting that the vaccine may be of some value for postexposure prophylaxis. Almost identical results were noted in a second trial among homosexual men who received 20-μg doses of vaccine (the calculated efficacy rate among those who produced anti-HBs of at least 10 RU being 98 per cent),[926] as well as in a trial involving staff members of hemodialysis units in the United States.[927] The latter study demonstrated another important finding, namely, that the vaccine used, of subtype ad, was equally effective in protecting against ad and ay HBV events, suggesting that it is antibody to the common a determinant that produces cross-protection.

Immunocompromised persons appear to be far less well protected. In a randomized, double-blind, placebo-controlled study that involved hemodialysis patients given 40 μg doses of the vaccine in the usual schedule,[938] approximately 50 per cent responded with adequate antibody production. The incidence of hepatitis over the following 25 months was the same, however, in recipients of vaccine and placebo; vaccine recipients who developed hepatitis either showed diminishing or nonexistent antibody production or were receiving immunosuppressive treatment. Similarly disappointing responses are noted in oncology patients treated with chemotherapy.[949]

Passive-Active Immunization

The particularly serious impact of perinatally transmitted hepatitis B has focused attention on the need to prevent maternal-infant transmission. Because studies with HBIG or the vaccine alone appear to provide only partial protection (70 to 75 per cent protective efficacy),[869a, 950–953] in part as a result of the delayed immune response, studies were undertaken to evaluate prophylaxis using both HBIG and the hepatitis B vaccine,[954, 955] so-called passive-active immunization. The evidence that the combination of the two agents produced appropriate protection without interfering with the immunogenic effects of each separately has led to a series of studies using this regimen for interruption of perinatal transmission.[869a, 950–953, 956, 957] The combination has markedly improved the efficacy rate to 90 to 95 per cent, reducing the carrier rate in newborns of HBeAg-positive mothers from an anticipated 90 per cent to 5 to 10 per cent. As a result, passive-active immunization has become the standard approach for postexposure prophylaxis, namely, perinatal and needle-stick exposure, and it is optional for sexual contact.

There are, at present, no trials of efficacy in adults with the recombinant vaccine. However, the high rate of immunogenicity, the evidence that vaccinated chimpanzees are protected when challenged with HBsAg, and the high protective efficacy rate (94 per cent) noted in studies of perinatal hepatitis together indicate that the efficacy of the recombinant vaccine equals that of the plasma vaccine.[957]

Safety

Both the plasma and the recombinant vaccines have a high margin of safety. In the original controlled trials of the plasma vaccine, the reported adverse reactions, occurring in about 20 per cent of recipients, were noted with equal frequency among recipients of the placebo, with the exception that pain at the injection site was reported more frequently in the vaccine recipients. The side effects have been relatively mild, consisting of arm soreness, fatigue, malaise, mild fever (<38° C), chills, headache, dizziness, myalgias, anorexia, nausea, rarely vomiting, abdominal cramps, and rash. The early concern regarding the development of the Guillain-Barré syndrome and the rare instances of other neurologic syndromes (e.g., aseptic meningitis, transverse myelitis, grand mal seizures) has faded because the frequency of these manifestations is no greater than in the general population. As noted earlier,[912–914] the inactivation steps applied in the production of the plasma vaccine are adequate for the eradication of all known viruses, including HIV-1, HIV-2, and HIV-3.

Long-term Booster Dose

The need for booster doses of vaccine beyond five years has not been fully established. Current data are derived primarily from one study in which vaccinated persons were followed for five years after completion of their vaccination schedule.[948] In this re-evaluation, anti-HBs was found to be lost entirely in 15 per cent of subjects and to have declined to less than 10 RU in an additional 27 per cent of vaccinees, an antibody attrition rate that is somewhat higher than that of another study performed in the United States with the same vaccine.[958] Subsequent infection was inversely related to the maximal anti-HBs level achieved: HBV infection occurred in 16.7 per cent of those in whom any anti-HBs developed, in 9 per cent of those whose peak levels were between 2.1 and 9.9 RU, in 9 per cent of those with levels of 10 to 49 RU, in 2.7 per cent of those with levels between 50 and 99 RU, and in 0.74 per cent of those whose levels exceeded 100 RU. Moreover, the same inverse relationship was noted between the degree of anti-HBs response and the severity of the infection that ensued: the rare events in the good responders consisted almost entirely of serologic rather than clinically manifested HBV infection. This suggests that good responders may remain protected even though evidence of humoral immunity wanes or disappears. These data contrast with those

from another study involving children living in a highly endemic area of the world.[959] In this uncontrolled study, previously vaccinated children were either revaccinated one year after completion of their initial series and then followed for an additional six years or were followed without receiving the booster dose. Hepatitis B occurred at a rate of 1.5 per cent/year in the former group and at a rate of 11.5 per cent/year in the latter group; all the infections of the former group developed in the fifth year. From this, the authors inferred that a second booster dose is required five years after the first.

Revaccination of Nonresponders

Only moderate success follows revaccination of nonresponders or poor responders.[948] In nonresponders, a three-dose revaccination series induced a good response (>10 RU) in 41 per cent of instances, but only 8 per cent of subjects maintained this response 18 months later. Revaccination of poor responders produced slightly better results; 79 per cent responded well to the third dose of vaccine and 29 per cent retained good levels of antibody 18 months later.

Alternative Vaccines

Efforts continue to develop vaccines that (1) bypass the need to rely on large numbers of human donors, (2) can be delivered in a more effective and convenient manner, and (3) will cost less to produce.[960] Attention has focused on the use of HBsAg derived from hepatoma cell lines,[961] the continued exploitation of recombinant DNA technology,[962, 963] efforts to further purify and enhance the immunogenicity of HBsAg,[964–971] and attempts to develop synthetic vaccines.[972–976]

CURRENT RECOMMENDATIONS FOR IMMUNOPROPHYLAXIS OF VIRAL HEPATITIS

HEPATITIS A

Passive

Prevention of hepatitis A begins with adherence to good sanitary habits coupled with avoidance of circumstances that promote transmission. Use of IG is recommended in certain circumstances (Table 37–16). It should be administered as soon as possible after exposure but preferably no later than two weeks after.[977] International travelers are now the prime target for pre-exposure prophylaxis; past recommendations also included persons working with nonhuman primates.[978] This may not be necessary if strict sanitation practices are applied. The primary group for postexposure prophylaxis is household contacts of an individual with acute illness. Although early administration increases the likelihood of protection, and efficacy beyond two weeks may be diminished, there are some authorities who have advocated its use as late as six weeks after exposure.[979] Another important circumstance for postexposure prophylaxis is outbreaks in day care centers, for which passive prophylaxis has been shown to be effective.[980] A consideration for all these situations is to prescreen the potential inoculee for anti-HAV, which if present precludes the need for prophylaxis.

TABLE 37–16. IMMUNE GLOBULIN (IG) FOR PREVENTION OF HEPATITIS A. RECOMMENDATIONS OF THE CENTERS FOR DISEASE CONTROL IMMUNIZATION PRACTICES ADVISORY COMMITTEE

Recommended for use	Type of Exposure	Circumstances of Exposure	Dose (ml/kg)	Frequency of Administration
Yes	Post-exposure	Contact with persons with acute hepatitis A All household and sexual contacts Day-care centers Institutions for mentally handicapped Prisons	0.02	Once
	Pre-exposure	Travelers to endemic areas outside of usual travel routes		
		≤2 months	0.02	Once
		>2 months	0.06	Every 5 months
		Handlers of imported primates	0.05	Every 4–6 months
No	Post-exposure	Casual school, hospital, office, factory Common source (food, water) unless identified in 2 wk		

Active

No vaccine is available for active immunization against hepatitis A at present. When it is released it will be useful for high-risk groups, such as regular travelers to endemic areas, certain institutionalized persons, children in day care centers, homosexual men, and military populations. General childhood immunization might also be considered.[895]

HEPATITIS B

Passive

Prior to the advent of the hepatitis B vaccine, HBIG was recommended as postexposure prophylaxis in the following circumstances: needle-stick (permucosal), maternal-neonatal (perinatal), and sexual exposures. Now that the vaccine is available, and in view of the short-lived immunity conferred by HBIG alone, combined passive-active immunization is considered the preferable method of prophylaxis. Indeed, this method is currently mandatory for perinatal exposure and will remain so unless vaccine immunogenicity can be greatly increased. If it is decided that passive prophylaxis alone should be used for the other two circumstances, the schedule is for percutaneous exposure—HBIG, 0.06 ml/kg body weight as soon as possible within 7 days of exposure and again 25 to 30 days later; for sexual contact—HBIG, 0.06 ml/kg within 14 days of contact.

Active

The Immunization Practices Advisory Committee, CDC, recommends certain groups receive vaccine prophylaxis, with or without HBIG (Table 37–17).[977, 978, 981] In the view of the CDC Advisory Committee, prophylaxis is deemed a recommendation for the groups in the table shown without parentheses but only a consideration for those shown in parentheses.

Among health care workers, the risk is higher in persons who have direct contact with blood, blood products, or other body fluids, (e.g., medical and dental surgeons, pathologists, technicians, emergency room staff, phlebotomists, hemodialysis nurses) than in those whose contact with blood is minimal (e.g., medical residents, ward nurses, psychiatrists, hospital administrative staff). Multitransfused groups at risk include hemophiliacs, persons with other clotting disorders, patients with refractory anemias, and

those with leukemias. All individuals who are susceptible should receive vaccine alone at zero, one, and six months in the doses listed in Table 37–18. Note the differing doses based on age, immune status of recipient, and type of vaccine (plasma or recombinant).

Postexposure prophylaxis for a needle stick is a complex situation. The following format has been devised by the Immunization Practices Advisory Committee:[977]

I. Unvaccinated Inoculee
   A. Source HBsAg-Positive: Give one dose of HBIG (0.06 ml/kg) immediately, but no later than seven days after exposure. Initiate hepatitis B vaccination in the usual three doses (plasma vaccine, 20 μg for adults, 10 μg for children; recombinant vaccine, 10 μg for adults, 5 μg for children).
   B. Known High-risk Source: Begin hepatitis B vaccine series and then test the source. If result is positive, administer one dose of HBIG.

TABLE 37–17. PERSONS RECOMMENDED FOR HEPATITIS B PROPHYLAXIS (VACCINE OR HBIG, OR BOTH) IN THE UNITED STATES*

Route of Exposure	Type of Exposure	
	Pre-exposure	Postexposure
Percutaneous	Health care workers Hemodialysis patients Parenteral narcotic addicts Regular blood recipients	Needle-stick exposure
Perinatal		Infants born to HBsAg-positive mothers
Sexual	Homosexually active men (Heterosexual contacts of HBsAg carriers)†	Sexual contacts of persons with acute hepatitis B
Miscellaneous	Clients, staff of institutions for mentally handicapped Household contacts of HBsAg carriers High-risk populations, e.g., Alaskan Eskimos, immigrants from Southeast Asia (Inmates of prisons)† (travelers to hepatitis B endemic areas)†	

*Source: Adapted from Stevens CE, Taylor PE. Sem Liver Dis 6:23, 1986, and the CDC Immunization Practices Advisory Committee.[977, 981]

†Vaccine listed as a consideration for these groups and as a recommendation for all the other groups.

TABLE 37–18. RECOMMENDED DOSE SCHEDULE FOR HEPATITIS B IMMUNOPROPHYLAXIS*

Type of Prophylaxis	Regimen	Dose	Schedule
Pre-exposure			
Adults	Plasma vaccine	20 µg IM	0, 1 and 6 months
	Recombinant vaccine	10 µg IM	0, 1 and 6 months
Children	Plasma vaccine	10 µg IM	0, 1 and 6 months
	Recombinant vaccine	5 µg IM	0, 1 and 6 months
Postexposure			
Adults	HBIG	0.06 ml/kg IM	Once
Neonates	HBIG	0.05 ml IM	Once at birth
Adults	Plasma vaccine	20 µg IM	Within 7–14 days and 1 and 6 months
	Recombinant vaccine	10 µg IM	Within 7–14 days and 1 and 6 months
Neonates	Plasma vaccine	10 µg IM	Within 7 days and 1 and 6 months
	Recombinant vaccine	5 µg IM	Within 7 days and 1 and 6 months

*Source: Adapted from Stevens CE, Taylor PE. Sem Liver Dis 6:23, 1986; Centers for Disease Control. Ann Int Med 107:353, 1987.

C. Known Low-risk Source: Begin hepatitis B vaccine series.

D. Unknown Source: Begin hepatitis B vaccine series.

II. Vaccinated Inoculee

A. Source HBsAg-positive: Test the inoculee for anti-HBs and if result is negative or less than 10 RU, administer HBIG immediately, together with a booster vaccine dose.

B. Known High-risk Source: Test source if inoculee is a known vaccine nonresponder. Give one dose of HBIG plus booster vaccine if source is HBsAg-positive.

C. Known Low-risk Source: No response.

D. Unknown Source: No response.

Perinatal exposure constitutes a special and critically important focus for immunoprophylaxis. All infants born to HBsAg-positive mothers, regardless of the HBeAg status, should receive appropriate protection. Current CDC recommendations indicate that women in known high-risk categories should have HBsAg testing during their prenatal visits in order to plan for immediate intervention if necessary. Recent reports indicating that women considered to be at low risk in fact test positive more frequently than anticipated has led to the authoritative suggestion that all pregnant women be tested routinely during the third trimester of pregnancy as close to the time of delivery as possible.[982–984] Exposed infants should receive HBIG, 0.5 ml/kg intramuscularly no later than 12 hours and preferably within 1 hour after birth. At the same time, plasma vaccine, 10 µg, or recombinant vaccine, 5 µg, should be administered also within 12 hours but no later than 7 days, to be repeated at one and six months.

Other circumstances of exposure listed in the table follow the routine vaccination schedule.

Pre- and Postvaccination Screening

Because of cost-estimate concerns,[979, 985] serologic testing prior to vaccination is believed warranted only for high-risk groups, such as homosexual men, parenteral drug addicts, persons of Asian origin, and so on. Although there is some controversy regarding the appropriate antibody to measure—anti-HBs or anti-HBc—most authorities select anti-HBs, accepting a result in excess of 10 RU as evidence of immunity. Given the fact that there is sometimes difficulty in interpreting the serologic findings following vaccination, the Immunization Practices Advisory Committee nevertheless accedes to postvaccination screening to aid in the decision regarding the need for booster doses. However, on the basis of present knowledge, they consider it unnecessary to administer routine booster doses at the end of five years in the immunocompetent person, even if anti-HBs levels have waned. In contrast, persons with immune deficiencies (e.g., hemodialysis patients) should receive a booster dose if the antibody level falls to less than 10 RU.

Finally, it must be noted that no adverse effect follows vaccine administration to HBsAg carriers or to those with pre-existing anti-HBs.[986] Also, in view of the serious consequences of infection in pregnant women, the fact that the vaccine is devoid of infectious virus, and the lack of evidence of unusual adverse reactions in these women, pregnancy does not constitute a contraindication to the use of hepatitis B vaccine.

DELTA HEPATITIS

No immunoprophylaxis for delta hepatitis is available, nor is it necessary if hepatitis B can be avoided in view of the total dependence of the delta virus on the presence of hepatitis B.

NON-A, NON-B HEPATITIS

The lack of a viral marker in this viral disease has hindered the development of specific preventive agents. However, in view of the equivocally positive data in the setting of post-transfusion hepatitis caused by this agent, the Immunization Practices Advisory Committee has concluded that the use of IG (0.06 ml/kg) as soon as possible after percutaneous exposure is a reasonable response.[977] Other circumstances in which IG prophylaxis for non-A, non-B hepatitis should be considered an option include perinatal and sexual exposure.[987, 988]

REFERENCES

1. Zuckerman AJ. Twenty-five centuries of viral hepatitis. Rush-Presbyterian-St. Lukes Med Bull 15:57, 1976.
2. Cockayne EA. Catarrhal jaundice, sporadic and epidemic, and its relation to acute yellow atrophy of the liver. Q J Med 6:1, 1912.
3. Bamberger H. Krankheiten des chylopoetischen Systems. Erlangen, Virchow's Handbuch der Pathologie und Therapie, 5, 1858.
4. Virchow R. Uber das Vorkommen und den Nachweis des Hepatogenen, insbesondere des Katarrhalischen Icterus. Virchows Arch Pathol Anat 32:117, 1865.

5. Heitler M. Zur Klinik des Ikterus Katarrhalis. Wien Klin Wochenschr 37:957, 1887.
6. Flindt N. Bemaerkninger med Hensyn til den Saakaldte Katarralske Ikterus's Aetiologi og Genese. Bibl F Laeger 7:420, 1890.
7. McDonald S. Acute yellow atrophy. Edinburgh Med J 15:208, 1918.
8. Blumer GB. Infectious jaundice in the United States. JAMA 81:353, 1923.
9. Williams H. Epidemic jaundice in New York State, 1921–1922. JAMA 80:532, 1923.
10. Pickles WN. Epidemiology in Country Practice. Bristol, John Wright and Sons Ltd 1939:331.
11. Havens WP Jr, Ward R, Drill VA, et al. Experimental production of hepatitis by feeding ictogenic materials. Proc Soc Exp Biol Med 57:206, 1944.
12. MacCallum FO, Bradley WH. Transmission of infective hepatitis to human volunteers. Lancet 2:228, 1944.
13. Paul JR, Havens WP Jr, Sabin AB, et al. Transmission experiments in serum jaundice and infectious hepatitis. JAMA 128:911, 1945.
14. Neefe JR, Gellis SS, Stokes J Jr. Homologous (serum) hepatitis and infectious (epidemic) hepatitis: studies of volunteers bearing on immunological and other characteristics of the etiological agents. Am J Med 1:3, 1946.
15. Roholm K, Iversen P. Changes in the liver in acute epidemic hepatitis (catarrhal jaundice) based on 38 aspiration biopsies. Acta Pathol Microbiol Scand 16:29, 1939.
16. Karmen A, Wroblewski F, LaDue JS. Transaminase activity in human blood. J Clin Invest 34:126, 1955.
17. Wroblewski F, LaDue JS. Serum glutamic oxalacetic transaminase activity as an index of liver cell injury. A preliminary report. Ann Intern Med 43:345, 1955.
18. Lurman A. Eine icterus epidemic. Berlin Klin Wochenschr 22:20, 1885.
19. Koff RS. Non-A, Non-B viral hepatitis. In: Koff RS, ed. Viral Hepatitis. New York, John Wiley & Sons 1978:35.
20. Flaum A, Malmros H, Persson E. Eine Moscocomiale Ikterus Epidemic. Acta Med Scand (Suppl) 16:54, 1926.
21. Droller H. An outbreak of hepatitis in a diabetic clinic. Br Med J 1:623, 1945.
22. Sherwood PM. Outbreak of syringe-transmitted hepatitis with jaundice in hospitalized diabetic patients. Ann Intern Med 33:380, 1950.
23. Soffer LJ. Post-arsphenamine jaundice. Am J Syph Gonorrhea Vener Dis 21:309, 1937.
24. Bigger JW. Jaundice in syphilitics under treatment. Lancet 1:457, 1943.
25. MacCollum FO. Transmission of arsenotherapy jaundice by blood. Lancet 1:342, 1945.
26. Sawyer WA, Meyer KF, Eaton MD. Jaundice in army personnel in the western region of the United States and its relation to vaccination against yellow fever. Am J Hyg 39:337, 1944.
27. Findlay GM, MacCallum FO. Note on acute hepatitis and yellow fever immunization. Trans R Soc Trop Med J 31:297, 1937.
27a. Seeff LB, Beebe GW, Hoofnagle JH, et al. A serologic follow-up of the 1942 epidemic of post-vaccinal hepatitis in the United States Army. N Engl J Med 36:965, 1987.
28. Beeson PB. Jaundice occurring one to four months after transfusion of blood or plasma. Report of 7 cases. JAMA 121:1332, 1943.
29. Morgan HV, Williamson DAJ. Jaundice following administration of human blood products. Br Med J 1:750, 1943.
30. Voeght H. Zur aetiologie der Hepatitis epidemica. Munchen Med Wochenschr 89:76, 1942.
31. Cameron JDA. Infective hepatitis. Q J Med 12:139, 1943.
32. Stokes J Jr, Neefe JR. The prevention and attenuation of infectious hepatitis by gamma globulin. JAMA 127:144, 1945.
33. Gellis SS, Stokes J Jr, Brother GM. The use of human immune serum globulin (gamma globulin) in infectious (epidemic) hepatitis in the Mediterranean theater of operations. I. Studies on prophylaxis in two epidemics of infectious hepatitis. JAMA 128:1062, 1945.
34. Havens WP Jr, Paul JR. Prevention of infectious hepatitis with gamma globulin. JAMA 129:270, 1945.
35. Stokes J Jr, Berk JE, Malamut LL, et al. The carrier state in viral hepatitis. JAMA 154:1059, 1954.
36. Neefe JR, Norris RF, Reingold JG, et al. Carriers of hepatitis virus in the blood and viral hepatitis in whole blood recipients. I. Studies on donors suspected as carriers of hepatitis virus and as sources of post-transfusion hepatitis. JAMA 154:1066, 1954.
37. MacCallum FO. Infectious hepatitis. Lancet 2:435, 1947.
38. Ward R, Krugman S, Giles JP, et al. Infectious hepatitis: studies of its natural history and prevention. N Engl J Med 258:407, 1958.
39. Krugman S, Ward R, Giles JP, et al. Infectious hepatitis: detection of virus during the incubation period and in clinically inapparent infections. N Engl J Med 261:729, 1959.
40. Krugman W, Ward R, Giles JP. Infectious hepatitis: studies on the effect of gamma globulin and on the incidence of inapparent infection. JAMA 174:823, 1960.

41. Krugman S, Ward R, Giles JP. The natural history of infectious hepatitis. Am J Med 32:717, 1962.
42. Krugman S, Giles JP, Hammond J. Infectious hepatitis: evidence for two distinctive clinical, epidemiological, and immunological types of infection. JAMA 200:365, 1967.
43. Krugman S, Giles JP. Viral hepatitis: new light on an old disease. JAMA 212:1019, 1970.
44. Krugman S, Giles JP, Hammond JP. Hepatitis virus: effect of heat on the infectivity and antigenicity of the MS-1 and MS-2 strain. J Infect Dis 122:432, 1970.
45. Krugman S, Giles JP, Hammond J. Viral hepatitis, type B (MS-2 strain): studies on active immunization. JAMA 217:41, 1971.
46. Krugman S, Giles JP, Hammond J. Viral hepatitis, type B (MS-2 strain): prevention with specific hepatitis B immune serum globulin. JAMA 218:1655, 1971.
47. Krugman S, Giles JP. Viral hepatitis, type B (MS-2 strain): further observations on natural history and prevention. N Engl J Med 288:755, 1973.
48. Krugman S. Effect of immune serum globulin on infectivity of hepatitis A virus. J Infect Dis 134:70, 1976.
49. Krugman S, Hoofnagle JH, Gerety RJ, et al. Viral hepatitis, type B: DNA polymerase activity and antibody to hepatitis B core antigen. N Engl J Med 290:1331, 1974.
50. Krugman S, Friedman H, Lattimer C. Viral hepatitis, type A: identification by specific complement fixation and immune adherence tests. N Engl J Med 292:1141, 1975.
51. Krugman S, Overby CR, Mushahwar IK, et al. Viral hepatitis type B: studies on the natural history and prevention re-examined. N Engl J Med 300:101, 1979.
52. Zuckerman AJ. Attempts to isolate the hepatitis virus by tissue culture methods. In: Virus Diseases of the Liver. London, Butterworths, 1970:46.
53. Provost PJ, Hilleman MR. Propagation of human hepatitis A virus in cell culture in vitro. Proc Soc Exp Biol Med 160:213, 1979.
54. Hillis WD. An outbreak of infectious hepatitis among chimpanzee handlers at a United States Air Force base. Am J Hyg 73:316, 1961.
55. Deinhardt F, Holmes AW, Capps RB, et al. Studies on the transmission of human viral hepatitis to marmoset monkeys. I. Transmission of disease, serial passages, and description of liver lesions. J Exp Med 125:637, 1967.
56. Holmes AW, Wolfe L, Rosenblate H, et al. Hepatitis in marmosets: induction of disease with coded specimens from a human volunteer study. Science 165:816, 1969.
57. Holmes AW, Wolfe L, Deinhardt F, et al. Transmission of human hepatitis to marmosets: further coded studies. J Infect Dis 124:520, 1971.
58. Lorenz D, Barker L, Stevens D, et al. Hepatitis in the marmoset, Saguinus mystax. Proc Soc Exp Biol Med 153:348, 1970.
59. Mascoli CC, Ittensohn OL, Villarejos VM, et al. Recovery of hepatic agents in the marmoset from human cases occurring in Costa Rica. Proc Soc Exp Biol Med 142:276, 1973.
60. Maynard JE, Bradley DW, Gravelle CR, et al. Preliminary studies of hepatitis A in chimpanzees. J Infect Dis 131:194, 1975.
61. Dienstag JC, Feinstone SM, Purcell RH, et al. Experimental infection of chimpanzees with hepatitis A virus. J Infect Dis 132:532, 1975.
62. Blumberg BS, Sutnick AK, London WT. Hepatitis and leukemia: their relation to Australia antigen. Bull NY Acad Med 44:1566, 1968.
63. Shulman NR, Barker LE. Virus-like antigen, antibody, and antigen-antibody complexes in hepatitis measured by complement fixation. Science 165:304, 1969.
64. Maynard JE, Hartwell WV, Berquist KR. Hepatitis-associated antigen in chimpanzees. J Infect Dis 123:660, 1971.
65. Maynard JE, Berquist KR, Krushack DH, et al. Experimental infection of chimpanzees with the virus of hepatitis B. Nature 237:514, 1972.
66. Barker LF, Chiari FV, McGrath PP, et al. Transmission of type B viral hepatitis to chimpanzees. J Infect Dis 127:648, 1973.
67. London WT, Alter HJ, Lander JJ, et al. Serial transmission to rhesus monkeys of an agent related to hepatitis-associated antigen. J Infect Dis 125:382, 1972.
68. Bancroft WH, Snitbhan R, Scott RM, et al. Transmission of hepatitis B virus to gibbons by exposure to saliva containing hepatitis B surface antigen. J Infect Dis 135:79, 1977.
69. Summers J, Smolec JM, Snyder RA. Virus similar to human hepatitis B virus associated with hepatitis and hepatoma in woodchucks. Proc Natl Acad Sci USA 75:4533, 1978.
69a. Marion PL, Oshiro L, Regney DC, et al. A virus in Beechey ground squirrels that is related to hepatitis B of man. Proc Natl Acad Sci USA 77:2941, 1980.
69b. Mason WS, Seal G, Summers J. Virus of Pekin ducks with structural and biological relatedness to human hepatitis B virus. J Virol 36:829, 1980.

70. Easton MD, Murphy WD, Hanford VL. Heterogenetic antibodies in acute hepatitis. J Exp Med 19:539, 1944.
71. Hoyt RE, Morrison LM. Reaction of viral hepatitis sera with M. rhesus erythrocytes. Proc Soc Exp Biol Med 93:547, 1956.
72. Havens WP Jr. Hemagglutination in viral hepatitis. N Engl J Med 259:1202, 1958.
73. Bolin VS, Chase BS, Alsener JB, et al. Viral hepatitis test. Fed Proc 24:159, 1965.
74. Weaver DR, King JW, Brown CH. A clinical evaluation of the "HIM" test. Am J Clin Pathol 49:647, 1960.
75. Mosley JW. Viral hepatitis. Recent studies of etiology. In: Popper H, Schaffner F, eds. Liver Diseases, Vol 3. New York, Grune & Stratton, 1970:252.
76. Rightsel WA, Keltsch RA, Tekushan FM, et al. Tissue-culture cultivation of cytopathogenetic agents from patients with clinical hepatitis. Science 124:226, 1956.
77. Davis EV. Isolation of viruses from children with infectious hepatitis. Science 133:2059, 1961.
78. Hartwell WV, Love CJ, Eidenboch MP. Adenovirus in blood clots from cases of infectious hepatitis. Science 152:1390, 1966.
79. Henson D. Cytomegalovirus hepatitis in an adult. Arch Pathol 88:199, 1969.
80. Schleissner LA, Portnoy B. Hepatitis and pneumonia associated with ECHO virus, type 9: infection in two adult siblings. Ann Intern Med 68:1315, 1968.
81. Flewett TH, Parker RGF, Philip WM. Acute hepatitis due to herpes simplex virus in an adult. J Clin Pathol 22:60, 1969.
82. Barker LF, Stevens DP, Hillis WD. Identification of reovirus type 2 in cell cultures inoculated with hepatitis sera. Proc Soc Exp Biol Med 131:262, 1969.
83. Hersey DF, Shaw ED. Viral agents in hepatitis, a review. Lab Invest 19:558, 1968.
84. Del Prete S, Constantino D, Doglia M, et al. Detection of a new serum-antigen in three epidemics of short-incubation hepatitis. Lancet 2:579, 1970.
85. Taylor PE, Almeida JA, Zuckerman AJ, et al. The relationship of the Milan antigen to abnormal serum lipoprotein. Am J Dis Child 123:329, 1972.
86. Blumberg BS, Alter HJ, Visnich S. A "new" antigen in leukemia sera. JAMA 191:541, 1965.
87. Feinstone SM, Kapikian AZ, Purcell RH. Hepatitis A: detection by immune electron microscopy of a virus like antigen associated with acute illness. Science 182:1026, 1973.
88. Blumberg G. Australia antigen and the biology of hepatitis B. Science 197:17, 1979.
89. Blumberg BS, Gerstley BJS, Hungerford DA, et al. A serum antigen (Australia antigen) in Down's syndrome, leukemia, and hepatitis. Ann Intern Med 66:924, 1967.
90. Prince AM. An antigen detected in the blood during the incubation period of serum hepatitis. Proc Natl Acad Sci USA 60:814, 1968.
91. Bayer ME, Blumberg BS, Werner B. Particles associated with Australia antigen in the sera of patients with leukemia, Down's syndrome, and hepatitis. Nature 218:1057, 1968.
92. Giles GP, McCollum RW, Berndtson LW Jr, et al. Viral hepatitis: relationship of Australia/SH antigen to the Willowbrook MS-2 strain. N Engl J Med 281:119, 1969.
93. Levene C, Blumberg BS. Additional specificities of Australia antigen and the possible identification of hepatitis carriers. Nature 221:195, 1969.
94. Dane DS, Cameron CA, Briggs M. Virus-like particles in serum of patients with Australia-antigen-associated hepatitis. Lancet 1:695, 1970.
95. Sherlock S, Fox RA, Niazi SP, et al. Chronic liver diseases and primary liver-cell cancer with hepatitis-associated (Australia) antigen in serum. Lancet 1:1243, 1970.
96. Walsh SH, Yalow RS, Berson SA. Detection of Australia antigen and antibody by radioimmunoassay technique. J Infect Dis 121:550, 1970.
97. Gocke DJ, Hsu K, Morgan C, et al. Association between polyarteritis and Australia antigen. Lancet 2:1149, 1970.
98. Gerin JL, Holland PV, Purcell RH. Australia antigen: large scale propagation from human serum and biochemical studies of its proteins. J Virol 7:569, 1971.
99. Almeida JD, Rubenstein D, Stott EJ. New antigen-antibody system in Australia antigen-positive hepatitis. Lancet 2:1225, 1971.
100. Hirschman SZ, Vernace R, Schaffner F. DNA-polymerase in preparations containing Australia antigen. Lancet 1:1099, 1971.
101. LeBouvier GL. The heterogenicity of Australia antigen. J Infect Dis 123:671, 1971.
102. Prince AM, Szmuness W, Woods KR, et al. Antibody against serum-hepatitis antigen. Prevalence and potential use as immune serum globulin in prevention of serum hepatitis infections. N Engl J Med 285:933, 1971.
103. Ling CA, Overby LR. Prevalence of hepatitis B virus antigen as revealed by direct radioimmune assay with 125I-antibody. J Immunol 109:834, 1972.
104. Magnius LO, Espmark JA. New specifications in Australia antigen positive sera distinct from the Le Bouvier determinants. J Immunol 109:1017, 1972.
105. Kaplan PM, Greenman RL, Gerin JL, et al. DNA polymerase associated with human hepatitis B antigen. J Virol 12:995, 1973.
106. Robinson WS, Greenman RL. DNA polymerase in the core of the human hepatitis B virus candidate. J Virol 13:1231, 1974.
107. Purcell RH, Gerin JL. Hepatitis B subunit vaccine: a preliminary report of safety and efficacy tests in chimpanzees. Am J Med Sci 270:395, 1975.
107a. Macnab GG, Alexander JJ, Lecatsas G, et al. Hepatitis B surface antigen produced by a human hepatoma cell line. Br J Cancer 34:509, 1976.
107b. Peterson DL, Roberts IM, Vyas GN. Partial amino-acid sequence of two major component polypeptides of hepatitis B surface antigen. Proc Natl Acad Sci USA 74:1530, 1977.
107c. Imai M, Yanase Y, Nojiri T, et al. A receptor for polymerized human and chimpanzee albumins on hepatitis B virus particles occurring with HBeAg. Gastroenterology 76:242, 1979.
107d. Szmuness W, Stevens CE, Harley EJ, et al. Hepatitis B vaccine: demonstration of efficacy in a controlled clinical trial in a high-risk population in the United States. N Engl J Med 303:833, 1980.
107e. Tiollais P, Charnay P, Vyas GN. Biology of hepatitis B virus. Science 213:406, 1981.
107f. Brechot L, Hadchouel M, Scotto J, et al. Detection of hepatitis B virus DNA in liver and serum: a direct appraisal of the chronic carrier state. Lancet 2:765, 1981.
107g. Melnick JL. Classification of hepatitis A virus as enterovirus 72 and of hepatitis B virus as hepadnavirus, type 1. Intervirology 18:105, 1982.
107h. Delius H, Gough NM, Cameron CH, et al. Structure of the hepatitis B virus genome. J Virol 47:337, 1983.
107i. McAleer WJ, Buynack EB, Margetter RZ, et al. Human hepatitis B vaccine from recombinant yeast. Nature 307:178, 1984.
107j. Neurath AR, Kent SBH, Strick N, et al. Hepatitis B virus contains pre-S gene-encoded domains. Nature 315:154, 1985.
107k. Sureau C, Romet-Lemonne J-L, Mullins JI, et al. Production of hepatitis B virus by differential human hepatoma cell line after transfection with cloned circular HBV DNA. Cell 47:37, 1986.
108. Burrell CJ, MacKay P, Greenway PJ, et al. Expression in Escherichia coli of hepatitis B virus DNA sequences cloned in plasmic pBR322. Nature 279:43, 1979.
109. Sninsky JS, Siddiqui A, Robinson WS, et al. Cloning and endonuclease mapping of the hepatitis B viral genome. Nature, 279:346, 1979.
110. Mascoli CC, Ittensohn OL, Villarejos VM, et al. Recovery of hepatitis agents in the marmoset from human cases occurring in Costa Rica. Proc Soc Exp Biol Med 142:276, 1973.
111. Gravelle CR, Hornbeck CL, Maynard JE, et al. Hepatitis A: report of a common source outbreak with recovery of a possible etiology agent. II. Laboratory studies. J Infect Dis 131:167, 1975.
112. Provost PJ, Wolanski BS, Miller WJ, et al. Biophysical and biochemical properties of CR 326 human hepatitis virus. Am J Med Sci 270:87, 1975.
112a. Provost PJ, Ittensohn OL, Villarejos VM, et al. A specific complement-fixation test for human hepatitis A employing CR326 antigen. Proc Soc Exp Biol Med 148:962, 1975.
113. Miller WH, Provost PJ, McAleer WJ, et al. Specific immune adherence assay for human hepatitis A antibody. Application to diagnostic and epidemiologic investigations. Proc Soc Exp Biol Med 149:254, 1975.
114. Hollinger FB, Bradley DW, Maynard JE, et al. Detection of hepatitis A viral antigen by radioimmunoassay. J Immunol 115:1464, 1975.
115. Feinstone SM, Kapikian AZ, Purcell RH, et al. Transfusion-associated hepatitis not due to viral hepatitis type A or B. N Engl J Med 292:767, 1975.
116. Szmuness W, Dienstag JL, Purcell RH, et al. Distribution of antibody to hepatitis A in urban adult populations. N Engl J Med 295:755, 1976.
117. Bradley DW, Maynard JE, Hindman SH. Serodiagnosis of viral hepatitis A: detection of acute-phase immunoglobulin M anti-hepatitis A virus by radioimmunoassay. J Clin Microbiol 5:521, 1977.
117a. Mathiesen LR, Feinstone SM, Wong DC, et al. Enzyme-linked immunosorbent assay for detection of hepatitis A antigen in stool and antibody to hepatitis A antigen in serum: comparison with solid-phase radioimmunoassay, immune electron microscopy, and immune adherence hemagglutination assay. J Clin Microbiol 7:184, 1978.
118. Provost PJ, Hilleman MR. An inactivated hepatitis A virus vaccine prepared from infected marmoset liver. Proc Soc Exp Biol Med 159:201, 1978.

118a. Mao JS, Go YY, Huang HJ, et al. Susceptibility of monkeys to human hepatitis A virus. J Infect Dis 144:55, 1981.

118b. LeDuc JW, Lemon SM, Keenan CM, et al. Experimental infection of the New World owl monkey (Aotus tringivatus) with hepatitis A virus. Infect Immunol 40:766, 1983.

118c. Ticehurst JR, Racaniello VR, Baroudy BM, et al. Molecular cloning and characterization of hepatitis A virus cDNA. Proc Natl Acad Sci USA 80:5885, 1983.

118d. Jansen RW, Newbold JE, Lemon SM. Combined immunoaffinity cDNA-RNA hybridization assay for detection of hepatitis A virus in clinical specimens. J Clin Microbiol 22:984, 1985.

119. Prince AM, Brotman B, Grady GF, et al. Long-incubation post-transfusion hepatitis without serological evidence of exposure to hepatitis-B serum. Lancet 2:241, 1974.

120. Villarejos VM, Kirsten PH, Visona KA, et al. Evidence for viral hepatitis other than A or type B among persons in Costa Rica. N Engl J Med 293:1350, 1975.

120a. Craske J, Dilling N, Stern D. An outbreak of hepatitis associated with intravenous injection of factor VIII concentrate. Lancet 2:221, 1975.

121. Mosley JW, Redeker AG, Feinstone SM, et al. Multiple hepatitis viruses in multiple attacks of acute viral hepatitis. N Engl J Med 296:75, 1977.

122. Hoofnagle JH, Gerety RJ, Tabor E, et al. Transmission of non-A, non-B hepatitis. Ann Intern Med 87:14, 1977.

123. Alter HJ, Purcell RH, Holland PV, et al. Transmissible agent in non-A, non-B hepatitis. Lancet 1:459, 1978.

124. Tabor E, Gerety RJ, Drucker JA, et al. Transmission of non-A, non-B hepatitis from man to chimpanzee. Lancet 1:463, 1978.

125. Shirachi R, Shiraishi H, Tateda A, et al. Hepatitis "C" antigen in non-A, non-B post-transfusion hepatitis. Lancet 2:853, 1978.

126. Kabiri M, Tabor E, Gerety RJ. Antigen-antibody system associated with non-A, non-B hepatitis detected by indirect immunofluorescence. Lancet 2:221, 1979.

127. Tabor E, Mitchell FD, Goudeua AM, et al. Detection of an antigen-antibody system in serum associated with human non-A, non-B hepatitis. J Med Virol 4:161, 1979.

127a. Shimizu YK, Feinstone SM, Purcell RH, et al. Non-A, non-B hepatitis: ultrastructural evidence for two agents in experimentally infected chimpanzees. Science 205:197, 1979.

127b. Bradley DW, Cook EH, Maynard JE, et al. Experimental infection of chimpanzees with antihemophilic-(factor VIII) materials: recovery of virus-like particles associated with non-A, non-B hepatitis. J Med Virol 3:253, 1979.

127c. Tabor E, Gerety RJ. Inactivation of an agent of human non-A, non-B hepatitis by formalin. J Infect Dis 142:767, 1980.

127d. Hollinger FB, Mosley JW, Szmuness W, et al. Transfusion-transmitted viruses study: experimental evidence for two non-A, non-B hepatitis agents. J Infect Dis 142:400, 1980.

127e. Tabor E, Seeff LB, Gerety RJ. Chronic non-A, non-B hepatitis carrier state: transmissible agent documented in one patient over a six-year period. N Engl J Med 303:140, 1980.

127f. Bradley DW, Maynard JE, Popper H, et al. Posttransfusion non-A, non-B hepatitis: physicochemical properties of two distinct agents. J Infect Dis 148:254, 1983.

127g. Seto B, Iwarson S, Coleman WG, et al. Detection of reverse transcriptase activity in association with the non-A, non-B hepatitis agent(s). Lancet 2:941, 1984.

127h. Prince AM, Williams BAA, Huima T, et al. Isolation of a virus from chimpanzee liver cell cultures inoculated with sera containing the agent of non-A, non-B hepatitis. Lancet 2:1071, 1984.

127i. Bradley DW, Maynard JE. Etiology and natural history of posttransfusion and enterically-transmitted non-A, non-B hepatitis. Semin Liver Dis 6:56, 1986.

127j. Viswanathan R. Infectious hepatitis in Delhi (1955–56): a critical study; epidemiologically. Indian J Med Res 45:1, 1957.

127k. Wong DC, Purcell RH, Sreenivasan MA, et al. Epidemic and endemic hepatitis in India: evidence for non-A/non-B hepatitis virus etiology. Lancet 2:876, 1980.

127l. Tandon BN, Joshi YK, Jain SK. An epidemic of non-A/non-B hepatitis in North India. Indian J Med Res 75:739, 1982.

127m. Balayan MS, Andjaparidze AG, Savinskaya SS, et al. Evidence for a virus in non-A/non-B hepatitis transmitted via the fecal-oral route. Intervirology 20:23, 1983.

127n. Rizzetto M, Canese MG, Arico S, et al. Immunofluorescence detection of a new antigen-antibody system (delta/anti-delta) associated with hepatitis B virus in liver and serum of HBsAg carriers. Gut 18:997, 1977.

127o. Rizzetto M, Shih JW-K, Gerin JL. The hepatitis B virus-associated antigen: isolation from liver, development of solid-phase radioimmunoassays for antigen and anti-δ, and partial characterization of antigen. J Immunol 125:318, 1980.

127p. Rizzetto M, Canese MG, Gerin JL, et al. Transmission of hepatitis B virus-associated delta antigen to chimpanzees. J Infect Dis 121:590, 1980.

127q. Rizzetto M, Hoyer B, Canese MG, et al. Delta antigen: the association of delta antigen with hepatitis B surface antigen and ribonucleic acid in the serum of delta infected chimpanzees. Proc Natl Acad Sci USA 77:6124, 1980.

127r. Smedile AG, Carci P, Verme G, et al. Influence of delta infection on severity of hepatitis B. Lancet 2:945, 1982.

127s. Rizzetto M, Verme G, Recchia S, et al. Chronic hepatitis in carriers of hepatitis B surface antigen with intrahepatic expression of the delta antigen: an active and progressive disease unresponsive to immunosuppressive treatment. Ann Intern Med 98:437, 1983.

127t. Ponzetto A, Cote PJ, Popper H, et al. Transmission of the hepatitis B virus-associated agent to the eastern woodchuck. Proc Natl Acad Sci USA 81:2208, 1984.

127u. Ponzetto A, Hoofnagle JH, Seeff LB. Antibody to the hepatitis B virus-associated delta-antigen in immune serum globulins. Gastroenterology 87:1213, 1984.

127v. Govindarajan S, Chin KP, Redeker SG, et al. Fulminant B viral hepatitis: role of delta antigen. Gastroenterology 8:1417, 1984.

127w. Denniston KJ, Hoyer BH, Smedile A, et al. Cloned fragments of the hepatitis delta virus RNA genome: sequence and diagnostic application. Science 232:873, 1986.

127x. Barbara JAJ, Howell DR, Briggs M, et al. Post-transfusion hepatitis A. Lancet 1:738, 1982.

127y. Hollinger FB, Khan NC, Oefinger PE, et al. Posttransfusion hepatitis type A. JAMA 250:2313, 1983.

128. Bryan JA, Gregg MB. Viral hepatitis in the United States: 1970–1973: an analysis of morbidity trends and the impact of HBsAg testing on surveillance and epidemiology. Am J Med Sci 270:271, 1975.

129. Alter HJ, Purcell RH, Feinstone SM, et al. Non-A/non-B hepatitis: a review and interim report of an ongoing prospective study. In: Vyas GN, Cohn SN, Schmid R, eds. Viral Hepatitis. Philadelphia, Franklin Institute Press, 1978:359.

129a. Ponzetto A, Seeff LB, Boskell-Bales Z, et al. Hepatitis B markers in United States drug addicts with special emphasis on one delta hepatitis virus. Hepatology 4:1111, 1984.

129b. Jacobson IM, Dienstag JL, Wernes BG, et al. Epidemiology and clinical impact of hepatitis D virus (delta) infection. Hepatology 5:188, 1985.

129c. De Cock KM, Govindarajan S, Chin KP, et al. Delta hepatitis in the Los Angeles area: a report of 126 cases. Ann Intern Med 105:108, 1986.

130. Conrad ME, Schwartz FA, Young AA. Viral hepatitis: a generalized disease. Am J Med 37:789, 1964.

131. Kudzma DJ, Peterson EW, Knudsen KB. Small intestinal morphology in infectious hepatitis. Arch Intern Med 124:32, 1969.

132. Williams CN, Sidorov JJ. Steatorrhea in patients with liver disease. Can Med Assoc J 105:1143, 1971.

133. Routenberg JA, Dienstag JL, Harrison WO, et al. Foodborne outbreak of hepatitis A: clinical and laboratory features of acute and protracted illness. Am J Med Sci 278:123, 1979.

134. Zimmerman HJ, Lowry CF, Uyeyama K, et al. Infectious hepatitis: clinical and laboratory features of 295 cases. Am J Med Sci 213:395, 1947.

134a. Turner RH, Snavely JR, Grossman EB, et al. Some clinical studies of acute hepatitis occurring in soldiers after inoculation with yellow fever vaccine; with especial consideration of severe attacks. Ann Intern Med 20:193, 1944.

135. Zimmerman HJ, Seeff LB. Enzymes in hepatic disease. In: Coodley EL, ed. Diagnostic Enzymology. Philadelphia, Lea & Febiger, 1970:1.

136. De Ritis F, Coltorti M, Giusti G. Attività transaminasia del siero umano nell'epatite virale. Minerva Med 46:1207, 1955.

137. Wroblewski F, La Due JS. Serum glutamic-pyruvic transaminase (SGP-T) in hepatic disease: a preliminary report. Ann Intern Med 45:801, 1956.

138. Wroblewski F, Jervis G, La Due JS. The diagnostic, prognostic and epidemiologic significance of alterations of serum glutamic oxaloacetic transaminase in hepatitis. Ann Intern Med 45:782, 1956.

139. Chinsky M, Sherry S. Serum transaminase as a diagnostic aid. Arch Intern Med 99:556, 1957.

140. West M, Zimmerman HJ. Serum enzymes in hepatic disease. Med Clin North Am 43:371, 1959.

141. De Ritis F, Mollochi L, Coltorti M, et al. Anicteric virus hepatitis in a closed environment as shown by serum transaminase activity. Bull WHO 20:589, 1959.

142. Schneider AJ, Mosley JW. Studies of variations of glutamic-oxaloacetic transaminase in serum and infectious hepatitis. Pediatrics 24:367, 1959.

143. Clermont RJ, Chalmers TC. The transaminase tests in liver disease. Medicine 46:197, 1967.

144. Barker LF, Murray R. Relationship of virus dose to incubation time

of clinical hepatitis and time of appearance of hepatitis-associated antigen. Am J Med Sci 263:27, 1971.

144a. Dienstag JL. Non-A, non-B hepatitis. I. Recognition, epidemiology, and clinical features. Gastroenterology 85:439, 1983.

144b. Hollinger FB, Mosley JW, Szmuness W, et al. Transfusion-transmitted viruses study: experimental evidence for two non-A, non-B hepatitis agents. J Infect Dis 142:400, 1980.

144c. Yoshizawa H, Itoh Y, Iwakiri S, et al. Demonstration of two different types of non-A, non-B hepatitis by reinjection and cross-challenge studies in chimpanzees. Gastroenterology 81:107, 1981.

144d. Bradley DW, Maynard JE, Popper H, et al. Posttransfusion non-A, non-B hepatitis: physicochemical properties of two distinct agents. J Infect Dis 148:254, 1983.

144e. Hruby MA, Schauf V. Transfusion-related short-incubation hepatitis in hemophiliac patients. JAMA 240:1355, 1978.

144f. Craske J, Spooner RJO, Vandervelde EM. Evidence for existence of at least two types of factor-VIII-associated non-B transfusion hepatitis. Lancet 2:221, 1978.

144g. Wong DC, Purcell RH, Sreenivarsan MA, et al. Epidemic and endemic hepatitis in India: evidence for a non-A, non-B hepatitis virus aetiology. Lancet 2:876, 1980.

144h. Khuroo MS. Study of an epidemic of non-A, non-B hepatitis: possibility of another human hepatitis virus distinct from post-transfusion non-A, non-B type. Am J Med 68:818, 1980.

144i. Balayan MS, Andjaparidze AG, Savinskaya SS, et al. Evidence of a virus in non-A, non-B hepatitis transmitted via the fecal-oral route. Intervirology 20:23, 1983.

145. Rozen P, Korn RJ, Zimmerman HJ. Computer analysis of liver function tests and their interrelationship in 347 cases of viral hepatitis. Isr J Med Sci 6:67, 1970.

146. Nielsen JO, Faber V, Poulsen H, et al. Acute viral hepatitis: a comparative study of clinical, biochemical, morphological, and immunological features in patients with and without Australia antigen. Scand J Infect Dis 7:173, 1975.

147. Berman M, Alter HJ, Ishak KG, et al. The chronic sequelae of non-A, non-B hepatitis. Ann Intern Med 91:1, 1979.

147a. Seeff LB, Cuccherini BA, Zimmerman HJ, et al. Acetaminophen hepatotoxicity in alcoholics: a therapeutic misadventure. Ann Intern Med 104:399, 1986.

148. De Ritis F, Giusti G, Piccinno F, et al. Biochemical laboratory tests in viral hepatitis and other hepatic diseases. Bull WHO 32:59, 1965.

149. De Ritis F, Coltorti M, Giusti G. Serum transaminase activities in liver disease. Lancet 1:685, 1972.

150. Skrede S, Blomhoff JP, Gjone E. Biochemical features of acute and chronic hepatitis. Ann Clin Res 8:182, 1976.

151. Harinasuta U, Chomet B, Ishak KG, et al. Steatonecrosis—Mallory body type. Medicine 46:141, 1967.

152. Cohen JA, Kaplan MM. The SGOT/SGPT ratio—an indicator of alcoholic liver disease. Dig Dis Sci 24:835, 1979.

153. Eshchar J, Korn RJ, Zimmerman HJ. Probable posttransfusion hepatitis during the course of cirrhosis. Arch Intern Med 120:193, 1967.

154. Pagliaro L, Gigli F, Le Moli S, et al. β-Glucuronidase and acid phosphatase activities of lysosomal preparations from human liver tissue obtained by liver biopsy from subjects with acute hepatitis and cirrhosis. J Lab Clin Med 63:977, 1964.

155. Schersten T, Bjorntorp P, Bjorkerud S, et al. Liver cell function in infectious hepatitis in man. Acta Hepatosplenol 17:375, 1970.

156. Bonini PA, Franzina C. Human urinary alpha-glucosidases in normal conditions and in acute hepatitis. J Biochem Biol Sperimentale 7:47, 1968.

157. Gamklou R, Iwarson S. Activity of α-1,4-glucosidase in extrahepatic cholestasis and acute viral hepatitis. Scand J Clin Lab Invest 31:327, 1973.

158. Tsou KC, McCoy MG, Lo KW, et al. 5′Nucleotide phosphodiesterase isoenzyme in patients with hepatitis B infection. Cancer Res 35:2361, 1975.

159. Lei-Injo LE, Tsou KC, Lo KW, et al. 5′Nucleotide phosphodiesterase isozyme-V in health, in cancer, and in viral hepatitis. Cancer 45:795, 1980.

160. Carella M, D'Arienzo A, Manzillo G, et al. An evaluation of urinary D-glucaric acid excretion during acute hepatitis in man. Am J Dig Dis 23:18, 1978.

161. Sorrell MF, Burnett DA, Tuma DJ, et al. Paradoxical urinary excretion of D-glucaric acid in acute viral hepatitis. Clin Pharmacol Ther 20:365, 1976.

162. Branch RA, Herbert CM, Read AE. Determinants of serum antipyrine half-lives in patients with liver disease. Gut 14:569, 1973.

163. Klotz U, Avant GR, Hoyumpa A, et al. The effects of age and liver disease on the disposition and elimination of diazepam in adult man. J Clin Invest 55:347, 1975.

164. Levi AJ, Sherlock S, Walker P. Phenylbutazone and isoniazid metabolism in patients with liver disease in relation to previous drug therapy. Lancet 1:125, 1968.

165. McHorse TS, Wilkinson GR, Johnson RF, et al. Effects of acute viral hepatitis in man on the disposition and elimination of meperidine. Gastroenterology 47:514, 1975.

166. Powell LW, Axelsen E. Corticosteroids in liver disease: studies on the biologic conversion of prednisone to prednisolone and plasma protein binding. Gut 13:690, 1972.

167. Burnett DA, Barak AJ, Tuma DJ, et al. Altered elimination of antipyrine in patients with acute viral hepatitis. Gut 17:341, 1976.

168. Blashke TF, Meffin PJ, Melman KL, et al. Influence of acute viral hepatitis on phenytoin kinetics and protein binding. Clin Pharmacol Ther 17:685, 1975.

169. Williams RL, Blashke TF, Meffin PF, et al. Influence of viral hepatitis on the disposition of two compounds with high hepatic clearance: lidocaine and indocyanine green. Clin Pharmacol Ther 20:219, 1976.

170. Held VH, Eisert R, Olderhausen HF. Pharmakokinetik von glymidine und tolbutamid bei acuten und chronischen Lieber. Schader Arzneim-Forsch 23:1801, 1973.

171. Zimmerman HJ. The differential diagnosis of jaundice. Med Clin North Am 52:1417, 1968.

172. Reinhold JG. Flocculation tests and their application to the study of liver disease. Adv Clin Chem 3:83, 1960.

173. Zimmerman HJ. Clinical and laboratory manifestations of hepatotoxicity. Ann NY Acad Sci 104:954, 1963.

174. Klatskin G. Bile pigment inactivation. Annu Rev Med 12:211, 1961.

175. Salen G, Goldstein F, Hairani R, et al. Acute hemolytic anemia complicating viral hepatitis in patients with glucose-6-phosphate dehydrogenase deficiency. Ann Intern Med 65:1210, 1966.

176. Clearfield HR, Brody JI, Tumen HJ. Acute viral hepatitis, glucose-6-phosphate dehydrogenase deficiency and hemolytic anemias. Arch Intern Med 123:689, 1969.

177. Chan TK, Todd D. Hemolysis complicating viral hepatitis in patients with glucose-6-phosphate dehydrogenase deficiency. Br Med J 1:131, 1975.

178. Hargrove MD Jr. Marked increase in serum bilirubin in sickle anemia: a report of six patients. Am J Dig Dis 15:437, 1970.

179. Kivel RM. Hematologic aspects of acute viral hepatitis. Am J Dig Dis 6:1017, 1961.

180. Hagler L, Pastore RA, Bergin JJ, et al. Aplastic anemia following viral hepatitis: report of two fatal cases and literature review. Medicine 54:139, 1975.

181. Havens WP Jr, March RE. The leukocyte response of patients with experimentally induced infectious hepatitis. Am J Med Sci 212:129, 1946.

182. Litwins J, Leibowitz S. Abnormal lymphocytes ("virocytes") in virus disease other than infectious mononucleosis. Acta Haematol 5:223, 1951.

183. Saunders SJ, Dowdle EB, Fiskerstrand C, et al. Serum factor affecting neutrophil function during acute viral hepatitis. Gut 19:930, 1978.

184. Vierucci A, de Martino M, London WT, et al. Neutrophil function in children who are carriers of hepatitis-B surface antigen. Lancet 1:157, 1977.

184a. Cawein MJ III, Hagedorn AB, Owen CA. Anemia of hepatic disease studied with radiochromium. Gastroenterology 38:324, 1960.

184b. Katz R, Velasco M, Guzman C, et al. Red cell survival estimated by radioactive chromium in hepatobiliary disease. Gastroenterology 46:399, 1964.

184c. Enk B, Friss T. Red cell survival in acute hepatitis. Nord Med 86:1148, 1971.

185. Conrad ME. Persistent hemolysis after infectious hepatitis. Gut 10:516, 1969.

186. Jones GP, Evans EG. Thrombocytopenic purpura in infective hepatitis. Br Med J 2:451, 1951.

187. Greenspan EM, Dreiling DA. Serum mucoprotein levels in differentiation of hepatogenic from obstructive jaundice. Arch Intern Med 91:189, 1961.

188. Owen JA, Padanyi R, Smith H. Serum haptoglobins and other tests in the diagnosis of hepatobiliary jaundice. Clin Sci 21:189, 1961.

189. Kindmark C-O, Laurell CB. Sequential changes of the plasma protein pattern in inoculation hepatitis. Scand J Clin Lab Invest 124:105, 1972.

190. Goldberg SJ, Smith CL, Caldwell AM. Abnormalities of haptoglobin in viral hepatitis. Gastroenterology 66:701, 1974.

191. Thalassinos N, Hatzioannou J, Scliros P, et al. Plasma α-lipoprotein pattern in acute viral hepatitis. Am J Dig Dis 20:148, 1975.

192. Lee FI. Immunoglobulins in viral hepatitis and active alcoholic liver disease. Lancet 2:1043, 1965.

193. Lo Grippo GA, Hayashi H, Sharpless N, et al. Effect of infectious hepatitis on the immunoglobulins in mentally retarded children. JAMA 195:155, 1966.

194. Peters RL, Ashcavai M. Immunoglobulin levels in detection of viral hepatitis. Am J Clin Pathol 54:102, 1970.

195. Wollheim FA. Immunoglobulins in the course of viral hepatitis and in

cholestatic and obstructive jaundice. Acta Med Scand 183:473, 1968.

195a. Mosley JW, Visona KA, Villarejos VM. Immunoglobulin M level in the diagnosis of type A hepatitis. Am J Clin Pathol 75:86, 1981.

196. Giles JP, Krugman S. Viral hepatitis: immunoglobulin response during the course of the disease. JAMA 208:497, 1969.

197. Peters CJ, Johnson KM. Serum immunoglobulin levels in Australia antigen positive and Australia antigen negative hepatitis. Clin Exp Immunol 11:381, 1972.

198. Charlesworth JA, Lennane RJ, Jones P, et al. Contrasting IgE levels in acute HBsAg positive and negative hepatitis. Aust NZ J Med 8:43, 1978.

199. Andersen P, Ladefoged K. Correlations between serum immunoglobulin concentrations and smooth-muscle antibodies in acute viral hepatitis. Scand J Infect Dis 11:107, 1979.

200. Bevan G, Taswell HF, Gleich GJ. Serum immunoglobulin levels in blood donors implicated in transmission of hepatitis. JAMA 203:92, 1968.

201. Fox RA, Dudley FJ, Sherlock S. The serum concentration of the third component of the complement $\beta_1 C/\beta_1 A$ in liver disease. Gut 12:574, 1971.

202. Kosmidis JC, Leader-Williams LK. Complement levels in acute infectious hepatitis and serum hepatitis. Clin Exp Immunol 11:31, 1972.

203. Alpert E, Schur PH, Isselbacher KJ. Sequential changes of serum complement in HAA related arthritis. N Engl J Med 287:103, 1971.

204. Baer GM, Walker JA, Yager PA. Studies of an outbreak of acute hepatitis A. I. Complement level fluctuations. J Med Virol 1:1, 1977.

205. Charlesworth JA, Lawrence S, Worsdale PA, et al. Acute hepatitis: significance of changes in complement components. Clin Exp Immunol 28:496, 1977.

206. Gitlin D, Perricelli A, Gitlin GM. Synthesis of α fetoprotein by liver, yolk sac and gastrointestinal tract of the human conceptus. Cancer Res 32:979, 1972.

207. Abelev GI. Alpha-fetoprotein in ontogenesis and its association with malignant tumors. Adv Cancer Res 14:295, 1971.

208. Ruoslahti E, Seppala M. α-Fetoprotein in normal human serum. Nature (Lond) 235:161, 1972.

209. Alpert E. Human alpha-fetoprotein. In: Popper H, Schaffner F, eds. Progress In Liver Diseases, Vol 5. New York, Grune & Stratton, 1976:337.

210. Smith JB. Occurrence of alpha-fetoprotein in acute viral hepatitis. Int J Cancer 8:421, 1971.

211. Akeyama T, Koyama T, Kamada T. Alpha-fetoprotein in acute viral hepatitis. N Engl J Med 287:989, 1972.

212. Kew MC, Purves LR, Bersohn I. Serum alpha-fetoprotein levels in acute viral hepatitis. Gut 14:939, 1973.

213. Ruoslahti E, Seppala M, Rasanen JA, et al. Alpha-fetoprotein and hepatitis B antigen in acute hepatitis and primary cancer of the liver. Scand J Gastroenterol 8:197, 1973.

214. Karvountsis GG, Redeker AG. Relation of alpha-fetoprotein in acute hepatitis to severity and prognosis. Ann Intern Med 80:156, 1974.

215. Bloomer JR, Waldmann TA, McIntire KR, et al. Serum α-fetoprotein in patients with massive hepatic necrosis. Gastroenterology 72:479, 1977.

216. Bloomer JR, Waldmann RA, McIntire KR, et al. Relationship of serum α-fetoprotein to the severity and duration of illness in patients with viral hepatitis. Gastroenterology 68:342, 1975.

217. Alpert E, Feller ER. α-Fetoprotein (AFP) in benign liver disease: evidence that normal liver regeneration does not induce AFP synthesis. Gastroenterology 74:856, 1978.

218. Chan D-S, Sung J-L. Relationship of hepatitis B surface antigen to serum alpha-fetoprotein in nonmalignant diseases of the liver. Cancer 44:984, 1979.

219. Villarejos VM, Arquembourg PC, Visona KA, et al. Antibodies to single-stranded DNA. An aid in diagnosis of viral hepatitis. J Med Virol 2:359, 1978.

219a. Wheelock EF, Schenker S, Combes B. Absence of circulating interferon in patients with infectious and serum hepatitis. Proc Soc Exp Biol Med 128:251, 1968.

219b. Hill DA, Walsh JH, Purcell RH. Failure to demonstrate circulating interferon during the incubation period and acute stage of transfusion-associated hepatitis. Proc Soc Exp Biol Med 136:853, 1971.

219c. Levin S, Halen T. Interferon system in acute viral hepatitis. Lancet 1:592, 1982.

219d. Kurane I, Binn LN, Bancroft WH, et al. Human lymphocyte response to hepatitis A virus-infected cells: interferon production of infected cells. J Immunol 135:2140, 1985.

219e. Vallbracht A, Gabriel P, Zahn J, et al. Hepatitis A virus infection and the interferon system. J Infect Dis 152:211, 1985.

220. McIntyre N, Calandra S, Pearson AJG. Lipid and lipoprotein abnormalities in liver disease: the possible role of lecithin: cholesterol

221. Epstein EZ. Cholesterol of the blood in hepatic and biliary diseases. Arch Intern Med 50:203, 1932.

222. Gjone E, Orning OM. Plasma phospholipids in patients with liver disease: a quantitative thin layer chromatographic study. Scand J Clin Lab Invest 18:209, 1966.

223. Phillips GB. The lipid composition of serum in patients with liver disease. J Clin Invest 39:1639, 1960.

224. Gjone E, Blomhoff JP, Mendie I. Plasma lecithin:cholesterol acyltransferase activity in acute hepatitis. Scand J Gastroenterol 6:161, 1971.

225. Simon JP. Lecithin:cholesterol esterification in liver disease. Scand J Clin Lab Invest (Suppl) 33(137):107, 1974.

226. Blomhoff JP, Skrede S, Rutland S. Lecithin:cholesterol acyltransferase and plasma proteins in liver disease. Clin Chim Acta 53:197, 1974.

227. Simon JB, Scheig R. Serum cholesterol esterification in liver disease: importance of lecithin:cholesterol acyltransferase. N Engl J Med 283:841, 1970.

228. Muller P, Fellin R, Lambrecht J, et al. Hypertriglyceridemia secondary to liver disease. Eur J Clin Invest 4:419, 1974.

229. Rudman D, Kendall FE. Bile acid content of human serum. I. Serum bile acids in patients with hepatic disease. J Clin Invest 36:530, 1957.

230. Carey JB Jr. The serum trihydroxy-dihydroxy bile acid ratio in liver and biliary tract disease. J Clin Invest 37:1494, 1958.

231. Makino I, Nakagawa S, Mashimo K. Conjugated and unconjugated serum bile acid levels in patients with hepatobiliary diseases. Gastroenterology 56:1033, 1969.

232. Osborn EC, Wootten IDP, Da-Silva LC, et al. Serum bile acid levels in liver disease. Lancet 2:1049, 1959.

233. Kaplowitz N, Kok E, Javitt NB. Post-prandial serum bile acid for the detection of hepatobiliary disease. JAMA 225:292, 1973.

234. Theodor E, Spritz N, Slesinger MH. Metabolism of intravenously injected isotopic cholic acid in viral hepatitis. Gastroenterology 55:183, 1968.

235. La Russo MF, Hoffmann NE, Hoffmann AF, et al. Validity and sensitivity of an intravenous bile acid tolerance test in patients with liver disease. N Engl J Med 292:1209, 1975.

236. Barnes S, Gallo GA, Trash BB, et al. Diagnostic value of serum bile acid estimations in liver disease. J Clin Pathol 28:506, 1975.

237. Fausa O, Gjone E. Serum bile acid concentrations in patients with liver disease. Scand J Gastroenterol 11:537, 1976.

238. Campbell CB, McGuffie C, Powell LW, et al. Postprandial changes in serum concentrations of individual bile salts in normal subjects and patients with acute viral hepatitis. Am J Dig Dis 23:599, 1978.

239. Balestreri WF, Tabor E, Gerety RJ, et al. Serum bile acids during experimentally induced hepatitis in chimpanzees. Clin Res 27:26A, 1979.

240. Cronholm T, Norman A, Sjovall J. Bile acids and steroid sulphates in serum of patients with infectious hepatitis. Scand J Gastroenterol 5:297, 1970.

241. Demers LM, Hepner G. Radioimmunoassay of bile acids in serum. Clin Chem 22:602, 1976.

242. Hoffmann AF, Korman MG, Krugman S. Sensitivity of serum bile acid assay for detection of liver damage in viral hepatitis, type B. Am J Dig Dis 19:908, 1974.

243. Korman MG, Hoffmann AF, Summerskill WHJ. Assessment of activity in chronic active liver disease: serum bile acids compared with conventional tests and histology. N Engl J Med 290:1399, 1974.

244. Gitnick GL, Brezina ML, Mullen RL. Application of alanine aminotransferase, carcinoembryonic antigen, and cholyl glycine levels to the prevention and evaluation of acute and chronic hepatitis. In: Vyas GN, Cohn SN, Schmid R, eds. Viral Hepatitis. Philadelphia, Franklin Institute Press, 1978:431.

245. Ducci H, Spoerer A, Katz R. Serum iron in liver disease. Gastroenterology 22:52, 1952.

246. Rumball JM, Stone CM, Hassett C. The behavior of serum iron in acute hepatitis. Gastroenterology 36:219, 1959.

247. Schamroth L, Edelston W, Politzer WL, et al. Serum iron in the diagnosis of hepato-biliary disease. Br Med J 1:960, 1956.

248. Ishak KG. Viral hepatitis: the morphologic spectrum. In: Gall EA, Mostofi FK, eds. The Liver. Baltimore, Williams & Wilkins, 1973:218.

249. Felton C, Lustbader ED, Morton C, et al. Serum iron levels and response to hepatitis B virus. Proc Natl Acad Sci USA 76:2438, 1979.

250. Turnberg LA. Iron absorption in acute hepatitis. Am J Dig Dis 11:20, 1966.

251. Bolin T, Davis AE. Iron absorption in infectious hepatitis. Am J Dig Dis 13:16, 1968.

252. Hult H. Posthepatitic siderosis of the liver. Acta Med Scand 142:113, 1952.

acyltransferase deficiency. Scand J Clin Lab Invest (Suppl) 33(137):115, 1974.

253. Scuro LA, Dobrilla G. Siderosis, hemolysis or hepatonecrosis in increasing post-desferrioxamine sideruria in acute viral hepatitis? Postgrad Med J 43:708, 1967.

254. Kahn AH, Helwig HL, Redeker AG, et al. Urine and serum zinc abnormalities in diseases of the liver. Am J Clin Pathol 44:426, 1965.

255. Henkin RI, Smith FR. Zinc and copper metabolism in acute viral hepatitis. Am J Med Sci 264:401, 1972.

256. Versieck J, Barbierie F, Speecke A, et al. Manganese, copper, and zinc concentrations in serum and packed blood cells during acute hepatitis, chronic hepatitis and posthepatitic cirrhosis. Clin Chem 20:1141, 1974.

257. Rachmilewitz M, Eliakim M. Serum B_{12}—a diagnostic test in liver disease. Israel J Med Sci 4:47, 1968.

258. Stein Y, Stein O, Aronovitch I, et al. Serum vitamin B_{12} in experimental liver injury. Bull Res Council Israel 6:5, 1956.

259. Rachmilewitz M, Moshkowitz B, Rachmilewitz B, et al. Serum vitamin B_{12} binding protein in viral hepatitis. Eur J Clin Invest 2:239, 1972.

260. Zimmerman HJ, Thomas LH, Scherr EH. Fasting blood sugar in hepatic disease with reference to infrequency of hypoglycemia. Arch Intern Med 91:577, 1953.

261. Felig P, Brown V, Levine RA, et al. Glucose homeostasis in viral hepatitis. N Engl J Med 283:1433, 1970.

262. Kelly M, Walsh H, Doyle C, et al. Glucose homeostasis in viral hepatitis. Digestion 6:286, 1973.

263. Record CO, Albert KGNM, Williamson DH, et al. Glucose tolerance and metabolic changes in human viral hepatitis. Clin Sci Mol Med 45:677, 1973.

264. Berkowitz D, Blinkoff B, Glassman S. Carbohydrate metabolism in jaundice. Gastroenterology 50:830, 1966.

265. Gioaminni P, Scalise G. Glucose tolerance in viral hepatitis. Acta Diabetica Latina 8:932, 1971.

266. Nieschlag E, Kremer GJ, Mussgung U. Insulin, Glucose-toleranz und freie Feltsauran wahrend und nach akuter Hepatitis. Klin Wochenschr 48:381, 1970.

267. Lucke B, Mallory T. The fulminant form of epidemic hepatitis. Am J Pathol 22:867, 1946.

268. Samson RI, Trey C, Timme AH, et al. Fulminating hepatitis with recurrent hypoglycemia and hemorrhage. Gastroenterology 53:291, 1967.

269. Preisig R, Williams R, Sweeting J, et al. Changes in sulfobromophthalein transport and storage by the liver during viral hepatitis in man. Am J Med 40:170, 1966.

270. Leevy CM, Smith F, Longueville S, et al. Indocyanine green clearance as a test for hepatic function: evaluation by dichromatic ear densitometry. JAMA 200:236, 1967.

271. Vahrman J. Viral hepatitis and ESR. Br Med J 1:466, 1971.

271a. Hadler SC, Webster HM, Erban JS, et al. Hepatitis A in day-care centers: a community-wide assessment. N Engl J Med 302:1222, 1980.

271b. Benenson MW, Takafuji ET, Bancroft WH, et al. A military community outbreak of hepatitis type A related to transmission in a child care facility. Am J Epidemiol 112:471, 1980.

271c. Lednar WM, Lemon SM, Kirkpatrick JW, et al. Frequency of illness associated with hepatitis A virus infection in adults. Am J Epidemiol 122:226, 1985.

271d. Dismukes WE, Bisno AL, Katz S, et al. An outbreak of gastroenteritis and infectious hepatitis attributed to raw clams. Am J Epidemiol 85:555, 1969.

271e. Kao HW, Ashcavai M, Redeker AG. The persistence of hepatitis A IgM antibody after acute clinical hepatitis A. Hepatology 4:933, 1984.

271f. Sjogren MH, Tanno H, Fay O, et al. Hepatitis A virus in stool during clinical relapse. Ann Intern Med 106:221, 1987.

271g. Gordon SC, Reddy KJ, Schiff ER, et al. Prolonged intrahepatic cholestasis secondary to acute hepatitis A. Ann Intern Med 101:635, 1984.

271h. Tavera C, Velasquez O, Avila C, et al. Enterically transmitted non-A, non-B hepatitis—Mexico. Morbid Mortal Weekly Rep 36:597, 1987.

271i. De Cock KM, Bradley DW, Sanford WL, et al. Epidemic non-A, non-B hepatitis in patients from Pakistan. Ann Intern Med 106:277, 1987.

271j. Khuroo MS, Teli MR, Skidmore S, et al. Incidence and severity of viral hepatitis in pregnancy. Am J Med 70:252, 1981.

271k. Resnick RH, Stone K, Antonioli D. Primary hepatocellular carcinoma after non-A, non-B posttransfusion hepatitis. Dig Dis Sci 28:908, 1983.

271l. Kiyosawa K, Akahane Y, Naguta A, et al. Hepatocellular carcinoma after non-A, non-B posttransfusion hepatitis. Am J Gastroenterol 79:777, 1984.

271m. Gilliam JH, Geisinger KR, Richter JE. Primary hepatocellular car-

cinoma after chronic non-A, non-B post-transfusion hepatitis. Ann Intern Med 101:794, 1984.

271n. Rizzetto M, Verme G, Gerin JL, et al. Hepatitis delta virus disease. Prog Liver Dis 8:417, 1986.

271o. Hadler SC, De Monzon M, Ponzetto A, et al. Delta virus infection and severe hepatitis: an epidemic in the Yucpa Indians of Venezuela. Ann Intern Med 100:339, 1984.

271p. Ljunggren KE, Pattarogo ME, Engle R, et al. Viral hepatitis in Colombia: a study of the "Hepatitis of the Sierra Nevada de Santa Maria." Hepatology 5:299, 1985.

271q. Rizzetto M, Verme G, Recchia S, et al. Chronic hepatitis in carriers of hepatitis B surface antigen with intrahepatic expression of the delta antigen: an active and progressive disease unresponsive to immunosuppressive treatment. Ann Intern Med 98:437, 1983.

271r. Govindarajan S, De Cock KM, Redeker AG. Natural course of delta superinfection in chronic hepatitis B virus-infected patients: histopathologic study with multiple liver biopsies. Hepatology 6:640, 1986.

272. Seeff LB, Zimmerman HJ, Wright EC, et al. A randomized, double-blind, controlled trial of the efficacy of immune serum globulin for the prevention of post-transfusion hepatitis. A Veterans Administration cooperative study. Gastroenterology 72:111, 1977.

273. Hampers S, Prager D, Senior JR. Post-transfusion anicteric hepatitis. N Engl J Med 271:747, 1964.

274. Shimizu Y, Kitamoto O. The incidence of viral hepatitis after blood transfusion. Gastroenterology 44:740, 1963.

275. National Transfusion Hepatitis Study. Risk of post-transfusion hepatitis in the United States—a prospective cooperative study. JAMA 220:692, 1972.

276. Cossart YE, Kirsch S, Ismay SL. Post-transfusion hepatitis in Australia: report of the Australian Red Cross study. Lancet 1:208, 1982.

276a. Alter HJ, Purcell RH, Femstone SM, et al. Non-A, non-B hepatitis; its relationship to cytomegalovirus, to chronic hepatitis, and to direct and indirect test methods. In: Szmuness W, Alter HJ, Maynard JE, eds. Viral Hepatitis: 1981 International Symposium. Philadelphia, Franklin Institute Press, 1982:279.

277. Morse LJ, Bryan JA, Hurley JP, et al. The Holy Cross College football team hepatitis outbreak. JAMA 219:706, 1972.

278. Wacker WEC, Riordin JF, Snodgrass PJ, et al. The Holy Cross hepatitis outbreak: clinical and chemical abnormalities. Arch Intern Med 113:357, 1972.

279. Mosley J. The epidemiology of viral hepatitis: an overview. Am J Med Sci 270:253, 1975.

280. Krugman S, Friedman H, Lattimer C. Hepatitis A and B: serologic screening of various population groups. Am J Med Sci 275:249, 1978.

281. Seeff LB, Zimmerman HJ, Wright EC, et al. Hepatic disease in asymptomatic parenteral narcotic drug abusers: a Veterans Administration collaborative study. Am J Med Sci 270:41, 1975.

282. Tabor E, Jones R, Gerety RJ, et al. Asymptomatic viral hepatitis types A and B in an adolescent population. Pediatrics 62:1026, 1979.

283. Chung WK, Moon SK, Gershon RK, et al. Anicteric hepatitis in Korea. I. Clinical and laboratory studies. Arch Intern Med 113:526, 1964.

284. Chung WK, Moon SK, Gershon RK, et al. Anicteric hepatitis in Korea. II. Serial histologic studies. Arch Intern Med 113:535, 1964.

285. Klatskin G. Subacute hepatitic necrosis and post-necrotic cirrhosis due to anicteric infections with the hepatitis virus. Am J Med 25:333, 1958.

286. Barker LF, Murray R. Acquisition of hepatitis-associated antigen: clinical features in young adults. JAMA 216:1971, 1971.

287. Sherlock S. Predicting progression of acute type-B hepatitis to chronicity. Lancet 2:354, 1976.

287a. Alward WLM, McMahon BJ, Hale DB, et al. The long-term serologic course of asymptomatic hepatitis B virus carriers and the development of primary hepatocellular carcinoma. J Infect Dis 151:604, 1985.

288. Garibaldi RA, Forrest JN, Bryan JA, et al. Hemodialysis-associated hepatitis. JAMA 225:384, 1973.

289. Szmuness W, Prince AM, Grady GF, et al. Hepatitis B infection: a point-prevalence study in 15 US hemodialysis centers. JAMA 227:901, 1974.

290. Ware AJ, Luby JP, Eigenbrodt EH, et al. Spectrum of liver disease in renal transplant recipients. Gastroenterology 68:755, 1975.

291. Anuras S, Piros J, Bonney WW, et al. Liver disease in liver transplant recipients. Arch Intern Med 137:42, 1977.

292. Cowan DH, Kouroupis GN, Leers W-D. Occurrence of hepatitis and hepatitis B surface antigen in adult patients with acute leukemia. Can Med Assoc J 112:693, 1975.

293. Wands JR, Chura CM, Roll FJ, et al. Serial studies of hepatitis-associated antigen and antibody in patients receiving anti-tumor

chemotherapy for myeloproliferative and lymphoproliferative disorders. Gastroenterology 68:105, 1975.

294. Blumberg BS, Gerstley BJS, Hungerford DA, et al. A serum antigen (Australia antigen) in Down's syndrome, leukemia and hepatitis. Ann Intern Med 66:924, 1967.

295. London WT, DiFiglia M, Sutnick AI, et al. An epidemic of hepatitis in a chronic hemodialysis unit. N Engl J Med 281:571, 1969.

296. London WT, Drew JS, Lustbader ED, et al. Host responses to hepatitis B infection in patients in a chronic hemodialysis unit. Kidney Int 12:51, 1977.

297. Dienstag JL, Routenberg JA, Purcell RH, et al. Food handler-associated outbreak of hepatitis A: an immune electron microscopic study. Ann Intern Med 83:647, 1975.

298. Redeker AG. Viral hepatitis: clinical aspects. Am J Med Sci 270:9, 1975.

299. Knodell RG, Conrad ME, Ishak KG. Development of chronic liver disease after acute non-A, non-B post-transfusion hepatitis. Role of λ-globulin prophylaxis in its prevention. Gastroenterology 79:902, 1977.

300. Strickland GT, Castell DO, Kromal RA. Prolonged observations on the liver function tests in infectious hepatitis. Am J Gastroenterol 55:257, 1971.

301. Schaffner F, Klion FM. Chronic hepatitis. Annu Rev Med 19:25, 1968.

302. Levine RA. Spectrum of liver disease after viral hepatitis. NY State J Med 68:1919, 1968.

303. Becker MD, Scheuer PJ, Baptista A, et al. Prognosis of chronic persistent hepatitis. Lancet 1:53, 1970.

304. Boyer JL. The diagnosis and pathogenesis of clinical variants in viral hepatitis. Am J Clin Pathol 65:898, 1976.

305. Popper H, Schaffner F. The vocabulary of chronic hepatitis. N Engl J Med 284:1154, 1971.

306. Wilkinson SP, Portmann B, Cochrane AMG, et al. Clinical course of chronic lobular hepatitis. Report of five cases. Q J Med 68:421, 1978.

306a. Liaw YF, Chu CM, Chen TJ, et al. Chronic lobular hepatitis: a clinicopathological and prognostic study. Hepatology 2:258, 1982.

306b. Seeff LB, Koff RS. Evolving concepts of the clinical and serologic consequences of hepatitis B virus infection. Semin Liver Dis 6:11, 1986.

307. Boyer JL, Klatskin G. Pattern of necrosis in acute viral hepatitis: prognostic value of bridging (subacute hepatic necrosis). N Engl J Med 283:1063, 1970.

308. Popper H, Schaffner F. Liver: Structure and Function. New York, Blakiston Division, McGraw-Hill, 1957:211.

309. Jersild M. Infectious hepatitis with subacute atrophy of the liver: an epidemic in women after the menopause. N Engl J Med 237:8, 1947.

310. Bjorneboe J, Raaschou F. The pathology of subchronic atrophy of the liver. Acta Med Scand (Suppl) 234:41, 1949.

311. Tisdale WA. Subacute hepatitis. N Engl J Med 268:85; 138, 1963.

312. Dietrichson O, Juhl E, Christoffersen P, et al. Acute viral hepatitis: factors possibly predicting chronic liver disease. Acta Pathol Microbiol Scand 83:183, 1975.

313. Nielsen JO, Dietrichson O, Elling P, et al. Incidence and meaning of persistence of Australia antigen in patients with acute viral hepatitis: development of chronic hepatitis. N Engl J Med 285:1157, 1971.

314. Vittal SBV, Thomas W, Thomas W, et al. Acute viral hepatitis: course and incidence in progression to chronic hepatitis. Am J Med 55:757, 1973.

315. Ware AJ, Eigenbrodt EH, Combes B. Prognostic significance of subacute hepatic necrosis in acute hepatitis. Gastroenterology 68:519, 1975.

316. Spitz ERD, Keren DF, Boitnott JK, et al. Bridging hepatic necrosis: etiology and prognosis. Am J Dig Dis 23:1076, 1978.

317. Ducci H, Katz R. Cortisone, ACTH and antibiotics in fulminant hepatitis. Gastroenterology 21:357, 1952.

318. Soloway RD, Summerskill WHJ, Baggenstoss AH, et al. Clinical, biochemical and histological remission of severe chronic active liver disease. A controlled study of treatment and early prognosis. Gastroenterology 63:820, 1972.

319. Gregory PB, Knauer CM, Kempson RL, et al. Steroid therapy in severe viral hepatitis: a double-blind, randomized trial of methylprednisolone versus placebo. N Engl J Med 294:681, 1976.

320. Ware A, Cuthbert J, Eigenbrodt E, et al. Controlled trial of corticosteroid therapy in severe acute viral hepatitis. Gastroenterology 75:992, 1978.

321. Karvountzis GG, Redeker AG, Peters RL. Long term follow-up studies of patients surviving fulminant viral hepatitis. Gastroenterology 67:870, 1974.

322. Petersen P, Christoffersen P, Elling P, et al. Acute viral hepatitis, a summary of 500 patients. Clinical, biochemical, immunological and morphology features at times of diagnosis. Scand J Gastroenterol 9:607, 1974.

323. Norkrans G. Clinical, epidemiological and prognostic aspects of hepatitis A, B and "non-A, non-B." Scand J Infect Dis (Suppl) 17:1, 1978.

324. Schweitzer IL. Vertical transmission of the hepatitis B surface antigen. Am J Med Sci 270:287, 1975.

325. Hasiba V, Spero JA, Lewis JH. Chronic hepatitis in hemophilia. Scand J Hematol 30:27, 1977.

326. Spero JA, Lewis JH, Van Thiel DH, et al. Asymptomatic structural liver disease in hemophilia. N Engl J Med 298:1373, 1978.

327. Norkrans G, Frosner G, Iwarson S. Determination of HBeAg by radioimmunoassay: prognostic implications in hepatitis B. Scand J Gastroenterol 14:289, 1979.

327a. Careoda F, De Francis R, D'Arminio Monforte A, et al. Persistence of antibody HBsAg/IgM complexes in acute viral hepatitis, type B: an early marker of chronic evolution. Lancet 2:358, 1982.

327b. Beasley RP, Hwang L-Y, Lin C-C, et al. Hepatitis B immune globulin (HBIG): efficacy in the interruption of perinatal transmission of the hepatitis B carrier state. Lancet 2:388, 1981.

327c. Stevens CE, Neurath RA, Beasley RP, et al. HBeAg and anti-HBe detection by radioimmunoassay: correlation with vertical transmission of hepatitis B virus in Taiwan. J Med Virol 3:237, 1979.

327d. Beasley RP, Hwang L-Y, Lin C-C, et al. Incidence of hepatitis B virus infection in preschool children in Taiwan. J Infect Dis 146:198, 1982.

327e. McMahon BJ, Alward WLM, Hall DB, et al. Acute hepatitis B virus infection: relation of age to the clinical expression of disease and subsequent development of the carrier state. J Infect Dis 151:599, 1985.

327f. Tassopolous NC, Papaevangelou GS, Sjogren MH, et al. Natural history of hepatitis B surface antigen-positive hepatitis in Greek adults. Gastroenterology 92:1844, 1987.

327g. Dienstag JL, Alter JH. Non-A, non-B hepatitis: evolving epidemiologic and clinical perspectives. Semin Liver Dis 6:67, 1986.

327h. Hay CRM, Preston FE, Triger DR, et al. Progressive liver disease in hemophilia: an understated problem? Lancet 1:1495, 1985.

328. Alter JH, Hoofnagle JH. Non-A, non-B: observation on the first decade. In: Vyas GN, Dienstag JL, Hoofnagle JH, eds. Viral Hepatitis and Liver Disease. Orlando, FL, Grune & Stratton, 1984:345.

329. Aledort LM, Levine PH, Hilgartner M, et al. A study of liver biopsies and liver disease among hemophiliacs. Blood 66:367, 1985.

330. Preston FE, Triger DR, Underwood JCE, et al. Percutaneous liver biopsy and chronic liver disease in haemophiliacs. Lancet 2:592, 1978.

331. Krarup NB, Roholm K. The development of cirrhosis of the liver after acute hepatitis, elucidated by aspiration biopsy. Acta Med Scand 108:306, 1941.

332. Chalmers TC. Viral hepatitis and its sequelae. Am J Dig Dis 6:189, 1961.

333. Nefzger MD, Chalmers TC. The treatment of acute infectious hepatitis: ten year follow up study of the effects of diet and rest. Am J Med 35:299, 1963.

334. Beebe GW, Simon AH. Cirrhosis of the liver following viral hepatitis: a twenty year mortality follow up. Am J Epidemiol 92:279, 1970.

335. Rakela J, Redeker AG, Edwards VM, et al. Hepatitis A virus infection in fulminant hepatitis and chronic active hepatitis. Gastroenterology 74:879, 1978.

336. Lundberg J, Frosner G, Hansson BG, et al. Serologic markers of hepatitis A and B in chronic active hepatitis. Scand J Gastroenterol 13:525, 1978.

337. Eppinger H. Die Leber krankheiten Allgemeine und spezialle pathologie und Therapie der Leber. Wein, Julius Springer, 1937.

338. Watson CJ, Hoffbauer FW. The problem of prolonged hepatitis with particular reference to the cholangiolitic type and to the development of cholangiolitic cirrhosis of the liver. Ann Intern Med 25:195, 1946.

339. Eliakim M, Rachmilewitz M. Cholangiolitic manifestations in virus hepatitis. Gastroenterology 31:369, 1956.

340. Sheldon S, Sherlock S. Virus hepatitis with features of prolonged bile retention. Br Med J 2:734, 1957.

341. Gall EA, Braunstein H. Hepatitis with manifestations simulating bile duct obstruction (so-called "cholangiolitic hepatitis"). Am J Clin Pathol 25:1113, 1955.

342. Dubin IN, Sullivan BH, LeGolvan PC, et al. The cholestatic form of viral hepatitis: experience with viral hepatitis at the Brooke Army Hospital during the years 1951 to 1953. Am J Med 29:55, 1960.

343. Gupta D, Smetana HF. The histopathology of epidemic viral hepatitis. Delhi 1955–1956. Report to the Indian Council of Medical Research, New Delhi, India, 1956.

344. Morrow RH Jr, Smetana HF, Edgcomb JH. Unusual features of viral hepatitis in Accra, Ghana. Ann Intern Med 68:1250, 1968.

345. Ishak KG. Light microscopic morphology of viral hepatitis. Am J Clin Pathol 65:787, 1976.

346. Dienstag JL, Popper H, Purcell RH. The pathology of viral hepatitis,

types A and B in chimpanzees: a comparison. Am J Pathol 85:131, 1976.

347. Seeff LB. Hepatitis in the drug abuser. Med Clin North Am 59:843, 1975.

348. Ishak BW, Ishak KG. Foreign-body reaction in the liver of a drug addict. J Forensic Sci 14:515, 1969.

349. Rappaport AM. Anatomic considerations. In: Schiff L, ed. Diseases of the Liver, 3rd ed. Philadelphia, JB Lippincott, 1969:1.

350. Scotto J, Opolon P, Eteve J, et al. Liver biopsy and prognosis in acute liver failure. Gut 14:1927, 1973.

351. Horney JT, Galambos JT. The liver during and after fulminant hepatitis. Gastroenterology 73:639, 1977.

352. Popper H. Pathology of viral hepatitis. Israel J Med Sci 15:240, 1979.

353. Schaffner F. The structural basis of altered hepatic function in viral hepatitis. Am J Med 49:658, 1970.

354. Hadziyannis S, Gerber MA, Vissoulis C, et al. Cytoplasmic hepatitis B antigen in "ground-glass" hepatocytes of carriers. Arch Pathol 96:327, 1973.

355. Klinge O, Bannasch P. Zur Vermehrung des glatten endoplasmatischen Reticulum in Hepatocyten menschlicher Leverbunktate. In: Verhandlungen der Deutschen Gesellschaft für Pathologie. Stuttgart, G. Fischer, 1968:568.

356. Klinge O, Kaboth U, Arnold R. Liver histology in healthy carriers of Australia SH antigen or antibodies. Germ Med Month 1:4, 1971.

357. Shikata T, Uzawa T, Yoshiwara N, et al. Staining methods of Australia antigen in paraffin sections: detection of cytoplasmic inclusion bodies. Jpn J Exp Med 44:25, 1974.

358. Gerber MA, Hadziyannis S, Vernace S, et al. Incidence and nature of cytoplasmic B antigen in hepatocytes. Lab Invest 32:251, 1975.

359. Deodhar KP, Tapp E, Scheuer PJ. Orcein staining of hepatitis B antigen in paraffin sections of liver biopsies. J Clin Pathol 28:66, 1975.

360. Sipponen P. Orcein positive hepatocellular material in long-standing biliary diseases. I. Histochemical abnormalities: II. Ultrastructural studies. Scand J Gastroenterol 11:545, 553, 1976.

361. Nakanuma Y, Karino T, Ohta G. Orcein positive granules in the hepatocytes in chronic intrahepatic cholestasis: morphological, histochemical, and electron x-ray microanalytical examination. Virchows Arch A Pathol Anat Histol 382:21, 1979.

362. Gerber MA, Hadziyannis S, Vissoulis C, et al. Electron microscopy and immunoelectron microscopy of cytoplasmic hepatitis B antigen in hepatocytes. Am J Pathol 75:489, 1974.

363. Yamada G, Nakane PK. Hepatitis B core and surface antigen in liver tissue: light and electron microscopic localization by the peroxidase labelled antibody method. Lab Invest 36:659, 1977.

364. Huang S-N. Immunohistochemical demonstration of hepatitis B core and surface antigens in paraffin sections. Lab Invest 33:88, 1975.

365. Huang S-N, Neurath AR. Immunologic demonstration of hepatitis B viral antigen in the liver with reference to its significance in liver injury. Lab Invest 40:1, 1979.

366. Gudat F, Bianchi L, Sonnabend W, et al. Pattern of core and surface expression in liver tissue reflects state of specific immune response in hepatitis B. Lab Invest 32:1, 1975.

367. Bianchi L, Gudat F. Immunopathology of hepatitis B. In: Popper H, Schaffner F, eds. Progress in Liver Diseases, Vol 6. New York, Grune & Stratton, 1979:371.

368. Lucke B. Pathology of fatal epidemic hepatitis. Am J Pathol 20:471, 1944.

369. Adler L, Lyon E. Cardiac disorders associated with infectious hepatitis. Cardiologia 11:111, 1947.

370. Saphir O, Amromin GD, Yokoo H. Myocarditis in viral (epidemic) hepatitis. Am J Med Sci 231:168, 1956.

371. Bell H. Cardiac manifestations of viral hepatitis. JAMA 218:387, 1971.

372. Eisen M, Markovich V. Fatal acute hepatitis: report of a case with massive hemorrhage in pericardial and pleural cavities. JAMA 146:141, 1951.

373. Adler R, Takahashi M, Wright HT Jr. Acute pericarditis associated with hepatitis B infection. Pediatrics 61:716, 1978.

374. Dehn H, Feil H, Rindersknecht RE. Electrocardiographic changes in cases of infectious hepatitis. Am Heart J 31:183, 1946.

375. Arnon R, Ehrlich R. Hepatitis, bradycardia, and the use of a cardiac pacemaker. JAMA 228:1024, 1974.

376. Gross P, Gerding DN. Pleural effusion associated with viral hepatitis. Gastroenterology 60:898, 1971.

377. Katsilabros L, Triandaffillon G, Kontoyiannis P, et al. Pleural effusion in hepatitis. Gastroenterology 63:718, 1972.

378. Sbosito M, Petroni VA, Veler L. Importanza diagnostica dei piccoli versamenti pleurici nella virus epatite. Epatologia, 12:228, 1966.

379. Owen RL, Shapiro H. Pleural effusion, rash, and anergy in icteric hepatitis. N Engl J Med 291:963, 1974.

380. Flacks CM, Lees D. A case of hepatitis B with pleural effusion. Aust NZ J Med 7:636, 1977.

381. Cocchi P, Silenzi M. Pleural effusion in HBsAg-positive hepatitis. J Pediatr 89:329, 1976.

382. Tabor E, Russell P, Gerety RJ, et al. Hepatitis B surface antigen and e antigen in pleural effusion. A case report. Gastroenterology 73:1157, 1977.

383. Bank J, Dixon CH. Gastroscopy in acute and chronic hepatitis. JAMA 131:107, 1946.

384. Loughead JR, Golding FC. The gastric mucosa in acute infectious hepatitis. Gastroenterology 20:471, 1952.

385. Havens WP Jr, Kushlan SD, Green MR. Experimentally induced infectious hepatitis: Roentgenographic and gastroscopic observations. Arch Intern Med 79:457, 1947.

386. Cirillo NB, Castell DO, Jacoby WS. Gastric acid secretion in infectious hepatitis. Milit Med 137:64, 1972.

387. Kravetz RE, Branzenis NV. Viral hepatitis associated with enteritis gravis. Arch Intern Med 112:179, 1963.

388. Astaldi G, Grandini V, Poggi C, et al. Intestinal biopsy in acute hepatitis. Am J Dig Dis 9:237, 1964.

389. Mondai N, Theodor E. Intestinal contents in patients with viral hepatitis after a liquid meal. Gastroenterology 58:379, 1970.

390. Mason JO, McLean WR. Infectious hepatitis traced to the consumption of raw oysters: an epidemiologic study. Am J Hyg 75:90, 1962.

391. Mathiesen LR, Feinstone SM, Purcell RH, et al. Detection of hepatitis A antigen by immunofluorescence. Infect Immun 18:524, 1977.

392. Mathiesen LR, Drucker J, Lorenz D, et al. Localization of hepatitis A antigen in marmoset organs during acute infection with hepatitis A virus. J Infect Dis 138:369, 1970.

392a. Pollack JS, Anders L, Gulumoglu A, et al. Direct measurement of hepatitis B viral antibody and antigen markers in gingival crevicular fluid. Oral Surg 57:499, 1984.

392b. Ward R, Borchert P, Wright A, et al. Hepatitis B in saliva and mouth washings. Lancet 2:726, 1972.

392c. Heathcote J, Cameron CH, Dane DS. Hepatitis-B antigen in saliva and semen. Lancet 1:71, 1974.

392d. Ogra PL. Immunologic aspects of hepatitis-associated antigen and antibody in human body fluids. J Immunol 110:723, 1973.

392e. Villarejos VM, Visona KA, Gutierrez A, et al. Role of saliva, urine and feces in the transmission of type B hepatitis. N Engl J Med 291:1375, 1974.

392f. Feinman SV, Krassinski O, Sinclair JL, et al. Hepatitis B surface antigen in saliva of HBsAg carriers. J Lab Clin Med 85:1042, 1975.

392g. Bancroft WH, Snitbhan R, Scott RM, et al. Transmission of hepatitis B virus to gibbons by exposure to human saliva containing hepatitis B surface antigen. J Infect Dis 135:79, 1977.

392h. Alter HJ, Purcell RH, Gerin JL, et al. Transmission of hepatitis B to chimpanzees by hepatitis-B surface antigen-positive saliva and semen. Infect Immunol 16:928, 1977.

392i. MacCallum FO, Bauer DJ. Homologous serum jaundice: transmission experiments with human volunteers. Lancet 1:622, 1944.

392j. Akdamar KA, Maumus L, Epps EC, et al. SH antigen in bile. Lancet 2:909, 1971.

392k. Serpeau D, Mannoni P, Dhumeaux D, et al. Hepatitis associated antigen in bile. Lancet 2:1266, 1971.

392l. Feinman SV, Berris B, Rebane A, et al. Failure to detect hepatitis B, surface antigen in feces of HBsAg-positive persons. J Infect Dis 140:407, 1979.

392m. Hoefs JC, Reiner IG, Ashcavai M, et al. Hepatitis B surface antigen in pancreatic and biliary secretions. Gastroenterology 79:191, 1980.

392n. Tripatzis I. Australia antigen in urine and feces. Am J Dis Child 123:400, 1972.

392o. Grob PJ, Jawalka H. Faecal SH (Australia) antigen in acute hepatitis. Lancet 1:206, 1971.

392p. Tiku ML, Bentner KR, Ramirez RI, et al. Distribution and characteristics of hepatitis B surface antigen in body fluids of institutionalized children and adults. J Infect Dis 134:342, 1976.

392q. Neefe JR, Gellis SS, Stokes J Jr. Homologous serum hepatitis and infectious (epidemic) hepatitis: studies in volunteers bearing on immunological and other characteristics of the etiologic agents. Am J Med 1:3, 1946.

392r. Neefe JR, Stokes J Jr, Reinhold JC. Oral administration to volunteers of feces from patients with homologous serum and infectious (epidemic) hepatitis. Am J Med Sci 210:29, 1945.

392s. Cossart YE, Vahrain D. Studies of Australia-SH antigen in sporadic viral hepatitis in London. Br Med J 1:403, 1970.

392t. Gust ID, Kaldor J, Nastasi M. Absence of Au antigen in faeces of patients with Au-positive sera. Lancet 1:797, 1971.

392u. Irwin GR, Allan AM, Bancroft WH, et al. Hepatitis B antigen in saliva, urine and stool. Infect Immunol 11:142, 1975.

392v. Mazzur S, Corbett J, Blumberg BS. Loss of immunologic reactivities of Australia antigen after incubation with bacteria. Proc Soc Exp Biol Med 142:327, 1973.

392w. Paizza M, Stasio GD, Maio G, et al. Hepatitis B antigen inhibitor in human feces and intestinal mucosa. Br Med J 2:334, 1973.

393. Moodie JW, Stannard LM, Kipps A. The problem of the demonstration

of hepatitis B antigen in faeces and bile. J Clin Pathol 27:693, 1974.

394. Grabow WOK, Prozesky OW, Applebaum PL, et al. Absence of hepatitis B antigens from feces and sewage as a result of enzymatic destruction. J Infect Dis 131:685, 1975.

395. Lisney AA. Discussion on infective hepatitis, recent field investigations. Proc R Soc Med 37:165, 1943.

396. Joske RA. The association of viral hepatitis and pancreatitis. R Melbourne Hosp Clin Res 25:20, 1955.

397. Achord JL. Acute pancreatitis with infectious hepatitis. JAMA 205:129, 1968.

398. Ham JM, Fitzpatrick P. Acute pancreatitis in patients with acute hepatic failure. Am J Dig Dis 18:1079, 1973.

399. Geokas MC, Olson H, Swanson V, et al. The association of viral hepatitis and acute pancreatitis. Calif Med 117:1, 1972.

400. Parbhoo SP, Welch J, Sherlock A. Acute pancreatitis in patients with fulminant hepatic failure. Gut 14:428, 1973.

401. Wands JR, Salyer DC, Boitnott JK, et al. Fulminant hepatitis complicated by pancreatitis. Johns Hopkins Med J 133:156, 1973.

402. Rake MO, Flute PT, Pannell G, et al. Intravascular coagulation in acute hepatic necrosis. Lancet 1:533, 1970.

403. Franzini C, Moda S. Human urinary amylolytic enzymes in acute hepatitis. J Clin Pathol 18:775, 1965.

403a. Karasawa T, Tsukagoshi S, Yoshimura M, et al. Light microscopic localization of hepatitis B virus antigens in the human pancreas: possibility of multiplication of hepatitis B virus in the human pancreas. Gastroenterology 81:998, 1981.

404. Laverdent C, Meunier J, Molini C. Functional involvement of the pancreas during virus hepatitis. Ann Med Intern (Paris) 122:343, 1971.

405. Adi FC. Diabetes mellitus associated with epidemic of infectious hepatitis in Nigeria. Br Med J 1:183, 1974.

406. Lorenz E, Quaiser K. Panmyelopathie nach Hepatitis epidemica. Wien Med Wochenschr 105:19, 1955.

407. Hagler L, Pastore RA, Bergin JJ, et al. Aplastic anemia following viral hepatitis. Report of two fatal cases and literature review. Medicine 54:139, 1975.

408. Rubin E, Gottlieb C, Vogen P. Syndrome of hepatitis in aplastic anemia. Am J Med 45:88, 1968.

409. Camitta BM, Nathan DG, Forman EN, et al. Post-hepatic severe aplastic anemia—an indication for early bone marrow transplantation. Blood 43:473, 1974.

410. Firkin FC, Nicholls K, Whelan G. Transient myeloid and erythroid aplasia associated with infectious hepatitis. Br Med J 2:1534, 1978.

411. Cascatoto DA, Klein CA, Kaplowitz N, et al. Aplastic anemia associated with type B viral hepatitis. Arch Intern Med 138:1157, 1978.

411a. Perrillo RP, Pohl DA, Roodman W, et al. Acute non-A, non-B hepatitis with serum sickness-like syndrome and aplastic anemia. JAMA 6:245, 1981.

411b. Zeldis JB. Aplastic anemia and non-A, non-B hepatitis. Am J Med 76:64, 1983.

412. Nagaraju M, Weitzman S, Baumann G. Viral hepatitis and agranulocytosis. Am J Dig Dis 18:247, 1973.

413. Bosset JF, Rozenbaum A, Flesch N, et al. Agranulocytose au cours de l'hepatite virale. Nouv Presse Med 8:130, 1979.

413a. Barton JL, Conrad ME. Beneficial effects of hepatitis in patients with acute myelogenous leukemia. Ann Intern Med 90:188, 1979.

413b. Cacciola E, Giustolisi R. Acute myelogenous leukemia and hepatitis. Ann Intern Med 92:127, 1980.

414. Raffensperger EC. Acute acquired hemolytic anemia in association with acute viral hepatitis. Ann Intern Med 48:1243, 1958.

415. Phillips SM, Silver MP. Glucose-6-phosphate dehydrogenase deficiency, infectious hepatitis, acute hemolysis and renal failure. Ann Intern Med 70:99, 1969.

416. Chan TK, Todd D. Hemolysis complicating viral hepatitis in patients with glucose-6-phosphate dehydrogenase deficiency. Br Med J 1:131, 1975.

417. Gassard BG, Henderson JM, Williams R. Factor VII levels as a guide to prognosis in fulminant hepatic failure. Gut 17:489, 1976.

418. Clark R, Rake MO, Flute PT, et al. Coagulation abnormalities in acute liver failure; pathogenetic and therapeutic implications. Scand J Gastroenterol 8 (Suppl 19):63, 1973.

418a. Gu JR, Chen YC, Jiang HQ, et al. State of hepatitis B virus DNA in leukocytes of hepatitis B patients. J Med Virol 17:73, 1985.

418b. Lie Injo LE, Balasegaram M, Lopez CG, et al. Hepatitis B virus DNA in liver and white blood cells of patients with hepatoma. DNA 2:301, 1983.

418c. Pontisso P, Poon MC, Tiollais P, et al. Detection of hepatitis B virus DNA in human blood mononuclear cells. Br Med J 288:1563, 1984.

418d. Laure F, Zagury O, Saimot AG, et al. Hepatitis B virus DNA sequences in lymphoid cells from patients with AIDS and AIDS-related complex. Science 229:561, 1985.

418e. Elfassi E, Romet Lemonne JL, Essex M, et al. Evidence of extra-chromosomal forms of hepatitis B viral DNA in bone marrow culture obtained from a patient recently infected with hepatitis B virus. Proc Natl Acad Sci USA 81:3526, 1984.

418f. Pontisso P, Locasciulli A, Schiarm E, et al. Detection of hepatitis B virus DNA sequences in bone marrow of children with leukemia. Cancer 59:292, 1987.

419. Apstein MD, Koff E, Koff RS. Neuropsychological dysfunction in acute viral hepatitis. Digestion 19:349, 1979.

420. Waring J. Acute lymphocytic meningitis in epidemic catarrhal jaundice. Br Med J 2:228, 1943.

421. Weinstein L, Davidson WT. Neurologic manifestations in the pre-icteric phase of infectious hepatitis. Am Practitioner 1:191, 1946.

422. Lescher FG. The nervous complications of infective hepatitis. Br Med J 1:554, 1944.

423. Thorling R. Neurologic complications in acute infectious hepatitis. Acta Med Scand 137:322, 1950.

423a. Bromberg K, Newhale DN, Peter G. Hepatitis A and meningoen-cephalitis. JAMA 247:815, 1982.

424. Byrne EAJ, Taylor GF. An outbreak of jaundice with signs in the nervous system. Br Med J 1:477, 1945.

425. Brooks BR. Viral hepatitis type B presenting with seizures. JAMA 237:472, 1977.

426. Klugman HB. Neurological manifestations of infectious hepatitis. S Afr Med J 35:681, 1961.

427. Friedlander WJ. Neurological signs and symptoms as a prodrome to virus hepatitis. Neurology 6:574, 1956.

428. Gortvai P, Hasan N. Status epilepticus in infectious hepatitis. Br J Clin Pract 27:139, 1973.

429. Zimmerman HJ, Lowery CM. Encephalomyeloradiculitis (Guillain-Barré syndrome) as a complication of infectious hepatitis. Ann Intern Med 26:934, 1947.

430. Plough IC, Ayerle RS. The Guillain-Barré syndrome associated with acute hepatitis. N Engl J Med 249:61, 1953.

430a. Tabor E. Guillain-Barré syndrome and other neurologic syndromes in hepatitis A, B, and non-A, non-B. J Med Virol 21:207, 1987.

430b. Johnston CLW, Schwartz M, Wansbrough-Jones MH. Acute inflammatory polyradiculoneuropathy following type A viral hepatitis. Postgrad Med 57:647, 1981.

430c. Dunk A, Jenkins WJ, Sherlock S. Guillain-Barré syndrome associated with hepatitis A in a male homosexual. Br J Vener Dis 58:269, 1982.

430d. Igarashi M, Tomono M, Uchida S, et al. Guillain-Barré syndrome associated with acute hepatitis A. Gastroenterol Jpn 18:549, 1983.

430e. Bosch VV, Dowling PC, Cook SD. Hepatitis A virus immunoglobulin M antibody in acute neurological disease. Ann Neurol 14:685, 1983.

430f. Grover B, Delassandro L, Sanders JG, et al. Severe viral hepatitis A infection, Landry-Guillain-Barré syndrome, and hereditary elliptocytosis. South Med J 79:251, 1986.

430g. Mares-Segura R, Sola-Lamoglia R, Soler-Singla L, et al. Guillain-Barré syndrome associated with hepatitis A. Ann Neurol 19:100, 1986.

430h. Neirmeiger P, Gipps CH. Guillain-Barré syndrome in acute HBsAg hepatitis. Br Med J 2:732, 1975.

430i. Ng PL, Powell L, Campbell B. Guillain-Barré syndrome in acute hepatitis. Br Med J 1:585, 1976.

430j. Huet P, Layrargues GP, Lebrun L, et al. Hepatitis B surface antigen in the cerebrospinal fluid in a case of Guillain-Barré syndrome. Can Med Assoc J 122:1157, 1980.

430k. Berger JR, Aygar DR, Sheremata WA. Guillain-Barré syndrome complicating acute hepatitis B: a case with detailed electrophysiological and immunological studies. Arch Neurol 38:366, 1981.

430l. Walle H, Lehmann H. Guillain-Barré syndrome and HBsAg-positive acute viral hepatitis (case report). Hepatogastroenterol 28:305, 1981.

430m. Penner E, Maida E, Mamoli B, et al. Serum and cerebrospinal fluid immune complexes containing hepatitis B surface antigen in Guillain-Barré syndrome. Gastroenterology 82:576, 1983.

431. Porst H, Hentschel R, Sauermann W, et al. Polyradikulitis Guillain-Barré bei akuter virushepatitis typ B. Fullbercht. Deutsche Zeitschrift fur Verdauungs und Stoffwechsel-Krankheiten. 43:146, 1983.

432. Fentren G, Gerbal J, Allinquant B, et al. Association of Guillain-Barré syndrome and B-virus hepatitis: simultaneous presence of anti-DS-DNA antibodies and HBs antigen cerebrospinal fluid. J Lab Clin Immunol 11:161, 1983.

433. Klippel M, Lhermitte T. Des névrites au cours des cirrhose du foie. Sem Med 28:13, 1908.

434. Fiqueredi R, Patel TG, Grosberg S, et al. Acute fulminant hepatitis: unusual neurological sequelae. Arch Intern Med 133:832, 1974.

435. Davison AM, Williams IR, Mawdsley C, et al. Neuropathy associated with hepatitis in patients maintained on hemodialysis. Br J Med 1:409, 1972.

436. Koff RS, Sax DS, Freiberger Z, et al. Peripheral motor neuropathy associated with viral hepatitis. Gastroenterology 65:A-29/553, 1973.
437. Farivar M, Wands JR, Benson GD, et al. Cryoprotein complexes and peripheral neuropathy in a patient with chronic active hepatitis. Gastroenterology 71:490, 1976.
438. Mandal BK, Allbeson M. Trigeminal sensory neuropathy and virus hepatitis. Lancet 2:1322, 1972.
439. Smith FR, Henkin RK, Dell RB. Disordered gustatory acuity in liver disease. Gastroenterology 70:568, 1976.
440. Henkin RI, Smith FS. Hyposmia in acute viral hepatitis. Lancet 1:823, 1971.
440a. Tsukada N, Koh C, Owa M, et al. Chronic neuropathy associated with immune complexes of hepatitis B virus. J Neurol Sci 61:193, 1983.
440b. Gocke DJ, Hsu K, Morgan C, et al. Vasculitis in association with Australia antigen. J Exp Med 134:330, 1971.
440c. Goudeau P, Trepo C, Herreman G, et al. Periarterite noueuse et antigene Australia: etude comparative a propos de 54 cas. Sem Hop Paris 53:613, 1977.
440d. Drucke T, Barbanel C, Jungers P, et al. Hepatitis B antigen-associated periarteritis nodosa in patients undergoing long-term hemodialysis. Am J Med 68:86, 1980.
441. Benjamin JE, Hoyt RC. Disability following post-vaccinial (yellow fever) hepatitis: study of 200 patients manifesting delayed convalescence. JAMA 128:319, 1945.
442. Sherlock S, Walshe V. The post-hepatitis syndrome. Lancet 2:482, 1946.
443. Martini GA, Strohmeyer G. Post-hepatitis syndromes. Clin Gastroenterol 3:377, 1975.
444. Ferguson SH, Arias DE. Hepatitis and neoplasia of the cervical epithelium. Am J Med Sci 246:459, 1963.
445. Ford JH Jr, Dudan RC, Averette HE. Hepatitis and positive cervical cytology. Obstet Gynecol 39:111, 1972.
446. Alpert E, Isselbacher KJ, Schur PH. The pathogenesis of arthritis associated with viral hepatitis: complement-component studies. N Engl J Med 285:185, 1971.
447. Koff RS. Immune-complex arthritis in viral hepatitis. N Engl J Med 285:229, 1971.
448. Fernandez R, McCarty DJ. The arthritis of viral hepatitis. Ann Intern Med 74:207, 1971.
449. Onion DK, Crumpacker CS, Gilliland BC. Arthritis of hepatitis associated with Australia antigen. Ann Intern Med 75:29, 1971.
450. Wenzel RP, McCormick DP, Busch HJ, et al. Arthritis and viral hepatitis: a patient with transient serum hepatitis-associated antigen, skin nodules, rash, and low serum complement. Arch Intern Med 130:770, 1972.
451. Stevens DP, Walker J, Crum E, et al. Anicteric hepatitis presenting as polyarthritis. JAMA 220:687, 1972.
452. Alacron GS, Towns AS. Arthritis in viral hepatitis. Report of two cases and review of the literature. Hopkins Med J 132:1, 1973.
453. McCarty DJ, Ormiste V. Arthritis and HBsAg-positive hepatitis. Arch Intern Med 132:264, 1973.
454. Schumacher HR, Gall EP. Arthritis in acute hepatitis and chronic active hepatitis. Pathology of the synovial membrane with the evidence for the presence of Australia antigen in synovial membranes. Am J Med 57:655, 1974.
455. Graves RJ. A System of Clinical Medicine. Dublin, Fannin and Company, 1843:564.
456. Wands JR, Mann E, Alpert E, et al. The pathogenesis of arthritis with acute-B surface antigen-positive hepatitis. Complement activation and characterization of circulating immune complexes. J Clin Invest 55:930, 1975.
457. Prestia AE, Lynfield YL. Scarlatiniform eruption in viral hepatitis. Arch Dermatol 101:353, 1970.
458. Steigman AJ. Rashes and arthropathy in viral hepatitis. Mt Sinai J Med 40:752, 1973.
459. Dienstag JL, Rhodes AR, Wands JR, et al. The pathogenesis of urticaria associated with acute viral hepatitis, type B. Gastroenterology 72:A-19/1217, 1977.
459a. Thorne EG, Krueger GG, Koehn GG, et al. Urticaria with hepatitis associated antigen (HAA) positive hepatitis. Cutis 10:705, 1972.
460. Veyre B, Brette R. L'hepatite B a la phase premonitoire: frequence des manifestations articulaires et cutanees, a propos de 100 cas. Nouv Presse Med 4:1349, 1975.
461. Weiss T, Tsai CC, Baldassare AR, et al. Skin lesions in viral hepatitis: histologic and immunofluorescent findings. Am J Med 64:269, 1978.
462. Duffy J, Lidsky MD, Sharp JT. Polyarthritis, polyarteritis and hepatitis B. Medicine 55:19, 1976.
463. Clark E, Kaplan BI. Endocardial, arterial, and other mesenchymal alterations associated with serum sickness in man. Arch Pathol 24:458, 1937.
464. Paull R. Periarteritis nodosa (panarteritis nodosa) with report of four previous cases. Calif Med 67:309, 1947.
465. Trepo CH, Girard M. Antigene Australia, hepatite virale et periarterite noueuse. Arch Fr Mal App Dig 60:687, 1971.
466. Prince AM, Trepo C. Role of immune complexes involving SH antigen in pathogenesis of chronic active hepatitis and polyarteritis nodosa. Lancet 1:1309, 1971.
467. Baker AL, Kaplan MM, Benz WC, et al. Polyarteritis associated with Australia antigen-positive hepatitis. Gastroenterology 62:105, 1971.
468. Trepo C, Thivolet J, Lambert J. Four cases of periarteritis nodosa associated with persistent Australia antigen. Digestion 5:100, 1972.
469. Koff RS, Widrich WC, Robbins AH. Necrotizing angitis in a methamphetamine user with hepatitis B—angiographic diagnosis, five-month follow-up results and localization of bleeding site. N Engl J Med 288:946, 1973.
470. Trepo C, Zuckerman AJ, Bird RC, et al. The role of circulating hepatitis B antigen-antibody immune complexes in the pathogenesis of vascular and hepatic manifestations in polyarteritis nodosa. J Clin Pathol 27:863, 1974.
471. Cosgriff TM, Arnold WJ. Digital vasospasm and infarction associated with hepatitis B antigenemia. JAMA 235:1362, 1976.
472. Boyer TD, Tong MJ, Rakela J, et al. Immunologic studies and clinical follow-up HBsAg-positive polyarteritis nodosa. Am J Dig Dis 22:497, 1977.
473. Sergent JS, Lockshin MD, Christian CL, et al. Vasculitis with hepatitis B antigenemia: long-term observations in nine patients. Medicine 55:1, 1976.
474. Michalak T. Immune complexes of hepatitis B surface antigen in the pathogenesis of periarteritis nodosa. Am J Pathol 90:619, 1978.
475. Fisher RG, Graham DY, Granmayeh M, et al. Polyarteritis nodosa and hepatitis-B surface antigen: role of angiography in diagnosis. Am J Roentgenol 129:77, 1977.
476. Farquhar JO. Renal studies in acute infectious (epidemic) hepatitis. Am J Med 210:291, 1949.
477. Combes B, Stastny P, Shorey J, et al. Glomerulonephritis with deposition of Australia antigen-antibody complexes in glomerular basement membrane. Lancet 2:234, 1971.
478. Myers BD, Griffel B, Naveh D, et al. Membrano-proliferative glomerulonephritis associated with persistent viral hepatitis. Am J Clin Pathol 59:222, 1972.
479. Eknoyan G, Gyorkey F, Dichoso C, et al. Renal morphological and immunological changes associated with acute viral hepatitis. Kidney Int 1:413, 1972.
480. Kohler PF, Cronin RE, Hammond WS, et al. Chronic membranous glomerulonephritis caused by hepatitis B antigen-antibody immune complexes. Ann Intern Med 81:448, 1974.
481. Kneiser MR, Jenis EH, Lowenthal DT, et al. Pathogenesis of renal disease associated with viral hepatitis. Arch Pathol 97:193, 1974.
482. Takekoshi Y, Tanaka M, Shida N, et al. Strong association between membranous nephropathy and hepatitis-B surface antigenemia in Japanese children. Lancet 1:1065, 1978.
483. Takekoshi Y, Tanaka M, Miyakawa Y, et al. Free "small" and IgG-associated "large" hepatitis B e antigen in the serum and glomerular capillary walls of two patients with membranous glomerulonephritis. N Engl J Med 300:814, 1979.
484. Brzosko WJ, Drawczynski R, Nazarewicz T, et al. Glomerulonephritis associated with hepatitis-B surface antigen immune complexes in children. Lancet 2:477, 1974.
485. Henson JB. Pathogenesis of the glomerular lesions in Aleutian disease of mink. Arch Pathol 87:21, 1969.
486. Oldstone MD, Dixon FJ. Pathogenesis of chronic disease associated with persistent lymphocytic choriomeningitis viral infection. J Exp Med 129:483, 1969.
486a. Conte JJ, Fourmie GJ. Antigène Australia et glomerulonephritis. Nouv Presse Med 4:49, 1975.
486b. Nagy J, Bajtai G, Brasch H, et al. The role of hepatitis B surface antigen in the pathogenesis of glomerulonephritis. Clin Nephrol 12:109, 1979.
486c. Ito H, Hattori S, Matsuda I, et al. Hepatitis B e antigen-mediated membranous glomerulonephritis: correlation of ultrastructural changes with HBeAg in the serum and glomeruli. Lab Invest 44:214, 1981.
486d. Knecht GL, Chisari FV. Reversibility of hepatitis B virus-induced glomerulonephritis and chronic active hepatitis after spontaneous clearance of serum hepatitis B surface antigen. Gastroenterology 75:1152, 1978.
487. Levo Y, Gorevic PD, Kassab HJ, et al. Liver involvement in the syndrome of mixed cryoglobulinemia. Ann Intern Med 87:287, 1977.
488. Levo Y, Gorevic PD, Kassab HJ, et al. Association between hepatitis B virus and essential mixed cryoglobulinemia. N Engl J Med 296:1501, 1977.

489. Popp JW, Dienstag JL, Wands JR, et al. Essential mixed cryoglobuli-nemia without evidence for hepatitis B virus infection. Ann Intern Med 92:379, 1980.

490. McIntosh RM, Koss MN, Gocke DJ. The nature and incidence of cryoproteins in hepatitis B antigen (HBsAg) positive patients. Q J Med 177:23, 1976.

491. Gianotti F. Papular acrodermatitis of childhood—an Australia antigen disease. Arch Dis Child 48:794, 1973.

492. Ishimaru Y, Ishimaru H, Toda G, et al. An epidemic of infantile papular acrodermatitis (Gianotti's disease) in Japan associated with hepatitis-B surface, subtype ayw. Lancet 1:707, 1976.

493. Colombo M, Gerber MA, Vernace SJ, et al. Immune response to hepatitis B virus in children with papular acrodermatitis. Gastro-enterology 73:1103, 1977.

494. Toda G, Ishimaru Y, Mayumi M, et al. Infantile papular acrodermatitis (Gianotti's disease) and intrafamilial occurrence of acute hepatitis B with jaundice: age dependency of clinical manifestations of hepatitis B virus infection. J Infect Dis 138:211, 1978.

495. Gianotti F. HBsAg and papular acrodermatitis of childhood. N Engl J Med 298:460, 1978.

496. Castellano A, Schweitzer R, Tong MJ, et al. Papular acrodermatitis of childhood and hepatitis B infection. Arch Dermatol 114:1530, 1978.

496a. Lee S, Kim KY, Hahn CS, et al. Gianotti-Crosti syndrome associated with hepatitis B surface antigen (subtype adr): J Am Acad Der-matol 12:629, 1985.

496b. Takata M, Fukui Y, Taketani T, et al. Papular acrodermatitis of childhood (Gianotti's disease). J Dermatol (Tokyo) 7:357, 1980.

497. Bacon PA, Doherty SM, Zuckerman AJ. Hepatitis-B antibody in polymyalgia rheumatica. Lancet 2:476, 1975.

498. Plouvier B, Wattre P, Cevulder B. HBsAg in superficial artery of a patient with polymyalgia rheumatica. Lancet 1:932, 1978.

499. Liang M, Greenberg H, Pincus T, et al. Hepatitis-B antibody in polymyalgia rheumatica. Lancet 1:43, 1976.

500. Bridgeford PH, Lowenstein M, Bocanegre TS, et al. Polymyalgia rheumatica and giant cell arteritis: histocompatibility typing and hepatitis-B infection states. Arthritis Rheum 23:516, 1980.

501. Zondek B, Branberg YM. Infectious hepatitis in pregnancy. J Mt Sinai Hosp 14:222, 1947.

502. Gelpi AP. Fatal hepatitis in Saudi Arabian women. Am J Gastroenterol 53:41, 1970.

503. Borhanmanesh F, Hagghighi P, Hekmat K, et al. Viral hepatitis during pregnancy: severity and effect on gestation. Gastroenterology 64:304, 1973.

504. Christie AB, Allan AA, Aref MK, et al. Pregnancy hepatitis in Libya. Lancet 2:827, 1976.

505. Naidu SS, Vismanathan R. Infectious hepatitis in pregnancy during Delhi epidemic. Indian J Med Res (Suppl) 45:71, 1957.

506. Malkani BK, Grewal AK. Observations on infectious hepatitis in pregnancy. Indian J Med Res (Suppl) 45:77, 1957.

507. Wahi PN, Arora MM. Epidemic hepatitis. N Engl J Med 248:451, 1953.

508. Phatak LV, Patel K. A study of infectious hepatitis in pregnancy. Indian J Med Sci 10:593, 1956.

508a. Tripathi BM, Misra NP. Viral hepatitis with pregnancy. J Assoc Phys India 29:463, 1981.

509. Ezes H, Bourdan R. Les hépatites ictérigènes graves d'allure virale au cours de la gestation. Gynecol Obstet (Paris) 55:288, 1956.

509a. Delons S, Berbich A, Raynaud R, et al. Contribution to the study of severe icterus of the pregnant woman in Morocco. Rev Medicho-chin Mal Foie 43:117, 1968.

509b. Tsega E. Viral hepatitis during pregnancy in Ethiopia. East Afr Med J 53:270, 1976.

510. Ingerslev M, Teilum G. Jaundice during pregnancy. Acta Obstet Gynecol Scand 31:74, 1951.

511. Roth LG. Infectious hepatitis in pregnancy. Am J Med Sci 225:139, 1953.

512. Thorling L. Jaundice in pregnancy: clinical study. Acta Med Scand (Suppl) 302, 1955.

513. Haemmerli UP. Jaundice during pregnancy. Acta Med Scand (Suppl) 444:23, 1966.

514. Adams RH, Combes R. Viral hepatitis during pregnancy. JAMA 192:195, 1965.

515. Hieber JP, Dalton D, Shorey J, et al. Hepatitis and pregnancy. J Pediatr 91:545, 1977.

515a. Shalev E, Bassan HM. Viral hepatitis during pregnancy in Israel. Int J Gynaecol Obstet 20:73, 1982.

515b. Peretz A, Paldi E, Brandstaeter S, et al. Infectious hepatitis in pregnancy. Obstet Gynecol 14:435, 1959.

516. Vincent CR. Jaundice in pregnancy. Obstet Gynecol 9:959, 1957.

517. Siegel M, Fuerst H, Peress N. Comparative fatal mortality in maternal virus diseases: a prospective study on rubella, measles, mumps, chickenpox, and hepatitis. N Engl J Med 274:768, 1966.

518. Hsia DV, Taylor RG, Gellis SS. Long-term follow up study of infectious hepatitis in pregnancy. J Pediatr 41:13, 1952.

519. Cahill KM. Hepatitis in pregnancy. Surg Gynecol Obstet 114:545, 1962.

520. Mickal A. Infectious hepatitis in pregnancy. Am J Obstet Gynecol 62:409, 1951.

521. Siegel M. Congenital malformation following chickenpox, measles, mumps and hepatitis: results of a cohort study. JAMA 226:1521, 1973.

522. Stoller A, Collman RD. Incidence of infectious hepatitis followed by Down's syndrome nine months later. Lancet, 2:1221, 1965.

523. Pantetakis SN, Chryssostomidou O, Alexiou D, et al. Sex chromatin and chromosomal abnormalities among 10,412 live-born babies. Arch Dis Child 45:87, 1970.

524. Kucera J. Down's syndrome and infectious hepatitis. Lancet 1:569, 1970.

524a. Singh DS, Balasubramanium M, Krishnaswami S, et al. Viral hepatitis during pregnancy. J Indian Med Assoc 73:90, 1979.

524b. Smithwick EM, Pascual E, Go SC. Hepatitis associated antigen: a possible relationship to premature delivery. J Pediatr 81:537, 1972.

525. Stark CR, Mantel N. Lack of seasonal- or temporal spatial clustering of Down's syndrome births in Michigan. Am J Epidemiol 86:199, 1967.

526. Kogan A, Kronmal R, Peterson DR. Relationship between infectious hepatitis and Down's syndrome. Am J Public Health 58:305, 1968.

527. Dietzman DE, Madden DL, Sever JL, et al. Lack of relationship between Down's syndrome and maternal exposure to Australia antigen. Am J Dis Child 124:195, 1972.

528. Sever JL, Kapikian AZ, Feinstone S. Hepatitis in Down's syndrome: lack of an association. J Infect Dis 134:198, 1976.

529. El-Alfi OS, Smith PM, Biesle JS. Chromosomal breaks in human leucocyte cultures induced by an agent in the plasma of infectious hepatitis patients. Hereditas 52:285, 1965.

530. Matsaniotis N, Kiossoglou K, Maounis F, et al. Chromosomal aber-rations in infective hepatitis. J Clin Pathol 23:553, 1970.

531. Mella B, Lang D. Leucocyte mitosis suppression in vitro associated with acute infectious hepatitis. Science 155:80, 1967.

532. Stokes J Jr, Wolman IJ, Blanchard MC, et al. Viral hepatitis in the newborn: clinical features, epidemiology and pathology. Am J Dis Child 82:213, 1951.

533. Gillespie A, Dorman D, Walker-Smith JA, et al. Neonatal hepatitis and Australia antigen. Lancet 2:1081, 1970.

534. Wright R, Perkins JR, Bower BD, et al. Cirrhosis associated with Australia antigen in an infant who acquired hepatitis from her mother. Br Med J 4:719, 1970.

535. Bancroft WH, Warkel RL, Talbert AA, et al. Family with hepatitis associated antigen. Spectrum of liver pathology. JAMA 217:1817, 1971.

536. Ohbayashi A, Okochi K, Mayumi M. Familial clustering of asympto-matic carriers of Australia antigen and patients with chronic liver disease or primary liver cancer. Gastroenterology 62:618, 1972.

537. Larouze B, London WT, Sarmot G, et al. Host responses to hepatitis-B infection in patients with primary hepatic carcinoma and their families. A case/control study in Senegal, West Africa. Lancet 2:534, 1976.

538. Schweitzer IL, Wing A, McPeak C, et al. Hepatitis and hepatitis-associated antigen in 56 mother-infant pairs. JAMA 220:1092, 1972.

539. Schweitzer IL, Mosley JW, Ashcavai M, et al. Factors influencing neonatal infection by hepatitis B virus. Gastroenterology 65:277, 1973.

540. Tong MJ, Thursby M, Rakela J, et al. Studies of the maternal-infant transmission of the viruses which cause acute hepatitis. Gastro-enterology 80:999, 1981.

540a. Gerety RJ, Schweitzer IL. Viral hepatitis, type B, during pregnancy, the neonatal period, and infancy. J Pediatr 90:368, 1977.

541. Merrill DA, Dubois RS, Kohler PF. Neonatal onset of the hepatitis-associated-antigen carrier state. N Engl J Med 287:1280, 1972.

542. Gerety RJ, Hoofnagle JH, Markenson JA, et al. Exposure to hepatitis B virus and development of the chronic HBsAg carrier state in children. J Pediatr 84:661, 1974.

543. Cossart YC, Hargraves D, March SP. Australia antigen and the human fetus. Am J Dis Child 123:376, 1972.

544. Skinhoj P, Sardemann H, Mikkelsen M, et al. Hepatitis associated antigen (HAA) in pregnant women and their newborn infants. Am J Dis Child 123:380, 1972.

545. Turner GC, Field AM, Lasheen RM, et al. SH (Australia) antigen in early life. J Clin Pathol 23:826, 1970.

546. Aziz MA, Khan G, Khanum T, et al. Transplacental and postnatal transmission of the hepatitis-associated antigen. J Infect Dis 127:110, 1973.

547. Papaevangelou G, Hoofnagle J, Kremastinou J. Transplacental trans-mission of hepatitis-B virus by symptom-free chronic carrier moth-ers. Lancet 2:746, 1974.

548. Schweitzer IL. Vertical transmission of hepatitis B surface antigen. Am J Med Sci 270:287, 1975.
549. Kew ML, Marcus RG, MacNab GM, et al. Hepatitis B (surface) antigen in mothers and their infants. S Afr Med J 49:1471, 1975.
550. Waterson AP, Almeida JD, Weeple PM, et al. Hepatitis B antigen-positive obstetric patients. Br J Obstet Gynecol 84:674, 1977.
551. Derso A, Boxall EH, Tarlow MJ, et al. Transmission of HBsAg from mother to infant in four ethnic groups. Br Med J 1:949, 1978.
551a. Woo D, Cummins M, Davies DH, et al. Vertical transmission of hepatitis B surface antigens in carrier mothers in two West London hospitals. Arch Dis Child 54:670, 1979.
552. Dupuy JM, Giraid P, Dupuy C, et al. Hepatitis B in children. J Pediatr 92:200, 1978.
553. Moroni GA, Cossu MM, Barbarani V. Vertical transmission of hepatitis B. Bol Ist Sieroter Milanese 57:1, 1978.
554. Okada K, Yamada T, Miyakawa Y, et al. Hepatitis B surface antigen in the serum of infants after delivery from asymptomatic carrier mothers. J Pediatr 87:360, 1975.
555. Stevens CE, Beasley RP, Tsui J, et al. Vertical transmission of hepatitis B antigen in Taiwan. N Engl J Med 292:771, 1975.
556. Anderson KE, Stevens CE, Tsui J, et al. Hepatitis B antigen in infants born to mothers with chronic hepatitis B antigenemia in Taiwan. Am J Dis Child 129:1389, 1975.
557. Okada K, Kamiyama I, Inomata M, et al. e Antigen and anti-e in the serum of asymptomatic carrier mothers as indicators of positive and negative transmission of hepatitis B virus to their infants. N Engl J Med 294:746, 1976.
558. Shiraki K, Yoshihara N, Kawana T, et al. Hepatitis B surface antigen and chronic hepatitis in infants born to asymptomatic carrier mothers. Am J Dis Child 131:664, 1977.
559. Lee AKY, Ip HMH, Wong VCN. Mechanisms of maternal-fetal transmission of hepatitis B virus. J Infect Dis 138:668, 1978.
560. Stevens CE, Neurath RA, Beasley RA, et al. HBeAg and anti-HBe detection by radioimmunoassay: correlation with vertical transmission of hepatitis B virus in Taiwan. J Med Virol 3:237, 1979.
560a. Beasley RP, Hwang LY, Lee GC, et al. Prevention of perinatally transmitted hepatitis B virus infection with hepatitis B immune globulin and hepatitis B vaccine. Lancet 2:1099, 1983.
561. Blumberg BS, Friedlander JS, Woodside A, et al. Hepatitis and Australia antigen: autosomal recessive inheritance of susceptibility to infection in humans. Proc Natl Acad Sci USA 62:1108, 1969.
562. Carbonara AO, Trinchieri J, Bedarida G, et al. A Caucasian population with a high frequency of Au "carriers": genetic analysis of the condition. Vox Sang 19:228, 1970.
563. Pertrakis N, Lederberg J. Genetic predisposition to hepatitis. In: Vyas, GN, Perkins HA, Schmidt R, eds. Hepatitis and Blood Transfusions. New York, Grune & Stratton, 1972:85.
564. Peters CJ, Reeves WC, Purcell RH. Disparate responses of monozygotic twins to hepatitis B virus infection. J Pediatr 91:265, 1977.
564a. Shiraki K, Yoshihara N, Sakurai M. Acute hepatitis B in infants born to carrier mothers with antibody to hepatitis B e antigen. J Pediatr 97:768, 1980.
564b. Sinatra FR, Shah P, Weissman JY, et al. Perinatally transmitted acute hepatitis B surface antigen positive and hepatitis B e-positive carrier mothers. Pediatrics 70:557, 1982.
564c. Nair PV, Weissman JY, Tong MJ, et al. Efficacy of hepatitis B immune globulin in prevention of perinatal transmission of the hepatitis B virus. Gastroenterology 87:293, 1984.
565. London WT, DiFiglia M, Rodgers J. Failure of transplacental transmission of Australia antigen. Lancet 2:900, 1969.
566. Smithwick EM, Go SC. Hepatitis-associated antigen in cord and maternal blood. Lancet 2:1080, 1970.
567. Schweitzer IL, Spears RL. Hepatitis-associated antigen (Australia antigen) in mother and infant. N Engl J Med 283:570, 1970.
568. Lyons KP, Guze LB. Australia antigen associated hepatitis: radioimmunoassay in mother and infant. JAMA 215:98, 1971.
569. Moronie GA, Constantino D, Zampieri G, et al. Do the hepatitis antigens cross the placenta? Lancet 2:376, 1971.
570. Holzbach RT. Australia antigen in pregnancy: evidence against transplacental transmission of Australia antigen in early and late pregnancy. Arch Intern Med 130:234, 1972.
571. Fujita K, Yamada T, Mayumi M, et al. Materno-fetal transport of Australia/SH antigen and antibody. Lancet 2:378, 1972.
572. Mollica F, Misumeci S, Rugolo S, et al. A prospective study of 18 infants of chronic HBsAg mothers. Arch Dis Child 54:750, 1979.
573. Cairns JM, Tabor E, Gerety RJ. Hepatitis B carriers in pregnancy: a preliminary report. Proc Assoc Surg E Africa 1:80, 1978.
574. Boxall EH, Davies H. Dane particles in cord blood. Lancet 2:1513, 1974.
574a. Goodeau A, Yvonnet B, Lesage G, et al. Lack of anti-HBc IgM in neonates with HBsAg carriers argues against transplacental transmission of hepatitis B virus infection. Lancet 2:110b, 1983.
575. Linnemann CC Jr, Goldberg S. HBsAg in breast milk. Lancet 2:155, 1974.
576. Boxall EH, Flewett TH, Dane DS, et al. Hepatitis B surface antigen in breast milk. Lancet 2:1007, 1974.
577. Beasley RP, Stevens CE. Vertical transmission of HBV and interruption with globulin. In: Vyas GN, Cohen SN, Schmid R, eds. Viral Hepatitis. Philadelphia, Franklin Institute Press, 1978:333.
577a. Botha JF, Ritchie MJJ, Dusheiko GM, et al. Hepatitis B virus carrier state in black children in Ovambaland: role of perinatal and horizontal infection. Lancet 1:1210, 1984.
577b. Dupuy JM, Kostewicz E, Alaqulle D. Hepatitis B in children. I. Analysis of 80 cases of acute and chronic hepatitis B. J Pediatr 92:17, 1978.
578. Jorge A, Diaz M, Sanchez D, et al. Vertical transmission of the virus of hepatitis B and neonatal hepatic cirrhosis in an Argentine family. Acta Hepato-Gastroenterol 24:162, 1977.
579. McCarthy JW. Hepatitis B antigen (HB-Ag)-positive chronic aggressive hepatitis and cirrhosis in an 8-month old infant. A case report. J Pediatr 83:638, 1973.
580. Dunn AEG, Peters RL, Schweitzer IL. An ultrastructural study of liver explants from infants with vertically transmitted hepatitis. Exp Mol Pathol 19:113, 1973.
581. Kattamis C, Demetriou D, Karambula K, et al. Neonatal hepatitis associated with Australia antigen (Au-1). Arch Dis Child 48:133, 1973.
582. Dupuy JM, Frommel D, Alagille D. Severe viral hepatitis, type B, in infancy. Lancet 2:191, 1975.
583. Fawaz KA, Grady GF, Kaplan MM, et al. Repetitive maternal-fetal transmission of fatal hepatitis B. N Engl J Med 293:1357, 1975.
584. Mollica F, Musumeci S, Fischer A. Neonatal hepatitis in five children of a hepatitis B surface carrier woman. J Pediatr 90:949, 1977.
585. Grady GF, cited by Beasley RP, Stevens CE. Vertical transmission of HBV and interruption with globulin. In: Vyas GN, Cohen SN, Schmid R, eds. Viral Hepatitis. Philadelphia, Franklin Institute Press, 1978:339.
586. Tong MJ, Rakela J, McPeak CM, et al. Studies in infants born to mothers with type B hepatitis and acute non-A, non-B hepatitis during pregnancy. Gastroenterology 75:991, 1978.
587. Gupta B, Agarwal S, Joshi VV. Maternal/fetal transmission of HBsAg-negative hepatitis. Lancet 2:740, 1978.
587a. Zanetti AR, Ferroni P, Magliano EM, et al. Perinatal transmission of the hepatitis B virus and of the HBV associated delta agent from mothers to offspring in Northern Italy. J Med Virol 9:139, 1982.
587b. Zanetti AR, Tanzi E, Ferroni P, et al. Vertical transmission of the HBV-associated delta agent. Prog Clin Biol Res 143:127, 1983.
588. Haemmerli UP, Wyss HI. Recurrent intrahepatic cholestasis of pregnancy: report of six cases and review of the literature. Medicine 46:299, 1967.
589. Bennett NM, Lehman NI, Speed BR. Viral hepatitis and intrahepatic cholestasis of pregnancy. Aust NZ J Med 9:54, 1979.
590. Ober WB, LeCompte PM. Acute fatty metamorphosis of the liver associated with pregnancy: a distinctive lesion. Am J Med 19:743, 1955.
591. Kunelis CT, Peters JL, Edmondson HA. Fatty liver of pregnancy and its relationship to tetracycline therapy. Am J Med 38:359, 1965.
592. Holzbach RT. Acute fatty liver of pregnancy with disseminated intravascular coagulation. Obstet Gynecol 43:470, 1974.
593. Aldercreutz H, Tenhunan R. Some aspects of the interaction between natural and synthetic female sex hormones and the liver. Am J Med 49:630, 1970.
594. Doar JWH. Metabolic side effects of oral contraceptives. Clin Endocrinol Metab 2:503, 1973.
595. Zimmerman HJ. Hormonal derivatives and other drugs used to treat endocrine disorders. In: Zimmerman HJ, ed. Hepatotoxicity. New York, Appleton-Century-Crofts, 1978:444.
596. Morrison AS, Jick H, Ory HW. Oral contraceptives and hepatitis: a report from the Boston Collaborative Drug Surveillance Program, Boston University Medical Center. Lancet 1:1142, 1977.
597. Jenny S, Markoff N. Oral contraceptives in liver disease. Schweiz Med Wochenschr 97:1502, 1967.
598. Schweitzer IL, Weiner JM, McPeak CM, et al. Oral contraceptives in acute viral hepatitis. JAMA 233:979, 1975.
599. Berk PD, Wolkoff AW, Berlin NI. Inborn errors of bilirubin metabolism. Med Clin North Am 59:803, 1975.
600. Hunter FM, Sparks RD, Flinner RL. Hepatitis with resulting mobilization of hepatic pigment in a patient with Dubin-Johnson syndrome. Gastroenterology 47:631, 1964.
601. Masuda M. On the relation between Dubin-Johnson syndrome and Rotor type: a case of Dubin-Johnson syndrome complicated with serum hepatitis. Rev Int Hepat 15:1229, 1965.
602. Varma RR, Grainger JM, Scheuer PJ. A case of the Dubin-Johnson syndrome complicated by acute hepatitis. Gut 11:817, 1970.
603. Dubin IN, Johnson FB. Chronic idiopathic jaundice with unidentified pigment in liver cells. Medicine (Baltimore) 33:155, 1954.
604. London RE. Multiple myeloma: report of a case showing unusual

remission lasting two years following severe hepatitis. Ann Intern Med 43:491, 1955.

605. Osserman EF, Takatsuki K. Considerations regarding the pathogenesis of the plasmocytic dyscrasias. Series Hematol 4:28, 1965.

606. Cohen RJ, Bohannon RA, Wallerstein RO. Waldenstrom's macroglobulinemia. A study of 10 cases. Am J Med 41:274, 1966.

607. Wolf RE, Riedel LO, Lein WC, et al. Remission of macroglobulinemia coincident with hepatitis: report of case and review of literature. Arch Intern Med 130:392, 1972.

608. Dymock IW, Tucker JS, Woolf IL, et al. Coagulation studies as a prognostic index in acute liver failure. Br J Hematol 29:385, 1975.

609. Barker MH, Capps RB, Allen FM. Acute infectious hepatitis in the Mediterranean theater, including acute hepatitis without jaundice. JAMA 128:997, 1945.

609a. Culbertson JW, Wilkins RW, Ingelfinger FJ, et al. The effect of the upright posture upon the hepatic blood flow in normotensive and hypertensive subjects. J Clin Invest 30:305, 1951.

610. Bradley SF. Variations in hepatic blood flow in man during health and disease. N Engl J Med 240:456, 1949.

610a. Rowell LB, Blackmon JR, Bruce RA. Indocyanine green clearance and estimated hepatic blood flow during mild to maximal exercise in upright man. J Clin Invest 43:1677, 1964.

611. Swift WE Jr, Gardner HT, Moore DJ, et al. Clinical course of viral hepatitis and the effect of exercise during convalescence. Am J Med 8:614, 1950.

612. Chalmers TC, Eckhardt RD, Reynolds WE, et al. The treatment of acute infectious hepatitis: controlled studies of the effects of diet, rest, and physical reconditioning on the acute course of the disease and on the incidence of relapses and residual abnormalities. J Clin Invest 34:1163, 1955.

613. Silverberg M, Wherrett B, Worden E, et al. An evaluation of rest and low-fat diet in the management of acute infectious hepatitis. J Pediatr 74:260, 1979.

614. Krikler DM, Zilberg B. Activity in hepatitis. Lancet 2:1046, 1966.

614a. Nelson RS, Sprinz H, Colbert JW, et al. Effect of physical activity on recovery from hepatitis. Am J Med 16:780, 1954.

615. Repsher LH, Freebern RK. Effects of early and vigorous exercise on recovery from infectious hepatitis. N Engl J Med 281:1393, 1969.

616. Edlund A. The effect of defined physical exercising in the early convalescence of viral hepatitis. Scand J Infect Dis 3:189, 1971.

617. Lundberg P, Strandell T. Changes in hepatic circulation at rest, during and after exercise in young males with infectious hepatitis compared with controls. Acta Med Scand 196:315, 1974.

618. Seeff LB, Zimmerman HJ. Acute viral hepatitis. In: Conn HF, ed. Current Therapy, 1977. Philadelphia, WB Saunders, 1977:384.

618a. Leone NC, Ratner F, Dietenbach WCL, et al. Clinical evaluation of a high-protein, high-carbohydrate, restricted fat diet in the treatment of viral hepatitis. Ann NY Acad Sci 57:948, 1954.

619. Shull HJ Jr, Wilkinson GR, Johnson R, et al. Normal disposition of oxazepam in acute viral hepatitis and cirrhosis. Ann Intern Med 84:420, 1976.

620. Gardner HT, Rovelstad RA, Moore DJ, et al. Hepatitis among American occupational troops in Germany: a follow-up study with particular reference to interim alcohol and physical activity. Ann Intern Med 30:1009, 1949.

620a. Galambos JT, Asada M, Shanks JZ. The effect of intravenous ethanol on serum enzymes in patients with normal or diseased liver. Gastroenterology 44:267, 1963.

621. Tabor E, Gerety RJ, Barker LF, et al. Effect of ethanol during hepatitis B virus infection in chimpanzees. J Med Virol 2:295, 1978.

622. Evans AS, Sprinz H, Nelson RS. Adrenal hormone therapy in viral hepatitis. I. The effect of ACTH on the acute disease. Ann Intern Med 38:1115, 1953.

623. Evans AS, Sprinz H, Nelson RS. Adrenal hormone therapy in viral hepatitis. II. The effect of cortisone in the acute disease. Ann Intern Med 38:1134, 1953.

623a. Sborov VM, Giges B, Plough IC, et al. ACTH therapy in acute viral hepatitis. J Lab Clin Med 43:48, 1954.

623b. Chalmers TC, Gill RJ, Jernigan TP, et al. Evaluation of a four day ACTH test in the differential diagnosis of jaundice. Gastroenterology 30:894, 1956.

624. DeRitis R, Giusti G, Molluci L, et al. Negative results of prednisone therapy in viral hepatitis. Lancet 1:533, 1964.

625. Blum AL, Stutz R, Haemmerli UP, et al. A fortuitously controlled study of steroid therapy in acute viral hepatitis. I. Acute disease. Am J Med 47:82, 1969.

626. Dudley FJ, Scheuer PJ, Sherlock S. Natural history of hepatitis-associated antigen-positive chronic liver disease. Lancet 2:1388, 1972.

626a. Redeker AG, Schweitzer IL, Yamahiro HS. Randomization of corticosteroid therapy in fulminant hepatitis. N Engl J Med 294:728, 1976.

626b. Acute Hepatic Failure Study Group, represented by Rakela J. A double-blinded, randomized trial of hydrocortisone in acute hepatic failure. Gastroenterology 76:1297, 1979.

626c. European Association for the Study of the Liver. Randomized trial of steroid therapy in acute liver failure. Gut 20:620, 1979.

626d. Lam KC, Lai CL, Ng RP, et al. Deleterious effect of prednisolone in HBsAg-positive chronic active hepatitis. N Engl J Med 304:380, 1981.

626e. European Association for the Study of the Liver. Steroids in chronic B-hepatitis: a randomized, double-blind, multinational trial on the effect of low-dose, long-term treatment on survival. Liver 6:227, 1986.

627. Leevy CM. Intrahepatic cholestasis. Am J Surg 97:132, 1959.

628. Harville DD, Summerskill WHJ. Surgery in acute hepatitis: cause and effects. JAMA 184:257, 1963.

629. Sidwell RW, Huffmann JH, Khare CP, et al. Broad-spectrum antiviral activity of virazole. Science 177:1705, 1972.

630. Sidwell RW, Huffmann JH, Campbell N, et al. Effect of ribavirin on viral hepatitis in laboratory animals. Ann NY Acad Sci 284:239, 1977.

631. Ayrosa-Galvao PA, Castro IO. The effect of 1-β-D-ribofuranosyl-1,2,4-triazole-3-carboxamide in acute viral hepatitis. Ann NY Acad Sci 284:278, 1977.

632. Lao LM, Alora BD, Tiu JB, et al. Infectious hepatitis. A comparative study of therapeutic methods. Philip J Micro Infect Dis 11:1, 1973.

633. Lam KC, Lin HJ, Lai CL, et al. Isoprinosine in classical acute viral hepatitis. Am J Dig Dis 23:893, 1978.

634. Blum AL, Berthet P, Doelle W, et al. Treatment of acute viral hepatitis with (+)-cyanidanol-3. Lancet 2:1153, 1977.

635. Par A, Barna K, Hollos I, et al. Levamisole in viral hepatitis. Lancet 1:702, 1977.

635a. Ellis-Pegler R, Sutherland DC, Douglas R, et al. Transfer factor and hepatitis B: a double-blind study. Clin Exp Immunol 36:221, 1979.

636. Acute Hepatic Failure Study Group. Failure of specific immunotherapy in fulminant type B hepatitis. Ann Intern Med 86:272, 1977.

637. Reed WD, Eddleston ALWF, Cullens H, et al. Infusion of hepatitis-B antibody in antigen-positive active chronic hepatitis. Lancet 2:1347, 1973.

638. Havens WP Jr. Infectious hepatitis. Medicine (Baltimore) 27:279, 1948.

639. Havens WP Jr. Period of infectivity of patients with experimentally induced infectious hepatitis. J Exp Med 83:2521, 1946.

640. Giles JP, Liebharber H, Krugman S, et al. Early viremia and viruria in infectious hepatitis. Virology 24:107, 1964.

640a. Havens WP Jr, Ward R, Drill LA, et al. Experimental production of hepatitis by feeding icterogenic materials. Proc Soc Exp Biol Med 57:206, 1944.

640b. Neefe JR, Stokes J, Reinhold JG. Oral administration to volunteers of feces from patients with homologous serum hepatitis and infectious (epidemic) hepatitis. Am J Med Sci 210:29, 1945.

640c. Dienstag JL, Feinstone SM, Kapikian AZ, et al. Fecal shedding of hepatitis-A antigen. Lancet 1:765, 1975.

641. Rakela J, Mosley JW. Fecal excretion of hepatitis A virus. J Infect Dis 135:933, 1977.

642. Hollinger FB, Bradley DW, Maynard JE, et al. Detection of hepatitis A viral antigen by radioimmunoassay. J Immunol 115:1464, 1975.

643. Knodell RG, Conrad ME, Dienstag JL, et al. Etiologic spectrum of post-transfusion hepatitis. Gastroenterology 69:1278, 1978.

644. Mosley JW, Speers JF, Chin TDY. Epidemiologic studies of a large urban outbreak of infectious hepatitis. Am J Public Health 53:1603, 1963.

645. Brooks BF, Hsia DY, Gellis SS. Family outbreak of infectious hepatitis: prophylactic use of gamma globulin. N Engl J Med 249:58, 1953.

646. Capps RB, Bennett AM, Stokes J Jr. Endemic infectious hepatitis in an infants' orphanage. I. Epidemiologic studies in student nurses. Arch Intern Med 89:6, 1952.

647. Neefe JR, Stokes J Jr. An epidemic of infectious hepatitis apparently due to a waterborne agent. JAMA 128:1063, 1945.

648. Mosley JW, Schrack WD Jr, Densham TW, et al. Infectious hepatitis in Clearfield County, Pennsylvania. I. A probable waterborne epidemic. Am J Med 26:55, 1959.

649. Poskanzer DC, Beadenkopf WG. Waterborne infectious hepatitis epidemic from chlorinated municipal supply. Public Health Rep 76:745, 1961.

649a. Bryan JA, Lehmann JD, Setiady IF, et al. An outbreak of hepatitis-A associated with recreational lake water. Am J Epidemiol 99:145, 1974.

650. Cliver DO. Implications of foodborne infectious hepatitis. Public Health Rep 80:173, 1965.

651. Denes AE, Smith JC, Hindman SH, et al. Foodborne hepatitis A infection: a report of two urban restaurant-associated outbreaks. Am J Epidemiol 105:156, 1977.

651a. Hadler SC, Webster HM, Erben JS, et al. Hepatitis A in day-care centers: a community-wide assessment. N Engl J Med 302:1222, 1980.

651b. Corey L, Holmes KK. Sexual transmission of hepatitis A in homosexual men: incidence and mechanism. N Engl J Med 302:435, 1980.

651c. Christenson B, Brostrom C, Bottiger M, et al. An epidemic outbreak of hepatitis A among homosexual men in Stockholm: hepatitis A, a special hazard for the male homosexual subpopulation in Sweden. Am J Epidemiol 116:599, 1982.

652. Whatley TR, Comstock GW, Garber HJ, et al. A waterborne outbreak of infectious hepatitis in a small Maryland town. Am J Epidemiol 87:138, 1968.

653. Reynolds RD, Summerville JJ, Shepard KS, et al. Freeze-ball hepatitis. Arch Intern Med 122:48, 1968.

654. Koff RS. Epidemiology of viral hepatitis. CRC Crit Rev Environ Control 1:383, 1970.

655. Murphy WJ, Petrie LM, Work SD. Outbreak of infectious hepatitis apparently waterborne. Am J Public Health 36:169, 1961.

656. Read MR, Bancroft H, Doull JA, et al. Infectious hepatitis—presumably foodborne outbreak. Am J Public Health 36:367, 1946.

657. Kaufmann GG, Shorov UM, Havens WP Jr. Outbreak of infectious hepatitis—presumably foodborne. JAMA 149:993, 1952.

658. Joseph PR, Miller JD, Henderson DA. An outbreak of hepatitis traced to food contamination. N Engl J Med 273:188, 1965.

659. Meyers JD, Romm FJ, Tihen WS, et al. Food-borne hepatitis A in a general hospital: epidemiologic study of an outbreak attributed to sandwiches. JAMA 231:1049, 1975.

660. Schoenbaum SC, Baker O, Jezek A. Common-source epidemic of hepatitis due to glazed and iced pastries. Am J Epidemiol 104:74, 1976.

661. Roos B. Hepatitis epidemic transmitted by oysters. Svenska Lakartidning 53:989, 1956.

662. Koff RS, Grady SG, Chalmers TC, et al. (Boston Inter-Hospital Liver Group). Viral hepatitis in a group of Boston hospitals. II. Importance of exposure to shellfish in a nonepidemic period. N Engl J Med 276:703, 1967.

663. Portnoy BL, Mackowiak PA, Caraway CT, et al. Oyster-associated hepatitis: failure of shellfish certification programs to prevent outbreak. JAMA 233:1065, 1975.

664. Cline AL, Mosley JW, Scovel FB. Viral hepatitis among American missionaries abroad. A preliminary study. JAMA 199:119, 1967.

665. Borg LA. Immune gamma globulin as a control for infectious disease in Bolivia. Milit Med 130:389, 1967.

666. Frame JD. Hepatitis among missionaries in Ethiopia and Sudan: susceptibles at high risk. JAMA 203:389, 1967.

667. Woodson RD, Clinton JJ. Hepatitis prophylaxis abroad: effectiveness of immune serum globulin protecting Peace Corp volunteers. JAMA 209:1053, 1969.

668. Woodson RD, Cahill KM. Viral hepatitis abroad. Incidence in Catholic missionaries. JAMA 219:1191, 1972.

669. Ruddy SJ, Mosley JW, Held JR. Chimpanzee-associated viral hepatitis in 1963. Am J Epidemiol 86:634, 1967.

670. Pattison CP, Maynard JE, Bryan JS. Subhuman primate-associated hepatitis. J Infect Dis 132:478, 1975.

671. Dienstag JL, Davenport FM, McCollum RW, et al. Nonhuman primate-associated viral hepatitis type A: serologic evidence of type A infection. JAMA 236:462, 1976.

671a. Friedmann CT, Dinnes MR, Bernstein JF, et al. Chimpanzee-associated hepatitis among personnel at an animal hospital. J Am Vet Med Assoc 159:541, 1971.

672. Mosley JW, Reinhardt HP, Hassler FR. Chimpanzee-associated hepatitis: an outbreak in Oklahoma. JAMA 199:695, 1967.

673. Mackowiak PA, Caraway CT, Portnoy BL. Oyster-associated hepatitis: lessons from the Louisiana experience. Am J Epidemiol 103:181, 1976.

674. Maynard JE. Viral hepatitis as an occupational hazard in the health care profession. In: Vyas GN, Cohen SN, Schmid R, eds. Viral Hepatitis. Philadelphia, Franklin Institute Press, 1978:321.

675. Szmuness W, Dienstag JL, Purcell RH, et al. Hepatitis type A and hemodialysis—a seroepidemiologic study in 15 US centers. Ann Intern Med 87:8, 1977.

676. Favero MS, Maynard JE, Leger RT, et al. Guidelines for the care of patients hospitalized with viral hepatitis. Ann Intern Med 91:872, 1979.

677. Broderson M, Steigmann S, Klein K-H, et al. Salivary HBAg detected by radioimmunoassay. Lancet 1:675, 1974.

678. Telectar H, Kayhan B, Kes S, et al. HBAg in sweat. Lancet 2:461, 1974.

679. Piazza M, Cacciatore L, Molinare V, et al. Presence of HBsAg in the bile of subjects with acute HBsAg viral hepatitis. Pathol Microbiol 43:307, 1975.

680. Dankert J, Postma A, DeVries JA, et al. HBsAg in spinal fluid from leukemic children. Lancet 1:690, 1975.

681. Denes AE, Ebert JW, Moncada RE, et al. Hepatitis-B surface antigen in cerebrospinal fluid. Lancet 2:1038, 1975.

682. Cacciatore L, Mollinari V, Guadagnino V, et al. Hepatitis B antigen in ascitic fluid in cirrhosis. Br Med J 3:172, 1973.

683. Mazzur S. Menstrual blood as a vehicle of Australia-antigen transmission. Lancet 1:749, 1973.

684. Darani M, Gerber M. Hepatitis B antigen in vaginal secretions. Lancet 2:1008, 1974.

685. Apostolov K, Bauer DJ, Selway JW, et al. Australia antigen in urine. Lancet 1:1274, 1971.

686. Scalise G, Mura MS. Australia antigen in urine. Lancet 2:1394, 1973.

687. Barker LF, Shulman NR, Murray R, et al. Transmission of serum hepatitis. JAMA 211:1509, 1970.

688. De Flora S. Thermal inactivation of hepatitis B surface antigen. J Immunol 120:40, 1978.

689. Havens WP Jr, Paul JR. Infectious hepatitis and serum hepatitis. In: Horsfall FL, Tamm I, eds. Viral and Rickettsial Infections of Man. Philadelphia, JB Lippincott, 1965:968.

690. Murray R, Diefenbach WCL. Effect of heat on the agent of homologous serum hepatitis. Proc Soc Exp Biol Med 84:230, 1953.

691. Gellis SS, Neefe JR, Stokes J Jr, et al. Chemical, clinical, and immunological studies on the products of human plasma fractionation. XXXVI. Inactivation of the virus of homologous serum hepatitis in solutions of normal human serum albumin by means of heat. J Clin Invest 27:239, 1948.

692. Soulier JP, Blatix C, Courouce AM, et al. Prevention of virus B hepatitis (SH hepatitis). Am J Dis Child 123:429, 1972.

693. Shikata T, Karasawa T, Abe K, et al. Incomplete inactivation of hepatitis B virus after heat treatment at 60° C for 10 hours. J Infect Dis 138:242, 1978.

694. Neefe JR, Baty JB, Reinhold JG, et al. Inactivation of infectious hepatitis in drinking water. Am J Public Health 37:365, 1947.

695. Barker LF. Australia antigen: isolation, purification, and physical properties. Proc Natl Acad Sci USA 66:229, 1970.

696. Schmidt NJ, Lennette EH. Safety precautions for performing tests for hepatitis-associated (Australia) antigen and antibodies. Am J Clin Pathol 57:526, 1972.

697. Bond WW, Peterson NJ, Favero MS. Viral hepatitis B: aspects of environmental control. Health Lab Sci 14:235, 1977.

698. Murray R, Oliphant JW, Tripp JT, et al. Effect of ultraviolet radiation on the infectivity of icterogenic plasma. JAMA 157:8, 1955.

699. Logrippo GA, Wolfram BR, Rupe CE. Human plasma treated with ultraviolet and tropmolactene. JAMA 187:722, 1964.

700. Kobagasliu H, Isuzuki M, Koshimizo K, et al. Susceptibility of hepatitis B virus to disinfectants or heat. J Clin Microbiol 20:214, 1984.

701. Feinstone SM, Mihalik KB, Kamimura T, et al. Inactivation of hepatitis B virus and non-A, non-B hepatitis by chloroform. Infect Immunol 41:816, 1983.

702. Tabor E, Buynack E, Smallwood CA, et al. Inactivation of hepatitis B virus by three methods: treatment with pepsin, urea, or formalin. J Med Virol 11:1, 1983.

703. Berry WR, Gottesfeld RL, Alter HJ, et al. Transmission of hepatitis B virus by artificial insemination. JAMA 257:1079, 1987.

704. MacQuarrie MB, Forghani B, Wolochow DA. Hepatitis B transmitted by a human bite. JAMA 230:723, 1974.

705. Jeffries DJ, James WH, Jefferiss FJG, et al. Australia (hepatitis-associated) antigen in patients attending a veneral disease clinic. Br Med J 2:455, 1973.

706. Fulford KWM, Danes DS, Caterall RD, et al. Australia antigen and antibody among patients attending a clinic for sexually transmitted diseases. Lancet 1:1470, 1973.

707. Szmuness W, Much MI, Prince AM, et al. On the role of sexual behavior in the spread of hepatitis B infection. Ann Intern Med 83:489, 1975.

707a. Dietzman DE, Harnish JP, Ray CG, et al. Hepatitis B surface antigen (HBsAg) and antibody to HBsAg: prevalence in homosexual and heterosexual men. JAMA 239:2625, 1977.

707b. Inaba N, Ohkawa R, Matsura A, et al. Sexual transmission of hepatitis B surface antigen: infection of husbands by HBsAg-carrier wives. Br J Vener Dis 55:366, 1979.

708. Kunin CM. Serum hepatitis from whole blood: incidence and relation to source of blood. Am J Med Sci 237:293, 1959.

709. Allen JG, Sayman WA. Serum hepatitis from transfusions of blood. JAMA 180:1079, 1962.

710. Grady GF, Chalmers TC, the Boston Inter-Hospital Liver Group. Risk of post-transfusion viral hepatitis. N Engl J Med 271:337, 1964.

711. Gocke DJ, Kavey NB. Hepatitis antigen: Correlation with disease and infectivity of blood donors. Lancet 1:1055, 1969.

712. Alter HJ, Holland PV, Purcall RH. The emerging pattern of post-transfusion hepatitis. Am J Med Sci 270:329, 1975.

712a. Aach RD, Lander JJ, Sherman LA, et al. Transfusion-transmitted viruses: interim analysis of hepatitis among transfused and non-transfused patients. In: Vyas GN, Cohen SN, Schmid R, eds. Viral Hepatitis. Philadelphia, Franklin Institute Press, 1978:383.

712b. Seeff LB, Wright EC, Zimmerman HJ, et al. Post-transfusion hepatitis, 1973–1975: a Veterans Administration cooperative study. In: Vyas GN, Cohen SN, Schmid R, eds. Viral Hepatitis. Philadelphia, Franklin Institute Press, 1978:371.

713. Grady GF, Lee VA. Hepatitis B immune globulin—prevention of hepatitis from accidental exposure among medical personnel. N Engl J Med 293:1067, 1975.

714. Seeff LB, Wright EC, Zimmerman HJ, et al. Type B hepatitis after needle-stick exposure: prevention with hepatitis B immune globulin. Ann Intern Med 88:285, 1978.

715. Kew MC. Possible transmission of serum (Australia-antigen-positive) hepatitis via the conjunctiva. Infect Immun 7:823, 1973.

716. Steigmann F, Hyman E, Goldbloom R. Infectious hepatitis (homologous serum type) in drug addicts. Gastroenterology 15:642, 1950.

717. Louria DB, Hensle T, Rose J. Major medical problems of heroin addiction. Ann Intern Med 67:1, 1967.

718. Sapira JD, Jasinski DR, Gorodeszky CW. Liver disease in narcotic addicts. II. The role of the needle. Clin Pharmacol Ther 9:725, 1968.

719. Cherubin CE, Hargrove RL, Prince AM. The serum hepatitis related antigen (SH) in illicit drug users. Am J Epidemiol 91:510, 1970.

720. Nordenfelt E, Kaij K, Ursing B. Presence and persistence of Australia antigen among drug addicts. Vox Sang 19:371, 1970.

721. Bewley TH, Ben-arie O, Marks V. Relation of hepatitis to self-injection techniques. Br Med J 1:703, 1967.

721a. Dismukes WE, Karchmer AW, Johnson RF, et al. Viral hepatitis associated with illicit parenteral use of drugs. JAMA 206:1048, 1968.

722. Roberts RH, Stul H. Homologous serum jaundice transmitted by a tattooing needle. Can Med Assoc J 62:75, 1950.

723. Hopkins GB, Gostling JUT, Hill I, et al. Hepatitis after tattooing: a fatal case. Br Med J 3:210, 1973.

724. Mowat NAG, Albert-Recht F, Brunt PW, et al. Outbreak of serum hepatitis associated with tattooing. Lancet 1:33, 1973.

725. Limentani AE, Elliott LM, Noah ND, et al. An outbreak of hepatitis B from tattooing. Lancet 2:86, 1979.

726. Johnson CJ, Anderson H, Spearman J, et al. Ear piercing and hepatitis: nonsterile instruments for ear piercing and the subsequent onset of viral hepatitis. JAMA 227:1165, 1974.

727. Carron H, Epstein BH, Grand B. Complications of acupuncture. JAMA 228:1552, 1974.

728. Boxall EH. Acupuncture hepatitis in the West Midlands, 1977. J Med Virol 2:377, 1978.

729. Larke RPB, Stewart IO. Neurologic examination and hepatitis B. Lancet 2:266, 1974.

729a. Mitch WE, Wands JR, Maddrey WC. Hepatitis B transmission in a family. JAMA 227:1043, 1974.

730. Snydman DR, Hindman SH, Wineland MD, et al. Nosocomial viral hepatitis B. A cluster among staff with subsequent transmission to patients. Ann Intern Med 85:573, 1976.

731. Prince AM, Metselaar D, Kafuko GW, et al. Hepatitis B antigen in wild-caught mosquitoes in Africa. Lancet 2:247, 1972.

732. Metselaar D, Blumberg BS, Millman I, et al. Hepatitis B antigen in colony mosquitoes. Lancet 2:758, 1973.

732a. Brotwan B, Prince AM, Godfrey H. Role of arthropods in transmission of hepatitis B virus in the tropics. Lancet 1:1305, 1973.

732b. Byron NA, Davidson CD, Draper CC, et al. Role of mosquitoes in transmission of hepatitis B antigen. J Infect Dis 128:259, 1973.

732c. Dick SJ, Tamburro OH, Leevy CM. Hepatitis B antigen in urban-caught mosquitoes. JAMA 229:1627, 1974.

733. Newkirk MM, Downe AER, Simon JB. Fate of ingested hepatitis B antigen in blood-sucking insects. Gastroenterology 69:982, 1975.

734. Berquist KR, Maynard FE, Francey DB, et al. Experimental studies on the transmission of hepatitis by mosquitoes. Am J Trop Med Hyg 25:730, 1976.

735. Ogston CW, Wittenstein FS, London WT, et al. Persistence of hepatitis B surface antigen in the bedbug, Cimex hemipterus. J Infect Dis 140:411, 1979.

736. Peterson MR, Barker LF, Schade DS. Detection of antibody to hepatitis-associated antigen in hemophilia patients and in voluntary blood donors. Vox Sang 24:66, 1973.

737. Lewis JH, Maxwell NG, Branden JM. Jaundice in hepatitis B antigen/antibody in hemophilia. Transfusion 14:203, 1974.

738. Hoofnagle JH, Aronson D, Roberts H. Serologic evidence for hepatitis B virus infection in patients with hemophilia B: a multicenter study. Thromb Diath Haemorrh 33:606, 1975.

739. Islam MN, Banatvala JE. The prevalence of hepatitis-B antigen (HBsAg) and its antibody (antiHBs) among London hemophiliacs and blood donors from London and two tropical areas. Transfusion 16:237, 1976.

740. Hansson BG. Antibodies to hepatitis B surface and core antigens in hemophiliacs and their contacts among hospital personnel. Scand J Infect Dis 9:167, 1977.

740a. Gerety RJ, Eyster ME. Hepatitis among hemophiliacs. In: Gerety RJ, ed. Non-A, Non-B Hepatitis. New York, Academic Press, 1981:97.

741. Leibowitz S, Greenwald L, Cohen I, et al. Serum hepatitis in a blood bank worker. JAMA 140:1331, 1949.

742. Byrne EB. Viral hepatitis: occupational hazard of medical personnel. Experience of the Yale-New Haven Hospital, 1952–1965. JAMA 195:362, 1966.

743. Kunst VAJM, Bloo JH. Australia antigen and antibody in laboratory and other hospital personnel. Vox Sang 24:61, 1973.

744. Devenyi P, Jourdain P. Viral hepatitis in health care personnel working with drug abusers. J Occup Med 15:779, 1973.

745. Lewis TL, Alter HJ, Chalmers TC, et al. A comparison of the frequency of hepatitis-B antigen and antibody in the hospital and non-hospital personnel. N Engl J Med 289:647, 1973.

746. Rosenberg JL, Jones DP, Lipitz LR. Viral hepatitis: an occupational hazard to surgeons. JAMA 223:395, 1973.

747. Pattison CP, Maynard JE, Berquist KR, et al. Epidemiology of hepatitis B in hospital personnel. Am J Epidemiol 101:59, 1975.

748. Eastwood JB, Curtis JR, Wing AJ, et al. Hepatitis in a maintenance hemodialysis unit. Ann Intern Med 69:59, 1968.

749. Snydman DR, Bregman D, Bryan JA. Hemodialysis-associated hepatitis in the United States, 1974. J Infect Dis 135:687, 1977.

750. Snydman DR, Bryan JA, Mason EJ. Hemodialysis-associated hepatitis: report of an epidemic with further evidence on mechanism of transmission. Am J Epidemiol 104:563, 1976.

751. Wands JR, Walker JA, Davis TT, et al. Hepatitis B in an oncology unit. N Engl J Med 291:1371, 1974.

752. Pattison CP, Boyer KM, Maynard EJ, et al. Epidemic viral hepatitis in a clinical laboratory: possible association with computer card handling. JAMA 230:854, 1974.

753. Sutnick AI, London WT, Millman I, et al. Ergasteric hepatitis: endemic hepatitis associated with Australia antigen in a research laboratory. Ann Intern Med 75:35, 1971.

754. Wetli CV, Heal AV, Miale JB. A previously unrecognized laboratory hazard: hepatitis B antigen-positive control and diagnostic sera. Am J Clin Pathol 59:684, 1973.

755. Gristi NR. Survey of hepatitis in laboratories. J Clin Pathol 27:84, 1974.

756. Lo Grippo GA, Hayashi H. Incidence of hepatitis and Australia antigenemia among laboratory workers. Health Lab Sci 10:157, 1973.

757. Berris B, Feinman SV, Richardson B, et al. Hepatitis in undertakers. JAMA 240:138, 1978.

758. Feldman RE, Schiff ER. Hepatitis in dental professionals. JAMA 232:1228, 1975.

759. Mosley JW, Edwards VM, Casey G, et al. Hepatitis B virus infection in dentists. N Engl J Med 293:729, 1975.

760. Williams SV, Pattison CP, Berquist KR. Dental infection with hepatitis B. JAMA 232:1231, 1975.

761. Levin MC, Maddrey WL, Wands JR, et al. Hepatitis B transmission by dentists. JAMA 228:1139, 1974.

762. Rimland D, Parker WE, Miller GB Jr, et al. Hepatitis B outbreak traced to an oral surgeon. N Engl J Med 296:954, 1977.

763. Hollinger FB, Grander JW, Nickel FR, et al. Hepatitis B prevalence within a dental student population. J Am Dent Assoc 94:521, 1977.

763a. Szmuness W, Prince AM, Grundy GF, et al. Hepatitis B infection: a point-prevalence study in 15 US hemodialysis centers. JAMA 227:901, 1974.

763b. Ware AJ, Luby JP, Hollinger FB, et al. Etiology of liver disease in renal-transplant patients. Ann Intern Med 91:364, 1979.

764. Westwood JCN, Chaudhary RK, Perry E. Short-term inapparent infection after accidental ingestion of hepatitis-B-positive serum. Lancet 2:1395, 1973.

765. Vitall SB, Dourdourekas D, Steigmann F. Hepatitis-B antigen in saliva, urine and tears. Am J Gastroenterol 61:133, 1974.

766. MacQuarrie MB, Forghani B, Wolodrow DA. Hepatitis transmitted by a human bite. JAMA 230:723, 1974.

767. Wong ML, Lehmann NI, Gust ID. Detection of hepatitis B surface antigen in the saliva of patients with acute hepatitis B, and of chronic carriers. Med J Aust 2:52, 1976.

768. Almeida JD, Chisholm GD, Kulatilake AE, et al. Possible airborne spread of serum hepatitis virus within a hemodialysis unit. Lancet 2:849, 1971.

769. Garibaldi RA, Hatch FE, Bisno AL, et al. Nonparenteral serum hepatitis: a report of an outbreak. JAMA 220:963, 1972.

770. Hersh T, Melnick JL, Goyal RK, et al. Nonparenteral transmission of hepatitis type B (Australia antigen-associated serum hepatitis). N Engl J Med 285:1363, 1971.

771. Heathcoate J, Sherlock S. Spread of acute type B hepatitis in London. Lancet 1:4168, 1973.

772. Lim KS, TaamWong V, Fulford KWM, et al. Role of sexual and non-

sexual practices in the transmission of hepatitis B. Br J Vener Dis 53:190, 1977.

773. Ellis WR, Murray-Lyon IM, Coleman JC, et al. Liver disease among homosexual males. Lancet 1:903, 1979.

774. Favero MS, Maynard JE, Peterson NJ, et al. Hepatitis-B antigen on environmental surfaces. Lancet 2:1455, 1973.

775. Favero MS, Bond WW, Peterson NJ, et al. Detection methods for study of the stability of hepatitis B on environmental surfaces. J Infect Dis 129:210, 1974.

776. Peterson NJ, Bond WW, Marshall JH, et al. An air sampling technique for hepatitis B surface antigen. Health Lab Sci 13:233, 1976.

777. Peterson NJ, Bond WW, Favero MS. Air sampling for hepatitis B surface antigen in a dental operatory. JAMA 99:465, 1979.

778. Redeker AG, Hopkins CE, Jackson B, et al. A controlled study of the safety of pooled plasma stored in the liquid state at 30–32° C for six months. Transfusion 8:60, 1968.

779. Barker LF, Hoofnagle JH. The transmission of hepatitis type B by plasma derivatives. Devel Biol Standards 27:178, 1973.

780. Biggs R. Jaundice and antibodies directed against factors VIII and IX in patients treated for haemophilia or Christmas disease in the United Kingdom. Br J Hematol 26:313, 1974.

781. Seeff LB, Zimmerman HJ, Wright EC, et al. (Members of VA Hepatitis Cooperative Study Group). VA cooperative study of post-transfusion hepatitis, 1969–1974: Incidence and characteristics of hepatitis and responsible risk factors. Am J Med Sci 270:355, 1975.

781a. Yoshizawa H, Akahane Y, Itoh Y, et al. Virus-like particles in a plasma fraction (fibrinogen) and in the circulation of apparently healthy blood donors capable of inducing non-A, non-B hepatitis in humans and chimpanzees. Gastroenterology 79:512, 1980.

782. Hoofnagle JH, Seeff LB, Bales ZB, et al, and the Veterans Administration Hepatitis Cooperative Study Group. Type B hepatitis after transfusion with blood containing antibody to hepatitis B core antigen. N Engl J Med 290:1379, 1978.

782a. Heimburger N, Schwinn H, Gratz P, et al. Factor VIII concentrate, highly purified and heated in solution. Arzneim Forsch 31:619, 1981.

782b. Hollinger FB, Dolana G, Thomas W, et al. Reduction in risk of hepatitis transmission by heat-treatment of a human factor VIII concentrate. J Infect Dis 150:250, 1984.

782c. Tabor E, Gerety RJ. The chimpanzee animal model for non-A, non-B hepatitis: new applications. In: Szmuness W, Alter HJ, Maynard JE, eds. Viral Hepatitis: 1981 International Symposium. Philadelphia, Franklin Institute Press, 1982:305.

782d. Tabor E, Aronson DL, Gerety RJ. Removal of hepatitis-B-virus infectivity in factor-IX complex by hepatitis-B-immune globulin. Lancet 2:68, 1980.

782e. Tabor E, Gerety RJ. Inactivation of an agent of non-A, non-B hepatitis by formalin. J Infect Dis 142:767, 1980.

782f. Yoshizawa H, Itoh Y, Iwakiri S, et al. Non-A, non-B (type 1) hepatitis agent capable of inducing tubular ultrastructures in the hepatocyte cytoplasm of chimpanzees: inactivation by formalin and heat. Gastroenterology 82:502, 1982.

782g. Tullis JL, Hinman J, Sproul MT, et al. Incidence of post-transfusion hepatitis in previously frozen blood. JAMA 214:719, 1970.

782h. Haugen RK. Hepatitis after the transfusion of frozen red cells and washed red cells. N Engl J Med 301:393, 1979.

782i. Alter HJ, Tabor E, Merryman HT, et al. Transmission of hepatitis B virus infection by transfusion of frozen-deglycerolized red blood cells. N Engl J Med 298:637, 1978.

782j. Bang NU, Ruegsegger P, Ley AB, et al. Detection of hepatitis carriers by serum glutamic oxalacetic transaminase activity. JAMA 171:2303, 1959.

782k. Brandt K-H, Meulendijk PN, Poulie NJ, et al. Data on the determination of SGOT and SGPT activity in donor blood for the possible prevention of post-transfusion hepatitis. Acta Med Scand 177:321, 1965.

782l. Otto-Servais M, Plonteux J, Brocteur J, et al. Interest of enzymatic determinations: OCT, GOT, GPT and observations of the presence of Australia antigen relating to viral hepatitis in blood donors. Vox Sang 19:338, 1970.

782m. Aach RD, Szmuness W, Mosley JW, et al. Serum alanine aminotransferase of donors in relation to the risk of non-A, non-B hepatitis in recipients: the Transfusion-Transmitted Viruses Study. N Engl J Med 304:989, 1981.

782n. Alter HJ, Purcell RH, Holland PV, et al. Donor transaminase and recipient hepatitis: impact on blood transfusion services. JAMA 246:630, 1981.

782o. Sherman KE, Dodd RY, the American Red Cross Alanine Aminotransferase Study Group. Alanine aminotransferase levels among volunteer blood donors: geographic variation and risk factors. J Infect Dis 145:383, 1982.

782p. Polesky HF, House K, Hanson M. Factors affecting ALT levels in blood donors. Transfusion 21:606, 1981.

782q. Alter HJ, Hoofnagle JH. Non-A, non-B hepatitis: observations on the first decade. In: Vyas GN, Dienstag JL, Hoofnagle JH, eds. Viral Hepatitis and Liver Disease. Orlando, FL, Grune & Stratton, 1984:345.

782r. Friedman LS, Dienstag JL, Watkins E, et al. Evaluation of blood donors with elevated serum alanine aminotransferase levels. Ann Intern Med 107:137, 1987.

782s. Stevens CE, Aach RD, Hollinger FB, et al. Hepatitis B virus antibody in blood donors and the occurrence of non-A, non-B hepatitis in transfusion recipients: an analysis of the Transfusion-Transmitted Viruses Study. Ann Intern Med 101:733, 1984.

782t. Koziol DE, Holland PV, Alling DW, et al. Antibody to hepatitis B core antigen as a paradoxical marker for non-A, non-B hepatitis agents in donated blood. Ann Intern Med 104:488, 1986.

783. Perkins JJ. Principles and Methods of Sterilization in Health Sciences. Springfield, IL, Charles C Thomas, 1970:342.

784. Spaulding EH. Chemical disinfection and antiseptics in the hospital. J Hosp Res 9:5, 1972.

785. Snydman DR, Bryan JA, Dixon RE. Prevention of nosocomial viral hepatitis, type B (hepatitis B). Ann Intern Med 83:838, 1975.

786. Miller WV, Walsh JH, Paskin S. Ethylene oxide sterilization to prevent post-transfusion hepatitis. N Engl J Med 280:386, 1969.

787. Bond WS, Favero MS, Peterson NJ, et al. Inactivation of hepatitis B virus by intermediate to high level disinfectant chemicals. J Clin Microbiol 18:535, 1983.

788. Garibaldi RA, Rasmussen CM, Holmes AW, et al. Hospital-acquired serum hepatitis. JAMA 219:1577, 1972.

789. Grob PJ, Moeschlin P. Risk to contacts of a medical practitioner carrying HBsAg. N Engl J Med 293:197, 1975.

790. Alter HJ, Chalmers TC, Freeman BM, et al. Health-care workers positive for hepatitis B surface antigen. N Engl J Med 292:454, 1975.

791. Acute Hepatitis B Associated with Gynecological Surgery. Report of a collaborative study by the Communicable Disease Surveillance Center and the Epidemiological Research Laboratory of the Public Health Service together with a district control-of-infection service. Lancet 1:1, 1980.

792. Alward WLM, McMahon BJ, Hall DB, et al. The long-term serologic course of asymptomatic hepatitis B virus carriers and the development of primary hepatocellular carcinoma. J Infect Dis 151:604, 1985.

793. Sampliner RE. The duration of hepatitis B surface antigenemia. Arch Intern Med 138:145, 1978.

794. Alter HJ, Seeff LB, Kaplan PM, et al. Type B hepatitis: the infectivity of blood positive for "e" antigen and DNA polymerase after accidental needle stick exposure. N Engl J Med 295:909, 1976.

795. US National Heart and Lung Institute Collaborative Study Group and Phoenix Laboratories Division, Bureau of Epidemiology, Center for Disease Control: Relation of "e" antigen to infectivity of HBsAg-positive inoculations among medical personnel. Lancet 2:492, 1976.

795a. Okada K, Kamiyama I, Inomata M, et al. e Antigen and anti-e in the serum of asymptomatic carrier mothers as indicators of positive and negative transmission of hepatitis B virus to their infants. N Engl J Med 294:746, 1976.

795b. Stevens CE, Neurath RA, Beasley RP, et al. HBeAg and anti-HBe detection by radioimmunoassay: correlation with vertical transmission of hepatitis B virus in Taiwan. J Med Virol 3:237, 1979.

795c. Lieberman HM, LaBrecque DR, Kew MC, et al. Detection of hepatitis B virus DNA directly in human serum by a simplified molecular hybridization test: comparison to HBeAg/anti-HBe status in HBsAg carriers. Hepatology 3:285, 1983.

795d. Hadziyannis SJ, Lieberman HM, Karvountzis GG, et al. Analysis of liver disease, nuclear HBcAg, viral replication, and hepatitis B virus DNA in liver and serum of HBeAg vs anti-HBe positive carriers of hepatitis B virus. Hepatology 3:656, 1983.

795e. Yokosuka O, Omata M, Imazeki F, et al. Active and inactive replication of hepatitis B virus deoxyribonucleic acid in chronic liver disease. Gastroenterology 89:610, 1985.

795f. Dusheiko GM, Bowyer SM, Sjogren MH, et al. Replication of hepatitis B virus in adult carriers in an endemic area. J Infect Dis 152:566, 1985.

796. Mosley JW. Epidemiology of viral hepatitis: an overview. Am J Med Sci 270:253, 1975.

797. Redeker AG, Mosley JW, Gocke DJ, et al. Hepatitis immune globulin as a prophylactic measure for spouses exposed to acute type B hepatitis. N Engl J Med 293:1055, 1975.

798. Koff RS, Slavin MS, Connelly LJD, et al. Contagiousness of acute hepatitis B: secondary attack rates in household contacts. Gastroenterology 72:297, 1977.

799. Alter HJ, Purcell RH, Holland PV, et al. Clinical and serological analysis of transfusion-associated hepatitis. Lancet 2:383, 1975.
800. Dienstag JL, Alaama A, Mosley JW, et al. Etiology of sporadic hepatitis B surface antigen-negative hepatitis. Ann Intern Med 87:1, 1977.
801. Craske J, Spooner RJD, Vandervelde EM. Evidence for the existence of at least two types of factor-VIII-associated non-B transfusion hepatitis. Lancet 2:1051, 1978.
802. Hruby MA, Schauf V. Transfusion-related short-incubation hepatitis in hemophilia patients. JAMA 240:1355, 1978.
803. Wyke RJ, Tsiquaye KN, Thornton A, et al. Transmission of non-A, non-B hepatitis to chimpanzees by factor-IX concentrates after fatal complications in patients with chronic liver disease. Lancet 1:520, 1979.
804. Karvountzis GG, Mosley JW, Redekder AG. Serologic characterization of patients with two episodes of acute viral hepatitis. Am J Med 58:815, 1975.
805. Tabor E, April M, Seeff LB, et al. Acute non-A, non-B hepatitis: prolonged presence of the infectious agent in the blood. Gastroenterology 76:680, 1979.
806. Norkrans G, Frosner G, Hermodsson S, et al. The epidemiological pattern of hepatitis A, B and non-A, non-B in Sweden. Scand J Gastroenterol 13:873, 1978.
807. Farrow LJ, Stewart JS, Lamb SGS, et al. Sporadic non-A, non-B hepatitis in West London. Lancet 2:300, 1979.
808. Aach RD, Lander JL, Sherman LA, et al. Transfusion-transmitted virus: interim analysis of hepatitis among transfused and non-transfused patients. In: Vyas GN, Cohen SN, Schmid R, eds. Viral Hepatitis. Philadelphia, Franklin Institute Press, 1978:383.
809. von Behring EA, Kitasoto S. Ueber die Zustander Kommen der Diphtherie-Immunitat und der Tetanus-Immunitat be Thieren. Deutsch Med Wochenschr 1:1113; 1145, 1890.
810. McKhann CF, Chu FT. Use of placental extract in prevention and modification of measles. Am J Dis Child 45:475, 1933.
811. Ordman CW, Jennings CG Jr, Janeway CA. The use of concentrated normal human serum gamma globulin (human immune globulin) in the prevention and attenuation of measles. J Clin Invest 23:541, 1944.
812. Cohn EJ, Oncley JL, Strong LE, et al. Chemical, clinical, and immunological studies on the products of human plasma fractionation. I. The characterization of the protein fractions of human plasma. J Clin Invest 23:417, 1944.
813. Enders JF. The concentration of certain antibodies in globulin fractions derived from human blood plasma. J Clin Invest 23:510, 1944.
814. Murray R, Ratner F. Safety of immune serum globulin with respect to homologous serum hepatitis. Proc Soc Exp Biol Med 83:554, 1953.
815. Schroeder DD, Mozen MM. Australia antigen: distribution during cold ethanol fractionation of human plasma. Science 168:1462, 1970.
816. Holland PV, Alter HJ, Purcell RH, et al. Hepatitis B antigen (HB Ag) and antibody (anti-HBAg) in cold ethanol fractions of human plasma. Transfusion 12:363, 1972.
817. Trepo C, Hantz O, Jacquier MF, et al. Different fates of hepatitis B markers during plasma fractionation: a clue to the infectivity of blood derivatives. Vox Sang 35:143, 1978.
818. Petrilli FC, Crovari P, De Flora S. Hepatitis B in subjects treated with a drug containing immunoglobulins. J Infect Dis 135:252, 1977.
819. Tabor E, Gerety RJ. Transmission of hepatitis by immune serum globulin. Lancet 2:1293, 1979.
820. Morgado AF, Da Fonte JG. An outbreak of hepatitis attributable to inoculation with contaminated gamma globulin. Bull Pan Am Health Org 13:177, 1979.
821. Nakamura S, Sato T. Acute hepatitis B after administration of gammaglobulin. Lancet 1:478, 1976.
822. John TJ, Nina GT, Rajagopalan MS, et al. Epidemic hepatitis B caused by commercial human immunoglobulin. Lancet 1:1074, 1979.
823. de Silva LC, Sette H, Antonacio F, et al. Commercial gamma globulin (CGG) as a possible vehicle of transmission of HBsAg in familial clustering. Rev Inst Med Trop Sao Paulo 19:352, 1977.
824. Hoofnagle JH, Gerety RJ, Barker LF. Antibody to hepatitis B surface antigen in immune serum globulin. Transfusion 50:408, 1975.
825. Frosner GG, Haas H, Hotz G. Hepatitis-A antibody in commercial lots of immune serum globulin. Lancet 1:432, 1977.
826. Hall WT, Mundon FK, Madden DL, et al. Distribution of antibody to hepatitis A antigen in a population of commercial plasma donors. J Clin Microbiol 6:132, 1977.
827. Hoofnagle JH, Waggoner JG. Hepatitis A and B virus markers in immune serum globulin. Gastroenterology 78:259, 1980.
828. Dixon FS, Talmage DW, Maurer PH. Half-life of homologous gamma globulin (antibody) in several species. J Exp Med 96:313, 1952.
829. Armstrong SH Jr, Kukral J, Hershman J, et al. Comparison of the persistence in the blood of gamma globulins labelled with S[35] and I[131] in the same subjects. J Lab Clin Med 44:762, 1954.
830. Volwiler W, Goldsworthy PD, MacMartin NP, et al. Biosynthetic determination with radioactive sulfur of turn-over rates of various plasma proteins in normal and cirrhotic man. J Clin Invest 34:1126, 1955.
831. Waldman TA, Strober W. Metabolism of immunoglobulins. Progr Allergy 13:1, 1969.
832. Janeway CA. Plasma fractionation. Adv Intern Med 3:295, 1949.
833. MacKenzie DL, Vlahcevic ZR. Adverse reaction to gamma globulin due to hypersensitivity to thiomerosal. N Engl J Med 290:749, 1974.
834. Vyas GN, Perkins AJ, Fudenberg HA. Anaphylactoid transfusion reactions associated with anti-IgA. Lancet 2:312, 1968.
835. Barandun S, Kistler P, Jeunet F, et al. Intravenous administration of human gamma globulin. Vox Sang 7:157, 1962.
836. Owings WBJ. Hypersensitivity to gamma globulin. J Med Assoc State Ala 23:74, 1953.
837. Baybutt JE. Hypersensitivity to immune serum globulin. JAMA 171:415, 1959.
838. Ellis EF, Henney CS. Adverse reactions following administration of human gamma globulin. J Allergy 43:45, 1969.
838a. Wells MA, Wittek AE, Epstein JS, et al. Inactivation and partition of human T-cell lymphotropic virus, type III, during ethanol fractionation of plasma. Transfusion 26:210, 1986.
838b. Centers for Disease Control. Safety of therapeutic immune globulin preparations with respect to transmission of human T-lymphotropic virus type III/lymphadenopathy-associated virus infection. Morbid Mortal Weekly Rep 35:231, 1986.
838c. Tedder RS, Uttley A, Cheinsong-Popov R. Safety of immunoglobulin preparation containing anti-HTLV-III (letter). Lancet 1:815, 1985.
839. Hsia DY, Lonsway M, Gellis SS. Gamma globulin in the prevention of infectious hepatitis: studies on the use of small doses in family outbreaks. N Engl J Med 250:417, 1954.
840. Ashley A. Gamma globulin: effect on secondary attack rates in infectious hepatitis. N Engl J Med 250:412, 1954.
840a. Centers for Disease Control, Department of Health and Human Services. Recommendations for protection against viral hepatitis: recommendation of the immunization practices advisory committee. Ann Intern Med 103:391, 1985.
841. Ashley A. Use of gamma globulin for control of infectious hepatitis in an institution for the mentally retarded. N Engl J Med 252:88, 1955.
842. Hall WT, Madden DL, Munden FK, et al. Preventive effect of immune globulin (ISG) against hepatitis A infection in a natural epidemic. Am J Epidemiol 106:72, 1977.
843. Stokes J Jr, Farquhar JA, Drake ME, et al. Infectious hepatitis: length of protection by immune serum globulin (gamma globulin) during epidemics. JAMA 147:714, 1951.
844. Drake ME, Ming C. Gamma globulin in epidemic hepatitis: comparative value of two dosage levels approximately near the minimal effective level. JAMA 155:1302, 1954.
845. Aach RD, Elsea WR, Lyerly J, et al. Efficacy of varied doses of gamma globulin during an epidemic of infectious hepatitis, Hoonah, Alaska, 1961. Am J Public Health 53:1623, 1963.
846. Fowinkle EW, Guthrie N. Comparison of two doses of gamma globulin in prevention of infectious hepatitis. Public Health Rep 79:634, 1964.
847. Stapleton JT, Jansen R, Lemon SM. Serum neutralizing antibody to hepatitis A virus in immune serum globulin and in the sera of common recipients of immune serum globulin. Gastroenterology 89:637, 1985
848. Brachott D, Mosley JW, Lipshitz I, et al. Fragmented IgG for postexposure prophylaxis of type A hepatitis. Transfusion. 12:389, 1972.
849. Mosley JW, Reisler DM, Brachott D, et al. Comparison of two lots of immune serum globulin for prophylaxis of infectious hepatitis. Am J Epidemiol 87:539, 1968.
850. Krasna V, Radkovsky J. Evaluation of the effectiveness of gamma globulin in the prevention of infectious hepatitis in Prague in 1953–1956. J Epidemiol Microbiol Immunol 6:295, 1957.
851. Mosley JW, Galambos J. Viral hepatitis. In: Schiff L, ed. Diseases of the Liver, 4th ed. Philadelphia, JB Lippincott, 1975:500.
852. Landrigan PJ, Huber DK, Murphy D III, et al. The protective efficacy of immune serum globulin in hepatitis A: a statistical approach. JAMA 223:74, 1973.
853. Andrews DA. Immunoglobulin prophylaxis of infectious hepatitis. NZ Med J 73:199, 1971.
854. Assessment of British gamma-globulin in preventing infectious hepatitis. A report to the Director of The Public Health Laboratory Service. Br Med J 3:451, 1968.
855. Werhle PF, Hammon WM. Absence of active immunization against infectious hepatitis: follow up study after administration of gamma globulin. JAMA 167:2062, 1958.
856. Stokes J Jr, Blanchard M, Neefe JR, et al. Methods of protection against homologous serum hepatitis. I. Studies on the protective value of gamma globulin in homologous serum hepatitis SH virus. JAMA 138:336, 1948.

857. Drake ME, Barondess JA, Bashe WJ Jr, et al. Failure of convalescent gamma globulin to protect against homologous serum hepatitis. JAMA 152:690, 1953.
858. A Cooperative Study. Prophylactic gamma globulin for prevention of endemic hepatitis. Effects of US gamma globulin on the incidence of viral hepatitis and other infectious diseases in US soldiers abroad. Arch Intern Med 128:723, 1971.
859. Ginsberg AL, Conrad ME, Bancroft WH, et al. Prevention of endemic HAA-positive hepatitis with gamma globulin: use of a simple radioimmune assay to detect HAA. N Engl J Med 286:562, 1972.
859a. Conrad ME, Lemon SM. Prevention of endemic icteric viral hepatitis by administration of immune serum gamma globulin. J Infect Dis 156:56, 1987.
860. Prince AM, Szmuness W, Woods KP, et al. Antibody against serum-hepatitis antigen: prevalence of protective use as immune serum globulin in prevention of serum-hepatitis infections. N Engl J Med 285:933, 1971.
861. Szmuness W, Prince AM, Goodman M, et al. Hepatitis-B-immune serum globulin in prevention of nonparenterally transmitted hepatitis B. N Engl J Med 290:701, 1974.
862. Desmyter J, Bradburne AF, Vermylen C, et al. Hepatitis-B immuno-globulin in prevention of HBs antigenemia in haemodialysis patients. Lancet 2:377, 1975.
863. Iwarson S, Ahlman J, Erickssen E, et al. Hepatitis B immune globulin in prevention of hepatitis B among hospital staff members. J Infect Dis 135:473, 1977.
864. Kleinknecht K, Courouce AM, Delons S, et al. Prevention of hepatitis B in hemodialysis patients using hepatitis B immunoglobulin: a controlled study. Clin Nephrol 8:373, 1977.
865. Prince AM, Szmuness W, Mann MK, et al. Hepatitis B immune globulin: final report of a controlled multicenter trial of the efficacy in prevention of dialysis-associated hepatitis. J Infect Dis 137:131, 1978.
866. Beasley RP, Stevens CE. Vertical transmission of HBV and interruption with globulin. In: Vyas GN, Cohen SN, Schmid R, eds. Viral Hepatitis. Philadelphia, Franklin Institute Press, 1978:333.
867. Public Health Laboratory Service Report. Decrease in the incidence of hepatitis in dialysis units associated with prevention programs. Br Med J 4:751, 1974.
868. Maynard JE. Passive immunization against hepatitis B. A review of studies and comment on current aspects of control. Am J Epidemiol 107:77, 1978.
869. Mosley JW. New information and invited discussion of unanswered questions. In: Vyas GN, Cohen SN, Schmid R, eds. Viral Hepatitis. Philadelphia, Franklin Institute Press, 1978:483.
869a. Beasley RP, Hwang LY, Stevens CE, et al. Efficacy of hepatitis B immune globulin for prevention of perinatal transmission of the hepatitis B virus carrier state: final report of a randomized, double-blind, placebo-controlled trial. Hepatology 3:135, 1983.
870. A Combined Medical Research Council and Public Health Laboratory Service Report. The incidence of hepatitis B infection after accidental exposure and anti-HBs immunoglobulin prophylaxis. Lancet 1:6, 1980.
871. Kohler PF, Dubois RS, Merrill DA, et al. Prevention of chronic neonatal hepatitis B virus infection with antibody to the hepatitis B surface antigen. N Engl J Med 291:1378, 1974.
872. Dosik H, Jhaveri R. Prevention of neonatal hepatitis infection by high dose immune globulin. N Engl J Med 298:602, 1978.
873. Iwarson S, Norkrans G, Hermodsson S, et al. Passive-active immunization in a neonate treated with repeated doses of high-titered hepatitis B immune globulin. Scand J Infect Dis 11:167, 1979.
874. Reesink HW, Reerink-Brongers E, Lafever-Schut BJT, et al. Prevention of chronic HBsAg carrier state in infants of HBsAg-positive mothers by hepatitis B immunoglobulin. Lancet 2:436, 1979.
875. Varma RR. Hepatitis B surface antigen carrier state in neonates. Prophylaxis with large doses of conventional immune human serum globulin. JAMA 236:2302, 1976.
876. Tong MJ, McPeak CM, Thursby MW, et al. Failure of immune serum globulin to prevent hepatitis B virus infection in infants born to HBsAg-positive mother. Gastroenterology 76:535, 1979.
877. Seeff LB, Zimmerman HJ, Wright EC, et al. Efficacy of hepatitis B immune globulin after accidental exposure: preliminary report of the Veterans Administration Cooperative Study. Lancet 2:939, 1975.
878. Hoofnagle JH, Seeff LB, Bales ZB, et al. (Veterans Administration Cooperative Study Group). Passive-active immunity from hepatitis B immune globulin: re-analysis of a Veterans Administration cooperative study of needle-stick hepatitis. Ann Intern Med 91:813, 1979.
879. Lemon SM, Gates N, Bancroft WH. Prevention of hepatitis with gamma globulin. Ann Intern Med 92:869, 1980.
880. Gateau PH, Opolon P, Nusinovici V, et al. Passive immunotherapy in HBsAg fulminant hepatitis: results on antigenemia and survival. Digestion 14:304, 1976.
881. Grady GF. New information and unanswered questions. In: Vyas GN, Cohen SN, Schmid R, eds. Viral Hepatitis. Philadelphia, Franklin Institute Press, 1978:599.
882. Grossman EB, Stewart SG, Stokes J Jr. Post-transfusion hepatitis in battle casualties. JAMA 129:991, 1945.
883. Csapo J, Budai J, Bartos A, et al. Prevention of transfusion hepatitis. Acta Paediatr Acad Sci Hung 4:195, 1963.
884. Mirick GS, Ward R, McCollum RW. Modification of post-transfusion hepatitis by gamma globulin. N Engl J Med 273:59, 1965.
885. Creutzfeldt W, Severidt H-J, Brachmann H, et al. Untersuchungen zur Prophylaxe der Transfusionhepatitis durch Gamma-Globulin. Deutsch Med Wochenschr 91:1905, 1966.
886. Katz R, Rodriguez R, Ward R. Post-transfusion hepatitis—effect of modified gamma globulin added to blood in vitro. N Engl J Med 285:925, 1971.
887. Knodell RG, Conrad ME, Ginsberg AL, et al. Efficacy of prophylactic gamma-globulin in preventing non-A, non-B post-transfusion hepatitis. Lancet 1:557, 1976.
888. Duncan GG, Christian HA, Stokes J Jr, et al. An evaluation of immune serum globulin as a prophylactic agent against homologous serum hepatitis. Am J Med Sci 213:53, 1947.
889. Holland PV, Rubinson RM, Morrow AG, et al. λ-Globulin in the prophylaxis of post-transfusion hepatitis. JAMA 196:471, 1966.
890. Spellberg MA, Berman PM. The incidence of post-transfusion hepatitis and the lack of efficacy of gamma globulin in its prevention. Am J Gastroenterol 55:564, 1971.
891. Kuhns WJ, Prince AM, Brotman B, et al. A clinical and laboratory evaluation of immune serum globulin from donors with a history of hepatitis: attempted prevention of post-transfusion hepatitis. Am J Med Sci 272:255, 1976.
892. Seeff LB, Wright EC, Zimmerman HJ, et al. Post-transfusion hepatitis, 1973–1975: A Veterans Administration Cooperative Study. In: Vyas GN, Cohen SN, Schmid R, eds. Viral Hepatitis. Philadelphia, Franklin Institute Press, 1978:371.
893. Provost PJ, Hilleman MR. Propagation of human hepatitis A virus in cell culture in vitro. Proc Soc Exp Biol Med 160:213, 1979.
894. Provost PJ, Giesa PA, McAleer WJ, et al. Isolation of hepatitis A virus in vitro in cell culture directly from human specimens. Proc Soc Exp Biol Med 167:201, 1981.
895. Lemon SM. Type A viral hepatitis: new developments in an old disease. N Engl J Med 313:1058, 1985.
896. Binn LN, Bancroft WH, Eckels KH, et al. Inactivated hepatitis A virus vaccine produced in human diploid MRC-5 cells. J Med Virol 21:25A, 1987.
897. Sjogren MH, Eckels KH, Binn LN, et al. Safety and immunogenicity of an inactivated hepatitis A vaccine in volunteers. J Med Virol 21:25A, 1987.
898. Provost PJ, Banker FS, Giesa PA, et al. Progress toward a live, attenuated human hepatitis A vaccine. Proc Soc Exp Biol Med 170:8, 1973.
899. Provost PJ, Conti PA, Giesa PA, et al. Studies in chimpanzees of live, attenuated hepatitis A vaccine candidates. Proc Soc Exp Biol Med 172:357, 1983.
900. Provost PJ, Buynack EB, McLean AA, et al. Progress toward a live attenuated human hepatitis A vaccine. In: Vyas GN, Dienstag JL, Hoofnagle JH, eds. Viral Hepatitis and Liver Disease. Orlando, FL, Grune & Stratton, 1984:467.
901. Flehmig B, Mauler RF, Noll G, et al. Progress towards developing an attenuated live hepatitis A vaccine. J Med Virol 21:26A, 1987.
902. Karron RA, Daemer RJ, Ticehurst JR, et al. Evaluation of attenuation of cell culture adapted hepatitis A virus in non-human primates. J Med Virol 21:26A, 1987.
903. Hu M, Scheid R, Deinhardt F, et al. Attenuated hepatitis A virus for vaccine development: attenuation and virulence for marmosets. J Med Virol 21:27A, 1987.
904. Baroudy BM, Ticehurst JR, Miele TA, et al. Sequence analysis of hepatitis A virus cDNA coding for capsid proteins and RNA polymerase. Proc Natl Acad Sci USA 82:2143, 1985.
905. Najarian R, Caput D, Gee W, et al. Primary structure and gene organization of human hepatitis A virus. Proc Natl Acad Sci USA 82:2627, 1985.
906. Linemeyer DL, Menke JG, Martin-Gallardo A, et al. Molecular cloning and partial sequencing of hepatitis A viral cDNA. J Virol 54:247, 1985.
907. Ticehurst JR. Hepatitis A virus: clones, cultures, and vaccines. Semin Liver Dis 6:46, 1986.
908. Widell A, Hansson BG, Nordenfelt E. A microcarrier cell culture system for large scale production of hepatitis A. J Virol Methods 8:63, 1984.
909. Siegl G, de Chastonay J, Kronauer G. Propagation and assay of hepatitis A virus in vitro. J Virol Methods 9:53, 1984.
910. Buynak EB, Roehm RR, Tytell AA, et al. Vaccine against human hepatitis B. JAMA 235:2832, 1976.
911. Buynak EB, Roehm RR, Tytell AA, et al. Development and chim-

panzee testing of a vaccine against human hepatitis B. Proc Soc Exp Biol Med 151:694, 1976.

912. Tabor E, Buynak EB, Smallwood LA, et al. Inactivation of hepatitis B virus by three methods: treatment with pepsin, urea or formalin. J Med Virol 11:1, 1983.

913. Hepatitis B virus vaccine safety: report of an interagency group. Morbid Mortal Weekly Rep 31:465, 1982.

914. Francis DP, Feorino PM, McDougal S, et al. The safety of the hepatitis B vaccine: inactivation of the AIDS virus during routine vaccine manufacture. JAMA 256:869, 1986.

915. Maupas P, Goudeau A, Coursaget P, et al. Immunization against hepatitis B in man: a pilot study of two years duration. In: Vyas GN, Cohen SN, Schmid R, eds. Viral Hepatitis. Philadelphia, Franklin Institute Press, 1978:539.

916. Reesink HW, Brummelhuis HGV, van Elven EH, et al. The preparation and evaluation of a hepatitis-B vaccine in the Netherlands. In: Vyas GN, Cohen SN, Schmid R, eds. Viral Hepatitis. Philadelphia, Franklin Institute Press, 1978:714.

917. Coutinho RA, Lelie N, Lent PA-V, et al. Efficacy of a heat inactivated hepatitis B vaccine in male homosexuals: outcome of a placebo-controlled double blind trial. Br Med J 286:1305, 1983.

918. Desmyter J, Colaert J, De Groote GH, et al. Efficacy of heat inactivated hepatitis B vaccine in haemodialysis patients and staff: double-blind, placebo-controlled trial. Lancet 1:797, 1983.

919. Burrell CJ, Mackay P, Greenaway PJ, et al. Expression in *Escherichia coli* of hepatitis B virus DNA sequences cloned in plasmid pBR322. Nature 280:815, 1979.

920. Valenzuela P, Medina A, Rutter WJ, et al. Synthesis and assembly of hepatitis B virus surface antigen particles in yeast. Nature 298:347, 1982.

921. Emini EA, Ellis RW, Miller WJ, et al. Production and immunological analysis of recombinant hepatitis B vaccine. J Infect (Suppl A) 13:3, 1986.

922. Purcell RH, Gerin JL. Hepatitis B vaccines: a status report. In: Vyas GN, Cohen SN, Schmid R, eds. Viral Hepatitis. Philadelphia, Franklin Institute Press, 1978:491.

923. Hilleman MR, Bertland AU, Buynak EB, et al. Clinical and laboratory studies of HBsAg vaccine. In Vyas GN, Cohen SN, Schmid R, eds. Viral Hepatitis. Philadelphia, Franklin Institute Press, 1978:539.

924. McAuliffe VJ, Purcell RH, Gerin JL. Type B hepatitis: a review of current prospects for a safe and effective vaccine. Rev Infect Dis 2:470, 1980.

925. Szmuness W, Stevens CE, Harley EJ, et al. Hepatitis B vaccine: demonstration of efficacy in a controlled clinical trial in a high-risk population in the United States. N Engl J Med 303:833, 1980.

926. Francis DP, Hadler SC, Thompson SE, et al. The prevention of hepatitis B with vaccine: report of the Centers for Disease Control multi-center efficacy trial among homosexual men. Ann Intern Med 97:362, 1982.

927. Szmuness W, Stevens CE, Zang EA, et al. Hepatitis B vaccine in medical staff of hemodialysis units: efficacy and subtype cross-protection. N Engl J Med 307:1481, 1982.

928. McLean AA, Shaw R Jr. Hepatitis B virus vaccine. Ann Intern Med 97:451, 1982.

929. Seeff LB, Koff RS. Passive and active immunoprophylaxis of hepatitis B. Gastroenterology 86:958, 1984.

930. Maupas P, Chiron J-P, Barin F, et al. Efficacy of hepatitis B vaccine in prevention of early HBsAg carrier state in children: controlled trial in an endemic area (Senegal). Lancet 1:289, 1981.

931. McLean AA, Hilleman MR, McAleer WJ, et al. Summary of worldwide experience with H-B-Vax (B, MSD). J Infect 7:95, 1983.

932. Prozesky OW, Stevens CE, Szmuness W, et al. Immune response in neonates to hepatitis B vaccine. J Infect Dis 7:53, 1983.

933. Maupas P, Goudeau A, Coursaget P, et al. Hepatitis B vaccine: efficacy in high-risk setting, a two-year study. Intervirology 10:196, 1978.

934. Deinhardt F. Aspects of vaccination against hepatitis B, passive-active immunization schedules and vaccination responses in different age groups. Scand J Infect Dis (Suppl) 38:17, 1983.

935. Crosnier J, Jongers P, Courouce A-M, et al. Randomised, placebo-controlled trial of hepatitis B surface antigen vaccine in French haemodialysis units. II. Haemodialysis patients. Lancet 2:797, 1981.

936. Grob P. Hepatitis B vaccination of renal transplant and hemodialysis patients. Scand J Infect Dis (Suppl) 38:28, 1983.

937. Stevens CE, Alter HJ, Taylor PE, et al. Hepatitis B vaccine in patients receiving hemodialysis: immunogenicity and efficacy. N Engl J Med 311:496, 1984.

938. Stevens CE, Szmuness W, Goodman AI, et al. Hepatitis B vaccine: immune response in haemodialysis patients. Lancet 2:1211, 1980.

939. Dienstag JL, Werner BG, Polk F, et al. Hepatitis B vaccine in health care personnel: safety, immunogenicity, and indicators of efficacy. Ann Intern Med 101:34, 1984.

940. Centers for Disease Control. Suboptimal response to hepatitis B vaccine given by injection into the buttock. Morbid Mortal Weekly Rep 34:105, 1985.

941. Jilg W, Schmidt M, Zoulek G, et al. Clinical evaluation of a recombinant hepatitis B vaccine. Lancet 2:1174, 1984.

942. Davidson M, Krugman S. Immunogenicity of recombinant yeast hepatitis B vaccine. Lancet 1:108, 1985.

943. Scolnick EM, McLean AA, West DJ, et al. Clinical evaluation in healthy adults of a hepatitis B vaccine made by recombinant DNA. JAMA 251:2812, 1984.

944. Dandalos E, Roumeliotou-Karayannis A, Richardson SC, et al. Safety and immunogenicity of a recombinant hepatitis B vaccine. J Med Virol 17:57, 1985.

945. Yamomoto S, Kuroki T, Kurai K, et al. Comparison of results for phase I studies with recombinant and plasma-derived hepatitis B vaccines, and controlled study comparing intramuscular and subcutaneous unjections of recombinant hepatitis B vaccine. J Infect 13A(Suppl):53, 1986.

946. Schalm SW, Heytink RA, Kruining H, et al. Immunogenicity of recombinant yeast hepatitis-B vaccine. Neth J Med 29:28, 1986.

947. Brown SE, Stanley C, Howard CR, et al. Antibody responses to recombinant and plasma derived hepatitis B vaccines. Br Med J 292:159, 1986.

948. Hadler SC, Francis DP, Maynard JE, et al. Long-term immunogenicity and efficacy of hepatitis B vaccine in homosexual men. N Engl J Med 315:209, 1986.

949. Weitberg AB, Weitzman SA, Watkins E, et al. Immunogenicity of hepatitis B vaccine in oncology patients receiving chemotherapy. J Clin Oncol 3:718, 1985.

950. Beasley RP, Hwang LY, Lee GCY, et al. Prevention of perinatally transmitted hepatitis B virus infections with hepatitis B immune globulin and hepatitis B vaccine. Lancet 2:1099, 1983.

951. Wong VCW, Ip HMH, Reesink HW, et al. Prevention of the HBsAg carrier state in newborn infants of mothers who are chronic carriers of HBsAg and HBeAg by administration of hepatitis-B vaccine and hepatitis-B immunoglobulin. Lancet 1:921, 1984.

952. Lo KJ, Tsai YT, Lee SD, et al. Immunoprophylaxis of infection with hepatitis B virus in infants born to hepatitis B surface antigen-positive carrier mothers. J Infect Dis 152:817, 1985.

953. Xu ZY, Liu CB, Francis DP, et al. Prevention of perinatal acquisition of hepatitis B virus carriage using vaccine: preliminary report of a randomized, double-blind placebo-controlled and comparative trial. Pediatrics 76:713, 1985.

954. Szmuness W, Stevens CE, Oleszko WR, et al. Passive-active immunization against hepatitis B: immunogenicity studies in adult Americans. Lancet 2:575, 1981.

955. Zachoval R, Deinhardt F, Frosner H, et al. Active and passive-active immunization against hepatitis B. In: Szmuness W, Alter HJ, Maynard JE, eds. Viral Hepatitis. Philadelphia: Franklin Institute Press, 1982:757.

956. Stevens CE, Toy PT, Tong MJ, et al. Perinatal hepatitis B virus transmission in the United States: prevention by passive-active immunization. JAMA 253:1740, 1985.

957. Stevens CE, Taylor PE, Tong MJ, et al. Yeast-recombinant hepatitis B vaccine: efficacy with hepatitis B immune globulin in prevention of perinatal hepatitis B virus transmission. JAMA 257:2612, 1987.

958. Stevens CE, Taylor PE, Tong MJ, et al. Hepatitis B vaccine: an overview. In: Vyas GN, Dienstag JL, Hoofnagle JH, eds. Viral Hepatitis and Liver Disease. Orlando, FL, Grune & Stratton, 1984:275.

959. Coursaget P, Yvonnet B, Chotard J, et al. Seven-year study of hepatitis B vaccine in infants from an endemic area (Senegal). Lancet 2:1143, 1986.

960. Purcell RH, Gerin JL. Prospects for second and third generation hepatitis B vaccines. Hepatology 5:159, 1985.

961. Hilleman MR, Buynack EB, Markus HZ, et al. Control of hepatitis B virus infection: vaccines produced from Alexander cell line and from recombinant yeast cells. In: Vyas GN, Dienstag JL, Hoofnagle JH, eds. Viral Hepatitis and Liver Disease. Orlando, FL, Grune & Stratton, 1984:307.

962. Smith GL, Mackett M, Moss B. Infectious vaccinia virus recombinants that express hepatitis B surface antigen. Nature 302:490, 1983.

963. Moss B, Smith GL, Gerin JL, et al. Live recombinant vaccinia virus protects chimpanzees against hepatitis B. Nature 311:67, 1984.

964. Dreesman GR, Hollinger FB, Sanchez Y, et al. Immunization of chimpanzees with hepatitis B virus-derived polypeptides. Infect Immunol 32:62, 1981.

965. Hollinger FB, Dreesman GR, Sanchez Y, et al. Experimental hepatitis B polypeptide vaccine in chimpanzees. In: Vyas GN, Cohen SN, Schmid R, eds. Viral Hepatitis. Philadelphia, Franklin Institute Press, 1978:557.

966. Sanchez Y, Ionescu-Matiu I, Melnick JL, et al. Comparative studies of the immunogenic activity of hepatitis B surface antigen (HBsAg) and HBsAg polypeptides. J Med Virol 11:115, 1983.

967. Hollinger FB, Troisi C, Heiberg D, et al. Response to a hepatitis B polypeptide vaccine in micelle form in a young adult population. J Med Virol 19:229, 1986.
968. Neurath AR, Kent SBH, Parker K, et al. Antibodies to a synthetic peptide from the preS 120–145 region of the hepatitis B virus envelope are virus-neutralizing. Vaccine 4:35, 1986.
969. Neurath AR, Kent SHB, Taylor P, et al. Hepatitis B virus contains pre-S gene-encoded domains. Nature 315:154, 1985.
970. Milich DR, Thornton GB, Neurath AR, et al. Enhanced immunogenicity of the pre-S region of hepatitis B surface antigen. Science 228:1195, 1985.
971. Neurath AR, Strick N, Kent SHB, et al. Enzyme-linked immunoassay of pre-S gene-encoded sequences in hepatitis B vaccines. J Virol Methods 12:185, 1985.
972. Hopp TP. A synthetic peptide with hepatitis B surface antigen reactivity. Mol Immunol 18:869, 1981.
973. Lerner RA, Green N, Alexander H, et al. Chemically synthesized peptides predicted from the nucleotide sequence of the hepatitis B virus genome elicit antibodies reactive with the native envelope protein in Dane particles. Proc Natl Acad Sci USA 78:3403, 1981.
974. Bhatnagar PK, Papas E, Blum HE, et al. Immune response to synthetic peptide analogues of hepatitis B surface antigen specific for the a determinant. Proc Natl Acad Sci USA 79:4400, 1982.
975. Gerin JL, Alexander H, Shih JW-KS, et al. Chemically synthesized peptides of hepatitis B surface antigen duplicate the d/y specificities and induce subtype-specific antibodies in chimpanzees. Proc Natl Acad Sci USA 80:2365, 1983.
976. Hollinger FB, Dreesman GR, Sparrow J, et al. Synthetic peptide vaccine for hepatitis B. In: Papaevangelou G, Hennessen W, eds. Viral hepatitis: standardization in immunoprophylaxis of infections by hepatitis viruses. Dev Biol Stand 54:113, 1983.
977. Centers for Disease Control. Recommendation of the Immunization Practices Advisory Committee. Recommendations for protection against viral hepatitis. Ann Int Med 103:391, 1985.
978. Centers for Disease Control. Immune globulins for protection against viral hepatitis. Recommendations of the Public Health Service Advisory Committee on Immunization Practices. MMWR 26:1977.
979. Mosley JW, Galambos J. In Schiff L, ed. Diseases of the Liver, 4th ed. Philadelphia, JB Lippincott Co., 1975:500.
980. Hadler SC, Erben JJ, Matthews D, et al. Effect of immunoglobulin on hepatitis A in day care centers. JAMA 249:48, 1987.
981. Centers for Disease Control. Recommendation of the Immunization Practices Advisory Committee. Update on hepatitis B prevention. Ann Int Med 107:353, 1987.
982. Kumar ML, Dawson NV, McCullough AJ, et al. Should all pregnant women be screened for hepatitis B? Ann Int Med 107:273, 1987.
983. Jonas MM, Schiff ER, O'Sullivan MJ, et al. Failure of Centers for Disease Control criteria to identify hepatitis B infection in a large municipal obstetrical population. Ann Int Med 107:335, 1987.
984. Stevens CE. Perinatal hepatitis B virus infection: screening of pregnant women and protection of the infant. Ann Int Med 107:412, 1987.
985. Mulley AG, Silverstein MD, Dienstag JL. Indications for use of hepatitis B vaccine, based on cost-effectiveness analysis. N Engl J Med 307:644, 1982.
986. Dienstag JL, Stevens CE, Bhan AK, et al. Hepatitis B vaccine administered to chronic carriers of hepatitis B surface antigen. Ann Int Med 96:644, 1982.
987. Seeff LB, Koff RS. Passive and active immunoprophylaxis of hepatitis B. Gastroenterology 86:958, 1984.
988. Stevens CE, Taylor PE. Hepatitis B vaccine: issues, recommendations, and new developments. Sem Liv Dis 6:23, 1986.
989. Kuo G, Choo Q-L, Alter HJ, et al. An assay for circulating antibodies to a major etiologic virus of human non-A, non-B hepatitis. Science 244:362, 1989.

38

Chronic Hepatitis

Willis C. Maddrey, M.D.

DEFINITIONS

CPH = Chronic persistent hepatitis. Histologic evidence of inflammation predominantly confined to the portal tract, with no disruption of the limiting plate around the portal tract. There may be evidence of minimal focal inflammation throughout the hepatic lobule. Generally considered to be a nonprogressive lesion.

CLH = Chronic lobular hepatitis. Inflammatory changes predominantly found throughout the hepatic lobule, with minimal portal and periportal inflammation.

CAH = Chronic active hepatitis. Histologic evidence of hepatocellular necrosis and fibrosis that often progresses to cirrhosis. The least severe form of chronic active hepatitis is characterized by disruption of the limiting plate around the portal tract and periportal (piecemeal) necrosis, often with evidence of trapping of hepatocytes around the portal tract. Bridging hepatic necrosis is a more severe form of chronic active hepatitis, characterized by linear areas of hepatocellular necrosis and drop-out linking portal tracts to each other or to terminal hepatic venules. Multilobular necrosis is the most severe form of chronic active hepatitis and is characterized by destruction of the entire lobule (panacinar).

Chronic hepatitis designates a group of disorders characterized by an unresolved inflammatory disease of the liver that has existed for more than six months.[1-4] This requirement (i.e., at least six months of inflammation) was chosen arbitrarily in order to exclude patients with acute hepatitis. It is well established that acute liver disease in the majority of patients resolves completely within three months of onset. Concern regarding possible chronicity begins between three and six months. Chronic active hepatitis is the preferred term for chronic hepatitis in a subgroup of patients in whom there is evidence of progressive injury with inflammatory and fibrotic changes that may lead to fibrosis. Before the availability and widespread use of diagnostic liver biopsy, chronic liver disease most often was recognized as cirrhosis during post-mortem examination of patients who had had advanced liver disease.

The criteria that are accepted most widely for classification of chronic hepatitis were developed in 1968 and divide chronic hepatitis into two broad categories based on histologic changes: *chronic persistent* and *chronic active hepatitis* (CAH).[3] This original system of classification has subsequently been reviewed and refined.[5] The major goal of the classification system is to differentiate those patients in whom chronic hepatitis is likely to proceed to cirrhosis from patients who have a more benign form of chronic inflammation and are unlikely to develop cirrhosis.

CPH is characterized histologically by portal inflammation and is basically a nonprogressive process. CAH is characterized by histologic evidence of hepatocellular necrosis and fibrosis and is considered a progressive, precirrhotic process.[3, 5] There has been a gradual evolution of concepts regarding the causes and histologic types of acute and chronic liver diseases. Subsequent to the initial classification, the category of *chronic lobular hepatitis* (CLH) was added to define a histologic lesion characterized by focal areas of inflammation and necrosis throughout the hepatic lobule, with minimal portal and periportal inflammation.[6]

There is no sharp line of demarcation between a slowly resolving episode of acute hepatitis and chronic hepatitis. Often the onset of the hepatitis is difficult to establish. In many instances, the patient has evidence of advanced chronic liver injury on initial evaluation even in the absence of a history of an acute injury, which would allow documentation of onset of the disorder. The availability of percutaneous liver biopsies from patients with clinical and laboratory evidence of hepatic inflammation led to the recognition of the frequency, types, and importance of chronic hepatitis. The development of aminotransferase tests as reliable indicators of hepatic inflammation assisted greatly in allowing recognition of chronic hepatitis in patients who either were asymptomatic or had only minimal evidence of liver injury. The use of sequential determinations of aminotransferase levels made it possible to follow the course of liver disease over time. Recognition that immunosuppressive therapy, especially corticosteroid therapy, could prolong life and decrease morbidity in at least some patients with chronic hepatitis was an additional stimulus to further study.

The discovery in 1967 of the Australia antigen (HBsAg) was followed by remarkable advances in the understanding of hepatitis B–induced liver disease that allowed identification of the large subgroup of patients with chronic hepatitis B. It has been established that 2 to 10 per cent of adult patients with acute hepatitis B do not completely recover and that many of these patients develop chronic hepatitis.[7, 8]

Over the two decades following the recognition of hepatitis B, it has become appreciated that patients with non-A, non-B hepatitis, especially those who acquire the disease following transfusion, often progress to chronic hepatitis and cirrhosis.[9] Whether more than one non-A, non-B viral agent is involved in the pathogenesis of chronic hepatitis will not be established until reliable viral markers are identified.

A further advance was the identification of the hepatitis A virus in 1973 and the subsequent demonstration that hepatitis A does *not* lead to chronic hepatitis.

DIFFERENTIAL DIAGNOSIS OF CHRONIC HEPATITIS

There are several established causes of chronic hepatitis. Hepatitis B and non-A, non-B hepatitis, are the most common etiologic agents in most studies of patients with chronic hepatitis. The relative contributions of these etiologies varies widely, usually depending on the frequency of hepatitis B in the particular area or population studied. Idiopathic autoimmune chronic active hepatitis (CAH) is the one type of hepatitis in which corticosteroid and other immunosuppressive therapies are beneficial.[10–12]

A number of therapeutic drugs, including methyldopa and nitrofurantoin, and laxative preparations containing

TABLE 38–1. DIFFERENTIAL DIAGNOSIS OF CHRONIC ACTIVE HEPATITIS (CAH) IN ADULTS

Hepatitis viruses
B
Non-A, Non-B
Idiopathic autoimmune
Therapeutic drug–induced
Methyldopa
Nitrofurantoin
Others
Wilson's disease
α_1-Antitrypsin deficiency

oxyphenisatin, which were formerly widely used, have been shown to cause chronic hepatitis indistinguishable from the idiopathic autoimmune variety.[13] Wilson's disease is a rare but important cause of chronic hepatitis in young individuals (Chap. 47).[14, 15] It has been recognized that patients with Wilson's disease may have chronic hepatitis in the absence of neurologic abnormalities. It has further been established that α_1-antitrypsin deficiency (see Chap. 50) may present as cirrhosis with features suggesting chronic hepatitis in adults with no evidence of pulmonary disease (Table 38–1).[16]

A variety of other disorders must be considered in the evaluation of a patient with chronic hepatic inflammation (Table 38–2). The diagnosis of chronic hepatitis is often considered in a patient whose illness is subsequently diagnosed as primary biliary cirrhosis (see Chap. 44), especially in the early stages of the disease. The clinical and histologic features of primary biliary cirrhosis may closely mimic those of CAH, especially the idiopathic autoimmune type.[17] The diagnosis of primary biliary cirrhosis is favored when the patient is a middle-aged woman who presents with pruritus, elevated alkaline phosphatase levels, high-titer antimitochondrial antibodies, and elevated serum IgM levels. Occasionally, it is not possible to differentiate primary biliary cirrhosis from idiopathic autoimmune CAH; in these situations, a short-term trial of corticosteroid therapy may be useful, since a response to treatment is evidence of idiopathic autoimmune CAH.[18]

Portal inflammation, often designated pericholangitis, may be found in patients with inflammatory bowel disease (see Chap. 43) and histologically may appear indistinguishable from CPH or CAH.[19] Most of these patients eventually will develop sclerosing cholangitis (Chap. 43), but the differentiation from CAH may not be possible except on long-term follow-up.[20] A careful history regarding bowel habits is indicated in the evaluation of chronic hepatitis, and sigmoidoscopy with biopsy may be required to confirm the diagnosis of inflammatory bowel disease. Endoscopic cholangiography or transhepatic cholangiography may be required to establish or exclude the diagnosis of sclerosing cholangitis. (Chaps. 43 and 59).

In chronic alcoholics with evidence of alcoholic liver disease, histologic features may suggest chronic active hepatitis, and evidence of liver injury may persist or even

TABLE 38–2. OTHER DISORDERS THAT SHOULD BE CONSIDERED IN PATIENT WITH CHRONIC HEPATIC INFLAMMATION

Primary biliary cirrhosis
Alcoholic liver disease
Inflammatory bowel disease
Steatonecrosis

increase following withdrawal of alcohol (Chap. 33).[21, 22] Whether alcohol-induced liver injury is in part mediated by an immunologic response to components of altered hepatocytes is unknown. Chronic alcoholics with portal hypertension have been reported to have a much higher incidence of antibodies to hepatitis B than a control population, suggesting a synergistic effect of the injuries.[23] Many chronic alcoholics also have a history of drug abuse or contact with drug abusers and other groups at increased risk for acquiring hepatitis B. A component of the chronic hepatitis found in alcoholic patients may result from superimposition of a viral infection.

Occasionally, patients with non–alcohol-induced fatty liver apparently related to obesity (see Chap. 33) may present with elevated aminotransferase levels and pathologic changes resembling those found in chronic hepatitis.[24] Patients with non–alcohol-induced fatty liver may progress to cirrhosis. The exact etiology of the disorder is not understood nor is the pathogenetic significance of obesity (Table 38–3).

In summary, the evaluation of a patient with chronic hepatitis must consider a number of possible etiologies for the hepatic injury; a careful assessment of the histologic extent of hepatic damage; and recognition of the limited outlook for effective therapy in most cases. The expansion of the list of underlying disorders that may cause chronic hepatitis has been impressive. Unfortunately, effective therapy to reverse the progression of chronic hepatitis to cirrhosis is available for only a small subgroup of these patients.

HISTOLOGIC MANIFESTATIONS AS THE BASIS FOR CLASSIFICATION OF CHRONIC HEPATITIS

As previously mentioned, the most widely accepted classification of chronic hepatitis, based on histologic findings, initially had two major subdivisions: chronic persistent hepatitis (CPH) (Fig. 38–1) and chronic active hepatitis (CAH) (Fig. 38–2).[3–5] Objectives of the classification system were to provide guidelines for predicting the eventual course of the chronic hepatitis and for distinguishing patients with benign, nonprogressive hepatitis (i.e., CPH) from those whose illness was likely to progress to cirrhosis (i.e., CAH). The fundamental histologic finding used initially to differentiate CPH from CAH was periportal, or

TABLE 38–3. DISORDERS ASSOCIATED WITH IDIOPATHIC AUTOIMMUNE CHRONIC ACTIVE HEPATITIS

Thyroiditis
Thyrotoxicosis (rare)
Hypothyroidism
Autoimmune hemolytic anemia
Polyarthritis
Capillaritis
Glomerulonephritis
Pulmonary disorders
   Fibrosing alveolitis
   Primary pulmonary hypertension
Amenorrhea and other menstrual abnormalities
Ulcerative colitis
Monoclonal gammopathy
Hyperviscosity syndrome
Lichen planus
Polymyositis
Uveitis

so-called piecemeal, hepatic necrosis in patients with CAH (Fig. 38–3). This lesion was defined as inflammatory invasion of the limiting plate of hepatocytes surrounding the portal triad and was considered the hallmark of CAH. The term chronic active hepatitis replaced the term chronic aggressive hepatitis, which was used earlier to designate the presence of piecemeal hepatic necrosis.[3, 5, 25] CPH is considered a benign lesion and is defined as chronic portal inflammation with no evidence of periportal piecemeal necrosis. A third category, *chronic lobular hepatitis* (CLH), was introduced to designate a group of patients with predominantly focal necrosis throughout the hepatic lobule and scant inflammation of the portal triads.[6]

It has become recognized and accepted that CAH with only periportal piecemeal necrosis is a relatively benign condition and that the histologic lesion called bridging hepatic necrosis identifies a more severe form of CAH (Figs. 38–4 and 38–5).[26–29] Bridging hepatic necrosis is characterized histologically by areas of confluent, often linear necrosis of hepatocytes and by connective tissue "bridges" between portal triads or between portal triads and terminal hepatic venules (central veins). These bridging lesions lead to remodeling of hepatic architecture. Further studies are needed to determine whether there is validity to the belief that portal to portal bridges are more benign findings than bridges linking portal areas to terminal hepatic venules (portal-central bridges).[29]

The importance of bridging hepatic necrosis as an adverse prognostic sign in a patient with acute hepatitis was first suggested by Boyer and Klatskin.[26] Results of subsequent studies indicated that bridging hepatic necrosis may be found in patients with acute hepatitis who later have complete resolution of the liver injury.[30, 31] Nevertheless, bridging hepatic necrosis is considered a definite adverse prognostic sign when found in a patient who has had signs or symptoms of liver disease or both for three to six months or longer. More extensive necrosis (i.e., destruction of entire lobules) is classified as *multilobular hepatic necrosis*; patients with this lesion have an even less favorable prognosis. At the Mayo Clinic, extensive follow-up studies of patients with severe CAH demonstrated that those with bridging or multilobular hepatic necrosis or both were at far greater risk for progression to cirrhosis than those with lesser evidence of hepatic injury.[12, 32–34] The adverse prognostic significance of bridging hepatic necrosis has been confirmed in studies from Japan.[28]

A major issue in the histopathologic evaluation of chronic hepatitis is whether a patient with periportal inflammation (piecemeal necrosis) and no evidence of bridging or multilobular hepatic necrosis should be grouped prognostically in the relatively benign category of CPH or in that of progressive CAH. Analysis of several series of patients with chronic hepatitis indicates that some patients with the classic CAH lesion of periportal piecemeal necrosis may progress to cirrhosis, with bridging hepatic necrosis developing as an intermediary lesion.[29, 32, 35]

Therefore, many questions remain as to the importance and prognostic significance of bridging hepatic necrosis found on liver biopsy. Factors to be considered in evaluation include duration of the illness before the lesion was diagnosed, type and number of bridging lesions, etiology of the chronic hepatitis, and previous corticosteroid or immunosuppressive therapy. It appears that chronic hepatitis with periportal necrosis and without bridging necrosis is a *relatively* benign lesion. As yet, there has been no controlled trial of corticosteroid versus placebo therapy in HBsAg-negative patients with periportal piecemeal necro-

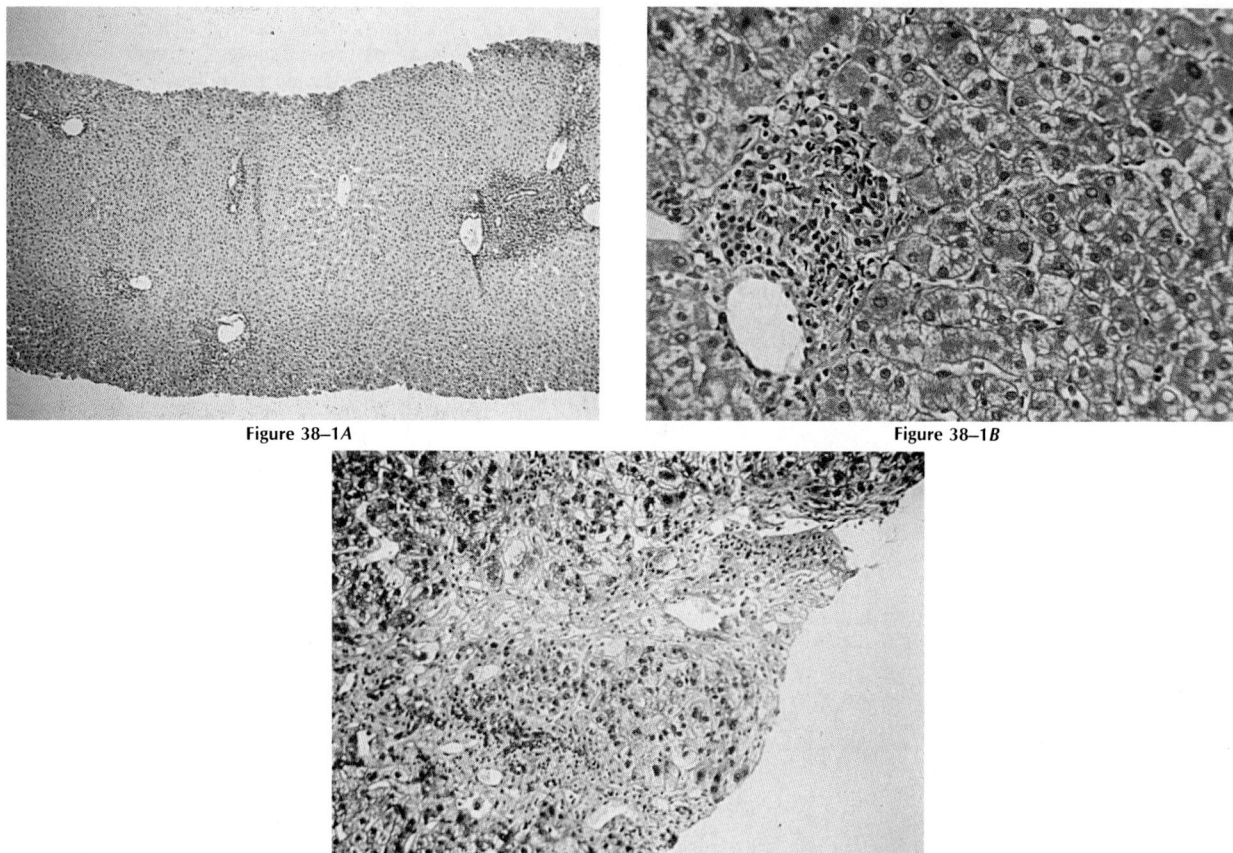

Figure 38–1A   Figure 38–1B

Figure 38–5

Figure 38–1. Chronic persistent hepatitis. *A,* Inflammatory infiltrate of portal tracts. Absence of periportal piecemeal necrosis and no evidence of fibrosis. H&E × 16. *B,* Portal inflammation with minimal disruption of limiting plate. H&E × 100.

Figure 38–5. Chronic active hepatitis with bridging hepatic necrosis. Masson trichrome × 100.

sis, in order to determine if treatment is warranted. To distinguish between the lesions of bridging hepatic necrosis, multilobular necrosis, and an active postnecrotic cirrhosis may be difficult (or impossible). The presence of well-developed regenerative nodules and inflammatory septae, which contain elastin, are evidence that cirrhosis has developed.

More recently, there has been a shift in emphasis from changes occurring in and around the portal triad to inflammatory changes occurring within the hepatic lobule.[36, 37] Popper has suggested that lobular necrosis may be the major determinant as to whether a patient with chronic hepatitis will develop cirrhosis, especially patients with chronic hepatitis caused by hepatitis B and non-A, non-B hepatitis.[36] Many patients with non-A, non-B hepatitis have a combination of periportal expansion and lobular inflammation.[9]

CLINICAL FEATURES OF CHRONIC HEPATITIS

The spectrum of clinical features of chronic hepatitis ranges from asymptomatic disease detected during evaluation of biochemical abnormalities found on a routine screen

to a rapidly deteriorating illness characterized by weakness, jaundice, bleeding, ascites, and hepatic encephalopathy. The clinical features of liver disease vary for each of the major subgroups of chronic hepatitis and will be discussed separately. Within each category there may be marked discrepancies between clinical evidence of liver disease and the histologic findings, emphasizing the need for liver biopsy in evaluation.

GENERAL PRINCIPLES OF MANAGEMENT AND TREATMENT OF CHRONIC HEPATITIS

The management and treatment of chronic hepatitis depend upon the availability of beneficial therapeutic approaches. Unfortunately, effective specific therapies are not available for the most prevalent forms of chronic liver disease, which result from viral infections. Also, no effective treatment is available for some of the most disabling symptoms of chronic hepatitis—fatigue, malaise, and anorexia,[38] nor are the causes for these symptoms known.

Patients with chronic hepatitis are often depressed and have problems sleeping. Right upper quadrant abdominal pain is frequent and is usually characterized by a dull, aching discomfort that is intermittent and increases late in

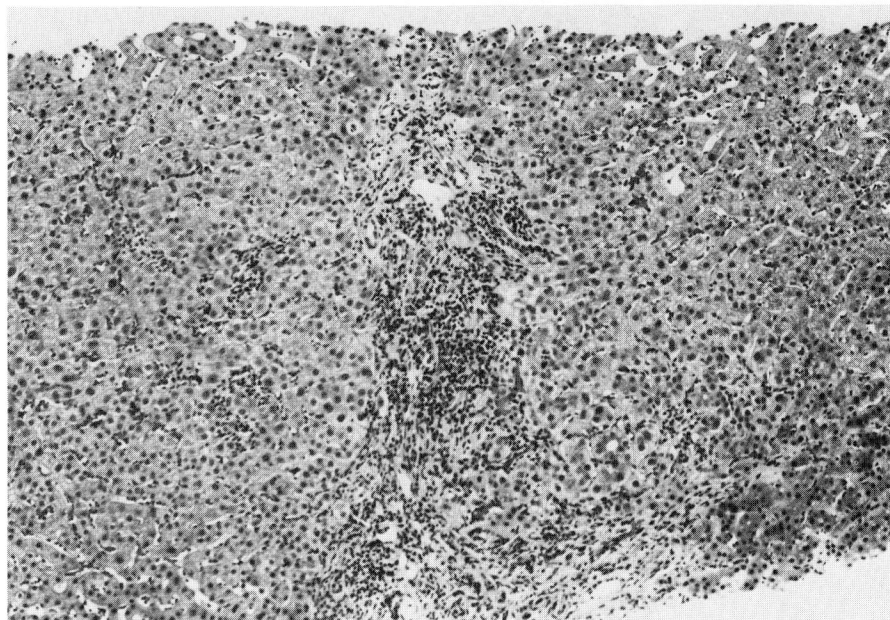

Figure 38–2. Chronic active hepatitis of mild to moderate severity with portal and periportal inflammation. Trapping of periportal hepatocytes and inflammation extending beyond portal tract. Focal lobular inflammation is also evident. H&E × 200.

the day or after strenuous activity. There is often little correlation between the level of symptoms and the biochemical and histologic evidence of disease. None of the usual medications for pain such as acetaminophen or nonsteroidal anti-inflammatory drugs (NSAIDs) are consistently effective.

Supportive care by the physician should include, insofar as possible, a hopeful prognosis with an emphasis on patient education about chronic hepatitis. Questions from patients regarding diet are frequent, and the range of unusual diets patients try, with an emphasis on "health foods" and supplemental vitamins, is remarkable. Some patients complain of afternoon nausea and anorexia. A rearrangement of meals to include a larger breakfast and lighter dinner may prove helpful in patients with anorexia. If fluid retention is a problem, salt restriction is necessary.

When symptoms include depression, decreased performance, or day-night reversal as an early manifestation of hepatic encephalopathy, lowering the protein in the diet with emphasis on vegetable protein and use of lactulose is warranted in a clinical trial to see whether improvement occurs. Beyond restriction of salt and protein, when these are specifically indicated, no other dietary changes have been of proven benefit. There is no evidence that lowering intake of fat or increasing protein to extraordinarily high levels affects the course of the liver disease. There also is no indication that supplemental vitamins are beneficial, although the concept of vitamin supplementation is so firmly entrenched that it is often better to suggest a specific multivitamin than to allow the patient to become involved in a potentially harmful megavitamin program. Excessive use of vitamin A in particular may lead to liver damage

Figure 38–3. Chronic active hepatitis. Extensive disruption of limiting plate of the portal tract and portal and periportal inflammation. H&E × 300.

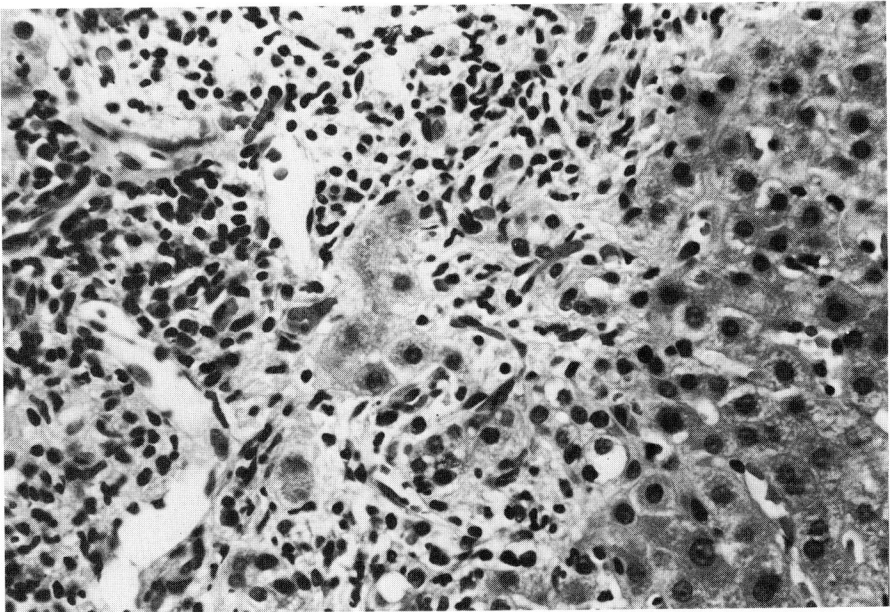

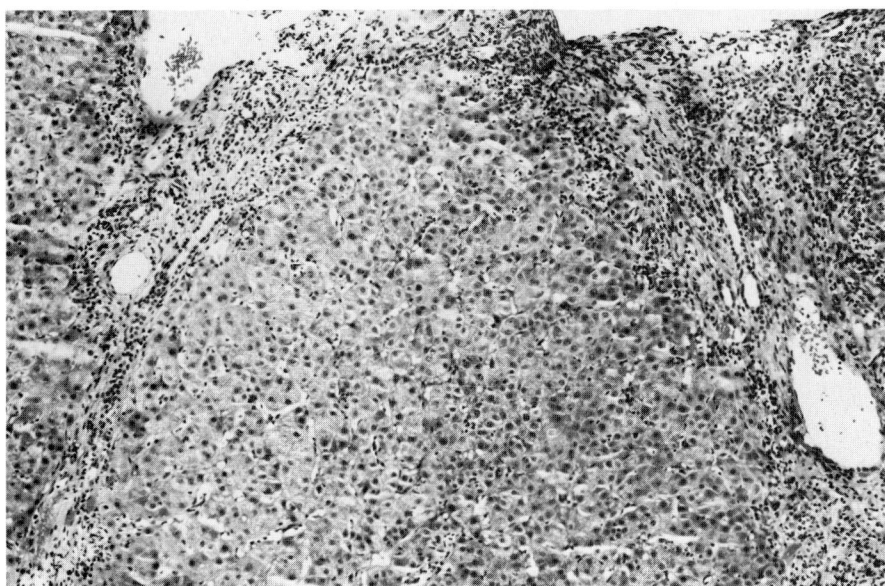

Figure 38–4. Chronic active hepatitis with bridging hepatic necrosis. Minimal lobular inflammation. H&E × 100.

and should be avoided. Patients who are deeply jaundiced and have considerable cholestasis and malabsorption may benefit from receiving supplements of vitamins A, D, and K, with appropriate biochemical monitoring of levels. When symptoms include malabsorption and weight loss, addition of medium-chain triglycerides to the diet may help maintain the patient's weight.

The question of whether alcohol ingestion should be allowed is one of particular concern to many patients. There is no evidence that small amounts (10 to 20 g) of ethanol are harmful in patients with chronic hepatitis. Patients should be advised not to drink large amounts of alcohol, and the physician must be especially vigilant in evaluating alcohol as a contributing factor when there is evidence of exacerbation of liver disease in a depressed patient with chronic hepatitis.

The recommendation of enforced bed rest in patients with liver disease fortunately has been replaced by policies designed to keep patients as active as possible. A regular program of walking or other exercise programs is beneficial to most patients.[39] We recommend exercising to the point of pleasant fatigue. Patients with chronic active hepatitis and cirrhosis should avoid heavy lifting, which leads to a Valsalva maneuver and possible initiation of bleeding from esophageal varices. Use of lower extremity stockings may be helpful in preventing swelling of the feet and lower legs throughout the day.

Patients with liver disease should be advised to exercise care in the use of both over-the-counter and prescription drugs. Aspirin may lead to gastrointestinal irritation. Acetaminophen in usual doses is generally safe, but patients with liver disease may have a decreased hepatic reserve of glutathione and at least the potential for liver damage.[40] There is no evidence that patients with chronic hepatitis cannot take oral contraceptives, but monitoring is advisable to detect any worsening of liver tests related to the use of these drugs. Agents known to have been associated with induction of chronic hepatitis such as methyldopa and nitrofurantoin either should not be used or use should be carefully monitored.[17]

Unless the patient has advanced chronic hepatitis with cirrhosis and portal hypertension, most other therapeutic drugs can be safely administered, at least initially, at the usual dose; however, the physician should be aware that reduction in dosage may be required depending on the response (see Chap. 10). There is no evidence that patients with chronic hepatitis are more likely than patients without liver disease to develop an adverse drug reaction, but any reaction that does occur may be more severe because of decreased hepatic reserve. We make every effort to avoid the use of tranquilizers or any medication to induce sleep. If surgery is needed, there is no reason to avoid the use of halogenated anesthetics since the incidence of halothane-induced liver injury (Chap. 34) is not increased in patients with chronic hepatitis.

ORTHOTOPIC LIVER TRANSPLANTATION IN PATIENTS WITH CHRONIC HEPATITIS

Orthotopic liver transplantation (see Chap. 55) has been performed in patients with cirrhosis caused by all known etiologies of chronic hepatitis. Generally, favorable results have been obtained, and with increasing experience, survival statistics are improving. The indications for liver transplantation are many; these can be summarized as evidence of end-stage, irreversible liver disease for which there is no effective alternative therapy. There should be no contraindications to the operation such as extreme age of the patient or evidence of multi-organ failure. As results improve, orthotopic liver transplantation will most likely be used earlier in the course of the disease (i.e., before severe wasting and other life-threatening manifestations of liver failure occur).

An issue that has been widely considered is whether the original liver disease will return in the liver graft after transplantation, especially in patients with the three most common causes of chronic hepatitis: idiopathic autoimmune CAH, hepatitis B, and non-A, non-B hepatitis. Evidence for a return of liver injury that resembled pre-transplant idiopathic autoimmune CAH has been reported.[41] In most patients with hepatitis B who have had orthotopic liver transplantation, there has been continuation of the hepatitis B infection with evidence of hepatitis in the transplanted liver.[42] Whether antiviral therapy will be effective in immunosuppressed post-transplant patients remains to be proved. Also, whether autoimmune idiopathic CAH will recur late after transplantation will not be established until many more patients have been followed.

Situations in which liver transplantation procedures have been life-saving include transplantation for patients with severe Wilson's disease in whom an episode of fulminant hepatitis has developed in a setting of chronic hepatic injury.[43, 44] In patients with α_1-antitrypsin disease and cirrhosis in the absence of advanced pulmonary disease, liver transplantation may not only cure the liver disease but the α_1-globulin produced by the new liver may protect the lungs from further damage.

In summary, the availability of orthotopic liver transplantation offers hope for large numbers of patients with end-stage liver disease from chronic hepatitis[43, 44] and may allow survival of many who would otherwise die from the liver disease or from complications of therapies (e.g., corticosteroids). The availability of orthotopic liver transplantation has led to reconsideration of the use of portacaval shunts and peritoneojugular shunts, which may make later transplantation difficult or impossible.

CHRONIC PERSISTENT HEPATITIS

DIAGNOSIS

Most instances of chronic persistent hepatitis (CPH) presumably result from viral infection. CPH is unusual in patients with idiopathic autoimmune chronic hepatitis who have not received corticosteroid therapy. The diagnosis of CPH is based on liver biopsy findings of portal inflammation, an intact periportal limiting plate, and occasionally isolated foci of intralobular necrosis, but no evidence of significant periportal inflammation, bridging necrosis, or fibrosis. Often the histologic distinction between CPH and mild CAH is difficult. Sampling error may be a problem, particularly when only a small amount of tissue is obtained, and within one specimen there may be separate areas compatible with CPH and CAH.[12] Attempts to differentiate CPH from asymptomatic or mildly symptomatic CAH by methods other than liver biopsy are not as reliable. For example, wedged hepatic venous pressures (WHVPs) are normal in patients with CPH, but a normal WHVP may occasionally be found in patients with mild CAH.[45] In one study, 22 of 23 patients with CPH had normal WHVPs, whereas 24 of 25 patients with CAH had elevated WHVPs.[45]

In our experience, technetium liver scans have been of no benefit in differentiating CPH from CAH. Three-hour postprandial bile salt determinations have been reported by Jones and associates to be useful in differentiation of CPH from asymptomatic or minimally symptomatic CAH.[45] Elevated levels (see Chap. 25) indicate the presence of CAH; normal levels indicate the presence of CPH when there is evidence of disease. However, there is some overlap of values in patients with CPH and in those with mild CAH. A combination of three-hour postprandial cholylglycine levels, total cholic acid conjugate, and the ALT may accurately differentiate CPH from CAH. In the study by Jones and co-workers, all 16 patients with asymptomatic CAH had cholylglycine levels as high as 200 mg/dL, a three-hour cholic acid level of 170 mg/dL, or an ALT level of 120 IU/L; in contrast, only 3 of 12 patients with CPH reached any of these levels.[46] These tests may be more valuable in following the course of a patient to determine if progression of disease has occurred than in making the initial diagnosis.

The diagnosis of CPH is often made when a liver biopsy is performed to evaluate abnormalities in serum aminotransferases that persist for months following apparent clinical recovery from an episode of acute viral hepatitis; or when a liver biopsy is performed in order to evaluate a patient with persistently elevated aminotransferase levels found initially during a screening examination. The elevations in aminotransferase levels may be trivial or as much as 10 to 15 times normal values. Hepatosplenomegaly is not found in CPH. Biochemical tests other than elevated aminotransferases are usually normal. A decreased serum albumin is almost never found in a patient with CPH. Hyperglobulinemia is not a feature, and the prothrombin time and other hematologic tests are normal.

Patients with CPH usually show no clinical signs of liver injury and are asymptomatic except for occasional instances of persistent fatigue and/or right upper quadrant abdominal pain. Symptoms may develop or increase once a patient is told of the possible presence of chronic liver disease.

ETIOLOGIES

The most frequent proven etiology of CPH is hepatitis B. Many chronic HBsAg carriers who are asymptomatic and who have modest elevations of aminotransferase levels or are only minimally symptomatic show the characteristic histologic changes of CPH on liver biopsy. CPH also may be found in patients with chronic non-A, non-B hepatitis, although in most of these patients, the histologic lesions are more compatible with CAH.[9] CPH is rarely found in patients with untreated idiopathic autoimmune CAH, but may be present in patients with idiopathic autoimmune CAH in whom successful remission has been induced by therapy with corticosteroids or other immunosuppressant agents.[47] In many patients with CPH, no etiology can be found for the liver abnormalities. Often a diagnosis of chronic non-A, non-B hepatitis is made, but at present this diagnosis is often an indication that no diagnosis has been established.

Other conditions to be considered when the histologic lesions characteristic of CPH are encountered include primary biliary cirrhosis, drug reactions from a variety of agents, the portal inflammatory lesion (pericholangitis) associated with inflammatory bowel disease, and portal inflammation secondary to extrahepatic tract disorders such as pancreatitis and choledocholithiasis.

PROGNOSIS

The prognosis of CPH is generally excellent.[48] In a long-term follow-up study of 26 patients with CPH, with an average observation period of 5.6 years, there was no evidence of progression to CAH in any patient.[25]

The prognosis is less favorable when a patient has developed CPH following therapy for idiopathic autoimmune CAH.[47] In these patients, a relapse with reappearance of histologic evidence of CAH may occur when immunosuppressive therapy is tapered or discontinued.

EVALUATION

The diagnosis of CPH is based on biopsy findings of portal inflammation with an intact limiting plate around the portal triad and no evidence of fibrosis. It is important to take a careful history regarding previous drug use (both illicit and therapeutic), sexual preferences and habits, alcohol use, blood transfusions, travel, and any change in bowel habits. The physical examination usually shows no evidence suggesting liver disease. HBsAg, anti-HBs, and anti-HBc determinations are necessary; sigmoidoscopy with biopsy should also be performed if there is any reason to suspect inflammatory bowel disease.

MANAGEMENT

No treatment beyond reassurance that no serious liver problem is present is indicated. There is no role for corticosteroid or immunosuppressant therapy.

CHRONIC LOBULAR HEPATITIS

The category chronic lobular hepatitis (CLH) was added to the histologic classification scheme for chronic hepatitis to define a group of patients with minimal portal inflammation, no piecemeal necrosis or periportal inflammation, and considerable focal lobular inflammation.[6, 49, 50] Most patients with CLH have a viral-induced illness. The histologic pattern often resembles that found in acute viral hepatitis. Bridging hepatic necrosis is not found.

In a series of five patients with CLH, all had an illness that closely resembled a prolonged acute viral hepatitis.[50] All of these patients had hepatomegaly, jaundice, and aminotransferase levels that suggested an acute hepatitis. On repeated liver biopsies of these patients, the changes were indistinguishable from those found in acute viral hepatitis, with spotty necrosis and collections of mononuclear cells throughout the lobule. There was no evidence of progression of CLH to chronic active hepatitis or cirrhosis.

In summary, patients with CLH have much more evidence of acute hepatitis than patients with CPH; however, the widespread acute-appearing lobular changes clearly differentiate CLH from CPH. The lack of progression to cirrhosis distinguishes CLH from CAH.

CHRONIC ACTIVE HEPATITIS

IDIOPATHIC AUTOIMMUNE CHRONIC ACTIVE HEPATITIS

Idiopathic autoimmune chronic active hepatitis (CAH) is a progressive, inflammatory liver disease of unknown etiology lasting at least six months, affecting women more frequently than men, and characteristically associated with abnormalities in immunoregulation.[51–58] Because the disorder is of unknown etiology, it is designated *idiopathic*; the remarkable array of immunologic abnormalities, often including autoantibodies, that usually characterizes this disease led to the designation *autoimmune*. However, in some patients with idiopathic CAH, none of the usual markers of an autoimmune process are found; thus the disorder is often classified as cryptogenic CAH, but it remains uncertain if this separate classification is warranted.[59] There are no absolute guidelines for distinguishing idiopathic autoimmune CAH from non-A, non-B hepatitis or from hepatitis B in which the usual serologic tests are not sufficiently sensitive to detect the virus; therefore, it is likely that further refinement of the syndrome will occur when a marker for one or more of the non-A, non-B hepatitis viruses is available and more sensitive tests for hepatitis B are in widespread use. The possibility that an unrecognized viral agent triggers the onset of idiopathic autoimmune CAH must be considered.

Evidence of persistence of part of the measles virus genome in lymphocytes was detected by molecular biologic techiques in 12 of 18 patients with idiopathic autoimmune CAH suggesting a possible role for measles infection in pathogenesis.[59a]

Idiopathic autoimmune CAH was initially described in 1950 by Waldenstrom.[60] Within several years the clinical and laboratory features of the disorder were well defined.[61–69] Most of the patients included in early series were young women with clinically severe disease characterized by the presence of serum autoantibodies and hyperglobulinemia.

Emphasis on the disordered immunologic aspects of idiopathic autoimmune CAH resulted from recognition in the 1950s and 1960s that idiopathic autoimmune CAH had all the classic markers of an autoimmune process: hyperglobulinemia; circulating autoantibodies; lymphoid infiltration of the liver; association with other presumed autoimmune disorders; and a therapeutic response to corticosteroid therapy.[84]

The recognition of positive LE cell tests in 10 to 15 per cent of patients with idiopathic autoimmune CAH further supported the concept of an autoimmune disorder and led to the designation *lupoid hepatitis*.[70–76] Subsequent investigations have indicated that LE cell–positive patients with idiopathic autoimmune CAH rarely have evidence of an associated classic lupus erythematosus, and the prognosis for the subgroup with LE cells is not different from that for patients without LE cells.[77, 78] It is now accepted that there is no association between idiopathic autoimmune CAH and classic systemic lupus erythematosus.[77–80]

The findings of an increased incidence of HLA B8 and DRw3 in patients with idiopathic autoimmune CAH, as well as an increased incidence of abnormal antibodies in relatives of patients with the syndrome, suggest that genetic predisposition may have a role in promoting the development of the disorder.[81–83]

CLINICAL FEATURES

Women have accounted for approximately 75 per cent of patients with idiopathic autoimmune CAH in large series, with the most frequent ages of onset between 10 and 40 years.[10, 12, 51, 57, 59, 66] In one series of patients with severe idiopathic autoimmune CAH, 72 per cent of 181 were women and the mean age of onset was 40 years.[85] However, the disorder may occur at any age and in both sexes.[51, 57, 64] Postmenopausal women with idiopathic autoimmune CAH are reported to represent a subset of patients with a lower incidence of associated autoimmune diseases and less benefit from corticosteroid therapy while having an increased incidence of complications from therapy when compared to younger patients.[86, 87]

The most characteristic clinical presentation of idiopathic autoimmune CAH is an insidious onset of malaise, anorexia, and fatigue in a young woman.[10, 12, 51, 59, 66] The onset of the illness is gradual in most patients, and in many (probably the great majority) the disease is well established at the time the diagnosis is made. Many patients have minimal symptoms and little physical evidence of liver disease, such as hepatosplenomegaly or jaundice. Other patients present with evidence of considerable liver injury, including severe fatigue, jaundice, hepatomegaly (which may be tender), splenomegaly, bleeding tendency, and ascites. Menstrual abnormalities are frequent, such as delayed onset or complete cessation of menses and irregular menstrual cycles. Gynecomastia may develop in males.[54, 57] Persistent fever may be a prominent feature, as may persistent arthralgias. Acne is often found. Abdominal pain, usually characterized by aching in the right upper quadrant, is present in approximately one third of patients.[52] Jaundice may be absent or barely detectable early in the illness. Spider angiomas are found on initial evaluation in most patients with idiopathic autoimmune CAH. Cutaneous striae may be found under the breasts, over the abdomen, or on the arms and thighs. The patient may have moon facies, a buffalo hump, truncal obesity with peripheral muscle wasting, and bruising prior to the initiation of corticosteroid therapy. Splenomegaly is found in most patients at the time of diagnosis, but ultrasonographic examination may be required to detect an enlarged spleen especially if the patient is obese or has ascites. In some patients, their illness is characterized by prominent hypercholesterolemia, pruritus, and markedly elevated levels of alkaline phosphatase, which may resemble primary biliary cirrhosis.[88–90]

In patients with *advanced* idiopathic autoimmune CAH and cirrhosis, bleeding from esophagogastric varices, ascites, and hepatic encephalopathy may dominate the presentation. However, the majority of patients with idiopathic autoimmune CAH present with only *mild* to *moderate* disease.[91]

In one large series, presentation of idiopathic autoimmune CAH as an acute hepatitis with jaundice was reported in less than one fourth of patients.[52, 66] In this subgroup, the diagnosis of chronic hepatitis may be established only after the patient has been observed to have continuing and often worsening hepatitis over a period of several months. Possibly, an apparent acute hepatitis-like illness represents an episode of activation of a chronic process that had previously been unrecognized. Acute onset for idiopathic autoimmune CAH has been documented in a few instances.[92, 93]

In the late 1960s, the Mayo Clinic established the following criteria for severe idiopathic autoimmune CAH:[12] an AST greater than ten times normal or an AST greater than five times normal plus a doubling of serum globulin levels; and evidence of CAH on liver biopsy in a patient in whom there had been documentation of liver disease for longer than 10 weeks. Cirrhosis should be suspected in a patient with idiopathic autoimmune CAH and thrombocytopenia, ascites, or hepatic encephalopathy.[94] Hypoalbuminemia and hyperglobulinemia are less specific indicators of cirrhosis.

With increased awareness and earlier diagnosis of idiopathic autoimmune CAH, there has been a considerable shift toward recognition of the disorder in asymptomatic or minimally symptomatic patients. The diagnosis is usually established in these patients when a liver biopsy is done as part of evaluating elevated aminotransferase levels, hyperglobulinemia, or both.

LABORATORY MANIFESTATIONS

Serum aminotransferase levels are elevated in almost every patient at the time of diagnosis of idiopathic autoimmune CAH. Occasionally, the levels of these enzymes are similar to those in patients with acute viral hepatitis.[92, 93] In most patients, aminotransferase levels at the time of diagnosis are 2 to 10 times the upper limit of normal. There is no significant correlation, however, between aminotransferase levels and histologic or clinical manifestations of disease.[92] Nevertheless, aminotransferase levels are the best available indicators of active inflammation, and elevations of more than twice normal are reliably associated with active inflammation.[95] The serum bilirubin is usually less than 10 mg/dL at the time of diagnosis; and many patients have normal bilirubin levels. A rising level of bilirubin is an adverse prognostic sign. Prolongation of the prothrombin time and falling serum albumin also are adverse prognostic signs. Alkaline phosphatase levels are usually normal or only slightly increased. Occasionally, a patient presents with a profile of obstructive jaundice with marked increases in alkaline phosphatase levels, suggesting bile duct blockage, primary biliary cirrhosis, or sclerosing cholangitis.[88–90] Serum levels of ceruloplasmin and alpha$_1$-antitrypsin are usually normal or increased. Decreased platelets and white blood cells may result from splenic enlargement. Many patients have a mild, normochromic, normocytic anemia.

Procollagen type III assays have been assessed in patients with idiopathic autoimmune CAH in order to determine possible correlations between hepatocellular inflammation, cirrhosis, and levels of type III procollagen.[96, 97] In a series of 47 patients with idiopathic autoimmune CAH evaluated during a therapeutic trial, mean levels of type III procollagen were elevated to a similar extent in cirrhotic and noncirrhotic patients on entry in the trial.[97] The type III procollagen levels returned to normal in both groups when remission was achieved. The levels did not correlate with histologic grade of inflammation or serum aminotransferase levels during active disease. It was concluded that assays of type III procollagen are useful in distinguishing patients with active disease from those in remission and in following the course of idiopathic autoimmune CAH.

IMMUNOLOGIC FEATURES AND POSSIBLE ROLE IN PATHOGENESIS

Many abnormalities of the immune system are found in patients with idiopathic autoimmune CAH.[98–103] The characteristic hyperglobulinemia is most often a polyclonal increase of IgG.[104] Elevated levels of IgG in serum are found in approximately 90 per cent of patients, with occasional remarkable elevations to greater than 5 g/dL. Hyperglobulinemia sufficient to cause a hyperviscosity syndrome has been observed.[105] Increases in serum IgM and IgA occur with less frequency and are usually found in association with an increased IgG. Increased titers of antibodies to several viral (e.g., measles and rubella) and bacterial (e.g., *Escherichia coli*, bacteroides, and salmonella) agents have been found in patients with idiopathic autoimmune CAH.[106, 107]

A defect in control of B cells by suppressor T cells, which allows uncontrolled production of immunoglobulins, may be important in the production of increased IgG.[108] Synthesis of IgG by mononuclear cells stimulated in vitro by pokeweed mitogen is increased in patients with idiopathic CAH, as compared with decreased synthesis in stimulated mononuclear cells from patients with hepatitis B–related CAH.[109]

Autoantibodies in patients with idiopathic autoimmune CAH include antinuclear antibody (ANA), antibody to double-stranded DNA (anti-ds-DNA), antiribosomal antibody, anti-liver/kidney microsomal antibody, and smooth muscle antibody (SMA).[110-117] Occasionally, antithyroid antibodies are detected.

The ANA found in 50 to 70 per cent of patients with idiopathic autoimmune CAH usually produces the homogeneous immunofluorescent pattern typically seen in patients with systemic lupus erythematosus, which results from reaction of the antibody with a DNA-histone complex.[118] The SMA found in greater than 60 per cent of patients with idiopathic autoimmune CAH is directed against actin.[110, 111, 115, 119, 120]

Antimitochondrial antibody (AMA) is found in 10 to 30 per cent of patients with idiopathic autoimmune CAH.[121] The AMA in idiopathic autoimmune CAH is usually found in low titers (less than 1:40). In a series comparing patients with idiopathic autoimmune CAH who had positive AMA tests with those with the disease who lacked the antibodies, patients with AMA had higher serum levels of alkaline phosphatase and more stainable iron.[121] The response to corticosteroid therapy in patients with idiopathic autoimmune CAH was not affected by the presence (or absence) of AMA. Differentiation of idiopathic autoimmune CAH from primary biliary cirrhosis is rarely a problem. Patients with primary biliary cirrhosis usually have high titers of AMA (greater than 1:160); IgM concentrations greater than 6.0 mg/mL; alkaline phosphatase elevations greater than fourfold; and cholesterol levels greater than 300 mg/dL.[121] If there is doubt as to the differential diagnosis of idiopathic autoimmune CAH and primary biliary cirrhosis, a short course of corticosteroid therapy may be warranted. A response can be expected in patients with idiopathic autoimmune CAH but not in patients with primary biliary cirrhosis.[18]

The detection of anti-ds-DNA has become an important diagnostic test in patients with systemic lupus erythematosus. The presence of these antibodies has been sought in patients with idiopathic autoimmune CAH.[122-124] Anti-ds-DNA was detected using a sensitive ELISA assay in patients with CAH of several etiologies and was not specific for the idiopathic autoimmune variety.[123] Anti-ds-DNA was found in 64 per cent of 99 patients with ANA-positive CAH; in contrast, 46 per cent of patients with CAH were negative for ANA.[123] However, anti-ds-DNA was also detected in 43 per cent of patients with chronic hepatitis B. The mean serum level of anti-ds-DNA was higher in patients who were ANA positive, but the differences in frequency or titer were not significant between the three groups. In five patients followed longitudinally, anti-ds-DNA disappeared when histologic remission was achieved. It was concluded therefore that the appearance of anti-ds-DNA is encountered frequently and is a nonspecific manifestation of hepatic inflammation. It does not otherwise correlate with a specific subtype of CAH as regards clinical manifestations or histologic extent of injury. However, in a study using a different technique, anti-ds-DNA was present in patients with systemic lupus erythematosus and absent in patients with autoimmune CAH.[124] In a third study using the Farr assay for detection, anti-ds-DNA was found in only low levels in patients with idiopathic autoimmune CAH. It was concluded that the antibodies detected were the result of the interaction of antibody to single-stranded DNA (anti-ss-DNA) or other serum components, with single-stranded DNA contaminating double-stranded DNA preparations.[122] The differences in the results from these several investigators remain unexplained and further studies are indicated.

Immune complexes that contain antinuclear antibodies, IgG, and histones, which are detected by the anti-antibody inhibition test, have been reported in patients with idiopathic autoimmune CAH.[125] Immune complexes containing nuclear antigens and IgG were found in six of nine patients with idiopathic autoimmune CAH and were not found in six patients with chronic hepatitis B or in normal controls. A role for immune complexes containing histones and other small nuclear components in the initiation or progression of idiopathic autoimmune CAH hepatitis remains to be established.

In a Mayo Clinic series of 126 patients with severe idiopathic CAH, 15 per cent were LE cell positive, 28 per cent were ANA positive, and 52 per cent were SMA positive (Fig. 38–6).[78] Both a positive LE cell test and ANA were found in 12 per cent; a positive LE cell test, ANA, and SMA were found in 8 per cent. It was noted that 81 per cent of the patients in the series had at least one marker, further emphasizing the frequency with which abnormal antibodies are found in patients with idiopathic CAH.

It has not been established whether there are subgroups within the broad category of idiopathic CAH that can be defined on the basis of specific patterns of autoantibodies and whether such subcategorizations will prove to be important. Several investigators have classified patients with idiopathic chronic active hepatitis into a subcategory of autoimmune CAH hepatitis characterized by the presence of ANA and anti-smooth muscle antibodies and another group who lack these autoantibodies but has anti-liver/kidney microsomal antibodies.[126] Both groups have a marked female predominance, hyperglobulinemia, evidence of autoimmune disease in many first-degree relatives, and a positive response to corticosteroid therapy.

Alterations in the numbers and ratios of OKT4 (helper cells) to OKT8 (suppressor/cytotoxic cells) are found in patients with idiopathic autoimmune CAH; however, there is no generally agreed-upon pattern.[127-130] In addition, impairment of suppressor lymphocyte activity has been demonstrated repeatedly in patients with idiopathic autoimmune CAH as well as in patients with hepatitis B–induced CAH.[108, 131-136] The defect in suppressor cell activity often found in idiopathic autoimmune CAH disappears when remission is induced by corticosteroid therapy.[136] Incubation

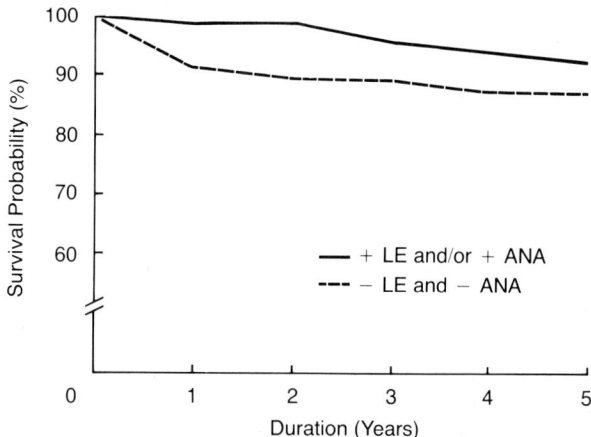

Figure 38–6. Survival of corticosteroid-treated HBsAg-negative patients with and without LE (lupus erythematosus) cell phenomenon or ANA (antinuclear antibody). (Reprinted with permission from Czaja AJ, et al. GASTROENTEROLOGY 85:713. Copyright 1983 by The American Gastroenterological Association.)

of lymphocytes, from patients with idiopathic autoimmune CAH, with prednisolone reversed the impaired suppressor function, whereas lymphocytes from patients with hepatitis B–induced CAH were unaffected, further indicating immunologic differences between the two disorders.[108, 131]

T lymphocytes and plasma cells are the major components of the mononuclear infiltrate in livers of patients with idiopathic autoimmune chronic active hepatitis.[127–130] Analysis of T lymphocyte subtype in the hepatic infiltrate in one study revealed a predominance of OKT4 over OKT8 in portal infiltrates from the majority of patients, whereas in another there was a preponderance of OKT8.[127, 129] The composition of the lymphocytic infiltration in the liver may vary with different stages of the chronic hepatitis, and the relative proportions of T lymphocytes in the liver may be unrelated to those found in the blood.[127]

LIVER-SPECIFIC ANTIGENS

The destruction of hepatocytes in a patient with idiopathic autoimmune CAH appears to result from an attack by lymphocytes on a cell that has had some alteration of the cell membrane. In patients with chronic hepatitis B (discussed later in the chapter), it appears that the hepatocyte membrane is changed by exhibition of HBcAg in conjunction with an HLA Type I glycoprotein. These alterations focus the attack of activated cytotoxic T cells. In idiopathic autoimmune CAH, the factors in the cell membrane that interact with T cells, leading to cell death, are not established, although several candidate alterations have been suggested. In the absence of an established etiology for idiopathic autoimmune CAH, the relation between intracellular events and changes on the hepatocyte membrane remain uncertain.

Considerable efforts have been directed toward identifying a liver-specific antigen that, if exhibited in the hepatocyte membrane, would serve as the target for immunologic reactions and especially for T cell attack. Two liver autoantigens have been identified: liver-specific protein (LSP) and liver membrane antigen (LMAg). Antibodies to both LSP and LMAg have been found in patients with idiopathic autoimmune CAH. The issues are whether LSP or LMAg are actually liver specific (unlikely) and whether there is any value in measuring the titer of antibodies to them (uncertain).

Liver-Specific Protein (LSP)

LSP is a complex material isolated from hepatocytes, which was detected initially through use of an assay for lymphokines in cell-mediated immunity.[137] LSP contains cell membrane and cytoplasmic components. It is not species specific. The material contains protein components as well as lecithin, sphingomyelin, fatty acids, and cholesterol. LSP as prepared by affinity chromatography has not been established to be liver specific.[138–141] Further work will be required to determine whether there is a true liver-specific antigen within the complex. Antibodies to LSP have been found in patients with viral-related and non-viral–related CAH.[142, 143] Anti-LSP antibodies have been found in other conditions, further suggesting a lack of specificity.[135, 144, 145]

Specific T cell populations directed against LSP have been suspected in patients with idiopathic autoimmune

CAH.[135] Incubation of mononuclear cells from the blood of patients with idiopathic autoimmune CAH with LSP led to release of migration inhibition factors in 26 of 29 patients, as compared to release of these factors in only one of 21 patients with hepatitis B–induced CAH and in none of 19 controls. The LSP-induced T cell production of migration inhibition factors was suppressed by co-culturing the T cells from patients with idiopathic autoimmune CAH with T cells from either normal controls or patients with hepatitis B virus–induced CAH. Membrane-bound IgG in idiopathic autoimmune CAH gives a linear fluorescent pattern, as compared to a granular pattern for membrane-bound IgG found in acute and chronic hepatitis B, further suggesting differences between the two disorders.[146]

Repeated injections of LSP into rabbits produced chronic liver injury, which in some progressed to cirrhosis.[147, 148] All animals developing chronic liver injury received injections of two liver-specific proteins, one of cytoplasmic origin and the other derived from hepatocyte membranes. The relevance of these observations to CAH in humans is unknown. No spontaneously occurring animal model resembling idiopathic autoimmune CAH has been identified. The persistence of antibodies to LSP in patients with idiopathic autoimmune CAH in remission induced by immunosuppressive therapy indicates a high likelihood of relapse when treatment is withdrawn.[136] This finding, which may be clinically relevant, needs to be confirmed.

Liver Membrane Antigen (LMAg)

LMAg is a hepatic membrane preparation that appears to have determinants separate from those of LSP.[140] LMAg was identified by immunofluorescence examination of isolated monkey hepatocytes. It has been suggested that LMAg may be a target for autoimmune reactions; however, as is the case with LSP, conclusive evidence is lacking.[103]

Patients with idiopathic autoimmune CAH have also been reported to have circulating T lymphocytes directed against the hepatic membrane asialoglycoprotein receptor.[149–151] The lymphocytes directed towards the asialoglycoprotein receptor are from a T4 subpopulation that includes helper cells as well as lymphocytes that induce T8 suppressor cells.[151] A defect in the subpopulation of T4 cells controlling the expression of T8 suppressor cells may be important in producing the characteristic reduction in T8 suppressor cells found in idiopathic autoimmune CAH.

Despite the lack of conclusive evidence, the findings in patients with idiopathic autoimmune CAH of IgG on the hepatocyte membrane and of antibodies in serum to LSP, LMAg, or the asialoglycoprotein receptor lends support to the concept that hepatocyte-specific antigens exposed by hitherto unidentified causes may be important in initiating or promoting hepatic injury in this group of patients.[142, 143, 146, 152, 153] The wide array of abnormalities of humoral and cellular abnormalities support the theory that immunologic mechanisms are important either in the initiation of idiopathic autoimmune CAH or in its perpetuation.[84] Alternatively, the immunologic abnormalities may be the result of alterations in the hepatocyte and may have little if any significance for pathogenesis.[99–101, 103] There is insufficient evidence to link directly any of the immunologic abnormalities found in patients with idiopathic autoimmune CAH to the pathogenesis of the hepatic injury. Therefore, conclusive evidence is lacking to support an immunologic basis for the *initiation* of injury in idiopathic autoimmune CAH.[100]

The occurrence of similar immunologic abnormalities in patients with drug-induced CAH, and the disappearance of these abnormalities when the drug is removed and the liver injury subsides, suggest that these immunologic abnormalities most likely are the result and not the cause of the liver injury.

On the other hand, it seems that much of the hepatocellular injury in idiopathic autoimmune CAH is related to membrane attack by cytotoxic T cells attracted by exposure of specific antigens on the cell membrane. Less certain is the contribution (if any) to injury from circulating ANA, AMA, SMA or other autoantibodies. The importance remains to be established of various liver- and serum-derived modulators of the immune response, including liver-derived inhibitory protein (LIP), rosette inhibitory factor (RIP), serum inhibitory factors (SIF), and immuno-regulatory low-density lipoproteins (LDL-In).[154–161]

HISTOLOGIC FINDINGS

Percutaneous liver biopsy is required to determine the extent and characteristics of liver damage in patients with idiopathic autoimmune CAH. There may be a patchy distribution to the hepatic injury, with extensively damaged areas adjacent to near normal lobules. In many patients with idiopathic autoimmune CAH, there is histologic evidence of considerably more extensive damage than was suspected from clinical evidence of liver injury. Sampling error leading to underestimation of the extent of disease may be a problem, especially in patients who have cirrhosis and in whom small, fragmented liver biopsies are obtained.[162] Percutaneous liver biopsy leads to reproducible staging of CAH and minimal observer variation in 90 per cent of patients with severe CAH but no cirrhosis.[32, 162] However, if cirrhosis is present, sampling error and observer variability increase markedly, with up to two thirds of liver biopsies not confirming the presence of cirrhosis.[162] Use of laparoscopy-guided biopsy reduces the number of instances of cirrhosis misdiagnosed by blind percutaneous biopsy.

Histologic patterns of CPH and CLH are infrequent in the idiopathic autoimmune variety of chronic hepatitis. Most patients with idiopathic autoimmune CAH have evidence of active periportal (piecemeal) necrosis and/or bridging hepatic necrosis. Many have a pattern of active cirrhosis even when the illness appears clinically to be at an early stage. In a series of 180 patients with severe idiopathic autoimmune CAH from the Mayo Clinic, 29 per cent had hepatocellular necrosis restricted to the portal and periportal areas with disruption of the limiting plate, 19 per cent had bridging necrosis, and 21 per cent had multilobular necrosis.[32, 163]

The inflammatory response in the liver in idiopathic autoimmune CAH consists almost exclusively of lymphocytes and plasma cells. Cellular infiltrates are found in portal areas and throughout the parenchyma. Rosettes of hepatocytes encircled by inflammatory cells may be found, especially around the portal areas, and disruption of the limiting plate encircling the portal tract is usual. Active fibrosis is characteristically present in and around areas of inflammation and cell necrosis. The terms *chronic active hepatitis with bridging hepatic necrosis* and *active cirrhosis* usually connote similar histologic patterns and often differ mainly depending on whether the pathologist has chosen to emphasize the inflammation (chronic active hepatitis) or the fibrosis and nodule formation (cirrhosis).

Specific immunofluorescent stains have demonstrated that the infiltrating plasma cells in idiopathic autoimmune CAH are predominantly producing IgG, as compared to predominant IgM production by plasma cells in patients with primary biliary cirrhosis. Occasionally the histologic pattern found in a patient with idiopathic autoimmune CAH is compatible with an acute hepatitis alone or superimposed on chronic hepatitis.[93, 164]

A numerical scoring system grading the liver biopsy for extent of periportal necrosis, intralobular necrosis, portal inflammation, and fibrosis has been developed in order to evaluate liver biopsies of patients with asymptomatic CAH.[165] Application of such a system in evaluating serial biopsies from patients with asymptomatic or minimally symptomatic idiopathic autoimmune CAH may be useful for evaluation of therapeutic efficacy in trials involving patients whose disease appears to be progressing slowly.

GENETIC PREDISPOSITION

Several lines of evidence indicate a genetic predisposition to the development of idiopathic autoimmune CAH.[83] In several series from around the world, an increased incidence of HLA-B8 and DRw3 has been reported in patients with idiopathic autoimmune CAH.[83, 93, 166–173] The strongest association is with HLA-B8, which is found in 62 to 79 per cent of patients with idiopathic autoimmune CAH, as compared to approximately 25 per cent in control individuals.[174] An association with HLA-DRw3 also was established; in one series, 68 per cent of patients with idiopathic autoimmune CAH had DRw3, compared to 24 per cent in controls.[172, 175] The DRw3 gene is considered a marker of susceptibility to autoimmunity, and the combination of DRw3 and HLA-B8 is found in association with many autoimmune disorders, including idiopathic autoimmune CAH.[82, 176]

It has been suggested that patients with HLA-B8/DRw3 may represent a specific subgroup within the category of idiopathic autoimmune CAH.[83, 169, 177] Patients with HLA-B8/DRw3 tend to be young women, have evidence of other immunologic abnormalities, and may require longer-term corticosteroid therapy, but the justification for making this group a separate subcategory is not established. An association has been noted between lymphocyte cytotoxicity directed against LSP-coated target cells and the presence of HLA-A1, B8, and DRw3.[178] Furthermore, it has been suggested that genetically determined low levels of C4 may predispose individuals to idiopathic autoimmune CAH.[179]

An increased incidence of autoantibodies and related autoimmune disorders has been reported in families of patients with idiopathic autoimmune CAH, supporting the probability of a genetic predisposition.[81] In one study, 165 relatives of 33 patients with idiopathic autoimmune CAH were tested for the presence of serum autoantibodies, and some abnormality was found in 42 per cent.[81] Abnormally elevated levels of immunoglobulin were found in 47 per cent of relatives; elevated levels of gamma globulin were found in 34 per cent. Three members of the family of one of the 33 patients had idiopathic autoimmune CAH; in another family, two members had the disease. Other autoimmune disorders found in families of patients in this series with idiopathic autoimmune CAH include pernicious anemia, Sjögren's syndrome, diabetes mellitus, thyroiditis, fibrosing alveolitis, autoimmune hemolytic anemia, and myxedema. In another series there was an increased frequency of hypergammaglobulinemia and positive ANA in relatives of patients with idiopathic autoimmune CAH.[68] Additional pedigrees have been extensively documented in which family members of patients with idiopathic autoimmune CAH have evidence of other immune-related diseases.[180-182]

ASSOCIATED DISORDERS

Many disorders with proven or suspected disturbances of immunoregulation (autoimmune disorders) have been found in association with idiopathic autoimmune CAH (see Table 38-3).[183-185] In a large series of patients with idiopathic autoimmune CAH, 63 per cent had evidence of involvement of at least one additional organ system.[183] Keratoconjunctivitis sicca (Sjögren's syndrome) was found in 35 per cent and renal tubular acidosis in 24 per cent. In addition, 10 per cent of these patients had peripheral neuropathy. Other disorders recognized included pulmonary diffusion defects, myopathy, arthropathy, skin disorders, and thyroiditis.[183] Idiopathic autoimmune CAH has also been reported in patients with mixed connective tissue syndrome.[186] In a series of 126 patients from the Mayo Clinic, an associated presumed autoimmune disorder was found in 17 per cent.[78] Thyroiditis was found in 7 per cent, ulcerative colitis in 4 per cent, and rheumatoid arthritis in 2 per cent, in addition to a variety of other disorders. Occasionally, the diagnosis of idiopathic autoimmune CAH is made following careful evaluation of a patient who presents with manifestations of another presumed immune related disorder.

The incidence of associated immunopathic disorders is similar for patients with and without autoimmune features, raising the question whether the disorder should be subdivided based on the presence of autoimmune features.[59] The presence of a concomitant autoimmune disorder in a patient with idiopathic autoimmune CAH does not appear to affect response to treatment.[78]

Uveitis. Rare instances of uveitis occurring in association with idiopathic autoimmune CAH have been reported.[187]

Thyroiditis. Hashimoto's thyroiditis has been reported in patients with idiopathic CAH.[59, 66, 183] CAH has been reported in two patients who had Graves's disease with hyperglobulinemia and a wide variety of abnormal antibodies.[188] Both patients had increased IgG levels and one had a monoclonal gammopathy that disappeared with corticosteroid therapy. The other patient had exophthalmos and high circulating levels of long-acting thyroid stimulator (LATS) as well as high antibody titers to several viruses.

Polyarthritis. Recurrent migratory polyarthritis with no evidence of joint deformity has been found in patients with idiopathic autoimmune CAH.[189]

Capillaritis. An allergic capillaritis characterized by active inflammatory papules with central crusting, which gradually progresses to pale depressed scars, has been reported in patients with idiopathic autoimmune CAH.[190]

Glomerulonephritis. Immune complexes containing small nuclear ribonucleoproteins and IgG were found in kidney eluates from two patients with idiopathic autoimmune CAH and membranous glomerulonephritis.[59, 125, 191] Another patient with CAH had selective IgA deficiency, focal glomerulonephritis, hemolytic anemia, and thrombocytopenic purpura.[192]

Ulcerative Colitis. Chronic ulcerative colitis has been reported in patients with idiopathic autoimmune CAH.[81, 193] In patients with evidence of chronic ulcerative colitis and liver disease, special attention must be directed to exclude pericholangitis or sclerosing cholangitis, which may closely resemble idiopathic autoimmune CAH (see Chap. 43).

Polymyositis. Rare instances of polymyositis and idiopathic autoimmune CAH have been reported.[194] In one patient, both the polymyositis and hepatitis responded to therapy with prednisolone and azathioprine.

Autoimmune Hemolytic Anemia. In a few instances, Coombs's positive autoimmune hemolytic anemia has been described in association with idiopathic autoimmune CAH.[66, 93, 195] A patient with a multisystemic disease including Coombs's positive hemolytic anemia, antiplatelet and anti-factor X antibodies has been reported.[196]

Lichen Planus. Several patients have been reported with lichen planus and idiopathic autoimmune CAH.[197] In one series of 44 patients with lichen planus evaluated in a dermatology clinic, five (11.3 per cent) were found to have histologic evidence of CAH.[197]

Monoclonal Gammopathy. Most often the hyperglobulinemia associated with idiopathic autoimmune CAH is polyclonal in nature, with the major increase in IgG. Occasionally, a monoclonal gammopathy has been observed.[198]

Hyperviscosity Syndrome. The hyperglobulinemia associated with idiopathic autoimmune CAH may be so severe as to cause signs and symptoms of a hyperviscosity state and resemble Waldenstrom's macroglobulinemia.[105, 199]

Pulmonary Disorders. Several types of pulmonary disorders including chronic fibrosing alveolitis and primary pulmonary hypertension have been described in patients with idiopathic autoimmune chronic active hepatitis.[59, 200] In one patient the constellation of fibrosing alveolitis, autoimmune hemolytic anemia and idiopathic autoimmune CAH was found.[201]

DIAGNOSIS

The diagnosis of idiopathic autoimmune CAH in the absence of a known etiology is one of exclusion. The basis for establishing the diagnosis depends on identification of compatible histologic findings in a patient with hyperglobulinemia and, often, positive ANA and SMA tests in whom there are no viral markers for hepatitis B. Additional important factors in establishing the diagnosis are absence of evidence of use of illicit drugs or therapeutic agents known to cause liver injury (such as methyldopa or nitrofurantoin), no history of transfusions or homosexual activity, and no evidence suggesting Wilson's disease or alpha-1 antitrypsin deficiency.

TREATMENT

Corticosteroid Therapy

The course of untreated idiopathic autoimmune CAH before the introduction of corticosteroid therapy was variable and unpredictable but usually one of progressive deterioration.[10-12] In some patients there were recurrent episodes of active hepatitis superimposed on a background of CAH. The occurrence of episodes of disease exacerbation is unpredictable, but fortunately, they are seen less frequently now that corticosteroid therapy is used almost universally. An occasional untreated patient enters a phase of spontaneous remission.[12]

The goals of therapy in idiopathic CAH are to decrease

mortality, diminish inflammation, and prevent the progression of the chronic hepatitis to cirrhosis. No regimen has achieved all these objectives. The value of corticosteroid therapy, with or without the addition of azathioprine, has been established for the patient with severe idiopathic autoimmune CAH in whom there is evidence of symptomatic disease associated with marked elevation of aminotransferases and hyperglobulinemia.[12, 202, 203] There is no question that patients with clinical and histologic evidence of severe idiopathic CAH and bridging hepatic necrosis should be treated with immunosuppressive therapy. The therapeutic decision for these patients is whether to use a corticosteroid alone or in combination with azathioprine. However, it must be recognized that benefits from therapy are established only for patients with well-defined, symptomatic severe chronic hepatitis characterized by considerable elevation of aminotransferase levels. There have been no controlled treatment trials demonstrating efficacy of therapy in the majority of patients with CAH in whom less severe illness is present.[91, 204, 205]

In general, immunosuppressant therapy is not used in asymptomatic or minimally symptomatic patients with evidence of only periportal piecemeal necrosis on liver biopsy. It is uncertain how frequently patients with histologically mild disease go on to develop more severe hepatitis or cirrhosis.[29] The risks of the side effects of the corticosteroid and azathioprine therapy must be considered in relation to possible therapeutic benefit. It is difficult to decide if and how to treat a patient with mild symptoms, moderate increases in aminotransferase levels, minimal or absent hyperglobulinemia, and bridging or multilobular necrosis on liver biopsy. In these borderline therapeutic situations, I have often used a three-month trial of corticosteroid therapy with a planned follow-up liver biopsy in order to make a decision regarding further therapy based on assessment of the post-treatment clinical status, the effects of therapy on aminotransferase levels, and histologic findings. It is even more uncertain whether corticosteroid therapy should be used in patients with mild symptoms or low levels of hepatic inflammation as assessed by determination of aminotransferase levels or in patients who have mild disease as evidenced by histologic findings of only periportal piecemeal necrosis, and most clinicians do not administer corticosteroids to such patients.

Evidence supporting the use of corticosteroid therapy in patients with severe idiopathic autoimmune CAH was derived from three prospective clinical trials reported in the early 1970s.[10-12, 206] These studies differed somewhat in entry criteria, corticosteroid dosage, methods of follow-up, and evaluation.[206] However, in general, patients with symptomatic severe disease were studied. The Mayo Clinic series evaluated patients who met pre-set standards to define severity, which included documentation of disease for at least ten weeks with an AST greater than 10 times normal or an AST greater than 5 times normal with a twofold elevation of serum globulin, and liver biopsy findings of CAH.[12, 207] Patients were excluded if there was evidence of hepatic encephalopathy, chronic alcoholism, alcoholic liver disease, or malignancy. Tests for HBsAg were not available when the three major therapeutic studies were performed. However, the trials were all performed in areas of the world with a low incidence of hepatitis B, and subsequent investigations have confirmed that few patients with hepatitis B were included. Detailed re-analysis, especially of the Mayo Clinic series, has not altered the initial conclusions of a benefit from corticosteroid therapy.[163] There was a decrease in mortality and morbidity associated with the use

of corticosteroids in all three trials. In the Mayo Clinic series there was a 30 per cent mortality in patients receiving placebo or azathioprine alone, compared with only 6 per cent in the groups receiving corticosteroid therapy.[12]

Patients generally feel better soon after initiation of corticosteroid therapy, with improved appetite, decreased fatigue, and reduction in arthralgias. Biochemical effects of corticosteroid therapy include decreases in serum bilirubin, aminotransferase and globulins and an increase in serum albumin. In some patients, corticosteroid treatment is associated with a loss of LE cells; these may return if the patient has a subsequent exacerbation of hepatitis.[12] It has not been established that corticosteroid therapy retards progression toward cirrhosis in patients with idiopathic autoimmune CAH, although there is generally a considerable decrease in hepatic inflammation (Fig. 38–7).[35]

The favorable effects on mortality induced by corticosteroid therapy are evident within the first several months to one year of therapy, and the benefits are sustained for many years (Fig. 38–8).[10, 208] In a follow-up study, of at least 10 years or until death, of 44 patients who participated in the initial Royal Free Hospital trial 63 per cent of treated patients were alive at 10 years, compared with only 27 per cent in the control group.[208] The median survival was 12.2 years in the treated group and 3.3 years in the control group. The conclusion was that corticosteroid therapy improves survival by reducing mortality early in the active phase of the hepatitis.

Many features of idiopathic autoimmune CAH have been evaluated for possible effects on the outcome of treatment (Table 38–4). However, these features are only relative indicators of treatment response. A trial of immunosuppressant therapy is warranted in all patients with evidence of severe idiopathic autoimmune CAH.

The treatment used in the Mayo Clinic trial included prednisone alone, prednisone in low dosage combined with azathioprine, azathioprine alone, and placebo. Approximately 25 per cent of patients receiving placebo or azathioprine alone achieved remission; thus, azathioprine alone was no better than placebo. The regimens with prednisone gave significantly better results.[12, 162, 207] The prednisone dosage regimen was 60 mg daily for one week, 40 mg daily for one week, 30 mg daily for two weeks, and then 20 mg

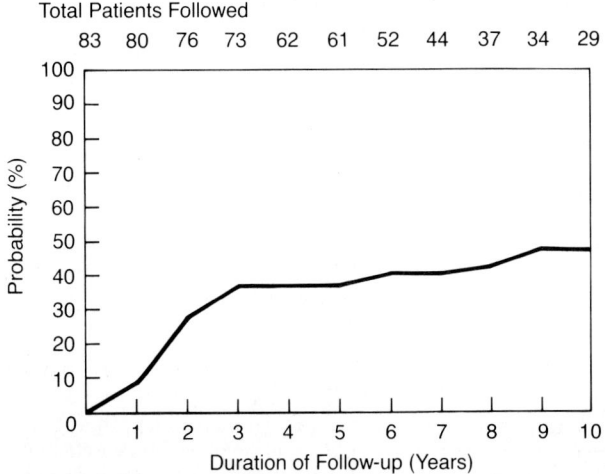

Figure 38–7. Probability of developing histologic manifestations of cirrhosis after diagnosis of chronic active hepatitis and institution of corticosteroid therapy. (Reprinted from Davis GL, Czaja AJ. In: Czaja AJ, Dickson ER, eds. Chronic Hepatitis: The Mayo Clinic Experience, p. 9 by courtesy of Marcel Dekker, Inc.)

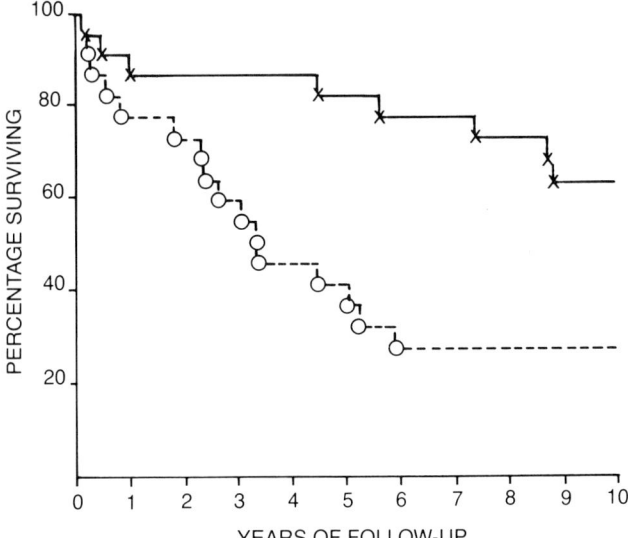

Figure 38–8. Life table survival curves of control and prednisolone-treated patients. o — o = controls; x — x = prednisolone. (Reproduced from Kirk AP, et al. Gut 21:78, 1980, with permission.)

daily as a maintenance dose. Patients on the regimen of lower doses of prednisone together with azathioprine received prednisone in doses of 30 mg daily for one week, 20 mg daily for one week, and 15 mg daily for two weeks, followed by a maintenance dose of 10 mg daily; the dose of azathioprine was 50 mg daily throughout.

An analysis by the Mayo Clinic of patients with severe disease and no evidence of hepatitis B clearly demonstrated the benefits of therapy with prednisone alone or prednisone plus azathioprine.[163] The patients were divided into four treatment groups. Twenty-four of the 28 patients receiving prednisone alone achieved remission, which was defined as resolution of clinical symptoms, AST less than twice normal, all other biochemical tests of the liver normal, and a liver biopsy that was normal or showed only CPH. The mean interval of therapy required to induce remission was 30.1 ± 5.9 months. Twenty-six of 29 patients treated with the combination of prednisone and azathioprine achieved remission, with a mean treatment interval of 21.9 ± 2.5 months. Seventeen of 28 patients treated with doses of prednisone that were gradually titrated and given on alternate days achieved remission. Only 6 of 14 patients in the control group entered a phase of remission. The results in patients receiving azathioprine alone did not differ from those found in the control group.

Long-term alternate-day treatment with prednisone also was evaluated. After an initial three months of daily treatment, 10 mg of prednisone was given every other day.[207] The dose was increased every two weeks, as necessary to stabilize biochemical tests. This regimen appeared less effective than daily prednisone or combination therapy.

TABLE 38–4. CORTICOSTEROID THERAPY IN IDIOPATHIC AUTOIMMUNE CHRONIC ACTIVE HEPATITIS

Appropriate	Uncertain	Inappropriate
Symptomatic	Portal	Asymptomatic
Premenopausal	expansion,	Postmenopausal
Bridging necrosis	piecemeal	Cirrhotic
Precirrhotic	necrosis	
Hyperglobulinemia		

A regimen of alternate-day corticosteroid and daily azathioprine therapy has not been studied. Oral pulse therapy of high-dose prednisone given in repeated three- to five-day courses at intervals of three to four weeks has been proposed but has not been employed in a large trial.[209]

Both prednisone and prednisolone have been used in the treatment of idiopathic autoimmune CAH. No differences in outcome were observed when prednisolone was used, although prednisone must undergo 11-oxo reduction by the liver to become the active corticosteroid prednisolone.[210-211] I prefer to use prednisolone.

In the absence of controlled trials to justify treatment in patients who are asymptomatic or have evidence of only mild disease, the clinician must depend on anecdotal experience.[91, 204, 205] My approach is not to use corticosteroid therapy if the patient has few or no symptoms. In the infrequently encountered patient with few symptoms but with aminotransferase levels five to ten times normal and evidence of bridging hepatic necrosis on liver biopsy, I have utilized a three- to six-month trial of moderate-dose therapy, beginning with 20 to 40 mg daily of prednisolone. A decision regarding continuation of therapy is based on the results of sequential improvement in laboratory studies (especially aminotransferase levels) and comparison of pretreatment liver biopsy with findings on follow-up biopsy.

A gradual reduction in dosage should follow initial therapy, depending on clinical improvement and decreased aminotransferase levels. No firm guidelines are available to determine when to begin tapering of the corticosteroid dosage or how much each reduction should be. My approach is to continue the initial daily dose (20 to 40 mg) for four to six weeks, followed by a gradual reduction of 5 mg every two weeks, so long as aminotransferase levels are decreasing and the patient is improving clinically.

In a Mayo Clinic trial, the presence or absence of autoimmune features (autoimmune versus cryptogenic) did not affect initial treatment response.[78] The five-year survival in patients with CAH characterized by autoimmune features was 93 per cent; in those whose disease had no autoimmune features, it was 87 per cent.

In an analysis of patients with CAH from King's College Hospital, 106 of 204 patients had autoimmune CAH; the disease of 69 patients was designated as cryptogenic, based on the absence of autoimmune markers or of a known etiology.[159] Those in the autoimmune group had a better prognosis (five-year survival on therapy of 87 per cent) than those in the cryptogenic group (65 per cent) (Fig. 38–9). The differences in survival were attributed to a higher incidence of cirrhosis at the time of diagnosis in the cryptogenic group than in those with autoimmune CAH (53 per cent and 38 per cent, respectively).

Complications

Major complications of corticosteroid therapy in patients with CAH include weight gain, hypertension, cataracts, diabetes mellitus, skeletal collapse, acne, and infections.[214, 215] Most complications develop within a year after beginning therapy. However, there are associations between the development of severe complications, such as bone disease, with duration of therapy and the dose of corticosteroid. Thrombocytopenia is the only significant side effect observed with azathioprine and is rarely seen with a dose of 50 to 75 mg daily.

Corticosteroid-induced side effects are usually mild and manageable if the prednisolone dosage is 15 mg daily

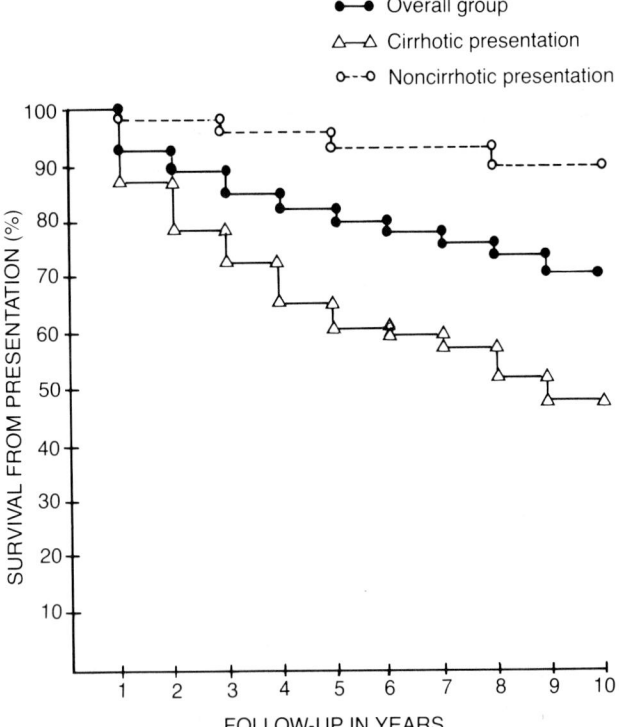

Figure 38–9. Comparison of survival rates of 204 patients with chronic active hepatitis presenting with and without cirrhosis. (Reproduced from Keating JJ, et al. Q J Med 237:58, 1987, with permission.)

or less. If side effects develop in a patient receiving corticosteroids as a single therapy, azathioprine (50 mg daily) may be added to the regimen and the pace of corticosteroid reduction accelerated. Azathioprine should be considered only as an adjunctive, corticosteroid-sparing agent for treating this disease.[12]

Results

Analysis of treatment results indicates that long-term immunosuppressant therapy may be required to induce remission in patients with idiopathic autoimmune CAH.[47, 212, 213] Outcomes are similar for men and women. For patients without cirrhosis or signs of hepatic failure at presentation in the Mayo Clinic series, survival was 98 per cent at ten years; for patients with cirrhosis at the time of diagnosis, survival was 80 per cent at five years and 65 per cent at ten years (Fig. 38–10).

Treatment should be discontinued once remission is achieved and liver biopsy shows no abnormalities or only evidence of CPH. However, in the Mayo Clinic series, only 24 of 52 patients with severe disease could be completely removed from corticosteroid therapy without relapse.[47] In 8 of 27 patients whose disease was in remission as a result of treatment with combined prednisolone and azathioprine therapy, relapse occurred within three years; however, relapse occurred in only 1 of 23 patients who continued combination therapy.[216]

In a long-term follow-up study of 66 patients with severe CAH who were withdrawn from corticosteroid therapy following induction of remission, 24 sustained remission for at least five years, and 42 (64 per cent) suffered a relapse and required re-treatment.[217] Factors associated with sustained remission included (1) a somewhat shorter dura-

tion of illness before therapy was begun and (2) more rapid improvement in laboratory test results during therapy. Patients had more side effects from therapy if re-treatment was required, although relapse apparently did not affect long-term prognosis. Possibly the use of tests to detect the presence of anti-LSP antibodies when planning withdrawal of treatment will identify patients who should be continued on corticosteroid therapy indefinitely.[136]

Follow-up liver biopsies are most helpful in following the long-term course of CAH during and following cessation of therapy. Many serious therapeutic exacerbations of hepatitis have resulted from premature reduction or discontinuation of corticosteroid therapy, with a resultant flare in hepatitis.[212, 213, 220] It also is important to recognize that long-term, even lifelong, immunosuppressive therapy may be required. It is important in regard to combined treatment with steroids and azathioprine that there is no evidence for an increased frequency of lymphoma or other malignancies after long-term use of azathioprine. This finding is in contrast to what has been found in renal transplant recipients receiving azathioprine.[218, 219]

Other Therapeutic Approaches

Cyclosporine therapy has been reported to be effective in treating a patient with idiopathic autoimmune CAH whose disease had become unresponsive to corticosteroid therapy and in whom drug sensitivity prevented the use of azathioprine.[221] However, no controlled trials of the use of cyclosporine in patients with idiopathic autoimmune CAH have been reported.

Thymic hormone extract, which has been shown to stimulate human suppressor T cell activity and inhibit immunoglobulin production, has been used in therapy of idiopathic autoimmune CAH.[222–224] In a preliminary study in patients with idiopathic autoimmune CAH, thymic hormone extract has no apparent effect on the clinical course of the chronic hepatitis or on the reoccurrence of the suppressor T defect following withdrawal of corticosteroid and azathioprine therapy.[224] A flavanoid substance, [+]-cyanidanol-3, which is a free radical scavenger and inhibitor of lipid peroxidation, was administered in a double-blind controlled trial in patients with CAH.[225] Patients

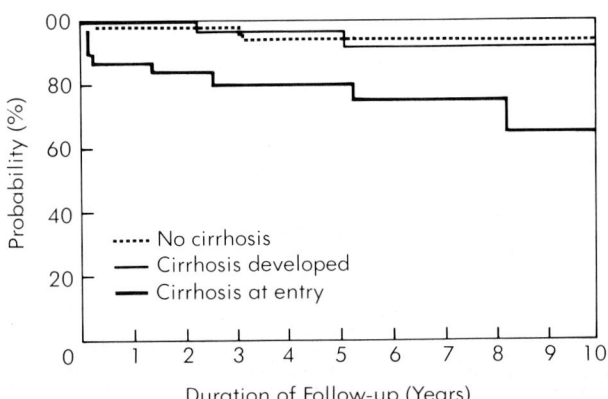

Figure 38–10. Probability of survival of patients with corticosteroid-treated severe idiopathic chronic active hepatitis with and without cirrhosis. (Reproduced from Davis GL, Czaja AJ. In: Czaja AJ, Dickson ER, eds. Chronic Active Hepatitis: The Mayo Clinic Experience. New York, Marcel Dekker, 1986, with permission.)

receiving [+]-cyanidanol fared no better than those receiving placebo and there has been little interest in further use of the drug. In addition, there is scant support for the use of D-penicillamine in the treatment of idiopathic autoimmune CAH.[226]

PREGNANCY IN PATIENTS WITH IDIOPATHIC AUTOIMMUNE CAH

Patients with idiopathic autoimmune CAH often have concerns regarding the ability to conceive, the effects of the liver disease on the pregnancy, and conversely the effects of the pregnancy on the liver disease. These patients may conceive and have a normal pregnancy and delivery (see Chap. 54).[227, 228] However, these patients often have amenorrhea or oligomenorrhea and fertility is reduced.

In an Australian series of 30 pregnancies in 16 patients with idiopathic autoimmune CAH, there was an increase in the incidence of prematurity (30 per cent), delivery by cesarean section (26 per cent), and perinatal mortality. Spontaneous abortion occurred in 10 per cent, which was not considered to be increased. Therefore, it appears that the patient with idiopathic autoimmune CAH has decreased fertility and an increased tendency to a stormy pregnancy with increased fetal loss and premature birth. Fortunately, pregnancy does not seem to cause major problems for the mother as regards the activity of the liver disease. Only 2 of 16 patients in the Australian series had an exacerbation of their liver disease during pregnancy; both responded to increased doses of corticosteroids.

A teratogenic effect of azathioprine has not been documented, although it would appear prudent to discontinue azathioprine in patients with idiopathic autoimmune CAH who wish to become pregnant. No evidence is available to warrant termination of pregnancy in a patient with idiopathic autoimmune CAH solely because the patient is receiving azathioprine. In fact, it is recommended that corticosteroid and azathioprine therapy be continued throughout the pregnancy. In the Australian series there were no maternal deaths related to the pregnancy, although more urinary tract infections (20 per cent) and postpartum hemorrhages (17 per cent) were found.[228] The increased plasma volume found in the third trimester of pregnancy may promote bleeding from esophagogastric varices in a patient who has idiopathic autoimmune CAH and cirrhosis.

LIVER TRANSPLANTATION IN PATIENTS WITH IDIOPATHIC AUTOIMMUNE CAH

Patients with idiopathic autoimmune CAH who develop advanced cirrhosis with life-threatening complications of portal hypertension, such as bleeding from esophageal varices, ascites, severe wasting, recurrent septicemia, and hepatic encephalopathy, are candidates for orthotopic liver transplantation. As results from orthotopic liver transplantation have improved (see Chap. 55), patients with idiopathic autoimmune CAH and cirrhosis are receiving transplants before multiple severe complications develop. In one patient, apparent recurrence of idiopathic autoimmune CAH developed in the liver graft.[41] Additional long-term studies will be required to determine whether there will be a recurrence of the idiopathic autoimmune CAH in the liver graft.

HEPATOCELLULAR CARCINOMA

Hepatocellular carcinoma is much less frequent in patients with idiopathic autoimmune CAH than in patients with chronic hepatitis B; however, occasionally tumors have been reported.[59, 229, 230]

CHRONIC HEPATITIS B

Chronic infection with hepatitis B is the most frequent cause of chronic hepatitis throughout the world and results from an inadequate immunologic response of the host to hepatocytes containing hepatitis B virus.[58, 231] In most patients with chronic hepatitis B, the clinical disease is mild and histologic changes are best categorized as either nonspecific changes, CPH, or CLH. The availability of serologic tests initially for HBsAg and subsequently for detection of other components of hepatitis B virus has allowed evaluation of the importance of hepatitis B in chronic hepatitis.[232]

Wide geographic variations in the frequency of hepatitis B infection and the resultant chronic hepatitis B are well recognized. In Asia and Africa, chronic hepatitis B accounts for the great majority of cases of chronic hepatitis. In Western Europe and the United States, hepatitis B infection is less prevalent and therefore the contribution of hepatitis B to the incidence of chronic hepatitis is less. Published reports from liver centers in Western countries as to the frequency of hepatitis B–related chronic hepatitis may be misleading regarding prevalence in the general population, with overrepresentation of groups with high hepatitis B carrier rates (i.e., male homosexuals, drug abusers, and several immigrant populations).

HISTORY

In follow-up studies of patients who acquired hepatitis during epidemics before and during World War II, some individuals developed severe injury and cirrhosis.[58, 233, 234] From 2 to 10 per cent of adults who acquire acute hepatitis B have some evidence of long-term sequelae, with 1 to 3 per cent developing chronic active hepatitis.[7, 8] Patient populations with a 10 per cent incidence of chronicity following acute hepatitis B included many individuals with underlying risk factors for developing chronic hepatitis B, such as male homosexuality or a history of drug abuse.[7] The risk of developing chronic disease in an adult population not drawn from high-risk groups is probably much lower than 10 per cent.[235, 236]

In follow-up of long-term survivors following injection of a contaminated lot of yellow-fever vaccine in 1942, Seeff and colleagues convincingly demonstrated that the epidemic, which affected more than 300,000 American soldiers, was from hepatitis B.[236] Ninety-seven per cent of 221 former soldiers who had developed jaundice following administration of the vaccine were positive for antibodies to hepatitis B, compared with 76 per cent of 171 soldiers who received the vaccine and did not become jaundiced. Only 13.1 per cent of 205 control soldiers who received another vaccine not implicated in the epidemic had antibodies to hepatitis B. Of particular note is that only 0.26 per cent of the recipients of contaminated vaccine were later found to be HBsAg positive, implying a very low hepatitis B carrier rate following the epidemic. These investigators suggest the risk of becoming a hepatitis B carrier is much lower in previously healthy young adults who acquire acute hepatitis B than in individuals from high risk groups such as male homosexuals, drug abusers, and in those who acquire infection while a neonate.

PATHOGENESIS

An effective and appropriate immune response, such as occurs in more than 90 per cent of adults who acquire hepatitis B, rids the liver of virus-containing cells; an overly vigorous immune response leads to fulminant hepatitis. Chronic hepatitis B develops when an ineffective immune response is mounted against hepatocytes containing hepatitis B virus, with incomplete eradication of infected hepatocytes.[237–239] It is important to keep in mind that the hepatitis B virus is not cytopathic for the hepatocyte and that liver damage does not occur in hepatitis B in the absence of viral replication.

A variety of factors with immunoregulatory properties, isolated from serum and from liver tissue, may affect the response of the body to hepatitis B infection.[154–161] Serum levels of rosette inhibiting factor (RIF) and serum inhibition factor (SIF) have been considered useful in judging prognosis in patients with chronic hepatitis B. In 25 of 27 patients with a limited, benign hepatitis B infection and complete elimination of HBsAg, RIF and SIF were found only transiently, whereas these factors were found persistently in two of three patients whose disease had a protracted course.[161] Persistence of RIF in the blood of patients with chronic viral hepatitis from either hepatitis B or non-A, non-B hepatitis has been seen in other studies as well.[240] Therefore, disappearance of RIF from the serum may be a good prognostic sign in a patient with virus-induced hepatitis.

In acute hepatitis B infection, cells containing the virus are destroyed by immunologic processes involving cytotoxic T cells directed in part against hepatitis B core antigen (HBcAg) expressed on the surface of the hepatocyte.[231, 237, 238, 241, 242, 244, 245] The histocompatibility system apparently is important in determining the course of disease in patients with chronic hepatitis B.[241, 242] For cytotoxicity to occur, there must be histocompatibility between the effector T cell and target hepatocyte.[241, 243] HBcAg found on the hepatocyte surface must be present in association with human HLA Class I glycoprotein to interact with cytotoxic T cells.[238, 239] One suggested mechanism leading to an incomplete clearance of hepatitis B and promotion of hepatitis B carrier state is diminished production of surface HLA Class I glycoprotein, which may be related to inadequate production of interferon.[237, 247, 248] Thus, interferons are important in inducing expression of HLA Class I glycoprotein, and an inability to produce adequate levels of interferon in response to hepatitis B infection may explain in part why hepatitis B becomes chronic in some patients.[248–252] An alternative but presently less favored explanation for the attack by lymphocytes on hepatocytes containing hepatitis B suggests that antibody-dependent cellular cytotoxicity is mediated by K lymphocytes directed against liver-specific protein (LSP) in the hepatocyte membrane, with the K lymphocytes binding to the Fc fragment of anti-LSP IgG.[131, 253]

There is no convincing evidence of an association between a specific HLA or DR subtype and a predilection to develop chronic hepatitis B, such as is the case with the associations of HLA-B8 and DRw3 and idiopathic autoimmune CAH.[83, 131]

STAGING

Chronic hepatitis B infection is divided broadly into *replicative* and *integrated* stages depending on whether there is evidence of production of complete hepatitis B.[100, 231, 232, 239] In the replicative phase, the patient is actively producing hepatitis B virus and has HBeAg, HBV DNA, and DNA polymerase in the serum in addition to HBsAg and anti-HBc. At some stage in the illness, many patients lose HBeAg, HBV DNA, and DNA polymerase and become anti-HBe positive. During the *integrated* phase, these patients usually continue to have HBsAg in the serum but do not produce complete hepatitis B (see Chap. 35). In anti-HBe positive patients, there is evidence that viral replication has ceased and part of the hepatitis B genome has become integrated into human DNA. If the integrated HBV DNA sequences code for HBsAg, the patient will continue to produce HBsAg. Patients with integrated hepatitis B apparently are those individuals at risk for later development of hepatocellular carcinoma (see Chaps. 36 and 45).

HISTOLOGIC MANIFESTATIONS

Liver biopsy is most useful in determining the extent of hepatic damage in a patient with chronic hepatitis B. Asymptomatic hepatitis B carriers have a normal liver biopsy or have only focal non-specific changes or mild disease.[254] Hepatocytes containing hepatitis B often have a ground-glass appearance resulting from viral accumulation, which may be identified by staining with orcein. There is an association between the degree of hepatic inflammation (especially lobular) and the presence of replicating virus.[255, 256]

The histologic changes in many patients with chronic hepatitis B are most satisfactorily classified as CPH with portal inflammation and absent or only scant periportal inflammation. Some patients are classified as having CLH with considerable lobular necrosis suggesting an ongoing necrotic process.[6] However, many patients have a combination of both portal and lobular inflammation.

The foci of inflammation throughout the lobule are characterized by cell drop-out and lymphocytic accumulation. In a study correlating markers of viral replication with histologic changes in 39 patients with chronic hepatitis B, there was a significant association between lobular inflammation and the presence of HBV DNA ($p > 0.02$) and HBeAg ($p > 0.001$).[255, 256] Patients with lobular inflammation had higher levels of serum aminotransferases, reflecting the inflammatory process. There was no correlation between the extent of periportal inflammation and viral replication. An increased display of beta$_2$-microglobulin on the surface of hepatocytes as an indication of the presence of HLA Type I proteins correlated with viral replication.[246] In addition, there was evidence of an increased display of HBcAg on the surface of hepatocytes containing replicating hepatitis B. These findings are consistent with the concept that hepatocytes containing replicating hepatitis B virus have enhanced membrane display of HLA Type I proteins, promoting recognition and attack of the virus-laden cell by cytotoxic T lymphocytes. These observations further underscore the need to evaluate portal, periportal, and lobular inflammation in assessing chronic hepatitis B.[36, 37, 165] Evidence is increasing that the lobular component of the hepatitis is of considerable importance in determining whether there will be progression of the viral hepatitis toward cirrhosis.[36, 37]

Clinical Manifestations

The spectrum of clinical signs and symptoms in patients with chronic hepatitis B ranges from a complete absence of evidence of any liver disease to a rapidly progressive illness characterized by jaundice, fluid retention, hepatic encephalopathy, and/or gastrointestinal bleeding, leading to rapid deterioration and death.[257, 258] The great majority of the estimated more than 200 million carriers of hepatitis B in the world have little evidence of liver injury. Most HBsAg carriers cannot recall an acute episode of hepatitis B and many (especially in the Far East) acquired the infection at or near the time of birth.[235, 259]

Many patients who develop chronic hepatitis B had an initial typical clinical course for acute hepatitis B with anorexia, nausea, and jaundice that persisted well beyond the usual two- to three-month course of resolution for acute hepatitis B. However, the majority of patients with chronic hepatitis B have an asymptomatic or relatively mild initial illness with persistent mild hepatomegaly and occasional right upper quadrant abdominal pain. Splenomegaly and occasionally jaundice may be present. Most of these patients with clinically mild disease have CPH or mild, nonspecific abnormalities found on liver biopsy. These patients tend to survive for many years and are at risk for development of hepatocellular carcinoma. However, patients with CAH B may pursue a stormy, rapidly deteriorating course characterized by progressive jaundice, extreme fatigue, wasting, fluid retention, bleeding, and development of cirrhosis.

The association between hepatitis B and polyarteritis nodosa is well established.[260-266] These patients often have fever, arthritis, myalgia, urticaria, rash, peripheral neuropathies, and hypertension. There is evidence that the manifestations of polyarteritis result from deposition of immune complexes containing HBsAg, anti-HBs, and immunoglobulin as well as complement. Many patients with polyarteritis in association with chronic hepatitis B have few if any manifestations of liver disease; however, instances of symptomatic CAH B and polyarteritis nodosa have been described.[266]

LABORATORY FINDINGS

Elevation of aminotransferase levels in patients with chronic hepatitis B correlates with the extent of active hepatic inflammation. A markedly elevated and rising serum bilirubin level indicates a subgroup of patients with a poor prognosis. Patients with chronic hepatitis B may have normal or only minimally abnormal routine tests and are diagnosed only after serologic tests detect HBsAg or anti-HBc. Gamma globulin levels are usually normal.[34] In patients with CAH B, 12 of 42 were found to have IgM anti-HBc, compared to an absence of IgM anti-HBc in 26 healthy hepatitis B carriers who did not have CAH.[267] No correlation was found between the presence of IgM anti-HBc and the degree of inflammation within the group of patients with CAH. Some patients with chronic hepatitis

have no serologic evidence of hepatitis B by conventional tests but have HBsAg or HBV DNA detected by monoclonal antibody tests.[268-270] It remains to be established whether these patients have chronic hepatitis related to the low levels of hepatitis B.

Markers suggesting autoimmunity, such as antinuclear antibodies, antimitochondrial antibodies and anti-smooth muscle antibodies, are much less frequent in patients with chronic hepatitis B than in patients with idiopathic autoimmune CAH.[34, 271-274] When present in patients with chronic hepatitis B, these antibodies are usually found in very low titers. The finding of LE cells in patients with chronic hepatitis B is extremely rare.[12, 275-276] Occasionally, elevated levels of alpha fetoprotein (AFP) are found in patients with chronic hepatitis B in whom there is no evidence of an underlying hepatocellular carcinoma.[277-282] Patients with elevated AFP levels and chronic hepatitis B often have evidence of active inflammatory disease, and the increased levels of AFP correlate with the presence of bridging necrosis.[282] In a series of 432 patients from Taiwan with chronic hepatitis B followed for 6 to 85 months, AFP levels were increased at least once in 45.6 per cent of the HBsAg positive patients; 19.4 per cent had AFP levels greater than 100 ng/ml.[282]

FACTORS PREDISPOSING TO CHRONIC HEPATITIS B

Host factors identified as important in promoting development of chronic hepatitis B infection include age at the time of infection, sex, immune status, and possibly ethnic origin.[33, 34, 231, 236, 237, 257, 283-285] Males appear to be far more susceptible than females to the development of hepatitis B infections of all varieties.[231, 237, 286] Drug abusers and male homosexuals appear to be particularly susceptible to the development of chronic hepatitis B. In addition, the women reported in large series of patients with chronic hepatitis B appear to have less severe disease. The reason males are apparently predisposed to develop chronic hepatitis B is not known. One suggestion is that there is an immunoregulatory gene on the X-chromosome that determines susceptibility.[287]

The increased prevalence of hepatitis B in male homosexuals and drug abusers, and to a lesser extent in medical personnel, is presumably related to exposure to infected individuals and blood products. Homosexual patients may have an acquired immunodeficiency state as a result of multiple infections, which promotes chronicity of the hepatitis B infection.[288] Age at acquisition appears to be the most important susceptibility factor; 90 to 95 per cent of neonates born to HBeAg-positive mothers develop chronic infection.[259, 289] Many of these neonates are asymptomatic from chronic hepatitis B infection and appear 20 to 40 years later with hepatocellular carcinoma (see Chap. 45). The effect of age on the rate of acquisition of hepatitis B was further demonstrated in Taiwan; only 1 of 39 (less than 3 per cent) university students who acquired acute hepatitis B became carriers.[290] An intermediate rate of acquisition of chronic hepatitis B (23 per cent) was found in follow-up of 98 infected preschool children.[235] Similar indications of an association of hepatitis B carrier state with age of acquisition was derived from studies of Yupik Eskimos in Alaska; in this population, the risk of becoming a hepatitis B carrier was inversely related to age at acquisition.[291]

It is fully established that patients with impaired immunity from a variety of causes are at increased risk of becoming hepatitis B carriers following an acute infection. Patients receiving cancer chemotherapy, or hemodialysis and patients with Down's syndrome and leprosy are all at considerably higher risk of becoming carriers of hepatitis B.[286, 292–294] One explanation for the high carrier rate for hepatitis B in male homosexuals and drug abusers is that frequent exposure to hepatitis and co-infection with other viral agents suppresses the immune system and increases the susceptibility to develop chronic hepatitis.[295–296] In a follow-up study of 16 homosexual males and 78 intravenous drug abusers who were chronic carriers of hepatitis B, there was a higher incidence of HBeAg positivity and evidence of more severe histologic damage in homosexuals than in drug abusers.[297] It also appears patients with a mild initial illness are more likely to develop a chronic hepatitis B carrier state and chronic hepatitis.[231–237] The mild initial illness may result from a blunted immunologic response to infection with hepatitis B.

ACUTE EPISODES OF HEPATITIS AND HEPATIC DECOMPENSATION

Many HBsAg carriers have little or no clinical, biochemical, or histologic evidence of liver disease. Some of these patients develop cirrhosis over many years and may present with bleeding esophagogastric varices or ascites as the first important manifestation of chronic hepatitis B. Others develop hepatocellular carcinoma following years of hepatitis B infection, and the manifestations of the tumor may be the initial indication of the underlying chronic viral infection.

Several causes of acute deterioration of previously asymptomatic carriers of hepatitis B have been recognized (Table 38–5). The causes and course of these *acute on chronic* situations have attracted considerable attention and investigation.

Superinfection with Additional Hepatitis Viruses

Patients with chronic hepatitis B may become superinfected with one or more additional hepatitis viruses.[298] Individuals in several high-risk groups for acquiring hepatitis viruses, such as male homosexuals and drug abusers, frequently have evidence of more than one hepatitis viral infection. Evidence for hepatitis A; non-A, non-B hepatitis; hepatitis D (delta hepatitis), Epstein-Barr viral infection; and cytomegalovirus infection may be found in patients with chronic hepatitis B. Often the major question is whether the patient has had an activation of the underlying chronic hepatitis B or superimposition of another virus.

TABLE 38–5. CAUSES OF ACUTE HEPATITIS AND HEPATIC DETERIORATION IN PATIENT WITH CHRONIC HEPATITIS B

Superinfection with other viral agents:
   Hepatitis D (delta hepatitis)
   Non-A, non-B hepatitis
   Hepatitis A
   Cytomegalovirus
   Epstein-Barr virus
Clearance of HBeAg:
   HBeAg → Anti-HBe
Spontaneous reactivation of hepatitis B
Corticosteroid withdrawal
Drug-induced hepatic injury
Hepatocellular carcinoma

Superimposition of hepatitis A may lead to a severe, even fulminant, hepatitis.[299–303] The titer of HBsAg generally decreases during infection with a superimposed acute hepatitis A.[304, 305] Acute hepatitis A superimposed on a chronic hepatitis B infection is especially prevalent among drug abusers and in individuals from areas endemic for hepatitis B.[304] Hepatitis A infection alone has not been implicated as a cause of chronic hepatitis.

Superinfection with non-A, non-B hepatitis in a patient with chronic hepatitis B remains a diagnosis of exclusion in the absence of a marker for non-A, non-B, hepatitis.[306] It is often difficult to decide whether a patient with chronic hepatitis B has a spontaneous reactivation of hepatitis B or a superimposed non-A, non-B hepatitis infection. A chronic hepatitis B carrier with superimposed non-A, non-B hepatitis should be negative for anti-HAV IgM, anti-HBc, and delta antibody. There is great promise for a newly developed serologic test for non-A, non-B hepatitis (hepatitis C).

Spontaneous Reactivation of Chronic Type B Hepatitis

Episodes of acute hepatitis occurring in chronic hepatitis B carriers in the absence of any evidence of superinfection with another virus or the appearance (or reappearance) of markers indicating hepatitis B replication have been observed and may be associated with severe illness.[307–309] In these patients either there was conversion from an integrated state (anti-HBe positive) to a replicative state (HBeAg positive) or a low level replicative state, which had been undetected by usual testing, had been unmasked. The diagnosis of reactivation of hepatitis B is based on demonstrating the reappearance of IgM anti-HBc in a patient who previously had IgG anti-HBc and anti-HBe.[310] Episodes of severe reactivation of hepatitis were observed in 3 of 150 patients with chronic hepatitis B, who were followed for an average of 2.4 years at the National Institutes of Health.[308] Evidence of mild to moderate hepatitis associated with reactivation of hepatitis B occurred in 8 of 25 HBsAg carriers who had previous anti-HBe, indicating an integrated (non-replicative) stage of hepatitis B.[307]

The factors associated with spontaneous reactivation of hepatitis B are unknown. The major evidence against superinfection with non-A, non-B hepatitis is the reappearance of the markers of hepatitis B viral replication. Hepatitis B may be reactivated in patients receiving antineoplastic, immunosuppressive, or corticosteroid drugs, presumably because of further impairment of the immune system.[311–319] However, other investigators have not found increased titers of hepatitis B markers during corticosteroid treatment in patients with chronic hepatitis B.[320] Reactivation of hepatitis B has been noted in renal transplant recipients, again presumably because immunosuppressive therapy promoted viral replication.[321, 322]

Reactivation of Hepatitis B Following Withdrawal of Immunosuppressant Therapy

Reactivation of hepatitis B has been observed following rapid withdrawal of corticosteroid or immunosuppressant therapy.[323, 324] In patients with chronic hepatitis B who develop reactivation upon withdrawal of corticosteroid therapy, there is a reappearance or increase in titer of IgM anti-HBc that correlates with an increase in DNA polymerase similar to that found in acute hepatitis B. These findings suggest increased hepatitis B viral replication related to the reappearance of acute hepatitis.

Superinfection with Delta Agent (Hepatitis D)

The superimposition of an acute infection with the delta agent (Hepatitis D virus [HDV]) in a patient who has chronic hepatitis B may lead to fulminant hepatitis or conversion of nonspecific or persistent hepatitis to severe CAH that progresses to cirrhosis.[325–333]

The delta agent has been well characterized as a transmissible, heterotropic, defective circular RNA satellite virus that depends on hepatitis B virus for its replication.[332, 334–337] Hepatitis D infection does not occur in the absence of hepatitis B.[332] Once HDV infection becomes established, there is partial inhibition of HBV synthesis, as evidenced by a decrease in hepatitis B markers.[338] HDV is invariably pathogenic. In the United States, in a series of 560 patients with chronic hepatitis B, 29 were seropositive for anti-HD.[334] The incidence of anti-HD was 26 per cent in patients with CAH, compared with no anti-HD in patients with CPH. Patients with CAH B who had symptomatic disease had a significantly higher incidence of anti-HD than those whose disease was asymptomatic. Studies have been reported in which HDV superinfection as a cause of exacerbation of chronic hepatitis B occurred more frequently in patients who were anti-HBe positive than in those who were HBeAg positive.[337] HDV infection may present as an acute co-infection with hepatitis B or as a superinfection in a patient with established chronic hepatitis B. It is the superinfection in the chronic hepatitis B carrier that often leads to severe liver disease.[339] In most patients, superinfection with HDV causes existing liver disease to become more severe, and in general there is an acceleration of the liver disease toward cirrhosis.[328] Patients at especially high risk of acquiring HDV superinfection include parenteral drug abusers and residents of highly endemic HDV areas such as Italy, parts of the Middle East, USSR, and South America.[331] Instances of HDV infection in male homosexuals are being reported with increasing frequency.[340, 341]

HDV infection is diagnosed by detection of anti-HD which is typically present in serum during acute and chronic delta hepatitis. Patients with a superinfection of HDV have a serologic profile of HBsAg, IgG anti-HBc, and anti-HD, whereas those with HDV co-infection will have HBsAg, IgM anti-HBc, and anti-HD.

Acute Hepatitis Associated with Clearance of HBeAg

The conversion (clearance) of HBeAg to anti-HBe in a patient with chronic hepatitis B is almost always associated with an exacerbation of hepatic inflammation and occasionally results in a tumultuous event with marked clinical deterioration and even death.[342] The reported annual rates of conversion of HBeAg to anti-HBe in hepatitis B carriers have been from 3 to 25 per cent per year.[231, 343–349] Following the clearance of HBeAg and appearance of anti-HBe, there is generally a decrease in aminotransferase levels and reduction in clinical symptoms.[343] The clearance of HBeAg signals a change in the course of the chronic hepatitis B from a replicative to an integrated status.[347] In the replicative phase, HBeAg, HBV DNA, DNA polymerase and IgM anti-HBc are present, whereas in the integrated phase production of whole virus ceases or at least falls to a low level, coinciding with the disappearance of HBeAg, HBV DNA, DNA polymerase, and IgM anti-HBc and the appearance of anti-HBe. An intermediate stage (low replicative phase) characterized by the presence of HBeAg or anti-HBe along with a low level of HBV DNA has been suggested from studies in the Orient.[255, 350]

Factors determining the timing of HBeAg clearance are unknown. The clearance of HBeAg may not be sustained, and HBeAg may reappear.[351] Presumably the flare in hepatitis occurring during conversion of HBeAg to anti-HBe is the result of a more effective attack by cytotoxic T lymphocytes on the infected hepatocyte.

In a study from Taiwan, HBeAg clearance occurred in 74 of 237 (31 per cent) HBeAg-positive patients with chronic hepatitis over a 6- to 72-month follow-up period (mean 24.5 months).[348] The rate of HBeAg clearance was 16.3 per cent per year, and no patient lost HBsAg during the study. There was a higher annual HBeAg clearance rate in males (18.7 per cent per year) than females (8.7 per cent per year). An increase in ALT to greater than 300 IU preceding the HBeAg clearance was found in 62 per cent of patients. Immunosuppressive therapy in these patients had no apparent effect on the rate of HBeAg clearance. An alpha fetoprotein (AFP) level greater than 100 ng/ml was a predictor that HBeAg would be cleared. Furthermore, it was noted that there was a higher clearance rate of HBeAg in patients with histologically more severe hepatitis, including those patients with CAH (15.6 per cent) and CLH (20.6 per cent), compared to patients with CPH (0 per cent) or nonspecific changes (8.8 per cent). The authors concluded that the more severe the hepatitis during the exacerbation, the more likely HBeAg would be cleared. In contrast to these findings from the Far East, a study from Alaska indicated a higher HBeAg clearance rate in women and also noted more rapid clearance in older patients.[349] Another study from Italy reported that immunosuppressive treatment delayed HBeAg seroconversion, in contrast to the absence of such an effect in patients from the Far East.[352]

Evaluation of Exacerbations of Hepatitis

When a patient who is a known chronic carrier of hepatitis B develops an episode of acute hepatitis or begins to show evidence of progressive deterioration, the diagnoses outlined in Table 38–5 should be investigated. Serologic tests are required for delta antibody (anti-HD), IgM anti-HAV, and antibodies to cytomegalovirus and Epstein-Barr virus, which may also superinfect these patients. Measurements of HBeAg, IgM anti-HBc, HBV DNA and/or DNA-polymerase are useful in determining if a patient is having a reactivation of hepatitis B. A careful history may yield evidence of use of a therapeutic drug known to cause liver damage or the concomitant excessive use of alcohol. As in so many other clinical situations, the diagnosis of non-A, non-B hepatitis remains a diagnosis of exclusion while development of a marker is awaited. Gallium scanning and determination of serum AFP levels may be useful in detecting hepatocellular carcinoma.

TREATMENT

It is important to remember that almost all patients with chronic hepatitis B–induced liver disease have detectable serum HBsAg. Sensitive tests for HBsAg with monoclonal antibodies may detect patients with low levels of hepatitis B infection whose disease is now diagnosed as chronic non-A, non-B hepatitis.[268, 269] A few patients have been recorded in whom HBsAg disappeared well after cirrhosis developed.[356, 357] If these patients had been initially evaluated at the HBsAg-negative stage, a diagnosis of non-A, non-B hepatitis or cryptogenic cirrhosis might have been made.

The two major approaches to the treatment of chronic hepatitis B are (1) directed toward eradication of the virus and (2) designed to modulate cellular and humoral immunity, thereby altering the host response to infection.[100, 237, 353–355] The treatment responses in chronic hepatitis B are affected by the age at which hepatitis B was acquired. Neonates are resistant to antiviral and interferon therapy.[259] It has been suggested that the immature immune system of the neonate allows tolerance to the hepatitis B virus to develop.[358] If maternal IgG anti-HBc crosses the placenta at a time that hepatitis B virus infection is developing, the IgG anti-HBc may interact with HBcAg in the membrane of the hepatocyte, thereby preventing subsequent recognition of an infected cell by cytotoxic T lymphocytes.[237]

Progress has been made in the development of antiviral chemotherapeutic agents for hepatitis B, but as yet no safe, reliably effective treatment or combinations of treatments are available. Features of an ideal therapeutic agent (or agents) are listed in Table 38–6. Immunosuppressive regimens to diminish the host immune response are based in large measure on observations that indicate that hepatitis B virus has little, if any, cytopathic effect, and that most of the chronic liver damage in chronic hepatitis B results from host immune response to hepatocytes transformed by the virus.[231, 237] The variety of approaches proposed and in many situations evaluated in the treatment of chronic hepatitis B attests to the ingenuity and imagination of clinical investigators attempting to eradicate hepatitis B.[231, 237] Unfortunately, there are as yet no randomized studies definitely indicating that any therapeutic agent has favorably and safely altered the course of chronic hepatitis B in patients, as measured by a disappearance of markers of replicating hepatitis B and by histologic improvement.[353]

It is important to establish the stage of the chronic hepatitis B (replicative or integrated) before considering therapy. Drugs directed against replicating virus will have no effect, for example, in a patient whose disease is in the integrated phase. Part of the difficulty in assessing the results of several reported treatment trials, therefore, relates to a failure to establish the stage of the chronic hepatitis B at the time of treatment.

Corticosteroid Therapy

The issue of whether or not to use corticosteroid therapy in patients with hepatitis B–related chronic hepatitis has been an area of considerable uncertainty for several years.[353, 359–361] Most evidence indicates that corticosteroids

TABLE 38–6. CRITERIA FOR SUCCESSFUL THERAPY OF CHRONIC HEPATITIS B

Well tolerated
Effects lasting beyond active therapy
Halt virus replication
Anti-inflammatory
Antifibrotic
Anticarcinogenic

are of no therapeutic value in chronic hepatitis B and may even be harmful. A study from the Far East reported that prednisolone therapy tended to delay the occurrence of remission in patients with CAH B.[359] The study included 51 patients randomized to receive either prednisolone (15 to 20 mg each day) or placebo. Patients receiving prednisolone had a higher death rate and a greater number of major complications. The only possible beneficial result noted was that patients receiving prednisolone had an early, transient decrease in serum bilirubin. A second controlled trial from the same group evaluated the effects of corticosteroid therapy on histologic manifestations of chronic hepatitis B.[361] Again, the corticosteroid-treated patients fared poorly, with histologic evidence of more frequent persistence, erosion of the limiting plate, and a higher titer of hepatitis B virus as evidenced by increases in HBsAg and anti-HBc titers. These observations were consistent with previous findings.[314, 315, 318] There was less intralobular inflammation in the corticosteroid-treated patients, but portal inflammation and fibrosis were not affected. Therefore, it appears that corticosteroid therapy worsened both histologic and clinical status. It must be noted that both trials involved small numbers of patients; many of the patients had acquired chronic hepatitis B as neonates; and follow-up liver biopsies were obtained at variable times after the onset of therapy.

A multicenter randomized double-blind trial of prednisolone therapy in patients with chronic hepatitis B was performed in 99 patients from 22 European centers.[362] Morbidity was 2.9 (95 per cent confidence limits, 0.9–9) times greater in the prednisolone-treated group than in the control group, supporting the concept that corticosteroids are not only useless but also dangerous in patients with chronic hepatitis B. Mortality in the prednisolone-treated group increased with age. In a long-term investigation of changes in HBV DNA levels in patients with chronic hepatitis B, those treated with corticosteroids had evidence of continuing HBV-DNA as an index of viral replication.[363]

In a large trial of prednisolone in patients with chronic viral hepatitis B, 204 patients with chronic hepatitis B were randomized to daily treatment with 20 mg of prednisolone, 100 mg of azathioprine, a combination of both drugs (20 mg of prednisolone and 50 mg of azathioprine), or no treatment.[364] No benefit from any of these therapeutic regimens was apparent in HBeAg-positive patients. Only 1 of 35 patients with HBeAg seroconverted to anti-HBe on any form of immunosuppressive therapy, whereas 4 of 12 untreated patients seroconverted. However, immunosuppressive therapy in this study appeared to result in improvement in patients who were anti-HBe positive as compared to no treatment. A major problem with interpretation of this study is the lack of a double-blind design.

Short-term Corticosteroid Therapy Followed by Withdrawal

Another approach to the management of chronic viral hepatitis B has been the use of short-term courses of corticosteroid therapy with the aim of promoting clearance of the virus when the corticosteroids are discontinued.[315, 323, 324] Clearance of whole virus as measured by disappearance of DNA polymerase occurred in 8 of 21 patients with CAH B after corticosteroid therapy was discontinued.[315] In three other patients treated prospectively, one cleared whole virus after a short course of prednisone. In six patients from another study, following withdrawal of corticosteroid therapy there was an increase in aminotransferase levels in association with a decrease in DNA polymerase activity.[323]

Fifteen patients with chronic hepatitis B were treated in a 28-day randomized, double-blind controlled trial comparing a placebo-treated group of patients with a group who received prednisolone beginning with 60 mg daily followed by tapering and then by withdrawal at day 28.[324] Serum aminotransferase levels decreased during treatment with prednisolone; however, a post-withdrawal rebound associated with exacerbation of symptomatic hepatitis was observed in several patients. Follow-up liver biopsies showed worsening of hepatitis in four of seven treated patients, with no changes noted in five control patients. It was concluded that a short course of corticosteroids was probably of no benefit and might be harmful. There have been reports of fulminant hepatitis occurring when corticosteroid therapy was withdrawn suddenly in patients with hepatitis B; any patient treated in this manner must be followed very carefully.[365] Therefore, results thus far indicate scant support for use of short-term corticosteroid therapy as a single agent in the treatment of chronic hepatitis B.

Interferon

The interferons are a family of glycoproteins with antiviral properties as well as multiple effects on the immune system.[249–252, 366–368] There are several types of interferons. Alpha interferon is produced by lymphocytes and monocytes, whereas beta interferon is produced by fibroblasts. Alpha and beta interferons are designated Type I interferons and are structurally similar. Both are produced in response to viral infections of many cell types and share a common receptor to enter cells.[369, 370] Gamma interferon is structurally different from alpha and beta interferons and is produced by T lymphocytes stimulated by mitogenic or antigenic stimuli. Gamma interferon is a lymphokine, which enters cells through a receptor separate from that for alpha and beta interferons.[371, 372]

Interferons stimulate increases in 2',5'-oligoadenylate synthetase (2',5'-AS) activity and enhance synthesis and expression of HLA Class I glycoproteins on the surface of cells, including hepatocytes, which normally have no HLA Class I display.[247, 373–379] Type II (gamma) interferon is much more potent than Type I (alpha and beta) in production of HLA Class I glycoproteins. Type I interferon is more potent in increasing activity of 2',5'-AS. The antiviral properties of interferons result in part from the activation of intracellular ribonucleases that destroy viral mRNA. Furthermore, interferons may inhibit entry of viruses into cells and interfere with subsequent steps relating to intracellular replication of viruses.[252, 366] Another effect of alpha interferon is to inhibit the differentiation of B cells into plasma cells, which produce and secrete immunoglobulins.[380]

Most trials of interferon in patients with chronic hepatitis B have employed alpha interferon.[381] Trials of beta interferon showed less effect on hepatitis B replication, although newer beta interferons produced by recombinant technology are under investigation. Beta interferon may have a lesser tendency to cause leukopenia.[382–384] In the future, combination therapies including alpha, beta, and gamma interferons may be shown to be more effective than a single agent. Of all the interferons, gamma interferon may prove to be the most useful in treatment of chronic hepatitis B because it enhances expression of membrane HLA Type I protein.

By use of polyclonal and monoclonal antibodies to detect interferon in patients with chronic hepatitis B, it has been demonstrated that interferon is produced by mononuclear cells infiltrating the liver and to a lesser extent by fibroblasts.[388] Alpha interferon, which is not produced by hepatocytes, is produced locally by cells near infected hepatocytes, which may explain why there may be no detectable serum interferon in patients with acute viral hepatitis.[373, 377] Treatment of chronic hepatitis B with alpha interferon leads to increased expression of membrane HBcAg and reduced expression of HBsAg.[389] A nucleotide sequence at the beginning of the HBc gene, which is similar to a sequence present upstream from genes induced by interferon in mammalian cells, has been identified, and the presence of the homologous sequence may influence the expression of viral genes.[389] It is suggested that integration of sequences of the hepatitis B virus may "neutralize" the interferon system and thereby facilitate the development of chronic infection as well as affect the response to interferon therapy.[389]

Administration of exogenous interferon leads to a decrease in alpha interferon production by peripheral blood mononuclear cells from patients with chronic hepatitis B when these cells are stimulated to produce interferon by exposure to Sendai virus.[390] No effect of exogenous alpha interferon on the production of gamma interferon was seen when cells were stimulated to produce gamma interferon by phytohemagglutinin.

It has been demonstrated that interferon is useful in suppressing hepatitis B viral replication.[237, 250, 376, 391–395] There has been definite evidence of reduction in hepatitis B replication when interferon was given to patients with chronic hepatitis B, but there is no evidence thus far of long-lasting benefit in the majority when interferon is used as a single therapy.[237, 346, 392]

An interesting study was reported in which the synthesis of 2',5'-oligonucleotides by peripheral blood monocytes was measured as an index of interferon activity in patients with a variety of types of hepatitis B.[251] The enzyme that catalyzes the reaction (2',5'-AS) is thought to be induced by all three classes of interferons, and the finding of 2'-5' AS is accepted as a marker of interferon activity.[396] Levels of 2',5'-AS activity were elevated in 77 per cent of patients with acute hepatitis B, in 56 per cent of healthy chronic carriers, and in 50 per cent of patients with CPH.[251] There were no differences in 2',5'-AS activity in peripheral blood mononuclear cells between patients with CAH B and controls, thereby implying an inability of CAH B-patients to respond to the viral infection. These investigators concluded there was an in vitro deficiency in interferon response in patients with chronic hepatitis B, and that the inadequate response might be important in the promotion of chronic hepatitis B.

A reduced capacity of peripheral blood lymphocytes to produce alpha and gamma interferon when given a standard viral stimulus with the Sendai virus has been observed in patients with chronic hepatitis B.[237] The reductions in response were significant and were unrelated to the level of viral replication or to the severity of liver disease in patients who were HBsAg and HBeAg positive. It is not known whether measuring serum interferon levels in patients early in the course of hepatitis B is useful in predicting the outcome of the hepatitis B.[252] It is possible that interferon is produced transiently in quantities sufficient to be detected in the serum early in acute hepatitis, and that later in the illness lesser amounts, which are not detectable in serum, are produced locally in areas adjacent to virus-laden cells. Several lines of evidence support the presence of a deficiency of interferon in patients with chronic hepatitis B. Peripheral blood mononuclear cells from patients with chronic hepatitis B lack the characteristic cytoplasmic tubuloreticular inclusions known to be induced by interferons.[397]

HLA Class 1 protein display and levels of hepatocellular 2′,5′-AS activity were compared in HBeAg and anti-HBe–positive patients with chronic hepatitis B.[398] Patients with HBeAg had no increase in HLA Class 1 protein display on the hepatocyte surface but had twice normal elevations of 2′,5′-AS activity, which is the response expected from Type I interferon (alpha and beta). In anti-HBe–positive patients, HLA Class I protein display was markedly increased and levels of 2′,5′-AS activity were normal, which is consistent with Type II (gamma) interferon activity. The gamma interferon leading to the enhanced display in the anti-HBe positive patients may be produced by circulating T cells.

Interferon Treatment Trials

A preliminary study utilized recombinant human alpha interferon therapy in nine patients with chronic hepatitis B and HBeAg and DNA polymerase in their sera.[394] Serum DNA polymerase activity decreased 15 to 30 per cent during treatment but returned to pretreatment levels within ten days following completion of interferon therapy. Two patients had a sustained remission during which HBV DNA, DNA polymerase, and HBeAg disappeared. Dose-related side effects were frequent and included fever, chills, fatigue, and neutropenia. The investigators considered the preliminary results sufficiently encouraging to warrant longer treatment trials.

Several generalizations regarding interferon therapy can be drawn from the available interferon treatment trials:

1. Prolonged (greater than 1 to 2 months) courses of interferon therapy will most likely be required.

2. Only 10 to 30 per cent of HBeAg-positive patients receiving alpha interferon as a single therapeutic agent have had conversion of HBeAg to anti-HBe, and in many of these patients there was a return of HBeAg after treatment was discontinued.

3. Doses of alpha interferon of 5 to 10 million units daily were as effective as higher doses (even up to 100 million units per day) with fewer side effects at lower doses.[384, 394]

4. Demographic factors are important in determining treatment outcome. Male homosexuals, Orientals, and patients who acquired hepatitis B as a neonate respond much less favorably.[231, 237]

5. Patients with HTLV-III antibody respond less favorably, presumably as the result of immunodeficiency.

6. The most important role of alpha interferon will most likely be in combination with other therapeutic agents.

Of great interest and potential therapeutic benefit for patients with chronic hepatitis have been observations that combinations of interferon with antiviral chemotherapy or corticosteroids may be more effective therapy than any single agent.

Antiviral Chemotherapy With or Without Interferon or Corticosteroids

A number of treatment trials using various preparations of adenine arabinosides with or without other therapy have been reported.[399–409] Adenine arabinoside (ara-A) is a synthetic nucleoside that inhibits replication of DNA viruses.[399] Because of poor solubility in water, the drug has to be administered intravenously. Arabinoside 5′-monophosphate (ara-AMP) is a water-soluble derivative that can be given intramuscularly. Both ara-A and ara-AMP are purine analogs that inhibit the synthesis of hepatitis B virus nucleic acid by acting as a faulty substrate. These drugs may act to inhibit HBV replication, allowing the immune system to recover and promote long-term control of hepatitis B.

In a study from the National Institutes of Health, ten HBeAg-positive patients received 28 days of ara-AMP at a dose of 10 mg per kg per day followed by 5 mg per kg per day for an additional 23 days. Results were compared to those in ten patients who received no treatment.[403] Complications from ara-AMP were many, and five of the ten patients receiving ara-AMP developed a dose-dependent neuropathic pain syndrome. However, despite the small numbers of patients in the trial, there was some suggestion of benefit. Six patients receiving ara-AMP had histologic improvement at 12 months, compared to improvement in three of ten individuals in the placebo group. Four treated patients cleared HBeAg at 12 months, compared to only one in the placebo group. Because of the considerable toxicity of ara-AMP, efforts have been initiated to utilize these drugs in intermittent dosing regimens.

Weller and colleagues conducted a randomized trial of four weeks of intramuscular ara-AMP in 29 hepatitis B carriers who had been HBeAg positive for at least six months.[399] Six of 15 treated patients lost HBV DNA polymerase, five patients developed anti-HBe, and one patient lost HBsAg. These investigators concluded that short-term use of ara-AMP was effective in reducing hepatic inflammation and in some patients led to long-term suppression of HBV replication.

In another study from the National Institutes of Health, ten male patients were given three ten-day courses of intramuscular ara-AMP monthly within three months.[407] There was marked decrease of DNA polymerase activity with each course of therapy. However, following the completion of therapy, all patients had a rapid return of DNA polymerase, indicating only transient benefit. Neuromuscular side effects from the therapy occurred in three patients. It was concluded that there was no long-term benefit in the use of ara-AMP for the treatment of chronic hepatitis B, and that the neuropathic side effects were sufficiently severe to prevent longer trials with this agent.

The efficacy of ara-AMP alone and in combination with prednisone has been compared in studies of 38 patients with chronic active hepatitis B.[405] In an initial trial, 22 patients were randomized to receive no treatment or treatment with a 28-day cycle of ara-AMP. Subsequently, 13 patients were randomized to receive no treatment or treatment with two 28-day cycles of ara-AMP separated by four-week intervals. In a third trial, 11 patients were treated for eight weeks with prednisone followed by 28 days with ara-AMP. The response rate was best with the regimen including prednisone (73 per cent); in the two trials not including prednisone, the response rates were 0 per cent and 15 per cent. The authors concluded that a combination of prednisone and ara-AMP offered more promise for successful treatment than ara-AMP alone. (It must be noted these studies were all of short duration.)

Important side effects have occurred in all clinical trials of ara-AMP. The most troublesome side effect has been a peculiar neuromuscular pain syndrome that developed in 70 to 80 per cent of patients treated with ara-AMP, characterized by severe muscle aches affecting large muscle groups such as the arms, thighs, and buttocks. The pain tends to be more severe while resting and during sleep and is partially relieved by exercise and analgesia. Searches are under way for antiviral chemotherapeutic agents less toxic than ara-AMP.

When evaluating the results of trials with ara-AMP (or any other therapy in chronic hepatitis B), the demographics of the patient population must be considered. Male homosexual patients rarely respond to ara-AMP, whereas response rates with loss of HBeAg as high as 45 per cent occurred in a heterosexual group of patients who acquired hepatitis B as adults.[237, 406] Furthermore, ara-AMP has not been effective in the treatment of patients who acquired hepatitis B while neonates. Therefore, overall results from several sources indicate that ara-AMP is effective in reducing viral replication, but in many instances benefits are transient and toxicities great.[353]

Acyclovir

Acyclovir is an anti-viral chemotherapeutic agent that is beneficial in the treatment of herpes viruses. The drug is relatively nontoxic and has been demonstrated to inhibit HBV DNA polymerase.[409] Schalm and colleagues reported results of administration of acyclovir to 12 patients with chronic hepatitis B who were positive for HBeAg and DNA polymerase for at least six months before the study.[410] There was a significantly greater fall in DNA polymerase and HBeAg when patients were treated with a combination of interferon and acyclovir than when they were treated with either agent alone. The combination of drugs appeared to be well tolerated, and further studies will undoubtedly be forthcoming. Deoxyacyclovir is an acyclovir prodrug that is converted by xanthine oxidase to acyclovir and has the advantage of oral administration. However, in preliminary trials, serum levels of acyclovir following oral administration of deoxyacyclovir were rather low, and some toxicity was associated with use of this drug. An oral, well-absorbed form of acyclovir is a therapeutic goal.

A randomized controlled trial of 28 days of intravenous acyclovir was carried out in 30 patients with chronic HBeAg-positive hepatitis B.[411] At 12 months, seroconversion of HBeAg to anti-HBe had occurred in 4 of 15 treated patients, compared to 1 of 15 untreated patients. Based on the low response rate, the authors concluded that the drug was of no significant benefit when administered as a single agent in the therapy of chronic hepatitis B.

Other Agents

A variety of other agents have been tried unsuccessfully in attempts to treat chronic hepatitis B. Suramin, an anti-viral chemotherapeutic agent, was given to three patients with chronic hepatitis B after the drug was shown to inhibit the activity in vitro of duck hepatitis B virus DNA polymerase.[412] Unfortunately, there was no in vivo suppression of human hepatitis B virus DNA polymerase, and the drug caused prolongation of the prothrombin time in all three patients, as well as a variety of other complications.

Levamisole is a synthetic anti-helminthic agent that augments cell-mediated immunity. No benefit was demonstrated in patients with chronic hepatitis B who were given the drug in hope of increasing immune competence and eradicating the virus.[413] However, in another randomized double-blind study involving 20 patients with chronic hepatitis B, those receiving levamisole tended to have a reduc-

tion in HBeAg and HBV DNA as well as a decrease in aminotransferase levels and improved histologic status, suggesting that further study of levamisole may be useful.[414] Transfer factor therapy has also been attempted with no benefit, and no trials are currently in progress.[415, 416] Little has come of attempts of the use of hepatitis B hyperimmune immunoglobulins or hepatitis B vaccine in attempts to augment the immune response.

The flavanoid (+)-cyanidanol-3 is a free radical scavenger that has been suggested as a useful agent in preventing toxic liver injury.[417] A number of studies from Europe evaluated cyanidanol in patients with acute and chronic hepatitis and reported little benefit; there is scant enthusiasm for continued study of this drug.[418] However, in a Japanese trial of cyanidanol therapy for chronic hepatitis B, there was at least a 50 per cent decrease in HBeAg titer in 44 of 144 treated patients with cyanidanol, with a similar decrease in titer in only 21 of 240 patients who received placebo.[419]

A further novel approach that also failed was the use of quinacrine hydrochloride in an attempt to inhibit DNA polymerase.[420] In a controlled trial, 10 patients received 100 mg per day of quinacrine for 3 months, whereas 12 patients received placebo in an identical double-blind fashion. All patients who received the drug developed a yellow color to the skin but none demonstrated any favorable effects on the titer of HBsAg or levels of DNA polymerase.

Interleukin-2 (IL-2) has been produced by recombinant DNA technology and trials of use of this agent will be available within the next several years.

PROGNOSIS

The prognosis for chronic hepatitis B is largely dependent on the histologic extent of the chronic hepatitis at the time of diagnosis.[257] It has been suggested that the prognosis for chronic hepatitis B is better than that for idiopathic autoimmune CAH, but the differences are not pronounced when patients are matched for clinical and histologic manifestations of severity.[34, 421] In a large series of 379 patients with chronic hepatitis B staged on the basis of liver biopsy, the estimated five-year survival rate was 97 per cent for patients with CPH; 86 per cent for patients with CAH; and 55 per cent for patients with CAH and cirrhosis[257] (Fig. 38–11). Factors associated with a poor prognosis in chronic hepatitis B were age greater than 40 years, serum bilirubin greater than 1.5 mg/dl, and presence of ascites and/or spider nevi. It was concluded that the prognosis for chronic hepatitis B does not differ from that for other forms of chronic hepatitis if the groups are matched for histologic severity. A further observation from the study was that women with chronic hepatitis B developed less serious sequelae than men.

HEPATOCELLULAR CARCINOMA

The development of hepatocellular carcinoma after many years of chronic hepatitis B virus (HBV) infection (see Chaps. 36 and 45) is an important problem in patients with long-standing hepatitis B.[349, 422, 423] A hepatitis B carrier is more than 200 times more likely than a non-carrier to develop hepatocellular carcinoma.[424, 425] The induction of hepatocellular carcinoma is attributed to alterations of human DNA by insertion of segments of HBV DNA.[426]

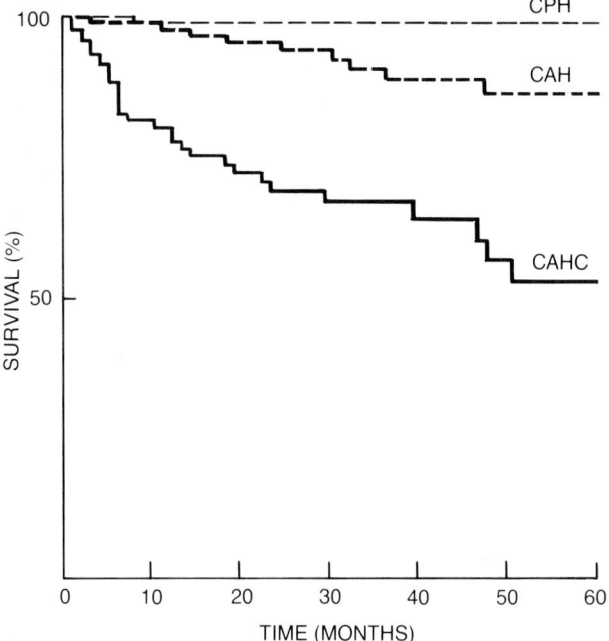

Figure 38–11. Five-year survival curves for 379 patients with chronic hepatitis B. The solid line indicates duration of survival for 130 patients with chronic active hepatitis and cirrhosis; the heavy dashed line represents duration of survival for 128 patients with chronic active hepatitis; the light dashed line represents survival for 121 patients with chronic persistent hepatitis. Each curve differs significantly from the others at p <0.001. (Reproduced from Weissberg JI, et al. Ann Intern Med 101:613, 1984, with permission.)

The time from onset of hepatitis B infection to the appearance of the tumor is usually several decades.

It remains to be proven whether any of the available experimental therapies will have an effect on the later development of hepatocellular carcinoma.

LIVER TRANSPLANTATION

Liver transplantation (see also Chap. 55) has been successfully performed in patients with chronic hepatitis B–related cirrhosis.[42] The indications for liver transplantation in patients with chronic hepatitis B are similar to those for patients with cirrhosis of other etiologies and include advanced wasting, portal hypertension with gastroesophageal bleeding, ascites, and uncontrollable hepatic encephalopathy. A major concern regarding liver transplantation of patients with hepatitis B is the likelihood of recurrence of the disease in the liver graft. In a series of patients with chronic hepatitis B who had liver transplants, all who survived more than two months after surgery had a recurrent hepatitis B infection.[42] The histologic evaluation indicated a predominantly lobular inflammation, a pattern somewhat distinct from rejection reactions, which more often involve portal areas. However, it may be difficult to determine if the hepatic inflammation is due to rejection, return of HBV infection, or both.

CHRONIC NON-A, NON-B HEPATITIS

Non-A, non-B hepatitis, especially when acquired as a result of transfusion, is an important and frequent cause of chronic hepatitis and cirrhosis.[9, 427–430] The presumed several agents that cause hepatitis non-A, non-B have not been identified, but as mentioned on page 1044 serologic testing for hepatitis C is now feasible. Nevertheless, the diagnosis of non-A, non-B hepatitis depends on exclusion of recognizable non-viral causes of hepatitis and of other hepatitis viruses including hepatitis A, hepatitis B, cytomegalovirus, herpesvirus, and Epstein-Barr virus; therefore, the prevalence of non-A, non-B hepatitis is uncertain.

Non-A, non-B hepatitis accounts for approximately 90 per cent of post-transfusion hepatitis.[9, 427–431] In addition to spread by blood and blood products, non-A, non-B hepatitis may be transmitted by non-percutaneous routes involving close personal contact. It is the cause of 20 to 40 per cent of sporadic hepatitis occurring in adults in the United States.[432] Non-A, non-B hepatitis, especially when acquired post-transfusion, often evolves into chronic hepatitis. In some series, as many as 50 to 60 per cent of patients who develop acute non-A, non-B hepatitis have elevated serum levels of aminotransferase one year after onset.[9, 427–433] Chronic hepatitis and cirrhosis may follow non-transfusion–related, sporadic non-A, non-B hepatitis, although the incidence appears to be lower than that of post-transfusion non-A, non-B hepatitis.[432, 434]

CLINICAL AND LABORATORY MANIFESTATIONS

The clinical illness associated with non-A, non-B hepatitis tends to be mild, with loss of energy and fatigue being the most prominent features.[9, 435] Aminotransferase levels are usually less than 800 IU, and a fluctuating pattern is often present, with wide variations in aminotransferase levels.[9] The majority of patients with chronic non-A, non-B hepatitis have evidence of mild CAH on liver biopsy. We have not observed a close correlation between aminotransferase levels and the histologic extent of injury. There are no clinical or biochemical findings during acute non-A, non-B hepatitis that are predictive of the subsequent development of chronic hepatitis.

HISTOLOGIC MANIFESTATIONS

The histologic lesions found in 72 patients with chronic non-A, non-B hepatitis in whom liver biopsies were performed after 6 to 12 months of elevated aminotransferase levels included CPH in 32 per cent, CAH in 46 per cent, and cirrhosis in 22 per cent.[9, 430, 436–440] The CAH resulting from non-A, non-B hepatitis is generally mild histologically and is characterized by moderate periportal piecemeal necrosis, with minimal disruption of the limiting plate and scattered foci of mononuclear cells in areas of necrosis throughout the lobule.[441–444] Bridging and multilobular necrosis are unusual. Approximately 10 to 20 per cent of patients with acute non-A, non-B hepatitis develop cirrhosis. The cirrhosis tends to be mild clinically.

Patients with sporadic non-A, non-B hepatitis usually have a histologically less severe injury than those with transfusion-related disease and are more likely to have a histologic pattern of CPH.[9, 430, 434] In a compilation of results from liver biopsies in 16 patients with sporadic non-A, non-B hepatitis, only 2 (12.5 per cent) patients had CAH. It is not known whether the substantially smaller incidence of chronic hepatitis in patients with sporadic non-A, non-B hepatitis than in those compared with transfusion-related disease results from infections with different viruses.

NON-A, NON-B HEPATITIS IN PATIENTS WITH HEMOPHILIA

Chronic non-A, non-B hepatitis is an important problem in patients with hemophilia because of the requirements for life-long administration of blood products.[445-448] Many patients with hemophilia have had multiple bouts of hepatitis caused by several viruses, including hepatitis B and non-A, non-B hepatitis, further complicating assignment of a specific etiology. In a compilation of results of hepatic histology from 155 hemophiliac patients, cirrhosis was found in 15 per cent and CAH in 7 per cent.[448] Many of these patients had chronic hepatitis secondary to infection with non-A, non-B hepatitis, hepatitis B, or (presumably, in many instances) infection with more than one viral agent.

THERAPY

There is no established specific treatment for non-A, non-B hepatitis. Corticosteroid therapy is not indicated, and there is at present no effective means for preventing the progression of the acute illness to chronic hepatitis and cirrhosis.[9] There is no convincing evidence that any form of immune globulin is useful in the prevention or treatment of non-A, non-B hepatitis.[449, 450] Treatment with low doses of recombinant human alpha interferon, in a preliminary trial, was associated with a decrease in aminotransferase levels and improvement in histology in three of ten patients after one year of therapy.[451] Patients with chronic non-A, non-B hepatitis who have manifestations of advanced liver failure or gastroesophageal bleeding are candidates for liver transplantation. Further follow-up evaluations are required to determine the frequency and importance of recurrent non-A, non-B hepatitis following transplantation.[452] There is no evidence that patients with chronic non-A, non-B hepatitis are at increased risk of developing hepatocellular carcinoma.

THERAPEUTIC AGENTS THAT INDUCE CHRONIC ACTIVE HEPATITIS
(see also Chapters 31, 32)

Several therapeutic drugs have been implicated in the production of chronic inflammatory liver disease (see also Chaps. 31 and 32).[13, 453-455] The diagnosis of drug-induced chronic liver injury is difficult because there are no specific clinical, biochemical, or histologic features. In the absence of specific diagnostic tests, the acceptance of a drug-induced etiology usually is based on improvement of the liver disease upon withdrawal of the implicated agent. Occasionally, strong support for drug-induced liver injury is provided by deliberate or inadvertent rechallenge with the drug.

Histologic findings in drug-induced chronic hepatitis may be indistinguishable from those of severe hepatic injury of other etiologies and may include dramatic portal and periportal inflammation with lymphocytes and plasma cells as well as bridging necrosis and multilobular necrosis.[30, 31] In some instances, eosinophils may be prominent.

Drug-induced chronic hepatitis from a number of diverse agents may closely resemble idiopathic autoimmune CAH.[13, 453-459] Oxyphenisatin, methyldopa, and nitrofurantoin have been incriminated most often. Less frequently, dantrolene, isoniazid, and halothane have produced histologic patterns consistent with idiopathic autoimmune CAH.

Several other drugs, including propylthiouracil and sulfonamides, have also been implicated, but less convincingly.

These drugs often have been taken for prolonged intervals, and the liver disease characteristically presents with an insidious onset. There is usually a striking predominance of females among affected patients. Serologic features that indicate autoimmune phenomena include antinuclear antibody, lupus erythematosus (LE) cells, smooth muscle antibody, anti–single-stranded DNA, and other antibodies against cell organelles. Often there is also marked hyperglobulinemia, which is largely IgG.

The treatment of drug-induced chronic hepatitis is twofold: (1) identification of the agent as the presumed cause of the liver injury and (2) removal of the agent. There is no indication that corticosteroid therapy is useful in drug-induced hepatic injury; and administration of corticosteroids while continuing the offending therapeutic drug may blunt the clinical manifestations of the illness but allow progression of the underlying process.

The major diagnostic problem in a patient with possible drug-induced hepatitis is differentiation of a drug-related injury from chronic non-A, non-B hepatitis. Often, evidence supporting a drug etiology for the illness is derived from observations following drug removal; a rapid improvement in levels of aminotransferase (deceleration) supports a drug as the cause of the injury. Most patients with drug-induced hepatic injury begin to improve clinically and biochemically within several days to weeks after withdrawal of the injurious agent.

SPECIFIC DRUGS

Oxyphenisatin

Oxyphenisatin, formerly a widely used component of laxative preparations, has been established as a cause of acute and chronic hepatic disease.[177, 456-462] More than 100 cases of hepatic injury have been identified. Once hepatoxicity from oxyphenisatin was recognized, the drug was removed from the market in the United States. Approximately two-thirds of affected patients presented with the syndrome of chronic hepatitis; the remainder had acute disease.[460]

The majority of patients with oxyphenisatin-induced liver injury were women and many had taken oxyphenisatin for longer than 6 months. In the majority of affected patients, signs and symptoms of liver disease appeared insidiously. Severe hepatic lesions were particularly likely in patients who continued taking the drug after onset of jaundice and other manifestations of liver disease.

Histologic manifestation in oxyphenisatin-induced disease ranged from those typical of acute hepatitis through the classic signs of idiopathic autoimmune CAH to frank cirrhosis. Corticosteroid therapy was not shown to be beneficial in oxyphenisatin-induced chronic hepatic injury. Resolution of the acute inflammation component of the hepatitis usually occurred rapidly following drug withdrawal. Chronic fibrotic changes and cirrhosis remained after the inflammatory component of the illness had subsided.

Nitrofurantoin

Most instances of hepatic injury from nitrofurantoin (a widely used urinary antiseptic) have been cholestatic, but hepatocellular damage has also been observed in recipients of this drug.[463–470] Histologic evidence of hepatic disease may include severe necrosis and inflammation with bridging and multilobular necrosis. More than 25 instances of CAH have been reported in recipients of nitrofurantoin.[470] Almost all patients with nitrofurantoin-induced chronic liver injury have been women. The syndrome may closely resemble idiopathic autoimmune CAH. Some patients had taken the drug for several months or up to 11 years.[463–470] The majority had taken the drug for longer than 6 months. Smooth muscle and antinuclear antibodies may be found and persist for long intervals after the drug is withdrawn. Hyperglobulinemia (especially increased IgG) may be a prominent feature. Most patients have a slow resolution of the CAH-type lesion upon withdrawal of the drug. At least three patients had HLA-B8 antigen; possibly patients with this particular HLA type are at increased risk of developing hepatic injury from nitrofurantoin.[177, 453]

Methyldopa

Methyldopa has been demonstrated to cause both acute and chronic hepatic injury.[471–477] Symptomatic hepatitis usually improves rapidly upon drug withdrawal. The majority of patients are women of middle age or older.[475, 476] In several studies, after withdrawal of methyldopa and return of biochemical studies to normal, the liver injury reappeared on rechallenge.[473, 475, 476] Methyldopa-induced hepatic necrosis may cause cirrhosis.[473] Hyperglobulinemia (especially IgG) and LE cells may be found, and Coombs' test may be positive. Because of the difficulty in differentiating methyldopa-induced injury from other types of chronic hepatitis, we recommend that the drug should not be used in any patient in whom liver injury is found.

Isoniazid (INH)

INH-induced hepatic injury occasionally may resemble idiopathic autoimmune CAH. There was scant evidence of INH-induced hepatic injury during the initial two decades of clinical use of the drug.[478–480] Despite the large number of recipients of INH, only a few instances of jaundice were attributed to the drug prior to 1972, and these were usually in patients who also had been taking other drugs.[478] In the late 1960s, INH began to be used alone as a prophylactic agent to prevent the later re-emergence of tuberculosis, and the spectrum of INH-induced hepatic injury was established. Clinical features of INH-induced liver injury usually are those typical of an acute viral hepatitis. Continued administration of INH after prodromal symptoms have appeared may enhance the severity of injury. Liver biopsy often reveals diffuse degeneration and necrosis. In a few patients, liver biopsy has shown changes consistent with CAH and cirrhosis.[478–480] Ongoing CAH after discontinuation of INH has not been reported; however, residual fibrosis may remain.

Acetaminophen

Acetaminophen in usual therapeutic doses taken over a prolonged interval has been reported to produce chronic liver damage in a few instances.[481] Bonkowsky and colleagues described chronic hepatic necrosis with inflammation and fibrosis in a man who had taken 4 grams of

acetaminophen daily for a year.[482] Following discontinuation of the drug, a fivefold elevation of aminotransferases returned to near normal. In another patient, a 59-year-old woman who had ingested 3 grams of acetaminophen daily for a year, evidence of acute and chronic liver injury was found on liver biopsy.[483] All biochemical tests returned to normal within five weeks following drug withdrawal.

Other Drugs

Other agents that have rarely been associated with chronic active hepatitis include etretinate, used to treat severe psoriasis, and dantrolene, used as a muscle relaxant.[484, 485]

WILSON'S DISEASE

Wilson's disease, *(hepatolenticular degeneration)*, a rare inherited disorder of copper metabolism, is a well-established cause of CAH and cirrhosis.[14, 15, 486–489] Patients may present with clinical and laboratory evidence of acute or chronic liver injury with no manifestations of tremor, dystonia, or other neurologic involvement. In the absence of neurologic symptoms, recognition of the correct etiology for the illness may be delayed. Wilson's disease should be considered in the differential diagnosis of CAH and cirrhosis, especially in patients who are HBsAg negative, have no history of blood transfusions or illicit drug use, and are less than 25 years of age.[14, 15] (The disease is discussed in detail in Chapter 47.)

ALPHA₁-ANTITRYPSIN DEFICIENCY AS A CAUSE OF CHRONIC LIVER DISEASE

In some adult patients, alpha$_1$-antitrypsin deficiency causes a syndrome similar in many clinical and biochemical features to CAH of other etiologies. (This disease is discussed in detail in Chapter 50.)

REFERENCES

1. Boyer JL. Chronic hepatitis—A perspective on classification and determinants of prognosis. Gastroenterology 70:1161, 1976.
2. Popper H, Schaffner F. Chronic hepatitis: Taxonomic, etiologic, and therapeutic problems. In: Popper H, Schaffner F eds. Progress in Liver Diseases, New York, Grune & Stratton, 1976:531.
3. DeGroote J, Desmet VJ, Gedigk P, et al. A classification of chronic hepatitis. Lancet 2:626, 1968.
4. Geall MG, Schoenfield LJ, Summerskill WHJ. Classification and treatment of chronic active liver disease. Gastroenterology 55:724, 1968.
5. Bianchi L, DeGroote J, Desmet VJ, et al. Morphological criteria in viral hepatitis. Review by an international group. Lancet 1:333, 1971.
6. Liaw Y-F, Chu C-M, Chen T-J, et al. Chronic lobular hepatitis: A clinicopathological and prognostic study. Hepatology 2:258, 1982.
7. Redeker AG. Viral hepatitis: Clinical aspects. Am J Med Sci 270:9, 1975.
8. Norkrans G, Hermodsson S, Lundin P, et al. The long-term outcome of hepatitis B. Infection 4:70, 1976.
9. Alter HJ. Resolved and unresolved issues in non-A, non-B hepatitis. In: Williams R, Maddrey WC, eds. Liver. Butterworths, 1984:165.
10. Cook GC, Mulligan R, Sherlock S. Controlled prospective trial of corticosteroid therapy in active chronic hepatitis. Q J Med 158:159, 1971.
11. Murray-Lyon IM, Stern RB, Williams R. Controlled trial of prednisone and azathioprine in active chronic hepatitis. Lancet 1:735, 1973.
12. Soloway RD, Summerskill WHJ, Baggenstoss AH, et al. Clinical,

biochemical, and histological remission of severe chronic active liver disease: A controlled study of treatments and early prognosis. Gastroenterology 63:820, 1972.

13. Maddrey WC, Boitnott JK. Drug-induced chronic liver disease. Gastroenterology. 72:1348, 1977.

14. Sternlieb I, Scheinberg IH. Chronic hepatitis as a first manifestation of Wilson's disease. Ann Int Med 76:59, 1972.

15. Scott J, Gollan JL, Samourian S, et al. Wilson's disease, presenting as chronic active hepatitis. Gastroenterology 74:645, 1978.

16. Sharp HL. Alpha-1 antitrypsin: An ignored protein in understanding liver disease. Sem Liv Dis 2:314, 1982.

17. Williamson JMS, Chalmers DM, Clayden AD, et al. Primary biliary cirrhosis and chronic active hepatitis: An examination of clinical, biochemical, and histopathologic features in differential diagnosis. J Clin Pathol 38:1007, 1985.

18. Geubel AP, Baggenstoss AH, Summerskill WHJ. Responses to treatment can differentiate chronic active liver disease with cholangitic features from the primary biliary cirrhosis syndrome. Gastroenterology 71:444, 1976.

19. Mistilis SP. Pericholangitis and ulcerative colitis. I. Pathology, etiology, and pathogenesis. Ann Int Med 63:1, 1965.

20. Chapman RWG, Arborgh BAM, Rhodes JM, et al. Primary sclerosing cholangitis: A review of its clinical features, cholangiography, and hepatic histology. Gut 21:870, 1980.

21. Zetterman RK, Sorrell MF. Immunologic aspects of alcoholic liver disease. Gastroenterology 81:616, 1981.

22. Zetterman RK. Alcoholic liver disease. In: Gitnick G, ed. Current Hepatology. Chicago, Year Book Medical Publishers, 1986:93–109.

23. Mills PR, Pennington TH, Kay P, et al. Hepatitis Bs antibody in alcoholic cirrhosis. J Clin Pathol 32:778, 1979.

24. Schaffner F, Thaler H. Nonalcoholic fatty liver disease. In: Popper H, Schaffner F, eds. Progress in Liver Diseases. New York, Grune & Stratton, 1986:283.

25. Chadwick RG, Galizzi J Jr, Heathcote J, et al. Chronic persistent hepatitis: Hepatitis B virus markers and histologic follow-up. Gut 20:372, 1979.

26. Boyer JL, Klatskin G. Pattern of necrosis in acute viral hepatitis. Prognostic value of bridging (subacute hepatic necrosis). N Engl J Med 283:1063, 1970.

27. Cooksley WGE, Bradbear RA, Robinson W, et al. The prognosis of chronic active hepatitis without cirrhosis in relation to bridging necrosis. Hepatology 6:345, 1986.

28. Okuno T, Okanoue T, Takino T, et al. Prognostic significance of bridging necrosis in chronic active hepatitis. Gastroenteral Jpn 18:577, 1983.

29. Combes B. The initial morphologic lesion in chronic hepatitis. Important or unimportant? Hepatology 6:518, 1986.

30. Ware AJ, Cuthbert JA, Shorey J, et al. A prospective trial of steroid therapy in severe viral hepatitis. Gastroenterology 80:219, 1981.

31. Spitz RD, Keren DF, Boitnott JK, et al. Bridging hepatic necrosis. Etiology and prognosis. Am J Dig Dis 23:1076, 1978.

32. Baggenstoss AH, Soloway RD, Summerskill WHJ, et al. The range of histologic lesions, their response to treatment, and evolution. Hum Pathol 3:183, 1972.

33. Schalm SW, Korman MG, Summerskill WHJ, et al. Severe chronic active liver disease. Prognostic significance of initial morphologic patterns. Am J Dig Dis 22:973, 1977.

34. Schalm SW, Summerskill WHJ, Gitnick GL, et al. Contrasting features and responses to treatment of severe chronic active liver disease with and without hepatitis Bs antigen. Gut 17:781, 1976.

35. Davis GL, Czaja AJ, Ludwig J. Development and prognosis of histologic cirrhosis in corticosteroid-treated hepatitis B surface antigen-negative chronic active hepatitis. Gastroenterology 87:1222, 1984.

36. Popper H. Changing concepts of the evolution of chronic hepatitis and the role of piecemeal necrosis. Hepatology 3:758, 1983.

37. Scheuer PJ. Changing views on chronic hepatitis. Histopathology 10:1, 1986.

38. Schaffner F. Management of chronic hepatitis. Sem Liv Dis 5:209, 1985.

39. Ritland S, Petlund CF, Knudsen T, et al. Improvement of physical capacity after long-term training in patients with chronic active hepatitis. Scand J Gastroenterol 18:1083, 1983.

40. Maddrey WC. Hepatic effects of acetaminophen. Enhanced toxicity in alcoholics. J Clin Gastroenterol 9:180, 1987.

41. Neuberger J, Portmann B, Calne R, et al. Recurrence of autoimmune chronic active hepatitis following orthotopic liver grafting. Transplantation 37:363, 1984.

42. Demetris AJ, Jaffe R, Sheahan DG, et al. Recurrent hepatitis B in liver allograft recipients. Differentiation between viral hepatitis B and rejection. Am J Pathol 125:161, 1986.

43. Sternlieb I. Wilson's disease: Indications for liver transplants. Hepatology 4:15S, 1984.

44. DuBois RS, Giles G, Rodgerson DO, et al. Orthotopic liver transplantation for Wilson's disease. Lancet 1:505, 1971.

45. Redeker AG. Advances in clinical aspects of acute and chronic liver disease of viral origin. In: Vyas GN, Cohen SN, and Schmid R, eds. Viral Hepatitis. Philadelphia, The Franklin Institute Press, 1978:425.

46. Jones MB, Weinstock S, Koretz RL, et al. Clinical value of serum bile acid levels in chronic hepatitis. Dig Dis Sci 26:978, 1981.

47. Czaja AJ, Ludwig J, Baggenstoss AH, et al. Corticosteroid-treated chronic active hepatitis in remission. Uncertain prognosis of chronic persistent hepatitis. N Engl J Med 304:5, 1981.

48. Becker MD, Scheuer PJ, Baptista A, et al. Prognosis of chronic persistent hepatitis. Lancet 1:53, 1970.

49. Popper H, and Schaffner F. The vocabulary of chronic hepatitis. N Engl J Med 284:1154, 1971.

50. Wilkinson SP, Portmann B, Cochrane AMG, et al. Clinical course of chronic lobular hepatitis. Report of five cases. Q J Med 188:421, 1978.

51. Mistilis SP, Skyring AP, and Blackburn CRB. Natural history of active chronic hepatitis. I. Clinical features, course, diagnostic criteria, morbidity, mortality, and survival. Aust Ann Med 17:214, 1968.

52. Mistilis SP, and Blackburn CRB. Active chronic hepatitis. Am J Med 48:484, 1970.

53. Tong MJ. Chronic hepatitis. In: Zakim D, and Boyer TD, eds. Hepatology: A Textbook of Liver Disease. Philadelphia, WB Saunders, 1982:972.

54. Czaja AJ. Natural history, clinical features, and treatment of autoimmune hepatitis. Sem Liv Dis 4:1, 1984.

55. Czaja AJ. Natural history of chronic active hepatitis. In: Czaja AJ, and Dickson ER, eds. Chronic Active Hepatitis: The Mayo Clinic Experience. New York, Marcel Dekker, Inc, 1986:9.

56. Mackinnon M, Cooksley WGE, and Smallwood RA. Chronic hepatitis: Pathogenesis and treatment. Aust NZ J Med 16:101, 1986.

57. Schaffner F. Autoimmune chronic active hepatitis: Three decades of progress. In: Popper H, and Schaffner F, eds. Progress in Liver Diseases. New York, Grune & Stratton, 1986:485.

58. Boyer JL, and Miller DJ. Chronic hepatitis. In: Schiff L, and Schiff ER, eds. Diseases of the Liver. Philadelphia, Lippincott, 1987:687.

59. Keating JJ, O'Brien CJ, Stellon AJ, et al. Influence of aetiology, clinical and histological features on survival in chronic active hepatitis: An analysis of 204 patients. Q J Med 237:59, 1987.

59a. Robertson DAF, Zhang SL, Guy EC, et al. Persistent measles virus genome in autoimmune chronic acute hepatitis. Lancet 2:9, 1987.

60. Waldenstrom J. Leber, Blutproteine und Nahrungeiweiss. Dtsch Z Verdau Stoffwechselkr 2:113, 1950.

61. Kunkel HG, Ahrens EH Jr, Eisenmenger WJ, et al. Extreme hypergammaglobulinemia in young women with liver disease of unknown etiology. J Clin Invest 30:654, 1951.

62. Zimmerman HJ, Heller P, and Hill RP. Extreme hyperglobulinemia in subacute hepatic necrosis. N Engl J Med 244:245, 1951.

63. Bearn AG, Kunkel HG, and Slater RJ. The problem of chronic liver disease in young women. Am J Med 21:3, 1956.

64. Willcox RG, and Isselbacher KJ. Chronic liver disease in young people. Am J Med 30:185, 1961.

65. Jones WA, and Castleman B. Liver disease in young women with hyperglobulinemia. Am J Pathol 40:315, 1962.

66. Read AE, Sherlock S, and Harrison CV. Active 'juvenile' cirrhosis considered as part of a systemic disease and the effect of corticosteroid therapy. Gut 4:378, 1963.

67. Reynolds TB, Edmondson HA, Peters RL, et al. Lupoid hepatitis. Ann Int Med 61:1064, 1964.

68. Maclachlan MJ, Rodnan GP, Cooper WM, et al. Chronic active ("lupoid") hepatitis. A clinical, serological, and pathological study of 20 patients. Ann Int Med 62:425, 1965.

69. Sherlock S. Waldenstrom's chronic active hepatitis. Acta Med Scand 179:426, 1966.

70. Joske RA, and King WE. The "L.E.-cell" phenomenon in active chronic viral hepatitis. Lancet 2:477, 1955.

71. Bettley FR. The "L.E. cell" phenomenon in active chronic viral hepatitis. Lancet 2:724, 1955.

72. Heller P, Zimmerman HJ, Rozengvaig S, et al. The L.E. cell phenomenon in chronic hepatic disease. N Engl J Med 254:1160, 1956.

73. Mackay IR, Taft LI, and Cowling DC. Lupoid hepatitis. Lancet 2:1323, 1956.

74. Bartholomew LG, Hagedorn AB, Cain JC, et al. Hepatitis and cirrhosis in women with positive clot tests for lupus erythematosus. N Engl J Med 259:947, 1958.

75. Aronson AR, and Montgomery MM. Chronic liver disease with a "lupus erythematosus-like syndrome." Arch Int Med 104:544, 1959.

76. Alarcon-Segovia D, Bartholomew LG, Cain JC, et al. Significance of the lupus erythematosus cell phenomenon in older women with chronic hepatic disease. Mayo Clin Proc 40:193, 1965.

77. Soloway RD, Summerskill WHJ, Baggenstoss AH, et al. "Lupoid"

hepatitis, a nonentity in the spectrum of chronic active liver disease. Gastroenterology 63:458, 1972.

78. Czaja AJ, Davis GL, Ludwig J, et al. Autoimmune features as determinants of prognosis in steroid-treated chronic active hepatitis of uncertain etiology. Gastroenterology 85:713, 1983.

79. Harvey AM, Shulman LE, Tumulty PA, et al. Systemic lupus erythematosus: Review of the literature and clinical analysis of 138 cases. Medicine 33:291, 1954.

80. Miller MH, Urowitz MB, Gladman DD, et al. The liver in systemic lupus erythematosus. Q J Med 211:401, 1984.

81. Galbraith RM, Smith M, Mackenzie RM, et al. High prevalence of seroimmunologic abnormalities in relatives of patients with active chronic hepatitis or primary biliary cirrhosis. N Engl J Med 290:63, 1974.

82. Mackay IR, Whittingham S, Mathews JD, et al. Genetic determinants of autoimmune chronic active hepatitis. Spring Sem Immunopath 3:285, 1980.

83. Mackay IR. Genetic aspects of immunologically mediated liver disease. Sem Liv Dis 4:13, 1984.

84. Mackay IR, and Wood IJ. Autoimmunity in liver disease. In: Popper H, and Schaffner F, eds. Progress in Liver Diseases. New York, Grune & Stratton, 1961:39.

85. Rakela J, and Czaja AJ. Clinical, biochemical, and histologic features of HBsAg-negative chronic active hepatitis. In: Czaja AJ, and Dickson ER, eds. Chronic Active Hepatitis: The Mayo Clinic Experience. New York, Dekker, 1986:69.

86. Lebovics E, Schaffner F, Klion FM, et al. Autoimmune chronic active hepatitis in postmenopausal women. Dig Dis Sci 30:824, 1985.

87. Martini GA, and Dolle W. Idiopathic liver cirrhosis in women during the menopause. Klin Wschr 38:13, 1960.

88. Datta DV, Sherlock S, and Scheuer PJ. Post-necrotic cirrhosis with chronic cholestasis. Gut 4:223, 1963.

89. Rodes J, Bruguera M, Bordas JM, et al. Chronic active hepatitis with features of primary biliary cirrhosis. Lancet 1:1184, 1971.

90. Cooksley WG, Powell LW, Kerr JF, et al. Cholestasis in active chronic hepatitis. Dig Dis Sci 17:495, 1972.

91. Koretz RL, Lewin KJ, Higgins J, et al. Chronic active hepatitis. Who meets treatment criteria? Dig Dis Sci 25:695, 1980.

92. Davis GL, Czaja AJ, Baggenstoss AH, et al. Prognostic and therapeutic implications of extreme serum aminotransferase elevation in chronic active hepatitis. Mayo Clin Proc 57:303, 1982.

93. Crapper RM, Bhathal PS, Mackay IR, et al. 'Acute' autoimmune hepatitis. Digest 34:216, 1986.

94. Czaja AJ, Wolf AM, and Baggenstoss AH. Clinical assessment of cirrhosis in severe chronic active liver disease. Specificity and sensitivity of physical and laboratory findings. Mayo Clin Proc 55:360, 1980.

95. Czaja AJ, Wolf AM, and Baggenstoss AH. Laboratory assessment of severe chronic active liver disease during and after corticosteroid therapy: Correlation of serum transaminase and gamma globulin level with histologic features. Gastroenterology 80:687, 1981.

96. Hahn EG. Blood analysis for liver fibrosis. J Hepatol 1:67, 1984.

97. McCullough AJ, Stassen WN, Weisner RH, et al. Serum type III procollagen peptide concentrations in severe chronic active hepatitis: Relationship to cirrhosis and disease activity. Hepatology 7:49, 1987.

98. Vento SV, Nouri-Aria KT, and Eddleston ALWF. Immune mechanisms in autoimmune chronic active hepatitis. Scand J Gastroenterol 20:91, 1985.

99. Klingenstein RJ, and Dienstag JL. Immunologic mechanisms in the initiation and maintenance of chronic active hepatitis. In: Cohen S, and Soloway RD, eds. Contemporary Issues in Gastroenterology—Chronic Active Liver Disease. New York, Churchill Livingstone, 1983:93.

100. Thomas HC, and Lok ASF. The immunopathology of autoimmune and hepatitis B virus-induced chronic hepatitis. Sem Liv Dis 4:36, 1984.

101. Meyer zum Buschenfelde KH, and Manns M. Mechanisms of autoimmune liver disease. Sem Liv Dis 4:26, 1984.

102. McFarlane IG. Autoimmunity in liver disease. Clin Sci 67:569, 1984.

103. Vogten AL, and Shorter RG. The immunologic features of chronic active hepatitis. In: Czaja AJ, and Dickson ER, eds. Chronic Active Hepatitis. The Mayo Clinic Experience. New York, Dekker, 1986.

104. Feizi T. Immunoglobulins in chronic liver disease. Gut 9:193, 1968.

105. Lee WM, Lebwohl O, and Chien S. Hyperviscosity syndrome attributable to hyperglobulinemia in chronic active hepatitis. Gastroenterology 74:918, 1978.

106. Laitinen O, and Vaheri A. Very high measles and rubella virus antibody titers associated with hepatitis, systemic lupus erythematosus and infectious mononucleosis. Lancet 1:194, 1974.

107. Triger DR. Bacterial, viral and autoantibodies in acute and chronic liver disease. Ann Clin Res 8:174, 1976.

108. Nouri-Aria KT, Hegarty JE, Alexander GJM, et al. Effect of cortico-

steroids on suppressor-cell activity in "autoimmune" and viral chronic active hepatitis. N Engl J Med 307:1301, 1982.

109. Triolo G, Nardiello S, Sagnelli E, et al. In vitro synthesis of IgG and IgM in patients with HBsAg-positive and HBsAg-negative chronic active hepatitis. Liver 3:207, 1983.

110. Holborow EJ, Asherson GL, Johnson GD, et al. Antinuclear factor and other antibodies in blood and liver diseases. Br Med J 2:656, 1963.

111. Johnson GD, Holborow EJ, and Glynn LE. Antibody to smooth muscle in patients with liver disease. Lancet 2:878, 1965.

112. Doniach D, Roitt IM, Walker JG, et al. Tissue antibodies in primary biliary cirrhosis, active chronic (lupoid) hepatitis, cryptogenic cirrhosis and other liver diseases and their clinical implications. Clin Exp Immunol 1:237, 1966.

113. Rizzetto M, Swana G, and Doniach D. Microsomal antibodies in active chronic hepatitis and other disorders. Clin Exp Immunol 15:331, 1973.

114. Gerber MA, Shapiro JM, Smith H Jr, et al. Antibodies to ribosomes in chronic active hepatitis. Gastroenterology 76:139, 1979.

115. Pedersen JS, Toh BH, Mackay IR, et al. Segregation of autoantibody to cytoskeletal filaments, actin, and intermediate filaments with two types of chronic active hepatitis. Clin Exp Immunol 48:527, 1982.

116. Kurki P, Gripenberg M, Teppo A-M, et al. Profiles of antinuclear antibodies in chronic active hepatitis, primary biliary cirrhosis and alcoholic liver disease. Liver 4:134, 1984.

117. Bernstein RM, Neuberger JM, Bunn CC, et al. Diversity of autoantibodies in primary biliary cirrhosis and chronic active hepatitis. Clin Exp Immunol 55:553, 1984.

118. Whittingham S, Morstyn G, Wilson JW, et al. An autoantibody reactive with nuclei of polymorphonuclear neutrophils: A cell differention marker. Blood 58:768, 1981.

119. Toh BH. Smooth muscle autoantibodies and autoantigens. Clin Exp Immunol 38:621, 1979.

120. Wiedmann KH, Melms A, and Berg PA. Anti-actin antibodies of IgM and IgG class in chronic liver diseases detected by fluorometric immunoassay. Liver 3:369, 1983.

121. Kenny RP, Czaja AJ, Ludwig J, et al. Frequency and significance of antimitochondrial antibodies in severe chronic active hepatitis. Dig Dis Sci 31:705, 1986.

122. Pollard KM, Steele R, Hogg S, et al. Measurement of serum DNA binding in chronic active hepatitis and systemic lupus erythematosus using the Farr assay. Rheumatol Int 6:139, 1986.

123. Wood JR, Czaja AJ, Beaver SJ, et al. Frequency and significance of antibody to double-stranded DNA in severe chronic active hepatitis. Hepatology 6:976, 1986.

124. Gurian LE, Rogoff TM, Ware AJ, et al. The immunologic diagnosis of chronic active "autoimmune" hepatitis: Distinction from systemic lupus erythematosus. Hepatology 5:397, 1985.

125. Penner E. Nature of immune complexes in autoimmune chronic active hepatitis. Gastroenterology 92:304, 1987.

126. Homberg J-C, Abuaf N, Bernard O, et al. Chronic active hepatitis associated with anti-liver/kidney microsome antibody type 1: A second type of "autoimmune" hepatitis. Hepatology 7:1333, 1987.

127. Si L, Whiteside TL, Schade RR, et al. Studies of lymphocyte subpopulations in the liver tissue and blood of patients with chronic active hepatitis (CAH). J Clin Immunol 3:408, 1983.

128. Montano L, Aranguibel F, Boffill M, et al. An analysis of the composition of the inflammatory infiltrate in autoimmune and hepatitis B virus-induced chronic liver disease. Hepatology 3:292, 1983.

129. Mariani E, Facchini A, Miglio F, et al. Analysis with OKT monoclonal antibodies of T-lymphocyte subsets present in blood and liver of patients with chronic active hepatitis. Liver 4:22, 1984.

130. Frazer IH, Mackay IR, Bell J, et al. The cellular infiltrate in the liver in auto-immune chronic active hepatitis: Analysis with monoclonal antibodies. Liver 5:162, 1985.

131. Eddleston ALWF. Immunology of chronic active hepatitis. Q J Med 55:191, 1985.

132. Kakumu S, Yata K, and Kashio T. Immunoregulatory T-cell function in acute and chronic liver disease. Gastroenterology 79:613, 1980.

133. Hotta R, Kuriki J, and Kakumu S. Loss of suppressor T-cell function and circulating immune complexes in chronic active liver diseases. Clin Exp Immunol 44:459, 1981.

134. Nonomura A, Tanino M, Kuruyama H, et al. Disordered immunoregulatory functions in patients with chronic active hepatitis. Clin Exp Immunol 47:595, 1982.

135. Vento S, Bottazzo G, Williams R, et al. Antigen specific suppressor cell function in autoimmune chronic active hepatitis. Lancet 1:1200, 1984.

136. McFarlane IG, Hegarty JE, McSorley CG, et al. Antibodies to liver-specific protein predict outcome of treatment withdrawal in autoimmune chronic active hepatitis. Lancet 2:954, 1984.

137. Meyer Zum Buschenfelde KH, and Miescher PA. Liver specific anti-

gens. Purification and characterization. Clin Exp Immunol 10:89, 1972.

138. McFarlane IG, Wojcicka BM, Zucker GM, et al. Purification and characterization of human liver-specific membrane lipoprotein (LSP). Clin Exp Immunol 27:381, 1977.

139. Riisom K, and Diederichsen H. Demonstration of organ-nonspecific antigens in liver-specific protein. Gastroenterology 85:1271, 1983.

140. Frazer IH, and Mackay IR. Antibodies to liver cell membrane antigens in chronic active hepatitis (CAH). III. Partial characterization of the liver cell membrane antigens and comparison of reactivities in sera from patients with various liver diseases. Clin Exp Immunol 57:429, 1984.

141. Frazer IH, Jordan TW, Colling EC, et al. Antibody to liver membrane antigens in chronic active hepatitis. IV. Exclusion of specific reactivity to polypeptide and glycolipids by immunoblotting. Hepatology 7:4, 1987.

142. Jensen DM, McFarlane IG, Portmann BS, et al. Detection of antibodies directed against a liver-specific membrane lipoprotein in patients with acute and chronic active hepatitis. N Engl J Med 299:1, 1978.

143. Manns M, Meyer Zum Buschenfelde KH, and Hess G. Autoantibodies against liver-specific membrane lipoprotein in acute and chronic liver diseases: Studies on organ, species, and disease specificity. Gut 21:955, 1980.

144. Mackay IR. Immunological aspects of chronic active hepatitis. Hepatology 3:724, 1983.

145. Gerber MA, Lebwohl N, and Thung SN. Liver-specific protein. How specific is it? In: Berk PD, and Chalmers TC, eds. Frontiers in Liver Disease. New York, Thieme-Stratton, 1981.

146. Hopf U, Meyer Zum Buschenfelde KH, and Dierich MP. Demonstration of binding sites for IgC Fc and the third complement component (C3) on isolated hepatocytes. J Immunol 117:639, 1976.

147. Hopf U, and Meyer Zum Buschenfelde KH. Studies on the pathogenesis of the experimental active chronic hepatitis (ACH) in rabbits. Digestion 10:306, 1974.

148. Feighery C, McDonald GSA, Greally JF, et al. Histological and immunological investigation of liver-specific protein (LSP) immunized rabbits compared with patients with liver disease. Clin Exp Immunol 45:143, 1981.

149. O'Brien CJ, Vento S, Donaldson PT, et al. Cell-mediated immunity and suppressor-T-cell defects to liver-derived antigens in families of patients with autoimmune chronic active hepatitis. Lancet 1:350, 1986.

150. Vento S, O'Brien CJ, McFarlane BM, et al. T-lymphocyte sensitization to hepatocyte antigens in autoimmune chronic active hepatitis and primary biliary cirrhosis. Gastroenterology 91:810, 1986.

151. Vento S, O'Brien CJ, McFarlane IG, et al. T-cell inducers of suppressor lymphocytes control liver-directed autoreactivity. Lancet 1:886, 1987.

152. Hopf U, Meyer Zum Buschenfelde KH, and Arnold W. Detection of a liver-membrane autoantibody in HBsAg-negative chronic active hepatitis. N Engl J Med 294:578, 1976.

153. Wiedmann KH, Bartholemew TC, Brown DJC, et al. Liver membrane antibodies detected by immunoradiometric assay in acute and chronic virus-induced and autoimmune liver disease. Hepatology 4:199, 1984.

154. Chisari FV, and Edgington TS. Lymphocyte E rosette inhibitory factor: A regulatory serum lipoprotein. J Exp Med 142:1092, 1975.

155. Chisari FV, Routenberg JA, and Edgington TS. Mechanisms responsible for defective human T lymphocyte sheep erythrocyte rosette function associated with hepatitis B virus infections. J Clin Invest 57:1227, 1976.

156. Brattig N, and Berg PA. Serum inhibitory factors (SIF) in patients with acute and chronic hepatitis and their clinical significance. Clin Exp Immunol 25:40, 1976.

157. Chisari FV, Routenberg JA, Fiala M, et al. Extrinsic modulation of human T-lymphocyte E rosette function associated with prolonged hepatocellular injury after viral hepatitis. J Clin Invest 59:134, 1977.

158. Curtiss LK, and Edgington TS. Differential sensitivity of lymphocyte subpopulations to suppression by low density lipoprotein inhibitor, an immunoregulatory human serum low density lipoprotein. J Clin Invest 63:193, 1979.

159. Sanders G, and Perrillo RP. Rosette inhibitory factor: T-lymphocyte subpopulation specificity and potential immunoregulatory role in hepatitis B virus infection. Hepatology 2:547, 1982.

160. Brattig N, and Berg PA. Immunosuppressive serum factors in viral hepatitis. I. Characterization of serum inhibition factor(s) as lymphocyte antiactivator(s). Hepatology 3:638, 1983.

161. Grauer W, Brattig NW, Schomerus H, et al. Immunosuppressive serum factors in viral hepatitis. III. Prognostic relevance of rosette inhibitory factor and serum inhibition factor in acute and chronic hepatitis. Hepatology 4:15, 1984.

162. Soloway RD, Baggenstoss AH, Schoenfield LJ, et al. Observer error

and sampling variability tested in evaluation of hepatitis and cirrhosis by liver biopsy. Dig Dis 16:1082, 1971.

163. Ammon HV. Assessment of treatment regimens. In: Czaja AJ, and Dickson ER, eds. Chronic Active Hepatitis: The Mayo Clinic Experience. New York, Dekker, 1986:33.

164. Lefkowitch JH, Apfelbaum TF, Weinberg L, et al. Acute liver biopsy lesions in early autoimmune ("lupoid") chronic active hepatitis. Liver 4:379, 1984.

165. Knodell RG, Ishak KG, Black WC, et al. Formulation and application of a numerical scoring system for assessing histological activity in asymptomatic chronic active hepatitis. Hepatology 1:431, 1981.

166. Mackay IR, and Morris PJ. Association of autoimmune active chronic hepatitis with HL-A1, 8. Lancet 2:793, 1972.

167. Galbraith RM, Eddleston ALWF, Smith MGM, et al. Histocompatibility antigens in active chronic hepatitis and primary biliary cirrhosis. Br Med J 3:604, 1974.

168. Page AR, Sharp HL, Greenberg LJ, et al. Genetic analysis of patients with chronic active hepatitis. J Clin Invest 56:530, 1975.

169. Morris PJ, Vaughan H, Tait BD, et al. Histocompatibility antigens (HLA): Associations with immunopathic diseases and with responses to microbial antigens. Aust NZ J Med 7:616, 1977.

170. Freudenberg J, Baumann H, Arnold W, et al. HLA in different forms of chronic active hepatitis. A comparison between adult patients and children. Digest 15:260, 1977.

171. Eddleston ALWF, and Williams R. HLA and liver disease. Br Med Bull 34:295, 1978.

172. Mackay IR, and Tait BD. HLA associations with autoimmune-type chronic active hepatitis: Identification of B8-DRw3 haplotype by family studies. Gastroenterology 79:95, 1980.

173. Nouri-Aria KT, Donaldson PT, Hegarty JE, et al. HLA A1-B8-DR3 and suppressor cell function in first-degree relatives of patients with autoimmune chronic active hepatitis. J Hepatol 1:235, 1985.

174. Paronetto F, and Sagnelli E. Immunologic observations in chronic active hepatitis: A disease of different etiologies. Pathobiol Ann 10:157, 1980.

175. Opelz G, Vogten AJM, Summerskill WHJ, et al. HLA determinants in chronic active liver disease: Possible relation of HLA-Dw3 to prognosis. Tiss Ant 9:36, 1977.

176. Ambinder JM, Chiorazzi N, Gibofsky A, et al. Special characteristics of cellular immune function in normal individuals of the HLA-DR3 type. Clin Immunol Immunopath 23:269, 1982.

177. Lindberg J, Lindholm U, Lundin P, et al. Trigger factors and HL-A antigens in chronic active hepatitis. Br Med J 4:77, 1975.

178. Vogten AJM, Shorter RG, and Opelz G. HLA and cell-mediated immunity in HBsAg negative chronic active hepatitis. Gut 20:523, 1979.

179. Vergani D, Larcher VF, Davies ET, et al. Genetically determined low C4: A predisposing factor to autoimmune chronic active hepatitis. Lancet 2:294, 1985.

180. Cavell B, and Leonhardt T. Hereditary hypergammaglobulinemia and lupoid hepatitis. Acta Med Scand 177:751, 1965.

181. Joske RA, and Laurence BH. Familial cirrhosis with autoimmune features and raised immunoglobulin levels. Gastroenterology 59:546, 1970.

182. Whittingham S, Mackay IR, and Kiss ZS. An interplay of genetic and environmental factors in familial hepatitis and myasthenia gravis. Gut 11:811, 1970.

183. Golding PL, Smith M, and Williams R. Multisystemic involvement in chronic liver disease. Studies of the incidence and pathogenesis. Am J Med 55:772, 1973.

184. Galbraith RM, and Fudenberg HH. Autoimmunity in chronic active hepatitis and diabetes mellitus. Clin Immunol Immunopath 8:116, 1977.

185. Culp KS, Fleming CR, Duffy J, et al. Autoimmune associations in primary biliary cirrhosis. Mayo Clin Proc 57:365, 1982.

186. Rolny P, Goobar J, and Zettergren L. HBsAg-negative chronic active hepatitis and mixed connective tissue disease syndrome. Acta Med Scand 215:391, 1984.

187. Bloom JN, Rabinowicz IM, and Shulman ST. Uveitis complicating autoimmune chronic active hepatitis. Am J Dis Child 137:1175, 1983.

188. Thompson WG, and Hart IR. Chronic active hepatitis and Graves' disease. Dig Dis 18:111, 1973.

189. Barnardo DE, Vernon-Roberts B, and Currey HLF. A case of active chronic hepatitis with painless erosive arthritis. Gut 14:800, 1973.

190. Sarkany I. Juvenile cirrhosis and allergic capillaritis of the skin. A hepato-cutaneous syndrome. Lancet 2:666, 1966.

191. Feizi T, and Gitlin N. Immune-complex disease of the kidney associated with chronic hepatitis and cryoglobulinaemia. Lancet 2:873, 1969.

192. Cuesta B, Fernandez J, Pardo J, et al. Evan's syndrome, chronic active hepatitis and focal glomerulonephritis in IgA deficiency. Acta Haemat 75:1, 1986.

193. Holdsworth CD, Hall EW, Dawson AM, et al. Ulcerative colitis in chronic liver disease. Q J Med 616:348, 1965.

194. Bradley JD, Pinals RS, and Gupta RC. Chronic active hepatitis associated with polymyositis. Association with precipitating mitochondrial M-B antibody. J Rheumatol 12:368, 1985.

195. Panush RS, Wilkinson LS, and Fagin RR. Chronic active hepatitis associated with eosinophilia and Coombs'-positive hemolytic anemia. Gastroenterology 64:1015, 1973.

196. Girino M, Riccardi A, Danova M, et al. Multisystemic disease with intracranial hypertension and autoimmune cytopenia in chronic active hepatitis. Clin Rheumatol 5:92, 1986.

197. Rebora A, and Rongioletti F. Lichen planus and chronic active hepatitis. A retrospective survey. Acta Dermatol Venereol 64:52, 1984.

198. Heer M, Joller-Jemelka H, Fontana A, et al. Monoclonal gammopathy in chronic active hepatitis. Liver 4:255, 1984.

199. Jensen DM, Papadakis M, and Payne JA. Chronic liver disease manifesting as Waldenstrom's macroglobulinemia. Arch Int Med 142:2318, 1982.

200. Turner-Warwick M. Fibrosing alveolitis and chronic liver disease. Q J Med 37:133, 1968.

201. Williams AJ, Marsh J, and Stableforth DE. Cryptogenic fibrosing alveolitis, chronic active hepatitis and autoimmune haemolytic anaemia in the same patient. Br J Dis Chest 79:200, 1985.

202. Summerskill WHJ. Chronic active liver disease reexamined: Prognosis hopeful. Gastroenterology 66:450, 1974.

203. Davis GL, and Czaja AJ. Immediate and long-term results of corticosteroid therapy for severe idiopathic chronic active hepatitis. In: Czaja AJ, and Dickson ER, eds. Chronic Active Hepatitis: The Mayo Clinic Experience. New York, Dekker, 1986:269.

204. Knodell RG. Natural history and management of asymptomatic chronic active hepatitis. In Cohen S, and Soloway RD, eds. Chronic Active Liver Disease. New York, Churchill Livingstone, 1983:33.

205. Fevery J, Desmet VJ, and DeGroote J. Long term follow-up and management of asymptomatic chronic active hepatitis. In: Cohen S, and Soloway RD, eds. Chronic Active Liver Disease. New York, Churchill Livingstone, 1983:51.

206. Wright EC, Seeff LB, Berk PD, et al. Treatment of chronic active hepatitis. An analysis of three controlled trials. Gastroenterology 73:1422, 1977.

207. Summerskill WHJ, Korman MG, Ammon HV, et al. Prednisone for chronic active liver disease: Dose titration, standard dose and combination with azathioprine compared. Gut 16:876, 1975.

208. Kirk AP, Jain S, Pocock S, et al. Late results of the Royal Free Hospital prospective controlled trial of prednisolone therapy in hepatitis B surface antigen negative chronic active hepatitis. Gut 21:78, 1980.

209. Chase WF, Winn RE, and Mayes GR. Oral pulse prednisone therapy in the treatment of HBsAg negative chronic active hepatitis. Gastroenterology 83:1292, 1982.

210. Schalm SW, Summerskill WHJ, and Go VLW. Prednisone for chronic active liver disease: Pharmacokinetics, including conversion to prednisone. Gastroenterology 72:910, 1977.

211. Renner E, Horber FF, Jost G, et al. Effect of liver function on the metabolism of prednisone and prednisolone in humans. Gastroenterology 90:819, 1986.

212. Hegarty JE, Nouri-Aria KT, Portmann B, et al. Relapse following treatment withdrawal in patients with autoimmune chronic active hepatitis. Hepatology 3:685, 1983.

213. Czaja AJ, Davis GL, and Ludwig J, et al. Complete resolution of inflammatory activity following corticosteroid treatment of HBsAg negative chronic active hepatitis. Hepatology 4:622, 1984.

214. Stellon AJ, Davies A, Compston J, et al. Bone loss in autoimmune chronic active hepatitis on maintenance corticosteroid therapy. Gastroenterology 89:1078, 1985.

215. Uribe M, Go VLW, and Kulge D. Prednisone for chronic active hepatitis: Pharmacokinetics and serum binding in patients with chronic active hepatitis and steroid major side effects. J Clin Gastroenterol 6:331, 1984.

216. Stellon AJ, Portmann B, Hegarty JE, et al. Randomised controlled trial of azathioprine withdrawal in autoimmune chronic active hepatitis. Lancet 1:668, 1985.

217. Czaja AJ, Beaver SJ, and Shiels MT. Sustained remission after corticosteroid therapy of severe hepatitis B surface antigen-negative chronic active hepatitis. Gastroenterology 92:215, 1987.

218. Czaja AJ, and Summerskill WHJ. Malignancy in chronic liver disease. Gastroenterology 73:192, 1977.

219. Hoover R, and Fraumeni JF Jr. Risk of cancer in renal-transplant recipients. Lancet 2:55, 1973.

220. McCullough AJ, and Czaja AJ. Relapse following treatment withdrawal in autoimmune chronic active hepatitis. Hepatology 4:747, 1984.

221. Mistilis SP, Vickers CR, Darroch MH, et al. Cyclosporin, a new treatment for autoimmune chronic active hepatitis. Med J Aust 143:463, 1985.

222. Wolf RE, Goldstein AL, and Ziff M. Suppression by thymosin of pokeweed mitogen-induced differentiation of human B cells. Clin Immunol Immunopath 11:303, 1978.

223. Wolf RE. Thymosin-induced suppression of proliferative response of human lymphocytes to mitogens. J Clin Invest 63:677, 1979.

224. Hegarty JE, Nouri-Aria KT, Eddleston ALWF, et al. Controlled trial of a thymic hormone extract (Thymostimulin) in 'autoimmune' chronic active hepatitis. Gut 25:279, 1984.

225. Bar-Meir S, Halpern Z, Gutman M, et al. Effect of (+)-cyanidanol-3 on chronic active hepatitis: A double blind controlled trial. Gut 26:975, 1985.

226. Stern RB, Wilkinson SP, Howorth PJN, et al. Controlled trial of synthetic D-penicillamine and prednisone in maintenance therapy for active chronic hepatitis. Gut 18:19, 1977.

227. Whelton MJ, and Sherlock S. Pregnancy in patients with hepatic cirrhosis. Management and outcome. Lancet 2:995, 1968.

228. Steven MM, Buckley JD, and Mackay IR. Pregnancy in chronic active hepatitis. Q J Med 192:519, 1979.

229. Burroughs AK, Bassendine MF, Thomas HC, et al. Primary liver cell cancer in autoimmune chronic liver disease. Br Med J 282:273, 1981.

230. Jakobovits AW, Gibson PR, and Dudley FJ. Primary liver cell carcinoma complicating autoimmune chronic active hepatitis. Dig Dis Sci 26:694, 1981.

231. Seeff LB, and Koff RS. Evolving concepts of the clinical and serologic consequences of hepatitis B virus infection. Sem Liv Dis 6:11, 1986.

232. Hoofnagle JH. Serodiagnosis of acute viral hepatitis. Hepatology 3:267, 1983.

233. Krarup NB, and Roholm K. The development of cirrhosis of the liver after acute hepatitis, elucidated by aspiration biopsy. Acta Med Scand 108:306, 1941.

234. Alsted G. Studies on malignant hepatitis. Am J Med Sci 213:257, 1947.

235. Beasley RP, Hwang L-Y, Lin C-C, et al. Incidence of hepatitis B virus infections in preschool children in Taiwan. J Inf Dis 146:198, 1982.

236. Seeff LB, Beebe GW, Hoofnagle JH, et al. A serologic follow-up of the 1942 epidemic of post-vaccination hepatitis in the United States Army. N Engl J Med 316:965, 1987.

237. Thomas HC, Lever AML, Scully LJ, et al. Approaches to the treatment of hepatitis B virus and delta-related liver disease. Sem Liv Dis 6:34, 1986.

238. Thomas HC, Montano L, Goodall A, et al. Immunological mechanisms in chronic hepatitis B virus infection. Hepatology 2:116S, 1982.

239. Thomas HC, Pignatelli M, and Scully LJ. Viruses and immune reactions in the liver. Scand J Gastroenterol S114:105, 1985.

240. Nakao M, Mizoguchi Y, Monna T, et al. Studies on an inhibitory factor to phytohemagglutinin-induced lymphocyte transformation found in the serum of patients with various liver diseases. Acta Hepato-Gastroenterol 25:335, 1978.

241. Thomas H, Shipton U, and Montano L. The HLA system: Its relevance to the pathogenesis of liver disease. In: Popper H, and Schaffner F, eds. Progress in Liver Diseases. New York, Grune & Stratton, 1982:517.

242. Doherty PC, and Zinkernagel RM. A biological role for the major histocompatibility antigens. Lancet 1:1406, 1975.

243. Montano L, Miescher GC, Goodall AH, et al. Hepatitis B virus and HLA antigen display in liver during chronic hepatitis B virus infection. Hepatology 2:557, 1982.

244. Eddleston ALWF, Mondelli M, Mieli-Vergani, G, et al. Lymphocyte cytotoxicity to autologous hepatocytes in chronic hepatitis B virus infection. Hepatology 2:122S, 1982.

245. Chu C-M, and Liaw Y-F. Intrahepatic distribution of hepatitis B surface and core antigens in chronic hepatitis B virus infection. Gastroenterology 92:220, 1987.

246. Nagafuchi Y, and Scheuer PJ. Expression of beta 2-microglobulin on hepatocytes in acute and chronic type B hepatitis. Hepatology 6:20, 1986.

247. Pignatelli M, Waters J, Brown D, et al. HLA Class I antigens on the hepatocyte membrane during recovery from acute hepatitis B virus infection and during interferon therapy in chronic hepatitis B virus infection. Hepatology 6:349, 1986.

248. Ikeda T, Lever AML, and Thomas HC. Evidence for a deficiency of interferon production in patients with chronic hepatitis B virus infection acquired in adult life. Hepatology 6:962, 1986.

249. Levin S, and Hahn T. Interferon system in acute viral hepatitis. Lancet 1:592, 1982.

250. Robinson WS, and Garcia G. Interferon and hepatitis B. Hepatology 5:336, 1985.

251. Poitrine A, Chousterman S, Chousterman M, et al. Lack of in vivo activation of the interferon system in HBsAg-positive chronic active hepatitis. Hepatology 5:171, 1985.

252. Davis GL, and Hoofnagle JH. Interferon in viral hepatitis: Role in pathogenesis and treatment. Hepatology 6:1038, 1986.

253. Eddleston ALWF, and Williams R. Inadequate antibody response to HBAg or suppressor T-cell defect in development of active chronic hepatitis. Lancet 2:1543, 1974.

254. Bianchi L, Zimmerli-Ning M, and Gudat F. Viral hepatitis. In: MacSween RNM, Anthony PP, and Scheuer PJ, eds. Pathology of the Liver. New York, Churchill Livingstone, 1979:164.

255. Chu C-M, Karayiannis P, Fowler MJF, et al. Natural history of chronic hepatitis B virus infection in Taiwan: Studies of hepatitis B virus DNA in serum. Hepatology 5:431, 1985.

256. Paz MOA, Brenes F, Karayiannis P, et al. Chronic hepatitis B virus infection. Viral replication and patterns of inflammatory activity: Serological, clinical and histologic correlations. J Hepatol 3:371, 1986.

257. Weissberg JI, Andres LL, Smith CI, et al. Survival in chronic hepatitis B. An analysis of 379 patients. Ann Int Med 101:613, 1984.

258. Bradbear RA, Robinson WN, Cooksley WGE, et al. Are the causes and presentation of chronic hepatitis changing? An analysis of 104 cases over 15 years. Q J Med 210:279, 1984.

259. Beasley RP, Hwang L-Y, Lin C-C, et al. Hepatitis B immune globulin (HBIG) efficacy in the interruption of perinatal transmission of hepatitis B virus carrier state. Initial report of a randomised double-blind placebo-controlled trial. Lancet 2:388, 1981.

260. Gocke DJ, Hsu K, Morgan C, et al. Association between polyarteritis and Australia antigen. Lancet 2:1149, 1970.

261. Baker AL, Kaplan MK, Benz WC, et al. Polyarteritis associated with Australia antigen-positive hepatitis. Gastroenterology 62:105, 1972.

262. Trepo CG, Zuckerman AJ, Bird RC, et al. The role of circulating hepatitis B antigen/antibody immune complexes in the pathogenesis of vascular and hepatic manifestations in polyarteritis nodosa. J Clin Path 27:863, 1974.

263. Duffy J, Lidsky MD, Sharp JT, et al. Polyarthritis, polyarteritis, and hepatitis B. Medicine 55:19, 1976.

264. Sergent JS, Lockshin MD, Christian CL, et al. Vasculitis with hepatitis B antigenemia: Long-term observations in nine patients. Medicine 55:1, 1976.

265. Drueke T, Barbanel C, Jungers P, et al. Hepatitis B antigen-associated periarteritis nodosa in patients undergoing long-term hemodialysis. Am J Med 68:86, 1980.

266. Naber AHJ, De Vlaam AM, and Breed WPM. Chronic active hepatitis and periarteritis nodosa in a patient with co-occurrence of circulatory hepatitis Bs antigen and anti-HBs. Neth J Med 29:189, 1986.

267. Surrenti C, Ambu S, Patussi V, et al. Diagnostic significance of anti-HBc IgM (RIA) in healthy HBsAg carriers and in chronic hepatitis B. J Med Virol 18:229, 1986.

268. Ben-Porath E, Wands J, Gruia M, et al. Clinical significance of enhanced detection of HBsAg by a monoclonal radioimmunoassay. Hepatology 4:803, 1984.

269. Brechot C, Degos F, Lugassy C, et al. Hepatitis B virus DNA in patients with chronic liver disease and negative tests for hepatitis B surface antigen. N Engl J Med 312:270, 1985.

270. Zeldis JB, Ben-Porath E, Enat R, et al. Correlation of HBV DNA and monoclonal reactivity with HBsAg in serum of patients with HBV infection. Virol Med 14:153, 1986.

271. Vischer TL. Australia antigen and autoantibodies in chronic hepatitis. Br Med J 2:695, 1970.

272. Wright R. Australia antigen and smooth-muscle antibody in acute and chronic hepatitis. Lancet 1:521, 1970.

273. Finlayson NDC, Krohn K, Anderson KE, et al. Interrelations of hepatitis B antigen and autoantibodies in chronic idiopathic liver disease. Gastroenterology 63:646, 1972.

274. Mackay IR, and Popper H. Immunopathogenesis of chronic hepatitis: A review. Aust NZ J Med 1:79, 1973.

275. Mathews JD, and Mackay IR. Australia antigen in chronic hepatitis in Australia. Br Med J 1:259, 1970.

276. Kater L, Van Den Tweel JG, Lourens J, et al. H.A.A. and A.N.A. in chronic active hepatitis. Lancet 1:598, 1971.

277. Kew MC, Purves LR, and Bersohn I. Serum alpha-fetoprotein levels in acute viral hepatitis. Gut 14:939, 1973.

278. Silver HKB, Gold P, Shuster J, et al. Alpha-fetoprotein in chronic liver disease. N Engl J Med 291:506, 1974.

279. Karvountzis GG, and Redeker AG. Relation of alpha-fetoprotein in acute hepatitis to severity and prognosis. Ann Int Med 80:156, 1974.

280. Bloomer JR, Waldmann TA, McIntire KR, et al. Serum alpha-fetoprotein in patients with massive hepatic necrosis. Gastroenterology 72:479, 1977.

281. Eleftheriou N, Heathcote J, Thomas HC, et al. Serum alpha-fetoprotein levels in patients with acute and chronic liver disease. J Clin Path 30:704, 1977.

282. Liaw Y-F, Tai D-I, Chen T-J, et al. Alpha-fetoprotein changes in the course of chronic hepatitis: Relation to bridging hepatic necrosis and hepatocellular carcinoma. Liver 6:133, 1986.

283. Blumberg BS, Sutnick AI, London WT, et al. Sex distribution of Australia antigen. Arch Int Med 130:227, 1972.

284. Klatskin G. Persistent HB antigenemia: Associated clinical manifestations and hepatic lesions. Am J Med Sci 270:33, 1975.

285. Peters RL. Viral hepatitis: A pathologic spectrum. Am J Med Sci 270:17, 1975.

286. Szmuness W, Prince AM, Grady GF, et al. Hepatitis B infection: A point-prevalence study in 15 US hemodialysis centers. JAMA 227:901, 1974.

287. Drew JS, London WT, Lustbader ED, et al. Cross reactivity between hepatitis B surface antigen and a male-associated antigen. Birth Defects 15:91, 1978.

288. Novick DM, Lok ASF, and Thomas HC. Diminished responsiveness of homosexual men to antiviral therapy for HBsAg-positive chronic liver disease. J Hepatol 1:29, 1984.

289. Stevens CE, Neurath RA, Beasley RP, et al. HBeAg and anti-HBe detection by radioimmunoassay: Correlation with vertical transmission of hepatitis B virus in Taiwan. J Med Virol 3:237, 1979.

290. Beasley RP, Hwayg L-Y, Lin C-C, et al. Incidence of hepatitis among students at a university in Taiwan. Am J Epidem 117:213, 1983.

291. McMahon BJ, Alward WLM, Hall DB, et al. Acute hepatitis B virus infection: Relation of age to the clinical expression of disease and subsequent development of the carrier state. J Inf Dis 151:599, 1985.

292. London WT, DiFiglia M, Sutnick AI, et al. An epidemic of hepatitis in a chronic hemodialysis unit: Australia antigen and differences in host response. N Engl J Med 281:571, 1969.

293. London WT, Drew JS, Lustbader ED, et al. Host reponses to hepatitis B infection in patients in a chronic hemodialysis unit. Kidney Int 12:51, 1977.

294. Dusheiko G, Song E, Bowyer S, et al. Natural history of hepatitis B virus infection in renal transplant recipients—A fifteen-year follow-up. Hepatology 3:330, 1983.

295. Dietzman DE, Harnisch JP, Ray CG, et al. Hepatitis B surface antigen (HBsAg) and antibody to HBsAg. Prevalence in homosexual and heterosexual men. JAMA 238:2625, 1977.

296. Shah N, Ostrow D, Altman N, et al. Evolution of acute hepatitis B in homosexual men to chronic hepatitis B: Prospective study of placebo recipients in a hepatitis B vaccine trial. Arch Int Med 145:881, 1985.

297. Moestrup T, Hansson BG, Widell A, et al. Long-term follow-up of chronic hepatitis B virus infection in intravenous drug abusers and homosexual men. Brit Med J 292:854, 1986.

298. Mosley JW, Redeker AG, Feinstone SM, et al. Multiple hepatitis viruses in multiple attacks of acute viral hepatitis. N Engl J Med 296:75, 1977.

299. Hindman SH, Maynard JE, Bradley DW, et al. Simultaneous infection with type A and B hepatitis viruses. Am J Epidem 105:135, 1977.

300. Willson RA. Intercurrent hepatitis A in B viral hepatitis. JAMA 245:2495, 1981.

301. Viola LA, Barrison IG, Coleman JC, et al. The clinical course of acute type A hepatitis in chronic HBsAg carriers—A report of 3 cases. Postgrad Med J 58:80, 1982.

302. Piazza M, Guadagnino V, Orlando R, et al. Acute B viral hepatitis becomes fulminant after infection with hepatitis A virus. Br Med J 284:1913, 1982.

303. Conteas C, Kao H, Rakela J, et al. Acute type A hepatitis in three patients with chronic HBV infection. Dig Dis Sci 28:684, 1983.

304. Zachoval R, Roggendorf M, and Deinhardt F. Hepatitis A infection in chronic carriers of hepatitis B virus. Hepatology 3:528, 1983.

305. Davis GL, Hoofnagle JH, and Waggoner JG. Acute type A hepatitis during chronic hepatitis B virus infection: Association of depressed hepatitis B virus replication with appearance of endogenous alpha interferon. J Med Virol 14:141, 1984.

306. Tsiquaye KN, Portmann B, Tovey G, et al. Non-A, non-B hepatitis in persistent carriers of hepatitis B virus. J Med Virol 11:179, 1983.

307. Davis GL, Hoofnagle JH, and Waggoner JG. Spontaneous reactivation of chronic hepatitis B virus infection. Gastroenterology 86:230, 1984.

308. Davis GL, and Hoofnagle JH. Reactivation of chronic type B hepatitis presenting as acute viral hepatitis. Ann Int Med 102:762, 1985.

309. Perrillo RP, Campbell CR, Sanders GE, et al. Spontaneous clearance and reactivation of hepatitis B virus infection among male homosexuals with chronic type B hepatitis. Ann Int Med 100:43, 1984.

310. Kryger P, Mathiesen LR, Aldershvile J, et al. Presence and meaning of anti-HBc IgM as determined by ELISA in patients with acute type B hepatitis and healthy HBsAg carriers. Hepatology 1:233, 1981.

311. Wands JR, Chura CM, Roll FJ, et al. Serial studies of hepatitis-associated antigen and antibody in patients receiving antitumor

chemotherapy for myeloproliferative and lymphoproliferative disorders. Gastroenterology 68:105, 1975.

312. Galbraith RM, Eddleston ALWF, Williams R, et al. Fulminant hepatic failure in leukaemia and choriocarcinoma related to withdrawal of cytotoxic drug therapy. Lancet 2:528, 1975.

313. Lightdale CJ, Ikram H, and Pinsky C. Primary hepatocellular carcinoma with hepatitis B antigenemia: Effects of chemotherapy. Cancer 46:1117, 1980.

314. Sagnelli E, Manzillo G, Maio G, et al. Serum levels of hepatitis B surface and core antigens during immunosuppressive treatment of HBsAg-positive chronic active hepatitis. Lancet 2:395, 1980.

315. Scullard GH, Smith CI, Merigan TC, et al. Effects of immunosuppressive therapy on viral markers in chronic active hepatitis B. Gastroenterology 81:987, 1981.

316. Villa E, Theodossi A, Portmann B, et al. Reactivation of hepatitis B virus infection in two patients: Immunofluorescence studies of liver tissue. Gastroenterology 80:1048, 1981.

317. Hoofnagle JH, Dusheiko GM, Schafer DF, et al. Reactivation of chronic hepatitis B virus infection by cancer chemotherapy. Ann Int Med 96:447, 1982.

318. Nowicki MJ, Tong MJ, Nair PV, et al. Detection of anti-HBc IgM following prednisone treatment in patients with chronic active hepatitis B virus infection. Hepatology 4:1129, 1984.

319. Locasciulli A, Santamaria M, Masera G, et al. Hepatitis B virus markers in children with acute leukemia: The effect of chemotherapy. J Med Virol 15:29, 1985.

320. Davis GL, Czaja AJ, Taswell HF, et al. Hepatitis B virus replication in steroid-treated severe HBsAg-positive chronic active hepatitis. Dig Dis Sci 30:97, 1985.

321. Nagington J, Cossart YE, and Cohen BJ. Reactivation of hepatitis B after transplantation operations. Lancet 1:558, 1977.

322. Duskeiko G, Song E, Bowyer S, et al. Natural history of hepatitis B virus infection in renal transplant recipients—A fifteen-year follow-up. Hepatology 3:330, 1983.

323. Rakela J, Redeker AG, and Weliky B. Effect of short-term prednisone therapy on aminotransferase levels and hepatitis B virus markers in chronic type B hepatitis. Gastroenterology 84:956, 1983.

324. Hoofnagle JH, Davis GL, Pappas SC, et al. A short course of prednisolone in chronic type B hepatitis. Ann Int Med 104:12, 1986.

325. Smedile A, Dentico P, Zanetti A, et al. Infection with the delta agent in chronic HBsAg carriers. Gastroenterology 81:992, 1981.

326. Smedile A, Farci P, Verme G, et al. Influence of delta infection on severity of hepatitis B. Lancet 2:945, 1982.

327. Farci P, Smedile A, Lavarini C, et al. Delta hepatitis in inapparent carriers of hepatitis B surface antigen: A disease simulating acute hepatitis B progressing to chronicity. Gastroenterology 85:669, 1983.

328. Govindarajan S, Kanel GC, and Peters RL. Prevalance of delta antibody among chronic hepatitis B-virus infected patients in the Los Angeles area: Its correlation with liver biopsy diagnosis. Gastroenterology 85:160, 1983.

329. Rizzetto M. The delta agent. Hepatology 3:729, 1983.

330. Rizzetto M, Verme G, Recchia S, et al. Chronic hepatitis in carriers of hepatitis B surface antigen, with intrahepatic expression of the delta antigen: An active and progressive disease unresponsive to immunosuppressive treatment. Ann Int Med 98:437, 1983.

331. Ponzetto A, Seeff LB, Buskell-Bales Z, et al. Hepatitis B markers in United States drug addicts with special emphasis on the delta hepatitis virus. Hepatology 4:1111, 1984.

332. Purcell RH, Rizzetto M, and Gerin JL. Hepatitis delta virus infection of the liver. Sem Liv Dis 4:340, 1984.

333. Govindarajan S, Valinluck B, and Peters L. Relapse of acute B viral hepatitis—Role of delta agent. Gut 27:19, 1986.

334. Shiels MT, Czaja AJ, Taswell HF, et al. Frequency and significance of delta antibody in acute and chronic hepatitis B. A United States experience. Gastroenterology 89:1230, 1985.

335. Chen L-K, Mathieu-Mahul D, Bach FH, et al. Recombinant interferon a can induce rearrangement of T-cell antigen receptor a-chain genes and maturation to cytotoxicity in T-lymphocyte clones in vitro. Proc Natl Acad Sci 83:4887, 1986.

336. Kos A, Dijkema R, Arnberg AC, et al. The hepatitis delta virus possesses a circular RNA. Nature 323:558, 1986.

337. Chu C-M, Parci P, Liaw Y-F, et al. The role of delta superinfection in acute exacerbations of chronic type B hepatitis. Liver 6:26, 1986.

338. Krogsgaard K, Kryger P, Aldershvile J, et al. Delta-infection and suppression of hepatitis B virus replication in chronic HBsAg carriers. Hepatology 7:42, 1987.

339. De Cock KM, Govindarajan S, and Redeker AG. Fulminant delta hepatitis in chronic hepatitis B infection. JAMA 252:2746, 1984.

340. Buti M, Esteban R, Jardi R, et al. Serological diagnosis of acute delta hepatitis. J Med Virol 18:81, 1986.

341. Aragona M, Macagno S, Caredda F, et al. Serological response to the hepatitis delta virus in hepatitis D. Lancet 1:478, 1987.

342. Sheen I-S, Liaw Y-F, Tai D-I, et al. Hepatic decompensation associated with hepatitis B e antigen clearance in chronic type B hepatitis. Gastroenterology 89:732, 1985.

343. Hoofnagle JH, Dusheiko GM, Seeff LB, et al. Seroconversion from hepatitis B e antigen to antibody in chronic type B hepatitis. Ann Int Med 94:744, 1981.

344. Viola LA, Barrison IG, Coleman JC, et al. The HBe antigen-antibody system and its relationship to clinical and laboratory findings in 100 chronic HBsAg carriers in Great Britain. J Med Virol 8:169, 1981.

345. Hoofnagle JH, Seeff LB. Natural history of chronic type B hepatitis. In: Popper H, Schaffner F, eds. Progress in Liver Diseases. New York, Grune & Stratton, 1982:469.

346. Schalm SW, Heijtink RA. Spontaneous disappearance of viral replication and liver cell inflammation in HBsAg-positive chronic active hepatitis: Results of a placebo vs. interferon trial. Hepatology 2:791, 1982.

347. Liaw Y-F, Chu C-M, Su I-J, et al. Clinical and histological events preceding hepatitis B e antigen seroconversion in chronic type B hepatitis. Gastroenterology 84:216, 1983.

348. Liaw Y-F, Chu CM, Huang M-J, et al. Determinants for hepatitis B e antigen clearance in chronic type B hepatitis. Liver 4:301, 1984.

349. Alward WLM, McMahon BJ, Hall DB, et al. The long-term serological course of asymptomatic hepatitis B virus carriers and the development of primary hepatocellular carcinoma. J Inf Dis 151:604, 1985.

350. Tong MJ, Stevenson D, Gordon I. Correlation of e antigen, DNA polymerase activity, and dane particles in chronic benign and chronic active type B hepatitis infections. J Inf Dis 135:980, 1977.

351. Perrillo RP, Campbell CR, Sanders GE, et al. Spontaneous clearance and reactivation of hepatitis B virus infection among male homosexuals with chronic type B hepatitis. Ann Int Med 100:43, 1984.

352. Realdi G, Alberti A, Rugge M, et al. Seroconversion from hepatitis B e antigen to anti-HBe in chronic hepatitis B virus infection. Gastroenterology 79:195, 1980.

353. Gregory PB. Treatment of chronic viral hepatitis. In: Vyas G, Dienstag JL, Hoofnagle JH, eds. Viral Hepatitis and Liver Disease. New York, Grune and Stratton, 1984:123.

354. Sherlock S, Thomas HC. Treatment of chronic hepatitis due to hepatitis B virus. Lancet 2:1343, 1985.

355. Thomas HC, Scully LJ. Antiviral therapy in hepatitis B infection. Br Med Bull 41:374, 1985.

356. Morgan TR, Redeker AG, Yamada S, et al. HBsAg clearance in chronic hepatitis B. A possible cause of cryptogenic cirrhosis. Dig Dis Sci 31:700, 1986.

357. Poralla T, Manns M, Hutteroth TH, et al. HBsAg clearance in patients with long-standing chronic active hepatitis B and hepatitis B virus-induced liver cirrhosis. Digestion 33:53, 1986.

358. Nash AA. Tolerance and suppression in virus diseases. Br Med Bull 41:41, 1985.

359. Lam KC, Lai CL, Trepo C, et al. Deleterious effect of prednisolone in HBsAg-positive chronic active hepatitis. N Engl J Med 304:380, 1981.

360. Conn HO, Maddrey WC, Soloway RD. The detrimental effects of adrenocorticosteroid therapy in HBsAg-positive chronic active hepatitis: Fact or artifact? Hepatology 2:885, 1982.

361. Wu PC, Lai CL, Lam KC, et al. Prednisolone in HBsAg-positive chronic active hepatitis: histologic evaluation in a controlled prospective study. Hepatology 2:777, 1982.

362. Tygstrup N, Andersen PK, Juhl E, et al. Steroids in chronic B-hepatitis. A randomized, double-blind, multinational trial on the effect of low-dose, long-term treatment on survival. Liver 6:227, 1986.

363. Alberti A, Pontisso P, Fattovich G, et al. Changes in serum hepatitis B virus (HBV) DNA positivity in chronic HBV infection: Results of a long-term follow-up study of 138 patients. J Inf Dis 154:562, 1986.

364. Sagnelli E, Piccinino F, Manzillo G, et al. Effect of immunosuppressive therapy on HBsAg-positive chronic active hepatitis in relation to presence or absence of HBeAg and anti-HBe. Hepatology 3:690, 1983.

365. Nair PV, Tong MJ, Stevenson D, et al. Effects of short-term, high-dose prednisone treatment of patients with HBsAg-positive chronic hepatitis. Liver 5:8, 1985.

366. Peters M, Davis GL, Dooley JS, et al. The interferon system in acute and chronic viral hepatitis. In: Popper H, Schaffner F, eds. Progress in Liver Diseases. New York, Grune & Stratton, 1986:453.

367. Stiehm ER, Kronenberg LH, Rosenblatt HM, et al. Interferon: Immunobiology and clinical significance. Ann Int Med 96:80, 1982.

368. Eddleston A. Interferons in the treatment of chronic hepatitis B virus infection. Med Clin North Am 5S:25, 1986.

369. Toy JL. The interferons. Clin Exp Immunol 54:1, 1983.

370. Grossberg SE. The interferons and their inducers: Molecular and therapeutic considerations. N Engl J Med 287:13, 1972.

371. Landolfo S, DiMatteo C, Capusso A, et al. Lymphokine production in primary mixed lymphocyte reactions. I. Characteristics of responding and stimulating cells. Exp Cell Biol 48:180, 1980.

372. Branca AA, Baglioni C. Evidence that types I and II interferons have different receptors. Nature 294:768, 1981.

373. Wheelock EF, Schenker S, Combes B. Absence of circulating interferon in patients with infectious and serum hepatitis. Proc Soc Biol Med 128:251, 1968.

374. Heron I, Hokland M, Berg K. Enhanced expression of beta-2 microglobulin and HLA antigens on human lymphoid cells by interferon. Proc Natl Acad Sci USA 75:6215, 1978.

375. Lengyel P. Mechanisms of interferon action: the $(2'5')$ $(A)_n$ synthetase-RNase L pathway. In: Gresser I, ed. Interferon 3. New York, Academic Press, 1981:77.

376. Dusheiko G, Dibisceglie A, Bowyer S, et al. Recombinant leukocyte interferon treatment of chronic hepatitis B. Hepatology 5:556, 1985.

377. Pirovino M, Aguet M, Huber M, et al. Absence of detectable serum interferon in acute and chronic viral hepatitis. Hepatology 6:645, 1986.

378. Mondelli MU, Alberti A, Realdi G, et al. In vitro effect of lymphoblastoid alpha-interferon on subpopulations of effector cells mediating cytotoxicity for autologous hepatocytes in hepatitis B and non-A, non-B. Int J Immunopharmac 8:887, 1986.

379. Nagafuchi Y, Scheuer PJ. Expression of Beta-2 microglobulin on hepatocytes in acute and chronic type B hepatitis. Hepatology 6:20, 1986.

380. Peters M, Walling DM, Kelly K, et al. Immunologic effects of interferon-a in man: Treatment with human recombinant interferon-a suppresses in vitro immunoglobulin production in patients with chronic type B hepatitis. J Immunol 137:3147, 1986.

381. Gregory PB. Interferon in chronic hepatitis B. Gastroenterology 90:237, 1986.

382. Weimar W, Heijtink RA, Schalm SW, et al. Fibroblast interferon in HBsAg-positive chronic active hepatitis. Lancet 2:1282, 1977.

383. Kingham JGC, Ganguly NK, Shaari ZD, et al. Treatment of HBsAg-positive chronic active hepatitis with human fibroblast interferon. Gut 19:91, 1978.

384. Eisenberg M, Rosno S, Garcia G, et al. Preliminary trial of recombinant fibroblast interferon in chronic hepatitis B virus infection. Antimicrob Ag Chemother 29:122, 1986.

385. Welsh RM, Hallenbeck LA. Effect of virus infections on target cell susceptibility to natural killer cell-mediated lysis. J Immunol 124:2491, 1980.

386. Dongworth DW, McMichael AJ. Inhibition of human T lymphocyte function with monoclonal antibodies. Br Med Bull 40:254, 1984.

387. Blackman MJ, Morris AG. The effect of interferon treatment of targets on susceptibility to cytotoxic T-lymphocyte killing: Augmentation of allogeneic killing and virus-specific killing relative to viral antigen expression. Immunology 56:451, 1985.

388. Jilbert AR, Burrell CJ, Gowans EJ, et al. Cellular localization of alpha-interferon in hepatitis B virus-infected liver tissue. Hepatology 6:957, 1986.

389. Thomas HC, Pignatelli M, Lever AML. Homology between HBV-DNA and a sequence regulating the interferon-induced antiviral system: Possible mechanism of persistent infection. J Med Virol 19:63, 1986.

390. Jicha DL, Davis GL, Peters MG, et al. Effects of recombinant human leukocyte interferon treatment of endogenous interferon production in patients with chronic type-B hepatitis. J Interfer Res 6:13, 1986.

391. Greenberg HB, Pollard RB, Lutwick LI, et al. Effect of human leukocyte interferon on hepatitis B virus infection in patients with chronic active hepatitis. N Engl J Med 295:517, 1976.

392. Lok ASF, Weller IVD, Karayiannis P, et al. Thrice weekly lymphoblastoid interferon is effective in inhibiting hepatitis B virus replication. Liver 4:45, 1984.

393. Omata M, Imazeki F, Yokosuka O, et al. Recombinant leukocyte A interferon treatment in patients with chronic hepatitis B virus infection. Gastroenterology 88:870, 1985.

394. Dooley JS, Davis GL, Peters M, et al. Pilot study of recombinant human alpha-interferon for chronic type B hepatitis. Gastroenterology 90:150, 1986.

395. Hess G, Meyer Zum Buschenfelde KH. Modification of hepatitis B virus infection by recombinant leukocyte alpha A interferon. Immunobiology 172:255, 1986.

396. Schattner A, Wallach D, Merlin G, et al. Variation of $(2'-5')$ oligo A synthetase level in lymphocytes and granulocytes of patients with viral infections and leukaemia. J Interferon Res 2:355, 1982.

397. Grimley PM, Davis GL, Kang Y-H, et al. Tubuloreticular inclusions in peripheral blood mononuclear cells related to systemic therapy with alpha interferon. Lab Invest 52:638, 1985.

398. Ikeda I, Pignatelli M, Lever AML, et al. Relationship of HLA protein display to activation of 2-5A synthetase in HBe antigen or anti-HBe positive chronic HBV infection. Gut 27:1498, 1986.

399. Weller IVD, Lok ASF, Mindel A, et al. Randomised controlled trial of adenine arabinoside 5'-monophosphate (ARA-AMP) in chronic hepatitis B virus infection. Gut 26:745, 1985.

400. Bassendine MF, Chadwick RG, Salmeron J, et al. Adenine arabinoside therapy in HBsAg-positive chronic liver disease: A controlled study. Gastroenterology 80:1016, 1981.

401. Scullard GH, Andres LL, Greenberg HB, et al. Antiviral treatment of chronic hepatitis B virus infection: Improvement in liver disease with interferon and adenine arabinoside. Hepatology 1:228, 1981.

402. Smith CI, Kitchen LW, Scullard GH, et al. Vidarabine monophosphate and human leukocyte interferon in chronic hepatitis B infection. JAMA 247:2261, 1982.

403. Hoofnagle JH, Hanson RG, Minuk GY, et al. Randomized controlled trial of adenine arabinoside monophosphate for chronic type B hepatitis. Gastroenterology 86:150, 1984.

404. Yokosuka O, Omata M, Imazeki F, et al. Combination of short-term prednisolone and adenine arabinoside in the treatment of chronic hepatitis B. A controlled study. Gastroenterology 89:246, 1985.

405. Perrillo RP, Regenstein FG, Bodicky CJ, et al. Comparative efficacy of adenine arabinoside 5' monophosphate and prednisone withdrawal followed by adenine arabinoside 5' monophosphate in the treatment of chronic active hepatitis type B. Gastroenterology 88:780, 1985.

406. Lok ASF, Novick DM, Karayiannis P, et al. A randomized study of the effects of adenine arabinoside 5' monophosphate (short or long courses) and lymphoblastoid interferon on hepatitis B virus replication. Hepatology 5:1132, 1985.

407. Hoofnagle JH, Davis GL, Hanson RG, et al. Treatment of chronic type B hepatitis with multiple ten-day courses of adenine arabinoside monophosphate. J Med Virol 15:121, 1985.

408. Guardia J, Esteban R, Buti M, et al. Prolonged inhibition of hepatitis-B virus replication with vidarabine monophosphate in chronic active type-B hepatitis. Liver 6:118, 1986.

409. Weller IVD, Carreno V, Fowler MJF, et al. Acyclovir in hepatitis B antigen-positive chronic liver disease: Inhibition of viral replication and transient renal impairment with iv bolus administration. J Antimicrob Chemother 11:223, 1983.

410. Schalm SW, Van Buuren HR, Heytink RA, et al. Acyclovir enhances the antiviral effect of interferon in chronic hepatitis B. Lancet 2:358, 1985.

411. Alexander GJM, Fagan EA, Hegarty JE, et al. Controlled clinical trial of acyclovir in chronic hepatitis B virus infection. J Med Virol 21:81, 1987.

412. Loke RHT, Anderson MG, Coleman JC, et al. Suramin treatment for chronic active hepatitis B—toxic and ineffective. J Med Virol 21:97, 1987.

413. Nilius R, Schentke U, Otto L, et al. Levamisole therapy in chronic hepatitis—Results of a multicentric double blind trial. Hepato-Gastroenterol 30:90, 1983.

414. Fattovich G, Brollo L, Pontisso P, et al. Levamisole therapy in chronic type B hepatitis. Results of a double-blind randomized trial. Gastroenterology 91:692, 1986.

415. Sodomann C-P, Maerker-Alzer G, Havemann K, et al. Transfer factor (TF) treatment of patients with HBsAg-positive chronic active hepatitis. Klin Wochenshrift 57:893, 1979.

416. Shulman ST, Hutto JH, Ayoub EM, et al. A double-blind evaluation of transfer factor therapy of HBsAg-positive chronic aggressive hepatitis: Preliminary report of efficacy. Cell Immunol 43:352, 1979.

417. Piazza M, De Mercato R, Guadagnino V, et al. Effect of (+)-cyanidanol-3 on chronic persistent and chronic active hepatitis. In: Conn HO, ed. (+)-Cyanidanol-3 in Diseases of the Liver, International Workshop. New York, Academic Press, 1981:123.

418. Keeling PWN, Viola L, Anderson MG, et al. Trial of (+)-cyanidanol-3 in patients with hepatitis B chronic liver disease. J Royal Soc Med 79:460, 1986.

419. Suzuki H, Yamamoto S, Hirayama C, et al. Cianidanol therapy for HBe-antigen-positive chronic hepatitis: A multicentre, double-blind study. Liver 6:35, 1986.

420. Bodenheimer HC Jr, Schaffner F, Vernace S, et al. Randomized controlled trial of Quinacrine for the treatment of HBsAg-positive chronic hepatitis. Hepatology 3:936, 1983.

421. Dudley FJ, Scheuer PJ, Sherlock S. Natural history of hepatitis-associated antigen-positive chronic liver disease. Lancet 2:1388, 1972.

422. Brechot C, Nalpas B, Courouce A-M, et al. Evidence that hepatitis B virus has a role in liver-cell carcinoma in alcoholic liver disease. N Engl J Med 306:1384, 1982.

423. Ohnishi K, Iida S, Iwama S, et al. The effect of chronic habitual alcohol intake on the development of liver cirrhosis and hepatocellular carcinoma. Relation to hepatitis B surface antigen carriage. Cancer 49:672, 1982.

424. Kew MC. The hepatitis-B virus and hepatocellular carcinoma. Sem Liv Dis 1:59, 1981.

425. Beasley RP, Lin C-C, Chien C-S, et al. Geographic distribution of HBsAg carriers in China. Hepatology 2:553, 1982.

426. Shafritz DA, Shouval D, Sherman HI, et al. Integration of hepatitis B virus DNA into the genome of liver cells in chronic liver disease and hepatocellular carcinoma: Studies in percutaneous liver biopsies and post-mortem tissue specimens. N Engl J Med 305:1067, 1981.

427. Dienstag JL. Non-A non-B Hepatitis. I. Recognition, epidemiology and clinical features. Gastroenterology 85:439, 1983.

428. Dienstag JL. Non-A non-B Hepatitis. II. Experimental transmission, putative virus agents and markers, and prevention. Gastroenterology 85:743, 1983.

429. Alter HJ. The dominant role of non-A, non-B in the pathogenesis of post-transfusion hepatitis: A clinical assessment. Clin Gastroenterol 9:155, 1980.

430. Shih W-K, Esteban Mur JI, Alter HJ. Non-A, non-B hepatitis: Advances and unfulfilled expectations of the first decade. In: Popper H, Schaffner F, eds. Progress in Liver Diseases. New York, Grune & Stratton, 1986:433.

431. Aach RD, Szmuness W, Mosley JW, et al. Serum alanine aminotransferase of donors in relation to the risk of non-A, non-B hepatitis in recipients: The transfusion-transmitted viruses study. N Engl J Med 304:989, 1981.

432. Alter MJ, Gerety RJ, Smallwood LA, et al. Sporadic non-A, non-B hepatitis: Frequency and epidemiology in an urban U. S. population. J Inf Dis 145:886, 1982.

433. Koretz RL, Stone O, Gitnick GL. The long-term course of non-A, non-B post-transfusion hepatitis. Gastroenterology 79:893, 1980.

434. Mathieson RD, Sampliner RE, Latham PS, et al. Chronic liver disease following community-acquired non-A, non-B hepatitis. Am J Clin Path 85:353, 1986.

435. Tabor E, Seeff LB, Gerety RJ. Chronic non-A, non-B hepatitis carrier state. N Engl J Med 303:140, 1980.

436. Knodell RG, Conrad ME, Ishak KG. Development of chronic liver disease after acute non-A, non-B post-transfusion hepatitis: role of gammaglobulin prophylaxis in its prevention. Gastroenterology 72:902, 1977.

437. Rakela J, Redeker AG. Chronic liver disease after acute non-A, non-B viral hepatitis. Gastroenterology 77:1200, 1979.

438. Omata M, Iwama S, Sumida M, et al. Clinico-pathological study of acute non-A, non-B post-transfusion hepatitis: Histological features of liver biopsies in acute phase. Liver 1:201, 1981.

439. Kujosawa K, Akahane Y, Nagata A, et al. The significance of blood transfusion in non-A non-B chronic liver disease in Japan. Vox Sang 43:45, 1982.

440. Realdi G, Alberti A, Rugge M, et al. Long-term follow-up of acute and chronic non-A, non-B post-transfusion hepatitis: Evidence of progression to liver cirrhosis. Gut 23:270, 1982.

441. Dienes HP, Popper H, Arnold W, et al. Histologic observations in human hepatitis non-A non-B. Hepatology 2:562, 1982.

442. Iwarson S, Lindberg J, Lundin P. Progression of hepatitis non-A non-B to chronic active hepatitis: A histological follow-up of two cases. J Clin Path 32:351, 1979.

443. Spero JA, Lewis JH, Van Thiel DH, et al. Asymptomatic structural liver disease in hemophilia. N Engl J Med 298:1373, 1978.

444. Marciano-Cabral F, Rublee KL, Carithers RL Jr, et al. Chronic non-A, non-B hepatitis: Ultrastructural and serologic studies. Hepatology 1:575, 1981.

445. Galbraith RM, Portmann B, Eddleston ALWF, et al. Chronic liver disease developing after outbreak of HBsAg-negative hepatitis in haemodialysis unit. Lancet 2:886, 1975.

446. Mannucci PM, Colombo M, Rizzetto M. Nonprogressive course of non-A, non-B chronic hepatitis in multitransfused hemophiliacs. Blood 60:655, 1982.

447. Colombo M, Rumi MG. Liver disease and pathology in hemophilia. Scand J Haematol 33:341, 1984.

448. Aledort LM, Levine PH, Hilgartner M, et al. A study of liver biopsies and liver disease among hemophiliacs. Blood 66:367, 1985.

449. Kuhns WJ, Prince AM, Brotman B, et al. A clinical and laboratory evaluation of immune serum globulin from donors with a history of hepatitis: Attempted prevention of post-transfusion hepatitis. Am J Med Sci 272:255, 1976.

450. Seeff LB, Zimmerman HJ, Wright EC, et al. A randomized double blind controlled trial of the efficacy of immune serum globulin for the prevention of post-transfusion hepatitis. A Veterans Administration cooperative study. Gastroenterology 72:111, 1977.

451. Hoofnagle JH, Mullen KD, Jones DB, et al. Treatment of chronic non-A, non-B hepatitis with recombinant human alpha interferon. N Engl J Med 315:1575, 1986.

452. Demetris AJ, Lasky S, Van Thiel DH, et al. Pathology of hepatic transplantation. Am J Pathol 118:151, 1985.

453. Maddrey WC. Drug-related acute and chronic hepatitis. Clin in Gastroenterol 9:213, 1980.

454. Seeff LB. Drug-induced chronic liver disease, with emphasis on chronic active hepatitis. Sem Liv Dis 1:104, 1981.

455. Wright R. Drug-induced chronic hepatitis. Spring Sem Immunopath 3:331, 1980.

456. Cooksley WGE, Cowen AE, Powell LW. The incidence of oxyphenisatin ingestion in active chronic hepatitis: A prospective controlled study of 29 patients. Aust NZ J Med 3:124, 1973.

457. Goldstein GB, Lam KC, Mistilis SP. Drug-induced active chronic hepatitis. Dig Dis 18:177, 1973.

458. Dietrichson O, Juhl E, Neilsen JO, et al. The incidence of oxyphenisatin-induced liver damage in chronic non-alcoholic liver disease. A controlled investigation. Scand J Gastroenterol 9:473, 1974.

459. Dietrichson O. Chronic active hepatitis. Aetiological considerations based on clinical and serological studies. Scand J Gastroenterol 10:617, 1975.

460. Reynolds TB, Peters RL, Yamada S. Chronic active and lupoid hepatitis caused by a laxative, oxyphenisatin. N Engl J Med 285:813, 1971.

461. Reynolds JDH, Wilber RD. Chronic active hepatitis associated with oxyphenisatin. Am J Gastroenterol 57:566, 1972.

462. Gjone E, Blomhoff JP, Ritland S, et al. Laxative-induced chronic liver disease. Scand J Gastroenterol 7:395, 1972.

463. Goldstein LI, Ishak KG, Burns W. Hepatic injury associated with nitrofurantoin therapy. Dig Dis 19:987, 1974.

464. Fagrell B, Strandberg I, Wengle B. A nitrofurantoin-induced disorder simulating chronic active hepatitis. A case report. Acta Med Scand 199:237, 1976.

465. Stromberg A, Wengle B. Chronic active hepatitis induced by nitrofurantoin. Br Med J 186:174, 1976.

466. Hatoff DE, Cohen M, Schweigert BF, et al. Nitrofurantoin: Another cause of drug-induced chronic active hepatitis? A report of a patient with HLA-B8 antigen. Am J Med 67:117, 1979.

467. Iwarson S, Lindberg J, Lundin P. Nitrofurantoin-induced chronic liver disease. Clinical course and outcome of five cases. Scand J Gastroenterol 14:497, 1979.

468. Tolman KG. Nitrofurantoin and chronic active hepatitis. Ann Int Med 92:119, 1980.

469. Sharp JR, Ishak KG, Zimmerman HJ. Chronic active hepatitis and severe hepatic necrosis associated with nitrofurantoin. Ann Int Med 92:14, 1980.

470. Black M, Rabin L, Schatz N. Nitrofurantoin-induced chronic active hepatitis. Ann Int Med 92:62, 1980.

471. Hoyumpa AM Jr, Connell AM. Methyldopa hepatitis: Report of three cases. Am J Dig Dis 18:213, 1973.

472. Rehman OU, Keith TA, Gall EA. Methyldopa-induced submassive hepatic necrosis. JAMA 224:1390, 1973.

473. Schweitzer IL, Peters RL. Acute submassive hepatic necrosis due to methyldopa: A case demonstrating possible initiation of chronic liver disease. Gastroenterology 66:1203, 1974.

474. Toghill PJ, Smith PG, Benton P, et al. Methyldopa liver damage. Br Med J 3:545, 1974.

475. Maddrey WC, Boitnott JK. Severe hepatitis from methyldopa. Gastroenterology 68:351, 1975.

476. Rodman JS, Deutsch DJ, Gutman SI. Methyldopa hepatitis: A report of six cases and review of the literature. Am J Med 60:941, 1976.

477. Thomas E, Bhuta S, Rosenthal WS. Methyldopa-induced liver injury. Arch Pathol Lab Med 100:132, 1976.

478. Maddrey WC, Boitnott JK. Isoniazid hepatitis. Ann Int Med 79:1, 1973.

479. Mitchell JR, Zimmerman HJ, Ishak KG, et al. Isoniazid liver injury: Clinical spectrum, pathology, and probable pathogenesis. Ann Int Med 84:181, 1976.

480. Black M, Mitchell JR, Zimmerman HJ, et al. Isoniazid-associated hepatitis in 114 patients. Gastroenterology 69:289, 1975.

481. Maddrey WC. Hepatic effects of acetaminophen. Enhanced toxicity in alcoholics. J Clin Gastroenterol 9:180, 1987.

482. Bonkowsky HL, Mudge GH, McCurtry RJ. Chronic hepatic inflammation and fibrosis due to low doses of paracetamol. Lancet 1:1016, 1978.

483. Johnson GK, Tolman KG. Chronic liver disease and acetaminophen. Ann Int Med 87:302, 1977.

484. Weiss VC, Layden T, Spinowitz A, et al. Chronic active hepatitis associated with etretinate therapy. Br J Dermatol 112:591, 1985.
485. Utili R, Boitnott JK, Zimmerman HJ. Dantrolene-associated hepatic injury. Gastroenterology 72:610, 1977.
486. Chalmers TC, Iber FL, Uzman LL. Hepatolenticular degeneration (Wilson's disease) as a form of idiopathic cirrhosis. N Engl J Med 256:235, 1957.
487. Walshe JM. Wilson's disease and chronic active hepatitis. Lancet 1:605, 1977.
488. Gollan JL. Copper toxicity and liver disease. In: Williams R, Maddrey WC, eds. Liver. London, Butterworths, 1984:76.
489. Scheinberg IH, Sternlieb I. Wilson's disease. In: Smith LH Jr, ed. Philadelphia, WB Saunders, 1984:70.

39

Parasitic Diseases of the Liver

Ira S. Goldman, M.D. • Lloyd L. Brandborg, M.D.

PROTOZOAN INFECTIONS

HEPATIC AMEBIC ABSCESS

General

Although various amebae normally inhabit the human colon, only *Entamoeba histolytica* is capable of tissue invasion. This ameba exists either as a trophozoite or as a cyst. The cyst, which is the infective form, usually contains four nuclei. Of the 5 to 10 per cent of the people in the United States who harbor *E. histolytica,* the vast majority are carriers or cyst passers, who have no symptoms as a result of the infection. Infection occurs via the fecal-oral route, food and drink becoming contaminated through exposure to human feces. Food-borne outbreaks of disease are due to unsanitary handling of food and its preparation by infected individuals. As might be expected, the disease is particularly prevalent where human feces are used for fertilizer. Incidences are high in institutional settings such as mental hospitals, prisons, and possibly day-care centers. Epidemics occur when raw sewage is discharged into water supplies. Flies have been incriminated in transmission of *E. histolytica* when they have access to fecal material and unprotected food, since viable cysts and trophozoites have been recovered from the intestine of the fly.

Pathophysiology

The cyst is resistant to gastric acid, and on ingestion it passes into the small intestine. The ameba within the cyst becomes active in the neutral or alkaline environment of the small intestine. The cyst wall is digested, probably by the digestive enzymes within the lumen of the gut. The ameba rapidly divides into the number of organisms corresponding to the number of nuclei present, usually four. This stage, the metacyst, develops into the form known as the metacystic trophozoite. These are carried in the intestinal chyme to the cecum, where they mature into trophozoites. In order to colonize the cecum, the amebae require the presence of enteric bacteria that can provide a low oxygen potential and probably supply other metabolic needs. This situation pertains to residence within the lumen of the colon prior to tissue invasion.

The living trophozoites range in diameter from 10 to about 60 μm. The cytoplasm of the organism has a clear outer ectoplasm. Centrally, there is granular endoplasm, which may contain food vacuoles. The nucleus is spherical, and its diameter is about one sixth the diameter of the entire ameba. It has a small, distinct, central karyosome surrounded by an unstained halo. The nuclear membrane is lined by small aggregations of chromatin, which appear to be small round granules.[1] As the amebae pass down the colon and the fecal stream becomes dehydrated, they assume a spherical shape known as a precyst. A thin, tough cyst wall is secreted, forming an unripe cyst. Two mitotic divisions occur, resulting in a cyst that contains four nuclei. This is evacuated in the stool and discharged into the environment.

The reason *E. histolytica* is the only ameba capable of tissue invasion is unknown. All strains of *E. histolytica* can hydrolyze guinea pig cecal epithelium, casein, gelatin, bovine hemoglobin, and fibrin. All strains also contain hyaluronidase and a mucopolysaccaridase, which probably are the enzymes permitting them to penetrate the mucosa.[2, 3] Invasion occurs first with a superficial lytic necrosis of the intestinal mucosa. The amebae divide by binary fission, increase in number, and spread superficially along the basement membrane of the mucosa. They also penetrate the interstitial tissue between the glandular cells. They may spread laterally or penetrate through the muscularis, resulting in perforation of the colon. It is presumed that they reach the liver by invasion of the mesenteric venules, from which they enter the portal vein. Most amebae reaching the liver fail to lodge there, instead passing into the systemic circulation. When they are retained by thrombi composed of fibrin and leukocytes in the liver, however, lytic digestion of the vessel wall occurs, allowing them to enter the hepatic sinusoids. When in the parenchyma of the liver, they produce lytic necrosis of hepatocytes, accompanied by an infiltration of leukocytes. Abscesses may be only a few millimeters to many centimeters in diameter. There are three gross divisions of the abscess: a necrotic center filled with thick fluid, a second zone composed of hepatic stroma, and a third, outer, area consisting of normal liver tissue being invaded by the organism. Most abscesses occur in the right lobe of the liver. Incidences of amebic abscesses of the left lobe range from 5 to about 21 per cent.[4, 5] At any one time more than 90 per cent of persons infected with *E. histolytica* have no bowel disease and are considered asymptomatic carriers since their infection is confined to the bowel lumen.[2] It is frequently impossible, however, to determine when the colon was infected.

Clinical Presentation

Durations of symptoms of hepatic amebic abscesses range from a few days to many months. Pain is the most common symptom, occurring in over 90 per cent of patients. It is located in the right upper quadrant of the abdomen, the epigastrium, the chest, or the right shoulder; it may occur singly or in various combinations. Pain occurs on the left side of the abdomen or left epigastrium with amebic abscess of the left lobe. Approximately 20 per cent of patients have past histories of dysentery. About 10 per cent of patients have diarrhea or dysentery at the time of diagnosis of amebic liver abscess. Eleven per cent of patients have cough, and 4 per cent have dyspnea.

The physical findings associated with hepatic amebic abscesses include tenderness in the right hypochondrium in 85 per cent of patients; a palpable, tender liver in 80 per cent; fever in 75 per cent; signs at the right lung base in about 50 per cent; localized intercostal tenderness in 40 per cent; epigastric tenderness in 22 per cent; and localized swelling over the liver in 10 per cent.[4]

The preceding clinical features are all important clues in the diagnosis of hepatic amebic abscess, particularly, point tenderness on palpation of the liver and intercostal tenderness. Hepatomegaly may not be detected in patients with amebic abscess of the dome of the liver, since the enlargement is upward. Amebic abscess and cirrhosis of the liver may coexist, so a hard liver does not exclude the diagnosis. Patients whose livers are not palpable may have unexplained pain in the epigastrium, right upper quadrant, or lower chest. Some patients have shoulder pain associated with an immobile diaphragm, and atelectasis or effusion in the right chest. An occasional patient with amebic abscess of the liver seeks treatment because of symptoms simulating an acute surgical abdomen. The usual clinical diagnosis in such a case is acute cholecystitis or appendicitis.[5, 6] Occasionally, the diagnosis of pneumonia or other primary pulmonary disease is entertained. In one recent series, the correct diagnosis was suspected less than 20 per cent of the time.[2, 5, 6]

Diagnosis

Laboratory Tests

Liver diagnosis tests are of little use in specifically diagnosing hepatic amebic abscesses. Jaundice occurs in fewer than 10 per cent of cases, and bilirubin rarely exceeds 2 mg/dl. Although results of liver tests occasionally may be abnormal, no characteristic pattern is found.[2, 4] Results of routine laboratory tests such as the serum albumin may be abnormal, but again, characteristic values are not observed. Leukocytosis with leukocyte counts greater than 10,000/mm[3] is common, as is anemia, with hemoglobin values of less than 12 g/dl being found in about 65 per cent of patients. The right diaphragm is elevated on the chest x-ray in 50 to 55 per cent of patients.

Radionuclide Imaging

Various methods for imaging the liver are available, but most experience has been accumulated with radionuclide imaging. Of the agents currently used, the most popular is ^{99m}Tc-sulfur colloid (Fig. 39–1). In one very large study,[7] 4,286 abscesses were detected on 3,379 liver scans of 2,500 patients. In that study, 79.6 per cent of the abscesses occurred in the right lobe and 20.4 per cent in the left lobe. The projection at which the liver is scanned greatly influences detection rates.[7] Recently, technitium-99m dimethyl iminodiacetic acid (^{99m}Tc-HIDA) has been used in both gallbladder and liver-spleen imaging. Cholescintigraphic rim enhancement around a photopenic liver defect has been shown to be highly suggestive of liver abscess.[8]

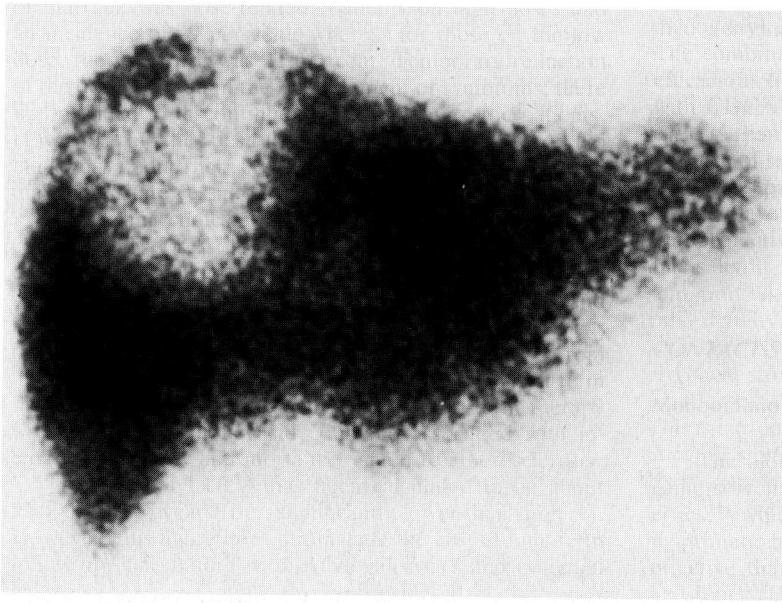

Figure 39–1. ^{99m}Tc-sulfur colloid liver scan, showing a large defect in the right lobe caused by an amebic abscess. (Courtesy of T. Boyer.)

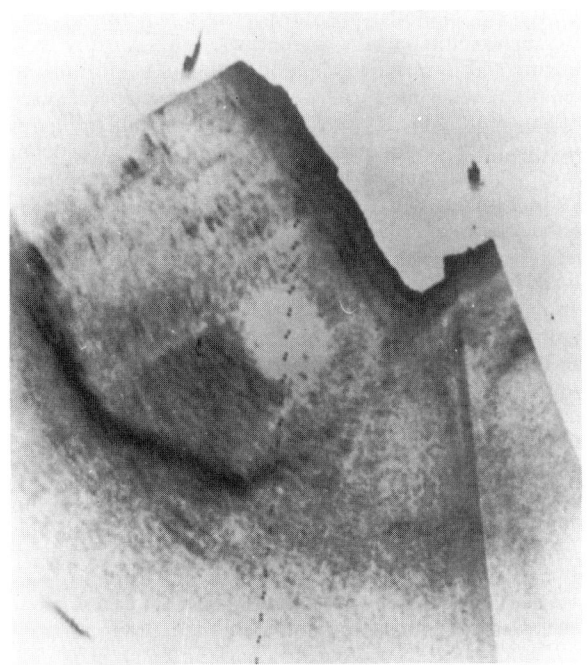

Figure 39–2. Ultrasonogram of the liver, showing a large defect caused by an amebic abscess. (Courtesy of G. Gooding.)

Radionuclide imaging has some disadvantages, including limited resolution. Interpretation of a mass within the liver may be incorrect when the portal area is prominent, when the gallbladder overlies the liver, or when there is a "defect" caused by a thin liver edge. An extrinsic lesion compressing the liver may also lead to an incorrect interpretation of a mass within the liver.[7]

Ultrasonography

Sonographic findings in hepatic amebic abscess have been well described. All amebic abscesses will not be detected by ultrasonography, but certain characteristics detectable by ultrasonography are highly suggestive of amebic abscess and are found in about one third of cases.[9] These include a peripheral location, predominantly fine, low-level echoes at high gain, slight distal sonic enhancement, and a well-defined lesion without a prominent abscess wall (Fig. 39–2).

Computed Tomographic (CT) Scanning

Computed tomographic (CT) scanning is probably the most accurate method of detecting intra-abdominal abscesses, although a distinct CT appearance of hepatic amebic abscesses has not been described.[9] Even though CT might identify smaller lesions than ultrasound or radioisotope imaging, the smallest abscesses in most series (about 3 cm) will easily be seen by these non-CT methods (Fig. 39–3).[5]

The use of magnetic resonance imaging (MRI) for liver imaging is increasing. However, the liver images still lack detail owing to respiratory artifacts. It is too early to assess their ultimate usefulness in the diagnosis of hepatic abscesses.

Aspiration

In the past, aspiration of amebic abscesses of the liver was almost routine, based on the rationale that diagnoses could often be made in this manner and that the procedure was therapeutic. Amebic pus is variable in color and appearance but is typically opaque, reddish, dirty brown, or pink. Amebic pus is almost always sterile. Bacterial infection can be introduced by repeated aspirations, however, or as a complication of surgical therapy. Some clinicians still advocate aspiration of virtually all abscesses,[4] but others believe that aspiration of amebic abscesses is no longer necessary for diagnosis because of the availability of sensitive and highly accurate serologic tests (see later).[10] It appears reasonable to aspirate amebic abscesses that are large and appear to be in imminent danger of rupture. It also seems logical to aspirate abscesses of the left lobe because of the possibility of rupture into the pericardium with subsequent development of amebic pericarditis.[4] This complication has a high fatality rate. Another indication for aspiration of abscesses occurs when the probability is high that the abscess may be pyogenic rather than amebic.

Serologic Tests

The availability of sensitive, specific serologic tests for the diagnosis of invasive amebiasis has virtually eliminated the need to aspirate for the sole purpose of diagnosis. These tests are generally positive in over 90 per cent of cases and include indirect immunofluorescence, indirect hemagglutination, enzyme-linked immunosorbent assay (ELISA), gel diffusion, latex agglutination, and others.[2, 11, 12] Since differ-

Figure 39–3. A CT scan of a liver, showing a large low-density mass with a rim around it that is less dense than the surrounding liver. The center of the mass appears to be dense, but this is because of a mechanical measuring device that gives the appearance of white dots. This appearance is typical for liver abscess. (Courtesy of H. Goldberg.)

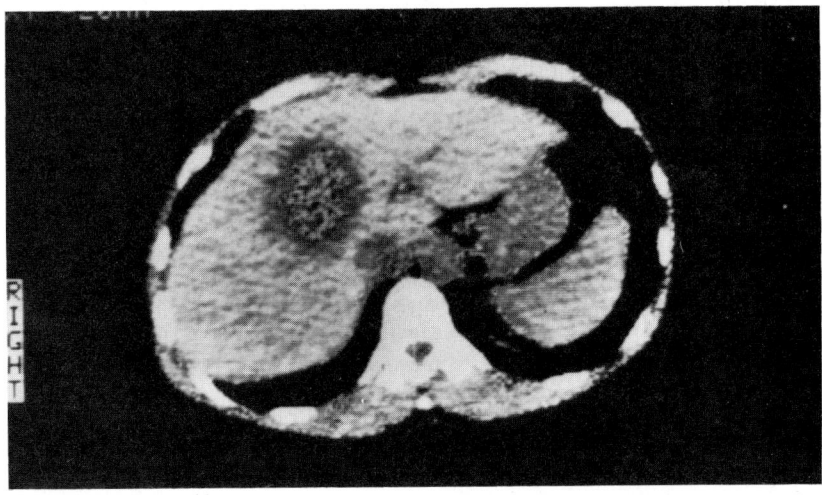

ent antibodies seem to be produced and each test is not always positive, the use of at least two different serologic tests is suggested for diagnostic purposes.[2] ELISA is probably the most sensitive test. Seropositivity, however, does not distinguish current from past disease. Several recent reports have used immunofluorescence techniques with IgM antibodies to indicate recent infection.[2, 11–13]

Complications

Rupture into the Chest

The commonest complication of hepatic amebic abscess is rupture into the chest.[4] This can lead to amebic empyema, consolidation, abscess formation, or hepatobronchial fistula. Rupture into a bronchus may result in expectoration of large quantities of amebic pus and rapid relief of the patient's symptoms. It offers the best chance of a spontaneous cure. With lesions of the lung that are remote from the diaphragm, diseases other than amebic abscess should be considered. Although right-sided pulmonary lesions are by far the commonest complication of amebic abscess of the liver, an amebic abscess of the left lobe occasionally perforates into the left chest.

The most common symptoms of extension into the chest are pleuritic chest pain, cough, hemoptysis, and dyspnea. Pain is located typically in the right lower chest or in the shoulder. Occasional patients do not have chest pain but only pain in the right upper quadrant of the abdomen. Left-sided pain is rare and frequently indicates pericardial involvement.[4] Cough, when present, is usually productive of small amounts of white sputum, except with hepatobronchial fistulas, when large quantities of amebic pus are expectorated. The physical signs of abscess rupture into the chest include an elevated right diaphragm and signs of consolidation or pleural effusion.

Peritonitis

Peritonitis is the next most common complication. It usually occurs as a sudden severe pain with signs of an acute abdomen. A history of previous hepatic pain is useful in making the diagnosis. In a minority of patients, the hepatic amebic abscess develops a slow leak, resulting in a walled-off intra-abdominal abscess.[4]

Amebic Pericarditis

This is the most ominous complication of hepatic amebic abscess.[4] There are three types of presenting symptoms: hepatic abnormalities, cardiac problems, and shock. With the first, the patient has signs and symptoms of hepatic amebic abscess, usually in the left lobe. The patient's condition deteriorates, with development of retrosternal pain in the left chest, dyspnea, elevation of the jugular venous pressure, an increasing pulse rate, a small pulse volume, and pulsus paradoxicus, with or without a pericardial friction rub.[4]

Those patients who have abnormal cardiac findings have pericarditis with effusion, congestive heart failure, or both. The hepatic amebic abscess is often inconspicuous.[4] Chest pain, left shoulder pain, a pericardial rub, and point tenderness over the liver in the midline or left hypochondrium suggest the correct diagnosis. In some cases, the diagnosis is made by direct aspiration of amebic pus from the pericardial sac.

Rarely, patients who have amebic pericarditis are in shock when first seen by the physician. The history is that of acute cardiac tamponade, and the main clinical features are an enlarged liver, cold extremities, nonpalpable pulses, and an unrecordable blood pressure. A pleural pericardial friction rub may be present. Acute cardiac tamponade may also complicate amebic liver abscess during treatment. It is almost always fatal.

Other Complications

Other (rare) complications include rupture into the bowel, which may be unsuspected and may lead to improvement in the patient's condition. Rarely, patients may have hemobilia with hematemesis and melena, usually from erosion of the abscess into an artery. Another rare complication is brain abscess, the signs and symptoms of which depend upon the size and the location of the abscess.

Therapy and Prognosis

Various drugs are effective in the treatment of hepatic amebic abscess.[4, 14] Metronidazole is the drug of choice, since it is also effective against intestinal amebiasis. The dose is 750 mg, three times a day for ten days. Some authorities recommend that an intestinal amebicide such as iodoquinol be given for 20 days at a dose of 650 mg, three times a day, following therapy with metronidazole or other tissue amebicides.[14] The pediatric dose of metronidazole is 35 to 50 mg/kg/day in three doses for ten days. The dose of iodoquinol is 30 to 40 mg/kg/day in three doses for 20 days, for a maximum of 2 g/day. Alternative regimens include dehydroemetine, 1 to 1.5 mg/kg/day (maximum 90 mg/day), given for as long as five days, followed by chloroquine phosphate, 1 g (600 mg base) daily for two days, then 500 mg (300 mg base) daily for two to three weeks. It is recommended that this regimen be followed by administration of iodoquinol in the dosage recommended above. Another alternative is emetine, 1 mg/kg/day (maximum 60 mg/day) given for as long as five days, again followed by chloroquine and iodoquinol in the regimen described (Table 39–1).

The regimens described are effective for treatment of thoracic amebiasis. Pleural effusions, if present, should be tapped frequently. It is recommended that the abscess be aspirated,[4] but there is little or no proof that aspiration of the abscess is therapeutic.[10]

Laparotomy or laparoscopy may be indicated for diagnosis of amebic peritonitis. If amebiasis is found, tissue amebicides as described for amebic abscess and thoracic disease are the treatment of choice.

In the management of amebic pericarditis, tissue amebicides are used as just described. The pericardial sac should be aspirated. It is also recommended that the hepatic amebic abscess be aspirated.[4]

Surgery is not indicated for uncomplicated hepatic amebic abscess. The indications for surgery are rupture or impending rupture; occasionally, failure of medical therapy; occasionally, a left lobe abscess; and diagnostic problems.[15] The diagnostic problems include acute abdominal conditions, e.g., rupture of the abscess, or, occasionally, a nonacute abdominal condition. However, most nonacute abdominal conditions are not indications for surgery, because of the availability of imaging techniques and sensitive and specific serologic tests for invasive amebiasis. The surgical mortality rates are very high, ranging from 17 per

TABLE 39–1. DRUGS AND TREATMENT REGIMENS FOR PARASITIC DISEASES

Infection	Drug	Adult Dose	Pediatric Dose
Amebic abscess			
Drug of choice	Metronidazole followed by iodoquinol	750 mg tid × 10 days	35–50 mg/kg/day in 3 doses × 10 days
		650 mg tid × 20 days	30–40 mg/kg/day in 3 doses × 20 days (max 2 g/day)
Alternatives	Dehydroemetine followed by chloroquine phosphate	1–1.5 mg/kg/day (max 90 mg/day) IM up to 5 days	1 to 1.5 mg/kg/day (max 90 mg/day) IM in 2 doses up to 5 days
		1 g (600 mg base) daily × 2 days; then 500 mg (300 mg base) daily × 2–3 weeks	10 mg base/kg/day × 21 days (max 300 mg base/day)
	Plus iodoquinol	650 mg tid × 20 days	30–40 mg/kg/day in 3 doses × 20 days (max 2 g/day)
	or Emetine followed by chloroquine phosphate	1 mg/kg/day (max 60 mg/day) IM up to 5 days	1 mg/kg/day in 2 doses (max. 60 mg/day) IM up to 5 days
		1 g (600 mg base) day × 2 days; then 500 mg (300 mg base) day × 2–3 weeks	10 mg base/kg/day × 21 days (max 300 mg base/day)
	plus iodoquinol	650 mg tid × 20 days	30–40 mg/kg/day in 3 doses × 20 days (max 2 g/day)
Malaria *(Plasmodium falciparum, P. ovale, P. vivax,*and *P. malariae)*			
Suppression or chemoprophylaxis of disease while in endemic area (all plasmodia except chloroquine-resistant *P. falciparum)*			
Drug of choice	Chloroquine phosphate	500 mg (300 mg base) once weekly; continued 6 weeks after last exposure in endemic area	<1 year, 37.5 mg base; 1–3 years, 75 mg base; 4–6 years, 100 mg base; 7–10 years, 150 mg base; 11–16 years, 225 mg base
Treatment of uncomplicated attack (all plasmodia except chloroquine-resistant *P. falciparum)*			
Drug of choice	Chloroquine phosphate	1 g (600 mg base); then 500 mg (300 mg base) in 6 hours; then 500 mg (300 mg base)/day × 2 days	10 mg base/kg (max 600 mg base); then half this dose one/day beginning 6 hours later × 2 days
Treatment of severe illness, parenteral dosage only if oral dose cannot be administered (regardless of severity) (all plasmodia except chloroquine-resistant *P. falciparum)*			
Drug of choice	Quinine dihydrochloride	600 mg in 300 ml normal saline IV over 2–4 hours; repeat every 8 hours (max 1,800 mg/day) until oral therapy can be started	25 mg/kg/day; administer one third of dose in 2- to 4-hour infusion, then every 8 hours if oral therapy still cannot be started (max 1,800 mg/day)
Plasmodium falciparum (chloroquine-resistant) suppression or chemoprophylaxis			
Drug of choice	Chloroquine phosphate plus	500 mg (300 mg base) once every week	<1 yr 37.5 mg base; 1–3 yrs 75 mg base; 4–6 yrs 100 mg base; 7–10 yrs, 150 mg base; 11–16 yrs, 225 mg base
	Pyrimethamine-sulfadoxine (Fansidar)	1 tablet (25 mg pyrimethamine, 500 mg sulfadoxine) once every week	6–11 months, ⅛ tablet; 1–3 yrs, ¼ tablet; 4–8 yrs, ½ tablet; 9–14 yrs, ¾ tablet; weekly

Table continued on following page

1066   INFECTIOUS AGENTS AND LIVER DISEASE

TABLE 39–1. DRUGS AND TREATMENT REGIMENS FOR PARASITIC DISEASES *Continued*

Infection	Drug	Adult Dose	Pediatric Dose
Treatment of uncomplicated attack (chloroquine-resistant *P. falciparum*)			
Drug of choice	Quinine sulfate plus	650 mg tid × 3 days	25 mg/kg/day in 3 doses × 3 days
	Pyrimethamine plus	25 mg bid × 3 days	<10 kg, 6.25 mg/day; 10–20 kg, 12.5 mg/day; 20–40 kg, 25 mg/day all × 3 days
	Sulfadiazine	500 mg qid × 5 days	100–200 mg/kg/day in 4 doses × 5 days (max 2 g/day)
Alternative	Quinine sulfate plus	650 mg tid × 3 days	25 mg/kg/day in 3 doses × 3 days
	Tetracycline	250 mg qid × 7 days	5 mg/kg qid × 7 days (max 2 g/day)
Treatment of severe illness, parenteral dosage (chloroquine-resistant *P. falciparum*)			
Drug of choice	Quinine dihydrochloride	600 mg in 300 ml normal saline IV over 2–4 hours; repeat every 8 hours (max 1,800 mg/day)	25 mg/kg/day; administer one-third of dose over 2–4 hours then every 8 hours if oral therapy still cannot be started (max 1,800 mg/day)
Alternative	Quinidine gluconate	unknown	unknown
Trypanosomiasis			
Trypanosoma cruzi (South American trypanosomiasis, Chagas' disease)			
Drug of choice	Nifurtimox	8–10 mg/kg/day orally in 4 divided doses for 120 days	1–10 yrs; 15–20 mg/kg/day in 4 divided doses in 90 days; 11–16 years; 12.5–15 mg/kg/day in 4 divided doses for 90 days
Alternative	Benzonidazole	5–7 mg/kg for 30–120 days	unknown
Trypanosoma gambiense, T. rhodesiense (African trypanosomiasis, sleeping sickness)			
Drug of choice	Suramin	100–200 mg (test dose) IV then 1 g IV on days 1, 3, 7, 14 and 21	20 mg/kg on days 1, 3, 7, 14 and 21
Alternative	Pentamidine isethionate	4 mg/kg/day IM × 10 days	4 mg/kg/day IM × 10 days
Late disease with CNS involvement			
Drug of choice	Melarsoprol	2–3.6 mg/kg/day IV × 3 doses; after 1 week 3.6 mg/kg/day IV × 3 doses; repeat again after 10–21 days	18–25 mg/kg total over 1 month; initial dose 0.36 mg/kg IV, increasing gradually to max. 3.6 mg/kg at intervals of 1–5 days for total 9–10 doses
Alternative	Tryparsamide plus	30 mg/kg IV in 1 injection every 5 days × 12 doses; may repeat in 1 month	unknown
	Suramin	10 mg/kg IV in 1 injection every 5 days × 12 doses; may repeat in 1 month	
Leishmaniasis			
Leishmania donovani (kala-azar, visceral leishmaniasis)			
Drug of choice	Stibogluconate sodium	20 mg/kg/day (max 800 mg/d) IM or IV × 20 days (may be repeated)	20 mg/kg/day IM or IV (max 800 mg/day) × 20 days
Alternative	Pentamidine	2–4 mg/kg/day IM up to 15 doses	2–4 mg/kg/day IM up to 15 doses
Toxoplasmosis (Toxoplasma gondii)			
Drug of choice	Pyrimethamine plus	25 mg/day × 3–4 weeks	1 mg/kg/day × 4 weeks after loading dose of 2 mg/kg/day × 3 days (max 25 mg/day)
	Trisulfapyrimidines	2–6 g/day × 3–4 weeks	100–200 mg/kg/day × 3–4 weeks
Alternative	Spiramycin	2–4 g/day × 3–4 weeks	50–100 mg/kg/day × 3–4 weeks

Table continued on following page

Table continued on following page

TABLE 39–1. DRUGS AND TREATMENT REGIMENS FOR PARASITIC DISEASES *Continued*

Infection	Drug	Adult Dose	Pediatric Dose
Schistosomiasis			
Schistosoma japonicum			
Drug of choice	Praziquantel	20 mg/kg tid × 1 day	20 mg/kg tid × 1 day
Schistosoma mansoni			
Drug of choice	Praziquantel	20 mg/kg tid × 1 day	20 mg/kg tid × 1 day
Alternative	Oxamniquine	15 mg/kg once	10 mg/kg bid. × 1 day
Echinococcus granulosus infestation			
Drug of choice	Mebendazole	40 mg/kg/day for 90 days or longer (if surgery contraindicated)	Unknown
Echinococcus multilocularis infestation			
Drug of choice	Mebendazole	40 mg/kg/day for 3 years or more	Unknown
Alternative	Albendazole	10 mg/kg/day for 90 days or longer	Unknown
Visceral larva migrans			
Drug of choice	Thiabendazole or	25 mg/kg bid × 5 days (max 3 g/day)	25 mg/kg bid × 5 days
	Diethylcarbamizine	2 mg/kg tid × 7–10 days	2 mg/kg tid × 7–10 days
Alternative	Mebendazole	200–400 mg/day × 5 days	Unknown
Hepatic capillariasis			
Drug of choice	Unknown		
Strongyloidiasis			
Drug of choice	Thiabendazole	25 mg/kg bid (max 3 g/day) × 2 days	25 mg/kg bid (max 3 g/day) × 2 days
Fascioliasis hepatica (sheep liver fluke) or *Fascioliasis gigantica* infestation			
Drug of choice	Bithionol	30–50 mg/kg on alternate days × 10–15 doses	30–50 mg/kg on alternate days × 10–15 doses
Ascaris lumbricoides (roundworm) infestation			
Drug of choice	Pyrantel pamoate Or	Single dose of 11 mg/kg (max 1 g)	Single dose of 11 mg/kg (max 1 g)
	Mebendazole	100 mg bid × 3 days	>2 years, 100 mg bid × 3 days
Alternative	Piperazine citrate	75 mg/kg (max 3.5 g)/day × 2 days	75 mg/kg (max 3.5 g)/day × 2 days
Hermaphroditic fluke infestation:			
Clonorchis sinensis (liver fluke)			
Drug of choice	Praziquantel	25 mg/kg tid × 2 days	25 mg/kg tid × 2 days
Cryptosporidiosis			
Cryptosporidium			
Drug of choice	Spiramycin	1 g tid × 14 days or more	Unknown

Source: Adapted from the Medical Letter, 30:15, 1988, with permission.

cent in patients operated on for failure of medical therapy to 48 per cent in patients with diagnostic problems.[15]

With uncomplicated hepatic amebic abscesses, the prognosis is good, with mortality rates in the range of 1 per cent.[4] With extension into the chest, the mortality rate is 6.2 per cent. With amebic pericarditis, the mortality rate is high, reaching approximately 30 per cent.[4]

MALARIA

Four species of plasmodium, *Plasmodium vivax, Plasmodium ovale, Plasmodium malariae,* and *Plasmodium falciparum,* cause malaria in humans. Infection is acquired when the female of any of a number of anopheline mosquitoes takes a blood meal and consequently injects the subject with one of the infective forms of malaria.

Pathophysiology

The mosquito is the definitive host, in which sexual reproduction of the parasite occurs; humans are the intermediate hosts, in which asexual reproduction occurs.[16] Mature microgametocytes (male) and macrogametocytes (female) are taken into the gut of the mosquito when it takes a blood meal from an infected individual. Fertilization occurs in the gut of the mosquito. The parasite grows into an oocyst, which matures and ultimately contains as many as a thousand of the infective forms, called sporozoites. The oocyst ruptures, and the sporozoites are dispersed throughout the insect's body.

Thereafter, when the mosquito takes a blood meal, it injects saliva containing sporozoites into the human host. They are rapidly cleared from the bloodstream and penetrate the parenchymal cells of the liver. Asexual reproduction, called primary exoerythrocytic schizogony, occurs in the liver. The sporozoite develops into a schizont. Its nucleus repeatedly divides, producing large numbers of exoerythrocytic merozoites. When the mature schizont ruptures, the merozoites, (now called trophozoites) invade the red blood cells. In the red cells, they undergo further schizogony, becoming mature schizonts and eventually releasing erythrocytic merozoites, which again invade the red cells. Some merozoites develop into microgametocytes or macrogametocytes, which are ingested by the mosquito, completing the cycle. *Plasmodium falciparum* has only one tissue stage, whereas *Plasmodium ovale, Plasmodium malariae,* and *Plasmodium vivax* have secondary hepatic cycles.[16, 17]

Malaria can also be transmitted by blood transfusion and by sharing of needles among drug addicts. Mosquitoborne outbreaks of malaria have occurred in the United States.[18]

The pathogenesis of symptoms in malaria is complex. Pathogenicity is seldom manifest until late in or after the incubation period.[16] A major factor is hypoxia caused by severe hemolysis of both parasitized and nonparasitized red cells. Some evidence exists that oxygen uptake by peripheral tissue may be deranged, leading to local cytotoxic hypoxia. In part, this hypoxia may be due to stasis and increased permeability of small blood vessels. In *P. falciparum* malaria, prolonged orthostatic hypotension and splenomegaly have been observed. Severely ill patients have hyponatremia, reversal of the urinary sodium-to-potassium ratio, increased urinary aldosterone excretion, and markedly elevated urinary osmolality. It is proposed that there is a decrease in hepatic and splanchnic blood flow. This may be an important factor in the pathogenesis of the hepatic abnormalities.[19] The symptoms of malaria coincide with the parasitemia. The diagnosis is made by identifying the parasites within red cells; usually, the largest numbers are found during the highest fever spikes. The differentiation of the various species is beyond the scope of this presentation.

Clinical Presentation

The classic clinical tetrad in malaria includes fever, usually with temperatures higher than 40° C, chills, headache, and variable gastrointestinal symptoms that include anorexia, nausea, vomiting, and diarrhea. The physical examination is often unrevealing, and does not lead to a diagnosis of malaria. The most common findings are tenderness to percussion over the liver or spleen, hepatomegaly, and splenomegaly.[20, 21] Hepatomegaly occurs in as many as 60 per cent of patients who have *P. vivax* or *P. falciparum* malaria.[20, 21] *P. falciparum* malaria may appear as jaundice and encephalopathy that simulates acute hepatic failure caused by fulminant hepatitis.[21]

Diagnosis

Most patients with malaria have liver test abnormalities during the course of their disease.[20-22] The most common abnormalities of liver tests are elevations of AST and ALT.[20, 21] Some patients have mild jaundice, with serum bilirubin rarely exceeding 5 mg/dl.[20, 21] These abnormalities have been observed in *Plasmodium falciparum* and *Plas-*

modium vivax malarias. Comparable data for *Plasmodium malariae* and *Plasmodium ovale* malarias are not available.

Pathology

Schizonts of *Plasmodium vivax* were observed in hepatocytes of a patient receiving therapeutic malaria for treatment of tertiary syphilis, on the basis of a liver biopsy seven days after the patient was infected. During the erythrocytic phase, parasites are not found in the liver on needle biopsy.[22] Abnormalities in the liver biopsy specimen are consistently seen during parasitemia and consist of Kupffer cell hyperplasia and lymphocytic infiltration of the periportal lymphatics with small groups of mononuclear cells near interlobular bile ducts. Occasionally, nonspecific granulomas containing cellular debris are seen. The hepatocytes have increased nuclear and cytoplasmic activity with little necrosis. Occasionally, individual cell death is present. Malarial pigment is present in the Kupffer cells in over 80 per cent of biopsy specimens. Stainable iron is present in Kupffer cells in the vast majority of specimens, sometimes in considerable amounts. Parasitized red cells are rarely observed in the sinusoids, and cholestasis is not present.

Therapy and Prognosis

The results of liver tests usually return to normal with successful treatment.[21] Chemoprophylaxis for all malarias except chloroquine-resistant *Plasmodium falciparum* malaria is advisable for travelers to endemic areas. The drug of choice is chloroquine phosphate, given to an adult in a dose of 500 mg once weekly and continued for six weeks after the last exposure in the endemic area. Pediatric chemoprophylaxis dosages are less: at 1 year of age, 37.5 mg of base; 1 to 3 years, 75 mg of base; 4 to 6 years, 100 mg of base; 7 to 10 years, 150 mg of base; 11 to 16 years, 225 mg of base (chloroquine phosphate 500 mg contains 300 mg of base).

The drug of choice for the treatment of all uncomplicated malarias except chloroquine-resistant *P. falciparum* malaria is chloroquine phosphate, 1 g (600 mg of base), then 500 mg in six hours, followed by 500 mg/day for two days. For children, the regimen is 10 mg of base/kg, then half the dose once daily, beginning six hours later, for two days. In severe illness, chloroquine hydrochloride may be administered intravenously, but this should be done only when the drug cannot be tolerated orally. (Table 39–1).

Chloroquine-resistant *Plasmodium falciparum* malaria is treated with quinine sulfate, 650 mg, three times a day for three days; pyrimethamine, 25 mg, twice a day for three days, and sulfadiazine, 500 mg, four times a day for five days. The dosage of quinine sulfate for children is 25 mg/kg/day, given in three divided doses for three days. The dosage of pyrimethamine depends upon the child's weight: less than 10 kg, 6.25 mg/day; 10 to 20 kg, 12.5 mg/day; 20 to 40 kg, 25 mg/day. Sulfadiazine is given in a dosage of 100 to 200 mg/kg/day in four divided doses for five days. The maximum dose for children should not exceed 2 g/day. For severe illness in an adult patient, quinine dihydrochloride, 600 mg, in 300 ml of normal saline is administered intravenously over two to four hours and repeated every eight hours (maximum 1800 mg/day). For children, the dose is 25 mg/kg/day. (see Table 39–1). Experimental work leading to the development of an antimalarial vaccine is in progress.[23]

AFRICAN TRYPANOSOMIASIS

Pathophysiology

In Africa, humans are parasitized by two species of trypanosomes, *Trypanosoma gambiense* and *Trypanosoma rhodesiense*. They are transmitted by bites of Glossina (tsetse) flies, the intermediate host. The trypanosome exists in three morphologic forms. The first, which occurs in the human blood stream and interstitial spaces, is a long, slender trypanosome having a flagellum measuring 14 to 33 μm by 1 to 3.5 μm. A broad form, without a flagellum, and an intermediate form are also seen in the blood stream. The trypanosome stage is ingested by the fly as it bites. This stage multiplies in the fly's midgut, followed by multiplication of a crithidial stage in salivary glands. The crithidial forms are transformed into metacyclic trypanosomes, which are introduced into the definitive host (human) by the fly on biting. The metacyclic trypanosomes develop into mature trypanosomes in the interstitial spaces in tissue and in the blood stream.[24] The life cycles of *T. gambiense* and *T. rhodesiense* are identical.

Clinical Presentation and Diagnosis

Trypanosoma gambiense produces a chronic disease; *Trypanosoma rhodesiense* produces a more acute disease that has a short course, usually ending fatally within a year when untreated. The incubation period is 2 to 23 days.[24] There are three stages following infection: (1) trypanosomes exclusively or predominantly in the circulation, (2) trypanosomes predominantly in lymph nodes, and (3) trypanosomes invading the central nervous system. Involvement of the central nervous system produces the major manifestations of *T. gambiense*. Since trypanosomiasis caused by *T. rhodesiense* has the more fulminant course, central nervous system involvement is not so prominent.

The parasite does not invade cells, but it produces lesions in every tissue and organ of the body. After an initial inflammatory reaction at the site of the bite, the parasite invades the interstitial spaces in the lymphatics, particularly the posterior cervical lymph nodes, but also the submaxillary, inguinal, and femoral nodes. During the febrile stage, these nodes are soft and swollen; in later stages, they become smaller and fibrous. The spleen is characteristically enlarged, and the liver may be enlarged and congested. A chronic leptomeningitis occurs in the central nervous system. The cerebrospinal fluid is turbid, the protein content is elevated, and trypanosomes are present. The pathologic features in the brain are basically those of lymphangitis and perivasculitis, consisting of plasma cells, lymphocytes, and macrophages.[24]

Diagnosis

The diagnosis is based on finding the parasite in the blood or aspirates of lymph nodes. An immunofluorescent serologic test is available for African trypanosomiasis.[25] It aids in diagnosis, but it is most useful for epidemiologic studies.

Most patients who have African trypanosomiasis are slightly jaundiced.[26-28] Serum alkaline phosphatase may be elevated, as may the AST, ALT, and bilirubin. The diagnosis of trypanosomiasis has been made in at least one case by finding the parasite in ascitic fluid.[28] Acute disease caused by *Trypanosoma rhodesiense* has been misdiagnosed as acute viral hepatitis.[27] Pathologically, in the acute stages, round cell infiltration of the portal tracts is seen in acute infections with *Trypanosoma rhodesiense*. There is some parenchymal cell death.[29]

Treatment

Treatment of the acute stages of African trypanosomiasis is with suramin. A 100- to 200-mg test dose is given intravenously, followed by 1 g intravenously on days 1, 3, 7, 14, and 21. The pediatric dose is 20 mg/kg on the same schedule.[14] An alternative drug is pentamidine, at a dose of 4 mg/kg/day, intramuscularly, for ten days. The pediatric dose is the same. For late disease with central nervous system involvement, the drug of choice is melarsoprol. The dose schedule is 2 to 3.6 mg/kg/day, intravenously, for three doses, and repeated after a week in a dose of 3.6 mg/kg/day, intravenously, for three doses, and again after 10 to 21 days. The pediatric dose is 18 to 25 mg/kg (total) given over a month. The initial dose is 0.36 mg/kg, intravenously, increased gradually to a maximum of 3.6 mg/kg at intervals of five days, for a total of nine to ten doses.[14]

SOUTH AMERICAN TRYPANOSOMIASIS

Pathophysiology

Chagas's disease (South American trypanosomiasis) is caused by *Trypanosoma cruzi*.[24, 30] The parasite exists as a trypanosome in the definitive vertebrate hosts, which include man and many other mammals. It is approximately 20 μm long by 2 μm wide and contains a large, round, subterminal blepharoplast. The trypanosome form invades tissues in virtually every organ of the body. It changes to a leishmanial form in this intracellular location and divides by successive binary fission. This leishmanial pseudocyst distends the cell, which ultimately ruptures, and the leishmanial form changes to the trypanosomal form.[24, 30] The insect vectors, certain reduviid bugs, ingest the trypanosomes while taking a blood meal from the infected host. In the gut of the reduviid bug, the trypanosomes are transformed into leishmanial forms and crithidia by binary division. The crithidia become metacyclic trypanosomes, which are the infective form. On taking a blood meal, the reduviid bug defecates, contaminating the site of the bite, which allows entry of the trypanosomes into the host, either through abrasions induced by scratching or through the conjunctiva.

The metacyclic trypanosomes are ingested by macrophages in the corium of the skin. They invade adjacent adipose tissue and nearby muscle cells. They multiply as leishmanial forms for three days. On rupture of the parasitized cells, infiltration with polymorphonuclear leukocytes, monocytes, and lymphocytes occurs. Regional lymph nodes are affected initially. On rupture of the leishmanial cysts, the organism assumes the trypanosome stage. It moves via blood and lymphatic channels to invade axillary and inguinal lymph nodes, lungs, spleen, liver, bone marrow, and mesenteric lymph nodes. It multiplies in these organs within fixed histiocytes. Leishmanial forms also invade muscle fibers, neuroglia, microglia, and pyramidal cells of the cerebral cortex. They have been found in the adrenal, thyroid, genitalia, and intestinal mucosa. The heart and brain are particularly vulnerable.[24, 30, 31]

Clinical Presentation and Diagnosis

Acute Chagas's disease may occur at any age, but it usually occurs in early childhood. It is manifested by malaise, fever, sweating, muscular pains, irritation, anorexia, and occasionally, vomiting and diarrhea. There is generalized edema and, occasionally, anasarca. Hepatomegaly is almost universal, and moderate splenomegaly occurs. The disease manifests most commonly by signs and symptoms of cardiac involvement or central nervous system invasion (acute meningoencephalitis).

Laboratory tests show leukocytosis with pronounced lymphocytosis, elevated sedimentation rates, coagulation defects, hypoalbuminemia, and hyperglobulinemia. The results of standard liver tests are usually abnormal.[24, 30, 31]

The diagnosis is made by the demonstration of *T. cruzi* in blood or tissues or by a positive serologic test.[24] Xenodiagnosis, allowing trypanosome-free laboratory-reared triatomids (reduviid bugs) to bite persons suspected of having the disease, had been widely used in the past. Examination of the intestinal tract of the bug ten to 30 days later revealed flagellated forms of the parasite if the patient had parasitemia when bitten.[24] Several serologic tests are available for the diagnosis of Chagas's disease, including direct agglutination, complement fixation, and indirect hemagglutination.[25]

The acute disease usually lasts 20 to 30 days. The liver is heavily parasitized; however, the signs and symptoms of the disease are due to cardiac and central nervous system involvement. Death occurs in two to four weeks, usually as a result of cardiac failure or meningoencephalitis. Survivors enter a chronic stage, which may last into adult life. In the chronic stages of the disease, abnormalities of liver function are due to chronic congestive heart failure and are the same as the abnormalities occurring with all other forms of chronic congestive heart failure (see Chapter 53).

Pathology

In the acute fatal cases, pathologic features of the liver include chronic passive congestion and, almost always, fatty infiltration.[31] Round cell infiltration of the portal areas is seen. Amastigote nests (leishmanial forms) are rarely seen in the Kupffer cells.[29] A lesion consisting of a nodule in the center of the liver lobule, composed of lymphocytes lying in a network of reticular histiocytes, is considered pathognomonic of Chagas's disease.[32]

In the chronic forms of the disease, the cardiac manifestations caused by the myocarditis, megaesophagus, and megacolon are the predominant manifestations. In fatal cases, the findings are those of chronic passive congestion and, occasionally, fatty infiltration of the liver. Leishmanial forms usually are not present.[31]

Therapy

The drug of choice for treatment of South American trypanosomiasis is nifurtimox.[14] The dose is 8 to 10 mg/kg/day, given orally in four divided doses for 120 days. The pediatric dose is 15 to 20 mg/kg/day in four divided doses for 90 days for children 1 to 10 years old. For those 11 to 16 years of age, it is 12.5 to 15 mg/kg/day in four divided doses for 90 days.[14] (see Table 39–1).

VISCERAL LEISHMANIASIS (KALA-AZAR)

Pathophysiology

Visceral leishmaniasis is caused by *Leishmania donovani*. The life cycle of *L. donovani* in the mammalian host consists of leishmanial forms that divide within reticuloendothelial cells by binary fission until the host cell is destroyed. The leishmanial forms are released and taken up by new macrophages, and the cycle is repeated. The insect vector consists of many species of sandflies, *Phlebotomus*. In the insect's intestine, the leishmanial forms become leptomonas forms, which divide by simple longitudinal fission into two individuals. Enormous numbers of the leptomonas forms are produced in the insect intestine. They are found first in the midgut and later in the pharynx and buccal cavity of the species of sandfly to which they are adapted.[24, 33] When the leptomonas stage of the parasite is injected into the victim's skin by the infected sandfly, it is ingested by nearby macrophages. Metamorphosis into the leishmanial stage occurs within the cytoplasm of these cells.

The incubation period may be as short as ten days but usually it is two to four months. Occasionally, it is a year or longer.[24, 33] The leishmanial forms multiply slowly at the site of infection and can remain dormant for weeks or months. Eventually, some of the parasitized macrophages rupture or are carried into the blood stream, whence they reach the viscera, where the parasite develops rapidly. The main organs parasitized are the spleen, liver, bone marrow, and other organs with reticuloendothelial activity.[24, 33]

Clinical Presentation

The disease may begin as an acute illness or may have an insidious onset. The most common symptoms of visceral leishmaniasis are fever, anorexia, abdominal pain, cough, weakness, marked weight loss, and diarrhea. Rare patients have jaundice.[24, 33-36] The physical findings include an undulant fever, occasionally with a double rise each 24 hours. The temperature may reach 40° C. Peripheral edema is frequently present. The patients appear emaciated, and there may be bleeding from the mucous membranes, the gums, and the nose. Splenomegaly and hepatomegaly are variable, with the splenic enlargement almost always being greater than the enlargement of the liver.[24, 33-36] Rarely, there may be ascites and, occasionally, intra-abdominal hemorrhage.[33]

Visceral leishmaniasis is often not diagnosed because of failure to consider the disease. If the patient has resided in or visited an endemic area and has intermittent fever, anemia, and marked hepatosplenomegaly, kala-azar must be considered. Endemic areas are widely spread throughout the Mediterranean basin, including Spain, France, Italy, Greece, and North Africa. Other endemic areas include southern Russia, eastern India, China, eastern Africa (including Kenya, Sudan, Uganda and Ethiopia), Brazil, Venezuela, and Paraguay.[37] An intact, T cell–dependent immune response seems to be necessary for successful host defense. There are several recent reports of progressive disease in the immunocompromised patient.[34]

Diagnosis

The routine clinical laboratory tests show pancytopenia, hypoalbuminemia, hypoprothrombinemia, and elevations of the AST, ALT, and serum alkaline phosphatase.[33, 34] The diagnosis is confirmed by establishing the presence of Leishman-Donovan bodies (leishmanial forms). This is done most usually by examination of sternal bone marrow. The leishmanial forms may also be demonstrated in splenic aspirates and liver biopsy specimens. There is some hazard of intra-abdominal hemorrhage from these latter procedures. Leishmanial forms may also be found occasionally in sputum, saliva, nasal scrapings, tonsillar exudate, urine, prostatic fluid, conjunctival secretions, feces, and chest effusions.[33] Sensitive immunoserologic tests such as the direct agglutination test and immunofluorescence antibody test are also available.[25]

Pathology

Examination of the spleen, liver, and involved lymph nodes shows marked reticuloendothelial hyperplasia. Phagocytic mononuclear cells contain large numbers of leishmanial forms. In the liver, there is marked hyperplasia of the Kupffer cells, whose cytoplasm contains numerous leishmanial forms. There may be phagocytic cells containing the organisms within portal areas, and there is degeneration of liver cells in the vicinity of the portal areas. There is atrophy of the parenchymal cells in the lobule caused by compression by the large numbers of Kupffer cells containing Leishman-Donovan bodies. Eosinophils may be present. There may be lymphocytes, monocytes, and even plasma cells in the sinusoids. Occasionally, bile stasis is observed.[33] Other organs involved include the kidneys, heart, and lungs, but muscle cells and the central nervous system are not usually involved.

Therapy

The drug of choice for visceral leishmaniasis is stibogluconate sodium. The adult dose is 20 mg/kg/day (maximum 800 mg/day) given intravenously or intramuscularly for 20 days. The course may be repeated. The pediatric dose is 20 mg/kg/day, given by the same routes, to a maximum of 800 mg/day for 20 days. An alternative drug is pentamidine at a dose of 2 to 4 mg/kg/day, intramuscularly, for as many as 15 doses. The adult and pediatric doses are the same (see Table 39–1).[14]

TOXOPLASMA HEPATITIS

Pathophysiology

Toxoplasma are ovoid in shape, resembling a banana with a motile anterior and a more blunted posterior end. This general shape occurs in trophozoites of the proliferative phase, merozoites from cysts, merozoites resulting from schizogony in the cat intestinal epithelium, and the sporozoites from the oocysts.[38] There are five stages in the life cycle, the proliferative phase, a cystic stage, a schizogonic form and a gametogonic form, and the oocyst. The asexual cycles consist of the proliferative phase and the cyst's stage in many hosts. Schizogony and gametogony occur only in the intestinal epithelium of the cat.[38] The parasite is a coccidian in the cat. It occurs only in the proliferative phase or the cystic phase in all other hosts. Carnivorism is one important mode of acquiring toxoplasmosis. The mature oocyst as excreted in cat feces is infective for many species, including humans.[38]

The parasites invade many organs. In the proliferative phase their size is approximately 4 to 7×2 to 4 μm. They develop intracellularly, ultimately destroying the host cell. The cyst develops in chronic infections. It appears to be distributed throughout many tissues and in extracellular locations. A tough cyst wall encloses the merozoites and part of the organ that is infected. The merozoites apparently can survive as cysts for long periods of time.[38]

Humans can acquire the infection through many routes, but most usually do so after ingesting raw or inadequately cooked meats. Lamb and pork appear to contain the infectious agent more often than does beef.[38] Infection exists in a chronic asymptomatic form in approximately 50 per cent of the infected population of the United States. There is an increasing incidence of the disease in immunocompromised patients.

Clinical Presentation

Hepatitis caused by acquired toxoplasmosis, although it has been reported, is rare.[39, 40] There are three clinical manifestations: (1) a long prodromal stage of several months heralded by lymphadenopathy, with or without fever, with the subsequent development of clinically apparent hepatitis; (2) primary liver disease without peripheral lymph node involvement and perhaps without lymphocytosis; (3) granulomatous hepatitis and generalized lymphadenopathy occurring together.[40]

The usual history of a patient with *Toxoplasma* hepatitis is one of lymphadenopathy, with or without fever. These symptoms are usually accompanied by fatigability, and anorexia and weight loss may occur. Symptoms may subside spontaneously; but weeks or months later, the increased tiredness may recur in association with headaches, nausea, and (rarely) vomiting. The patient may then be noticed to be jaundiced.[39] Some patients develop a skin rash, which is reported to be a generalized, red-brown, confluent, papular eruption.[40] Physical examination discloses jaundice, lymphadenopathy, hepatomegaly, and splenomegaly.

Diagnosis

Routine laboratory studies show no anemia. Leukocyte counts may range from 5,500 to 16,000mm^3, and there is usually a lymphocytosis. There may be slight hypoalbuminemia and elevation of serum globulins. The AST and ALT are elevated, in some cases markedly, to 1500 to 2000 IU/ml. Serum bilirubin may also be elevated, and there may be hypoprothrombinemia.[39, 40]

The Sabin-Feldman dye test is specific and positive at high titer.[38, 39] Other serologic tests include direct agglutination, latex agglutination, complement fixation, indirect hemagglutination, indirect immunofluorescence, and ELISA. Positive serologic tests do not necessarily indicate acute infection.

Pathology

Liver biopsy shows a picture of acute generalized hepatitis. There is degeneration, with necrosis of hepatocytes and infiltration by lymphocytes, histiocytes, and granulocytes, including eosinophils. Staining with specific fluorescent antibodies may demonstrate T. gondii.[39, 40] Rarely, granulomas not related to the nests of parasites are present.[40]

Congenital Toxoplasmosis

Acute or subacute congenital toxoplasmosis is accompanied by jaundice, purpura, and hepatosplenomegaly. Pathologic examination of the liver demonstrates giant cell hepatitis and extramedullary hematopoiesis.[38] Affected infants also have meningoencephalitis, chorioretinitis, convulsions, hydrocephalus, and intracerebral calcifications. Approximately 3000 cases of congenital toxoplasmosis occur per year in the United States.[41]

Therapy

Some patients recover spontaneously. The drugs of choice for adult toxoplasmosis are pyrimethamine, 25 mg/day, given for three to four weeks, plus trisulfapyrimidines, 2 to 6 g/day, given for three to four weeks. The pediatric dose of pyrimethamine is 1 mg/kg/day for four weeks after a loading dose of 2 mg/kg/day for three days to a maximum of 25 mg/day. The trisulfapyrimidine dosage is 100 to 200 mg/kg/day for three to four weeks (see Table 39–1).[14]

HELMINTHIC INFESTATIONS

SCHISTOSOMIASIS

Pathophysiology

Liver involvement with schistosomiasis is due to Schistosoma mansoni and Schistosoma japonica. Humans are the definitive hosts, but the parasite has a phase of its life cycle in suitable snails.[42–45] There are several important differences between infections caused by the two parasites, including biologic and ecologic differences in the snails, differences in cercarial outputs and in distributions of cercariae in water, different locations of adult worms in the intestines, different patterns of egg-laying and host responses to the eggs, varying disease syndromes, and different responses to therapy. Nevertheless, the two diseases may be considered together.

The life cycle of schistosomes in man is initiated when the fork-tailed cercariae penetrate the skin or mucosa. Penetration, which occurs in less than a minute, may be aided by lytic enzymes. On penetration, the cercariae lose their tails to become schistosomulae, which migrate through the lymphatics of the skin to the circulation. In the circulation, they travel first to the lungs and subsequently to the liver. Only a small proportion of the cercariae invading humans mature to adult worms in various branches of the portal venous system. The rest are destroyed by host defense mechanisms. Schistosoma mansoni lives in the portal venous system, primarily in the branches of the inferior mesenteric vein, whereas Schistosoma japonicum resides primarily in the superior mesenteric vessels. About 30 days after infection, the worms begin to lay eggs in the small venules in the wall of the intestine. A pair of Schistosoma mansoni worms can release 1000 eggs per day

and a pair of Schistosoma japonicum, 1500 to 3000. The newly laid eggs are immature and develop in about six days into miracidia, which may live in tissue for as long as 30 days. The eggs begin to appear in feces 40 days after cercarial infection.

The ova in feces contain mature miracidia that hatch under the proper conditions of temperature, humidity, and light. The miracidium is a larval form that swims actively for some hours searching for the suitable intermediate snail host. Two days after penetration of the snail's tissues, a mother sporocyst develops, which in turn gives rise to many daughter sporocysts and large numbers of cercariae. After departing the snail host, the cercariae live only a few hours unless they find a suitable definitive host. Schistosoma mansoni is found only in humans, but Schistosoma japonicum has a number of definitive hosts in addition.[42–45]

The pathogenesis of disease in schistosomal infection is complex. The adult worms are well tolerated by the host; they do not produce irritation, inflammation, or mechanical effects.[44] The adult worms also incorporate human antigens into their integument and are not recognized by the host as a foreign antigen.[46] Dead worms, on the other hand, promote local inflammatory lesions, with necrosis, vessel obstruction, and eventual scarring. These changes occur primarily in the lung and liver.

The clinical and pathologic manifestations of schistosomal infection are due to the host's immune response to the eggs trapped in the tissues. The basic reaction on the part of the host is granuloma formation in response to the ova. There is a delayed hypersensitivity reaction to soluble antigens released from the mature ovum. The reaction becomes more intense on repeated exposure.[47] Cellular sensitization to worm, egg, and cercarial antigens has been demonstrated by lymphocyte transformation and migration inhibition factor studies. Circulating immune complexes and increased suppressor T-cell populations may be responsible for perpetuation of liver injury.[48, 49] In addition, lymphocytes sensitized by cercarial antigen may stimulate collagen synthesis.[50] The worm load influences the severity of the disease. By use of extracorporeal filtration of portal venous blood, as many as 1000 worms have been recovered from a single patient. The worm burden gradually decreases with age, and male patients generally harbor more parasites than do female patients. An indirect technique for assessing the worm burden is by quantitating eggs in feces. There generally is a correlation between severe forms of the disease and large numbers of eggs in the feces.[44] A genetic factor seems to be present, demonstrated by the association between HLA B_1 and B_5 with hepatosplenic schistosomiasis.[51]

Clinical Presentation and Diagnosis of Acute Schistosomiasis

On penetration of the skin, the cercariae produce an irritating maculopapular rash that may last several days. This response is more common in reinfections than in first infections. The magnitude of the cutaneous response is not related, however, to the numbers of cercariae penetrating the skin but appears to be an immune response on the part of the host.[44] After an incubation period of one to two months, some patients develop asthenia, headache, anorexia, lassitude, and nausea. This is followed by the abrupt onset of fever, headache, chills, sweating, weakness, anorexia, muscle pains, cough, and diarrhea. Fever is intermittent, with temperatures reaching 39° C. It may persist for one to two months and disappear by lysis. The sweating and chills may be marked. Bronchospasm may be so severe as to lead to status asthmaticus and to be associated with pneumonia. Nausea and vomiting are frequent. Diarrhea and dysentery may be prolonged. There is associated epigastric discomfort, with abdominal pain and distention. Rarely, patients may have serious complications such as coma or an acute abdomen with jaundice when first seen, but in endemic areas the infection usually does not progress to this acute toxemic phase. This form of the disease is seen primarily in nonimmune visitors to endemic areas.[47]

Physical examination shows hepatomegaly and evidence of weight loss. The spleen is palpable but soft. It never attains the large size seen with chronic schistosomiasis (see later). There is generalized lymphadenopathy. On sigmoidoscopy, the rectum and sigmoid are edematous and hyperemic, with fine granulations; there also are petechial hemorrhages and small ulcerations that are not necessarily related to the worm or the egg burden.[44] In fatal cases, granulomas with exudate and necrosis are found in the liver, intestines, peritoneum, abdominal and pulmonary lymph nodes, pleura, lungs, and pancreas. Hepatocellular necrosis has also been observed. The diagnosis is made by demonstrating the presence of ova in the stool. Early in the disease the rectal biopsy may be negative, but as the disease progresses, and more and more ova are trapped within the submucosal tissues, rectal biopsy becomes a sensitive technique for establishing the diagnosis. It is a reliable method of diagnosing both *Schistosoma mansoni* and *Schistosoma japonicum* schistosomiasis. Serologic tests, including radioimmunoassay (RIA) and ELISA, are available, but they are not yet entirely reliable.[47]

Clinical Presentation and Diagnosis of Chronic Schistosomiasis

The majority of patients with chronic schistosomiasis are asymptomatic. Approximately 10 per cent of patients in hyperendemic areas develop hepatosplenic schistosomiasis, which is one of the more ominous complications of the chronic illness. It is found most often in the 6- to 20-years age group, occurring 5 to 15 years after acquisition of the infection. The first manifestation is an increase in blood leukocytes and lymphocytes, followed by a progressive hepatosplenomegaly. Most patients are unaware of this complication until variceal hemorrhage occurs. Ascites occurs in about 15 per cent of patients who have hepatosplenic schistosomiasis and is more common in Egypt than in Brazil. Variceal hemorrhage is the most important complication. Hemorrhage may be preceded by asthenia or epigastric discomfort or may be seen without any antecedent symptom. Melena without hematemesis is uncommon. With the onset of variceal hemorrhage, these patients develop hypothermia, somnolence, thirst, sweating, and anemia, and splenic size decreases. Fever and melena appear next, and if the hemorrhage is massive, edema and ascites may develop.

The most prominent physical finding is hepatosplenomegaly. Other signs of chronic liver disease, such as jaundice, muscle atrophy, spider angiomas, palmar erythema, and gynecomastia, are absent. Some of these signs may be found, however, with extremely advanced disease or may appear after portacaval shunting. Abdominal collaterals are present in some patients, particularly those who have ascites.

Hypersplenism is common, manifested by leukopenia, neutropenia, and thrombocytopenia. Almost all patients have significant eosinophilia. Anemia is common, even when not preceded by hemorrhage. Hypoalbuminemia occurs, perhaps because of reduced synthesis, protein-losing enteropathy, or both. Hyperglobulinemia, particularly hypergammaglobulinemia is present. The AST and ALT are usually normal or minimally elevated. Serum alkaline phosphatase may be elevated, and hypoprothrombinemia is occasionally seen.[44] There is an increased incidence of hepatitis B surface antigenemia in those with chronic schistosomiasis.[47] The diagnosis of chronic schistosomiasis is based principally on examination of feces for ova. With advanced disease, rectal biopsy often shows no abnormality.[44] Characteristic findings on radionuclide scanning and ultrasonography of the liver have been described.[47]

Another complication of hepatosplenic schistosomiasis is pulmonary hypertension. This occurs because collaterals between the portal circulation and the lungs allow large numbers of eggs to reach the pulmonary vascular bed and to lodge there. Terminally, these patients can develop cyanotic pulmonary hypertension and severe right-sided congestive heart failure.[44] Other forms of chronic schistosomiasis include a pseudo-neoplastic form affecting the gut. The lesions are composed of confluent schistosomal granulomas, may attain very large size, and are mistaken for polyps within the intestine or tumors in the mesentery or pericolic areas. The central nervous system can be involved. Affected patients can have a transverse myelitis or the cauda equina syndrome or both. There have been several well-described cases of myocarditis in patients with dissemination of ova.[44]

Yet another complication of chronic schistosomiasis is prolonged Salmonella infection. It is characterized by fever that may persist as long as 12 months. Laboratory tests reveal leukocytosis with neutrophilia and eosinophilia, and blood cultures for salmonella are consistently positive. This form of salmonellosis is cured only by specific treatment for schistosomiasis.

Pathology of Acute and Chronic Schistosomiasis

Needle biopsy of the liver in acute schistosomiasis discloses an intense eosinophilic infiltration, as well as the presence of an occasional ovum. Granulomas are not seen until about 80 days after infection, by which time the eosinophilic infiltration has disappeared or diminished markedly.[42] In patients who have an explosive onset of acute schistosomiasis within 15 to 25 days after exposure, only schistosomulae are present in sinusoids and vascular spaces. These patients have relatively intense hepatitis associated with foci of inflammation in the liver that are not necessarily related to the presence of the schistosomulae. When schistosomiasis is present but not hepatic fibrosis, ova and granuloma are distributed randomly throughout the liver lobule. With Symmers's fibrosis, there is a marked concentration of eggs in the portal spaces. Vascular lesions are common. Small intrahepatic portal veins are occluded by granulomas and, occasionally, by dead worms.[42] Thrombophlebitis of the larger portal vein branches with destruction of all layers of the vessel wall, in association with preservation of the hepatic artery and bile duct, is pathognomonic of schistosomiasis even when ova are absent.[42] A few patients with far advanced hepatosplenic shistosomiasis may have frank cirrhosis. It is not clear whether this is due to the infection.

Therapy

The treatment for *Schistosoma japonicum* schistosomiasis is praziquantel, 20 mg/kg, three times a day for one day. The pediatric and adult doses are the same. Oxamniquine, 15 mg/kg as a single oral dose, is an alternative for *S. mansoni*. The pediatric dose is 10 mg/kg twice a day for one day (see Table 39–1). The use of colchicine as an antifibrotic agent in cirrhosis has been suggested. The pattern of collagen deposition in schistosomiasis is similar to that of alcoholic cirrhosis.[47]

Management of patients who have portal hypertension and bleeding varices is difficult. Many of these patients have recurrent hemorrhage for many years.[42, 44] In general, treatment should be conservative.[45] Following reports of reduced gastrointestinal bleeding in cirrhotics treated with propranalol, preliminary evidence showed decreased portal pressure and spleen size in a group of patients with schistosomiasis treated with propranalol.[47] Injection sclerotherapy has been shown to be effective in the control of bleeding esophageal varices in these patients. Portacaval shunting is accompanied by an unacceptably high incidence of hepatic encephalopathy and the risk of systemic dissemination of ova. When surgery is necessitated by hypersplenism in nonbleeders, splenectomy alone may be performed. This will reduce the portal venous pressure by about 40 per cent. Splenectomy is also indicated when portal hypertension is due to a hyperdynamic spleen.[52] Splenectomy and gastroesophageal variceal devascularization may be done in patients who have hemorrhaged. The distal splenorenal shunt has been advocated as the shunt of choice for treating portal hypertension in patients who have chronic schistosomiasis.[47, 53] This shunt has the advantage of a lower incidence of hepatic encephalopathy, and it does not allow ova to enter the systemic circulation (see Chap. 23).

ECHINOCOCCOSIS

Echinococcosis in man is caused by *Echinococcus granulosus* and *Echinococcus multilocularis*. These are small tapeworms that live in the intestine of the definitive host, usually the dog. Other definitive hosts include wolves, jackals, dingoes, hyenas, pumas, jaguars, arctic foxes, and domestic cats.[54] *Echinococcus multilocularis* differs from *Echinococcus granulosus* in that herbivores do not play any part in its life cycle. The usual definitive hosts are various foxes; the intermediate hosts are usually a series of rodents. *Echinococcus granulosus* has a worldwide distribution from the arctic to the tropics but is most common in sheep- and cattle-raising areas.

Pathophysiology of Echinococcosis Caused by *Echinococcus granulosus*

Echinococcus granulosus is a small tapeworm, 3 to 6 mm long. The scolex contains a rostellum with 20 to 50 hooks, and has four suckers extending into a narrow neck. It consists of an immature proglottid, a mature proglottid, and a gravid proglottid; the gravid proglottid contains 400 to 800 eggs.[54] The gravid proglottid ruptures, either in the lumen of the bowel or after passage in the feces, and the eggs are swallowed as a contaminant by the intermediate host, which may be a human or any of a large number of other mammals. The external shell of the egg is digested in the duodenum, and the embryo is freed. The embryo moves actively into the intestinal mucosa until it enters a blood vessel through which it is transported by the blood until held up by narrowing of the capillaries. Most of the embryos are trapped in the liver, but lungs, spleen, kidneys, central nervous system, and bone can be involved. Other organs are infected only rarely.

Many of the embryos are destroyed by host defense mechanisms. A surviving embryo develops into the hydatid stage in four to five days while trapped within a capillary. The growing hydatid consists of connective tissue, adventitial membrane from host tissues, a laminated cuticle (which has no nuclei), and a germinal layer from which the scoleces develop. The definitive host is infected by ingesting infected viscera of the intermediate host. The scoleces develop into adult worms in the intestine of the definitive host, thereby completing the life cycle.[54]

Clinical Presentation

The signs and symptoms of echinococcal infection are determined by the size of the cyst and its location. Since an echinococcal cyst enlarges at a rate of approximately 1 cm per year, the clinical manifestations of echinococcosis occur many years after acquisition of the infection.[54, 55] Often, patients are asymptomatic, and the mass is discovered on a routine physical examination, or by the patient himself. However, large cysts can obstruct blood and bile flow, causing portal hypertension and jaundice, respectively. Cysts may become infected or rupture into the biliary tract and lead to cholangitis. Cysts that are close to the liver capsule grow away from the liver and may become pedunculated. Those growing toward the diaphragm sometimes perforate into the pleural or pericardial cavities, pulmonary parenchyma, or bronchi. Cysts growing toward the peritoneal cavity may perforate into the duodenum, colon, right renal pelvis, or peritoneum. Those near the porta hepatis produce obstructive jaundice.[54, 55] The fluid in echinococcal cysts is highly antigenic; hence, a rupture can produce anaphylactic shock and even death.

The only prominent physical findings due to cysts are abdominal masses, particularly in the liver, which may be tender to palpation. If there has been peritoneal seeding, there may be a number of palpable masses. With pulmonary involvement, solitary or multiple, sharply circumscribed masses may be visible on chest radiographs and other imaging studies.

Diagnosis

The routine laboratory tests are of little use in making a diagnosis of echinococcosis. Anemia is not present, although there may be slight leukocytosis with eosinophilia. Eosinophilia is seen, particularly with cysts that have ruptured. Obstructive jaundice may be present, and AST, ALT, and alkaline phosphatase have been observed to be elevated. Indirect hemagglutination, dot immunobinding, and ELISA are positive in more than 80 per cent of cases and are diagnostic of echinococcosis.

Routine radiologic investigations of the abdomen or chest may disclose a mass that occasionally is calcified around its rim.[56] Echinococcal cysts may also be diagnosed by radionuclide scanning, ultrasonography, CT, and MRI. The CT scan characteristics are those of a parenchymal, sharply circumscribed defect with a low attenuation value and a rim that may enhance.[56] An echinococcal cyst cannot

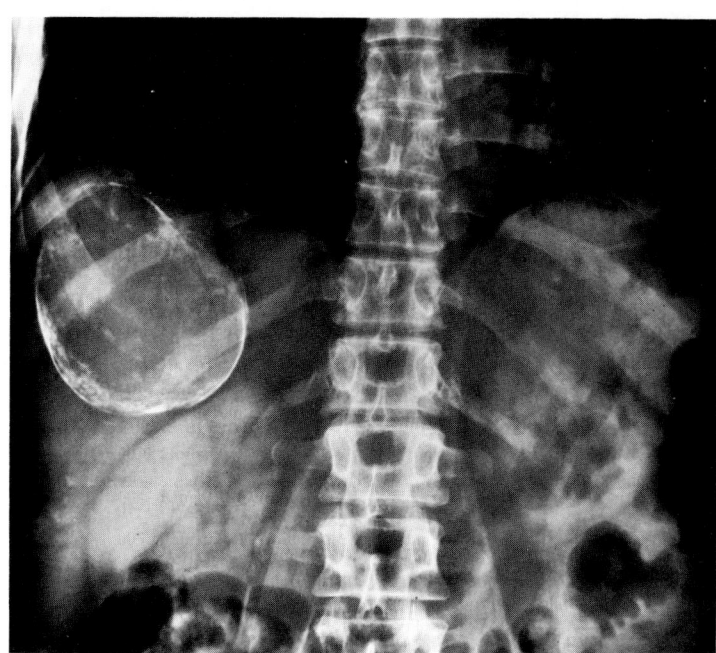

Figure 39–4. Plain radiograph of the abdomen, showing a large echinococcal cyst with a calcified wall. (Courtesy of M. Federle.)

be differentiated from a simple solitary cyst of the liver, however, unless there are daughter cysts within it and calcifications of the cyst wall are present (Figs. 39–4 and 39–5).

Pathology

The liver's initial inflammatory reaction to the embryo, which occurs a few hours after ingestion, is infiltration with eosinophils and mononuclear cells. The growing hydatid stimulates the formation of a connective tissue adventitial membrane on the part of the host. This is composed of a dense, hyalinized inner zone, a middle zone of fibroblastic granulomatous tissue, and an outer layer of neutrophils, lymphocytes, and eosinophils. There is pressure atrophy of the surrounding hepatocytes, and bile stasis may be present.

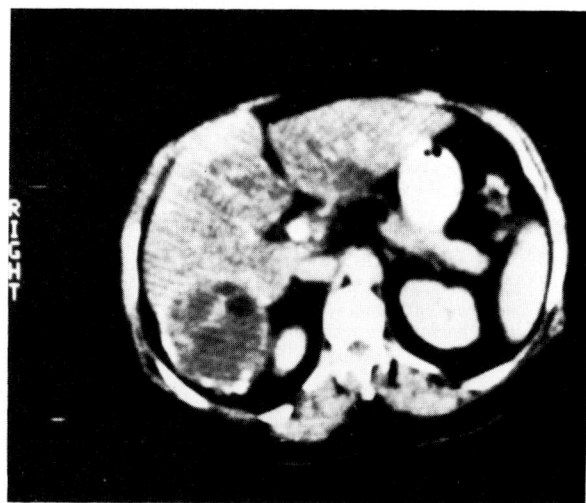

Figure 39–5. A CT scan showing an echinococcal cyst with a calcified wall and two daughter cysts. (Courtesy of M. Federle.)

Therapy

The treatment of hydatid disease of the liver is primarily surgical. Since cyst fluid is usually under pressure, percutaneous puncture should be avoided since this may allow leakage of cyst fluid into the peritoneal cavity. Small cysts less than 5 cm in diameter at the edge of the liver may be excised with a wedge of surrounding tissue. Larger cysts are isolated from the peritoneal cavity by appropriate surgical packs soaked in sterile 20 per cent saline. Such a cyst is penetrated and the hydatid fluid and sand (brood capsules) are evacuated. The fluid removed from the cyst is replaced by 20 per cent sterile saline, which is lethal to the scoleces. The cyst is opened, and any fluid in the dependent part is suctioned until it is empty. Daughter cysts, if present, are removed. Uncomplicated cysts that do not communicate with the biliary tree may be closed without drainage if they are deep within the liver. Superficial cysts may be unroofed so that the remaining space is left open in the peritoneal cavity. In complicated cysts, drainage of the residual cavity is recommended.[57] Heavy calcification of a cyst usually indicates that it is dead, in which instance therapy is not indicated unless the cyst is symptomatic.

Several cases of sclerosing cholangitis have been reported after use of hypertonic saline as a scolicidal agent. This probably occurs from the caustic effect of the hypertonic saline, which diffuses from the cyst into the biliary tree.[58]

Rupture of a hepatic hydatid cyst into the biliary tract occurs in 5 to 17 per cent of cases with hepatic involvement and may produce a clinical picture similar to that of choledocholithiasis.[59] Endoscopic retrograde cholangiography (ERCP) has been used to make this diagnosis preoperatively. ERCP may demonstrate dilation of the common bile duct with hydatid membranes or daughter cysts. Endoscopic sphincterotomy has been used both preoperatively and postoperatively to remove hydatid material from the bile ducts and relieve obstruction.[59]

If surgery is contraindicated, or if a cyst ruptures during surgery, or if patients have nonresectable alveolar hydatid disease caused by *Echinococcus multilocularis,* drug therapy is used. Most recent experience has been with mebendazole 40 mg/kg/day with the length of treatment varying from weeks to over ten years.[60] Mebendazole seems to prevent progression of the primary lesion as well as to suppress or to prevent metastatic activity. It is appropriate therapy both preoperatively and postoperatively. Albendazole, 400 mg twice a day, was recently shown to be effective against both *Echinococcus granulosa* and *Echinococcus multilocularis.* The major metabolite, albendazole sulphoxide, achieves higher tissue and cyst levels than mebendazole, so albendazole shows promise of even better long-term efficacy than mebendazole.[60, 61]

Pathophysiology of Echinococcosis Caused by Echinococcus Multilocularis

Echinococcosis caused by *Echinococcus multilocularis* differs from that caused by *Echinococcus granulosus.* In the former, the germinal membrane is not confined by a cyst wall within a single cyst. Scoleces develop in an uncontrolled manner, invading adjacent tissue. The hydatids also may metastasize to distant organs. The liver is the primary site, however, in 90 per cent of cases of infection caused by *Echinococcus multilocularis.* Cysts of *Echinococcus multilocularis* behave like slowly growing malignant lesions. Echinococcosis caused by *Echinococcus multilocularis* usually is not curable by surgery because of the multicystic, invasive properties of the cysts.

Diagnosis

Routine laboratory data are of little use in making a diagnosis of infection by *Echinococcus multilocularis.* Serologic testing can be positive, but this does not differentiate between infection due to *Echinococcus granulosus* and that caused by *Echinococcus multilocularis.* This determination must be made on other grounds, such as radiologic studies. The ultrasound or CT appearance of *Echinococcus multilocularis* infection may resemble that of polycystic disease.[56] Cysts of *Echinococcus multilocularis* are often initially identified at laparotomy.

TOXOCARIASIS

Pathophysiology

Toxocariasis is caused by *Toxocara canis,* a common roundworm of dogs or less often by *Toxocara cati,* a common roundworm of cats.[62–64] In natural hosts such as domestic and wild dogs, cats, and foxes, infection is acquired by the fetus in utero or shortly after birth. In the natural hosts, infections acquired by ingesting infective eggs lead to a life cycle similar to that of *Ascaris lumbricoides* in man (see later). Unnatural hosts, such as humans, acquire the infection by ingesting infective eggs. Children between the ages of one and four years are most often infected, because of their habit of placing foreign objects and dirt in their mouths. Dogs are the most common source of infective eggs, as they are indiscriminate defecators, unlike the cat, which is more fastidious in covering up its feces.

Once ingested, larvae in the eggs excyst in the upper small intestine and penetrate the wall of the gut, gaining access to the portal venous circulation. When larvae are detained by the diminution of blood vessels within the liver and other organs, they bore their way out of the vascular lumen to enter parenchymal tissues. Larvae move actively through these tissues, leaving a trail of tissue disorganization, cytolysis, interstitial edema, hemorrhage, and a predominantly eosinophilic exudate.[62] The initial lesions in the liver are eosinophilic abscesses, which subsequently develop into granulomas. These consist of radially arranged epithelioid cells mixed with multinucleated giant cells. The epithelioid cells are gradually replaced by fibroblasts, which ultimately surround the larvae with a hyalinized connective tissue. When thus encapsulated, the larvae may survive for months or even years.

Other organ systems invaded include the heart, lymphatic systems, central nervous system, and eye.[62–64]

Clinical Presentation

Mild forms of the disease are characterized by episodes of wheezing, colds, cough, rhinorrhea, asthmatic attacks, or urticarial rashes. There may be a brief febrile illness, mild gastrointestinal upsets, anorexia, failure to gain weight, and moderate lymphadenopathy. A few patients have only persistent eosinophilia and hepatomegaly without apparent systemic manifestations. In older children and young adults, the disease manifests as an insidious development of fever, coughing, nausea, and vomiting, occurring mainly at night. There may be dyspnea, orthopnea, chest pain, and fever with temperatures as high as 39° to 40° C. Night sweats are common. Younger patients have a greater probability of having hepatomegaly and generalized lymphadenopathy. The most severe infections occur mainly in toddlers or young children, who may experience anorexia, muscle aches, joint pains, weakness, lassitude, and failure to gain weight or even weight loss. Gastrointestinal symptoms, present in addition to the respiratory symptoms, include vomiting and occult blood in the stool. Abdominal pain may be sufficient to suggest an acute abdomen and indicate surgical exploration. Occasionally, patients have exfoliative dermatitis and subcutaneous nodules suggesting erythema nodosum. These lesions may be intensely pruritic.

Physical examination shows slight scleral icterus with lymphadenopathy, a moderately to markedly enlarged liver, and splenomegaly. There may be exquisite pain on palpation over the enlarged liver, and some patients have abdominal distention.

Diagnosis

Routine laboratory tests disclose moderate to marked leukocytosis, with leukocyte counts of 20,000 to more than 100,000/mm^3. The eosinophil count may be greater than 90 per cent. There is an increase in the IgM fraction of the gamma globulins. The transaminases are seldom increased, and hyperbilirubinemia, when present, is slight.

Most serologic tests that have been used for toxocariasis are nonspecific because of cross-reactivity with other roundworms. ELISA, using a larva-specific antigen, has been found to be positive for more than 85 per cent of infected patients. The predictive value of a negative test was greater than 85 per cent. Thus, ELISA, using the larval antigen, appears to be the serologic diagnostic method of choice for toxocariasis.[65]

Pathology

Liver biopsy has been suggested as a method of diagnosis. Granulomas may be found, but the larvae may be extraordinarily difficult to identify. It has been suggested that laparoscopy may be worthwhile, since the subcapsular granulomas can be identified and biopsied under direct vision.[63]

In human infections seen at surgery or autopsy, the liver is enlarged, and the capsule has scattered nodules ranging from 0.1 to 1 cm or more in diameter. These vary from soft to firm and cut with increased resistance. The gross appearance suggests multiple metastases from a neoplastic process. The granulomatous process predominates histologically, although larvae are difficult to identify without serial or subserial sectioning. This may be so because larvae often depart the granulomas and migrate to other areas within the liver. Larvae may occasionally be found in areas where the granulomas have undergone fibrinoid necrosis or have hyalinized. Blood vessels are often involved in the inflammatory processes adjacent to the granulomas. The portal areas are infiltrated with plasma cells, lymphocytes, and eosinophils. The hepatocytes are normal in areas not directly affected by granulomas.[62] Similar lesions occur in the lungs and other organs. The heart may be involved by diffuse interstitial myocarditis consisting of eosinophils, histiocytes, and plasma cells. There is fragmentation of the myocardial fibers. The most serious complication of toxocariasis is ocular involvement. Funduscopic examination of infected patients reveals retinal granulomas. When living larvae are present, they may be seen to move. With ocular toxocariasis, leukocytosis, eosinophilia, and serologic evidence of infection may be lacking. Concurrent ocular involvement and visceral involvement are uncommon.[62] Many eyes infected with Toxocara organisms have needlessly been enucleated because of the suspicion of retinoblastoma, which may clinically mimic ocular toxocariasis.

Therapy

The drug used for toxocariasis is thiabendazole, 25 mg/kg, given twice daily for five days. The adult and pediatric doses are the same. An alternative is diethylcarbamazine, 2 mg/kg, given three times daily for 7 to 10 days; the pediatric dose is the same (Table 39–1).[14]

HEPATIC CAPILLARIASIS

Pathophysiology

Capillaria hepatica is a common parasite in the livers of rats. It is less frequently found in squirrels, muskrats, mice, hares, dogs, pigs, beavers, and some species of monkeys.[66] When humans acquire the infection by eating uncooked or poorly cooked livers of rodents such as squirrels, beavers, or muskrats, the ova are passed in the feces without damage. Another mode of infection is ingestion of food or dirt containing embryonated ova. The ova hatch in the cecum, and the larvae penetrate the mucosa, entering the tributaries of the portal vein. On reaching the liver, they mature in approximately three weeks. A week later the adults disintegrate, releasing large numbers of ova. In the liver, the ova stimulate formation of granulomas and cause formation of large numbers of abscesses.

Clinical Presentation

Infection of man with *C. hepatica* is rare. Infected patients are acutely ill, dehydrated, undernourished, and lethargic. Symptoms may be of several months' duration. Temperatures as high as 41° C are common, occurring mainly in the evening, and associated with night sweats. Infected patients have anorexia, postprandial nausea and vomiting, with occasional hematemesis. Some have constipation; others have diarrhea. Occult blood is often found in the stool.

Physical examination shows abdominal distention and edema of the hands and lower extremities. The hands and feet may have a reddish discoloration and be painful on motion or to palpation. There is massive hepatomegaly. The liver is tender and smooth. Splenomegaly is also present.

Diagnosis and Pathology

Routine laboratory tests show leukocytosis, with leukocyte counts of 30,000 to 80,000/mm³ and eosinophil counts as high as 85 per cent. Hypochromic anemia is a consistent finding, and there may be marked hypergammaglobulinemia. The AST, ALT, and alkaline phosphatase are frequently elevated.[66, 67]

The diagnosis is made by needle biopsy of the liver. Because of the severity and extent of the granulomatous process, large numbers of ova are usually present. Needle biopsy of the liver is also used in differentiating hepatic capillariasis from toxocariasis (with which it may be confused).

At autopsy, the liver is greatly enlarged. The surface is salmon pink to purple, covered with myriad pearly white to yellowish-gray nodules, ranging in diameter from 0.1 to 0.2 cm. The nodules may coalesce, creating lesions 2 to 3 cm in diameter. The ultrastructure of the liver is markedly distorted by abscess-like lesions and granulomas. The abscesses contain masses of necrotic cells with adult parasites and ova. The adult worms may be well preserved or partly disintegrated. Some lesions consist of a fibrinoid material without apparent adult worms. The granulomas consist of palisading epithelioid cells and multinucleated giant cells surrounding either the parasites or the ova. The vessels in involved areas are distended and thrombosed. There is a heavy infiltration of plasma cells, eosinophils, and macrophages at the periphery of these granulomas. Considerable hepatic necrosis and interstitial inflammation are present in the vicinity of the granulomas. In areas of the liver not involved by the granulomatous process, parenchymal cells are normal. Some of the portal areas contain eosinophils, plasma cells, and histiocytes.

Therapy

The disease carries a poor prognosis; patients die either from complications or from liver failure. There is no known effective therapy for hepatic capillariasis. Mebendazole 200 mg twice a day for 20 days or thiabendazole 25 mg/kg/day for 30 days are considered investigational drugs for this indication by the US Food and Drug Administration.[14] (Table 39–1). However, killing the adult worms might aggravate the disease by releasing large numbers of ova.

STRONGYLOIDIASIS

Pathophysiology

Strongyloides stercoralis has two modes of existence. Under appropriate conditions in soil, the free-living adult males and females copulate and produce rhabditiform larvae. These larvae undergo several moults and become filariform larvae, which are the infective form for humans. They penetrate the skin or, occasionally, the mucous membranes and enter the lymphatic and venous circulations. They are carried to the right heart, then to the lungs, where they lodge and penetrate into the alveolar spaces. They then migrate up the trachea and are swallowed, thus reaching their usual site of residence in the duodenum and proximal jejunum. The filariform larvae burrow into the intestinal mucosa and become hermaphroditic adult females, each of which lays as many as 40 eggs per day. The ova develop into rhabditiform larvae, which are nonparasitic and are expelled in the feces. In transit through the intestinal tract, however, some of the rhabditiform larvae become infective filariform larvae. These larvae can reinvade the intestinal wall or penetrate the perianal skin, establishing an endogenous cycle.[68, 69] This autoinfection results in the passage of the parasite to the lungs and into the intestine by the usual route. It accounts for the persistence of the parasite for decades in some patients who have left the geographic areas in which they acquired the infection.

Clinical Presentation

Probably, most patients infected with Strongyloides organisms are asymptomatic. Others have symptoms that are confined to the intestines, such as abdominal pain, weight loss, diarrhea, and, occasionally, malabsorption.

An occasional patient will have massive systemic invasion by a larval stage of the parasite.[68, 69] Patients at risk for this complication include those with protein-calorie malnutrition, leukemia, lymphoma, and systemic connective tissue diseases, as well as renal transplant recipients. At the time of systemic dissemination, most of these patients are receiving cancer chemotherapeutic agents or immunosuppressive drugs. In some patients, dissemination has occurred in a setting of treatment with corticosteroids for such conditions as nephrotic syndrome, chronic glomerulonephritis, and ulcerative colitis.[69] Others have had chronic infections such as leprosy and tuberculosis. Fatal dissemination has been observed in chronic alcoholism, with malignancies, in chronic renal failure, and in some cases of achlorhydria.[69]

Patients with systemic invasion have severe abdominal pain, diarrhea, vomiting, shock, cough, fever, dyspnea, meningitis, and bacteremia.[68–70]

Physical examination occasionally discloses mild jaundice. Other physical findings include shock, nuchal rigidity, altered sense of consciousness, and hyperpnea. There is usually abdominal tenderness, and in some cases, peritoneal signs are present, especially voluntary guarding. The liver may be enlarged, but splenomegaly has not been described.

Diagnosis

The laboratory findings usually include eosinophilia unless the patient has received sufficient corticosteroids to suppress any eosinophilic response. Hypoalbuminemia is almost always seen and is caused by a protein-losing enteropathy. Liver tests may reveal a slight hyperbilirubinemia and elevations of AST, ALT, serum alkaline phosphatase, and lactate dehydrogenase (LDH). Blood cultures frequently demonstrate gram-negative organisms.

The diagnosis of strongyloidiasis is made on the basis of identification of the larvae, adult worms, or ova.[71] Ova are rarely present in the feces unless diarrhea is massive, but adult worms, rhabditiform larvae, and filariform larvae may be found in feces. Duodenal aspiration gives a much higher diagnostic yield. The Enterotest, a gelatin capsule containing 140 cm of white nylon line, is swallowed by the patient and withdrawn after four hours. The fluid expressed from the line is examined for the parasite. The test is positive for more than 90 per cent of individuals harboring the parasite. Larvae may be found in the sputum, peritoneal fluid, lymph nodes, cutaneous cysts, and urine. They have been found in gastric ulcers and in the appendix as well.[69] Serologic tests and skin tests have not been widely used because of their lack of specificity and the unavailability of an appropriate antigen.

Pathology

Needle biopsy studies of the liver in disseminated strongyloidiasis have not been reported. However, pathologic features of the liver in fatal cases coming to autopsy have been well described.[68, 70, 72] Strongyloides larvae are found in the portal tracts and throughout the lobule. Some larvae do not provoke any cellular reaction, but dead worms, on the other hand, are always surrounded by an inflammatory reaction. The portal tracts are infiltrated with plasma cells, lymphocytes, eosinophils, and, occasionally, neutrophils. Granulomas consisting of macrophages, giant cells, plasma cells, lymphocytes, eosinophils, and (rarely) neutrophils, are found in portal tracts and in the lobule. A diffuse, moderate fatty change appears to occur in most livers.[70, 72] Cholestasis is common and is seen as fine bile droplets in hepatocytes and small bile thrombi in canaliculi. Evidence of obstruction of larger biliary ducts is not seen.

Therapy

The drug of choice for treatment of strongyloidiasis is thiabendazole 25 mg/kg given twice daily (maximum 3 gm day) for two days (Table 39–1).[14] In disseminated strongyloidiasis, the regimen is continued for at least five days. Some immunosuppressed human hosts may not clear the organism or may be subject to repeated reinfection, particularly when they live in unhygienic situations. Other situations that may predispose to failure to eradicate the parasite include blind loops, which might occur with gastrectomy and gastrojejunostomy. The parasite may reside in the afferent loop of the duodenum in a patient so treated.[69] It has been recommended that the immunosuppressed patient who has a history of previous strongyloidiasis be treated prophylactically with thiabendazole, 1 g/day, for two days every month.[69]

FASCIOLIASIS

Pathophysiology

Fasciola hepatica, a large, hermaphroditic, leaf-shaped trematode, 30 mm × 13 mm resides in the intrahepatic biliary tree. The eggs are large, ovoid, operculate, and yellowish-brown, measuring 130 to 150 × 63 to 90 μm. They pass in the bile into the intestinal tract and are evacuated in the feces. Ova mature in 10 to 15 days. Miracidia escape from the egg and must invade a suitable snail within a few hours. On entering the snail's tissue they transform into sporocysts. In approximately three weeks, the sporocysts produce first-generation rediae and in the fourth week, second generation rediae, in which the cercariae develop. The cercariae adhere to surfaces of aquatic plants, grass, stones, and so forth, shedding their tails and encysting as metacercariae. Humans acquire the infection by the ingestion of aquatic plants, particularly watercress, or by drinking water containing the metacercariae.

The metacercariae excyst in the duodenum, penetrate the wall, and enter the peritoneal cavity. They then penetrate the capsule of the liver. They migrate through the hepatic parenchyma, producing burrows with ragged walls of damaged parenchyma; hemorrhage; and infiltration with leukocytes, eosinophils, and macrophages. As the parasite grows, it produces larger defects within the liver. The flukes reach the bile ducts, where they mature into adults within three to four months after the initial infection. At this time, ova are found in the feces. The tracts through the liver heal by granulation tissue and finally fibrosis, which leaves linear scars throughout the hepatic parenchyma.[73]

Several epidemics of fascioliasis have been described. The disease has two phases, an acute invasive phase, during which the parasite is migrating through the liver, and a chronic or latent phase, during which it resides in the biliary tract.[73]

Clinical Presentation of Acute Fascioliasis

The acute phase usually begins with a transitory period of dyspepsia, followed by high temperatures (39 to 40° C). Most patients have abdominal pain that varies in intensity and is localized to the right hypochondrium or epigastrium. Other symptoms include prostration, anorexia, sweating, myalgias, joint and bone pains, violent headaches, nausea, and vomiting. Weight loss may be marked,[73] and in some patients, diarrhea is severe.[74] Others have jaundice, allergic manifestations, and urticaria and are pale. Hemobilia from direct injury to the common bile duct by the flukes has been reported.[75] A few patients have intense abdominal pain and shock due to hepatic rupture or rupture of subcapsular hematomas when first seen by the physician.[73]

The most prominent physical findings is an enlarged liver, which may be markedly tender. Almost all patients are febrile, and some have splenomegaly.

Diagnosis

Leukocytosis, with leukocyte counts as high as 35,000/mm³ or higher, is observed in many patients. The eosinophil count may be 80 to 90 per cent. Serum alkaline phosphatase, AST, ALT, and bilirubin are frequently elevated. Hypergammaglobulinemia is common. The major elevations are in the IgG and IgM fractions.

Pathology

Pathologic features of the acute invasive phase depend upon the number of parasites present and their growth rates. The necrotic tracts are involved by coagulation ne-

crosis of the hepatocytes and contain numerous neutrophils, lymphocytes, and erythrocytes. Adjacent hepatocytes are also undergoing necrosis. The portal areas are infiltrated with round cells and are edematous. There may be small areas of infarction caused by thrombosis of blood vessels. Healing occurs by scarring and regeneration.[73] Rarely, ova are present in the parenchyma and are surrounded by granulomas.

Clinical Presentation of Chronic Fascioliasis

Many patients with chronic fascioliasis are asymptomatic. Symptoms, when present, are those of biliary obstruction or cholangitis. Pigment gallstones have been found in the common bile duct. Patients with symptoms usually have diffuse pain in the right upper quadrant or epigastrium, nausea, vomiting, and diarrhea. Some are jaundiced.[73, 75]

Physical findings can include hepatomegaly and splenomegaly. There is frequently tenderness in the epigastrium and right upper quadrant. Patients may be pale as a result of anemia.

Diagnosis and Pathology

Approximately half the patients have eosinophilia, although eosinophil counts are not as high as those found in the acute invasive phase. There are fluctuating elevations of alkaline phosphatase, bilirubin, AST, and ALT. Some patients have profound iron-deficiency anemia and a few have hypoprothrombinemia.

Liver biopsy may disclose portal inflammation with eosinophils, lymphocytes, neutrophils, plasma cells, and macrophages. There may be small or large areas of focal hepatic necrosis. Retained bile is frequently present in hepatocytes, and bile thrombi in canaliculi. Kupffer cells are often prominent. The gross pathologic features of the liver include moderate hepatomegaly, increased consistency, and cholestasis. There are small nodules and linear scars beneath the capsule. The common bile duct may be markedly dilated and fibrotic. The adult parasite may be present in association with choledocholithiasis. Marked adenomatous hyperplasia of the biliary ductal epithelium has been observed. An association with carcinoma of the bile duct has not been established.

The diagnosis of fascioliasis is made by finding the ova in either feces or duodenal drainage. Standard radiologic imaging tests are not particularly helpful, although low-density areas have been demonstrated on CT scanning. Both ERCP and percutaneous cholangiography have been useful in defining changes in the bile ducts as well as in demonstrating the parasite directly.[76, 77] Laparoscopic abnormalities, including raised, vermiform nodules have been well described.[78] The serologic tests available are immunoelectrophoresis and complement fixation, indirect hemagglutination, and indirect immunofluorescence tests.[25]

The parasite has been found in other organs, including the lungs and bronchi, peritoneum, muscles, orbit of the eye, brain, and subcutaneous tissues.

Therapy

The drug of choice for hepatic fascioliasis is bithionol, 30 to 50 mg/kg, giver on alternate days for 10 to 15 doses.

The adult and pediatric doses are the same (Table 39–1).[14, 77]

Fasciola gigantica is a common parasite of cattle in Africa, Asia, and Hawaii. A few instances of infection in humans have been reported. The life cycle of the parasite and the pathogenesis, symptoms, and pathologic characteristics of the infection are similar to those found for *Fasciola hepatica*.

ASCARIASIS

Pathophysiology

Ascariasis is caused by the large intestinal roundworm *Ascaris lumbricoides*. It is estimated that approximately 650 million people throughout the world are infected by this parasite.[79]

The normal habitat of the adult parasite is the small intestine. The female is 20 to 35 cm long and 0.3 to 0.6 cm in diameter; the male varies from 15 to 31 cm in length and from 0.2 to 0.4 cm in diameter. The fertile female deposits an average of 200,000 ova daily. The life span of the adult in the intestine is estimated to be approximately a year.

Ova shed in feces may be fertilized or unfertilized. Fertilized ova are ovoid, mamillated, and golden-brown, and are 45 to 75 μm long and 35 to 50 μm in diameter. Unfertilized ova are longer (88 to 95 μm) and are 44 μm in diameter. They have a thin shell and an irregular shape. Ova passed in feces are unsegmented, but under the proper conditions cell division begins promptly. The larval stage is reached within 9 to 12 days. The rhabditiform larvae will be infective about one week later. On ingestion by the human host, the outer coats of the ova are digested in the stomach. The larvae excyst in the small intestine and penetrate the epithelium of the intestine, eliciting a moderate eosinophilic response in the lamina propria. They enter the small veins of the portal system and lymphatic vessels on their way to the liver and regional lymph nodes. They reach the thoracic duct, and thus the lungs. In the hepatic sinusoids, the larvae move actively without stimulating any inflammatory response, but dead larvae in the liver stimulate a granulomatous reaction. In the pulmonary capillaries, the larvae are surrounded by eosinophils and neutrophils. Dead larvae in the lung stimulate a granulomatous reaction similar to that in the liver. The surviving larvae break through the capillary wall and enter the bronchi, where they moult twice and grow considerably in length and width. In the lumens of the bronchi, the third- and fourth-stage larvae are surrounded by mucus, edema fluid, and inflammatory cells. They ascend the tracheobronchial tree and larynx to the hypopharynx, where they are swallowed. On reaching the small intestine they attain sexual maturity in two to three months.

Clinical Presentation

The most severe complications of ascariasis are due to the large numbers of parasites in the intestinal lumen, their tendency to wrap themselves into tight bundles, and their propensity for entering small orifices.[79] Intestinal obstruction is the most common complication. Penetration into the appendix may produce acute appendicitis, and perforation into the peritoneal cavity may be followed by localized or generalized peritonitis.

Biliary ascariasis is one of the more severe complications. The incidence is much greater in children and young adults than in more mature individuals. The clinical manifestations vary in severity, depending upon the number of parasites in the biliary system and whether they remain in the duct or return to the intestine.

Patients who have biliary ascariasis have sudden onset of severe, colicky pain in the epigastrium or right upper quadrant. The pain radiates to the shoulder, back, or hypogastrium. It may last 10 to 20 minutes or longer and then slowly remit. The attacks of pain may stop after a number of hours, or they may persist for days. Nausea and vomiting are common, and there is frequent vomiting of worms. In patients who have symptoms of long duration, fever is common. A change in the character of the pain from paroxysmal and colicky to continuous, dull, and less severe may indicate the parasite has died. In patients in whom the parasite migrates and is trapped in the intrahepatic ducts, the symptoms become much more severe and persistent. The right upper quadrant pain is continuous and unremittent. Anorexia and nausea are common. There may be septic fever and rapid weight loss.[79–82] Jaundice occurs in 10 to 20 per cent of patients.

Hepatomegaly is found in approximately 50 per cent of patients who have uncomplicated biliary ascariasis. The liver may be exquisitely tender to palpation. The greatest tenderness is in the epigastrium, just to the right of the xiphoid process. There is little or no guarding or rigidity. When the parasite has migrated into the intrahepatic bile ducts, the temperature may reach 38 to 41° C. The liver is enlarged, nodular and tender. In some cases a well-defined mass is connected to the liver.[79, 80] There is tenderness over the gallbladder, and sometimes the gallbladder is palpable.

Complications

Complications of biliary ascariasis include rupture of the hepatic or common bile duct with bile peritonitis. Abscesses may rupture into the peritoneal cavity. Worms in abscesses of the dome of the liver may rupture into the subdiaphragmatic space, whence they can burrow through the diaphragm into the pleural space and cause empyema.[79] One of the most ominous complications of ascarid cholangitis is extension of the inflammatory process to the hepatic or portal veins, leading to pylephlebitis, which is almost always fatal. Worms can penetrate into the lumens of these vessels to enter the circulation. If they reach the inferior vena cava, they are propelled to the right ventricle, whence they embolize to the pulmonary artery. This leads to infarction or sudden death.[79]

Diagnosis

With uncomplicated biliary ascariasis, the laboratory data are frequently normal. There may be elevations of serum alkaline phosphatase and in some cases, slight hyperbilirubinemia. Biliary ascariasis of long duration is associated with leukocytosis, with leukocyte counts as high as 20,000/mm³. Eosinophilia usually is not prominent, eosinophil counts being less than 5 per cent. Patients who have acute or chronic suppurative cholangitis resulting from migration of *Ascaris* into the intrahepatic bile ducts or into the liver parenchyma have pronounced leukocytosis, with a marked leftward shift and hypoalbuminemia.[79] The AST, ALT, and alkaline phosphatase may be elevated. Approximately 25 per cent of patients with common bile duct ascariasis, particularly when the worm has not completely entered the common duct, have hyperamylasemia without evidence of pancreatitis. Conversely, approximately 25 per cent of patients with pancreatitis due to ascariasis have biliary obstruction with slight hyperbilirubinemia (serum bilirubin 3 to 5 mg/dl).[80]

The diagnosis of ascariasis is made by finding ova or the adult worm. A history of vomiting worms or passage of worms in the feces further supports the diagnosis. Duodenal drainage after the administration of magnesium sulfate may recover ova from the biliary tract. Plain radiographs of the abdomen may demonstrate air in the biliary tree. Ultrasonography may demonstrate dilated bile ducts and liver abscesses. On real-time scanning, live worms have been seen moving within liver cavities.[82] CT scanning has also been useful in demonstrating hepatic abscesses and dilated bile ducts. Further support for the diagnosis of biliary ascariasis is the demonstration of worms in the duodenum on barium studies. Occasionally, a worm may be seen fluoroscopically to be protruding from the ampulla of Vater or maybe visualized directly in the duodenum or biliary tree with the use of endoscopy and ERCP.[83, 84]

Pathology

The common bile duct is the most common location for the parasite. Most patients have only one worm in the common bile duct, but 20 to 30 have been observed. If the worms are all living, the only operative finding is a dilated common bile duct.[79] The presence of dead and disintegrating worms in the biliary ducts causes destruction of the mucosa, exudation of eosinophils, and fibrosis, which may lead to stricture of the ducts. This predisposes to calculus formation and infection.[80] When the worms are trapped in the intrahepatic ducts, thousands of eggs are released upon their disintegration, resulting in an acute and chronic suppurative cholangitis. At autopsy or surgery, the adult parasite may be seen under Glisson's capsule or burrowing through the capsule under the surface. The liver is markedly enlarged and contains many irregular abscesses filled with foul-smelling pus. Both living and dead parasites may be seen.[79, 85] The material within the abscesses is composed of cellular debris, neutrophils, and eosinophils. Fragments of degenerated adult worms and ova in various stages of preservation are also present. Peripheral to the abscesses are zones of granulomatous inflammation, including epithelioid and multinucleated giant cells, eosinophils, plasma cells, and lymphocytes. Many ova are usually present. Immediately around the granulomatous tissue, a dense layer of fibrosis delimits the focus of inflammation from the adjacent liver parenchyma.[79] Some patients have numerous hard, pale yellow nodules in the liver that resemble metastatic neoplasms. Ascaris ova are found surrounded by a chronic granulomatous reaction, which is usually centered around a distended and often destroyed biliary duct. The portal areas are widened and infiltrated by eosinophils, plasma cells, and macrophages. Eventually, these lesions undergo extensive fibrosis containing only a few multinucleated giant cells, a few plasma cells, and some eosinophils. In this late chronic stage ova are no longer apparent.

Therapy

The treatment of hepatic abscesses caused by ascariasis is surgical, with drainage and evacuation of all worms,

followed by specific drug therapy.[80-82] Uncomplicated biliary ascariasis may be managed by medical therapy.[80] Obstructive cholangitis caused by biliary ascariasis has been treated by ERCP with endoscopic sphincterotomy and removal of worms with an endoscopic basket.[84]

The drugs of choice for A. lumbricoides ascariasis are pyrantel pamoate given as a single dose of 11 mg/kg (maximum 1 g; the adult dose and the pediatric dose for children older than two years of age are the same) or mebendazole, 100 mg, given twice a day for three days. An alternative treatment is with piperazine citrate, 75 mg/kg (maximum 3.5 g) per day, given for two days. The pediatric and adult doses are the same (Table 39–1).[14]

CLONORCHIASIS AND OPISTHORCHIASIS

Pathophysiology

All adult liver flukes are similar, and the clinical manifestations, pathogenetic features, and pathologic characteristics of infestations with the various species resemble each other. Clonorchis sinensis is a flat, leaf-shaped, transparent fluke 10 to 25 mm long, 3 to 5 mm broad, and about 1 mm thick. It parasitizes the biliary tracts of a number of animals, but humans are considered to be the definitive hosts. Opisthorchis felineus and Opisthorchis viverrini are common liver flukes of cats, for which humans are accidental hosts. The cat flukes are somewhat smaller than C. sinensis.[86-88] The lancet fluke Dicrocoelium dendriticum is an unusual biliary tract fluke in humans.[89]

The mature flukes live in biliary ducts, pancreatic ducts, and, occasionally, the gallbladder. The life cycle requires two intermediate hosts. The first intermediate hosts are various species of snails; the second intermediate hosts are freshwater fish. Ova are carried down the common bile duct and excreted in the feces. On reaching water, the eggs are operculated and contain fully developed miracidia. When ingested by the appropriate snail host, the miracidia develop into sporocysts, from which rediae develop and emerge. The redial stage traverses the lymphatic spaces of the snail and develops in tissues to the cercarial stage. The mature cercariae rupture into the tissues of the host and are shed in the water. A free-swimming cercaria, on making contact with a suitable freshwater fish, penetrates the skin and sheds its tail. The organism then encysts in the muscle of the fish and becomes a metacercaria. Humans and other hosts acquire the infection by the ingestion of raw or incompletely cooked fish. The metacercariae excyst in the duodenum through peptic and tryptic digestion. They migrate to the ampulla of Vater, biliary ducts, pancreatic ducts, and the gallbladder. They tend to reside in the smallest biliary ducts that can accommodate them. The worm begins laying eggs three to four weeks after infestation.[86]

Clinical Presentation

The stages of the disease correlate with worm burden, duration of infestation, and condition of the host. Patients with mild infections (less than 100 flukes) may have no symptoms. Patients with moderate infections (up to 1000 flukes) have anorexia, nausea, epigastric distress, fullness, and various other nonspecific upper abdominal complaints. In severe infections (up to 20,000 flukes), symptoms are due to the direct effect of the worms' causing intrahepatic and extrahepatic biliary duct obstruction. Some patients have associated cholangitis as a result of bacterial infections. Toxic metabolites of the worms may contribute to the clinical picture. Occasionally, worms migrate into the hepatic parenchyma.

The signs and symptoms in liver fluke infestation depend upon the number of worms present and whether there is secondary bacterial infection. With opisthorchiasis, jaundice is common and is usually slight to moderate.[88] Anorexia, nausea, and weight loss are also prominent. Jaundice is not so common in clonorchiasis, although some patients have deep jaundice with acholic stools and itching. Patients with associated cholangitis have fever, chills, and deep jaundice. A few patients have symptoms suggesting cholecystitis. In the very late stages of the illness, patients may develop secondary biliary cirrhosis and portal hypertension. A few manifest hepatic coma and gastrointestinal bleeding. Secondary infection may be the terminal event.

Physical examination usually shows slight to moderate jaundice, hepatomegaly, and splenomegaly. With obstructive jaundice, the gallbladder is frequently palpable. With cholangitis, there may be cystic dilation of the intrahepatic biliary ducts, and the liver is enlarged and tender to palpation. The cystic enlargement reflects a biliary abscess secondary to ascending cholangitis. Some patients have enlarged, nontender, cystic livers. Aspiration of the cysts may disclose fluid that is white, yellow, yellowish-brown, bile-stained, serosanguineous, transparent, or turbid. The cysts usually contain liver fluke ova, which are numerous at times. Occasionally, adult worms are aspirated as transparent reddish parasites.

Some patients seek medical aid because of a mass in the region of the liver. Cholangiocarcinoma is the most common concomitant malignancy with liver fluke infestations.[88-91] Hepatocellular carcinoma has been associated with these parasites, but the hepatitis B surface antigen status of affected patients has not been reported. These patients have weight loss, fever, severe anorexia, and jaundice. On physical examination, the liver is markedly enlarged, has an irregular consistency, and contains a mass. There are usually cystic areas. These patients die rapidly. The terminal complications are usually hematemesis, melena, hypoglycemia, ascites, and hepatic coma.

Diagnosis

The diagnosis of liver fluke infestations should be suspected in patients residing in endemic areas who have jaundice, hepatomegaly, enlarged gallbladders, or obscure liver disease. However, recent surveys have revealed that up to 26 per cent of Asian immigrants to the United States have an active liver fluke infestation.[90, 91] The definitive diagnosis is made by identification of eggs in the feces or in the duodenal aspirate. The results of liver tests may be normal in mild infections. In severe cases, there are variable elevations of bilirubin, AST, ALT, cholesterol, alkaline phosphatase, and γ-glutamyl transpeptidase. Hypoalbuminemia and hyperglobulinemia are frequent. Serologic tests have been of little use in diagnosis, because other parasites possess the same group antigens.

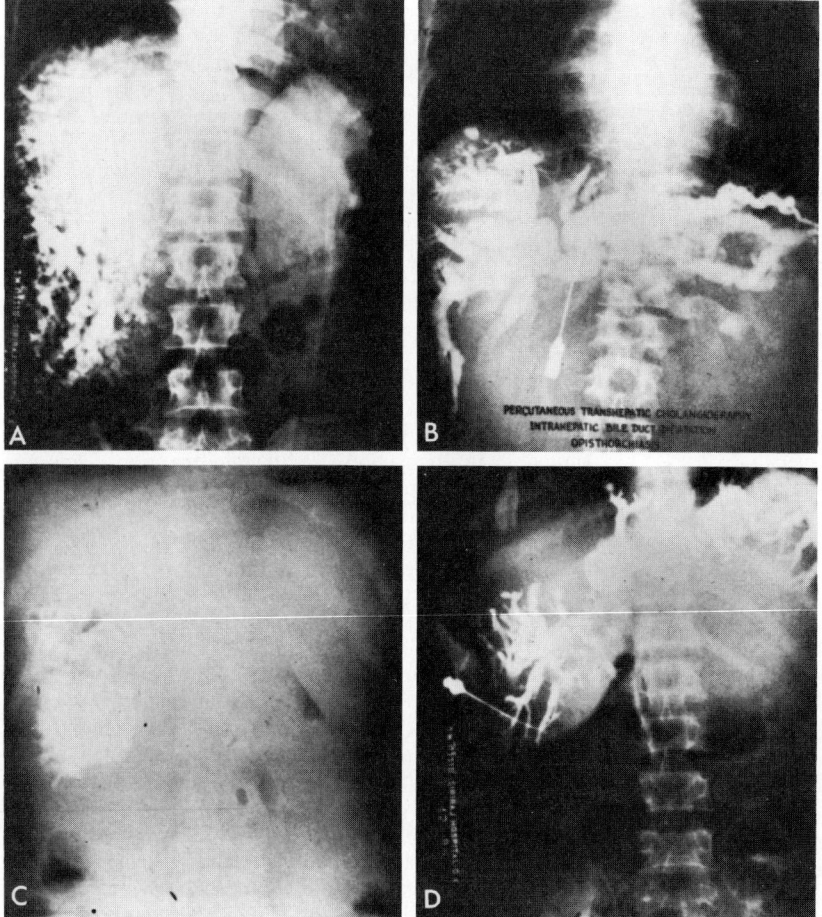

Figure 39–6. A–C, Percutaneous transhepatic cholangiograms in patients with opisthorchiasis. A shows typical fine mulberry-like dilation of the interhepatic bile ducts. In B, saccular dilation of bile ducts is seen. In C, there is a large cystic dilation of the bile duct on the left. D shows a combination of large cystic dilation and small cystic ectasia of a bile duct, pathognomonic of liver fluke infestation. (Reproduced from Tansurat P. In: Marcial Rojas RA, ed. Pathology of Protozoal and Helminthic Diseases, with Clinical Correlation, p. 536. © 1971, The Williams & Wilkins Co., Baltimore.)

In mild infestations, laparoscopic examination may disclose a normal liver, but the liver is extremely enlarged when liver fluke infestation is associated with malignancy. Jaundiced patients have green livers with markedly dilated subcapsular biliary ducts. When secondary biliary cirrhosis is present, the surface of the liver is granular. The gallbladder may be markedly enlarged when adult worms block the common bile duct.[92]

Endoscopic retrograde cholangiography and percutaneous transhepatic cholangiography are useful in the diagnosis of patients with jaundice. Four patterns have been observed: (1) diffuse tapering of the intrahepatic ducts with dilation indistinguishable from that associated with extrahepatic obstruction; (2) a solitary cyst similar to a liver abscess cavity or retention cyst; (3) multiple cystic dilations of the intrahepatic ducts, producing a mulberry-like appearance that is characteristic of liver fluke infestation; (4) a combination of these findings, with extensive cystic dilation in some areas of the liver and biliary duct ectasia in others (Fig. 39–6, *A–D*). In heavy infections, ultrasonography or CT scanning may show intrahepatic defects in addition to dilated bile ducts.

TABLE 39–2. GEOGRAPHIC DISTRIBUTION OF PARASITES AFFECTING THE LIVER

Parasite	Distribution	Parasite	Distribution
Entamoeba histolytica	Worldwide	*Toxoplasma gondii*	Worldwide; low rates of infection in cold climates and arid areas
Plasmodium (malaria)	Central and South America, Africa, southern Europe, Turkey, Iraq, Iran, Afghanistan, India, Ceylon, Burma, China, Cambodia, Vietnam, Laos, Thailand, Malaysia, Indonesia, Formosa, Philippines, and many Pacific islands	*Schistosoma mansoni*	Nile Delta, Upper Sudan, Eritrea through Kenya, Tanzania, Malawi, Zambesi River, Rhodesia, Zambia, Congo basin, Senegal, the Cameroons, Dahomey, Guinea to Lake Chad, Sierra Leone, Liberia, Libya, Yemen, Natal, and the Transvaal; Western hemisphere: Brazil, Venezuela, Surinam, Antigua, Guadeloupe, Martinique, St. Lucia, Nevis, Monserrat, Viegues, and Puerto Rico (control measures have reduced prevalences in Puerto Rico and Venezuela)
Trypanosoma gambiense	Senegal to Lakes Victoria, Albert, Banguelo, and Tanganyika in the east to North Angola in the south		
Trypanosoma rhodesiense	East and Central Africa from South Sudan to Mozambique		
Trypanosoma cruzi	Brazil, Argentina, Uruguay, Chile, and Venezuela; rare cases in all South and Central American countries except Surinam and Guyana; a few cases in the United States and Mexico	*Schistosoma japonicum*	Japan, China, Philippines, Celebes, Laos, Cambodia (China has virtually eliminated *S. japonicum* by control measures)
Leishmania donovani	Asia, Middle East, Mediterranean littoral, Africa, South America; occasional cases in Central America and Mexico	*Echinococcus granulosus*	South Australia, Tasmania, New Zealand, northern and southern Africa, Argentina, Paraguay, Chile, Uruguay, southern Brazil, Europe, Siberia, Turkestan, Mongolia, North China, southern Japan, North Vietnam, Philippines, Syria, Lebanon, Iraq, Israel, Arabia, northern Canada, Alaska, Ireland, western United States
Fascioliasis hepatica	Venezuela, Uruguay, Argentina, Chile, Puerto Rico, Cuba, Costa Rica, Syria, Turkey, China, U.S.S.R., Poland, Madeira, England, France, Italy, Corsica, Spain, Hungary, Roumania, Salonika, the Dardanelles, Algeria, Somaliland, South Africa, and Hawaii		
		Echinococcus multilocularis	Southern German, Switzerland, the Tyrol, U.S.S.R., Iceland, northern Germany, Italy, France, Poland, the Balkans, Uruguay, Argentina, Australia, New Zealand, Japan, England, Canadian western Arctic, Alaska, North Dakota, Turkey
Fascioliasis gigantica	Important liver fluke in cattle and other herbivores, North America and Northern Europe; rare in humans		
Ascaris lumbricoides	Worldwide; more common in warm, moist climates		
		Toxocara	Eastern and southern United States, Puerto Rico, Holland, England, Hawaii, Philippines, Australia, South Africa, Turkey, Roumania, Colombia, Israel
Clonorchis sinensis	Japan, Korea, Taiwan, nearly all of China, and Vietnam		
Opisthorchis felineus	Southern, central and eastern Europe, Siberia, East Prussia, Poland, India, North Vietnam, North Korea, Japan, and the Philippines	*Capillaria hepatica*	India, New Orleans, Baltimore, Hawaii, Johannesburg, Durban, Mexico, Brazil (rare)
Opisthorchis viverrini	Thailand and Laos	*Strongyloides stercoralis*	Worldwide, primarily in areas with warm climates, but has been reported from temperate and cold regions

Pathology

At autopsy or laparotomy, the liver may be small to markedly enlarged, and examination of the surface shows dilation of the subcapsular biliary ducts. At autopsy, the cut surface of the liver demonstrates markedly dilated biliary ducts with extremely thick walls. Flukes are usually visible. The gallbladder may be enlarged and contains white bile and flukes. In some cases, the worms are found in pancreatic ducts. Clonorchiasis predisposes to intrahepatic gallstone formation, whereas this is a rare finding in opisthorchiasis. Microscopically, the biliary duct epithelium is markedly proliferated, a finding referred to as adenomatous hyperplasia. Periductal fibrosis and eosinophilic infiltration are present. Occasional ova and granulomatous lesions are seen in the connective tissue of the liver, associated with infiltration of many eosinophils. In patients dying of suppurative cholangitis, the infection may extend into the liver parenchyma, causing micro- and macro-abscesses. Free ova have been observed in the exudates in these abscesses.

Therapy

Chemotherapy of liver fluke infestation is unsatisfactory. Praziquantel, 25 mg/kg three times a day for two days, is considered an investigational drug for this condition (Table 39–1).[14] Surgical approaches have been unsuccessful.

OTHER PARASITIC DISEASES

A number of other parasites have been reported to infrequently infect the liver. Microfilariae of *Wucheria bancrofti* have been found in hepatic sinusoids in a patient presenting with hepatomegaly and inferior vena cava obstruction.[93] Elevations in the ALT and AST in patients with other forms of filariasis have been described.

New opportunistic infections have been seen in patients with the acquired immunodeficiency syndrome (AIDS). Cryptosporidiosis usually involves the gastrointestinal tract, causing protracted, watery diarrhea. Cryptosporidium organisms have been seen in the gallbladder and biliary tract. A recent case of cryptosporidial hepatitis associated with cytomegalovirus hepatitis had cryptosporidia present on liver biopsy.[94] Microsporidian hepatitis caused by *Encephalitozoon cuniculi* has also been found in a patient with AIDS. Although serologic tests exist, diagnosis depends on the proper identification of the protozoan on electron microscopic examination of tissue sections.[95] (See Chap. 53 for discussion of AIDS.)

CONCLUSIONS

A travel history is obviously necessary in the management of a patient who has a parasitic disease involving the liver. Table 39–2 outlines the endemic areas of the world where the various parasites described in this chapter are acquired.

REFERENCES

1. Beaver PC, Jung RC, Cupp EW. Amebae inhabiting the alimentary canal. In: Clinical Parisitology. Philadelphia, Lea & Febiger, 1984:101.
2. Knight R. Hepatic amebiasis. Semin Liv Dis 4:277, 1984.
3. Jarumilinta R, Maegraith BG. Hyaluronidase activity in *Entamoeba histolytica*. Trans R Soc Trop Med Hyg 54:5, 1960.
4. Adams EB, Macleod IN. Invasive amebiasis. II. Amebic liver abscess and its complications. Medicine 56:325, 1977.
5. Thompson JE Sr, Glasser AJ. Amebic abscess of the liver: diagnostic features. J Clin Gastroenterol 8:550, 1986.
6. Krettek JG, Goldstein LI, Busutill RW. The symptoms of an amebic abscess of the liver simulating an acute surgical abdomen. Surg Gynecol Obstet 148:552, 1979.
7. Cuarón A, Gordon F. Liver scanning, analysis of 2500 cases of amebic hepatic abscesses. J Nucl Med 11:435, 1970.
8. Remedios PA, Colletti PM, Ralls PW. Hepatic amebic abscess: cholescintigraphic rim enhancement. Radiology 160:395, 1986.
9. Ralls PW, Colletti PM, Quinn MF, et al. Sonographic findings in hepatic amebic abscess. Radiology 145:123, 1982.
10. Reynolds TB. Amoebic abscess of the liver (editorial). Gastroenterology 60:952, 1971.
11. Gandhi BM, Irshad M, Chawla TC, et al. Enzyme-linked protein A: an ELISA for detection of amebic antibody. Trans Royal Soc Trop Med Hyg 81:183, 1987.
12. Patterson M, Healy GR, Shabor SM. Serologic testing for amebiasis. Gastroenterology 78:136, 1980.
13. Jackson TFHG, Anderson CB, Simjee HE. Serological differentiation between past and present infection in hepatic amebiasis. Trans Royal Soc Trop Med Hyg 78:342, 1984.
14. Drugs for parasitic infection. Med Lett 30:15, 1988.
15. Eggleston FC, Verghese M, Handa AK, et al. The results of surgery in amebic liver abscess: experiences in eighty-three patients. Surgery 83:536, 1978.
16. Beaver PC, Jung RC, Cupp EW. Malaria parasites and piroplasms. In: Clinical Parisitology. Philadelphia, Lea & Febiger, 1984:174.
17. Tan JS. Common and uncommon parasitic infections in the United States. Med Clin North Am 62:1059, 1978.
18. Heineman HS. The clinical syndrome of malaria in the United States. A current review of diagnosis and treatment for American physicians. Arch Intern Med 129:607, 1972.
19. Warrell DA. Pathophysiology of severe falciparum malaria in man. Parasitology 94:S53, 1987.
20. Ramachandrans S, Perera MV. Jaundice and hepatomegaly in primary malaria. J Trop Med Hyg 79:207, 1976.
21. Joshi YK, Tandon BN, Acharya SK, et al. Acute hepatic failure due to *Plasmodium falciparum* liver injury. Liver 6:357, 1986.
22. White LG, Doerner AA. Functional and needle biopsy of the liver in malaria. JAMA 155:637, 1954.
23. Hollingdale M. Malaria and the liver. Hepatology, 5:327, 1985.
24. Beaver PC, Jung RC, Cupp EW. The blood and tissue flagellates. In: Clinical Parasitology. Philadelphia, Lea & Febiger, 1984:55.
25. Kagan IG. Diagnostic, epidemiologic, and experimental parasitology: immunologic aspects. Am J Trop Med Hyg 28:429, 1979.
26. Robertson DHH, Jenkins AR. Hepatic dysfunction in human trypanosomiasis. I. Abnormalities of excretory function, seroflocculation phenomena and other tests of hepatic function with observations on the alterations of these tests during treatment and convalescence. Trans R Soc Trop Med Hyg 53:511, 1959.
27. Gelfand M, Friedlander J. Jaundice in Rhodesian sleeping sickness. Report on two European cases. Trans R Soc Trop Med Hyg 57:290, 1963.
28. Francis TI. Visceral complications of Gambian trypanosomiasis in a Nigerian. Trans R Soc Trop Med Hyg 66:140, 1972.
29. Marsden PD. Parasitic diseases of the liver. In: Schiff L, ed. Diseases of the Liver, 4th ed. Philadelphia. JB Lippincott, 1975:1078.
30. Andrade ZA, Andrade SG. Chagas' disease (American trypanosomiasis). In: Marcial-Rojas RA, ed. Pathology of Protozoal and Helminthic Diseases with Clinical Correlation. Baltimore, Williams & Wilkins, 1971:69.
31. Laranja FS, Dias E, Nobrega G, et al. Chagas' disease. A clinical, epidemiologic and pathologic study. Circulation, 14:1035, 1956.
32. Mazza D. Inexistencia de un sintoma patognomonico enformas agudas de enfermad de Chagas. Prens Med Argent 26:1569, 1939. [Cited in Reference 24.]
33. Winslow DJ. Kala-azar (visceral leishmaniasis). In: Marcial-Rojas RA, ed. Pathology of Protozoal and Helminthic Diseases with Clinical Correlation. Baltimore, Williams & Wilkins, 1971:56.
34. Badaro R, Carvalho EM, Rocha H, et al. Leishmania donovani: an opportunistic microbe associated with progressive disease in three immunocompromised patients. Lancet 1:647, 1986.
35. Maru M. Clinical and laboratory features and treatment of visceral leishmaniasis in hospitalized patients in northwestern Ethiopia. Am J Trop Med Hyg 28:15, 1979.
36. Most H, Lavietes PH. Kala-azar in American military personnel. Medicine 26:221, 1947.
37. Marsden PD. Current concepts in parasitology. Leishmaniasis. N Engl J Med 300:350, 1979.
38. Frenkel JK. Toxoplasmosis. In: Marcial-Rojas RA, ed. Pathology of

Protozoal and Helminthic Diseases with Clinical Correlation. Baltimore, Williams & Wilkins, 1971:254.

39. Vischer TL, Bernheim C, Engelbrecht E. Two cases of hepatitis due to *Toxoplasma gondii*. Lancet 2:919, 1967.

40. Weitberg AB, Alper JC, Diamond I, et al. Acute granulomatous hepatitis in the course of acquired toxoplasmosis. N Engl J Med 300:1093, 1979.

41. Krick JA, Remington JS. Current concepts in parasitology. Toxoplasmosis in the adult—an overview. N Engl J Med 298:550, 1978.

42. Marcial-Rojas RA. Schistosomiasis mansoni. In: Marcial-Rojas RA, ed. Pathology of Protozoal and Helminthic Diseases with Clinical Correlation. Baltimore, Williams & Wilkins, 1971:373.

43. Miyake M. Schistosomiasis japonicum. In: Marcial-Rojas RA, ed. Pathology of Protozoal and Helminthic Diseases with Clinical Correlation. Baltimore, Williams & Wilkins, 1971:414.

44. Prata A. Schistosomiasis mansoni. Clin Gastroenterol 7:49, 1978.

45. Warren KS. Schistosomiasis japonica. Clin Gastroenterol 7:77, 1978.

46. Clegg JA, Smithers SR, Terry RI. Acquisition of human antigens by *Schistosoma mansoni* during cultivation *in vitro*. Nature 232:653, 1971.

47. El-Rooby A. Management of hepatic schistosomiasis. Semin Liver Dis 5:263, 1985.

48. Colley DG, Cook GL, Freeman JR, et al. Immune response during human schistosomiasis mansoni. I. *In vitro* lymphocyte blastogenic response to heterogenous antigenic preparations from schistosome eggs, worms and cercariae. Int Arch Allergy Appl Immunol 53:420, 1977.

49. Colley DG, Lewis FA, Goodgame RW. Immune response during human schistosomiasis. IV. Induction of suppressor cell activity by schistosome antigen populations and concanavalin A J Immunol 118:648, 1977.

50. Kanagasundaram N, Leevy CM. Immunologic aspects of liver disease. Med Clin North Am 63:631, 1979.

51. Warren K. The kinetics of hepatosplenic schistosomiasis. Semin Liver Dis 4:293, 1984.

52. El-Gendi MA. Radiographic and haemodynamic patterns of portal hypertension in hepatosplenic schistosomiasis: selection of surgical procedure. Gut 20:177, 1979.

53. DaSilva LC, Macedo AL, Fermanian J, et al. A randomized trial for the study of the elective surgical treatment of portal hypertension in mansonic schistosomiasis. Ann Surg 204:148, 1986.

54. Poole JB, Marcial-Rojas RA. Echinococcosis. In: Marcial-Rojas RA, ed. Pathology of Protozoal and Helminthic Diseases with Clinical Correlation. Baltimore, Williams & Wilkins, 1971:635.

55. Lewis JW Jr, Koss N, Kerstein MD. A review of echinococcal disease. Ann Surg 181:390, 1975.

56. Beggs I. The radiological appearances of hydatid disease of the liver. Clin Radiol 34:555, 1983.

57. Langer B. Surgical treatment of hydatid disease of the liver. Br J Surg 74:237, 1987.

58. Belghiti J, Benhamou JP, Houry S, et al. Caustic sclerosing cholangitis. Arch Surg 121:1162, 1986.

59. Ponchon T, Bory R, Chavaillon A. Endoscopic retrograde cholangiography and sphincterotomy for complicated hepatic hydatid cyst. Endoscopy 19:174, 1987.

60. Rausch RL, Wilson JF, McMahon BJ, et al. Consequences of continuous mebendazole therapy in alveolar hydatid disease with a summary of a ten-year clinical trial. Ann Trop Med Parasitol 80:403, 1986.

61. Wilson JF, Rausch RL, McMahon BJ, et al. Albendazole therapy in alveolar hydatid disease: a report of favorable results in two patients after short-term therapy. Amer J Trop Med 37:162, 1987.

62. Areán VM, Crandall CA. Toxocariasis. In: Marcial-Rojas RA, ed. Pathology of Protozoal and Helminthic Diseases with Clinical Correlation. Baltimore, Williams & Wilkins, 1971:808.

63. Marsden PD. Other nematodes. Clin Gastroenterol 7:219, 1978.

64. Schantz PM, Glickman LT. Toxocaral visceral larva migrans. N Engl J Med 298:436, 1978.

65. Glickman L, Schantz P, Dombroske R, et al. Evaluation of serodiagnostic tests for visceral larva migrans. Am J Trop Med Hyg 27:492, 1978.

66. Areán VM. Capillariasis. In: Marcial-Rojas RA, ed. Pathology of

Protozoal and Helminthic Diseases with Clinical Correlation. Baltimore, Williams & Wilkins, 1971:666.

67. Attah EB, Nagarajan S, Obineche EN, et al. Hepatic capillariasis. Amer J Clin Pathol 79:127, 1983.

68. Marcial-Rojas RA. Strongyloidiasis. In: Marcial-Rojas RA, ed. Pathology of Protozoal and Helminthic Diseases with Clinical Correlation. Baltimore, Williams & Wilkins, 1971:711.

69. Scowden EB, Schaffner W, Stone WJ. Overwhelming strongyloidiasis: an unappreciated opportunistic infection. Medicine 57:527, 1978.

70. Poltera AA, Katsimbura N. Granulomatous hepatitis due to *Strongyloides stercoralis*. J Pathol 113:241, 1974.

71. Grove DI, Warren KS, Mahmoud AA. Algorithms in the diagnosis and management of exotic diseases. III. Strongyloidiasis. J Infect Dis 131:755, 1975.

72. DePaola D, Braga-Diaz L, Rodrigues da Silva J. Enteritis due to *Strongyloides stercoralis*. A report of 5 fatal cases. Am J Dig Dis 7:1086, 1962.

73. Náquira-Vidoso F, Marcial-Rojas RA. Fascioliasis. In: Marcial-Rojas RA, ed. Pathology of Protozoal and Helminthic Diseases with Clinical Correlation. Baltimore, Williams & Wilkins, 1971:477.

74. Jones EA, Kay JM, Milligan HP, et al. Massive infection with *Fasciola hepatica*. in man. Am J Med 63:836, 1977.

75. Acuna-Soto R, Braun-Roth G. Bleeding ulcer in the common bile duct due to fasciola hepatica. Am J Gastroenterol 82:560, 1987.

76. Wong RK, Peura DA, Mutter ML, et al. Hemobilia and liver flukes in a patient from Thailand. Gastroenterology 88:1958, 1985.

77. Condomines J, Rene-Espinet JM, Espinos-Perez JC, et al. Percutaneous cholangiography in the diagnosis of hepatic fascioliasis. Am J Gastroenterol 80:384, 1985.

78. Uribarrena R, Borda F, Munoz M, et al. Laparoscopic findings in eight cases of liver fascioliasis. Endoscopy 17:137, 1985.

79. Areán VM, Crandall CA. Ascariasis. In: Marcial-Rojas RA, ed. Pathology of Protozoal and Helminthic Diseases with Clinical Correlation. Baltimore, Williams & Wilkins, 1971:769.

80. Louw JH. Abdominal complications of *Ascaris lumbricoides* infestation in children. Br J Surg 53:510, 1966.

81. Wright RM, Dorrough RL, Ditmore HB. Ascariasis of the biliary system. Arch Surg 86:72, 1963.

82. Lloyd DA. Hepatic ascariasis. S Afr J Surg 20:297, 1982.

83. VanSeveren M, Lengele B, Dureuil J, et al. Hepatic ascaridiasis. Endoscopy 19:140, 1987.

84. Jessen K, Al Mofleh I, Al Mofarreh M. Endoscopic treatment of ascariasis causing acute obstructive cholangitis. Hepatogastroenterol 33:275, 1986.

85. Piggott J, Hansbarger EA Jr, Neafie RC. Human ascariasis. Am J Clin Pathol 53:223, 1970.

86. Gibson JB, Sun T. Clonorchiasis. In: Marcial-Rojas RA, ed. Pathology of Protozoal and Helminthic Diseases with Clinical Correlation. Baltimore, Williams & Wilkins, 1971:546.

87. Tansurat P. Opisthorchiasis. In: Marcial-Rojas RA, ed. Pathology of Protozoal and Helminthic Diseases with Clinical Correlation. Baltimore, Williams & Wilkins, 1971:536.

88. Viranuvatti V, Stitnimankarn T. Liver fluke infection and infestation in southeast Asia. Progr Liver Dis 4:537, 1972.

89. Chan CW, Lam SK. Diseases caused by liver flukes and cholangiocarcinoma. Ballieres Clin Gastroenterol 1:297, 1987.

90. Lin AC, Chapman SW, Turner HR, et al. Clonorchiasis: an update. South Med J 80:919, 1987.

91. Schwartz D. Cholangiocarcinoma associated with liver fluke infection: a preventable source of morbidity in Asian immigrants. Am J Gastroenterol 81:76, 1986.

92. Hitanant S, Trong DT, Damrongsak C, et al. Peritoneoscopic findings in 203 patients with *Opisthorchis viverrini* infection. Gastrointest Endosc 33:18, 1987.

93. Sanjeeva CJ, Rao MH, Rao B, et al. Filariasis with visceral involvement and inferior vena caval obstruction. J Indian Med Assoc 74:114, 1980.

94. Kahn DG, Garfinkel JM, Klonoff DC, et al. Cryptosporidial and cytomegaloviral hepatitis and cholecystitis. Arch Pathol Lab Med 111:879, 1987.

95. Terada S, Reddy KR, Jeffers LJ, et al. Microsporidian hepatitis in the acquired immunodeficiency syndrome. Ann Int Med 107:61, 1987.

40

Bacterial and Miscellaneous Infections of the Liver

Lloyd L. Brandborg, M.D. • Ira S. Goldman, M.D.

PYOGENIC ABSCESS OF THE LIVER

Incidence and Pathogenesis

Pyogenic abscesses of the liver are relatively uncommon and account for between 0.007 and 0.016 per cent of hospital admissions.[1-7] The prevalence in autopsy series ranges from 0.29 to 1.47 per cent.[4] Although the incidence seems to have increased slightly in recent series, perhaps because of better imaging methods,[4] the clinical presentation and associated findings have changed significantly since Ochsner reported his classic series in 1938.[3] Prior to the antibiotic era, liver abscesses were most often associated with pyelophlebitis secondary to appendicitis. They occurred most frequently in individuals in the third to fourth decades of life.[3] Currently, the most common association of pyogenic abscess is with benign or malignant obstruction of the biliary tract and cholangitis.[1, 2, 4-7] The incidence is highest in the fifth and sixth decades of life and later.

Pyogenic bacteria reach the liver through several routes, the usual one being direct extension of infection from contiguous organs. Biliary tract disease accounts for the largest number of cases, with extrahepatic obstruction leading to cholangitis and abscess formation. Choledocholithiasis, benign or malignant tumors of the biliary tract and pancreas, and postsurgical stricture are potential sources of obstruction. Abscesses can form in metastatic tumor nodules within the liver. Direct extension of infection from contiguous organs—such as in lobar pneumonia, pyelonephritis, subphrenic abscess, or perforated gastric ulcer—may allow entry of bacteria into the liver.

Some liver abscesses occur because of seeding or embolization through the portal venous system of bacteria that originate in infectious processes within the abdomen, such as appendicitis, diverticulitis, inflammatory bowel disease, proctitis, infected hemorrhoids, pancreatitis, and splenitis. Fortunately, these sources of hepatic abscesses are now rare. In infancy and childhood, pyogenic abscesses occur most often in the setting of umbilical infection or sepsis.[8] Older children with hepatic abscesses have associated defects in host defenses, such as chronic granulomatous disease and leukemia. Staphylococci are the organisms most commonly isolated from hepatic abscesses in children. Infection through the hepatic artery may result from septicemia secondary to osteomyelitis, infective endocarditis, pneumonitis, or any other source from which septicemia may arise.

Trauma is rarely followed by pyogenic hepatic abscesses, but penetrating injuries from knife and bullet wounds and blunt trauma with contusion of the liver can cause such abscesses.

No cause is found for approximately half the instances of hepatic abscesses. There is an increased incidence in patients with diabetes mellitus and metastatic cancer.[4, 5]

Clinical Features

The clinical features of pyogenic liver abscess are variable and at times nonspecific. The most common symptoms are fever, malaise, weakness, rigors, diaphoresis, and anorexia. Many patients have substantial weight losses, amounting to 4.5 kg or more. Many patients have diarrhea, and abdominal pain, particularly in the right upper quadrant, is common. Pain also occurs in the left upper quadrant with abscesses of the left lobe, and the pain is diffuse in patients who have peritonitis. Many patients have a cough. Pleuritic chest pain and pain in the right shoulder also are seen (Table 40–1).[1, 2, 4-10]

The most common physical finding is hepatomegaly. Some patients have a palpable mass in the liver, and right upper quadrant abdominal tenderness is present in many. There are frequently abnormal physical findings in the chest, including pleuropericardial friction rubs, rales, pleural effusions, and signs of consolidation. Jaundice is seen in about a fourth to half of the patients. Splenomegaly occurs in approximately 25 per cent of patients (Table 40–2).[1, 2, 4, 5, 7, 10]

The laboratory abnormalities are nonspecific and, with the exception of a negative amebic serologic picture, they are similar to those in amebic liver abscesses.

TABLE 40–1. SYMPTOMS ASSOCIATED WITH PYOGENIC LIVER ABSCESSES[1, 2, 4, 5, 7, 10]

Symptom	No. of Patients (%)
Fever	87–100
Weakness	30–96
Rigors	38–88
Diaphoresis	11–84
Anorexia	38–80
Abdominal pain	48–80
Malaise	30–68
Weight loss	25–68
Nausea and vomiting	28–53
Diarrhea	17–48
Cough	11–28
Pleuritic pain	9–24

TABLE 40–2. SIGNS ASSOCIATED WITH PYOGENIC LIVER ABSCESSES[1, 2, 4, 5, 7, 10]

Sign	No. of Patients (%)
Hepatomegaly	51–92
Right upper quadrant tenderness	41–72
Mass in liver	17–18
Jaundice	23–43
Splenomegaly	21–24
Chest findings	11–48
Rales	21–24
Effusion	11–12
Friction rub	4–8
Consolidation	4–8

Many patients have anemia. Leukocyte counts are increased to more than 10,000/mm³ in the vast majority of cases. The level of serum alkaline phosphatase is elevated in most patients, and half of the patients, or more, have elevations of aminotransferases. A substantial number of patients have elevated bilirubin levels, and hypoalbuminemia is common. Hyperglobulinemia is seen in about a third of patients. The prothrombin time is usually prolonged (Table 40–3).[1, 8, 9]

Pathologic Features

Pyogenic liver abscesses may be single or multiple and are found in about equal frequency in most series.[4, 5, 7] Most are found in the right lobe, although multiple abscesses may be found in both lobes. Most abscesses of biliary tract origin are multiple, whereas most having their source in the portal system are single and in the right lobe.[2] Abscesses may be divided by size into macroscopic and microscopic groups. Microscopic abscesses are almost always multiple and are more difficult to diagnose. In one series, only 22 per cent of patients with hepatic microabscesses were diagnosed before death.[1]

Diagnosis

The diagnosis of pyogenic liver abscess is often delayed. More than one third of patients in a recent series had been symptomatic for at least two weeks before seeking medical therapy.[5] The delay in diagnosis may reflect, in part, that these patients are often elderly, with underlying diseases that can mask their symptoms due to the liver abscess. The mistaken initial diagnoses in patients with pyogenic liver abscesses usually are cholangitis, fever of

TABLE 40–3. LABORATORY FINDINGS ASSOCIATED WITH PYOGENIC LIVER ABSCESSES[1, 2, 4, 5, 7, 10]

Laboratory Finding	No. of Patients (%)
Anemia	50–80
Leukocyte count > 10,000/mm³	75–96
Alkaline phosphatase level elevated	95–100
Aspartate or alanine aminotransferase (AST; ALT) elevated	48–60
Bilirubin elevated	28–73
Albumin <3.0 g/dl	33–87
Globulin >3.0 g/dl	33
Prothrombin time prolonged	71–87

unknown origin, perforated viscus or mesenteric artery occlusion, pneumonia, bacteremia, metastatic malignancy, pulmonary emboli, and pancreatitis. In some cases, significant delays in diagnosis may be related to previous administration of antibiotics, which may prevent recovery of the infecting organisms.[10] Avoiding delay in arriving at a correct diagnosis may be critical for the patient's survival.

In routine roentgenologic examinations, the chest x-ray film is abnormal in approximately half of the cases. Included in the findings are pneumonitis, consolidation, pleural effusions, and immobility of the diaphragm. In the presence of gas-forming organisms, plain films of the abdomen may show a hepatic mass with an air-fluid level within it. Unless the abscess is in the left lobe, which is relatively uncommon, there is no displacement of the barium column on upper gastrointestinal studies.[2, 4, 10]

Radionuclide scanning with ⁹⁹ᵐTc sulfur colloid was the first widely used imaging test to reliably detect mass lesions more than 2 cm in diameter within the liver. The sensitivity ranges from approximately 50 to 85 per cent and often lacks specificity. Specificity is increased only slightly when ⁶⁷Ga- or ¹¹¹In-labeled leukocyte scanning is used. Although early reviews of scanning by computerized tomography (CT) showed its sensitivity to be similar to that of radionuclide scanning,[11] ultrasonography and CT scanning have largely replaced radionuclide scanning as the diagnostic procedures of choice for liver imaging. Real-time gray scale ultrasonography shows pyogenic abscesses to be round or oval areas within the liver that are usually less echogenic than the surrounding liver.[12] The sensitivity of sonography in detecting pyogenic abscesses ranges from 80 to 100 per cent.[5] Lesions high in the dome of the liver can be difficult to image, as can multiple microabscesses, which can mimic other diffuse liver diseases such as cirrhosis or metastases.[5] CT images are usually less dense (low attenuation) than surrounding normal liver tissue (Fig. 40–1). Intravenous contrast usually improves detection of pyogenic abscesses, since they do not enhance, whereas the surrounding liver tissue does.[11, 13, 14] CT scanning is as sensitive as ultrasonography in the detection of pyogenic abscesses.[5, 7] Since CT images also lack specificity, the addition of sonographic or CT-guided aspiration of suspected abscesses may help iden-

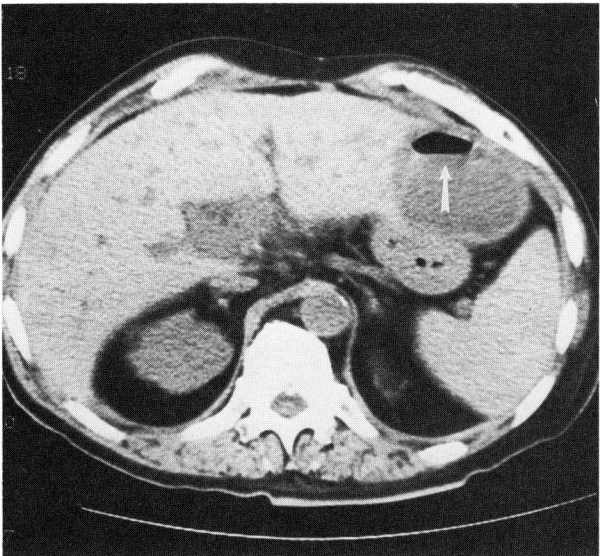

Figure 40–1. A CT scan, showing a pyogenic liver abscess in the left lobe of the liver. The arrow points to an air-fluid level within the abscess. (Courtesy of I. Goldman.)

tify the type of abscess with little added risk.[5] Angiography is rarely used today in the diagnosis of pyogenic abscesses because of the wide availability of noninvasive imaging techniques, but angiography shows displacement of the intrahepatic blood vessels and the presence of an avascular mass. The diagnosis of pyogenic hepatic abscess has also been made by percutaneous transhepatic cholangiography and endoscopic retrograde cholangiography.[15, 16] If these procedures are contemplated in the presence of cholangitis, the patient should receive antibiotics intended to be effective against both anaerobic and aerobic organisms. Contrast-enhanced magnetic resonance imaging has been used in animals to effectively demonstrate pyogenic abscesses as small as 3 mm.[17]

Bacteriology

Fifty per cent of liver abscesses were considered in the past to be sterile.[3] This was almost certainly the result of failure to obtain adequate anaerobic cultures and failure to transport the specimens in oxygen-free containers.[10] With strict anaerobic techniques, approximately 50 per cent of pyogenic liver abscesses are found to be caused by anaerobic organisms or mixed anaerobic and aerobic organisms.[5, 9, 10] The organisms recovered from pyogenic liver abscesses vary greatly (Table 40–4). Facultative gram-negative enteric bacilli, anaerobic gram-negative bacilli, and microaerophilic streptococci are isolated most frequently.[7] In some series, Escherichia coli has been the organism isolated most commonly. Blood culture results are positive for the responsible bacteria in 33 to 64 per cent of cases, compared with 73 to 100 per cent positive results from cultures of the abscess. The cultures are frequently polymicrobial.[4, 5, 7] The chances of obtaining a positive blood culture are better with multiple abscesses than with solitary abscesses.

Gram's stain may give clues to the presence of specific bacteria, as well as to their identities.[10] Bacteroides species are pleomorphic, pale, irregularly staining gram-negative rods. Bacteroides fragilis often look like safety pins because of their bipolar staining. Bacteroides melaninogenicus are small coccobacillary forms. Fusobacterium species are thin, delicate, pale-staining, gram-negative rods with tapered ends, which may resemble needle-like crystals. Sphaerophorus species are long filaments with central swellings. Anaerobic cocci are often smaller than aerobic cocci. Actinomyces organisms are thin, gram-positive, branching rods. They may be filamentous. Clostridia, except for Clostridium perfringens, frequently have detectable spores. Gram's stain also is important for quality control in that if organisms are seen on smear and not grown, it is probable that the transport or the cultural method was inadequate.[10]

TREATMENT

Until recently, open surgical drainage plus antibiotics was the treatment of choice for pyogenic liver abscesses. Multiple liver abscesses posed difficult technical problems for the surgeon, and the mortality rate was often as high as 70 per cent.[18] Although diagnostic aspiration was suggested as early as 1898,[7] it was not until 1953 that the first successful treatment of pyogenic abscess by percutaneous aspiration and antibiotics was reported.[19] This technique, however, did not become widely accepted until the late 1970s. In 1979, a small, highly selected series of six patients demonstrated successful medical treatment of pyogenic abscesses with antibiotics alone.[20] With the growth of ultrasonography and CT imaging, a number of series have demonstrated that many, if not most, pyogenic abscesses can be effectively treated with antibiotics, alone or in combination with percutaneous drainage.[5, 7, 20–25] A recent retrospective literature review of several selected, nonrandomized series of percutaneous needle aspiration and percutaneous catheter drainage in 139 cases of pyogenic liver abscess showed a success rate of 90 per cent.[25] Relative contraindications to percutaneous drainage include ascites and coagulopathy. Perforation of other abdominal organs, pneumothorax, hemorrhage, and leakage of abscess contents into areas including the peritoneum are potential complications of percutaneous drainage (see Complications).

Initial antibiotic therapy should provide coverage against aerobic gram-negative bacilli, microaerophilic streptococci, and anaerobes including B. fragilis.[5] The use of ampicillin, an aminoglycoside, and metronidazole or clindamycin should provide such coverage. Third-generation cephalosporins can be substituted for the aminoglycoside in patients at risk for renal toxicity.[5] When culture results are available, antibiotic coverage can be more specifically directed. Parenteral antibiotics are usually given for 10 to 14 days, followed by oral antibiotics to complete a six-week course. Most patients show improvement within a few days to a week after initiation of treatment.[5]

Therapy must also be directed at the underlying cause of the liver abscess. If a surgical cause for the abscess is identified outside the liver, it is an indication for early surgical drainage of the abscess and correction of the underlying problem. Surgery should generally be reserved for the clinically stable patient who has remained febrile for more than two weeks while on antibiotic therapy and percutaneous catheter drainage. If the clinical course deteriorates, surgical drainage should be initiated sooner.

COMPLICATIONS

Rapid diagnosis of pyogenic liver abscess with noninvasive imaging has decreased the incidence of complica-

---

TABLE 40–4. ORGANISMS CULTURED FROM PYOGENIC LIVER ABSCESSES

Aerobic
Escherichia coli
Klebsiella
Streptococcus viridans group
Streptococcus pneumoniae
Staphylococcus aureus
Enterococcus
Proteus species
Pseudomonas species
Enterobacter
Listeria
Yersinia

Anaerobic
Anaerobic streptococci
Microaerophilic streptococci
Bacteroides species
Bacteroides fragilis
Fusobacterium species
Clostridium species
Actinomyces
Eubacterium
Proprionobacterium
Unidentified anaerobic gram-negative rods

tions. The complications of pyogenic liver abscesses result from rupture of the abscesses or extension into adjacent structures. The most common complication is pleuropulmonary involvement, which in early series occurred in 15 to 20 per cent of patients. It develops by direct extension through the diaphragm or by embolization. Most often, pleuropulmonary complications are seen with solitary pyogenic abscesses. With septicemia, involvement of other organs is common. If the abscess enlarges rapidly before obliterative, adherent pleuritis develops, it may rupture through the diaphragm, with resulting empyema. Slowly enlarging abscesses lead to pleurisy with adhesions and obliteration of the pleural cavity. In this setting, the abscess may rupture directly into the lung. Peritonitis may result from rupture of the abscess cavity or contamination of the peritoneal space when the abscess is surgically drained. A subphrenic abscess develops in 2 to 5 per cent of cases. Rarely, such an abscess may rupture into the pericardium, vena cava, hepatic veins, thoracic ducts, or abdominal wall.

The mortality associated with untreated pyogenic hepatic abscesses is close to 100 per cent. Even with treatment, mortality is high. Patients who will die are likely to have elevations of bilirubin and AST levels, hypoalbuminemia, and more than 80 per cent polymorphonuclear leukocytes.[18] Mortality is also influenced by the number of abscesses present, in that patients with multiple abscesses have a much greater mortality rate than do patients with solitary abscesses. Abscesses of biliary origin, whether benign or malignant, also carry a high mortality rate because most of these abscesses are multiple. Mortality is also greater in patients more than 70 years old. Sex and race appear to have no influence on mortality.

Patients who have polymicrobial infections have a higher mortality rate than do patients with infections due to single organisms.[18] In one series, all of 14 patients who had two or more organisms isolated from the blood died.[2] Significantly lower mortality rates in patients with pure anaerobic infections and in those with mixed anaerobic and aerobic infections seem to reflect that these abscesses are most often solitary.[18]

Even treated pyogenic hepatic abscesses carry high mortality, the rates ranging from 11 to 58 per cent.[5] With early diagnosis, appropriate drainage, and long-term antibiotic therapy, the prognosis improves substantially, and the rate may be reduced. A high index of suspicion must be maintained. Early use of imaging techniques in examining patients who have mysterious febrile illnesses will probably detect many more pyogenic hepatic abscesses and lead to substantially less mortality.

HEPATIC DYSFUNCTION ASSOCIATED WITH SYSTEMIC INFECTIONS

The normal human liver is very effective in removing bacteria from the blood in the presence of bacteremia,[26] but bacteria can rarely be grown from liver biopsy specimens.[27] In one study in which 86 biopsy specimens from 66 patients were cultured, organisms grew in only 3 specimens. One specimen had a Klebsiella-like organism, which was not further identified. Another grew a fungus. In the third case, positive culture results were obtained from a biopsy specimen obtained 30 minutes after death. Streptococcus pyogenes, Escherichia coli, Proteus vulgaris, and Proteus mirabilis were cultured from this specimen. All three of the patients with positive culture results had cirrhosis. Cultures of biopsy specimens from patients with acute hepatitis, chronic hepatitis, fatty liver, hemolytic jaundice, and amebic hepatitis, and cultures from healthy subjects, were uniformly sterile. In contradistinction to this, clostridia are found in a significant proportion of biopsy specimens from dog livers.[27]

Transient bacteremia occurred in 12 of 89 patients following liver biopsy in one study. Identical organisms were found in five of six biopsy specimens that were positive on culture of the liver tissue coincidental with the bacteremia.[28] Seven patients who had negative culture results from the liver biopsy specimens also developed bacteremia. The bacteremia was of short duration, not exceeding 30 minutes. The organisms cultured from the liver biopsy specimens included an alpha-hemolytic streptococcus from a patient with viral hepatitis, Staphylococcus aureus from a patient with leukemia, Escherichia coli from a patient with a cholangitis, and diphtheroids from two patients with viral hepatitis.

Alterations of liver structure and function occur in many systemic infections.[29–34] Jaundice occurs occasionally. The hepatic disease is rarely severe enough to increase the morbidity or mortality. However, in the presence of jaundice, diagnostic errors may occur, and the patient may be considered to have primary hepatic or biliary tract disease. These diagnostic errors may lead to inappropriate treatment.

The pathogenesis of hepatic injury in systemic infections is not known. The following mechanisms may contribute in some cases: (1) direct invasion of the parenchyma and Kupffer cells by blood-borne or lymph-borne infectious agents, (2) hepatocellular injury by circulating toxins, and (3) nonspecific injury to the liver related to fever, malnutrition, and hypoxia.[29] It has been suggested that hemolysis may play a part in the pathogenesis of jaundice. However, except in specific circumstances, such as glucose-6-phosphate dehydrogenase deficiency and Clostridium perfringens infection, hemolysis does not seem to be important. It has been suggested that the jaundice of infection is caused by a rather selective defect in the transport and excretion of conjugated bilirubin.[32]

HEPATIC DYSFUNCTION IN BACTERIAL SEPSIS

Jaundice with liver function abnormalities as a complication of severe bacterial infections in newborns and young infants is well recognized.[35–39] A few reports have described this complication in adults.[29–34, 40] In one series of 1150 patients with bacteremia, jaundice was observed in only 7 individuals. This is probably an underestimate, since only overtly jaundiced patients were described. Prospective data delineating the incidence of hepatic dysfunction in bacteremia are not available.

Numerous organisms have been associated with hepatic dysfunction in bacteremia. Included are Escherichia coli, Klebsiella pneumoniae, Pseudomonas aeruginosa, Hemophilus influenzae, Proteus species, Bacteroides species, aerobic and anaerobic streptococci, and Staphylococcus aureus.[29–34, 40] The sites of infection include areas involved by appendicitis, diverticulitis, pyelonephritis, pneumonia, endocarditis, and pelvic, subphrenic, pulmonary, and soft tissue abscesses.[29–34, 40] Small numbers of jaundiced patients have also been described as having peritonitis, meningitis, bronchiectasis, and septic abortion.[32]

Clinical Features

The clinical manifestations and laboratory findings are sufficiently characteristic to separate the underlying disease from jaundice of other causes. Jaundice due to generalized sepsis must be differentiated from primary infections of the liver, such as cholangitis and hepatic abscess.

When it occurs in the presence of septicemia, jaundice is usually cholestatic. Jaundice usually develops within a few days of the onset of bacteremia. The manifestations of the underlying infection usually dominate the clinical picture. Pruritis and abdominal pain are rare, but hepatomegaly is found approximately 50 per cent of the time. The level of serum bilirubin is usually between 5 and 10 mg/dl, although levels as high as 30 to 50 mg/dl have been reported.[34] Levels of serum alkaline phosphatase, AST, and alanine aminotransferase (ALT) may be slightly elevated. Usually they are not more than two to three times that of normal. A small series has been reported showing marked elevation in the alkaline phosphatase level up to ten times normal.[31] The albumin concentration is occasionally low. Successful therapy of the underlying infection usually results in prompt resolution of the liver function abnormalities.

Pathologic Features

The pathologic features of the septic liver associated with abnormal results of liver function tests have been well described.[29–34, 40, 41] The most prominent feature is intrahepatic cholestasis. There is usually little or no necrosis of hepatocytes. Kupffer cell hyperplasia, a nonspecific hepatitis, an increase in inflammatory cells in the portal areas, and slight fatty changes have been described. Transmission electron microscopy shows marked dilation of some of the bile canaliculi. Microvilli are flattened and reduced in numbers. The Golgi complex is prominent and contains bile, and the endoplasmic reticulum is somewhat dilated. Some of the mitochondria are larger than normal and contain a lamellar system running either longitudinally or transversely.[33]

Prognosis

Jaundice resulting from sepsis, seen only in severe infections, may portend a poor prognosis. Mortality rates as high as 90 per cent have been reported.[40] These patients do not succumb from hepatic failure. Rather, they die of their underlying diseases. The high mortality rate does not correlate with the severity or duration of hyperbilirubinemia. Minor abnormalities of alkaline phosphatase, ALT, and AST determinations when there is no jaundice apparently carry a much better prognosis, being associated with a mortality rate of approximately 10 per cent.[41]

LIVER DYSFUNCTION IN GRAM-POSITIVE INFECTIONS

PNEUMOCOCCAL INFECTIONS

Jaundice associated with lobar pneumonia was first described in 1836.[42] Most patients with pneumococcal pneumonia have abnormalities of liver function tests whether they are jaundiced or not.[29, 30, 34, 43, 44] The incidence of jaundice in patients with pneumococcal pneumonia has been reported to be 3 to 67.7 per cent.[29, 34] The ratio of males to females who develop jaundice with pneumococcal pneumonia is 10:1. The reason for this difference is not known. Jaundice is more likely to occur when the pneumonic process involves the right lung.

Pathogenesis

It is likely that hepatocellular injury is responsible for the liver function abnormalities and the development of jaundice. It is probable, too, that toxic effects of the pneumococcal infection are responsible.[29, 30, 34, 43] Conversely, it has been suggested that increased hemolysis contributes to the development of jaundice, though most investigators discount hemolysis as a major contributing factor in the development of jaundice in pneumococcal pneumonia.[34] The severity and extent of the pneumonia and the presence of bacteremia do not appear to be important in the pathogenesis of the jaundice.[43] The introduction of effective antibiotic therapy does not appear to have decreased the incidence of jaundice.[43] Antecedent liver disease may be an important factor in the development of jaundice, as chronic alcoholics are more likely to develop jaundice in the presence of pneumonia than are nonalcoholics.

Clinical and Pathologic Features

The pulmonary and systemic manifestations of the pneumonia dominate the clinical picture. Jaundice usually appears on the fifth or sixth day of the disease. It may occur as early as the second day or as late as the twelfth day.[29] It is usually associated with bilirubinuria and increased excretion of urobilinogen. The jaundice subsides promptly as the pneumonia resolves.[43]

In a study of patients with lobar pneumonia, 76.8 per cent of jaundiced patients had abnormal AST determinations, 21.4 per cent had abnormal ALT determinations, 32.1 per cent had abnormal alkaline phosphatase determinations, and 35.7 per cent had hypoalbuminemia. Patients without jaundice had similar abnormalities, but they occurred less often than in the jaundiced patients.[44]

The pathologic features of the liver in pneumococcal pneumonia have been well described. The most prominent finding is marked swelling of the hepatocytes, to the extent of obliteration of the hepatic sinusoids. Bile stasis may or may not be present. Small areas of focal necrosis are observed. Inflammatory cells are increased in the portal areas. Some patients have marked hyperplasia of the Kupffer cells, whereas others do not. On electron microscopy, the most prominent feature is dilation of the bile canaliculi with disappearance of microvilli. Intracellular bile pigment, dilation of the rough endoplasmic reticulum, and increased numbers of free ribosomes and polysomes are found. Paracrystalline inclusions are seen in mitochondria. Increased numbers of cells containing fat are found within the space of Disse. Intracytoplasmic vacuoles are present.[44, 45]

STREPTOCOCCAL INFECTIONS

Streptococcal infections occasionally are associated with liver function abnormalities and, very rarely, with jaundice.[29, 30, 46, 47] Jaundice occurs in fewer than 3 per cent of patients with streptococcal bacteremia. Hepatic abscesses resulting from streptococcal involvement of the liver have been described. Jaundice has been observed as an early manifestation of scarlet fever,[46] with bilirubin levels as high as 8 or 9 mg/dl, whereas the serum alkaline phosphatase level is usually normal. The liver is slightly enlarged and tender to palpation. These abnormalities resolve with resolution of the infection.

The pathologic features include infiltration of the portal areas with polymorphonuclear leukocytes and lymphocytes. Focal necrosis is present, with lymphocytes, polymorphonuclear leukocytes, histiocytes, eosinophils, and occasional plasma cells surrounding the necrotic areas. In some instances, numerous streptococci can be demonstrated in the liver by Gram's stain.[46, 48] Other lesions include centrilobular hepatocellular degeneration and necrosis. Rarely, the process may be diffuse and resemble massive hepatic necrosis. Occasionally the lesions are zonal, but they tend to be periportal or midzonal in the presence of demonstrable streptococci.[29]

There is a report describing the case of a patient with a prolonged fever of unknown origin. *Streptococcus viridans* was cultured from two needle biopsy specimens of the liver and from three of four wedge biopsy specimens obtained at laparotomy. Biopsy specimens of both kidneys and many lymph nodes were sterile on culture. Numerous blood cultures also had been sterile prior to laparotomy. The alkaline phosphatase level was elevated to three times that of normal. The patient's fever responded to high doses of penicillin.[49]

STAPHYLOCOCCAL INFECTIONS

The liver is rarely involved in staphylococcal infection or in staphylococcal septicemia, but pyogenic abscesses due to *Streptococcus aureus* have been reported. Fibrin ring granulomata similar to those seen in Q fever were recently seen in a patient with *Staphylococcus epidermidis* septicemia. There were mild elevations in the levels of alkaline phosphatase, γ-glutamyl transpeptidase (GGTP), AST, and ALT, which returned to normal after antibiotic therapy.[50] One instance of staphylococcal osteomyelitis associated with granulomatous hepatitis has been described.[30]

Jaundice is found in more than 50 per cent of patients with the toxic shock syndrome but does not seem to affect the outcome of the illness.[51] Elevations in AST and ALT levels are common.

GONOCOCCAL INFECTIONS

The liver is commonly involved in gonococcal bacteremia as occurs in gonococcal endocarditis. Approximately 50 per cent of patients have abnormal liver function tests. The level of serum alkaline phosphatase is elevated in almost all patients, and the AST concentration is elevated in approximately 30 to 40 per cent of patients.[52] Jaundice occurs only rarely, probably in fewer than 10 per cent of patients. Biopsy of the liver in gonococcal hepatitis discloses focal necrosis of hepatocytes. There is an inflammatory infiltrate that is particularly striking and is dense in the portal areas.[52] Perihepatitis (Fitz-Hugh-Curtis syndrome) is the most common hepatic complication of gonococcal infection.[29, 30, 52, 53] The vast majority of patients with this syndrome are women. It usually has a sudden onset, causing sharp pain in the right upper quadrant that can be confused with pleurisy, cholelithiasis, or acute cholecystitis. The liver is usually tender, and a friction rub may be heard. Occasionally, oral cholecystography reveals a nonfunctioning gallbladder.[54] Most patients have histories of previous pelvic infection, occasionally many years prior to the perihepatitis. The diagnosis may be made by isolation of gonococci from a vaginal swab. The organism has been isolated from liver biopsy specimens.[55]

Gonococcal infection is thought to reach the liver by spread from the pelvic organs through the peritoneal cavity. There have been cases in men, in whom it is presumed that the liver was seeded during a bacteremic phase.[29, 30, 55] The hepatitis of gonococcal infection does not seem to affect morbidity or mortality. Arthritis—including septic arthritis—cutaneous manifestations, myocarditis and pericarditis, and occasionally, meningitis, dominate the clinical picture.

With the exception of infections caused by resistant *Neisseria gonorrhoeae*, gonococcal infections respond dramatically to parenteral administration of penicillin G. Erythromycin and third-generation cephalosporins also may be used. The results of liver function tests may continue to become increasingly abnormal during therapy, although the major clinical manifestations respond to penicillin. Usually, results of hepatic tests return to normal within a month.

CLOSTRIDIUM PERFRINGENS INFECTION

Severe jaundice occurs in as many as 20 per cent or more of patients with gas gangrene caused by *Clostridium perfringens* or other species of *Clostridium*. It is almost certain that most of the jaundice is due to hemolysis caused by the release of an exotoxin from the organisms. Most cases are associated with cholecystitis or biliary tract obstruction, though the liver may be involved directly in the infectious process. Plain x-ray films of the area can show collections of gas within the liver and in the portal venous system. The gas usually is contained within abscess cavities.[29, 30, 56]

The prognosis of a patient who has gas gangrene is poor. Treatment consists of hyperbaric oxygen, debridement, and broad-spectrum antibiotics. In fatal cases, clostridia can be recovered from every organ in the body.[56]

LIVER DYSFUNCTION IN GRAM-NEGATIVE BACTERIAL INFECTIONS

Jaundice with hepatic dysfunction as a result of gram-negative bacterial infections is well recognized (Table 40–5).[29–40] Jaundice is much more common in infants and very young children than in adults.[35–39] Reported frequencies of jaundice range from 6 to 60 per cent.[35–39] The rare instances of jaundice in adults are usually mild. Exceptions occur in

TABLE 40–5. GRAM-NEGATIVE BACTERIA ASSOCIATED WITH LIVER DYSFUNCTION WITH OR WITHOUT JAUNDICE

Escherichia coli
Pseudomonas
Proteus
Bacteroides
Enterobacter
Klebsiella
Salmonella
Shigella
Legionella pneumophila

patients who have severe sepsis. In neonates and young infants, the urinary tract is the most usual site of infection. The organism most often identified is *Escherichia coli*. In addition to urinary tract infections, adults may have many types of severe intra-abdominal infections causing liver dysfunction.[34] The syndrome in infants is associated with a very high mortality rate, particularly when the infection occurs during the first week of life. The prompt recognition of the cause of the jaundice in an infant and the administration of appropriate antibiotics will lead to recovery in almost all cases.[38]

Jaundice may be the only clinical sign of infection in infants. Fever may not be present, and the relationship to infection may be overlooked. The failure to recognize the underlying infection is almost certainly the cause of the high mortality rate. Early diagnosis and appropriate treatment with antibiotics will cure almost all patients.[38]

When jaundice is present, almost all of the bilirubin is in the conjugated form. Alkaline phosphatase levels vary widely and may be minimally or markedly elevated. The AST and ALT levels are usually only slightly or moderately elevated.

At postmortem examination of infants with *Escherichia coli* infection, pathologic hepatic findings include central bile stasis and foci of hepatocellular necrosis. Regeneration is evidenced by double-nucleated cells and occasional mitoses. Giant cell transformation of hepatocytes is occasionally seen, and there is a minimal inflammation of the portal areas.[35, 36] Kupffer cell hyperplasia may also be present. Electron microscopy shows bile within hepatocytes, dilation of the canaliculi, and loss of microvilli.[33]

The pathogenesis of cholestasis in gram-negative bacterial infections is not entirely understood, but there is good evidence that the changes in liver structure and function are due to circulating endotoxin.[34] Thus, endotoxins from *Escherichia coli* and *Salmonella enteritidis* produce dose-dependent decreases in bile flow and excretion of sulfobromophthalein in the isolated, perfused rat liver system. The same effect is seen in bile salt-free systems, suggesting a selective decrease in bile salt–independent bile flow.[34]

Patients who have decompensated alcoholic or nonalcoholic cirrhosis occasionally develop *Escherichia coli* septicemia. It is almost always accompanied by peritonitis. Typically, these patients have abdominal pain, chills, fever, tenderness, and hypoactive bowel sounds or none at all.[57, 58] Hypotension or frank shock as well as hepatic encephalopathy may develop. Virtually all patients are jaundiced.[57, 58] There are variable elevations of serum alkaline phosphatase and AST. Serum albumin levels are low in most patients, and the prothrombin time is prolonged.[58] Appropriate antibiotic therapy usually will cure the peritonitis. However, these patients succumb to progressive deterioration of their liver disease in a few weeks or a few months. In one series of 15 patients, only 2 left the hospital alive.[58] It is unclear how the bacterial infection contributes to the progressive hepatic deterioration.

LEGIONNAIRE'S DISEASE

The bacillus *Legionella pneumophila* causes legionnaire's disease. The abnormal physical findings are primarily confined to the chest.[59] Hepatomegaly and splenomegaly have not been reported. Results of liver function tests frequently are abnormal, with elevations of AST in 50 per cent of patients, serum alkaline phosphatase in 45 per cent

of patients, and total bilirubin in 20 per cent of patients.[34] The elevations of bilirubin are slight (less than 5.0 mg/dl). Pathologic changes in the liver are minor and include focal necrosis and microvesicular steatosis. The organism has been identified on liver biopsy specimens. The hepatic involvement does not appear to influence mortality or morbidity. After the diagnosis is made, rapid improvement occurs with the administration of erythromycin. Rifampin is sometimes used in addition to erythromycin.

TYPHOID FEVER

Enteric fever is an acute systemic bacterial infection known since the late 1800s to involve the liver. It may be caused by each of the three species of *Salmonella* and occurs throughout the world. *Salmonella typhi*, which causes typhoid fever, is the most common type. Hepatomegaly is found in 13 to 65 per cent of patients who have typhoid fever.[29, 30, 60–65] In one series, 43 per cent of patients also had splenomegaly.[60] Clinical jaundice occurs in 4 to 16 per cent of patients. Hyperbilirubinemia, however, may be detected in as many as 23 per cent of cases. The aminotransferase levels are elevated in approximately 50 per cent of cases.[60] In one recent series, 90 per cent of patients had elevations in the fasting and postprandial serum bile acid levels, which returned to normal after appropriate antibiotic treatment.[64] A few patients may present with a hepatitis-like illness, consisting of fever, tender hepatomegaly, and jaundice.[65] Hepatomegaly is not a prerequisite for abnormal liver function tests, as many patients with abnormal test results did not have enlarged livers.

Pathologic examination of the liver shows focal cellular necrosis, mononuclear cell infiltration, and marked hyperplasia of Kupffer cells. The Kupffer cells tend to aggregate, and the aggregations have been called typhoid nodules. The typhoid nodules appear to be characteristic of typhoid fever and are randomly distributed throughout the lobule.[60, 63] There is also mild cholestasis.[29, 30, 34, 60, 63]

The pathogenesis of the hepatic lesion in typhoid fever is not entirely clear, but it appears to be caused by the endotoxin of the organism. Intact fluorescent *Salmonella* bacilli have been found in the liver of patients with hepatitis associated with typhoid fever.[66] The limulus test for endotoxin was positive in all 21 patients with typhoid fever in a recent study.[64] Observations in rabbits have shown that injection of *Salmonella typhi* endotoxin produces focal areas of liver cell necrosis, infiltration of mononuclear phagocytes in the areas of necrosis, and hyperplastic Kupffer cells that are filled with debris.[67] These lesions closely resemble the pathologic findings in patients with typhoid hepatitis. A recent case in which intact bacilli were demonstrated within the liver suggests that liver injury may occur by local release of cytotoxins or local inflammatory reactions within the reticuloendothelial cells. The electron microscopic changes are similar to those seen in bacterial sepsis.[67]

The abnormal liver function tests, hepatomegaly, and splenomegaly usually resolve within two to three weeks after successful treatment of the infection. The chronic carrier state for typhoid is thought to be caused by persistence of the infection in the liver or gallbladder.

PARATYPHOID FEVER

Other species of *Salmonella* may produce changes in liver function similar to those seen in typhoid fever. The organisms most often responsible for the complication of hepatitis are members of the paratyphoid group, *Salmonella paratyphi*, types A and B.[29, 30, 68] As in typhoid fever, the infection is largely confined to the reticuloendothelial system. Following establishment of the organism in the reticuloendothelial system, continuous bacteremia develops,[68] which initiates the clinical manifestations.

In one series of patients with paratyphoid fever, 16 per cent had hepatomegaly and 2 per cent had splenomegaly. There was elevation of serum bilirubin in 18 per cent, AST in 82 per cent, and serum alkaline phosphatase in 39 per cent.[68] The hepatic pathology features are not as well described as in typhoid fever, but the liver is said to show a nonspecific hepatitis.[30]

In epidemics of salmonellosis, the jaundice is frequently due to concomitant infection with a hepatitis virus. This is particularly true in epidemics in which more jaundice develops in more patients than have evidence of *salmonella* infection. In some patients with paratyphoid fever suppurative cholangitis develops to cause jaundice. In others, such as those infected with *Salmonella typhimurium* and *Salmonella enteritidis*, the hepatic manifestations are probably caused by endotoxin.[29]

SHIGELLOSIS

Jaundice that occurs in association with epidemics of shigellosis is well recognized. Most often it is due to concurrent infection with hepatitis A virus. However, a few sporadic case reports seem to indicate that *Shigella* infection will produce functional and morphologic alterations in the liver.[69, 70] Hepatomegaly has been reported. The abnormalities disclosed by liver function tests have included mild jaundice and elevations of AST, ALT, and serum alkaline phosphatase levels. One patient also had hypoprothrombinemia.[70]

The pathologic findings in the liver in one case in which liver biopsy was done included prominent cholestasis, a few areas of focal necrosis, and portal inflammation. Portal inflammation was predominantly caused by polymorphonuclear leukocytes, with involvement of bile ductules. The portal and periportal inflammation and necrosis produced destruction of the limiting plate. The portal tracts contained mononuclear cells in addition to the polymorphonuclear leukocytes.[69] This lesion is distinctly different from that in acute hepatitis.

MELIOIDOSIS

Melioidosis is endemic to Southeast Asia and is caused by the organism *Pseudomonas pseudomallei*. There is a wide spectrum of disease, including asymptomatic infection. The acute form of the disease may be fulminant, with septicemia and involvement of the lungs, gastrointestinal tract, and liver. Multiple small liver abscesses, focal hepatic necrosis, and inflammatory infiltrates are seen on liver biopsy. The organisms can usually be seen when sections are stained with Giemsa stain.[30, 71, 72] In the chronic form of the disease, the liver may be the only organ affected, with granulomatous inflammatory areas commonly found on biopsy specimens.[72] Serologic diagnosis can be made by a fourfold or greater rise in antibody titers.[71]

LISTEROSIS

Listeria monocytogenes is an unusual cause of liver dysfunction in humans. Most cases occur in immunocompromised adults or in neonates, resulting in miliary granulomata and small focal areas of necrosis seen on liver biopsy specimens.[73]

BRUCELLOSIS

Brucellosis is generally found in individuals who work with cattle, goats, sheep, or pigs.[30] Liver involvement by one of the three main species of *Brucella* is common during the acute phase of infection. Liver function tests are frequently abnormal, and jaundice may occur in severe cases. Noncaseating granulomata are the most frequent finding in liver biopsy specimens, though an inflammatory infiltrate without granulomata may be found.[74–76]

SPIROCHETAL INFECTIONS

SYPHILIS

Congenital Syphilis

Congenital syphilis, which is highly lethal, is rare in countries in which mothers are routinely screened for syphilis with appropriate serologic tests. The liver is involved in approximately 80 per cent of cases.[29, 30] The spirochete probably penetrates the placenta, entering the umbilical vein and subsequently the liver. At autopsy, the liver is enlarged, and in some patients splenomegaly is present. Jaundice is relatively uncommon but may be present at birth. Congenital syphilis may be confused with erythroblastosis in these jaundiced patients.[29] Serologic test results in infants with congenital syphilis are always positive. The stigmata of congenital syphilis disappear following appropriate penicillin therapy.

The hepatic pathologic findings in congenital syphilis include a fine, diffuse fibrosis extending from the portal triads into the lobules. The liver cells may be atrophic, and there may be a diffuse round cell inflammatory reaction in the fibrous septa and hepatic parenchyma. A few patients have granulomatous lesions in the septa and evidence of arteritis.[29] In silver-stained sections, numerous *Treponema pallidum* organisms are seen. The organisms are present in connective tissue, in the walls of small blood vessels, and in the parenchymal cells.

SECONDARY SYPHILIS

Some patients with secondary syphilis have an associated hepatitis that may closely mimic viral hepatitis.[29, 30, 77–83] The incidence of hepatitis in some series has been as low as 1 per cent. However, in one series in which 175 patients with secondary syphilis were examined, liver damage was found in 10 per cent of all subjects.[80] In another study of 18 randomly selected patients with secondary syphilis, 9 individuals had significantly abnormal liver function test results without jaundice being present.[82]

The most common symptoms of secondary syphilis are malaise, anorexia, weight loss, fever, and a nonpruritic rash. Patients with rectal syphilis may have painful defecation, with or without diarrhea and bleeding.[79, 81, 83] Many patients do not give a history of a primary chancre.

About 80 per cent of patients with secondary syphilis have rashes. The rashes vary considerably in appearance. The lesions are usually widespread and symmetric in distribution and are pink, coppery, or dusky red. The early lesions are macules seen at the margins of the ribs and on the trunk. The lesions later spread to the rest of the body. Occasionally, lesions occur around the mouth. The macular lesions develop into a generalized papular rash that particularly affects the palms of the hands and soles of the feet. In warm, moist areas, such as the perineum, the papules may coalesce to form flat condylomata (condylomata lata). Occasionally, condylomata occur in the axilla. Mucous membrane lesions are common. Almost all patients have a generalized lymphadenopathy, including the epitrochlear lymph nodes. Most have hepatomegaly and tenderness to palpation over the liver. A few have splenomegaly.[78–81]

The most usual laboratory abnormalities include elevations of AST, ALT, GGTP, and lactate dehydrogenase levels and a disproportionate elevation of the level of serum alkaline phosphatase. The results of liver function tests may remain abnormal for several weeks after successful treatment of syphilis. The serum alkaline phosphatase concentration is usually last to return to normal.

Hepatic histologic abnormalities include Kupffer cell hyperplasia, focal necrosis, occasional areas of necrosis that extend from portal areas to central veins,[77, 81, 83] and foci of necrosis with inflammatory infiltrates around the central veins. The portal areas are infiltrated with polymorphonuclear leukocytes, lymphocytes, plasma cells, and histiocytes. In some patients, there is damage to bile ductules.[83] Spirochetes are difficult to demonstrate in biopsy material. However, with appropriate silver stains, they can be found in as many as 50 per cent of patients.[80, 83] Many patients who have been cured of their infection have collagen deposition in the sinusoids and between parenchymal cells.[80] There also may be thickening of the wall of the central vein. The ultrastructural changes include reduced glycogen content, electron-dense material in the mitochondria, increases in the size and number of lysosomes, and degranulated and tubularized endoplasmic reticulum. Bile droplets are occasionally found in some cells.[80]

Late Syphilis

Tertiary syphilis has not been common since the introduction of effective antisyphilitic therapy. The lesion present in the liver is a gumma, which may be single or multiple. Gummas are focal lesions with central necrosis resembling caseation. They are surrounded by granulation tissue, fibrosis, and marked endarteritis. Plasma cell infiltration and lymphocytic infiltration surround the gumma. On healing, a dense contracted scar is formed.

The gumma is usually asymptomatic and is found only incidentally at laparotomy or at autopsy. Some patients complain of anorexia, weight loss, and abdominal pain with or without fever. Rare patients may have jaundice, ascites, and portal hypertension.[29, 30] In some patients, the liver is large and tender, and its nodular character may cause the disease to be confused with metastatic malignancy.

LEPTOSPIROSIS

Epidemiology

Leptospires parasitize wild and domestic animals. Man is infected only incidentally. Leptospires are distributed worldwide, and virtually any animal may become infected. Rodents are clearly the most important reservoirs in transmitting the disease to humans. Of domestic animals, dogs, cattle, and swine are the most important vectors. The organism is regularly excreted in the urine of many species of animals. Humans become infected by direct contact with either the urine or infected animal tissue. Those in certain occupations, such as veterinarians, farmers, and workers in slaughterhouses, are at risk. Sewer and dock workers who are exposed to infected rats are also considered to be at risk. Another mode of infection is exposure to water that has become contaminated by excretion of the organisms into the soil and water by infected animals.[84–87] Although certain occupational groups are at higher risk, it has been found that the disease occurs in urban and suburban areas in patients without such occupational histories.[88, 89]

Leptospires are tightly coiled spirochetes that are 6 to 20 μm long and approximately 0.1 μm in diameter. The genus consists of only one species, *Leptospira interrogans*. The species is divided into two complexes. Organisms of the biflexa complex are saprophytic and rarely cause disease in humans. Those of the interrogans complex are responsible for infection in humans and in animals.[86] There are more than 150 serotypes in the interrogans complex.[86] The serotypes most commonly pathogenic to humans include *Leptospira autumnalis*, *Leptospira canicola*, *Leptospira grippotyphosa*, *Leptospira hebdomidis*, *Leptospira icterohaemorrhagiae*, and *Leptospira pomona*. Other serotypes that have caused sporadic infection in humans include *Leptospira australis*, *Leptospira pyrogenes*, *Leptospira bataviae*, and *Leptospira tarassovi*.[90]

Leptospires gain entrance to the body through breaks in the skin or through mucous membranes. The incubation period is 5 to 20 days, with an average of about 10 days. The majority of patients with leptospirosis are anicteric. Jaundice develops in only 5 to 10 per cent.

Most patients with leptospirosis have a biphasic illness. The first phase is a septicemic or leptospiremic phase. During this period, leptospires can be isolated from the blood and cerebrospinal fluid. The second phase has been called the immune phase, since it is thought to be caused by the body's immune response to the leptospiral infection.

The first phase is characterized by an onset that is usually abrupt. A few patients have nonspecific malaise for two to three days before the onset of the more characteristic symptoms. The septicemic phase begins with a rapidly rising temperature, chills, headache, severe myalgias, and malaise. High spiking fevers continue, the headache is usually unrelenting, and the myalgias may be severe. Many patients have abdominal complaints, including pain, nausea, and vomiting. A few individuals may have constipation or diarrhea. Conjunctival suffusion without conjunctivitis is characteristic. Other signs and symptoms include cough, hemorrhage, rashes, retrobulbar pain, and arthralgias. Some patients have hepatosplenomegaly. Lymphadenopathy is somewhat less common. Occasionally, patients have altered states of consciousness. Rare manifestations of the first phase include acute arthritis, parotitis, epididymitis, orchitis, myocarditis, and pancreatitis.[86] The first phase lasts four to seven days, followed by defervescence and symptomatic improvement. At this time, leptospires can no longer be found in the blood. After a period of one to three days, any or all of the signs of the first phase recur in 85 to 90 per cent of cases. The most common manifestation is a recurrence of fever and the onset of aseptic meningitis. The fever during the second phase is usually not as high as that during the first phase. Headache is the most common symptom. The myalgias may be generalized or localized in specific muscle groups, such as the calf, thigh, and abdomen. In a few patients, the abdominal myalgias are so severe they can mimic an acute abdomen, and surgical procedures have been performed. In addition to the central and peripheral nervous system manifestations during the second phase, some patients have an anterior uveitis. They also regularly excrete leptospires in the urine.

One or more liver function test abnormalities may be seen in association with anicteric leptospirosis, including mild to moderate elevations of the aminotransferase and alkaline phosphatase levels. By definition, there is no hyperbilirubinemia.[90] Little is known about the pathologic characteristics of the liver in anicteric leptospirosis, since recovery is almost universal. No recorded biopsy studies or autopsy data are available.

The various species of *Leptospira* are sensitive to antibiotics in vitro. However, antibiotics have limited value in the treatment of the infection. If antimicrobial drugs are to have effect, they must be given within four days of the onset of illness.[87] Doxycycline (200 mg orally once a week) has been shown to be effective prophyllaxis.[91] When taken daily at a dose of 100 mg twice a day it reduced the severity of the disease.[92] However, the diagnosis rarely is suspected, and treatment is not usually initiated this early in the course of the illness.

WEIL'S DISEASE

Clinical Features

Weil's disease, a severe form of leptospirosis, is characterized by jaundice, renal insufficiency, hemorrhagic diathesis, hypotension, and confusion. It is an uncommon illness, accounting for only 5 to 10 per cent of all leptospiral infections. Several serotypes of *Leptospira* are capable of producing this severe form of the disease.

The onset of Weil's disease is similar or identical to that of the milder forms of anicteric leptospirosis. Jaundice and renal insufficiency usually occur on the second or third day of illness. The hepatic manifestations and renal failure reach a peak during the second week. Although the illness tends to be biphasic, its severity often obscures this aspect. Extreme hyperbilirubinemia may be seen; bilirubin levels as high as 60 to 80 mg/dl have been observed. It has been speculated that a subcellular defect in bilirubin metabolism and transport, in addition to possible hemolysis, accounts for the marked hyperbilirubinemia.[86]

Severe renal insufficiency and anuria are seen only in Weil's disease, although patients with anicteric leptospirosis may have slight abnormalities of renal function. In a few patients, prerenal factors result in renal insufficiency, which responds to fluid administration. Others have acute tubular necrosis with histologic changes identical to those seen in acute tubular necrosis from other causes. Mortality in Weil's disease is almost exclusively due to renal failure. Supportive measures and dialysis lead to recovery without residual kidney abnormalities.

The severity of hemorrhage is directly related to the severity of the disease. In the more severe forms of disease, hemoptysis, melena, hematuria, or epistaxis may occur. It is thought that an underlying vasculitis is responsible for the hemorrhage. Some patients have prolonged bleeding times and prolongation of the prothrombin time. A few patients have thrombocytopenia.[84, 86] Although serum bilirubin levels may be extremely high, the results of other liver function tests are usually only slightly deranged. Slight

to moderate elevations of serum transaminases and alkaline phosphatase levels are most commonly observed.

Pathologic Features

In fatal cases, the liver is large and has a yellowish green discoloration and subcapsular hemorrhages. There is a marked discrepancy between the severity of the jaundice and the pathologic findings in the liver. The lobule is usually well preserved, although there may be disorganization of the centrilobular architecture. Mitosis and binucleate liver cells are frequent, suggesting regeneration. However, there is little or no observable necrosis, and the hepatocytes show only minimal degenerative changes. Bile stasis is seen in the centrilobular canaliculi. There may be a mononuclear infiltration in the portal areas. The changes observed on electron microscopy suggest a toxic process.[30, 87]

Diagnosis and Treatment

The diagnosis of leptospirosis in anicteric disease may be made by direct culture of the organism from blood and cerebrospinal fluid during the first four to seven days after infection. A number of serologic tests are available for use in the immune phase. Although there is some cross-reactivity among the various species, species-specific tests are available. Asymptomatic infections do occur, as demonstrated by serologic surveys.[71, 86-88]

The treatment of Weil's disease is supportive. It has been suggested that doxycycline or tetracycline may be of use during the anicteric phase; however, antibiotics are ineffective after the onset of jaundice. Treatment of the renal insufficiency offers the best hope for survival.

RELAPSING FEVER (BORRELIOSIS)

Two types of relapsing fever occur; one is tick-borne and endemic, and the other is louse-borne and epidemic. The majority of cases are louse-borne and occur outside of the United States. Most cases occurring in the United States are tick-borne.[93] The disease is transmitted by ticks of the species of *Ornithodoros*. *Ornithodoros hermsi* transmits disease in the western United States, and *Ornithodoros turicata* is responsible for the disease in the southwestern United States. Once the tick becomes infected with a *Borrelia* spirochete, it probably remains infective for life.

Most cases occur in forested, high, arid regions of the 13 western states of the United States. The patient may not recall the bite, since it is nearly painless and the tick has a short feeding time.[93] The incubation period after the tick bite is approximately a week. The onset of symptoms is abrupt. Typical symptoms include fever, rigors, severe headaches, and profound malaise. Some patients have severe myalgias. The latter occur particularly in the lumbar area. A few patients have weakness and arthralgias. Abdominal symptoms include pain in the right and left upper quadrants, nausea and vomiting, and diarrhea.

On physical examination, most patients have temperatures higher than 39.5° C. Some patients have rashes, which vary from a nonspecific macular rash to one that resembles the rose spots of typhoid fever. Others have frank petechiae. Meningeal signs may be present; some patients have abdominal tenderness. Tender hepatosplenomegaly is found in approximately half of the cases (with splenomegaly being slightly more common). About 40 to 50 per cent of patients have jaundice.[29, 30, 93, 94]

The diagnosis is best made on the basis of examination of stained peripheral blood smears. Spirochetes may be found in approximately 70 per cent of cases. The yield may be increased slightly by examining serial blood smears, including thick and thin preparations.[93]

The laboratory data may show many abnormalities. There is usually a mild normocytic normochromic anemia. The liver function tests usually show slight to moderate elevations of the transaminases, although very high levels of AST have been reported.[94] The hyperbilirubinemia is usually mild, although bilirubin levels as high as 33 mg/dl have been reported. Coagulation studies may disclose various abnormalities. There may be hypoprothrombinemia, prolongation of the partial thromboplastin time, and circulating fibrin monomers. There is usually thrombocytopenia. These events occur even in patients without evidence of bleeding.

Few data are available regarding the hepatic pathologic features in nonfatal cases. In fatal cases, petechial hemorrhages are present over the surfaces of the meninges, pleura, heart, kidneys, and mesentery. Splenomegaly is a regular finding. The spleen contains multiple microabscesses. The liver is enlarged because of congestion and edema. There are small scattered foci of necrosis and hemorrhage in the midzonal regions. Sometimes there is Kupffer cell hyperplasia, and the sinusoids contain many polymorphonuclear leukocytes. Intracanalicular bile stasis is uncommon.[94] In one series, all of the patients who died had an interstitial histiocytic myocarditis, which is probably the most common cause of death in fatal cases of relapsing fever.[94] In this series, one patient died in hepatic coma.

In untreated patients, recurrent fever is the most common symptom. The number of febrile episodes may exceed five. Ultimate recovery is usual, though death may occur in up to 5 per cent of cases. When the diagnosis is made during the first cycle of fever, tetracycline is effective. Defervescence will occur within 24 hours, with rapid resolution of other symptoms. Erythromycin and penicillin G may also be effective.

LYME DISEASE

Lyme disease is caused by the tick-borne spirochete *Borrelia burgdorferi* and is most often associated with a characteristic rash (erythema chronicum migrans) and arthritis. Rash, lymphadenopathy, and liver abnormalities occur most often in the first stage of the disease, whereas later in the disease (second stage), neurologic abnormalities and myocarditis are more frequent. Months to years later (third stage) a more persistent arthritis develops.[95] Approximately 20 per cent of patients have early elevations of AST and ALT levels, which usually return to normal after antibiotic treatment.[96] Jaundice does not seem to occur frequently. There is a case report describing the organism in the liver of an infected newborn.[97] Tetracycline or doxycycline are the drugs of choice. Erythromycin, ceftriaxone, and penicillin have also been used successfully in the treatment of the disease.[98]

ROCKY MOUNTAIN SPOTTED FEVER

Rocky Mountain spotted fever, caused by *Rickettsia rickettsii*, is transmitted to humans by several species of ticks. The disease initially was encountered in Montana and Idaho but has been recognized in at least 46 states in the United States. It is more prevalent in the southern Atlantic states than it is in the western states. It is seen only in the western hemisphere.

The disease begins as an acute prostrating illness, with fever, headache, malaise, and generalized myalgias. A rash generally appears on the second or third day of fever, beginning distally and extending centrally. In fulminant disease, extensive vascular damage causes purpura and severe central nervous system dysfunction. Jaundice is rare, occurring mainly in fatal cases.[99]

On physical examination, the rash is prominent. Depending on the duration of illness, there may be pink macules, which progress to a fixed dark red or purplish maculopapular rash. Petechiae also appear. Hemorrhagic rashes may have coalesced. Some patients have tender hepatomegaly. Splenomegaly has not been described.

The diagnosis is usually made on the basis of a high index of suspicion and the history of the patient's being bitten by a tick. The complement fixation test is the best serologic test, but the diagnostic fourfold increase in antibody titer occurs in the second or third week of illness and thus is not useful in making clinical decisions. About 70 to 80 per cent of patients have positive Weil-Felix tests. Because of cross-reactivity with other *Rickettsiae* and *Proteus*, the test is not specific, but it is clinically useful as a confirmatory test.

Jaundice is inapparent in the majority of patients. Results of liver function tests have not been reported for anicteric patients. In two patients with bilirubin levels between 7 and 9 mg/dl, AST and ALT levels were elevated, as was the level of serum alkaline phosphatase. Liver biopsy specimens show portal inflammation with large mononuclear cells and neutrophils and focal cholestasis. Sinusoidal erythrophagocytosis is common. Hepatocellular necrosis is not usually seen. *Rickettsia* is frequently demonstrated in portal areas using immunofluorescence microscopy.[100, 101] In fatal cases, periportal round cell infiltration, fatty infiltration, Kupffer cell swelling, intracapillary leukocytosis, and focal necrosis are found.[99]

Early recognition and therapy of Rocky Mountain spotted fever may be lifesaving. Tetracycline, 250 to 500 mg orally every six hours, is an effective regimen in adults. Chloramphenicol is also effective and is the drug of choice in children less than 8 years of age.[102]

MYCOBACTERIA

In the 1980s, mycobacterial infections are seen predominantly in immunocompromised hosts, specifically those with T-cell defects. *Mycobacterium tuberculosis*, *Mycobacterium avium*, *Mycobacterium intracellulare*, and *Mycobacterium kanasasii* are most common. Liver involvement has been reported in 37 to 57 per cent of cases with mycobacterial involvement in other organs, most commonly the lung and lymph nodes.[103] The *Mycobacterium avium* complex (*Mycobacterium avium* and *Mycobacterium intracellulare*) has been particularly common in patients with acquired immunodeficiency syndrome (AIDS). Fever and hepatomegaly are the most common physical findings. The alkaline phosphatase, ALT, and AST levels may be elevated. Whereas *Mycobacterium tuberculosis* is characterized histologically by rare periodic acid-Schiff (PAS)-negative acid-fast bacilli in well-formed caseous granulomata, *Mycobacterium avium* complex granulomata are composed of foamy histiocytic cells with little inflammatory response.[103] PAS-positive acid-fast organisms are commonly seen in granulomata and in or around sinusoids in those infected with the *Mycobacterium avium* complex. Routine culturing and use of special stains for mycobacteria should be done in all AIDS patients undergoing liver biopsy, since myco-bacterial infection may not be seen on routine stains.[103]

REFERENCES

1. Rubin RH, Swartz MN, Malt R. Hepatic abscess: changes in clinical, bacteriologic and therapeutic aspects. Am J Med 57:601, 1974.
2. Lazarchick J, deSouza e Silva NA, Nichols DR, et al. Pyogenic liver abscess. Mayo Clin Proc 48:349, 1973.
3. Ochsner A, DeBakey M, Murray S. Pyogenic abscess of the liver. Am J Surg 40:292, 1938.
4. Greenstein AJ, Lowenthal D, Hammer GS, et al. Continuing changing patterns of disease in pyogenic liver abscess: a study of 38 patients. Am J Gastroenterol 79:217, 1984.
5. Barnes PF, DeCock KM, Reynolds TN, et al. A comparison of amebic and pyogenic abscess of the liver. Medicine 66:472, 1987.
6. Conter RL, Pitt HA, Tompkins RK, et al. Differentiation of pyogenic from amebic hepatic abscesses. Surg Gynecol Obstet 162:114, 1986.
7. McDonald MI, Corey GR, Gallis HA, et al. Single and multiple pyogenic liver abscesses; natural history, diagnosis and treatment, with emphasis on percutaneous drainage. Medicine 63:291, 1984.
8. Chusid MJ. Pyogenic hepatic abscess in infancy and childhood. Pediatrics 62:554, 1978.
9. Lee FS, Block GE. The changing clinical patterns of hepatic abscesses. Arch Surg 104:465, 1972.
10. Sabbaj J, Sutter VL, Finegold SM. Anaerobic pyogenic liver abscess. Ann Intern Med 77:629, 1972.
11. Rubinson HA, Isikoff MB, Hill MC. Diagnostic imaging of hepatic abscesses: a retrospective analysis. Am J Roentgenol 135:735, 1980.
12. Newlin N, Silver TM, Stuck KJ, et al. Ultrasonic features of pyogenic liver abscesses. Radiology 139:155, 1981.
13. Halverson RA, Korobkin M, Foster WL, et al. The variable CT appearance of hepatic abscesses. Am J Radiol 14:941, 1984.
14. Callen PW. Computed tomographic evaluation of abdominal and pelvic abscesses. Radiology 131:171, 1979.
15. Grossman RI, Ring EJ, Oleaga JA, et al. Diagnosis of pyogenic hepatic abscesses by percutaneous transhepatic cholangiography. Am J Roentgenol 132:919, 1979.
16. Ascione A, Elias E, Scott J, et al. Endoscopic retrograde cholangiography (ERC) in nonamebic liver abscesses. Am J Dig Dis 23:39, 1978.
17. Weissleder R, Saini S, Stark DD, et al. Pyogenic liver abscess: contrast-enhanced MR imaging in rats. AJR 150:115, 1988.
18. Pitt HA, Zuidema GD. Factors influencing mortality in the treatment of pyogenic hepatic abscess. Surg Gynecol Obstet 140:228, 1975.
19. McFadzean AJS, Chang KPS, Wong C. Solitary pyogenic abscess of the liver treated by closed aspiration and antibiotics. Br J Surg 41:141, 1953.
20. Maher JA Jr, Reynolds TB, Yellin A. Successful medical treatment of pyogenic liver abscess. Gastroenterology 77:618, 1979.
21. Kraulis JE, Bird BL, Colapinto ND. Percutaneous catheter drainage of liver abscess: an alternative to open drainage. Br J Surg 67:400, 1980.
22. Herbert DA, Rotham J, Simmons F, et al. Pyogenic liver abscesses: successful non-surgical therapy. Lancet 1:134, 1982.
23. Johnson RD, Mueller PR, Ferrucci JT, et al. Percutaneous drainage of pyogenic liver abscesses. Am J Roentgenol 144:463, 1985.
24. Gerzof SG, Johnson WC, Robbins AH, et al. Intrahepatic pyogenic abscesses: treatment by percutaneous drainage. Am J Surg 149:487, 1985.
25. Bertel CK, VanHeerden JA, Sheedy PF. Treatment of pyogenic hepatic abscesses; surgical vs percutaneous drainage. Arch Surg 121:554, 1986.
26. Beeson PE, Brannon ES, Warren JV. Observations on the sites of removal of bacteria from the blood in patients with bacterial endocarditis. J Exp Med 81:9, 1945.
27. Sborov VM, Morse WC, Giges B, et al. Bacteriology of the human liver. J Clin Invest 31:986, 1952.
28. LeFrock JL, Ellis CA, Turchik JB, et al. Transient bacteremia associated with percutaneous liver biopsy. J Infect Dis (Suppl) 131:S104, 1975.
29. Klatskin G. Hepatitis associated with systemic infections. In: Schiff L,
30. Holdstock G, Balasegaram M, Millwarf-Sadler GH, et al. The liver in infection. In: Wright R, Millward-Sadler GH, Alberti K, et al., eds. Liver and Biliary Disease. London, WB Saunders, 1985:1077.
31. Fang MH, Ginsberg AL, Dobbins WO. Marked elevation in serum alkaline phosphatase activity as a manifestation of systemic infection. Gastroenterology 78:592, 1980.
32. Miller DJ, Keeton GR, Webber RL, et al. Jaundice in severe bacterial infection. Gastroenterology 71:94, 1976.
33. Fahrlander H, Huber F, Gloor F. Intrahepatic retention of bile in severe bacterial infections. Gastroenterology 47:590, 1964.
34. Zimmerman HJ, Fang M, Utili R, et al. Jaundice due to bacterial infection. Gastroenterology 77:362, 1979.
35. Bernstein J, Brown AK. Sepsis and jaundice in early infancy. Pediatrics 29:873, 1962.
36. Hamilton JR, Sass-Kortsak A. Jaundice associated with severe bacterial infections in young infants. J Pediatr 63:121, 1963.
37. Seeler RA, Hahn K. Jaundice in urinary tract infection in infancy. Am J Dis Child 118:553, 1969.
38. Rooney JC, Hill DJ, Danks DM. Jaundice associated with bacterial infection in the newborn. Am J Dis Child 122:39, 1971.
39. Escobedo MB, Barton LL, Marshall RE. The frequency of jaundice in neonatal bacterial infections. Clin Pediatr 13:656, 1974.
40. Vermillion SE, Gregg JA, Baggenstoss AH. Jaundice associated with bacteremia. Arch Intern Med 124:611, 1969.
41. Neale G, Caughey DE, Mollin DL, et al. Effects of intrahepatic and extrahepatic infection on liver function. Br Med J 1:382, 1966.
42. Garvin IP. Remarks on pneumonia biliosa. South Med Surg 1:536, 1936.
43. Zimmerman HJ, Thomas LJ. The liver in pneumococcal pneumonia. Observations in 94 cases on liver function and jaundice in pneumonia. J Lab Clin Med 35:556, 1950.
44. Tugwell P, Williams AO. Jaundice associated with lobar pneumonia. Q J Med 46:97, 1977.
45. Theron JJ, Pepler WJ, Mekel RCPM. Ultrastructure of the liver in Bantu patients with pneumonia and jaundice. J Pathol 106:113, 1972.
46. Fishbein WN. Jaundice as an early manifestation of scarlet fever. Report of three cases in adults and review of the literature. Ann Intern Med 57:60, 1962.
47. Reid TMS, Davidson AI. Streptococcus liver abscesses. Lancet 1:648, 1976.
48. Kotin P, Butt EM. Streptococcus hepatitis. Arch Pathol 52:288, 1951.
49. Weinstein L. Bacterial hepatitis. A case report on an unrecognized cause of fever of unknown origin. N Engl J Med 299:1052, 1978.
50. Font J, Bruguera M, Perez-Villa F, et al. Hepatic fibrin-ring granulomas caused by *Staphylococcus epidermidis* generalized infection (letter). Gastroenterology 93:1449, 1987.
51. Shands KN, Schmid GP, Dan BB, et al. Toxic-shock syndrome in menstruating women: association with tampon use and *Staphylococcus aureus* and clinical features in 52 cases. N Engl J Med 303:1436, 1980.
52. Holmes KK, Counts GW, Beaty HN. Disseminated gonococcal infection. Ann Intern Med 74:979, 1971.
53. Lightfoot RW, Gotschlich E. Gonococcal disease. Am J Med 56:347, 1974.
54. Vickers FN, Maloney PJ. Gonococcal perihepatitis. Arch Intern Med 114:120, 1964.
55. Kimble MW, Knee S. Gonococcal perihepatitis in a male. The Fitz-Hugh-Curtis syndrome. N Engl J Med 282:1082, 1970.
56. Danke SG, King AM, Slack WK. Gas gangrene and related infection: classification, clinical features and etiology, management and mortality: a report of 88 cases. Br J Surg 64:104, 1977.
57. Conn HO, Fessel JM. Spontaneous bacterial peritonitis in cirrhosis: variations on a theme. Medicine 50:161, 1971.
58. Curry N, McCallum RW, Guth PH. Spontaneous peritonitis in cirrhotic ascites. A decade of experience. Am J Dig Dis 19:685, 1974.
59. Kirby BD, Snyder KM, Meyer RD, et al. Legionnaire's disease: clinical features of 24 cases. Am J Med 89:297, 1980.
60. Nasrallah SM, Nassar VH. Enteric fever. A clinicopathologic study of 104 cases. Am J Gastroenterol 69:63, 1978.
61. Ayham A, Gokot A, Karacadag S, et al. The liver in typhoid fever. Am J Gastroenterol 59:141, 1973.
62. Stuart BM, Pullen RL. Typhoid: clinical analysis of three hundred and sixty cases. Arch Intern Med 78:629, 1946.
63. Khosla SN, Singh R, Singh GP, et al. The spectrum of hepatic injury in enteric fever. Am J Gastroenterol 83:413, 1988.
64. Adinolfi LE, Utili R, Gaeta GB, et al. Presence of endotoxemia and its relationship to liver dysfunction in patients with typhoid fever. Infection 15:359, 1987.
65. Pais P. A hepatitis like picture in typhoid fever. Br Med J 289:226, 1984.

ed. Diseases of the Liver. Philadelphia, Toronto, JB Lippincott, 1975:711.

66. Calva JJ, Ruiz-Palacios GM. *Salmonella* hepatitis: detection of *Salmonella* antigens in the liver of patients with typhoid fever. J Infect Dis 154:373, 1986.
67. Schwartz A, Rubinstein HS, Coons AH. Electron microscopy of cellular responses following immunization with endotoxin. Am J Pathol 19:135, 1968.
68. Meals RA. Paratyphoid fever. A report of 62 cases with several unusual findings and a review of the literature. Arch Intern Med 136:1422, 1976.
69. Hornsey JT, Schwarzmann SW, Galambos JY. *Shigella* hepatitis. Am J Gastroenterol 66:146, 1976.
70. Stern MS, Gitnick GL. *Shigella* hepatitis. JAMA 235:2628, 1976.
71. Vainrub B. Bacterical infections of the liver and biliary tract: laboratory studies to determine etiology. Lab Res Methods Biol Med 7:119, 1983.
72. Greenawald KA, Nash G, Foley FD. Acute systemic melioidosis. Autopsy findings in four patients. Am J Clin Pathol 52:188, 1969.
73. Ray CJ, Wedgewood RJ. Neonatal listerosis: six case reports and a review of the literature. Pediatrics 34:378, 1964.
74. Buchanan TM, Faber LC, Feldman RA. Brucellosis in the United States, 1960–1972. An abattoir-associated disease. Medicine 53:403, 1974.
75. Joske RA, Finckh ES. Hepatic changes in human brucellosis. Med J Aust 1:266, 1955.
76. Young EJ. *Brucella melitensis* hepatitis: the absence of granulomas. Ann Intern Med 91:414, 1979.
77. Baker AL, Kaplan MM, Wolfe HJ, et al. Liver disease associated with early syphilis. N Engl J Med 284:1422, 1971.
78. Lee RV, Thornton GF, Conn HO. Liver disease associated with secondary syphilis. N Engl J Med 284:1423, 1971.
79. Sobel HJ, Wolf EH. Liver involvement in early syphilis. Arch Pathol 93:565, 1972.
80. Feher J, Somogy T, Timmer M, et al. Early syphilitic hepatitis. Lancet 2:896, 1975.
81. Haburchak DR, Davidson H. Anorectal lesions and syphilitic hepatitis. West J Med 126:64, 1978.
82. Parcek SS. Liver involvement in secondary syphilis. Dig Dis Sci 24:41, 1979.
83. Romeu J, Rybak B, Pradyuman D, et al. Spirochetal vasculitis and bile ductular damage in early hepatic syphilis. Am J Gastroenterol 74:752, 1980.
84. Edwards GE, Domm BM. Human leptospirosis. Medicine 39:117, 1960.
85. Heath CW, Alexander AD, Galton MM. Leptospirosis in the United States. Analysis of 483 cases in man, 1949–1961. N Engl J Med 273:857, 915, 1975.
86. Jacobs R. Leptospirosis—Medical Staff Conference. University of California, San Francisco, West J Med 132:440, 1980.
87. Sanford J. Leptospirosis. In: Schiff L, Schiff ER, eds. Diseases of the liver. Philadelphia, JB Lippincott, 1987:1197.
88. Fegin RD, Lobes LA Jr, Anderson D, et al. Human leptospirosis from immunized dogs. Ann Intern Med 79:777, 1973.
89. Fraser DW, Glosser JW, Francis DP, et al. Leptospirosis caused by serotype, Fort Bragg. A suburban outbreak. Ann Intern Med 79:786, 1973.
90. Berman JJ, Che-Chung T, Holmes K, et al. Sporadic anicteric leptospirosis in South Vietnam. Ann Intern Med 79:167, 1973.
91. Takafuji ET, Kirkpatrick JW, Miller RN, et al. An efficacy trial of doxycycline chemoprophylaxis against leptospirosis. N Engl J Med 310:497, 1984.
92. McClain JB, Ballou WR, Harrison SM, et al. Doxycycline therapy for leptospirosis. Ann Intern Med 100:696, 1984.
93. Fihn J, Larson EB. Tick-borne relapsing fever in the Pacific Northwest: an underdiagnosed illness. West J Med 133:203, 1980.
94. Judge DM, Samuel I, Perine PL, et al. Louse-borne relapsing fever in man. Arch Pathol 97:136, 1974.
95. Steere AC, Bartenhagen NH, Craft JE, et al. Clinical manifestations of Lyme disease. Zentralb Bakteriol Mikrobiol Hyg 263:201, 1986.
96. Steere AC, Bartenhagen NH, Craft JE, et al. The early clinical manifestations of Lyme disease. Ann Intern Med 99:76, 1983.
97. Weber K, Neubert U. Clinical features of early erythema migrans disease and related disorders. Zentralbl Bakteriol Mikrobiol Hyg 263:209, 1986.
98. Treatment of Lyme disease. Med Lett Drugs Ther 30:65, 1988.
99. Ramphal R, Kluge R, Cohen V, et al. Rocky Mountain spotted fever and jaundice. Two consecutive cases acquired in Florida and a review of the literature on this complication. Arch Intern Med 138:260, 1978.
100. Jackson MD, Kirkman C, Bradford WD, et al. Rocky Mountain spotted fever: hepatic lesions in childhood cases. Pediatr Pathol 5:379, 1986.
101. Adams JS, Walker DH. The liver in Rocky Mountain spotted fever. Am J Clin Pathol 75:156, 1981.
102. Kamper CA, Chessman KH, Phelps SJ. Rocky Mountain spotted fever. Clin Pharm 7:109, 1988.
103. Palmer M, Braly LF, Schaffner F. The liver in acquired immune deficiency disease. Semin Liver Dis 7:192, 1987.

41

Hepatic Granulomata

Telfer B. Reynolds, M.D. • *Jose L. Campra, M.D.*
• *Robert L. Peters, M.D.**

DEFINITION AND PATHOLOGIC FEATURES OF GRANULOMA

A granuloma is a proliferative inflammatory reaction that results in a granular, circumscribed lesion that is clearly distinct from the adjacent uninvolved tissue.[1, 2] It is a compact, organized collection of chronic inflammatory cells, predominantly consisting of mature mononuclear phagocytes (macrophages). Lymphocytes, fibroblasts, and lesser numbers of other types of inflammatory cells may be found in a rim in the periphery of the granuloma (Fig. 41–1). In granulomata characterized as epithelioid, macrophages that have no phagocytosed material or have disposed of phagocytosed matter tend to evolve into epithelioid cells, thus named because of their polygonal shape, abundant pale-stained cytoplasm, and ill-defined interlocking cytoplasmic processes (Fig. 41–2). In a further stage of maturation, contiguous macrophages fuse together to form multinucleated giant cells. The morphologic characteristics of giant cells are not uniform, and two types have been described: (1) the foreign-body type, which tends to develop in response to foreign materials and usually has its nuclei in a

*Deceased 2/16/85.

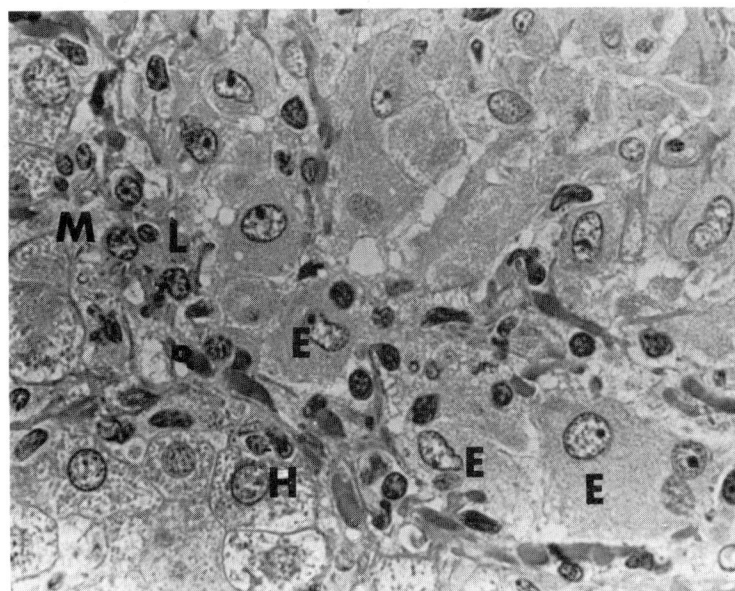

Figure 41–1. High-power photomicrograph of margin of epithelioid granuloma. Note the thin layer of lymphocytes and the large epithelioid cells at the margin (hematoxylin and eosin, × 480).

M = monocytes; L = lymphocytes; E = epithelioid cells; H = hepatocyte.

central position or scattered throughout the cytoplasm and (2) the Langhans' cell type, with nuclei arranged in the periphery of the cell. Giant cells may be as large as 40 or 50 μm in diameter, and some contain as many as 50 nuclei, although most contain a dozen or fewer (Fig. 41–3). Granulomata may be found with accessory features such as amorphous, caseous, suppurative, or gummatous necrosis. Paramyloid material may be found. Older lesions tend to be surrounded by a fibrous capsule. Healing may be accompanied by hyaline changes or calcification. Inclusion bodies or foreign material (asteroids, talc, beryllium, silica) may be found in special circumstances.

LIPOGRANULOMATA

Patients who have fatty livers may, on occasion, have focal areas of hepatocytolysis with fat droplets in histiocytes

(Fig. 41–4). Occasionally, the areas of necrosis will be rather large, will be composed of histiocytes, and will even contain giant cells that on rare occasions engulf fat globules and appear to be reacting directly to them. It is unclear what part the fat droplet plays in this lesion. Lack of close correlation between lipogranulomata and hepatic steatosis in some series has suggested that they may be reactions to ingested mineral oil.[3] It is quite possible that the focal hepatocytolysis, which is nonspecific and often resembles that seen in persistent viral hepatitis, only fortuitously affects a fat-laden hepatocyte and that the lipid released into tissues is engulfed by histiocytes in exactly the same way as are glycoprotein, lipofuscin, and hemosiderin when hepatocytes undergo destruction. Christoffersen and associates found such lesions in 64 per cent of liver biopsy specimens sectioned serially, which otherwise had only fatty changes.[4] There is no evidence that such lipogranulomata are part of progressive alcoholic liver disease.

Figure 41–2. High-power photomicrograph of epithelioid cells (hematoxylin and eosin, × 960).

E = epitheliod cell.

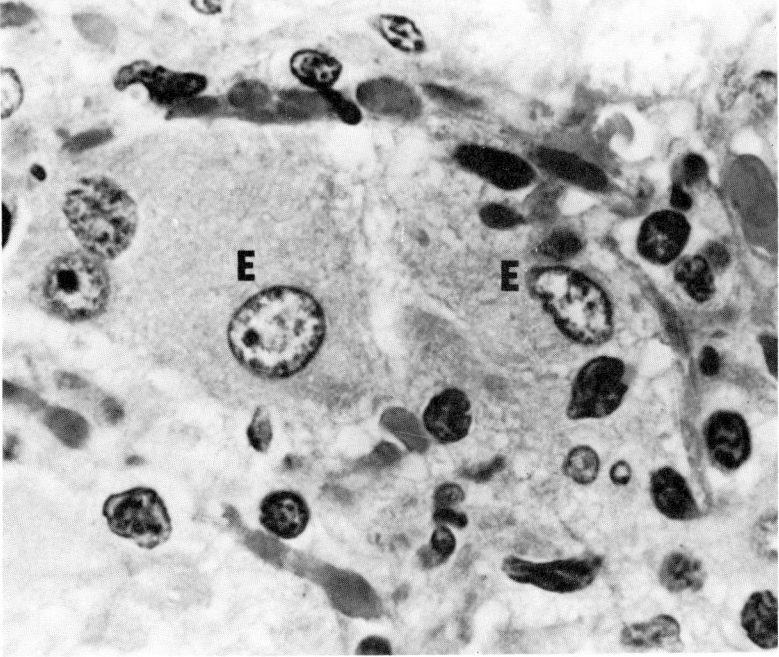

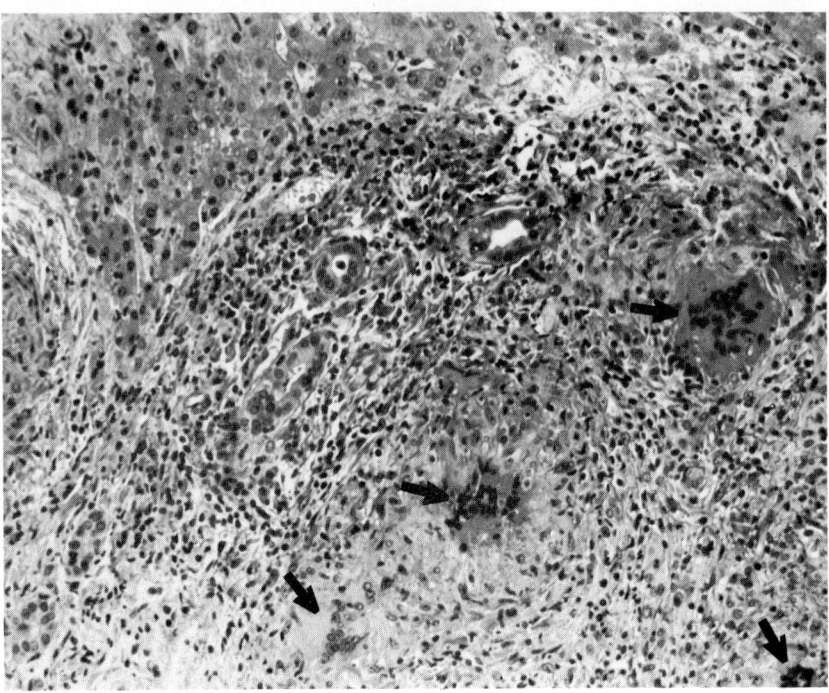

Figure 41–3. Multiple foreign body giant cells (*arrows*). Note the multiple nuclei (hematoxylin and eosin, × 92).

IMPLICATIONS OF HEPATIC GRANULOMATA

Widespread use of needle biopsy has led to awareness that the liver often contains granulomatous lesions.[5–9] This is not surprising, since the liver is the largest organ in the body and contains a highly developed system of reticulo-endothelial cells whose function is to clear the circulation of alien elements such as microorganisms, antigens, foreign bodies, and immune complexes. The hepatic granuloma is nonspecific and represents a pathologic reaction induced by any of a number of factors. From the pathophysiologic standpoint, its presence implies that the liver is engaged in the process of destroying or removing antigenic or foreign material by means of cellular or immune reactions.[10, 11] From the standpoint of hepatic function, the identification of granulomata is usually irrelevant, since only in advanced sarcoidosis or primary biliary cirrhosis is there any important structural damage (resulting in portal hypertension). The finding of hepatic granulomata is, instead, important as a clue to the recognition of systemic disorders. The liver biopsy findings in granulomatous diseases are generally similar, although subtle differences in the appearance of the specimens may suggest specific causes.[12–14] Only in rare instances can the pathogenesis of a granuloma be established unequivocally on histologic grounds alone (acid-fast bacilli in leprosy or tuberculosis, ova in visceral larva migrans, and spherules in coccidioidomycosis). The recog-

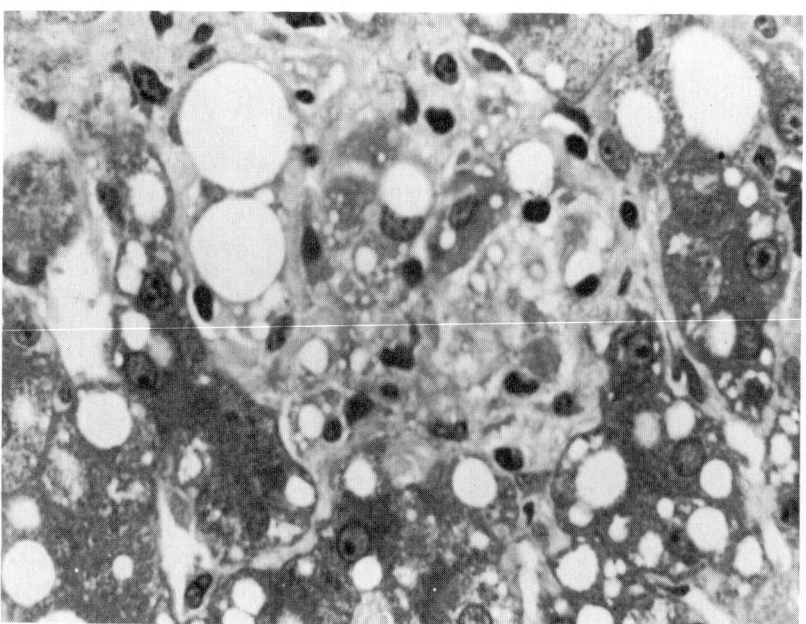

Figure 41–4. Lipogranuloma. Note small lipid droplets in histiocytes (hematoxylin and eosin, × 480).

nition of hepatic granulomata should suggest a step by step comprehensive diagnostic approach that should lead to the identification of the primary cause in most cases. However, even after the most comprehensive investigation there will still be a significant number of cases in which the causative factors remain unknown.[15-17]

CAUSES OF HEPATIC GRANULOMATA

Table 41–1 shows the most frequent causes of hepatic granulomata as listed in various reviews.[5, 10, 13, 15-22] Table 41–2 shows the frequencies of various diseases found in a review of 169 cases in the liver unit at the University of Southern California. There is regional variation in the frequencies of the different diseases causing granulomata. For example, at the University of Southern California there has been no granuloma caused by schistosomiasis in a liver biopsy specimen, reflecting the rarity of this disease on the West Coast of the United States, whereas leprosy related granulomata are not rare, owing to the proximity to Mexico, where leprosy is endemic. Tuberculosis and sarcoidosis are the most common causes of hepatic epithelioid granulomata in all series in the United States. Next in frequency are some infectious diseases that are relatively rare but almost invariably include hepatic granulomata in their manifesta-

TABLE 41–1. REPORTED CAUSES OF HEPATIC GRANULOMA[4, 9, 12, 14-21]*

INFECTIONS
Bacterial
  Tuberculosis
  Leprosy
  Brucellosis
  (Salmonellosis, tularemia, granuloma inguinale, melioidosis, listerosis)
Mycotic
  Histoplasmosis
  Coccidioidomycosis
  (Blastomycosis, toxoplasmosis, nocardiosis, cryptococcosis, candidiasis, actinomycosis)
Parasitic
  Schistosomiasis
  Toxocariasis
  (Tongueworm, strongyloides, ascariasis)
Viral
  (Mononucleosis, cytomegalovirus infection, lymphogranuloma venereum, psittacosis, cat-scratch fever)
Rickettsial
  Q fever
Spirochetal
  (Secondary syphilis)
DRUGS AND FOREIGN SUBSTANCES
  Beryllium, phenylbutazone, allopurinol, sulfonamides, chlorpropamide, quinidine
  (Methyldopa, hydralazine, cephalexin, phenytoin, procainamide, halothane, zirconium, penicillin, silica, quinine, diltiazem, tocainide, gold, carbamazepine)
OTHER DISORDERS
  Sarcoidosis
  Primary biliary cirrhosis
  Crohn's disease
  Hodgkin's disease and non-Hodgkin's lymphoma
  Jejunoileal bypass
  Wegener's granulomatosis
  Polymyalgia rheumatica
  Hypogammaglobulinemia
  Carcinoma

*Less common causes are enclosed in brackets.

TABLE 41–2. CAUSES OF HEPATIC GRANULOMAS IN PATIENTS SEEN AT THE UNIVERSITY OF SOUTHERN CALIFORNIA LIVER UNIT*

Disorder	No. Patients
Sarcoidosis	49
Tuberculosis	46
Leprosy	9
Brucellosis	9
Hodgkin's disease	7
Q fever	6
Mycoses	5
Jejunoileal bypass	4
Syphilis	2
Toxoplasmosis	2
Drug-related	2
Psittacosis	1
Infectious mononucleosis	1
Wegener's granulomatosis	1
Unknown causes	25
9 protracted course	
7 acute, self-limited	
2 associated with carcinoma	
2 incidental, with other liver disease	
TOTAL	169

*Cases of primary biliary cirrhosis have been excluded.

tions. These diseases include brucellosis and leprosy, as well as Q fever, which produces distinctive nonepithelioid granulomata. Certain other infectious diseases are more common but only occasionally result in hepatic granulomata; when present, the granulomata are typically nonepithelioid. They include secondary syphilis, toxoplasmosis, cytomegalovirus infection, infectious mononucleosis, and salmonellosis. Systemic mycoses (coccidioidomycosis and histoplasmosis) sometimes produce hepatic granulomata, but we have seen no example of hepatic cryptococcal granulomata. As in other parts of the body, cryptococcal involvement is diffuse when it occurs in the liver. Various drugs have been associated with hypersensitivity reactions that include granulomatous lesions in the liver. Widespread use of staging liver biopsy in Hodgkin's disease has revealed unexplained granulomata in as many as 5 per cent of patients. Whether they are part of the Hodgkin's disease itself or reflect an unusual reaction of the body to some infectious agent is uncertain. Biopsy specimens of the livers of jejunoileal bypass patients have shown a surprising frequency of hepatic granulomata. Whether they are related directly to the bypass surgery or indicate susceptibility to infections such as tuberculosis is unknown. Parasites, including *Toxocara* and *Bilharzia*, may induce granulomatous reactions surrounding worm parts in the liver. In primary biliary cirrhosis, there are often granulomatous lesions in the portal areas. Because of the associated pathologic and clinical pictures, they are rarely confused with the other granulomatous lesions of the liver. Eliakim and co-workers described an acute, febrile, self-limited disease with respiratory symptoms, splenomegaly, lymphocytosis, and hepatic granulomata.[23] We have seen similar cases. Whether this represents a new disease or simply failure to diagnose one of the known infectious diseases that causes hepatic granulomata is uncertain. Simon and Wolff have described a prolonged febrile disease with hepatic granulomata.[22] Their patients had severe systemic symptoms that responded remarkably well to prednisone treatment. It is unclear whether these patients had sarcoidosis or another disease.

The overall frequency of the finding of hepatic granulomata in liver biopsy specimens varies widely, ranging from 3 to 10.5 per cent.[5-8, 13, 14] This variability is related to several different factors: (1) the incidence of certain diseases in different geographic areas, (2) the frequency with which needle biopsies of the liver is performed in diagnosing fevers of unknown cause, (3) the frequency of performing liver biopsies for staging and evaluation in diseases such as Hodgkin's disease, sarcoidosis, tuberculosis, and leprosy.

CLINICAL FEATURES

Clinical findings in patients with hepatic granulomata depend on the underlying disease. Fever is the most common symptom, being present in tuberculosis, most cases of sarcoidosis, and all of the infectious diseases that result in granulomata. Nonspecific systemic features that commonly accompany fever include night sweats, asthenia, weight loss, leg pains, and nonspecific digestive symptoms. Disorders associated with hepatic granulomata that do not cause fever include primary biliary cirrhosis, parasitic infestations, and berylliosis.

Palpability of the liver and splenomegaly are common in most of the conditions causing hepatic granulomata. Infrequently, the liver is tender. Moderate lymphadenopathy is common in sarcoidosis, tuberculosis, and secondary syphilis and may be found in any of the other infectious diseases causing granulomata. Skin lesions are sometimes found in sarcoidosis, leprosy, and syphilis and may be relatively specific on the biopsy specimen. Erythema nodosum may accompany hepatic granulomata arising from sarcoidosis, leprosy, tuberculosis, and syphilis. Jaundice is uncommon with hepatic granulomatous disorders; when present, it suggests tuberculosis or sarcoidosis. Occasional patients with sarcoidosis have moderate to deep jaundice, and differentiating it from primary biliary cirrhosis is difficult.[24-27] Evidence of portal hypertension is found only in chronic sarcoidosis, primary biliary cirrhosis, schistosomiasis, or in the coincidental occurrence of alcoholic liver disease and tuberculosis.

LABORATORY TEST ABNORMALITIES

There is no pathognomonic pattern of hepatic biochemical test abnormalities in the granulomatous diseases. The most common pattern is a moderate to marked elevation of the serum alkaline phosphatase level with slight increases in the levels of serum transaminases (to two to eight times normal). Minor elevations of total and direct serum bilirubin are common, but levels greater than 3 mg/dl are unusual, except in primary biliary cirrhosis and in some cases of sarcoidosis. Sulfobromophthalein retention is frequently abnormal. Hepatic synthetic function is usually well preserved, with relatively small changes in prothrombin times and albumin levels. Serum gamma globulin is often increased in sarcoidosis but rarely in the other granulomatous disorders. Table 41–3 shows the means and ranges of the results of standard liver status tests of our patients with sarcoidosis (49 cases) and tuberculosis (46 cases). A higher proportion of patients with sarcoidosis had bilirubin values of more than 3 mg/dl, and the mean and range of the alkaline phosphatase values were higher.

Other laboratory test abnormalities that may be associated with the diseases causing hepatic granulomata are nonspecific anemia and an increased sedimentation rate.

TABLE 41–3. HEPATIC TEST RESULTS (MEANS AND RANGES) AT THE TIME OF DIAGNOSIS IN PATIENTS WITH GRANULOMAS DUE TO SARCOIDOSIS AND TUBERCULOSIS SEEN AT THE UNIVERSITY OF SOUTHERN CALIFORNIA LIVER UNIT

	Sarcoidosis (49 Patients)	Tuberculosis (46 Patients)
Bilirubin		
Total (mg/dl)	2.1 (0.1–9.2)	2.4 (0.2–20.4)
Direct (mg/dl)	0.9 (0.1–4.7)	1.1 (0.1–12.2)
Per cent of patients with bilirubin > 3 mg/dl	22	17
Alkaline phosphatase (Bessey-Lowry units/ml; normal 1–3)	15.4 (2.0–72.5)	6.8 (1.9–25)
Aspartate aminotransferase (AST; SGOT) (Reitman-Frankel units/ml; normal <40)	96 (20–470)	99 (13–362)
Alanine aminotransferase (ALT; SGPT) (Reitman-Frankel units/ml; normal <40)	58 (5–244)	69 (6–470)
Albumin (g/dl, normal 3.9–5.0)	3.4 (1.8–4.8)	3.1 (1.5–4.7)
Globulin (g/dl, normal 2.6–3.8)	4.3 (2.8–6.4)	4.4 (2.8–8.1)
Prothrombin (%)	94 (65–100)	70 (19–100)

Leukocyte counts vary according to the underlying diseases. Eosinophilia, when present, suggests sarcoidosis, drug hypersensitivity, Hodgkin's disease, or parasitic infestation.

DIFFERENTIAL DIAGNOSIS

One should bear in mind that tuberculosis and sarcoidosis together account for 50 to 75 per cent of hepatic granulomata, and that from a therapeutic standpoint, tuberculosis is the most important of all of the lesions to detect.

HISTOLOGIC DIFFERENTIATION

Although accurate assessment of the pathogenesis of hepatic granulomata by histologic study alone is only occasionally possible, there are features that allow the pathologist to favor one cause over another. The first step is to separate epithelioid granulomata from granulomatous necrosis. Tuberculosis, sarcoidosis, leprosy, chronic histoplasmosis, coccidioidomycosis, and chronic brucellosis belong to the former category. The latter category includes Q fever, acute brucellosis, infectious mononucleosis, cytomegalovirus infection, typhoid fever, tularemia, and most granulomata associated with drugs. Many other disorders, such as primary biliary cirrhosis and Hodgkin's disease, may be associated with either epithelioid granulomata or non-epithelioid granulomatous necrosis.

When there are large numbers of epithelioid granulomata in the liver, the most frequent cause in the United States is sarcoidosis. Sarcoid granulomata tend to become segmented as they enlarge, forming multilobulated granulomata (Fig. 41–5, p. 1103). Tuberculous granulomata are usually portal and rarely perivenular; tuberculosis is present

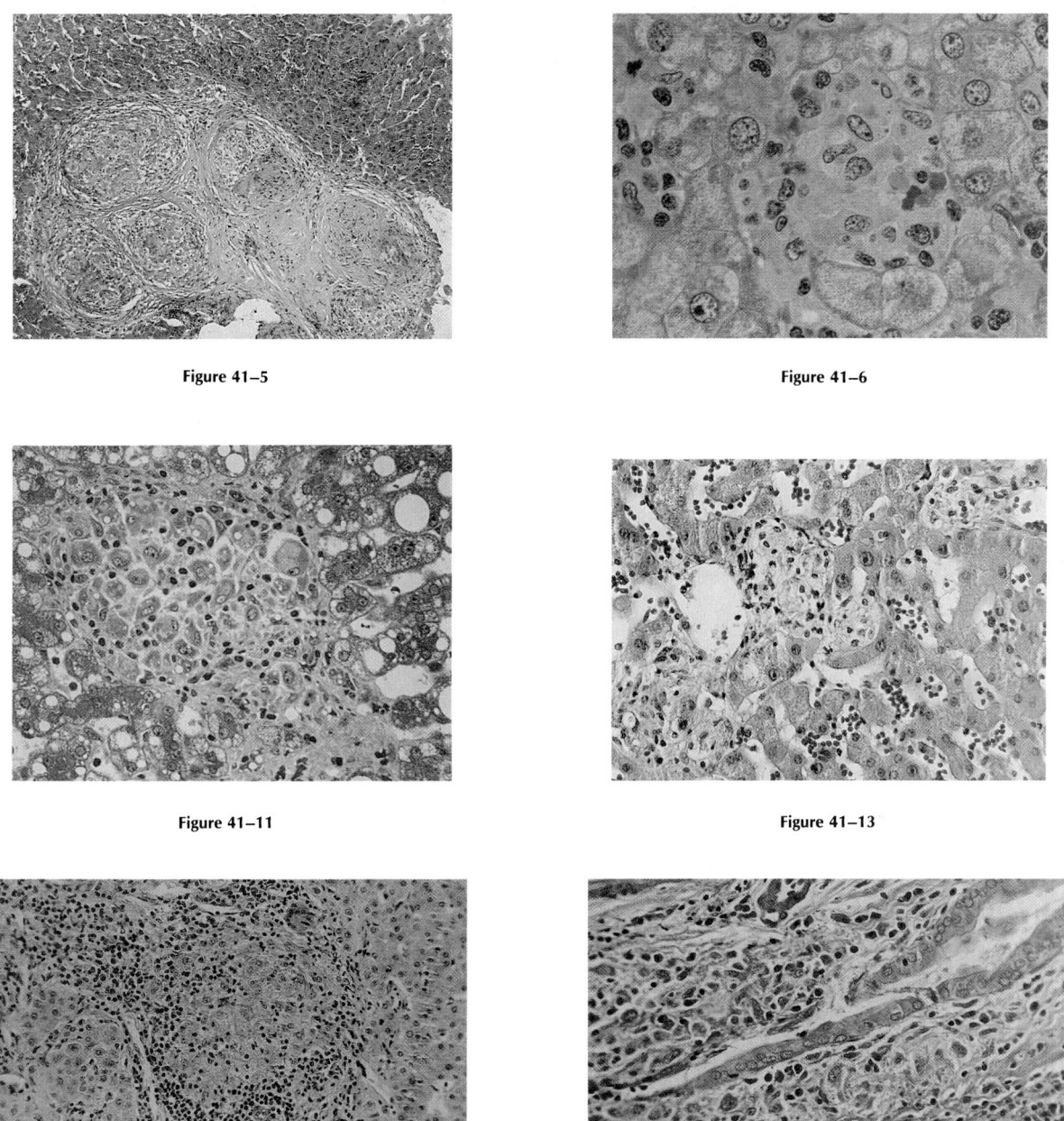

Figure 41–5

Figure 41–6

Figure 41–11

Figure 41–13

Figure 41–17

Figure 41–18

Figure 41–5. Segmentation occurs in sarcoid granulomas as they enlarge (hematoxylin and eosin, × 55).

Figure 41–6. Granulomatous necrosis. Note that the punched-out lesion is made up of histiocytes but not epithelioid cells in a patient with infectious mononucleosis (see Fig. 41–2) (hematoxylin and eosin, × 250).

Figure 41–11. Histiocytic granuloma in patient who has undergone an earlier jejunoileal bypass (hematoxylin and eosin, × 92).

Figure 41–13. Numerous small foci of foamy histiocytes near terminal hepatic venule in patient with lepromatous leprosy (hematoxylin and eosin, × 150).

Figure 41–17. Portal granulomas in patient with primary biliary cirrhosis (hematoxylin and eosin, × 55).

Figure 41–18. Granulomatous destruction of interlobular duct in patient with PBC (hematoxylin and eosin, × 150).

more often when the granuloma is found in a setting of alcoholic liver disease. Granulomata in leprosy are made up to a large extent of foamy histiocytes, as well as epithelioid cells, and may vary in size and location. Tuberculosis, sarcoidosis, histoplasmosis, and coccidioidomycosis granulomata may be associated with caseation. Three of our patients with sarcoidosis have had areas of necrosis in large granulomata.

Many diseases may be associated with punched-out clusters of histiocytes or lymphocytes. We prefer to call such lesions *granulomatous necrosis*, in contradistinction to *epithelioid granulomata* (Fig. 41–6, p. 1103). Granulomatous necrosis may be seen in diseases not usually considered to be generalized granulomatous disorders (infectious mononucleosis, cytomegalovirus, healing viral hepatitis, typhoid fever, and other salmonelloses and tularemia, to name a few). It may also be seen as the early lesion of any of the more classic granulomatous disorders (tuberculosis, sarcoid, Q fever, brucellosis).

SPECIAL HISTOLOGIC STAINS

The yield of positive results from acid-fast stains in studies of granulomata in liver biopsy specimens is disappointing, although when a granuloma is caseous, tubercle bacilli may be demonstrated by acid-fast stains or by the fluorescent auramine stain.

Mycobacterium leprae are very numerous in noncaseating epithelioid lepromatous granulomata, and may be demonstrated by either acid-fast stains or the fluorescent auramine stain.

Histoplasmosis and coccidioidomycosis organisms may be recognized on hematoxylin and eosin staining, but periodic acid-Schiff (PAS) or methanamine silver stains that demonstrate the glycoprotein components of the capsules are more sensitive tests. Spirochetes may be identified in the liver by Levaditi's method or by other stains in syphilitic hepatitis of the secondary stage of syphilis, but the organisms are not necessarily located in the rare granulomata. Because of the spirochetemia of secondary syphilis, it is questionable whether demonstration of the organism in the liver reflects hepatic involvement or simply intravascular localization of organisms.

CULTURES

Demonstration of *M. tubrculosis* by culture is the most valuable of all the potential findings in the evaluation of a patient who has granulomatous liver disease. For this reason, cultures on special media of all available materials are indicated. These materials include sputum, gastric washings, urine, and bone marrow aspirates. The authors have had several instances of positive culture results from liver biopsy specimens and so recommend that a portion of the initial specimen be cultured for *M. tuberculosis,* and, if this was not considered at the time of the initial biopsy, a second biopsy should be performed specifically for culture. Others have reported successful culture of *M. tuberculosis* from liver biopsy samples.[28–30] Fungi may be grown on the same medium. Standard blood cultures are indicated for the demonstration of brucellosis; the yield may be increased by the use of Castaneda's medium. If there is accessible lymphadenopathy, lymph node biopsy and culture may be very helpful.

SKIN TESTS

The purified protein derivative (PPD) skin test result usually is positive in tuberculosis and negative in sarcoidosis. However, there are exceptions to these general rules; with widespread tuberculosis or with an additional disorder such as alcoholic liver disease, the PPD skin test result of a patient with tuberculosis may be negative. The axiom is that sarcoid patients have negative reactions to tuberculin skin tests. A recent review maintains that fewer than 50 per cent of patients with sarcoidosis are negative reactors to 100 TU tuberculin.[31] A few patients with sarcoid have high degrees of tuberculin sensitivity. Additional skin tests can be used to assess anergy; they include tests of reactivity to mumps antigen, *Candida, Trichophyton,* and streptokinase-streptodornase. The Kveim test for sarcoidosis is a delayed granulomatous reaction at the site of injection of an extract of sarcoid spleen. Much has been written about the specificity of this test. Recent reports point out a sizable number of false-negative Kveim test results in sarcoidosis because of inadequate antigenic material or because of inactive disease, lack of lymph node involvement, or intercurrent steroid therapy.[32, 33] False-positive reactions have also been found in patients with Crohn's disease.[32] The original Silzbach antigen that was successfully used in the United States for the diagnosis of sarcoidosis is no longer available in most centers. Antigen from the Commonwealth Serum Laboratories in Melbourne has been discredited because of large numbers of false-negative and false-positive reactions.[34]

Fungal skin tests for reactivity to *Coccidioides, Histoplasma,* and *Blastomyces* are readily available, but their usefulness is questionable. False-negative skin test results are known to occur in a high proportion of cases of disseminated mycoses. Lot to lot reproducibility of coccidioidin and histoplasmin material has not been proved. Skin testing may interfere with fungal serologic tests. Healthy patients often have positive skin test results. For these reasons, fungal skin tests cannot be recommended for use in diagnosing the acute illness.[35, 36]

SEROLOGIC TESTS

Reliable agglutination or complement-fixation tests are available for brucellosis, Q fever, mononucleosis, cytomegalovirus infection, toxoplasmosis, coccidioidomycosis, histoplasmosis, and blastomycosis. Depending on the duration of the illness, these tests may have to be repeated after a two- to four-week interval to demonstrate a rising titer. *Brucella* agglutinins can be missed if there are blocking antibodies and the serum is not sufficiently diluted. Most good laboratories are aware of this potential pitfall and take steps to avoid it. A false-positive serologic test result for syphilis should be excluded by the fluorescent treponemal antibody-absorption (FTA-ABS) test, and the heterophil antibody should be confirmed by a differential absorption test with sheep red cells or, in some cases, by immunofluorescent testing of sera for antibody to specific Epstein-Barr virus antigens in cell culture. Serologic tests for both schistosomiasis and toxocariasis are available from the Centers for Disease Control, Atlanta, Georgia. They are moderately reliable. Ova can be detected in the stools in active schistosomiasis. In later stages of disease biopsy of rectal mucosa is more effective.

ANCILLARY TESTS

Levels of angiotensin-converting enzyme in serum are elevated in a high proportion of patients with active sarcoidosis.[37-39] Ophthalmoscopy and slit-lamp examination may show ocular involvement in either sarcoidosis or tuberculosis. Serum calcium levels are elevated in a small proportion of patients with sarcoidosis.

THERAPEUTIC TRIAL

When a patient has fever and clinical illness that have not resolved after three to four weeks, a therapeutic trial should be considered if the diagnosis remains uncertain. Presupposing that none of the serologic tests provides a diagnosis and that appropriate cultures have been done, the therapeutic trial for tuberculosis can be started with a combination of isoniazid and ethambutol. Rifampicin is avoided because a therapeutic response could be caused by its action against other bacteria. Fever should subside and clinical improvement begin in two to six weeks if the patient has tuberculosis. Illness will continue if sarcoidosis is present. If there has been no response to antituberculous treatment by the end of six weeks, and all of the cultural material is negative for *Mycobarterium tuberculosis,* therapy for sarcoidosis is warranted. This consists of a moderate dosage of prednisone (15 to 25 mg daily), which causes very rapid clinical improvement and abatement of fever in sarcoidosis. If a response is seen after a short period, the dosage of prednisone can be reduced to between 7.5 and 15 mg daily for prolonged therapy. Most authorities consider it wise to continue giving isoniazid as a prophylactic measure during prednisone therapy in such a patient. Prednisone therapy may be needed for one to three years, since the fever usually will return when prednisone is discontinued within the first few months. If the therapeutic trials as described are instituted too early in the course of a febrile syndrome with hepatic granulomata, there is danger that spontaneous improvement will be misinterpreted as a response to either antituberculous therapy or to prednisone. The patients with self-limited febrile granulomatosis of unknown cause described by Eliakim and colleagues had spontaneous disappearance of fever in three to four weeks.[23] Granulomata were not found in the livers of these patients on follow-up biopsy.

DISORDERS ASSOCIATED WITH HEPATIC GRANULOMATA

SARCOIDOSIS

Sarcoidosis, a systemic inflammatory disease of uncertain cause, is characterized by epithelioid cell granulomata involving many organs. In the United States there is a markedly greater incidence in blacks than in other races. In about two thirds of cases, the liver contains numerous granulomata. The clinical features of sarcoidosis are remarkably variable, depending on the organ or organs that show the major involvement. Often the hepatic involvement seems incidental, and there are no symptoms or laboratory abnormalities directly attributable to liver disease. Conversely, a sizable proportion of patients seek treatment because of fever and nonspecific systemic manifestations and are found from liver biopsy specimens to have numerous non-caseating granulomata in the liver. A few patients with hepatic sarcoidosis have symptoms and signs of serious hepatic dysfunction, with jaundice, ascites, and esophageal varices. A very few have jaundice, pruritus, and a clinical syndrome that is indistinguishable from primary biliary cirrhosis. Since portal granulomata are also a feature of primary biliary cirrhosis, the major diagnostic distinction between the two diseases is the result of the mitochondrial antibody test result, which is negative in sarcoidosis and usually positive in primary biliary cirrhosis. The ranges and means of liver tests for 49 patients with hepatic sarcoidosis from the liver unit at the University of Southern California are shown in Table 41–3. The most consistently abnormal value is that for serum alkaline phosphatase. In addition, there is often a nonspecific, moderate anemia. In approximately 5 per cent of patients, the serum calcium level is elevated. The serum angiotensin-converting enzyme level is increased in 50 to 80 per cent of cases, depending on the extent of disease activity.[37-39] Gallium-67 (^{67}Ga) citrate scanning often reveals areas of active disease by abnormal uptake of the isotope in the involved organs.[40] There is depression of delayed-type hypersensitivity, and skin reactivity to tuberculin, mumps antigen, *Trichophyton,* dinitrochlorobenzene, and other antigens is lacking or decreased. Humoral immunity is unimpaired. There is characteristic skin reactivity (granuloma formation) to some preparations of Kveim antigen but not to others. Reliable preparations are not readily available, and the test is no longer widely used.

Abnormality of the uveal tract may be evident on slit-lamp examination. Chest x-ray films may show pulmonary infiltrates or evidence of hilar or paratracheal adenopathy. Various nodular skin lesions may be present.

Sarcoid granulomata may appear anywhere within the hepatic lobule, although many are in the portal area. The granulomata are made up of epithelioid cells, often with a thin rim of lymphocytes (Fig. 41–1). Giant cells of either the foreign-body type or the Langhans' cell type may be present (Fig. 41–3); occasionally the giant cells contain stellate or laminated concretions (asteroid or Schaumann's bodies, respectively). A sarcoid granuloma within the lobule starts as a cluster of histiocytes in the sinusoids that crowds aside the hepatocytes as it grows. After reaching about 50 μm in diameter, the sarcoid granuloma tends to become segmented (Fig. 41–5); occasionally, the clustering of granulomata so characteristic of sarcoidosis in lymph nodes may also be seen in the liver. Sarcoid granulomata are numerous enough to make it unlikely that they could be missed in a liver biopsy sample of even moderate size. In one study, the average density of granulomata was one/0.51 mm^2 of liver tissue (the average needle liver biopsy specimen is 7 to 15 mm^2 in area).[41]

As the sarcoid granuloma ages, there may be deposition of collagen arranged in a lamellar fashion at the periphery of the granuloma. Occasionally, only small fibrous nodules may be found as the residua of sarcoid granulomata (Fig. 41–7).

An occasional patient with sarcoidosis has features of cholestasis; here, the histologic distinction from primary biliary cirrhosis may be difficult. In livers of such patients, interlobular ducts may be destroyed, and the limiting plates of the portal areas become unrecognizable. Of five male patients with chronic cholestasis related to sarcoidosis studied by Rudzki and colleagues,[25] cirrhosis of a biliary type developed in three of them, whereas the other two patients developed biliary fibrosis. Hepatic fibrosis and cirrhosis

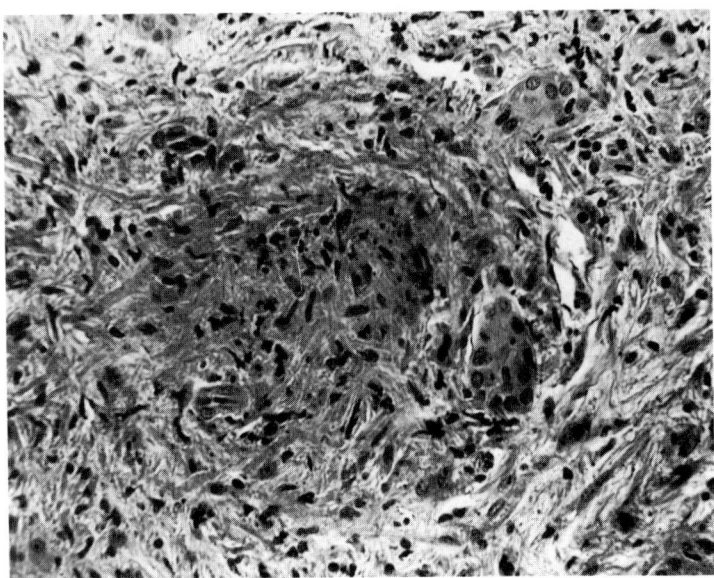

Figure 41–7. Liver from patient with longstanding sarcoidosis. Note the bundles of partly hyalinized connective tissue (hematoxylin and eosin, × 184).

associated with portal hypertension also develop in some patients with sarcoidosis.[42, 43] The fibrous septa that develop seem in excess of simple fibrous conversions of healing granulomata.

Some authorities require that granulomata be demonstrated in more than one organ before a confident diagnosis of sarcoidosis is made.[44] Other tissues from which positive biopsy specimen results often are obtained include scalene fat pads, skeletal muscle, conjunctiva, mediastinal lymph nodes, and lung.

A characteristic feature of sarcoid hepatic granulomata is their persistence for long periods. Whereas the granulomata of tuberculosis disappear rapidly with antituberculous treatment, and the granulomata from other infectious diseases such as Q fever, brucellosis, and secondary syphilis disappear as the patient recovers, the granulomata of sarcoidosis tend to remain for years, whether or not the patient receives corticosteroid treatment. Some patients have progressive fibrosis of the granulomata, and in a few cases granulomata have disappeared as fibrous scarring and progressive liver disease developed.

Treatment of symptomatic hepatic sarcoidosis with corticosteroids is very effective, as in the case of symptomatic involvement of other organs. Fever and systemic symptoms disappear rapidly, often with dosages of prednisone as small as 15 mg daily. Hypercalcemia, if present, soon disappears, and results of liver tests usually improve substantially, although there may be persistent moderate elevation of serum alkaline phosphatase levels. Fever often recurs as soon as corticosteroid therapy is discontinued, and it may be necessary to continue treatment for many months to prevent relapse. A major unsettled question is whether corticosteroid treatment delays or prevents progression to fibrosis and portal hypertension. This, of course, is particularly important in deciding whether or not to treat patients who have extensive hepatic granulomata and are afebrile and asymptomatic. The same dilemma exists with regard to treatment of asymptomatic pulmonary sarcoidosis.

The authors' belief is that when thorough investigation discloses no other diagnosis, and when therapeutic trials of antituberculous drugs are ineffective, hepatic granulomata that persist for several months are almost certainly due to sarcoidosis.

TUBERCULOSIS

Hepatic granulomata are present in virtually all cases of miliary tuberculosis, in approximately three fourths of cases of extrapulmonary tuberculosis, and in a small proportion of cases of pulmonary infections. Involvement of the liver is presumably by hematogenous dissemination. Often, the site of primary tuberculosis infection is asymptomatic and inapparent, and the patient seeks medical attention with symptoms and signs of nonspecific illness, including fever, night sweats, malaise, fatigue, anorexia, and weight loss (fever of unknown origin). The liver may be moderately enlarged and palpable, and there may be minimal splenomegaly and lymphadenopathy. Rarely, with extensive liver involvement, there will be slight jaundice. Concomitant alcoholic liver disease may result in prominent hepatic manifestations. Occasionally, white spots (tubercles) are visible on the retina at funduscopy. Very rarely there is extensive involvement of the biliary tree by tuberculosis, with a clinical picture resembling bacterial cholangitis. With hepatic tuberculosis, liver test abnormalities vary greatly. In the authors' series, alcoholic liver disease coexisting with hepatic tuberculosis no doubt contributed to the abnormalities of liver test results (Table 41–3). When there is extensive tuberculous involvement of the bone marrow, the patient may have anemia, neutropenia, polycythemia, or a leukemoid reaction.

Tuberculous granulomata are found most frequently within the portal areas; they may develop within the hepatic lobules but rarely near the hepatic veins. Tuberculous granulomata start as a cluster of monocytes, usually surrounded by a thin rim of necrosis or edema. As the monocytes transform into epithelioid cells, there is often a thin rim of lymphocytes. Tuberculous granulomata do not typically segment, as do sarcoid granulomata; they appear to reach only a size comparable to that of a portal area, unless they caseate. The presence of hepatic noncaseating epithelioid granulomata, which may be found in some cases of pulmonary tuberculosis, should not be equated with miliary tuberculosis. Miliary tuberculosis refers to widespread multiple granulomata the size of millet seeds, that is, 1 to 2 mm in diameter. Microscopically, miliary granulomata are caseous and represent a life-threatening form of tuberculosis.

In managing the febrile patient who has hepatic granulomata of uncertain cause, a therapeutic trial with isoniazid and ethambutol should be carried out. This should be preceded by cultures for *Mycobacterium tuberculosis* of all available material (nebulized sputum or fasting gastric contents, urine, and bone marrow). Since the authors have obtained several positive culture results from aspiration biopsy of the liver, they advocate taking a portion of the first liver biopsy sample for culture if granulomatous disease is suspected, or repeating the biopsy to obtain material for culture after hepatic granulomata are discovered.

The response to therapy for tuberculosis may be evident after a week or, in exceptional cases, may take six to eight weeks; therefore, it is recommended that therapy continue for a maximum of eight weeks if a response is not obvious. Most undiagnosed patients who remain febrile this long will be found to have sarcoidosis, which will respond rapidly to small doses of prednisone.

BRUCELLOSIS

In the United States, brucellosis can be acquired by contact with swine, cattle, or goats (e.g., by farmers, abattoir workers, and veterinarians) or by ingestion of unpasteurized dairy products (including goat cheese), usually on trips outside the United States.[45, 46] Recently, a few cases of human infection by *Brucella canis*, acquired from contact with dogs, have been identified.[45] The *Brucella* organisms (*B. suis*, *B. abortus*, *B. melitensis*, and *B. canis*) tend to cause granulomatous reactions in the reticuloendothelial system, including the liver.[47-50] Symptoms are nonspecific and consist of fever, sweats, and fatigue. Some patients have severe aches and pains, often in the back, that mimic musculoskeletal disease. Excessive weakness and depression are often present during the acute illness and for prolonged periods after objective evidence of active disease is gone. Remissions and relapses (undulant fever) are common. Physical findings include slight enlargement of the liver, spleen, and lymph nodes. The leukocyte count usually is normal or low, with relative lymphocytosis. Slight abnormalities of liver test results (elevated levels of serum transaminases and alkaline phosphatase) are common, although jaundice is unusual. Complications of brucellosis include orchitis, osteomyelitis, arthritis of the hip or knee, renal abscess, endocarditis, meningoencephalitis, and pulmonary nodule formation. The diagnosis can be made by identification of increasing serum agglutinins in response to a standard strain of *B. abortus*. Positive reactions in titers of 1:320 or more are considered diagnostic. A prozone phenomenon due to blocking antibody is relatively common and is overcome by appropriate serum dilution. Blood or bone marrow culture is the most reliable method of establishing the diagnosis. The organisms are relatively fastidious, and repeated cultures may be necessary. Castaneda's medium is helpful, and the addition of 10 per cent carbon dioxide is useful for culturing *B. abortus*. *B. melitensis* may be mistaken for *Moraxella phenylpyruvica* because the two have similar biochemical characteristics.[51]

When brucellosis is untreated, the usual course is recovery within 3 to 12 months. Fatalities are rare. Antibiotic therapy is considered helpful, but the results are rarely dramatic. Tetracycline (21-day course) is the antibiotic of choice; streptomycin sometimes is used concomitantly.

The granulomatous reactions associated with *Brucellosis abortus* generally have been encountered in the chronic form of the disease. The granulomata are sparse, punched out, and epithelioid. They may appear particularly bland because of the frequent lack of a rim of lymphocytes or a mixture of lymphoid forms within the granulomata. The granulomata are typically within the lobules rather than within the portal areas. More acute forms of brucellosis, usually characterized by infection with *B. melitensis*, feature a striking Kupffer cell hyperplasia, reminiscent of that produced by typhoid fever or other salmonelloses, but more elongated forms of Kupffer cells predominate, instead of the round monocytoid forms of typhoid fever. Occasionally, in the more acute reaction, the histiocytes cluster together to form non-epithelioid granulomata (Fig. 41–8).

Figure 41–8. Areas of granulomatous necrosis in patient with acute infection with *Brucella melitensis* (hematoxylin and eosin, × 460).

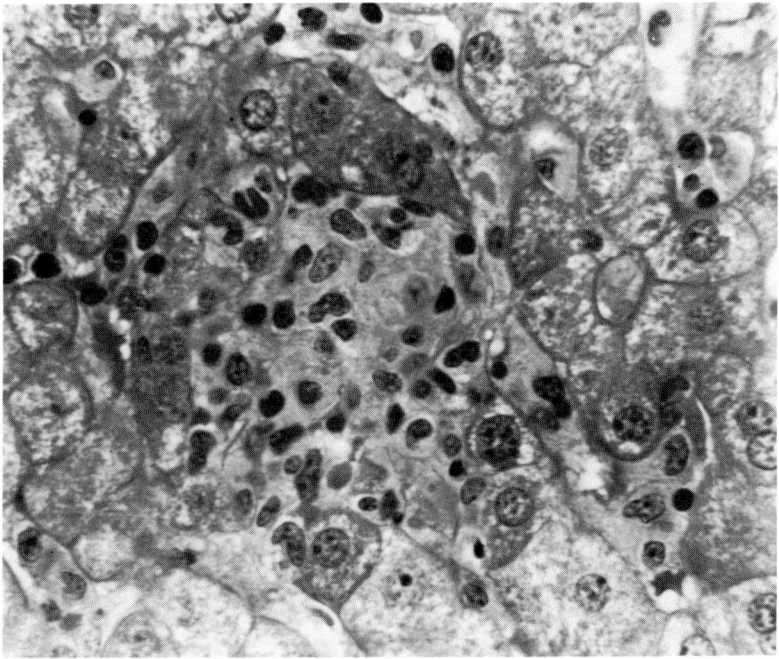

Q FEVER

Q fever, an infectious disease caused by a rickettsia, *Coxiella burnetii,* spreads to humans from infected cows, sheep, and goats, or from their ticks. The organism is resistant to drying and is easily aerosolized, so it can be acquired by inhalation near dairies in which there are infected cows. Other routes of infection include the drinking of raw milk, the handling of infected meat or placentae, and, rarely, tick bites. The incubation period is one to two weeks. The primary site of infection is the respiratory tract, with an illness resembling viral pneumonia. Headache, fever, and myalgias are prominent. There is no rash. The pulse is often unusually slow, as in typhoid fever. Chest x-ray films show patchy infiltrates or nodular densities. Mild to moderate leukocytosis is common. Occasionally, there is involvement of the joints, the central nervous system, the kidneys, the epididymis, the pericardium, or the heart valves. Ten to 15 per cent of patients have clinical evidence of hepatic involvement, with prolonged fever, hepatic enlargement and tenderness, and jaundice (usually slight).[52-56] Hepatic test abnormalities are minimal and include increases in serum alkaline phosphatase and transaminase activity, reductions of the albumin level and prothrombin activity, and increases in direct and indirect bilirubin. In some reported cases of Q fever hepatitis, the patients have had no history of pulmonary symptoms and have had normal chest x-ray films.

The hepatitis reaction of Q fever is more exudative than are those observed with most other granulomatous disorders. The portal areas of involved livers have striking lymphoid hyperplasia and exudates, with destruction of the limiting plates. Kupffer cells are hyperplastic, and there are numerous foci of necrosis with clusters of lymphocytes and histiocytes (Fig. 41–9). Some of the foci of necrosis are large enough to be considered granulomatous, and many of the granulomata have a pattern nearly unique to Q fever. The most characteristic feature of the Q fever granuloma is a ring of fibrinoid necrosis surrounded by lymphocytes

and histiocytes. The fibrinoid ring often encloses a clear space, which has given rise to the terms *doughnut* and *fibrin-ring* granuloma (Fig. 41–10). These lesions are not pathognomonic for Q fever, since they have been seen rarely in lymphoma,[57] allopurinol hypersensitivity,[58] and in our experience in several patients with acquired immune deficiency syndrome (AIDS) who had negative serologic test results for *C. burnetii.* Nevertheless, this type of lesion is highly suggestive of Q fever.[59, 60]

Diagnosis is made by demonstration of a rising titer of complement-fixing antibodies to *C. burnetii* that appears two to three weeks after infection. Treatment of Q fever with tetracycline or chloramphenicol is considered helpful, although not dramatically so.

HODGKIN'S DISEASE

Extensive use of staging laparotomy with multiple liver biopsies in Hodgkin's disease has disclosed that as many as 12 per cent of patients have isolated epithelioid cell granulomata in the liver.[61-63] Experience from the Stanford University series shows that they are found prior to treatment for Hodgkin's disease, that they are not dependent on prior lymphangiography, and that patients with granulomata have about the same incidence of symptoms and cutaneous anergy as do patients without granulomata.[63] Special staining for organisms and cultures for bacteria and fungi have yielded negative results when performed. The granulomata are epithelioid without caseation and occasionally contain Langhans' giant cells. They do not resemble lipogranulomata. Their location is usually but not exclusively portal. In 23 of 31 patients in the Stanford University series, the granulomata were not located close to the lesions of Hodgkin's disease, and their presence in liver tissue has not been considered pertinent for staging the disease.[63] Similar granulomata have been found in the spleen, bone marrow, and abdominal lymph nodes, although less frequently than in the liver. They were found in about 2 per

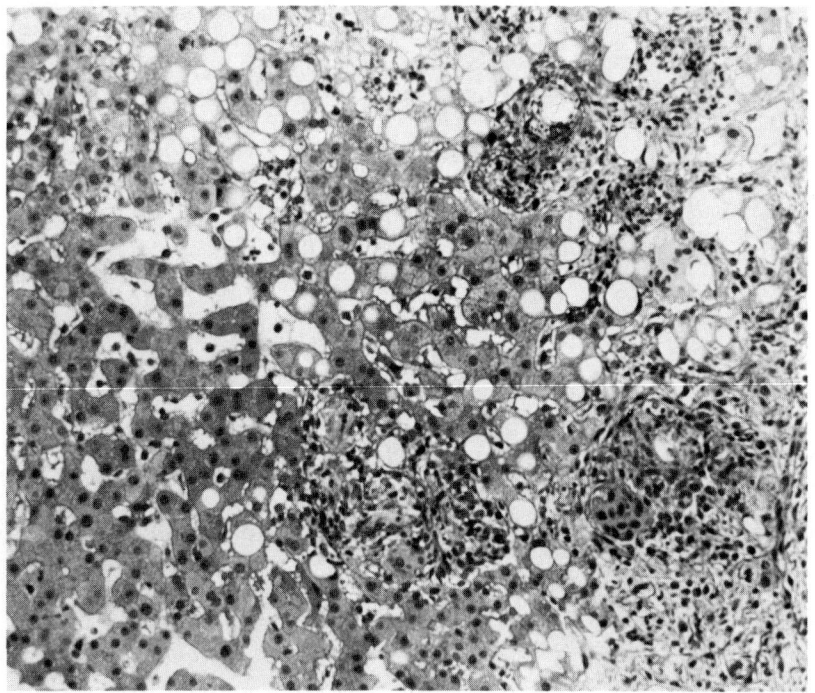

Figure 41–9. Numerous foci of granulomatous necrosis in Q fever (hematoxylin and eosin, × 92).

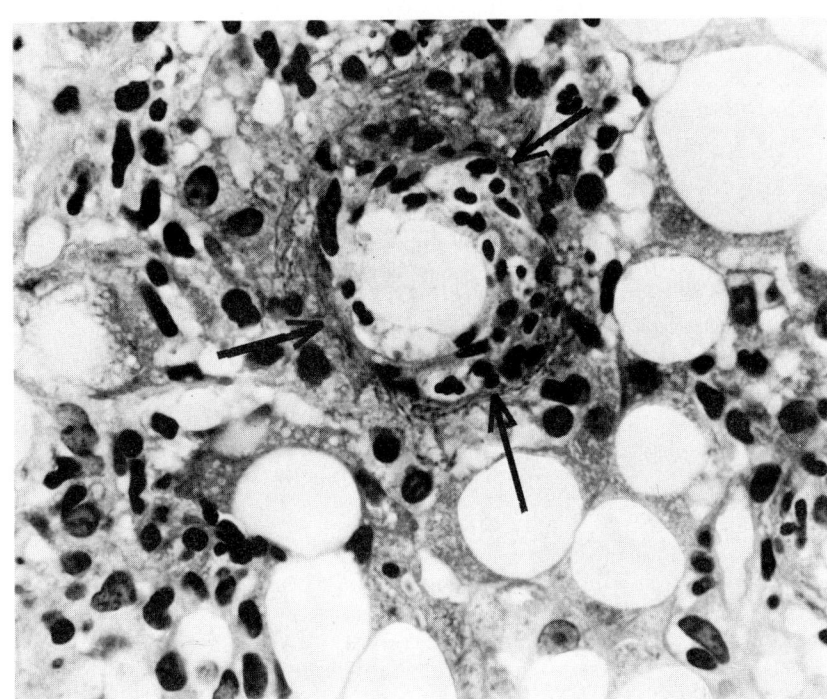

Figure 41–10. "Doughnut" granuloma of Q fever. Note the fibrinoid ring (*arrows*) around the margin of the doughnut hole (hematoxylin and eosin, × 460).

cent of patients with non-Hodgkin's lymphoma.[64] Braylan and co-workers found extensive, unexplained granulomata in three patients with non-Hodgkin's lymphoma.[64] There is no indication from the reports of others or from our own experience that these granulomata are due to tuberculosis. Concomitant sarcoidosis has been suggested,[65] but for several reasons this seems unlikely. Present opinion is that the granulomata represent a host response to the presence of a nearby neoplastic process, or that they are morphologic evidence of an abnormal immune response.[66] In febrile patients with hepatic granulomata of uncertain cause, Aderka and colleagues suggested that the following criteria should raise suspicion of the presence of lymphoma: fever persisting beyond four weeks, liver or spleen enlarged more than 4 cm below the costal margin, and eosinophilia greater than 4 per cent.[67]

INTESTINAL BYPASS SURGERY

Several investigators have reported the finding of single or multiple epithelioid, noncaseating granulomata in liver biopsy specimens after intestinal bypass surgery, and this is consistent with the authors' experience. This has been too frequent a finding to be explained by coincidence; for example, Halverson and colleagues, at Washington University, found a 7 per cent incidence in 101 patients,[68] and Banner and Banner found granulomata in 6 of 40 postshunt biopsy specimens.[69] Although tuberculosis has also been reported to occur after intestinal bypass,[70] the hepatic granulomata are probably not due to tuberculosis. No suitable explanation has been found for them.

The granulomata found in intestinal bypass patients are usually punched-out nodules of histiocytes that have nuclei larger than those of typical epithelioid cells. There is usually no peripheral lymphocytic rim in the individual granuloma (Fig. 41–11, p. 1103).

LEPROSY

Hepatic granulomata are very common in patients with leprosy, even though clinical signs and symptoms of liver disease are unusual. After the mucocutaneous system and lymph nodes, the liver is the organ most commonly found to be involved at necropsy.[71] From 62 to 84 per cent of patients with lepromatous leprosy have hepatic granulomata,[72, 73] which are especially likely to be found when erythema nodosum is present, whereas hepatic involvement is the exception in tuberculoid leprosy. According to Chen and co-workers,[73] the presence of hepatic granulomata correlates well with the frequency and intensity of bacteremia. As many as 10^5 *Mycobacterium leprae* organisms/ml of blood may be present in untreated lepromatous leprosy. The granulomata may be composed primarily of epithelioid cells or histiocytes (tuberculoid leprosy) or foam cells (lepromatous leprosy) (Fig. 41–12). The foam cell collections with scant inflammatory elements consist of distinctive Kupffer cells swollen with myriad *M. leprae* organisms (Fig. 41–13).[74] The organisms, which are acid-fast and easily visible on Fite staining, are much less common in epithelioid and histiocytic granulomata. Although the organisms are visible, they cannot be cultured, but they may be infective for the mouse footpad. An occasional leprosy patient has accompanying amyloid deposition.[75]

Abnormalities in hepatic biochemical tests in leprosy are usually minor and not consistently present and correlate poorly with the presence of granulomata.[72] Symptoms and signs referable to the liver are rare, though both liver and spleen often are palpable.

SYSTEMIC MYCOSES

Coccidioides immitis and *Histoplasma capsulatum* are fungi that may cause human infection. The organisms are

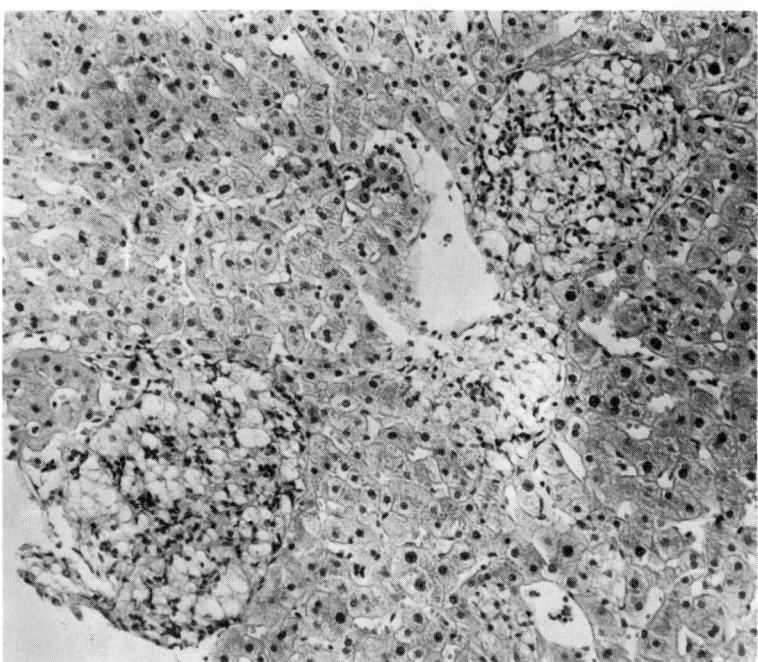

Figure 41–12. Granulomata made up of foam cells in patient with lepromatous leprosy (hematoxylin and eosin, × 92).

found in a mycelial phase in soil. In the United States, *Coccidioides* is prevalent in the dry valleys in the Southwest coastal area and *Histoplasma* is prevalent in the east-central plains. Both organisms become yeast forms in human tissue. Humans are infected by inhalation of organisms, with primary infection in the lungs. Most patients recover completely, chronic pulmonary lesions develop in a few, and in a very few there is widespread dissemination to many organs, including the liver. The hepatic reaction to these fungi is usually granuloma formation.

Dissemination of *Coccidioides* infection occurs in 0.5 to 1 per cent of infected patients, notably in blacks and Filipinos. The disease is slowly progressive, with meningeal involvement being the most prominent clinical problem. In 40 to 50 per cent of cases in which necropsies are done, the liver is found to contain granulomata,[76, 77] but only rarely is there a significant disturbance in hepatic biochemical tests or liver function. Palpability of the liver can be a clue to hepatic involvement, and liver biopsy can be diagnostic if characteristic spherules of *Coccidioides immitis* are found in hepatic granulomata[78] (Fig. 41–14). Serial sectioning and PAS staining help in visualizing the organisms. Eosinophilia is often present when there is dissemination.[79, 80] The skin test with coccidioidin usually produces negative results, but the complement-fixation test gives reliably positive results in almost all cases of disseminated disease. Recognition of disseminated coccidioides is important, since moderately effective therapy with amphotericin and 5-fluorocytosine is available.

Dissemination of *Histoplasma* infection is considerably less frequent than is that found with *Coccidioides* infection. This event is more common in infants and children than in adults and in patients who are being treated with corticosteroids or who have T-lymphocyte dysfunction. Disseminated disease usually manifests as fever and debility of unknown cause, often with hepatosplenomegaly and oral ulcers. Development of Addison's disease from adrenal destruction is remarkably common. When the liver is enlarged, it usually contains granulomatous lesions, sometimes with central caseation necrosis that resembles tuberculosis.[81-83] Organisms can often be found in the granulomatous foci by hematoxylin and eosin staining, but use of special stains (methenamine silver, Hotchkiss-McManus) makes identification easier. There is no consistent pattern of abnormalities in hepatic biochemical tests. Diagnosis is best confirmed by culture of the organism from blood, bone marrow, sputum, and oral ulcers (scrapings or biopsy material). Culture results of liver biopsy specimens were positive in two of three cases reported by Sarosi and colleagues.[81] Both skin testing and serologic testing are unreliable and often produce negative results in disseminated disease. As with *Coccidioides* infection, treatment with amphotericin or 5-fluorocytosine may be lifesaving in disseminated disease and may be very helpful when there are progressive pulmonary lesions. Corticosteroid therapy is necessary when adrenal insufficiency develops.

SCHISTOSOMIASIS

Human infestation with *Schistosoma* is prevalent in many areas of the world, including Africa, the Middle East, South America, and the Caribbean (*Schistosoma mansoni*), Japan, China, and Southeast Asia (*Schistosoma japonicum*) (See also Chap. 39). Thin adult male and female schistosomes 1 to 2 cm long live together in the venules and capillaries of the mesenteric veins; the females lay as many as 3000 ellipsoidal eggs daily during life spans as long as ten years.[84, 85] About half of the eggs reach the intestine by migration through the tissues with the aid of secreted enzymes. Many of the non-excreted eggs are swept to the liver in the portal vessels, at which point they embolize in the portal venules. Granulomatous reactions to egg components, possibly mediated by T-cell lymphokines,[85] may result in large portal-area granulomata containing macrophages, lymphocytes, and eosinophils. Fibrosis accompanies and surrounds the granulomata, giving the appearance of clay pipe–stem fibrosis to the cut surface of the liver in advanced cases. Patients who have only a few lesions have no symptoms or abnormal findings. However, a large worm

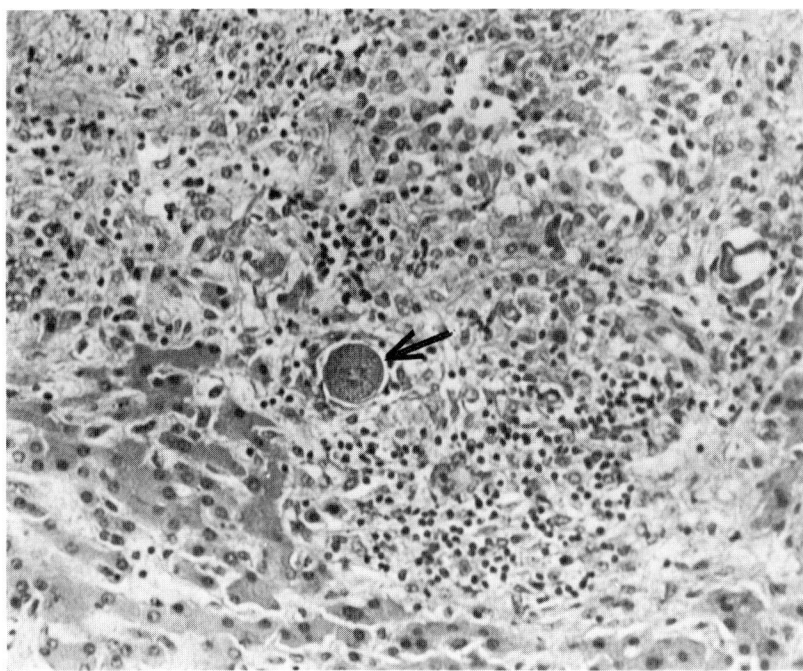

Figure 41–14. Coccidioides (*arrow*) in hepatic granuloma (hematoxylin and eosin, × 92).

burden results in the development of portal hypertension with hepatomegaly, especially of the left lobe, and splenomegaly.

Liver biopsy in a patient with schistosomiasis who has emigrated from another country to the United States usually reveals only dense portal fibrosis surrounding dead, occasionally calcified, ova (Fig. 41–15). In early lesions, the cellular reaction is more prominent (Fig. 41–16). The diagnosis can be made by finding eggs in the feces, in a biopsy specimen of the rectal mucosa, or in a hepatic granuloma. Wedged hepatic venous pressure is normal or nearly normal even in the presence of severe portal hypertension.

PRIMARY BILIARY CIRRHOSIS

About 25 per cent of cases of primary biliary cirrhosis are associated with either granulomatous necrosis or granulomata with giant cells. The granulomata may be either within the lobules or in the portal areas (Fig. 41–17, p. 1103). When they are in the portal areas, granulomata may be confused with follicular centers of lymphoid follicles, which are also common in primary biliary cirrhosis. Occasionally, granulomatous destruction of bile ducts may be seen (Fig. 41–18, p. 1103), but the typical epithelioid granulomata seem to be distinct from the ducts.

Primary biliary cirrhosis has a relatively distinctive

Figure 41–15. *Schistosoma japonicum* fibrosis in liver. By the time of autopsy, granulomata are apparently uncommon (hematoxylin and eosin, × 92).

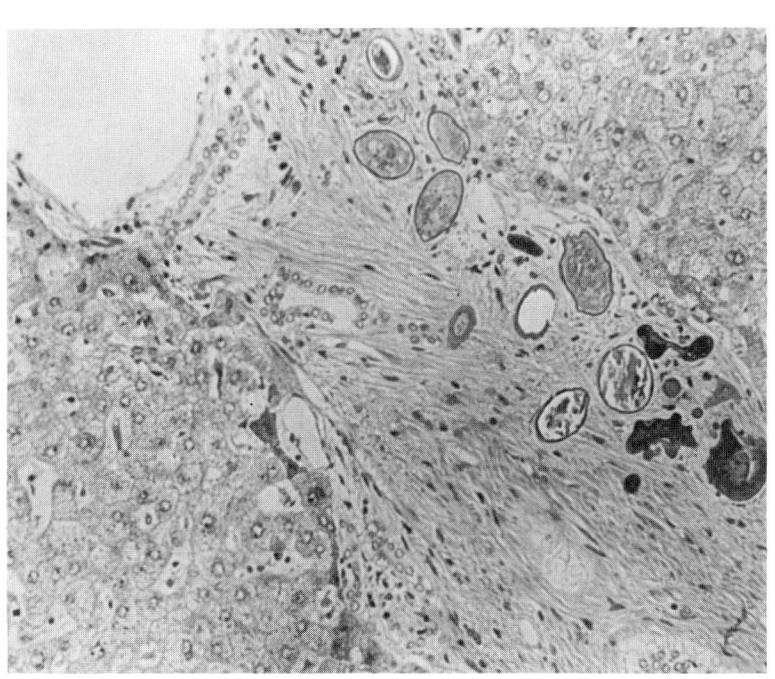

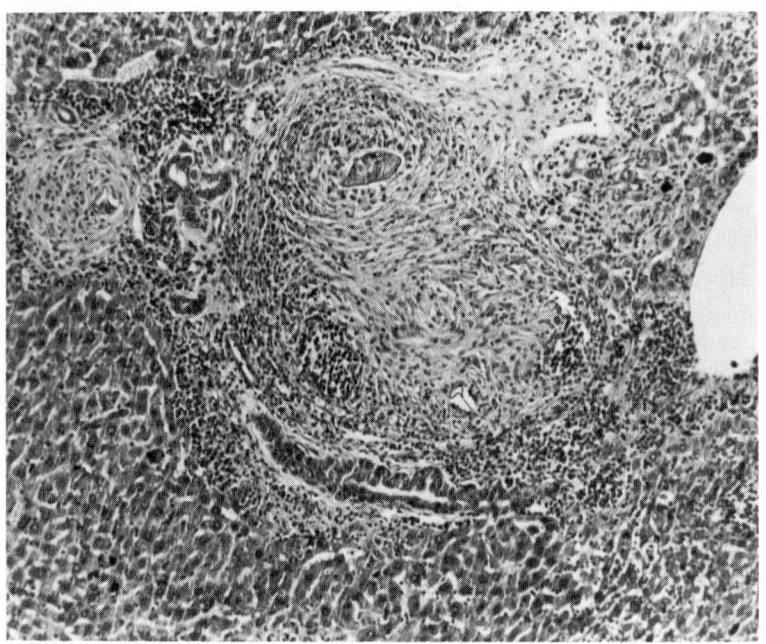

Figure 41–16. Earlier stage of hepatic schistosomiasis with exuberant inflammatory reaction (hematoxylin and eosin, × 55).

clinical picture and rarely is confused with the other disorders that are accompanied by hepatic granulomata (see Chap. 44). There is no fever. Jaundice, pruritus, markedly elevated serum alkaline phosphatase levels and hypercholesterolemia, increased IgM levels, and a positive antimitochondrial antibody test are typically found. Only in an occasional instance of sarcoidosis is there difficulty with the differential diagnosis.[24-26]

DRUG HYPERSENSITIVITY

A wide variety of drugs have been reported to cause granulomatous reactions in the liver (see Table 41–1). In most instances, identification of drugs as causative factors has been based on circumstantial evidence, since drug challenge has been carried out only infrequently. McMaster and Hennigar reported that 28 of 95 hepatic granulomata encountered during a ten-year period were potentially drug-related.[86] This proportion is far higher than usually reported.

Features that favor a drug-related pathogenesis are peripheral eosinophilia, tissue eosinophilia, and a portal location of the granulomata. Since there is no pathognomonic characteristic of drug-related hepatic granulomata, it seems sensible to discontinue all medications that are not necessary for life support in patients who have hepatic granulomata of uncertain cause.

ACQUIRED IMMUNE DEFICIENCY SYNDROME

Patients with AIDS have a greatly increased prevalence of disseminated infections with organisms that ordinarily cause hepatic granulomata. They include *Mycobacterium avium-intracellulare*, *M. tuberculosis*, *Cryptococcus*, and *Histoplasma*.[87-90] Presumably because of impaired immunity, granulomata are often poorly formed or lacking in the AIDS patient with these infections. Instead there may be only collections of foamy histiocytes or simply enlarged Kupffer cells with minimal inflammatory response. All of

the lesions tend to contain large numbers of organisms which, in the case of the mycobacteria, are easily visualized with acid-fast stains, as in leprosy. The fungi are seen best with PAS or methenamine silver stains. Cultures of liver biopsy fragments on appropriate media usually give positive results as do blood cultures. Unfortunately, response to treatment is poor.

The clues to hepatic involvement by these infections include substantial elevation in serum alkaline phosphatase levels along with a mild increase in serum transaminase levels, and moderate hepatomegaly. Other hepatic lesions that are relatively common in AIDS patients include chronic hepatitis B, cytomegalovirus infection, Kaposi's sarcoma, non-Hodgkin's lymphoma, and biliary infection with *Cryptosporidium* or cytomegalovirus (see Chapter 53).

REFERENCES

1. Wilhelm DL. Inflammation and healing. In: Anderson WAD, Kissane JM, eds. Pathology, 7th ed. Vol. 1. St. Louis, CV Mosby, 1977:67.
2. Adams DO. The granulomatous inflammatory response. A review. Am J Pathol 84:164, 1976.
3. Wanless IR, Geddie W-R. Mineral oil lipogranulomata in liver and spleen. A study of 465 autopsies. Arch Pathol Lab Med 109:283, 1985.
4. Christoffersen P, Braendstrup O, Juhl E, et al. Lipogranulomas in human liver biopsies with fatty change. Acta Pathol Microbiol Scand A 79:150, 1971.
5. Wagoner GP, Anton AT, Gall EA, et al. Needle biopsy of the liver. VIII. Experiences with hepatic granulomas. Gastroenterology 25:487, 1953.
6. Schiff L. The clinical value of needle biopsy of the liver. Ann Intern Med 34:948, 1951.
7. Rubin E. Interpretation of the liver biopsy. Gastroenterology 45:400, 1963.
8. Edmondson HA. Needle biopsy in differential diagnosis of acute liver disease. JAMA 191:480, 1965.
9. Baggenstoss AH. Morphologic and etiologic diagnoses from hepatic biopsies without clinical data. Medicine (Baltimore) 45:435, 1966.
10. Fauci AS, Wolff SM. Granulomatous hepatitis. In: Popper H, Schaffner F, ed. Progress in Liver Disease, Vol. 5. New York, Grune & Stratton, 1976:609.
11. Robbins SL, Cotran RS. Pathologic Basis of Disease, 2nd ed. Philadelphia, WB Saunders, 1979:84.

12. Popper H, Schaffner F. Liver: Structure and Function. New York, McGraw Hill, 1957:551.

13. Klatskin G. Hepatic granulomata: problems in interpretation. Ann NY Acad Sci 278:427, 1976.

14. Edmondson HA, Peters RI. Diagnostic problems in liver biopsies. Pathol Annu 2:213, 1967.

15. Guckian JC, Perry JE: Granulomatous hepatitis. An analysis of 63 cases and review of the literature. Ann Intern Med 65:1081, 1966.

16. Neville E, Piyasena KHG, James GD. Granulomas of the liver. Postgrad Med J 51:361, 1975.

17. Scalises G, Boggiano CA, Pippi L, et al. I Processi Granulomatosi Epatici. Omina Med Ter 47:357, 1969.

18. Mir-Madjlessi SH, Farmer RG, Hawk WA. Granulomatous hepatitis. A review of 50 cases. Am J Gastroenterol 60:122, 1973.

19. Hughes M, Fox H. A histological analysis of granulomatous hepatitis. J Clin Pathol 25:817, 1972.

20. Gelb AM, Brazenas N, Sussman H, et al. Acute granulomatous disease of the liver. Am J Dig Dis 15:842, 1970.

21. Klatskin G, Yesner R. Hepatic manifestations of sarcoidosis and other granulomatous diseases. Yale J Biol Med 23:207, 1950.

22. Simon HB, Wolff SM. Granulomatous hepatitis and prolonged fever of unknown origin: a study of 13 patients. Medicine (Baltimore) 52:1, 1973.

23. Eliakim M, Eisenberg S, Levij IS, et al. Granulomatous hepatitis accompanying a self-limited febrile disease. Lancet 1:1348, 1968.

24. Iversen K, Christoffersen P, Poulsen H. Epithelioid cell granulomas in liver biopsies. Scand J Gastroenterol (Suppl) 7:61, 1970.

25. Rudzki C, Ishak KG, Zimmerman HJ. Chronic intrahepatic cholestasis of sarcoidosis. Am J Med 59:373, 1975.

26. Fagan EA, Moore-Gilon JC, Turner-Warwick M. Multiorgan granulomas and mitochondrial antibodies. N Engl J Med 308:572, 1983.

27. Maddrey WC. Sarcoidosis and primary biliary cirrhosis. Associated disorders? N Engl J Med 308:588, 1983.

28. Rumball JM, Baum GL. Liver biopsy culture in the diagnosis of miliary tuberculosis: a case report. Gastroenterology 22:124, 1952.

29. Healey RJ, Leff AH, Rosenak BD. Needle biopsy in tuberculosis of the liver, with culture of acid-fast bacilli: a case report. Am J Dig Dis 4:638, 1959.

30. Alexander JF, Galambos JT. Granulomatous hepatitis. The usefulness of liver biopsy in the diagnosis of tuberculosis and sarcoidosis. Am J Gastroenterol 59:23, 1973.

31. Mitchell DN, Scadding JG. Sarcoidosis. Am Rev Resp Dis 110:774, 1974.

32. The Kveim Controversy (editorial). Lancet 2:750, 1971.

33. James DG. Kveim revisited, reassessed. N Engl J Med 292:859, 1975.

34. Hurley TH, Sullivan JR, Hurley JV. Reaction to Kveim test material in sarcoidosis and other diseases. Lancet 1:494, 1975.

35. Levin S. The fungal skin test as a diagnostic hindrance (editorial). J Infect Dis 122:343, 1970.

36. Sbarbaro JA. Skin test antigens: an evaluation whose time has come (editorial). Am Rev Dis 118:1, 1978.

37. Lieberman J. Elevation of serum angiotensin-converting-enzyme (ACE) level sarcoidosis. Am J Med 59:365, 1975.

38. Schweisfurth H, Wernze H. Changes of serum angiotensin I converting enzyme in patients with viral hepatitis and liver cirrhosis. Acta Hepato-Gastroenterol 26:207, 1979.

39. Silverstein E, Friedland J, Lyons HA, et al. Elevation of angiotensin-converting enzyme in granulomatous lymph nodes and serum in sarcoidosis: clinical and possible pathological significance. Ann NY Acad Sci 278:498, 1976.

40. Nosal A, Schleissner LA, Mishkin FS, et al. Angiotensin-I-converting enzyme and gallium scan in non-invasive evaluation of sarcoidosis. Ann Intern Med 90:328, 1979.

41. Hercules HD, Bethlem NM. Value of liver biopsy in sarcoidosis. Arch Pathol Lab Med 108:831, 1984.

42. Maddrey WC, Johns CJ, Boitnott JK, et al. Sarcoidosis and chronic hepatic disease: clinical and pathologic study of 20 patients. Medicine (Baltimore) 49:375, 1970.

43. Porter GH. Hepatic sarcoidosis. A cause of portal hypertension and liver failure. A review. Arch Intern Med 108:483, 1961.

44. Israel HL, Margolis ML, Rose LJ. Hepatic granulomatosis and sarcoidosis. Further observations. Dig Dis Sci 29:353, 1984.

45. Fox MD, Kaufman AF. Brucellosis in the United States, 1965–1974. J Infect Dis 136:312, 1977.

46. Young EJ, Suvannoparrat U. Brucellosis outbreak attributable to ingestion of unpasteurized goat cheese. Arch Intern Med 135:240, 1975.

47. Barrett GM, Rickards AG. Chronic brucellosis. Q J Med 22(85):23, 1953.

48. Joske RA, Finckh ES. Hepatic changes in human brucellosis. Med J Aust 1:266, 1955.

49. Fogel R, Lewis S. Diagnosis of *Brucella melitensis* infection by percutaneous needle biopsy of the liver. Ann Intern Med 53:204, 1960.

50. Cervantes F, Bruguera M, Carbonell J, et al. Liver disease in brucellosis. A clinical and pathological study of 40 cases. Postgrad Med J 58:346, 1982.

51. D'Auria A. A case of brucellosis and a problem in the identification of the etiologic agent. Am J Med Technol 44:751, 1978.

52. Clark WH, Lennette EH, Railsback OC, et al. Q fever in California. VII. Clinical features in 180 cases. Arch Intern Med 88:155, 1951.

53. Picchi J, Nelson AR, Waller EE, et al. Q fever associated with granulomatous hepatitis. Ann Intern Med 53:1065, 1960.

54. Bernstein M, Edmondson HA, Barbour BH. The liver lesion in Q fever. Clinical and pathologic features. Arch Intern Med 116:491, 1965.

55. Dupont HL, Hornick RB, Levin HS, et al. Q fever hepatitis. Ann Intern Med 74:198, 1971.

56. Hofmann CE, Heaton JW. Q fever hepatitis. Clinical manifestations and pathological findings. Gastroenterology 83:474, 1982.

57. Voigt JJ, Delsol G, Fabre J. Liver and bone marrow granulomas in Q fever (letter). Gastroenterology 84:887, 1983.

58. Vanderstigel M, Zaframi ES, Lejonc JL, et al. Allopurinol hypersensitivity syndrome as a cause of hepatic fibrin-ring granulomas. Gastroenterology 90:188, 1986.

59. Qizilbash AH. The pathology of Q fever as seen on liver biopsy. Arch Pathol Lab Med 107:364, 1983.

60. Pellegrin M, Delsol G, Auvergnat JC, et al. Granulomatous hepatitis in Q fever. Hum Pathol 11:51, 1980.

61. Bagley CM Jr, Roth JA, Thomas LB, et al. Liver biopsy in Hodgkin's disease. Clinicopathologic correlations in 127 patients. Ann Intern Med 76:219, 1972.

62. Kim H, Dorfman RF, Rosenberg SA. Pathology of malignant lymphomas in the liver: application in staging. In: Popper H, Schaffner F, ed. Progress in Liver Diseases, Vol. 5. New York, Grune & Stratton, 1976:683.

63. Kadin ME, Donaldson SS, Dorfman RF. Isolated granulomas in Hodgkin's disease. N Engl J Med 283:859, 1970.

64. Braylan RC, Long JC, Jaffe ES, et al. Malignant lymphoma obscured by concomitant extensive epithelioid granulomas: report of three cases with similar clinicopathologic features. Cancer 39:1146, 1977.

65. Goldfarb BL, Cohen SS. Coexistent disseminated sarcoidosis and Hodgkin's disease. JAMA 211:1525, 1970.

66. Nadel EM, Ackerman LV. Lesions resembling Boeck's sarcoid in lymph nodes draining an area containing a malignant neoplasm. Am J Clin Pathol 20:952, 1950.

67. Aderka D, Kraus M, Weinberger A, et al. Parameters which can differentiate patients with "idiopathic" from patients with lymphoma-induced liver granulomas. Am J Gastroenterol 80:1004, 1985.

68. Halverson JD, Wise L, Wazna MF, et al. Jejunoileal bypass for morbid obesity. A critical appraisal. Am J Med 64:461, 1978.

69. Banner BF, Banner AS. Hepatic granulomas following ileal bypass for obesity. Arch Pathol Lab Med 102:655, 1978.

70. Pickleman JR, Evans LS, Kane JM, et al. Tuberculosis after jejunoileal bypass for obesity. JAMA 234:744, 1975.

71. Powell CS, Swan LL. Leprosy: pathological changes observed in 50 consecutive necropsies. Am J Pathol 31:1131, 1955.

72. Karat ABA, Job CK, Rao PSS. Liver in leprosy: histological and biochemical findings. Br Med J 1:307, 1971.

73. Chen TSN, Drutz DJ, Whelan GE. Hepatic granulomas in leprosy. Their relation to bacteremia. Arch Pathol Lab Med 100:182, 1976.

74. Kramarsky B, Edmondson HA, Peters RL, et al. Lepromatous leprosy in reaction. A study of liver and skin lesions. Arch Pathol 85:516, 1968.

75. Contreras F Jr, De las Aquas JT, Contreras F. Hepatic lesions in lepromatous patients. Int J Leprosy 37:270, 1969.

76. Forbus WD, Bestebreurtje AM. Coccidioidomycosis: a study of 95 cases of the disseminated type with special reference to the pathogenesis of the disease. Surgeon 99:653, 1946.

77. Huntington RW Jr. Diagnostic and biologic implications of the histopathology of coccidioidomycosis. In: Proceedings of a Symposium on Coccidioidomycosis. U.S. Department of Health, Publication No. 575, 1957:38.

78. Craig JR, Hillberg RH, Balchum OJ. Disseminated coccidioidomycosis. Diagnosis by needle biopsy of liver. West J Med 122:171, 1975.

79. Ward JR, Hunter RC. Disseminated coccidioidomycosis demonstrated by needle biopsy of the liver. Ann Intern Med 48:157, 1958.

80. Coodley EL. Disseminated coccidioidomycosis: diagnosis by liver biopsy. Gastroenterology 53:947, 1967.

81. Sarosi GA, Voth DW, Dahl BA, et al. Disseminated histoplasmosis: results of long-term follow-up. A Center for Disease Control cooperative mycosis study. Ann Intern Med 75:511, 1971.

82. Silverman FN, Schwarz J, Lakey ME, et al. Histoplasmosis. Am J Med 19:410, 1955.

83. Reddy P, Gorebick DF, Brasher CA, et al. Progressive disseminated histoplasmosis as seen in adults. Am J Med 48:629, 1970.

84. Mahmoud AA. Schistosomiasis. N Engl J Med 297:1329, 1977.
85. Warren KS. Hepatosplenic schistosomiasis: a greatly neglected disease of the liver. Gut 19:572, 1978.
86. McMaster KR, Hennigar GR. Drug-induced granulomatous hepatitis. Lab Invest 44:61, 1981.
87. Lebovics E, Thung SN, Schaffner F, et al. The liver in the acquired immunodeficiency syndrome: A clinical and histologic study. Hepatology 5:293, 1985.
88. Glasgow BJ, Anders K, Layfield LJ, et al. Clinical and pathologic findings of the liver in the acquired immune deficiency syndrome (AIDS). Am J Clin Pathol 83:582, 1985.
89. Orenstein MS, Tavitian A, Yonk B, et al. Granulomatous involvement of the liver in patients with AIDS. Gut 26:1220, 1985.
90. Nakanuma Y, Liew CT, Peters RL, et al. Pathologic features of the liver in acquired immune deficiency syndrome (AIDS). Liver 6:158, 1986.

IV C.   Liver Disease in Association with Disorders of Immunity

42

Immunologic Mechanisms in Chronic Liver Disease

Howard C. Thomas, B.Sc., Ph.D., M.D., F.R.C.P.

The immune system has two limbs (Fig. 42–1). The *afferent limb* of the system differentiates foreign antigens from self-antigens and "presents" the former to specialized B and T lymphocytes. This leads in turn to "priming," or activation, of the *efferent limb* (or effector limb) of the immune system.

AFFERENT LIMB OF THE IMMUNE SYSTEM

Soluble antigens are taken up by a variety of antigen-presenting cells.[1] After intracellular processing, they are presented, in association with the MHC Class II molecules on the cell surface, to helper T and B lymphocytes within the germinal centers of the lymph nodes and spleen. This process results in priming and proliferation of antigen-specific B cells and ultimately in production of specific antibodies. Similar complexes between antigen and MHC class II molecules on the surface of Langerhans cells in the skin are presented to CD4 helper T cells in the paracortical areas of the lymph nodes and spleen. This results in the priming of CD8 cytotoxic T cells, which then will recognize the antigen in association with MHC class I molecules.

An important characteristic of the afferent limb of the immune system is amplification of the signal produced by antigen in order to increase the number of primed cells. Interleukin 1 (IL 1) produced by macrophages, stimulates proliferation of helper T cells. These cells in turn produce interleukin 2 (IL 2), which stimulates further expansion of the population of helper T cells (Fig. 42–2).

The activity of the helper T cells is modulated by the activity of suppressor T cells. The balance between the function of these two populations of T cells determines the level of proliferation and differentiation of the primed B or cytotoxic T cells. These regulator cells may be concerned with the responses to specific antigens[2] or with the overall level of responsiveness of the immune system to a variety of antigens.[3]

EFFERENT LIMB OF THE IMMUNE SYSTEM

It is convenient to divide the efferent limb into two parts: the antibody-dependent limb and the T cell–dependent limb.

Antibody-Dependent Limb. Antibodies interact with monocytes, macrophages and polymorphs. For example, they facilitate phagocytosis of foreign microbes or cells, or in conjunction with K cells they cause lysis of foreign or infected cells. In some cases, antibodies, particularly when present in high density on the surface of a microorganism, result in activation of complement, leading to lysis or accelerated phagocytosis of the microorganisms. The complement system is composed of a complex series of enzymes that, in analogy with blood clotting, become activated in sequence. This leads ultimately to the activation of the third component of complement (C3) (Fig. 42–3). Activation of the complement system occurs by two different processes designated the classic and alternative pathways. The classic pathway usually is activated by an antibody-antigen complex; the alternate pathway can be activated directly by microorganisms or foreign cells, without the binding of antibody. In addition, the alternative pathway amplifies the level of activation of the classic pathway by a series of regulated enzyme actions. It should be remembered that complement serves not only to lyse or enhance the phagocytosis of foreign microorganisms and cells, but also to solubilize circulating immune complexes so that they do not deposit in the vascular endothelium and cause an inflammatory reaction.

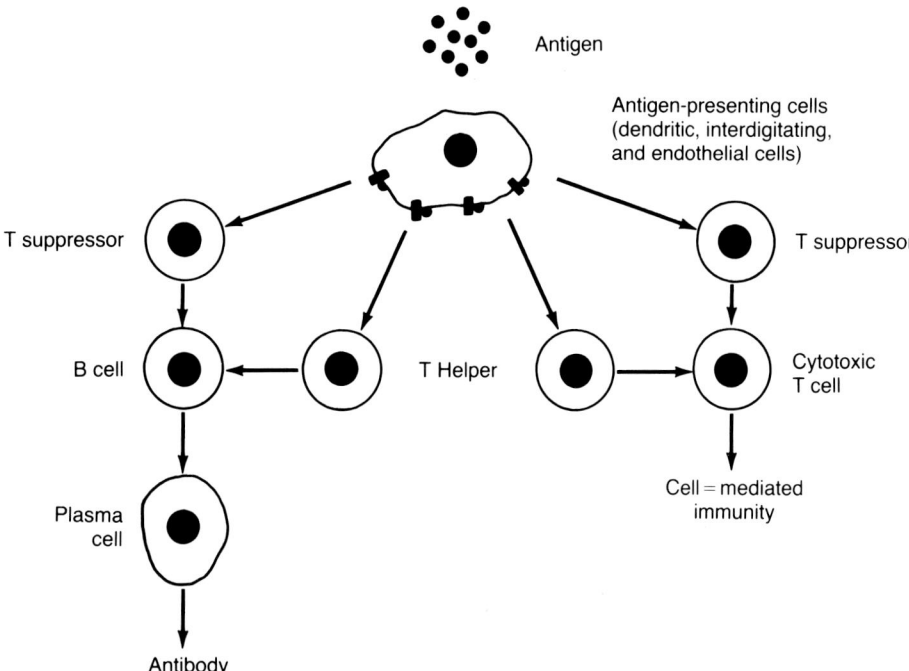

Figure 42–1. Antigen-presenting cells are involved in the induction of cytotoxic T cells and sensitized B cells. The level of proliferation of these cells is influenced by regulatory helper and suppressor T cells.

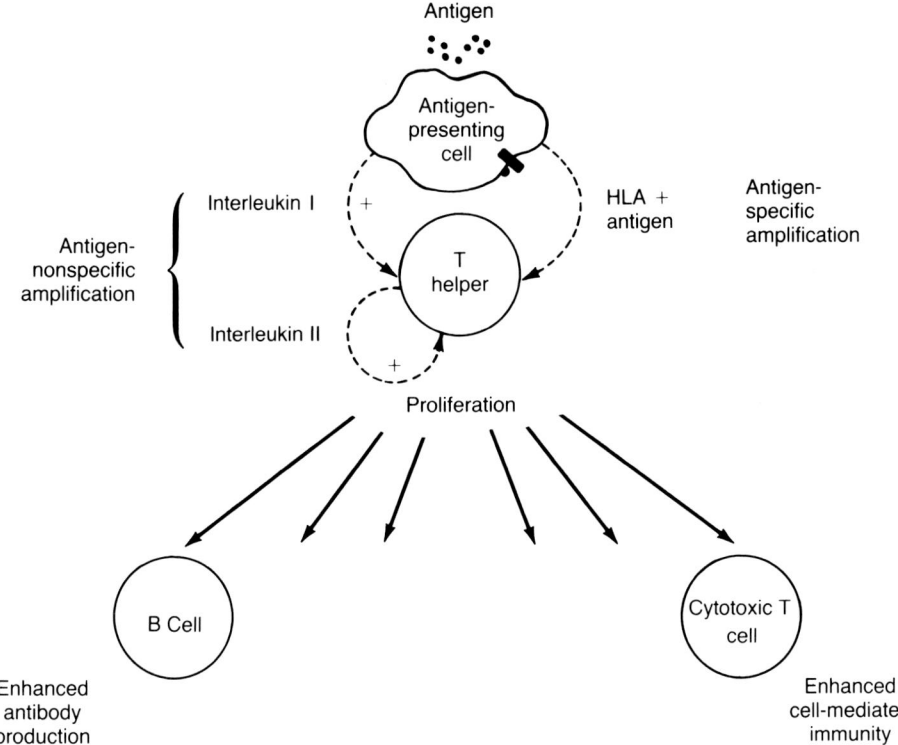

Figure 42–2. Amplification of the immune response is dependent on the production of soluble intercellular regulatory proteins (interleukins).

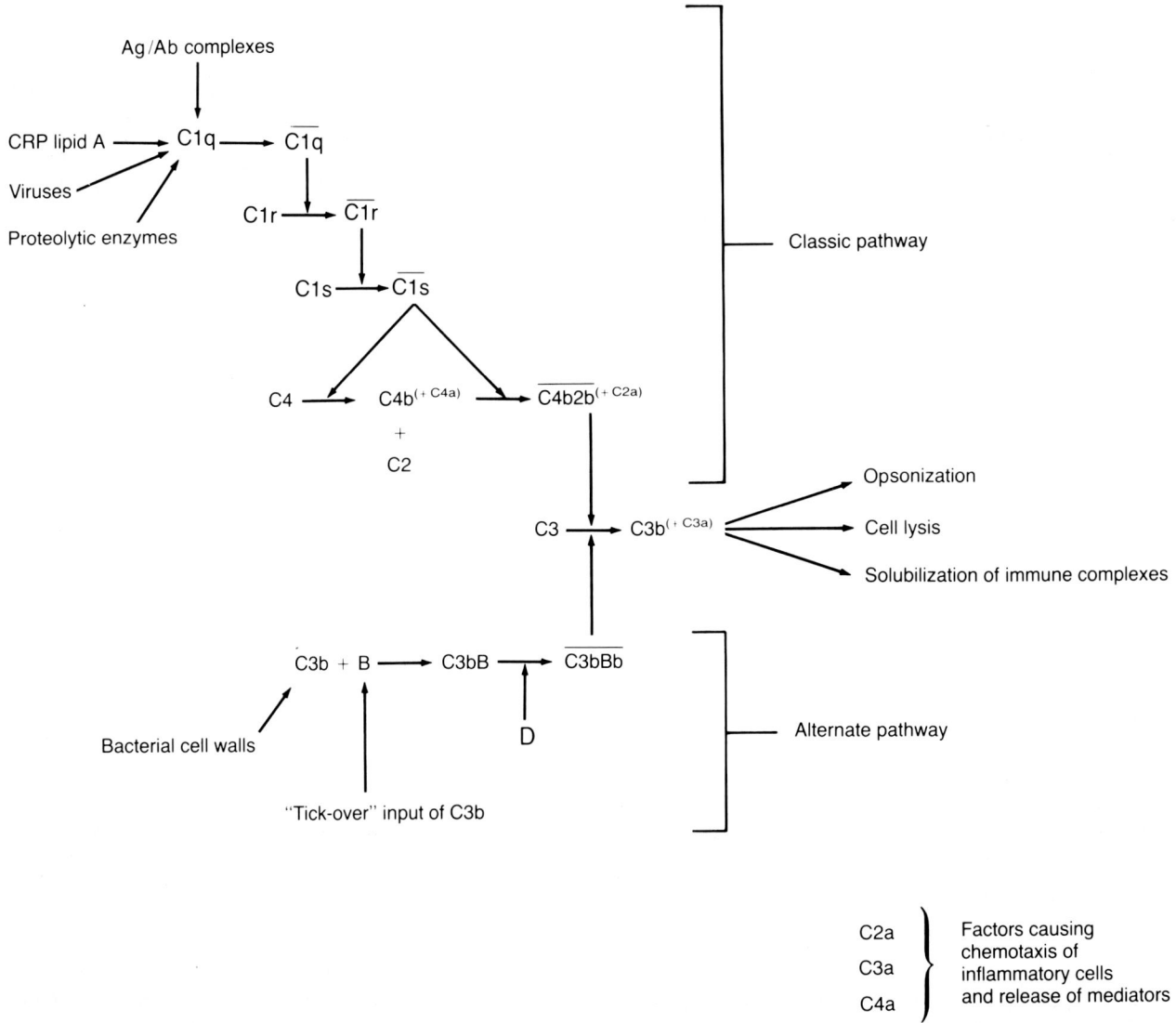

Figure 42–3. The complement system is a complex cascade of plasma proteins with two activation pathways. Note that certain substances may activate complement directly; in other cases, fixation of antibody is necessary. Some viruses activate complement directly (e.g., retroviruses).

T Cell–Dependent Limb. The function of cytotoxic T cells is to eliminate virus-infected and neoplastic (also homografted) tissues. Cytotoxic T cells are activated by complexes between a foreign protein and the MHC glycoproteins of the host (Fig. 42–4).[4] The cytotoxic T cell, when activated in this way, can kill target cells directly. In addition, the complex between antigen and MHC glycoprotein stimulates the cytotoxic T cell to produce a variety of lymphokines that attract polymorphonuclear and mononuclear cells of the inflammatory system. The production of lymphokines by the cytotoxic T cell is an important process for recruiting non–antigen-specific cells to the site of immune activity. These lymphokines are also important in the activation of macrophages to deal with intracellular parasites.

In some situations the response of epithelial cells to gamma interferon, which is released from sensitized T lymphocytes, will induce the display of MHC class II glycoproteins.[5] The association of this glycoprotein with other membrane-displayed autoantigens will prime helper T cells, leading to an immune response against these auto-antigens.[6] Such transient responses to autoantigens may occur during a vigorous immune response to foreign antigens.

IMMUNOLOGIC ABNORMALITIES IN AUTOIMMUNE CHRONIC ACTIVE HEPATITIS

The immune system in normal subjects permits responses to foreign antigens but suppresses those directed to self-components. Autoimmune disease occurs when this system fails because of either a primary defect in the regulatory apparatus (primary autoimmunization) or a change in the antigenicity of the tissues (e.g., induction of MHC class II proteins on epithelial cells[6]) (secondary autoimmunization).

Autoaggressive reactions are associated with the presence of autoantibodies. When these antibodies are directed to antigens displayed on membranes, they are probably important in the lysis of cells. Those directed to cytoplasmic antigens may be useful diagnostically but are of unknown

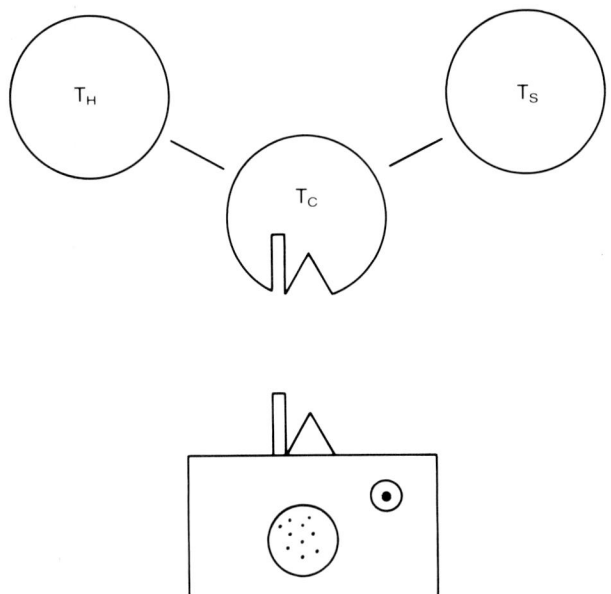

Figure 42–4. Cytotoxic T cells recognize foreign MHC proteins or foreign proteins associated with the body's own MHC class I proteins. These cells are capable of destroying transplanted tissue and virus-infected cells. T_H = helper T cells, T_C = cytotoxic T cells, T_S = suppressor T cells.

pathogenic significance. When no extrinsic etiologic factor can be identified in patients with presumed autoimmune diseases, the process is assumed to result from a failure of the regulatory system, which allows the expansion of a clone of autoreactive lymphocytes. This defect may be general or it may be restricted to certain specific groups of self-antigens. Thus, the autoimmune attack may be generalized or specific, (i.e., several or a single tissue may be affected). The recent development of techniques to enumerate and measure the functional activity of the regulatory lymphocytes controlling the effector limbs of the immune system enables us to test whether various putative autoimmune diseases are due to a generalized defect in immunoregulatory function.

EVIDENCE FOR A DEFECT IN THE IMMUNOREGULATORY SYSTEM

Defects in the mechanisms of regulation of immunoglobulin synthesis[7, 8] and the responsiveness of T cells to mitogens[9] have been identified. The T lymphocytes derived from the peripheral blood of patients with autoimmune chronic active hepatitis (CAH) do not suppress the synthesis of immunoglobulins by B cells in peripheral blood. In contrast, T cells from normal individuals demonstrate significant suppressor activity.[9] The T lymphocytes in peripheral blood contain both helper and suppressor T cells. It was unknown at first whether the defect in patients with autoimmune CAH resulted from enhanced helper or diminished suppressor activity.[10] With the availability of monoclonal antibodies to differentiate functional helper from cytotoxic/suppressor T lymphocytes, it became possible to enumerate these cell populations.[11] Several groups demonstrated an increased ratio of helper to cytotoxic/suppressor T cells[12, 13] in affected patients, and it became evident that this altered ratio reflected changes in populations of both helper and suppressor cells.[14] Therefore, the

defect in immunity in patients with autoimmune CAH is heterogeneous. The abnormal ratios of helper to cytotoxic/suppressor cells return to normal as the liver disease improves during therapy with prednisolone.[12] The administration of prednisolone to normal subjects (without liver disease) also produces a fall in the ratio of helper cells to cytotoxic/suppressor T cells, suggesting a direct effect of the drug on the lymphoid system,[12] rather than changes in the immune system secondary to improved liver function produced by other effects of prednisolone.

TARGET ANTIGENS ON THE HEPATOCYTE MEMBRANE

Autoimmune CAH is characterized by the presence of non–organ-specific antibodies, including antinuclear factors and smooth muscle antibodies. How these antibodies relate to the pathogenesis of the disease is unknown.

The description of antibodies directed to liver-specific determinants[15] is of special interest because it provides a possible link between the immunologic phenomena and the liver cell damage. Liver-specific protein (LSP) (Fig. 42–5), first isolated in 1972,[16] is part of a large lipoprotein complex derived from a crude liver homogenate. This complex contains an antigen localized on the plasma membrane of hepatocytes, which can be shown by immunofluorescence using isolated hepatocytes and heterologous anti-LSP sera. Antibodies[15] and sensitized T lymphocytes[17] to LSP are present in the blood of patients with autoimmune CAH, but they are also present in the blood of patients with other forms of acute and chronic liver disease. Thus it is unclear whether this antibody is of primary pathogenic significance or whether it is present because of liver damage due to other, possibly nonimmunologic, reasons. Furthermore, the antigenic complexity of the lipoprotein complex designated as LSP is considerable.[18] It is possible, therefore, that there is considerable heterogeneity of the immune response to this protein complex.

In addition to the LSP determinants, other antigens have been identified in the plasma membranes of hepatocytes using naturally occurring antibodies obtained from the sera of patients with autoimmune CAH.[19] Unlike the antibodies to LSP, these liver membrane antibodies are found predominantly in sera of patients with autoimmune CAH and rarely in patients with other types of liver disease. This antibody activity was detected initially by indirect

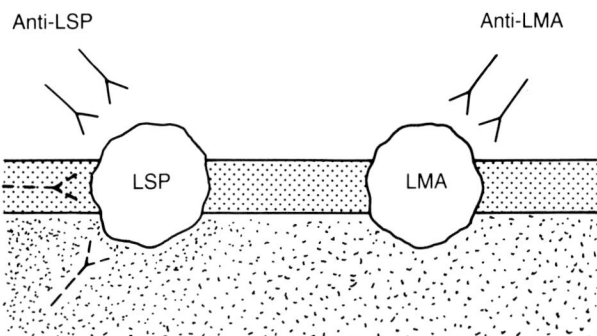

Figure 42–5. Liver-specific protein (LSP) and liver membrane antigens (LMA) are independent complexes within the liver cell membrane. Antibodies to LSP (anti-LSP) are measured by radioimmunoassay using extracted LSP and may bind to surface or cryptic determinants. Antibodies to LMA (anti-LMA) are measured by binding to intact hepatocytes and include only surface specificities.

immunofluorescence using rabbit or human hepatocytes as targets. More recently, radioimmunometric assays, using rat hepatocytes as targets, have been developed.[20, 21] This procedure provides an objective measure of autoantibody response and, by further modification,[21] allows the differentiation between liver membrane antibodies and immune complexes binding to Fc receptors on hepatocytes. Use of this assay confirms that the liver membrane antibody response is found predominantly in patients with autoimmune CAH and in some patients with primary biliary cirrhosis who have piecemeal necrosis. The antibody to liver membrane antigen (LMA) is found rarely, and at low titer, in patients with hepatitis B virus–induced chronic active liver disease. Once again, it is likely that the LMA is complex and that the antibody response to it is heterogeneous.

In order to examine further the specificity of the immune response directed to antigens in the plasma membrane of the liver, attempts have been made to demonstrate liver-specific epitopes using murine monoclonal antibodies.[22] Some liver-specific epitopes have been identified, but the majority are also found in other tissues. Some of these, but not all, are species specific. The specificity for liver of the humoral and cellular responses to LSP reported in the literature[15, 17] must be questioned.

One of the murine monoclonal antibodies to LSP reacts with antigens in microsomes from liver and kidney[23] and also binds to the plasma membrane of the liver cell. This antibody is present in the sera from patients with autoimmune CAH.[23] The above technique is being extended to determine, in different patient groups, the specificities of other naturally occurring antibodies to liver plasma membranes. Although all sera contain anti-LSP reactivity, some specificities may be restricted to certain diseases.

NATURE OF EFFECTOR MECHANISMS

A variety of effector mechanisms may be involved in the mediation of liver cell damage in patients with autoimmune CAH (Fig. 42–6). Investigators have followed two paths in studying the problem. The first is to examine the cytotoxicity of lymphocytes in peripheral blood against the patient's own hepatocytes.[24] These studies point to antibody-dependent, cell-mediated cytotoxicity as a significant mechanism in the lysis of hepatocytes. Cell-mediated immune mechanisms, independent of antibody, have a lesser role. The second experimental approach utilizes monoclonal antibodies to examine the composition of mononuclear

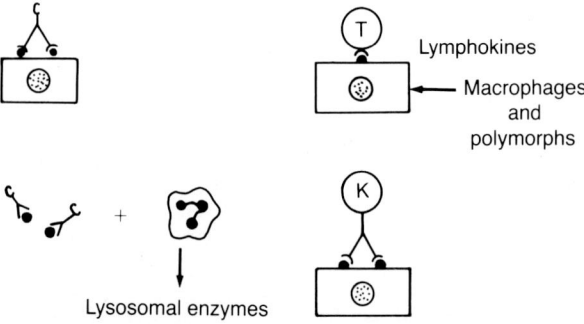

Figure 42–6. Mechanism of humoral and cell-mediated effectors. Antibodies may bind to the autoantigen and either fix complement or initiate K-cell killing (antibody-assisted cellular cytotoxicity) or bind to soluble antigen resulting in formation of immune complexes. Sensitized T cells may lyse the cell directly or secrete lymphokines that attract macrophages and polymorphs. T = T cell, C = complement, K = killer cell.

cells infiltrating the liver tissue. These investigations demonstrate a predominance of B lymphocytes and helper T cells with relatively fewer cytotoxic/suppressor T cells.[25] The pattern of B lymphocytes with helper T cells, in conjunction with interdigitating and dendritic reticulum cells (i.e., antigen-presenting cells), in the periportal areas of the lobule[26] suggests that there is local production of antibody. Studies of the catabolism of Clq and C3[27, 28] and of the concentration of C3d in serum[29] indicate that C3 activation is not increased in these patients because of a deficiency of C4,[29] an early component of the classical activation pathway. Cytotoxic T cells, macrophages, and natural killer (NK) cells are less common components of the infiltrates.

APPROACHES TO THERAPY

Once the target antigens of the abnormal immune response have been identified, it will be possible to examine the regulatory system further for antigen-specific defects. Anti-idiotypic or clonal deletion approaches to therapy may then be possible (Fig. 42–7).

IMMUNOPATHOLOGY OF ACUTE AND CHRONIC HEPATITIS B INFECTION

During acute viral hepatitis, the liver is infiltrated with NK and cytotoxic/suppressor HNK1-positive and CD8-positive cells.[30] NK cells, which are stimulated by interferon, selectively eliminate cells supporting viral replication. It is likely that they are important in the clearance of hepatocytes infected with hepatitis B virus (HBV) during the early phase of the acute infection. Alpha interferons are present in the serum during the prodromal phase of acute hepatitis B both in man and chimpanzees,[31] and NK activity in peripheral blood increases during this phase of the disease. The role of cytotoxic T cells during acute hepatitis B is currently unknown. Activated T cells are present in the hepatic infiltrate,[30] but the target antigens have not been identified. Viral determinants, including HBsAg and HBc/e, are displayed on the hepatocyte membrane during chronic HBV infection,[32] and cytotoxic T cells directed to HBc and HBe are present in the peripheral blood.[33, 34] It seems probable that similar cells contribute to the elimination of virus-infected hepatocytes during the acute illness. Recent studies, using monoclonal antibodies that are known to bind to specific regions on the nucleocapsid protein, suggest that the cytotoxic T-cell response is directed to HBeAg,[34] a non-conformational determinant containing aminoacids 120–160 in the HBc gene product (unpublished observations). The humoral immune response is directed to conformational determinants containing the sequence 74–89.[35] Further studies show that helper T cells (CD4 + ve) reactive with HBcAg are present in the peripheral blood of HBV-infected patients[36, 36a]; these presumably amplify the humoral response. The epitopes involved in the stimulation of helper T cells have not been identified.

Cytotoxic T cells recognize viral determinants in association with MHC glycoproteins. In the absence of infection, there is a low density of HLA A, B, and C proteins on the hepatocyte plasma membrane, but the amount of these proteins increases rapidly during the early phase of acute HBV infection, induced initially by alpha interferons[31] and then sustained by gamma interferon (Fig. 42–8). It seems probable that the cytotoxic T-cell response to the

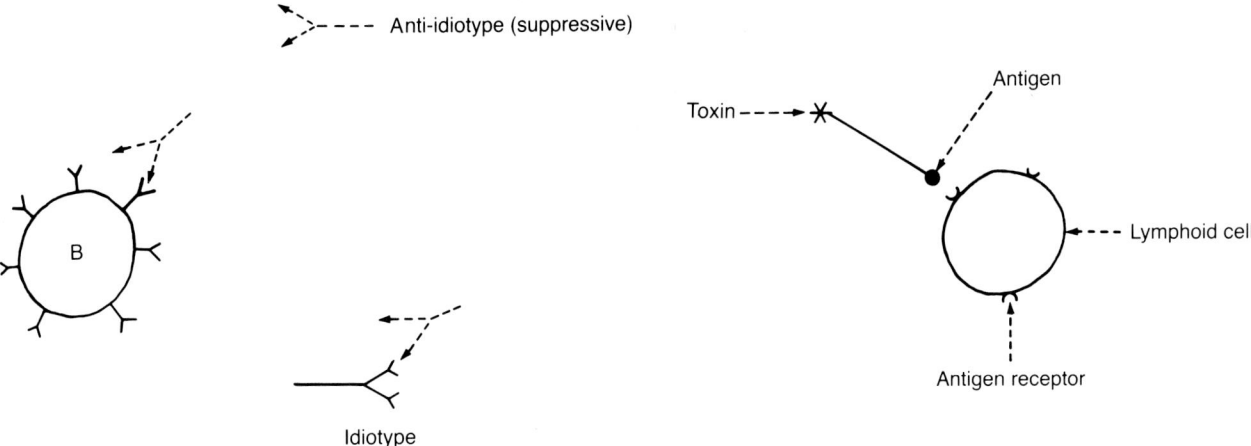

Figure 42–7. New approaches to the treatment of autoimmune chronic hepatitis. Autoreactive clones (left) may be suppressed by some types of anti-idiotype (antibody to antigen binding site of autoantibody) antibodies. Deletion of autoreactive clones (right) is achieved with toxin-labeled antigen that binds specifically to the antigen receptor on the B lymphocyte (B).

infected hepatocyte is modulated, to some extent, by the effect of interferon on the display of MHC class I protein[31] and by antibodies to the determinants on the nucleocapsid of the virus.[34] It is of considerable interest that the anti-HBc and anti-HBs responses are oligoclonal.[35, 37] This restricted clonality of the immune response raises the possibility that genetic factors may be important in determining whether the virus is cleared.

European patients with chronic HBV infection have increased levels of hepatic 2-5A oligoadenylate synthetase, indicating exposure of the infected cells to interferon.[38] However, increased levels of MHC class I protein are not seen on the plasma membranes of infected hepatocytes[39] and NK cells are almost absent from the hepatic infiltrate.[30] These data suggest that the concentration of interferon is insufficient to stimulate NK activity and synthesis of MHC proteins[38] or that the infected cell is unable to respond to interferon.[40] Transfection studies, in which copies of the HBV genome are introduced into various cell lines, indicate that the virus has the capacity to reduce the responsiveness of the cell to alpha, beta, and gamma interferons.[40] This may result from the presence of sequences in the HBV genome that are homologous to cellular sequences regulating the induction of the antiviral state and the display of

HLA by interferon.[41] Thus, when HBV infects an individual with a suboptimal capacity to produce alpha interferon[41a] and replicates to a high number of genomes per cell, the cell is rendered unable to enhance its display of HLA on the plasma membrane and is not subject to efficient lysis by NK and cytotoxic T cells. Studies of the viral proteins in the plasma membranes at this stage of the infection indicate the presence of HBsAg[39] and HBc.[34] It appears, therefore, that failure of the immune system to clear virus-infected cells may be related to a failure of the interferon system to enhance the display of MHC class I protein on the plasma membrane and allow T-cell cytolysis. This concept is supported by the observation that exogenous interferon, in supra-physiologic doses, produces a rapid increase in MHC class I protein on the hepatocyte plasma membrane. This is followed, in the majority of patients, by lysis of virus-infected hepatocytes (see Fig. 42–5).[31] A proportion of patients show a less than normal increase in the display of MHC class I protein in response to interferon; these patients, in general, fail to respond to treatment with interferon.[31] There may be additional immunological defects in other patients or a failure of the hepatocyte to respond to interferon, accounting for the failure to respond to interferon therapy. Currently, 30 to 40 per cent of adult

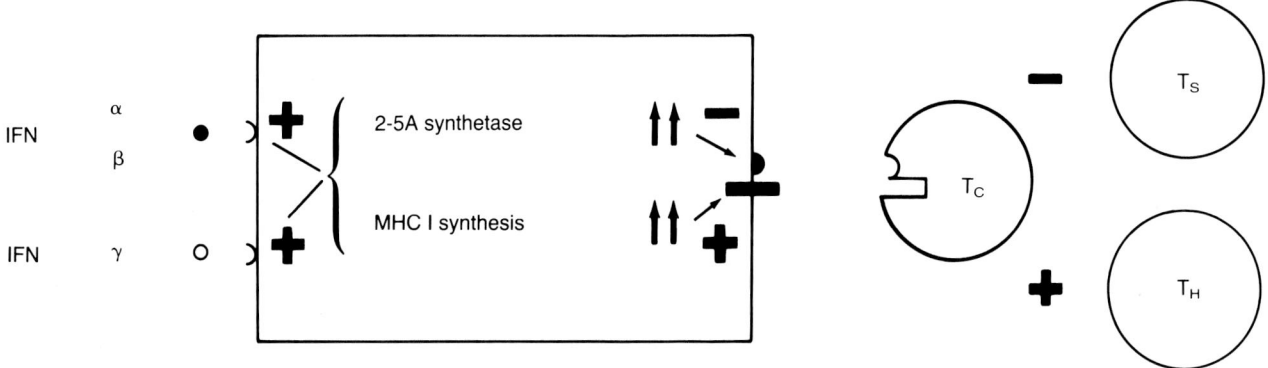

ENHANCEMENT OF MHC I SYNTHESIS

Figure 42–8. Cytotoxic T-cell killing of infected cells may be modulated by alpha and gamma interferon (IFN α & γ) induction of MHC class I proteins. T_S = suppressor T cell, T_H = helper T cell, T_C = cytotoxic T cell.

CARRIER MOTHER

(HBs + ve, HBeAg + ve)

NEONATE

Blood   Placenta   Blood   Liver

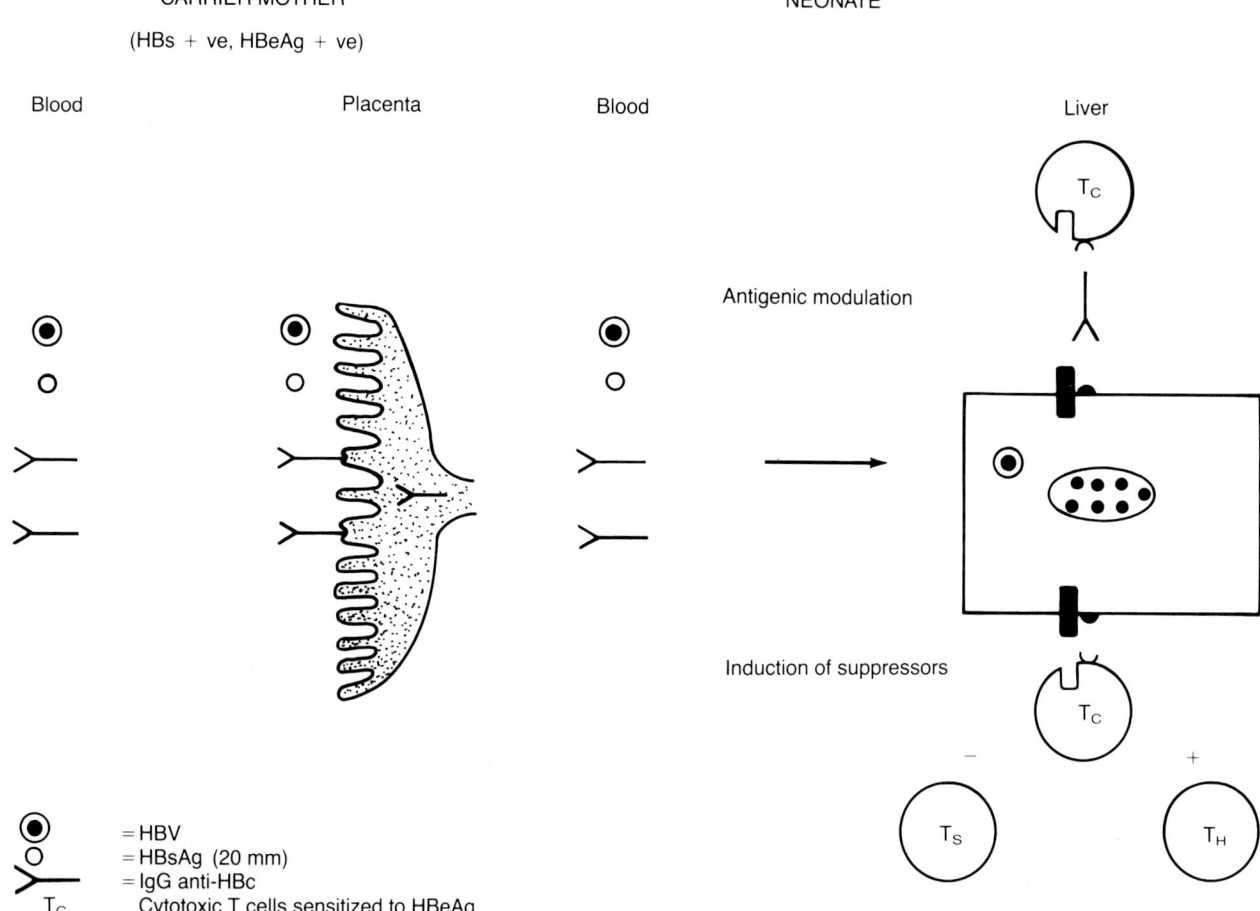

Antigenic modulation

Induction of suppressors

= HBV
= HBsAg (20 mm)
= IgG anti-HBc
T_C   Cytotoxic T cells sensitized to HBeAg

Figure 42–9. Transfer of maternal IgG anti-HBc or soluble HBe antigen across the placenta to the fetus results in the modulation in display of HBc antigen on the hepatocyte and the modification of the cell-mediated immune response to HBe (tolerance). In both cases, there is failure of clearance of HBV-infected cells by cytotoxic T cells (T_C) sensitized to HBc and HBe antigens. T_H = helper T cells, T_S = suppressor T cells.

patients of Northern European and Mediterranean origins respond to a three-month course of thrice weekly lymphoblastoid interferon.[42] The majority of these patients are heterosexual, but homosexual patients also show a high response rate.

In marked contrast, Chinese patients do not usually respond to lymphoblastoid interferon.[42] This suggests that the cause of the carrier state in these patients is different from that in European patients. One difference is that Chinese carriers usually acquire the infection at birth, whereas European carriers are infected in childhood or adult life. In addition, whereas only 5 to 10 per cent of patients infected in adult life develop a chronic carrier state, more than 95 per cent of those infected at birth become long-term carriers. Several factors may influence the ability of the infected child to clear the virus. First, it is possible that the immune system of the child is immature. The NK activity of peripheral blood mononuclear cells from children less than 12 years old is decreased compared to adults (43 to 49 years of age), and recovery from acute hepatitis B does involve the NK-interferon system. Second, transfer of the soluble nucleocapsid protein HBe across the placenta may induce nonresponsiveness of the fetal or neonatal immune system to this protein, which is one target of the cytotoxic T lymphocytes involved in immune clearance of HBV-infected hepatocytes. Third, maternal IgG anti-HBc may pass across the placenta and modify the

nucleocapsid protein display on the infected hepatocytes, preventing recognition by NK and cytotoxic T cells (Fig. 42–9). This hypothesis is supported by the observation that monoclonal anti-HBc against an immunodominant HBc epitope,[35] when injected with the virus into a chimpanzee, resulted in protracted HBV infection.[34] Therapeutic maneuvers directed toward restoring a state of immunity to HBc and HBe might allow clearance of HBV-infected cells in these individuals. The demonstration that the immune response to HBc and HBe is restricted to relatively few epitopes raises the possibility that active immunomodulation may be possible using anti-idiotype systems.

PRIMARY BILIARY CIRRHOSIS

In primary biliary cirrhosis (PBC), a chronic granulomatous inflammatory process, results in destruction of the intrahepatic biliary tree (see Chap. 43).[50, 51] Patients also exhibit lesions of the salivary, lacrimal, and pancreatic glands, scleroderma, rheumatoid arthritis, and thyroid disease.[52, 53] The finding of mitochrondrial antibody in the serum of these patients led to the conclusion that the disease was probably of autoimmune origin.[54]

PBC occurs commonly in middle-aged women who present with symptoms of cholestasis. The rate of progression is variable. Many patients remain anicteric for 10 to

20 years. Once jaundice develops, life expectancy is considerably reduced.[55]

IMMUNOLOGIC ASPECTS OF PATHOGENESIS

Recent studies report evidence of an abnormality in the immunoregulatory system in these patients. Both the concentrations and the functions of suppressor T-cells are markedly reduced.[56, 57] It is hypothesized that this abnormality allows the expansion of a clone of autoreactive lymphocytes with the potential to mount an autoimmune response to both hepatic and nonhepatic ductular antigens.[58] Similarity of the syndrome to chronic graft-versus-host disease, in which transplanted lymphoid cells attack tissues with a high density of MHC antigens, has led to the suggestion that the target antigen in PBC may be either a native or an altered MHC protein.[58]

One result of the reduced suppressor T-cell activity is an increased rate of synthesis of IgM,[57] with failure of polymerization leading to release of monomeric IgM.[59] An additional abnormality of the humoral immune system is failure to convert from IgM to IgG antibody production.[60] The protracted IgM response may be the result of failure of feedback inhibition because of the poor IgG antibody response.

MITOCHONDRIAL ANTIBODY

Mitochondrial antibody (MA) was first described in 1966 by Doniach et al.[61] The pattern in indirect immuno-fluorescence studies is coarsely granular, and mitochondria of all tissues are reactive. However, renal tubular cells rich in mitochondria are the usual substrate. The antibody can be found in the three main immunoglobulin classes, but IgM antibody predominates.[62] The antibody is present in more than 95 per cent of cases.[63] It is detectable in only a few other conditions, including Sjögren's disease.[64] The antibody is not found in jaundice due to extrahepatic biliary obstruction.[65]

The antigen, which has been localized to the inner membrane of mitochondria, is a lipoprotein of 180,000 to 200,000 daltons.[66] The "classic" mitochondrial antibody of PBC is one of four types.[67] The group of antibodies includes (1) anticardiolipin (M1), (2) antibody of PBC (M2), (3) antibody of the pseudolupus syndrome (M3), and (4) antibody of the CAH-PBC "overlap" disease (M4). Labro and coworkers recently described another type (M5) seen in patients with systemic lupus erythematosus.[68] The use of immunoblotting has shown that the M-2 antigen consists of at least three polypeptides of molecular weights 70, 45, and 39 kd.[68a] The gene encoding for the large protein has been cloned and sequenced[68b] and identified as the E2 component of pyruvate dihydrogenase.[68c]

IMMUNE COMPLEXES AND COMPLEMENT ACTIVATION

Patients with PBC have large amounts of "immune complex-like" material in their sera.[69, 70] This results in activation of the classic and alternative pathways of complement.[70, 71] These complexes are cleared abnormally slowly because of the presence of circulating antibodies to the C3b receptor in the patient's serum.[72, 73] The complexes may be responsible for certain extrahepatic manifestations

of the disease, including arthritis, arteritis, and glomerulonephritis.[74] Their role in the genesis of hepatic granulomas is unknown.

ABNORMALITIES OF CELL-MEDIATED IMMUNITY

Patients with PBC are severely anergic in delayed hypersensitivity skin tests.[75] Serum factors appear to be important.[76] Recently, evidence has focused on the contribution of abnormal high- and low-density lipoproteins in the anergic state.[77, 78]

IMMUNOLOGIC ASPECTS OF TREATMENT

Penicillamine, a copper chelating and anti-inflammatory compound, has been shown in some studies to produce biochemical and histologic improvement, but its effect on survival has not been established.[79, 80] This drug has been shown to reduce the ratio of helper to suppressor T cells.[56] Cyclosporin produces similar changes in the subsets of T cells and a marked improvement in liver biochemistry.[81] Clinical trials with this agent are currently under way.

ALCOHOL-INDUCED LIVER DISEASE

Several factors contribute to the liver damage that occurs in alcoholics. The alcohol or its metabolites are undoubtedly directly hepatotoxic, producing ultrastructural changes within a few hours after ingestion (see Chap. 31). Because persons with histories of similar exposure may respond with widely different degrees of liver damage, it is suspected that factors other than the amount of alcohol consumed influence susceptibility.[82, 83] It is likely that alcohol ingestion induces steatosis in all persons, but progression to hepatitis and cirrhosis does not always occur. Some investigations suggest that all patients with cirrhosis have gone through a stage of hepatitis; however, in other studies this progression is less clear. The factors that determine the rate of progression of the disease are not understood.

Recent studies have revealed an increased incidence of HLA-B8 in a group of patients with alcohol-induced hepatitis.[84, 85] The incidence in patients with steatosis is similar to that found in the normal population; persons who have cirrhosis without obvious hepatitis exhibit a low incidence of this phenotype. The authors suggest that in individuals who have progressed to cirrhosis with or without hepatitis, the mechanism of liver damage may be similar, but the presence of the gene or genes linked to HLA-B8 predispose the patient to a more florid hepatitic component of the disease. Other investigators have found linkage with other HLA phenotypes or no linkage at all.[86–90]

IMMUNE RESPONSE TO LIVER CELL ANTIGENS

Some features of the histology in alcohol-induced liver disease are compatible with an immunologically mediated component of the disease process. Although a major feature is central necrosis and polymorphonuclear cell infiltration, in some cases the portal zones reveal a mononuclear cell infiltrate and stellate fibrosis. This periportal infiltrate is similar to that seen in CAH and may represent an immunologic reaction to hepatocytes at the point of entry of lymphocytes to the hepatic lobule. This possibility is supported by the observation that lymphocytes from patients with alcohol-induced hepatitis are sensitized to liver cell antigens and are cytotoxic for rabbit hepatocytes.[91, 92] Recently, antibodies to alcohol-altered hepatocytes have been found in sera of patients with alcohol-induced hepatitis.[93]

The involvement of immune mechanisms in alcohol-induced liver disease is further supported by studies of the hepatic inflammatory infiltrate. Approximately 80 per cent of the cells in the livers of patients with alcoholic hepatitis are T lymphocytes; the remainder are B lymphocytes.[94] This contrasts with other forms of liver disease, in which the ratio of T to B lymphocytes is nearer 50:50. These findings are consistent with the suggestion that T lymphocytes have become sensitized to liver antigens and are mediating a tissue-damaging reaction.[91]

The role of an immune response to Mallory's hyalin in the pathogenesis of alcohol-induced hepatitis is more difficult to determine. Hyalin is found in about 50 per cent of cirrhotic patients with a history of alcohol abuse; however, it is also found in patients with Indian childhood cirrhosis, Wilson's disease, and PBC. Hyalin is a highly refractile, eosinophilic, cytoplasmic inclusion that probably represents a condensation of intracellular contractile filaments. Interest in this material has increased following the demonstration that patients with alcohol-induced hepatitis and cirrhosis are sensitized to the purified material.[95] These patients also exhibit low-titer antibodies to smooth muscle antigens and aggregated albumin.[96, 97] It is probable that these antibodies reflect an immune response to intracellular proteins released from degenerating hepatocytes.

ALTERED HUMORAL IMMUNITY

Although many of the immunologic features of alcohol-induced liver disease are common to other types of liver injury and presumably result from changes in hepatic phagocyte functions, some features are peculiar to the disease.[98] In alcohol-induced liver disease, one of the earliest changes is an increase in serum IgA concentration.[85] This occurs at a stage when the liver is either normal or exhibits only a mild degree of steatosis. Since this class of antibody is produced in the intestinal wall, one explanation of this increase would be that alcohol exposure results in an increase in permeability of the mucosa, thereby allowing increased access of intestinal antigens to the IgA immunocytes of the lamina propria and mesenteric lymph nodes. This change may represent merely an epiphenomenon; however, it is also possible that the change in permeability allows absorption of factors that contribute to the induction of hepatic damage. Increased titers of antibody to *Escherichia coli* occur at this early stage, suggesting that endotoxin-containing bacteria are absorbed and may be one of the intestine-derived factors contributing to the ongoing liver damage.[99, 100]

ALTERED CELL-MEDIATED IMMUNITY

Cell-mediated immunity is altered in patients with alcohol-induced liver disease.[101] Since many of the changes are also found in other types of liver disease and in animal models of cirrhosis,[102, 103] it is probable that they are the result of liver damage rather than of the chemical effect of alcohol.

Eighty per cent of patients with alcohol-induced liver disease fail to develop a delayed hypersensitivity reaction to a challenge with dinitrochlorobenzene and exhibit a significant decrease in responsiveness to streptokinase and to mumps, antigens to which the subjects are likely to have been sensitized previously.[101] This demonstrates a defect in the efferent limb of the delayed hypersensitivity response but does not exclude a coexisting defect in the afferent limb. The normal response to croton oil rules out a defect in the inflammatory response.[101] In these patients, the in vitro response of T cells to mitogens is normal, but inhibitors of this response can be demonstrated in serum.[102]

IMMUNOLOGIC ASPECTS OF TREATMENT

Withdrawal of alcohol is the main goal of therapy. In florid alcohol-induced hepatitis, corticosteroid therapy has been tried, but without significant beneficial effect.[104–110] In poorly nourished alcoholics, some immunologic abnormalities may respond to improved diet.

INFLUENCE OF LIVER DISEASE ON THE IMMUNE RESPONSE

Hyperglobulinemia[111–113] and depressed cell-mediated immunity[103, 112] are common in most forms of chronic liver disease, and it seems probable that these changes are a result of liver damage. This is supported by the fact that similar changes can be induced in rats that are made cirrhotic.[98, 103]

PHAGOCYTIC FUNCTION

Phagocytic function is markedly altered in patients with hepatic cirrhosis.[98, 113, 114] This results in changes in antigen distribution, which is a major factor in determining the characteristics of the ensuing humoral and cellular immune responses.[98] Antigens enter the circulation from the gastrointestinal tract, the larger ones via the mesenteric lymphatics and the smaller ones via the mesenteric venous circulation.[112] The liver, which is an important phagocytic organ, may therefore receive intestinally derived antigen, directly via the portal circulation when it acts as a "filter interposed in series" with the rest of the body, or it may receive antigen from the systemic circulation via its arterial supply; in this situation it acts as a "filter in parallel." The hepatic phagocytes render antigens nonimmunogenic, whereas splenic and lymph node–derived macrophages enhance immunogenicity.[98] Thus the distribution of antigens between liver and spleen (and other lymphoid organs) will influence the magnitude of the immune response (i.e., diversion of antigen from liver to spleen enhances the immune response).[98] Changes in the phagocytic function of the liver affect both portal and systemic routes of immunization.[112]

Immune complexes are cleared from the portal and systemic blood by the hepatic sinusoidal phagocytes. Large complexes that fix complement are avidly cleared by the liver, whereas smaller complexes, which do not fix complement, are cleared by the spleen.[115] In hepatic cirrhosis, these functions are impaired and complexes accumulate in the plasma.[114] In most cases, these complexes do not result in significant activation of C3 and do not cause tissue damage. The composition of such complexes is unknown, but it is probable that many contain antigens derived from food and bacteria in the gut.

Endotoxins are phagocytosed and detoxified by the liver. In normal subjects they can be demonstrated in portal blood but not in systemic blood.[116] Systemic endotoxemia has been demonstrated during fulminant hepatic failure and in some subjects with established cirrhosis, presumably as a result of impaired hepatic clearance of this substance.[117, 118]

HUMORAL IMMUNITY

The altered processing of antigen in patients with hepatic cirrhosis has a significant effect on the humoral immune response.[98, 113, 119] This is seen most clearly in the response to putative thymus-independent antigens,[99, 113, 120] which are not influenced by the changes in cell-mediated immunity that accompany the development of chronic liver disease. It is probable that the increased titers of antibodies to *E. Coli* found in patients with alcohol-induced cirrhosis, chronic active liver disease, and PBC are the result of this phenomenon.[99, 120, 121]

The response to thymus-dependent antigens is more complex, involving the cooperation not only of antigen-presenting cells and B lymphocytes but also of T lymphocytes. When patients with alcohol-induced cirrhosis, chronic active liver disease, or PBC were immunized intravenously with the bacteriphage ϕX174 (a thymus-dependent antigen), the primary and secondary responses were significantly decreased compared with the responses of normal subjects.[60] In the presence of increased responses to thymus-independent antigens, this implies that the cooperating functions of T cells are reduced, so that B cells challenged with thymus-dependent antigens cannot respond to the increased antigenic stimulus.

In addition to the quantitative changes in the humoral response of patients with hepatic cirrhosis, there are qualitative changes. In normal subjects, during a secondary response more than 90 per cent of the antibody is IgG; however, in patients with PBC, CAH, or alcohol-induced cirrhosis, the percentage of IgM antibody is greatly increased.[60] This relative failure to change from IgM to IgG antibody production during the evolution of the immune response is compatible with a defect in T-cell switching function.

The relation of the increased titers of viral antibodies, which have been described in chronic liver disease, to altered mononuclear phagocytic function is not clear.[122–126] Small increases in titers to lipoprotein-coated viruses such as herpes simplex, cytomegalovirus, influenza A, rubella, and measles in patients with HBsAg-positive CAH, alcohol-induced cirrhosis, and PBC are probably due to changes in hepatic phagocytic function.[124] There is a sixfold increase in titers to measles and rubella virus in patients with lupoid chronic active liver disease, which is peculiar to this disease.[124] Defects in the early classic pathway of complement activation have been described in this disease.[127]

The cumulative effect of these increased humoral responses is readily seen in the hypergammaglobulinemia that accompanies any form of experimental[83, 87] or naturally occurring chronic liver disease.[83, 87, 118, 128]

CELL-MEDIATED IMMUNITY

The incidence of positive delayed hypersensitivity skin tests to common bacterial and viral antigens is decreased in patients with alcohol-related liver disease, CAH, and PBC. This occurrence in all types of liver disease suggests that it is in part secondary to chronic liver disease.

The delayed hypersensitivity response involves the cooperation of macrophages and T cells in the presence of various serum factors that may enhance or inhibit the response. The afferent limb of the system, whereby cells become sensitized to the antigens concerned, has not been evaluated in patients with chronic liver disease because of the limitations of available test systems. The effectiveness of the efferent limb requires that T lymphocytes are present in adequate concentrations, are sensitized to and recognize the antigen under test, and are capable of producing lymphokine mediators of the delayed hypersensitivity reaction. The concentration of T lymphocytes in blood, measured by rosetting techniques, is diminished in HBsAg-positive and HBsAg-negative chronic active liver disease, alcohol-related liver disease, or PBC.[101, 129–132] The presence of plasma or serum inhibitors of T-lymphocyte function also may contribute to the anergy in patients with chronic liver disease. Serum factors that inhibit mitogen transformation of lymphocytes have been demonstrated in patients with PBC or alcohol-induced liver disease as well as in an animal model of hepatic cirrhosis.[76, 102, 103] Increased macrophage suppressor cell activity, which is dependent on the level of antigenic stimulation, has also been described in animals with cirrhosis.[103] Although the humoral and cellular inhibitors of T-lymphocyte function are readily demonstrated in vitro, their functional importance in vivo remains uncertain. Many of the inhibitors appear to be common to several types of liver disease and therefore are probably a reflection of the altered metabolic state in these conditions.

IMMUNOLOGICALLY ACTIVE PLASMA PROTEINS

The liver is the major site of synthesis for many plasma proteins, some of which have either a regulatory or effector role in the immune response.

Alpha-fetoprotein. Alpha-fetoprotein (AFP) is produced by the entodermal cells of the foregut, particularly the liver. It is present in high concentrations in the plasma of the fetus and mother. Within a few hours after birth, the concentration starts to fall; by one year of age, adult levels are attained (10 to 20 ng/ml). The immunosuppressant properties of AFP have been shown to be dependent on the induction of a suppressor cell.[133–135] The presence of sialic acid residues on the protein appears to be essential for these biologic effects. Recently, however, other investigators have failed to confirm these observations.[136]

Alpha Globulins. Alpha globulins are a complex group of proteins produced by the liver that have immunoregulatory properties.[137, 138] Pregnancy-associated alpha globulin inhibits T-cell functions.[139, 140] Alpha globulin is increased in pregnancy, but is also increased in patients with chronic liver disease and with cancer. An important inhibitor of both the complement and coagulation systems is α_2 macroglobulin.[141] It has been suggested that α_2 macroglobulin has immunoregulatory properties in relation to K-cell function.[137] Increased concentrations are found in patients with PBC and HBsAg-negative CAH.[142]

Complement Components. These components are produced by either mononuclear phagocytes or hepatocytes. Levels often are reduced in patients with acute or chronic liver disease.[143]

REFERENCES

1. Review of antigen-presenting cells. Immunobiology 16:345, 1984.
2. Taussig MJ. Antigen specific T-cell factors. Immunology 41:759, 1980.
3. Interleukins and lymphocyte activation. In: Muller G, ed. Immunological Reviews, No. 63. Copenhagen, Munksgaard, 1982:1.
4. Doherty PC, Zinkernagel RM. A biological role for major histocompatibility antigens. Lancet 1:1406, 1975.

5. Todd I, Pujol-Borrel R, Hammond LJ, et al. Interferon gamma induces HLA-Dr expression by thyroid epithelium. Clin Exp Immunol 61:265, 1985.
6. Londei M, Lamb JR, Bottazzo GF, et al. Cells expressing aberrant MHC class II-determinants can present antigen to clonal human T-cells. Nature 312:639, 1984.
7. James SP, Elson CO, Jones EA, et al. Abnormal regulation of immunoglobulin synthesis in vitro in primary biliary cirrhosis. Gastroenterology 79:242, 1980.
8. Nouri-Aria KT, Hegarty JE, Alexander GJM, et al. Effect of corticosteroids on suppressor cell activity in autoimmune and viral chronic active hepatitis. N Engl J Med 307:1300, 1982.
9. Hodgson HJ, Wands JR, Isselbacher KJ. Alteration in suppressor cell activity in active chronic hepatitis. Proc Nat Acad Sci (USA) 75:1549, 1978.
10. Reinherz EL, Rubinstein A, Seha RS, et al. Abnormalities of immunoregulatory T-cells in disorders of immune function. N Engl J Med 301:1018, 1979.
11. Reinherz EL, Scholssman SF. Regulation of the immune response: Inducer and suppressor T lymphocyte subsets in human beings. N Engl J Med 303:370, 1980.
12. Thomas HC, Brown D, LaBrooy J, et al. T-cell subsets in autoimmune and HBV-induced chronic liver disease: A review of the abnormalities and the effects of treatment. Liver 2:266, 1982.
13. Bach MA, Bach JF. Imbalance in T-cell subsets in human diseases. Int J Immunopharmacol 3:269, 1981.
14. Bach MA, Bach JF. The use of monoclonal anti-T-cell antibodies to study T-cell imbalances in human diseases. Clin Exp Immunol 45:449, 1981.
15. Jensen DM, McFarlane IG, Portmann BS, et al. Detection of antibodies directed against a liver-specific membrane lipoprotein in patients with acute and chronic active hepatitis. N Engl J Med 229:1, 1978.
16. Meyer zum Buchenfelde KH, Miescher PA. Liver specific antigens: Purification and characterisation. Clin Exp Immunol 10:89, 1972.
17. Thestrup-Peterson K, Ladefoged K, Andersen L. Lymphocyte transformation test with liver specific protein and phytohaemagglutinin in patients with liver disease. Clin Exp Immunol 24:1, 1976.
18. McFarlane IG, Wojcictea BM, Zucker GM, Eddleston ALWF. Purification and characterisation of human LSP. Clin Exp Immunol 27:381, 1977.
19. Hopf U, Meyer zum Buschenfelde KH, Arnold W. Detection of a liver membrane autoantibody in HBs antigen negative CAH. N Engl J Med 294:578, 1976.
20. Thomas HC, Montano L, Goodall A, et al. Immunological mechanisms in chronic hepatitis B infection. Hepatology 2:1162S, 1982.
21. Wiedmann KH, Bartholomew TC, Brown DJC, et al. Liver membrane antibodies detected by immunoradiometricassay in acute and chronic virus induced and autoimmune liver disease. Hepatology 4:199, 1984.
22. Wiedmann KH, Trejdosiewicz LK, Goodall AH, et al. An analysis of the antigenic composition of liver specific lipoprotein (LSP) using murine monoclonal antibodies. Gut 26:510, 1985.
23. Wiedmann KH, Thomas HC. Microsomal antigens in liver specific lipoprotein complex (LSP): Characterisation by monoclonal antibodies. (In press.)
24. Mieli-Vergani G, Eddleston ALWF. Autoimmunity to liver membrane antigens in acute and chronic hepatitis. Clin Immunol Allergy 1:181, 1981.
25. Montano L, Arnaguibel F, Boffill M, et al. An analysis of the composition of the inflammatory infiltrate in autoimmune and hepatitis B virus–induced chronic liver disease. Hepatology 3:292, 1983.
26. Bardadin KA, Desmet VJ. Interdigitating and dendritic reticulum cells in chronic active hepatitis. Histopathology 8:657, 1984.
27. Potter BJ, Elias E, Thomas HC, Sherlock S. Complement metabolism in chronic liver disease: Catabolism of C1q in chronic active liver disease and primary biliary cirrhosis. Gastroenterology 78:1034, 1980.
28. Thomas HC, Potter BJ, Elias E, et al. Metabolism of the third component of complement in acute type B hepatitis, HBs antigen positive glomerulonephritis, polyarteritis nodosum and HBs antigen positive CALD. Gastroenterology 76:673, 1979.
29. Munoz LE, deVilliers D, Markham D, et al. Complement activation in chronic liver disease. Clin Exp Immunol 47:548, 1982.
30. Eggink HF, Houthoff HJ, Huitema S, et al. Cellular and humoral immune reactions in chronic active liver disease II. Lymphocytes subsets and viral antigens in the liver of patients with acute or chronic HBV. Clin Exp Immunol 56:121, 1984.
31. Pignatelli M, Waters J, Brown D, et al. HLA class I antigens on the hepatocyte membrane during recovery from acute hepatitis B virus infection and during interferon therapy in chronic HBV infection. Hepatology 6:349, 1986.

32. Naumov NV, Mondelli M, Alexander GJM, et al. Relationship between expression of hepatitis B virus antigens in isolated hepatocytes and autologous lymphocyte cytotoxicity in patients with chronic hepatitis B virus infection. Hepatology 4:63, 1984.
33. Mondelli M, Mieli-Vergani G, Alberto A, et al. Specificity of T-lymphocyte cytotoxicity to autologous hepatocytes in chronic hepatitis B virus infection: Evidence that T-cells are directed against HBV core antigen expressed on hepatocytes. J Immunol 129:2773, 1982.
34. Pignatelli M, Waters J, Lever A, et al. Cytotoxic T-cell responses to the nucleocapsid proteins of HBV in chronic hepatitis: Evidence that antibody modulation causes protracted infection. J Hepatol 4:15, 1987.
35. Salfeld J, Pfaff E, Noah M, et al. Antigenic determinants and functional domains in HBc antigen and HBe antigen from HBV. J Virol. (In press.)
36. Ferrari C, Amalia P, Sansoni P, et al. Selective sensitisation of peripheral blood T-lymphocytes to hepatitis B core antigen in patients with chronic active hepatitis type B. Clin Exp Immunol 67:497, 1986.
36a. Milich DR, McLachlan A, Stahl S, et al. Comparative immunogenicity of hepatitis B virus core and e antigens. J Immunol 141:3617, 1988.
37. Waters J, Pignatelli M, Galpin S, et al. Viral neutralising antibodies to hepatitis B virus: the nature of an important immunogenic epitope on the S gene peptide. J Gen Virol 67:2457, 1986.
38. Ikeda T, Pignatelli M, Lever AML, et al. Relationship of HLA protein display to activation of 2-5A synthetase in HBe antigen or anti-HBe–positive chronic HBV infection. Gut 27:1498, 1986.
39. Montano L, Miescher GC, Goodall AH, et al. Hepatitis B virus and HLA antigen display in the liver during chronic hepatitis B infection. Hepatology 2:557, 1982.
40. Onji M, Lever AML, Thomas HC. Transfection of HBV into cell lines reduces their responsiveness to interferon. Hepatology 9:92, 1989.
41. Thomas HC, Pignatelli M, Lever AML. Homology between HBV-DNA and a sequence regulating the interferon induced antiviral system: a possible mechanism of persistent infection. J Med Virol 19(1):63, 1986.
41a. Ikeda I, Lever AML, Thomas HC. Evidence for a defective production of interferon in chronic HBV carriers. Hepatology 6:962, 1986.
42. Thomas HC, Scully LJ. Antiviral therapy in chronic hepatitis B virus infection. Br Med Bull 41:374, 1985.
43. Nair MPN, Shwartz SA, Memon M. Decreased natural and antibody dependent cellular cytotoxicity is associated with decreased production of natural killer cytotoxic factors and interferon in neonates. Pediatr Res 19(4) (Pt 2; abstr 1011):297a, 1985.
44. Kuhls TL, Pineda E, Garratty E. Deficient immune interferon production by lectin induced leukocytes due to the absence of a macrophage derived soluble mediator. Pediatr Res 20(4) (Pt 2; abstr 1384):391a, 1986.
45. Abo T, Miller CA, Gartland L, Balch CM. Differentiation stages of human natural killer cells in lymphoid tissues from foetal to adult life. J Exp Med 157:273, 1983.
46. Kaplan J, Shope TC, Bollinger RO, et al. Human newborns are deficient in natural killer activity. J Clin Immunol 2(4):350, 1982.
47. Bryson YJ, Winter HS, Gard SE. Deficiency of immune interferon production by lymphocytes of normal newborns. Cell Immunol 55:191, 1980.
48. Uksila J, Lassila O, Hirvonen T, et al. Development of natural killer function in the human foetus. J Immunol 130:153, 1983.
49. Uksila J, Lassila O, Hirvonen T. Natural killer cell function of human neonatal lymphocytes. Clin Exp Immunol 48:649, 1982.
50. Scheuer PJ. Biliary disease and cholestasis. In Scheuer PJ, ed. Liver Biopsy Interpretation, 3rd ed. London, Ballière Tindall, 1985.
51. Sherlock S, Scheuer PJ. The presentation and diagnosis of 100 patients with primary biliary cirrhosis. N Engl J Med 289:674, 1973.
52. Golding PL, Smith M, Williams R. Multisystem involvement in chronic liver disease. Am J Med 55:772, 1973.
53. Golding PL, Smith M, Williams R. Sicca complex in liver disease. Br Med J 4:340, 1970.
54. Walker JG, Doniach D, Roitt IM. Serological tests in diagnosis of primary biliary cirrhosis. Lancet 1:827, 1965.
55. Shapiro JM, Smith H, Schaffner F. Serum bilirubin: a prognostic factor in primary biliary cirrhosis. Gut 20:137, 1979.
56. Thomas HC. T-cell subsets in patients with acute and chronic HBV infection, primary biliary cirrhosis, and alcohol-induced liver disease. J Immunopharmacol 3:301, 1981.
57. James SP, Elson CO, Jones EA, et al. Abnormal regulation of immunoglobulin synthesis in vitro in primary biliary cirrhosis. Gastroenterology 79:242, 1980.
58. Epstein O, Thomas HC, Sherlock S. Primary biliary cirrhosis is a dry

gland syndrome with features of chronic graft-versus-host disease. Lancet 1:1166, 1980.

59. Fakunle YM, Aranguibel F, de Villiers D, et al. Monometric (7S) IgM in chronic liver disease. Clin Exp Immunol 38:204, 1979.

60. Thomas HC, Holden R, Verner-Jones J, et al. Immune response to X174 in man. 5. Primary and secondary antibody production in primary biliary cirrhosis. Gut 16:836, 1976.

61. Doniach D, Roitt IM, Walker JG, et al. Tissue antibodies in primary biliary cirrhosis, active chronic (lupoid) hepatitis, cryptogenic cirrhosis, and other liver diseases and their clinical implications. Clin Exp Immunol 1:237, 1966.

62. Baum H, Berg PA. The complex nature of mitochondrial antibodies and their relationship to primary biliary cirrhosis. Semin Liver Dis 1(4):309, 1981.

63. Munoz LE, Doniach D, Scheuer PJ, et al. Is mitochondrial antibody diagnostic of primary biliary cirrhosis? Gut 22:136, 1981.

64. Whaley K, Webb J, McAvoy BA, et al. Sjögren's syndrome. 2. Clinical associations and immunological phenomena. Q J Med 42:513, 1973.

65. Whittingham S. Immunofluorescence reactions in patients with prolonged extrahepatic biliary obstruction. Gastroenterology 66:169, 1974.

66. Berg PA, Doniach D, Roitt IM. Mitochondrial antibodies in primary biliary cirrhosis. I. Localisation of the antigen to mitochondrial membranes. J Exp Med 126:277, 1967.

67. Berg PA, Sayers T, Wiedmann KH, et al. Serological classification of chronic cholestatic liver disease by the use of two different types of antimitochondrial antibodies. Lancet 2:1329, 1980.

68. Labro MT, Andrieu MC, Weber M, et al. A new pattern of non-organ and non-species–specific anti-organelle antibody detected by immunofluorescence: the mitochondrial antibody number 5. Clin Exp Immunol 31:357, 1978.

68a. Frazer IH, MacKay IR, Jordan S, et al. Reactivity of anti-mitochondrial antibodies in PBC: definition of two novel mitochondrial polypeptide autoantigens. J Immunol 135:1739, 1985.

68b. Gershwin ME, MacKay IR, Sturgess A, et al. Identification and specificity of a cDNA encoding the 70-kd mitochondrial antigen recognized in PBC. J Immunol 138:3525, 1987.

68c. Yeoman SJ, Fussey SPM, Donner DJ, et al. Primary biliary cirrhosis: identification of two major M2 mitochondrial autoantigens. Lancet 1:1067, 1988.

69. Thomas HC, de Villiers D, Potter BJ, et al. Immune complexes in acute and chronic liver disease. Clin Exp Immunol 31:150, 1978.

70. Wands JR, Dienstag JL, Bhan AT, et al. Circulating immune complexes and complement activation in primary biliary cirrhosis. N Engl J Med 298:233, 1978.

71. Potter BJ, Elias E, Jones EA. Hypercatabolism of the third component of complement in patients with primary biliary cirrhosis. J Lab Clin Med 88:427, 1976.

72. Jones EA, Frank MM, Jaffe CJ. Primary biliary cirrhosis and the complement system. Ann Intern Med 90:72, 1979.

73. Minuti GY, Jones EA. IgM anti-complement receptor antibodies in serum of patients with primary biliary cirrhosis. Abstract No. 212, American Association for Study of Liver Disease, Hepatology, p 725, 1982.

74. Thomas HC, Potter BJ, Sherlock S. Is primary biliary cirrhosis an immune complex disease? Lancet 2:1261, 1977.

75. Fox RA, Scheuer PJ, James DG, et al. Impaired delayed hypersensitivity in primary biliary cirrhosis. Lancet 1:959, 1969.

76. MacSween RNM, Thomas MA. Lymphocyte transformation by phytohaemagglutinin (PHA) and purified protein derivative (PPD) in primary biliary cirrhosis: Evidence of serum inhibitory factors. Clin Exp Immunol 15:523, 1973.

77. Owen JS. Plasma lipoproteins and the regulation of cellular function. In: Reid E, Cook GMW, Morre DJ, eds. Investigation of Membrane-Located Receptors. New York, Plenum Press, 1984:311.

78. Owen JS, Brown D, Chu P, et al. The effect of high-density lipoprotein from patients with liver disease on erythrocyte morphology and lymphocyte transformation. Gastroenterology 79:1118, 1980.

79. Epstein O, Jain S, Lee R, et al. D-Penicillamine treatment improves survival in primary biliary cirrhosis. Lancet 1:1275, 1984.

80. Routhier G, Goldstein G, Tidman N, et al. Effects of cyclosporin A on suppressor and inducer T-lymphocytes in primary biliary cirrhosis. Lancet 2:1223, 1980.

82. Leevy CM, Chen T, Luisada-Opper A, et al. Liver disease of the alcoholic: the role of immunologic abnormalities in pathogenesis, recognition, and treatment. Prog Liver Dis 5:516, 1976.

83. Leevy CM, Chen T, Zetterman R. Alcoholic hepatitis, cirrhosis and immunologic reactivity. Ann NY Acad Sci 252:106, 1975.

84. Bailey RJ, Krasner N, Eddleston ALWF, et al. Histocompatibility antigens, autoantibodies and immunoglobulins in alcoholic liver disease. Br Med J 2:727, 1976.

85. Morgan MY, Ross MGR, Ng CM, et al. HLA-B8 viral antibodies,

86. Bell H, Nordhagen R. Association between HLA-BW40 and alcoholic liver disease with cirrhosis. Br Med J 1:822, 1978.

87. Bell H, Nordhagen R. HLA antigens in alcoholics with special reference to alcoholic cirrhosis. Scand J Gastroenterol 15:453, 1980.

88. Melendez M, Vargas-Tank L, Fuentes C, et al. Distribution of HLA compatibility antigens, ABO groups and Rh antigens in alcoholic liver disease. Gut 20:288, 1979.

89. Scott BB, Rajah SM, Losowsky MS. Histocompatibility antigens in chronic liver disease. Gastroenterology 72:122, 1972.

90. Simon M, Bourel M, Genetet B, et al. Idiopathic hemochromatics and iron overload in alcoholic liver disease: Differentiation by HCA phenotype. Gastroenterology 73:655, 1977.

91. Mihas AA, Bull DM, Davidson CS. Cell-mediated immunity to liver in patients with alcoholic hepatitis. Lancet 1:951, 1975.

92. Kakumu S, Leevy CM. Lymphocyte cytotoxicity in alcoholic hepatitis. Gastroenterology 72:594, 1977.

93. MacSween RN, Anthony RS, Farquharson M. Liver antibodies in alcohol-related liver disease and antibodies to alcohol-altered hepatocytes. Lancet 2:803, 1981.

94. Sanchez-Tapias J, Thomas HC, Sherlock S. Lymphocyte populations in liver biopsy specimens from patients with chronic liver disease. Gut 18:472, 1977.

95. Kanagasundaram N, Kakumu S, Chen T, et al. Alcoholic hyalin antigen (AHAg) and antibody (AHAb) in alcoholic hepatitis. Gastroenterology 73:1368, 1977.

96. French SW, Sim JS, Franks KE, et al. Alcoholic hepatitis. In: Fisher MM, Rankin JG, eds. Alcohol and the Liver. New York, Plenum, 1977:261.

97. Hauptman S, Tomasi TB. Antibodies to human albumin in cirrhosis sera. J Clin Invest 54:122, 1974.

98. Thomas HC, McSween RNM, White RG. The role of the liver in controlling the immunogenicity of commensal bacteria in the gut. Lancet 1:1288, 1973.

99. Simjee AE, Hamilton-Miller JMT, Thomas HC, et al. Antibodies to Escherichia coli in chronic liver diseases. Gut 16:871, 1975.

100. Rutenberg AM, Sonnenblick E, Koven I, et al. The role of intestinal bacteria in the development of dietary cirrhosis in rats. J Exp Med 106:1, 1957.

101. Berenyi MR, Straus B, Cruz D. In vitro and in vivo studies of cellular immunity in alcoholic cirrhosis. Am J Dig Dis 19:199, 1974.

102. Hsu CCS, Leevy CM. Inhibition of PHA-stimulated lymphocyte transformation by plasma from patients with advanced cirrhosis. Clin Exp Immunol 8:749, 1971.

103. Thomas HC, Singer CRJ, Tilney NL, et al. The immune response in cirrhotic rats: Antigen distribution, humoral immunity, cell-mediated immunity, and splenic suppressor cell activity. Clin Exp Immunol 26:574, 1976.

104. Blitzer BL, Mutchnick MG, Joshi PH, et al. Adrenocorticosteroid therapy in alcoholic hepatitis: A prospective, double-blind randomized study. Am J Dig Dis 22:477, 1977.

105. Campra JL, Hamlin EM, Kirshbaum RJ, et al. Prednisone therapy of acute alcoholic hepatitis. Ann Intern Med 79:625, 1973.

106. Helman RA, Temko MH, Nye SW, et al. Alcoholic hepatitis: natural history and evaluation of prednisolone therapy. Ann Intern Med 74:311, 1971.

107. Maddrey WC, Boitnott JK, Bedine MS, et al. Corticosteroid therapy of alcoholic hepatitis. Gastroenterology 75:193, 1978.

108. Rennick RH, Iber FL. Progress report: Treatment of acute alcoholic hepatitis. Gut 13:68, 1972.

109. Schlichting P, Juhl E, Poulsen H, et al. Alcoholic hepatitis superimposed on cirrhosis: Clinical significance and effect of long-term prednisone treatment. Scand J Gastroenterol 11:305, 1976.

110. Shumaker JB, Resnick RH, Galambos JT, et al. A controlled trial of 6-methyl-prednisolone in acute alcoholic hepatitis. With a note on published results in encephalopathic patients. Am J Gastroenterol 69:443, 1978.

111. Feizi T. Immunoglobulins in chronic liver disease. Gut 9:193, 1968.

112. Thomas HC. The role of the liver in immunological disease. Proc Roy Soc Med (Lond) 70:521, 1977.

113. Triger DR, Alp MH, Wright R. Bacterial and dietary antibodies in liver disease. Lancet 1:60, 1972.

114. Thomas HC, Vaez-Zadeh F. A homeostatic mechanism for the removal of antigen from the portal circulation. Immunology 26:375, 1974.

115. Mannik M, Arend WP. Fate of preformed immune complexes in rabbits and rhesus monkeys. J Exp Med 134:19s, 1971.

116. Braude AI, Carey FJ, Zalesky M. Studies with radioactive endotoxin, II. Correlation of physiological effects with distribution of radioactivity in rabbits injected with lethal doses of E. Coli endotoxin labeled with radioactive sodium chromate. J Clin Invest 34:858, 1955.

117. Wilkinson SP, Arroyo VA, Moodie H, et al. Abnormalities of sodium

excretion and other disorders of renal function in fulminant hepatic failure. Gut 17:501, 1976.

118. Liehr H, Grun M, Brunswig D, et al. Endotoxaemia in liver cirrhosis, treatment with polymyxin B. Lancet 1:810, 1975.

119. Souhami RL. The effect of colloidal carbon on the organ distribution of sheep red blood cells and the immune response. Immunology 22:685, 1972.

120. Bjorneboe M, Prytz H, Orskov F. Antibodies to intestinal microbes in serum of patients with cirrhosis of the liver. Lancet 1:58, 1972.

121. Triger DR. Bacterial, viral and autoantibodies in acute and chronic liver disease. Ann Clin Res 8:174, 1976.

122. Closs O, Haukenes G, Blomhoff JP, et al. High titers of antibodies against rubella and morbilli virus in patients with chronic hepatitis. Scand J Gastroenterol 8:523, 1973.

123. Closs O, Hawkenes G, Gjone E, et al. Raised antibody titers in chronic liver disease. Lancet 2:1202, 1971.

124. Crimmins FB, Adams D, Ross M, et al. Viral antibody titers in HBs antigen–positive and negative chronic active hepatitis. Scand J Gastroenterol 15:107, 1980.

125. Thomas HC, Grimmonds F, Sherlock S. Measles, rubella and lymphocyte antibodies in chronic active hepatitis. Clin Sci Med 49:27, 1975.

126. Triger DR, MacCallum FO, Kurtz JB, et al. Raised antibody titers to measles and rubella viruses in chronic active hepatitis. Lancet 1:665, 1972.

127. Munoz LE, DeVilliers D, Markham D, et al. Complement activation in chronic liver disease. Clin Exp Immunol 47:548, 1982.

128. Bjorneboe M, Jensen KB, Scheibel I, et al. Tetanus anti-toxin production and gamma globulin levels in patients with cirrhosis of the liver. Acta Med Scand 188:541, 1970.

129. Colombo M, Vernace SJ, Paronetto F. T and B lymphocytes in patients with chronic active hepatitis (CAH). Clin Exp Immunol 30:4, 1977.

130. De Horatius RJ, Strickland RG, Williams RC. T and B lymphocytes in acute and chronic hepatitis. Clin Immunol Immunopathol 2:353, 1974.

131. Bernstein IM, Williams RC, Webster KH, et al. Reduction in circulat-

ing T lymphocytes in alcoholic liver disease. Lancet 2:488, 1974.

132. Thomas HC, Freni M, Sanchez-Tapias J, et al. Peripheral blood lymphocyte populations in chronic liver disease. Clin Exp Immunol 26:222, 1976.

133. Murgita RA, Tomasi TB. Suppression of the immune response by alpha-fetoprotein, II. The effect of mouse alpha-fetoprotein on mixed lymphocyte reactivity and mitogen-induced lymphocyte transformation. J Exp Med 141:440, 1975.

134. Murgita RA, Tomasi TB. Suppression of the immune response by alpha-fetoprotein, I. The effect of mouse alpha-fetoprotein on the primary and secondary antibody response. J Exp Med 141:269, 1975.

135. Murgita RA, Goidl EA, Kontiainen S, et al. Alpha-fetoprotein induces suppressor T-cells in vitro. Nature 267:257, 1977.

136. Littman BM, Alpert E, Rocklin RE. The effect of purified alpha-fetoprotein on in vitro assays of cell-mediated immunity. Cell Immunol 30:35, 1977.

137. Calder EA, Urbaniak SJ, Irvine WJ, et al. The effect of alpha$_2$-macroglobulin on K-cell cytolysis and T and B-cell rosette formation. Immunology 22:112, 1975.

138. Cooperband SR, Badger AM, Davis RC, et al. The effect of immunoregulatory globulin (IRA) upon lymphocytes in vitro. J Immunol 109:154, 1972.

139. Stimson WH. Studies on the immunosuppressive properties of a pregnancy-associated macroglobulin. Clin Exp Immunol 25:199, 1976.

140. Stimson WH. Variations in the level of a pregnancy-associated macroglobulin in patients with cancer. J Clin Pathol 28:868, 1975.

141. In Steinbuch M, Audran R, Fritz H, et al, eds. Biology and Pathology of Plasma Proteinase Inhibitors. Proceedings of the 2nd International Research Conference (5th Bayer Symposium) Berlin, Springer-Verlag, 1974:78.

142. MacSween RNM, Horne CHW, Moffat AJ, et al. Serum protein levels in primary biliary cirrhosis. J Clin Pathol 25:789, 1972.

143. Potter BJ, Elias E, Fayers PM, et al. Profiles of serum complement in patients with heptobiliary diseases. Digestion 18:371, 1978.

43

Hepatobiliary Complications of Ulcerative Colitis and Crohn's Disease

John M. Vierling, M.D

Extraintestinal complications of inflammatory bowel disease, including diseases of the liver and biliary tract, affect a large number of patients with ulcerative colitis or Crohn's disease.[1] Indeed, hepatobiliary complications may affect as many as 10 per cent of patients with inflammatory bowel disease. The occurrences of specific hepatobiliary diseases associated with inflammatory bowel disease (Table 43–1), however, vary widely; some disorders occur commonly and others rarely. The clinical significances of individual hepatobiliary disorders also vary, ranging from inconsequential to life-threatening. The purpose of this chapter is to review the spectrum, diagnosis, management, and concepts of pathogenesis of the hepatobiliary diseases associated with ulcerative colitis and Crohn's disease.

OVERVIEW AND CRITICAL COMMENTS

The association between ulcerative colitis and liver disease was first described in the late nineteenth century.[2, 3] The number of patients reported prior to 1950, however, was small and reflected the biases of autopsy studies. During this period, several studies of large numbers of patients with ulcerative colitis showed either no hepatobiliary complications[4, 5] or the infrequent occurrence of hepatic abscess,[6, 7] hepatitis,[8, 9] or cirrhosis.[9] Moreover, reviews of extraintestinal complications of inflammatory bowel disease tended to ignore hepatobiliary disorders.[4] It is understandable, therefore, that there was skepticism as to whether hepatobiliary diseases occurred in patients with inflamma-

TABLE 43–1. HEPATOBILIARY COMPLICATIONS OF ULCERATIVE COLITIS AND CROHN'S DISEASE

Diseases of the liver
    Pericholangitis
    Fatty liver
    Chronic hepatitis
    Fibrosis and cirrhosis
    Amyloidosis
    Hepatic granulomas
    Primary biliary cirrhosis
    α_1-Antitrypsin deficiency

Miscellaneous disorders
    Hepatic abscess
    Portal vein thrombosis
    Hepatic infarction
    Hepatic sinusoidal dilatation
    Hemosiderosis
    Sarcoidosis
    Benign neoplasia of bile ducts

Diseases of the biliary tract
    Primary sclerosing cholangitis
    Carcinoma of the biliary tract
    Cholelithiasis

tory bowel disease more frequently than could be expected by chance.[10]

From 1950 to the present, numerous reports have verified an association between inflammatory bowel disease and hepatobiliary complications. Such reports originally suggested that hepatobiliary disorders were more frequent in ulcerative colitis than in Crohn's disease. This misconception was due, in part, to the fact that patients with Crohn's disease mistakenly were reported as having ulcerative colitis[11] prior to the comprehensive description of the colitis of Crohn's disease in 1960.[12] In addition, there was little evidence initially that Crohn's disease of the small intestine was complicated by hepatobiliary disease. For example, early studies of selected patients with Crohn's disease of the small intestine either did not note hepatobiliary complications[13, 14] or found them infrequently.[15] Subsequent studies have shown that hepatobiliary complications occur in patients with Crohn's disease of the small intestine, colon, or intestine and colon.[16-23] It is now recognized, therefore, that hepatobiliary complications occur with comparable frequencies in male and female patients with ulcerative colitis and those with Crohn's disease,[11, 16, 20, 21] although certain differences in frequencies exist for specific complications (discussed later). The relationship between hepatobiliary complications and other extraintestinal complications in inflammatory bowel disease remains unclear.[1] Patients who have hepatobiliary complications of ulcerative colitis and Crohn's disease, however, commonly have other extraintestinal complications.[11, 20, 24]

In the absence of experimental animal models of inflammatory bowel disease, the reports of hepatobiliary complications have been purely descriptive. Furthermore, they have been published over a span of four decades in which substantial progress has occurred in the design and interpretation of human studies, the histologic classification of liver diseases, the techniques of cholangiography, and the use and interpretation of laboratory tests. Consequently, many of the published reports contain weaknesses that confront the critical reader interested in analyzing the subject. Several of these weaknesses deserve specific discussion in order to define the appropriate limitations of the published information and the extent to which valid conclusions can be made concerning the hepatobiliary complications of inflammatory bowel disease.

Since each of the disorders listed in Table 43–1 also occurs in patients without inflammatory bowel disease, it is important to define the relationship between inflammatory bowel disease and specific hepatobiliary diseases. To verify a true association between hepatobiliary disease and inflammatory bowel disease requires comparison of the prevalences and incidences of the hepatobiliary disease in patients with and without inflammatory bowel disease. Unfortunately, neither the prevalence nor the incidence of hepatobiliary complications in ulcerative colitis or Crohn's disease is known. The data from both retrospective and prospective studies do suggest, however, that hepatobiliary diseases occur more often in patients with inflammatory bowel disease than in the general population.[25, 38] The most common disorders currently recognized in practice are pericholangitis, primary sclerosing cholangitis, chronic hepatitis, and cryptogenic cirrhosis.[38]

Early estimates of prevalence were based on the frequency of abnormal values for alkaline phosphatase and sulfobromophthalein (Bromosulfophthalein [BSP]) retention. These tests were abnormal in 38 to 86 per cent of patients with ulcerative colitis[39-41] and in as many as 58 per cent of patients with Crohn's disease.[42] Subsequent studies showed that the frequency of histologic abnormalities of the liver could be either overestimated or underestimated on the basis of the results of liver tests. For example, Perrett and associates found that 45 of 300 patients with ulcerative colitis had abnormal results in one or more liver tests (aspartate aminotransferase [AST; GOT], alkaline phosphatase, and BSP retention).[11] However, biopsies of the livers of these 45 patients showed abnormalities in only 65 per cent. Thus, the finding of abnormal liver tests could overestimate the frequency of histologic liver disease in patients with ulcerative colitis[21, 39, 43, 44] and Crohn's disease.[15, 19-21] Conversely, liver biopsies performed in patients with normal liver tests have shown an appreciable frequency of histologic abnormalities in patients with ulcerative colitis[11, 21, 45, 46] or Crohn's disease.[15, 19, 20] In the study of patients with ulcerative colitis by Perrett and colleagues, 54 per cent of patients with normal liver tests had abnormal biopsy findings.[11] In the study of Crohn's disease by Dordal and co-workers, BSP retention was normal in 9 per cent of patients with cirrhosis, 24 per cent of patients with pericholangitis and 33 per cent of patients with fatty liver.[19] A recent retrospective study indicates that up to 55 per cent of patients with ulcerative colitis have abnormal liver tests, but in 30 per cent of this group the abnormalities are mild and transient.[33]

The findings just described suggest that calculation of the true prevalence and incidence of hepatobiliary complications requires a prospective histologic study of the livers of patients with inflammatory bowel disease. The results of studies using modern techniques of cholangiography in patients with inflammatory bowel disease also suggest that a prospective cholangiographic study would be necessary for diagnostic accuracy.[31, 32-38, 47-49] In the absence of such data, the term frequency is used in this chapter to discuss the hepatobiliary disorders associated with inflammatory bowel disease. This term represents the percentage of patients *specifically* evaluated for the presence of hepatobiliary disease who were found to have a particular lesion. Thus, frequency cannot be interpreted as an estimate of prevalence or incidence. It does avoid, however, the bias present in estimates of prevalence and incidence calculated as the percentage of patients with documented hepatobiliary disease among all patients with inflammatory bowel disease seen over extended periods of time.[11, 20, 21, 27, 50] The latter estimates are inaccurate because all patients with inflammatory bowel disease were not subjected to the same clinical, laboratory, or biopsy evaluations used to detect the presence of hepatobiliary disease.

Biases in the selection of patients, differences in the designs of the studies, and variability in the reporting of clinical details restrict our understanding of the hepatobiliary complications of inflammatory bowel disease. Biases in the selection of patients range from those inherent in autopsy and retrospective studies to those found in prospective studies of patients who have been preselected by virtue of their referral to an academic center. Marked differences in the designs of studies are common and often make comparison of results difficult. The designs of studies range from prospective evaluations of consecutive patients to retrospective reviews of the records of patients with overt, symptomatic hepatobiliary disease. The reporting of the clinical features of hepatobiliary diseases also varies, and sometimes it is impossible to match clinical features with a specific histologic diagnosis. In contrast, most studies describe the pertinent features of the inflammatory bowel disease, although older studies often do not subdivide patients with Crohn's disease on the basis of the anatomic site of involvement. Overall, the data suggest that the severity, duration, and extent of the inflammatory bowel disease correlate poorly with the type or severity of the hepatobiliary disease.[19, 23, 39, 42, 45, 46, 51–54] However, a recent retrospective study of 202 patients with ulcerative colitis indicates that pancolitis was significantly more frequent in patients with marked abnormalities in liver tests than in patients whose test results were normal or mildly abnormal.[33] Duration, unlike severity, was unrelated to liver test abnormalities.[33]

It is equally important to recognize the limitations imposed by the lack of precise definitions and diagnostic criteria for the hepatobiliary disorders associated with inflammatory bowel disease.[38] Many reports use diagnostic terms now discarded or terms without precise definitions.[55] The latter is particularly true of the term *pericholangitis*. Criteria for the diagnosis of hepatobiliary disease in the available reports often are incomplete, inconsistent, or not stated. Tests currently available to assess biochemical, serologic, virologic, and cholangiographic features of hepatobiliary diseases have been employed only in the most recent studies.[31–38, 49]

In the following section, individual hepatobiliary complications of inflammatory bowel disease are reviewed. In the text and accompanying tables, the effects of the factors just discussed are considered. Recognition of the limitations of our current knowledge may be useful in the design and execution of future studies in this area.

DISEASES OF THE LIVER

PERICHOLANGITIS

Prospective and retrospective studies have shown that patients with inflammatory bowel disease frequently have chronic inflammatory lesions of the portal tracts.[11, 16–23, 26, 28, 31–38, 43, 44, 46, 49, 56, 58] Such lesions represent the most common hepatobiliary abnormality in biopsy specimens from living patients with inflammatory bowel disease, although the exact prevalence of the disorder remains unknown. Table 43–2 summarizes the frequency and clinical features of these lesions in patients with inflammatory bowel disease reported in selected series. Currently, the appropriate terminology for these lesions remains controversial,[38, 51, 55, 59] and our knowledge of their natural history and prognosis remains incomplete. Recent reports of cholangiographic studies challenge the arbitrary concept that the process is primarily a disease of the liver[22, 23, 38, 51, 56, 59] rather than of the biliary tract by demonstrating the presence of sclerosing lesions of the bile ducts in at least a subpopulation of patients.[31–38, 48, 49, 59, 60]

Pathology

There is general agreement on the histologic features of the inflammatory hepatic lesion most frequently seen in patients with ulcerative colitis and Crohn's disease. Morphologically, it is characterized by infiltration of the portal tracts with lymphocytes, plasma cells, macrophages, up to 15 per cent neutrophils, and a variable but small number of eosinophils.[23, 28] The involved portal tracts are expanded and edematous. Proliferation of bile ductules often is present. Most often, the bile duct epithelium is normal, even in chronic lesions when periductular fibrosis is present.[45] In a minority of patients, however, the bile duct epithelium is conspicuously abnormal.[25, 34, 38, 59] An exception to this feature was found in the series reported by Mistilis, in which abnormalities of the bile ducts such as swelling, edema, inflammatory infiltration of the bile ductules, and occasional desquamation of the epithelium were common.[28] Although the term pericholangitis has been used most often to describe the portal inflammation, it may be inappropriate, since it implies that the bile duct is the focus of the inflammatory response. There is no definitive evidence to support this concept and some believe there is reason to doubt it.[21, 26, 56]

Within a single biopsy specimen, the intensity and distribution of inflammation may vary from one portal tract to another, making it impossible to determine the focus of inflammation. For this reason, histologic features referred to as "pericholangitis" by some investigators have been referred to by others as interlobular hepatitis, portal tract inflammation, portal triaditis, chronic periportal inflammation, increased cellularity of the portal tracts, and intrahepatic cholangiolitic hepatitis. These designations reflect a reluctance to ascribe the focus of inflammation to one specific element within the portal tract; instead they emphasize that the main characteristic of the inflammation is its diffuse and nonfocal nature. Still others eschew both the term pericholangitis and the concept that the inflammation is nonfocal. They believe instead that the inflammation focuses primarily on the portal veins (periphlebitis).[23, 26, 56] Mistilis, a proponent of the concept that the bile duct is the focus of the inflammatory infiltrate, acknowledges that inflammation of both the portal venules and lymphatics is a common feature of pericholangitis.[28] Inflammation of lymphatics complicates the interpretation of the significance of periductular inflammation, since the bile ducts are surrounded by the space of Mall, which is in continuity with the lymphatics (see Chapter 1).[61]

The problems of nomenclature are compounded further by features of pericholangitis that overlap the morphologic features of chronic persistent and chronic active hepatitis.[62] Indeed, many reported descriptions of pericholangitis in association with inflammatory bowel disease are indistinguishable from chronic persistent hepatitis. Some patients reported to have features of pericholangitis may have had chronic persistent hepatitis.[59] Alternately, piecemeal necrosis, suggestive of chronic active hepatitis, has

TABLE 43–2. PERICHOLANGITIS AND SYNONYMOUS LESIONS IN SELECTED SERIES OF PATIENTS WITH INFLAMMATORY BOWEL DISEASE

Series	Type of Inflammatory Bowel Disease*	No. of Patients with Liver Biopsy	Histologic Term	Frequency (%)	Features of Hepatic Disease Clinical	Features of Hepatic Disease Laboratory†	Comments
Kimmelstiel et al.[26]	UC	93	Interlobular hepatitis	10	—	—	Retrospective autopsy study excluding patients with defined cause for hepatic disease
Kleckner et al.[46]	UC	32	Chronic pericholangitis	19	Three patients asymptomatic, three patients jaundiced with hepatomegaly or splenomegaly	Normal ↑ AP and bili	Prospective study of patients undergoing percutaneous liver biopsy regardless of evidence suggesting hepatic disease
Boden et al.[43]	UC	10	Pericholangitis (with and without fibrosis)	70	Most jaundiced, some with episodes of "cholangitis," hepatomegaly, splenomegaly, portal venous hypertension	↑ AP	Retrospective study of patients with symptomatic liver disease
Ross et al.[50]	UC	17	Pericholangitis	29	—	—	Retrospective study, criteria for liver biopsy not stated; laboratory data not matched to histology
Eade[56]	UC	132	Inflammatory celllular infiltration	47	—	↑ AP, ↑ globulin, ↓ alb	Prospective study of 132 surgical liver biopsies in 138 consecutive patients undergoing colectomy; clinical and laboratory data not matched to histology
Palmer et al.[27]	UC	51	Cholangiolitic hepatitis	4	—	—	Retrospective autopsy study
Mistilis[28] Mistilis and Goulston[53]	UC	49 living 34 autopsy	Pericholangitis	49 24	Asymptomatic, cholestatic, and cholangitic forms Hepatomegaly common, splenomegaly rare; occasional portal venous hypertension	↑ AP, bili, abnormal BSP retention, ↑ choles	Liver biopsy study of 49 living patients selected because of symptoms, signs, or laboratory evidence of liver disease; concurrent study of 34 patients undergoing autopsy
Vinnik et al.[44]	UC	8	Pericholangitis	50	Asymptomatic	↑ AP. 5'-NT, ↑ AST, abnormal BSP retention in some patients	Prospective study of liver tests in 37 consecutive patients, liver biopsies in 5 of 10 with abnormal and 3 of 27 with normal liver tests
de Dombal et al.[57]	UC	58	Increased cellularity of portal tracts	83	—	—	Prospective study of surgical liver biopsies in 58 consecutive patients undergoing colectomy
Stauffer et al.[59]	UC	30	Portal triaditis	73	Jaundiced, rare pruritus; hepatosplenomegaly common; occasional portal venous hypertension	↑ AP, bili, AST: abnormal BSP retention; occasional ↑ choles, gammaglobulin	Retrospective study of liver biopsies in 30 patients with overt liver disease
Perrett et al.[11]	UC	50	Pericholangitis	30	—	↑ AP in some	Prospective study of 100 patients; liver biopsies performed in 50 patients; clinical and laboratory data not matched to histology
Chapin et al.[16]	CD of small bowel	39	Portal tract inflammation	36	—	—	Retrospective autopsy study
Palmer et al.[18]	CD of small bowel	8	Periportal infiltration	12	Asymptomatic	—	Retrospective autopsy study

Table continued on following page

TABLE 43–2. PERICHOLANGITIS AND SYNONYMOUS LESIONS IN SELECTED SERIES OF PATIENTS WITH INFLAMMATORY BOWEL DISEASE *Continued*

Series	Type of Inflammatory Bowel Disease*	No. of Patients with Liver Biopsy	Histologic Term	Frequency (%)	Features of Hepatic Disease — Clinical	Features of Hepatic Disease — Laboratory†	Comments
Cohen et al.[131]	CD of small bowel	19	Pericholangitis	80	None jaundiced	↑ AP, abnormal BSP retention	Prospective study employing percutaneous biopsy in the presence of abnormal liver tests or surgical biopsy during bowel resection; laboratory data not matched to histology
Kleckner[15]	CD of small bowel	20	Pericholangitis	0	Asymptomatic	Abnormal BSP retention in 1 patient	Prospective percutaneous biopsy study of 20 consecutive patients
Perrett et al.[20]	CD	39	Pericholangitis	21	—	↑ AP, ↑ ALT, abnormal BSP retention	Prospective study of 100 patients; liver biopsy performed in 39 patients
Eade et al.[20]	CD of small bowel, colon, or bowel and colon	49	Inflammatory cellular infiltration	46	—	—	Retrospective and prospective study of 100 patients; surgical liver biopsies performed during bowel resection in 49 patients; clinical and laboratory data not matched to histology
Eade et al.[22]	CD of colon	20	Inflammatory cellular infiltration	35	Asymptomatic; past medical history of jaundice in 4 patients	—	Prospective study of 20 surgical liver biopsies obtained in 21 consecutive colectomies for CD; laboratory data not matched to histology
Dordal et al.[19]	CD of small bowel or small bowel and colon	27	Pericholangitis	41	—	↑ AP, ↑ bili, ↑ AST, abnormal BSP retention	Retrospective study of surgical and percutaneous liver biopsies in 103 patients with inflammatory bowel disease; laboratory data not matched to histology
	UC	76	Pericholangitis	29			
Dew et al.[21]	CD	Approx 32	Portal triaditis	26	—	↑ AP	Retrospective and prospective study of 58 patients with UC and 43 patients with CD selected on the basis of ↑ AP; the number of liver biopsies is an approximation since only a small number of patients with a perioperative ↑ AP had biopsy
	UC	Approx 51	Portal triaditis	25	—	↑ AP	
Monto[17]	UC	100	Chronic periportal inflammation	17	—	—	Retrospective autopsy study
	CD of small bowel	4	Chronic periportal inflammation	75	—	—	Clinical and laboratory data not matched to histology
Perold et al.[34]	UC	10	Pericholangitis	10	Jaundice, cholangitis	↓ AP, Bili, ALT, AST, NT, ERCP	Prospective study of 20 consecutive patients; all 10 with abnormal liver tests were biopsied
Wee and Ludwig[38]	UC	107	Small-duct primary sclerosing cholangitis	35	—	↓ AP, AST	Retrospective study of histology; of 37 patients, primary sclerosing cholangitis was excluded in only 11
Ludwig et al.[59]	UC	19	—	68	—	↑ AP, AST	Retrospective study of patients without primary sclerosing cholangitis (PSC); emphasizes that histopathology was similar to that observed in PSC and that cirrhosis occurred in 42%

*UC = ulcerative colitis; CD = Crohn's disease.

†AP = alkaline phosphatase; bili = bilirubin; BSP = Bromsulphalein (sulfobromophthalein); ALT = alanine aminotransferase (SGPT); alb = albumin; AST = aspartate aminotransferase (SGOT); choles = cholesterol; 5′ NT = 5%-nucleotidase.

been present in biopsy specimens from some patients with pericholangitis.[26, 28] Inclusion of patients with conspicuous piecemeal necrosis and intralobular inflammation with hepatocellular necrosis under the term pericholangitis may be inappropriate, because these features do not typify the majority of patients diagnosed as having pericholangitis.[25] The issue is further complicated by unequivocal evidence that typical features of chronic active hepatitis occur in patients with primary sclerosing cholangitis[33, 35, 36–39, 59] and that the morphologic features of pericholangitis and primary sclerosing cholangitis are often indistinguishable.[59] Based on morphologic criteria, the term pericholangitis as a designation for a particular disease entity is untenable. Indeed, the recent classification of standardized nomenclature eliminates the term, prefering the definition chronic active hepatitis associated with inflammatory bowel disease.[62] Unfortunately, the absence of a suitable alternative term to distinguish early nonspecific inflammatory lesions and more chronic lesions from true chronic active hepatitis and primary sclerosing cholangitis necessitates an arbitrary choice of terms. For the purpose of discussion, the term pericholangitis is used in this chapter. It is important to remember, however, that this term may encompass a heterogeneous array of pathologic processes in patients with inflammatory bowel disease. Furthermore, it also should be noted that the term pericholangitis has been used to describe histologic features in patients with chronic obstruction of the extrahepatic biliary tract, pancreatitis, diverticulitis, typhoid fever, septicemia, chronic hepatitis, primary biliary cirrhosis, benign recurrent intrahepatic cholestasis, drug-induced hepatitis, and primary sclerosing cholangitis.[63]

Mistilis has defined and subdivided the histologic features of pericholangitis into three stages: acute, subacute, and chronic.[28] Progression through these stages has been documented in a small number of patients with inflammatory bowel disease and substantiates the view that pericholangitis can be a progressive lesion.[21, 28, 43, 45, 53, 58, 59, 64] The *acute* stage is characterized by inflammation of the portal tracts and proliferation of bile ducts, as already described (Fig. 43–1). In this stage, Mistilis also has found extension of the inflammatory infiltrate into the hepatic lobule and occasional desquamation of the bile duct epithelium resulting in the formation of an obstructing plug. Although bile ducts of all sizes may be involved, the most severe inflammation appears to surround the small to medium-sized interlobular ducts. Prominent dilatation and inflammation of lymphatic channels and portal venules also characterize this stage.

Changes characteristic of the *subacute* stage are an increase in connective tissue in the portal tracts, accumulation of hyaline-like material in the walls of bile ducts, and a decrease in the inflammatory infiltrates and edema seen in the acute stage. These changes often coexist in the same biopsy specimen with lesions that could be classified as either acute or chronic, thus emphasizing the patchy and overlapping nature of the process.

The *chronic* lesion is defined by the presence of concentric fibrosis surrounding the bile ducts, periportal fibrosis extending into the lobule in a stellate pattern, lymphangiectasia, and some phlebosclerosis (Fig. 43–2). Even Eade, who argues strongly against the use of the term pericholangitis, has noted the presence of circumductal fibrosis in his series.[22, 23, 56] Inflammatory infiltration of the portal tract is less intense in this stage, and inflammatory cells may breech the limiting plate with frank piecemeal necrosis. The concentric fibrosis around bile ducts appears to be characteristic of the chronic lesion in patients with inflam-

matory bowel disease and differentiates this process from chronic active hepatitis. The epithelium of the bile duct is generally normal and the ducts are not obliterated. Periductal and periportal fibrosis may be present in the absence of inflammation.[25] The distribution of such lesions may be patchy, and they may not be evident in small biopsy specimens.[39] In a minority of patients, pericholangitis progresses to cirrhosis.[11, 28, 46, 50, 52, 58, 59, 64]

As mentioned, the histologic features of pericholangitis have been reported to occur in a variety of other conditions, including primary diseases of the biliary tract. Most of the studies summarized in Table 43–2, however, did not evaluate the biliary tract. Only rarely have investigators specified that their criteria for the diagnosis of pericholangitis include a normal biliary tract.[26, 45, 59] Using modern techniques of cholangiography, the intra- and extra-hepatic portions of the biliary tract recently have been studied in patients with typical pericholangitis.[35, 36, 38, 41–43, 47–49, 59] These studies demonstrate sclerosing lesions of the biliary tract in a substantial proportion of patients with pericholangitis. Cholangiographic evidence of primary sclerosing cholangitis also has been found in other patients with inflammatory bowel disease, whose histologic diagnosis was pericholangitis.[31, 32, 35, 36, 38, 59, 65] Based on these findings, there is reason to doubt that pericholangitis is an entity separate from the spectrum of sclerosing cholangitis.[38, 59] (See Primary Sclerosing Cholangitis.)

Recent introduction by Wee and Ludwig of the term *primary sclerosing cholangitis of the small bile ducts* to replace the term *pericholangitis* reflects this view but remains controversial.[38, 59] In their retrospective study of 107 patients with ulcerative colitis and hepatobiliary disease, the term primary sclerosing cholangitis of the small bile ducts was applied to 37 patients whose disease was previously labeled pericholangitis but whose histopathologic features were similar to those of patients with classic primary sclerosing cholangitis involving the extrahepatic ducts.[38] Only 11 of the 37 patients had exclusion of large-duct sclerosis. Six of 18 patients who ultimately developed large-duct sclerosing cholangitis had biopsy evidence of small-duct disease 1 to 12 years earlier and negative *intravenous* cholangiograms 1 to 4 years earlier; this observation suggests (but does not prove) that small-duct disease may evolve into classic primary sclerosing cholangitis. Intravenous cholangiography is too insensitive a test, however, to exclude the possibility that these patients had early lesions of primary sclerosing cholangitis when the biopsies were performed. The finding that 10 of the 37 patients with small-duct disease had no evidence of primary sclerosing cholangitis 7 to 31 years after diagnosis clearly indicates that progression does not occur in all such patients. Further support for a relationship between pericholangitis and primary sclerosing cholangitis will require prospective study of patients serially evaluated by both liver biopsy and retrograde cholangiography. Histopathology alone cannot discriminate between the conditions.[35, 36, 38, 59, 65]

Recent studies have begun to clarify the relationship between the histopathological entity pericholangitis and the cholangiographic appearance of the intra- and extrahepatic bile ducts. Blackstone and Nemchausky performed endoscopic retrograde cholangiography in eight patients with ulcerative colitis complicated by pericholangitis.[48] Five of the eight were asymptomatic, two had pruritus for more than a year, and one was jaundiced. Lesions resembling sclerosing cholangitis were found in seven patients in whom the intra- and extrahepatic bile ducts were visualized. All seven patients had abnormalities of the intrahepatic ducts;

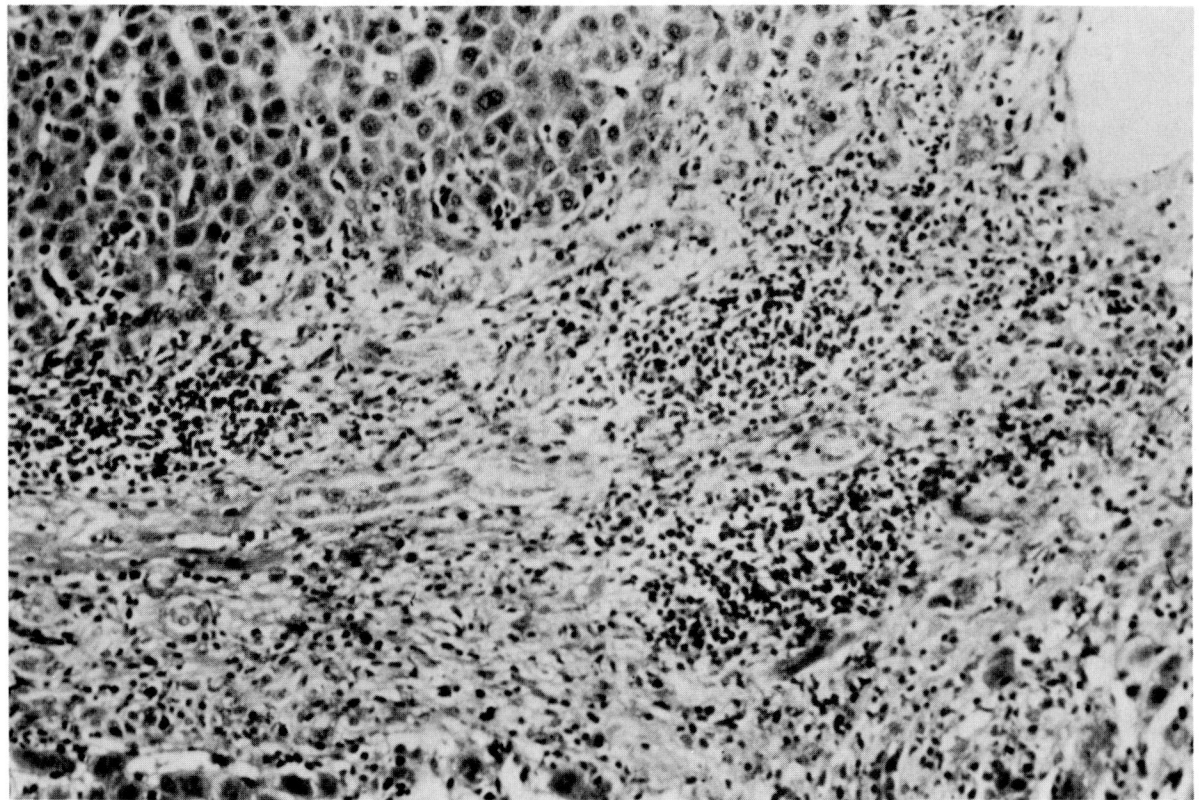

Figure 43–1. Acute pericholangitis in ulcerative colitis. Diffuse (nonfocal) chronic inflammation confined to the portal tract with bile ductular proliferation.

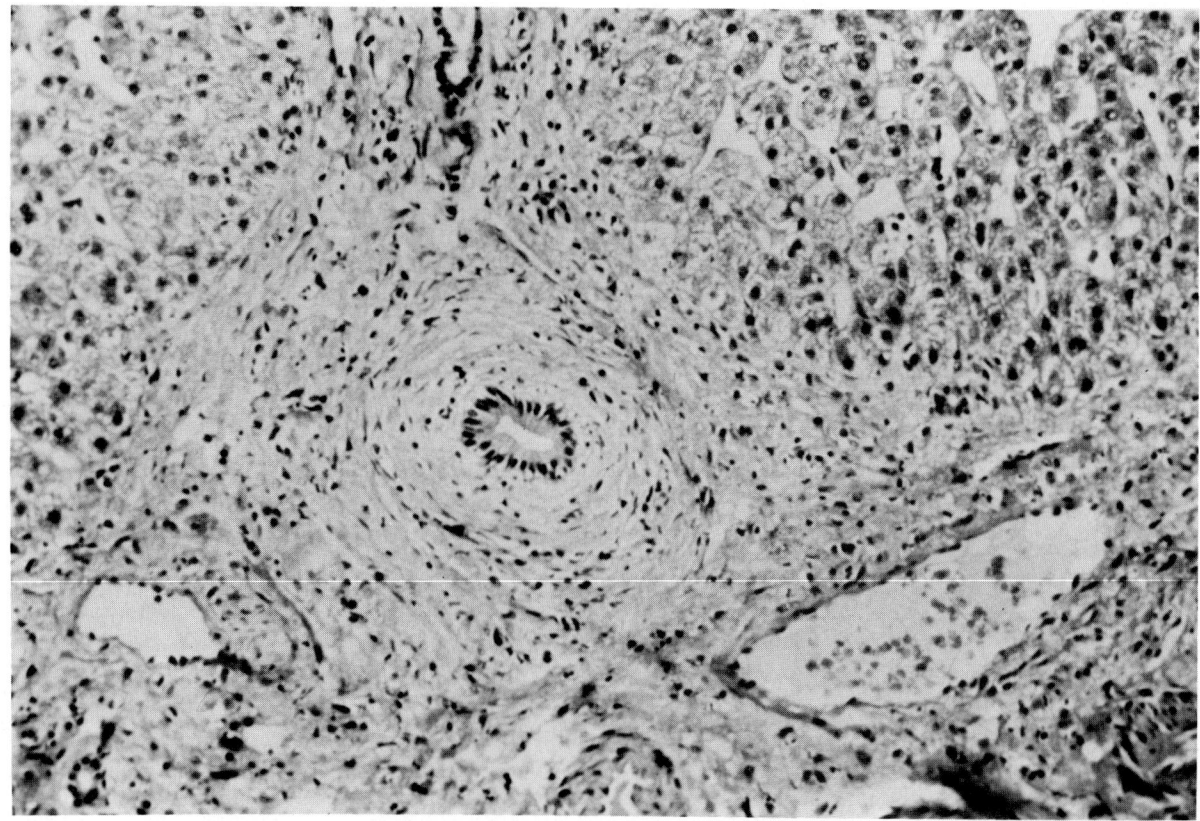

Figure 43–2. Chronic pericholangitis in ulcerative colitis. Concentric fibrosis around a bile duct with intact epithelium.

two had involvement of the common bile duct. In the remaining patient, only the common bile duct was visualized, and it was normal. In another study using endoscopic retrograde cholangiography to assess patients with ulcerative colitis and biopsy-proven liver disease, Schrumpf et al. demonstrated sclerosing cholangitis in 5 of 18 patients with pericholangitis, 4 of 13 patients with portal inflammation and fibrosis, 1 of 8 patients with nonspecific reactive changes, and 2 of 4 patients with cirrhosis.[49] Among 21 patients with abnormal liver tests in a group of 681 patients followed for ulcerative colitis, 17 were found to have sclerosing cholangitis.[35] In 6 of the 17, a histologic diagnosis of either chronic hepatitis or pericholangitis had been made prior to cholangiography. It is important to note that the natural history of patients with histologic evidence of pericholangitis and cholangiographic evidence of sclerosis limited to *intrahepatic* bile ducts[35, 48] has not been adequately defined. It is unknown whether all patients with intrahepatic duct involvement progress to classic primary sclerosing cholangitis with extrahepatic duct sclerosis.

From the preceding discussion, it is apparent that there is a high potential for diagnostic confusion. Lesions referred to as pericholangitis in the literature actually may reflect a heterogeneous mixture of hepatobiliary disorders encompassing chronic hepatitis and sclerosing cholangitis as well as a process resulting in circumductal fibrosis without biliary obstruction. The possible existence of distinct subgroups of patients with pericholangitis has important implications for our understanding of the clinical features and natural history of pericholangitis in inflammatory bowel disease and requires further study and refinement of nomenclature. It is imperative to know whether a subgroup of patients exists in the pericholangitis category that is unassociated with both chronic active hepatitis and classic primary sclerosing cholangitis.

Clinical Features and Frequency

Both the prevalence and the clinical features of pericholangitis are difficult to define. This is a direct result of the variability in the terminology used to report the morphologic lesion, the selection biases in the reported series, the paucity of published clinical details, and the variability in the performances and reporting of the results of biochemical, serologic, and organic anion clearance tests of liver function. The frequency of lesions fulfilling morphologic criteria for pericholangitis in selected reports from 1950 to the present ranges from zero to 83 per cent (see Table 43–2). Based on these data, pericholangitis represents the most common hepatic disease associated with inflammatory bowel disease, and occurs with comparable frequency in ulcerative colitis and Crohn's disease. In most reports, pericholangitis is as frequent in Crohn's colitis and ileocolitis as it is in Crohn's disease limited to the small bowel.[16, 17, 19, 20, 23]

Symptoms and signs of liver disease in patients with pericholangitis vary considerably and have not been described in all reported series. In several studies, patients were asymptomatic and had no evidence of liver disease on physical examination, whereas in others, patients were selected on the basis of presence of signs or symptoms of liver disease (Table 43–2). Mistilis has identified three clinical presentations in patients with pericholangitis: asymptomatic, cholestatic, and cholangitic.[28, 53] The term asymptomatic applies to the absence of signs and symptoms of liver disease only; the inflammatory bowel disease may

be active. Jaundice, the most frequent sign of cholestasis, either develops insidiously or occurs as abrupt, intermittent episodes of icterus. Pruritus has been reported in a minority of patients in association with jaundice. Patients with intermittent episodes of jaundice occasionally have fever and abdominal pain, simulating acute cholangitis. Rarely have such patients been evaluated rigorously to exclude the presence of obstructing lesions of the biliary tract. Some patients with pericholangitis have a clinical picture typical of acute viral hepatitis.

Results of physical examination usually are normal or only moderately abnormal. Hepatomegaly, when present, is slight to moderate. Splenomegaly infrequently is present and most often occurs in association with hepatomegaly. In reports emphasizing patients with overt, symptomatic liver disease, the frequencies of these findings are increased. A minority of patients with pericholangitis have stigmata of chronic liver disease, including vascular spiders, ascites, and edema.[46, 53]

Results of biochemical, serologic and organic anion clearance tests have not been reported in all series. In those series in which such tests have been utilized, they have often been performed in only selected patients (see Table 43–2). As discussed previously, patients with pericholangitis may have normal liver test results.[11, 20] The abnormality most frequently found in patients with pericholangitis is an elevated alkaline phosphatase,[19, 21, 44, 53] substantiated to be hepatic in origin by concomitant elevation of 5'-nucleotidase.[44] The 5'-nucleotidase may be normal, however, in patients with Crohn's disease, who have an elevated alkaline phosphatase,[20, 23] which has been attributed to osteomalacia.[23] The serum bilirubin may be elevated to levels causing jaundice, and slight elevations are not infrequent in asymptomatic, nonicteric individuals. Both the direct- and indirect-reacting components are increased. Aminotransferases may be normal or moderately elevated. Clearance of BSP has been impaired in some patients, but has been entirely normal in others with comparable morphologic lesions.[11, 20] Several patients reported to have abnormal BSP retention at 45 minutes were febrile, and the presence of fever raises the possibility of a false-positive test.[68] Measurements of serum proteins and lipids have been performed in several studies. Hypergammaglobulinemia and elevated cholesterol have been found in some patients,[11, 19, 20, 53, 58] but there is no characteristic alteration of either test in pericholangitis. Limited serologic testing of organ nonspecific autoantibodies (e.g., mitochondrial, smooth muscle, nuclear) has shown a low frequency of positivity in patients with ulcerative colitis or Crohn's disease, regardless of the presence or absence of hepatobiliary complications.[11, 19, 20, 22, 23]

Natural History and Prognosis

In the majority of patients, the clinical onset of the inflammatory bowel disease precedes the diagnosis of pericholangitis. The reported interval from the onset of inflammatory bowel disease to the diagnosis of pericholangitis is an imperfect estimate of the time required for the development of liver disease, since most patients in published series had not been tested previously for liver disease and could have had abnormalities of liver function for variable periods prior to liver biopsy. Recognizing this bias, the average duration of inflammatory bowel disease before performance of a liver biopsy in the series by Dordal and colleagues (including ulcerative colitis and Crohn's disease) was 8 years, with a range of 1 to 32 years.[19] In contrast, Schrumpf and co-workers reported that the median time from the onset of symptomatic ulcerative colitis necessitating hospitalization to the diagnosis of hepatobiliary disease was only a year.[49] In the latter series, laboratory tests of liver function were performed systematically in all patients, and all patients with abnormal tests had liver biopsies. In a minority of patients with pericholangitis, evidence of liver disease precedes the onset of inflammatory bowel disease by periods of months to years.[20, 53] In other patients, the liver and bowel diseases occur simultaneously.[11, 50]

The severity, extent, and duration of inflammatory bowel disease do not correlate with the presence of pericholangitis, the histologic or clinical severity of the liver disease, or the liability for progression of the liver disease.[11, 19, 20, 53] Although many patients with ulcerative colitis and pericholangitis have pancolitis,[19, 46, 53, 56–58] a substantial number of patients have only limited colonic disease,[11, 19, 53, 56, 57] including involvement of the rectum alone.[19, 57] For example, in the series of Perrett and co-workers the frequencies of pericholangitis were similar regardless of whether the extent of ulcerative colitis was categorized as distal, substantial, or universal.[11] Pericholangitis occurs in patients with Crohn's disease limited to the small bowel,[16–21, 23] the colon,[20–23] or the small bowel and colon.[20, 21, 23] The majority of patients have moderately active inflammatory bowel disease and a course characterized by remissions and relapses. The duration of inflammatory bowel disease is not related to the frequency of pericholangitis or to its prognosis.[19, 22, 53]

The question of prognosis is fundamentally related to the frequency with which pericholangitis progresses to cirrhosis. In the majority of patients with acute pericholangitis, the course is benign[38] and spontaneous histologic resolution is frequent.[19, 25, 28] For example, Dordal and associates reported that serial biopsies of the livers of five patients with pericholangitis showed histologic improvement during a period of several weeks to more than five years.[19] Some patients with acute pericholangitis progress, however, to a subacute or chronic picture (see section on Pathology).[28] In the majority of these patients, either the typical histologic changes persist or the inflammation ultimately subsides, leaving a clinically unimportant residue of hepatic fibrosis. Only a minority of patients progress to cirrhosis.[11, 18, 27, 28, 38, 43, 46, 58, 59, 64, 66]

The types of cirrhosis vary; some pathologists report a micronodular,[27, 58] and others a macronodular, pattern.[11, 28, 46] Less frequently, "biliary cirrhosis" has been described,[18, 27, 43, 64] and rarely a specific diagnosis of primary biliary cirrhosis has been made.[18, 27, 35, 46] Mistilis has argued that the diagnosis of primary biliary cirrhosis represents a histologic overinterpretation, since in other respects these patients are dissimilar to those with typical primary biliary cirrhosis (see Chap. 44).[28] It should be re-emphasized that the progression of pericholangitis to cirrhosis could be explained partially by the unrecognized inclusion of patients with chronic active hepatitis, partial mechanical obstruction of the biliary tract, or sclerosing cholangitis. The histologic lesions in these diseases can be indistinguishable from those of pericholangitis,[38, 59, 63] and each can progress to cirrhosis.[62]

Portal venous hypertension and its complications have been reported in association with pericholangitis.[53, 58, 67, 68] In some patients it represents a consequence of cirrhosis.[28, 58, 67, 68] In other patients it may represent a presinusoidal process,[28, 53, 58] which has been attributed to phlebosclerosis of the portal veins within the portal tracts. This concept is supported by evidence in some patients of normal wedged hepatic vein pressures and patency of the extrahepatic portal venous system.[53]

Pathogenesis

The pathogenesis of pericholangitis associated with inflammatory bowel disease is unknown. Factors postulated to be involved include portal bacteremia, toxins released from the inflamed bowel, changes in bile acid composition, hepatotoxicity of lithocholic acid, enhanced permeability of inflamed bowel to noxious factors, hepatotoxicity of medications, immune complexes, and autoimmunity.

Portal Bacteremia. Portal venous blood and the liver parenchyma are sterile in normal humans.[69] Uncontrolled studies by Brooke and colleagues support the possibility that bacteremia of the portal vein resulting from disruption of mucosal barriers in the bowel may produce pericholangitis.[70–72] In the most rigorous study, Eade and Brooke cultured, aerobically and anaerobically, portal venous blood obtained at the time of colectomy from 100 patients with ulcerative colitis.[72] Biopsy specimens of the livers were cultured in the same manner. The culture of portal venous blood was positive for 24 patients, and the culture of the liver specimen was positive for 11. These results exclude cultures positive for *Staphylococcus albus*, a contaminant in an additional nine specimens of either portal venous blood or liver. Organisms of potential pathogenic significance included fecal aerobes and, in four instances, anaerobes. Although results of liver tests were not reported, the frequencies of histologic lesions (fatty infiltration, inflammatory cell infiltration, fibrosis, bile duct proliferation, and hepatocellular necrosis) were similar in patients with and without positive cultures.

In contrast to these results, Perrett and associates cultured aerobically 45 liver biopsy specimens from 42 patients with ulcerative colitis and found 41 negative and 4 positive cultures.[11] Each positive culture was ascribed to contamination. An unsuccessful attempt was made to culture L forms in specimens from 20 patients. Dordal and colleagues obtained similar results of aerobic and anaerobic cultures with 69 needle biopsy specimens obtained from a group of 103 patients with either ulcerative colitis or Crohn's disease.[19] Fifty-two cultures were negative, 15 were considered contaminated, and the remaining 2 grew *Paracolobactrum aerogenoides* and nonhemolytic anaerobic streptococcus, respectively. Cultures of a second biopsy specimen from one of the last 2 patients were negative. The types of inflammatory bowel disease were not specified for the patients whose biopsy specimens were cultured; thus, the specific numbers of patients with ulcerative colitis and Crohn's disease are unknown. At the time of colectomy for Crohn's disease, Eade et al. cultured portal venous blood prior to handling the bowel in 9 of 21 cases.[22] *Proteus vulgaris* was present in a single specimen. Perrett et al. aerobically cultured needle biopsy specimens of liver from 34 patients with Crohn's disease.[20] Cultures of 30 of the specimens were negative, and the remainder were considered to be contaminated.

Based on the above results, the role of portal bacteremia in the pathogenesis of pericholangitis remains moot. One interpretation of these studies is that the prevalence of positive cultures is too low to suggest that portal bacteremia is a factor in pathogenesis. Alternatively, portal bacteremia could have injurious effects, but by occurring only intermittently, may not be detected readily by a single culture. The question of the possible role of anaerobic bacteria has not been settled. Even though anaerobic culture conditions were employed in some studies,[19, 70] the techniques of handling specimens prior to incubation were inferior to those now recommended.

Experimental evidence for hepatic injury induced by portal venous bacteremia is scant but intriguing. Hektoen found inflammation, bile duct proliferation, and fibrosis of portal tracts in guinea pigs after a single intraperitoneal injection of pseudodiphtheriae.[73] Weaver produced identical lesions in guinea pigs by injecting *Escherichia coli.*[74] MacMahon and Mallory showed that a single injection of hemolytic streptococci into the mesenteric vein of rabbits produced acute inflammation of the portal triads, bile duct proliferation, and focal necrosis.[75] Wachstein et al. produced focal degenerative changes and Kupffer cell proliferation by intraperitoneal injection of *Salmonella typhimurium* into rats.[76] Vinnik et al. evaluated the effect of chronic portal venous bacteremia in calves.[77] In three of six animals, they found edema of the portal tract with inflammation, focal necrosis, bile duct proliferation, and Kupffer cell hyperplasia in association with elevated aspartate aminotransferase, alkaline phosphatase, and 5'-nucleotidase. Results of similarly designed studies to evaluate chronic portal bacteremia have not been reported.

Bacterial Toxins. Endotoxin has not been measured systematically in the portal venous blood of patients with inflammatory bowel disease or in the systemic circulation of patients with hepatic lesions associated with inflammatory bowel disease. The presence of endotoxin in the portal venous blood of patients undergoing elective abdominal surgery (including patients with ulcerative colitis) suggests that it may be a normal constituent.[78] Endotoxin, however, is not found normally in the systemic circulation because it is removed by the liver. In cirrhosis, endotoxin has been detected in the peripheral venous blood,[79, 80] but the validity of these results has been questioned.[81] It is postulated that systemic endotoxemia in patients with cirrhosis represents either Kupffer cell dysfunction or significant portal-systemic venous shunting. In models of experimental liver injury producing Kupffer cell dysfunction, subsequent injections of normally innocuous quantities of endotoxin can produce hepatic necrosis.[82] This raises the question of whether endotoxin could be a primary factor in the pathogenesis of liver disease in patients with inflammatory bowel disease or could adversely affect the liver after some other mechanism had caused Kupffer cell dysfunction. Utili et al. have shown that endotoxin produces cholestasis in perfused rat livers by inhibiting bile salt–independent flow.[83] This represents a possible mechanism for the intermittent episodes of cholestasis observed in patients with pericholangitis whose histologic lesions may or may not fluctuate in severity concurrent with the clinical episodes of jaundice.[28, 53]

It is also plausible that products of bacterial metabolism in the gut, produced normally in healthy humans or uniquely in inflammatory bowel disease, could be hepatotoxic.[28] Such hepatotoxicity might be facilitated in patients with inflammatory bowel disease if there were increased absorption of toxic products across an injured mucosa. Studies have been performed to quantitate the absorption of ^3H_2O[84] and ^{131}I-albumin[85] across the rectal mucosa in patients with ulcerative colitis and in normal controls. Absorption was not increased in patients with ulcerative colitis as compared with controls. Even in the absence of evidence for increased permeability of the inflamed bowel, recent studies of enzyme induction in intestinal flora and the potentially adverse effects of products of bacterial catabolism make the basic hypothesis attractive.[86, 87] Future

investigation in this area may provide insight into the mechanisms of hepatobiliary disease and the increased incidence of carcinoma of the bowel associated with ulcerative colitis and Crohn's disease.

Toxicity of Bile Acids. Changes in bile acid composition or bile acid–mediated hepatotoxicity have been suggested as causes of pericholangitis.[88] It is postulated that hepatotoxicity results from the effects of secondary bile acids that are present in abnormally large amounts because of increased production and/or increased absorption. This hypothesis is not supported by available evidence. The types and proportions of bile acids in the sera of patients with ulcerative colitis and Crohn's disease who have associated hepatic disease are identical to those in patients with hepatic disease unassociated with inflammatory bowel disease.[89] Moreover, patients who have inflammatory bowel disease unassociated with hepatic abnormalities have the same proportions and concentrations of bile acids in gallbladder bile[89] and portal venous blood[89, 90] as do normal controls. Postprandial levels of serum bile acids in patients with uncomplicated inflammatory bowel disease also are normal, which argues against the presence of subclinical hepatic dysfunction.[89] The initial interest in lithocholic acid as a hepatotoxin has abated with recognition of the capacity of humans to sulfate and detoxify this secondary bile acid.[91] Thus, there is no direct evidence that the composition of the bile acid pool, the metabolism of bile acids in the intestine, or the intestinal absorption of bile acids contributes to pericholangitis.

Drug Toxicity. The possibility that pericholangitis represents drug toxicity has been commented on with particular reference to a hypersensitivity reaction to sulfonamides, especially sulfasalazine.[11, 20, 60] Hepatic lesions in patients with inflammatory bowel disease that are compatible with sulfonamide toxicity include hepatocellular necrosis, focal necrosis, granulomatous hepatitis, and chronic hepatitis.[92] Reports of hepatotoxicity due to sulfasalazine in patients with inflammatory bowel disease, however, are rare.[52, 93–95] The best substantiated case of hepatocellular injury due to sulfasalazine in a patient with ulcerative colitis was associated with fever and jaundice and an initially mixed hepatocellular-cholestatic biochemical profile that became decidedly more hepatocellular after rechallenges with the drug.[94] Unfortunately, liver biopsy was not performed. No report suggests that the chronic use of sulfasalazine causes intermittent or chronic biochemical or clinical cholestasis, the feature most characteristic of pericholangitis. Sulfasalazine, however, may cause acute worsening of jaundice in patients with coexistent inflammatory bowel disease and liver disease.[58] The relatively constant frequencies of pericholangitis reported in large series of patients over the past 30 years argues against a pathogenic role for several drugs used in therapeutic regimens that subsequently have been modified or abandoned.

Autoimmunity. As with other chronic inflammatory lesions of the liver, the possibility has been considered that autoimmunity is involved in the pathogenesis of pericholangitis. Plausible arguments have been advanced that humoral or cellular immunity could produce injury, either as a result of sensitization to bowel or fecal antigens that cross-react with hepatobiliary antigens or as a result of primary sensitization to hepatobiliary antigens alone. There is no direct evidence to support or refute these hypotheses in patients with inflammatory bowel disease. In a rabbit model of ulcerative colitis induced by dinitrochlorobenzene sensitivity, however, hepatic lesions characterized by infiltration of the portal tracts with leukocytes and plasma cells and focal infiltration of the parenchyma were found in eight of ten animals.[96] Whether the hepatic lesions in these animals were related to the sensitized T lymphocytes mediating delayed-type hypersensitivity is unknown.

The role of the immune complexes in inflammatory bowel disease associated with hepatic disease is the subject of debate. Several investigators have detected immune complexes in patients with inflammatory bowel disease by the use of indirect assays.[97] Others, using similar methods, have failed to detect immune complexes.[98] Interest in the possibly pathogenic role of immune complexes in inflammatory bowel disease has been stimulated by recent reports of immune complex-induced acute and chronic colitis in rabbits.[99, 100] Whether or not immune complexes are pathogenic in chronic inflammatory diseases of the liver also is the subject of controversy and speculation. Although immune complexes have been detected in chronic hepatitis and primary biliary cirrhosis,[97] similar studies have not been performed in patients with pericholangitis (see discussion of Primary Sclerosing Cholangitis).

Therapy

A rational approach to therapy rests on understanding the natural history of the specific disease and its pathogenesis. Neither criterion has been fulfilled for pericholangitis in association with inflammatory bowel disease. This situation is complicated further by our inability to recognize the minority of patients who are prone to progression of the hepatic lesion. The possibility exists, therefore, that a specific therapy might be falsely considered efficacious for patients in whom the natural history of the disease is benign. That the natural history of pericholangitis in most patients is benign[19, 25, 28, 38] suggests that treatment is unnecessary except in patients whose clinical courses and serial liver biopsies indicate progressive liver disease. As discussed above, some of the reported patients with progressive liver disease attributed to pericholangitis actually may have had chronic hepatitis or sclerosing cholangitis. This possibility makes interpretation of the reported effects of different therapies in pericholangitis even more difficult.

The principal therapies employed for pericholangitis have been antimicrobials, corticosteroids, and resection of the diseased bowel. The use of antimicrobials is based on the concept that portal venous bacteremia causes the lesion or contributes to its perpetuation. Tetracycline, initially reported to be beneficial in a small number of patients,[101] was ineffective in later studies.[102] The failure of tetracycline might be related to its ineffectiveness against anaerobic bacteria, which quantitatively are dominant in the fecal flora. The efficacy of antimicrobials effective against anaerobic bacteria in the treatment of patients with pericholangitis has not been reported.

Corticosteroids have been used for patients with pericholangitis and have had only a limited effect. In most instances, corticosteroids have been used to treat the active inflammatory bowel disease rather than the pericholangitis. In the study of Mistilis, the long-term treatment with prednisone of patients with pericholangitis and hepatic symptoms had no effect on the clinical course, morphologic features of the hepatic lesion, or results of laboratory tests.[102] Episodes of cholestasis or cholangitis continued and elevated alkaline phosphatase persisted. Histologic progression from acute to chronic pericholangitis was noted, and in three patients macronodular cirrhosis developed.

The most perplexing therapeutic question is whether resection of the diseased bowel arrests or alleviates pericholangitis. Resection of diseased bowel theoretically should abolish or significantly decrease the effects of unspecified toxins, the generation of immune complexes, and the continued sensitization of lymphocytes. The largest study to address this question in patients with ulcerative colitis has been that of Eade et al.[56, 67] Wedge biopsies of the livers revealed abnormalities in 94 per cent of 132 patients undergoing colectomy for severe ulcerative colitis.[56] The frequency of "inflammatory change" (preferred by Eade over the term pericholangitis) was 73 per cent. Biopsies of the livers of 33 of 117 survivors were repeated three to seven years after colectomy. These 33 patients were selected because of abnormal results of liver tests and represented a majority of patients with significant histologic lesions at the time of colectomy. The frequency of histologic abnormalities disclosed by the follow-up biopsies was substantially reduced, with decreases in inflammatory infiltration (42 per cent reduced to 15 per cent), bile duct proliferation (54 per cent reduced to 30 per cent), and fibrosis (57 per cent reduced to 18 per cent). In every patient whose repeat biopsy showed the continued presence of a specific lesion, there was no evidence of progression. In each of three patients with active proctitis in the unresected rectum, however, the liver disease progressed. The authors concluded that total colectomy was beneficial in the management of inflammatory disease of the liver associated with ulcerative colitis.

Others dispute the effectiveness of colectomy in the management of pericholangitis in patients with ulcerative colitis.[60, 102] Stauffer et al. reported variable results after colectomy in seven patients with hepatobiliary complications of ulcerative colitis.[58] In three patients, two of whom had portal triaditis, there was lessening of jaundice. Of three other patients with portal triaditis, two did not improve and one died postoperatively. The authors concluded that colectomy might benefit some but not all patients. In the series reported by Mistilis et al., colectomy had no beneficial effect on the clinical course, liver tests, or histologic lesions in patients with ulcerative colitis and pericholangitis.[102] Current evidence indicates that colectomy has no role in the management of patients with ulcerative colitis and pericholangitis.

The effect of colectomy in Crohn's colitis is even less well defined. In a study by Eade et al. of 21 patients undergoing colectomy for Crohn's colitis,[22] the frequency of "inflammatory change" in the liver biopsy was comparable to that found in patients with ulcerative colitis. The number of patients who had repeat biopsies three to seven years later was insufficient, however, to permit drawing conclusions about the usefulness of colectomy as a treatment for the inflammatory lesions. Similarly, the usefulness of small bowel resection in the management of patients with Crohn's disease and pericholangitis remains unknown.[21, 23]

FATTY LIVER

Fatty liver, the term preferred by the committee on standardization of nomenclature, is defined as an acquired disorder of metabolism resulting in accumulation of triglycerides within hepatocytes in quantities sufficient to be visible by light microscopy.[63] Many processes may lead to such accumulations,[38] and several are associated with progressive hepatic disease. The accumulation of fat within the liver per se does not result in necrosis, inflammation, fibrosis, or cirrhosis and is a potentially reversible lesion. The biochemical features and pathophysiology of this lesion are discussed in Chapter 5.

Pathology

Accumulation of fat has been found in livers from patients with both ulcerative colitis and Crohn's disease (Table 43–3). The fat appears to be contained in large vesicles and typically is diffusely distributed in the lobule, although some report preferential distribution in the centrilobular or periportal areas.[11, 20, 22, 56] Rarely, Mallory's hyaline has been found.[28] Fat often is present concurrently with other histologic lesions, which makes interpretation of the clinical and biochemical significance of fatty liver more difficult.[19, 23, 28, 56, 57]

Frequency and Clinical Features

Fatty liver has been described in most reports of large series of patients. Reported frequencies range from 0 to 80 per cent, with a mean of 33 per cent (see Table 43–3). Analysis of the individual studies is complicated by variations in the diagnostic criteria. These range from the inclusion of all patients with any evidence of fat in the biopsy specimen to inclusion of only patients considered to have "severe" fatty changes. Based on autopsy studies, fatty liver is the hepatobiliary disorder most frequently associated with inflammatory bowel disease. This impression probably is erroneous, because the frequency of fatty liver often is much lower in liver biopsy specimens from living patients as compared with liver obtained at autopsy.[28, 59]

Individual investigators debate the relationship between fatty liver and the severity, duration, or extent of ulcerative colitis or Crohn's disease. Many reported patients have been chronically ill and often severely malnourished. This is especially true for patients in whom the fatty change is most extensive and for patients in autopsy series. The possibility that terminal illness and malnutrition contribute to the production of fatty liver led to a comparison of the frequency of fatty liver in patients dying from ulcerative colitis and those dying from other causes.[26, 27] In one study, 15 per cent of autopsies in the ulcerative colitis group

TABLE 43–3. FATTY LIVER IN SELECTED SERIES OF PATIENTS WITH INFLAMMATORY BOWEL DISEASE

Series	Type of Inflammatory Bowel Disease*	Number of Patients with Liver Biopsy	Frequency (Percentage)	Features of Hepatic Disease		Comments‡
				Clinical	Laboratory†	
Kimmelstiel et al.[26]	UC	93	15		—	Reports only *severe* fat accumulation
Kleckner et al.[46]	UC	32	28	No physical findings of hepatic disease	Abnormal BSP retention	Reports all instances of fat accumulation
Boden et al.[43]	UC	10	0	Jaundice, hepatosplenomegaly frequent	↑ AP, bili, abnormal BSP	—
Ross et al.[50]	UC	17	0	Hepato-splenomegaly frequent	—	—
Eade[56]	UC	132	45	—	↑ AP	Reports all instances of fat accumulation; fat present with other lesions; severe fatty liver present in 14%
Palmer et al.[27]	UC	51	54	—	—	Fat present with other lesions
Mistilis[28]	UC	49 living	12	—	—	Fat frequently associated with pericholangitis
Mistilis and Goulston[53]		34 autopsy	47	—	—	Frequency in autopsy groups may reflect effects of terminal illness
Vinnik et al.[44]	UC	8	0	—	—	—
de Dombal et al.[57]	UC	58	83	—	—	Fat associated with portal tract inflammation
Stauffer et al.[58]	UC	30	0	—	—	—
Perrett et al.[11]	UC	50	38	—	↑ AP, abnormal BSP retention	Most severe fat accumulation in patients requiring emergency colectomy
Chapin et al.[16]	CD of small bowel	39	51	—	—	Patients severely debilitated with high frequency of terminal infections; reports all instances of fat accumulation
Palmer et al.[18]	CD of small bowel	8	25	Hepato-splenomegaly	—	Patients severely malnourished
Cohen et al.[131]	CD of small bowel	19	37	—	—	Fat accumulation focal in 66%; fat present with other lesions

Table continued on following page

TABLE 43–3. FATTY LIVER IN SELECTED SERIES OF PATIENTS WITH INFLAMMATORY BOWEL DISEASE *Continued*

Series	Type of Inflammatory Bowel Disease*	Number of Patients with Liver Biopsy	Frequency (Percentage)	Features of Hepatic Disease		Comments‡
				Clinical	*Laboratory†*	
Kleckner[15]	CD of small bowel	20	15	Asymptomatic, no physical signs	Abnormal BSP retention in 1 patient	—
Perrett et al.[20]	CD	39	21	—	—	Fat present with other lesions
Eade et al.[23]	CD of small bowel, colon or small bowel and colon	49	38	—	—	Reports all instances of fat accumulation
Eade et al.[22]	CD of colon	20	40	—	—	—
Dordal et al.[19]	CD of small bowel or small bowel and colon	27	26	—	↑ AP; abnormal BSP retention in some, rare; ↑ bili	Fat present with other lesions
	UC	76	20	—	—	
Dew et al.[21]	CD	Approx 32	0	—	↑ AP (criterion for selection)	—
	UC	Approx 51	0	—		
Monto[17]	UC	100	80	—	—	Clinical and laboratory data not matched to histology
	CD of small bowel	4	75	—	—	
Perold, et al.[34]	UC	10	20	—	↑ AST or BSP retention	Prospective study; mild fat deposition in centrolobular areas without other histopathologic lesions
Wee and Ludwig[38]	UC	107	24	—	↑ AP, AST	Retrospective study; inconspicuous fat present in 43% of patients with small or large-duct sclerosis; 2 other patients had true steatohepatitis
Ludwig et al.[59]	UC	42	10	—	↑ AP, AST	Retrospective study; of 23 patients with PSC, 9% had fat; of 19 patients with abnormal liver tests and normal bile ducts, 11% had fat

*UC = ulcerative colitis; CD = Crohn's disease.
†AP = alkaline phosphatase; bili = bilirubin; BSP = Bromsulphalein (sulfobromophthalein).
‡See Table 43–2 for general comments regarding each study.

showed fatty liver, as compared with only 1.4 per cent of 1000 unselected autopsies.[26] In the other study, the frequency of fatty liver was 54 per cent in patients with ulcerative colitis, 26 per cent in unselected control patients, and 41 per cent in patients dying from "debilitating causes."[27] These studies suggest that factors other than malnutrition are important in the development of fatty liver in patients with inflammatory bowel disease.

In general, most patients with fatty liver are asymptomatic with respect to symptoms of liver disease. Examples to the contrary often represent patients in whom fatty liver occurs concomitantly with other hepatic lesions.[28] It is not possible to ascribe clinical or biochemical abnormalities to the presence of fat alone in such patients. The physical examination usually shows no abnormality but hepatomegaly may be present. Results of laboratory investigations of patients with fatty liver tend to be normal, but abnormal tests have been reported, especially for patients with histologic evidence of additional diseases. The specific patterns of laboratory abnormalities in such patients are those associated with the additional diseases.

Natural History and Prognosis

The fatty infiltration may subside in seriously ill patients who respond to therapy for their inflammatory bowel disease and malnutrition.[11, 19, 28] Persistence of fat, however, has been documented in several instances when repeat biopsies have been obtained.[11, 19] The presence of fat alone is not associated with progressive hepatic damage in patients with inflammatory bowel disease, but progression to fibrosis may occur when fatty liver coexists with severe inflammatory lesions.[28] Therefore, the finding of fat without hepatic inflammation in a liver biopsy specimen from a patient with inflammatory bowel disease is generally of no clinical consequence.

Pathogenesis

The pathogenesis of fatty liver in inflammatory bowel disease is not known, but circumstantial evidence suggests that it is multifactorial (see Chapter 5). Patients who have severe, debilitating illness and malnutrition may have protein-calorie malnutrition, a known cause of fatty liver.[62] A possible relationship between malnutrition and fatty liver is suggested by the finding that patients with ulcerative colitis or Crohn's disease and fatty livers have lower serum levels of carotene than do patients with either pericholangitis or cirrhosis.[19] Both tetracyclines and corticosteroids have been implicated in the pathogenesis of fatty liver. Tetracycline is an unlikely cause since other characteristic features, such as hepatocellular necrosis, are absent. Moreover, the frequency of fatty liver far exceeds that predicted by the reported use of tetracycline in inflammatory bowel disease. Corticosteroids may contribute to the production of fatty liver,[103] and have been used in the treatment of most of reported patients with severe inflammatory bowel disease. Fatty liver occurs, however, in a substantial number of patients not receiving corticosteroids. The possible role of unrecognized alcohol abuse is undefined. Several studies have attempted to exclude patients with alcoholism, but these have relied solely on a negative history. The possibility that some bacterial metabolite or chemical toxin induces fatty change in patients with inflammatory bowel disease remains speculative.

Therapy

Treatment should be directed toward the inflammatory bowel disease itself and restoration of protein-calorie nutrition. Resection of the bowel is neither beneficial nor indicated for the hepatic lesion. Eade et al. showed that the frequency of fatty liver was the same three to seven years after colectomy for ulcerative colitis as it had been at the time of the bowel resection.[67] Comparable data have not been reported for patients with Crohn's disease.

CHRONIC HEPATITIS

There is substantial confusion regarding the occurrence of chronic hepatitis in association with inflammatory bowel disease.[33-36, 38, 59] This confusion, in part, reflects the evolution during the past three decades of a complex, changing nomenclature and unsuccessful attempts to derive a single classification that is accurate simultaneously for clinical, histologic, and pathogenic features. Current definitions of chronic hepatitis emphasize morphologic characteristics and can be subdivided into chronic persistent hepatitis and chronic active hepatitis.[62] These definitions have been used in reviewing the literature and have been applied as strictly as possible to reported patients.

It is important to emphasize that morphologic features of chronic hepatitis may occur in patients with pericholangitis and primary sclerosing cholangitis, confusing the diagnosis.[33-36, 38, 59] Thus, definition of the true frequency of chronic hepatitis in patients with inflammatory bowel disease would require exclusion of sclerotic lesions by cholangiography. Indeed, recent reports indicate that a proportion of patients with primary sclerosing cholangitis are incorrectly diagnosed as having chronic active hepatitis by liver biopsy.[35, 36, 38] However, application of strict histopathologic and cholangiographic criteria continues to reveal an association between inflammatory bowel disease and true chronic hepatitis.[38]

Pathology

The two morphologic subtypes of chronic hepatitis differ in severity and thus in their tendencies to progress to cirrhosis (see Chapter 38). *Chronic persistent hepatitis* is a nonspecific morphologic lesion characterized by chronic inflammatory infiltrates in the portal tracts with absent or, at most, minimal piecemeal necrosis. It may be associated with focal necrosis similar to that seen in acute viral hepatitis. Although rare patients have been reported to progress to chronic active hepatitis, chronic persistent hepatitis is considered to be a benign, nonprogressive lesion.

Chronic active hepatitis (CAH) is also a nonspecific morphologic lesion, caused by several different agents.[104] It is characterized by chronic inflammatory infiltrates in the portal tracts, with moderate to severe piecemeal necrosis. Necrosis may bridge the lobule, connecting portal tracts to portal tracts or portal tracts to central veins, or diffusely involve adjacent lobules. The presence of significant piecemeal necrosis, however, may not be diagnostic of chronic active hepatitis in patients with inflammatory bowel disease, since it has been considered a feature of pericholangitis[28] and occurs frequently in patients with sclerosing cholangitis (see section on Primary Sclerosing Cholangitis).[31, 32, 35, 36, 38] Chronic active hepatitis may progress to macronodular cirrhosis with or without the continued presence of active necrosis. This situation is particularly relevant because several reports identify patients with inflammatory bowel disease as having chronic hepatitis with cirrhosis.[33-36, 38, 59, 105, 106]

Frequency

The frequency with which chronic persistent hepatitis occurs in association with inflammatory bowel disease cannot be determined. As discussed earlier, features of chronic persistent hepatitis are present in many reported patients referred to as having pericholangitis. With the exception of two patients with ulcerative colitis,[49, 107] one of whom had eosinophilia, autoimmune thyroid disease, and sulfasalazine hypersensitivity,[107] the term chronic persistent hepatitis has not been applied to patients with inflammatory bowel disease.

The frequency of chronic active hepatitis in association with inflammatory bowel disease varies. In several large series of patients with ulcerative colitis and Crohn's disease, chronic active hepatitis was either absent or rare.[11, 19-23, 56] In contrast, Mistilis and colleagues reported that 16 per cent of biopsied patients had chronic active hepatitis.[28] One prospective study of patients with ulcerative colitis showed chronic active hepatitis in 1 per cent,[49] whereas another prospective study of ulcerative colitis showed a frequency of 20 per cent.[34] Estimates of the frequency of chronic active hepatitis associated with inflammatory bowel disease have also been made by determining the prevalence of inflammatory bowel disease in groups of patients selected because of the presence of liver disease.[29, 105, 106, 108-110] These estimates, ranging from 4 to 28 per cent, are biased by the selection of patients with moderate to severe symptomatic liver disease. Similar studies of the prevalence of inflammatory bowel disease have not been made in patients with chronic active hepatitis who are asymptomatic or who have only moderately abnormal liver tests.

Willcox and Isselbacher found ulcerative colitis in 7 of 33 patients less than 40 years old with chronic hepatitis,[29] but in none of 143 patients more than 40 years old with chronic hepatitis. Gray and co-workers reported 8 patients with chronic active hepatitis and inflammatory bowel disease with concurrent evidence of autoimmune phenomenon.[109] MacKay and Wood reported that 5 of 22 patients with "lupoid hepatitis" (chronic active hepatitis) had ulcerative colitis.[108] Read and associates reported 5 instances of ulcerative colitis among 81 patients with cirrhosis presumed to be secondary to chronic active hepatitis.[105] Holdsworth et al. reported 22 patients with ulcerative colitis and chronic hepatitis seen over a four-year period, 20 of whom had cirrhosis.[106] In keeping with the observation of Willcox and Isselbacher, these cirrhotic patients were significantly younger than those in a group of 200 patients with cirrhosis not related to alcohol abuse, who did not have ulcerative colitis. Olsson and Hulten reported 25 patients with chronic active hepatitis, 7 of whom had coexisting ulcerative colitis.[110] Mistilis, in the description of 14 patients with chronic pericholangitis, noted piecemeal necrosis in 11 and bridging necrosis in 7.[28] In his series, chronic active hepatitis was diagnosed on the initial biopsy in an additional eight of 49 patients.

In a recent retrospective analysis from the Johns Hopkins Hospital, 8 patients with postnecrotic cirrhosis attributed to chronic active hepatitis were identified among 202 patients with ulcerative colitis (4 per cent).[33] In each patient, primary sclerosing cholangitis was excluded during laparotomy for portal systemic shunting or colectomy. In a prospective study of 10 consecutive patients with ulcerative colitis and abnormal liver tests, two (20 per cent) had histologic chronic active hepatitis, but cholangiography was not performed to exclude primary sclerosing cholangitis.[34] Continued observation of patients with ulcerative colitis at Oxford revealed that 23 per cent of patients with primary sclerosing cholangitis had been incorrectly diagnosed as having chronic active hepatitis.[35] One patient (6 per cent of the population with persistently abnormal liver tests) had steroid-responsive, autoimmune chronic active hepatitis, and 2 additional patients were found to have heterozygous α_1-antitrypsin deficiency. In a comprehensive retrospective analysis of ulcerative colitis patients at the Mayo Clinic, 14 of 107 patients (13 per cent) with concurrent hepatobiliary disease had chronic active hepatitis.[38] One patient had hepatitis B and 3 had changes suggestive of post-transfusion non-A, non-B hepatitis. In the remaining 9 patients the chronic active hepatitis was considered idiopathic.

To date, the majority of reported patients with inflammatory bowel disease and chronic active hepatitis have had ulcerative colitis. Chronic active hepatitis has not been reported in most studies of patients with Crohn's disease.[16, 18, 19, 22, 23] Perrett et al. described a single such patient with chronic active hepatitis,[20] whereas Dew et al. omitted chronic hepatitis as a diagnostic category in their study.[21] The complex effects of changing nomenclature, morphologic overlap with the definition of pericholangitis, and biases in patient selection make it impossible to define the true incidence of chronic hepatitis in association with inflammatory bowel disease. It appears, however, that chronic hepatitis is associated with ulcerative colitis more frequently than would be expected by chance. The data for Crohn's disease do not support a similar conclusion.

Clinical Features

The duration of inflammatory bowel disease before recognition of chronic hepatitis is variable. In most reports, there are examples of patients with documented ulcerative colitis preceding chronic hepatitis, instances of concurrent onset, and examples of chronic hepatitis preceding the onset of ulcerative colitis. Crohn's disease (sites of involvement unspecified) preceded symptoms leading to the diagnosis of chronic active hepatitis in the patient reported by Perrett et al.[20]

The majority of reported patients have had symptomatic liver disease, which reflects the use of diagnostic criteria emphasizing symptoms. The symptoms and signs of liver disease are similar to those associated with chronic active hepatitis in the absence of inflammatory bowel disease (see Chapter 38). Specific autoimmune features have included polyarthritis,[109] thyroiditis,[107] glomerulonephritis,[106, 109] thrombocytopenic purpura,[109] nonthrombocytopenic purpura,[111] and pericarditis.[109] Physical findings generally include hepatomegaly, cutaneous stigmata of chronic liver disease, and occasionally splenomegaly, ascites, and edema. This again reflects the severity of the hepatic disease in these selected patients, many of whom had "active cirrhosis" at the time of biopsy.

Reporting of laboratory tests has not been uniform. The abnormalities, as expected, include moderate to marked elevations of aminotransferase activity and variable elevations of total bilirubin and alkaline phosphatase. The majority of reported patients had elevated gamma globulins, and tests for lupus erythematosus cells or antinuclear antibodies were frequently positive for patients with associated autoimmune features. Tests for hepatitis B surface antigen (HBsAg), performed in only a minority of patients, were negative,[107, 110, 111] with the exception of one patient.[38] Positive tests for antibodies against nuclear and smooth muscle antigens were common, whereas there were no positive tests for antimitochondrial antibodies.[49, 110]

Natural History and Prognosis

The activity and progression of chronic hepatitis do not correlate with the extent of involvement or severity of the inflammatory bowel disease.[49, 105, 111] Indeed, the activities of the liver and bowel diseases vary independently.[110] Chronic active hepatitis associated with inflammatory bowel disease progresses to cirrhosis[29, 38, 105, 106, 109, 110] in accordance with the natural history of chronic active hepatitis alone. The mortality of untreated patients with chronic active hepatitis and inflammatory bowel disease has been low; however, it should be emphasized that the durations of follow-up were short in most studies. As mentioned before, patients with chronic persistent hepatitis may have been included mistakenly in reports of pericholangitis.

Pathogenesis

Virtually all the mechanisms postulated as causes of pericholangitis have been considered by investigators describing the association of chronic active hepatitis and inflammatory bowel disease. The factor initiating chronic hepatitis, assuming a similarity to chronic hepatitis occurring in the absence of inflammatory bowel disease, is most likely a hepatitis virus or a toxic reaction to an exogenous substance or medication.[104] The nature of the mechanism(s) responsible for perpetuation of chronic hepatitis, however, remains unknown. One hypothesis states that both inflammatory bowel disease and chronic hepatitis occur as a consequence of abnormal "autoimmune" responsiveness. Although several immunopathogenic mechanisms have been proposed,[110, 111, 112] there is no direct evidence that they occur. The role of drug-induced injury, especially the possibility of chronic hepatitis induced by sulfonamides,[113] remains undefined.

Since chronic hepatitis may be caused by hepatitis B and non-A, non-B viruses, it is particularly important to assess the prevalence of acute viral hepatitis in patients with inflammatory bowel disease. Whereas there is no evidence to suggest that patients with inflammatory bowel disease are more susceptible to acute viral hepatitis, many patients have had repeated exposures to blood products. Edwards and Truelove, reporting on the complications in 624 patients with ulcerative colitis, described 30 patients with acute icteric viral hepatitis (4.8 per cent); two of these cases were related to blood transfusions.[114] Sixteen instances of "chronic liver disease" were noted (2.6 per cent) in their series. Greenstein et al. found acute icteric hepatitis following surgery or blood transfusion in 10 of 202 patients with ulcerative colitis, 3 of 6 patients with Crohn's colitis, 7 of 223 patients with Crohn's ileocolitis, and 4 of 213 patients with Crohn's disease of the ileum.[115] In the series of Holdsworth et al., 7 of 18 patients with "active" cirrhosis had an onset resembling acute viral hepatitis.[106] Palmer et al. described a patient with ulcerative colitis who presented with acute viral hepatitis, improved, and then progressed to death nine months later with lesions of chronic active hepatitis and multilobular necrosis.[27] Three other patients with cirrhosis had histories of antecedent acute viral hepatitis and subsequent episodes of jaundice. Despite the presumed risk of post-transfusion hepatitis in patients with inflammatory bowel disease, most authors feel post-transfusion hepatitis uncommonly leads to chronic liver disease.[38] Eade comments, for example, that the role of post-transfusion hepatitis in the production of chronic liver disease is negligible, since no instance of cirrhosis occurred in 225 patients with Crohn's disease, 80 per cent of whom had had blood transfusions.[22] The information just summarized relates only to patients with acute hepatitis, and may not be indicative of the true relationship between post-transfusion hepatitis, which is often anicteric, and the development of chronic hepatitis in patients with inflammatory bowel disease.

In the Mayo Clinic experience, 3 of 14 patients with chronic active hepatitis had histopathologic features of post-transfusion non-A, non-B hepatitis, and one had hepatitis B.[38] Two of the former patients had been transfused prior to the onset of liver dysfunction. Since 7 of 9 patients with "idiopathic" chronic active hepatitis received transfusions after the onset of liver dysfunction, superinfection with non-A, non-B viruses also may have played a role.

Therapy

Corticosteroids have been used in symptomatic patients with chronic active hepatitis associated with inflammatory bowel disease. Gray et al. reported responses to steroids that were moderate to excellent in five and poor in three of eight patients with ulcerative colitis and chronic active hepatitis with autoimmune features.[109] In the report of Read et al., 43 of 81 patients with chronic active hepatitis and "active" cirrhosis were treated with corticosteroids.[105] It is difficult to determine whether all five of the patients with ulcerative colitis in this series were treated; however, one patient developed ulcerative colitis while receiving corticosteroids for chronic active hepatitis. Overall, corticosteroids reduced symptoms in the treated patients, but did not

prevent progression of the liver disease or prolong life. Harris and Neugarten described an excellent response to corticosteroids in a woman with chronic active hepatitis, nonthrombocytopenic purpura, hypergammaglobulinemia and positive tests for rheumatoid factor and VDRL.[111] Czaja and Wolf compared the results of corticosteroid therapy in eight patients with chronic active hepatitis and ulcerative colitis with the results in 141 patients, including 25 patients who had associated immunopathic diseases.[116] Although corticosteroids alleviated the ulcerative colitis in each patient, their effect on the chronic active hepatitis was consistently unsatisfactory. Indeed, a statistically significant decrease in remissions of chronic active hepatitis and an increase in treatment failures were found in these patients. The implication that ulcerative colitis adversely affects the responsiveness of chronic active hepatitis to corticosteroids needs further study.

The effect of colectomy on chronic active hepatitis has been assessed in patients with severe ulcerative colitis.[29, 110] In one series, six patients had received corticosteroids or azathioprine for durations of more than a year prior to surgery.[110] Colectomy was performed on five patients because of exacerbations of colitis and was needed in one case because of colonic carcinoma. The activity of liver disease was assessed as mild to moderate at the time of operation. Following colectomy, spontaneous improvement in abnormal results of liver tests was found for four of the six patients. Further studies of larger numbers of patients are needed to assess the role of colectomy in the treatment of chronic active hepatitis associated with inflammatory bowel disease.

FIBROSIS AND CIRRHOSIS

Conspicuous fibrosis and cirrhosis have been found in most large series of patients with inflammatory bowel disease (Table 43–4). As discussed above, both "pericholangitis" and chronic hepatitis have been associated with progression to fibrosis and cirrhosis.

Pathology

Fibrosis, a sequela of several hepatic disorders, may result either from collapse of pre-existing collagen or from formation of new collagen. Cirrhosis is characterized by extensive fibrosis and the presence of regenerative parenchymal nodules.[62] Regenerative nodules may contain hepatocytes from one or more than one lobule and are separated from adjacent nodules by fibrous tissue. The diagnosis of cirrhosis remains difficult, especially when based on percutaneous needle biopsy specimens, which may be too small to permit differentiation between fibrosis and cirrhosis. Thus, the potential exists for either under- or overestimating the presence of cirrhosis in such specimens. A more accurate diagnosis is possible from wedge biopsies that have been performed in selected patients with inflammatory bowel disease. Because of problems in distinguishing fibrosis and cirrhosis in many reports, the data for fibrosis and cirrhosis have been combined in Table 43–4.

Currently, the preferred morphologic classification of cirrhosis is based on the sizes of regenerative nodules (micronodular, macronodular, and mixed macro- and micronodular).[62] These terms replace most of the terms employed in the series summarized in Table 43–4 but offer no heuristic advantage. For clarity, both the current terms and

TABLE 43–4. FIBROSIS AND CIRRHOSIS IN SELECTED SERIES OF PATIENTS WITH INFLAMMATORY BOWEL DISEASE

Series	Type of Inflammatory Bowel Disease*	Number of Patients with Liver Biopsy	Histologic Term	Frequency (Percentage)	Features of Hepatic Disease		Comments‡
					Clinical	*Laboratory†*	
Kimmelstiel et al.[26]	UC	93	Fibrosis Cirrhosis	1 1	Hepatomegaly Jaundiced terminally	— —	Fibrosis described as pseudolobulation; possibly true cirrhosis
Kleckner et al.[46]	UC	32	Portal cirrhosis (micronodular); postnecrotic cirrhosis (macronodular); biliary cirrhosis	19	Hepato-splenomegaly; occasional jaundice, edema, ascites	Abnormal BSP retention, ↑ bili, nl choles	—
Boden et al.[43]	UC	10	Biliary cirrhosis	20	Jaundice, hepato-splenomegaly, ascites	↑ AP, bili, abnormal BSP retention	One patient with pericholangitis progressing to cirrhosis
Ross et al[50]	UC	17	Portal cirrhosis (micronodular); postnecrotic cirrhosis (macronodular); biliary cirrhosis	76	Jaundice, hepato-splenomegaly	—	—
Eade[56]	UC	132	Fibrosis Cirrhosis	51 4.5	—	↑ AP, ↑ globulin, ↓ alb	Inflammatory infiltrates frequently present with fibrosis
Palmer et al.[27]	UC	51	Fibrosis Portal cirrhosis (micronodular); postnecrotic cirrhosis (macronodular); biliary cirrhosis	8 12	— Jaundice, hepato-splenomegaly, portal venous hypertension	— ↑ AP, bili, abnormal BSP retention	Two patients with cirrhosis secondary to biliary obstruction; 1 with choledocholithiasis, 1 with benign cholangioma
Mistilis[28]	UC	49 living 34 autopsy	Fibrosis Postnecrotic cirrhosis (macronodular) Fibrosis	29 12 24	— —	— —	Fibrosis associated with subacute and chronic pericholangitis; cirrhosis preceded by pericholangitis in 50% Fibrosis associated with chronic pericholangitis
de Dombal et al.[57]	UC	58	Portal cirrhosis (micronodular)	2	—	—	Cirrhosis associated with fatty liver
Stauffer et al.[58]	UC	30	Fibrosis Portal cirrhosis (micronodular); postnecrotic cirrhosis (macronodular); primary biliary cirrhosis	3 20	Jaundice, hepato-splenomegaly, portal venous hypertension	↑ AP, bili, AST, abnormal BSP retention	Patient with "primary biliary cirrhosis" had sclerosis of the common bile duct at surgery
Perrett et al.[11]	UC	50	Postnecrotic cirrhosis (macronodular)	6	Jaundice	↑ AP, bili, ALT, abnormal BSP retention	—
Chapin et al.[16]	CD of small bowel	39	Portal cirrhosis (micronodular)	8	—	—	66% with cirrhosis had a past medical history of alcohol abuse
Palmar et al.[18]	CD of small bowel	8	Portal cirrhosis (micronodular) Biliary cirrhosis	43	Hepato-splenomegaly	—	—
Cohen et al.[131]	CD of small bowel	19	Fibrosis	26	—	—	—
Perrett et al.[20]	CD	39	Fibrosis Portal cirrhosis (micronodular)	16 5	—	—	All fibrosis associated with chronic pericholangitis; cirrhotic liver contained hemosiderin
Eade et al.[23]	CD of small bowel, colon or small bowel and colon	49	Fibrosis	54	—	—	Fibrosis frequently associated with inflammatory infiltration of portal tracts; cirrhosis not present

Table continued on opposite page

TABLE 43–4. FIBROSIS AND CIRRHOSIS IN SELECTED SERIES OF PATIENTS WITH INFLAMMATORY BOWEL DISEASE *Continued*

Series	Type of Inflammatory Bowel Disease*	Number of Patients with Liver Biopsy	Histologic Term	Frequency (Percentage)	Features of Hepatic Disease		Comments‡
					Clinical	*Laboratory†*	
Eade et al.[22]	CD of colon	20	Fibrosis	35	Jaundice in 1 cirrhotic	—	—
			Micronodular cirrhosis	10			
Dordal et al.[19]	CD of small bowel or of small bowel and colon	27	Cirrhosis or "bridging portal hepatofibrosis"	19	—	—	—
	UC	76	Same as above	20	—	—	One cirrhotic patient developed a cholangiocarcinoma
Dew et al.[21]	CD	Approx 32	Cirrhosis	9	Portal venous hypertension	↑ AP (criterion for selection)	—
	UC	Approx 51	Cirrhosis	22	Portal venous hypertension	↑ AP (criterion for selection)	
Monto[17]	UC	100	Fibrosis "Early" cirrhosis	7 1	—	—	Fibrosis frequently associated with bile duct proliferation and fatty infiltration
	CD of small bowel	4	Fibrosis	75	—	—	
Lupinetti, et al.[33]	UC	Unstated	Cirrhosis	?	Mid to severe portal hypertension	—	Retrospective study; 5 of 8 required portal systemic shunts
Shepard, et al.[35]	UC	21	Cirrhosis	5	—	—	Prospective study; 1 cirrhotic
Steckman, et al.[36]	UC	6	Fibrosis	100	Jaundice, hepatomegaly	↑ AP, AST	Prospective study; 3 with progressive fibrosis, 3 with cirrhosis; All patients had liver disease prior to onset of UC
Wee and Ludwig[38]	UC	107	Cirrhosis	31	—	↑ AP, AST	Retrospective study of referred patients; 10 patients had small- or large-duct sclerosing cholangitis; 11 had chronic active hepatitis; 12 had cryptogenic cirrhosis
Ludwig, et al.[59]	UC	23	Cirrhosis	22	—	↑ AP, AST	Retrospective study; Cirrhosis in 22% of 23 patients with primary sclerosing pericholangitis (PSC)
	—	20	Cirrhosis	45	—	↑ AP, AST	Cirrhosis in 45% of 20 patients with PSC in the absence of UC
	UC	19	Cirrhosis	42	—	↑ AP, AST	Cirrhosis in 42% of 19 patients with UC in the absence of PSC

*UC = ulcerative colitis; CD = Crohn's disease.

†AP = alkaline phosphatase; bili = bilirubin; BSP = Bromsulphalein (sulfobromophthalein); AST = aspartate aminotransferase (SGOT); ALT = alanine aminotransferase (SGPT); alb = albumin; choles = cholesterol.

‡See Table 43–2 for general comments regarding each study.

those used in the individual reports have been tabulated. Cirrhosis in the majority of patients has been described as "postnecrotic" (macronodular),[11, 18, 27, 28, 33, 35, 36, 38, 46, 50, 54, 57, 59, 117] with occasional examples of "portal or Laennec's" (micronodular) cirrhosis,[20, 21, 27, 54, 58, 117] and "biliary cirrhosis,"[18, 19, 27, 50, 64] including "primary biliary cirrhosis."[27, 43, 58] In addition, Dordal et al. and Eade et al. use the term "bridging portal hepatofibrosis" to describe cirrhosis characterized by fibrosis extending between adjacent portal areas, distorted lobular architecture, regenerative nodules, and proliferation of bile ducts.[19, 56] In general, this is similar to biliary cirrhosis.

Frequency and Clinical Features

The reported frequency of cirrhosis among patients with inflammatory bowel disease undergoing biopsy varies widely (see Table 43–4). The range in ulcerative colitis is from zero to 45 per cent, with an average of 12 per cent. The range in Crohn's disease is from zero to 29 per cent, with an average of 12 per cent. Overall, the prevalence of cirrhosis appears to be between 1 and 5 per cent in both ulcerative colitis and Crohn's disease. The prevalence was 1.2 per cent in a prospective study of patients with ulcerative colitis.[49] The prevalence of cirrhosis in patients with inflammatory bowel disease appears to exceed that expected in the general population. In one study by Kimmelstiel et al., the prevalence of cirrhosis was identical for patients with ulcerative colitis and control patients.[26] On the other hand, the autopsy study of Palmer et al. showed that the frequency of cirrhosis in patients with ulcerative colitis was increased 12-fold over that in the control group.[27] In patients selected solely on the basis of cirrhosis, the prevalence of ulcerative colitis is five to six times greater than that in the general population.[105, 106] Cirrhosis associated with Crohn's disease limited to the small bowel was not evident in some studies[17, 23] but was present in others.[16, 18] In general, cirrhosis occurs more commonly in patients with extensive ulcerative colitis[11, 21, 33] or Crohn's colitis.[21, 22] The frequency of cirrhosis appears to be comparable for patients with ulcerative colitis and those with Crohn's colitis, although fewer of the latter patients have been reported.[22]

The clinical features attributable to fibrosis alone are minimal in patients with inflammatory bowel disease. The fibrosis primarily involves the portal tract and rarely is associated with portal venous hypertension (see the section on Pericholangitis). The clinical features of the lesions associated with fibrosis, pericholangitis and chronic hepatitis have been discussed above. The clinical and laboratory features of patients with inflammatory bowel disease and cirrhosis vary. Some patients are asymptomatic and have minimal abnormalities of liver tests.[21] Other patients have overt symptoms and signs of liver disease and marked abnormalities in liver tests. The clinical and laboratory features in symptomatic patients are similar to those seen in patients with chronic pericholangitis or chronic hepatitis (discussed earlier). In more advanced cases, complications of portal venous hypertension[21, 33, 68] or hepatic decompensation[21] may occur.

Natural History

Life expectancy is decreased by cirrhosis. However, in the majority of reports the follow-up periods have not been long enough to allow definite conclusions. The presence of inflammatory bowel disease does not appear to influence the course of patients with cirrhosis as compared with that of cirrhotic patients without inflammatory bowel disease. Hemorrhage from esophageal varices may occur in the former group, and recurrence can be prevented by portal-systemic shunting.[33, 68] In patients with cirrhosis and ulcerative colitis or Crohn's colitis, bleeding can occur from varices of the ileal stoma following colectomy.[21, 108-121] In severe cases, portal-systemic shunt surgery has controlled the ileal bleeding.[119-121] In one patient, liver transplantation resulted in decompression of peristomal varices.[121] Risk factors for the development of peristomal bleeding following colectomy in patients with hepatobiliary disease include cirrhosis, splenomegaly, esophageal varices, low serum albumin, prolonged prothrombin time, and thrombocytopenia.[121] In such patients, a proctocolectomy with ileoanal anastomosis should be considered, since perirectal bleeding has not been observed.[121] Hepatoma has been reported to occur in patients with ulcerative colitis as a late complication of macronodular cirrhosis.[21, 56, 122]

Pathogenesis

The relationship of pericholangitis and chronic hepatitis to the development of cirrhosis in patients with inflammatory bowel disease is unknown. Most authors postulate that these disorders cause the majority of cases of cirrhosis in association with inflammatory bowel disease. Cholangiography or surgery has been performed in only a small proportion of patients with cirrhosis to assess the presence of mechanical biliary obstruction or sclerosing cholangitis.[31, 49, 58]

In recent series employing cholangiography and liver biopsy for the diagnosis of primary sclerosing cholangitis,

cirrhosis has been very common.[36, 38, 59, 123] The series of Steckman et al. is notable because five patients were evaluated for hepatobiliary disease before the clinical onset of ulcerative colitis.[36] Each of the five had primary sclerosing cholangitis; one had cirrhosis at initial presentation, one developed cirrhosis during follow-up, and in two patients their disease progressed to severe fibrosis. Eight of 18 patients (44 per cent) with classic large-duct sclerosing cholangitis studied at the Mayo Clinic had cirrhosis.[38] Among an additional group of patients with primary sclerosing cholangitis and ulcerative colitis at the same institution, 5 of 23 (22 per cent) had cirrhosis.[59] Over a period of two to eight years, Schrumpf et al. noted progression of disease in 14 patients with primary sclerosing cholangitis and ulcerative colitis.[123] Thus, primary sclerosing cholangitis appears to be the most important disease contributing to cirrhosis in patients with inflammatory bowel disease.

As mentioned in the discussion of pericholangitis, the histologic features of mechanical obstruction and sclerosing cholangitis can be indistinguishable from those of pericholangitis, and both can progress to cirrhosis. The diagnosis of primary biliary cirrhosis in early reports of patients with inflammatory bowel disease is probably erroneous.[28] There is no evidence that primary biliary cirrhosis contributes to the incidence of cirrhosis in patients with inflammatory bowel disease, although coincidental occurrence of primary biliary cirrhosis has been reported.[124, 125]

Therapy

There is no effective treatment for established fibrosis or cirrhosis. Therapy should be directed instead against the process(es) responsible for continued hepatocellular necrosis and fibrogenesis (see the sections on Pericholangitis, Chronic Hepatitis, and Primary Sclerosing Cholangitis). Colectomy has been advised, but its effectiveness is unproved.[21, 22, 33, 56]

AMYLOIDOSIS

Amyloid infiltration of the liver has been reported to occur in patients with both ulcerative colitis and Crohn's disease.[11, 16, 18, 19, 22, 23, 56, 115, 126-128] The amyloidosis has been suspected generally on the basis of extrahepatic manifestations such as nephropathy, although in several reports amyloidosis was disclosed by liver biopsy in the absence of any previous clinical suspicion.

Pathology

Hepatic amyloid has been detected in patients with inflammatory bowel disease on the basis of its affinity for Congo red. The distribution of the amyloid includes the media of vessels in the portal tract and the reticulin framework of the hepatic cords. Atrophy of hepatocytes may occur as a secondary consequence of compression. It is now recognized that the major protein components of amyloid fibrils vary in different organs, and that specific protein components are related to distinct clinicopathologic conditions.[129] Currently, the term reactive systemic amyloidosis is preferred over the older term secondary amyloidosis[129] to describe the type of amyloidosis seen in patients with inflammatory bowel disease. The major fibrillar protein in reactive systemic amyloidosis is AA, and the characteristic sites of deposition are the liver, spleen, and kidney (see Chapter 53).

Frequency and Clinical Features

Amyloidosis of the liver or other organs is rare among patients with inflammatory bowel disease and occurs more often in patients with Crohn's disease.[11, 16, 18, 19, 22, 23, 56, 128] Shorvon, in a recent review of the association between amyloidosis and inflammatory bowel disease, summarized the findings in 41 patients reported since 1936.[128] He excluded 9 patients because of inadequate diagnostic information. Of the remaining 33 patients, 18 had Crohn's disease and 15 were reported to have ulcerative colitis. The majority of the 15 cases of ulcerative colitis, however, were diagnosed prior to the clinical recognition of Crohn's colitis and 14 had features suggesting the diagnosis of Crohn's colitis. These features included jejunal or ileal disease, fistulae, perianal disease, rectal sparing, and inflammation of the full thickness of the colon. Eade, using pathologic changes in colectomy specimens as the diagnostic criterion for ulcerative colitis, found one case of hepatic amyloidosis among 132 consecutive patients with ulcerative colitis undergoing colectomy and liver biopsy.[56] Others have also noted that reactive systemic amyloidosis is rare in ulcerative colitis.[127] Amyloidosis occurs in patients with Crohn's disease regardless of the site of anatomic involvement. For example, amyloidosis was found in 1 of 62 patients with Crohn's colitis, 3 of 223 with ileocolitis, and 1 of 213 with exclusive small bowel involvement.[115] All 5 of these patients had renal involvement; hepatic involvement, although anticipated, was not mentioned.

Clinical features have not been reported in most articles describing amyloidosis in inflammatory bowel disease, except for the frequent occurrence of proteinuria. It is important to note, however, that the majority of patients with amyloidosis also have foci of chronic suppuration as extraintestinal complications of their inflammatory bowel disease.[128] In addition, some patients have chronic rheumatic diseases such as rheumatoid arthritis or ankylosing spondylitis.[126, 127] The results of laboratory tests of patients with amyloidosis and inflammatory bowel disease have not been reported. Based on the general experience with hepatic amyloidosis, evidence of hepatocellular necrosis is rare even with extensive deposition. Slight elevations of alkaline phosphatase, and, rarely, of bilirubin may occur.

Pathogenesis

Amyloid deposition in the liver is presumed to be secondary to chronic inflammation analogous to the amyloidoses associated with other chronic suppurative processes. The mechanism is unknown. The rare occurrence of amyloidosis in patients without extraintestinal foci of chronic suppuration or rheumatic disease suggests that inflammation of the bowel alone generally is insufficient to produce amyloidosis.

Prognosis and Treatment

Progressive amyloidosis is fatal if untreated. In reactive systemic amyloidosis, the nature of the underlying disease and the rate of amyloid deposition determine the prognosis. Control of the underlying disease, in certain circumstances,

has led to clinical recovery,[129] but the applicability of this observation to patients with inflammatory bowel disease remains undefined. In experimental models of reactive systemic amyloidosis, deposition can be increased by corticosteroids.[129] Despite these data, it seems unreasonable to withhold the use of corticosteroids if they are needed for the management of the inflammatory bowel disease. There is no information concerning the possible usefulness of either colchicine or dimethyl sulfoxide in the treatment of hepatic amyloidosis associated with inflammatory bowel disease.[129] Attempts to control extraintestinal foci of inflammation are rational, but may be difficult or impossible to accomplish.

HEPATIC GRANULOMAS

Hepatic granulomas (see Chapter 41) have been reported in several series.[16, 19, 21–23, 27, 118, 119] The majority have been found in patients with Crohn's disease, although they also are seen in association with ulcerative colitis.[34, 38, 56] Frequencies in reported series range from zero to 15 per cent. The reports of Eade et al. describing patients with ulcerative colitis or Crohn's disease of either the small bowel or the colon suggest a frequency of approximately 8 per cent.[22, 23, 56] In the series of Wee and Ludwig, granulomas were present in 4 per cent and were most frequently attributed to sarcoidosis.[38]

Pathology

The term hepatic granulomatosis describes the pathologic features more accurately than does the term granulomatous hepatitis. The granulomas are noncaseating and are located in both the portal tracts and the parenchyma. Epithelioid giant cells have been present occasionally. In several instances, aggregates of lymphocytes and histiocytes have been described as "granuloma-like."[22, 23] Granulomas may be found alone or in association with fibrosis, fatty liver, pericholangitis, or cirrhosis.[19] Only one patient reported as having primary biliary cirrhosis in association with inflammatory bowel disease had hepatic granulomas.[125]

Clinical Features and Prognosis

Available clinical detail is insufficient to assess whether patients with hepatic granulomatosis and inflammatory bowel disease have any pathognomonic features. The majority are asymptomatic, and the abnormality found most commonly on laboratory testing is elevation of alkaline phosphatase. The prognosis for patients with hepatic granulomas and inflammatory bowel disease is good. Such patients have not developed progressive liver disease or cirrhosis. One cirrhotic patient with ulcerative colitis, however, was found to have granulomas on repeat biopsy two years after the diagnosis of cirrhosis.[27] Another patient with hepatic granulomas and mild pericholangitis at the time of colectomy for ulcerative colitis subsequently developed a cholangiocarcinoma of the common bile duct.[47] Granulomas also were noted in a patient with chronic active hepatitis associated with ulcerative colitis.[34]

Pathogenesis

The cause of hepatic granulomas in association with inflammatory bowel disease remains unknown, and may be multifactorial. Obvious infectious factors in the causation of granulomas have not been reported, and four patients in one series were thought to have sarcoidosis.[21, 38] It is plausible that granulomas result from an infrequent immune reaction to substances in portal venous blood or to deposits of immune complexes. The possibility of a drug-related pathogenesis is intriguing, since hepatic granulomas may occur as a consequence of sulfonamide hepatotoxicity.[132] Callen and Soderstrom reported one case of documented sulfasalazine-induced hepatic granulomas in a patient with ulcerative colitis,[133] but no other example has been published.

Therapy

No specific therapy has been proposed for hepatic granulomas in patients with inflammatory bowel disease. Treatment should be directed toward the inflammatory bowel disease itself. The role of colectomy in the management of hepatic granulomas in patients with colitis is unknown. Eade et al. reported the results of repeat liver biopsies of two patients with hepatic granulomas three and six years after colectomy for Crohn's colitis.[22] Granulomas were decreased in number in one biopsy specimen and absent in the other.

MISCELLANEOUS DISORDERS

Several hepatic disorders have been reported to occur in only a few patients with inflammatory bowel disease. The associations between most of these disorders and the inflammatory bowel disease, therefore, appear to be coincidental. Pyogenic hepatic abscess represents a specific exception.

Hepatic Abscess. Prior to the availability of broad-spectrum antimicrobial therapy, pylephlebitis and pyogenic liver abscess were associated frequently with severe inflammatory bowel disease. Today, hepatic abscesses in patients with inflammatory bowel disease are rare.

Portal Vein Thrombosis. Chapin et al. reported four patients with Crohn's disease who developed thrombosis of the portal vein,[16] and Stauffer et al. found this complication in a patient with ulcerative colitis.[52]

Hepatic Infarction. Two patients dying of Crohn's disease had evidence of acute hepatic infarction and portal vein thrombosis at autopsy.[16]

Hepatic Venous Occlusion. Hepatic venous occlusion has been reported to occur in several patients with ulcerative colitis.[134] In one patient, acute Budd-Chiari syndrome was the result of extrinsic compression of the hepatic veins by an anaplastic carcinoma of the bile duct.

Hepatic Sinusoidal Dilatation. Sinusoidal dilatation has been found rarely in patients with Crohn's disease.[135, 136] Two reported patients were using oral contraceptives, which have been implicated in the pathogenesis of this lesion.[137]

Hepatoma. Hepatoma has been reported to occur in patients with macronodular cirrhosis and ulcerative colitis.[21, 56, 122]

Hemosiderosis. Perrett et al. reported that hemosiderosis was present in one patient with ulcerative colitis[11] and two patients with Crohn's disease.[20] Iron was present both in the hepatocytes and in the Kupffer cells in the patient with ulcerative colitis, who had a history of anemia and repeated transfusions. One of the patients with Crohn's disease had cirrhosis.

Sarcoidosis. Sarcoidosis of the liver has been reported in four patients with ulcerative colitis.[21, 38]

Benign Neoplasia of the Bile Ducts. Palmer et al. reported one patient with ulcerative colitis and secondary biliary cirrhosis who had a benign cholangioma.[27]

Primary Biliary Cirrhosis. Early reports of primary biliary cirrhosis in association with inflammatory bowel disease may have been erroneous because rigorous diagnostic criteria were unavailable and primary sclerosing cholangitis was not excluded.[28] However, recently two patients with unequivocal primary biliary cirrhosis and ulcerative colitis have been described.[124, 125]

α_1-Antitrypsin Deficiency. Two patients with heterozygous α_1-antitrypsin deficiency were identified among 681 patients followed for ulcerative colitis in Oxford.[35] Both had persistently abnormal liver tests and low serum concentrations of α_1-antitrypsin. Each had the PiM$_1$Z phenotype, and immunoreactive granules of α_1-antitrypsin were identified in both biopsy specimens. Typical PAS-positive, diastase-resistant granules, however, were present in only one patient.

DISEASES OF THE BILIARY TRACT

PRIMARY SCLEROSING CHOLANGITIS

Primary sclerosing cholangitis is a chronic cholestatic liver disease characterized by fibrosing inflammation of segments of the extrahepatic bile ducts, with or without involvement of the intrahepatic ducts.[35, 38, 59, 124, 138–140] It results in progressive narrowing or obliteration of the bile duct lumens, associated with clinical and biochemical evidence of cholestasis and progression to secondary biliary cirrhosis, portal hypertension, and hepatic failure. Introduction of endoscopic retrograde cholangiography in the early 1970s has resulted in a marked increase in the frequency of diagnosis[141] and has greatly contributed to the understanding of the clinical, radiologic, and histologic features of the disease. Despite these advances, the cause remains unknown, and no curative therapy has been identified.

Disease Associations

Inflammatory bowel disease occurs in 50 to 75 per cent of patients with primary sclerosing cholangitis.[31, 32, 138–141] The vast majority have ulcerative colitis; a small minority have Crohn's disease. In addition to inflammatory bowel disease, primary sclerosing cholangitis is associated with a variety of other conditions, including thyroiditis (Riedel's struma),[142] retroperitoneal fibrosis,[142, 143] mediastinal fibrosis,[144] pseudotumor of the orbit,[145] vasculitis,[143] immunodeficiency states,[146] porphyria cutanea tarda,[147] Peyronie's disease,[148] pyoderma gangrenosum,[149] bronchiectasis,[150] angioblastic lymphadenopathy,[151] histiocytosis X,[152, 153] chronic pancreatitis,[154, 155] Sjögren's syndrome,[154] massive intra-abdominal adenopathy,[156] hypereosinophilia,[157] immune thrombocytopenia purpura,[158] and lupus anticoagulant.[159] The majority of these reported associations appear to be coincidental.

Twenty-five to 50 per cent of cases of primary sclerosing cholangitis occur in otherwise healthy individuals. Despite the legitimate question of whether primary sclerosing cholangitis in association with inflammatory bowel disease represents the same pathologic process seen in healthy individuals or patients with other associated illnesses, no compelling evidence suggests that the processes are different. The clinical, biochemical, histologic, and cholangiographic features of primary sclerosing cholangitis appear to be identical in patients with or without inflammatory bowel disease.

Diagnostic Criteria

Classic criteria for the diagnosis of primary sclerosing cholangitis include (1) absence of previous biliary tract surgery, (2) absence of cholelithiasis, (3) diffuse involvement of the extrahepatic biliary tract, and (4) exclusion of cholangiocarcinoma. Warren has argued that strict adherence to these criteria will lead to a correct diagnosis in many cases of primary sclerosing cholangitis, but that indiscriminate application of the first three will exclude some cases of primary sclerosing cholangitis and hence underestimate both the frequency and the clinicopathologic spectrum of the disease.[160] Currently, the diagnostic criteria have been modified to include patients with cholelithiasis confined to the gallbladder.[31, 38, 59, 138-141] In each patient, primary sclerosing cholangitis must be distinguished from secondary sclerosing cholangitis, which may occur as a consequence of biliary surgery, choledocholithiasis, or cholangiocarcinoma. Differentiating benign strictures of primary sclerosing cholangitis from sclerosis due to cholangiocarcinoma is not always possible and represents the major diagnostic difficulty. Utilizing prolonged follow-up to exclude cholangiocarcinoma is inappropriate since cholangiocarcinoma develops de novo in approximately 10 per cent of patients with primary sclerosing cholangitis.[161, 162] Cholangiographic features suggestive of cholangiocarcinoma include (1) excessive dilatation of ducts, (2) polypoid masses, (3) and progression of ductular dilatation or stricturing.

The lack of standardized nomenclature contributes to continued confusion regarding the relationship between pericholangitis, chronic active hepatitis and primary sclerosing cholangitis. As discussed earlier, the term pericholangitis has been omitted from recently standardized nomenclature even though its spectrum of features is poorly encompassed by the designation "chronic active hepatitis associated with inflammatory bowel disease."[62] In primary sclerosing cholangitis, cholangiographic diagnostic criteria are well established,[139, 162] but nomenclature has not been devised for the hepatic histopathology.[59] In early studies, some investigators describe pericholangitis concurrent with sclerosing cholangitis,[65, 164] whereas others accept the diagnosis of pericholangitis only in the presence of normal bile ducts.[45] It is now well established that many patients with inflammatory bowel disease diagnosed as having pericholangitis actually had primary sclerosing cholangitis.[35, 38, 48, 49, 58, 59, 65] Cholangiography of additional patients with pericholangitis demonstrated sclerosis of the intrahepatic bile ducts without involvement of the extrahepatic bile ducts.[35, 48] The relationship between sclerosing lesions limited to the intrahepatic ducts and typical primary sclerosing cholangitis remains debatable. Some authors believe the sclerosis limited to the intrahepatic bile ducts is a variant of primary sclerosing cholangitis.[32, 35, 38, 48, 59, 143, 165, 166] Thorpe and colleagues suggest that pericholangitis may reflect the intrahepatic component of a syndrome in which typical primary sclerosing cholangitis represents the extrahepatic component,[58, 65] and Wee and Ludwig suggest that intrahepatic ("small-duct") sclerosing cholangitis may progress to large-duct sclerosing cholangitis.[59] Thus, some investigators now

doubt whether pericholangitis exists as a clinical entity distinct from primary sclerosing cholangitis.[32, 59] It is important to note, however, that the frequency of primary sclerosing cholangitis in patients with inflammatory bowel disease remains substantially less than the reported frequency of pericholangitis. Moreover, the bile ducts have been reported to be normal in several well-studied patients with pericholangitis,[43, 64] and serial evaluations show that the majority of such patients do not progress to primary sclerosing cholangitis.[59] These findings suggest either that primary sclerosing cholangitis is a distinct entity or that, if it is a consequence of pericholangitis, it develops in only a fraction of patients with pericholangitis. Further studies employing both liver biopsy and cholangiography are needed to clarify the relationship between pericholangitis, chronic active hepatitis, and sclerosing cholangitis. Thus, all patients with liver biopsies consistent with the diagnosis of pericholangitis or chronic active hepatitis should have endoscopic retrograde cholangiography to evaluate the extra- and intrahepatic bile ducts.

Pathology

Fibrosing inflammation of the common bile duct, hepatic ducts, and intrahepatic ducts result in stenosis of the lumens and thickening of the walls without dilatation.[139, 163] Stenosis may be present throughout the course of the common bile duct or only in isolated segments. Involvement of the intrahepatic ducts is characterized most commonly by segmental stenosis. Involved segments of bile ducts in strictured areas show diffuse fibrotic thickening and infiltration of the submucosal and subserosal areas with mononuclear inflammatory cells.[167] The mucosal surface appears relatively normal by light microscopy. Electron microscopy of ductular epithelial cells in interlobular bile ducts has shown decreases in the numbers of organelles, fibrils, and intercellular junctions. Moreover, reduplication of the basement membrane has been present,[167] and finger-like projections have been observed on the basal surface of the bile ducts.[168] Point contacts between lymphocytes and biliary epithelial cells occasionally have been seen.

The histologic appearances of the liver in primary sclerosing cholangitis may be quite variable in specimens obtained by percutaneous needle biopsy, depending on the presence or absence of involvement of the intrahepatic bile ducts, the duration of the disease, and the number of sections examined.[38, 59, 139, 168] The range of findings includes relatively normal-appearing interlobular ducts, portal tract inflammation with a predominantly periductular distribution, sclerosis of the bile ducts, formation of bile lakes, periportal fibrosis, intrahepatic cholestasis, bile ductopenia, and hepatocellular (piecemeal) necrosis.[31, 32, 38, 59, 139, 169] Thus, the histologic findings may encompass features of "pericholangitis," extrahepatic biliary obstruction, chronic active hepatitis, or rarely, primary biliary cirrhosis.[31, 32] In cases of long-standing biliary obstruction, secondary biliary cirrhosis is common.[38, 59, 139, 169] Accumulation of hepatic copper in primary sclerosing cholangitis results from biliary obstruction.[31, 32, 59, 139, 169, 170] The copper is confined primarily within lipolysosomes.[59]

Given the wide spectrum of histopathologic abnormalities and the absence of defined nomenclature, it is not surprising that liver biopsies are not diagnostic for primary sclerosing cholangitis. The most characteristic histopathologic features observed in primary sclerosing cholangitis (in order of frequency) are (1) bile duct proliferation,

(2) periductal fibrosis, (3) periductal inflammation, and (4) loss of bile ducts.[59] The presence of fibrous obliterative cholangitis is strongly associated with the diagnosis, but is observed infrequently in needle biopsy specimens.[59, 139] In the absence of diagnostic features, Ludwig et al. have proposed a classification subdividing the disease into four stages.[59] Stage I is characterized by changes confined to the portal tract such as portal inflammation, connective tissue expansion, and cholangitis. Stage II is characterized by extension of the fibrosis and inflammation into the periportal parenchyma, resulting in piecemeal necrosis and periportal fibrosis. Stage III is characterized by the formation of fibrous septa extending from the portal tract or bridging necrosis. Stage IV is characterized by biliary cirrhosis. Despite prolonged necroinflammatory disease of the liver and the development of cirrhosis, hepatocellular carcinoma does not occur.[31, 38, 59]

Gallstones are present infrequently in the gallbladders of patients with primary sclerosing cholangitis,[51, 65, 160, 171] although histologic changes of chronic cholecystitis have been found in more than 20 per cent of such patients.[65, 160, 171] Occasionally choledocholithiasis is found in the absence of stones in the gallbladder; this may occur as a secondary consequence of bile stasis caused by the sclerosing process.[166] Lymph nodes in the porta hepatitis frequently are enlarged as a result of hyperplasia.

The pancreatic duct may also be involved with sclerosis,[139, 172] and chronic pancreatitis has been reported.[154, 155] The frequency of pancreatic duct involvement is unknown but appears to be rare. In a recent study of 38 patients with primary sclerosing cholangitis evaluated by retrograde pancreatography, none had abnormalities of the pancreatic duct.[173]

Frequency

Primary sclerosing cholangitis is predominantly associated with ulcerative colitis,[31, 38, 54, 65, 138–141, 166]. It has also been found in several patients with Crohn's disease.[21, 31, 174] In patients with Crohn's disease, primary sclerosing cholangitis has been associated almost exclusively with either colitis or ileocolitis.[21, 31] An association with Crohn's disease limited to the small bowel has been reported in only a single case.[174]

In early reports, the prevalence of inflammatory bowel disease in patients with primary sclerosing cholangitis was approximately 30 per cent.[160] Results of recent studies suggest that the prevalence of inflammatory bowel disease in patients with primary sclerosing cholangitis may be as high as 54 to 72 per cent.[31, 32] Primary sclerosing cholangitis, however, remains uncommon. The frequency of primary sclerosing cholangitis in patients with inflammatory bowel disease has been estimated to be less than 1 per cent,[160] although a prospective study of 336 patients with ulcerative colitis demonstrated a prevalence of 4 per cent.[49] Serial study of 681 patients with ulcerative colitis has shown a prevalence of primary sclerosing cholangitis of 2.4 per cent.[35]

Clinical Features

Primary sclerosing cholangitis can affect any age group, having been reported in infancy,[175] in childhood,[176, 177] and throughout adult life.[139] Currently, 60 to 70 per cent of patients are male and two thirds are less than 45 years of age at the time of diagnosis.[31, 138–140] In patients with inflammatory bowel disease and primary sclerosing cholangitis, the clinical features do not differ from those in patients without inflammatory bowel disease. At presentation, patients may be asymptomatic with respect to their hepatobiliary disease or may exhibit persistent or intermittent symptoms and signs of cholestatic liver disease. Common presenting features include intermittent, fluctuating jaundice, pruritus, nausea, abdominal pain, vomiting, and fever.[31, 32, 160] These occur with fatigue, malaise, diminished appetite, and, usually, weight loss. Symptoms of cholangitis usually are not found when the patients are first examined[31, 32, 138–141] because bacterial cholangitis prior to surgical exploration is rare.[178] Symptoms have been present for periods ranging from weeks to more than ten years prior to the diagnosis;[160] the majority of patients have had symptoms for two years before diagnosis.[138–141] Asymptomatic patients are being recognized with increasing frequency.[138–141, 179] Results of initial physical examinations are normal for approximately 50 per cent of patients.[31, 138] Patients with abnormal findings frequently have jaundice and hepatomegaly with or without splenomegaly. Less than 50 per cent show tenderness to palpation of the right upper quadrant.[160] Vascular spiders, ascites, and clubbing are unusual.

Laboratory Tests

The results of laboratory tests in primary sclerosing cholangitis are variable.[31, 32, 49, 138–141, 160] During clinical episodes of cholestasis or cholangitis, leukocytosis may be present. Alkaline phosphatase activity usually is elevated, often to very high levels, but it can be normal even in advanced histologic stages of disease.[180] In the study by Schrumpf et al., alkaline phosphatase activity was found to be significantly greater in patients with primary sclerosing cholangitis than in patients with other hepatobiliary diseases complicating ulcerative colitis.[49] Total bilirubin is increased in approximately 50 per cent of patients.[31, 138] Aminotransferase activities may be normal or moderately elevated; mild elevations occur in more than 90 per cent of patients.[138] Hypoalbuminemia and abnormal prothrombin times are infrequently present, having been found in 17 per cent and 6 per cent of patients, respectively, in a recent study.[31] Hypergammaglobulinemia occurs in approximately 30 per cent of patients, and IgM is increased selectively in 45 per cent of patients.[32] Three recent series[31, 32, 138] confirm the earlier findings of Thorpe et al.[65] that autoantibodies are rare in patients with primary sclerosing cholangitis. Antimitochondrial, antinuclear, and anti–smooth muscle antibodies are present in only 5 to 10 per cent of patients, and the titers are low. Primary sclerosing cholangitis is associated with secondary abnormalities similar to those accompanying other syndromes of obstructive cholestasis (see Chapter 12).[181] These include increased levels of unesterified cholesterol and phospholipid, abnormal low-density lipoproteins, liability for the formation of pigmented gallstones, changes in the proportions of primary bile acids and the urinary excretion of sulfated bile acid, and malabsorption of fat and fat-soluble vitamins.

Diagnosis

Primary sclerosing cholangitis is diagnosed by exclusion. The most important diagnostic test is cholangiography. The pathologic process favors the use of endoscopic retrograde cholangiography over the percutaneous transhepatic approach.[32, 33, 38, 59, 138-141] The use of intravenous cholangiography for the subgroup of patients with only slight elevations of bilirubin is unjustified because of the inferior quality of the detail obtained.[182] In approximately 75 per cent of patients, the process diffusely involves the extra- and intrahepatic ducts, often segmentally. Involvement of intrahepatic ducts results in stenotic areas with adjacent areas of ectasia (Fig. 43–3). This appearance often is reminiscent of Caroli's disease (see Chapter 52).[183] Sclerosis of the bile ducts also may occur in cholangiocarcinoma, and differentiation between carcinoma and sclerosing cholangitis can be difficult. It is especially important to consider the possibility of cholangiocarcinoma in patients with inflammatory bowel disease because the incidences of malignancies of the bile ducts and gallbladder are increased in these patients (discussed later), and cholangiocarcinoma may develop de novo in patients with primary sclerosing cholangitis.[162] Other diseases such as metastatic carcinoma, lymphoma, cirrhosis, and polycystic liver disease may cause narrowing and deformity of bile ducts; however, they do not cause the characteristic beaded appearance of primary sclerosing cholangitis.[163]

The role of the liver biopsy in the diagnosis of primary sclerosing cholangitis is equivocal. The disease is segmental and, as mentioned earlier, the histologic features overlap those seen in pericholangitis, extrahepatic biliary obstruction, chronic active hepatitis, and primary biliary cirrhosis.[31, 32, 33, 38, 59] The results of biopsy are often consistent only with the diagnosis.

Natural History and Prognosis

The natural history of primary sclerosing cholangitis is incompletely understood. This is especially true for asymptomatic patients and the subgroup of patients with disease confined to the intrahepatic ducts. Recent recognition of patients without elevations of alkaline phosphatase[180] and large groups of asymptomatic patients suggests that the disease may evolve through four sequential phases.[183] The earliest, or preclinical, phase occurs in the absence

of hepatobiliary symptoms or cholestatic abnormalities of standard liver tests. Patients in this phase of disease would be virtually undetectable unless evaluated for nonspecific complaints. Indeed, patients reported by the Mayo Clinic had cholangiography primarily to evaluate chronic abdominal pain. The patients evaluated were five men and five women with a mean age of 46 years. Cholangiographic evidence of extra- and intrahepatic duct sclerosis was present in each, and eight of the ten patients had inflammatory bowel disease. Serial evaluation confirmed that the alkaline phosphatase and bilirubin remained normal, and causes of alkaline phosphatase reduction were excluded (e.g., hypophosphatasia, pernicious anemia, hypothyroidism, and substances that can interfere with the assay). Similarly, causes of secondary sclerosing cholangitis were also excluded. Despite the absence of hepatobiliary symptoms or elevated alkaline phosphatase, the disease in three of the ten patients was in advanced histological stages on liver biopsy: two had stage III lesions and one had biliary cirrhosis. Further follow-up is required to assess the duration of this phase. The second sequential phase is characterized by asymptomatic cholestatic abnormalities of liver tests with elevation of alkaline phosphatase. Modest elevations of aminotransferases also may occur, but the bilirubin is usually normal. Physical examination may be normal; however, up to 45 per cent of patients have hepatomegaly and occasional patients have stigmata of advanced disease. Recent reports emphasize that primary sclerosing cholangitis is being diagnosed with increasing frequency in this phase.[31, 35, 123, 140, 141, 184, 185] It remains unclear whether this primarily reflects increased physician awareness and application of cholangiography or an increase in incidence. This phase can be quite prolonged; in a recent retrospective analysis, asymptomatic patients did not develop symptomatic disease during an average of 4.7 years of observation.[141] The third, or symptomatic, phase refers to that period when patients exhibit a variety of hepatobiliary symptoms. The most frequent symptoms are fatigue, pruritus, jaundice, dark urine, and light stools. Fever, abdominal pain, episodic jaundice, and acute ascending cholangitis occur in a minority of patients. Physical examination frequently reveals jaundice, hepatomegaly, and splenomegaly. The

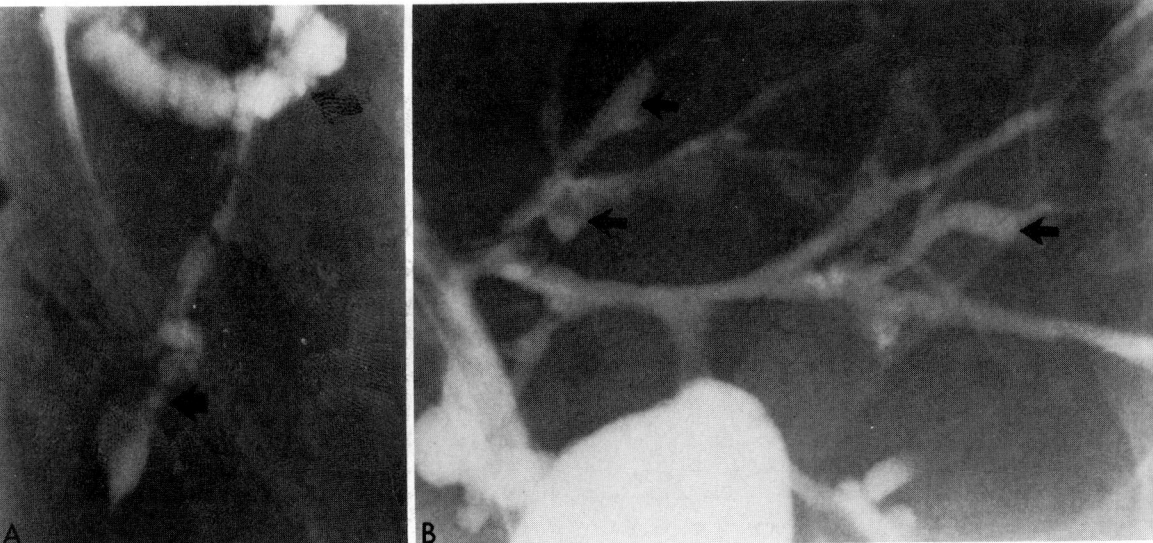

Figure 43–3. Cholangiogram from a patient with ulcerative colitis complicated by sclerosing cholangitis. *A,* The common bile duct (straight arrow) is narrowed and irregular. The cystic duct (curved arrow) is normal. *B,* Intrahepatic bile ducts are irregular, with stenotic areas alternating with areas of saccular dilatation (arrows). (Courtesy of Dr. Thomas Boyer.)

clinical features in patients with associated inflammatory bowel disease do not differ from those in patients without inflammatory bowel disease. In addition, the pattern of bile duct involvement does not differ in symptomatic and asymptomatic patients with primary sclerosing cholangitis.[31, 138, 141, 184, 185] Prospective and retrospective analyses indicate that symptoms and biochemical abnormalities progress with time.[31, 138, 139, 141, 184]

IV) The fourth or terminal phase of the disease is characterized by decompensated cirrhosis, complication of portal hypertension, and hepatic failure. In adults, partial biliary obstruction leads to cirrhosis over variable periods of time, generally taking 5 to 11 years. In the study by Warren et al., 7 of 12 patients had clinical evidence of portal venous hypertension at the time of laparotomy for jaundice. Nine of 12 patients progressed to cirrhosis in an average follow-up period of 4.5 years.[160] Secondary biliary cirrhosis may develop or progress despite apparent surgical relief of biliary strictures.

The prognosis of patients with primary sclerosing cholangitis differs in recent reports, depending on the proportion of symptomatic patients within the study group.[31, 32, 35, 38, 123, 138, 141, 184] Of 39 symptomatic patients, 13 (33 per cent) died between 5 and 108 months after diagnosis.[31] Ten of the 13 patients had portal venous hypertension, and 6 of the 13 had cirrhosis. Of interest, 7 of these 13 patients had inflammatory bowel disease. Liver failure was the most common cause of death and occurred in 11 of the 13 patients. Of 26 survivors followed for 6 to 110 months after diagnosis, 12 had clinical evidence of portal venous hypertension and cirrhosis. Chapman et al. reported a similarly high mortality rate in symptomatic patients with primary sclerosing cholangitis and inflammatory bowel disease.[32] In their series, 10 of the 11 patients who died had ulcerative colitis. A recent retrospective study of 38 patients (29 symptomatic at presentation) showed a poor prognosis in 45 per cent during a mean follow-up period of 6.3 ± 4.9 years.[184] During this period, 11 patients (29 per cent) died and 6 (16 per cent) developed variceal hemorrhage or encephalopathy or required hepatic transplantation. It is noteworthy that a poor outcome was not confined to symptomatic patients; 5 of 9 asymptomatic patients had a similar outcome.

In contrast, other studies of asymptomatic patients suggest a much better prognosis. During prolonged observation, Schrumpf et al. observed only 2 deaths in 18 asymptomatic patients with primary sclerosing cholangitis; 1 died of cholangiocarcinoma, the other from nonhepatic causes.[123] The remaining 16 were observed for an average of 6 years (range 3 to 13 years). Ten remained asymptomatic, four had intermittent symptoms, and two developed signs and symptoms of advanced disease. The majority of laboratory tests were stable, but bilirubin elevation progressed in four patients. Progressive worsening of cholangiographic findings were observed, but was unassociated with worsening of clinical, biochemical or histopathological features. During a mean follow-up of 6.8 years, asymptomatic patients had a significantly better prognosis than symptomatic patients.[185] Among 136 symptomatic patients, death occurred in 31 (23 per cent) compared to a single death among 38 asymptomatic patients (2.6 per cent). Ten-year actuarial survival was calculated to be 93 per cent in asymptomatic patients and 47 per cent in symptomatic patients. Recently, Helzberg et al. reported a retrospective analysis of 53 patients, indicating an improved survival among both symptomatic and asymptomatic patients.[141] During a mean follow-up of 4.7 years, most patients did not progress symptomatically. Calculation of actuarial survival indicated that 75 per cent of patients survived for nine years. Multivariate analysis showed that elevated bilirubin and hepatomegaly at presentation independently correlated with a poor prognosis, although the cholangiographic pattern of duct involvement, the presence or absence of inflammatory bowel disease, advanced histologic stages, and age did not. Unique features of this population included a higher percentage of older, asymptomatic females and a substantial number of patients with disease confined to the intrahepatic ducts.

Continued study of the natural history of different subgroups is imperative to define positive and negative prognostic features. These are needed to determine the appropriate time for hepatic transplantation and to design rational, controlled clinical trials of therapy.

Pathogenesis

The cause of primary sclerosing cholangitis and the mechanisms responsible for its progression are unknown.[138] The significant association with inflammatory bowel disease, especially colitis, raises the same speculations discussed in the section on Pericholangitis. Several caveats are required for discussion of current theories of pathogenesis. First, despite identification of several mechanisms of possible pathogenetic significance, our current knowledge is inadequate to interpret the significance of many observations, particularly those related to the putative role of the host's immune response. Second, the postulated mechanisms are not mutually exclusive and, therefore, could act in concert or sequentially during different phases of the disease. Third, it is likely that mechanisms responsible for initiation of disease may differ from those responsible for perpetuation. Fourth, postulated mechanisms should account for the diffuse infiltration of the portal tracts with T lymphocytes, the characteristic periductular fibrosis resulting in atrophy and obliteration of bile ducts, the focal nature of the diffuse annular fibrosis of extra- and intrahepatic ducts, and the occurrence of periportal fibrosis and piecemeal necrosis of hepatocytes. Fifth, the noxious effects of retained bile may contribute independently to progressive fibrosis and the development of biliary cirrhosis.

Table 43–5 summarizes the pathogenetic mechanisms postulated in primary sclerosing cholangitis. The frequent association of ulcerative colitis has suggested a role for portal bacteremia or absorbed bacterial or colonic toxins in the development of the disease (see section on Pericholangitis). Yet, portal bacteremia is infrequent in ulcerative colitis, experimental lesions are dissimilar from primary sclerosing cholangitis, and there is no correlation between the duration and severity of colitis and the frequency or severity of primary sclerosing cholangitis. Thus, there is no support for this hypothesis, which also fails to account for the occurrence of primary sclerosing cholangitis in the

TABLE 43–5. FACTORS POSTULATED IN THE PATHOGENESIS OF PRIMARY SCLEROSING CHOLANGITIS

Portal bacteremia
Absorption of toxins
Abnormal or toxic bile acids
Hepatotoxicity of copper
Viral infection
Genetic predisposition
Immunologic mechanisms
Arteriolar injury

absence of colonic inflammation or in patients years after colectomy. A similar hypothesis suggests a noxious role for increased quantities of secondary bile acids that might result from increased intestinal production or absorption. No abnormalities have been detected in portal venous bile acids in inflammatory bowel disease to support this hypothesis.[186]

The potential toxic effects of accumulated hepatic copper also have been postulated as a pathogenetic mechanism. Although copper accumulates in the livers of patients with primary sclerosing cholangitis,[139, 140] it does so as the secondary consequence of the process leading to chronic cholestasis and not as a primary event.[187] Even if excessive copper contributed to hepatocyte injury, it would not account for the focal nature of bile duct lesions or the characteristic involvement of the extrahepatic biliary tract.

Infection of biliary epithelial cells or hepatocytes by unidentified viruses also has been postulated. Reports that Reovirus type 3 can induce cholangitis and biliary atresia in weanling mice,[188, 189] primates, and possibly human neonates[190] led to its proposal as an etiologic agent in primary sclerosing cholangitis. Despite evidence that it can induce experimental fibrosis and obliterative cholangitis, infection of human liver has not been substantiated. Moreover, recent data show that neither the prevalence nor the titer of antibodies to Reovirus type 3 differ between normal adults and patients with primary sclerosing cholangitis.[191] The possibility that hepatitis viruses are involved in the pathogenesis is unsupported by data. Although cytomegalovirus infection affects intrahepatic bile ducts, the histopathology is distinct from that of primary sclerosing cholangitis.[192]

Genetic and familial factors have been postulated to play a role in pathogenesis. Recent studies indicate a strong association between primary biliary cirrhosis and the HLA haplotype B8, DR3, which is known to be associated with a variety of autoimmune diseases.[193, 194] HLA-B8 was present in 60 per cent of patients with primary sclerosing cholangitis with and without ulcerative colitis, compared to 25 per cent of a large control group.[193] An independent study found HLA-B8 in 80 per cent and DR3 in 70 per cent of patients with ulcerative colitis and hepatobiliary disease; the majority had primary sclerosing cholangitis.[194] The occurrence of primary sclerosing cholangitis and ulcerative colitis in siblings from four families supports the concept that genetic factors may influence susceptibility.[140, 155]

Several features of primary sclerosing cholangitis suggest the possibility of an immunopathogenesis. These include the presence of histopathologic lymphoctytic infiltrates, the prevalence of hypergammaglobulinemia, elevations of IgM, and the presence of circulating antibodies reactive with colonic epithelial cells and proliferating bile ductules.[140, 195] The strong association between primary sclerosing cholangitis and inflammatory bowel disease and the increased prevalence of the HLA B8, DR3 haplotype (associated with other autoimmune diseases) have provided circumstantial support for the concept of an immunopathogenesis. Recent studies have demonstrated a variety of immunologic abnormalities in patients with primary sclerosing cholangitis, but their relevance to pathogenesis remains speculative. Specifically, it is unclear whether they are primary events or secondary consequences of the disease process.

Several reports indicate the possibility that biliary epithelial cells may be targets of an immune response. In ulcerative colitis, antibodies bound to an autoantigen present on the surface membranes of colonic epithelium have been identified and used to isolated the antigen.[196] Subsequent studies indicate that a similar antigen also is expressed on the surface of extra- and intrahepatic biliary epithelial cells.[197] Inhibition of leukocyte migration by biliary antigens suggests that patients have been sensitized to these antigens.[198] Recently, enhanced expression of HLA class II antigens on biliary epithelia has been observed in primary sclerosing cholangitis,[199] suggesting that these cells may present self-antigens to host T lymphocytes. Studies of the inflammatory cells infiltrating the portal tracts are consistent with this notion and demonstrate the presence of both CD4 (helper phenotype) and CD8 (cytotoxic/suppressor phenotype), with an increased proportion of the latter.[200] Such findings suggest that biliary epithelial cells are targets of the immune response. However, these findings offer no explanation for the focal nature of biliary injury, the periductular fibrosis with atrophy and obliteration of ducts without nonsuppurative destructive cholangitis, or the involvement of the extrahepatic biliary tract. It is attractive to speculate that the pathology may result from cytokines secreted by inflammatory cells.

Other studies indicative of immunologic abnormalities provide circumstantial support for the concept that alterations of immune function are involved in pathogenesis. Evidence for increased catabolism of C3 suggests activation of the humoral immune system in patients with primary sclerosing cholangitis.[201] In addition, circulating immune complex–like materials have been identified,[202] and diminished clearance of exogenously administered immune complexes suggests a defective reticuloendothelial function.[203] Quantitative abnormalities of T lymphocyte subsets have been identified,[204] and increased reactivity of CD8 (cytotoxic/suppressor) cells to autologous stimuli has been observed in vitro.[205]

Recent reports indicate that direct injury to the peribiliary arteriolar plexus can result in injury to the biliary tract.[206, 207] Figure 43–4 illustrates the anatomic relationship between the bile ducts and the peribiliary arteriolar plexus. Intra-arterial infusion of floxuridine[207] produces diffuse, focal strictures of the extra- and intrahepatic bile ducts and fibrous inflammation of the portal tracts. This lesion is indistinguishable from primary sclerosing cholangitis. Interestingly, strictures most commonly occur in both extra- and intrahepatic ducts, but may also occur in either site exclusively. Experimental embolization of alcohol into the hepatic arteries of Rhesus monkeys resulted in diffuse, focal intrahepatic biliary strictures, mild dilatation of the intervening segments of the bile ducts, and chronic inflammation and fibrosis of the portal tracts.[206] Again, the cholangiographic picture was similar to that seen in primary sclerosing cholangitis. In addition, periarteritis nodosa of the hepatic artery has been associated with cholangiographic findings similar to those in primary sclerosing cholangitis.[206] These data strongly suggest that a pathologic process with many features similar to primary sclerosing cholangitis may be initiated by arterial injury. It is attractive to speculate that immunologic mechanisms may subsequently perpetuate the process.

Treatment

The treatment of primary sclerosing cholangitis has three major goals: (1) symptomatic management of chronic cholestasis, (2) management of complications, and (3) retardation or reversal of the disease process. Despite major progress in the past decade, our ability to fulfill these goals

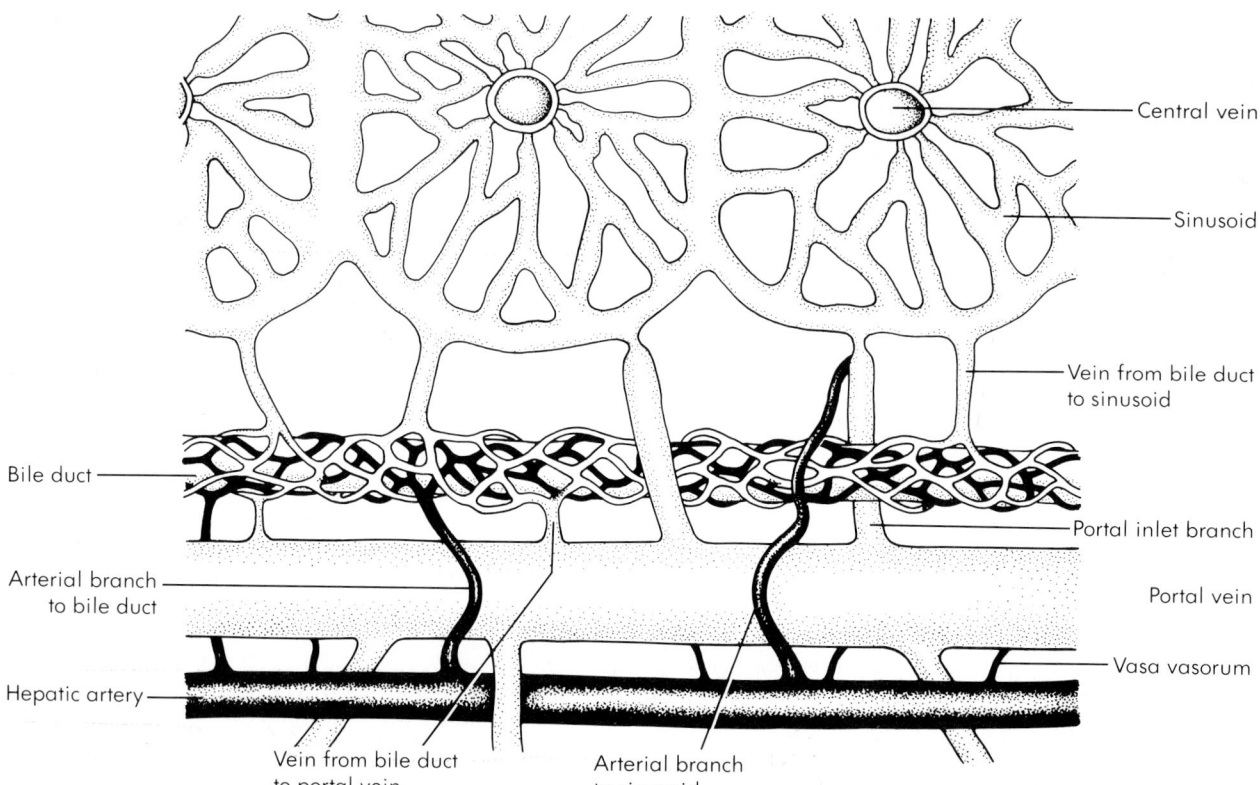

Figure 43–4. Diagram showing vascular plexus and venous drainage of the bile duct. The hepatic artery gives off its branches to the sinusoid, the bile duct, and the portal vein (vasa vasorum). The venous plexus of the bile duct (light vessels) is drained into the portal vein via the interlobular vein and into the sinusoids via the lobular vein. (Reproduced from Cho KJ, Lunderquist A. The peribiliary vascular plexus: The microvascular architecture of the bile duct in the rabbit and in clinical cases. Radiology, 147:357, 1983, with permission.)

remains limited, and curative therapy for the disease process has not been identified.

Management of Chronic Cholestasis

Pruritus is most often controlled by cholestyramine. When cholestyramine is ineffective, the regimen should be supplemented with phenobarbital given at bedtime. For difficult cases, activated charcoal capsules may be added to the regimen. If pruritus is intractable despite intense therapy, plasmapheresis[208] or plasma perfusion over charcoal-coated beads[209] may be beneficial.

All patients are at risk for development of fat-soluble vitamin deficiencies, and the risk increases with the duration and severity of cholestasis. Vitamin A deficiency occurs in approximately 50 per cent of patients, in association with jaundice and steatorrhea.[210] It is generally asymptomatic but can cause night blindness. Hepatic osteodystrophy is less frequent in primary sclerosing cholangitis than in primary biliary cirrhosis. When present, bone biopsies have shown osteoporosis rather than osteomalacia.[211] Even in the absence of evidence of symptomatic deficiency of vitamin D, supplementation with oral vitamin D and calcium appears to be prudent. Vitamin K deficiency may result in bruising, bleeding, and worsening coagulation tests. Supplementation is required to distinguish deficiency from severe hepatocellular disease causing coagulopathy. Vitamin E deficiency has not been detected in patients with primary sclerosing cholangitis.[212] To control symptoms of steatorrhea, dietary fat should be restricted.

Management of Complications

Cholangitis most commonly occurs after surgical manipulation of the bile ducts and less often as a spontaneous event.[31, 32, 36, 138, 139] Prompt treatment with broad-spectrum antibiotics should be instituted to prevent hepatic abscesses and septicemia. Prophylactic antibiotics are of unproven benefit and may predispose to the development of resistant flora. Patients with recurrent episodes of cholangitis should have antibiotics available at home to initiate therapy at the onset of symptoms.

Focal sclerosis of bile ducts may result in dominant strictures and abrupt worsening of clinical and biochemical cholestasis.[140] Cholangiography should be performed to identify strictured areas amenable to dilatation. Balloon dilatation performed percutaneously or endoscopically is the preferred method of treatment.[213]

Prospective studies indicate that cholangiocarcinoma develops in 10 to 15 per cent of patients with long-standing primary sclerosing cholangitis.[162] Since the tumor is often associated with insidious clinical and biochemical deterioration indistinguishable from the basic disease process, early detection is unusual. When suspected, retrograde cholangiography should be performed and bile samples obtained for cytology. As discussed earlier, differentiation from the primary disease may be difficult.

Cholelithiasis and choledocholithiasis may occur in patients with chronic disease.[138, 211] Chronic cholestasis predisposes to the formation of lithogenic bile and the development of cholesterol gallstones, whereas bile stasis and recurrent ascending cholangitis predispose to the formation of pigmented stones. Cholecystitis should be considered in patients with primary sclerosing cholangitis and right upper quadrant abdominal pain, even though many patients experience pain as a result of the primary disease alone. Impaction of intraductal stones may worsen cholestasis or cholangitis and should be excluded by retrograde cholangiography. Once the stones are identified, an endoscopic sphincterotomy should be performed and the stones removed.

Portal venous hypertension may result in hemorrhage from esophageal or gastric varices. Local measures such as injection of sclerosants or ligation are preferable to surgical shunts, since shunt surgery compromises the ability to perform liver transplantation. As discussed earlier (see section on Cirrhosis), patients with portal venous hypertension undergoing colectomy for their inflammatory bowel disease are at risk for developing peristomal varices at the ileostomy site.[121] If colectomy is necessary, an ileoanal anastomosis should be considered, since preliminary experience indicates that the risk of bleeding is less.[121]

Management of the Primary Disease

Although a variety of specific therapies have been investigated (Table 43–6), no specific therapy except for liver transplantation has been identified that is capable of curing or arresting the disease. In early reports, surgery to relieve biliary obstruction did not retard the progress of disease,[31, 32, 160] and secondary biliary cirrhosis developed despite surgical relief of strictures.[160] More recently, internal and external biliary drainage through stents has been advocated, but studies have been uncontrolled and anecdotal. Overall, there is no compelling evidence that such therapy is of long-term benefit, since it would not be expected to alter the pathogenetic mechanisms of the primary disease.

The effect of colectomy has been evaluated in uncontrolled series.[139] As discussed earlier, there is no evidence that colectomy influences the course of primary sclerosing cholangitis. Its lack of efficacy is best demonstrated by reports of primary sclerosing cholangitis occurring in patients after colectomy.[140]

Based on the concept that primary sclerosing cholangitis was caused by portal bacteremia or bacterial toxins, uncontrolled trials with a variety of antibiotics were performed.[181] Antibiotics were ineffective. They should not be used for primary treatment but reserved for treatment of ascending cholangitis.

Hepatic copper concentrations progressively increase in primary sclerosing cholangitis as the result of chronic cholestasis.[187, 232] A preliminary report of a randomized, double-blind, placebo-controlled therapeutic trial of D-penicillamine indicates that cupruesis occurred in the treatment group but was unassociated with improvement in clinical,

biochemical, or histopathologic features or with increased survival.

A variety of therapies have been employed to suppress inflammation and immunologic reactions. Corticosteroids have been administered systemically and by nasobiliary lavage in primary sclerosing cholangitis, but results are uninterpretable because of the small numbers of patients and lack of suitable controls.[140] Randomized, controlled trials will be required to assess the efficacy and role of corticosteroid therapy. Preliminary results with combined prednisone and colchicine therapy have recently been reported.[218, 219] Based on the favorable report of combined therapy in a man with primary sclerosing cholangitis and ulcerative colitis,[218] a small controlled trial was instituted at the Mayo Clinic.[219] Comparison of 12 treated and untreated patients matched for age, sex, initial biochemical values, and histologic stage showed significant improvement in the treated group for bilirubin, alkaline phosphatase, and aminotransferases at 6 and 12 months. This study, however, was small, and further experience is required with this combination of drugs.

Azathioprine therapy has been reported in two patients: one improved and the other deteriorated.[220, 221] A randomized, double-blind controlled trial of cyclosporine was begun at the Mayo Clinic in an attempt to modify the disease by reducing the activation and proliferation of T lymphocytes.[140] No results have been reported.

Finally, the effect of methotrexate therapy in two patients has recently been published.[222] Improvement in biochemical tests and histologic features was notable. Controlled trials are required to assess this preliminary success. The evidence supporting a possible immunopathogenesis, although incomplete, is sufficient to warrant continued controlled trials of immunosuppressive agents alone or in combination. The results of these trials should provide additional insights into the pathogenesis of the disease and its management.

Until definitive therapies are established, orthotopic liver transplantation offers the only prospect for cure and survival of patients in the terminal phase of disease. Marsh et al. have recently reported the results of transplantation in 55 patients with primary sclerosing cholangitis.[223] The indications for transplantation included hepatic failure in 25, variceal bleeding in 15 and recurrent bacterial cholangitis in 15. After a follow-up of up to four years, 67 per cent are alive. Of the 18 patients who died, 11 (61 per cent) expired within three months of transplantation. Nine deaths were due to graft failure and 2 were related to immunosuppression. Between six months and two years, 2 patients died of recurrent cholangiocarcinoma. To date, the primary disease has not recurred in the allograft. Of interest is the observation that the inflammatory bowel disease has been inactive during treatment with immunosuppression including steroids and cyclosporine.

TABLE 43–6. TREATMENTS EMPLOYED IN PRIMARY SCLEROSING CHOLANGITIS

Surgery of bile ducts
Biliary drainage
Colectomy
Antibiotics
Cupruresis
Immunosuppression
   Corticosteroids
   Steroids plus colchicine
   Azathioprine
   Methotrexate
Liver transplantation

CARCINOMA OF THE BILIARY TRACT

Carcinoma of the biliary tract occurs in association with ulcerative colitis[21, 30, 162, 224, 225] with an estimated frequency of 0.4 per cent, which is ten times greater than that in the general population.[30] Carcinoma of the biliary tract in association with Crohn's disease has not been reported. In a comprehensive analysis of the association between carcinoma of the biliary tract and ulcerative colitis, Ritchie et al. reviewed the cases of 67 patients.[30] The male-to-female ratio of 1.6 to 1 in patients with ulcerative colitis and carcinoma of the biliary tract is in accord with the observation of a male predominance in patients with cholangiocarcinoma who do not have ulcerative colitis.

Pathology

The majority of tumors are adenocarcinomas and are associated with an extensive desmoplastic reaction. An anaplastic tumor with a squamous cell component has been found in one patient.[134] The tumors occur most frequently in the extrahepatic ducts, but may involve the intrahepatic ducts or occur at the bifurcation of the hepatic ducts. Adenocarcinoma can develop in patients with long-standing primary sclerosing cholangitis (discussed earlier).[31, 32] In nine of 67 patients reviewed by Ritchie et al., the tumors arose in the gallbladder.[30]

Clinical Features

Pancolitis was present in 87 per cent of patients for whom the extent of colitis was reported.[30] The mean duration of ulcerative colitis prior to the diagnosis of carcinoma was 15 years, but the range was wide and included instances of carcinoma diagnosed within a year of the onset of symptoms of ulcerative colitis. In 19 patients, carcinoma of the biliary tract occurred after colectomy for ulcerative colitis. In these patients, the durations of illness prior to surgery ranged from 2 to 22 years, with a mean of 11 years. The operations included proctocolectomy performed as a one- or two-stage procedure in 18 and subtotal colectomy in 1 patient. Thus, the complete excision of the inflamed bowel in the majority did not protect against the development of carcinoma 1 to 20 years after surgery (mean 8 years). Compared with an unselected patient population with carcinoma of the biliary tract, the tumors occur 20 or more years earlier in patients with ulcerative colitis.

Patients most often seek medical advice because of obstructive jaundice.[30] In 15 patients studied in detail, 9 had no associated liver disease. In the remaining 6, the presence of cirrhosis in 4 and pericholangitis in 2 complicated the evaluation and interpretation of the jaundice. Cholangiocarcinoma is infrequently associated with cholelithiasis in patients with ulcerative colitis, in contradistinction to a 30 to 50 per cent prevalence of cholelithiasis in patients without colitis who have cholangiocarcinoma. Tumors also have been found incidentally during colectomy or at autopsy.

Results of laboratory tests have been reported for only a few patients. As expected, the predominant abnormalities are increased total and direct-reacting bilirubin and alkaline phosphatase. Slight elevations of aminotransferases also may occur.

Pathogenesis

The nature of the association between carcinoma of the biliary tract and ulcerative colitis is unknown. Any hypothesis relating the occurrence to the extent, duration, or severity of the disease must be tempered, since tumors can develop many years after proctocolectomy. The observation that patients with primary sclerosing cholangitis may be particularly predisposed to develop carcinoma of the biliary tract[31, 32] suggests that chronic inflammation or bile

stasis may contribute to the development of cholangiocarcinoma.

Prognosis and Therapy

The prognosis generally is poor for carcinoma of the biliary tract. Small tumors of the bile ducts and tumors localized to the gallbladder may be excised surgically.[226] When resection is impossible, a biliary drainage procedure proximal to the tumor is recommended. This may involve a choledocho- or cholecystoenterostomy or hepaticoenterostomy. In the latter case, cholecystectomy is recommended to prevent obstruction of the cystic duct. When the extent of the tumor precludes a drainage procedure, operative dilatation and placement of a stent may achieve adequate drainage. Percutaneous, transhepatic placement of stents also has been performed.[227] The roles of chemotherapy[228] and radiotherapy[229] are unclear at the present time.

CHOLELITHIASIS

In the United States, an estimated 25 million individuals have gallstones representing a prevalence of approximately 11 per cent. It is not unexpected, therefore, that some patients with inflammatory bowel disease will have cholelithiasis coincidentally. Indeed, patients with ulcerative colitis and Crohn's colitis appear to have gallstones with frequencies compatible with the age-related prevalence in the general population.[115, 230] However, patients with extensive or long-standing Crohn's disease of the ileum and patients who have had ileal resection have significantly increased frequencies of cholelithiasis.[115, 131, 228, 229] The prevalence of cholelithiasis in such patients was approximately 30 per cent in three independent studies.[131, 228, 231] The increased frequency of cholelithiasis in patients with Crohn's disease is correlated directly with the duration and extent of the ileal disease or the interval following ileal resection.[131, 230, 231]

Pathogenesis

The stones reported in association with Crohn's disease of the ileum typically have been cholesterol gallstones.[131, 229] This is the expected consequence of the physiologic derangement. In the presence of diffuse ileal disease or following ileal resection, inadequate absorption of bile acids in the ileum results in their fecal loss. If the hepatic synthesis of bile acids is insufficient to solubilize cholesterol in bile acid-lecithin micelles, then lithogenic bile results. Subsequent precipitation of cholesterol crystals results in the formation of cholesterol gallstones (see Chapter 11).

Therapy

The therapy for symptomatic gallstones is cholecystectomy. The use of chenodeoxycholic acid or ursodeoxycholic acid to prevent the production of lithogenic bile has not been evaluated in patients with Crohn's disease of the ileum or in patients following ileal resection.

REFERENCES

1. Kirsner JB. The local and systemic complications of inflammatory bowel disease. JAMA 242:1177, 1979.

2. Thomas GH. Ulceration of the colon with enlarged fatty liver. Trans Pathol Soc Philadelphia 4:87, 1874.

3. Lister TD. A specimen of diffuse ulcerative colitis with secondary diffuse hepatitis. Trans Pathol Soc London 50:130, 1899.

4. Jankelson IR, McClure CW, Sweetsir FN. Chronic ulcerative colitis. II. Complications outside the digestive tract. Rev Gastroenterol 9:99, 1942.

5. Banks BM, Korelitz BI, Zetsel L. The course of non-specific ulcerative colitis: review of 20 years experience and late results. Gastroenterology 32:983, 1957.

6. Bargen JA. The Management of Colitis. New York, National Medical Book Company, 1935.

7. Jackman RJ, Bargen JA, Helmholz HF. The life histories of 95 children with chronic ulcerative colitis. Am J Dis Child 59:459, 1940.

8. Comfort MW, Bargen JA, Morlock CG. The association of chronic ulcerative colitis (colitis gravis) with hepatic insufficiency: report of 4 cases. Med Clin North Am 22:1089, 1938.

9. Logan AH. Chronic ulcerative colitis. A review of 117 cases. Northwest Med 18:1, 1919.

10. Cirrhosis and colitis (editorial). Br Med J 1:189, 1949.

11. Perrett AD, Higgins G, Johnston HH, et al. The liver in ulcerative colitis. Q J Med 40:211, 1971.

12. Lockhart-Mummery HE, Morson BC. Crohn's disease (regional enteritis) of the large intestine and its distinction from ulcerative colitis. Gut 1:87, 1960.

13. Van Patter WN, Bargen JA, Dockerty MB, et al. Regional enteritis. Gastroenterology 26:347, 1954.

14. Crohn BB. Regional Ileitis. New York, Grune & Stratton, 1949.

15. Kleckner MS. The liver in regional enteritis. Gastroenterology 30:416, 1956.

16. Chapin LE, Scudamore HH, Baggenstoss AH, et al. Regional enteritis: associated visceral changes. Gastroenterology 30:404, 1956.

17. Monto AS. The liver in ulcerative disease of the intestinal tract: functional and anatomic changes. Ann Intern Med 50:1385, 1959.

18. Palmer WL, Kirsner JB, Goldgraber MB, et al. Disease of the liver in regional enteritis. Am J Med Sci 246:663, 1963.

19. Dordal E, Glagov S, Kirsner JB. Hepatic lesions in chronic inflammatory bowel disease. I. Clinical correlations with liver biopsy diagnoses in 103 patients. Gastroenterology 52:239, 1967.

20. Perrett AD, Higgins G, Johnston HH, et al. The liver in Crohn's disease. Q J Med 40:187, 1971.

21. Dew MJ, Thompson H, Allain RN. The spectrum of hepatic dysfunction in inflammatory bowel disease. Q J Med 48:113, 1979.

22. Eade MN, Cooke WT, Brooke BN, et al. Liver disease in Crohn's colitis. A study of 21 consecutive patients having colectomy. Ann Intern Med 74:518, 1971.

23. Eade MN, Cooke WT, Williams JA. Liver disease in Crohn's disease. A study of 100 consecutive patients. Scand J Gastroenterol 6:199, 1971.

24. Rankin GB, Watts HD, Melnyk CS, et al. National cooperative Crohn's disease study: extraintestinal manifestations and perianal complications. Gastroenterology 77:914, 1979.

25. Kern F. Hepatobiliary disorders in inflammatory bowel disease. In: Popper H, Schaffner F, eds. Progress in Liver Diseases. Vol 5. New York, Grune & Stratton, 1976:575.

26. Kimmelstiel P, Large HL, Verner HD. Liver damage in ulcerative colitis. Am J Pathol 28:259, 1952.

27. Palmer WL, Kirsner JB, Goldgraber MB, et al. Disease of the liver in chronic ulcerative colitis. Am J Med 36:856, 1964.

28. Mistilis SP. Pericholangitis and ulcerative colitis. I. Pathology, etiology, and pathogenesis. Ann Intern Med 63:1, 1965.

29. Willcox RG, Isselbacher KJ. Chronic liver disease in young people. Am J Med 30:185, 1961.

30. Ritchie JK, Allan RN, Macartney J, et al. Biliary tract carcinoma associated with ulcerative colitis. Q J Med 43:263, 1974.

31. Wiesner RH, La Russo NF. Clinicopathologic features of the syndrome of primary sclerosing cholangitis. Gastroenterology 79:200, 1980.

32. Chapman RWG, Marborgh BA, Rhodes JM, et al. Primary sclerosing cholangitis: a review of its clinical features, cholangiography, and hepatic histology. Gut 21:870, 1980.

33. Lupinetti M, Mehigan D, Cameron JL. Hepatobiliary complications of ulcerative colitis. Am J Surg 139:113, 1980.

34. Perold JG, Bezuidenhout DJJ, Erasmus TD, et al. The association between ulcerative colitis and chronic liver disease at Tygerberg Hospital. S Afr Med J 61:186, 1982.

35. Shepard HA, Selby WS, Chapman RWG, et al. Ulcerative colitis and persistent liver dysfunction. Q J Med 208:503, 1983.

36. Steckman M, Drossman DA, Lesesne HR. Hepatobiliary disease that precedes ulcerative colitis. J Clin Gastroenterol 6:425, 1984.

37. Christophi C, Hughes ER. Hepatobiliary disorders in inflammatory bowel disease. Surg Gynecol Obstet 160:187, 1985.

38. Wee A, Ludwig J. Pericholangitis in chronic ulcerative colitis: Primary sclerosing cholangitis of the small bile ducts? Ann Intern Med 102:581, 1985.

39. Kanin HJ, Levin JJ, Lindert MCF. The association of liver disease with ulcerative colitis. Am J Gastroenterol 25:172, 1956.

40. Pollard HM, Block M. Association of hepatic insufficiency with chronic ulcerative colitis. Arch Intern Med 82:159, 1948.

41. Bendandi A. Liver function in ulcerative colitis. Gastroenterologia 86:658, 1956.

42. Dyer NH, Dawson AM. The incidence and significance of liver dysfunction in Crohn's disease. Digestion 5:317, 1972.

43. Boden RW, Rankin JG, Goulston SJM, et al. The liver in ulcerative colitis. The significance of raised serum-alkaline-phosphatase levels. Lancet 2:245, 1959.

44. Vinnik IE, Kern F, Corley WD. Serum 5-nucleotidase and pericholangitis in patients with chronic ulcerative colitis. Gastroenterology 45:492, 1963.

45. Vinnik IE, Kern F. Liver diseases in ulcerative colitis. Arch Intern Med 112:87, 1963.

46. Kleckner MS, Stauffer MH, Bargen JA, et al. Hepatic lesions in the living patient with chronic ulcerative colitis as demonstrated by needle biopsy. Gastroenterology 22:13, 1952.

47. Elias E, Summerfield JA, Sherlock S. Endoscopic retrograde cholangiopancreatography in the diagnosis of jaundice associated with ulcerative colitis. Gastroenterology 67:907, 1974.

48. Blackstone MO, Nemchausky BA. Cholangiographic abnormalities in ulcerative colitis associated pericholangitis which resemble sclerosing cholangitis. Dig Dis 23:579, 1978.

49. Schrumpf E, Elgjo K, Fausa D, et al. Sclerosing cholangitis in ulcerative colitis. Scand J Gastroenterol 15:689, 1980.

50. Ross JR, Nugent FW, Hajjar J-J, et al. Liver disease in chronic ulcerative colitis. Lahey Clin Found Bull 15:93, 1966.

51. Liver disease in ulcerative colitis (editorial). Lancet 2:402, 1970.

52. Bargen JA. Disease of the liver associated with ulcerative colitis. Ann Intern Med 39:285, 1953.

53. Mistilis SP, Goulston SJM. Pericholangitis and ulcerative colitis. II. Clinical aspects. Ann Intern Med 63:17, 1965.

54. Olhagen L. Ulcerative colitis in cirrhosis of the liver. Acta Med Scand 162:143, 1958.

55. Ludwig J. Some names hang on like leeches (editorial). Dig Dis Sci 24:967, 1979.

56. Eade MN. Liver disease in ulcerative colitis. I. Analysis of operative liver biopsy in 138 consecutive patients having colectomy. Ann Intern Med 72:475, 1970.

57. de Dombal FT, Goldie W, Watts J McK, et al. Hepatic histological changes in ulcerative colitis. A series of 58 consecutive operative liver biopsies. Scand J Gastroenterol 1:220, 1966.

58. Stauffer MH, Sauer WG, Dearing WH, et al. The spectrum of cholestatic hepatic disease. JAMA 191:125, 1965.

59. Ludwig J, Barham SS, LaRusso NF, et al. Morphologic features of chronic hepatitis associated with primary sclerosing cholangitis and chronic ulcerative colitis. Hepatology 1:632, 1981.

60. Geisse G, Melson GL, Tedesco FJ, et al. Stenosing lesions of the biliary tree. Am J Roentgenol 123:378, 1975.

61. Bloom W, Fawcett DW. A Textbook of Histology, 10th ed. Philadelphia, WB Saunders, 1975:711.

62. Leevy CM, Popper H, Sherlock S. Diseases of the Liver and Biliary Tract. Standardization of Nomenclature, Diagnostic Criteria, and Diagnostic Methodology. Washington DC, US Government Printing Office, 1976.

63. Mistilis SP. Liver disease in bowel disorders. In: Schiff L, ed. Diseases of the Liver. 4th ed. Philadelphia, JB Lippincott, 1975:1373.

64. Vinnik IE, Kern F. Biliary cirrhosis in a patient with chronic ulcerative colitis. Gastroenterology 45:529, 1963.

65. Thorpe MEC, Scheuer PJ, Sherlock S. Primary sclerosing cholangitis, the biliary tree, and ulcerative colitis. Gut 8:435, 1967.

66. Blaschke TF, Elin RJ, Berk PD, et al. Effect of induced fever on sulfobromophthalein kinetics in man. Ann Intern Med 78:221, 1973.

67. Eade MN, Cooke WT, Brooke BN. Liver disease in ulcerative colitis. II. The long-term effect of colectomy. Ann Intern Med 72:489, 1970.

68. McCarthy CF, Read MD. Bleeding esophageal varices in ulcerative colitis. Gastroenterology 42:325, 1962.

69. Orloff MJ, Peskin GW, Ellis HL. A bacteriologic study of human portal blood: implications regarding hepatic ischemia in man. Ann Surg 148:738, 1958.

70. Brooke BN, Slaney G. Portal bacteremia in ulcerative colitis. Lancet 1:1206, 1958.

71. Brooke BN, Dykes PW, Walker FC. A study of liver disorders in ulcerative colitis. Postgrad Med J 37:245, 1961.

72. Eade MN, Brooke BN. Portal bacteremia in cases of ulcerative colitis submitted to colectomy. Lancet 1:1008, 1969.

73. Hektoen L. Experimental bacillary cirrhosis of the liver. J Pathol Bacteriol 7:214, 1901.

74. Weaver GH. Cirrhosis by injecting portal vein with E. coli. Johns Hopkins Hosp Rep 9:297, 1900.

75. MacMahon HE, Mallory FB. Streptococcus hepatitis. Am J Pathol 7:299, 1931.
76. Wachstein M, Meisel E, Falcon C. Enzymatic histochemistry in the experimentally damaged liver. Am J Pathol 40:219, 1962.
77. Vinnik IE, Kern F, Struthers JE, et al. Experimental chronic portal vein bacteremia. Proc Soc Exp Biol Med 115:311, 1964.
78. Jacob AI, Goldberg PK, Bloom N, et al. Endotoxin and bacteria in portal blood. Gastroenterology 72:1268, 1977.
79. Pryta H, Hoest-Christensen J, Korner B, et al. Portal liver disease and systemic endotoxemia in patients with cirrhosis. Scand J Gastroenterol 11:857, 1976.
80. Tarao K, So K, Moroi T, et al. Detection of endotoxin in plasma and ascitic fluid of patients with cirrhosis: its clinical significance. Gastroenterology 73:539, 1977.
81. Fulenwider JT, Sibley C, Stein SF, et al. Endotoxemia of cirrhosis: an observation not substantiated. Gastroenterology 78:1001, 1980.
82. Grün M, Liehr H. Biological significance of altered von Kupffer cell function in experimental liver disease. In: Wisse E, Knook DL, eds. Kupffer Cells and Other Liver Sinusoidal Cells. Amsterdam, Elsevier/North-Holland Biomedical Press, 1977:437.
83. Utili R, Abernathy CO, Zimmerman HJ. Studies on the effects of E. coli endotoxin on canalicular bile formation in the isolated perfused rat liver. J Lab Clin Med 89:471, 1977.
84. Levitan R, Brudno S. Permeability of the rectosigmoid mucosa to tritiated water in normal subjects and in patients with mild idiopathic ulcerative colitis. Gut 8:15, 1967.
85. Dalmark M. Plasma radioactivity after rectal instillation of radioiodine labelled human albumin in normal subjects and in patients with ulcerative colitis. Scand J Gastroenterol 3:490, 1968.
86. Hill MJ. Role of colon anaerobes in the metabolism of bile acids and steroids, and its relation to colon cancer. Cancer 36:2387, 1975.
87. Goldin BR, Gorbach SL. The relationship between diet and rat fecal bacterial enzymes implicated in colon cancer. J Natl Cancer Inst USA 57:371, 1976.
88. Palmer RH. Bile acids, liver injury, and liver disease. Arch Intern Med 130:606, 1972.
89. Siegel JH, Barnes S, Morris JS. Bile acids in liver disease associated with inflammatory bowel disease. Digestion 15:469, 1977.
90. Holzbach RT, Marsh ME, Freedman MR, et al. Portal vein bile acids in patients with severe inflammatory bowel disease. Gut 21:428, 1980.
91. Gadacz TR, Allan RN, Mack E, et al. Impaired lithocholate sulfation in the rhesus monkey: a possible mechanism for chenodeoxycholate toxicity. Gastroenterology 70:1125, 1976.
92. Zimmerman HJ. Hepatotoxicity: The Adverse Effects of Drugs and Other Chemicals on the Liver. New York, Appleton-Century-Crofts, 1978:481.
93. Caravati CM, Hooker TH. Acute massive hepatic necrosis with fatal liver failure. Am J Dig Dis 16:803, 1971.
94. Kanner RS, Tedesco FJ, Kalser MH. Azulfidine-induced hepatic injury. Dig Dis 23:956, 1978.
95. Mihas AA, Goldenberg DJ, Slaughter RL. Sulfasalazine toxic reactions. Hepatitis, fever, skin rash with hypocomplementemia and immune complexes. JAMA 239:2590, 1978.
96. Rabin BS, Rogers SJ. A cell-mediated immune model of inflammatory bowel disease in the rabbit. Gastroenterology 75:29, 1978.
97. Lawley TJ, James SP, Jones EA. Circulating immune complexes: their detection and potential significance in some hepatobiliary and intestinal diseases. Gastroenterology 78:626, 1980.
98. Soltis RD, Hasz D, Morris MJ, et al. Evidence against the presence of circulating immune complexes in chronic inflammatory bowel disease. Gastroenterology 76:1380, 1979.
99. Hodgson HJF, Potter BJ, Skinner J, et al. Immune-complex mediated colitis in rabbits. Gut 19:225, 1978.
100. Mee AS, McLaughlin JE, Hodgson HJF, et al. Chronic immune colitis in rabbits. Gut 20:1, 1979.
101. Rankin JG, Boden RW, Goulston SJ, et al. The liver in ulcerative colitis. Lancet 2:1110, 1959.
102. Mistilis SP, Skyring AP, Goulston SJM. Effect of long-term tetracycline therapy, steroid therapy and colectomy in pericholangitis associated with ulcerative colitis. Aust Ann Med 14:286, 1965.
103. Hill RB, Droke WE, Harp AP. Hepatic lipid metabolism in the cortisone-treated rat. Exp Molec Pathol 4:320, 1965.
104. Boyer JL. Chronic hepatitis. A perspective on classification and determinants of prognosis. Gastroenterology 70:1161, 1976.
105. Read AE, Sherlock S, Harrison CV. Active "juvenile" cirrhosis considered as part of a systemic disease and the effect of corticosteroid therapy. Gut 4:378, 1963.
106. Holdsworth CD, Hall EW, Dawson AM, et al. Ulcerative colitis in chronic liver disease. Q J Med 34:211, 1965.
107. Kane SP. Ulcerative colitis with chronic liver disease, eosinophilia and auto-immune thyroid disease. Postgrad Med J 53:105, 1977.
108. MacKay IR, Wood IJ. Lupoid hepatitis: a comparison of 22 cases with other types of chronic liver disease. Q J Med 31:485, 1962.
109. Gray N, MacKay IR, Taft LI, et al. Hepatitis, colitis, and lupus manifestations. Am J Dig Dis 3:481, 1958.
110. Olsson R, Hulten L. Concurrence of ulcerative colitis and chronic active hepatitis. Clinical courses and results of colectomy. Scand J Gastroenterol 10:331, 1975.
111. Harris AI, Newgarten J. Chronic active hepatitis and ulcerative colitis associated with eosinophilia, nonthrombocytopenic hypergammaglobulinemia purpura and serological abnormalities. Am J Gastroenterol 69:191, 1978.
112. Fiocchi C, Farmer RG. Autoimmunity in inflammatory bowel disease. Clin Aspects Autoimmunity 1:12, 1987.
113. Ronder M, Norday A, Elgjo K. Sulfonamide-induced chronic liver disease. Scand J Gastroenterol 9:93, 1974.
114. Edwards FC, Truelove SC. The course and prognosis of ulcerative colitis. Part III. Complications. Gut 5:1, 1964.
115. Greenstein AJ, Janowitz HD, Sachar DB. The extraintestinal complications of Crohn's disease and ulcerative colitis: a study of 700 patients. Medicine 55:401, 1976.
116. Czaja AJ, Wolf AM. Immunopathic disease associated with severe chronic active liver disease: determinants of treatment response? (abstr). Gastroenterology 78:1152, 1980.
117. Hoffbauer FW, McCartney JS, Dennis C, et al. The relationship of chronic ulcerative colitis and cirrhosis. Ann Intern Med 39:267, 1953.
118. Eade MN, Williams JA, Cooke WT. Bleeding from an ileostomy caput medusae. Lancet 2:1166, 1969.
119. Cameron AD, Fone DJ. Portal hypertension and bleeding varices after colectomy and ileostomy for chronic ulcerative colitis. Gut 11:755, 1970.
120. Adson MA, Fulton RE. The ileal stoma and portal hypertension. An uncommon site of variceal bleeding. Arch Surg 112:501, 1977.
121. Wiesner RH, LaRusso NF, Dozois RR, et al. Peristomal varices after proctocolectomy in patients with primary sclerosing cholangitis. Gastroenterology 83:316, 1986.
122. Smith PM. Hepatoma associated with ulcerative colitis. Dis Colon Rectum 17:554, 1974.
123. Schrumpf E, Fausa O, Kolmannskog F, et al. Sclerosing cholangitis in ulcerative colitis. A follow-up study. Scand J Gastroenterol 17:33, 1982.
124. Kato Y, Morimoto H, Unoura M, et al. Primary biliary cirrhosis and chronic pancreatitis in a patient with ulcerative colitis. J Clin Gastroenterol 5:425, 1985.
125. Ludwig J, LaRusso NF. Primary biliary cirrhosis in a patient with chronic ulcerative colitis. In: Ishak KG, ed. Hepatopathology 1985. American Association for the Study of Liver Diseases, New Jersey, 1985:197.
126. Werther JL, Schapira A, Rubenstein O, et al. Amyloidosis in regional enteritis: a report of five cases. Am J Med 29:416, 1960.
127. Benedek TG, Zawadzki ZA. Ankylosing spondylitis with ulcerative colitis and amyloidosis. Am J Med 40:431, 1966.
128. Shorvon PJ. Amyloidosis and inflammatory bowel disease. Dig Dis 22:209, 1977.
129. Glenner GG. Amyloid deposits and amyloidosis: the β-fibrilloses. N Engl J Med 302:1282 and 1333, 1980.
130. Maurer LH, Hughes RW, Folley JH, et al. Granulomatous hepatitis associated with regional enteritis. Gastroenterology 53:301, 1967.
131. Cohen S, Kaplan M, Gottlieb L, et al. Liver disease and gallstones in regional enteritis. Gastroenterology 60:237, 1971.
132. Espiritu CR, Kim TS, Levine RA. Granulomatous hepatitis associated with sulfadimethoxine hypersensitivity. JAMA 202:985, 1967.
133. Callen JP, Soderstrom RM. Granulomatous hepatitis associated with salicylazosulfapyridine therapy. South Med J 71:1159, 1978.
134. Lytton DG, McCaughan G. Hepatic venous occlusion from carcinoma of bile duct in ulcerative colitis. Aust NZ J Med 7:404, 1977.
135. Bruguera M, Aranguibel F, Ros E, et al. Incidence and clinical significance of sinusoidal dilatation in liver biopsies. Gastroenterology 75:474, 1978.
136. Camilleri M, Schafler K, Chadwick VS, et al. Periportal sinusoidal dilatation, inflammatory bowel disease, and the contraceptive pill. Gastroenterology 80:810, 1981.
137. Winkler K, Poulsen H. Liver disease with periportal sinusoidal dilatation. A possible complication of contraceptive steroids. Scand J Gastroenterol 10:699, 1975.
138. Wiesner RH, LaRusso NF, Ludwig J, et al. Comparison of the clinicopathologic features of primary sclerosing cholangitis and primary biliary cirrhosis. Gastroenterology 88:108, 1985.
139. Lefkowitch JH, Martin ED. Primary sclerosing cholangitis. Prog Liver Dis 8:557, 1986.
140. Lindor KD, Wiesner RH, LaRusso NF. Recent advances in the management of primary sclerosing cholangitis. Semin Liver Dis 7:322, 1987.
141. Helzberg JH, Petersen JM, Boyer JL. Improved survival with primary sclerosing cholangitis. A review of clinicopathologic features and comparison of symptomatic and asymptomatic patients. Gastroenterology 92:1869, 1987.

142. Bartholomew LG, Cain JC, Woolner LB, et al. Sclerosing cholangitis: its possible association with Riedel's struma and fibrous retroperitonitis—report of two cases. N Engl J Med 269:8, 1963.

143. Hellstrom HR, Perez-Stable EC. Retroperitoneal fibrosis with disseminated vasculitis and intrahepatic sclerosing cholangitis. Am J Med 40:184, 1966.

144. Hawk WA, Hazard JB. Sclerosing retroperitonitis and sclerosing mediastinitis. Am J Clin Pathol 32:321, 1959.

145. Wenger J, Gingrich GW, Mendeloff J. Sclerosing cholangitis—manifestation of systemic disease. Arch Intern Med 116:509, 1965.

146. Record CO, Eddleston ALWF, Shilkin KB, et al. Intrahepatic sclerosing cholangitis associated with a familial immunodeficiency syndrome. Lancet 2:18, 1973.

147. Danzi JT, Makipour H, Farmer RG. Primary sclerosing cholangitis: a report of nine cases and clinical review. Am J Gastroenterol 65:109, 1976.

148. Viteri AL, Hardin WJ, Dyck WP. Peyronie's disease and sclerosing cholangitis in a patient with ulcerative colitis. Am J Dig Dis 24:490, 1979.

149. Bretagne J-F, Tassou R, Ramee M-P, et al. Colite aigue grave, cholangite sclerosante primitive et pyoderma gangrenosum. Gastroenterol Clin Biol 6:448, 1982.

150. Pang JA, Vicary FR. Carcinoma of the colon, sclerosing cholangitis, pericholangitis, and bronchiectasis in a patient with chronic ulcerative colitis. J Clin Gastroenterol 6:361, 1984.

151. Bass NM, Chapman RW, O'Reilly A, et al. Primary sclerosing cholangitis associated with angioimmunoblastic lymphadenopathy. Gastroenterology 85:420, 1983.

152. Roge J, Testas P, Durand B, et al. L'histiocytose X: Une nouvelle etiologie de la cholangite sclerosante? Gastroenterol Clin Biol 5:620, 1981.

153. Thompson HH, Pitt HA, Lewin KJ, et al. Sclerosing cholangitis and histiocytosis X. Gut 25:526, 1984.

154. Montefusco PP, Geiss AC, Bronzo RL, et al. Sclerosing cholangitis, chronic pancreatitis, and Sjögren's syndrome: A syndrome complex. Am J Surg 147:822, 1984.

155. Waldram R, Kopelman H, Tsantoulas D, et al. Chronic pancreatitis, sclerosing cholangitis and sicca complex in two siblings. Lancet 1:550, 1975.

156. Alberti-Flor JJ, Kalemeris G, Dunn GD, et al. Primary sclerosing cholangitis associated with massive intraabdominal lymphadenopathy. Am J Gastroenterol 81:55, 1986.

157. Mir-Madjlessi SH, Sivak MV, Farmer RG. Hypereosinophilia, ulcerative colitis, sclerosing cholangitis, and bile duct carcinoma. Am J Gastroenterol 81:483, 1986.

158. Gupta S, Saverymuttu SH, Marsh JCW, et al. Immune thrombocytopenic purpura, neutropenia and sclerosing cholangitis associated with ulcerative colitis in an adult. Clin Lab Haemat 8:67, 1986.

159. Kirby DF, Blei AT, Rosen ST, et al. Primary sclerosing cholangitis in the presence of lupus anticoagulant. Am J Med 81:1077, 1986.

160. Warren KW, Athanassiades S, Monge JI. Primary sclerosing cholangitis. A study of forty-two cases. Am J Surg 111:23, 1966.

161. Thompson HH, Pitt HA, Tompkins RK, et al. Primary sclerosing cholangitis: A heterogeneous disease. Ann Surg 196:127, 1982.

162. Wee A, Ludwig J, Coffey RJ, et al. Hepatobiliary carcinoma associated with primary sclerosing cholangitis and chronic ulcerative colitis. Hum Pathol 16:719, 1985.

163. Li-Yeng D, Goldberg HI. Sclerosing cholangitis: Broad spectrum of radiographic features. Gastrointest Radiol 9:39, 1984.

164. Smith MP, Loe RH. Sclerosing cholangitis: review of recent case reports and associated diseases and four new cases. Am J Surg 110:239, 1965.

165. Bhathal PS, Powell IW. Primary intrahepatic obliterating cholangitis: a possible variant of sclerosing cholangitis. Gut 10:886, 1969.

166. Warren KW, Tan EGC. Diseases of the gallbladder and bile ducts. In: Schiff L, ed. Diseases of the Liver. 4th edition. Philadelphia, JB Lippincott, 1975:1319.

167. Smuckler EA. Pathology. In: Cello JP, moderator. Cholestasis in ulcerative colitis. Gastroenterology 73:357, 1977.

168. Nakanuma Y, Hirai N, Kono N, et al. Histological and ultrastructural examination of the intrahepatic biliary tree in primary sclerosing cholangitis. Liver 6:317, 1986.

169. Ludwig J. New concepts in biliary cirrhosis. Semin Liver Dis 7:293, 1987.

170. Ritland S, Elgio K, Johansen O, et al. Liver copper content in patients with inflammatory bowel disease and associated liver disorders. Scand J Gastroenterol 14:711, 1979.

171. Schwartz SI, Dale WA. Primary sclerosing cholangitis: review and report of six cases. Arch Surg 77:439, 1958.

172. Epstein O, Chapman RWG, Lake-Bakaar G, et al. The pancreas in primary biliary cirrhosis and primary sclerosing cholangitis. Gastroenterology 83:1177, 1982.

173. Fausa O, Kolmannskog F, Ritland S. The pancreatic ducts in primary biliary cirrhosis and sclerosing cholangitis. Scand J Gastroenterol 20(suppl):32, 1985.

174. Atkinson AJ, Carroll WW. Sclerosing cholangitis, association with regional enteritis. JAMA 188:183, 1964.

175. Amedee-Manesme O, Brunelle F, Hadchouel M, et al. Sclerosing cholangitis in infancy. Hepatology 4:786, 1984.

176. El-Shabrawi M, Wilkinson ML, Portmann B, et al. Primary sclerosing cholangitis in childhood. Gastroenterology 92:1226, 1987.

177. Classen M, Goetze H, Richter H-J, et al. Primary sclerosing cholangitis in children. J Ped Gastroenterol Nutr 6:197, 1987.

178. Way LW. Surgical management in sclerosing cholangitis. In: Cello JP, moderator. Cholestasis in ulcerative colitis. Gastroenterology 73:357, 1977.

179. Wiesner RH, Beaver SJ, Ludwig J, et al. The natural history of symptomatic and asymptomatic primary sclerosing cholangitis. (Abstr) Gastroenterology 90:1780, 1986.

180. Balasubramaniam K, Wiesner RH, LaRusso NF. Can serum alkaline phosphatase levels be normal in primary sclerosing cholangitis? (Abstr) Gastroenterology 92:1303, 1987.

181. Cello JP. Long term complications and medical therapy. In: Cello JP, moderator. Cholestasis in ulcerative colitis. Gastroenterology 73:357, 1977.

182. Goodman MW, Ansel HJ, Vennes JA, et al. Is intravenous cholangiography still useful? Gastroenterology 79:642, 1980.

183. Vierling JM. Natural history and pathogenesis of primary biliary cirrhosis and primary sclerosing cholangitis. In: Van Thiel D, ed. Advances in Hepatobiliary Diseases Seen in Practice. American Association for the Study of Liver Diseases, New Jersey, 1987:9.

184. Lebovics E, Palmer M, Woo J, et al. Outcome of primary sclerosing cholangitis. Analysis of long-term observation of 38 patients. Arch Intern Med 147:729, 1987.

185. LaRusso NF, Wiesner RH, Ludwig J, et al. Primary sclerosing cholangitis. N Engl J Med 310:899, 1984.

186. Holzbach RT, Marsh ME, Freedman MR, et al. Portal vein bile acids in patients with severe inflammatory bowel disease. Gut 21:428, 1980.

187. Gross JB, Ludwig J, Wiesner RH, et al. Abnormalities in tests of copper metabolism in primary sclerosing cholangitis. Gastroenterology 89:272, 1985.

188. Phillips PA, Keast D, Papadimitious JM, et al. Chronic obstructive jaundice induced by Reovirus type e in weanling mice. Pathology 1:193, 1969.

189. Bangaru B, Morecki R, Glaser JH, et al. Comparative studies of biliary atresia in the human newborn and reovirus-induced cholangitis in weanling mice. Lab Invest 43:456, 1980.

190. Morecki R, Glaser JH, Cho S, et al. Biliary atresia and reovirus type 3 infection. N Engl J Med 307:481, 1982.

191. Minuk GY, Paul RW, Lee PWK. The prevalence of antibodies to reovirus type 3 in adults with idiopathic cholestatic liver disease. J Med Virol 16:55, 1985.

192. Finegold MJ, Carpenter RJ. Obliterative cholangitis due to cytomegalovirus: A possible precursor of paucity of intrahepatic bile ducts. Hum Pathol 13:662, 1982.

193. Chapman RW, Varghese Z, Gaul R, et al. Association of primary sclerosing cholangitis with HLA-B8. Gut 24:38, 1983.

194. Schrumpf E, Fausa O, Forre O, et al. HLA antigens and immunoregulatory T cells in ulcerative colitis associated with hepatobiliary disease. Scand J Gastroenterol 17:187, 1982.

195. Chapman RWG, Jewell DP. Primary sclerosing cholangitis—An immunologically mediated disease? West J Med 143:193, 1985.

196. Takahashi F, Das KM. Isolation and characterization of a colonic autoantigen specifically recognized by colon tissue-bound immunoglobulin G from idiopathic ulcerative colitis. J Clin Invest 76:311, 1985.

197. Vecchi M, Sakamski S, Das KM. The Mr 40,000 colonic protein, an autoantigen associated with ulcerative colitis: Recognition of similar epitope(s) in skin and biliary tree by anti-Mr 40,000 antibodies. Gastroenterology 92:1682, 1987. (Abstract.)

198. McFarlane JG, Wojcicka BM, Tsantoulas DC, et al. Leukocyte migration inhibition in response to biliary antigens in primary biliary cirrhosis, sclerosing cholangitis and other chronic liver diseases. Gastroenterology 76:1333, 1979.

199. Chapman RW, Kelly P, Heryat A, et al. Expression of HLA-DR antigens on bile duct epithelium in primary sclerosing cholangitis. Gastroenterology 92(Abstr):1724, 1987.

200. Whiteside TL, Lasky S, Si L, et al. Immunologic analysis of mononuclear cells in liver tissues and blood of patients with primary sclerosing cholangitis. Hepatology 5:468, 1985.

201. Brinch L, Teisberg P, Schrumpf E, et al. The in vivo metabolism of C3 in hepatobiliary disease associated with ulcerative colitis. Scand J Gastroenterol 17:523, 1982.

202. Bodenheimer HC, LaRusso NF, Thayer WR, et al. Elevated circulating immune complexes in primary sclerosing cholangitis. Hepatology 3:150, 1983.

203. Minuk GY, Angus M, Brickman CM, et al. Abnormal clearance of immune complexes from the circulation of patients with primary sclerosing cholangitis. Gastroenterology 88:166, 1985.
204. Lindor KD, Wiesner RH, Katzmann JA, et al. Lymphocyte subsets in primary sclerosing cholangitis. Dig Dis Sci 32:720, 1987.
205. Lindor KD, Wiesner RH, LaRusso NF, et al. Enhanced autoreactivity of T-lymphocytes in primary sclerosing cholangitis. Hepatology 7:884, 1987.
206. Doppman JL, Girton ME. Bile duct scarring following ethanol embolization of the hepatic artery: An experimental study in monkeys. Radiology 152:621, 1984.
207. Dikengil A, Siskind BN, Morse SS, et al. Sclerosing cholangitis from intra-arterial floxuridine. J Clin Gastroenterol 8:690, 1986.
208. Gomez RL, Griffin JW, Squires JE. Prolonged relief of intractable pruritus in primary sclerosing cholangitis by plasmapheresis. J Clin Gastroenterol 8:301, 1986.
209. Lauterburg BH, Taswell HF, Pineda AA, et al. Treatment of pruritus of cholestasis by plasma perfusion through USP-charcoal-coated beads. Lancet 2:53, 1980.
210. Sartin JS, Wiesner RH, LaRusso NF. Fat-soluble vitamin deficiency in primary sclerosing cholangitis. Gastroenterology 92:1615, 1987. (Abstract.)
211. Wiesner RH, Ludwig J, LaRusso NF, et al. Diagnosis and treatment of primary sclerosing cholangitis. Semin Liver Dis 5:241, 1985.
212. Munoz SJ, Heubi JE, Balistreri WF, et al. Vitamin E deficiency in primary biliary cirrhosis: Mechanism and relation to deficiency in other lipid soluble vitamins. Gastroenterology 92:1758, 1987. (Abstract.)
213. May GR, Bender CE, Williams HJ. Radiologic approaches to the treatment of benign and malignant biliary tract disease. Semin Liver Dis 7:334, 1987.
214. Wood RAB, Cusheri A. Is sclerosing cholangitis complicating ulcerative colitis a reversible condition? Lancet 2:716, 1980.
215. Collier NA, Armitage NC, Hadjis NS, et al. Surgical approaches in primary sclerosing cholangitis. Aust NZ J Surg 55:437, 1895.
216. Salaspuro MP, Sipponen P, Makkonen H. The occurrence of orcein-positive hepatocellular material in various liver diseases. Scand J Gastroenterol 11:677, 1976.
217. LaRusso NF, Wiesner RH, Ludwig J, et al. Randomized trial of penicillamine in primary sclerosing cholangitis. Hepatology 6:1205, 1986. (Abstract.)
218. Leiser A, Kadish U. Beneficial effect of colchicine in a case of sclerosing cholangitis. Am J Med Sci 291:416, 1986.
219. LaRusso NF, Wiesner RH, Beaver SJ. Combined antifibrogenic and immunosuppressive therapy in primary sclerosing cholangitis. Gastroenterology 92:1493, 1987. (Abstract.)
220. Javett SL. Azathioprine in primary sclerosing cholangitis. Lancet 1:810, 1971.
221. Wagner A. Azathioprine treatment in primary sclerosing cholangitis. Lancet 2:663, 1971.
222. Kaplan MM, Arora S, Pincus SH. Primary sclerosing cholangitis and low-dose oral pulse methotrexate therapy. Clinical and histologic response. Ann Intern Med 106:231, 1987.
223. Marsh JW, Iwatsuki S, Makowka L, et al. Orthotopic liver transplantation for primary sclerosing cholangitis. Ann Surg 207:21, 1988.
224. Converse CF, Reagan JW, DeCosse JJ. Ulcerative colitis and carcinoma of the bile ducts. Am J Surg 121:39, 1971.
225. Ross AP, Braasch JW. Ulcerative colitis and carcinoma of the proximal bile ducts. Gut 14:94, 1973.
226. Black K, Hanna SS, Langer B, et al. Management of carcinoma of the extrahepatic bile ducts. Can J Surg 21:542, 1978.
227. Pereiras RV, Rheingold OJ, Hutson D, et al. Relief of malignant obstructive jaundice by percutaneous insertion of a permanent prosthesis in the biliary tree. Ann Intern Med 89:589, 1978.
228. Hall SW, Benjamin RS, Murphy WK, et al. Adriamycin, BCNU, FTORAFUR chemotherapy of pancreatic and biliary tract cancer. Cancer 44:2008, 1979.
229. Pilepich MV, Lambert PM. Radiotherapy of carcinomas of the extrahepatic biliary system. Radiology 127:767, 1978.
230. Baker AL, Kaplan MM, Norton RA, et al. Gallstones in inflammatory bowel disease. Dig Dis 19:109, 1974.
231. Heaton KW, Read AE. Gallstones in patients with disorders of the terminal ileum and disturbed bile salt metabolism. Br Med J 3:494, 1969.
232. Ritland S, Eigjo K, Sohansen O, et al. Liver copper content in patients with inflammatory bowel disease and associated liver disorders. Scand J Gastroenterol 14:711, 1979.

44

Primary Biliary Cirrhosis

John M. Vierling, M.D.

DEFINITION

PBC = primary biliary cirrhosis

Primary biliary cirrhosis is a chronic, progressive cholestatic liver disease of unknown cause. It is characterized by inflammatory destruction of intrahepatic bile ducts, periportal hepatitis with piecemeal necrosis, and progression to cirrhosis with portal hypertension. Addison and Gull, writing about xanthomatous skin lesions in 1851,[1] have been credited with the first description of a patient with this disorder. Hanot, in 1875, recognized this cholestatic disease as a distinct entity.[2] Subsequent investigators referred to this liver disease either as Hanot's cirrhosis or as "xanthomatous biliary cirrhosis,"[3] in recognition of its association with cutaneous xanthomas. The term primary biliary cirrhosis (PBC) was introduced in 1949 to distinguish biliary cirrhosis in the absence of extrahepatic biliary obstruction from that associated with obstruction of the large bile ducts.[4] A year later, Ahrens et al. reported the first comprehensive description of the clinical features of PBC.[5] Until that time PBC has been considered to be rare; fewer than 100 cases had been reported.

Recognizing that the disease is characterized by inflammatory destruction of interlobular and septal bile ducts, Sherlock proposed in 1959 that the term "chronic intrahepatic obstructive jaundice" was more descriptive than the term PBC.[6] In 1965, Rubin et al. described the characteristic histologic process resulting in the destruction of intrahepatic bile ducts as "nonsuppurative destructive cholangitis."[7] Finally, in 1967, Scheuer described the evolution of hepatobiliary lesions in PBC in terms of four overlapping histologic stages, with only the last stage representing true cirrhosis.[8]

During the past two decades, numerous investigations have advanced our understanding of PBC and have contributed to the evolution of our concepts concerning pathogenesis and therapy. Prominent recent contributions to our knowledge include the recognition of asymptomatic patients, a more precise description of the natural history and complications of the disease, a more accurate estimate of the prevalence of PBC, an appreciation of the association between PBC and putative immunologic diseases, an investigation of the role of immune function in the pathogenesis of PBC, and the results of controlled trials of therapy. The purpose of this chapter is to examine the clinical and pathologic features of PBC and to discuss the current concepts of pathogenesis and therapy. Even though PBC is a misnomer prior to the development of cirrhosis, the term PBC continues to be favored[9-13] over the histologically more accurate term chronic nonsuppurative destructive cholangitis. In this chapter, the term PBC refers to the disease process without regard to the presence or absence of cirrhosis.

ETIOLOGY

The cause of PBC remains unknown, but several etiologic agents have been postulated. These include hepatotropic viruses, fungi, bacteria, unspecified environmental toxins, abnormal or toxic bile acids, hepatotoxic medications and selenium deficiency. Studies of families with more than one affected member and relatives of patients with PBC suggest that genetically determined host susceptibility may be involved in the initiation of disease. Similarly, the preponderance of adult women with PBC suggests that female sex hormones may play a role in susceptibility. In discussing the postulated causes of PBC, it is important to distinguish between the concept of etiologic factors that initiate disease and the actual pathogenetic mechanisms that perpetuate disease (see the section on Pathogenesis).

VIRAL INFECTION

The hypothesis that viral infection of the liver causes PBC remains speculative. To date, studies of viral markers in PBC have been confined to the hepatitis B virus.[14-16] This virus appears to play no role, since the prevalence of positive tests for HBsAg or anti-HBs is no greater in patients with PBC than in control populations. Furthermore, in a recent report, HBsAg was not detected in 150 consecutive patients with PBC.[11] Evaluation of etiologic roles for other viruses, such as non-A, non-B hepatitis viruses, awaits the development of specific tests. A preliminary report suggests that up to 15 per cent of patients may have false-positive ELISA tests for antibodies reactive with human immunodeficiency virus.[17]

FUNGAL INFECTION

Berg and Baum speculated that PBC might be initiated by infection with the Neurospora species of yeast.[18] Previous work by these investigators suggested that the antigen specificity of the antimitochondrial antibody found in PBC differed from that of mitochondrial antibodies found in other hepatic and nonhepatic diseases (see the section on Laboratory Tests). They believe that the characteristic specificity of the antimitochondrial antibody in PBC, which is for a normally inaccessible component of the inner mitochondrial membrane, is not explained readily by the release of mitochondria from necrotic hepatobiliary tissue or by a specific alteration of immunoregulation. Since the mitochondria of some eukaryotes, including Neurospora, contain the specific antigen(s) recognized by the antimitochondrial antibody found in the sera of patients with PBC, Berg and Baum propose that infection of the liver with such an organism could result in the production of antibody that would cross-react with host mitochondria. Although

this hypothesis can explain the production of antimitochondrial antibody of a certain specificity, it does not explain the way in which inflammatory destruction of bile ducts and hepatocytes is initiated. Presumably, the latter mechanism would be independent of the production of antimitochondrial antibody, since circulating antibody may not be present in all patients with PBC (see Laboratory Tests).

BACTERIAL INFECTION

Recent studies have demonstrated that circulating antimitochondrial antibodies react with mitochondrial antigens of specific molecular weights (see section on Antimitochondrial Antibodies). Investigators questioned whether antimitochondrial antibodies in PBC are stimulated by antigens in bacterial membranes because the bacterial antigens cross react with mitochondrial antigens. The reactivity of sera from patients with PBC, patients with other liver diseases, and normal controls was assessed against mitochondrial and bacterial cell wall antigens.[40] The PBC sera exclusively reacted with specific mitochondrial antigens with molecular weights of 50 and 70 Kd. Similar reactions were observed using bacterial antigens, and absorption of the sera with these antigens eliminated reactivity with mitochondrial antigens. The bacterial antigens recognized by the PBC sera were also recognized by experimental rabbit antisera produced against specific R-mutant bacteria. These observations suggested that R-mutants, expressing PBC-specific antigens on their surface, could incite the production of antimitochondrial antibodies in PBC. Since neither the presence nor the titer of antimitochondrial antibodies has been directly related to hepatobiliary injury in PBC, the mechanism responsible for organ injury following bacterial stimulation of antibody production is unknown. However, it should be noted that an analogous situation has been postulated to explain the increased risk of ankylosing spondylitis in patients with ulcerative colitis who are HLA-B27 positive.[41] Since HLA-B27–positive lymphocytes express antigens that are cross-reactive with antigens on Klebsiella pneumoniae, it has been postulated that disease could result from production of antimicrobial antibodies that also recognize host antigen or that the microbial antigens bind to the HLA complex, rendering it susceptible to immunologic attack.

ENVIRONMENTAL TOXINS

The existence of undefined, transmissible environmental factors (either viral or nonviral) has been suggested. Geographic clustering of patients with PBC (90 per cent of patients were from an area containing only 4 per cent of the population) in a large epidemiologic survey suggested a relationship between PBC and a specific municipal water supply.[20] Similar observations of urban clustering have been reported by others.[21] In another study, an individual developed PBC shortly after having served as a nurse for a patient with the disease.[22] More research is needed to explore the possibility that viral or other transmissible agents in the environment cause PBC.

TOXICITY OF BILE ACIDS

The hypothesis that PBC results from an abnormality of bile acid metabolism is unsupported by experimental data. Also, interest in lithocholic acid as a hepatotoxin has abated with recognition that in humans this secondary bile acid is sulfated and detoxified.[23] Abnormal or unusual bile acids have not been identified in patients with PBC.[24] Elevations of total bile acids in the serum, which are seen even in the early stages of PBC, appear to be the secondary consequence of the inflammatory destruction of bile ducts rather than the result of an abnormality of bile acid metabolism.

TOXICITY OF MEDICATIONS

The possibility that medications might initiate PBC in susceptible individuals has been suggested by the occurrence of clinical and biochemical cholestasis resembling PBC following the use of phenothiazines,[25] tolbutamide,[26] organic arsenicals,[27] thiobendazole,[28] methyltestosterone,[29, 30] and contraceptive steroids.[31] The cholestatic syndrome caused by these drugs may include pruritus, jaundice, xanthomas, and very high levels of alkaline phosphatase and cholesterol. The hepatic injury induced by these drugs usually resolves completely after the medication is discontinued, but in rare instances persistence of cholestasis has suggested the development of PBC. For example, in a detailed investigation of patients with cholestasis induced by phenothiazines, 17 per cent were found to have clinical and biochemical features similar to those seen in PBC for as long as 36 months after discontinuation of the drugs.[25] Moreover, hepatic histologic features were similar to those seen in PBC. In another report, tolbutamide was administered for a prolonged period after the onset of jaundice. The liver biopsy from this patient showed chronic portal inflammation, destruction of interlobular bile ducts, and ductopenia, reminiscent of the findings in PBC.[28]

Although it is possible that drug-induced hepatic injury may initiate some cases of PBC, an attractive alternative explanation is that drugs capable of producing cholestasis act to unmask asymptomatic, pre-existing disease. The latter mechanism may explain the occasional onset of symptomatic PBC during pregnancy, when the levels of estrogen are increased.

SELENIUM DEFICIENCY

The hypothesis that initiation of PBC is the result of selenium deficiency has been proposed recently.[34] Since selenium is essential for glutathione peroxidase activity, which provides protection against toxic hydroperoxides, a deficiency of selenium might result in free radical–mediated lipid peroxidation and biliary injury. In accord with this hypothesis are observations that the incidence of PBC is increased in northern Sweden,[35] where selenium deficiency is endemic,[36] and that serum selenium levels are significantly reduced in a substantial number of PBC patients.[32, 33] Evidence against the hypothesis is the report that seven of eight PBC patients with normal serum selenium levels had normal serum levels of octadeca-9-11 dienoic acid (a reflection of hepatic free radical activity).[34] Also, there is no evidence that hepatic cytochrome P-450 microsomal enzyme activity (the postulated source of reactive metabolites) is abnormal in PBC regardless of the histologic stage.[37]

MULTIPLE FACTORS

In the absence of a defined etiology in PBC, it seems prudent to consider the possibility that more than one factor may initiate the pathologic process responsible for the characteristic clinical and histologic features of the disease. Our understanding of chronic active hepatitis provides a precedent for this idea, since it is now evident that diverse causative factors can result in both the characteristic morphologic lesion and the progressive course of this disease. These factors include infection with hepatitis B virus[38] and non-A, non-B viruses,[39] hepatotoxic medications,[40] Wilson's disease,[41] and heterozygous α_1-antitrypsin deficiency.[42] Further investigations are needed to define the etiologic factor(s) responsible for PBC. Research in this area should complement investigations of the pathogenetic mechanisms in PBC, and could help to resolve the dilemma of deciding which features of PBC are important in its pathogenesis and which are merely secondary consequences of the disease.

INCIDENCE OF EPIDEMIOLOGY

PBC occurs worldwide and has been found in all races. It has been estimated to account for 0.6 to 2 per cent of deaths from cirrhosis throughout the world.[43] In a study from England, an annual incidence of 5.8 cases per million population and a point prevalence (number of cases in a community at a particular time) of 5.4 cases per 100,000 population were found.[20] Remarkably similar estimates of incidence and point prevalence have been reported independently throughout the United Kingdom.[44] Similar epidemiologic studies of prevalence have been conducted worldwide.[35, 45, 46] The yearly incidence of PBC in a defined area of Sweden from 1976 to 1983 was 1.4 per 100,000, and the prevalence has been calculated as 6.4 per 100,000.[45] Continued observation of this area showed an unexplained increase in point prevalence on December 31, 1983 to 12.8 per 100,000, which represents the highest figure reported in the world.[35] Recent data[45, 46] indicate that the prevalence per 100,000 population is: 0.7 in West Germany, 0.7 to 1.2 in Eire, 1.2 to 5.0 in France, 2.3 in Denmark, 2.5 to 6.4 in Great Britain, 4.4 in Finland, 7.4 in Portugal, and up to 7.5 in Spain. Comparable studies have not been performed in the United States. In developed nations the prevalence appears to be increasing. Whether this apparent increase in prevalence reflects an actual increase in the incidence of PBC or is merely the result of diagnosing more cases of PBC at an earlier stage of disease is unknown.

The possible roles of environmental factors and the effects of socioeconomic factors on the epidemiology of PBC have been the subject of limited investigation. One English epidemiologic study found that PBC predominantly affected middle-aged women from an upper-middle-class background, and was more common in urban than in rural areas.[34] Further epidemiologic surveys from other countries are necessary to appraise this interesting finding. Future surveys also are needed to assess the significance of the recent findings of a geographic clustering of patients with PBC,[20, 21] and the striking increase in prevalence noted recently in Sweden.[35]

CLINICAL FEATURES

The disease primarily affects middle-aged women.[11, 43, 45, 46] In recent reports, the sex ratio in PBC has been nine to ten females to one male.[11, 43, 45–49] Although most symptomatic patients seek treatment between the ages of 40 and 60 years,[45] reported ages at diagnosis have ranged from 23[50] to 78[46] years. Many of the patients less than 40 years old now have their disease diagnosed prior to the onset of symptoms of hepatobiliary disease.

SYMPTOMS AND SIGNS

Classic descriptions of patients with PBC emphasize the presence of clinical cholestasis and the stigmata of chronic liver disease at the time of presentation.[5, 6] Such descriptions reflect that prior to 1960 PBC was diagnosed most often in patients who had far-advanced, icteric disease. Subsequent studies of symptomatic patients with earlier stages of PBC led to the recognition of a spectrum of symptoms and signs. More recently, asymptomatic patients with PBC have been detected with increasing frequency.

The presenting symptoms and signs in 100 patients with PBC reported by Sherlock and Scheuer during the period 1965 to 1972[45] are summarized in Table 44–1. Pruritus was present in 82 per cent of patients and most often had been insidious in onset. Typically, patients experience intermittent pruritus, which tends to be worse at night. Pruritus may be noticed initially in an acral or perianal distribution, but with time it usually becomes generalized. In the absence of jaundice, pruritus may be attributed mistakenly to a dermatologic or psychiatric disorder before appropriate hepatic tests are performed.[10] In 5 to 10 per cent of patients with PBC, the initial symptom of pruritus appears during pregnancy.[45, 51] Whereas the pruritus of pregnancy typically resolves rapidly in the postpartum period, pruritus often persists in patients with PBC. In other pregnant patients with PBC, the pruritus resolves spontaneously after delivery, only to recur months or even years later. It appears likely, therefore, that the cholestatic effects of high levels of estrogens in pregnancy[52] provoke symptoms in patients with asymptomatic PBC. Thus, not unexpectedly, oral contraceptives containing estrogen also may precipitate pruritus in women with PBC.[12]

Jaundice may precede pruritus, but it is unusual (6 per cent of patients) for jaundice to occur alone.[45] In patients with pruritus, jaundice may occur simultaneously or be delayed for variable periods ranging from months to more than ten years.[11, 45] Once present, jaundice tends to persist and does not resolve spontaneously. There are exceptions to this rule, however; jaundice in three patients with PBC resolved completely over periods of one to four months.[49] The diagnosis of PBC was suspected only after values for total serum bilirubin became normal while the levels of alkaline phosphatase remained elevated.

Table 44–2 lists the frequencies of symptoms at the time of referral for 151 patients enrolled in the Mayo Clinic's controlled trial of D-penicillamine therapy in the

TABLE 44–1. CLINICAL FEATURES OF 100 CONSECUTIVE PATIENTS WITH PRIMARY BILIARY CIRRHOSIS AT THE TIME OF PRESENTATION

Sign or Symptom	% Affected
Insidious onset of pruritus	57
Simultaneous onsets of pruritus and jaundice	20
Postpartum persistence of pruritus of pregnancy	5
Jaundice preceding pruritus	2
Jaundice without pruritus	6
Portal venous hypertension	4
Hepatosplenomegaly	3
Discovery during evaluation of another condition	4

Source: Data compiled from Sherlock S, Scheuer PJ. N Engl J Med 289:674, 1973.

TABLE 44–2. SYMPTOMS PRESENT AT THE TIME OF REFERRAL IN 151 PATIENTS WITH PRIMARY BILIARY CIRRHOSIS

Symptom	% Affected
Fatigue	70
Pruritus	66
Jaundice	47
Dark urine	52
Light stools	44
Easy bruising	31
Bone pain	16
Abdominal pain	16
Anorexia	22
Weight loss	28
Amenorrhea	5
Gastrointestinal bleeding	13
Hepatic encephalopathy	1

Source: Data compiled from Dickson ER, Summerfield J. Primary biliary cirrhosis. In: Current Concepts in Gastrointestinal Disease. Am Gastroenterol Assoc Postgraduate Course, Thorofare, NJ, Charles B Slack, 1979.

treatment of PBC.[53] The most frequent symptoms of cholestasis were pruritus and jaundice. It is noteworthy that individual patients frequently had two or more symptoms, including complaints of fatigue in 70 per cent. In a recently reported series of 236 patients with PBC,[46] the first symptom or sign was tabulated. Of symptoms or signs attributed to hepatobiliary disease, pruritus was reported by 47 per cent of patients, jaundice by 12 per cent, gastrointestinal hemorrhage by 6 per cent, and ascites by 2 per cent. Symptoms or signs classified as nonspecific included fatigue in 8 per cent of cases, abdominal pain in 7 per cent, and dyspepsia, weight loss, steatorrhea, xanthelasma, abdominal mass, and vertebral collapse, in less than 3 per cent each. Symptoms or signs of an associated collagen vascular disease were the initial complaints of 5 per cent of the patients (see the section on Associated Diseases).

PBC may be diagnosed prior to the onset of symptoms of hepatobiliary disease, and such patients often are referred to as asymptomatic.[11, 35, 45, 47649, 54–56] It is important to note, however, that many of these patients have symptoms or signs of disorders unrelated to hepatic disease. Thus, the designation *asymptomatic* often is accurate only in regard to symptoms of hepatobiliary disease. For example, in the series of 20 asymptomatic patients reported by Long et al., eight were seen as a result of investigations for other disorders, including keratoconjunctivitis sicca, rheumatoid arthritis, arthropathy, cervical spondylitis, hyperparathyroidism, pernicious anemia, telangiectasia, abdominal pain, and alcoholism.[52] Fleming et al. reported 21 asymptomatic patients among 103 patients enrolled in a controlled trial of D-penicillamine therapy.[54] Fourteen patients (67 per cent) had sought medical attention for nonhepatic conditions. Three patients had previously diagnosed diseases, including rheumatoid arthritis and scleroderma, and 11 had complaints ascribed to dyspepsia, peptic ulcer disease, esophageal reflux, irritable bowel syndrome, hypertension, or pneumonia. Analysis of the presenting symptom or sign in a series of 236 patients enrolled in a controlled trial of azathioprine therapy[46] revealed that a minimum of 52 patients could be considered asymptomatic in regard to hepatobiliary disease. Forty of these patients had sought medical attention for nonhepatic symptoms, related in 11 instances to collagen vascular diseases. Two of 10 patients with asymptomatic PBC reported by Hanik and Eriksson had symptoms of nonhepatic diseases at presentation.[55] In a recent study of Tornay of 40 consecutive patients with

PBC diagnosed since 1970, 24 had sought treatment without symptoms of liver disease.[49] In another recent series, reported by James et al., 45 of 93 consecutive patients with PBC were asymptomatic.[56] Studies of the incidence and prevalence of PBC in a defined area of Sweden indicate that approximately 50 per cent of patients are asymptomatic at the time of diagnosis.[35]

Virtually all the patients with PBC just mentioned had abnormal biochemical tests of hepatic function, including elevations of serum alkaline phosphatase. Indeed, in many instances the biochemical abnormalities prompted the diagnostic evaluation for the presence of liver disease. Two independent reports described the clinical features of patients with positive screening tests for antimitochondrial antibody, normal levels of alkaline phosphatase, and findings on liver biopsy consistent with the diagnosis of PBC.[56, 57] In the study of James et al.,[56] antimitochondrial antibody (titers 1:40 to 1:320) was discovered in 13 patients during immunologic screening tests for other diseases, such as arthritis, thyroid disease, and pernicious anemia. These patients thus were similar to the asymptomatic patients with PBC just described. Although all their biochemical tests of liver function were normal, the histologic features of the livers of the 13 patients were consistent with the diagnosis of PBC. The diagnosis of PBC would appear to have been accurate, since six of these patients developed abnormal hepatic biochemical tests and one developed pruritus during follow-up periods of two to five years. In another report, Munoz et al.[57] evaluated three patients who had positive tests for antimitochondrial antibody (titers 1:10 to 1:1000) and normal levels of alkaline phosphatase. The first patient (the daughter of a patient with PBC) had premenstrual pruritus, the second had Hashimoto's thyroiditis, and the third had unexplained hepatomegaly. Hepatic biochemical tests were normal except for a minimal elevation of aspartate aminotransferase (AST) in one patient. In all three patients, liver biopsy revealed classic changes of early PBC.

Recently, James and colleagues reported on an additional 16 patients with positive antimitochondrial antibody tests (titers $\geq$ 1:40) detected during screening for other autoimmune diseases in the absence of symptoms of liver disease or abnormal tests for bilirubin, alkaline phosphatase, or aminotransferases.[58] Autoantibodies were screened in the combined total of 29 patients (28 females) because of concern about thyroid disease in 9, pernicious anemia in 4, arthropathy in 7, lupus erythematosus in 2, and scleroderma, urticaria, abdominal pain, and hepatomegaly in 1 patient per disorder. An additional patient was identified in a population survey. Of note, 2 patients were a mother and daughter who were detected independently; none of the other patients had relatives with PBC. Although alkaline phosphatase levels were normal by definition, 14 of 28 patients had modest elevations of γ-glutamyltransferase that were not attributable to alcohol consumption. Liver biopsies were performed in each patient, and each patient was prospectively observed. Of the 29 liver biopsies, 12 were highly consistent with the diagnosis of PBC with inflammatory injury of interlobular and segmental bile ducts with or without portal granulomas. In these biopsies, piecemeal necrosis was present in five and fibrosis in four. Twelve additional biopsies were consistent with the diagnosis of PBC with portal inflammation centered around bile ducts or portal lymphoid aggregates. Two other biopsies showed granulomatous changes exclusively in the portal tracts. One biopsy showed nonspecific hepatitis, whereas two biopsies were normal.

During a mean of 8.7 years of observation, five patients developed symptoms compatible with PBC: pruritus in four and severe malaise in one. Two of the patients who developed pruritus did so in less than four years. Twelve of 16 women observed for four years or longer developed abnormal liver tests; in 11 the alkaline phosphatase has been transiently or permanently elevated. The antimitochondrial antibody has remained positive in all patients, without significant increases in titer. Thirteen of the 16 have had elevated serum levels of IgM. The combined data indicate that an early phase of PBC exists in which neither symptoms nor abnormalities of routine liver tests are present. Detection of patients on the basis of a positive test for antimitochondrial antibody supports the view that the presence of such antibodies (with reactivity against specific mitochondrial antigens) is virtually diagnostic of PBC (see section on Antimitochondrial Antibodies). Therefore, it would be of great interest to study the antigenic specificities of the antimitochondrial antibodies in these patients. Since the age of the patients in this preclinical phase of PBC does not differ substantially from that of patients diagnosed with PBC on the basis of symptoms or abnormalities of liver tests,[59, 60] it is debatable that this is a phase of the natural history through which all patients pass. If this is true, patients detected at this preclinical stage would be expected to be younger. However, the findings of histologically advanced lesions in this phase are compatible with the observation that a substantial proportion of asymptomatic patients with abnormal liver tests have advanced histologic stages of disease when first detected. Continued observation of patients in this preclinical phase of disease is necessary to define the frequency of progression and relationship to the classic phases of PBC.

Based on the combined observations of several reports, it is now clear that a substantial proportion of patients with PBC are asymptomatic with respect to liver disease when their disease is first diagnosed. However, less than 40 per cent of patients with PBC referred to as asymptomatic actually are free of all symptoms. Symptoms associated with collagen vascular diseases or thyroid disease are particularly common and most likely reflect the strong association between PBC and putative autoimmune diseases (see section on Associated Diseases). The true frequency of asymptomatic patients within a population of patients with PBC is difficult to determine, since estimates range from 20[46] to 77[55] per cent. In two large reported series, a similar frequency of approximately 20 per cent was noted,[46, 54] but prospective studies in Sweden indicate that 50 per cent of patients whose disorder was recently diagnosed as PBC were asymptomatic.[35] The recent identification of additional asymptomatic patients with PBC, who were detected solely on the basis of a positive test for antimitochondrial antibody, suggests that the true frequency of asymptomatic patients may be higher.

The majority of data regarding the clinical features of PBC reflect the signs and symptoms of women, rather than of men, who constitute a minority of patients with PBC. Recently, studies have been conducted to evaluate the similarity of clinical and histologic features in men and women with PBC.[47, 48] In the initial retrospective study of Rubel et al.,[48] the clinical and histologic features of 30 with PBC were compared in 30 men and of 30 women matched for age. It was concluded that there was little difference between the groups, except that men tended to have higher levels of alkaline phosphatase and a lower frequency of piecemeal necrosis on liver biopsy. However, the preponderance of women with PBC and the wide variation in clinical symptoms suggest that comparison of so few patients may have masked true differences. This is substantiated by another study[47] that compared the presentation and course of PBC in all patients followed prospectively during a 15-year period. Of 230 patients with PBC, 39 (16 per cent) were male. The mean age of men and women at diagnosis, the frequency of early and advanced histopathology, and the levels of serum bilirubin were similar. Although a larger proportion of men were symptomatic (23 per cent versus 12 per cent), this difference was not statistically significant. Among symptomatic patients, significantly fewer men exhibited pruritus than did women. Despite progressive increases in the frequency of pruritus in both sexes during follow-up, the significant difference between men and women persisted and was most pronounced between men and premenopausal women. These data are compatible with the hypothesis that the frequency of pruritus is influenced by levels of circulating female sex steroids and not solely by the degree of cholestasis.

The clinical description of PBC is also heavily weighted in favor of middle-aged patients with asymptomatic and symptomatic disease. With the increasing frequency of diagnosis in PBC, a substantial number of patients have been detected at an advanced age. To evaluate potential differences among young and old patients, the presenting features and clinical course of 35 patients who were more than 65 years of age at presentation were compared with those of 86 younger patients.[60] The frequency of asymptomatic disease in these patients was comparable: 31 per cent in elderly patients versus 20 per cent in younger patients. The frequency of pruritus, fatigue, jaundice, abdominal pain, weight loss, bone pain, gastrointestinal hemorrhage, and encephalopathy was also comparable in both groups. The prevalence of associated autoimmune disorders was similar in both groups, except for the presence of the CREST (Calcinosis cutis, Raynaud's phenomenon, Esophageal dysfunction, Sclerodactyly, and Telangiectasia) syndrome, which was significantly more frequent among younger patients. Thus, PBC diagnosed in patients after the age of 65 is very similar to the disease in younger patients.

PHYSICAL EXAMINATION

The findings on physical examination when patients first seek medical advice vary widely. At one extreme the examination may show no abnormality, whereas at the other extreme nonspecific stigmata of chronic liver disease may predominate. Abnormal physical findings are reported most often for symptomatic patients but also may occur in asymptomatic patients. For example, stigmata of liver disease were found in 43 per cent of asymptomatic patients.[54] Hepatomegaly or hepatosplenomegaly was present on presentation in 35 per cent of such patients described by Long et al.[50] and 40 per cent of those reported by Hanik and Eriksson.[55] In addition to organomegaly, abnormal features found in asymptomatic patients with PBC include spider angiomas, hyperpigmentation, and xanthelasma.[54] In symptomatic patients, excoriations due to severe pruritus are seen frequently. Table 44–3 lists the abnormal physical findings in PBC, with estimates of the frequencies of individual findings at presentation. No significant differences between men and women have been noted in the frequency of jaundice, hepatomegaly, splenomegaly, ascites, or xanthomata.[47] However, hyperpigmentation and the sicca complex occur significantly more often in women

TABLE 44–3. PHYSICAL FINDINGS IN PATIENTS WITH PRIMARY BILIARY CIRRHOSIS AT THE TIME OF PRESENTATION

	% of Affected Patients
Skin	
Hyperpigmentation*	59
Lichenification	—
Excoriations	25
Xanthelasma	21
Xanthoma	6
Vascular spiders	32
Jaundice	50
Purpura	Rare
Eyes	
Pigmented corneal rings	Rare
Jaundiced bulbar conjunctivae	50
Abdomen	
Hepatomegaly	55
Splenomegaly	33
Ascites	5
Musculoskeletal system	
Bone tenderness	Rare
Clubbing	8
Edema	14
Neurologic	
Peripheral neuropathy	Rare
Portosystemic encephalopathy	Rare

Source: Data compiled from references 11, 39, 50, 53, and 54.
*May precede, occur simultaneously with, or follow clinical cholestasis.

than in men.[47] Comparison of young and elderly patients with PBC reveals no significant differences in the frequency of hepatomegaly, splenomegaly, hyperpigmentation, xanthomata, or ascites.[60] The progression of physical findings during the course of the disease is discussed under Natural History.

LABORATORY TESTS

SERUM BIOCHEMICAL TESTS

With rare exception,[56–58] routine biochemical tests of hepatic function are abnormal and show a cholestatic rather than a hepatocellular pattern. Table 44–4 summarizes the results of laboratory tests performed on symptomatic and asymptomatic patients with PBC at the time of referral to the Mayo Clinic. Alkaline phosphatase almost always is elevated in PBC and is of hepatobiliary origin, as can be shown by concomitant elevations of 5'-nucleotidase, leucine aminopeptidase, or γ-glutamyltranspeptidase. Even early in the course of PBC, substantial elevations of alkaline phosphatase are so prevalent that they have been used as a criterion for patient selection in recent studies.[46] Values for alkaline phosphatase at presentation are generally more than twofold greater than the upper limit of normal; such elevations were found in 96 per cent of patients reported by Sherlock and Scheuer.[45] Very high values of alkaline phosphatase are not infrequent. The mean value for patients studied at the Mayo Clinic represented a fivefold elevation (see Table 44–4).[54]

As discussed earlier, some asymptomatic patients with PBC have normal levels of alkaline phosphatase at the time of diagnosis. Until recently, such patients usually were discovered by chance because of liver biopsy performed for other indications.[59] However, reports now indicate that

TABLE 44–4. MEAN LABORATORY VALUES OF SYMPTOMATIC AND ASYMPTOMATIC PATIENTS WITH PRIMARY BILIARY CIRRHOSIS

	Normal	Symptomatic	Asymptomatic
Alkaline phosphatase	87–250 IU/l	1695 IU/l	1395 IU/l
Total bilirubin	<1 mg/dl	4.4 mg/dl	0.9 mg/dl
Asparate aminotransferase (AST; SGOT)	8–20 IU/l	85 IU/l	78 IU/l
Albumin	3.5–4.7 g/dl	3.5 g/dl	3.8 g/dl
Cholesterol	218–300 mg/dl	377 mg/dl	285 mg/dl
Triglycerides	101–150 mg/dl	133 mg/dl	96 mg/dl
Gamma-globulin	0.8–1.6 g/dl	1.9 g/dl	2.1 g/dl
IgM	0.2–1.4 mg/ml	6.0 mg/ml	7.1 mg/ml
Prothrombin time	10–12 sec	11.3 sec	11.1 sec
Erythrocyte sedimentation rate	<40 mm/1 hr	65 mm/1 hr	56 mm/1 hr

Source: Data compiled from Dickson ER, Summerfield J. Primary biliary cirrhosis. In: Current Concepts in Gastrointestinal Disease. Am Gastroenterol Assoc Postgraduate Course. Thorofare, NJ, Charles B Slack, 1979, and from Fleming CR, et al. Mayo Clin Proc 53:587, 1978.

pruritic or asymptomatic patients with positive tests for antimitochondrial antibody and normal levels of alkaline phosphatase may have histologic lesions of the liver consistent with the diagnosis of PBC.[56–58] In one recent report, some of these patients had abnormalities of γ-glutamyltransferase.[58]

Values for total serum bilirubin vary, depending on the clinical stage of the disease. Early in the course of the disease total bilirubin may be normal, especially in asymptomatic patients.[54–58] At the time of presentation, even symptomatic patients may have normal values or only modest elevations. In one report, approximately 50 per cent of patients had bilirubin values of less than 2 mg/dL at presentation.[45] Thus, the total bilirubin values often seem disproportionately low in comparison with the clinical evidence of severe cholestasis (e.g., pruritus, excoriations, lichenification, hyperpigmentation). During the later stages of the disease the levels of birirubin progressively rise, but they generally do not exceed 20 mg/dL even in the terminal phase of the disease[46, 61, 62] (see section on Natural History). Fractionation of elevated values of total bilirubin shows a direct-reacting component of ≥ 50 per cent. Increases in the direct-reacting fraction also may be found in patients whose total bilirubin values are normal, and the usefulness of fractionating the total bilirubin is further limited by the fact that commercially available tests for direct-reacting bilirubin vary in accuracy.[61]

Except in rare instances,[56–58] levels of aminotransferases are elevated in patients with PBC at presentation. Mean values generally are no higher than four to five times the upper limit of normal[54]; values greater than 250 IU/L are rare.[46, 53] Alanine aminotransferase activity is comparable to or slightly exceeds that of aspartate aminotransferase.

Asymptomatic patients with PBC may have milder biochemical abnormalities than do symptomatic patients. In two series, values for alkaline phosphatase and total bilirubin were generally less in asymptomatic than in symptomatic patients.[50, 55] However, others reported that values for alkaline phosphatase in asymptomatic and symptomatic patients were comparable.[62] In the same study, values for total bilirubin, cholesterol, and triglycerides were significantly lower in the asymptomatic group, compared with the symptomatic group.

Men and women with PBC do not differ with respect to levels of bilirubin or alkaline phosphatase.[47] Similarly, young and elderly patients with PBC have comparable levels of bilirubin, alkaline phosphatase, and albumin.[60]

Lipids

Total serum lipids are increased in PBC. Total serum cholesterol is elevated in approximately 50 per cent of patients at presentation,[11] and the mean values are higher in symptomatic patients.[54] Less information is available regarding serum triglyceride levels in PBC. In general, serum triglycerides are normal or only moderately increased. The levels tend to be higher in patients with symptomatic disease.[54]

Nonspecific abnormalities of lipoproteins seen in other types of liver disease also occur in PBC[64] (see Chap. 5). Lipoprotein electrophoresis shows abnormalities in all types of liver disease involving hepatocellular injury, characterized by the lack of α and pre-β bands and the presence of a dense β fraction. Although such bands can be equaled, respectively, with high-density lipoprotein, low-density lipoprotein, and very low-density lipoprotein in health, this is not true for patients with hepatocellular disease. For example, presence of an abnormal high-density lipoprotein may be associated with absence of an α band, and very low-density lipoprotein can be present in blood even in the absence of a pre-β band.

Two abnormal lipoproteins are detectable in the plasma of patients with cholestatic liver disease.[64–67] Lipoprotein-X migrates in the β position on electrophoresis, and contains unesterified cholesterol, phospholipid, apolipoprotein C and E, minor amounts of apolipoproteins B and A-I, and albumin as its major protein. Lipoprotein-X appears as bilamellar disks on electron microscopy (see Fig. 5–2, Chap. 5). Lipoprotein-X appears to accumulate as the result of regurgitation of biliary lipid into plasma and/or as the result of deficiency of lecithin:cholesterol acyltransferase (LCAT).[65] Lipoprotein-X is found no more frequently in patients with extrahepatic biliary obstruction than in patients with intrahepatic cholestasis.[68] Lipoprotein-X may be present in patients with PBC even early in the course of their disease[64, 68] but is more common after prolonged cholestasis.[65, 66] High-density lipoprotein rich in apolipoprotein E also is observed and appears similar to that seen in familial deficiency of LCAT.[65, 66] Thus, it may be a nascent high-density lipoprotein that persists in the circulation because of LCAT deficiency.

An abnormal low-density lipoprotein migrating in the α position has been detected in the sera of 40 of 77 patients with PBC.[11] This α_1 low-density lipoprotein is distinct from lipoprotein-X and was present in the sera of only 5 of 120,000 patients with diseases other than PBC. Four of these patients had either chronic active hepatitis or sclerosing cholangitis associated with ulcerative colitis. It is of interest that this α_1 low-density lipoprotein was found in 71 per cent of patients with PBC who had negative tests for antimitochondrial antibody. In another study, this lipoprotein was termed "slow α-lipoprotein" because of its retarded mobility on agarose gel electrophoresis.[65] Its density by ultracentrifugation was between the ranges of low-density lipoprotein and high-density lipoprotein, and apolipoprotein E was a major constituent, even though it is not a major apolipoprotein of either normal low- or high-density lipoproteins. The slow α-lipoprotein was present in 80 per cent of patients and occurred exclusively in histologic stages greater than stage II.

Recent studies have assessed the relationship between abnormalities of lipids and the duration and clinical phase of disease.[65–67] In patients with early and intermediate histologic stages, high-density lipoproteins were markedly elevated,[66, 69] whereas very low-density and low-density lipoproteins were mildly elevated.[66] In patients with advanced disease, low-density lipoproteins were markedly elevated, lipoprotein-X was present, and high-density lipoproteins were decreased.[66] In patients with early- and late-stage disease, hepatic lipase activity was decreased significantly. The inverse correlation between hepatic lipase activity and elevated high-density lipoprotein$_2$ (HDL$_2$) in early stages of disease suggested that decreased lipase activity resulted in the elevation of HDL$_2$.[66] Decreased concentrations of high-density lipoproteins observed in advanced disease (despite decreased hepatic lipase activity) appeared to be related to concomitant LCAT deficiency.

In patients with early stages of disease, an abnormal high-density lipoprotein which is distinct from HDL$_2$ has been identified, and contains apolipoprotein A-I and greater than expected amounts of apolipoprotein E and phospholipid.[67] A similar abnormal high-density lipoprotein can be generated by incubating normal serum with liposomes containing large amounts of phospholipids, indicating a role for phospholipid in the formation of this high-density lipoprotein.[67]

The effect of PBC on apolipoprotein levels remains unclear, although a relationship to the duration and stage of disease appears likely.[66, 67, 69] In a study of patients with predominantly early disease, levels of apolipoproteins A-I, B, and C-III were normal, levels of apolipoproteins E and C-II were markedly increased, and levels of apolipoprotein A-II were decreased.[65] The increase in apolipoprotein E was the most distinctive feature. In another study comparing early and late stages of disease, levels of apolipoproteins A-I, A-II, and C-II were significantly increased in early stages (E was not studied).[66] Among patients with a wide variation in the degree of hyperbilirubinemia, levels of apolipoproteins A-I, A-II, and E were decreased and levels of apolipoprotein A-I were inversely correlated with the serum bilirubin.[69] Further studies of well-defined patient groups reflecting the entire spectrum of disease are required to distinguish the specific effects of PBC on lipid metabolism from nonspecific effects of chronic cholestasis and altered nutrition.

Bile Acids

Serum bile acids are increased in all cholestatic conditions, including PBC.[22, 70–73] Fasting concentrations of serum bile acids are elevated in 93 to 100 per cent of patients with PBC.[70, 71] Moreover, bile acid levels are increased in approximately 80 per cent of patients with PBC who have normal total serum bilirubin.[71] Cholic acid is the predominant bile acid in the sera of patients with PBC, and the ratio of cholic to chenodeoxycholic acid is greater than 1.[72] An initial report of elevated levels of monohydroxy bile acids[70] has not been substantiated.[23, 72] Taurine conjugates generally exceed glycine conjugates. With progression of the disease, the levels of total bile acids increase and the ratio of cholic to chenodeoxycholic acid decreases.[71] Abnormal bile acids have not been found in patients who have intense pruritus, suggesting that abnormal pathways of bile acid metabolism do not occur in PBC.[23] During therapy with cholestyramine, total bile acids decrease and the ratio of cholic to chenodeoxycholic acid increases.[70] In contrast to the effects of cholestyramine, phenobarbital therapy, which reduces total bile acids in some patients with PBC, decreases the ratio of cholic to chenodeoxycholic acid.[23]

In one study, biliary and fecal bile acids were measured in nine patients with PBC.[73] The composition of biliary lipid was normal, as was the concentration of chenodeoxycholic acid. The relative amount of biliary deoxycholic acid was much less than normal in patients with PBC, whereas the amount of cholic acid was increased. Similar results have been found in other studies of chronic liver diseases associated with cholestasis.[74, 75] Recent assessment of the biliary output of bilirubin, phospholipids, and bile acids in eight patients with variable stages of PBC showed that biliary bilirubin output was identical to that in control subjects.[76] The biliary output of bilirubin was high in comparison to either phospholipid or bile acids. Thus, the data indicate a decrease in the biliary output of phospholipids and bile acids with maintenance of bilirubin output in PBC. The relative excess of bilirubin could contribute to an increased risk of pigment stone formation.

IMMUNOSEROLOGIC TESTS

Antimitochondrial Antibodies

The discovery of complement-fixing autoantibodies reactive with tissue extracts by McKay in 1957 led to the proposal that PBC was an autoimmune disease.[78] In 1965, Walker et al. reported that patients with PBC had serum antibodies that reacted with mitochondria.[77] Since that time the validity of this observation and the value of this test have been confirmed repeatedly.[18, 79–86] Yet it remains uncertain whether antimitochondrial antibodies are related to the pathogenesis of PBC or are a consequence of the disease. Recent work has clarified the spectrum of mitochondrial antigens recognized by antimitochondrial antibodies, identified specific antigens recognized by antibodies present in PBC sera, and provided more accurate methods for detection of antimitochondrial antibodies.[84–86] Cloning of the rat liver cDNA that encodes the autoantigen most specific for PBC provides unparalleled opportunities to evaluate the relationship between antimitochondrial antibodies and disease pathogenesis.[86]

Mitochondrial Antigens

Mitochondria contain hundreds of proteins, the majority of which are encoded by nuclear rather than mitochondrial DNA.[86] These proteins are produced in the cytosol and transported to mitochondria. Currently, nine separate mitochondrial antigens have been identified that react with antimitochondrial antibodies.[84, 86] These antigens and their disease associations are summarized in Table 44–5.

Antimitochondrial antibodies are detected most commonly by indirect immunofluorescent microscopy; several tissues, including kidney, thyroid, gastric mucosa, and liver, have been used as antigen substrates.[18, 79, 81] Rat kidney is used by most laboratories, although studies suggest that human kidney may be preferable as a substrate because of

TABLE 44–5. MITOCHONDRIAL AUTOANTIGENS

Antigen	Clinical Association	Biochemical Definition	Molecular Weight	Organ Specificity	Mitochondrial Membrane
M1	Syphilis	Cardiolipin	Unknown	No	Inner
M2	Very specific for PBC	Sequenced	70, 45, 39 kD complex	No	Inner
M3	Pseudolupus	Unknown	Unknown	No	Outer
M4	"Overlap" PBC and CAH	Unknown	Unknown	No	Outer
M5	Connective tissue disease	Unknown	Unknown	No	Outer
M6	Drug-induced hepatitis	Unknown	Unknown	Liver	Outer
M7	Cardiomyopathies	Unknown	Unknown	Myocardium	Inner
M8	PBC (may correlate with severity)	Unknown	Unknown	No	Outer
M9	PBC (but not specific)	Unknown	Unknown	No	Outer

Source: Modified from Gershwin ME et al. Hepatology 8:147, 1988 © by Am Assoc for the Study of Liver Diseases.

less nonspecific immunofluorescence.[79] The strongest immunofluorescent reactions occur within renal tubular epithelial cells located in the distal convoluted tubule or in the ascending loop of Henle.[18, 79] In the thyroid,[18] oxyphil cells stain more intensely than other cells. Gastric parietal cells stain uniformly, whereas liver cells show a weak, granular pattern of fluorescence.[18] Antigens designated M1, M2, and M7 are located on the inner membrane of mitochondria, whereas the others are on the outer membrane. The antigens are located in all organs, with the exception of M6 and M7, which are preferentially located in the liver and myocardium, respectively. In addition to immunofluorescence, mitochondrial antigens can be detected by complement fixation (except for M9) and are suitable for radioimmunoassays and ELISA.

Serum samples are routinely diluted 1:10 for immunofluorescence testing to avoid false-positive and false-negative results.[81] Undiluted sera from normal individuals may give false-positive reactions because of nonspecific immunofluorescence. Conversely, undiluted sera with high titers of antimitochondrial antibody may give false-negative reactions as a result of a prozone effect. Results of tests for antimitochondrial antibody have been variously reported either as positive or negative or as the greatest dilution (titer) of serum yielding a positive result.

The mitochondrial antigen most specifically associated with PBC is designated M2.[84–91] The M2 antigen is composed of at least three polypeptides with apparent molecular weights of 39, 45, and 70 Kd, although some discrepancies in apparent molecular weights have been reported.[92–94] Structurally, M2 has not been identified; earlier reports that it represented a component of ATPase or the adenine translocator enzyme were erroneous.[86, 87] The majority of patients with PBC have antibodies that react with the 70 Kd antigen, and reactivity to the 39- or 45-Kd antigens is rare in the absence of reactivity to the 70 Kd antigen.[84, 87] Gershwin et al. recently isolated a cDNA from rat liver that encodes the 70 Kd antigen.[85] A clone of cells transfected with a vector containing this cDNA expressed a fused polypeptide of 160 Kd that corresponded antigenically to the 70-Kd M2 mitochondrial antigen. The fused polypeptide reacted with 100 per cent of sera from patients with PBC and with none of the sera from healthy controls or patients with chronic active hepatitis, rheumatoid arthritis, or systemic lupus erythematosus. Extensive control experiments demonstrated that the fused polypeptide contained the epitopes recognized by the antimitochondrial antibodies in PBC sera.

Three other mitochondrial antigens (M4, M8, and M9) apparently localized to the outer membrane are recognized by antibodies in the sera of patients with PBC. M4 has been reported to react with sera of patients with PBC and patients with histologic features of an "overlap" syndrome of both PBC and chronic active hepatitis.[95] It is not disease specific, however, since sera from patients with systemic lupus erythematosus also react with M4.[84] The presence of antibodies reactive with M8 (always found concomitantly with antibodies to M2) appears to be related to a poor prognosis.[46] Antibodies reacting with M9 have been identified not only in PBC but also in family members of patients with PBC, in 15 per cent of normal controls, and in 63 per cent of technicians handling PBC sera.[86] Further studies are required to assess the specificity and frequency of reactions with these three antigens and to study the possibility that M4, M8, and M9 antigens actually may represent cytoplasmic antigens recognized by nonmitochondrial antibodies present in high titer in sera of patients with PBC.[97, 98]

Relationship to Pathogenesis

Currently, neither the presence nor the titers of mitochondrial antibodies have been shown to be related to the pathogenetic mechanisms responsible for PBC. This conclusion is supported by the fact that the presence and titers of antimitochondrial antibodies do not correlate with the duration of disease or with the clinical, biochemical, or histologic severity of disease.[11, 46, 99] In addition, the clinical course of PBC in patients who have negative tests for antimitochondrial antibodies is no different from that in patients whose tests are positive.[11, 99] Furthermore, antimitochondrial antibodies occur in other hepatic and nonhepatic diseases and have been found in an appreciable proportion of apparently healthy relatives of patients with PBC.[100, 101] Finally, antimitochondrial antibodies with specificities for M2, M4, and M8 continue to be present following successful liver transplantation for PBC in the absence of disease recurrence.[102]

Although compelling, the above observations do not refute the possibility that antimitochondrial antibodies are related to disease pathogenesis. The specific association between antimitochondrial antibodies in PBC and the M2 antigen counters evidence that the reactivities of other antimitochondrial antibodies are nonspecific for PBC. The explanation that antimitochondrial antibodies arise as a consequence of bile duct injury does not adequately explain the absence of such antibodies in other diseases in which the bile duct epithelia are destroyed. Recent evidence that antigens "cross-reactive" with antimitochondrial antibodies are present on the cell surface membrane of bacteria and rat hepatocytes[18, 103] suggests that epitopes of the M2 antigen could serve as targets for immunologic attack. This is in accord with recent evidence that specific epitopes with amphipathic helical configuration are necessary for reaction with T-cell receptors.[84, 104] Since T cells might react with epitopes on the M2 antigen distinct from those recognized by antimitochondrial antibodies, the antimitochondrial antibodies could be associated indirectly with a T-cell–mediated pathogenesis.

Frequency

Table 44–6 compares the frequencies of positive immunofluorescent tests for antimitochondrial antibodies in PBC and several other liver diseases. The test is positive in approximately 83 to 99 per cent of patients with PBC. In two large series of patients, the prevalence of positive tests for antimitochondrial antibodies was 95 per cent and 91 per cent, respectively.[11, 105] It should be noted, however, that in both series the groups of patients were selected by the process of referral.

Negative tests for antimitochondrial antibodies were reported in 1 to 17 per cent of patients with PBC (see Table 44–6). However, with serial testing or the use of undiluted serum in the assay, positive tests were found in these patients.[55] A positive test discriminates most precisely between patients with PBC and patients with extrahepatic biliary obstruction[82] or primary sclerosing cholangitis.[106, 107] Positive tests in patients with extrahepatic biliary obstruction[79, 80, 83, 108] have been attributed to technical differences in the performance of the tests[81, 82] or to the coexistence of liver disease, such as PBC, and extrahepatic biliary obstruction. Demonstration of appreciable numbers of positive tests in patients with chronic active hepatitis (8 to 28 per cent), cryptogenic cirrhosis (6 to 31 per cent), and collagen vascular diseases (2 to 29 per cent) underscores the importance of interpreting a positive test for antimitochondrial antibody in the light of all available clinical, biochemical, and histologic information. Although it has been suggested that the titers of antimitochondrial antibodies may help to distinguish patients with PBC (titer >1:160) from patients with chronic active hepatitis who have positive tests (titer <1:40), this has been questioned by others.[57, 58] It is interesting to speculate that some patients with cryptogenic cirrhosis and positive tests for antimitochondrial antibody[79, 107] actually may have had PBC. This possibility is suggested by the preponderance of middle-aged women in this group, by the presence of features of cholestasis, and by the presence of histologic features now considered compatible with diagnosis of PBC.[18, 81]

It is important to exercise special care in the interpretation of positive immunofluorescence tests in chronic active hepatitis, since many of these patients have antibodies that react with antigens of the endoplasmic reticulum. Immunofluorescence caused by these antimicrosomal antibodies can be distinguished from true antimitochondrial antibody by scrutinizing the renal medullary tissue, where antimitochondrial antibody stains the loop of Henle but antimicrosomal antibody does not. Development of tests utilizing highly purified, disease specific mitochondrial antigens should obviate the concerns imposed by reliance on immunofluorescent methods. The availability of a recombinant source of M2 antigen should also make standardization to a reference antigen feasible.[85, 86]

Other Autoantibodies

Patients who have PBC also may have antibodies that react against other non–organ-, non–species-specific tissue or cellular antigens.[46, 79, 81, 97, 98, 109, 110] The types and reported frequencies of positive tests include the following: antinuclear, 5 to 54 per cent; anti–smooth muscle, 26 to 49 per cent; rheumatoid factor, 24 to 60 per cent; anti-thyroid, 15 to 26 per cent; and anti–bile canalicular, 35 per cent. In series where healthy, matched controls were tested, the frequency of positive tests was generally less than 5 per cent. Among patients with chronic active hepatitis or cryptogenic cirrhosis, the frequency of positive tests was comparable to or greater than that seen in PBC.[109] Antibodies reacting with cytoplasmic antigens (e.g., microsomes) also are present in high titer in PBC sera[97, 98] and have been implicated in reactions with the putative mitochondrial antigens M4, M8, and M9 (see section on Antimitochondrial Antibodies). These autoantibodies are thought not to be of pathogenic significance, since they are not specific for diseases of the liver and their presence and titers do not correlate with the duration or severity of disease.

Studies of the isotypes and antigen specificities of anti–smooth muscle antibodies have shown several differences between patients with PBC and those with chronic active hepatitis.[111] In patients with chronic active hepatitis, anti–smooth muscle antibody was predominantly of the IgG isotype, in contrast to a predominance of the IgM isotype in patients with PBC. In patients who had an atypical, cholestatic variant of chronic active hepatitis, the anti–smooth muscle antibodies were of the IgM class. The specificities of anti–smooth muscle antibodies for actin also differed for PBC and chronic active hepatitis, being more common in the latter.

OTHER IMMUNOLOGIC TESTS

Hypergammaglobulinemia may develop any time during the course of PBC but is most common in the later

---

TABLE 44–6. REPORTED FREQUENCIES OF ANTIMITOCHONDRIAL ANTIBODY IN PATIENTS WITH HEPATOBILIARY DISEASES*

	Frequency (%) in the Series of:						
	Doniach et al.[79]	Klatskin and Kanton[80]	Richer and Viallet[82]	Ward et al.[83]	Munoz et al.[57]	Wiesner and LaRusso[106]	Chapman et al.[107]
Primary biliary cirrhosis	98 (41)	84 (188)	100 (5)	83 (24)	99 (218)	—	—
Extrahepatic biliary obstruction	7 (28)	2 (180)	0 (36)	9 (57)	—	—	—
Chronic active hepatitis	28 (43)	10 (77)	12 (25)	8 (38)	—	—	—
Acute viral hepatitis	—	0 (332)	0 (100)	—	—	—	—
Cryptogenic cirrhosis	31 (32)	6 (33)	—	—	—	—	—
Alcoholic liver disease	—	—	0.6 (159)	5 (59)	—	—	—
Miscellaneous liver diseases	—	0.9 (230)	0 (56)	—	—	—	—
Primary sclerosing cholangitis	—	—	—	—	—	9 (23)	0 (25)

*Reported frequencies of positive tests in the general population range from 0 to 0.7 per cent. The numbers in parentheses are numbers of patients studied.

histologic stages of the disease. A polyclonal increase in IgM often is present, however, even in the early stages of disease. The disproportionate elevation of IgM is a feature that distinguishes PBC from other liver diseases associated with hypergammaglobulinemia. Elevated IgM has been found in approximately 90 per cent of patients with PBC seen at the Mayo Clinic.[11] IgM was elevated in 56 of 76 patients (74 per cent) reported by Sherlock and Scheuer, occasionally to values as high as 14-fold greater than the upper limit of normal.[45] The median value for IgM was increased for a series of 236 patients with PBC; however, the proportion of patients with elevations was not reported.[46] The presence of a polyclonal increase in IgM may be regarded as supporting evidence for a diagnosis of PBC in the appropriate clinical setting.

The presence of monomeric IgM in sera of patients with PBC has been reported recently.[112, 113] Monomeric IgM can result in falsely elevated measurements of IgM by radial immunodiffusion, and may contribute to the magnitude of the IgM elevation reported in PBC.[114] Indeed, quantitative crossed immunoelectrophoresis does not confirm the elevation of IgM demonstrated by immunodiffusion.[115] Monomeric IgM is found in several autoimmune disorders, but its significance remains unknown.

HEMATOLOGIC TESTS

Abnormalities of the hematopoietic system are nonspecific. Patients generally have mild to moderate normocytic, normochromic anemia. Changes in osmotic fragility and target cells have been found in both PBC and other chronic liver diseases. The most prevalent abnormality is an increased erythrocyte sedimentation rate, which is found in 90 per cent of patients (see Table 44–4).[11] An elevated erythrocyte sedimentation rate was the cause of referral of eight of the ten asymptomatic[11] patients reported by Hanik and Eriksson.[55]

ROENTGENOGRAPHY

Cholangiography reveals a normal extrahepatic biliary system and larger than normal distal intrahepatic bile ducts.[117, 118] The small, proximal intrahepatic radicles seen during retrograde cholangiography may appear normal or diffusely or focally narrowed with shortening and diminished branching. Postmortem cholangiography performed at the Mayo Clinic showed that two patients had unexplained, segmental dilation of the intrahepatic bile ducts.[11] Cholelithiasis is not uncommon; in one selected series, more than 35 per cent of patients with PBC had radiographic evidence of gallstones.[118]

Chest radiographs of patients with PBC are almost always normal. They show abnormal interstitial patterns in less than half of the patients with PBC who have concurrent pulmonary fibrosis.[109, 119] A reticulonodular pattern has been described in atypical patients with PBC, who had granulomas in several sites, including the lungs.[120, 121] Recent studies indicate that a high proportion of patients with PBC have subclinical inflammatory alveolitis despite normal chest radiographs.[119] The radiographic findings in patients with hepatic osteodystrophy are discussed under Complications.

TESTS OF COPPER METABOLISM

Primary biliary cirrhosis is associated with excessive quantities of copper in the liver as well as in certain other organs (see the section on Pathogenesis).[123] Abnormalities of copper metabolism in patients with PBC include elevations of levels of ceruloplasmin and serum copper and increased urinary excretion of copper.

QUANTITATIVE TESTS OF HEPATIC FUNCTION

Quantitative tests of hepatic function in PBC have not been evaluated systematically. Studies of small numbers of patients show a reduction in antipyrine clearance when expressed per unit volume of liver[124a] and abnormalities of the first and second exponential components of the plasma disappearance curve for sulfobromophthalein (Bromsulphalein [BSP]).[125a] Serial assessment of true tests of hepatic function could be of great benefit in assessing the progression of disease, the effectiveness of experimental therapies, and timing of liver transplantation.

PATHOLOGY

GROSS FEATURES

In advanced disease, the liver is enlarged and bile-stained.[12] The surface is smooth prior to the development of cirrhotic nodules. The calibers of the distal intrahepatic and extrahepatic bile ducts are normal. The gallbladder is usually normal but may contain stones in a few patients.[118] Hyperplastic lymph nodes may be seen in the porta hepatis or adjacent to the common bile duct.[120] The spleen is enlarged, and hyperplasia is present in advanced disease. Vascular changes of portal venous hypertension are frequent and may antedate the development of cirrhotic nodules.[126, 127a] Rarely, patients may have widespread granulomas in organs other than the liver.[84]

HISTOLOGIC FEATURES AND CLASSIFICATIONS USED IN STAGING

The application of liver biopsy in the diagnostic evaluation of cholestatic liver diseases and evaluation of serial biopsy specimens from large numbers of patients have led to an increased understanding of the histologic spectrum and progression in PBC. In an attempt to categorize the histologic lesions and the sequence of their progression, three systems of staging have been proposed (Table 44–7). Insufficient studies of serial biopsies performed in large numbers of patients have been performed to prove or refute the staging systems.[123] Variability in the distribution of portal lesions within the liver and the absence of proof that disease in all patients evolves sequentially through the different stages, raises questions about the utility of staging.[124] However, available data have never refuted the correlation between staging criteria and the course of disease. This correlation is most evident when staging is subdivided into (1) early, characterized by the absence of significant portal fibrosis, and (2) late, characterized by the presence of advanced fibrosis and ultimately cirrhosis.

Most hepatopathologists employ the staging system of Scheuer[125] or that of Popper and Schaffner.[126a] Both systems describe four histologic stages in the pathologic evolution of the disease. The histologic diagnosis of early stages may be difficult, since lesions of stages I and II are not distributed uniformly in the liver and frequently are absent in percutaneous needle biopsy specimens.[125] Also, morpho-

TABLE 44–7. COMPARISON OF SYSTEMS FOR HISTOLOGIC STAGING IN PRIMARY BILIARY CIRRHOSIS

Author	Morphologic Features			
	Stage 1	*Stage 2*	*Stage 3*	*Stage 4*
Scheuer (1967)	Florid duct lesion	Ductular proliferation	Scarring	Cirrhosis
Popper and Schaffner (1970)	Cholangitis	Ductular proliferation	Pre-cirrhotic stage	Cirrhosis
Ludwig, Dickson and MacDonald (1978)	Portal hepatitis	Periportal hepatitis	Bridging necrosis or fibrous septa or both	Cirrhosis

Source: Reprinted with permission from MacSween RNM, Burt AD. Molec Asp Med 8:269, 1985, Pergamon Press plc.

logic features of more than one stage may occur in the same specimen. In such an instance, staging should be based on the most advanced lesion present in the specimen.[44]

Ludwig et al. feel that these limitations compromise[127] the value of both systems of staging in the serial evaluation of patients enrolled in controlled therapeutic trials. Accordingly, Ludwig et al. have proposed an alternative system of four stages that is based on histologic features consistently present in needle biopsy specimens.[11, 127] The histologic features in their system are not based on diagnostic features of PBC, and thus their system requires that the diagnosis of PBC be established on combined clinical, biochemical, serologic, radiographic, and histologic grounds before staging. Table 44–8 compares the frequency of morphologic features in the four histologic stages in Ludwig's classification.

Recently, a new classification was proposed, based on the histopathologic patterns observed in 605 biopsy specimens from 209 patients.[129] The classification, based on the type of piecemeal necrosis, was divided into four patterns: (1) biliary piecemeal necrosis, characterized by invasion of vacuolated periportal hepatocytes by foamy macrophages, (2) lymphocytic piecemeal necrosis, characterized by the presence of lymphocytes and plasma cells among hydropic periportal hepatocytes, (3) ductular piecemeal necrosis, characterized by proliferation of ductules or ductular transformation of hepatocyte cords extending from portal areas into the lobules, and (4) fibrotic piecemeal necrosis, characterized by extension of fibrous tissue from the portal areas into the periportal tissue. Biliary piecemeal necrosis appeared to increase in intensity and frequency from stage II to stage IV. Lymphocytic piecemeal necrosis was most frequent in stage II. Ductular piecemeal necrosis was evenly distributed in stages II through IV, whereas fibrotic piecemeal necrosis was observed in stages III and IV. It is not known whether this classification reflects different stages of disease or variations in the patterns observable in PBC.[123, 124, 129] The degree to which the histologic type of piecemeal necrosis persists or changes during the course of the disease appears to be variable, and mixtures of types were noted.

Thus, the relationship of the type of piecemeal necrosis to the evolution of disease remains unclear. This provocative classification, however, suggests the possibility that different histogenetic pathways may exist in PBC that are inadequately classified by the three major staging systems (Table 44–7).

Major Staging Systems (see Table 44–7)

Stage I: Florid Duct Lesion (Scheuer[125]); Nonsuppurative Destructive Cholangitis (Popper and Schaffner[126a]); Portal Stage (Ludwig et al.[127])

Stage I is characterized by the inflammatory destruction of intrahepatic bile ducts in the classifications of Scheuer and Popper and Schaffner (Fig. 44–1). The initial destruction preferentially involves septal and interlobular bile ducts ranging in diameter from 45 to 100 μm. Ducts of this size may not be present on needle biopsy specimens but are present consistently in wedge biopsy specimens obtained at laparotomy. Early lesions involve only segments of individual bile ducts and tend to be focal within the liver. Lesions of stage I may be seen alone or may coexist with features characteristic of stages II to IV. The epithelial cells of involved ducts show nuclear pyknosis, karyorrhexis, ballooning of the cytoplasm, slight vacuolation, and loss of their usual cuboidal arrangement as a result of crowding or frank necrosis of a portion of the bile duct. The resulting discontinuity of the epithelium is referred to as "rupture" by Scheuer. The term florid duct lesion refers to the presence of a necrotic, ruptured bile duct. Histologically normal ducts may be seen in the same specimen. Multiple sections of each portal tract must be scrutinized to detect lesions that may be present over only a small portion of the length of the bile duct.

An inflammatory infiltrate surrounds the bile ducts; mononuclear inflammatory cells may breach the basement membrane and be present in the epithelial layer (see Fig. 44–1). This is the lesion of chronic, nonsuppurative destructive cholangitis in the classification of Popper and Schaffner.

TABLE 44–8. FREQUENCIES OF SELECTED MORPHOLOGIC FEATURES IN THE FOUR HISTOLOGIC STAGES OF PRIMARY BILIARY CIRRHOSIS DESCRIBED BY LUDWIG et al.[127]

	% of Patients			
	Stage I	*Stage II*	*Stage III*	*Stage IV*
Florid lesion of interlobular bile ducts	38	45	19	15
Cholestasis	0	10	20	36
Decreased interlobular ducts	5	45	75	90
Bile ductular proliferation	0	55	84	93
Stainable copper	15	72	93	100

Source: Modified from data in Dickson ER, et al. Primary biliary cirrhosis. In: Popper H, Schaffner F, eds. Progress in Liver Diseases, Vol. 6. New York, Grune & Stratton 1978:487, and Ludwig J, et al. Virch Arch A Path Anat Histol 379:103, 1978.

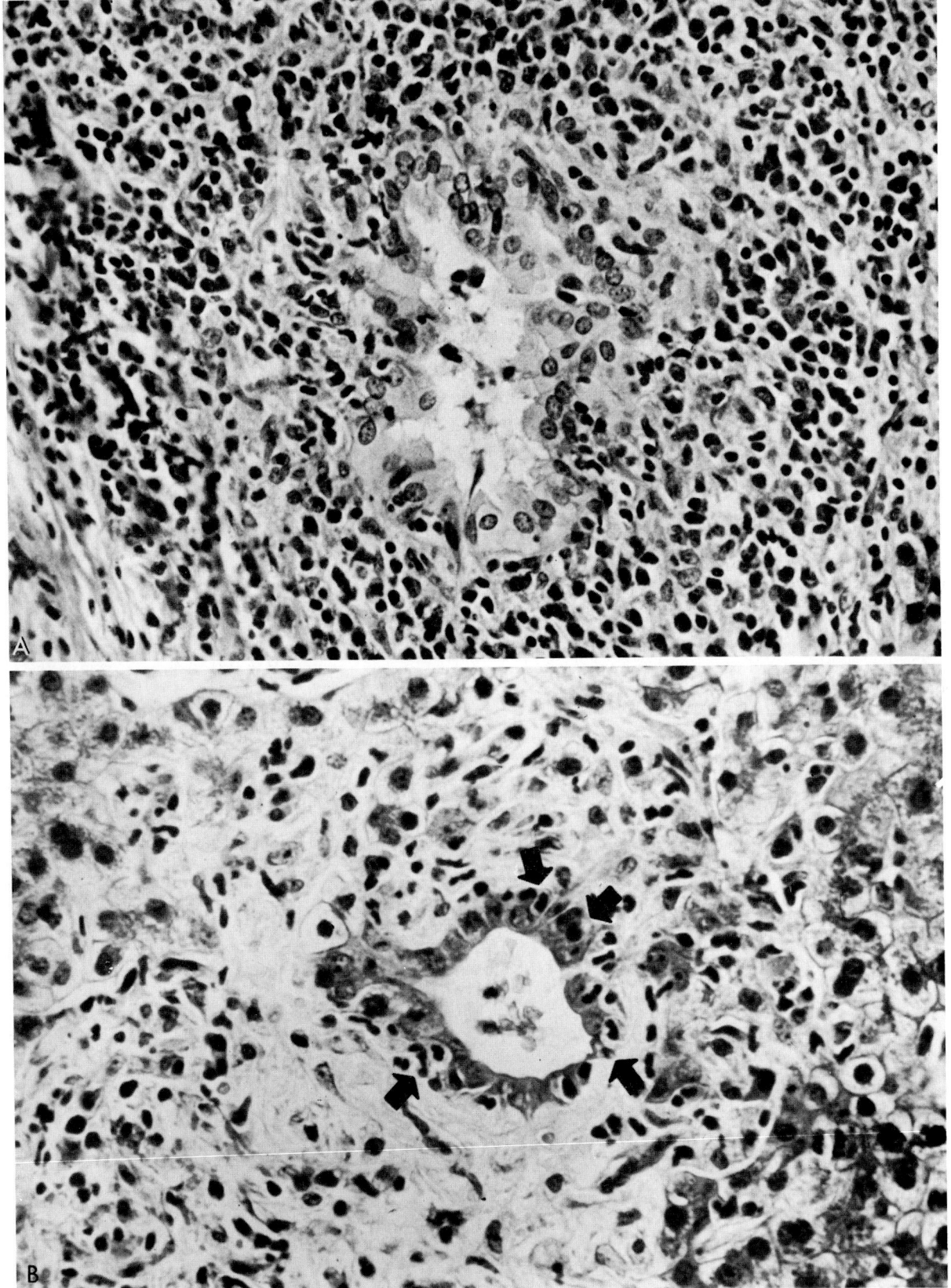

Figure 44–1. Histologic stage I of primary biliary cirrhosis (PBC). *A,* Florid duct lesion; *B,* nonsuppurative destructive cholangitis. Note the inflammatory infiltration of the bile duct epithelium (arrows) by mononuclear cells. X 320.

Mononuclear inflammation of the epithelium of bile ducts is seen more commonly than are the frankly necrotic bile ducts (florid duct lesion) that result from this process.[7] The presence of florid duct lesions has been considered pathognomonic of PBC.[8, 125] They must be distinguished, however, from similar lesions of bile ducts that may occur in chronic active hepatitis.[130–132] This distinction can be difficult or impossible to make, especially when features of PBC and chronic active hepatitis overlap.[133, 134] Important distinguishing features of lesions associated with chronic active hepatitis are discussed under Differential Diagnosis.

The portal tracts in PBC are expanded by an inflammatory infiltrate predominantly composed of lymphocytes, monocyte-macrophages, and plasma cells (see Fig. 44–1). A few eosinophils or neutrophils may be present. Dense aggregates of lymphocytes, some with germinal centers, may be seen. Granulomas identifiable either as aggregates of histiocytes or as fully developed noncaseating lesions are present in some portal tracts, usually adjacent to damaged bile ducts (Fig. 44–2).[135] The collagen content of the portal tracts is increased. In the classification of Scheuer, the limiting plate need not be intact, but Popper and Schaffner restrict stage I to expanded portal tracts with intact limiting plates. This distinction is considered crucial in the classification of Ludwig et al.[127] discussed later. Parenchymal changes are not conspicuous in stage I. The hepatocytes are generally intact, although small foci of mononuclear inflammation may be present, primarily within the sinusoids. Kupffer cells appear activated and contain abundant cytoplasm. Rarely, periportal macrophages have a foamy cytoplasm. Cholestasis (bile pigment within hepatocytes, canalicular plugs) is usually absent.

Since it is recognized that the florid duct lesions are spotty, are restricted to ducts of a particular caliber, and may be present in histologic stages II to IV, Ludwig et al. have proposed an alternative definition of stage I. They refer to this stage as the portal stage or stage of portal hepatitis to emphasize the invariant finding of inflammation confined to the portal tract with "little or no periportal inflammation" or piecemeal necrosis.[127] These features are indistinguishable from those seen in chronic persistent hepatitis. Only 38 percent of needle-biopsy specimens classified as stage I by Ludwig et al.[127] contained florid duct lesions.

Stage II: Ductular Proliferation (Scheuer[125]; Popper and Schaffner[126a]); Periportal Stage (Ludwig et al.[127])

Proliferation of the bile ductules within the portal tracts is the principal morphologic feature of stage II according to the classifications of Scheuer and of Popper and Schaffner (Fig. 44–3). The newly formed ductules tend to be tortuous and to have poorly defined lumens. Periductal inflammatory lesions are more widespread in stage II compared with stage I, but the intensity of inflammation is often less than that of stage I. The proportions of histiocytes, lymphocytes, and plasma cells in the inflammatory infiltrate are quite variable. The neutrophilic component of the inflammation is often more prominent in stage II than in stage I. Florid duct lesions may or may not be seen in stage II. Interlobular bile ducts are diminished in number as a result of their replacement by aggregates of lymphoid cells and fibrosis. Irregular fibrosis is present within the expanded portal tracts. Granulomas are less frequent in stage II than in stage I. Histiocytes engorged with lipid may form xanthomatous nodules. Inflammation frequently extends past the limiting plate in stage II to involve the adjacent parenchyma (piecemeal necrosis). Histologic evidence of cholestasis, if

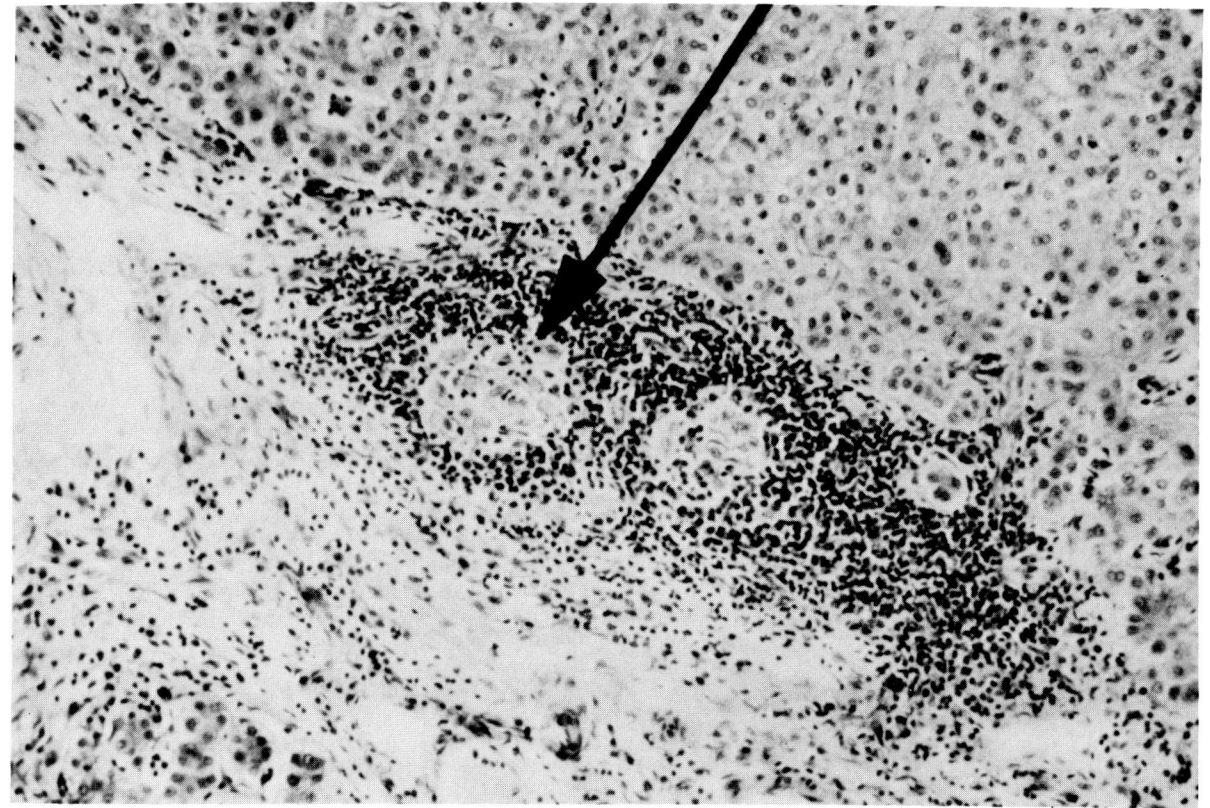

Figure 44–2. Granulomas within a portal lymphoid aggregate. X 150. (Courtesy of E. A. Jones.)

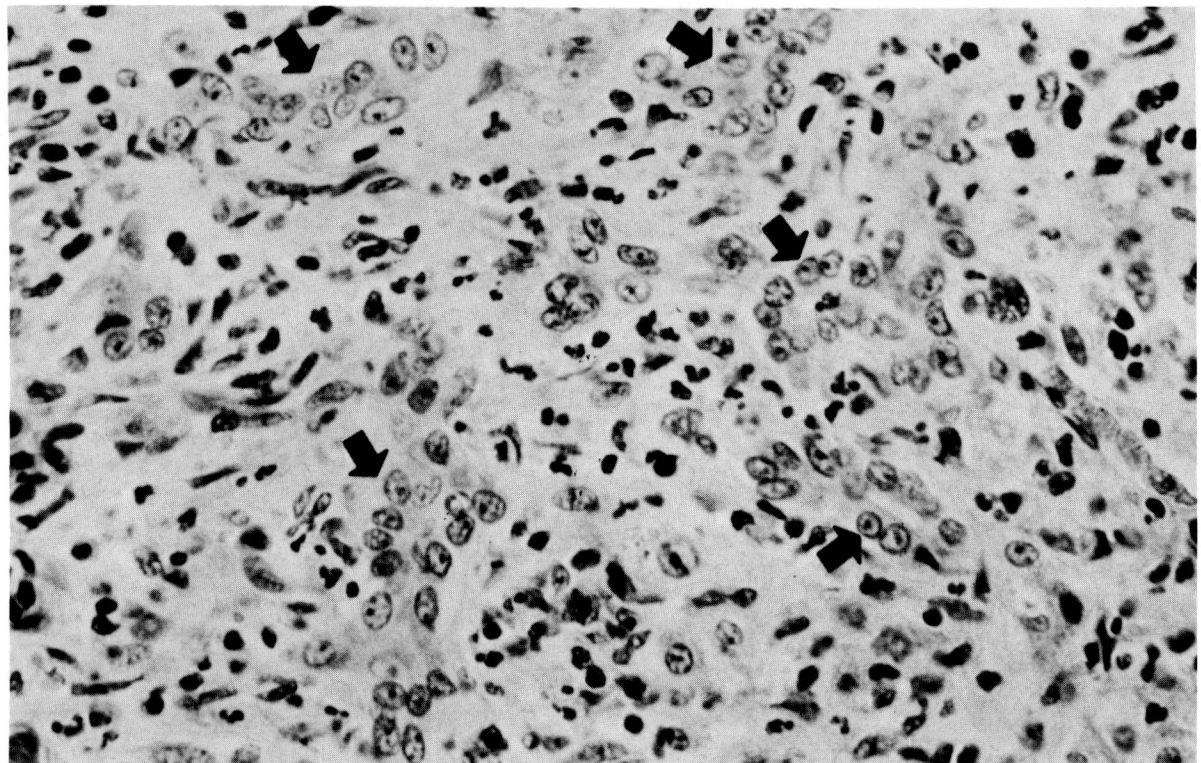

Figure 44–3. Histologic stage II of primary biliary cirrhosis (PBC). Proliferation of bile ductules within a portal tract. X 350.

present at all, is characterized by the presence of bile pigment within periportal hepatocytes and bile canalicular plugs. The lesions of stage II have features also seen in chronic active hepatitis and extrahepatic biliary obstruction that are principal considerations in the differential diagnosis at this stage (see section on Differential Diagnosis). The biopsy findings must be interpreted, therefore, in the light of the combined clinical, biochemical, serologic, and radiographic findings. Lesions of stage II disease are generally consistent or compatible only with the diagnosis of PBC.

Ludwig et al. define stage II as the periportal stage to emphasize the presence of "periportal hepatitis." The histologic features of periportal hepatitis are indistinguishable from those found in chronic active hepatitis. In the classification of Ludwig and colleagues, the presence or absence of bile ductular proliferation, inflammatory destruction of bile ducts, or granulomas is inconsequential for purposes of staging. Thus, they emphasize the extension of the necroinflammatory process to the parenchyma as the important histopathogenetic link to the development of stage III lesions.

Stage III: Scarring or Fibrosis (Scheuer[8, 125]; Popper and Schaffner[126a]); Septal Stage (Ludwig et al.[127])

In stage III, the intensity of the portal inflammatory process is decreased, and the dominant feature is conspicuous fibrosis extending as septa from the portal tracts (Fig. 44–4). The hepatic architecture may be severely distorted ("precirrhosis"), but, by definition, regenerative nodules are absent. Aggregates of lymphoid cells are still present in the portal tracts, whereas the septa are usually acellular. Bile ducts are frequently absent from portal tracts (Fig. 44–5); florid duct lesions, however, may be seen in this stage. Periportal cholestasis may be severe and presumably

is the result of the local obstruction to bile flow. The features of stage III are not diagnostic for PBC and must only be considered to be compatible with the diagnosis.

Ludwig et al.[127] classify stage III as the septal stage. The essential feature is the presence of acellular fibrous septa, bridging necrosis (referred to as "active septa"), or both. As discussed earlier in reference to stage II, the presence or absence of other histologic features does not influence the assignment of this stage in this classification.

Stage IV: Cirrhosis (Scheuer[8, 125]; Popper and Schaffner[126a]; Ludwig et al.[127])

Each of the classifications recognizes cirrhosis (fibrous septa and regenerative nodules) as the final stage of morphologic progression in PBC (Fig. 44–6). Although cirrhosis in the biopsy specimen at this stage may be difficult to distinguish from cirrhosis from other causes, the diagnosis of PBC frequently is suggested by the absence of bile ducts in portal tracts and the presence of mononuclear inflammation. However, interlobular bile ducts may be preserved and florid duct lesions may continue to be seen.

The advantages and disadvantages of each system of staging continue to be debated.[123, 124, 129] In fact, it has been suggested that the concept of staging in PBC may have only limited value in the assessment of (1) progression of the disease in an individual patient and (2) the response to therapy. The focal, segmental nature of the inflammatory lesions of the bile ducts, the finding of characteristic features of different stages in the same biopsy specimen, and the variability in the natural rates of progression of histologic lesions in individual patients all serve to limit the usefulness of staging. The evidence from all investigators confirms the variability in finding fully developed florid duct lesions in early stages of the disease, as well as the propensity to find

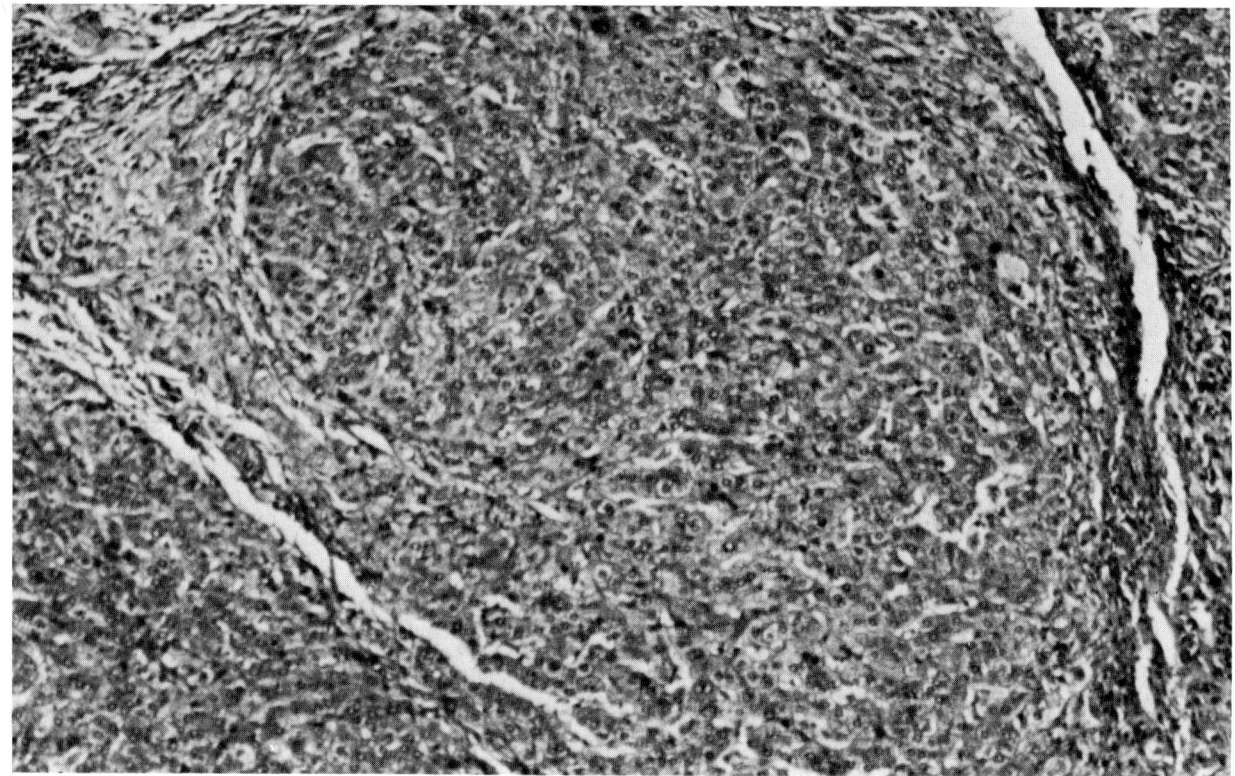

Figure 44–4. Histologic stage III of primary biliary cirrhosis (PBC). Conspicuous fibrous septa. X 120.

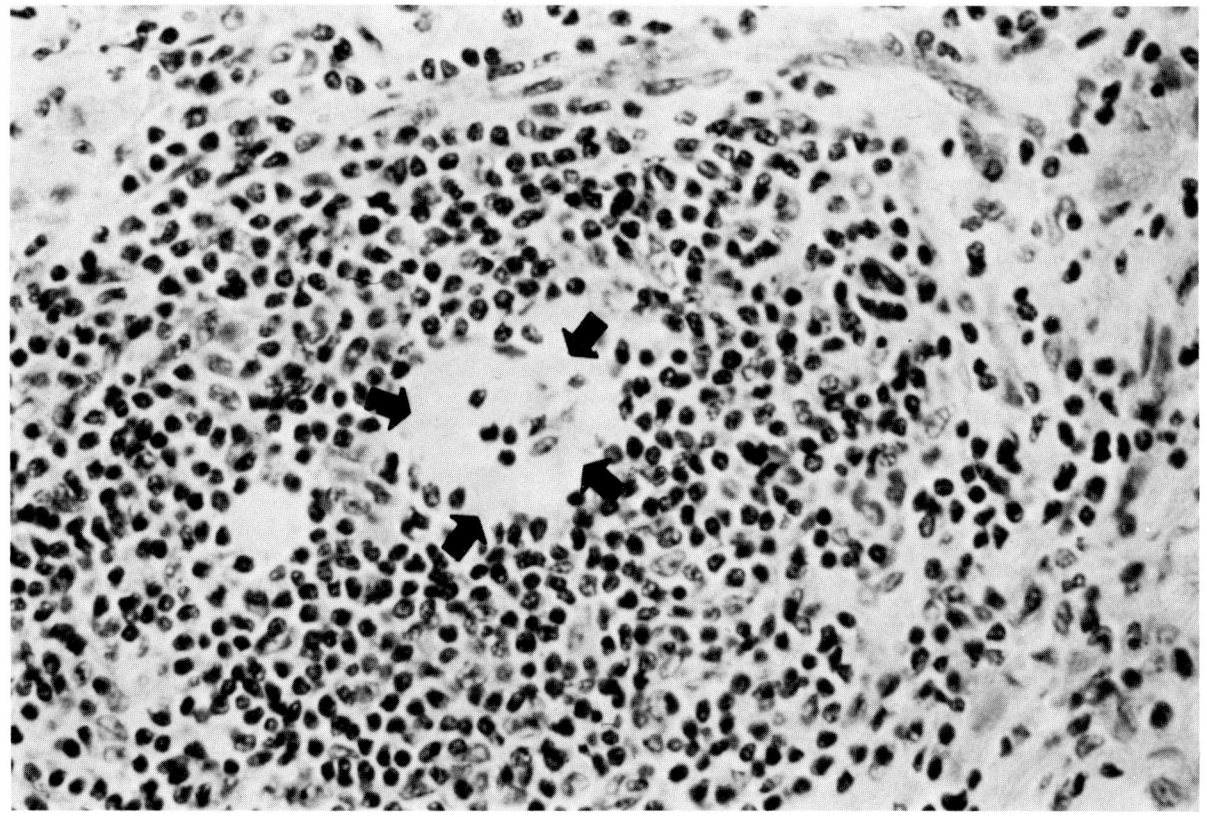

Figure 44–5. Fibrotic remnant of interlobular bile duct (arrows) surrounded by a dense inflammatory infiltrate of mononuclear cells. X 320.

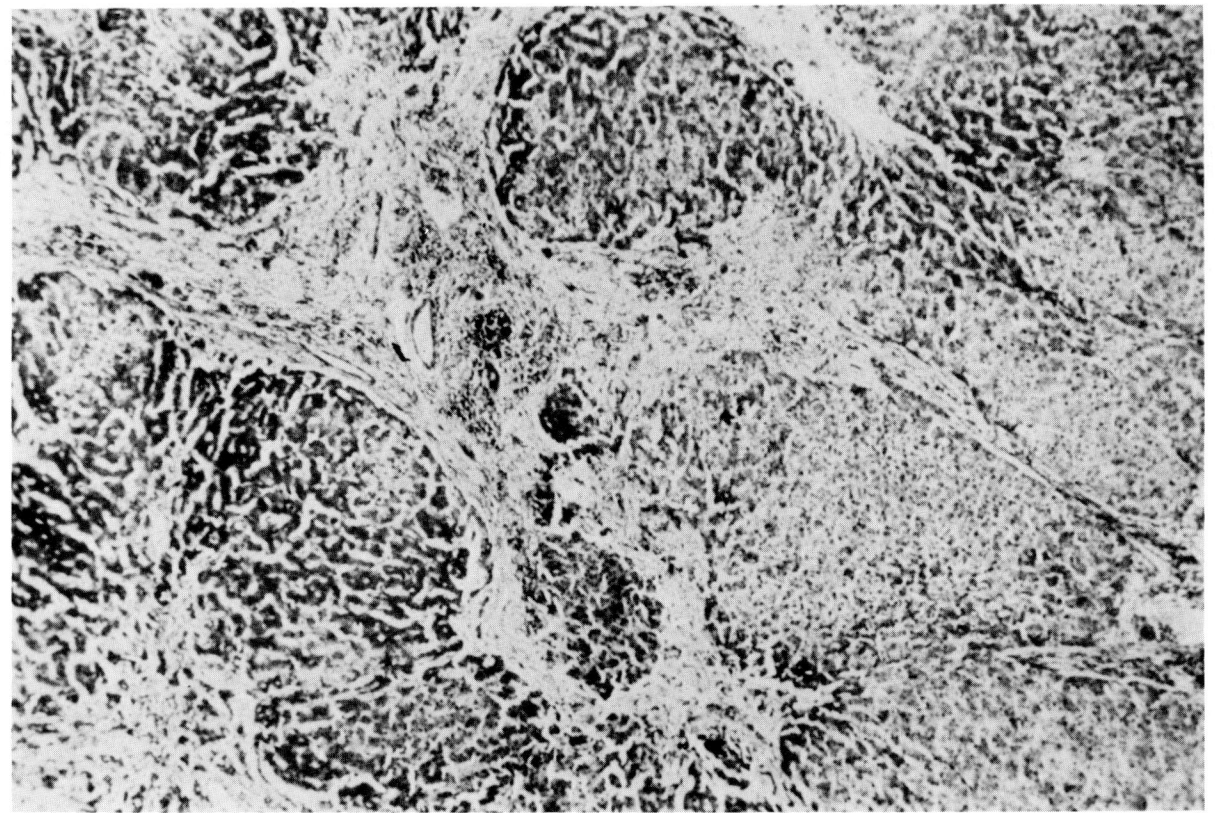

Figure 44–6. Histologic stage IV of primary biliary cirrhosis (PBC). X 80.

such lesions in more advanced stages, including cirrhosis. This suggests that staging cannot be assigned on the basis of this particular lesion. If the development of cirrhosis is dependent upon invasion and destruction of parenchymal cells adjacent to the inflamed portal tracts, as is postulated for chronic active hepatitis, then the classification of Ludwig et al.[127] may be the most advantageous for the purpose of staging. Their classification, however, relies on general features that de-emphasize the specificity of the histologic findings for PBC. It is interesting to note the frequencies with which the morphologic features of PBC emphasized in other systems of staging occur in the four stages of Ludwig and colleagues (see Table 44–6).

OTHER HISTOLOGIC FEATURES

Granulomas

Granulomas have been found in all stages of the disease. They are most prevalent in stage I[8, 135] (see Fig. 44–2). Sectioning of wedge biopsy specimens reveals an inverse relationship between the frequency of granulomas and the histologic stage: 86 per cent in stages I and II, 75 per cent in stage III, and 0 per cent in stage IV.[135] Even in early stages they are not invariably present. Recognizing semantic differences among pathologists regarding the definition of granuloma, 60 to 86 per cent of patients (all four stages) are found to have granulomas when serial biopsies are done[46] or when multiple sections of wedge biopsies are evaluated.[135] Granulomas frequently are adjacent to or replace inflamed bile ducts in the portal tracts but also may be found in the parenchyma. Initial indications that patients

with granulomas have a better prognosis[137] have not been confirmed by larger studies.[129]

Hyaline and Mucoprotein Deposits

Periportal hepatocytes, especially those with bile pigment, may contain fibrillar material indistinguishable from Mallory's hyalin.[136] The frequency of this finding may be as high as 26 per cent,[136] and this material is often found in biopsy specimens that show histologic evidence of cholestasis.[127] Adjacent to damaged bile ducts, periodic acid–Schiff (PAS)-positive material may be present. This material has properties of a mucoprotein and presumably originates from the epithelium of bile ducts.[7] Histiocytes in the portal tracts may contain non-glycogen, PAS-positive material; similar material occurs within multinucleated giant cells in granulomas.[7]

Copper Deposits

Primary biliary cirrhosis and other types of chronic cholestasis are associated with the accumulation of copper in the liver.[122] Stainable copper may be important diagnostically in PBC since other types of cholestatic disease often have negative staining reactions for copper despite quantitative increases in total hepatic copper. As is discussed later under Pathogenesis, this finding may relate to the absolute quantity of hepatic copper in PBC or to the types of copper-protein complexes found in the liver.

Staining with Shikata's orcein is the most reliable histochemical method for detecting excessive copper in PBC, even though the stain reacts only with a copper-associated protein rather than with copper itself. Stainable copper, however, is not always demonstrable in stage I and II lesions, even though the quantity of hepatic copper is increased. In stage II, copper is present predominantly in periportal hepatocytes, especially those adjacent to macrophages. In stage III lesions, stainable copper is located in both periportal and periseptal hepatocytes. In stage IV lesions, stainable copper is even more prominent, especially within periportal hepatocytes and those adjacent to fibrous septa or at the periphery of regenerative nodules. Copper is consistently evident in hepatocytes containing Mallory's hyalin in PBC. Table 44–8 summarizes the frequencies of positive orcein stains found in association with different histologic stages of PBC. Scanning proton microprobe analysis shows that copper is preferentially located in periportal hepatocytes in association with sulfur, which is consistent with the presence of aggregates of copper-loaded metallothionein.

Histomorphometry

Histometric observations of serial sections of the intrahepatic bile ducts in PBC have shown that bile ducts with diameters of less than 70 to 80 μ (diameter = distance between epithelial basement membranes) are preferentially destroyed in PBC.[124, 139] Three distinct types of periductal lesions precede the disappearance of bile ducts: (1) periductal inflammation, including chronic nonsuppurative cholangitis, (2) periductal edema, and (3) periductal fibrosis. The first and third types of lesions are more common in histologic stages I and II. The first and second types occur more frequently in stage III, and the third type of lesion most often occurs alone in stage IV. Serial sections reveal the presence of cholangitis adjacent to areas of disruption and dissolution along the courses of individual bile ducts. Earlier studies of three-dimensional reconstructions of the liver confirmed the finding of segmental destruction along the courses of individual bile ducts.[140]

Nodular Hyperplasia

Nodular hyperplastic changes of hepatocytes have recently been noted in patients with PBC in the absence of cirrhosis or bridging fibrosis.[141] In a systematic review of biopsies from 26 patients all with stage I and II lesions, nodular hyperplasia was present in 9 (35 per cent). The lesions were indistinguishable from those observed in nodular regenerative hyperplasia of the liver, and were associated with esophageal varices in six of the nine patients. The unrecognized presence of nodular hyperplasia may explain the occurrence of significant portal venous hypertension reported in some patients with PBC without cirrhosis.[126, 127a, 141, 143]

Immunohistochemical Studies

The proportions of T cell subsets, B cells, and monocyte/macrophages in the inflammatory infiltrates of biopsy specimens have been quantitated using monoclonal antibody reagents.[144–148] The inflammatory infiltrates within portal tracts predominantly contain T cells, with lesser numbers of B cells, natural killer cells, and monocyte/macrophages. T cells with a helper/inducer phenotype exceed those with a suppressor/cytotoxic phenotype, and the latter are signif-

icantly enriched in liver tissue compared to peripheral blood. A similar composition of inflammatory cells has been observed in chronic active hepatitis and primary sclerosing cholangitis and thus is not specific for PBC.[147, 148] In some reports, T helper/inducer cells were more prevalent in the portal tracts, whereas T suppressor/cytotoxic cells were more prevalent in the areas of piecemeal necrosis. Others have found comparable mixtures of both T cell phenotypes in both locations.[144] In most studies, B cells and natural killer cells have been present in small numbers, whereas monocyte/macrophages compose about 20 to 30 per cent of the infiltrates.[144–148] Only small numbers of natural killer cells have been identified.[144, 145] The majority of T cells, regardless of phenotype, express HLA class II antigens and/or interleukin 2 receptors, which are indicative of an activated functional state.[144, 146] T cells present in granulomas exhibit a helper/inducer phenotype.[147]

Recent studies have evaluated the phenotypes of T cells abutting and penetrating the bile duct epithelium.[145–147] By light and electron microscopy, the majority of cells in intimate contact with bile duct epithelial cells are T suppressor/cytotoxic cells.[145, 147] Using double labeling techniques, the cells penetrating the bile duct epithelium were predominantly T cytotoxic cells, although T helper/inducer and natural killer cell phenotypes also were observed.[145] By electron microscopy, pseudopods were observed projecting from the T cells to the biliary epithelial cells. In other studies, activated T helper/inducer cells have been most prominent adjacent to injured bile ducts.[146] These results indicate involvement of certain types of T cells in the inflammatory destruction of bile-duct epithelial cells; yet it must be noted that phenotypes are imperfectly related to the function of T cells, and studies of the function of T cells isolated from inflamed bile duct epithelium have not been performed (see section on Immunologic Pathogenesis).

ULTRASTRUCTURAL FEATURES

The electron microscopic appearance of hepatocytes is altered minimally in the early stages of PBC.[149] As in other cholestatic conditions, occasional mitochondria have curled cristae, and Golgi vesicles may contain electron-opaque material. The canaliculi and microvilli are usually normal, although edema of the microvilli may be seen. Rhomboid crystals, probably cholesterol, may be present intracellularly. In the presence of the progressive destruction of bile ducts and ductular proliferation of stage II, the hepatocytes may contain cytoplasmic material with the electronmicroscopic appearance of Mallory's hyalin. Bile canaliculi are often dilated, with shortened, swollen or ablated microvilli. Increased numbers of microfilaments and an increase in the thickness of microfilament bundles have been found adjacent to canaliculi regardless of the presence or absence of canalicular dilatation.[149] These changes are nonspecific in that they are found in association with other cholestatic conditions.

Normal bile duct epithelial cells have a fine network of microfilaments adjacent to the basilateral membranes. In PBC and other forms of cholestasis, the microfilaments form dense, interconnecting bundles adjacent to the luminal surface membrane.[149] Microvilli of the luminal membrane are decreased in number and are edematous. Cytoplasmic blebs devoid of filaments occasionally protrude into the true lumens of the bile ducts. The basement membranes of bile ducts are thickened and may show invasion by leukocytes.

Recently, results of ultrastructural studies of the bile ducts in patients with PBC have been reported.[145, 150, 151] In each instance, bile ducts with recognizable lumens and intact basement membranes were present. Bile ductules lined with both hepatocytes and biliary epithelial cells were seen frequently. Abnormalities of the bile duct epithelial cells included irregularity of the nuclei, dilatation of the endoplasmic reticulum, and swelling of the mitochondria. Membrane-bound vacuoles frequently were present in the cytoplasm. Certain biliary cells showed a peculiar form of necrosis (apoptosis), with condensation of the cytoplasm and fragmentation of nuclear chromatin. In some instances bile ducts were severely disrupted and isolated biliary epithelial cells were observed with fragments of their original basement membranes. Detachment of one or more biliary cells from the basement membrane of the bile duct and from adjacent epithelial cells also was prominent.[151]

Occasionally lymphocytes were present within dilated intercellular spaces between necrotic-appearing cells. The basement membrane was disrupted at the sites of penetration by the lymphocytes. Lymphocytes also were numerous in the vicinity of disrupted bile ducts. Pseudopods projected from the surfaces of the lymphocytes and formed contacts with the membranes of biliary epithelial cells. In addition, striking abnormalities of the basement membranes of the bile ducts were present. The abnormal features included irregular thickening of the basement membrane, areas of rarefaction within the basement membrane, reduplication of the membrane with multiple layers, and deposits of amorphous basement membrane–like material in the interstitial spaces.

Similar features also were seen in patients with graft-versus-host disease.[150] The similarity of the findings in the two conditions is compatible with the concept that PBC, like graft-versus-host disease, is immunologically mediated (see the section on Pathogenesis).

The ultrastructural appearance of granulomas in PBC also has been reported recently.[152] Adjacent to injured bile ducts, activated macrophages were commonly observed. In contrast, granulomas contained vesicular epithelioid cells with numerous membrane-bound vesicles and specialized phagosomes. The presence of such epithelioid cells suggests that activated macrophages may transform into vesicular forms with time. The granulomas resembled those observed in sarcoidosis rather than in tuberculosis.

DISEASES ASSOCIATED WITH PBC

PBC is associated with a variety of disorders (Table 44–9). Some associations, seen repeatedly in independent series, are well substantiated and have suggested possible pathogenetic relationships between PBC and the associated diseases. Other associations have been reported less frequently and may be coincidental. The frequency with which associated diseases were found in selected groups of patients with PBC was reported to be 100 per cent in one series.[153] In another study, 69 per cent of 47 patients with PBC had an associated disorder. The experience of most clinicians seeing patients with PBC is that associated diseases occur in most of them some time in the course of their illness. As noted earlier, symptoms of associated diseases, in particular collagen vascular diseases, often lead to the diagnosis of PBC in asymptomatic patients.

TABLE 44–9. DISORDERS REPORTED IN ASSOCIATION WITH PRIMARY BILIARY CIRRHOSIS

Scleroderma
Sjögren's syndrome
Arthropathy
    Rheumatoid arthritis
    Psoriatic arthritis
    Chondrocalcinosis
    Hypertrophic osteodystrophy
    Avascular necrosis
Thyroiditis
Renal tubular acidosis
Breast carcinoma
Urinary tract infection
Celiac disease
Miscellaneous conditions
    Mixed connective tissue disease
    Polymyositis
    Polymyalgia rheumatica
    Rash
    Pulmonary fibrosis
    Neuropathy
    Glomerulonephritis
    Hemolytic anemia
    Cardiomyopathy
    Concurrent Hashimoto's thyroiditis and myasthenia gravis
    Progressive ophthalmoplegia
    Choledochal cyst
    Multiple myeloma
    Systemic lupus erythematosus
    Pernicious anemia
    Ulcerative colitis
    Pancreatic insufficiency
    Graves' disease
    Retroperitoneal fibrosis
    Menstrual abnormalities

SCLERODERMA

The association of scleroderma and PBC has been reported repeatedly.[58, 154–158] In one series of 83 consecutive patients with PBC, scleroderma was present in 17 per cent.[156] Only two of these patients had the CREST variant.[156] This is in contrast to earlier findings suggesting that the CREST variant of scleroderma was extraordinarily common in patients with PBC and scleroderma.[154, 155] Since 72 of the 83 patients were enrolled in a therapeutic trial comparing azathioprine and placebo, the possibility exists that the therapy may have influenced the development of the CREST syndrome. A recent evaluation of 26 consecutive patients diagnosed with PBC showed complete or incomplete CREST syndrome in 4 (16 per cent).[48] Anticentromere antibodies were present in each patient.

The association between scleroderma and PBC appears to be dependent on the presence of PBC. Liver disease is rare in large series of patients with scleroderma; the prevalence of liver disease in patients with scleroderma often does not exceed that in controls.[159, 160] Scleroderma in PBC is generally mild; the prognosis is not dependent on the scleroderma but rather on the progression of the liver disease. The skin may be involved alone or the disease may be systemic. Even with systemic disease, involvement often is limited to a loss of peristalsis in the esophagus or to a reduction in the diffusion capacity of carbon monoxide in the lung.[156] Raynaud's phenomenon may occur alone without evidence of cutaneous involvement. Polymyositis and scleroderma have been found concomitantly in PBC, suggesting the presence of a mixed connective tissue.[161] The frequency of HLA haplotype A1,B8 has been reported to be increased in patients with PBC associated with sclero-derma.[156] The significance of this finding is unclear, since the frequency of this haplotype is normal in populations of patients with PBC[162] and is not increased in association with scleroderma alone.[156]

SJÖGREN'S SYNDROME

This syndrome has been defined by the presence of at least two of the following: (1) keratoconjunctivitis sicca, (2) xerostomia, and (3) connective tissue disease, chronic hepatitis, or PBC.[163] By this definition the presence of (1) or (2) establishes the diagnosis in a patient with PBC. Based on Schirmer's test of lacrimation, 27 to 41 per cent of patients with PBC have xerophthalmia.[109, 153, 164, 165] The prevalences of keratoconjunctivitis sicca, xerostomia, or the combination of both (sicca complex), however, range from 72 to 100 per cent in patients with PBC who undergo specific testing.[109, 153] Symptoms are generally mild or even absent despite the presence of abnormal tests of lacrimal and salivary gland function. Neither the presence nor the extent of the abnormalities of the lacrimal and salivary glands correlates with the duration or severity of liver disease, the presence of autoantibodies, or levels of serum immunoglobulins.[98, 153, 166]

The sicca complex is associated with the HLA haplo-types B8 and Dw3 when it occurs alone, but this HLA association is not evident when the sicca complex occurs in association with another disease.[164] As might be expected, no HLA association is present in patients with PBC who have the sicca complex.[164]

Although the sicca complex occurs most commonly in association with PBC, the prevalence also is substantial in patients with chronic hepatitis (35 per cent) and those with cryptogenic cirrhosis (24 per cent).[109] Liver disease, how-ever, is infrequent in patients selected because of the presence of Sjögren's syndrome. In one study of patients with Sjögren's syndrome who had positive tests for anti-mitochondrial antibody, only 6 per cent had biochemical or histologic evidence of liver disease.[168]

ARTHROPATHY

The reported prevalences of symptomatic inflammatory arthropathy in PBC ranges from 4 to 50 per cent.[45, 54, 58, 97, 98, 109, 156, 169-171] Approximately 5 per cent of patients with PBC in three independent series also had arthritis.[45, 109, 156] Among four patients with arthritis reported by Clarke et al.,[156] two had seronegative destructive arthritis of the hands and ankles, one had polyarthritis of the small joints of the hands and feet with a low titer of rheumatoid factor, and the fourth patient had scleroderma and psoriatic arthritis. In another study, 24 per cent of patients had arthritis.[170] The majority of patients with seropositive polyarthritis had elevated C1q-binding activity in their sera (a putative measure of immune complexes), whereas patients with mild seronegative arthritis associated with scleroderma and Ray-naud's phenomenon did not. Two recent studies of consec-utively diagnosed patients rigorously analyzed the fre-quency and type of arthropathy.[97, 98] In one study 18 of 26 consecutive patients with PBC had arthropathy.[97] Of these 18, the arthropathy (gout and osteoarthritis) in 5 was not considered to be associated with PBC. Of the remaining 13 patients, 7 met the criteria for rheumatoid arthritis. All patients were symptomatic; most had chronic pain, whereas

a few had episodic symptoms. Seven patients were positive for HLA B27, and four had arthritis. In the second study, 9 of 26 consecutive patients (35 per cent) had arthropathy, but only 1 patient had rheumatoid arthritis.[98] Symptoms of arthritis were acute in 3 patients and chronic in the remain-der. No association with HLA types was observed.

Arthritis is a frequent complaint in otherwise asymp-tomatic patients and also has been observed in the preclin-ical phase of PBC associated with normal levels of alkaline phosphatase.[58] Among 29 patients found to have positive tests for antimitochondrial antibodies, normal levels of alkaline phosphatase, and liver biopsies consistent with a diagnosis of PBC, 5 (17 per cent) sought medical attention because of arthritis. The prevalence of arthritis in PBC may be underestimated by relying on the presence of symptoms. For example, non-deforming, erosive arthritis was evident on radiographs of the hands of 12 of 13 patients with PBC, although only three had symptoms.[169] The three symptom-atic patients were seronegative, whereas three of the asymp-tomatic patients were seropositive. The erosive arthritis involved the distal interphalangeal joint in ten patients, the proximal interphalangeal joint in six, the metacarpophalan-geal joint in four, the intercarpal joint in four, and the ulnar styloid process in two. Soft-tissue changes were com-mon, especially swelling of the distal interphalangeal and proximal interphalangeal joints. Seven of the patients had hepatic osteodystrophy. Interestingly, two patients had radiographic evidence of hyperparathyroidism, two had chondrocalcinosis, and one had hypertrophic osteoarthrop-athy.

Four patients evaluated by Clarke et al. had a striking destructive arthropathy of the shoulders or hips that resem-bled avascular necrosis.[156] Histologically, the femoral heads at the time of total hip replacement showed only osteoar-thritic changes. No patient had received corticosteroids or had significant hypercholesterolemia to account for the skeletal lesions. It is relevant that in a series of patients with avascular necrosis, 13 per cent had chronic liver disease of an unspecified type.[156]

These reports indicate that PBC may be associated with several types of arthropathy. The frequencies of ar-thritis in the individual reports vary, but generally are less than the frequency of arthritis associated with chronic active hepatitis (28 per cent).[109] In some series the frequency of symptomatic arthritis in PBC is comparable to the fre-quency of approximately 6 per cent in the general popula-tion, whereas recent prospective studies indicate a substan-tially increased frequency of 35 to 50 per cent in PBC.[97, 98]

THYROIDITIS

Autoimmune thyroiditis occurs in association with PBC.[45, 56, 172, 173] Thyroiditis was present in 6 per cent of patients with PBC reported by Sherlock and Scheuer.[45] In another large series, 17 per cent of patients with PBC had evidence of thyroid disease at presentation.[56] As mentioned earlier, anti-thyroid antibodies occur in at least 15 per cent of patients with PBC.[110] The presence of such antibodies correlates imperfectly both with lymphocytic thyroiditis (since antibodies are not always detected in this disease) and with clinical or biochemical evidence of hypothyroid-ism. A proportion of patients who have thyroid antibodies but no evidence of thyroid dysfunction may develop dys-function with time.[173] The pathologic features are those of a focal, lymphocytic thyroiditis. These pathologic findings may be present in autopsy even in patients with PBC who had no clinical evidence of thyroid disease.[172]

In one study, 95 patients with PBC (76 females, 19 males) were evaluated for subtle or overt evidence of thyroid disease.[172] Twenty-four females and one male had thyroid antibodies; 21 had antimicrosomal, 16 had anti-thyroglobulin, and 12 had both types of antibodies. Thyroid antibodies in 36 per cent of older women with PBC can be compared with a frequency of 12 per cent in healthy age- and sex-matched controls. Antibody-positive patients with PBC did not differ from antibody-negative patients with PBC with respect to age, the duration of liver disease, biochemical tests, or the presence of anti-mitochondrial antibody. Thirteen female patients with thyroid antibodies had thyroid dysfunction. The abnormalities included hypothyroidism in eight, elevated thyroid-stimulating hormone in two, and an abnormal response to thyrotropin-releasing hormone in three. Among antibody-negative patients, three clinically euthyroid individuals had low thyroxine levels and two had an abnormal response to thyroid-releasing hormone. Thyroid dysfunction was not correlated with the histologic stage of the liver disease, and the distributions of stages in the antibody-positive and antibody-negative groups were comparable. Xerophthalmia was evident disproportionately in antibody-positive patients (81 per cent) as compared with antibody-negative patients (22 per cent). This statistically significant association with xerophthalmia does not occur with either Hashimoto's thyroiditis or hypothyroidism alone, which suggests that the association is the result of the presence of PBC.

RENAL TUBULAR ACIDOSIS

Renal tubular acidosis occurs frequently in chronic liver diseases, including PBC.[109, 174] Available data suggest that the prevalence of renal tubular acidosis in PBC exceeds its prevalence in other liver diseases. Renal tubular acidosis was present in 25 per cent of patients with chronic active hepatitis, 21 per cent of patients with cryptogenic cirrhosis, and 1 per cent of patients with alcoholic cirrhosis.[109] In one study, 53 per cent of patients with PBC had a defect in urinary acidification.[109] Both overt renal tubular acidosis and a latent form, detected with an acid-loading test, were found. Twice as many patients had the latent form as had the overt form. Patients with overt renal tubular acidosis had symptoms that included muscular weakness, nausea, vomiting, polyuria, and polydipsia. Renal tubular acidosis was of the distal tubular type except in one patient who had a combined proximal and distal tubular type. In another study, 33 per cent of patients with PBC had renal tubular acidosis[174]; however, none of these patients had classic renal tubular acidosis associated with systemic acidosis. Instead, defects in urinary acidification were found only after administration of an acid load. As anticipated, glycosuria and aminoaciduria were absent. Hypouricemia and hyperuricosuria due to defective postsecretory reabsorption of uric acid in the renal tubule also occur in PBC.[175]

The pathogenesis of renal tubular acidosis in liver disease is unknown. Osteomalacia complicating PBC has been suggested as one cause.[176] However, this should result in a proximal tubular lesion associated with aminoaciduria and glycosuria, which is seen only rarely in PBC.[109] The possibility that copper deposition in the kidney might cause renal dysfunction has been suggested by the presence of renal tubular acidosis in Wilson's disease.[177] Recently, a close association between the presence of abnormal copper metabolism and renal tubular acidosis in PBC was reported.[174] Elevations of the plasma concentrations of copper as well as the urinary excretion of copper were significantly greater in patients with PBC and renal tubular acidosis than in patients with PBC who did not have renal tubular acidosis. Moreover, the ability to acidify the urine after an acid load correlated with both the plasma copper concentration and the urinary excretion of copper. The possibility that renal tubular acidosis is the result of an autoimmune process also has been suggested.[109, 178] This concept is supported by observations that patients with PBC may be sensitized to Tamm-Horsfall glycoprotein[178] and the finding of serum antibodies that react against the loop of Henle.[179]

Breast Carcinoma and Extrahepatic Malignancy

Evaluation of patients with PBC referred to specialized centers indicates that PBC is associated with an increased incidence of breast carcinoma.[180, 181] A retrospective review of 195 patients with PBC revealed six instances of breast carcinoma, representing a statistically significant increase compared to the expected incidence in the general population.[180] An independent retrospective study of 208 patients with PBC found the incidence of breast carcinoma to be increased 4.4 times.[181] The incidence of other extrahepatic malignancies did not exceed that predicted for the general population.[180, 181]

Urinary Tract Infection

Women with PBC have an increased, unexplained susceptibility to urinary tract infections.[182] Among 87 women with PBC, 19 per cent developed urinary tract infections during one year of observation, compared with 7 per cent of women with other chronic liver diseases and 8 per cent of women with rheumatoid arthritis. The prevalence of bacteriuria rose to 35 per cent during a subsequent two-year observation of 144 consecutive women with PBC. Bacteriuria was correlated with the presence of advanced histologic stages. Reinfection also was significantly more prevalent in PBC than in controls. The bacterial species were similar to those observed in other groups with urinary tract infections.

Celiac Disease

Several reports indicate an association between PBC and celiac sprue.[183–187] In the original reports, investigation of intestinal complaints led to the diagnosis of PBC.[186, 187] In a recent prospective study, 5 out of 26 consecutive patients with PBC had intestinal villous atrophy.[182] These patients were predominantly male and had a high prevalence of HLA B8, which is not a feature of populations of patients with PBC. Intestinal symptoms responded to a gluten-free diet, but the liver disease was unaffected. Two other patients with PBC and celiac sprue also had dermatitis herpetiformis. Thus, celiac sprue should be considered in the differential diagnosis of diarrhea and malabsorption that commonly occurs in patients with PBC and chronic cholestasis.

INFREQUENTLY ASSOCIATED CONDITIONS

Several conditions or diseases have been reported to occur in small numbers of patients with PBC. Many of these have features of autoimmune diseases, which no doubt explains the enthusiasm for reporting their association with PBC. It is unclear at present, however, whether these represent true associations or mere coincidences. In instances where more than one rare disease is present concurrently with PBC, it is attractive to speculate that the association is not fortuitous.

Mixed Connective Tissue Disease

Mixed connective tissue disease occurred in 5 per cent of patients reported by James et al.[56] All of the patients had the CREST variant of scleroderma and antibody to extractable nuclear antigen. Unfortunately, the nature of the mixed connective tissue disorder was not specified. An earlier report of a patient with PBC, scleroderma, and polymyositis also suggested the presence of mixed connective tissue disease.[161, 188]

Polymyositis

Polymyositis has been reported infrequently in association with PBC.[56, 161, 188]

Polymyalgia Rheumatica

Polymyalgia rheumatica has been reported in association with PBC.[189] Abnormalities of liver tests reflecting cholestasis and hepatic histologic abnormalities (portal inflammation and granulomas), however, have been found in patients with polymyalgia rheumatica alone.[190, 191] It is difficult to assess, therefore, whether the patients reported by Robertson et al.[189] actually had PBC.

Skin Lesions

Skin lesions are uncommon in PBC. Several patients have had maculopapular lesions suggesting an allergic capillaritis.[56, 192] Papular lesions or petechiae and evidence of vasculitis with deposition of IgM and complement have been reported.[192, 193] Bullous pemphigoid has been reported in association with membranous glomerulonephritis in one patient,[194] and pemphigus erythematosus developed in a patient receiving D-penicillamine.[195] Other reported lesions include: dermatitis herpetiformis,[183, 184] generalized morphea,[196, 197] lichen sclerosus et atrophicus,[196, 198] vitiligo,[199] and telangiectasias of the skin and mucous membranes resembling those found in Osler-Weber-Rendu syndrome.[200]

Pulmonary Fibrosis

Pulmonary fibrosis has been diagnosed in patients with PBC on the basis of abnormal pulmonary function tests and chest radiographs.[109, 119] The most frequent finding is a reduced diffusion capacity for carbon monoxide. Chest radiographs are abnormal for less than half the patients who have abnormal diffusion capacities. A recent study suggests that pulmonary fibrosis occurs most often in pa-

tients with PBC who also have Sjögren's syndrome.[119] Subclinical inflammatory alveolitis also has been detected by bronchoalveolar lavage in patients with PBC in the absence of pulmonary symptoms or abnormal chest roentgenograms.[201] Their alveolar lavage fluid contained increased quantities of activated macrophages and T cells of a helper/inducer phenotype compared to controls or patients with alcoholic liver disease.

Neurologic Disease

Several patients with PBC and neurologic syndromes have been reported.[56, 202-204] Peripheral neuropathy occurs in less than 5 per cent of patients who have PBC.[56] One patient with PBC had a sensory neuropathy due to axonal degeneration of large myelinated fibers.[202] One patient developed severe neurologic consequences of vitamin E deficiency including weakness, muscle wasting, areflexia, and decreased vibratory and proprioceptive sensation.[203] Another patient with PBC and Sjögren's syndrome experienced recurrent transverse myelitis associated with vasculitis and necrotizing myelopathy of the cervical and thoracic spinal cord.[204]

Nephropathy

Several patients with nephropathy in association with PBC have been reported.[11, 174, 192, 194] In one patient, membranous glomerulonephritis associated with renal deposits of IgM and IgG was reported.[192] This patient had both renal tubular acidosis and the nephrotic syndrome. Mild proteinuria has been found in association with PBC,[11] and one patient had evidence of glomerulosclerosis.[174] An additional patient with PBC and bullous pemphigoid had the nephrotic syndrome associated with membranous glomerulonephritis.[194] Interstitial nephritis also has been reported in a patient evaluated for sodium- and potassium-losing nephropathy.[205]

Hemolytic Anemia and Thrombocytopenia

Cold autoimmune hemolytic anemia has been found in a single patient with PBC.[206] Autoimmune thrombocytopenia has been described in a patient with autoantibodies to insulin receptors and episodic hypoglycemia.[207] In a prospective study of 62 patients with PBC, increased amounts of platelet-bound IgG were found in 40 per cent.[208] Nine of these patients had thrombocytopenia, and eight were cirrhotics with splenomegaly. The presence of platelet-bound antibodies suggests that the thrombocytopenia resulted from both the autoantibodies and hypersplenism.

Cardiomyopathy

Hypertrophic and restrictive types of cardiomyopathy have been reported to occur in patients with PBC.[109]

Concurrence of Hashimoto's Thyroiditis and Myasthenia Gravis

One patient with PBC who had both thyroiditis and myasthenia gravis has been described.[209]

Progressive Ophthalmoplegia

Primary biliary cirrhosis was diagnosed in one patient ten years after the onset of progressive ophthalmoplegia.[210]

Choledochal Cyst

A large choledochal cyst involving the common hepatic and proximal common bile ducts in a patient with PBC has been reported.[211]

Multiple Myeloma

Multiple myeloma and PBC were detected in one patient.[212]

Systemic Lupus Erythematosus

Anecdotal reports of patients with PBC and systemic lupus erythematosus[45] are difficult to interpret, since anti–double-stranded DNA antibodies are found in as many as 26 per cent of patients with PBC.[213]

Pernicious Anemia

Rare patients with PBC and pernicious anemia have been reported by several groups.[50, 54, 56, 58]

Ulcerative Colitis

Several patients with PBC have been reported with ulcerative colitis in whom the diagnosis of primary sclerosing cholangitis was rigorously excluded.[214, 215] The coexistence of PBC and ulcerative colitis appears to be coincidental, in contrast to the strong association between primary sclerosing cholangitis and ulcerative colitis (see Chap. 43).

Pancreatic Insufficiency

Chronic pancreatitis has been reported infrequently in association with PBC.[215] However, subclinical damage of the exocrine pancreas may be relatively frequent.[216] Either immunoreactive trypsin or pancreatic lipase was elevated in 73 per cent of patients in one study; the elevations were not correlated with the age of the patients, histologic stage, or severity of cholestasis.[216] In another study, pancreatic fluid output and bicarbonate content were found to be normal in patients with PBC.[217]

Graves' Disease

Graves' disease has been reported in several patients with PBC.[59, 218]

Retroperitoneal Fibrosis

In one patient, idiopathic retroperitoneal fibrosis associated with obstructive uropathy was diagnosed 20 years prior to the development of symptomatic PBC.[219]

Menstrual Abnormalities

In a study of 87 female patients with PBC, the incidence of dilatation and curettage and of hysterectomy was significantly increased.[220] The menstrual abnormalities necessitating these procedures usually preceded the diagnosis of PBC by more than a decade, suggesting an abnormality in the metabolism of female sex hormones.

NATURAL HISTORY AND PROGNOSIS

Available information indicates that the natural history of PBC can be subdivided into four sequential phases (Table 44–10). The earliest, or *preclinical phase*, has been identified on the basis of positive screening tests for antimitochondrial antibodies in the absence of hepatobiliary symptoms or cholestatic abnormalities of routine liver tests.[56–58] It is important to note that these patients underwent serologic screening because of symptoms of nonhepatic diseases known to be associated with autoimmunity or PBC. Over a mean of 8.7 years of observation, 5 of 29 patients developed symptoms of PBC, and 12 of 16 women observed for 4 years or longer also developed liver test abnormalities.[58] The duration of this phase, from the time of recognition until evidence of progression, appears to be 2 to 10 years. However, the length of this phase from its true onset until recognition is unknown. The *asymptomatic phase* denotes a period characterized by cholestatic abnormalities of liver tests and the absence of hepatobiliary symptoms.[11, 35, 50, 54, 59, 60, 221] The earliest abnormality is an isolated elevation of hepatic alkaline phosphatase. Although aminotransfer-

TABLE 44–10. SEQUENTIAL PHASES IN THE NATURAL HISTORY OF PRIMARY BILIARY CIRRHOSIS

	Estimated Duration	References
1. "Preclinical" phase with normal hepatic biochemical tests	Unknown; at least 2 to 10 years	James et al.[56] Munoz et al.[57]
2. Asymptomatic phase with abnormal hepatic biochemical tests	Indefinite in some; 2 to 20 years in others	Mitchison et al.[58] Dickson et al.[11] Long et al.[50] Fleming et al.[54] Balasubramaniam et al.[221]
3. Symptomatic phase	3 to 11 years	Christensen et al.[39] Blade et al.[212]
4. Terminal phase with portal venous hypertension and hepatic failure	0 to 2 years	Haeki et al.[125a] Kew et al.[126]

ases may be elevated, total bilirubin is usually normal. The course of disease in this phase is variable. One subgroup of patients may remain asymptomatic indefinitely; another subgroup of patients ultimately develops hepatobiliary symptoms after a period of 2 to 20 years. The existence of subgroups among asymptomatic patients also is supported by studies of actuarial survival, indicating differences in prognosis (see section on Prognosis below).[50, 59, 221] The *symptomatic phase* is characterized by the presence of hepatobiliary symptoms (see Tables 44–1 and 44–2). Long-term observation indicates that patients with symptomatic disease continue to progress, but at highly variable rates. Ultimately, symptomatic patients enter a *terminal phase* of disease characterized by decompensated cirrhosis, complications of portal venous hypertension, and hepatic failure.

The large, multicenter, longitudinal study of Christensen et al.[46] has provided the most complete information regarding the natural history of patients with PBC. In this study, the classification of Popper and Schaffner[126a] was used for histologic staging. At the time of referral, the frequencies of individual stages were I (14 per cent), II (40 per cent), III (19 per cent), and IV (27 per cent). The lifetable method was used to analyze the data in order to overcome bias due to the loss of more severely ill patients as a result of withdrawal or death. Individual signs and symptoms were evaluated serially, and cumulative percentages of patients with each were calculated yearly. Liver biopsy was performed yearly.

The cumulative percentage of patients with symptoms and signs of hepatic disease increased progressively with time. For example, pruritus (the presenting complaint of 42 per cent of patients) was present in 75 per cent of patients by the time of entry into the study. The median duration of disease before pruritic patients entered the study was less than three years. During the next five years, the cumulative percentage of patients with pruritus increased from 75 to 95 per cent. Similarly, over the same five-year period the percentage of patients with hyperpigmentation increased from 53 to 82 per cent and the percentage with jaundice rose from 58 to 79 per cent. The percentage of patients experiencing gastrointestinal bleeding also increased, from 5 to 46 per cent, over a period of five years.

The presenting symptoms of 11 patients were the result of collagen vascular diseases. By the time of referral to the study (median duration of disease = two years), many additional patients had developed signs or symptoms of collagen vascular diseases. For example, scleroderma was the initial complaint of only one patient, but was present in a total of 11 patients on entry into the study. Over the next two years, scleroderma was diagnosed in another four patients. Sjögren's syndrome, the initial complaint of two patients, was present in nine patients at the time of referral. Two more patients had this diagnosis made during the subsequent two years. In the same interval, seven patients developed hypothyroidism associated with anti-thyroid antibodies.

The prevalence of abnormal physical findings also progressed with time. Over a five-year period of follow-up, the percentage of patients with hepatomegaly increased from 55 to 83 per cent. Similar increases were found for splenomegaly (34 to 65 per cent), xanthomas (27 to 50 per cent), and ascites (5 to 49 per cent). Based on the number of patients who needed diuretics, 76 per cent of patients experienced fluid retention during the five-year period. Vertebral collapse, a flagrant sign of hepatic osteodystrophy, was present as a presenting sign in only one patient,

but was found in 20 per cent of patients after five years of observation.

In contrast to the progression of symptoms and signs in patients with PBC, the median values of laboratory tests did not vary in a significant way. Even though median values for individual laboratory tests tended to remain stable, increasing proportions of patients developed values that fell within the upper (or lower in the case of albumin) 15th percentiles calculated from values for all patients at the time of entry. Thus, over a five-year period, 60 per cent of the values for albumin, 52 per cent of the values for bilirubin, 43 per cent of the values for alkaline phosphatase, 40 per cent of the values for alanine aminotransferase (ALT; SGPT), and 25 per cent of the values for cholesterol fell in this range.

At the time of entry into the study, autoantibodies were detected frequently. Ninety-one per cent of patients had antimitochondrial, 26 per cent anti-thyroid, 31 per cent antinuclear, and 33 per cent anti-smooth muscle antibodies. Although the percentage of patients with each antibody did not change with time, the titers of antimitochondrial antibody increased to values greater than the level of the upper 15th percentile at entry. After five years, the titers of antimitochondrial antibody were equal to or greater than 1:1200 in 82 per cent of patients. Similar progressions were found for the serum concentrations of IgM, IgG, and IgA.

The progression of histologic features from the time of entry was striking. The cumulative percentage of patients with proliferation and destruction of ductules rose from 78 to 100 per cent in three years. In the same period, the percentage of patients with piecemeal necrosis rose from 69 to 100 per cent. Loss of bile ducts was found in 31 per cent of biopsies initially and 62 per cent after five years. Histologic evidence of cholestasis increased with time, and was most marked in a periportal distribution. Other features showing cumulative progression over five years included lymphoid follicles (38 to 88 per cent), fibrosis (58 to 85 per cent), cirrhosis (29 to 82 per cent), and granulomas (24 to 56 per cent).

Information is incomplete regarding the natural history of patients with preclinical and asymptomatic phases of disease. Such patients are underrepresented in therapeutic trials requiring referral to a treatment center; thus, systematic assessment of large numbers of patients in these groups has been impossible. Careful study of these patients with serial testing of quantitative liver function may provide important information regarding progression that might be inapparent using actuarial survival methods.

PROGNOSIS

No spontaneous remission of PBC has been documented; hence, the long-term prognosis is poor. The short-term prognosis, however, is extremely variable.[46, 50, 54, 57, 59, 60, 221, 222] For patients presenting with cholestatic symptoms and jaundice, in the past the average life expectancy from the time of diagnosis was 5.5 years (range 3 to 11 years).[222] Similar patients in whom PBC is diagnosed today actually may have an average life expectancy of more than this, since they are unlikely to undergo surgical exploration of the bile ducts, which some feel reduces the life span of the patient with PBC.[126a]

The short-term prognosis for asymptomatic patients with PBC is excellent.[11, 49, 54, 56, 57, 59, 60, 221] The prognosis for asymptomatic patients with positive tests for antimitochondrial antibody and normal hepatic biochemical tests[56–58] has not been defined adequately. During an observation period of at least 4 years, 12 of 16 women developed abnormalities of liver tests but remained asymptomatic.[58] Over a mean observation period of 8.7 years, 5 of the 29 patients developed hepatobiliary symptoms typically associated with PBC. Thus, some patients in the preclinical phase progressed to the more classically recognized asymptomatic and symptomatic phases of the disease within a decade. Once hepatic tests become abnormal, the future course is likely to be similar to that described for asymptomatic patients with abnormal hepatic biochemical tests.[49, 50, 54, 56, 57, 59, 60, 221] and for symptomatic patients.[46, 222]

The prognosis for asymptomatic patients with abnormal hepatic biochemical tests has been defined partially and is the subject of controversy. Based on observations of 20 such patients, Long et al. retrospectively identified two groups.[50] Patients in group I (n = 10), with an average age of 44 years at presentation, remained asymptomatic for an average of 4.5 years (range 2 to 10 years), whereas patients in group II (n = 10), with an average age of 51 years at presentation, remained asymptomatic for an average of only 2.2 years after presentation. The two groups were comparable in terms of the histologic stage of disease, the prevalence of antimitochondrial antibody, and the mean values for most hepatic biochemical tests. Patients in group I, however, were younger and had significantly lower values for total bilirubin (see below) than did patients in group II.

Eight of ten patients in group I were alive 2 to 10 years after the diagnosis of PBC, and four remained asymptomatic. The two deaths in this group were not caused by liver failure. Interestingly, the symptoms that developed included only fatigue and xerostomia. It could be argued that these symptoms, albeit new, do not constitute a significant change from the designation "asymptomatic," since at the time of inclusion into the study eight of the 20 asymptomatic patients were being investigated for other diseases, including keratoconjunctivitis sicca. On the other hand, all ten patients in group II developed pruritus as their initial symptom 1 to 4 years after presentation. Seven patients were alive after a mean period of 2.7 symptomatic years, and three died of hepatic failure after 4 symptomatic years. Thus, patients with asymptomatic PBC may remain free of hepatobiliary symptoms for 10 years or more following diagnosis. Once symptoms develop, the life expectancy was similar to that reported for symptomatic patients.[46, 222] The report of Fleming et al. suggests that asymptomatic patients with stage III or IV histologic lesions may have had the disease for 10 years or more prior to diagnosis.[54] Thus, depending on the time of diagnosis, an asymptomatic course of 10 to 20 years appears to be possible in PBC.[11, 54]

Progression and ultimately decreased survival may not occur in all patients with asymptomatic disease. Retrospective actuarial analysis of survival in PBC by Roll et al. indicated that the survival of "asymptomatic" patients followed for a median period of 6 years did not differ from that of age- and sex-matched individuals in the general population.[59] In contrast, the mean survival of symptomatic patients was 11.9 years. Observation of the asymptomatic group for an additional 5 years (median period of 11.4 years) showed that their survival continued to be comparable to the general population. During the observation period, however, 15 of the 36 patients developed symptoms and 6 of 8 deaths were due to liver disease. Portal granulomas correlated with normal survival and continuation of a asymptomatic status, whereas associated autoimmune disorders correlated with decreased survival. No other clinical, laboratory, or histologic features correlated with either survival or development of symptoms. In a recent study of elderly patients diagnosed with PBC, the survival of asymptomatic and symptomatic patients was comparable to age- and sex-matched controls in the general population.[60] Recently, the actuarial survival of 44 asymptomatic patients with PBC referred to the Mayo Clinic was reported to be less favorable.[221] During a mean observation period of 7.1 years, 77 per cent developed hepatobiliary symptoms, 34 per cent developed esophageal varices, and 13 patients (30 per cent) died. Nine of the 13 deaths were due to liver failure. Actuarial analysis indicated that survival was comparable to that of the general population for the first 5 years and then decreased sharply.

The combined reports suggest that asymptomatic patients represent a heterogeneous group. One subgroup appears to remain asymptomatic and has a normal life expectancy.[59, 223] Another subgroup may develop hepatobiliary symptoms with time but also has a normal survival.[223] Yet another subgroup may develop symptoms, experience progression of disease, and succumb to liver failure.[50, 221] Clearly, reliance on the absence of symptoms elicited during a careful history is inadequate to differentiate between benign and severe outcomes. Further studies are required to determine more objective prognostic criteria for patients identified in the asymptomatic phase.

Several clinical, biochemical, and histologic features have prognostic significance in PBC. In the report of Christensen et al.[46] age and sex were not important determinants of prognosis following age adjustment of mortality rates. As expected from the discussion above, the nature of the initial symptom or sign was related to prognosis. Patients presenting with pruritus, jaundice, ascites, or gastrointestinal hemorrhage were older, had shorter durations of symptoms and higher levels of serum bilirubin, and were more likely to have cirrhosis. Asymptomatic patients presenting without any symptoms or with only symptoms of a collagen vascular disease or an intercurrent, unrelated process had lower levels of serum bilirubin, aminotransferases, and cholesterol. Histologically, their disease was characterized by bile duct destruction and granulomas; cirrhosis was infrequent.

The level of serum bilirubin at the time of entry was an important prognostic variable and showed a significant correlation with the presence of histologic evidence of cholestasis. The total bilirubin at the time of entry into the study correlated significantly with the rates of occurrence for jaundice, ascites, and death. The correlation of total bilirubin and a progressive course was independent of the prognostic influence of the histologic stage. This finding substantiates the observations in a group of 55 patients that indicated the level of total serum bilirubin is prognostic in PBC.[61] In that series, the following mean survivals were found for specific values of total bilirubin (two determinations more than 6 months apart): > 2 mg/dl, 49 months; > 6 mg/dl, 25 months; > 10 mg/dl, 17 months.

The histologic stage at the time of the first biopsy has prognostic significance.[46, 59, 224] In the study of Christensen et al.,[46] mortality rates were similar for patients with disease in histologic stages I, II, and III but 2.8 times greater for patients with cirrhosis. In the study of Kloppel et al.,[224] patients with stage III and IV disease had higher mortality also. The presence of granulomas also is reported to be a favorable prognostic histopathologic feature,[137, 223] but larger studies have failed to confirm this impression.[129] Since the presence of granulomas is inversely related to the histopathologic stage of disease,[135] the apparent prognostic relationship between granulomas and survival may actually reflect the prognostic relationship with the histologic stage.

The frequencies of certain clinical features at the time of entry were significantly greater in patients who died of hepatic failure (with or without gastrointestinal hemorrhage) than in patients who survived.[46] Features characteristic of patients with a poor prognosis included hyperpigmentation, jaundice, ascites, a requirement for diuretics, elevated serum bilirubin, low serum albumin, and the histologic presence of periportal cholestasis, cirrhosis, and bile ductopenia. Even though the group with a high mortality rate did not have symptoms for longer periods than did other patients, the progression of disease was much more rapid. The influence of the clinical features just described on prognosis was independent of the influence of advanced histologic stage or the value of total bilirubin.

Using the time of death as a reference point, the cumulative percentage of patients with a particular abnormal feature prior to death was calculated. From five to three years prior to death, the only feature increasing substantially was jaundice (from 40 to 59 per cent). In the two-year period prior to death, the frequency of jaundice increased from 65 to 100 per cent, the frequency of hepatomegaly from 70 to 97 per cent, and the frequency of ascites from 15 to nearly 100 per cent. Histologic progression was characterized by peripheral cholestasis preceding cirrhosis and cirrhosis preceding the development of centrilobular cholestasis.

Multiple regression analysis was performed on all clinical, biochemical, and histologic variables in 216 patients with PBC to assess their relationship to prognosis.[225, 226] In these 216 patients, who were enrolled in a placebo-controlled trial of azathioprine,[46] six variables had prognostic significance: serum bilirubin, age, cirrhosis, serum albumin, centrilobular cholestasis on liver biopsy, and therapy with azathioprine. From these variables a prognostic index (PI) could be calculated by the following formula: $PI = 2.52 \times \log_{10}$, serum bilirubin μmol/L $+ 0.0069 \times \exp$. ([age yrs $- 20$]/10) $- 0.05 \times$ serum albumin g/L $\times 0.88$ (if cirrhosis present) or $+ 0.68$ (if centrilobular cholestasis present) $+ 0.52$ (if not treated with azathioprine). Using the PI, a survival estimate can be calculated that has been validated by comparing the calculated survival with the observed survival in three groups of patients receiving a placebo in a controlled trial.[225] Further refinement of calculated prognostic indexes should be beneficial in determining the optimal timing of liver transplantation in patients with PBC.[226]

COMPLICATIONS

Advancing disease results in increasing cholestasis, decreased hepatocellular function, and the development of portal venous hypertension. As a consequence, patients with PBC may experience a variety of complications ranging in severity from mild to life-threatening.

GENERAL

The complications of cholestasis include pruritus, hyperpigmentation, hyperlipidemia, and the formation of xanthomas, steatorrhea, diarrhea, and neuropathy. Pruritus may increase during the course of disease until the preterminal phase, when it may subside. Excoriations resulting from intense pruritus are prone to secondary bacterial infection. Hyperlipidemia in PBC is not associated with an obvious increase in atherosclerotic complications. As total serum lipids increase, however, patients frequently develop xanthelasma. Xanthomas occur less frequently; often they are planar and involve the flexion creases of the palms, fingers, and elbows. They also appear in creases beneath the breasts and about the neck. Tuberous xanthomas involving extensor surfaces of the upper and lower extremities, buttocks, and pressure points also occur.

Steatorrhea in PBC occurs primarily in patients who have advanced cholestasis.[73, 227] The severity of steatorrhea was related to decreased output of bile acids, the magnitude of cholestasis, and advanced histologic stages.[227] In patients with mild cholestasis, the fecal fat is either normal[73, 227] or only modestly elevated.[228, 229] The major consequence of steatorrhea is the malabsorption of fat-soluble vitamins, especially vitamin D (discussed later) and vitamin A.[229] Although weight loss is the presenting complaint of some patients with PBC,[46, 53] significant weight loss and malnutrition are unusual before the terminal stages of the disease. In a recent report of six patients with PBC who had lost weight, significant steatorrhea was associated with an abnormal D-xylose absorption test even though the small bowel was normal radiographically and histologically.[230] In other studies, D-xylose aborption was normal in all patients even though steatorrhea was common.[227, 229] Patients with PBC infrequently complain of diarrhea. When present, it has been presumed to be related to steatorrhea. It should be recalled that celiac disease has been found in association with PBC.[182–187]

Sensory neuropathy occurs in approximately 5 per cent of patients with PBC.[109] The major complaint in these patients is painful dysesthesias of the hands and feet. In some instances, the neuropathy is caused by xanthomatous deposits in the peripheral nerves.[231] Recently, the case of a patient who had a sensory neuropathy caused by axonal degeneration of the nerves was reported.[202]

PORTAL VENOUS HYPERTENSION

Portal venous hypertension frequently is demonstrable in PBC, even early in the course of the disease.[126, 127, 141–143] For example, esophagrams of 109 patients with PBC revealed esophageal varices in 50.[126] Four of these patients presented with variceal hemorrhage, and an additional 17 bled within two years of developing hepatobiliary symptoms. Portal venous hypertension may precede true cirrhosis[126, 127a, 141–143] and may be related to nodular hyperplasia[141] or may be due to obstruction at a presinusoidal level by the inflamed and fibrotic portal tracts. The extent of portal inflammation and fibrosis, however, appears to be similar for patients with and without esophageal varices. Moreover, normal numbers of patent portal veins appear to be present. When portal venous hypertension occurs secondary to true cirrhosis in PBC, hepatocellular function often is well preserved. Consequently, portal-systemic vascular shunts may be tolerated quite well.[126, 127a] As expected, surgical shunts prevent further hemorrhage but do not alter the progression of the liver disease. In 23 patients with PBC undergoing portal-systemic shunts, there was no operative mortality; survivals ranged from 1 to 8 years, with a mean of 3.4 years.[127a] Despite the effectiveness of portal-systemic shunting, it should be avoided in all patients who are candidates for liver transplantation in order to preserve the portal venous system for surgical anastomoses.

HEMORRHAGE FROM VARICES

Hemorrhage from esophageal varices is primarily a late complication of PBC,[46, 120] but may occur as the presenting feature. The reported frequencies of this presentation range from 3 to 65 per cent.[45, 127a] The latter figure represents a selected series of patients referred for portal-systemic shunts. In another series of 109 cases of PBC, 4 per cent of the patients presented with hemorrhage from varices.[126] In the series reported by Christensen et al.,[46] 6 per cent of patients presented with "gastrointestinal bleeding," and presumably some of these episodes were due to esophageal varices. Overall, between 25 and 50 per cent of patients with PBC bleed from varices at some time in the course of their disease.[46]

CHOLELITHIASIS

Cholelithiasis was found in 39 per cent of 23 patients with PBC studied by endoscopic retrograde cholangiography.[118] In one autopsy study of cirrhotic patients, 31 per cent of those who had PBC had gallstones, compared with 13 per cent of individuals without cirrhosis.[232] In cirrhosis due to any cause, most gallstones are of the pigmented type. Cholecystitis due to the impaction of a gallstone in the cystic duct or choledocholithiasis should be considered in the differential diagnosis when patients with PBC develop typical symptoms of abdominal pain or show abrupt increases in the biochemical indices of cholestasis.

HEPATOCELLULAR CARCINOMA

Compared with the incidence of hepatocellular carcinoma in other forms of cirrhosis, this malignancy is a rare complication of PBC.[129, 144, 181] In several series it has not been found,[46, 126a] whereas in one series 3 of 52 patients with PBC (6 per cent) had hepatocellular carcinoma.[233] In the Mayo Clinic series, 2 patients who were not enrolled in the controlled trial of D-penicillamine therapy developed hepatocellular carcinoma.[11] None of the 124 patients enrolled in the study at that time had developed this complication. In a retrospective review of 208 patients, only one hepatocellular carcinoma was noted.[181]

MISCELLANEOUS

Other complications associated with cirrhosis, decreased hepatocellular function, and portal venous hypertension include coagulopathy, portal-systemic encephalopathy, and peptic ulcer disease. Each has been found in association with PBC.[46, 50, 53, 54]

FAT–SOLUBLE VITAMIN DEFICIENCY

Recent studies indicate that patients with advanced PBC may suffer effects from deficiencies of vitamin A[234–237] and vitamin E.[203, 238, 239] Patients with vitamin A deficiency have low serum levels and impaired dark adaptation. Vitamin A deficiency has been attributed to steatorrhea and malabsorption as well as to ineffective mobilization from hepatocytes.[237] Some patients with vitamin A deficiency also are deficient in zinc.[234] Less is known about the consequences of vitamin E deficiency in PBC except for well-documented reports of neurologic effects.[203, 239] In one study of 80 patients with PBC, 64 per cent had vitamin E deficiency, and the 12 most profoundly deficient patients underwent extensive neurologic testing.[239] Five of these patients had a mixed sensorimotor neuropathy that was incompatible with the neurologic syndrome expected in vitamin E deficiency. In another recent study of 45 patients, 13 per cent had abnormally low serum vitamin E levels, but neurologic examinations and red blood cell peroxide hemolysis tests were uniformly normal.[238] Vitamin E absorption was significantly impaired.[238]

HEPATIC OSTEODYSTROPHY

Manifestations of hepatic osteodystrophy in PBC include bone pain, tenderness, and fractures involving the hips, pelvis, thoracic cage, and vertebrae.[240–246] Both osteomalacia and osteoporosis occur, but osteoporosis is considered to be more common in PBC, especially in the United States.[242–246] Differentiation between osteomalacia and osteoporosis in PBC is important, since only the former responds to currently available therapy.

Osteomalacia is the consequence of vitamin D deficiency. Factors leading to the deficiency of vitamin D in PBC include malabsorption of vitamin D,[244, 247, 248, 250] poor dietary intake,[241, 249] renal wasting of vitamin D metabolites,[244, 247, 250] and inadequate synthesis of vitamin D_3 in the skin.[240, 250] In addition to symptoms related to bone demineralization, proximal muscular weakness may occur in osteomalacia. Radiographic findings in osteomalacia range from pathognomonic pseudofractures in advanced disease to normal-appearing bones in less advanced disease. Indeed, until mineralization is decreased by 30 to 40 per cent, radiographic examination of bones shows no abnormality.[255] Thus, negative skeletal roentgenograms are not uncommon even when symptoms are prominent. Patients with PBC complicated by osteomalacia generally have normal serum levels of calcium, phosphorus, and parathyroid hormone.[240, 241] Elevations of alkaline phosphatase most often are attributed to cholestasis, but no studies have been performed to assess the relative contributions of hepatic and bone isoenzymes to the total activity present in the serum.

Recent studies indicate that osteoporosis is the most common metabolic bone disease in PBC.[242–246] The etiology of osteoporosis complicating PBC remains undefined. The roles of vitamin D and calcium metabolism in its pathogenesis are debated,[240, 242–246, 256] and recent evidence of impaired osteoblastic function suggests that reduced stimulation of osteoblastic activity may play a primary role.[242, 243] Osteoporosis commonly involves the vertebrae, and patients usually are asymptomatic prior to vertebral collapse.[241] Radiographic findings may be normal prior to significant demineralization. Even when osteopenia is present radiographically, it is impossible to differentiate between osteoporosis and osteomalacia.

Biopsy with examination of an undecalcified specimen of bone is the only reliable way to differentiate osteomalacia from osteoporosis.[242–246] In osteomalacia, the osteoid seam is increased and calcification front is deficient; in osteoporosis and cortex is thin and the trabecular bone is decreased. In several series in which bone biopsies were performed, an average of 30 per cent of patients with PBC had osteomalacia.[248, 250, 257, 258] In contrast, all recent studies using rigorous histologic criteria for the classification of metabolic bone disease have shown a lack of osteomalacia and a high frequency of osteoporosis.[242-246] Among 33 patients with PBC, findings consistent with osteoporosis included significant decreases in trabecular bone volume, osteoid volume, osteoid surface, and appositional rate of mineralization.[245] These findings, combined with normal values for serum calcium, phosphorus, and 25-(OH)D, exclude the possibility of osteomalacia. Other independent studies have confirmed the high prevalence of osteoporosis,[242-244, 246] although the interpretation of the results of one study suggested a novel form of bone disease[246] that has not been confirmed by others.[242, 243]

Two studies indicate that the primary defect in PBC is reduced osteoblastic function resulting in a state of low bone turnover.[242, 243] In the study of Stellon et al.,[242] 30 female patients underwent iliac crest biopsy following double tetracycline labeling. Trabecular plate thinning, rather than removal of whole trabecular plates, resulted in a significant decrease in the mean trabecular bone volume in pre- and postmenopausal subjects. Impaired osteoblast function was inferred from measurements of wall thickness, osteoid seam width, findings compatible with a defect in matrix synthesis, and a low bone formation rate in the postmenopausal patients. In addition, the presence of increased total resorption surfaces and urinary calcium creatinine ratios in premenopausal patients suggested that bone resorption also might contribute to bone loss. In the study of Hodgson et al.,[243] histomorphometric examination showed a reduced rate of bone formation and a significantly decreased level of serum osteocalcin, a specific marker of bone turnover. Although their results confirmed a defect in osteoblast function, urinary hydroxyproline excretion did not confirm the presence of increased bone resorption. These data confirm the impression that osteoporosis is the dominant pathologic process and suggest that therapy should be directed toward inhibiting currently undefined toxic cholestatic factors that might impair osteoblast function[243] or toward stimulating osteoblastic activity with agents such as sodium fluoride.[242]

Ergocalciferol (vitamin D_2) and cholecalciferol (vitamin D_3) are the two primary forms of vitamin D. Vitamin D_3 is synthesized in the skin as the result of ultraviolet irradiation of 7-dehydrocholesterol, whereas vitamin D_2 is absorbed from the diet. The metabolism of vitamin D_2 is identical to the metabolism of vitamin D_3. However, in normal humans, circulating metabolites of vitamin D are predominantly derived from vitamin D_3.[240, 244] Both vitamin D_2 and vitamin D_3 are taken up by hepatocytes and hydroxylated at the 25 position by enzymes in the endoplasmic reticulum. The resultant 25-(OH)D is the major circulating metabolite of vitamin D. It is bound in the serum to a specific binding globulin, which is synthesized by the liver.[259] Subsequent metabolism of 25-(OH)D varies quantitatively, depending upon the presence or absence of vitamin D deficiency. In non-deficient subjects, much of the 25-(OH)D undergoes additional hydroxylation in the kidney to form 24,25-$(OH)_2$D, 25,26-$(OH)_2$D, and small amounts of 1,25,26-$(OH)_3$D.[240, 241, 244] In vitamin D deficiency, most 25-(OH)D is metabolized by 1α-hydroxylase in the kidney to form 1,25-$(OH)_2$D, the most biologically active metabolite of vitamin D.

Serum 25-(OH)D levels (combined 25-$(OH)D_2$ and D_3) have been measured in PBC.[241, 244, 247, 249, 250, 256, 258, 260, 261] Although abnormally low concentrations have been found in some patients not receiving vitamin D supplements,[247, 248, 260, 261] normal levels of 25-(OH)D are found in the vast majority of patients,[242-246, 256] especially early in the course of their disease.[262] Abnormally low levels of 25-(OH)D also

have been found in association with other chronic liver diseases, and thus, they are not specific for PBC. Low 25-(OH)D levels of PBC cannot be explained by defective hydroxylation of orally administered vitamin D. The liver is able to hydroxylate vitamin D_3 synthesized in the skin or vitamin D administered orally or parenterally.[244, 247, 250, 260] When injected parenterally, radiolabeled vitamin D_3 is readily converted to 25-$(OH)D_3$ in patients with PBC, and the percentage of serum radioactivity in the form of 25-$(OH)D_3$ is inversely related to the initial level of 25-(OH)D.[247] This is consistent with other studies showing that vitamin D deficiency is associated with a preferential metabolism of vitamin D to 25-(OH)D. Repetitive doses of vitamin D over a prolonged time may be required, however, to increase serum 25-(OH)D levels.[260] For example, serum 25-(OH)D levels did not increase in patients with PBC after a single intramuscular injection of vitamin D_2, but did rise to normal when monthly injections were given over periods of 3 to 16 months.[260] Following simultaneous intravenous injection of labeled D_2 and D_3 into patients with PBC, normal amounts of 25-$(OH)D_2$ and D_3 were formed.[244] In both controls and patients with PBC, D_2 was preferentially converted to 24,25-(OH)D while D_3 was preferentially converted to 25,26-(OH)D. Urinary excretion of D_2 and D_3 derivatives was strikingly increased compared to controls and was significantly correlated with the level of serum bilirubin. Thus, patients with PBC can form 25-(OH)D if the supply of substrate is adequate and can carry out subsequent hydroxylations.[24] Excessive urinary losses of polar metabolites indicate an increased requirement for vitamin D in patients with PBC.

These data suggest that vitamin D deficiency, not abnormal metabolism, is responsible for occasional cases of osteomalacia in PBC. The relationship between vitamin D deficiency and the development of osteoporosis in PBC remains speculative. One study indicates that osteoporosis in PBC is not the result of deficient quantities of 25-(OH)D or 1,25-$(OH)_2$D, but instead may be related to low levels of 24,25-$(OH)_2$D or yet undefined factors.[256] Evidence of impaired osteoblastic function suggests that malabsorption or deficiencies of vitamin D and calcium may be largely unrelated to the pathogenesis of osteoporosis in PBC.[242, 243]

As already mentioned, many factors can contribute to deficiencies of vitamin D. These include dietary deficiency or malabsorption of vitamin D, lack of exposure to ultraviolet light, increased urinary excretion of vitamin D, decreased amounts of specific serum-binding protein, and the formation of inactive metabolites as a result of enzyme induction. Each of these factors has been assessed to some extent in patients with PBC.

Dietary intake of vitamin D undoubtedly varies among patients with PBC. When vitamin D intake is assessed by a dietary history, it is often found to be subnormal.[241] Compounding the effects of a potentially inadequate intake, there is definitive evidence of vitamin D malabsorption in some patients with PBC.[247, 250] This appears to be the consequence of the malabsorption of fat-soluble vitamins that results from the decreased intraluminal concentrations of bile acids. The negative correlation of vitamin D absorption with fecal fat excretion is in accord with this explanation.[247] Treatment with cholestyramine, which binds bile acids and promotes their fecal loss, may worsen steatorrhea and increase the malabsorption of vitamin D.[248] Malabsorption not only of dietary vitamin D but also of metabolites of vitamin D entering the gut in the bile could contribute to vitamin D deficiency. In normal man a large amount of vitamin D_3 administered intravenously enters the duodenum, and 85 per cent is reabsorbed.[263] The significance in PBC of potential losses of vitamin D caused by disruption of this enterohepatic circulation has not been studied adequately.

Reduced exposure to ultraviolet light also may contribute to increased requirements for vitamin D in PBC.[240] In a recent study, the response to ultraviolet light was measured in three patients with PBC.[250] The levels of 25-(OH)D were normal in two patients and reduced in the third. In each patient, ultraviolet light increased 25-(OH)D levels to the high-normal range. A ninefold increase was seen in the patient whose 25-(OH)D level was initially low. In this patient concomitant rises in serum calcium, phosphate, and alkaline phosphatase were found. These observations suggest that exposure to artificial ultraviolet light or sunlight can increase 25-(OH)D in PBC.

In patients with PBC, excessive urinary excretion of vitamin D also may contribute to increased vitamin D requirements.[244, 248, 250] The metabolites of vitamin D in the urine appear to be more polar than the usual di- and trihydroxy derivatives. The mechanism responsible for the formation and urinary excretion of these metabolites is unknown. Theoretically, diminished hepatic synthesis of vitamin D–binding globulin could contribute to abnormal metabolism of vitamin D. This seems unlikely, since concentrations of the binding globulin are only slightly decreased in PBC.[250] Furthermore, the capacity of the remaining globulin to bind vitamin D should be adequate, since only 5 per cent of the binding sites are occupied normally.[240]

The possibility that induction of enzymes in the endoplasmic reticulum of hepatocytes might promote the formation of inactive metabolites of vitamin D in patients with PBC has been suggested.[241] Although inactive metabolites are produced in patients receiving phenytoin, there is no direct evidence that inactive metabolites are formed in patients with PBC. Patients who have PBC, however, may be exposed to drugs such as spironolactone or phenobarbital that induce enzymes of the endoplasmic reticulum.

Parenteral administration of vitamin D$_2$ to patients with PBC and vitamin D deficiency improves the absorption of calcium[257] and restores serum levels of 25-(OH)D to normal.[260] Parenteral vitamin D$_2$, however, has little effect on the skeletal symptoms of osteomalacia or osteoporosis in patients with PBC and does not promote healing. In fact, patients with PBC actually may develop osteomalacia while receiving prophylactic injections of vitamin D$_2$.[264] In contrast to the poor clinical results observed with parenteral vitamin D$_2$, several metabolites of vitamin D$_3$ can promote healing of osteomalacia in patients with PBC.[240] The therapeutically effective metabolites include 25-(OH)D$_3$,[258] 1,25-(OH)$_2$D$_3$,[264] and 1α-(OH)D$_3$.[265] Vitamin D, including metabolites of vitamin D$_3$, is not therapeutically effective in the treatment of osteoporosis.[242, 243, 256] The reason for the effectiveness of the derivatives of vitamin D$_3$ over vitamin D$_2$ in the treatment of osteomalacia is unknown. Recently, Shike et al. reported that parenteral vitamin D$_2$ actually may promote the development of metabolic bone disease in patients receiving long-term parenteral nutrition.[266] This possibly could explain the new onset of osteomalacia in some patients with PBC who have received long-term courses of parenteral vitamin D$_2$.

Based on our current understanding of the metabolism of vitamin D and of the prevalence of hepatic osteodystrophy in PBC, the following recommendations are reasonable. All patients with PBC should have periodic measurements of serum calcium, phosphate, and 25-(OH)D to detect vitamin D deficiency. If the level of 25-(OH)D is low and skeletal symptoms are absent, roentgenograms should be obtained to assess the status of bone mineralization, and bone densitometry should be performed. Vitamin D therapy then should be commenced (see section on Treatment). If skeletal symptoms are present, radiographs should be evaluated for features pathognomonic of osteomalacia. In the absence of such features, a bone biopsy after tetracycline labeling should be considered to establish the diagnosis of osteomalacia or osteoporosis.[242, 243, 245, 255] This distinction is important, since vitamin D therapy promotes healing in osteomalacia[233] but is of no benefit in osteoporosis.[256]

Prophylaxis of hepatic osteodystrophy in patients with PBC who have normal levels of 25-(OH)D and who do not have skeletal symptoms has not been adequately studied. Clearly, parenteral vitamin D$_2$ is not uniformly effective[264, 266] and possibly may be deleterious. However, excessive urinary losses of vitamin D metabolites suggests that patients with PBC have increased requirements for vitamin D.[244] Based on the evidence that vitamin D$_3$ and its derivatives are effective in the treatment of osteomalacia (discussed earlier), exposure to sunlight or ultraviolet lamps[250] may be an important prophylactic measure. Since dietary vitamin D$_2$ is malabsorbed, oral supplements of vitamin D$_2$ or of more polar derivatives also may be given.

DIFFERENTIAL DIAGNOSIS

The differential diagnosis of PBC may be considered from several perspectives. Differential diagnoses based on the histologic features of PBC or on the occurrence of cholestasis in adults include many conditions that are irrelevant to the clinician considering a diagnosis of PBC based on a combination of clinical, biochemical, serologic, and histologic information. Several specific diseases, however, may cause diagnostic confusion, and are discussed here.

EXTRAHEPATIC BILIARY OBSTRUCTION

Incomplete obstruction of the distal biliary tract may be difficult to distinguish from PBC, especially if dilated ducts are not seen on ultrasonography or computerized tomography. It is essential to diagnose mechanical obstruction, since it may be remediable and can result in secondary biliary cirrhosis if untreated. The presence of symptoms of cholangitis or rapidly occurring elevations of total bilirubin should suggest the possibility of extrahepatic biliary obstruction. As discussed above, the antimitochondrial antibody test is usually negative in patients with biliary obstruction.[79, 80, 82]

Cholangiography, the definitive test to assess the patency of the biliary tract (see section on Diagnostic Evaluation), should be performed promptly when extrahepatic obstruction is suspected.

A liver biopsy may or may not show features suggestive of obstruction, such as bile infarcts (uncommon but pathognomonic), concentric periductular fibrosis, or a significant neutrophilic component in the portal inflammatory infiltrate. The presence of bile ductular proliferation and portal inflammation in both obstruction and PBC can cause diagnostic difficulties.

PRIMARY SCLEROSING CHOLANGITIS

The features of this disease and its prevalence as a complication of inflammatory bowel disease are discussed in detail elsewhere (Chap. 43). Although the clinical, biochemical, and histologic features of primary sclerosing cholangitis may be indistinguishable from those of PBC,[106, 107, 267] application of multifactorial diagnostic criteria (Table 44–10) permits accurate distinction. A history of inflammatory bowel disease strongly suggests the possibility of sclerosing cholangitis. Tests for antimitochondrial antibody are typically negative.[107, 267]; however, up to 5 per cent of patients with primary sclerosing cholangitis had positive tests with low titers (< 1:20).[267]

The histologic features of primary sclerosing cholangitis are variable and not diagnostic.[106, 207, 267] Inflammation of the portal tracts and abnormal-appearing interlobular bile ducts may be confused with lesions seen in the early stages of PBC. Piecemeal necrosis, bridging necrosis, fibrosis, and cirrhosis are other features seen in both primary sclerosing cholangitis and PBC. Florid duct lesions, however, are not seen in primary sclerosing cholangitis.

In primary sclerosing cholangitis, cholangiography shows sclerosis and ectasia of the bile ducts. The extrahepatic ducts are involved, either alone or in combination with the intrahepatic ducts. As discussed earlier, the extrahepatic bile ducts are normal in PBC.[118]

PERICHOLANGITIS

This confusing histologic lesion also is discussed in detail elsewhere (Chap. 43). It is the most common hepatic lesion associated with inflammatory bowel disease, and thus should be considered when inflammatory bowel disease is present. Biochemical abnormalities, as in PBC, are predominantly cholestatic; an elevated alkaline phosphatase is the most prevalent abnormality. Tests for antimitochondrial antibody are negative in patients with pericholangitis.

Lesions of pericholangitis may be spotty. Some of the histologic features of these lesions are similar to those seen in PBC.[124] Both show mononuclear inflammation of the portal tracts and distortion of the interlobular bile ducts. Florid duct lesions are not seen in pericholangitis, however. In advanced pericholangitis, there is concentric fibrosis around the involved bile ducts. This is in contrast to the progressive obliteration of bile ducts seen in PBC.

DRUG-INDUCED CHOLESTASIS

Clinical and biochemical cholestasis may be caused by a variety of medications.[30, 40] A careful history regarding medications, including those that have been discontinued, should be obtained for every patient suspected of having PBC. The physician should discontinue all nonessential drugs and substitute different agents for any essential agent known to be hepatotoxic.

Agents causing intrahepatic cholestasis that closely resembles PBC include methyltestosterone,[28, 29] phenothiazines,[24] tolbutamide,[25] organic arsenicals,[26] thiobendazole,[27] and contraceptive steroids.[30] The clinical features of the hepatotoxicities of these agents are discussed in detail in the section on Etiology. Tests for antimitochondrial antibody usually are negative in drug-induced cholestasis, but rare positive tests have been reported.[80] Histologic features that help to differentiate PBC from hepatotoxicity due to the just mentioned drugs are the marked cholestasis seen with phenothiazines, tolbutamide, and arsenicals; the paucity of portal inflammation seen with methyltestosterone; and the portal infiltration with eosinophils seen with arsenicals.

SARCOIDOSIS

The presence of hepatic granulomas and chronic intrahepatic cholestasis in sarcoidosis[120, 268] may result in diagnostic confusion. Distinction is generally possible on clinical and histologic grounds, since florid duct lesions and destruction of bile ducts are not seen in sarcoidosis. In hepatic sarcoidosis, tests for antimitochondrial antibodies are negative, but the Kveim test may be positive. Positive Kveim tests do not occur in PBC.

HBsAg-NEGATIVE CHRONIC ACTIVE HEPATITIS AND OVERLAP SYNDROMES

It may be difficult in some situations to differentiate between PBC and chronic active hepatitis.[269] This is a particular problem in the management of those patients with chronic active hepatitis who have cholestasis, systemic features of autoimmune diseases, histologic abnormalities of bile ducts, and positive tests for antimitochondrial antibody. Cholangiography is normal in these patients. Such patients are representative of an "overlap syndrome" in that the combination of clinical, biochemical, serologic, histologic, and cholangiographic findings is insufficient to establish a definitive diagnosis. Although it may be possible to differentiate such patients on the basis of the antigen specificity of their antimitochondrial antibodies in the future, this is not possible at present.[84, 86, 132]

Histologic abnormalities of interlobular bile ducts may be seen in chronic active hepatitis.[130, 132, 269] These lesions of the bile ducts show subtle differences, however, from those seen in PBC. These differences include prominent vacuolation of the ductular epithelial cells, absence of rupture of the epithelium, and the consistent presence of stratification of the ductular epithelial cells in chronic active hepatitis. When the patient has conspicuous fibrosis or cirrhosis, the distinction between PBC and chronic active hepatitis may be easier since interlobular bile ducts are frequently absent in PBC but are preserved in chronic active hepatitis. Granulomas are absent in chronic active hepatitis. It must be emphasized, however, that even experienced hepatopathologists may not be able to distinguish between the two diseases.[269] Of interest is the postulate that HBsAg-negative chronic hepatitis and PBC are part of a spectrum of liver diseases.[110, 257]

It has been proposed that the response to a three- to six-month course of corticosteroids or corticosteroids plus azathioprine may help differentiate patients with chronic active hepatitis from those with PBC.[271] In one study, only patients with chronic active hepatitis responded to immunosuppression. In contrast, other workers have reported that not all patients with chronic active hepatitis and cholestasis respond to immunosuppressive therapy. Patients whose biopsy specimens stain positively with orcein are not responsive to immunosuppression, whereas patients whose biopsy specimens do not stain with orcein are responsive to immunosuppression.[272] Moreover, patients with PBC, especially in early histologic stages, may respond dramatically to corticosteroids (see section on Treatment).

DIAGNOSTIC EVALUATION

The clinician may be called upon to establish a diagnosis of PBC during any phase of the disease (Table 44–11).[273] Today, increasing proportions of patients with PBC are referred because biochemical abnormalities of cholestasis are detected by multiphasic blood-screening tests. Most of these patients have no symptoms of hepatobiliary disease, but they often have symptoms of other disorders. Other patients may present with symptoms of cholestasis. In the management of either the asymptomatic or the symptomatic patient, the history should include questions about (1) symptoms or signs of diseases commonly associated with PBC, (2) the use of medications, (3) symptoms or signs of inflammatory bowel disease, (4) symptoms or signs of acute hepatitis, (5) a personal or family history of gallstones, and (for women) (6) symptoms of cholestasis associated with pregnancy or the use of oral contraceptives. This information should help to establish the clinical differential diagnosis, and may suggest a need for specific investigations. As discussed earlier, the physical findings are quite variable in patients with PBC. A normal physical examination must not dissuade the clinician from performing further tests.

To establish the diagnosis of PBC, the most discriminating combination of biochemical and serologic tests is (1) an elevation of alkaline phosphatase activity to more than twice the upper limit of normal, (2) the presence of antimitochondrial antibody (especially in high titer), and, (3) an elevation of IgM. The hepatic origin of an elevation of alkaline phosphatase must be confirmed by the concomitant elevation of 5'-nucleotidase, γ-glutamyl transpeptidase, or leucine aminopeptidase. This is particularly important in patients with complaints of skeletal pain, since elevated levels of alkaline phosphatase can originate from bone. The presence of antimitochondrial antibody makes the diagnosis of PBC more likely but is not pathognomonic.[86, 269] Conversely, the absence of antimitochondrial antibody does not exclude the diagnosis. Other tests, such as determination of erythrocyte sedimentation rate, bilirubin, bile acids, cholesterol, triglycerides, and autoantibodies other than antimitochondrial antibody, are less specific. Both the erythrocyte sedimentation rate and the level of ceruloplasmin, an acute-phase reactant, are generally elevated. At presentation, the level of total serum bilirubin is usually normal or only modestly elevated. Serum bile acids are elevated in a variety of cholestatic diseases and are of little diagnostic value in PBC. Elevated levels of serum cholesterol and triglycerides tend to be seen in late stages of the disease.

Liver biopsy is mandatory in the evaluation of a patient suspected of having PBC.[273] It is most commonly performed by percutaneous needle aspiration. The size of the specimen must be adequate (approximately 2 cm); two passes should be made if the initial specimen is small. The size of the specimen is important because lesions of the bile ducts may be spotty. Also, the probability of observing the lesions increases with the number of portal tracts present in the biopsy specimen. Multiple sections should be reviewed, since lesions may be localized to only a short segment of

TABLE 44–11. COMPARISON OF DIAGNOSTIC FEATURES IN PRIMARY BILIARY CIRRHOSIS (PBC) AND PRIMARY SCLEROSING CHOLANGITIS (PSC)

Feature	PBC	PSC
Clinical		
Predominant sex	Female	Male
Age	Middle-age	Children-Adult
Symptomatic	> 65%	> 75%
Pruritus	> 70%	> 70%
Fever	< 2%	> 30%
Cholangitis	Absent	< 15%
Physical Findings		
Hepatomegaly	> 50%	> 50%
Splenomegaly	> 25%	> 25%
Jaundice	> 40%	> 40%
Hyperpigmentation	> 50%	< 25%
Xanthomata	> 15%	< 5%
Laboratory Tests		
Alkaline phosphatase	+ + + +	+ + + +
Bilirubin	+ +	+ +
↑ IgM	+ + + +	+ +
Aminotransferases	+ +	+ +
Serologic Tests		
Antimitochondrial antibodies	> 90%	< 5% (low titer)
Associated Disorders		
Inflammatory bowel disease	< 0.04%	> 65%
Sicca syndrome	> 65%	< 2%
Arthritis	> 15%	< 10%
Thyroid disease	> 15%	< 2%
Histologic Features		
Florid duct lesion	Diagnostic	Absent
Fibrosing cholangitis	Absent	Diagnostic
Cholangiography	Frequently normal	Diagnostic
Complications		
Hepatocellular carcinoma	Rare	Absent
Cholangiocarcinoma	Absent	Rare

an individual bile duct. Since most biopsy specimens can be interpreted only as "compatible" with the diagnosis of PBC, a special effort should be made to have the specimen reviewed by an experienced hepatopathologist skilled in the recognition of PBC. Special stains for copper may provide additional support for the diagnosis of PBC.[122, 269] The orcein stain is the most sensitive of these, but positive reactions are not specific for PBC.[272]

The biliary tract should be evaluated in every patient suspected of having PBC. Since the extrahepatic and distal intrahepatic bile ducts are patent and of normal caliber in PBC, ultrasonography and computerized tomography usually show no abnormality. Cholangiography is indicated to exclude the presence of primary sclerosing cholangitis or an unsuspected partial mechanical obstruction of the biliary tract. Intravenous cholangiography is not recommended because the visualization of the bile ducts often is suboptimal.[274] Both endoscopic retrograde cholangiography and percutaneous transhepatic cholangiography with a "skinny" needle have been successful in patients with PBC.[118, 275] Endoscopic retrograde cholangiography is preferred for the assessment of the extrahepatic biliary system.

In special circumstances, laparotomy may be necessary in the diagnostic evaluation of a patient suspected of having PBC. This is particularly true when a patient has unusual or atypical clinical features, a test for antimitochondrial antibody is negative, and attempts at cholangiography have been unsuccessful. Laparotomy permits operative cholangiography, wedge biopsy of the liver, and direct inspection of the gallbladder.

PATHOGENESIS

The pathogenesis of PBC is undefined. Several factors of possible pathogenetic significance have been identified, and studies have been performed to elucidate these areas. Our knowledge, however, remains incomplete, and our ability to interpret the significance of any observation remains limited. As a result, the following discussion of the postulated mechanisms of pathogenesis in PBC is largely speculative.

PERSISTENT VIRAL INFECTION

Following the discovery of markers for the hepatitis B virus, several investigations established that the prevalence of HBsAg and anti-HBs in patients with PBC was comparable to that in control populations.[14–16] Thus, PBC appeared not to be related to infection with the hepatitis B virus. Little further attention has been paid to the possibility of a viral pathogenesis because no candidate virus has been identified. Recent advances in our understanding of latent or persistent viral infections and the role of the host response in diseases resulting from such infections make reconsideration of a viral pathogenesis attractive.

Persistence of viral infection depends upon a balance between virus and host responses.[276] Those related to the virus include its cytopathogenicity and its susceptibility to host defenses. Immunologic factors of the host that predispose to persistent or latent viral infection include immunosuppression, ineffective antibody production, failure of an adequate T cell response to the virus, or failure to detect latent virus in a protected, intracellular location. Studies with murine lymphocytic choriomeningitis virus, a virus of low cytopathogenicity, have shown that disease is produced

by the host's cytotoxic T cells and that a deficient immune response can result in the persistence of viral infection and the development of chronic disease.[277] Thus, genetic predisposition to an abnormal immune response could increase susceptibility to chronic infection and result in chronic, immune-mediated injury of tissue. The possibility of a latent or persistent viral mechanism in PBC is intriguing in light of many observations indicating that immune function is defective in this disease (discussed later). Indeed, recent studies indicate that intracellular viruses may not even replicate in order for their host cells to be recognized by cytotoxic T cells.[178]

GENETIC FACTORS

Primary biliary cirrhosis is not an inherited disease. However, the rare occurrence of PBC in more than one member of the same family and the results of studies of unaffected relatives of patients with PBC suggest that genetically determined susceptibility may be involved in PBC. Familial occurrences of PBC have been documented in mothers and daughters,[21, 55, 58, 279, 280] brothers,[100] sisters,[11, 80, 281–284] a brother and sister,[10] and identical twin brothers.[285] In one report of two sisters with chronic liver disease, one had PBC and hypothyroidism and the other had chronic active hepatitis.[282] In a case report of a mother and daughter with PBC, an unrelated friend who had taken care of the daughter during her illness developed PBC less than two years later.[21] Such an event suggests the possibility of an inciting environmental agent. In this regard, a history of jaundice at age 5 in twin sisters with PBC, and a similar history among six sisters, four of whom developed PBC, are of interest.[286] Whether these histories indicate a common exposure to an environmental agent or coincidental hepatitis is conjectural.

Whether or not an environmental agent exists, family studies suggest the presence of a genetically based abnormality of the immune system in apparently healthy relatives of patients with PBC.[100, 287] In a large study of asymptomatic relatives, Galbraith et al. found that 49 per cent had one or more autoantibodies and 48 per cent had abnormal immunoglobulin levels.[100] The prevalences of the different autoantibodies were antimitochondrial, 7.4 per cent; anti-smooth muscle, 11 per cent; anti-nuclear, 16 per cent. The specificity of antimitochondrial antibodies among relatives is not for the M2 antigen.[84, 86]

Several studies have attempted to define the role of genetics in the abnormal immune responses of patients with PBC and their relatives.[162, 163] Until recently, no association between PBC and genetic markers such as ABO blood groups,[288] Rh groups,[288] or HLA antigens[162, 163, 289–291] had been described. Ercilla et al., however, found an increased frequency of the HLA-D locus antigen DR3 in a study of 21 patients with PBC.[289] This association is somewhat surprising since this locus is linked frequently with HLA-B8, and previous studies had not shown an increased frequency of HLA-B8 antigen in PBC,[162, 163] except in patients who also had scleroderma[156] or celiac sprue.[183–187] Subsequent studies of HLA-D antigens have not confirmed an association with HLA-DR3.[290, 291] An English study of HLA-DR antigens in 75 patients with PBC failed to show any association.[290] In contrast, a study of 114 consecutive, unrelated Caucasian patients with PBC evaluated in the United States showed a significant sixfold increase in the frequency of HLA-DRw8 in patients compared to controls.[291] Although discrepancies between the reported findings have not been resolved, further studies are indicated, since products of the HLA-D loci are involved in antigen presentation and in genetic regulation of immune responses.

IMMUNOLOGIC MECHANISMS

Several features of PBC suggest a possible role for the immune system in its pathogenesis. These include the histologic findings of chronic inflammatory cells and granulomas in apposition to necrotic hepatobiliary tissue, the high prevalence of autoantibodies, chronic activation of complement, and the association of PBC with other diseases suspected of having an autoimmune basis. The concept of an immunopathogenesis in PBC is predicated on the belief that etiologic or initiating factors result in an abnormally regulated immune response that is responsible for the perpetuation of hepatobiliary necrosis and fibrosis.

Numerous studies have been performed to assess the immune status and function of patients with PBC. Many of the resulting observations are compatible with the concept that one or more immune mechanisms may cause cellular damage to bile ducts, but such a relationship has not been proven. Several recent reviews summarize the numerous studies of immunologic function in PBC.[292-295]

Critics have noted that the disorders in PBC that are related to the immune system could be secondary consequences of the PBC rather than factors related to its pathogenesis. Indeed, the prevalence of autoantibodies and abnormal levels of immunoglobulins in asymptomatic relatives suggest that some features may not be either primary or secondary, but instead are markers of a genetic predisposition or susceptibility. At present the issue of which features are related to pathogenesis and which are consequences of the disease remains unresolved. Thus, the role of immunologic mechanisms in the pathogenesis of PBC remains speculative.

A prominent hypothesis postulates that the immunopathogenic mechanism responsible for hepatobiliary necrosis in PBC results from the sensitization of autologous lymphoid cells to hepatobiliary antigens. These sensitized cells then mediate cytotoxicity against hepatobiliary tissue. The theoretical possibility exists that the sensitizing antigens, rather than being hepatobiliary, are associated with infectious agents[18, 86, 276, 296] and elicit an immune response that cross-reacts with hepatobiliary tissue. In either instance, an implicit assumption in this hypothesis is dysfunction of immunoregulatory mechanisms normally responsible for maintaining tolerance to self.

The concept that lymphocytes from patients with PBC are sensitized to hepatobiliary antigens is supported by the demonstration that peripheral blood lymphocytes from patients with PBC produce lymphokines when exposed to such antigens. This has been shown using homogenates of normal human liver,[297] isolated, hepatospecific, cell-surface antigens,[298, 299] antigens derived from normal human bile,[300, 301] and salivary antigens that share antigens with biliary epithelial cells.[302] These studies indicate that lymphocytes from some, but not all, PBC patients have been sensitized to one or more hepatobiliary antigens; however, similar findings were noted in other liver disease, and thus these were not specific for PBC. Furthermore, none of the antigens eliciting reactions was present on biliary epithelial cells, the earliest target of histologic destruction in PBC. Finally, it is impossible to ascertain whether the observed antigen sensitization was a primary event or merely secondary to chronic hepatobiliary injury.

Initial attempts to demonstrate circulating cytotoxic effector cells in patients with PBC yielded mixed results. When rabbit hepatocytes were used as target cells, peripheral blood mononuclear cells from two of six patients with PBC showed cytotoxicity in vitro.[303] On the other hand, cytotoxicity against isolated rat hepatocytes was reported to be increased in each of nine patients with PBC.[304] Using cultured Chang cells (originally derived from human hepatocytes) as targets, the cytotoxic capacity of mononuclear cells from patients with PBC was shown to be significantly decreased compared with the cytotoxic capacity of normal individuals or patients with IBsAg-negative chronic hepatitis.[305] The cytotoxicity in these experiments was not specific for Chang cells, since similar results were obtained using a nonhepatic, xenogeneic cell. The relevant effector cells mediating cytotoxicity against these targets were lymphocytes that lacked surface immunoglobulin, bore Fc receptors, and did not spontaneously form significant quantities of rosettes with sheep erythrocytes. These characteristics are identical to those of nonimmune, cytotoxic cells referred to as natural killer cells.

Studies in which autologous hepatic tissue obtained from percutaneous liver biopsies was used as a source of target cells were next reported.[306] The results of a single study in patients with PBC were reported as the ratio of cytotoxicity induced by patients' cells divided by the cytotoxicity induced by normal control cells. No clear conclusion regarding antigen-specific cytotoxicity could be drawn from this study because ratios of greater and lesser than unity were observed. Although the use of biopsy specimens of liver as a source of target cells poses many problems,[305] the rationale for using an autologous target cell is sound.

The importance of using autologous target cells in assays of antigen-specific cytotoxicity has been demonstrated by studies in animals[307] and humans.[308] The results indicate that an antigen-specific cytotoxic T cell is capable of killing *only* target cells that bear both the relevant antigen and homologous determinants coded for by the major histocompatibility complex (HLA in humans). Thus, in humans an antigen-specific cytotoxic T cell can lyse an autologous target bearing antigen but cannot lyse a xenogenic cell or an allogeneic cell of a different HLA type even though it bears the relevant antigen. Future studies of the antigen-specific cytotoxicity in PBC, therefore, must employ autologous target cells. To do this, the technical problems of working with autologous hepatobiliary tissue must be overcome or circumvented. One promising approach is to study nonhepatic autologous cells to which hepatobiliary antigens have been coupled.

Recent observations in mice suggest that natural killer cells may mediate cytotoxicity against hepatobiliary tissue in PBC. It is now clear that natural killer cells, once considered an artifact of in vitro assays of cytotoxicity, can mediate cytotoxicity in vivo and may participate in the host defense against viral infection. Of particular interest is the fact that natural killer cells are stimulated by interferon. Although natural killer cell activity of circulating mononuclear cells is significantly decreased in PBC,[305, 310] it can be restored by either interferon or interleukin 2,[310] which should be present in the portal inflammatory milieu.[144-149]

Further assessment of the role of cytotoxic mechanisms in hepatobiliary tissue injury requires studies of inflammatory cells isolated directly from the diseased liver at different histologic stages of progression. Recently, T cell lines and clones exhibiting cytotoxic function in vitro have been prepared directly from liver biopsies of patients with PBC.[311] Rigorous studies of cytotoxicity await development of techniques to prepare autologous target cells from biliary epithelia and hepatocytes. This endeavor should be aided by the availability of PBC livers obtained at transplantation.

Despite the absence of definitive proof, circumstantial evidence strongly supports the hypothesis that destruction of bile duct epithelial cells is mediated by T lymphocytes. Before discussing this evidence, it is prudent to review several facts about T cells. In humans, two types of T cells are identified on the basis of phenotypic antigens on the cell surface. T cells with the CD4 phenotype exhibit specificity for antigen in the context of HLA class II determinants encoded by the HLA-D locus. The primary function of CD4 T cells is to provide help to other T cells and to B cells by secretion of lymphokines. Thus, they are commonly referred to as T helper/inducer cells. In contrast, T cells of the CD8 phenotype exhibit specificity for antigen in the context of self-HLA class I determinants encoded by the HLA-A, -B, and -C loci. CD8 T cells primarily function as suppressor T cells or as antigen-specific cytotoxic T cells and are commonly referred to as T suppressor/cytotoxic cells. Three caveats, however, are important when reviewing the data regarding T cells in PBC. First, neither the HLA class I or II specificity nor the functions of CD4 and CD8 cells are absolute. Approximately 1 per cent of the cells overlap in HLA class I and II specificity, and 10 per cent overlap in function. Thus, CD4 cells can be cytotoxic or suppressive, whereas CD8 cells can mediate helper functions; therefore, inferences of function based solely on cell surface phenotype may be inaccurate. Second, T cells recognize antigen only in the context of HLA class I or II determinants present on the surface of antigen-presenting cells or target cells. Third, aberrant expression of HLA class II antigens on cells normally devoid of these determinants (e.g., biliary epithelial cells) may elicit an alloimmune T cell response in certain circumstances.[313, 314]

Compelling evidence for the role of T cells in the pathogenesis of the bile duct destruction comes from immunohistochemical studies of liver biopsies (see section on Pathology).[144-149] Inflammatory infiltrates adjacent to bile ducts are composed predominantly of T cells with lesser numbers of monocyte/macrophages and B cells. Activated CD4 and CD8 cells are both present, and CD4 cells predominate. By light and electron microscopy, the majority of cells penetrating the bile duct epithelia were CD8 cells, although CD4 cells also were observed. Electron microscopic evidence of cellular connections between T cells and biliary epithelial cells suggests a cytotoxic function for T cells. Recent studies also indicate that in PBC, biliary epithelial cells express increased amounts of HLA class I and II determinants, compared to normal bile ducts which express only small amounts of Class I antigens.[315, 316] Thus, biliary epithelial cells express HLA determinants required for T cell recognition of antigen.[317] Moreover, dense expression of HLA-DR, -DQ, and -DP on bile ducts in early stages of the disease[316] suggests that biliary cells may act as antigen-presenting cells for direct activation of T cells that then recognize the biliary antigens as targets. Interferon produced locally in the liver could account for the hepatobiliary specificity of the necrosis seen in PBC.

Recent studies of chronic graft-versus-host disease[150, 318, 319] and chronic rejection of liver allografts[320-322] provide additional circumstantial support for the concept that bile duct destruction is immunologically mediated in PBC. In both situations, nonsuppurative destructive cholangitis and disappearance of interlobular, but not septal, bile ducts have been demonstrated. The precise mechanism of injury and the reason that damage is restricted to the interlobular bile ducts remain unexplained. Since injury is mediated by sensitized T cells in experimental models of graft-versus-host disease and in the rejection of homografts, these observations are consistent with the hypothesis that sensitized lymphocytes also mediate the necrosis of bile ducts in PBC.

Pathogenetic mechanisms in PBC other than antigen-specific T cell cytotoxicity also have been proposed. For instance, it is possible that sensitization to antigens might also induce a humoral antibody response. Such antibodies could mediate cytotoxicity against hepatobiliary tissue either alone or in concert with complement. Indeed, injured bile ducts surrounded by immunoglobulin and complement have been found in PBC,[323] but this finding has not been substantiated by others.[324] Even if the antibodies were not cytotoxic or capable of fixing complement, they could promote destruction of the target cell through the mechanism of antibody-dependent cellular cytotoxicity.[292, 305] It is important to note, however, that antibody-dependent cellular cytotoxicity has not been documented to occur in vivo in human beings and antigens unique to the surface membrane of biliary epithelial cells have not been identified.

Several studies have demonstrated the presence of serum antibodies in PBC that react with hepatic antigens.[329-329] In one study, antibodies bound to cultured human hepatocytes in vitro but were not cytotoxic.[325] Although the antigen specificities of the antibodies reacting against hepatic tissue have not been studied thoroughly, several studies have demonstrated antibodies that react with a complex of lipoprotein antigens present in the plasma membrane of hepatocytes.[299, 326-329] This finding is not specific for PBC, since similar antibodies are present in the sera of patients who have chronic active hepatitis.[299, 328, 329] The reported prevalences of these antibodies in patients with PBC vary considerably. One report indicates that they are present exclusively in patients with disease of histologic stages III and IV.[327] Studies to assess whether patients with PBC have antibodies that react with the epithelium of bile ducts have not been successful.

Based on the studies of human graft-versus-host disease, Epstein et al.[330] have postulated that PBC may be a forme fruste of graft-versus-host disease, either caused by the effects of a chronic viral infection, as documented in animals, or resulting from the persistence of maternal lymphocytes (graft) in the newborn (host). Similarities between PBC and graft-versus-host disease in addition to the lesions of the bile ducts include the sicca complex, hyperpigmentation, scleroderma-like skin lesions, autoantibodies, hypergammaglobulinemia, immune complexes, and anergy. Dissimilarities also exist, and it must be stressed that the hepatic lesions and clinical features of graft-versus-host disease are not identical to those of PBC. For example, the lesions of nonsuppurative destructive cholangitis in graft-versus-host disease are confined to interlobular bile ducts that have diameters of less than 45 μm.[128] Bile ducts with diameters as large as 100 μm are affected in PBC.[13] Nevertheless, the study of chronic graft-versus-host disease may provide new insight into the immune mechanisms responsible for specific necrosis of bile ducts. As noted above, it is interesting to speculate that aberrant expression of HLA class II antigens might directly elicit an alloimmune response.

The recent demonstration of putative "immune complexes" in the sera of patients with PBC has incited great interest. It should be emphasized, however, that conclusive proof that the materials reacting in the indirect assays are immune complexes has been verified in only a few studies.[292, 331] Using several assays, approximately 60 to 95 per cent of patients with PBC have been shown to have "immune complexes."[170, 332-335] The immune complexes vary in size but a substantial proportion are quite large (coefficient of sedimentation > 19S),[332, 334] exceeding in size immune complexes found in other diseases. Using the Raji cell immunoassay, which detects immune complexes containing complement, one group found that 95 per cent of patients with PBC had such immune complexes.[332] Analysis of cryoglobulins (anti-immunoglobulin immune complexes) in PBC demonstrated the presence of IgM complexed with IgG, IgA, or IgM.[332] Complement components were not present in the cryoglobulins despite the ability of the cryoglobulins to activate complement. A unique cryoprecipitable IgM capable of activating complement and of reacting like an immune complex in some assays also has been described.[336]

The relationship of immune complexes to the pathogenesis of PBC is unknown. The presence of immune complexes, however, is not unique to PBC, since they also are found in other chronic liver diseases.[337] One hypothesis is that an unknown initiating event results in immune recognition of an altered bile duct antigen, production of IgM, and formation of large immune complexes near bile ducts.[338] These immune complexes then evoke a granulomatous response. Excessive production of immune complex results in a spillover into the circulation, where the complexes are involved in the pathogenesis of associated autoimmune disease. In addition, it is postulated that the circulating immune complexes cause abnormal immune regulation by interacting with receptors for C3 or the Fc portion of immunoglobulin molecules. Both receptors are present on B cells and macrophages; Fc receptors are present on T cells. Except for one report,[323] evidence of the deposition of immune complexes in bile ducts is lacking. Moreover, granulomas are neither uniformly seen in PBC nor restricted to the portal areas. Thus, this hypothesis lacks experimental support.

The nature of the "antigen(s)" contained in the immune complexes present in PBC remains poorly defined. One preliminary report suggested that the immune complex contains antigens identical to or cross-reactive with those present in the epithelium of bile ducts.[339] In another study, antimitochondrial antibodies were found to be enriched in immune complexes from patients with PBC, suggesting that the complexes contained mitochondrial antigens.[340] Subsequent studies have not confirmed these results.[336, 341] Although the hypothesis of Thomas et al.[338] depends upon the presence of biliary antigens in the immune complexes, it is possible that the actual antigen is irrelevant. The mere presence of circulating immune complexes might affect adversely immunoregulation and the competence of the reticuloendothelial system.[342] Available data do not support a role for immune complexes in the primary pathogenesis of PBC.

The complement system has been evaluated extensively in PBC. Several defects have been defined that apparently are specific for this disease.[343] Early studies demonstrated that the serum levels of immunoreactive C3 were increased in PBC[343] as a result of the presence of both native C3 and conversion products of C3 activation.[344] Subsequent studies confirmed that the rate of catabolism of C3 is accelerated in patients with PBC compared with the rate in normal controls or patients with HBsAg-negative chronic active hepatitis.[336, 345, 346] Since the serum concentration of C3 was constant, these data suggested that the hypercatabolism of C3 was accompanied by an accelerated synthesis of C3.

The classical pathways of complement activation appear to mediate the hypercatabolism of C3.[336, 346] A role for the alternative pathway of complement activation has been suggested by the evidence that cryoprecipitates in PBC can cleave factor B.[332] In addition, accelerated kinetics of the alternative pathway of complement activation in vitro have been demonstrated in PBC.[347] The kinetics of the alternative pathway of complement activation were not accelerated in patients with chronic active hepatitis or sclerosing cholangitis. Recent studies of 18 patients with PBC revealed no evidence of alternative pathway activation in vivo.[346]

The presence of large, circulating immune complexes in PBC indicates that the functional capacity of the reticuloendothelial system to clear such complexes is abnormal in this disease.[343] However, using radiolabeled aggregated albumin, the nonspecific phagocytic function of the reticuloendothelial system was found to be normal in PBC.[342] On the other hand, in vivo studies of the immunoreceptor-mediated clearance functions of the reticuloendothelial system showed a marked decrease in the C3b-receptor–mediated function of hepatic macrophages in patients with PBC.[342] This defect was specific for PBC. In the same patients, the Fc-receptor–mediated clearance function of the splenic macrophages was normal. It is not known whether the defective C3b-receptor function results from decreased numbers of receptors, from reduced affinity of the receptors, or from competitive inhibition of these receptors by circulating conversion products of C3 or immune complexes that contain complement.[343] In vitro studies of monocytes from patients with PBC suggest that C3b-receptor blockade is due to a circulating factor, possibly IgM.[348, 349]

A common feature of the proposed immunopathogenic mechanisms discussed earlier is the implicit assumption that regulation of the immune response is abnormal in PBC.[292] Even though it is not yet possible to discern which immunologic features are related to pathogenesis and which are secondary consequences of the disease, it is constructive to note the numerous abnormalities of the immune system in PBC. These abnormalities include a high prevalence of anergy,[350, 351] decreased primary[351] and secondary[352] responses to immunization, a failure to convert from IgM to IgG synthesis following immunization,[352] a suboptimal proliferative response of circulating lymphocytes to plant mitogens,[305, 353] decreased numbers of total circulating T cells with a disproportionate reduction of helper T cells,[354, 355] defective function of suppressor T cells in vitro,[356, 357] reduction of the proliferative response to autologous cells in vitro,[358, 359] reduced cytotoxic capacity of natural killer cells[305, 310] and the presence of numerous autoantibodies[292] and of activated T cells and B cells in peripheral blood.[359, 360]

Evidence of abnormalities of immunoregulation in relatives of patients with PBC (see section on Genetic Factors) suggests an underlying genetic predisposition for inadequate generation of T cell suppression of immune responses. The reduced proliferation of T cells in PBC patients to autologous stimuli[292, 353] is consistent with this view, since the ultimate result of the autologous stimulation is the production of T suppressor cells. Generalized failure to suppress immune responses adequately could explain the extreme variety of immunologic abnormalities noted in PBC, most of which appear to be unrelated to pathogenesis. Specific failure to regulate T cell responses to biliary antigens and to control effector cells generated by these responses may represent the primary pathogenetic mechanism of PBC.

COPPER METABOLISM

Primary biliary cirrhosis is associated with excessive deposits of copper in the liver.[122] The finding of increased amounts of hepatic copper in other chronic liver diseases, however, suggested that excess hepatic copper was a non-specific, secondary phenomenon in PBC. Fleming et al[361] re-evaluated this concept in 1974 by quantitating copper in specimens of liver, kidney, spleen, and brain obtained at autopsy from patients with PBC and other chronic hepatobiliary diseases. The amounts of hepatic copper in PBC were comparable to those in Wilson's disease. An unexpected finding, unique to patients with PBC, was an increased quantity of copper in extrahepatic organs, such as the kidney and spleen. This suggested a further analogy between PBC and Wilson's disease, although copper deposition was not found in the brains of patients with PBC. These observations suggested that an abnormality of copper metabolism in PBC might be involved in the pathogenesis of the disease.

The absolute quantity of hepatic copper in patients with PBC is directly proportional to the histologic stage of the disease and the duration of cholestasis.[362] Table 44–12 compares the concentrations of hepatic copper in normal individuals and patients with chronic liver disease. It is apparent that the mean concentration of hepatic copper in PBC is exceeded routinely only in Wilson's disease and Indian childhood cirrhosis. It should be noted, however, that the values summarized in Table 44–12 are most representative of patients with advanced histologic stages of PBC.

Demonstration of hepatic copper by histochemical techniques does not correlate always with the presence of a quantitative increase in hepatic copper. Thus, false-negative stains for copper may occur in as many as 44 per cent of patients.[362] Shikata's orcein is the most reliable histochemical stain. Since it reacts with copper-associated protein in lysosomes rather than with copper directly, positive stains vary with the intracellular distribution of copper in hepatocytes. The results of histochemical staining for copper in the different histologic stages of PBC are discussed in the section on Pathology.

The majority of patients with PBC, regardless of the histologic stage of their disease, have abnormal concentrations of copper and ceruloplasmin in their sera.[122] For example, serum copper was elevated in 70 per cent of patients enrolled in the Mayo Clinic trial of D-penicillamine therapy.[11] The elevation was due primarily to an increased quantity of copper found to ceruloplasmin. Ceruloplasmin levels were elevated in 90 per cent of patients with PBC.

TABLE 44–12. CONCENTRATIONS OF HEPATIC COPPER IN PRIMARY BILIARY CIRRHOSIS AND OTHER CONDITIONS

	Mean Concentration of Hepatic Copper (μg/g Dry Weight)
Primary biliary cirrhosis	411
Wilson's disease	728
Indian childhood cirrhosis	1832
Primary sclerosing cholangitis	244
Extrahepatic biliary obstruction	128
Chronic active hepatitis	40
Alcoholic and cryptogenic cirrhosis	39
Normal controls	31

Source: From Vierling JM. *Seminars in Liver Disease*, Volume 1, Number 4, New York, 1981, Thieme Medical Publishers, Inc. Reprinted by permission.

The urinary excretion of copper also was increased in 75 per cent of patients with PBC, and this increase is assumed to reflect the glomerular filtration of copper that is not bound to ceruloplasmin.

As already mentioned, some patients with PBC have excessive amounts of copper in extrahepatic organs.[361] Recently, pigmented corneal rings have been found in several patients with PBC.[363, 364] These pigmented corneal rings differ from Kayser-Fleischer rings in Wilson's disease in that they tend to be greenish or tan rather than golden brown.[123] Pigmented corneal rings also have been found in association with chronic active hepatitis and cirrhosis[364] and intrahepatic cholestasis of childhood.[365]

The metabolism of copper has been evaluated in patients with PBC using radiocopper.[122] In one study, the metabolic fates of two isotopes of copper (^{64}Cu and ^{67}Cu) were assessed after simultaneous administration of one isotope orally and the other intravenously.[366, 367] The metabolism of each isotope was studied over a 12-day period by whole-body counting, by probe counting over the liver, and by measuring the content of radiocopper in the blood, plasma, ceruloplasmin, urine, and feces. The results of these studies indicate that in PBC (1) the intestinal absorption of copper is normal, (2) the hepatic uptake of absorbed dietary copper is normal, (3) the size of the initial mixing pool for copper is reduced (consistent with the concept that extravascular tissue sites are occupied by copper in this disease), (4) copper is incorporated into ceruloplasmin by both a rapid route and a slow route, and (5) the biliary excretion of copper is impaired.

Excessive hepatic copper is known to cause liver injury in domestic animals and in patients with Wilson's disease.[122] Whether excessive copper is hepatotoxic in PBC is a fundamental but unanswered question. Several mechanisms have been proposed to explain the hepatotoxicity of copper. These include deleterious effects of copper on intracellular enzymes, plasma membranes, organelles (such as lysosomes), the cytoskeleton, and nucleic acids. Based on incomplete knowledge, it appears that the hepatotoxic potential of copper is determined by both its physical-chemical state and its intracellular distribution. If copper is hepatotoxic in PBC, this toxicity must be regarded as a secondary event, since the pathologic process of PBC *precedes* the accumulation of copper.

CONCEPT OF A MULTIFACTORIAL PATHOGENESIS

The potentially pathogenetic mechanisms discussed earlier are not mutually exclusive. Thus, it is interesting to consider the possibility that several independent pathogenetic mechanisms might act in concert in PBC.[13] This concept is particularly appealing with regard to histologic stages III and IV, where loss of bile ducts results in progressive histologic cholestasis and the accumulation of copper within hepatocytes. In these stages it is possible that the putative immune-mediated injury may be augmented by the hepatotoxicity of retained bile and copper.

TREATMENT

THERAPY OF COMPLICATIONS

Nutrition and Activity

Studies to show the advantages of one diet over another in PBC have not been performed. In patients with absent or minimal signs or symptoms of cholestasis, the only stipulation should be that the diet contain adequate calories, vitamins, calcium, phosphorus, and protein. As cholestasis progresses, decreases in the intraluminal concentrations of bile acids result in the malabsorption of fat-soluble vitamins and reduction in calcium absorption. On theoretical grounds, restriction of dietary fat to 40 g/day and substitution of medium-chain triglycerides have been recommended,[12] but this appears indicated only in patients with steatorrhea. Vitamin K (10 mg/month) and vitamin A (100,000 IU/month) should be given intramuscularly as a prophylactic measure in advanced disease. Vitamin A should not be given to women of childbearing age since it is teratogenic. Supplementary vitamin D and calcium should be taken orally. Currently, the necessity for vitamin E supplementation is debatable. Even though the role of copper in the pathogenesis of PBC remains undefined, it seems prudent to recommend a diet low in copper. Foods rich in copper include nuts, shellfish, corn oil margarine, kidney, liver, and dried legumes; most can be avoided easily.

Normal activities should be encouraged. The fact that normal activities can be continued for many years following the diagnosis of PBC should be stressed to patients and their families.

Pruritus

Cholestyramine is the most effective agent for the control of pruritus. It is believed to reduce pruritus by binding bile acids in the small intestine so that they are subsequently lost in the feces. For patients who have intact gallbladders, the resin should be given prior to meals in order to take advantage of the meal-stimulated discharge of stored gallbladder bile into the intestine. Since storage of bile is maximum after the prolonged overnight fast, the largest proportion of the daily dose should be given at breakfast.[368] Patients must be advised that cholestyramine therapy is not effective immediately and that it must be continued even when no immediate benefit has been noticed. The dosages required to control pruritus vary and may be quite large. Cholestyramine has no apparent effect on the progression of the primary disease. Sherlock[12] has suggested, however, that the use of cholestyramine in the management of all patients (regardless of the presence of pruritus) might help to reduce the injurious effects of retained bile within the liver, but this view remains unsubstantiated. The prolonged use of cholestyramine may increase the malabsorption of vitamin D and provides an additional rationale for vitamin D and calcium supplements.[241]

When patients are intolerant of cholestyramine or do not benefit from it, other therapies may be useful in controlling pruritus. Phenobarbital, at doses of 2 to 4 mg/kg/day, has controlled pruritus in some patients with PBC.[23] Lower doses also may be effective in individual patients; the soporific effects can be exploited by giving the drug as a single dose at bedtime.

Occasionally, pruritus becomes intractable and may be devastating both to patients and to their families. Although methyltestosterone can relieve pruritus in such patients it causes a marked elevation of serum bilirubin and virilization; thus, it should be abandoned. Rifampin has been evaluated in the treatment of intractable pruritus with promising results.[369, 370] In the original report, rifampin resulted in a marked decrease in pruritus in five of six

patients, all of whom exhibited induction of oxidative microsomal drug metabolism.[369] Subsequently, a randomized, double-blind, placebo-controlled, cross-over trial was undertaken in nine patients.[370] Rifampin induced a significant reduction in pruritus that was independent of the order of treatment. Neither the mechanism nor the duration of rifampin's beneficial effect has been determined. In another study, a patient refractory to high-dose cholestyramine therapy appeared to benefit from a short course of ultraviolet phototherapy.[371] Following successful phototherapy, symptomatic relief was sustained by low-dose cholestyramine treatment. Temporary relief of severe pruritus has been obtained following subcutaneous administration of naloxone, which may act on central receptors involved in the sensation of itching.[372] Perfusion of plasma through charcoal-coated glass beads was reported to reduce bile acid levels and relieve intractable pruritus.[373] By separating the formed elements of the blood from plasma before perfusion, the substantial losses of leukocytes and platelets that occur with perfusion of whole blood over charcoal-coated surfaces were prevented. Perfusion of between 1000 and 6000 ml of plasma resulted in the mean extraction of 81 per cent of the bile acids and in prompt relief of pruritus. This effect lasted 24 hours to five months. Since bile acids would be expected to reaccumulate over approximately five days, the prolonged relief in some patients suggests the possibility that an absorbable factor other than bile acids may be responsible for pruritus.

Hyperlipidemia and Xanthomatous Complications

Dietary regimens low in cholesterol or high in polyunsaturated fat have not had consistent or long-term beneficial effects in reducing serum lipids. Cholestyramine therapy may initially lower the serum cholesterol level, but the effect is transient. Clofibrate is contraindicated, as it paradoxically raises cholesterol levels in patients with PBC, may worsen xanthomas, and increases the formation of gallstones.[374, 375] In a few patients with xanthomatous neuropathy (a rare complication), plasma exchange and plasmapheresis have been beneficial.[376]

Hepatic Osteodystrophy

As discussed earlier, patients with PBC have a multifactorial liability for vitamin D deficiency and calcium malabsorption. General measures potentially may be of benefit in preventing osteomalacia, but their efficacy as prophylaxis has not been studied. These would include a regimen of exposure to sunlight for 10 to 20 minutes per day; dietary supplementation with vitamin D (4000 IU/day), since intake is often low; and provision for extra calcium in the diet. To achieve maximum absorption of supplemental vitamin D and calcium, they should not be given at the same time as cholestyramine.

Healing of osteomalacia in PBC has been demonstrated in a small number of patients treated primarily with orally or parenterally administered derivatives of vitamin D_3 (see section on Complications). Therapeutically effective metabolites of vitamin D_3 include 25-$(OH)D_3$,[258] 1,25-$(OH)_2D_3$,[284] and 1α-$(OH)D_3$.[265] The possibility that derivatives of vitamin D_3 are more effective than derivatives of vitamin D_2 in the prevention and treatment of osteomalacia needs further evaluation. Medium-chain triglycerides may also benefit patients with symptomatic osteomalacia.[377] Patients receiving this therapy had decreased steatorrhea and relief of bone pain.

No effective therapy exists for patients with established osteoporosis.[242, 243] Therapeutic trials of sex hormones and calcitonin have not been performed in patients with PBC. Intravenous infusions of calcium may be effective in relieving severe bone pain in patients with osteoporosis or osteomalacia.[378] Measures that theoretically may be helpful in preventing osteoporosis include a diet rich in protein, supplemental ascorbic acid, avoidance of ethanol ingestion, and avoidance of immobilization. Corticosteroids are contraindicated for patients with hepatic osteodystrophy, because they accelerate the development of osteopenia.

Gallstones

Cholelithiasis is generally asymptomatic in patients who have PBC. Cholecystectomy should be performed on such a patient only when symptoms develop. If choledocholithiasis is present, endoscopic sphincterotomy and removal of stones should be performed to prevent obstruction, pancreatitis, cholangitis, and the development of secondary biliary cirrhosis.

Steatorrhea

Steatorrhea in PBC primarily results from decreased concentrations of bile acids in the intestine. The resulting fat malabsorption requires supplementation with fat soluble vitamins and calcium as discussed above. In severe cases, weight loss and diarrhea due to the secretory stimulus of malabsorbed fatty acids may require specific therapy. Reduction of dietary fat to ≤ 40 g/day should be tried first. If this is unsuccessful, medium-chain triglycerides should be substituted for approximately 60 per cent of the estimated dietary intake of fat. It must be emphasized that malabsorption in PBC occasionally results from celiac sprue or pancreatic insufficiency, and they must be considered in the differential diagnosis (see section on Complications). The former responds to a gluten-free diet and the latter to pancreatic enzyme supplements.

Xerophthalmia

In patients with sicca syndrome, which is a common complication of PBC, xerophthalmia is a frequently annoying symptom (see section on Complications). Xerophthalmia responds readily to administration of artificial tears (methylcellulose).

Esophageal Variceal Hemorrhage

Initial therapy for esophageal variceal hemorrhage (see Chap. 23) should include intravenous vasopressin with Sengstaken-Blakemore balloon tamponade if bleeding persists. Although emergent sclerotherapy has not been specifically studied in PBC, it should be considered to prevent the necessity of an emergent shunting procedure. Such procedures should be avoided in all patients who are candidates for liver transplantation. The role of propranolol in prophylaxis has not been adequately studied in patients with PBC. In one report, propranolol precipitated hepatic encephalopathy in a patient with PBC, which resolved after its discontinuation.[379]

THERAPY OF THE DISEASE PROCESS

No specific therapy has been identified that is capable of curing or arresting the disease. Since both the etiology and the pathogenetic mechanisms responsible for PBC remain unknown, the choice of therapeutic agents has been based largely on the assumption that the disease is immunologically mediated or is aggravated by retention of copper or toxins normally eliminated in the bile. More recently, antifibrotic therapy has been evaluated.

Interpretation and design of therapeutic trials in PBC is confounded by several factors. First, the efficacy of any therapy must be compared to the expected and the observed prognosis of untreated patients in controlled trials. As discussed earlier, the prognosis of PBC is quite variable and may depend on factors that remain to be defined. The existence of subgroups of patients in different phases of the natural history of the disease suggests that studies should be carefully stratified, a requirement that substantially increases the size of the populations required for meaningful analysis. Second, the unresolved issue of the prognosis of asymptomatic patients also is problematic. If life expectancy in this group is normal, trials of potentially toxic therapies may be unwarranted; if life expectancy is reduced, the risk of such therapies may be appropriate. Third, the choice of therapeutic agents is further complicated by the realization that multifactorial pathogenetic mechanisms may be involved (see discussion of Multifactorial Pathogenesis above). In the earliest stages of disease, when immunologically mediated destruction of interlobular bile ducts is most likely, immunosuppressive therapies appear most reasonable. In later stages, characterized by fibrosis, cirrhosis and progressive effects of cholestasis, immunosuppressive therapies may be incapable of arresting the disease or affecting nonimmunologic pathogenetic factors. In such patients, antifibrotic therapy or therapy to nullify noxious effects of cholestasis may be more appropriate. Fourth, application of any requirement that a controlled trial be exclusively performed in patients with early histologic stages (prefibrotic stages) of PBC is limited by the limited availability of such patients. Despite recognition of preclinical phases of disease and of asymptomatic patients with early histologic lesions, up to 50 per cent of asymptomatic patients have advanced histologic lesions at the time of diagnosis. Fifth, survival as the measure of efficacy of treatment is untenable. Although survival of patients in early reports was only 5 to 8 years, current studies indicate the potential for a normal survival in at least a subgroup of asymptomatic patients and a *median* survival of 8 to 11.9 years in symptomatic patients with advanced histologic stages of PBC. Thus, the time required for therapeutic trials based on survival is excessive, and the low frequency of PBC in the population significantly limits the number of agents that can be tested. Moreover, the success of liver transplantation in PBC must limit the duration of experimental therapies and makes survival an inappropriate end point of therapeutic trials.

The design of future therapeutic trials and the rational choice of therapeutic agents requires a greater understanding of the pathogenetic mechanisms responsible for the initiation and progression of PBC. Discovery of the immunologic mechanisms putatively responsible for the earliest injury may permit highly specific therapy. However, until that time, therapeutic trials will be largely empiric and based on theoretical rationales. Wiesner has proposed that future trials adhere to specific guidelines.[380] These include (1) a convincing rationale for the therapeutic agent; (2) enrollment of appropriate numbers of patients, stratified for different phases of disease; (3) an adequate period of observation; (4) use of objective criteria for decisions regarding the timing of analyses and publication; and (5) monitoring of drug toxicities. In addition, a concerted effort is necessary to validate prognostic indicators such as serial quantitative tests of liver function and clinical formulae for estimating survival in order to provide end points that will not interfere with referral for transplantation if the experimental therapy is ineffective.

Corticosteroids

Corticosteroids were used initially in uncontrolled therapeutic trials because of the perceived analogy between certain features of PBC and features of chronic active hepatitis and autoimmune diseases. Corticosteroids had no beneficial effect on the progression of PBC, but they promoted the development of osteoporosis in the majority of patients receiving chronic therapy.[381] This led to the dictum that corticosteroids should not be used in PBC. It should be stressed, however, that at the time of these trials, the patients studied were representative only of that subpopulation with advanced symptomatic disease.

With the recognition of increasing numbers of patients with early, asymptomatic disease[56] and serial histologic studies showing the importance of piecemeal necrosis in the development of fibrosis and cirrhosis,[46] the issue of corticosteroid therapy has been re-evaluated.

Thomas and Epstein described two patients with early PBC who had therapeutic responses to prednisolone.[295] Both patients were asymptomatic, and lesions of stage I PBC were present on biopsy. Each patient was initially evaluated after at least four months of prednisolone therapy, which had been given because of the mistaken diagnosis of chronic active hepatitis. Liver biopsy, repeated in both patients, showed marked improvement as compared with the original biopsies. In one patient the biopsy specimen was nearly normal. This evidence of histologic improvement was corroborated by improvements in biochemical tests of hepatic function and reductions in the levels of IgM. When prednisolone was discontinued, the levels of alkaline phosphatase, aminotransferases, and IgM again became abnormal. Six months later, the liver of the patient whose biopsy specimen had reverted to normal in response to steroids was again biopsied. Stage I histologic features similar to those seen on her original biopsy were found, indicating that the disease had relapsed. The anecdotal experience with these two patients, as well as with others (H. Popper, personal communication), suggests that prednisolone therapy may be beneficial in PBC, if given in the earliest stage of disease. This is consistent with the notion that the early phase of the disease is mediated by an immune process that is responsive to immunosuppressive drugs.

Recently, the results of the first controlled trial of prednisolone therapy in PBC were reported.[382] Thirty-six patients were randomized to either prednisolone or placebo. The two groups were similar with respect to levels of serum bilirubin and histologic stages. After one year of therapy, patients treated with prednisolone had significant improvement in pruritus, fatigue, and levels of bilirubin, alkaline phosphatase, aminotransferase, immunoglobulin,

and procollagen III. Prednisolone therapy also was associated with histologic improvement with reduction in inflammatory infiltrates, piecemeal necrosis, and the degree of fibrosis. Serial measurements of bone densitometry, however, showed a marked decrease in trabecular bone volume in the prednisolone-treated group. The authors concluded that the beneficial effects of prednisolone warranted further evaluation but that acceleration of osteopenia might be an unacceptable side effect of long-term use. Further controlled studies are necessary to evaluate the risks and benefits of corticosteroids; this is especially true for patients with the earliest stages of disease, when osteopenia is absent.[262]

Azathioprine

Azathioprine, an immunosuppressive drug of proven benefit in the prevention of renal allograft rejection and in the treatment of autoimmune chronic active hepatitis, has been evaluated in two prospective, randomized, controlled trials.[46, 105, 225, 382] In the first study, 22 patients with symptomatic, precirrhotic disease were treated with azathioprine (2 mg/kg); their clinical courses were compared with those of 23 other patients. No placebo was used in the control group. Progression to cirrhosis was the same in both groups, and no improvement was evident in biochemical or serologic tests of the group treated with azathioprine. The small size of the series prevented an assessment of efficacy based on survival. In the second study, 236 patients were enrolled in an international, cooperative, double-blind, randomized study of azathioprine (1 mg/kg to a maximum of 100 mg/day) versus a placebo. In a preliminary report of the results after a median follow-up of 18 months, no significant difference was found between the groups with respect to survival, clinical progression, histology, or biochemical and serologic tests.[105] The incidence of complications such as infections, gastrointestinal bleeding, and malignancies was not increased in patients receiving azathioprine.

In 1985, the results of this multicenter trial were updated.[225] Of the 248 patients enrolled, 127 had received azathioprine and 121 had received placebo. The dose of azathioprine varied from 0.5 to 1.5 mg/kg/day. Actuarial analysis again showed no significant differences in survival between the groups. However, identification of prognostic indicators by Cox multiple regression analysis led them to conclude that at randomization the treatment group had contained a disproportionate number of patients with bilirubin elevations indicative of a poorer prognosis than the placebo group. By readjusting the data to compensate for this imbalance, they concluded that azathioprine significantly improved survival after 20 months of therapy (p <0.01). In addition, azathioprine appeared to retard progression of clinical symptoms. The authors' conclusion that azathioprine should be used for all patients with PBC has not been widely accepted because of several shortcomings. First, a substantial number of patients (63) were lost to follow-up and 20 patients were withdrawn from the study because of adverse effects. Second, azathioprine appeared to have little effect on the progression of liver tests, including bilirubin, which has definite prognostic significance. Third, azathioprine did not retard histologic progression of the disease. Thus, their survival estimate based on statistical reanalysis of the original data should be interpreted with caution. On the basis of available information, further demonstration of unequivocal efficacy is required before azathioprine should be recommended for the treatment of PBC.

D-Penicillamine

Based on an analogy with Wilson's disease, in which hepatotoxicity is prevented by D-penicillamine, randomized, controlled therapeutic trials of D-penicillamine therapy for PBC were initiated. Since PBC is associated with progressive accumulation of copper within hepatocytes, the primary rationale for the use of D-penicillamine was its cupruretic action. It should be noted that D-penicillamine also has potent effects on the immune system and an antifibrogenic action.

The results of eight controlled trials of D-penicillamine therapy in PBC have been published.[383-392] Seven of the eight were placebo-controlled trials, and one was dose-controlled. The original report suggested that D-penicillamine improved both survival and liver function.[383] However, the duration of observation was inadequate for a meaningful conclusion. In the eight trials, 823 patients were studied, and those in the experimental groups received doses of D-penicillamine varying from 250 to 1000 mg/day. In each trial, D-penicillamine caused a substantial cupruresis and decrease in the quantity of hepatic copper. However, D-penicillamine did not result in any beneficial effects with respect to symptoms, liver biochemical tests, histologic progression, or survival. Significant side effects,[393, 394] including fatality, occurred in 29 to 46 per cent of patients. Thus, D-penicillamine is an ineffective therapy associated with serious side effects and should be abandoned.

Triethylene Tetramine Dihydrochloride (Trien)

Trien was used in four patients with PBC as an alternative chelator of copper, in an attempt to circumvent the problems of D-penicillamine toxicity.[393a] Trien promoted cupruresis in each patient but also produced significant side effects. Three patients had gastrointestinal toxicity (two had gastritis and one, anorexia), one patient had a rash, and the final patient developed acute rhabdomyolysis. As a result of toxicity, the trial was abandoned.

Zinc

Oral zinc competes with dietary copper for absorption and can induce negative copper balance.[122] In order to retard the accumulation of copper resulting from chronic cholestasis, eight patients have been evaluated in uncontrolled trials using oral zinc.[396, 397] No improvements in liver biochemical tests or histopathology were noted in seven patients, and hepatic copper concentrations were not reduced in the course of these short studies. Since copper does not appear to play a significant role in the pathogenesis of PBC and reductions of hepatic copper had no effect in the D-penicillamine trials, zinc therapy cannot be recommended.

Chlorambucil

Chlorambucil is an alkylating agent that has been beneficial in the treatment of immunologically mediated diseases such as systemic lupus erythematosus, membranous glomerulonephritis, and rheumatoid arthritis. Its effect in PBC has been evaluated in one small, unblinded, controlled trial.[395] Twenty-four patients were randomized to receive either chlorambucil or no therapy. Both groups were comparable with respect to age, serum bilirubin, and immunoglobulins. However, the disease in only 23 per cent of patients randomized to chlorambucil was in advanced histologic stages III and IV, whereas in 64 per cent of patients randomized to no therapy the disease had advanced histopathology. Of 13 patients treated with chlorambucil, the initial dose was 10 mg/day for 10 days and then the dose was adjusted to maintain the leukocyte count at 50 per cent of its initial value. The maintenance doses varied from 0.5 to 4 mg/day. During a mean observation period of 4.1 years (range 2 to 6 years), serum levels of bilirubin, aspartate aminotransferase, and albumin remained stable or improved in the chlorambucil group and worsened in the untreated group. Improvement in the degree of hepatic inflammation also was noted in the chlorambucil group, but there was no significant changes in the degree of fibrosis or histologic stages between the two groups. Bone marrow suppression required discontinuation of the drug in 4 patients; also, a trend toward more viral and bacterial infections was noted in the chlorambucil group but did not reach statistical significance. Survival could not be analyzed, since only 2 patients died (both in the untreated group). Although the study suggests that chlorambucil may improve liver biochemical tests and reduce hepatic inflammation, the disproportionate number of patients with advanced disease in the untreated group may have influenced this conclusion. Further controlled studies are required to assess the value of chlorambucil. The high incidence of infection, bone marrow suppression, and risk of developing nonlymphocytic leukemia indicate that chlorambucil should not be used outside of a controlled trial.

Colchicine

Colchicine, an agent with anti-inflammatory and antifibrotic actions, has long been used for the treatment of acute gout. It has also been reported to be beneficial in long-term therapy for alcoholic and cryptogenic cirrhosis.[398] Based on preliminary work by Koldinger in PBC patients,[399] three controlled trials have been undertaken.[400-402] The first, reported in abstract form in 1984,[400] randomized 34 patients to receive colchicine (1 mg/day) and 30 to receive placebo. The groups were matched for clinical, laboratory, and histologic features. After one year of therapy, the disease in 60 per cent of the placebo group had advanced one or more histologic stages compared to only 41 per cent of the colchicine group. After 18 months of treatment, survival was improved in the colchicine group (84 per cent) compared to the placebo group (69 per cent), but these values were not statistically significant. Diarrhea occurred as a side effect in 25 per cent of the colchicine group.

In 1986, another group reported the results of a controlled trial of colchicine in 60 patients with PBC.[401] In this study, 30 patients with disease in early histologic stages I and II and 30 patients with disease in late histologic stages III and IV were randomized to receive colchicine (1.2 mg/day) or an identical-appearing placebo. At entry, the treatment and placebo groups were comparable with respect to clinical, laboratory, and histologic parameters. After two years of observation, all patients remaining in the placebo group were switched to colchicine therapy. Patients treated with colchicine showed significant improvement in levels of bilirubin, alkaline phosphatase, cholesterol, aminotransferase, and albumin compared to the placebo group. However, there was no improvement in the severity of signs or symptoms. Also, histologic progression occurred in 50 per cent of patients in both the colchicine and placebo group. The cumulative mortality due to liver failure in the colchicine group (21 per cent) was significantly less (p <0.05) than that in the placebo group (47 per cent). However, this apparent benefit should be viewed with reservation. Two patients died in the colchicine group due to causes other than liver failure, and a third patient with stage IV disease was excluded from analysis because of discontinuation of therapy after one week. If these three patients were included in the survival analysis, the results would not show a significant difference. In addition, the mortality in the placebo group (47 per cent) was considerably higher than the mortality reported for the placebo group (35 per cent) in large trials of D-penicillamine therapy,[389, 390] whereas the mortality in the colchicine group (21 per cent) was lower than that reported in the D-penicillamine studies. Finally, the anticipated benefit of a truly efficacious therapy was not observed in the placebo group after switching to colchicine therapy. Indeed, the cumulative mortality in the original placebo group continued unabated following the addition of colchicine.

In the most recent study of colchicine therapy, which was reported in abstract form in 1986,[402] 57 patients were randomized to colchicine (1.2 mg/day) or an identical-appearing placebo. Improvements were noted for alkaline phosphatase and aminotransferase in the colchicine group, but only after four years of therapy. No differences were noted in serum bilirubin levels, and comparable histologic progression was noted in both groups. Toxicity was minimal, and colchicine was withdrawn in only 3 patients because of diarrhea. However, 27 patients (47 per cent) were withdrawn from the study for noncompliance or other reasons. Although survival was not analyzed by acturarial methods, six deaths occurred in the placebo group, and 2 patients receiving colchicine died or underwent transplantation.

The combined data suggest that colchicine has little effect on clinical signs or symptoms and does not retard histologic progression of PBC. It is, however, associated with improvements in laboratory tests. The conclusion that colchicine improves survival should be viewed with caution (see discussion above) until further results of controlled trials are available.

Cyclosporin A

Cyclosporin A, a potent immunosuppressive that inhibits interleukin 2 production by T cells, was evaluated in a pilot study of six patients with PBC.[404] Improvements in laboratory tests were offset by frequent nephrotoxicity, which prevented continuation of therapy. Further studies of this agent are important because it has been useful in the prevention of hepatic allograft rejection and chronic graft-versus-host disease after bone marrow transplantation. Since both of these alloimmune processes are associated with bile duct lesions similar to those observed in PBC, treatment of patients with early stages of PBC appears most rational. Indeed, a controlled therapeutic trial of low-dose cyclosporin A in precirrhotic patients is being performed at the Mayo Clinic. Preliminary results of biochemical improvement and reduction of pruritus are encouraging, but analysis of histologic effects has not been reported.

The frequency of nephrotoxicity (58 per cent) and hypertension (47 per cent) has been substantial and is disturbing in patients whose short-term survival (based on early stage of disease) cannot be predictably improved.

Levamisole

A pilot study of levamisole was begun to assess its immunostimulatory effects in PBC.[405] No benefit was evident after six months and the trial was abandoned.

Ursodeoxycholic Acid

As discussed above, the progressive accumulation of noxious substances, such as toxic endogenous bile acids, may contribute to liver injury in PBC. Therefore, a prospective, uncontrolled trial of ursodeoxycholic acid was performed in 15 patients with PBC.[406] After two years of therapy, the proportion of patients with significant pruritus was substantially reduced, and there were significant decreases in alkaline phosphatase, gamma glutamyltransferase, bilirubin, aminotransferases, and gamma globulin. Three patients who agreed to discontinue the drug after two years of therapy experienced deterioration of liver biochemical tests that promptly improved with reinstitution of therapy. These encouraging results warrant investigation, including correlation of clinical improvement with hepatic histology, in randomized, controlled trials that are being developed.

Plasmapheresis

Plasmapheresis, a therapy known to benefit patients with immune complex disease, was used in five patients with PBC.[407] After a mean number of 63 plasmaphereses per patient, there was no improvement in liver biochemical tests or in histology. As discussed earlier, plasmapheresis has been beneficial in the treatment of pruritus and xanthomatous neuropathy. Thus, it was not surprising that all of the patients experienced transient relief of pruritus and partial or complete resolution of xanthomata.

Plasma Exchange

Eriksson and Lindgren have described the effects of plasma exchange in four patients with PBC.[408] Exchange of 1.5 to 2 liters of plasma, twice or three times per week, reduced the levels of IgM, cryoprecipitable material, and urinary copper. The ^{14}C-aminopyrine breath test improved in each patient. The effects of this therapy on PBC have not been evaluated in large-scale, controlled trials.

Liver Transplantation

For patients in the terminal phase of PBC, liver transplantation affords the only opportunity for cure and survival. Criteria for candidacy and absolute and relative contraindications are identical to those used in adult patients with other nonalcoholic forms of cirrhosis (see Chap. 55). Refinement of systems to predict prognosis in individual patients should result in enhanced ability to select the appropriate time of transplantation.

In a recent review of 819 patients transplanted in eight different centers in the United States and Europe, the one-year survival for adult patients with nonalcoholic cirrhosis, including PBC, was 60 per cent for the cohort transplanted between May, 1983 and August, 1984.[409] Esquivel et al. recently reported the results of transplantation in 76 patients with PBC ranging in age from 31 to 68 years.[410] The male:female ratio was 1:10 and 98 per cent were positive for antimitochondrial antibodies. The mean preoperative bilirubin was 20.1, although one patient was transplanted with a bilirubin of 1.5 mg/dl because of numerous pathologic fractures and recurrent variceal hemorrhage. Retransplantation was required in 25 per cent of patients and was performed as early as three days and as late as three years following the original operation. Fifty-two of the 76 patients (68 per cent) survived, with a follow-up period ranging from one to 6.5 years. The five-year survival based on actuarial analysis was 66 per cent, which indicates that survival is prolonged once patients survive the first year. Overall the quality of life has been judged as good. As anticipated, antimitochondrial antibodies persisted in 43 of 45 tested. No recurrences of PBC have been observed.

REFERENCES

1. Addison T, Gull, W. On a certain affection of the skin vitiligoidea—α plana, β tuberosa. Guy's Hosp Rep 7:265, 1851.
2. Hanot, V. Etude sur une Forme de Cirrhose Hypertrophique du Foie (Cirrhose Hypertrophique avec Ictere Chronique) Paris, J. B. Balliere, 1876.
3. MacMahon HE, and Thannhauser SJ. Xanthomatous biliary cirrhosis (a clinical syndrome). Ann Intern Med 30:121, 1949.
4. Dauphinee JA, and Sinclair JC. Primary biliary cirrhosis. Can Med Assoc J 61:1, 1949.
5. Ahrens EH, Payne MA, Kunkel HG, et al. Primary biliary cirrhosis. Medicine 29:299, 1950.
6. Sherlock S. Primary biliary cirrhosis (chronic intrahepatic obstructive jaundice). Gastroenterology 37:574, 1959.
7. Rubin E, Schaffner F, and Popper H. Primary biliary cirrhosis. Chronic non-suppurative destructive cholangitis. Am J Pathol 46:387, 1965.
8. Scheuer PJ. Primary biliary cirrhosis. Proc R Soc Med 60:1257, 1967.
9. Popper H. Primary biliary cirrhosis. Rev Int Hepatol 16:239, 1966.
10. Schaffner F. Primary biliary cirrhosis. Clinics Gastroenterol 4:351, 1975.
11. Dickson ER, Fleming CR, Ludwig J. Primary biliary cirrhosis. In: Popper H, Schaffner F, eds. Progress in Liver Diseases, Vol. 6, New York, Grune & Stratton, 1978: 487.
12. Sherlock S. Primary biliary cirrhosis. In: Wright R, Alberti KG MM, Karran S, and Millward-Sadler GH, eds. Liver and Biliary Disease. Philadelphia, WB Saunders, 1979: 715.
13. Popper H, and Paronetto F. Clinical, histologic, and immunopathologic features of primary biliary cirrhosis. Springer Semin Immunopathol 3:339, 1980.
14. Maddrey WC, Saito S, Shulman NR, et al. Coincidental Australia antigenemia in primary biliary cirrhosis. Ann Intern Med 76:705, 1972.
15. MacSween RNM, Yeung Laiwah AAC, Busuttil AA, et al. Australia antigen and primary biliary cirrhosis. J Clin Pathol 26:335, 1973.
16. Grady GF, Kaplan MM, and Vyas GN. Antibody to hepatitis B core antigen in chronic hepatitis and primary biliary cirrhosis: evaluation by a new autologous solid phase radioimmunoassay. Gastroenterology 72:590, 1977.
17. Munoz SJ, Ballas SK, Norberg R, Maddrey WC. Antibodies to human immunodeficiency virus in primary biliary cirrhosis. Gastroenterology (Abstract). In Press.
18. Stemerowicz R, Hopf U, Moeller B, et al. Are mitochondrial antibodies in primary biliary cirrhosis induced by R-mutants of gram-negative bacteria? Lancet 2:1166, 1988.
18a. Berg PA, and Baum H. Serology of primary biliary cirrhosis. Springer Semin Immunopathol 3:355, 1980.
19. Ebringer RW. HLA-B27 and the link with rheumatic diseases: Recent developments. Clin Sci 59:405, 1980.
20. Triger DR. Primary biliary cirrhosis: an epidemiological study. Br Med J 281:772, 1980.
21. Mayberry JF, Giggs J, Smart HL. Urban clustering of primary biliary cirrhosis. Gut 27:A1265, 1986 (Abstract).
22. Douglas JG, and Finlayson NDC. Are increased individual susceptibility and environmental factors both necessary for the development of primary biliary cirrhosis? Br Med J 2:419, 1979.
23. Gadacz TR, Allan RN, Mack E, et al. Impaired lithocholate sulfation in the rhesus monkey: a possible mechanism for chenodeoxycholate toxicity. Gastroenterology 70:1125, 1976.
24. Stellaard F, Bolt MG, Boyer JL, et al. Phenobarbital treatment in primary biliary cirrhosis: differences in bile acid composition between responders and non-responders. J Lab Clin Med 94:853, 1979.
25. Ishak KG, and Irey NS. Hepatic injury asociated with the phenothiazines. Arch Pathol 93:283, 1972.
26. Gregory DH, Zaki GF, Sarcosi GA, et al. Chronic cholestasis following prolonged tolbutamide administration. Arch Pathol 84:194, 1967.
27. Haubrich WS, and Sacetta SM. Spontaneous recovery from hepatobiliary disease with xanthomatosis. Gastroenterology 26:658, 1954.
28. Jalota R, and Freston JW. Severe intrahepatic cholestasis due to thiobendazole. Am J Trop Med Hyg 23:676, 1974.
29. Foss GL, and Simpson SL. Oral methyltestosterone and jaundice. Br Med J 1:259, 1959.
30. Glober GA, and Wilkerson JA. Biliary cirrhosis following the administration of methyltestosterone. JAMA 204:170, 1968.
31. Zimmerman HJ. Hepatotoxicity. Adverse Effects of Drugs and Other Chemicals on the Liver. New York, Appleton-Century Crofts, 1978, p. 447.
32. Valimaki MJ, Harju KJ, Ylikarhri RH. Decreased serum selenium in alcoholics. A consequence of liver dysfunction. Clin Chim Acta 130:291, 1983.
33. Thuluvath PJ, Triger DR. Selenium in primary biliary cirrhosis. Lancet 2:219, 1987 (Letter).
34. Braganza JM, Day JP. Serum octadeca-9-11 dienoic acid concentrations in primary biliary cirrhosis. Lancet 1:987, 1987 (Letter).
35. Lofgren J, Jarnerot G, Danielsson D, Hemdal I. Incidence and prevalence of primary biliary cirrhosis in a defined population in Sweden. Scand J Gastroenterol 20:647, 1985.
36. Neve J, Vertongen F, Molle L. Selenium deficiency. Clin Endocrinol Metab 14:629, 1985.
37. Woodhouse KW, Mitchison HC, Mutch E, et al. The metabolism of 7-ethoxycoumarin in human liver microsomes and the effect of primary biliary cirrhosis: Implications for studies of drug metabolism in liver disease. Br J Clin Pharmacol 20:77, 1985.
38. Nielson JO, Dietrischen O, Elling P, et al. Incidence and meaning of persistence of Australia antigen in patients with acute viral hepatitis: development of chronic hepatitis. N Engl J Med 285:1157, 1971.
39. Berman M, Alter HG, Ishak KG, et al. The chronic sequelae of non-A, non-B hepatitis. Ann Intern Med 91:1, 1979.
40. Zimmerman HJ. Drug-induced chronic hepatic disease. Med Clin North Am 63:567, 1979.
41. Scott J, Gollan JL, Samourian S, et al. Wilson's disease presenting as chronic active hepatitis. Gastroenterology 74:645, 1978.
42. Hodges JR, Millward-Sadler GH, Barbatis C, et al. Heterozygous MZ alpha-1-antitrypsin deficiency in adults with chronic active hepatitis and cryptogenic cirrhosis. N Engl J Med 304:557, 1981.
43. Hamlyn AN, and Sherlock S. The epidemiology of primary biliary cirrhosis: a survey of mortality in England and Wales. Gut 15:473, 1974.
44. Anon. Primary biliary cirrhosis (editorial). Br Med J 283:514, 1981.
45. Sherlock S, and Scheuer PJ. The presentation and diagnosis of 100 patients with primary biliary cirrhosis. N Engl J Med 289:674, 1973.
46. Christensen E, Crowe J, Doniach D, et al. Clinical pattern and course of disease in primary biliary cirrhosis based on an analysis of 236 patients. Gastroenterology 78:236, 1980.
47. Lucey MR, Neuberger JM, Williams R. Primary biliary cirrhosis in men. Gut 27:1373, 1986.
48. Rubel LR, Rabin L, Seeff LB, et al. Does primary biliary cirrhosis in men differ from primary biliary cirrhosis in women? Hepatology 4:671, 1984.
49. Tornay AS. Primary biliary cirrhosis. Natural history. Am J Gastroenterol 73:223, 1980.
50. Long RG, Scheuer PJ, and Sherlock S. Presentation and course of asymptomatic primary biliary cirrhosis. Gastroenterology 72:1204, 1977.
51. Foulk WT, Baggenstoss AH, and Butt HR. Primary biliary cirrhosis: reevaluation by clinical and histologic study of 49 cases. Gastroenterology 47:354, 1964.
52. Simon FR. Effects of estrogens on the liver. Gastroenterology, 75:512, 1978.
53. Dickson ER, and Summerfield J. Primary biliary cirrhosis, In: Current Concepts in Gastrointestinal Disease. American Gastroenterological Association Postgraduate Course. Thorofare, NJ, Charles B Slack, 1979.
54. Fleming CR, Ludwig J, and Dickson ER. Asymptomatic primary

biliary cirrhosis—presentation, histology, and results with D-penicillamine. Mayo Clin Proc 53:587, 1978.

55. Hanik L, and Eriksson S. Presymptomatic primary biliary cirrhosis. Acta Med Scand 202:277, 1977.

56. James O, Macklon AF, and Watson AJ. Primary biliary cirrhosis—A revised clinical spectrum. Lancet 1:1278, 1981.

57. Munoz LE, Thomas HC, Scheuer PJ, et al. Is mitochondrial antibody diagnostic of primary biliary cirrhosis? Gut 22:136, 1981.

58. Mitchison HC, Bassendine MF, Hendrick A, et al. Positive antimitochondrial antibody but normal alkaline phosphatase: Is this primary biliary cirrhosis? Hepatology 6:1279, 1986.

59. Roll J, Boyer JL, Barry D, et al. The prognostic importance of clinical and histological features in asymptomatic and symptomatic primary biliary cirrhosis. N Engl J Med 308:1, 1983.

60. Lehmann AB, Bassendine MF, James OFW. Is primary biliary cirrhosis a different disease in the elderly? Gerontology 31:186, 1985.

61. Shapiro JM, Smith H, and Schaffner F. Serum bilirubin, a prognostic factor in primary biliary cirrhosis. Gut 20:137, 1979.

62. Epstein O, Jain S, Lee RG, et al. D-Penicillamine treatment improves survival in primary biliary cirrhosis. Lancet 1:1275, 1981.

63. Killenberg PG, Stevens RD, Wilderman RF, et al. The laboratory method as a variable in the interpretation of serum bilirubin fractionation. Gastroenterology 78:1011, 1980.

64. Sabesin SM, Bertram PD, and Freeman MR. Lipoprotein metabolism in liver disease, In: Stollerman GH, eds. Advances in Internal Medicine. Vol. 26. Chicago, Year Book Medical Publishers, 1979, p. 487.

65. Koga S, Miyata Y, Ibayashi H. Plasmal lipoproteins and apoproteins in primary biliary cirrhosis. Hepatology 5:286, 1985.

66. Jahn CE, Schaefer EJ, Taam LA, et al. Lipoprotein abnormalities in primary biliary cirrhosis. Gastroenterology 89:1266, 1985.

67. Teramoto T, Kato H, Hashimoto Y, et al. Abnormal high density lipoprotein of primary biliary cirrhosis analyzed by high performance liquid chromatography. Clin Chim Acta 149:135, 1985.

68. Simon JB, and Poon RWM. Lipoprotein-X levels in extrahepatic versus intrahepatic cholestasis. Gastroenterology 75:177, 1978.

69. Floren C-H, Gustafson A. Apolipoproteins A-I, A-II and E in cholestatic liver disease. Scand J Clin Lab Invest 45:103, 1985.

70. Murphy GM, Ross A, and Billing BH. Serum bile acids in primary biliary cirrhosis. Gut 13:201, 1972.

71. Bloomer JR, Allen RM, and Klatskin G. Serum bile acids in primary biliary cirrhosis. Arch Intern Med 136:57, 1976.

72. Bremmelgaard A, and Almé B. Analysis of plasma bile acid profiles in patients with liver diseases associated with cholestasis. Scand J Gastroenterol 15:593, 1980.

73. Kesaniemi YA, Miettinen TA, and Salaspuro MP. Biliary lipids, faecal steroids and liver function in patients with chronic active hepatitis and primary biliary cirrhosis: significance of hepatic orcein-stained complexes. Gut 22:579, 1981.

74. Turnberg LA, and Grahame G. Bile salt secretion in cirrhosis of the liver. Gut 11:126, 1970.

75. Vlachevic ZR, Buhac I, Bell CC, et al. Abnormal metabolism of secondary bile acids in patients with cirrhosis. Gut 11:420, 1970.

76. Kesaniemi YA, Miettinen TA. Biliary secretion of bilirubin and lipids in chronic cholestatic liver disease. Scand J Gastroenterol 20:433, 1985.

77. Walker JG, Doniach D, Roitt IM, et al. Serological tests in the diagnosis of primary biliary cirrhosis. Lancet 1:827, 1965.

78. Mackay IR. Primary biliary cirrhosis sharing a high titer of autoantibody. N Engl J Med 258:185, 1958.

79. Doniach D, Roitt IM, Walker JG, et al. Tissue antibodies in primary biliary cirrhosis, active chronic (lupoid) hepatitis, cryptogenic cirrhosis and other liver diseases and their clinical implications. Clin Exp Immunol 1:237, 1966.

80. Klatskin G, and Kantor FS. Mitochondrial antibody in primary biliary cirrhosis and other diseases. Ann Intern Med 77:533, 1972.

81. Doniach D, and Walker G. Progress report. Mitochondrial antibodies. (AMA). Gut 15:664, 1974.

82. Richer G, and Viallet A. Mitochondrial antibodies in extrahepatic biliary obstruction. Dig Dis 19:740, 1974.

83. Ward AM, Ellis G, and Goldberg DM. Serum immunoglobulin concentration and autoantibody titers in diseases of the liver and biliary tree. Am J Clin Pathol 70:352, 1978.

84. Berg PA, Klein R, Lindenborn-Fotinos J. Antimitochondrial antibodies in primary biliary cirrhosis. J Hepatol 2:123, 1986.

85. Gershwin ME, Mackay IR, Sturgess A, et al. Identification and specificity of a cDNA encoding the 70-kd mitochondrial antigen recognized in primary biliary cirrhosis. J Immunol 138:3525, 1987.

86. Gershwin ME, Coppel RL, Mackay IR. Primary biliary cirrhosis and mitochondrial autoantigens—Insights from molecular biology. Hepatology 8:147, 1988.

87. Frazer IH, Mackay IR, Jordan TW, et al. Reactivity of antimitochondrial autoantibodies in primary biliary cirrhosis: Definition of two novel mitochondrial polypeptide autoantigens. J Immunol 135:1739, 1985.

88. Lindenborn-Fotinos J, Baum H, Berg PA. Mitochondrial antibodies in primary biliary cirrhosis: Species and nonspecies specific determinants of M2 antigen. Hepatology 5:763, 1985.

89. Mendel-Hartvig I, Nelson BD, Loof L, et al. Primary biliary cirrhosis. Further biochemical and immunological characterization of mitochondrial antigens. Clin Exp Immunol 62:371, 1985.

90. Baum H, Palmer C. The PBC specific antigen. Mol Aspects Med 8:201, 1985.

91. Ishii H, Saifuku K, Namihisa T. Multiplicity of mitochondrial inner membrane antigens from beef heart reacting with antimitochondrial antibodies in sera of patients with primary biliary cirrhosis. Immunol Lett 9:325, 1985.

92. Manns M, Gerken G, Kyriatsoulis A, et al. Two different subtypes of antimitochondrial antibodies are associated with primary biliary cirrhosis: Identification and characterization by radioimmunoassay and immunoblotting. Hepatology 7:893, 1987.

93. Ishii H, Saifuku K, Namishisa T. Reactivities and clinical relevance of antimitochondrial antibodies to four mitochondrial inner membrane proteins in sera of patients with primary biliary cirrhosis. Hepatology 7:134, 1987.

94. McMillan SA, Alderdice JM, McKee CM, et al. Diversity of autoantibodies in patients with antimitochondrial antibody and their diagnostic value. J Clin Pathol 40:232, 1987.

95. Berg PA, Wiedmann KH, Sayer T, et al. Serological classifications of chronic cholestatic liver disease due to two different types of antimitochondrial antibodies. Lancet 2:1329, 1980.

96. Weber P, Brenner J, Stechemesser E, et al. Characterization and clinical relevance of a new complement fixing antibody antipM8 in patients with primary biliary cirrhosis. Hepatology 6:553, 1986.

97. Uddenfeldt P, Danielsson A. Evaluation of rheumatic disorders in patients with primary biliary cirrhosis. Ann Clin Res 18:148, 1986.

98. Modena V, Marengo C, Amoroso A, et al. Primary biliary cirrhosis and rheumatic diseases: A clinical, immunological and immunogenetical study. Clin Exp Rheum 4:129, 1986.

99. Hadziyannis S, Scheuer PJ, Feizi T, et al. Immunological and histological studies in primary biliary cirrhosis. J Clin Pathol 23:95, 1970.

100. Galbraith RM, Smith M, MacKenzie RM, et al. High prevalence of seroimmunologic abnormalities in relatives of patients with active chronic hepatitis or primary biliary cirrhosis. N Engl J Med 290:63, 1974.

101. Feizi T, Naccarato R, Sherlock S, et al. Mitochondrial and other tissue antibodies in relatives of patients with primary biliary cirrhosis. Clin Exp Immunol 10:609, 1972.

102. Haagsma EB, Manns M, Klein R, et al. Subtypes of antimitochondrial antibodies in primary biliary cirrhosis before and after orthotopic liver transplantation. Hepatology 7:129, 1987.

103. Ghadiminejad I, Baum H. Evidence for the cell-surface localization of antigens cross-reacting with the "mitochondrial antibodies" of primary biliary cirrhosis. Hepatology 7:743, 1987.

104. Delisi C, Berzofsky JA. T cell antigenic sites tend to be amphipathic structures. Proc Natl Acad Sci 82:7048, 1985.

105. Crowe J, Christensen E, Smith M, et al. Azathioprine in primary biliary cirrhosis: a preliminary report of an international trial. Gastroenterology 78:1005, 1980.

106. Wiesner RH, and LaRusso NF. Clinicopathologic features of the syndrome of primary sclerosing cholangitis. Gastroenterology 79:200, 1980.

107. Chapman RWG, Marborgh BA, Rhodes JM, et al. Primary sclerosing cholangitis: a review of its clinical features, cholangiography, and hepatic histology. Gut 21:870, 1980.

108. Lam KC, Mistilis SP, and Perrott N. Positive tissue antibody tests in patients with prolonged extrahepatic biliary obstruction. N Engl J Med 286:1400, 1972.

109. Golding PL, Smith M, and Williams R. Multisystem involvement in chronic liver disease. Studies on the incidence and pathogenesis. Am J Med 55:772, 1973.

110. Doniach D, and Walker G. Immunopathology of liver disease, In: Popper, H., and Schaffner, F. eds. Progress in Liver Diseases. Volume 4. New York, Grune & Stratton, 1972, p. 381.

111. Kurki P, Miettinen A, Linder E, et al. Different types of smooth muscle antibodies in chronic active hepatitis and primary biliary cirrhosis: their diagnostic and prognostic significance. Gut 21:878, 1980.

112. Fakunle YM, DeVilliers D, Thomas HC, et al. Monomeric IgM in chronic liver disease. Clin Exp Immunol 38:204, 1979.

113. Taal BG, Schalm SW, DeBruyn AM, et al. Serum IgM in primary biliary cirrhosis. Clin Chim Acta 108:457, 1980.

114. Lindgren S, Eriksson S, Lofberg H, McKay J. IgM deposition in skin biopsies from patients with primary biliary cirrhosis. Acta Med Scand 210:317, 1981.

115. Vierling JM, Emmett M, Rosandich M, Crowle AT. Serum proteins in primary biliary cirrhosis and chronic active hepatitis by crossed immunoelectrophoresis. Fed Proc 44:1396, 1985.

116. Harris-Dang Kul V, McDougal JS, Knapp M, et al. Naturally occurring

low molecular weight IgM in patients with rheumatoid arthritis, systemic lupus erythematosus, and macroglobulinemia. Purification and immunological studies. J Immunol 116:216, 1975.

117. Legge DA, Carlson HC, Dickson ER, et al. Cholangiographic findings in cholangiolitic hepatitis: syndrome of primary biliary cirrhosis. Am J Roentgenol 113:16, 1971.

118. Summerfield JA, Elias E, Hungerford GD, et al. The biliary system in primary biliary cirrhosis: a study by endoscopic retrograde cholangiopancreatography. Gastroenterology, 70:240, 1976.

119. Rodriguez-Roisin R, Pares A, Bruguera M, et al. Pulmonary involvement in primary biliary cirrhosis. Thorax 36:208, 1981.

120. Stanley NN, Fox RA, Whimster WF, et al: Primary biliary cirrhosis or sarcoidosis—or both. N Engl J Med 287:1282, 1972.

121. Fagan EA, Moore-Gillon JC, Turner-Warwick M. Multiorgan granulomas and mitochondrial antibodies. N Engl J Med 308:572, 1983.

122. Vierling JM: Copper metabolism in primary biliary cirrhosis. Sem Liver Dis 1:293, 1981.

123. Peters RL. Primary biliary cirrhosis. Gastroenterology 88:1998, 1985 (Editorial).

124. Ludwig J. New concepts in biliary cirrhosis. Sem Liver Dis 7:293, 1987.

124a. Homeida M, Roberts CJC, Halliwell M, et al. Antipyrine clearance per unit volume liver: an assessment of hepatic function in chronic liver disease. Gut 20:596, 1979.

125. Scheuer PJ. Liver Biopsy Interpretation. Second edition. Baltimore, Williams and Wilkins, 1973.

125a. Haeki W, Bircher J, and Preisig R. A new look at the plasma disappearance of sulfobromophthalein (BSP): correlation with the BSP transport maximum and the hepatic plasma flow in man. J Lab Clin Med 88:1019, 1976.

126. Kew MC, Varma RR, Dos Santos HA, et al. Portal hypertension in primary biliary cirrhosis. Gut 12:830, 1971.

126a. Popper H, Schaffner F. Nonsuppurative destructive chronic cholangitis and chronic hepatitis. In: Popper H, and Schaffner F, eds. Progress in Liver Diseases. Vol 3. New York, Grune & Stratton, 1970, p. 336.

127. Ludwig J, Dickson ER, McDonald GSA. Staging of chronic nonsuppurative destructive cholangitis (syndrome of primary biliary cirrhosis). Virchows Arch A Path Anat Histol 379:103, 1978.

127a. Zeegan R, Stansfield AG, Dawson AM, et al. Bleeding esophageal varices as the presenting feature in primary biliary cirrhosis. Lancet 2:9, 1969.

128. MacSween RNM, Sumithran E. Histopathology of primary biliary cirrhosis. Sem Liver Dis 1:282, 1981.

129. Portmann B, Popper H, Neuberger J, Williams R. Sequential and diagnostic features in primary biliary cirrhosis based on serial histologic study in 209 patients. Gastroenterology 88:1777, 1985.

130. Poulsen H, and Christoffersen P. Abnormal bile duct epithelium in chronic aggressive hepatitis and cirrhosis: a review of morphology and clinical, biochemical, and immunological features. Hum Pathol 3:217, 1972.

131. Christoffersen P, Poulsen H, Scheuer PJ. Abnormal bile duct epithelium in chronic aggressive hepatitis and primary biliary cirrhosis. Hum Pathol 3:227, 1972.

132. Klöppel G, Seifert G, Lindner H, et al. Histopathological features in mixed types of chronic aggressive hepatitis and primary biliary cirrhosis. Correlations of liver histology with mitochondrial antibodies of different specificity. Virchows Arch (Pathol Anat) 373:143, 1977.

133. Skrede S, Solberg HE, Ritland S, et al. Follow-up and prospective studies of the classification of liver disease. Scand J Gastroenterol 20(Suppl):40, 1985.

134. Okuno T, Seto Y, Okanoue T, Takino T. Chronic active hepatitis with histological features of primary biliary cirrhosis. Dig Dis Sci 32:775, 1987.

135. Nakanuma Y, Ohta G. Quantitation of hepatic granulomas and epithelioid cells in primary biliary cirrhosis. Hepatology 3:423, 1983.

136. MacSween RN. Mallory's (alcoholic) hyaline in primary biliary cirrhosis. J Clin Pathol 26:340, 1973.

137. Lee G, Epstein O, Jauregui H, et al. Granulomas in primary biliary cirrhosis. Gastroenterology 81:983, 1981.

138. Vaux DJT, Watt F, Grime GW, Takacs J. Hepatic copper distribution in primary biliary cirrhosis shown by the scanning proton microprobe. J Clin Pathol 38:653, 1985.

139. Nakanuma Y, and Ohta G. Histometric and serial section observations of the intrahepatic bile ducts in primary biliary cirrhosis. Gastroenterology 76:1326, 1979.

140. Lévy VG, Opolon P, and Caroli J: Cirrhoses biliaires primitives. Contribution au diagnostic. Etude anatomopathologique par la methode de reconstruction. Sem Hop Paris 40:1749, 1964.

141. Nakanuma Y, Ohta G. Nodular hyperplasia of the liver in primary biliary cirrhosis of early histological stages. Am J Gastroenterol 82:8, 1987.

142. Arora S, Kaplan M. Portal hypertension in early-stage primary biliary cirrhosis: A possible explanation. Am J Gastroenterol 82:90, 1987 (Editorial).

143. Navasa M, Pares A, Bruguera M, et al. Portal hypertension in primary biliary cirrhosis. Relationship with histological features. J Hepatol 5:292, 1987.

144. MacSween RNM, Burt AD. The cellular pathology of primary biliary cirrhosis. Molec Aspects Med 8:269, 1985.

145. Yamada G, Hyodo I, Tobe K, et al. Ultrastructure and immunocytochemical analysis of lymphocytes infiltrating bile duct epithelia in primary biliary cirrhosis. Hepatology 6:385, 1986.

146. Colucci G, Schaffner F, Paronetto F. In situ characterization of the cell surface antigens of the mononuclear cell infiltrate and bile duct epithelium in primary biliary cirrhosis. Clin Immunol Immunopathol 41:35, 1986.

147. Shimizu M, Yuh K, Ichihara AI, et al. Immunohistochemical characterization of inflammatory infiltrates at the site of bile duct injury in primary biliary cirrhosis. Liver 6:1, 1986.

148. Whiteside TL, Lasky S, Si L, Van Thiel DH. Immunologic analysis of mononuclear cells in liver tissues and blood of patients with primary sclerosing cholangitis. Hepatology 5:468, 1985.

149. Adler M, Chung KW, and Schaffner F. Pericanalicular hepatocytic and bile ductular microfilaments in cholestasis in man. Am J Pathol 98:603, 1980.

150. Bernuau D, Feldmann G, Degott C, et al. Ultrastructural lesions of bile ducts in primary biliary cirrhosis. A comparison with the lesions observed in graft versus host disease. Hum Pathol 12:782, 1981.

151. Nakanuma Y, Ohta G, Kono N, et al. Electron microscopic observation of destruction of biliary epithelium in primary biliary cirrhosis. Liver 3:238, 1983.

152. Tobe K, Itoshima T, Tsuchiya T, et al. Electron microscopy of granulomatous lesions of the liver in primary biliary cirrhosis. Acta Pathol Japan 35:1309, 1985.

153. Alarcon-Segovia D, Diaz-Jouanen E, and Fishbein E. Features of Sjögren's syndrome in primary biliary cirrhosis. Ann Intern Med 79:31, 1973.

154. Murray-Lyon IM, Thompson RPH, Ansell ID, et al. Scleroderma and primary biliary cirrhosis. Br Med J 3:258, 1970.

155. Reynolds TB, Denison EK, Frankl HD, et al. Primary biliary cirrhosis with scleroderma, Raynaud's phenomenon and telangiectasia. Am J Med 50:302, 1971.

156. Clarke AK, Galbraith RM, Hamilton EBD, et al. Rheumatic disorders in primary biliary cirrhosis. Ann Rheum Dis 37:42, 1978.

157. Miller F, Lane B, Soterakis J, et al: Primary biliary cirrhosis and scleroderma. The possibility of a common pathogenetic mechanism. Arch Pathol Lab Med 103:505, 1979.

158. Medd WL, and Sodhi HS. Primary biliary cirrhosis and scleroderma variant. A case presentation. J Maine Med Assoc 71:308, 1980.

159. Medsger TA, and Masi AT. Epidemiology of systemic sclerosis. Ann Intern Med 74:714, 1971.

160. Tuzzanelli DL, and Winklemann RK. Systemic scleroderma: a clinical study of 727 cases. Arch Dermatol 84:359, 1961.

161. Uhl GS, Baldwin JL, and Arnett FC. Primary biliary cirrhosis in systemic sclerosis (scleroderma) and polymyositis. Johns Hopkins Med Bull 135:191, 1974.

162. Galbraith RM, Eddleston ALWF, Smith MEM, et al. Histocompatibility antigens in active chronic hepatitis and primary biliary cirrhosis. Br Med J 3:604, 1974.

163. Kassan SS, and Gandy M. Sjögren's syndrome: an update and overview. Am J Med 64:1037, 1978.

164. Hamlyn AN, Adams D, and Sherlock S: Primary or secondary sicca complex? Investigation in primary biliary cirrhosis by histocompatibility testing. Br Med J 281:425, 1980.

165. McFarlane IG, Wojcicka BM, Tsantoulas DC, et al. Cellular immune responses to salivary antigens in autoimmune liver disease with sicca syndrome. Clin Exp Immunol 25:389, 1976.

166. Giovanni A, Ballardini G, Amatetti S, et al. Patterns of lacrimal dysfunction in primary biliary cirrhosis. Brit J Ophthalmol 69:832, 1985.

167. Moutsopoulos HM, Mann DL, Johnson AH, et al. Genetic differences between primary and secondary sicca syndrome. N Engl J Med 301:761, 1979.

168. Whaley K, Goudie RB, Williamson J, et al. Liver disease in Sjögren's syndrome and rheumatoid arthritis. Lancet 1:861, 1970.

169. Marx WJ, and O'Connell DJ. Arthritis of primary biliary cirrhosis. Arch Intern Med 139:213, 1979.

170. Crowe JP, Malloy MG, Wells I, et al. Increased C1q binding and arthritis in primary biliary cirrhosis. Gut 21:418, 1980.

171. Child DL, Mathews JA, and Thompson RPH. Arthritis and primary biliary cirrhosis. Br Med J 2:557, 1977.

172. Crowe JP, Christensen E, Butler J, et al. Primary biliary cirrhosis and the prevalence of hypothyroidism and its relationship to thyroid autoantibodies and sicca syndrome. Gastroenterology 78:1437, 1980.

173. Gordin A, and Lamberg BA. Natural course of symptomless autoimmune thyroiditis. Lancet 2:1234, 1975.

174. Pares A, Rimola A, Bruguera M, et al. Renal tubular acidosis in primary biliary cirrhosis. Gastroenterology 80:681, 1981.
175. Izumi N, Haumura Y, Takeuchi J. Hypouricemia and hyperuricosuria as expressions of renal tubular damage in primary biliary cirrhosis. Hepatology 3:719, 1983.
176. Muldowney FP, Freaney R, and McGeeney D. Renal tubular acidosis and aminoaciduria in osteomalacia of dietary or intestinal origin. Q J Med 37:517, 1968.
177. Leu ML, and Strickland GT. Renal tubular acidosis in Wilson's disease: characteristics, mechanisms and implications. J Formosan Med Assoc 76:829, 1977.
178. Tsantoulas DC, McFarlane IG, Portmann B, et al. Cell mediated immunity to human Tamm-Horsfall glycoproteins in autoimmune liver disease with renal tubular acidosis. Br Med J 4:491, 1974.
179. Chanarin I, Loewii G, Tavill AS, et al. Defect of renal tubular acidification with antibody to loop of Henle. Lancet 2:317, 1973.
180. Goudie BM, Burt AD, Boyle P, et al. Breast cancer in women with primary biliary cirrhosis. Br Med J 291:1597, 1985.
181. Wolke AM, Schaffner F, Kapelman B, Sacks HS. Malignancy in primary biliary cirrhosis. Increased incidence of breast cancer in affected women. Am J Med 76:1075, 1984.
182. Burroughs AK, Rosenstein IJ, Epstein O, et al. Bacteriuria and primary biliary cirrhosis. Gut 25:133, 1984.
183. Olsson R, Kagevi I, Rydberg L. On the concurrence of primary biliary cirrhosis and intestinal villous atrophy. Scand J Gastroenterol 17:625, 1982.
184. Gabrielsen TO, Hoel PS. Primary biliary cirrhosis associated with coeliac disease and dermatitis herpetiformis. Dermatologica 170:31, 1985.
185. Behr W, Barnert J. Adult celiac disease and primary biliary cirrhosis. Am J Gastroenterol 81:796, 1986.
186. Logan RFA, Ferguson A, Finlayson NDC, et al. Primary biliary cirrhosis and celiac disease. Lancet 1:230, 1978.
187. Iliffe GD, Owen DA. An association between primary biliary cirrhosis and jejunal villous atrophy resembling celiac disease. Dig Dis Sci 24:802, 1979.
188. Willson RA. Therapeutic quandary. Asymptomatic primary biliary cirrhosis associated with polymyositis. Dig Dis Sci 26:372, 1981.
189. Robertson JC, Batstone GF, Loebl WY. Polymyalgia rheumatica and primary biliary cirrhosis. Br Med J 2:1128, 1978.
190. von Knorring J, Wasastjerna C. Liver involvement in polymyalgia rheumatica. Scand J Rheumatol 5:197, 1976.
191. Long R, James O. Polymyalgia rheumatica and liver disease. Lancet 1:77, 1974.
192. Rai GS, Hamlyn AN, Dahl MGC, et al. Primary biliary cirrhosis, cutaneous capillaritis, and IgM-associated membranous glomerulonephritis. Br Med J 1:817, 1977.
193. Diederichsen H, Sorensen PG, Mickley H, et al. Petechiae and vasculitis in asymptomatic primary biliary cirrhosis. Acta Derm Venereol (Stockh) 65:263, 1985.
194. Singhal PC, Scharschmidt LA. Membranous nephropathy associated with primary biliary cirrhosis and bullous pemphigoid. Ann Allergy 55:484, 1985.
195. Gibson LE, Dicken CH. Pemphigus erythematosus, primary biliary cirrhosis, and D-penicillamine: Report of a case. J Am Acad Derm 12:883, 1985.
196. Natarajan S, Green ST. Generalized morphoea, lichen sclerosus et atrophicus and primary biliary cirrhosis. Clin Exp Derm 11:304, 1986.
197. Suyama Y, Murawaki Y, Horie Y, et al. A case of primary biliary cirrhosis associated with generalized morphea. Hepatogastroenterology 33:199, 1986.
198. Graham-Brown RAC, Sarkany I. Lichen sclerosus et atrophicus. Int J Dermatol 25:317, 1986.
199. Enat R, Gilhar A. Vitiligo and primary biliary cirrhosis. Am J Gastroenterol 79:804, 1984.
200. Hays SB, Camiso C. Rendu-Osler-Weber–like telangiectasia associated with primary biliary cirrhosis. Cutis 35:152, 1985.
201. Wallaert B, Bonniere P, Prin L, et al. Primary biliary cirrhosis. Subclinical inflammatory alveolitis in patients with normal chest roentgenograms. Chest 90:842, 1986.
202. Charron L, Peyronnard J, Marchand L. Sensory neuropathy associated with primary biliary cirrhosis—histologic and morphometric studies. Arch Neurol 37:84, 1980.
203. Knight RE, Bourne AJ, Newton M, et al. Neurologic syndrome associated with low levels of vitamin E in primary biliary cirrhosis. Gastroenterology 91:209, 1986.
204. Rutan G, Martinez AJ, Fieshko JT, et al. Primary biliary cirrhosis, Sjögren's syndrome, and transverse myelitis. Gastroenterology 90:206, 1986.
205. Macdougall IC, Isles CG, Whitworth JA, et al. Interstitial nephritis and primary biliary cirrhosis: A new association? Clin Nephrol 27:1136, 1987.
206. Orlin JB, Berkman EM, Matloff DS, et al. Primary biliary cirrhosis

207. and cold autoimmune hemolytic anemia: effect of partial plasma exchange. Gastroenterology 78:576, 1980.
207. Selinger S, Tsai J, Pulini M, et al. Autoimmune thrombocytopenia and primary biliary cirrhosis with hypoglycemia and insulin receptor autoantibodies. Ann Intern Med 107:686, 1987.
208. Bassendine MF, Collins JD, Stephenson J, et al. Platelet associated immunoglobulins in primary biliary cirrhosis: A cause of thrombocytopenia? Gut 26:1074, 1985.
209. Rajaraman S, Deodhar SD, Carey WD, et al. Hashimoto's thyroiditis, primary biliary cirrhosis, and myasthenia gravis. Am J Clin Pathol 74:831, 1980.
210. Remacle J, Pellissier J, Chamlian A, et al. Progressive ophthalmoplegia associated with asymptomatic primary biliary cirrhosis—histologic, histochemical, cytochemical, and ultrastructural studies of muscle and liver biopsy specimens. Hum Pathol 11:540, 1980.
211. Douglas JG, Feek CM, Irvine WJ, et al. A choledochal cyst in association with primary biliary cirrhosis. Scott Med J 26:65, 1981.
212. Bladé J, Montserrat E, Bruguera M, et al. Multiple myeloma in primary biliary cirrhosis. Scand J Haematol 26:14, 1981.
213. Jain S, Markham R, Thomas HC, et al. Double stranded DNA binding capacity of serum in acute and chronic liver diseases. Clin Exp Immunol 26:35, 1976.
214. Bush A, Mitchison H, Walt R, et al. Primary biliary cirrhosis and ulcerative colitis. Gastroenterology 92:2009, 1987.
215. Kato Y, Morimoto H, Unouri M, et al. Primary biliary cirrhosis and chronic pancreatitis in a patient with ulcerative colitis. J Clin Gastroenterol 7:425, 1985.
216. Fonseca V, Epstein O, Katrak A, et al. Serum immunoreactive trypsin and pancreatic lipase in primary biliary cirrhosis. J Clin Pathol 39:638, 1986.
217. Shanahan F, Stack J, Maguire S, et al. The pancreas, primary biliary cirrhosis and the dry gland syndrome. IMJS 154:387, 1985.
218. Nieri S, Riccardo GG, Salvadori G, et al. Primary biliary cirrhosis and Graves' disease. J Clin Gastroenterol 7:434, 1985.
219. Sevenet F, Capron-Chivrac D, Delcenserie R, et al. Idiopathic retroperitoneal fibrosis and primary biliary cirrhosis. A new association: Arch Intern Med 145:2124, 1985.
220. Stellon AJ, Williams R. Increased incidence of menstrual abnormalities and hysterectomy preceding primary biliary cirrhosis. Br Med J 293:297, 1986.
221. Balasubramaniam K, Grambsch PM, Wiesner RH, et al. Asymptomatic primary biliary cirrhosis: Patients have a diminished survival. Hepatology 7:1025, 1987 (Abstract).
222. Sherlock S, Datta DV, Walker JG. Prognosis and treatment of primary biliary cirrhosis. Rev Int Hepatol 16:217, 1966.
223. Beswick DR, Klatskin G, Boyer JL. Asymptomatic primary biliary cirrhosis. Gastroenterology 89:267, 1985.
224. Kloeppel G, Kirchhof M, Berg PA. Natural course of primary biliary cirrhosis. I. A morphological, clinical and serological analysis of 103 cases. Liver 2:141, 1982.
225. Christensen E, Neuberger J, Crowe J, et al. Beneficial effect of azathioprine and prediction of prognosis in primary biliary cirrhosis. Gastroenterology 89:1084, 1985.
226. Neuberger J, Altman DG, Christensen E, et al. Use of a prognostic index in evaluation of liver transplantation for primary biliary cirrhosis. Transplantation 41:713, 1986.
227. Lanspa SJ, Chan AT, Bell JS, et al. Pathogenesis of steatorrhea in primary biliary cirrhosis. Hepatology 5:837, 1985.
228. Miettinen TA. Lipid absorption, bile acids, and cholesterol metabolism in patients with chronic liver disease. Gut 13:682, 1972.
229. Herlong HF, Russell RM, Garrett M, et al. Vitamin A deficiency in primary biliary cirrhosis: an additional role for zinc. Gastroenterology 77:A16, 1979 (Abstract).
230. Beckett GJ, Dewhurst N, Finlayson NDC, et al. Weight loss in primary biliary cirrhosis. Gut 21:734, 1980.
231. Thomas PK, Walker JG. Xanthomatous neuropathy in primary biliary cirrhosis. Brain 88:1079, 1965.
232. Bouchier IAD: Postmortem study of the frequency of gallstones in patients with cirrhosis of the liver. Gut 10:705, 1969.
233. MacSween RNM, Berg PA. Autoimmune diseases of the liver, In: Ferguson A, MacSween RNM, eds. Immunological Aspects of the Liver and Gastrointestinal Tract. Baltimore, University Park Press, 1976, p. 366.
234. Herlog FH, Russell RM, Maddrey WC. Vitamin A and zinc therapy in primary biliary cirrhosis. Hepatology 1:348, 1981.
235. Walt RP, Kemp CM, Bird AC, et al. Vitamin A treatment for night blindness in primary biliary cirrhosis. Br Med J 288:1030, 1984.
236. Shepherd AN, Dedford GJ, Hill A, et al. Primary biliary cirrhosis, dark adoptometry, electro-oculography, and vitamin A state. Br Med J 289:1484, 1984.
237. Nyberg A, Berne B, Nordlinder H, et al. Impaired release of vitamin A from liver in primary biliary cirrhosis. Hepatology 8:136, 1988.
238. Munoz SJ, Heubi JE, Balistreri WF, et al. Vitamin E deficiency in primary biliary cirrhosis: Mechanism and relations to deficiency in

other lipid soluble vitamins. Gastroenterology 92:1758, 1987 (Abstract).
239. Jeffrey GP, Muller DPR, Burroughs AK, et al. Vitamin E deficiency and its clinical significance in adults with primary biliary cirrhosis and other forms of chronic liver disease. J Hepatol 4:307, 1987.
240. Long RC. Hepatic osteodystrophy: outlook good but some problems unsolved (editorial). Gastroenterology 78:644, 1980.
241. Long RC, Sherlock S. Vitamin D in chronic liver disease, In: Popper H, Schaffner F, eds. Progress in Liver Diseases. Volume 6. New York, Grune & Stratton, 1979:539.
242. Stellon AJ, Webb A, Compston J, et al. Low bone turnover state in primary biliary cirrhosis. Hepatology 7:137, 1987.
243. Hodgson SF, Rolland E, Wahner HW, et al. Bone loss and reduced osteoblast function in primary biliary cirrhosis. Ann Intern Med 103:855, 1985.
244. Mawer EB, Klass HJ, Warnes TW, et al. Metabolism of vitamin D in patients with primary biliary cirrhosis and alcoholic liver diseases. Clin Sci 69:561, 1985.
245. Stellon AJ, Webb A, Compston J, et al. Lack of osteomalacia in chronic cholestatic liver disease. Bone 7:181, 1986.
246. Cuthbert JA, Pak CYC, Zerwekh JE, et al. Bone diseases in primary biliary cirrhosis: Increased bone resorption and turnover in the absence of osteoporosis or osteomalacia. Hepatology 4:1, 1984.
247. Krawitt EL, Grundman MJ, and Mawer EB. Absorption, hydroxylation, and excretion of vitamin D3 in primary biliary cirrhosis. Lancet 2:1246, 1977.
248. Compston JE, Thompson RPH. Intestinal absorption of 25-hydroxyvitamin D and osteomalacia in primary biliary cirrhosis. Lancet 1:721, 1977.
249. Barragry JM, Long RG, France MW, et al. Intestinal absorption of cholecalciferol in alcoholic liver disease and primary biliary cirrhosis. Gut 20:559, 1979.
250. Jung RT, Davie M, Siklos P, et al. Vitamin D metabolism in acute and chronic cholestasis. Gut 20:840, 1979.
251. Personal communication.
252. Personal communication.
253. Personal communication.
254. Personal communication.
255. Chase L, Murphy W, Whyte M, et al. Osteopenia. Am J Med 69:915, 1980.
256. Kaplan MM, Goldberg MJ, Matloff DS, et al. Effect of 25-hydroxyvitamin D3 on vitamin D metabolites in primary biliary cirrhosis. Gastroenterology 81:681, 1981.
257. Kehayoglou AK, Holdsworth CD, Agnew JE, et al. Bone disease and calcium absorption in primary biliary cirrhosis—with special reference to vitamin D therapy. Lancet 1:715, 1968.
258. Reed JS, Meredith SC, Nemchausky BA, et al. Bone disease in primary biliary cirrhosis: reversal of osteomalacia with oral 25-hydroxyvitamin D. Gastroenterology 78:512, 1980.
259. Imawari M, Akanuma Y, Itakura H, et al. The effects of diseases of the liver on serum 25-hydroxy-vitamin D and on the serum binding protein for vitamin D and its metabolites. J Lab Clin Med 93:171, 1979.
260. Skinner RK, Long RG, Sherlock S, et al. Hydroxylation of vitamin D in primary biliary cirrhosis. Lancet 1:720, 1977.
261. Wagonfeld JB, Memchausky BA, Bolt M, et al. Comparison of vitamin D and 25-hydroxy-vitamin D in the therapy of primary biliary cirrhosis. Lancet 2:391, 1976.
262. Mitchison HC, Malcolm AJ, Bassendine MF, et al. Metabolic bone disease in primary biliary cirrhosis at presentation. Gastroenterology 94:463, 1988.
263. Arnaud SB, Goldsmith RS, Lambert PW, et al. 25-hydroxyvitamin D3: evidence of an entero-hepatic circulation in man. Proc Soc Exp Biol Med 149:570, 1975.
264. Long RG, Varghese Z, Meinhard EA, et al. Parenteral 1,25-dihydroxycholecalciferol in hepatic osteomalacia. Br Med J 1:75, 1978.
265. Compston JE, Crowe JP, Horton LWL. Treatment of osteomalacia associated with primary biliary cirrhosis with oral 1-alpha-hydroxyvitamin D3. Br Med J 2:309, 1979.
266. Shike M, Sturtridge WC, Tam CS, et al. A possible role of vitamin D in the genesis of parenteral-nutrition-induced metabolic bone disease. Gastroenterology 95:560, 1981.
267. Wiesner RH, LaRusso NF, Ludwig J, et al. Comparison of the clinicopathologic features of primary sclerosing cholangitis and primary biliary cirrhosis. Gastroenterology 88:108, 1985.
268. Rudzki C, Ishak KG, and Zimmerman HJ. Chronic intrahepatic cholestasis of sarcoidosis. Am J Med 59:373, 1975.
269. Williamson JMS, Chalmer DM, Clayden AD, et al. Primary biliary cirrhosis and chronic active hepatitis: An examination of clinical, biochemical, and histopathological features in differential diagnosis. J Clin Pathol 38:1007, 1985.
270. Doniach D, Walker JG. A unified concept of autoimmune hepatitis. Lancet 1:813, 1969.
271. Geubel AP, Baggenstoss AH, and Summerskill WHJ. Responses to

treatment can differentiate chronic active liver disease with cholangitic features from the primary biliary cirrhosis syndrome. Gastroenterology 71:444, 1976.
272. Salaspuro MP, Sipponen P, Ikkala E, et al. Clinical correlations and significance of orcein positivity in chronic active hepatitis and primary biliary cirrhosis. Ann Clin Res 8:206, 1976.
273. Crowe J, Christensen E, Doniach D, et al. Early features of primary biliary cirrhosis: An analysis of 85 patients. Am J Gastroenterol 80:466, 1985.
274. Goodman MW, Ansel HJ, Vennes JA, et al. Is intravenous cholangiography still useful? Gastroenterology 79:642, 1980.
275. Jain S, Scheuer PJ, Samourian S, et al. A controlled trial of D-penicillamine therapy in primary biliary cirrhosis. Lancet 1:831, 1977.
276. Dienstag JL. Summary of immunological interactions, In: Popper H, Bianchi L, Gudat F, Reutter W, eds. Communications of Liver Cells. Lancaster, England, MTP Press, 1980, p 305.
277. Zinkernagel RM. T-cell-mediated antiviral protection versus immunopathology: a question of balance, In: Popper HG, Bianchi, L, Gudat F, Reutter W, eds. Communications of Liver Cells. Lancaster, England, MTP Press, 1980, p. 279.
278. Yewdell JW, Bennink JR, Hosaka Y. Cells process exogenous proteins for recognition by cytotoxic T lymphocytes. Science 239:637, 1988.
279. Fagan E, Williams R, Cox S. Primary biliary cirrhosis in mother and daughter. Br Med J 2:1195, 1977.
280. Tong MJ, Nies KM, Reynolds TB, et al. Immunological studies in familial primary biliary cirrhosis. Gastroenterology 71:305, 1976.
281. Walker JG, Bates D, Doniach D, et al. Chronic liver disease and mitochondrial antibodies: a family study. Br Med J 1:146, 1972.
282. Chohan MR. Primary biliary cirrhosis in twin sisters. Gut 14:213, 1973.
283. Williams M, Smith PM, Doniach D. Primary biliary cirrhosis and chronic active hepatitis in two sisters. Br Med J 2:566, 1976.
284. James SP, Jones EA, Schafer DF, et al. Selective immunoglobulin A deficiency associated with primary biliary cirrhosis in a family with liver disease. Gastroenterology 90:283, 1986.
285. Kogan MH, Hammond DD, Vierling JM. Proliferation and immunoglobulin secretion to autologous stimuli in siblings of patients with primary biliary cirrhosis. Gastroenterology 92:1744, 1987 (Abstract).
286. Jaup BH, Zetergren SW. Familial occurrence of primary biliary cirrhosis associated with hypergammaglobulinemia in descendants: a family study. Gastroenterology 78:549, 1980.
287. Salaspuro MP, Laitinen OI, Lehtola J, et al. Immunological parameters, viral antibodies, and biochemical and histological findings in relatives of patients with chronic active hepatitis and primary biliary cirrhosis. Scand J Gastroenterol 11:313, 1976.
288. Hamlyn AN, Morris JS, Sherlock S. ABO blood groups, Rhesus negativity, and primary biliary cirrhosis. Gut 15:480, 1974.
289. Ercilla G, Pares A, Arriaga F, et al. Primary biliary cirrhosis associated with HLA-DRw 3 Tiss. Antigens 14:449, 1979.
290. Bassendine MF, Dewar PJ, James OFW. HLA-DR antigens in primary biliary cirrhosis: Lack of association. Gut 26:625, 1985.
291. Gores GJ, Moore SB, Fisher LD, et al. Primary biliary cirrhosis: Associations with class II major histocompatibility complex antigens. Hepatology 7:889, 1987.
292. James SP, Hoofnagel JH, Strober W, et al. Primary biliary cirrhosis: A model autoimmune disease. Ann Intern Med 99:500, 1983.
293. Epstein O. The pathogenesis of primary biliary cirrhosis. Mol Aspects Med 3:293, 1985.
294. Kaplan MM. Primary biliary cirrhosis. N Engl J Med 316:521, 1987.
295. McFarlane IG. Autoreactivity against biliary tract antigens in primary biliary cirrhosis. Mol Aspects Med 3:249, 1985.
296. Uzoegwu PN, Baum H, Williamson J. Detection of an antigen to primary biliary cirrhosis in wild type and petite mutant Saccharomyces cerevisiae. Cell Biol Int Rept 11:987, 1984.
297. Smith MGM, Golding PL, Eddleston ALWF, et al. Cell-mediated immune responses in chronic liver diseases. Br Med J 1:527, 1972.
298. Miller J, Mitchell CG, Eddleston ALWF, et al: Cell-mediated immunity to a human liver-specific antigen in patients with active chronic hepatitis and primary biliary cirrhosis. Lancet 2:296, 1972.
299. Vento S, O'Brien CJ, McFarlane BM, et al. T-lymphocytes' sensitization to hepatocyte antigens in autoimmune chronic active hepatitis and primary biliary cirrhosis. Gastroenterology 91:810, 1986.
300. McFarlane IG, Wojcicka BM, Tsantoulas DC, et al. Leukocyte migration inhibition in response to biliary antigens in primary biliary cirrhosis, sclerosing cholangitis, and other chronic liver diseases. Gastroenterology 76:1333, 1979.
301. Fujiwara R, Tobe K, Nagahima H. Studies on cellular immunity against bile proteins in primary biliary cirrhosis by the leukocyte migration inhibition test (microdroplet method) Acta Med Okayama 40:17, 1986.
302. MacFarlane IG, Wojcicka BM, Tsantoulas DC, et al. Cellular immune responses to salivary antigens in autoimmune liver disease with sicca syndrome. Clin Exp Immunol 25:389, 1976.

303. Thompson AD, Cochrane MAG, McFarlane IG, et al. Lymphocyte cytotoxicity to isolated hepatocytes in chronic active hepatitis. Nature 252:721, 1974.

304. Fernandez-Cruz E, Escartin P, Bootello A, et al. Hepatocyte damage induced by lymphocytes from patients with chronic liver diseases, as detected by LDH release. Clin Exp Immunol 31:436, 1978.

305. Vierling JM, Nelson DL, Strober W, et al. In vitro cell-mediated cytotoxicity in primary biliary cirrhosis and chronic hepatitis. J Clin Invest 60:1116, 1977.

306. Geubel AP, Keller RH, Summerskill WHJ, et al. Lymphocyte cytotoxicity and inhibition studies with autologous liver cells: observations in chronic active liver disease and primary biliary cirrhosis syndrome. Gastroenterology 71:450, 1976.

307. Doherty PC, Zinkernagel RM. H-2 compatibility is required for T-cell mediated lysis of target cells infected with lymphocytic choriomeningitis virus. J Exp Med 141:502, 1975.

308. McMichael AJ, Ting A, Zweerink HJ, et al. HLA restriction of cell-mediated lysis of influenza virus-infected human cells. Nature 270:524, 1977.

309. Personal communication.

310. James SP, Jones EA. Abnormal natural killer cytotoxicity in primary biliary cirrhosis: Evidence for a functional deficiency of cytolytic effector cells. Gastroenterology 89:165, 1985.

311. Hoffman RM, Pape GR, Rieber EP, et al. Generation of T-cell clones and lines from liver biopsies of patients with primary biliary cirrhosis. Hepatology 6:1115, 1986 (Abstract).

312. Pasternack MS. Cytotoxic T-lymphocytes. Adv Intern Med 33:17, 1988.

313. Bottazzo GF, Putol-Borrel R, Hanafusa T. Role of aberrant HLA-DR expression and antigen presentation in induction of endocrine autoimmunity. Lancet 2:1115, 1983.

314. Bevan MJ. High determinant density may explain the phenomenon of alloreactivity. Immunol Today 5:128, 1984.

315. Ballardini G, Mirakian R, Bianchi FB, et al. Aberrant expression of HLA-DR antigens on bile duct epithelium in primary biliary cirrhosis: Relevance to pathogenesis. Lancet 2:1009, 1984.

316. Spengler U, Pape GR, Hoffman RM, et al. Differential expression of MHC class II subregion products on bile duct epithelial cells and hepatocytes in patients with primary biliary cirrhosis. Hepatology 8:459, 1988.

317. Zinkernagel RM, Doherty PC. MHC-restricted cytotoxic T cells: Studies on the biological role of polymorphic major transplantation antigens determining T-cell restriction—specificity, function, and responsiveness. Adv Immunol 27:51, 1979.

318. Shulman HM, Sullivan KM, Weiden PL, et al. Chronic graft-versus-host syndrome in man—a long-term clinicopathologic study of 20 Seattle patients. Am J Med 69:204, 1980.

319. Sloane JP, Farthing MJG, and Powles RL. Histopathological changes in the liver after allogeneic bone marrow transplantation. J Clin Pathol 33:344, 1980.

320. Vierling JM, Fennell RH Jr. Histopathology of early and late human hepatic allograft rejection: Evidence of progressive destruction of interlobular bile ducts. Hepatology 5:1076, 1985.

321. Fennell RH Jr, Vierling JM. Electron microscopy of rejected human liver allografts. Hepatology 5:1083, 1985.

322. Demetris AJ, Lasky S, van Thiel DH, et al. Pathology of hepatic transplantation: A review of 62 adult allograft recipients immunosuppressed with a cyclosporine/steroid regimen. Am J Pathol 118:151, 1985.

323. Paronetto F, Popper H. Hetero-, iso- and autoimmune phenomena in the liver, In: Miescher PA, Müller-Eberhard HJ, eds. Textbook of Immunopathology, Vol. 2. New York, Grune & Stratton, 1976, p. 789.

324. Goldberg M, Kaplan M, Matloff D, et al. Evidence against an immune complex pathogenesis of primary biliary cirrhosis. Gastroenterology 78:1306, 1980 (Abstract).

325. Paronetto F, Gerber M, Vernace SJ. Immunologic studies in patients with chronic active hepatitis and primary biliary cirrhosis. I. Cytotoxic activity and binding of sera to human liver cells grown in tissue culture. Proc Soc Exp Biol Med 143:756, 1973.

326. Kakumu S, Arakawa Y, Goji H, et al. Occurrence and significance of antibody to liver-specific membrane lipoprotein by double-antibody immunoprecipitation method in sera of patients with acute and chronic liver diseases. Gastroenterology 76:665, 1979.

327. Tsantoulas D, Perperas A, Portmann B, et al. Antibodies to a human liver membrane lipoprotein (LSP) in primary biliary cirrhosis. Gut 21:557, 1980.

328. Behrens UJ, Vernace S, Paronetto F. Studies on "liver-specific" antigens. II. Detection of serum antibodies to liver and kidney cell membrane antigens in patients with chronic liver disease. Gastroenterology 77:1053, 1979.

329. Meyer zum Büschenfelde KH, Hütteroth TH, Manns M, et al. The role of liver membrane antigens as targets in autoimmune type liver disease. Springer Sem Immunopathol 3:297, 1980.

330. Epstein O, Thomas HC, Sherlock S. Primary biliary cirrhosis is a dry gland syndrome with features of chronic graft-vs-host disease. Lancet 1:1166, 1980.

331. Penner E. Demonstration of immune complexes containing the ribonucleoprotein antigen Ro in primary biliary cirrhosis. Gastroenterology 90:724, 1986.

332. Wands JR, Dienstag JL, Bhan AK, et al. Circulating immune complexes and complement activation in primary biliary cirrhosis. N Engl J Med 298:233, 1978.

333. Thomas HC, DeVilliers D, Potter BJ, et al. Immune complexes in acute and chronic liver disease. Clin Exp Immunol 31:150, 1978.

334. Gupta RC, Dickson ER, McDuffie FC, et al. Circulating IgG complexes in primary biliary cirrhosis. A serial study in forty patients followed for two years. Clin Exp Immunol 34:19, 1978.

335. Lawley TJ, James SP, Jones EA. Circulating immune complexes: their detection and potential significance in some hepatobiliary and intestinal diseases. Gastroenterology 78:626, 1980.

336. Lindgren S, Eriksson S. IgM in primary biliary cirrhosis: Physicochemical and complement activating properties. J Lab Clin Med 99:636, 1982.

337. Abrass C, Border WA, Hepner G. Non-specificity of circulating immune complexes in patients with acute and chronic liver disease. Clin Exp Immunol 40:292, 1980.

338. Thomas HC, Potter BJ, Sherlock S. Is primary biliary cirrhosis an immune complex disease? Lancet 2:1261, 1977.

339. Amoroso D, Vergani D, Wojcicka BM, et al. Identification of biliary antigens in circulating immune complexes in primary biliary cirrhosis. Clin Exp Immunol 42:95, 1980.

340. Gupta RC, Tan EM. Isolation of circulating immune complexes by conglutinin and separation of antigen from dissociated complexes by immobilized protein A. Clin Exp Immunol 46:9, 1981.

341. Goldberg MJ, Kaplan MM, Mitamura T, et al. Evidence against an immune complex pathogenesis of primary biliary cirrhosis. Gastroenterology 83:677, 1982.

342. Jaffe CJ, Vierling JM, Jones EA, et al. Receptor specific clearance by the reticuloendothelial system in chronic liver diseases. J Clin Invest 62:1069, 1978.

343. Jones EA, Frank MM, Jaffe CJ, et al. Primary biliary cirrhosis and the complement system. Ann Intern Med 90:72, 1979.

344. Tiesberg P, Gjone E. Circulating conversion products of C3 in liver disease. Evidence for in vivo activation of the complement system. Clin Exp Immunol 14:509, 1973.

345. Potter BJ, Elias E, Jones EA. Hypercatabolism of the third component of complement in patients with primary biliary cirrhosis. J Lab Clin Med 88:427, 1976.

346. Lindgren S, Laurell A-B, Eriksson S. Complement components and activation in primary biliary cirrhosis. Hepatology 4:9, 1984.

347. Vierling JM, Johnston RB, Jones EA. Accelerated kinetics of the alternative pathway of complement activation in primary biliary cirrhosis. Gastroenterology 80:1309, 1981 (Abstract).

348. Al-Aghbar MNA, Neuberger J, Williams R. Mononuclear cell complement receptor blockade in primary biliary cirrhosis. Gut 26:20, 1985.

349. Minuk GY, Vergalla J, Hanson RG, et al. Anticomplement receptor activity in the serum of patients with primary biliary cirrhosis. Gut 27:324, 1986.

350. Fox RA, James DG, Scheuer PJ, et al. Impaired delayed hypersensitivity in primary biliary cirrhosis. Lancet 1:959, 1969.

351. Fox RA, Dudley RJ, Sherlock S. The primary immune response to haemocyanin in patients with primary biliary cirrhosis. Clin Exp Immunol 14:473, 1973.

352. Thomas HC, Holden R, Jones JV, et al. Immune response to Φ X 174 in man. 5. Primary and secondary antibody production in primary biliary cirrhosis. Gut 17:884, 1976.

353. Fox RA, Dudley RJ, Samuels M, et al. Lymphocyte transformation in response to phytohaemagglutinin in primary biliary cirrhosis: the search for a plasma inhibitory factor. Gut, 14:89, 1973.

354. Cancellieri V, Scaroni C, Vernace SJ, et al. Subpopulations of T lymphocytes in primary biliary cirrhosis. Clin Immunol Immunopathol 20:255, 1981.

355. Routhier G, Epstein O, Janossy G, et al. Effects of cyclosporin A on suppressor and inducer T lymphocytes in primary biliary cirrhosis. Lancet 2:1223, 1980.

356. James SP, Elson CO, Jones EA, et al. Abnormal regulation of immunoglobulin synthesis in vitro in primary biliary cirrhosis. Gastroenterology 79:242, 1980.

357. Zetterman RK, Woltjen JA. Suppressor cell activity in primary biliary cirrhosis. Dig Dis Sci 25:104, 1980.

358. James SP, Elson CO, Waggoner JG, et al. Deficiency of the autologous mixed lymphocyte reaction in patients with primary biliary cirrhosis. J Clin Invest 66:1305, 1980.

359. Scudeletti M, Indiveri F, Pierri I, et al. T cells from patients with chronic liver diseases: Abnormalities in PHA-induced expression of HLA class II antigens and in autologous mixed-lymphocyte reactions. Cell Immunol 102:227, 1986.

360. James SP, Jones EA, Hoofnage JH, Strober W. Circulating activated B cells in primary biliary cirrhosis. J Clin Immunol 5:254, 1985.

361. Fleming CR, Dickson ER, Baggenstoss AH, et al. Copper and primary biliary cirrhosis. Gastroenterology 67:1182, 1974.

362. Ludwig J, McDonald GSA, Dickson ER, et al. Copper stains and the syndrome of primary biliary cirrhosis. Evaluation of staining methods and their usefulness for diagnosis and trials of penicillamine treatment. Arch Pathol Lab Med 103:467, 1979.

363. Fleming CR, Dickson ER, Wahner HW, et al. Pigmented corneal rings in non-Wilsonian liver disease. Ann Intern Med 86:285, 1977.

364. Fleming CR, Dickson ER, Hollenhurst RW, et al. Pigmented corneal rings in a patient with primary biliary cirrhosis. Gastroenterology 69:220, 1975.

365. Jones EA, Rabin L, Buckley CH, et al. Progressive intrahepatic cholestasis of infancy and childhood. A clinicopathologic study of a patient surviving to the age of 18 years. Gastroenterology 71:675, 1976.

366. Vierling JM, Rumble WF, Aamodt RL, et al. Kinetics of oral and intravenous radio copper in normal subjects and patients with primary biliary cirrhosis. Gastroenterology 72:1185, 1977 (Abstract).

367. Vierling JM, Shrager R, Rumble WF, et al. Incorporation of radiocopper into ceruloplasmin in normal subjects and patients with primary biliary cirrhosis and Wilson's disease. Gastroenterology. 74:652, 1978.

368. Javitt NB. Timing of cholestyramine doses in cholestatic liver disease. (Letter.) N Engl J Med 290:1328, 1974.

369. Hoensch HP, Balzer K, Dylewicz P, et al. Effect of rifampicin treatment on hepatic drug metabolism and serum bile acids in patients with primary biliary cirrhosis. Eur J Clin Pharmacol 28:475, 1985.

370. Ghent CN, Carruthers SG. Treatment of pruritus in primary biliary cirrhosis with rifampin. Gastroenterology 94:488, 1988.

371. Cerio R, Murphy GM, Sladen GE, et al. A combination of phototherapy and cholestyramine for the relief of pruritus in primary biliary cirrhosis. Br J Dermatol 116:265, 1987.

372. Bernstein JE, Swift R. Relief of intractable pruritus with naloxone. Arch Dermatol 115:1366, 1979.

373. Lauterburg BH, Pineda AA, Burgstaler EA, et al. Treatment of pruritus of cholestasis by plasma perfusion through USP-charcoal-coated glass beads. Lancet 2:53, 1980.

374. Schaffner F. Paradoxical elevation of serum cholesterol by clofibrate in patients with primary biliary cirrhosis. Gastroenterology 57:253, 1969.

375. Summerfield JA, Elias E, Sherlock S. Effects of clofibrate on primary biliary cirrhosis, hypercholesterolemia and gallstones. Gastroenterology 69:998, 1975.

376. Turnberg LA, Mahoney MP, Gleeson MH, et al. Plasmaphoresis and plasma exchange in the treatment of hyperlipaemia and xanthomatous neuropathy in patients with primary biliary cirrhosis. Gut 13:976, 1972.

377. Kehayoglou K, Hadziyannis S, Kostamis P, et al. The effect of medium-chain triglyceride on ^{47}calcium absorption in patients with primary biliary cirrhosis. Gut 14:653, 1973.

378. Ajdukiewicz AB, Agnew JE, Byers PD, et al. The relief of bone pain in primary biliary cirrhosis with calcium infusion. Gut 15:788, 1974.

379. Wiesner RH. Does propranolol precipitate hepatic encephalopathy? J Clin Gastroenterol 8:74, 1986.

380. Wiesner RH. New and evolving therapies for primary biliary cirrhosis. In: Advances in Hepatobiliary Diseases Seen in Practice. Am Assoc for the Study of Liver Diseases, NJ: 1987:19.

381. Howat HT, Ralston AJ, Varley H, et al. The late results of long-term treatment of primary biliary cirrhosis by corticosteroids. Rev Int Hepatol 16:227, 1966.

381a. Thomas HC, Epstein O. Immunological aspects of the pathogenesis and treatment of primary biliary cirrhosis. In: Berk PD, Chalmers TC, eds. Frontiers in Liver Disease. New York, Grune & Stratton, 1981:269.

382. Heathcote J, Ross A, Sherlock S. A prospective controlled trial of azathioprine in primary biliary cirrhosis. Gastroenterology 70:656, 1976.

382a. Mitchison HC, Bassendine MF, Record CO, et al. Controlled trial of prednisolone for primary biliary cirrhosis: Good for the liver, bad for the bones. Hepatology 6:1211, 1986 (Abstract).

383. Epstein O, Jain S, Lee RG, et al. D-Penicillamine treatment improves survival in primary biliary cirrhosis. Lancet 1:1275, 1981.

384. Triger D, Manifod IN, Cloke P, et al. D-Penicillamine in primary biliary cirrhosis: Two year results. Gut 21:919, 1980 (Abstract).

385. Matloff DS, Alpert E, Resnick RH, et al. A prospective trial of D-Penicillamine in primary biliary cirrhosis. N Engl J Med 306:319, 1982.

386. Bassendine MF, Macklon AF, Mulcahy R, James OFW. Controlled trial of high and low dose D-penicillamine in primary biliary cirrhosis. Gut 23:909, 1982 (Abstract).

387. Taal BF, Schalm SW, Tenkate FW, et al. Therapeutic value of D-Penicillamine in short-term prospective trial in primary biliary cirrhosis. Liver 3:345, 1983.

388. Epstein O, Cook DG, Jain S, et al. D-Penicillamine and clinical trials in primary biliary cirrhosis. Hepatology 4:1032, 1984 (Abstract).

389. Dickson ER, Fleming TR, Weisner RH, et al. Trial of penicillamine in advanced primary biliary cirrhosis. N Engl J Med 312:1011, 1985.

390. Neuberger J, Christensen E, Portmann B, et al. Double-blind controlled trial of D-Penicillamine in patients with primary biliary cirrhosis. Gut 26:114, 1985.

391. Bodenheimer HC, Schaffner F, Sternlieb I, et al. A prospective clinical trial of D-Penicillamine in the treatment of primary biliary cirrhosis. Hepatology 5:1139, 1985.

392. Epstein O, Cook DG, Jain S, et al. D-Penicillamine in primary biliary cirrhosis—An untested and untestable treatment. J Hepatol 1(Suppl):49, 1985 (Abstract).

393. Sternlieb I. The beneficial and adverse effects of penicillamine, In: Popper H, Becker K, eds. Collagen Metabolism in the Liver. New York, Stratton Intercontinental, 1975:183.

393a. Epstein O, Sherlock S. Triethylene tetramine dihydrochloride. Gastroenterology 78:1442, 1980.

394. Matloff DS, Kaplan MM. D-Penicillamine-induced Goodpasture's-like syndrome in primary biliary cirrhosis. Successful treatment with plasmapheresis and immunosuppressives. Gastroenterology 78:1046, 1980.

395. Hoofnagel JH, Davis GL, Schafer DF, et al. Randomized trial of chorambucil for primary biliary cirrhosis. Gastroenterology 91:1327, 1986.

396. Olsson, R. Oral zinc treatment in primary biliary cirrhosis. Acta Med Scand 212:191, 1982.

397. Kaplan MM, Matloff DS. Oral zinc in primary biliary cirrhosis. N Engl J Med 307:123, 1982.

398. Kirshenobich P, Uribe M, Suarez GI, et al. Treatment of cirrhosis with colchicine: Double-blind, randomized trial. Gastroenterology 77:532, 1979.

399. Koldinger RE. Treatment of primary biliary cirrhosis with colchicine. 78:1309, 1980 (Abstract).

400. Warnes TW, Smith A, Lee F. A controlled trial of colchicine in primary biliary cirrhosis. Hepatology 4:1022, 1984 (Abstract).

401. Kaplan MM, Alling DW, Zimmerman HJ, et al. A prospective trial of colchicine for primary biliary cirrhosis. N Engl J Med 315:1448, 1986.

402. Bodenheimer H, Schaffner F, Pezzullo J. Colchicine therapy in primary biliary cirrhosis. 6:1172, 1986 (Abstract).

404. Wiesner RH, Dickson ER, Lindor KD, et al. A controlled clinical trial evaluating cyclosporin in the treatment of primary biliary cirrhosis: A preliminary report. Hepatology 7:1025, 1987 (Abstract).

405. Hishon S, Tobin G, Ciclitira PJ. A clinical trial of levamisole in primary biliary cirrhosis. Postgrad Med J 58:701, 1982.

406. Poupon R, Poupon RE, Calmus V, et al. Is ursodeoxycholic acid an effective treatment for primary biliary cirrhosis? Lancet 1:834, 1987.

407. Ambinder EP, Cohen LB, Wolke AM, et al. The clinical effectiveness and safety of chronic plasmapheresis in patients with primary biliary cirrhosis. J Clin Apheresis 2:219, 1985.

408. Eriksson S, Lindgren S. Plasma exchange in primary biliary cirrhosis (Letter.) N Engl J Med 302:809, 1980.

409. Scharschmidt BF. Human liver transplantation: An analysis of 819 patients from 8 centers. In: Jones EA, ed. Recent Advances in Hepatology, Vol. 2. London, Churchill Livingstone, 1986.

410. Esquivel CO, Bernardos A, Iwatsuki S, et al. Liver transplantation for primary biliary cirrhosis in 76 patients during the cyclosporine era. Gastroenterology 94:1207, 1988.

IV D.   Hepatic Tumors

45

Tumors of The Liver

Michael C. Kew, M.D., D.Sc., F.R.C.P.

Tumors of the liver are either primary or metastatic, although occasionally the liver is involved by direct spread of a neoplasm from an adjacent organ, particularly the gallbladder. Primary hepatic tumors, whether benign or malignant, may arise from hepatic parenchymal cells, bile duct epithelium, or the supporting mesenchymal tissue, or from more than one of these tissues (Table 45–1).

The types and relative incidences of hepatic tumors encountered in clinical practice depend to a large extent on geographic location and the age of the patients. Benign tumors are, with one exception, rare in all age groups and in all geographic locations, but the types seen and their relative incidences differ considerably between adults and children. In children of all countries, primary malignant tumors, although rare, are more common than either hepatic metastases or benign hepatic tumors. In highly industrialized Western countries metastases (particularly from

TABLE 45–1. CLASSIFICATION OF PRIMARY TUMORS OF THE LIVER

Benign	Malignant
Epithelial tumors	
Hepatocellular adenoma	Hepatocellular carcinoma
Bile duct adenoma	Cholangiocarcinoma
Biliary cystadenoma	Biliary cystadenocarcinoma
Carcinoid tumor	—
—	Squamous carcinoma
—	Mucoepidermoid carcinoma
Mesenchymal tumors	
Cavernous hemangioma	—
Infantile	Angiosarcoma
hemangioendothelioma	
—	Epithelioid
	hemangioendothelioma
—	Undifferentiated (embryonal)
	sarcoma
Fibroma	Fibrosarcoma
Lipoma	—
Leiomyoma	Leiomyosarcoma
—	Epithelioid leiomyoma
	(leiomyoblastoma)
Benign mesenchymoma	Malignant mesenchymoma
Mixed tumors	
—	Hepatoblastoma
—	Mixed hepatic tumor
—	Carcinosarcoma
Teratoma	—
Tumor-like lesions	
Focal nodular hyperplasia	
Mesenchymal hamartoma	
Microhamartoma	
(von Meyenburg complex)	

primary tumors in the gastrointestinal tract, breast, and lung) are the most prevalent form of malignant hepatic disease in adults, and hepatocellular carcinoma is uncommon. In contrast, in developing countries in sub-Saharan Africa and the Far East, hepatocellular carcinoma is the dominant tumor, and relatively less metastatic disease is seen. Other primary malignant tumors are generally rare and, with the exception of cholangiocarcinoma, have no particular geographic distribution. In addition to these tumors, certain tumor-like lesions, most notably focal nodular hyperplasia, may occur in the liver. The nature of these lesions is not known, and they are considered separately in this chapter.

One quarter of a million people develop and die from hepatocellular carcinoma each year. This incidence alone qualifies hepatocellular carcinoma as one of the major malignant diseases in the world today. Hepatocellular carcinoma presents one of the most crucial and potentially rewarding challenges in the whole field of hepatic disease. The peculiar geographic and cultural distribution of this tumor provides strong circumstantial evidence for an environmental cause, and the opportunity, indeed the necessity, to identify the causative agent(s). When this has been accomplished, it should be possible to introduce appropriate programs of intervention aimed ultimately at eliminating this common and devastating tumor. Until such time as this is a reality, the present low rate of resectability and the poor response to chemotherapy and radiation therapy of patients with hepatocellular carcinoma make it essential that the tumor be diagnosed at an early stage in its natural history, when surgical resection is still possible. For patients in whom operative treatment is not feasible, the need is for effective new cancer chemotherapeutic agents. In addition to these practical considerations, hepatocellular carcinoma may have considerable theoretical importance. Investigation of the many and diverse manifestations of this tumor may lead to a better understanding of the basic biology of neoplasia.

PRIMARY MALIGNANT TUMORS

HEPATOCELLULAR CARCINOMA

Incidence and Geographic Distribution

Hepatocellular carcinoma occurs commonly (age-adjusted incidences greater than 20 per 100,000 per annum) throughout Africa south of the Sahara and in many parts of the Far East; the highest frequencies have been recorded in Mozambique (103.8 per 100,000 per annum in males), Taiwan, and southeast China.[1–3] Moderately high incidences

(10 to 20 per 100,000 per annum) are encountered in Japan, southern Europe, Switzerland, and Bulgaria.[1-3] Hepatocellular carcinoma is uncommon or rare (less than 5 and usually less than 3 per 100,000 per annum) in North America, Canada, Britain, Australia, New Zealand, Scandinavia, Israel, Latin America, India, and Sri Lanka and in South African Caucasians.[1-3] In the remaining countries there is either an intermediate frequency of the tumor (5 to 9 per 100,000 per annum in Poland, Germany, Romania, Austria, Belgium, Czechoslovakia, Hungary, France, and Yugoslavia) or the incidence has not been documented.[1-3]

Even in countries with high incidences of hepatocellular carcinoma, the tumor is not uniformly common. This is seen, for example, in China,[4] Japan[5] and Mozambique, where the tumor occurs nine times more often in the eastern or coastal regions than in the inland areas.[6]

There is some evidence that in recent years the frequency rates of hepatocellular carcinoma in North America and parts of Europe have increased slightly.[7-10] This change may reflect larger numbers of patients with alcoholic cirrhosis, improved treatment of this condition with more prolonged survival, or the emergence of new pathogenetic factors.

Individuals of African or Asian descent who migrate to countries with low incidences of hepatocellular carcinoma have lower incidences of the tumor compared with individuals remaining in their lands of origin.[1, 7] However, when people migrate from countries with low incidences of hepatocellular carcinoma to areas where the tumor is common, they retain their low frequency rates.[1, 7] People migrating from a region with a high incidence to one with a low incidence of this tumor usually adopt the life style and practices of their new environment, whereas individuals migrating from sophisticated, industrialized countries to under-developed countries retain most of their own habits and customs. These observations suggest that environmental factors rather than racial or genetic predisposition play the key role in the pathogenesis of hepatocellular carcinoma.

Age

The age of onset of hepatocellular carcinoma varies with geographic location. In sub-Saharan Africa the tumor develops at a relatively young age, the peak incidence being in the third, fourth, and fifth decades of life.[1, 11-14] Hepatocellular carcinoma frequently is encountered in the second decade of life in southern African blacks. The youngest patients with this tumor are Mozambican Shangaans, 50 per cent of whom are less than 30 years old (mean age 33 years).[11] In the Far East, hepatocellular carcinoma generally develops at an older age, with most cases occurring in the fifth and sixth decades of life (mean age 52 to 59 years).[5, 15, 16] In populations with low incidences, the elderly are affected predominantly, with a peak occurrence in the sixth, seventh, and eighth decades of life (mean age 55 to 62 years).[1, 3, 17] Hepatocellular carcinoma is rare in children.[18] When it does occur, the children are usually between the ages of 5 and 15 years.

Sex

Hepatocellular carcinoma occurs predominantly in men in almost all parts of the world. In those populations in which the tumor is common, male to female incidence ratios range from 4:1 to 8:1.[5, 13, 16, 19, 20] The male preponderance is less striking in populations with low incidences, e.g., 2.5:1 in the United States.[17] In many of these countries, the incidence in the age group 15 to 45 years is slightly higher for females than for males. In patients from Western countries who do not have cirrhosis, the sex ratio is approximately equal.[21] Women are affected slightly more often than men, in all age groups, in a few countries with low incidences of hepatocellular carcinoma, notably Iceland.[19]

Clinical Presentation

In populations that have high incidences of hepatocellular carcinoma, the tumor usually develops in individuals who were previously apparently healthy, even though the majority are found to have cirrhosis in the nontumorous parts of the liver. In contrast, in low-incidence populations the tumor often supervenes in a patient known to have had cirrhosis for some time.[22] Clinical recognition of the tumor depends primarily on an awareness of the condition and its various manifestations.

Symptoms

Hepatocellular carcinoma is insidious in onset and runs a silent course during the early stages of the disease. For this reason patients usually are unaware of its presence until the cancer has reached an advanced stage.[22] African patients particularly tend to seek treatment late in the course of the disease, when the diagnosis is usually obvious to a clinician who has had some experience with hepatocellular carcinoma. When discovered in most of these patients the tumor is too far advanced for resection or for effective cancer chemotherapy.[12-14] The most common and often the first complaint is upper abdominal pain or discomfort.[12-14, 16, 17, 22] The pain initially is a dull ache, although it frequently becomes severe in the late stages of the illness. It is continuous but may be aggravated by jolting or in certain positions. The pain is experienced most commonly in the right hypochondrium or epigastrium, but it may occasionally be felt in the left hypochondrium or in the back. Rarely it may radiate to the right shoulder. Pain is almost invariable in black and Chinese patients (Table 45–2), but it is less frequent in other populations. A sudden increase in pain, accompanied by tenderness of the liver and perhaps by an increase in its size, may indicate hemorrhage into the tumor.

Another frequent symptom is weight loss. This may be accompanied by weakness, which has often been present for a surprisingly short time in black and Oriental patients when one considers the extent of the tumor. A not uncommon symptom may be a feeling of fullness in the upper abdomen after eating. Anorexia also may be present. The patient also may have become aware of an upper abdominal mass, or he may complain of generalized swelling of the abdomen when ascites is present. Intermittent nausea and vomiting are occasional complaints, as is constipation. Jaundice is an infrequent presenting symptom. Patients, especially in developing countries, may be admitted to the hospital because of an acute abdominal catastrophe,[12, 16, 23, 24] which results from sudden intraperitoneal hemorrhage caused by rupture of the tumor. These patients have a particularly poor prognosis. In patients already known to have hepatocellular carcinoma, rupture of the tumor is a frequent terminal event.[23-25] Hepatocellular car-

TABLE 45–2. MAIN SYMPTOMS AND SIGNS IN 550 SOUTHERN AFRICAN BLACKS WITH HEPATOCELLULAR CARCINOMA

Symptoms	Per Cent Affected
Abdominal pain	91
Weight loss	35
Weakness	31
Feeling of fullness after meals/anorexia	27
Swelling of the abdomen/abdominal mass	43
Jaundice	7
Vomiting	8
Acute hemoperitoneum	11.6
Physical signs	
Hepatomegaly	89
Hepatic arterial bruit	28
Ascites	52
Splenomegaly	45
Jaundice	41
Wasting	
Mild to moderate	15
Severe	10
Fever	38

cinoma is the most common cause of nontraumatic acute hemoperitoneum in males in countries with a high incidence of hepatocellular carcinoma. This presentation is less frequent in those parts of the world where hepatocellular carcinoma is uncommon.[17, 22] Rarely, the patient seeks treatment for bone pain caused by skeletal metastases or for gastrointestinal bleeding.

The duration of symptoms is often surprisingly short, particularly in populations in which this tumor is common: African and Oriental patients frequently admit to symptoms of only four to six weeks' duration.[14, 16]

Physical Findings

The physical findings depend on the stage of the disease when the patient seeks treatment.[12–14, 16, 17, 22] Early on, the only abnormality may be a slightly or moderately enlarged liver. Frequently, however, the disease is advanced when the patient is first seen. The liver is then almost invariably enlarged, particularly in African and Oriental patients, and may be massively so (Table 45–2). One or both lobes may be enlarged. The surface of the liver is frequently irregular or nodular, but it may be smooth. Although the consistency of the liver is typically stony-hard, it may just be firm and may even fluctuate in some areas. Liver tenderness is frequent and may be severe, particularly when hemorrhage into or necrosis of the tumor has occurred. An arterial bruit can be heard over the liver in 7 to 29 per cent of patients.[12, 14, 22, 26] While not pathognomonic of hepatocellular carcinoma, this sign is an extremely valuable pointer to its diagnosis. It is thought to reflect the highly vascular nature of the tumor, with turbulence occurring in the dilated and irregular vessels within it. The bruit usually is systolic in timing but may be continuous with systolic accentuation. It is harsh and is distinguished easily from a venous hum. Rarely, a friction rub can be heard over the liver. However, this sign is more common in metastatic hepatic disease and amebic hepatic abscesses.

On admission to the hospital, 20 to 50 per cent of patients have ascites, which becomes more prominent as the disease progresses. It is more likely to be present in the early stages in patients with underlying cirrhosis. Ascites is caused by either portal hypertension or malignant inva-

sion of the peritoneum. Ascitic fluid may be bloodstained in the latter case. Bloodstained ascitic fluid may result also from bleeding from the primary tumor. Ascites developing late in the course of the disease may be caused by tumor invasion of either the portal veins or the hepatic veins with superimposed thrombosis. Frequent paracenteses may be needed for symptomatic relief. The superficial abdominal veins may be dilated because of portal hypertension or neoplastic obstruction of the inferior vena cava. Splenomegaly is found in 28 to 48 per cent of patients. Splenic enlargement usually is modest and is the result of portal hypertension. The presence of tense ascites or a very large liver prevents palpation of an enlarged spleen in some patients.

The patient usually is not jaundiced when first seen. When present, jaundice is almost always slight or moderate in degree, although it may deepen during the late stages of the illness. Early, deep jaundice should suggest the possibility of a cholangiocarcinoma, although in some instances an obstructive type of jaundice may be seen as a result of invasion of the intrahepatic biliary system by the tumor or compression of the common hepatic duct by tumorous glands in the porta hepatis.[23] Rarely, jaundice is caused by hemobilia.[27] Persistent fever is present in 6 to 54 per cent of patients.[12, 14, 15, 17, 22] The fever is slight or moderate and is intermittent or remittent. Although low-grade fever can occur in patients with cirrhosis,[28] the finding of a persistently elevated temperature should suggest the possibility of malignant change.

A minority of patients are wasted when first seen. However, progressive weight loss and wasting occur, and the patients often become emaciated during the terminal phases of the illness. Stigmata of chronic hepatic disease, such as gynecomastia, are present often in patients in low-incidence areas (e.g., 51 per cent in a study from the United Kingdom)[22] but are rare in African and Oriental patients.

In some black and Oriental patients[16] who have short histories of acute right hypochondrial or epigastric pain, high temperatures, and enlarged tender livers, it may be difficult to distinguish between acute amebic hepatic abscesses and hepatocellular carcinoma.

In those countries in which hepatocellular carcinoma arises as a late complication of cirrhosis, it may be difficult to distinguish the symptoms and signs of the tumor from those of the underlying disease.[22] One circumstance that should alert the clinician to the possibility of hepatocellular carcinoma is a sudden and unexplained deterioration in the condition of a patient known to have cirrhosis or hemochromatosis. Such a patient may complain of abdominal pain or weight loss; ascites may become a problem or become bloodstained; the liver may enlarge suddenly or develop a bruit; or hepatic failure may supervene.

Paraneoplastic Manifestations

Many of the deleterious effects of hepatocellular carcinoma are not caused either by the local effects of the tumor or by metastases but result because the tumor produces substances that enter the blood stream and exert effects on distant tissues. Clinically recognizable syndromes result from ectopic synthesis and secretion of hormones. The tumor also may produce carcinofetal proteins, such as α-fetoprotein and carcinoembryonic antigen, and carcinofetal or carcinoplacental isoenzymes. These proteins cause no clinically apparent disorder and are discovered only by laboratory testing of blood. Paraneoplastic manifestations may have important clinical and therapeutic implications; since they may antedate the local effects of the tumor, they may direct attention to its presence.

Although not all of the paraneoplastic phenomena of hepatocellular carcinoma can be explained by a single mechanism, many of the apparently diverse sequelae may share a common pathogenesis.[29] The many morphologic and functional cell types of a multicellular organism contain identical data coded into the nuclear nucleic acid.[30] More than 90 per cent of this information is repressed in the differentiated cell. However, any or all such data may be derepressed with neoplastic transformation, allowing the appearance of functions attributed usually to other types of cells.

A classification of the paraneoplastic manifestations of hepatocellular carcinoma is shown in Table 45–3.

Ectopic Hormonal Syndromes

Erythrocytosis. Erythrocytosis is one of the most common of the paraneoplastic phenomena in hepatocellular carcinoma. Based on values of the hematocrit or hemoglobin, its incidence ranges from 2.8 to 11.7 per cent.[31–33] However, these figures are likely to be an underestimate because the presence of an expanded plasma volume resulting from the associated cirrhosis falsely lowers the hematocrit and reduces the concentration of hemoglobin.

The pathogenesis of the erythrocytosis has not been elucidated. Erythropoietin (or an erythropoietin-like substance) may be synthesized and secreted by the tumor.[32] Erythropoietic activity frequently has been demonstrated in patients' sera, but assay of tumor tissue usually has failed to show such activity.[32] Alternatively, the tumor could be secreting increased quantities of the globulin that interacts normally with erythropoiesis-stimulating factor synthesized by the kidney to produce excessive quantities of erythropoietin.[32] Other postulated explanations are that hypoxia of hepatic tissue adjacent to the hepatocellular carcinoma caused by growth of the tumor stimulates the kidney to secrete erythropoietin (or erythropoiesis-stimulating factor)[34] or that increased erythropoiesis results from failure of inactivation of erythropoietin by the liver.[32]

TABLE 45–3. PARANEOPLASTIC MANIFESTATIONS OF HEPATOCELLULAR CARCINOMA

Ectopic hormonal syndromes
  Erythrocytosis
  Hypercalcemia
  Sexual changes
  Carcinoid syndrome
  Hypertrophic osteoarthropathy
  Thyroxine-binding globulin
Metabolic changes
  Hypoglycemia
  Hypercholesterolemia
  Porphyria cutanea tarda
Carcino-fetal proteins
  Alpha-fetoprotein
  Carcinoembryonic antigen
  Isoferritins
  Dysfibrinogenemia
Carcino-placental or carcino-fetal isoenzymes
  Variant alkaline phosphatase
  Gamma-glutamyl transferase
  5'-nucleotide phosphodiesterase
Miscellaneous
  Vitamin B_{12} binding protein
  Fever
  Cachexia

Hypercalcemia. A few patients with hepatocellular carcinoma and hypercalcemia in the absence of osseous metastases have been reported, but the frequency of this complication has not been determined. More than one pathogenetic mechanism may be responsible for hypercalcemia in the absence of metastatic osteolysis. Each involves a hormone or a hormone-like substance that is produced by the tumor and alters bone metabolism, with release of calcium. Ectopic production of a peptide with parathormone-like immunoreactivity has been found in a few malignancies, including cholangiocarcinoma,[35] but not in hepatocellular carcinoma.[36] Prostaglandins of the E series stimulate bone resorption in vitro.[37] A metabolite of prostaglandin E_2 (PGE-M) has been found in increased amounts in the sera of patients with breast and renal carcinomas who are hypercalcemic.[38] After treatment with inhibitors of prostaglandin synthetase, the serum calcium concentrations returned to normal. The importance of prostaglandins in the hypercalcemia associated with hepatocellular carcinoma remains to be determined. Other humoral factors that may be responsible for hypercalcemia in malignant disease by enhancing osteoclastic activity are interleukin 1 and several growth factors derived from tumors, some of which are similar to epidermal growth factor. However, at present there is no evidence that any of these factors are produced by hepatocellular carcinoma.

Sexual Changes. Three types of sexual change—isosexual precocious puberty, gynecomastia, and feminization—can occur in patients with hepatocellular carcinoma.[39] Isosexual precocity has been reported in several boys with this tumor.[40] Gonadotropin was found in sera, urines, and samples of tumor tissue from some of these patients, and the sexual change was attributed to ectopic production and secretion of this substance. The apparent limitation of the syndrome to males points to elaboration of a substance possessing mainly interstitial cell-stimulating properties. Serum concentrations of human chorionic gonadotropin were found to be increased in 17 per cent of adult Ugandan patients with hepatocellular carcinoma.[41] However, these patients showed no obvious endocrine disturbances.

Feminization (or gynecomastia alone) is rare in patients who have hepatocellular carcinoma without cirrhosis. In the only well-studied case, feminization was shown to be caused by the tumor acting as trophoblastic tissue.[42] The patient's serum estrone, estradiol, estriol, and human placental lactogen concentrations were increased. In vitro assay of tumor tissue showed estrogenic activity and high levels of beta subunits of human chorionic gonadotropin. The tumor tissue was shown in vitro to convert dehydroepiandrosterone sulfate and dehydroepiandrosterone to estrone and estradiol. The serum levels of the hormones returned to normal, and all signs of feminization disappeared after surgical removal of the tumor. Two other patients with hepatocellular carcinoma were found to have high concentrations of human placental lactogen but showed no endocrine disturbance.[43]

One patient with carcinoid syndrome[44] and two with hypertrophic osteoarthropathy[45] complicating hepatocellular carcinoma have been reported. Elevated serum concentrations of thyroxine-binding globulin have been found in a few patients, but they have not had clinically evident disturbances of thyroid function.[46, 47]

Metabolic Changes

Hypoglycemia. Hypoglycemia is probably the most common and certainly the most dangerous of the paraneoplastic syndromes associated with hepatocellular carcinoma. However, its exact prevalence is uncertain; reported incidences in different populations range from 4.6 to 27 per cent.[39] Hypoglycemia occurs in two distinct clinical circumstances in Chinese patients with hepatocellular carcinomas.[48] In the majority the tumor is poorly differentiated and grows rapidly. Hypoglycemia occurs in about 20 per cent of these patients. It develops during the terminal two weeks of the illness and is relatively mild (type A). In the remaining patients the tumor is well differentiated and grows more slowly. Profound hypoglycemia occurs in all of these patients, and develops early in the course of the disease (type B).

The pathogenesis of hypoglycemia in hepatocellular carcinoma is not fully understood.[39] There is no evidence for the production by the tumor of either immunoreactive insulin or an insulinotropic substance. In one study, two of four patients were reported to have raised serum concentrations of insulin-like growth Factors I and II, but this was not confirmed in a larger series of black patients with hypoglycemia.[49] Although hepatocellular carcinomas grow rapidly, there is no evidence yet that enhanced glycolysis and glucose utilization by the tumor are responsible by themselves for hypoglycemia.

It has been suggested that glucose might enter malignant cells in the absence of insulin, and that this might contribute to a large hepatocellular carcinoma acting as a "sponge" for glucose.[50] However, hepatic tissue is capable of an enormous increase in glucose output, which would normally compensate for increased glucose utilization by the tumor. In the terminal stages of the illness replacement of hepatic tissue by the tumor may be so extensive that there is insufficient unaffected tissue to meet the glucose requirements of the large, rapidly growing carcinoma, as well as the other tissues of the body (type A). In type B hypoglycemia, hepatic glycogenolysis is impaired, as shown by a subnormal response to glucagon and substantially reduced phosphorylase activity.[51] This affects normal hepatic tissue and the tumor, both of which can be shown to have an increased glycogen content. In addition to this acquired defect in glycogenolysis, enzymes concerned with gluconeogenesis, e.g., glucose-6-phosphatase, are reduced in amount or completely absent. It is possible that some substance secreted by or released from the tumor might inhibit glycogenolysis or gluconeogenesis, or both.

Hypercholesterolemia. Hypercholesterolemia occurs in 11 to 38 per cent of African patients who have hepatocellular carcinoma.[12, 52] Both animal and human studies of hepatocellular carcinomas have shown an association of an elevated serum cholesterol concentration with increased cholesterol synthesis by the tumor.[52] This in turn appears to result from a complete absence in the malignant cells of the normal negative-feedback system. More than 90 per cent of the sterols produced as a result of deletion of this control are released into the circulation. Experiments in animal hepatomas have not detected any abnormality in β hydroxy-β-methylglutaryl coenzyme A reductase, the rate-limiting enzyme in cholesterol biosynthesis.[39] However, studies on experimental hepatomas in animals have shown that malignant hepatocytes lack receptors for chylomicron remnants (in spite of having coated pits on the cell surfaces).[53] Chylomicron remnants, and hence cholesterol, therefore, do not enter the malignant hepatocytes and thus do not exert an inhibitory effect on β-hydroxy-β-methylglutaryl coenzyme A reductase.[53]

Porphyria cutanea tarda has been reported to develop rarely in patients with hepatocellular carcinoma.[54]

Carcinofetal Proteins

Alpha-Fetoprotein. Alpha-fetoprotein is an α_1-globulin normally present in high concentration in fetal serum but present in only minute amounts thereafter. In adulthood, reappearance of α-fetoprotein in high concentrations in the serum is a strong pointer to the diagnosis of hepatocellular carcinoma, and in childhood, to either hepatoblastoma or hepatocellular carcinoma.[55, 56] Using a relatively insensitive immunodiffusion method, between 28 and 87 per cent of patients with hepatocellular carcinoma will have demonstrable α-fetoprotein in the serum. Using radioimmunoassay, the number of patients with raised serum values increases significantly; for example, the "positivity rate" in Chinese patients increased from 69 per cent with immunodiffusion to 93 per cent with radioimmunoassay. However, with the more sensitive assay there is inevitably a lessening of the diagnostic specificity of the test, with slightly elevated levels being recorded in association with acute and chronic hepatitis, cirrhosis, and other tumors. Even with the most sensitive techniques available, it appears that in some patients hepatocellular carcinoma does not produce α-fetoprotein. Synthesis of the globulin is therefore not essential for oncogenesis. It is not known whether tumors that do not produce α-fetoprotein are biologically different from the majority of hepatocellular carcinomas. The serum concentrations of α-fetoprotein in hepatocellular carcinoma range over six orders of magnitude, the highest values being about 7 mg/ml and the lowest concentrations only slightly above the normal adult levels of less than 20 ng/ml.[55]

There is no obvious correlation between the serum α-fetoprotein concentration and any of the clinical or biochemical features of the disease, the size and stage of the tumor, or survival time after diagnosis.[55] Attempts to relate the extent of differentiation of the tumor to production of the globulin have produced conflicting results. Synthesis of α-fetoprotein by hepatocellular carcinoma appears to be permanent. However, with effective chemotherapy the serum concentrations decrease. They return to normal after successful surgical resection.[56]

Carcinoembryonic Antigen. Serum concentrations of carcinoembryonic antigen were found to be elevated in 39 per cent of 72 southern African blacks who had hepatocellular carcinoma.[57] However, in only 4 per cent of the patients were the elevations in the "cancer range," (i.e., greater than 20 ng/ml), so that estimation of serum carcinoembryonic antigen concentrations is of no value in the diagnosis of hepatocellular carcinoma. There was no correlation between serum carcinoembryonic antigen and α-fetoprotein concentrations in individual patients.[57]

Isoferritins. Serum ferritin concentrations are frequently increased in patients who have hepatocellular carcinoma.[58-60] Acidic isoferritins have been demonstrated in human hepatocellular carcinoma tissue,[58, 59] and these acidic isoferritins, as well as the usual more basic isoferritins, were found in the serum of one patient.[60] An isoferritin similar to that found in hepatocellular carcinoma has been isolated from fetal liver.[61] It is therefore conceivable that isoferritin production by the tumor represents a dedifferentiation of function of the malignant hepatocyte. An inverse correlation between serum ferritin and α-fetoprotein concentrations has been shown, although the significance of this finding is not known.[59]

Dysfibrinogenemia. Dysfibrinogenemia, as evidenced by a prolonged reptilase test time, may occur in patients with hepatocellular carcinoma.[62, 63] Gralnick believes the functional defect to be one of delayed polymerization of the fibrin monomer.[64] The fibrinogen found in the sera of patients with hepatocellular carcinomas is similar in many respects to fetal fibrinogen, and may represent ectopic production of the fetal form by the tumor.

Vitamin B$_{12}$-Binding Protein. Increased concentrations of vitamin B$_{12}$-binding proteins have been demonstrated in the sera of a few patients with hepatocellular carcinomas.[65] These patients usually have been less than 20 years old, and all have been "α-fetoprotein-negative." Waxman et al. have suggested that the tumor-associated vitamin B$_{12}$-binding protein is leukocyte-derived but is sialated during transit through the malignant hepatocytes.[65] The abnormal vitamin B$_{12}$-binding protein appears to be associated specifically with the fibrolamellar variant of hepatocellular carcinoma.[66, 67] This may also be true of the hormone neurotensin. Four out of five patients with hepatocellular carcinoma found to have raised serum concentrations of neurotensin had the fibrolamellar variant of the tumor.[68]

Carcinoplacental or Carcinofetal Isoenzymes

In fast-growing, undifferentiated, transplantable hepatomas, the enzymes glucose-ATP-phosphotransferase, aldolase, pyruvate kinase, and glycogen phosphorylase that are characteristic of adult liver and under host, dietary and hormonal control practically disappear, and are replaced by their fetal counterparts.[69] The latter are suited for efficient utilization of metabolic fuel but are no longer subject to host regulation. This fetal glycolytic mechanism is largely responsible for the high glycolytic rates of transplantable hepatomas.

The best known of the carcinofetal or carcinoplacental isoenzymes in human hepatocellular carcinoma is a variant alkaline phosphatase.[70] This enzyme resembles the D-variant of placental alkaline phosphatase in some respects. It has been demonstrated in tumor tissue as well as in serum and appears to be virtually specific to hepatocellular carcinoma. Variant alkaline phosphatase differs from the placental alkaline phosphatases (Regan and Nagao isoenzymes), which are produced by other types of cancer. Isoenzymes of γ-glutamyl transferase[71] and 5'-nucleotide phosphodiesterase[72] have also been found in the sera of patients with hepatocellular carcinomas.

Diagnosis

The diagnosis of hepatocellular carcinoma generally is made late in the course of the disease, and sometimes only at necropsy. In Africa and, to a lesser extent, the Far East, this is because the patients tend to seek medical attention only when the disease is already far advanced. In Western countries there are other reasons: because of the large size of the liver, the tumor usually has to reach a considerable size before it invades adjacent structures; the liver is relatively inaccessible to the examining hand; hepatocellular carcinoma frequently arises in an already diseased liver; the hepatic reserves are such that a large proportion of the liver must be replaced before jaundice or other signs of hepatic failure appear; distant metastases usually appear late in the course of the disease; and there are no specific biochemical changes. However, with a greater awareness of the disease and the use of modern diagnostic techniques, it is now possible to make the diagnosis of hepatocellular carcinoma in the great majority of instances.

Alpha-Fetoprotein Determination

In those geographic regions where hepatocellular carcinoma is common, the most useful diagnostic test is unquestionably the serum α-fetoprotein determination. Generally speaking, the immunodiffusion method for detecting α-fetoprotein is used for diagnostic purposes, whereas the more sensitive (but more expensive) radioimmunoassay technique is used for assessing response to therapy, completeness of surgical resection, or recurrence after operation.[55, 56] The immunodiffusion method is performed easily even in small, peripheral laboratories and yields positive results in about 75 per cent of the patients in populations with a high incidence of hepatocellular carcinoma.[55, 56] A positive result almost always indicates the presence of hepatocellular carcinoma, because false-positive results are rare. In populations with a low incidence of the tumor, α-fetoprotein determination is less useful because of the large number of false-negative results obtained by immunodiffusion (50 per cent or more).[55, 56] The use of radioimmunoassay significantly increases the number of positive results in these populations. However, when α-fetoprotein is present only in low concentrations (less than 500 ng/ml), it is difficult to distinguish hepatocellular carcinoma from acute and chronic hepatic parenchymal disease and other tumors (i.e., the number of false-positive results will increase).

In surveillance programs of individuals at high risk for developing hepatocellular carcinoma, serial estimations of α-fetoprotein levels have proved to be a useful although not infallible means of detecting small tumors. A sustained rise in the concentration of α-fetoprotein occurs in about 50 per cent of cases. However, in up to 30 per cent of the subjects, the values remain in the normal range; in the remainder, the concentrations are raised, but not to diagnostic levels.[73]

Tumor-Associated Isoenzymes of Gamma-Glutamyl Transferase

Three tumor-associated isoenzymes of γ-glutamyl transferase have been described in the serum of patients with hepatocellular carcinoma.[71, 74] One or more of these isoenzymes are present in 60 per cent of Japanese and southern African blacks with this tumor: I' is present in about 55 per cent, I'' in about 27 per cent, and II' in about 34 per cent. These isoenzymes have not been described in normal serum and are present only occasionally in association with other tumors or benign hepatic disease. Although these isoenzymes are less useful than α-fetoprotein as a marker of hepatocellular carcinoma, the two can be used in conjunction. For example, only 4 per cent of southern African blacks with this tumor have neither of the two markers.

Des-Gamma-Carboxy Prothrombin

This abnormal prothrombin was found in high concentration in the serum of 90 per cent of Taiwanese and American patients with hepatocellular carcinoma.[75] The mean serum concentration was 900 ng/ml, compared with 10 ng/ml in patients with chronic active hepatitis and 42 ng/ml in those with hepatic metastases. If these findings are confirmed, des-γ-carboxy prothrombin may prove to be an additional marker of hepatocellular carcinoma.

Tissue Polypeptide Antigen

Tissue polypeptide antigen is a polypeptide that has been isolated from malignant cells and is present in high concentration in the serum of patients with various tumors.

Raised values were found in 96 per cent of patients with hepatocellular carcinoma, but also in 61 per cent of patients with amebic hepatic abscesses, 86 per cent with chronic hepatic parenchymal disease, and 90 per cent with acute hepatitis.[76] Tissue polypeptide antigen is comparable in sensitivity with alpha-fetoprotein as a marker of hepatocellular carcinoma, but its lack of specificity severely limits its clinical usefulness.

Biochemical Changes

The biochemical changes in hepatocellular carcinoma are nonspecific and, in the main, indistinguishable from those found in cirrhosis.[12, 13, 15, 16, 22, 77] They are therefore of little value in the diagnosis of hepatocellular carcinoma. At best they may suggest the presence of a space-occupying or infiltrative lesion in the liver, but they provide no indication as to its nature. A significantly elevated serum alkaline phosphatase concentration with a normal or only a slightly increased serum bilirubin and a normal or slightly higher than normal serum aminotransferase level, suggestive of a space-occupying or infiltrative hepatic lesion,[78] is present in as many as 50 per cent of cases. In a patient known to have cirrhosis, an abrupt and significant increase in the serum alkaline phosphatase concentration should suggest the possibility of malignant change. The serum albumin concentration is frequently subnormal. The serum bilirubin concentration is usually normal early in the development of the tumor, but may rise in the later stages. In a minority of cases the biochemical picture is that of obstructive jaundice.

In Africa and the Far East, low hemoglobin and hematocrit values are found in about half of the patients who have hepatocellular carcinomas.[15, 32] However, anemia is less frequent in Western populations. Severe anemia is observed rarely, and then only in patients with hematemesis or intraperitoneal hemorrhage. A mild or moderate leukocytosis may be present (in 21 per cent of southern African blacks), but leukopenia also may be found (in 6.5 per cent of southern African blacks).[14, 15, 22]

Radiologic Investigations

Plain radiographs of the abdomen usually show an enlarged liver and, in rare instances, calcification in the tumor.[5] Pulmonary metastases may be seen at the time of admission to the hospital (e.g., in 19 per cent of southern African blacks),[79] or they may become apparent during the ensuing weeks or months[80] (in 6 per cent of southern African blacks).[79] These metastases are almost always multiple, they tend to be of more or less the same size, and they often enlarge rapidly. The right hemidiaphragm may be significantly raised (more than 2.5 cm higher than the left hemidiaphragm on a posteroanterior chest film).[79, 80] This radiologic sign is present in 30 per cent of southern African blacks.[79] There may be an associated right basal pleural effusion, and linear atelactases may be present in the right lower lobe. Skeletal metastases are occasionally seen.

A barium meal may show esophagogastric varices, and indentation or displacement of the stomach by the enlarged liver.

Hepatic Arteriography. Hepatocellular carcinoma derives its blood supply from the hepatic artery.[81] Hepatic arteriography therefore may be extremely useful in the diagnosis of this tumor, and is essential in delineating the hepatic arterial anatomy when planning surgical resection, dearterialization of the liver, embolization of the tumor, or infusion of cytotoxic drugs directly into the hepatic artery.

Hepatocellular carcinoma is often highly vascular, in contradistinction to hepatic metastases, which usually have a poor blood supply[82–84] (Fig. 45–1). In hepatocellular carcinoma, the arteries are irregular in caliber and do not taper normally. The smaller branches may show a bizarre pattern[82–84] (Fig. 45–1). There is early filling of the hepatic veins and retrograde filling of portal vein branches. This results from the presence of arteriovenous anastomoses in the tumor. In addition, there is a delay in capillary emptying, which is seen as a "blush." In some instances the center of a large tumor is avascular as a result of necrosis or, less often, hemorrhage. Multinodular tumors may be hypovascular.

Examination of the portal veins during recirculation after celiac axis arteriography or during portal venography may show the presence of tumor within the portal venous system.[85] Less often, tumorous invasion of the hepatic veins can be demonstrated. Vena cavography may show extension of the tumor into the inferior vena cava. These observations have important implications when considering the possibility of surgical resection.

Isotopic Hepatic Scanning. Isotopic scanning of the liver is useful in confirming or establishing the presence of a mass in the liver and in indicating the optimal site for percutaneous biopsy[86, 87] (Fig. 45–2). It may also be of value in assessing operability of the tumor. Small lesions (less than 3 cm in diameter) are not visible on the scan. In the great majority of cases one or more defects are seen on the standard ^{99m}Tc-sulfur colloid scan.[86, 87] However, the scintiscan picture is not diagnostic, and other radiopharmaceuticals have been used to increase the diagnostic accuracy of hepatic scanning. ^{75}Se-selenomethionine is metabolized by the liver in the same way as is methionine.[88] As the morphology and function of well-differentiated hepatocellular carcinoma may closely resemble those of normal hepatic tissue, the uptake of this radiopharmaceutical by the tumor might be expected to approach that of surrounding normal hepatic tissue, a property not shared by other hepatic lesions. Unfortunately, false-negative results are frequent, at least in southern African blacks.[88] This has been attributed to the anaplastic nature of the tumor in some patients and the frequency with which tumor necrosis occurs. Another tumor-seeking agent, ^{57}Co-bleomycin, was also found to be of limited value, as only 31 per cent of the defects attributable to hepatocellular carcinoma concentrated this radiopharmaceutical.[89] Difficulty may be experienced in differentiating between defects caused by cirrhosis and those produced by a superimposed hepatocellular carcinoma. Because ^{67}Ga-citrate is not taken up by cirrhotic defects, it has been used for this purpose. However, the tumor also may fail to concentrate ^{67}Ga-citrate, as occurred in 30 per cent of southern African blacks with hepatocellular carcinomas so examined.[90] Dynamic blood flow scintigraphy using ^{99m}Tc-pertechnetate may be used to differentiate between highly vascular hepatocellular carcinomas and avascular hepatic masses. Disappearance of the defect shown on the ^{99m}Tc-sulfur colloid scan favors a diagnosis of hepatocellular carcinoma (Fig. 45–3); however, as the tumor may be hypovascular, failure of the defect to do so does not exclude this diagnosis.

Ultrasonography. Ultrasonography will differentiate between solid and cystic hepatic mass lesions but does not distinguish hepatocellular carcinoma from other solid lesions. Features suggestive of hepatocellular carcinoma are harsh echoes in a lesion with irregular and sometimes ill-defined margins[91] (Fig. 45–4). About two thirds of the tumors are uniformly echogenic; the remainder are partly

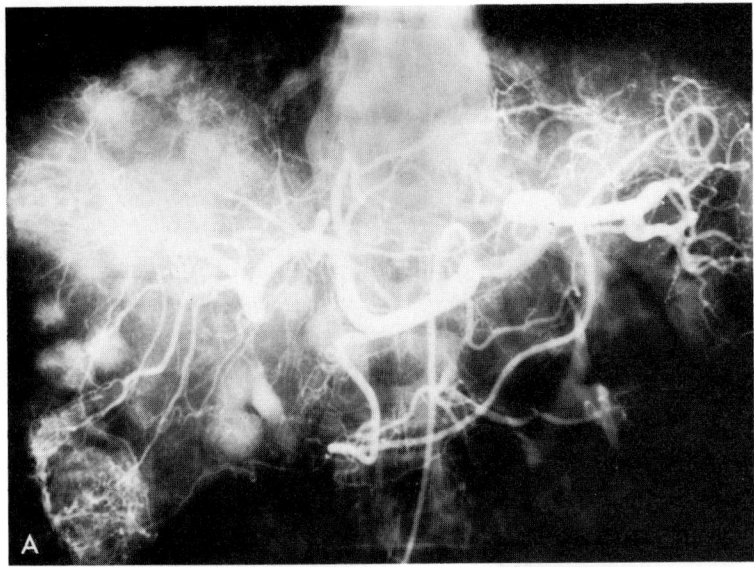

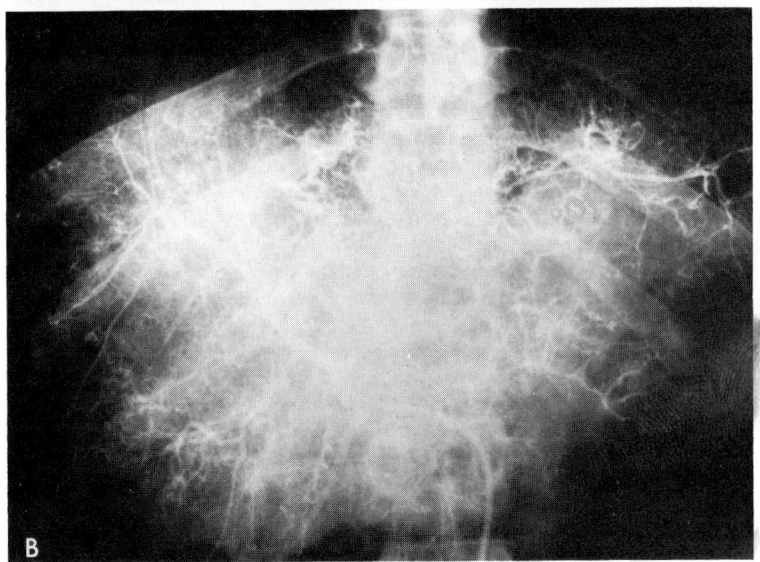

Figure 45–1. *A,* Celiac axis arteriogram, showing the features of a highly vascular multinodular hepatocellular carcinoma. *B,* Selective hepatic arteriogram, showing a highly vascular hepatocellular carcinoma involving almost the whole liver (massive variety).

echogenic and partly transonic. The transonic areas are thought to result from necrosis within the tumor.[91] Small tumors detected in surveillance programs are frequently transonic. Ultrasonography can be used to assess the patency of the portal vein and its larger branches and of the inferior vena cava.[92] Ultrasonography is particularly useful in differentiating between hepatocellular carcinomas and amebic hepatic abscesses in those patients who have short histories of severe right hypochondrial pain, high fevers, and enlarged, tender livers.

Computerized Axial Tomography. Plain or dynamic computerized tomography is capable of detecting and defining the extent of the tumor in the great majority of patients. The images obtained are not specific, however, for hepatocellular carcinoma (Fig. 45–5). Lesions too small to be seen with plain computerized tomograms may be visualized by infusing contrast material intravenously or intra-arterially.[93, 94]

Magnetic Resonance Imaging. Hepatocellular carcinoma typically appears as one or more masses of increased intensity on spin echo images and of diminished intensity on inversion recovery images.[94] Because all or most of these tumors have prolonged T_1 and T_2 times, they are best visualized using spin echo techniques with a long interval between excitations. Magnetic resonance imaging is of particular value in demonstrating the internal architecture of the tumor and in defining the relation of the hepatic blood vessels to the malignancy.

Laparoscopy. Laparoscopy can be used to visualize the size and extent of the tumor, to see whether the nontumorous liver is cirrhotic, to look for peritoneal spread, and to obtain a needle biopsy under direct vision.

Definitive diagnosis of hepatocellular carcinoma depends on the demonstration of the histologic features of the tumor. This usually can be achieved by percutaneous biopsy. Significant bleeding from the biopsy site is rare. The risk is greater, however, than it is in non-neoplastic conditions. Because of the risk of local or systemic spread of the tumor by needle biopsy, we refrain from doing a percutaneous biopsy as long as we believe the tumor to be resectable. In those cases in which laparotomy is performed with a view to possible resection, biopsy is done during the operation, and a frozen section is examined.

Pathology

Gross Appearance. Although hepatocellular carcinoma may arise in a small liver, it is found more usually in an

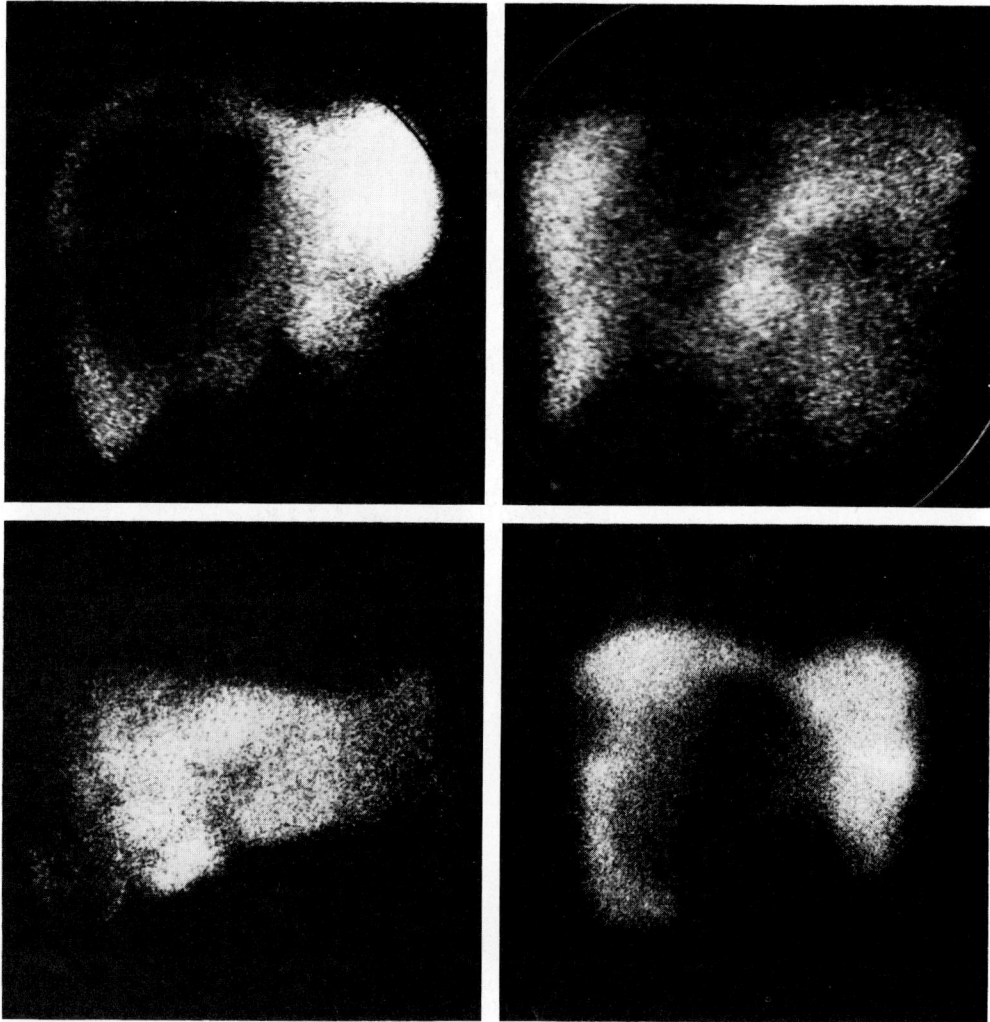

Figure 45–2. Four examples of types of defects seen on isotope liver scanning in patients with hepatocellular carcinoma (gamma camera pictures after an intravenous injection of ^{99m}Tc-sulfur colloid).

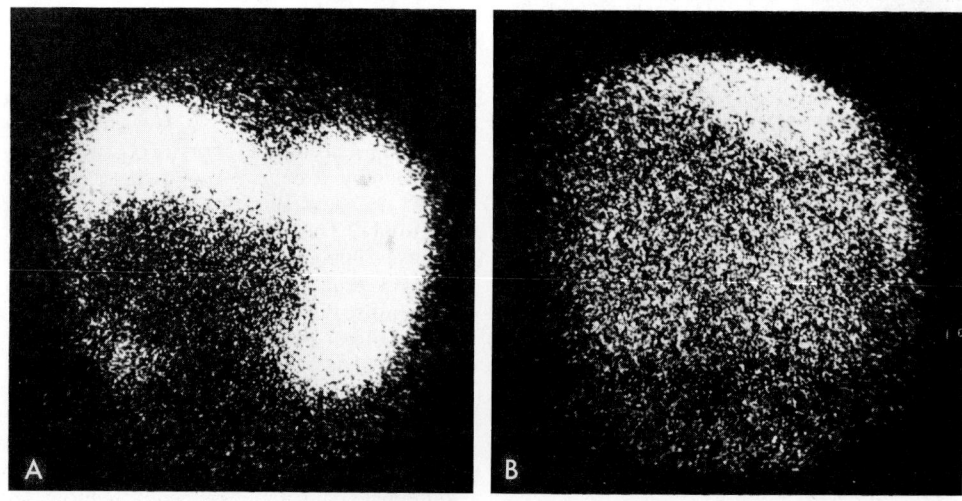

Figure 45–3. A large defect visible in the liver on a ^{99m}Tc-sulfur colloid scan (A) is not seen during dynamic blood flow scintigraphy using technetium pertechnetate (B), indicating the highly vascular nature of the hepatocellular carcinoma in this patient.

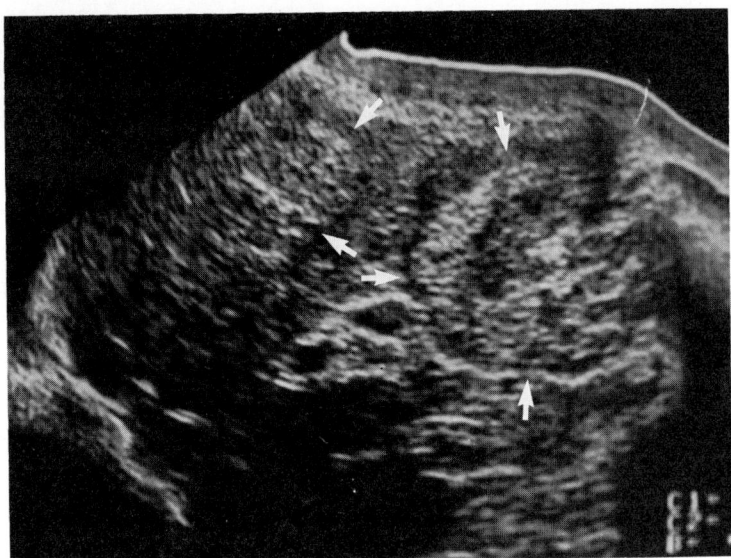

Figure 45-4. Longitudinal sonogram of a patient with hepatocellular carcinoma, showing two large echogenic masses (arrows).

obviously enlarged liver. This is particularly so in black patients, in whom the tumorous livers often weigh 500 to 1000 grams more than those in Caucasian patients. The large size of the liver results mainly from the bulk of the tumor, although cirrhosis, when present, contributes.[95] Three basic types of hepatocellular carcinoma are described—nodular, massive, and diffuse.[95–98] The nodular variety is the most common, accounting for about 75 per cent of all cases, and is usually found in cirrhotic livers. It consists of numerous round or irregular nodules of various sizes scattered throughout the liver, although one nodule is often larger than all the others. Some of the smaller nodules are tumor foci within vessels. Umbilication of subcapsular tumor masses in hepatocellular carcinoma is rare.

The massive type of hepatocellular carcinoma is most common in the noncirrhotic livers of younger individuals. It consists of a large, circumscribed mass occupying a significant proportion of the liver, often with smaller satellite nodules. The right hepatic lobe is affected more often, although this probably reflects the difference between the sizes of the two lobes. This form of hepatocellular carcinoma is the most prone to rupture.

The diffusely infiltrating variety is rare. A large part of the liver is homogeneously and widely infiltrated with indistinct minute tumor nodules, which may be difficult to distinguish from the regenerating nodules of the cirrhosis that almost invariably is present.

In the nodular and massive types, the tumor tissue is usually soft and bulges above the surrounding cut surface of the liver. Areas of necrosis and hemorrhage frequently are present. Well-differentiated tumors are light brown, whereas anaplastic tumors are yellowish-white or gray. Bile production may make the tumor greenish-brown. The portal vein and its tributaries frequently are occluded by the tumor. This occurs less often with the hepatic veins, but in these cases the tumor may grow into the inferior vena cava and even into the right atrium. In some livers the intrahepatic bile ducts are occluded by tumor.

Whether hepatocellular carcinoma is unicentric (with intrahepatic spread) or multicentric in origin is not known.

Microscopic Appearance. Hepatocellular carcinoma may be divided histologically into well-differentiated, moderately differentiated, and undifferentiated (anaplastic) forms.[95–98]

WELL-DIFFERENTIATED FORM. Despite the aggressive nature and poor prognosis of hepatocellular carcinomas, the majority are well differentiated. Well-differentiated hepatocellular carcinoma may be subdivided into a trabecular (or sinusoidal) subgroup and an acinar (or tubular) subgroup, although both growth patterns may be seen in the same tumor.

Trabecular. In the trabecular subgroup, the tumor cells grow in irregular, anstomosing plates separated by sinusoids, which are lined by flat endothelial cells that resemble Kupffer cells. The trabeculae resemble those in the normal adult liver (Fig. 45–6), but frequently they are thicker and may be composed of several layers. The sinusoids may be inconspicuous. Scanty collagen fibers may be present in relation to the sinusoidal walls. The malignant hepatocytes are polygonal, with an abundant slightly granular cytoplasm that is less eosinophilic than that of normal hepatocytes.

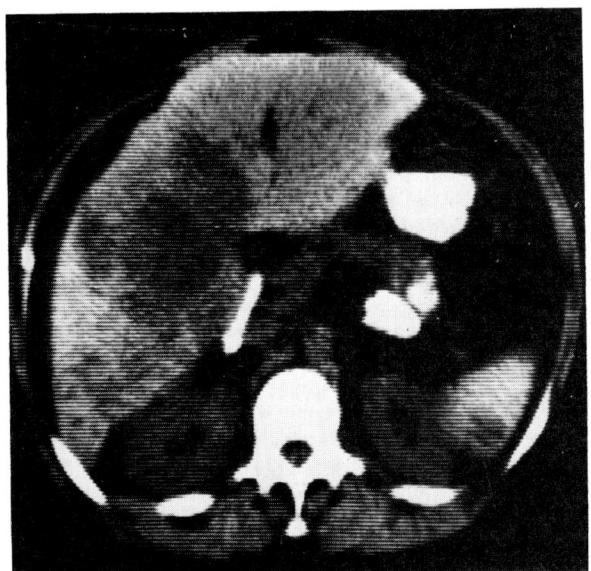

Figure 45-5. Computerized tomographic scan of a patient with a massive hepatocellular carcinoma, showing a large tumor mass in the right lobe of the liver. The left hepatic lobe appears to be free of tumor, and this was confirmed on hepatic arteriography. Surgical resection was not undertaken because macronodular cirrhosis was present in the non-tumorous liver.

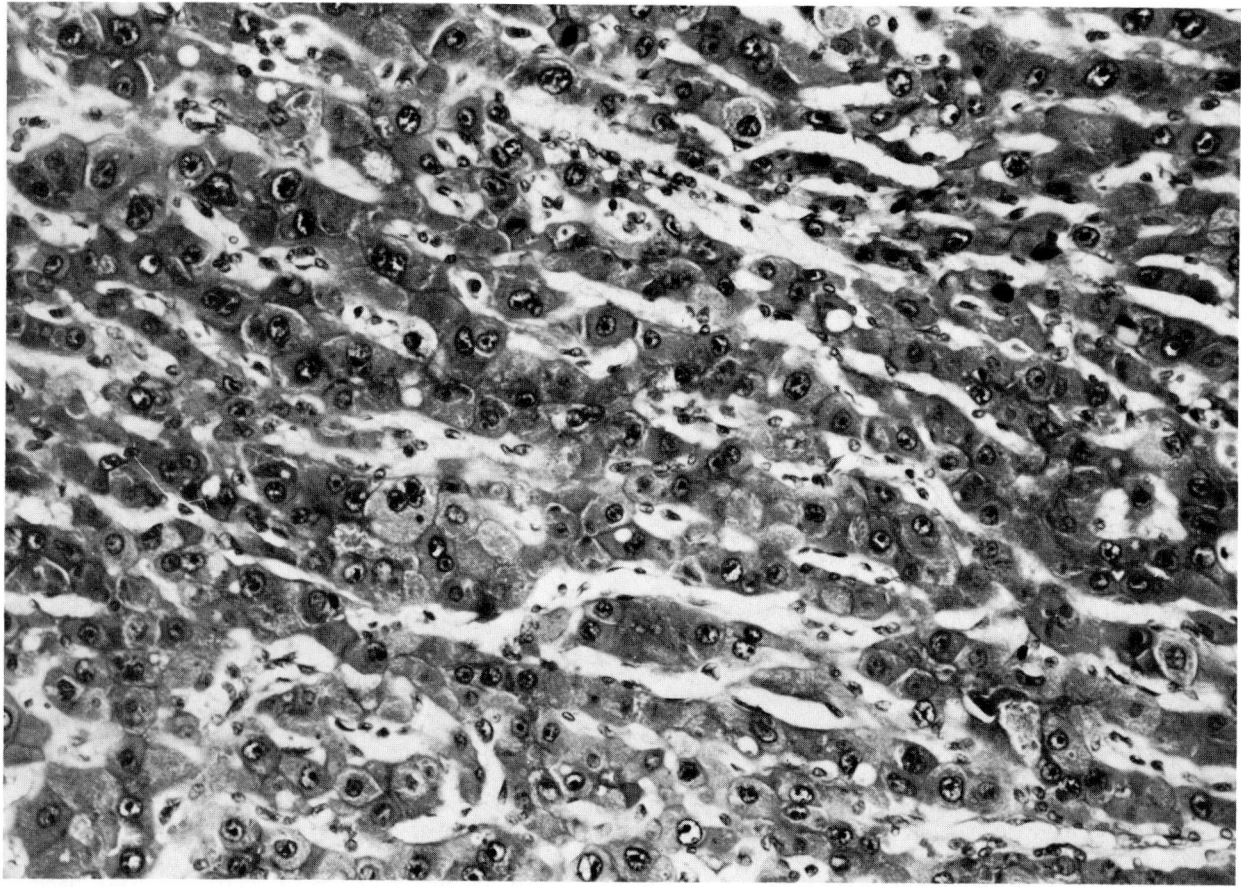

Figure 45–6. Trabecular hepatocellular carcinoma. The tumor cells are arranged in irregular anastomosing cords one or two cells thick. The sinusoids are lined by flattened endothelial cells. Hematoxylin and eosin, × 250.

The nuclei are large and hyperchromatic with well-defined nuclear membranes and prominent nucleoli (Fig. 45–6).

Acinar. In this form a variety of gland-like structures are present (Fig. 45–7). These are composed of layers of malignant hepatocytes surrounding the lumen of a bile canaliculus, which may be distended and may contain inspissated bile. Bile production is the hallmark of hepatocellular carcinoma, whatever the pattern. The individual cells resemble those of the trabecular form, although they may be more elongated and cylindrical (Fig. 45–7). A tubular or pseudopapillary appearance may be produced by degeneration and loss of cells, or cystic spaces may form in otherwise solid trabeculae. Occasionally, a follicular, thyroid-like appearance is produced.

MODERATELY DIFFERENTIATED FORM. Solid, scirrhous, and clear cell variants are described. In the *solid* form the cells are usually small, although they show marked variation in shapes, sizes, and staining qualities. The cytoplasm may contain small amounts of glycogen. Pleomorphic multinucleate giant cells are seen rarely. The tumor grows in solid masses or cell nests devoid of architectural arrangement. Bile canaliculi or signs of bile secretion are rare. Connective tissue is inconspicuous, and as the tumor grows, central ischemic necrosis is often found. In the *scirrhous* form, the malignant hepatocytes grow in narrow bundles separated by abundant fibrous stroma. Duct-like structures, which may be difficult to differentiate from real ducts, are present occasionally. In most cases the tumor cells resemble hepatocytes, although the resemblance varies with the degree of differentiation. Hepatocellular carcinoma may

also contain areas of *clear cells*; rarely, the tumor is predominantly or wholly composed of these cells. The clear appearance usually results from a high glycogen content but in some cases may be caused by fat.

UNDIFFERENTIATED FORM. The cells are pleomorphic, varying greatly in size, shape, and staining properties. The nuclei are likewise extremely variable. Large numbers of bizarre giant cells are present. The cells may be spindle-shaped, resembling those seen in sarcomas.

Globular hyaline structures may be seen in all forms of hepatocellular carcinoma. These may reflect the presence of α-fetoprotein, α_1-antitrypsin, or perhaps other proteins. Occasionally, Mallory's hyaline is seen.

Extrahepatic metastases are found frequently at necropsy. They are present in 40 to 57.5 per cent of all cases, but are more common in patients without cirrhosis (about 70 per cent) than in those with cirrhosis (about 30 per cent).[95–98] The most common sites are the lungs (about 50 per cent in some series) and the regional lymph nodes (about 20 per cent). Less frequent sites are bone and the adrenal glands.

FIBROLAMELLAR HEPATOCELLULAR CARCINOMA. This type of hepatocellular carcinoma typically occurs in young patients, has an approximately equal sex distribution, is not associated with α-fetoprotein secretion or with chronic hepatitis B virus infection, almost always arises in a noncirrhotic liver, is often amenable to resection, and carries a relatively good prognosis.[99, 100] Histologically it is characterized by plump, deeply eosinophilic hepatocytes encompassed by an abundant fibrous stroma composed of thin

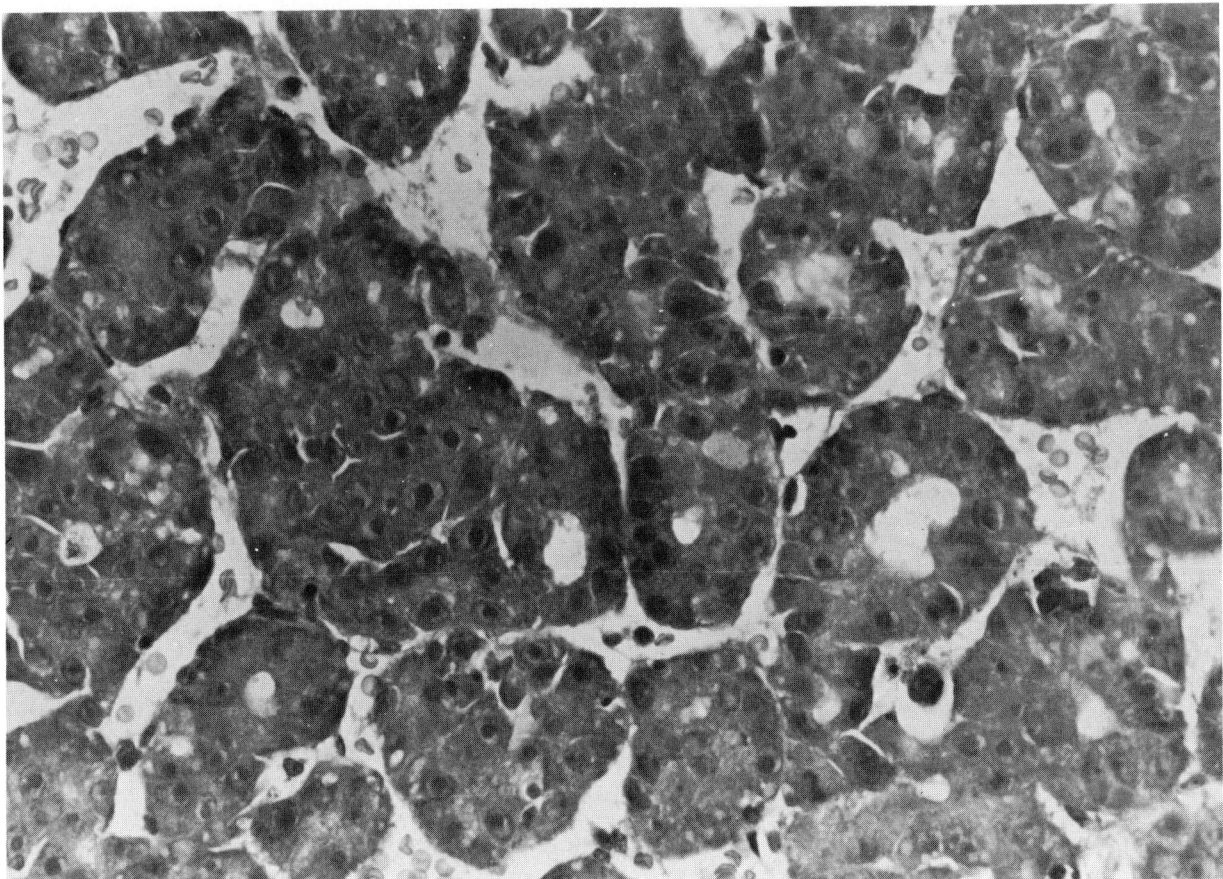

Figure 45–7. Well-differentiated hepatocellular carcinoma (acinar pattern), in which the tumor cells are arranged in small acini around a central lumen. The lumen is formed by a bile canaliculus, which may be distended and may contain bile. Hematoxylin and eosin, × 500.

parallel fibrous bands that separate the epithelial cells into trabeculae or large nodules[99, 100] (Fig. 45–8). The cytoplasm is packed with swollen mitochondria. In about one half of the tumors, the hepatocytes contain pale cytoplasmic bodies and hyaline bodies. Nucleoli are prominent, and mitoses are rare.

MIXED HEPATOCELLULAR CARCINOMA AND CHOLANGIOCARCINOMA. In about 4 per cent of hepatic carcinomas the histologic features of both hepatocellular carcinoma and cholangiocarcinoma are present in the same tumor.[101] This is not surprising, because hepatocytes and small bile ducts have a common origin, and the ability of each cell type to form the other is retained. Grossly, these tumors usually resemble hepatocellular carcinoma. The clinical features, natural history, and responses to treatment are also the same as those of hepatocellular carcinoma.

CHOLANGIOLOCELLULAR CARCINOMA. Higginson and Steiner described a carcinoma arising from the cholangioles (canals of Hering) under the term "cholangiolocellular carcinoma."[102] These tumors have been regarded, at least embryologically, as a subgroup of hepatocellular carcinoma, and they resemble the cholangiomatous part of the mixed tumor. In pure form, cholangiolocellular carcinoma is extremely rare, constituting only 1 per cent of primary hepatic carcinomas. Histologically, the tumor cells resemble the epithelial cells of cholangioles. They form double-layered, cuboidal epthelial cell cords with tiny lumens. The cytoplasm is scanty and pale and the nuclei are dark and oval without prominent nucleoli. However, in some parts of the tumor the cells resemble those of hepatocellular carcinoma, while in others they are like cholangiocarcinoma cells or

appear to be intermediate between the two. The malignant cells may grow along sinusoids.

Pathogenesis

Although the pathogenesis of hepatocellular carcinoma has not been elucidated, the available evidence suggests that more than one factor is involved and that the tumor has different causes in different parts of the world. Hepatocellular carcinoma seems to exist in two forms. In the industrialized, Western world this tumor is not common; it occurs predominantly in elderly people, with a slight male preponderance; it almost always arises as a complication of long-standing cirrhosis; the immunodiffusion test for α-fetoprotein is positive infrequently; and the tumor tends to be insidious in onset, runs a relatively benign course, may be resectable, and may respond at least partially to cancer chemotherapy.

On the other hand, in developing countries in sub-Saharan Africa and the Far East, where hepatocellular carcinoma is extremely common, it occurs in younger adults, with a more striking male predominance; it arises less frequently in a cirrhotic liver; the immunodiffusion test for α-fetoprotein is usually positive; onset is more acute; the tumor frequently develops extremely rapidly, does not appear to respond to cancer chemotherapeutic agents and rarely is resectable. It would not be surprising if different pathogenetic factors were operative in the two forms of the disease.

The peculiar geographic and cultural distribution of

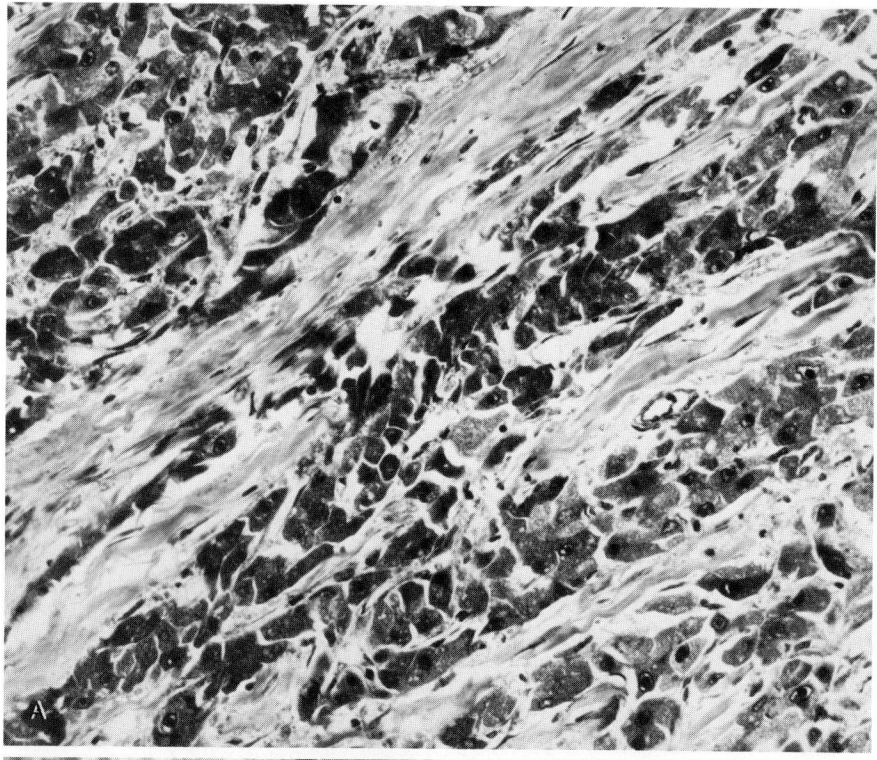

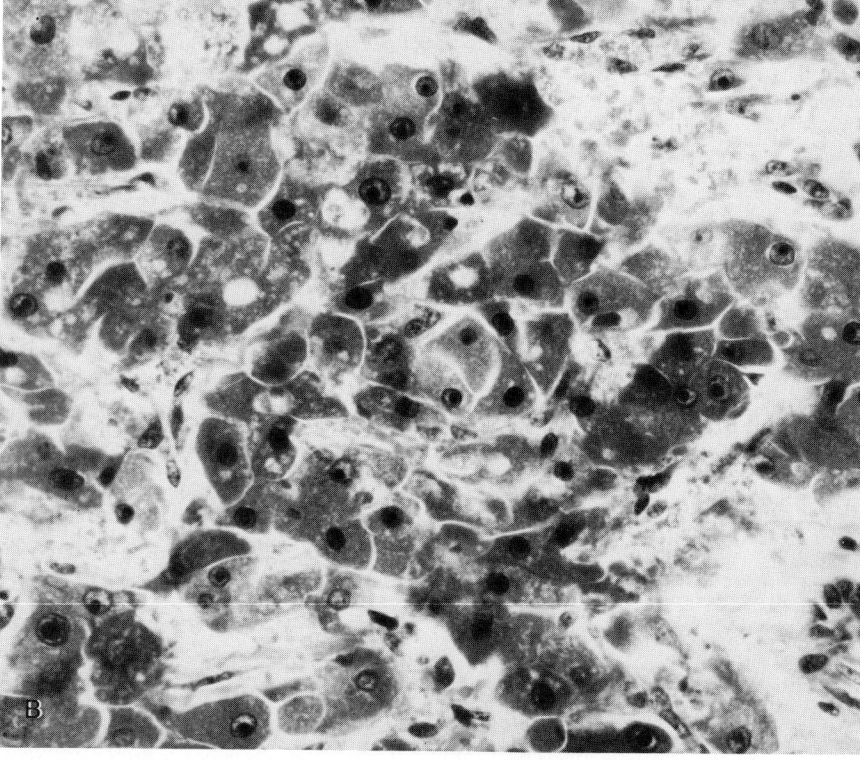

Figure 45–8. Fibrolamellar hepatocellular carcinoma. *A*, The tumor cells are encompassed by an abundant fibrous stroma composed of thin, parallel fibrous bands. Hematoxylin and eosin, × 250. *B*, The malignant hepatocytes are plump and have deeply eosinophilic cytoplasm. Cytoplasmic bodies are common, and nucleoli are prominent. Hematoxylin and eosin, × 400. (Courtesy Dr. A. Paterson.)

hepatocellular carcinoma, as well as the results of studies of incidences in migrant populations, suggests that the tumor is caused by one or more environmental carcinogens. There is no evidence for a major inherited component in human hepatocellular carcinoma, although genetic, immunologic and nutritional factors may play a contributory role or act indirectly by increasing susceptibility to environmental carcinogens.[103] Isolated cases of hepatocellular carcinoma in regions of low incidence have been reported in individuals with α_1-antitrypsin deficiency; but when large series of cancer patients have been studied, this inherited abnormality has not proved to be a significant pathogenetic factor.[104, 105] Patients with another rare inherited metabolic disorder, hemochromatosis, often develop hepatocellular carcinoma if they live long enough.[106] However, the neoplastic transformation appears to be related directly to the presence of cirrhosis, and it may be no more common in patients with hemochromatosis than in other cirrhotic male patients.[107] The related condition, hemosiderosis, which is common in southern African blacks, does not play a causative role in the high incidence of hepatocellular carcinomas in that population.[108] Hepatocellular carcinoma occurs rarely in patients with the inherited disorders of tyrosinemia, galactosemia, type I glycogenosis (see Chap. 49), or hereditary hemorrhagic telangiectasia.

The nature of the environmental pathogenetic agent or agents has not been established, but several minor and three major (chronic hepatitis B virus infection, aflatoxin ingestion, and cirrhosis) etiological associations have been identified.

Hepatitis B Virus Infection

Compelling evidence incriminates persistent hepatitis B virus (HBV) infection in the etiology of about 80 per cent of cases of hepatocellular carcinoma worldwide. This evidence can be summarized as follows.[109, 110]

There is a close geographical parallel between the incidence of hepatocellular carcinoma and the prevalence of the HBV carrier state. In regions of high incidence of the tumor, there are no exceptions to the correlation with a high HBV carrier rate, but in regions of low incidence there are one or two possible exceptions (Greenland and Chile) of relatively high HBV carrier rates and low incidences of hepatocellular carcinoma. We have shown recently in southern African blacks that when the HBV carrier rate decreases as a result of urbanization, the incidence of hepatocellular carcinoma shows a corresponding decrease.[111]

The great majority of Chinese and blacks with hepatocellular carcinoma show serologic markers of current HBV infection; almost all of the remainder have markers of past infection. In populations with a low incidence of the tumor, a lesser but still significant proportion of patients show these markers. Persistent HBV infection precedes the development of hepatocellular carcinoma by several years. Indeed, the HBV carrier state in both Chinese and blacks is established in the early years of childhood.[112, 113] Chinese infants are infected predominantly by perinatal transmission of the virus, with fewer children being infected later by "horizontal" means, whereas comparatively few black babies are infected perinatally. The majority of blacks become carriers as a result of horizontal infection, starting at about 11 months of age. This difference seems to be related to the replicative state of HBV in pregnant women; 40 per cent or more of Chinese women still have replicative infection (HBeAg-positive) at this time and are therefore

highly infectious,[112] compared with only about 14 per cent of black women.[113]

In a prospective study, Beasley and colleagues[114] showed that Taiwanese male carriers of HBV have a lifetime relative risk of developing hepatocellular carcinoma of 217, and that 40 per cent of these carriers will die as a result of the tumor or cirrhosis or both. Institutionalized mentally retarded HBV carriers in California have been shown to have a similar relative risk of developing hepatocellular carcinoma.[115]

During the past few years, molecular hybridization and gene cloning techniques have been used to demonstrate that HBV DNA is integrated into the human genome in the malignant cells of most (but not all) patients with HBV-related hepatocellular carcinoma.[116] (See Chap. 36). Integration is known to precede the development of the tumor. Although the sequence of cellular events leading to human hepatocellular carcinoma is not yet understood, these findings are consistent with, but do not prove, that HBV acts as a genotoxic initiator of hepatocarcinogenesis.

Indirect evidence for the hepatocarcinogenicity of HBV is provided by recent observations in the hepadna group of viruses (of which HBV is one). The American woodchuck, the Beechey ground squirrel, and the Pekin duck have been shown to be chronically infected with a virus that is morphologically and immunologically almost identical to HBV.[116] Chronically infected woodchucks in particular, and the ground squirrel and Pekin duck less frequently, develop hepatocellular carcinoma very similar to that which develops in human HBV carriers (See Chaps. 35 and 36).

The delta hepatitis virus plays no part in the pathogenesis of hepatocellular carcinoma,[117] possibly because patients with combined delta and hepatitis B virus infections die as a result of chronic hepatic parenchymal disease before the tumor has had time to develop. There is no evidence that the hepatitis A virus is implicated as a cause of hepatocellular carcinoma, although it is possible that the non-A, non B-hepatitis viruses may share the oncogenic potential of HBV.

Aflatoxins

Evidence of chemical hepatocarcinogenesis in man often remains indirect because no biologic stigmata have been identified that can be measured years after exposure. There is no unequivocal evidence at present that any single chemical agent causes human hepatocellular carcinoma.[118] Nevertheless, some data suggest that aflatoxin B_1, a metabolite of the fungus *Aspergillus flavus*, may play, either in combination with the hepatitis B virus or independently, an etiologic role in this tumor.[118, 119] Aflatoxin B_1 is the most potent known experimental hepatocarcinogen. Doses of the order of a few parts per billion produce liver cancers in susceptible animals. Aflatoxins B_2, G_1, and G_2 are also carcinogenic.[118, 119]

Aflatoxin B_1

Aspergillus flavus is ubiquitous in nature and contaminates many foodstuffs, including ground nuts, wheat, soya bean, corn, rice, barley, and cottonseed. The risk of contamination is greatest where storage conditions favor the growth of fungi. These conditions are found in many parts of the tropical world. Field studies in several parts of Africa and the Far East have shown a direct correlation between high incidences of hepatocellular carcinoma and contamination of staple foodstuffs by this mycotoxin.[118, 119] These studies assume that it is legitimate to compare current exposure to aflatoxin with present cancer rates on the basis that diet, food storage, and cooking habits have not changed in these rural areas. No correlation between aflatoxin ingestion and hepatocellular carcinoma incidence could be found, however, in studies in Hong Kong and Greece.[120, 121] Urinary excretion of aflatoxin M_1, a metabolite of aflatoxin B_1, is greatly increased in inhabitants of high tumor–risk areas in China, compared with people living in low-risk areas.[122] However, proof of a cause-and-effect relationship between ingestion of aflatoxin and the development of hepatocellular carcinoma is still lacking. This may be provided only by a study aimed at reducing aflatoxin exposure by lessening the fungal contamination of staple foods and observing the effect on the incidence of hepatocellular carcinoma.[123] Even if aflatoxin is shown to be pathogenetically important in developing countries, it seems unlikely that it plays a significant role in the "western" world.

Cirrhosis

The majority of patients who develop hepatocellular carcinoma in low-incidence regions do so against a background of long-standing cirrhosis (a few have chronic active hepatitis). Cirrhosis per se is without doubt the most important etiologic association of the tumor in these populations.[124, 125] In low-risk populations, alcohol abuse has long been considered to be the commonest cause of cirrhosis that is complicated by hepatocellular carcinoma.[124] Micronodular cirrhosis, which is most often caused by excessive alcohol consumption, is complicated by malignant transformation in 3 to 10 per cent of cases. However, macronodular cirrhosis also may occur with alcohol abuse; when hepatocellular carcinoma develops in chronic alcoholics, this type of cirrhosis is likely to be present. Abstinence after the onset of alcoholic cirrhosis was associated in one study with a higher frequency of macronodular cirrhosis and an increased risk of tumor formation,[126] compared with continued alcohol abuse and attendant micronodular cirrhosis. The likelihood of malignant transformation is related to the severity of the cirrhosis.[127] Alcohol has not been shown experimentally to be mutagenic and is unlikely to be an initiator of hepatocarcinogenesis. However, it could function as a promotor, acting in conjunction, for example, with the hepatitis B virus or with chemicals such as vinyl chloride. Alternatively, the apparent role of alcohol as a co-carcinogen could be explained by excessive alcohol ingestion causing cirrhosis.[124]

In developing countries with a high incidence of hepatocellular carcinoma, the associated cirrhosis almost always is the macronodular type,[124] but there is no evidence that the high incidence of the tumor in these areas can be explained solely by the high frequency of cirrhosis. Thus, hepatocellular carcinoma in the absence of cirrhosis is common in these regions.[14] The pathogenesis of malignant transformation in cirrhosis is not known. Two explanations have been suggested.[124] The first is that cirrhosis is itself a premalignant condition (i.e., hyperplasia leads to neoplasia

in the absence of additional factors). The second possible explanation is that the accelerated turn-over rate of hepatocytes in cirrhosis renders these cells more susceptible to environmental carcinogens (i.e., replication of DNA may take place before carcinogen-induced damage to it is repaired, resulting in permanently altered progeny).

Liver-Cell Dysplasia. Large parenchymal cells with bizarre hyperchromatic nuclei may be found commonly in cirrhotic livers and rarely in noncirrhotic livers.[128] These cells may be scattered randomly or may occur in groups. Sometimes, they occupy whole cirrhotic nodules. They occur more commonly in cirrhotic livers associated with hepatocellular carcinoma than in those without this complication. Moreover, patients who have dysplasia and cirrhosis are on the average ten years older than those with cirrhosis alone. Like hepatocellular carcinomas, dysplastic cells are more common in males. They may or may not be associated with the presence of markers of the hepatitis B virus in the liver tissue. The evidence available indicates that the presence of liver cell dysplasia reflects an increased likelihood of malignant change in cirrhosis.[128]

Steroids

In regions of low incidence of hepatocellular carcinoma, a few patients with aplastic anemia or hypogonadism, who have been treated with anabolic androgenic steriods for long periods, have developed hepatocellular carcinomas.[129, 130] There is also experimental evidence that male hormones may have etiologic significance in the causation of primary liver tumors.[131] The significance of recent reports of young women developing hepatocellular carcinomas while or after taking contraceptive steroids has yet to be evaluated. Certainly there is no evidence that either of these exogenous steroids plays a significant causative role in hepatocellular carcinoma in those parts of the world where this tumor is common.

Summary

The pathogenesis of hepatocellular carcinoma is almost certainly multifactorial, and the roles played by the various etiologic factors may vary in different parts of the world. In countries with high incidences, the dominant environmental carcinogens may be the hepatitis B virus and aflatoxins, which may act as cocarcinogens. The early onset of the disease in areas with high rates of hepatocellular carcinoma probably reflects a high intensity of exposure to environmental carcinogens from an early age. In the regions of low incidence alcoholic cirrhosis seems to be the most common predisposing condition, although the hepatitis B virus may be the causative agent in those cases not related to alcoholic cirrhosis.[124] Other chemicals, such as anabolic androgenic steroids and contraceptive steroids or industrial chemicals not yet identified, may be important in some cases, as may other factors such as α_1-antitrypsin deficiency and other inherited disorders. The male hormonal environment seems to play a promotive or permissive role.

Natural History

The natural history of the tumor in its florid form is one of rapid progression, with increasing pain and hepatomegaly, anorexia and profound cachexia, the development of tense ascites, and deepening jaundice. The cause of death is usually malignant cachexia, although the terminal event is not infrequently rupture of the tumor with massive hemoperitoneum.[16, 23–25] In some series liver failure or hematemesis has been a frequent cause of death.[28] In African and Oriental patients, death frequently ensues within four months of the onset of symptoms (the mean survival period in southern African blacks is 11.2 weeks from the onset of symptoms and 6.0 weeks from the time of diagnosis).[14] In Western countries the tumor has a somewhat more benign course, and prolonged survival may occur.[17, 22] In some instances the tumor is first detected either at laparotomy (done usually for some complication of cirrhosis) or at necropsy.

Treatment and Prognosis

Hepatocellular carcinoma has been regarded as a disease with a dismal prognosis. This view has arisen largely because the diagnosis is made at an advanced stage of the tumor, usually too late to allow for surgical resection, and the tumor burden is too massive for nonsurgical therapy to have a reasonable chance of succeeding. Some improvement in prognosis could be expected with earlier diagnosis.

The treatment of hepatocellular carcinoma depends on the extent of the disease and the presence or absence of underlying cirrhosis.

Surgical Resection

At present, surgical resection (segmentectomy, partial hepatectomy, hemihepatectomy, or extended hemihepatectomy) offers the only chance of cure of hepatocellular carcinoma (see Chap. 46). For resection to be possible, the tumor must be confined to one hepatic lobe, and the nontumorous liver should be free of cirrhosis. Segmentectomy or more extensive resections can be performed if the lesion is confined to the left lobe and if the cirrhosis in the right lobe is not considered severe.[132] Unfortunately, the proportion of patients with potentially resectable tumors is relatively small. Certainly, in sub-Saharan Africa fewer than 5 per cent of patients prove to have resectable tumors,[133] and the figure is 7 per cent in Malaysia.[134] This is so because the following features, singly or in combination, militate against resectability: involvement by tumor of both lobes of the liver; distant spread, particularly pulmonary metastases; invasion of portal veins, hepatic veins, or the inferior vena cava; ascites; poor liver function; poor general condition; and severe cirrhosis in the nontumorous part of the liver. The situation is less bleak in Taiwan[132] and Western countries,[135] where 9 to 37 per cent of patients are considered to have resectable tumors. Five-year survival rates of 16 to 23 per cent are recorded for hepatocellular carcinomas in these areas. In significant numbers of patients in the latter countries surgical resection is precluded by the underlying cirrhosis or other factors such as advanced age rather than by the extent of the tumor.

When rupture of the tumor has occurred, resection is the recommended treatment if it is possible. Unfortunately, at least in African patients, this is seldom the case. If resection is not feasible, ligation of the hepatic artery can be life-saving in the short term. However, the prognosis for patients in whom the tumor ruptures is especially grave.

In the case of small, early hepatocellular carcinomas detected in surveillance programs of individuals at high risk for developing this tumor, resection often is possible. Less extensive resections can be performed, making surgery feasible even in the presence of well-established cirrhosis.

Liver Transplantation

Liver transplantation (see Chap. 55) has been performed on patients in whom both lobes of the liver have been tumorous, when there was no evidence of spread beyond the liver.[136] A number of technical problems exist in the conduct of this operation, but the main problem has been recurrence of tumor in the transplanted liver in 70 per cent of cases.

Hepatic Dearterialization

Hepatic artery ligation or complete hepatic dearterialization has been tried when the tumor was considered to be unresectable.[134] The latter procedure involves ligating the hepatic artery close to the porta hepatis and completely dearterializing the liver by tying off all the peripheral feeding arteries. The technique originally was performed once. More recently, repeated devascularization procedures have been carried out so that the collateral vessels that form can be ligated. Prolonged survival has been reported for some patients.[134] This operation may be technically impossible when the liver is enlarged massively. Both of these procedures are contraindicated in the presence of cirrhosis because of the poor functional reserve of the cirrhotic liver and its inability to regenerate, and because of the diversion of portal venous blood from the liver through portal-systemic collateral vessels.

Direct Hepatic Arterial Infusion of Drugs

This form of therapy is based also on the fact that hepatocellular carcinoma derives its blood supply from the hepatic artery.[81] Many problems are associated with this mode of treatment, including a high incidence of technical difficulties (maintaining the catheter in position and patent; avoiding infection), frequent toxic effects, and the need for continuous hospitalization and close monitoring of the patient.[137–139] However, worthwhile palliation can be achieved with intra-arterial chemotherapy.[137, 139] The drugs used have been 5-fluorouracil, methotrexate, 5-fluorodeoxyuridine, adriamycin, and mitomycin C.

External Irradiation

Early results in patients from areas with a low incidence of hepatocellular carcinoma suggested that the tumor might be radiosensitive. For example, Ariel[140] claimed symptomatic improvements lasting 9 to 50 months in five of ten patients. However, radiotherapists in Africa and the Far East have not been able to reproduce these encouraging results, even using telecobalt therapy.[141] Even when radiotherapy has been combined with chemotherapy in the form of procarbazine or hydroxyurea, the survival rates have not been greater than those achieved with placebo therapy.[141] In a recent study in the United Kingdom, patients receiving radiotherapy followed by quadruple chemotherapy did not survive as long as patients receiving the quadruple chemotherapy alone.[142]

Immunotherapy

There is no clinical role for immunotherapy at present.

Chemotherapy

5-Fluorouracil given intravenously and quadruple parenteral chemotherapy with 5-fluorouracil, cyclophosphamide, methotrexate, and vincristine have produced some prolongation of life in patients in Western countries.[142] However, a whole host of alkylating agents and antimetabolites, alone and in combination, have been tried in Africa and the Far East, without significant response.[141] Orally administered 5-fluorouracil universally has been shown to be of no value. Adriamycin was reported by Olweny et al. to produce remissions in 11 of 11 Ugandan patients (median survival time, eight months).[143] Although an anti-tumor effect was confirmed, response rates were substantially lower in two studies in the United States and in two others in which the subjects were American and African patients.[144–146] In the United Kingdom, adriamycin has been reported to induce clinical remission in 32 per cent of patients.[147] More recently, VP 16 has been shown to have a similar response rate (18%) to adriamycin, although the duration of response was shorter with VP 16.[148] The addition of methyl—CCNU to adriamycin did not increase either response rate or survival compared with adriamycin alone.[149] Disappointing results were obtained with m-AMSA.[150] In a non-randomized trial in Greece it was found that urea given orally increased the survival times of patients with hepatocellular carcinomas,[151] but these results could not be confirmed in black patients.

In a few patients, selective embolization, with gelatin foam, of the arteries supplying the tumor has been used to reduce the viable tumor mass before the initiation of cancer chemotherapy.[152]

CHOLANGIOCARCINOMA

Cholangiocarcinomas may arise from either small peripheral intrahepatic bile ducts (peripheral cholangiocarcinoma) or large bile ducts. Both the major intrahepatic bile ducts (hilar cholangiocarcinoma) and the extrahepatic bile ducts (bile duct carcinoma) can be the sites of origin.

Occurrence and Pathogenesis

Incidences of cholangiocarcinoma differ in different parts of the world, although not to the same extent as incidences of hepatocellular carcinoma.[153] Frequency rates relative to hepatocellular carcinoma range from 5 to 30 per cent.[153] The higher ratios occur in parts of the Far East where this tumor has been shown to be associated with chronic infestation of the biliary tree with *Chlonorchis sinensis* and *Opisthorchis viverrini*.[154, 155] Cholangiocarcinoma occasionally has developed years after the administration of thorium dioxide,[156] and a few cases in patients with α_1-antitrypsin deficiency[157] have been described. Hilar cholangiocarcinoma has occurred in patients with long-standing ulcerative colitis, Crohn's disease,[158] congenital biliary atresia[159] or other developmental abnormalities of the bile ducts[160] and has been associated with gallstones in the intrahepatic bile ducts.[161] Cholangiocarcinoma is associated with cirrhosis in the nontumorous parts of the liver less often than is the case with hepatocellular carcinoma.[162, 163] There is no known association with chronic hepatitis B virus infection or exposure to mycotoxins.

Cholangiocarcinoma occurs particularly in older individuals, the average age at onset being about 60 years; it is rare before the age of 40 years.[164–166] Although men are affected more often than women, the male predominance is not as striking as that associated with hepatocellular carcinoma.[164, 167]

Presentation

The signs and symptoms of the peripheral type of cholangiocarcinoma are similar to those of hepatocellular carcinoma, except that jaundice may be an earlier, more prominent, and more frequent feature in the former.[153, 164] Other differences are that the liver tends to be less enlarged, a bruit is not heard, ascites is less common, signs of portal hypertension are absent, and fever and extrahepatic metastases are less frequent in the patients with cholangiocarcinoma. With hilar cholangiocarcinoma the clinical presentation is one of progressive obstructive jaundice, with or without weight loss.[153, 164, 168]

Investigations

Neither type of cholangiocarcinoma produces α-fetoprotein.[164, 165] Peripheral cholangiocarcinoma may be characterized biochemically by higher concentrations of bilirubin and alkaline phosphatase in serum, but is otherwise similar to hepatocellular carcinoma.[164] With hilar cholangiocarcinoma the biochemical picture is that of obstructive jaundice.[164] By isotopic hepatic scanning and computerized axial tomography, peripheral cholangiocarcinoma is similar to hepatocellular carcinoma. Larger hilar lesions may also be seen with these techniques. Ultrasonography may show dilated intrahepatic ducts with hilar cholangiocarcinoma, and transhepatic or endoscopic retrograde cholangiography will localize the site of the tumor. A characteristic picture is seen on hepatic arteriography in the peripheral type of cholangiocarcinoma. The marked desmoplastic reaction that often occurs with this tumor causes the branches of the hepatic artery to appear scanty, stretched out, and attenuated.[169]

Cholangiocarcinoma occasionally produces hypercalcemia in the absence of osseous metastases. This has been shown, in one patient at least, to result from ectopic production of immunoreactive parathormone by the tumor.[35]

Pathology

Peripheral cholangiocarcinoma usually forms a large solitary tumor, but a multinodular type may occur. Because of the fibrous stroma, peripheral cholangiocarcinoma is grayish-white in color and firm in consistency.[153, 162, 167] The tumor is not well vascularized, and hemorrhage into it is uncommon. It rarely ruptures. Vascular invasion and tumor necrosis are seen less commonly than in hepatocellular carcinoma. Cirrhosis is present infrequently in the nontumorous parts of the liver. Hilar cholangiocarcinoma may take the form of a firm, intramural, annular tumor encircling the bile duct, a bulky hard mass centered on the duct or hilar region and radiating into the hepatic substance, or a spongy, friable mass within the lumen of the bile duct.[168] Metastatic nodules may be distributed irregularly through the liver. The bile ducts peripheral to the tumor may be dilated, and in long-standing cases biliary cirrhosis may be present.

Microscopically, cholangiocarcinomas have acinar or tubular structures resembling those of other adenocarcinomas[153, 162, 167, 168] (Fig. 45–9). Most are well differentiated, although not to the extent seen in bile duct adenoma. The cells are cuboidal or columnar. The cytoplasm is eosinophilic and usually clear, but it may be granular. The

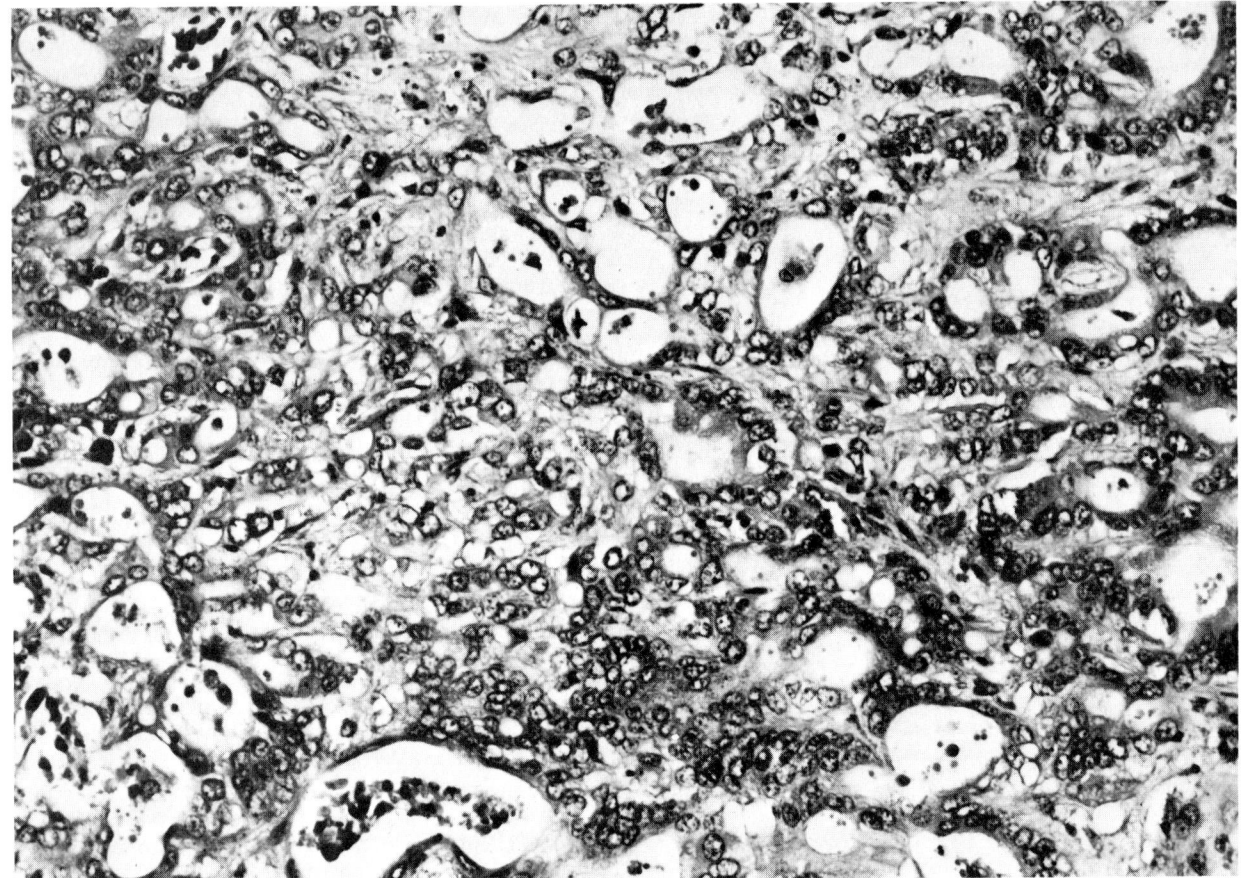

Figure 45–9. Peripheral cholangiocarcinoma, showing acinar structures. A moderate amount of collagenous stroma is present between the duct-like structures. Hematoxylin and eosin, × 250.

nuclei are smaller and more uniform in size than are those in hepatocellular carcinoma. There may be papillary infolding in some tumors. Secretion of mucus may be demonstrable, but bile production is never seen. Mitotic figures are infrequent. The tumor cells provoke a variable desmoplastic reaction, and in many cases, collagenized stroma may be the most prominent feature. In patients infected chronically with hepatic flukes, premalignant changes in the bile ducts consist of hyperplasia and adenomatous proliferation of the epithelial lining.

Peripheral cholangiocarcinoma often is complicated by intrahepatic metastases and tumor growth along the biliary tracts.[153] Metastases in hilar and peripancreatic lymph nodes occur in about 50 per cent of cases.[153, 167] Spread via the blood stream occurs less commonly than in hepatocellular carcinoma.[153]

Treatment and Prognosis

Early diagnosis of peripheral cholangiocarcinoma is seldom achieved. This tumor carries the same poor prognosis as does hepatocellular carcinoma.[153, 164] Surgical resection is rarely possible. The results of radiation therapy and cancer chemotherapy are poor. Surgical resection of hilar cholangiocarcinoma may be feasible, depending upon its position and size. Even when inoperable, hilar cholangiocarcinoma tends to progress more slowly than does peripheral cholangiocarcinoma.[170] In inoperable cases, biliary drainage with a U-tube or biliary stent should be performed to relieve the obstructive jaundice.

HEPATOBLASTOMA

Occurrence

Hepatoblastoma, a malignant embryonal tumor of the liver, occurs almost exclusively in the first three years of life.[171–173] Ocasionally, the tumor attains a considerable size in the fetus and is detected at birth. Hepatoblastoma is the most common hepatic tumor in children but is exceedingly rare in adults.[174] Boys are affected about twice as often as girls.

Presentation

The great majority of patients with hepatoblastoma are brought to the physician because of abdominal swelling.[171–173] Other complaints include loss of weight or failure to gain weight, poor appetite, abdominal pain, irritability, and intermittent vomiting and diarrhea. The liver is almost invariably enlarged. The tumor is usually felt in the right hypochondrium or epigastrium, but more massive tumors may occupy the right upper and lower quadrants or even the whole abdomen. The liver feels firm and has a smooth or nodular surface; it may be tender. Pallor is common, but the patient is seldom jaundiced. Hepatoblastomas occasionally rupture, producing the symptoms and signs of an abdominal emergency. The tumor rarely causes isosexual precocious puberty in boys as a result of ectopic secretion of human chorionic gonadotropin.[40] Developmental malformations such as hemihypertrophy, macroglossia, or cardiac defects may coexist with the tumor.[175]

Investigations

Alpha-fetoprotein is present in high concentrations in the sera of 80 to 90 per cent of patients who have hepatoblastomas and serves as a useful diagnostic pointer.[176] Changes in hepatic function are slight and nonspecific.[171, 173] Rarely, plain abdominal radiographs show mottled calcification in the tumor. Pulmonary metastases may be seen on chest radiography. The tumor is visualized as a defect on isotopic hepatic scanning, and as an avascular mass on hepatic arteriography. In neither instance is the appearance specific to hepatoblastoma. Anemia is common[171–173] and both high[175] and low[173] platelet counts have occasionally been recorded.

Pathology

Hepatoblastomas are classified morphologically as (1) an epithelial type, composed predominantly of epithelial cells varying in maturity, and (2) a mixed epithelial and mesenchymal type that contains, in addition, tissues of mesenchymal derivation.[171] Both types occur in an otherwise normal liver.[171–173, 177]

The tumors, which are usually solitary, range in largest diameters from 5 to 25 cm, and arise most often in the right lobe of the liver.[171–173, 177, 178] Hepatoblastomas are always well circumscribed, and about half are encapsulated. Microscopic intravascular spread beyond an encapsulated tumor may be found. The epithelial type of hepatoblastoma is usually surrounded by a pseudocapsule composed of reticulin and collagen fibers. Collagenous septa contain vessels, lymphatics, and small immature bile ducts. Mixed hepatoblastomas are frequently lobulated, the lobules being separated by white bands of collagenous tissue. The lobules vary in color from tan to grayish-white and contain foci of hemorrhage, necrosis, or calcification. Prominent vascular channels may be present on the capsular surface. The cut surfaces of epithelial hepatoblastomas are more uniform. These tumors are solid, similar in color to mixed hepatoblastomas, and they, too, show areas of hemorrhage or necrosis.

Two types of epithelial cells are present in hepatoblastomas.[171, 172, 177] The first resembles fetal hepatocytes (Fig. 45–10). These cells are smaller than normal hepatocytes and are arranged in irregular plates, usually two cells thick, with bile canaliculi between individual cells and sinusoids between the plates. Their cytoplasm is eosinophilic and appears slightly granular or vacuolated. Few mitotic figures are seen. Extramedullary hematopoiesis usually is present in areas containing fetal-type cells. The embryonal type of epithelial cell is far more poorly differentiated (Fig. 45–11). These cells show weak cohesiveness and are usually arranged in sheets or ribbons; acinar, pseudorosette, or papillary formations are sometimes present. The cells are small, fusiform, and dark-staining with irregular, poorly defined outlines. The cytoplasm is scanty and amphophilic. Nuclei contain abundant chromatin, and large nucleoli may

be present. The embryonal cells show far more mitotic activity than do fetal-type cells.

In addition to collagenous septa, supporting reticulin fibers, blood vessels supplying the tumor, and hematopoietic foci, mixed hepatoblastomas contain other mesenchymal elements. These include areas of a highly cellular "primitive" type of mesenchyme intimately admixed with the epithelial elements (Fig. 45–10). The cells are elongated and spindle-shaped, with delicate processes arising from the tapering ends. Cytoplasm is scanty and the nuclei are elongated but plump with rounded ends. These tumors also contain areas in which the cells are intermediate between primitive mesenchyme and the acellular collagen of the fibrous septa. These areas include an "immature" type of mesenchyme of moderate cellularity, in which the cells show a parallel orientation and resemble young fibroblasts. Collagen fibers are present between the cells. Very occasionally the cells are arranged loosely and have a myxomatous appearance. Osteoid tissue is present in most mixed hepatoblastomas, often in large amounts (Fig. 45–12). Cartilage may be present, as may striated muscle. Hepatoblastomas may show foci of squamous cells with or without keratinization, and giant cells of the foreign-body type may occur in relation to these foci. Vascular invasion may be seen. Metastases, when present, most commonly involve the lung, abdominal lymph nodes, and brain.

Treatment and Prognosis

Hepatoblastoma is a rapidly progressive tumor. The pure fetal hepatoblastoma has the least favorable prognosis, with the embryonal and mixed types carrying equally grave prognoses.[178] If the lesion is solitary and is sufficiently localized to be resectable, surgery may be curative.[173, 178] In some patients in whom the tumor is regarded initially as being unresectable, chemotherapy (cyclophosphamide, vincristine, 5-fluorouracil, adriamycin, and cisplatin have been used) with or without radiotherapy has resulted in sufficient reduction in the size of the tumor for resection to become possible.[179, 180] If surgery is not feasible, the prognosis is very poor, as hepatoblastomas do not respond consistently to radiotherapy or to currently available cancer chemotherapeutic drugs.

ANGIOSARCOMA

Occurrence

Angiosarcoma (also known as hemangiosarcoma, malignant hemangioendothelioma, or Kupffer cell sarcoma) is an extremely rare hepatic tumor. Only one hepatic angiosarcoma was found in 50,000 necropsies,[162] and it has been estimated that each year fewer than 25 cases occur in North America[181] and only one or two in Britain.[182] Nevertheless, angiosarcoma is the most common of the malignant mesenchymal tumors of the liver. It occurs almost exclusively in adults and reaches its greatest incidence in the sixth and seventh decades of life.[183, 184] Men are affected four times more often than women.[183, 184]

Pathogenesis

In spite of its rarity, hepatic angiosarcoma is of special interest because specific carcinogens have been identified.

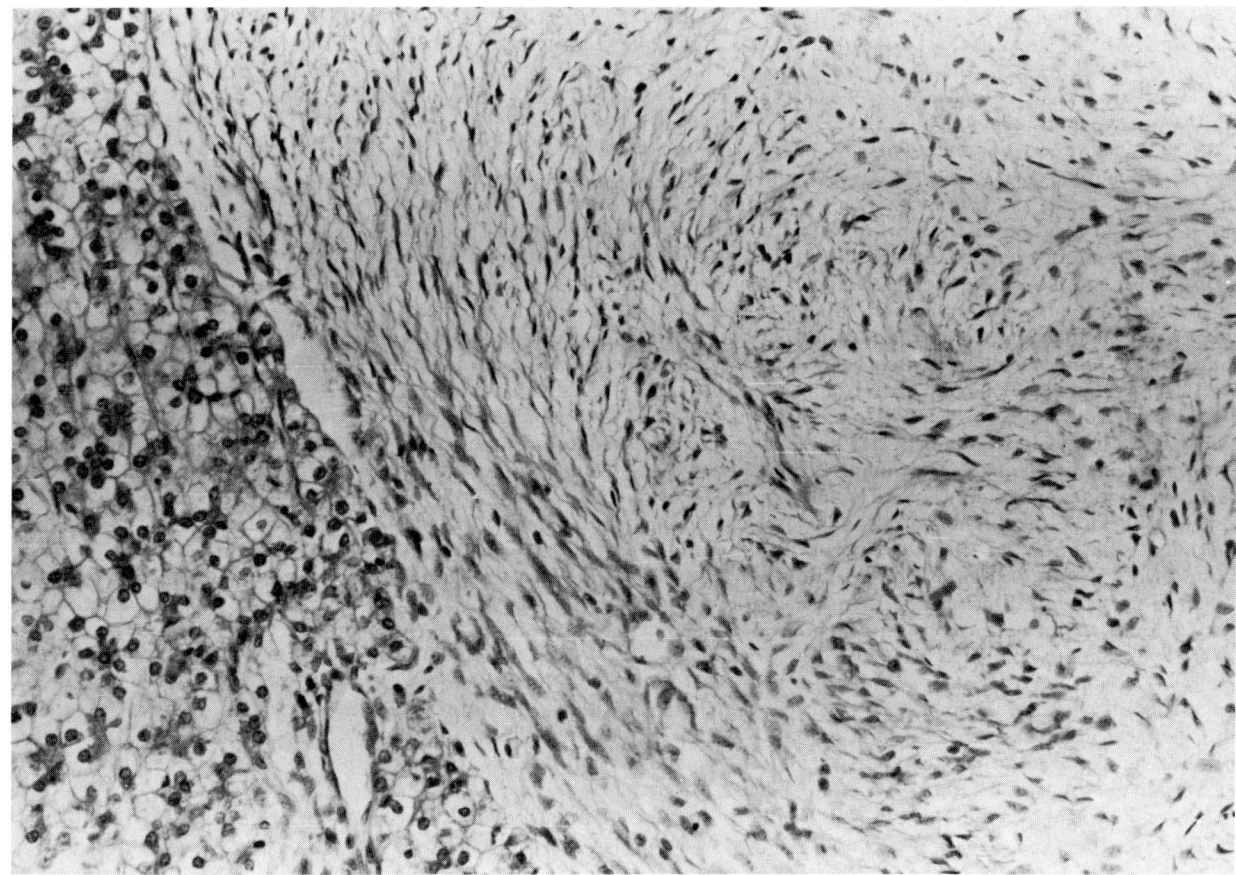

Figure 45–10. Mixed hepatoblastoma, showing a fetal type of epithelial cell on the left side of the photomicrograph, with an area of primitive mesenchymal tissue immediately adjacent. Hematoxylin and eosin, × 250.

In many of the recorded cases of hepatic angiosarcoma, particularly in the early literature, the tumor appeared about 20 years after the patient had been exposed to thorium dioxide.[185, 186] Thorotrast, a 20 per cent solution of thorium dioxide, was used extensively as a radiographic contrast material between 1930 and the mid-1950s, and at least 50,000 patients received injections of this substance. Thorium dioxide was deposited throughout the reticuloendothelial system, but especially in the liver. Its rate of excretion was negligible, the calculated biological half-life being around 400 years. Thorium and its daughter nuclides emit substantial amounts of alpha, beta, and gamma radiation over many years.

Angiosarcoma of the liver also occurred in German vintners who, until 1942, made use of arsenic-containing insecticides and who also drank wine adulterated with arsenic.[187] A few patients with angiosarcoma of the liver had taken potassium arsenite (Fowler's) solution for many years as treatment of psoriasis.[188]

The first cases of hepatic angiosarcoma occurring in vinyl chloride workers were reported in North America in 1974.[189] Since then, cases in Germany, Sweden, Canada, and Great Britain, as well as additional cases from North America, have been described. Vinyl chloride ($H_2C=CHC1$), a gaseous chemical, is used in the manufacture of synthetic rubber, spray paints, and insecticide aerosols. It is polymerized to polyvinyl chloride resin, paste, and latex. Vinyl chloride is transformed by enzymes of the endoplasmic reticulum to mutagenic and potentially oncogenic metabolites, which bind covalently to DNA.

In many of the recently reported cases, patients with hepatic angiosarcoma had been involved in the polymerization of vinyl chloride monomers for periods ranging from 11 to 37 years or had had initial periods of heavy exposure some years before.[181, 190, 191] The mean age at diagnosis was 48 years. It has been estimated that the incidence of hepatic angiosarcoma is 400 times greater in exposed than in nonexposed individuals. A cause-and-effect relationship between exposure to vinyl chloride monomers and angiosarcoma of the liver is supported by the experimental finding that these tumors can be induced in rats by exposing them to gaseous vinyl chloride.[192] There is at present no evidence to incriminate the finished polymer, polyvinyl chloride, in the pathogenesis of the tumor.

In addition to angiosarcoma, a variety of other disturbances, including acro-osteolysis, scleroderma-like skin lesions, Raynaud's phenomenon, circulatory disturbances, and hepatic fibrosis with consequent portal hypertension, have been reported to occur in vinyl chloride workers.[193–195] There appears also to be an increased incidence of tumors in other tissues such as the lung and brain.[183]

Other substances that have been implicated in the causation of hepatic angiosarcoma are radium,[196] inorganic copper,[197] and the monoamine oxidase inhibitor, phenethylhydrazine.[198] The tumor also has been reported to develop in patients with idiopathic hemochromatosis.[199] Although progress has been made in identifying pathogenetic factors in angiosarcoma, the majority of cases still have no discernible cause.

Presentation

The main initial symptom is abdominal pain or discomfort, but other frequent complaints are abdominal swelling,

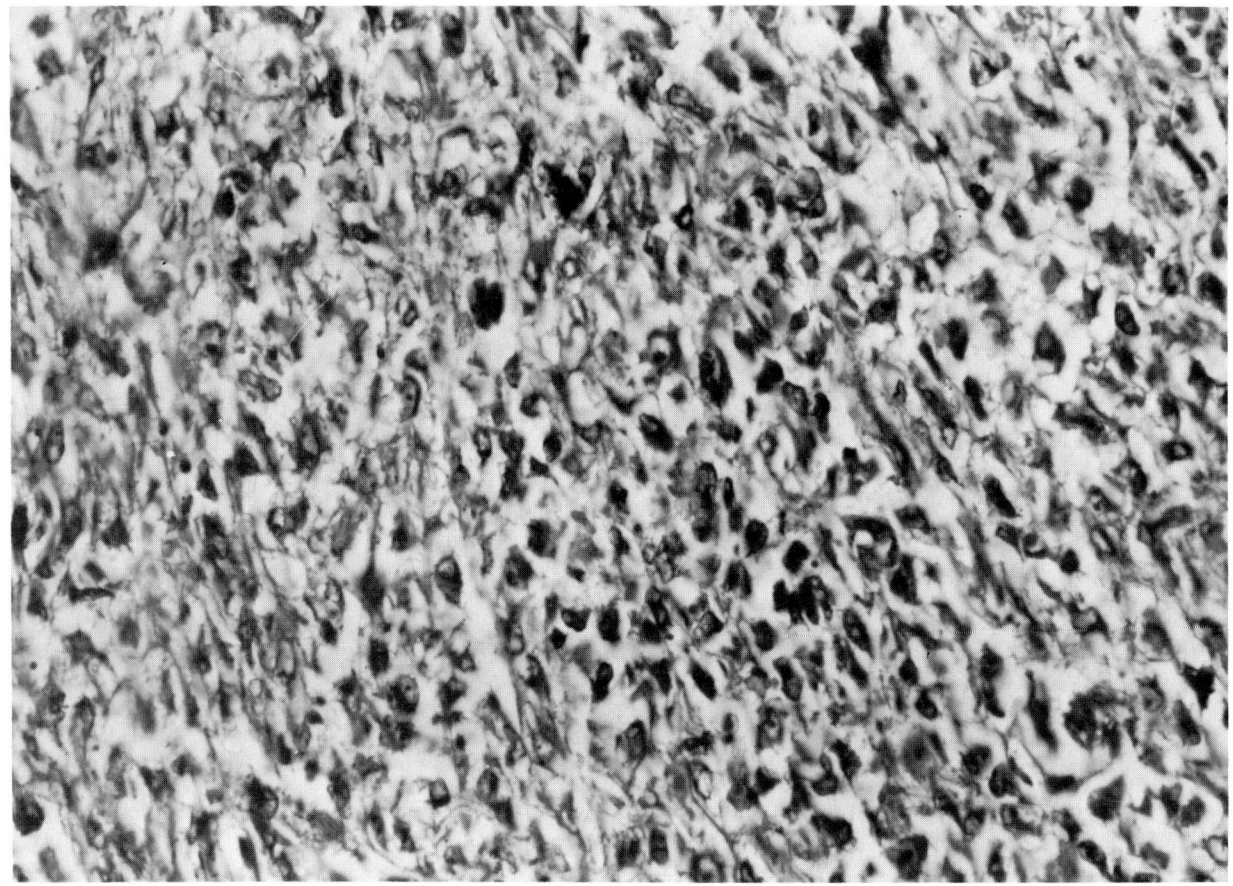

Figure 45–11. Embryonal epithelial cells in a mixed hepatoblastoma (from the same case illustrated in Figs. 41–10 and 41–12). Hematoxylin and eosin, × 500.

rapidly progressive liver failure, malaise, weakness, weight loss, anorexia, and nausea.[183, 184, 200, 201] Vomiting is present occasionally. The duration of symptoms usually is one week to six months, but a few patients have been symptomatic for as long as two years.

The liver is almost always enlarged. The surface may be nodular or a definite mass may be felt in the liver, which usually is tender.[183, 184, 200, 201] An arterial bruit occasionally is heard over the liver. Splenomegaly may be present, although this is attributable to the associated hepatic fibrosis and portal hypertension rather than to the tumor itself. Ascites is not infrequent, and the fluid may be bloodstained. The patient is often jaundiced. Fever and dependent edema are found less frequently. A few patients (about 15 per cent) seek treatment because of acute hemoperitoneum caused by rupture of the tumor. Rarely, pulmonary or skeletal metastases are present.

Investigations

A rising serum bilirubin concentration and other evidence of progressive hepatic dysfunction may be present, particularly in the later stages of the disease. Rarely, plain radiographs of the abdomen show flecks of calcification in the tumor; in those patients in whom the hepatic angiosarcoma has followed exposure to thorium dioxide, radiopaque deposits of this material may be seen in the liver and spleen. Chest radiographs may show pulmonary metastases or an elevated right hemidiaphragm. Skeletal metastases are seen occasionally. One or more defects may be present

on a hepatic scan, but with the diffusely infiltrating variety of angiosarcoma the picture may be one of patchy uptake of the isotope.[202] Hepatic arteriography reveals a characteristic appearance.[203] The hepatic arteries are normal in size but may be displaced by the tumor. The tumor shows a blush and "puddling" during the middle of the arterial phase, persisting for many seconds, except in the central area, which may be hypovascular.

Percutaneous biopsy is contraindicated because of the vascular nature of the tumor and because of the possibility of a complicating thrombocytopenia or disseminated intravascular coagulation.

Complications and Prognosis

Angiosarcoma of the liver grows rapidly and carries a poor prognosis.[183, 184, 200, 201] Untreated, most patients die within six months of admission to the hospital. The only long-term survivors have had the tumor resected. The cause of death usually is hepatic failure or malignant cachexia, although patients may die as a result of rupture of the tumor. Distant metastases occur in about 50 per cent of patients. The diagnosis is made before the patient's death in only about a third of cases.

Patients with hepatic angiosarcoma often have thrombocytopenia[183, 199, 203] caused by entrapment of platelets within the tumor. Rarer complications are disseminated intravascular coagulation with secondary fibrinolysis[203, 204] and a microangiopathic hemolytic anemia resulting from fragmentation of erythrocytes within the tumor circula-

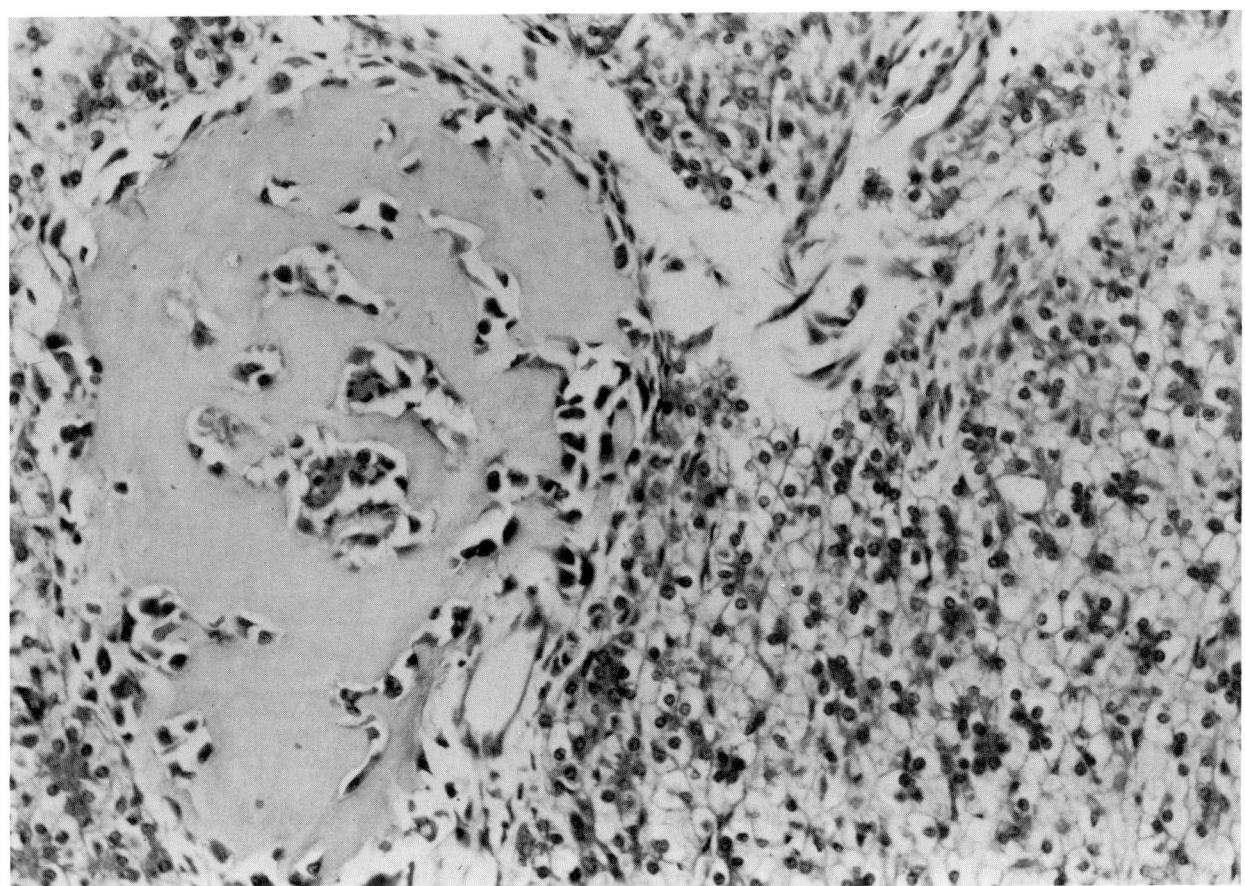

Figure 45–12. Mixed hepatoblastoma, showing osteoid formation in an area of fetal-type epithelial cells. Hematoxylin and eosin, × 250.

tion.[203, 205, 206] An occasional patient has had hypercalcemia in the absence of osseous metastases.[183]

Pathology

Angiosarcomas are usually multicentric and involve both lobes of the liver.[183, 184, 200, 201, 203] The hallmark of these tumors, visible to the unaided eye, is blood-filled cysts, which may be as large as several centimeters in diameter. Thus, the tumor can be mistaken for peliosis hepatis. However, solid tumor growth is always present, varying from minute foci to large nodules. Although fairly well circumscribed, the lesions are not encapsulated. The larger masses are spongy and may bulge beneath Glisson's capsule.

The earliest microscopic change is the appearance of hypertrophied sinusoidal epithelial lining cells with hyperchromatic nuclei.[162, 184, 201, 203] These are usually seen as ill-defined foci but may occur diffusely throughout the liver. With progression of the lesion, the size and the extent of nuclear polychromasia of the cells, sinusoidal dilatation, and disruption of the pattern of the hepatic plates increase. As the plates become separated by the malignant endothelial cells, larger sinusoidal spaces are formed. Hepatocytes surrounded by sarcomatous cells undergo progressive atrophy. Initially the malignant cells are supported by a single layer of reticulin fibers, but as the tumor nodule grows the deposition of collagen increases. The collagen eventually completely replaces the atrophied hepatocytes. With enlargement of the vascular spaces, lined by malignant cells,

the tumor becomes obviously cavernous. The cells lining these spaces may form a single layer, but more frequently they are multilayered or project into the cavity in intricate fronds and tufts supported by fibrous tissue.

The malignant endothelial cells are usually elongated and have ill-defined borders. The cytoplasm is clear and faintly eosinophilic. The nuclei are hyperchromatic and vary greatly in size and shape. Chromatin granules are fine, and the nucleoli small and amphophilic. Bizarre cells with irregular, intensely hyperchromatic nuclei or multinucleated cells may be present. The cells may show evidence of phagocytic properties.[207]

Neoplastic invasion of the portal vein or central veins is seen in the majority of cases. This occurs within the tumor nodules but also in distant hepatic lobules. Foci of extramedullary hematopoiesis are seen frequently.[162, 184] Hemosiderosis secondary to a microangiopathic hemolytic anemia may be present.[205] Angiosarcomas induced by thorium dioxide, arsenic, or vinyl chloride often show fibrosis or cirrhosis in the non-neoplastic tissue. Concomitant cirrhosis is present in a third of the idiopathic cases. There is no morphologic difference between the tumors associated with definite causative agents and idiopathic tumors.

Treatment

Attempts to treat hepatic angiosarcomas have been unsuccessful.[184] Operative treatment frequently is precluded by the advanced stage of these tumors when the patients are first seen for treatment. There are occasional reports of long-term survival after partial hepatectomy, but more usually the patient survives only one to three years after the operation.[184] Results of radiation therapy and chemotherapy have been disappointing.[184]

EPITHELIOID HEMANGIOENDOTHELIOMA

This rare tumor pursues a course intermediate between those of hepatic angiosarcoma and hemangioma. Metastases occur in about 20 per cent of patients. The tumor affects adults, especially women, and presents with upper abdominal discomfort or pain, weight loss, or nonspecific gastrointestinal symptoms. An upper abdominal mass is the usual finding, and about 20 per cent of patients are jaundiced.[208] The tumors are often multiple and are generally firm and white. Microscopically, two types of malignant cells are observed—dendritic and epithelioid. They are set in a myxoid matrix, but in time this becomes hyalinized and sclerotic and may undergo calcification. The tumor cells infiltrate hepatic sinusoids and intrahepatic veins. They are vasoformative and synthesize Factor VIII–related antigen.[208]

SQUAMOUS CARCINOMA

Squamous carcinoma occurs rarely in the liver. It arises from congenital hepatic cysts, presumably as a result of squamous metaplasia of the lining epithelium.[209, 210]

MUCOEPIDERMOID CARCINOMA

One such tumor has been reported.[211] It was composed of nests of epidermoid and mucus-secreting cells, sometimes with central cystic spaces. Intercellular bridges and keratinization were present in the epidermoid parts of the tumor. The tumor is believed to arise from the terminal ramifications of the bile canaliculi that have undergone squamous metaplasia.

UNDIFFERENTIATED (EMBRYONAL) SARCOMA

Because they show no evidence of differentiation, these very rare sarcomas defy categorization. Undifferentiated sarcomas may be the malignant counterpart of the mesenchymal hamartoma. They occur predominantly in children between the ages of 6 and 15 years, and the two sexes are affected equally.[162, 212]

Presentation and Investigations

An abdominal mass and pain are the usual presenting symptoms.[162, 212, 213] Other complaints include fever, weight loss, anorexia, and vomiting. Hemorrhage into or rupture of the tumor occurs occasionally.

Special investigations are singularly unhelpful in the diagnosis of undifferentiated sarcomas.[162, 212] A nonspecific defect may be seen on an isotope liver scan, and an avascular mass may be observed on hepatic arteriography.

Description

The tumor occurs as a large, solitary lesion that is usually globular and well demarcated with a fibrous pseudocapsule.[162, 212] The cut surface has a variegated, gelatinous, or glistening appearance and ranges in color from yellowish-gray to tan. In more than half of the cases many cystic areas containing necrotic debris, clotted blood, or gelatinous material can be seen. There also may be extensive areas of necrosis and hemorrhage. The sarcomatous cells are stellate or spindle-shaped with ill-defined outlines.[162, 212] They are arranged in whorls, or sheets, or scattered loosely in a ground substance that is rich in acid mucopolysaccharides. Reticulin and collagen fibers are present between the cells. Dense bundles of collagen can be found in localized areas. The nuclei are round, elongated, or highly irregular, with finely stippled chromatin granules and inconspicuous nucleoli. Multinucleated cells, as well as bizarre cells with large hyperchromatic nuclei and atypical mitotic figures, are present in all tumors. The cytoplasm is lightly eosinophilic and finely granular or vesicular. Periodic acid–Schiff (PAS)-positive, diastase-resistant globules may be seen in the cells adjacent to the pseudocapsule. Foci of hematopoiesis are seen in about half of cases. Clusters or cords of hepatocytes and cystic structures resembling bile ducts frequently are found within the pseudocapsule or at the periphery of the tumor. Multiple vessels, mostly thin-walled veins, are scattered throughout the tumor. Recent and organizing thrombi frequently are identified in the gelatinous, hemorrhagic, and necrotic portions of the tumor. Pulmonary metastases may be present.

Prognosis and Treatment

The prognosis for a patient with undifferentiated sarcoma of the liver is poor. The usual survival time is less than a year.[162, 212] The lesions seldom are resectable, and treatment with radiotherapy and chemotherapy has produced disappointing results.

FIBROSARCOMA AND LEIOMYOSARCOMA

These rare tumors occur particularly in middle-aged and elderly men. The majority of patients have an abdominal mass. Before designating a leiomyosarcoma as a primary hepatic tumor, the possibility of hepatic metastases from a gastrointestinal or uterine leiomyosarcoma must be excluded. A few patients with fibrosarcoma have hypoglycemia.[201] The gross and microscopic features resemble those of similar tumors arising in other sites. The prognosis is poor if the tumor cannot be resected.

MALIGNANT MESENCHYMOMA

This rare tumor arises from the pluripotential mesenchyme.[162, 214] It occurs almost exclusively in children, and grows rapidly. The tumor is composed of mesenchymal tissues, often associated with extramedullary hematopoiesis, smooth or striated muscle fibers, and fibroblastic and myxoid connective tissue.[162, 201, 213, 214] Any of the spindle cell elements may be sarcomatous.

CARCINOSARCOMA

Malignant hepatic tumors in adults rarely may contain both liver cell carcinoma and a spindle cell component having the characteristics of sarcoma.[162] The two elements may be admixed or occur as separate tumors. Carcinosarcomas often arise in cirrhotic livers.

BENIGN HEPATIC TUMORS

HEPATOCELLULAR ADENOMA

The importance of this rare benign hepatic tumor lies mainly in its probable etiologic association with the long-term use of oral contraceptive steroids.

Occurrence and Relation to Contraceptive Steroids

Hepatocellular adenoma was extremely rare before the use of oral contraceptive agents became widespread. For example, Edmondson could find only two such tumors in 50,000 necropsies performed at the Los Angeles County General Hospital from 1918 to 1954.[162] The tumor occurred almost exclusively in women of childbearing age and was practically unknown in men. However, since the early 1970s there has been a remarkable increase in the number of reports of hepatocellular adenoma in the medical literature.[215-226] Moreover, the vast majority of the recently described patients have been women taking contraceptive steroids. Occasional cases have also occurred in women receiving conjugated equine estrogens.[219] This phenomenon may be explained partly by a tendency to report "pill-associated" tumors but not to report tumors occurring in women not using this form of contraception. Furthermore, the same cases have been described by more than one group of authors.[222, 223] Formal studies of the relation between oral contraceptive steroids and hepatocellular adenoma are few, and most have not been of rigorous design.[224] Even allowing for these reservations, the number of women developing hepatocellular adenoma while or after receiving contraceptive steroids is impressive and strongly suggests a cause-and-effect relation. This conclusion is supported by reports of recurrence of hepatocellular adenoma after surgical resection when the patient has continued to take "the pill"[222, 227] and of regression of the tumors when the pill has been discontinued.

Because many patients who have a hepatocellular adenoma are asymptomatic, show no specific laboratory abnormalities, and are recognized only when the tumor ruptures or becomes large enough to be felt, there are undoubtedly a substantial number of unrecognized cases in the population.

The association between oral contraceptive agents and hepatocellular adenoma is particularly strong with prolonged usage. Reported patients usually have taken oral contraceptive steroids for more than four years.[216, 219, 220, 222, 225] However, periods as short as six months have been recorded. Women who use oral contraceptive agents continuously for five to seven years have been estimated to run five times the normal risk of developing a benign hepatic tumor. This figure rises to 25 times with usage for longer than nine years.[216] The use of contraceptive steroids with high hormonal potency and an age of more than 30 years seem to increase further the risk of hepatocellular adenoma formation.[226] When one realizes that in North America alone as many as 50 million women either have used or are currently taking contraceptive steroids, these figures sound daunting, but the actual number of women likely to be affected is probably extremely small. After combining data from two family planning surveys based on 45,000 woman-years, and two population surveys involving six million individuals, Vessey et al.[228] could find only one woman with a benign hepatic neoplasm that might have been attributable to oral contraceptive steroids. This suggests that some form of genetic predisposition to the development of hepatocellular adenoma may be operative in patients taking oral contraceptives.

Hepatocellular adenoma has been associated with both types of synthetic estrogen and all forms of progestogen contained in the many preparations of oral contraceptives on the market.[215-226] Consequently, it is not known whether it is the estrogenic or the progestogenic component, or the combination, that is implicated in the causation of the tumor. Estrogens are known to be carcinogenic in other organs, and they promote hepatic regeneration in rats.[229] The occurrence of hepatocellular adenoma in women during treatment with conjugated equine estrogens,[219] during pregnancy[230] or in the postpartum period,[230] and in association with estrogen-producing tumors,[231] suggests that estrogens may be the culprit. Progestogens are enzyme inducers,[219] and enzyme induction increases the carcinogenicity of certain compounds. Furthermore, progestogens are structurally similar to anabolic androgenic steroids, which have been incriminated in the pathogenesis of hepatocellular carcinoma[129, 130] and have occasionally been associated with liver cell adenoma.[233] All contraceptive steroids are C17 alkyl–substituted and therefore are mildly cholestatic.[234] This property might enhance the potentially carcinogenic action of substances normally secreted in bile. Intimal thickening and hyperplasia of the media of arteries and veins, as well as neovascularization and peliosis hepatis, are found in hepatocellular adenoma. These findings raise the possibility that loss of vascular elasticity with intravascular thrombosis and consequent hypoxia of liver cells may play a role in the causation of liver cell adenoma.

Even if contraceptive steroids do not play a part in causing these tumors, hepatocellular adenomas appear to be hormone-dependent, as evidenced by regression of the tumor after cessation of oral contraceptive therapy[222, 235] and by an increase in size of the tumor during pregnancy.[230] The appearance of a second tumor in a young woman who continued to take the pill may also be explained on this basis.[236] Hepatocellular adenomas also occur in patients with glycogenosis type IA (see Chap. 49) and in individuals taking anabolic androgenic steroids.[232]

Presentation

Hepatocellular adenomas can present in several ways.[218, 220, 222, 223, 225, 227] The tumor is sometimes asymptomatic, but the woman or her physician feels a mass in the upper abdomen. About one fourth of patients experience pain in the right hypochondrium or epigastrium. This is usually slight and ill-defined, but it may be severe as a result of bleeding into or infarction of the tumor. The pain or discomfort may be accompanied by anorexia, nausea, vomiting, and fever. The surface of the enlarged liver is smooth and may be slightly tender. The most alarming manifestation occurs when the tumor ruptures, producing a hemoperitoneum. This complication is not uncommon (31 per cent of patients in one large series[236]), and carries an appreciable mortality. Tumors that rupture are usually large and are often solitary.[236] The woman is often menstruating when rupture occurs,[216] and it has been suggested that the vessels in the adenoma behave like endometrial spiral arteries. Rupture is most common when hepatocellular adenomas are associated with the use of contraceptive steroids. A minority of the tumors are found incidentally at laparotomy or necropsy. This obviously applies particularly to small lesions and occurs more commonly in women not taking contraceptive steroids.

Investigations

Liver tests are usually normal, but even when they are not, the changes are slight and nonspecific.[219, 222, 225, 236] Serum alkaline phosphatase and aminotransferase concentrations may be elevated slightly. Alpha-fetoprotein is not present in the serum in abnormally high concentrations. If the adenoma is more than 3 cm in diameter, it probably will show as a defect on an isotopic hepatic scan.[237] However, the picture obtained is not diagnostic. Hepatic arteriography is the most useful aid to diagnosis.[223, 238] About one half of hepatocellular adenomas are hypovascular, with draping of hepatic arteries around the lesion; the remainder are hypervascular. The lesion has a clearly defined margin, and frequently has approximately parallel vessels entering from the periphery ("spoke-wheel" appearance). Alternatively, it may contain tortuous vessels coursing irregularly through the tumor. When hypervascular, the lesion may have avascular areas caused by hemorrhage or necrosis.

Open biopsy is preferred to percutaneous biopsy because of the vascular nature of the tumor.

Pathology

Hepatocellular adenoma usually occurs as a solitary, relatively soft, light brown-to-yellow tumor which is sharply circumscribed but may or may not be encapsulated.[216, 218, 221, 236, 239, 240] It arises in an otherwise normal liver. Occasionally, two or more lesions are present. The tumors range from 1 to 30 cm in diameter, but the majority are 8 to 15 cm in diameter. Hepatocellular adenomas tend to be larger in women taking oral contraceptive steroids. They are more common in the right lobe, and usually occupy a subcapsular position, projecting slightly from the surface; occasionally, they are pedunculated. The cut surface may show ill-defined lobulation but is never nodular or fibrotic. Foci of hemorrhage or necrosis are frequently present, and bile-staining may be noted.

Microscopically, the tumor may mimic normal liver tissue to an astonishing extent. It is composed of sheets or cords of normal-looking or slightly atypical hepatocytes that show no features of malignancy. The cells occasionally have an acinar arrangement. There are few or no portal tracts or central veins (Fig. 45–13).[216, 218, 221, 222, 236, 239, 240] Only an infrequent vascular, fibrous septum traverses the lesion. A more or less normal reticulin pattern is demonstrable throughout the tumor. Bile ducts are conspicuously absent, and Kupffer cells are either markedly reduced in number or absent. Bile stasis may be present. The hepatocytes may be slightly larger and paler than normal, with cytoplasm that is finely vacuolated or granular. Eosinophilic inclusions, consisting of α_1-antitrypsin, are often present.[236] The nuclei show minimal variation in structure (see Fig. 45–13). Nucleoli are often present and are small and regular. The

sinusoids are dilated focally, and arteries and veins show thickening of their walls. Some of the areas with vascular abnormalities are infarcted, and thromboses may be seen. Peliosis hepatitis may be found in relation to the tumor.

Treatment and Prognosis

Because of the danger of rupture of the tumor, surgical treatment is recommended whenever possible. Resection is usually feasible in the uncomplicated case. When rupture has occurred, emergency resection should be performed if possible (it may be necessary to clamp the hepatic artery first to stop the bleeding). If resection cannot be accomplished, the hepatic artery should be ligated. The threat of rupture is determined more by a superficial position of the tumor than by its size. With smaller and deeper asymptomatic lesions, it may be difficult to decide whether to resect the tumor. It is important, however, that the patient discontinue taking contraceptive steroids, whether or not the adenoma is resected. If the adenoma is not resected, pregnancy should be avoided.

That hepatocellular carcinoma has been reported to occur in a small number of women taking contraceptive steroids has led to speculation that in some cases liver cell adenomas may undergo malignant transformation. This has occurred in a few reported instances;[222, 241] therefore, a risk is involved in treating adenomas by merely stopping the medication.

CAVERNOUS HEMANGIOMA

Occurrence

Cavernous hemangioma is the most common benign tumor of the liver, with incidences in necropsy series ranging from 0.4 to 7.4 per cent.[162, 201, 242] Some idea of its relative frequency can be obtained from the necropsy study at the Los Angeles County General Hospital, which included 176 cavernous hemangiomas, compared with only 2 hepatocellular adenomas.[162] Cavernous hemangiomas have a uniform worldwide distribution. They occur at all ages, although they are commonest in the older age groups and are rare in young children.[162, 201, 243] The tumor affects women predominantly, the sex ratio being 4 to 6:1.[162] In addition, the onset of cavernous hemangioma tends to occur at a younger age and the tumor tends to be larger and is more likely to become clinically manifest in women than in men.[162, 244] Cavernous hemangiomas may increase in size with pregnancy or with the administration of estrogens, and they are more common in multiparous women.[177] These observations suggest an etiologic role for female sex hormones in this tumor. Clearly, the tumor is hormone-dependent.

Presentation

The great majority of cavernous hemangiomas are small and asymptomatic, and are discovered incidentally at necropsy or laparotomy.[245, 246] Large or multiple lesions produce symptoms. Abdominal pain or discomfort is the most common complaint; however, anorexia, nausea, and vomiting may also occur[201] and are caused by pressure on or displacement of abdominal viscera by the tumor. These symptoms may have been present for months or years.

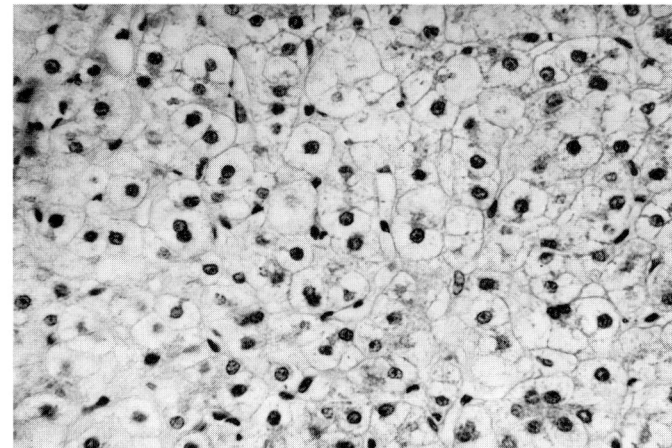

Figure 45–13. Liver cell adenoma, composed of sheets of normal or slightly atypical hepatocytes without bile ducts or ductules. Hematoxylin and eosin, × 300. (Reproduced from Fechner R E. Hum Pathol 8:255, 1977, with permission.)

Episodes of acute abdominal pain may be caused by thrombosis or hemorrhage in the tumor. A small proportion of patients seek treatment as a result of acute hemoperitoneum following rupture of the hemangioma.[246] In some cases an enlarged liver is found unexpectedly. An arterial bruit is heard occasionally over the tumor.

Investigations

As with other benign hepatic tumors, hepatic tests are of little help in the diagnosis of cavernous hemangiomas.[244] Rarely, plain abdominal radiographs show calcification in the tumor,[247] particularly in elderly patients, and very rarely a calcified phlebolith can be seen.[242] The findings on isotopic hepatic scanning are not specific. However, dynamic hepatic blood flow scintigraphy will show the lesion or lesions to be vascular. The features on ultrasonography are suggestive rather than diagnostic.[248] Almost all cavernous hemangiomas greater than 3 cm in diameter can be diagnosed by bolus-enhanced computed tomography with sequential scans.[249] Magnetic resonance imaging may be useful in the diagnosis of small cavernous hemangiomas.[249] A most useful investigation is hepatic arteriography.[249, 250] With large or multiple lesions, the celiac and hepatic arteries are enlarged and may be displaced. The branches of the hepatic artery are displaced and crowded together; they may be stretched around the lesion. However, they taper normally. There is early opacification of irregular areas or lakes, and the contrast material remains in these vascular lakes long after arterial emptying. With small hemangiomas, the contrast material may be arranged in rings or be C-shaped, with avascular centers resulting from fibrous obliteration of the center of the lesion. This finding is pathognomonic of cavernous hemangiomas.

Thrombocytopenia, attributed to sequestration and destruction of platelets in large hemangiomas (Kasabach-Merritt syndrome), although sometimes found in infants, is rare in adults with cavernous hemangiomas.[251] Hypofibrinogemia may also occur.[252] This is thought to result from deposition of fibrin in the tumor with secondary fibrinolysis.

Percutaneous biopsy is contraindicated because of the danger of hemorrhage.

Pathology

Cavernous hemangiomas vary in size from a few millimeters to many centimeters.[162, 243, 244, 246, 253] The larger lesions may be pedunculated. They are usually solitary, but two or more tumors occur in 10 per cent of patients. Hemangiomas are found more often in the right lobe. Reddish-purple or bluish masses are seen under Glisson's capsule or deep in the substance of the liver. The vascular spaces may contain thrombi. The lesions are well circumscribed, but seldom encapsulated. Hemangiomas may show central fibrosis, and in some instances, the whole tumor has a firm grayish-white appearance.

Microscopically, the tumor is composed of many vascular channels of different sizes, lined by a single layer of flattened endothelium, separated and supported by fibrous septa (Fig. 45–14).[162, 202, 243, 244, 246, 253] The vascular spaces may contain thrombi.

Cavernous hemangiomas of the liver occasionally are associated with hemangiomas in other organs. They may also coexist with cysts in the liver or pancreas,[253] bile duct hamartomas (von Meyenburg complexes),[254] or focal nodular hyperplasia.[255]

Treatment

When the hemangioma is large and symptomatic, yet localized, it should be resected.[244, 246] When resection is not feasible, reduction in the size of the hemangioma with relief of symptoms has been achieved with radiation therapy.[245] If the hemangioma has ruptured, it may be necessary to clamp the hepatic artery to stop bleeding before proceeding to resect. This maneuver also may be necessary prior to resection of a very large hemangioma.

INFANTILE HEMANGIOENDOTHELIOMA

Occurrence and Presentation

Benign hemangioendothelioma (also known as multinodular hepatic hemangiomatosis) is a rare but important tumor of the liver in infants. Its importance stems from the high incidence of congestive cardiac failure in patients with this tumor and the high mortality rate (70 per cent) that results therefrom.[256, 257] The tumor is thought to be of embryonal origin and almost always manifests in the first six months of life.[256, 257] Children of both sexes are affected, although the tumor is twice as common in girls.[256, 257]

Hepatic hemangioendothelioma is frequently associated with hemangiomas in other organs or tissues, partic-

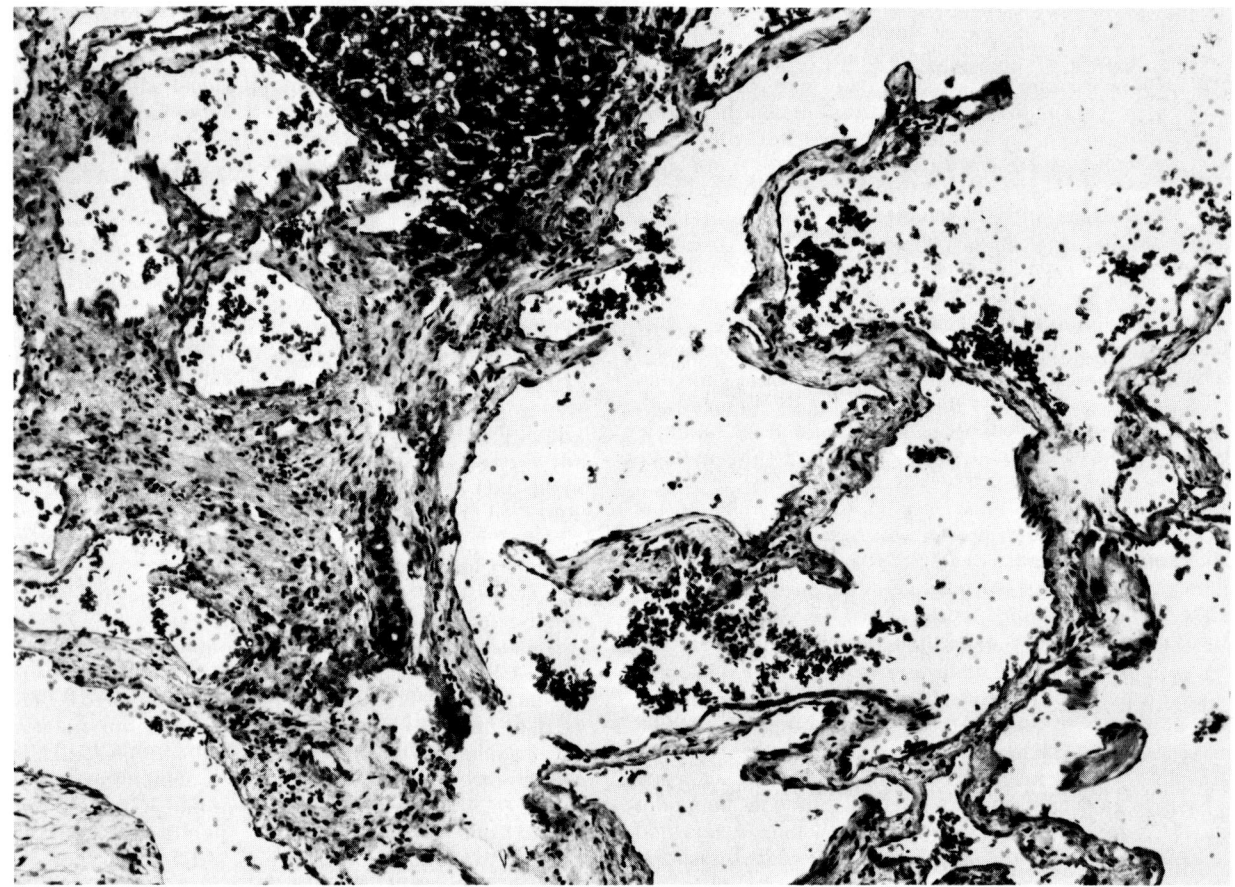

Figure 45–14. Cavernous hemangioma. Multiple vascular channels of various sizes are present. They are lined by a single layer of flattened endothelium and supported by fibrous septa. Hematoxylin and eosin, × 250.

ularly the skin. Cutaneous hemangiomas are present in about half of the patients.

Small hemangioendotheliomas are asymptomatic.[244] The presence of a large lesion is recognized clinically by the diagnostic triad of an enlarged liver, high-output cardiac failure, and multiple cutaneous hemangiomas.[256, 257] The size of the liver is disproportionate to the severity of cardiac failure, and hepatomegaly persists after the cardiac failure has been treated successfully. When small hemangiomas occur diffusely throughout the liver, as they usually do, their combined effect is to act as a massive peripheral arteriovenous shunt. Shunts of this magnitude cause high-output cardiac failure.[256, 257] An arterial bruit is occasionally heard over the liver.[257] Jaundice is present in about a third of patients.[243] The tumors occasionally rupture. When they do, the prognosis is poor.[258]

Anemia is sometimes present. This results partly from a dilutional effect of the increased circulating blood volume that develops with large peripheral arteriovenous fistulas,[243] but a microangiopathic hemolytic anemia may occur.[243] Hepatic hemangioendotheliomas can be complicated by thrombocytopenia.[243] This is thought to be caused by the sequestration and destruction of platelets within the tumor circulation as occurs with large hemangiomas in other organs (Kasabach-Merritt syndrome).

Investigations

Hepatic tests are of no diagnostic value. Isotopic scans may show one or more defects in the liver, or uptake of

the isotope may be generally poor. The most useful investigation is hepatic arteriography.[258] This shows dilated celiac and hepatic arteries. The intrahepatic branches may be stretched, but are not displaced. Abnormal vessels arise from the hepatic arteries and promptly opacify the liver, giving rise to the characteristic blush of an arteriovenous shunt. The circulation time through the liver is very fast. Avascular areas may be present when hemorrhage into or infarction of the tumor has occurred. Tiny flecks of calcification in the tumor occasionally are seen radiologically.

Percutaneous biopsy is contraindicated because of the danger of bleeding.

Pathology

Benign hemangioendotheliomas may be solitary but are typically multicentric and produce a nodular deformity of the whole liver.[243, 256] The nodules vary in size from a few millimeters to many centimeters and are well demarcated although not encapsulated. They have a reddish-purple appearance. At laparotomy they can be seen to pulsate. Large tumors are gray to tan, and may show hemorrhages, fibrosis, or calcification. Microscopically, the tumor is composed of anastomosing vascular channels lined by one or more layers of plump endothelial cells. A single layer is referred to as a type I pattern; several layers represent the type II pattern. Solid masses of mesoblastic primordial cells with early differentiation into vascular structures are observed in some areas of the tumor. Nuclei may vary in size and staining, but mitoses are rare. Fibrous septa may be prominent, and extramedullary hematopoiesis often is present. Thrombosis and infarction occur and may be followed by scarring and calcification.

Treatment and Prognosis

The natural history of these tumors is one of growth during the early months of life, followed by gradual involution.[256] If the child survives, the tumor may disappear completely. The life-threatening aspect of the condition is intractable congestive cardiac failure and, to a lesser extent, tumor rupture.[256, 257] Heart failure should be treated in the first instance with digitalis, diuretics, and oxygen.[257] If these measures fail, more drastic forms of treatment can be tried. The use of corticosteroids has been successful in many but not all patients,[259] whereas irradiating the liver has seldom been beneficial.[256] In some cases ligating the hepatic artery has resulted in disappearance of the cardiac failure.[260] When the lesion has been confined to one lobe, surgical resection has been accomplished, even in the presence of heart failure. Evaluation of the results of these forms of therapy is complicated by the tendency of these tumors to involute spontaneously with the passage of time.

BILE DUCT ADENOMA

This benign tumor is very rare, only four cases being found in 50,000 necropsies.[162] It occurs more commonly in males than females, and two thirds of the patients are more than 50 years of age.[162, 239]

Bile duct adenomas do not manifest clinically but are incidental findings at either necropsy or laparotomy.[162, 177, 239] They are almost always solitary and are found predominantly in the right lobe of the liver; they frequently occupy a subcapsular position. The lesions are usually small, and only 10 per cent have diameters greater than 1 cm. Bile duct adenomas are grayish-white, firm, and well circumscribed but not encapsulated. Microscopically, the tumor is seen to be composed of many small, normal-looking ductules with cuboidal or low columnar epithelium.[162, 177, 239] The lesion is believed by some to be a hamartoma.[239]

The chief significance of the bile duct adenoma is its possible confusion at laparotomy with metastatic carcinoma, cholangiocarcinoma, or other focal hepatic lesions.

BILIARY CYSTADENOMA AND CYSTADENOCARCINOMA

Occurrence and Presentation

Biliary cystadenoma and cystadenocarcinoma are rare tumors that arise in the liver or, less frequently, in the extrahepatic bile ducts.[162, 261, 262] They occur in adulthood, and women are affected more often than men.[162, 261, 262]

A patient with a biliary cystadenoma or cystadenocarcinoma usually complains of an upper abdominal mass but also may experience abdominal pain, indigestion, or anorexia.[261] These symptoms may have been present for several years.

Description

Both the benign and the malignant tumors are always large.[162, 261] They have a globular shape and a smooth external surface. The cut surface reveals locules of different sizes. In biliary cystadenomas the walls are thin and the lining is smooth and glistening. In cystadenocarcinomas the walls vary in thickness, and the lining may have numerous papillary projections as large as 2 cm in diameter.

Microscopically, the cysts in the cystadenoma are lined by a biliary type of epithelium supported by dense cellular fibrous stroma that resembles ovarian stroma, in which smooth muscle fibers may be identified.[162] This layer in turn is surrounded by a looser and less cellular layer of collagen that contains vessels, nerve fibers, and bile ducts. A characteristic feature is the presence of macrophages with phagocytosed lipofuscin, presumably a reaction to degeneration and inflammation in the cyst wall. In biliary cystadenocarcinomas the lining epithelium is multilayered and has numerous papillary projections. The cells show pleomorphism and anaplasia with infiltration through the basement membrane into the underlying stroma. The cysts frequently contain blood or chocolate-colored material. With both the adenoma and adenocarcinoma, abnormal "hamartomatous" bile ducts may surround the main tumor.

Biliary cystadenocarcinomas may invade adjacent tissues, and they may metastasize.[162, 261] Nevertheless, the prognosis is better than that associated with cholangiocarcinoma.

Treatment

Although benign lesions have been aspirated, drained, or marsupialized, surgical resection is the treatment of choice.[261] This should not be delayed, because malignant transformation of the cyst lining may occur.[263] Cystadenocarcinomas should be resected if possible.

CARCINOID TUMOR

This exceedingly rare benign liver tumor arises from the scattered argentaffin cells that are found in the walls of intrahepatic bile ducts.[162] It manifests clinically with the carcinoid syndrome. In one report, a patient with a hepatic carcinoid tumor sought treatment for intractable hypoglycemia.[264]

TERATOMA

The liver is an unusual site for teratomas.[265] In most of the few cases reported, the patients have been female and less than 3 years old.[265-267] The mode of origin is not completely understood, but the tumors may arise from foci of totipotential cells.[265] Teratomas contain tissues of tridermal derivation; the presence of ectodermal elements separates them from hepatoblastomas.[265-267] Macroscopically, they have a bizarre lobulated structure. Microscopically, they show benign differentiated mesodermal elements together with epithelial components such as hepatocytes, ductular structures, brain, skin, and teeth. They may be benign or malignant.[265-267] Even the histologically benign tumors may prove fatal because of their enormous size. Surgical resection is indicated but may be difficult because of the large size of the teratomas.[265-267]

TUMOR-LIKE LESIONS

FOCAL NODULAR HYPERPLASIA

Considerable uncertainty exists as to the precise nature of focal nodular hyperplasia. It has at various times been regarded as a regenerative phenomenon, a hamartoma, or a benign tumor. During recent years most interest in focal nodular hyperplasia has been directed toward a possible association with the long-term use of contraceptive steroids.

Occurrence and Relation to Contraceptive Steroids

Although a rare condition, focal nodular hyperplasia is more common than hepatocellular adenoma. Thus, in the necropsy series from the Los Angeles County General Hospital, which included two hepatocellular adenomas, there were 14 cases of focal nodular hyperplasia.[162] A review of the Anglo-Saxon, German, French, and Scandinavian medical literature for the years 1923 to 1974 revealed 141 cases of focal nodular hyperplasia, compared with 69 cases of hepatocellular adenoma.[268] Although the lesion is more common in women, the sex difference is less striking than that found for hepatocellular adenoma.[219, 222, 224] Focal nodular hyperplasia reaches a peak incidence in the third, fourth, and fifth decades of life but occurs at all ages, sometimes in children.[219, 222, 224]

Several authors have suggested a role for oral contraceptive steroids in the pathogenesis of focal nodular hyperplasia. In some reports a clear distinction between hepatocellular adenoma and focal nodular hyperplasia was not made,[226] and it was concluded that the incidence of "benign liver tumors" has increased substantially since the use of contraceptive steroids became widespread. In addition to confusion over diagnosis, the problem of selective reporting already alluded to in respect to hepatocellular adenoma applies equally to focal nodular hyperplasia. When hospital records have been analyzed without this bias, no unequivocal evidence of a recent increase in incidence of focal nodular hyperplasia has been found.[219, 222, 224, 240, 269] Moreover, in half of the cases reported by Vana et al.,[221] focal nodular hyperplasia was discovered after less than two years of exposure to oral contraceptives, whereas the great majority of the patients who had hepatocellular adenoma had been taking the pill for at least four years. There is, however, considerable evidence that focal nodular hyperplasia may be hormone-dependent, such as reports of regression of the lesion after stopping the use of oral contraceptive agents.[223, 228, 270] Contraceptive steroids may accentuate the vascular abnormalities in focal nodular hyperplasia, causing the lesion to enlarge, to become more symptomatic, and even to rupture.[223, 271]

The histologic features almost always make it possible to distinguish between focal nodular hyperplasia and hepatocellular adenoma, but the distinction may be extremely difficult in a few instances.

Presentation

About three fourths of these lesions are asymptomatic and are discovered incidentally during laparotomy or necropsy. However, focal nodular hyperplasia in women taking oral contraceptive steroids is likely to be symptomatic (only 50 per cent of these patients are asymptomatic[219, 222]). Either the patient or a physician may feel a mass in the upper abdomen. The lesion may be felt lower in the abdomen when it is pedunculated. The mass is usually not tender. The patient may complain of pain in the upper abdomen resulting from hemorrhage into or necrosis of the lesion. This presentation is more common in patients taking oral contraceptive steroids.[219, 222, 228] Focal nodular hyperplasia seldom ruptures in patients not taking contraceptive steroids; however, this presentation is significantly more common in those using this form of contraception (21 per cent) than in those not doing so (1 per cent).[219, 222, 228] In a few documented instances nodules of hyperplasia located in the perihilar region of the liver (reported as "partial nodular transformation of the liver") have been responsible for long-standing portal hypertension with splenomegaly and bleeding esophageal varices.[272]

Diagnosis

Hepatic function is well preserved with focal nodular hyperplasia, and conventional biochemical tests are of little value in its diagnosis.[223, 271] Alpha-fetoprotein is not present in the serum in abnormally high concentration. Isotopic hepatic scans show an area of defective uptake in about two thirds of cases, but the picture is in no way specific.[220] Selective hepatic arteriography shows a dilated hepatic artery with one or more highly vascular lesions.[224, 238] The vessels within the lesions are very tortuous. In about half of the cases, septation of the tumor mass is visible during the capillary phase, which is also characterized by an irregular granularity. However, it is frequently not possible to distinguish between focal nodular hyperplasia and hepatocellular adenoma on the basis of arteriographic features. Open liver biopsy is preferred because of the vascular nature of the lesion.

Pathology

Focal nodular hyperplasia usually presents as a firm, coarsely nodular mass of variable size with a dense, central, stellate scar and radiating fibrous septa that divide the lesion into lobules[219, 222, 223, 239-241] (Fig. 45–15). The nodules may be small, resembling cirrhotic nodules, or extremely large. The lesion is light brown or yellowish-gray. It is usually solitary but may be multiple, and it usually occupies a superficial position. It may be pedunculated. Focal nodular hyperplasia can arise in either lobe of the liver. The larger lesions may show foci of hemorrhage or necrosis, although these are less frequently seen than in hepatocellular adenomas.[230] The fibrous septa are sometimes poorly developed and the central scar absent. The lesion is sharply demarcated from the surrounding liver tissue, which is normal, but there is no true capsule.

Microscopically, focal nodular hyperplasia closely resembles an inactive cirrhosis.[219, 222, 223, 239-241] The hepatocytes are indistinguishable from those of normal liver. However, they lack the normal cord arrangement in relation to sinusoids, central veins, and portal tracts. In large nodules the hepatocytes may be somewhat smaller. The cytoplasm is finely granular but may be vacuolated. Kupffer cells are present. Characteristically, the fibrous septa contain numerous bile ductules and vessels. In addition, heavy infiltrations of lymphocytes and, to a lesser extent, plasma cells and histiocytes, are present. Branches of the hepatic artery and portal vein show various combinations of intimal and smooth muscle hyperplasia, subintimal fibrosis, thickening

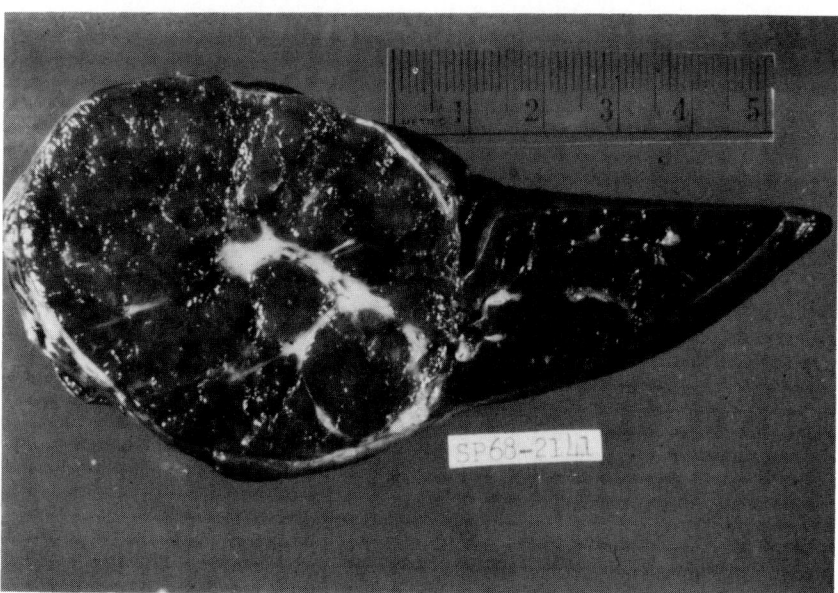

Figure 45–15. Solitary nodule of focal nodular hyperplasia with a central stellate scar. (Courtesy of Dr. C. Montgomery.)

of the wall and occlusive luminal lesions and, at times, occluding thrombosis. Whether these vascular changes are primary or secondary is not known. Peliosis hepatis may be an associated lesion.

Treatment

Small or complicated lesions should be resected. If this is not possible and the patient is taking contraceptive steroids, these should be discontinued. Pregnancy should also be avoided in the latter circumstance.

There is no evidence to suggest that focal nodular hyperplasia is a premalignant condition.

MESENCHYMAL HAMARTOMA

Occurrence

Mesenchymal hamartoma of the liver is a rare lesion.[172, 239, 273–275] It may be a fibrodysplasia of the liver rather than a true tumor. The patients are almost always less than 2 years of age, and the oldest reported child was 8 years old. One case in a young adult has been described.[276] The two sexes are affected equally often.

Presentation

The affected infant or young child has progressive swelling of the abdomen and a palpable mass.[172, 239, 273–275] The tumor may grow rapidly and cause life-threatening respiratory embarrassment. Other possible symptoms are abdominal pain, weight loss, vomiting, diarrhea, and constipation. The serum α-fetoprotein level may be increased.

Description

Mesenchymal hamartomas are usually solitary and large (the average diameter is 16 cm).[172, 239, 273–276] In a third of cases the lesion is pedunculated. It is gray or dark red,

and the cut surface shows numerous cysts in an edematous stroma. Areas of necrosis and hemorrhage are rarely present. The cysts contain colorless or yellow, watery, or gelatinous fluid. The lesion is not encapsulated but merges gradually with the adjacent liver tissue.

Microscopically, mesenchymal hamartomas are characterized by an admixture of ductal structures in a copious, loose, connective tissue stroma.[172, 239, 273–275] Less conspicuous elements include hepatocytes and hematopoietic cells. The stroma has a peculiar propensity to accumulate fluid in quantities sufficient to create microscopic and macroscopic acellular spaces suggestive of lymphangiomatous channels but without an endothelial lining. The histologic findings differ widely from site to site in the tumor. The loose collagenous tissue is considered to arise from primitive mesenchyme. Proliferation or cystic dilation of bile ducts is prominent. Islands of hepatic parenchyma lie between the edematous mesenchymal areas. Cysts may have either a single layer of lining cells or no lining.

Prognosis and Treatment

The prognosis is generally good.[172, 239, 273–275] Treatment consists of surgical resection, which should be undertaken before the tumor becomes too large.[172, 239, 273–275]

Malignant change has not been reported to occur, although the undifferentiated (embryonal) sarcoma is thought to be the malignant equivalent of the mesenchymal hamartoma.

MICROHAMARTOMAS (VON MEYENBURG COMPLEXES)

Microhamartomas, which are considered to be part of the spectrum of adult polycystic liver disease, are commonly present in the liver. The lesions are small and usually multiple; they are grayish-white or green in color. Each complex is composed of cystically dilated bile ducts lying in a fibrous tissue stroma.[277] They occur adjacent to or in portal tracts. The ducts are lined by cuboidal epithelium and may contain bile.

Microhamartomas rarely give rise to symptoms, but occasionally multiple lesions are associated with portal hypertension, and these cases merge imperceptibly with congenital hepatic fibrosis.[277] This latter lesion is discussed in detail in Chapter 52. They may possibly undergo malignant transformation into cholangiocarcinoma.[267, 278] Microhamartomas occasionally are found in association with cavernous hemangiomas.[255]

REFERENCES

1. Higginson J. The geographical pathology of primary liver cancer. Cancer Res 23:1624, 1963.
2. Dunham LJ, Bailar JC. World maps of cancer mortality rates and frequency rates. J Natl Cancer Inst 41:155, 1968.
3. Waterhouse J, Muir C, Correa P, et al. Cancer Incidence in Five Continents. Lyon, World Health Organization, 1977.
4. Terry WD. Primary cancer of the liver. In: Kaplan HS, Tsuchitani PJ, eds. Cancer in China. New York, Alan R. Liss, Inc., 1978:101.
5. Okuda K. Clinical aspects of hepatocellular carcinoma—analysis of 134 cases. In: Okuda K, Peters RL, eds. Hepatocellular Carcinoma. New York, John Wiley and Sons, 1976:387.
6. Harington JS, McGlashan ND, Bradshaw E, et al. A spatial and temporal analysis of four cancers in African gold-miners from southern Africa. Br J Cancer 31:665, 1976.
7. Linsell DA, Higginson J. The geographic pathology of liver cell cancer. In: Cameron HM, Linsell DA, Warwick GP, eds. Liver Cell Cancer. Amsterdam, Elsevier, 1976:1.
8. Saracci R, Repetto F. Time trends of primary liver cancer. Indication of increased incidence in selected cancer registry populations. J Natl Cancer Inst 65:241, 1980.
9. Manderson WG, Patrick RS, Peters EE. Primary carcinoma of the liver. A survey of cases admitted to Glasgow Royal Infirmary during 1949–1963. Scot Med J 10:60, 1965.
10. Sandler DP, Sandler RS, Horney LF. Primary liver cancer mortality in the United States. J Chronic Dis 3:227, 1983.
11. Prates MD. Cancer and cirrhosis of the liver in the Portugese East African. Acta Un Int Contra Cancrum 17:718, 1961.
12. Alpert ME, Hutt MSR, Davidson CS. Primary hepatoma in Uganda. Am J Med 46:794, 1969.
13. Bagshaw A, Cameron HM. The clinical problem of liver cell cancer in a high incidence area. In: Cameron HM, Linsell DA, Warwick GP, eds. Liver Cell Cancer. Amsterdam, Elsevier, 1976:45.
14. Kew MC, Geddes EW. Hepatocellular carcinoma in rural southern African Blacks. Medicine (Balt) 61:98, 1982.
15. Chan CH. Primary carcinoma of the liver. Med Clin North Am 59:989, 1975.
16. Sung J-L, Wang T-H, Yu J-Y. Clinical study on primary carcinoma of the liver in Taiwan. Am J Dig Dis 12:1036, 1967.
17. Ihde DC, Sherlock P, Winawer SJ, et al. Clinical manifestations of hepatoma. Am J Med 56:83, 1974.
18. Shorter RG, Baggenstoss AH, Logan GB, et al. Primary carcinoma of the liver in infancy and childhood. Pediatrics 25:191, 1960.
19. Hutt MSR. Epidemiology of human primary liver cancer. In: Liver Cancer. Lyon, IARC Scientific Publications, No. 1, 1970:21.
20. Higginson J. The epidemiology of primary carcinoma of the liver. In: Pack GT, Islami AH, eds. Tumors of the Liver. Berlin, Springer, 1970:38.
21. Edmondson HA, Peters RL. Neoplasms of the liver. In: Schiff L, Schiff ER, eds. Diseases of the Liver, 5th ed. Philadelphia, Lippincott, 1982:1101.
22. Kew MC, Dos Santos HA, Sherlock S. Diagnosis of primary cancer of the liver. Br Med J 4:408, 1971.
23. Kew MC, Paterson AC. Unusual clinical presentations of hepatocellular carcinoma. Trop Gastroenterol 6:10, 1985.
24. Chearanai O, Plengvanit U, Asavanich C, et al. Spontaneous rupture of primary hepatoma. Cancer 51:1532, 1983.
25. Lai CL, Lam KC, Wu PC, et al. Clinical features of hepatocellular carcinoma. Cancer 47:2746, 1981.
26. Clain D, Wartnaby K, Sherlock S. Abdominal arterial murmurs in liver disease. Lancet 2:516, 1966.
27. Johns WA, Zimmerman A. Biliary obstruction due to hemobilia caused by liver carcinoma. Ann Surg 153:706, 1961.
28. MacDonald R. Primary carcinoma of the liver. Arch Intern Med 99:266, 1957.
29. Ellison ML. Cell differentiation and the biological significance of inappropriate tumor products. Proc R Soc Med 70:845, 1977.
30. Gordon JB. Adult frogs derived from nuclei of single somatic cells. Devel Biol 4:256, 1962.
31. Kan YW, McFadzean AJS, Todd D, et al. Further observations on polycythemia in hepatocellular carcinoma. Blood 18:592, 1961.
32. Jacobson RJ, Lowenthal MN, Kew MC. Erythrocytosis in hepatocellular cancer. S Afr Med J 53:658, 1978.
33. Brownstein MH, Ballard HS. Hepatoma associated with erythrocytosis. Am J Med 40:204, 1966.
34. Tso SC, Hua ASP. Erythrocytosis in hepatocellular carcinoma: a compensatory phenomenon. Br J Haematol 28:497, 1974.
35. Knill-Jones RP, Buckle RM, Parsons V, et al. Hypercalcemia and increased parathyroid activity in primary hepatoma. N Engl J Med 282:704, 1970.
36. Riggs BL, Arnaud CD, Reynolds LC, et al. Immunologic differentiation of primary hyperparathyroidism with hyperparathyroidism due to non-parathyroid cancer. J Clin Invest 50:2079, 1971.
37. Klein DC, Raisz LG. Prostaglandins: stimulation of bone resorption in tissue culture. Endocrinology 86:1436, 1970.
38. Seyberth HW, Segre GV, Morgan JL, et al. Prostaglandins as mediators of hypercalcemia associated with certain types of cancer. N Engl J Med 293:1278, 1975.
39. Kew MC, Dusheiko GM. Paraneoplastic manifestations of hepatocellular carcinoma. In: Chalmers TC, Berk PD, eds. Frontiers of Science in Liver Disease. New York, Thieme-Stratton, Inc, 1981:305.
40. McArthur JW, Toll GD, Russfield AB, et al. Sexual precocity attributable to ectopic gonadotropin secretion by hepatoblastoma. Am J Med 54:390, 1973.
41. Braunstein GD, Vogel CL, Vaitukaitis MD, et al. Ectopic production of human chorionic gonadotropin in Ugandan patients with hepatocellular carcinoma. Cancer 32:223, 1973.
42. Kew MC, Kirschner MA, Abrahams GE, et al. Mechanism of feminization in primary liver cancer. N Engl J Med 296:1084, 1977.
43. Weintraub BD, Rosen SW. Ectopic production of human chorionic somatomammotropin by non-trophoblastic cancers. J Clin Endocrinol 32:94, 1971.
44. Primack A, Wilson J, O'Connor GT, et al. Hepatocellular carcinoma with carcinoid syndrome. Cancer 27:1182, 1971.
45. Morgan AG, Walker WC, Mason MK, et al. A new syndrome associated with hepatocellular carcinoma. Gastroenterology 63:340, 1972.
46. Kalk WJ, Kew MC, Danilewitz MD, et al. Thyroxin-binding globulin and thyroid function tests in patients with hepatocellular carcinoma. Hepatology 2:72, 1982.
47. Gershengorn MC, Larsen PR, Robbins J. Radioimmunoassay for serum thyroxine-binding globulin: results in normal subjects and in patients with hepatocellular carcinoma. J Clin Endocrinol Metab 42:907, 1976.
48. McFadzean AJS, Yeung RTT. Further observations on hypoglycemia in hepatocellular carcinoma. Am J Med 47:220, 1969.
49. Widmer U, Zapf J, Froesch ER, et al. Insulin-like growth factor levels measured by radioimmunoassay and radioreceptor assay in various forms of tumor hypoglycemia. In: Spencer M, ed. Insulin-like Growth Factors/Somatomedins. New York, Walter de Gruyter & Co, 1983:317.
50. Horecker BL, Hiatt HH. Pathways of carbohydrate metabolism in normal and neoplastic cells. N Engl J Med 258:177, 1958.
51. Landau BR, Wills N, Craig JW, et al. The mechanism of hepatoma-induced hypoglycemia. Cancer 15:1088, 1962.
52. Goldberg RB, Bersohn I, Kew MC. Hypercholesterolaemia in primary cancer of the liver. S Afr Med J 49:1464, 1975.
53. Danilewitz MD, Herrerra GA, Kew MC, et al. Autonomous cholesterol biosynthesis in murine hepatoma. A receptor defect with normal coated pits. Cancer 54:1562, 1984.
54. Thompson RPH, Nicholson DC, Farnan T, et al. Cutaneous porphyria due to a malignant primary hepatoma. Gastroenterology 59:779, 1970.
55. Kew MC. Alpha-fetoprotein. In: Read AE, ed. Modern Trends in Gastroenterology. Volume 5. London, Butterworths, 1975:91.
56. Alpert E. Human alpha-1 fetoprotein. In: Okuda K, Peters RL, eds. Hepatocellular Carcinoma. New York, John Wiley and Sons, 1976:353.
57. Macnab GM, Urbanowicz JM, Kew MC. Carcinoembryonic antigen in hepatocellular carcinoma. Br J Cancer 38:51, 1978.
58. Niitsu Y, Ohtsuka SD, Kohgo Y, et al. Human ferritin in the tissue and serum. Tumor Res 10:31, 1975.
59. Kew MC, Torrance JD, Derman D, et al. Serum and tumor ferritins in primary liver cancer. Gut 19:294, 1978.
60. Powell LW, Halliday JW, McKeering LV. Studies of serum ferritin with emphasis on its importance in clinical medicine. In: Crichton RR, ed. Proteins of Iron Storage and Transport in Biochemistry and Medicine. Amsterdam, North Holland, 1975:215.
61. Alpert E, Coston RL, Drysdale JW. Carcinofetal human liver ferritins. Nature (Lond) 242:194, 1973.
62. Barr RD, Ouna H, Simpson JG, et al. Dysfibrinogenaemia and primary hepatocellular carcinoma. Q J Med 180:647, 1976.

63. van der Walt JA, Gomperts ED, Kew MC. Hemostatic factors in primary hepatocellular cancer. Cancer 40:1593, 1977.
64. Gralnick HR, Gwelber H, Abrams E. Dysfibrinogenemia associated with hepatoma. N Engl J Med 299:221, 1978.
65. Waxman S, Liu C-K, Schreiber C, et al. The clinical and physiological implications of hepatoma B_{12} binding proteins. Cancer Res 37:1908, 1977.
66. Paradinas FJ, Melia WM, Wilkinson ML, et al. High serum vitamin B_{12} binding capacity as a marker of the fibrolamellar variant of hepatocellular carcinoma. Br Med J 285:840, 1982.
67. van Tonder S, Kew MC, Hodkinson J, et al. Serum vitamin B_{12} binders in South African Blacks with hepatocellular carcinoma. Cancer 56:789, 1985.
68. Collier NA, Weinbren K, Bloom SR, et al. Neurotensin secretion by fibrolamellar carcinoma of the liver. Lancet 1:538, 1984.
69. Weinhouse S. Metabolism and isoenzyme alterations in experimental hepatomas. Fed Proc 32:2162, 1973.
70. Warnock ML, Reisman R. Variant alkaline phosphatases in human hepatocellular cancers. Clin Chim Acta 24:5, 1969.
71. Kew MC, Wolf P, Whittaker D, et al. Tumour-associated isoenzymes of gamma-glutamyl transferase in the serum of patients with hepatocellular carcinoma. Br J Cancer 50:451, 1984.
72. Tsou KC, Ledis S, McCoy MG. 5'Nucleotide phosphodiesterase isoenzyme pattern in the serum of human hepatoma. Cancer Res 33:2215, 1973.
73. Okuda K, Kotoda K, Obata H, et al. Clinical observations during a relatively early stage of hepatocellular carcinoma, with special reference to serum alpha-fetoprotein levels. Gastroenterology 69:226, 1975.
74. Kojima J, Kanatani M, Nakamura N, et al. Electrophoretic fractionation of serum gamma-glutamyl transpeptidase in human hepatic cancer. Clin Chim Acta 106:165, 1980.
75. Liebman HA, Furie BC, Tong MJ, et al. Des-gamma-carboxy (abnormal) prothrombin as a serum marker of primary hepatocellular carcinoma. N Engl J Med 310:427, 1984.
76. Kew MC, Berger EL. The value of serum concentrations of tissue polypeptide antigen in the diagnosis of hepatocellular carcinoma. Cancer 58:127, 1986.
77. Bersohn I, Purves LR, Geddes EW. Liver function tests in primary liver cancer in the Bantu. In: Liver Cancer. Lyon, International Agency for Research on Cancer, 1971:158.
78. Ross RS, Iber FL, Harvey AM. The serum alkaline phosphatase in chronic infiltrative disease of the liver. Am J Med 21:850, 1956.
79. Levy LI, Geddes EW, Kew MC. The chest radiograph in primary liver cancer. S Afr Med J 50:1323, 1976.
80. Sanders CF. The plain chest radiograph in seventy-five cases of primary carcinoma of the liver. Clin Radiol 19:341, 1968.
81. Breedis C, Young G. Blood supply of neoplasms in liver. J Pathol 30:969, 1954.
82. Kido C, Sasaki T, Kaneko M. Angiography of primary liver cancer. Am J Radiol 113:70, 1971.
83. Okuda K, Obata H, Jinnouchi S, et al. Angiographic assessment of gross anatomy of hepatocellular carcinoma: comparisons of celiac angiograms and liver pathology in 100 cases. Radiology 123:21, 1977.
84. Marks WM, Jacobs RP, Goodman PC, et al. Hepatocellular carcinoma: clinical and angiographic findings and predictability for surgical resection. Am J Radiol 132:7, 1979.
85. Okuda K, Musha H, Yoshida T, et al. Demonstration of growing casts of hepatocellular carcinoma in the portal vein by celiac angiography. Radiology 117:305, 1975.
86. Levin J, Geddes EW, Kew MC. Radionuclide scanning of the liver in primary hepatic cancer: an analysis of 202 cases. J Nucl Med 15:296, 1974.
87. Bieler EU, Meyer BS, Jansen CR. Liver scanning as a method for detecting primary liver cancer. Report on 100 cases. Am J Radiol 115:709, 1972.
88. Kew MC, Geddes EW, Levin J. False-negative ^{75}Se-selenomethionine scans in primary liver cancer. J Nucl Med 15:234, 1974.
89. Kew MC, Allan J, Levin J. [57]Co-Bleomycin as a tumor scanning agent in primary hepatocellular cancer. Eur J Nucl Med 1:247, 1976.
90. Levin J, Kew MC. [67]Gallium citrate scanning in primary cancer of the liver: diagnostic value in the presence of cirrhosis and relation to alpha-fetoprotein. J Nucl Med 16:949, 1975.
91. Boultbee JE. Gray scale appearances in hepatocellular carcinoma. Clin Radiol 30:547, 1979.
92. Miller EL, Thomas RH. Portal vein invasion demonstrated by ultrasound. J Clin Ultrasonogr 7:57, 1979.
93. Itai Y, Nishikawa J, Tasaka A. Computerised tomography in the evaluation of hepatocellular carcinoma. Radiology 131:165, 1979.
94. Moss AM, Goldberg HI, Stark DB, et al. Hepatic tumors. Magnetic resonance and computerized tomographic appearance. Radiology 150:142, 1984.
95. Lapis K, Johannessen JT. Pathology of primary liver cancer. J Toxicol Environ Health 5:315, 1979.
96. Peters RL. Pathology of hepatocellular carcinoma. In: Okuda K, Peters RL, eds. Hepatocellular Carcinoma. New York, John Wiley and Sons, 1976:107.
97. Cameron HM. Pathology of liver cell cancer. In: Cameron HM, Linsell DA, Warwick GP, eds. Liver Cell Cancer. Amsterdam, Elsevier, 1976:17.
98. Anthony PP. Hepatic neoplasms. In: MacSween RHM, Anthony PP, Scheuer PJ, eds. Pathology of the Liver. Edinburgh, Churchill Livingstone, 1979:387.
99. Craig JR, Peters RL, Edmondson HA, et al. Fibrolamellar carcinoma of the liver: a tumor of adolescents and young adults with distinctive clinico-pathologic features. Cancer 46:372, 1980.
100. Berman MM, Libbey P, Foster JH. Hepatocellular carcinoma: Polygonal cell type with fibrous stroma. An atypical variant with favorable prognosis. Cancer 46:1448, 1980.
101. Allen RA, Lisa IR. Combined liver cell and bile duct carcinoma. Am J Pathol 25:647, 1949.
102. Higginson J, Steiner PE. Definition and classification of malignant epithelial neoplasms of the liver. Acta Un Int Contra Cancrum 17:593, 1961.
103. Kew MC, Newberne PM, Popper H. Other aetiological processes in hepatocellular carcinoma—genetic factors. In: Okuda K, Mackay I, eds. Hepatocellular Carcinoma. Geneva, U.I.C.C., 1982:108.
104. Kew MC, Turnbull R, Prinsloo I. Alpha$_1$-antitrypsin deficiency and hepatocellular carcinoma. Br J Cancer 37:635, 1978.
105. Kelly JK, Davies JS, Jones AW. Alpha$_1$-antitrypsin deficiency and hepatocellular carcinoma. J Clin Pathol 32:373, 1979.
106. Bomford A, Williams R. Long-term results of venesection therapy in idiopathic haemochromatosis. Q J Med 80:611, 1976.
107. MacSween RNM. A clinicopathological review of 100 cases of primary malignant tumors of the liver. J Clin Pathol 27:669, 1974.
108. Oettle GA. The aetiology of primary carcinoma of the liver in Africa: a critical appraisal of previous ideas with an outline of the mycotoxin hypothesis. S Afr Med J 39:817, 1965.
109. Kew MC. The hepatitis B virus and hepatocellular carcinoma. Sem Liver Dis 1:59, 1981.
110. Beasley RP, Blumberg B, Popper H, et al. Hepatitis B virus and hepatocellular carcinoma. In: Okuda K, Mackay I, eds. Hepatocellular Carcinoma. Geneva, U.I.C.C., 1982:60.
111. Kew MC, Kassianides C, Hodkinson J, et al. Hepatocellular carcinoma in urban-born Blacks: Frequency and relation to hepatitis B virus infection. Br Med J 293:1339, 1986.
112. Stevens CE, Szmuness W. Vertical transmission of hepatitis B and neonatal hepatitis B. In: Bianchi L, Gerock W, Sickinger K, et al., eds. Virus and the Liver. Lancaster, England, MTP Press, 1980:285.
113. Botha JF, Ritchie MJJ, Dusheiko GM, et al. Hepatitis B virus carrier state in Black children in Ovamboland: Role of perinatal and horizontal infection. Lancet 2:1209, 1984.
114. Beasley RP, Hwang LY, Lin CC, et al. Hepatocellular carcinoma and hepatitis B virus. A prospective study of 22,707 men in Taiwan. Lancet 2:1129, 1981.
115. Lohiya G, Pirkle H, Hoefs J, et al. Hepatocellular carcinoma in young mentally-retarded HbsAg carriers without cirrhosis. Hepatology 5:824, 1985.
116. Sherman M, Shafritz DA. Hepatitis B virus and hepatocellular carcinoma: Molecular biology and mechanistic considerations. Sem Liver Dis 4:98, 1984.
117. Kew MC, Dusheiko GM, Hadziyannis SJ, et al. Does delta infection play a part in the pathogenesis of hepatitis B virus–related hepatocellular carcinoma? Br Med J 288:1727, 1984.
118. Newberne PM. Chemical carcinogenesis: Mycotoxins and other chemicals to which humans are exposed. Sem Liver Dis 4:122, 1984.
119. Linsell A. Liver cancer and mycotoxins. In: Williams AO, O'Conor GT, De-The GG, et al., eds. Virus-associated Cancers in Africa. Lyon, I.A.R.C., 1984:161.
120. Lam KC, Yu MC, Leung JW, et al. Hepatitis B virus and cigarette smoking: Risk factors for hepatocellular carcinoma in Hong Kong. Cancer Res 42:5246, 1982.
121. Trichopoulos D. The causes of primary hepatocellular carcinoma in Greece. Progr Med Virol 27:14, 1981.
122. Harris CC, Sun TT. Multifactorial etiology of human liver cancer. Carcinogenesis 5:677, 1984.
123. Linsell DA, Peers FG. Aflatoxin and liver cell cancer. Trans R Soc Trop Med Hyg 71:471, 1977.
124. Kew MC, Popper H. Relationship between hepatocellular carcinoma and cirrhosis. Sem Liver Dis 4:136, 1984.
125. Zaman SN, Melia MW, Johnson RD, et al. Risk factors in the development of hepatocellular carcinoma in cirrhosis: Prospective study of 613 patients. Lancet 2:1357, 1985.
126. Lee FI. Cirrhosis and hepatoma in alcoholics. Gut 7:77, 1966.
127. Leevy CM, Gellene R, Ning M. Primary liver cancer in cirrhosis of the alcoholic. Ann NY Acad Sci 114:1026, 1964.
128. Anthony PP. Pre-cancerous changes in the human liver. J Toxicol Environ Health 15:301, 1979.

129. Johnson LF, Feagler JR, Lerner KG, et al. Association of anabolic androgenic steroid therapy with development of hepatocellular carcinoma. Lancet 2:123, 1972.

130. Kew MC, van Coller B, Prowse CM, et al. Occurrence of primary hepatocellular cancer and peliosis hepatis after treatment with androgenic steroids. S Afr Med J 50:1233, 1976.

131. Reuber MD. Influence of hormones on N-2-fluorenyldiacetamide-induced hyperplastic hepatic nodules in rats. J Natl Cancer Inst 43:445, 1969.

132. Lin T-Y. The results of hepatic lobectomy for primary carcinoma of the liver. Surg Gynecol Obstet 123:289, 1966.

133. Harrison NW, Dhru D, Primack A, et al. The surgical management of primary hepatocellular carcinoma in Uganda. Br J Surg 60:565, 1973.

134. Balasegaram M. Management of primary liver cancer. Am J Surg 130:33, 1975.

135. Foster JA, Berman MM. Solid liver tumors. Maj Probl Clin Surg 22:1, 1977.

136. Calne RY, Williams R. Orthotopic liver transplantation: experience with the first 60 patients treated. Br Med J 1:471, 1977.

137. Bern MM, McDermott W, Cady B, et al. Intra-arterial hepatic infusion and intravenous adriamycin for treatment of hepatocellular carcinoma. Cancer 42:399, 1978.

138. Lange M, Falkson G, Geddes EW. Intra-arterial chemotherapy in the treatment of primary liver cancer. S Afr J Surg 12:245, 1974.

139. Wellwood JM, Cady B, Oberfield RA. Treatment of primary liver cancer: response to regional chemotherapy. Clin Oncol 5:25, 1979.

140. Ariel LM. The treatment of primary and metastatic cancer of the liver. Surgery 39:70, 1956.

141. Falkson G. The treatment of liver cell cancer. In: Cameron HM, Linsell DA, Warwick GP, eds. Liver Cell Cancer. Amsterdam, Elsevier, 1976:81.

142. Cochrane AMG, Murray-Lyon IM, Brinkley DM, et al. Quadruple chemotherapy versus radiotherapy in treatment of primary hepatocellular carcinoma. Cancer 40:609, 1977.

143. Olweny CLM, Toya T, Katongole-Mbidde E, et al. Treatment of hepatocellular carcinoma with adriamycin. Cancer 36:1250, 1975.

144. Ihde DC, Kane RC, Cohen MH, et al. Adriamycin therapy in American patients with hepatocellular carcinoma. Cancer Res 17:159, 1976.

145. Vogel CL, Bayley AC, Brooker RJ, et al. A phase II study of Adriamycin (NSC 123127) in patients with hepatocellular carcinoma from Zambia and the United States. Cancer 39:1929, 1977.

146. Falkson G, Moertel CG, Lavin P, et al. Adriamycin chemotherapy studies in primary liver cancer. A prospective randomized clinical trial. Cancer 42:2149, 1978.

147. Johnson PJ, Williams R, Thomas H, et al. Induction of remission of hepatocellular carcinoma with doxorubicin. Lancet 1:1006, 1978.

148. Melia WM, Johnson PJ, Williams R. Induction of remission in hepatocellular carcinoma. A comparison of VP 16 with adriamycin. Cancer 51:206, 1983.

149. Chlebowski RT, Chan KK, Tong MT, et al. Adriamycin and methyl-CCNU combination therapy in hepatocellular carcinoma. Cancer 48:1085, 1981.

150. Bukowski RM, Legha S, Saiki J, et al. Phase II trial of m-AMSA in hepatocellular carcinoma: A Southwest Oncology Group study. Cancer Treat Rep 66:1651, 1982.

151. Danopoulos ED, Danopoulo IE. The results of urea treatment in liver malignancies. Clin Oncol 1:341, 1975.

152. Wheeler PG, Melia W, Jones B, et al. Non-operative arterial embolization in primary liver tumors. Br Med J 2:242, 1979.

153. Mori W, Nagasako K. Cholangiocarcinoma and related lesions. In: Okuda K, Peters RL, eds. Hepatocellular Carcinoma. New York, John Wiley and Sons, 1976:227.

154. Hou PC. The relationship between primary carcinoma of the liver and infestation with Clonorchis sinensis. J Pathol Bacteriol 72:239, 1956.

155. Purtilo DT. Clonorchiasis and hepatic neoplasms. Trop Geog Med 28:21, 1976.

156. Wogan GN. The induction of liver cancer by chemicals. In: Cameron HM, Linsell DA, Warwick GP, eds. Liver Cell Cancer. New York, John Wiley & Sons, 1976:6.

157. Eriksson S, Hagerstrand I. Cirrhosis and malignant hepatoma in alpha$_1$-antitrypsin deficiency. Acta Med Scand 195:451, 1974.

158. Stauffer MH, Sauer WG, Dearing WH, et al. The spectrum of cholestatic hepatic disease. JAMA 191:829, 1965.

159. Kulkarni PB, Beatty EC. Cholangiocarcinoma associated with biliary atresia. Am J Dis Child 131:442, 1977.

160. Gallagher PJ, Millis RR, Mitchison MJ. Congenital dilatation of the intrahepatic bile ducts with cholangiocarcinoma. J Clin Pathol 25:804, 1972.

161. Sane S, MacCallum JD. Primary carcinoma of the liver: cholangioma in hepatolithiasis. Am J Pathol 18:675, 1942.

162. Edmondson HA. Atlas of Tumor Pathology: Tumors of the Liver and Intrahepatic Bile Ducts. Section VII. Fascicle 25. Washington, DC, Armed Forces Institute of Pathology, 1958.

163. Omata M, Aschavai M, Liew CT, et al. Hepatocellular carcinoma in the U.S.A. Etiologic considerations. Gastroenterology 76:280, 1979.

164. Okuda K, Kubo Y, Okazaki N, et al. Clinical aspects of intrahepatic bile duct carcinoma including hilar carcinoma. Cancer 39:232, 1977.

165. Anthony PP. Primary carcinoma of the liver. Ann R Coll Surg Engl 58:285, 1976.

166. MacDonald RA. Cirrhosis and primary carcinoma of the liver. Changes in their occurrence at the Boston City Hospital 1897–1954. N Engl J Med 255:1179, 1956.

167. Cruickshank AH. The pathology of 111 cases of primary hepatic malignancy collected in the Liverpool area. J Clin Pathol 14:120, 1961.

168. Klatskin G. Adenocarcinoma of the hepatic duct at its bifurcation within the porta hepatitis. Am J Med 38:241, 1965.

169. Kaude J, Rian R. Cholangiocarcinoma. Radiology 100:573, 1971.

170. Meyerowitz BR, Aird I. Carcinoma of the hepatic ducts within the liver. Br J Surg 50:178, 1962.

171. Ishak KG, Glunz PR. Hepatoblastoma and hepatocarcinoma in infancy and childhood. Cancer 20:396, 1967.

172. Keeling JW. Liver tumours in infancy and childhood. J Pathol 103:69, 1971.

173. Exelby PR, Filler RM, Grosfield JL. Liver tumors in children with particular reference to hepatoblastoma and hepatocellular carcinoma. American Academy of Pediatrics, Surgical Section Survey. J Pediatr Surg 10:329, 1975.

174. Carter R. Hepatoblastoma in the adult. Cancer 23:191, 1969.

175. Napoli VM, Campbell WG. Hepatoblastoma in infant sister and brother. Cancer 39:2647, 1977.

176. Hasegawa H, Mukojima T, Hattori N, et al. Embryonal carcinoma and alpha-fetoprotein. Gann Monogr Cancer Res 14:129, 1973.

177. Baggenstoss AH. The pathology of tumors of the liver in infancy and childhood. In: Pack GT, Islami AH, eds. Tumours of the Liver. London, William Heinemann, 1970:249.

178. Landing BH. Tumors of the liver in childhood. In: Okuda K, Peters RL, eds. Hepatocellular Carcinoma. New York, John Wiley and Sons, 1976:212.

179. Ikeda K, Suita S, Nakagawara A, et al. Preoperative chemotherapy for initially irresectable hepatoblastoma in children. Arch Surg 114:203, 1979.

180. Siegel MM, Siegel SE, Isaacs H, et al. Primary chemotherapeutic management of irresectable and metastatic hepatoblastoma in children. Med Pediatr Oncol 4:297, 1978.

181. Falk H, Greech JL, Heath CW, et al. Hepatic disease among workers at a vinyl chloride polymerization plant. JAMA 230:59, 1974.

182. Baxter PJ, Anthony PP, MacSween RMN, et al. Angiosarcoma of the liver in Great Britain, 1963–73. Br Med J 4:919, 1977.

183. Locker GY, Doroshaw JH, Zwelling LA, et al. The clinical features of hepatic angiosarcoma: a report of four cases and a review of the English literature. Medicine (Balt) 58:48, 1979.

184. Makk L, Delmore F, Creech JL, et al. Clinical and morphological features of hepatic angiosarcoma in vinyl chloride workers. Cancer 37:149, 1976.

185. Visfeldt J, Poulsen H. On the histopathology of liver and liver tumours in thorium-dioxide patients. Acta Pathol Microbiol Scand 80A:97, 1972.

186. Tesluk H, Nordin WA. Hemangioendothelioma of the liver following thorium dioxide administration. Arch Pathol 60:493, 1955.

187. Roth F. Arsen-Leber-Tumoren (Hemangioendotheliom). Z Krebsforsch 61:468, 1957.

188. Regelson W, Kim U, Ospina J, et al. Hemangioendothelial sarcoma of the liver from chronic arsenic intoxication by Fowler's solution. Cancer 21:514, 1968.

189. Greech JL, Johnson MN. Angiosarcoma of the liver in the manufacture of polyvinyl chloride. J Occup Med 16:150, 1974.

190. Lloyd JW. Angiosarcoma of the liver of vinyl chloride/polyvinyl chloride workers. J Occup Med 17:333, 1975.

191. Falk H, Waxweiler RJ. Epidemiological studies of vinyl chloride health effects in the United States. Proc R Soc Med 69:303, 1976.

192. Maltoni C, Lefemine G. Carcinogenicity bioassays of vinyl chloride. Environ Res 7:387, 1974.

193. Dinman BD, Cook WA, Whitehouse WM, et al. Occupational acro-osteolysis. I. An epidemiological study. Arch Environ Health 22:61, 1971.

194. Lange CE, Jühe S, Stein G, et al. Vinylchloridkrankheiteine berufsbedingte systems klerose. Int Arch Arbeitmed 32:1, 1974.

195. Thomas LB, Popper H, Berk PD, et al. Vinyl chloride-induced liver disease. N Engl J Med 292:17, 1975.

196. Ross JM. A case illustrating the effects of prolonged action of radium. J Pathol Bacteriol 35:899, 1932.

197. Pimentel JC, Menezes AP. Liver disease in vineyard sprayers. Gastroenterology 72:275, 1977.

198. Daneshmend TK, Scott GL, Bradfield JWB. Angiosarcoma of the liver associated with phenelzine. Br Med J 1:1679, 1979.
199. Sussman EB, Nydick J, Gray G. Hemangioendothelial sarcoma of the liver and hemochromatosis. Arch Pathol 97:39, 1974.
200. Ludwig J, Hoffman HN. Hemangiosarcoma of the liver. Mayo Clin Proc 50:255, 1975.
201. Ishak KG. Mesenchymal tumors of the liver. In: Okuda K, Peters RL, eds. Hepatocellular Carcinoma. New York, John Wiley and Sons, 1976:286.
202. Whelan JG, Creech JL, Tamburro CH. Angiographic and radionuclide characteristics of hepatic angiosarcoma found in vinyl chloride workers. Radiology 118:549, 1976.
203. Pollard SM, Millward-Sadler GH. Malignant hemangioendotheliama involving the liver. J Clin Pathol 27:214, 1974.
204. Truell JE, Peck SD, Reiguam CW. Hemangiosarcoma of the liver complicated by disseminated intravascular coagulation. Gastroenterology 65:936, 1973.
205. Alpert LI, Benisch B. Hemangioendothelioma of the liver associated with microangiopathic hemolytic anemia. Am J Med 48:624, 1970.
206. Donald D, Dawson AM. Microangiopathic hemolytic anemia associated with malignant hemangioendothelioma. J Clin Pathol 24:456, 1971.
207. Burston J. Kupffer cell sarcoma. Cancer 11:798, 1958.
208. Ishak KG, Sesterhen IA, Goodman ZD, et al. Epithelioid hemangioendothelioma of the liver. Hum Pathol 15:839, 1984.
209. Bloustein PA, Silverberg SG. Squamous cell carcinoma originating in an hepatic cyst. Cancer 38:2002, 1976.
210. Greenwood H, Orr WN. Primary squamous cell carcinoma arising in a solitary non-parasitic cyst of the liver. J Pathol 107:145, 1972.
211. Pianzola LE, Drut R. Mucoepidermoid carcinoma of the liver. Am J Clin Pathol 56:758, 1971.
212. Stocker JT, Ishak KG. Undifferentiated (embryonal) sarcoma of the liver. Cancer 42:336, 1978.
213. Lorimer WS Jr. Right hepatolobectomy for primary mesenchymoma of the liver. Am Surg 141:246, 1955.
214. Sumiyoshi A, Niho Y. Primary osteogenic sarcoma of the liver—Report on an autopsy case. Acta Pathol Jpn 21:973, 1971.
215. Baum JK, Holtz F, Bookstein JJ, et al. Possible association between benign hepatomas and oral contraceptives. Lancet 2:926, 1973.
216. Edmondson HA, Henderson B, Benton B. Liver cell adenomas associated with the use of oral contraceptives. N Engl J Med 294:470, 1976.
217. Ameriks JA, Thompson NW, Norman W, et al. Hepatic adenomas, spontaneous liver rupture, and oral contraceptives. Arch Surg 110:548, 1975.
218. Fechner RE. Benign hepatic lesions and orally administered contraceptives. Hum Pathol 8:255, 1977.
219. Christopherson WM, Mays ET. Liver tumors and contraceptive steroids: experience with the first 100 registry patients. J Natl Cancer Inst 58:167, 1977.
220. Vana J, Murphy GP, Aronoff BL, et al. Primary liver tumors and oral contraceptives. JAMA 238:2154, 1977.
221. Guzman IJ, Gold JH, Rosai J, et al. Benign hepatocellular tumors. Surgery 82:495, 1977.
222. Klatskin G. Hepatic tumors: possible relation to use of oral contraceptives. Gastroenterology 73:386, 1977.
223. Knowles DM, Casarella WJ, Johnson PM, et al. The clinical, radiologic and pathologic characterization of benign hepatic neoplasms. Alleged association with oral contraceptives. Medicine 57:223, 1978.
224. Aungst CW. Benign liver tumors and oral contraceptives. NY State J Med 78:1933, 1978.
225. Nissen ED, Kent DR, Nissen SE. The role of oral contraceptive agents in the pathogenesis of liver tumors. J Toxicol Environ Health 5:231, 1979.
226. Rooks JB, Ory HW, Ishak KG, et al. Epidemiology of hepatocellular adenoma. The role of oral contraceptive use. JAMA 242:644, 1979.
227. Mays ET, Christopherson WM, Mahr MM, et al. Hepatic changes in young women ingesting contraceptive steroids. JAMA 235:730, 1976.
228. Vessey MP, Kay CR, Baldwin JA, et al. Oral contraceptives and benign liver tumours. Br Med J 1:164, 1977.
229. Adlercreutz A, Tenhunen R. Some aspects of the interaction between natural and synthetic female sex hormones and the liver. Am J Med 49:630, 1970.
230. Malt RA, Hershberg RA, Miller WL. Experience with benign tumors of the liver. Surg Gynecol Obstet 130:285, 1970.
231. Grabowski M, Stenram U, Bergvist A. Focal nodular hyperplasia of the liver, benign hepatomas, oral contraceptives and other drugs affecting the liver. Acta Pathol Microbiol Scand (A) 93:615, 1975.
232. Hernandez-Nieto L, Bruguera M, Bombi SA, et al. Benign liver cell adenoma associated with long-term administration of an androgenic-anabolic steroid (Methandienone). Cancer 40:1761, 1977.
233. Carrasco D, Prieto M, Pallardo L, et al. Multiple hepatic adenomas after long-term therapy with testosterone enanthenate. J Hepatol 1:573, 1985.
234. Schaffner F. The effect of oral contraceptives on the liver. JAMA 198:1010, 1966.
235. Edmondson HA, Reynolds TB, Henderson B, et al. Regression of liver cell adenomas associated with oral contraceptives. Ann Intern Med 86:180, 1977.
236. Mays ET, Christopherson W. Hepatic tumors induced by sex steroids. Sem Liver Dis 4:147, 1984.
237. Salvo AF, Schiller A, Athanasoulis A, et al. Hepatoadenoma and focal nodular hyperplasia. Pitfalls in radiocolloid imaging. Radiology 125:451, 1977.
238. Knowles DM, Wolff M, Johnson PM. Focal nodular hyperplasia and liver cell adenoma: radiologic and pathologic differentiation. Am J Radiol 131:393, 1978.
239. Ishak KG, Rabin L. Benign tumors of the liver. Med Clin North Am 59:995, 1975.
240. Christopherson WM, Mays ET. Relation of steroids to liver oncogenesis. J Toxicol Environ Health 5:207, 1979.
241. Davis M, Portmann B, Searle M, et al. Histological evidence of carcinoma in a hepatic tumour associated with oral contraceptives. Br Med J 4:496, 1975.
242. Ochsner JL, Halpert B. Cavernous hemangiomas of the liver. Surgery 43:577, 1958.
243. Dehner LP, Ishak KG. Vascular tumors of the liver in infants and young children. Arch Pathol 92:101, 1971.
244. Henson SW, Gray HK, Dockerty MB. Benign tumors of the liver. II. Hemangiomas. Surg Gynecol Obstet 103:327, 1956.
245. Park WC, Phillips R. The role of radiation therapy in the management of hemangiomas of the liver. JAMA 212:1496, 1970.
246. Schumacker HB. Hemangioma of the liver. Discussion of symptomatology and report of patient treated by operation. Surgery 11:209, 1942.
247. Plachta A. Calcified cavernous hemangioma of the liver. Radiology 79:783, 1962.
248. Freeny PC, Vimant TR, Barnett DC. Cavernous hemangioma of the liver: ultrasonography, arteriography and computed tomography. Radiology 132:143, 1979.
249. Yamauchi T, Minami M, Yashiro N. Non-invasive diagnosis of small cavernous hemangioma of the liver: Advantage of magnetic resonance imaging. Am J Radiol 145:1195, 1985.
250. McLaughlin MJ. Angiography in cavernous hemangioma of the liver. Am J Radiol 113:50, 1971.
251. Cooper WH, Martin JF. Hemangioma of the liver with thrombocytopenia. Am J Radiol 88:751, 1962.
252. Martinez J, Shapiro SS, Halburn RR, et al. Hypofibrinogenemia associated with hemangioma of the liver. Am J Clin Pathol 60:192, 1973.
253. Feldman M. Hemangioma of the liver. Special reference to its association with cysts of the liver and pancreas. Am J Clin Pathol 29:160, 1958.
254. Chung EB. Multiple bile duct hamartomas. Cancer 26:287, 1970.
255. Benz EJ, Baggenstoss AH. Focal cirrhosis of the liver: its relation to the so-called hamartoma (adenoma, benign hepatoma). Cancer 6:743, 1953.
256. McLean RH, Moller JH, Warwick J, et al. Multinodular hemangiomatosis of the liver in infancy. Pediatrics 49:563, 1972.
257. Braun P, Ducharme JC, Riopelle JL, et al. Hemangiomatosis of the liver in infants. J Pediatr Surg 10:121, 1975.
258. Mortensson W, Petersson H. Infantile hemangioendothelioma. Angiographic considerations. Acta Radiol (Diag) (Stockh)20:161, 1979.
259. Fost NC, Esterly NB. Successful treatment of juvenile hemangiomas with prednisone. J Pediatr 72:351, 1968.
260. Rake MO, Liberman MM, Dawson JL. Ligation of the hepatic artery in the treatment of heart failure due to hepatic hemangiomatosis. Gut 11:512, 1970.
261. Ishak KG, Willis GW, Cummins SD, et al. Biliary cystadenoma and cystadenocarcinoma. Cancer 39:322, 1977.
262. More JRS. Cystadenocarcinoma of the liver. J Clin Pathol 19:470, 1966.
263. Cruickshank AH, Sparshott SM. Malignancy in natural and experimental hepatic cysts. Experiments with aflatoxin in rats and the malignant transformation of cysts in human livers. J Pathol 104:185, 1971.
264. Ali M, Fayeuci AO, Braun EV. Malignant apudoma of the liver with symptomatic intractable hypoglycaemia. Cancer 42:686, 1978.
265. Willis RA. Teratomas. In: Atlas of Tumor Pathology. Section III, Fascicle 9. Washington, DC, Armed Forces Institute of Pathology, 1951:10.
266. Misugi K, Reiner CB. A malignant true teratoma of childhood. Arch Pathol 80:409, 1965.
267. Kiryabwire JWM, Mugerwa JW. Teratoma of the liver in an African child. Br J Surg 54:585, 1967.
268. Sorensen TIA, Baden H. Benign hepatocellular tumors. Scand J Gastroenterol 10:113, 1975.

269. O'Sullivan JP. Oral contraceptives and liver tumors. Proc R Soc Med 69:351, 1976.
270. Ross D, Pina J, Mirza M, et al. Regression of focal nodular hyperplasia after discontinuation of oral contraceptives. Ann Intern Med 85:203, 1976.
271. Mays ET, Christopherson WM, Barrows GH. Focal nodular hyperplasia of the liver. Possible relationship to oral contraceptives. Am J Clin Pathol 61:735, 1974.
272. Sherlock S, Feldman CA, Moran B, et al. Partial nodular transformation of the liver with portal hypertension. Am J Med 40:195, 1966.
273. Edmondson HA. Differential diagnosis of tumors and tumor-like lesions of liver in infancy and childhood. Am J Dis Child 91:168, 1956.
274. Sutton CA, Eller JL. Mesenchymal hamartoma of the liver. Cancer 22:29, 1968.
275. Srouji MN, Chatten J, Schulman WM, et al. Mesenchymal hamartoma of the liver in infants. Cancer 42:2483, 1978.
276. Grases PJ, Matos-Villalobos M, Arcia-Romero F, et al. Mesenchymal hamartoma of the liver. Gastroenterology 76:1466, 1979.
277. Scheuer PJ. Liver Biopsy Interpretation. Baltimore, Williams & Wilkins, 1968:93.
278. Homer LW, White HJ, Read RC. Neoplastic transformation of von Meyenburg complexes. J Pathol Bacteriol 96:499, 1968.

46

The Surgical Management of Primary Hepatocellular Carcinoma and Metastatic Liver Cancer

James H. Foster, M.D.

In the United States before 1970, few elective liver resections were attempted for the cure or palliation of patients with primary or metastatic liver cancer. The natural history of these diseases was believed to be so grim and the danger of major liver resection so high that only a few centers were willing to undertake the necessary pioneering efforts. Two decades later, much has changed. Modern radiologic imaging and the use of tumor markers have allowed earlier diagnosis; refinements in technique and increasing experience have allowed safer operation. Today, resection provides the only chance for cure for most patients with either metastatic or primary carcinoma of the liver. Resection occasionally may play a role in palliation.

Hundreds of operations have been done, and enough experience has accumulated to allow a firm basis for recommending indications for operation and assigning prognosis. Asian surgeons continue to pioneer in the field of resection for primary cancer, and their results in both the discovery and treatment of patients with subclinical disease are outstanding. In contrast, resection has not been important in the control of primary hepatocellular carcinoma in sub-Saharan Africa. This difference may reflect a variation in the disease or may be related to late case-finding.

This chapter will attempt to outline those diagnostic and prognostic features that aid the clinician in selecting patients for operation. A brief comparison of the results of resection with the natural history of the disease and with the results of other therapeutic methods will be made. For details of operative technique, the reader is referred elsewhere. Etiology, epidemiology, incidence, and pathology of primary cancer are covered in Chapter 45. Liver transplantation in patients with hepatoma is discussed in Chapter 55.

DIAGNOSTIC AIDS CONTRIBUTING TO SURGICAL DECISIONS

Primary and secondary liver cancers may grow to large size before they cause symptoms. Dull pain, epigastric fullness, and early satiety occur with large tumors, often together with vague feelings of fatigue and anorexia. Sharp pain usually connotes rapid stretching of Glisson's capsule, often due to necrosis and hemorrhage within the tumor. Jaundice, shoulder pain, and weight loss are ominous symptoms of both primary and metastatic disease.

There are many biochemical tests used as aids in the diagnosis of liver tumors, but the alanine aminotransferase (ALT) and aspartate aminotransferase (AST) are as reliable as any in picking up early lesions. Diminished synthetic function usually accompanies more massive involvement. Ultrasonography and computerized tomography have replaced radionuclide scanning and angiography in the discovery of liver cancer and the delineation of its geography (Chap. 26). Angiography, however, may be helpful in the differentiation of cavernous hemangiomas and focal nodular hyperplasia from liver cancer. The accuracy of computerized tomography may be augmented by the use of oily solutions, late imaging, or both.[1] The screening of high-risk populations with alpha-fetoprotein or carcinoembryonic antigen (CEA) may lead to a diagnosis of liver cancer many months before clinical signs appear but has not proved to be cost-effective in general populations. In patients without hepatomegaly who have had resection of primary cancers outside of the liver and who are at risk for liver metastasis, a normal alkaline phosphatase, AST, and CEA plus *either* a normal ultrasonogram or a computerized tomogram will rule out spread to the liver in most patients.[48] Additional tests will add cost more rapidly than benefit.

To make an appropriate decision about resection, the surgeon needs to know about the general condition of the patient, the histology of both the liver tumor and the adjacent nontumorous liver, the geography of the tumor, the benefits of nonresective therapy, and the natural history of the disease without treatment.

Percutaneous needle biopsy is often but not always helpful and may be dangerous. Lesions that may be hemangiomas or hydatid cysts should never be biopsied. Needle biopsy of benign tumors such as liver cell adenoma and focal nodular hyperplasia may result in misleading diagnoses of normal liver and cirrhosis, respectively. If laparotomy is necessary in any case, tissue diagnosis should be delayed until a generous open biopsy can be obtained. On the other hand, if the result of a percutaneous needle biopsy will alter a decision about laparotomy, then percutaneous biopsy should be done, even in patients with vascular neoplasms. In patients with probable primary cancer and possible cirrhosis, a needle biopsy of the nontumorous liver may be safer and help more with decision making than a biopsy of the tumor itself. Fine-needle aspiration biopsy may be helpful in the patient with metastatic carcinoma but in the author's experience has been misleading (in both directions) with hepatocellular carcinoma, particularly in cirrhotic patients.

The most useful and efficient tool to detect liver metastases or the location and number of primary tumors in a noncirrhotic liver (with the possible exception of intraoperative ultrasonography) is the surgeon's hand. If laparotomy is inevitable for a patient with cancer of the gastrointestinal tract, the preoperative demonstration of metastatic liver disease is seldom warranted. On the other hand, demonstration of massive liver metastasis in a patient with a nonobstructing colon cancer may spare the patient an unnecessary operation. Each patient presents a different problem and requires different diagnostic tactics, but in general, only those tests should be done that will contribute directly to a decision about therapy.

DETERMINING RESECTABILITY

A liver tumor is resectable if it can be removed without interfering with the inflow and outflow vessels of enough residual liver tissue to support life. For the patient without cirrhosis, the inferior vena cava and the area of the hilar bifurcations must not be involved. Hepatocellular carcinoma has a marked propensity for growing down into the portal vein and its branches and up into the major hepatic veins. Angiography and radionuclide scanning often are misleading about hilar or caval involvement, whereas real-time ultrasonography and computerized tomography have proved to be remarkably accurate.

The question of resectability of hepatocellular carcinoma in a cirrhotic patient needs special discussion. As we will see later, the results after early recognition and resection of hepatocellular carcinoma from Asian patients with chronic active hepatitis B and cirrhosis have been surprisingly encouraging.[15] These patients most commonly present with symptoms from their tumors, not from cirrhosis, and they tolerate limited resection reasonably well. A significant proportion have long disease-free survivals after "curative" resection (see later). In contrast, Western patients with hepatocellular carcinoma and cirrhosis are usually alcoholics who are symptomatic and subsequently develop a liver tumor. These patients tolerate operation poorly, and their tumor seems to recur rapidly—perhaps caused by multicentricity. With few exceptions, primary cancers should probably not be resected from Western patients with diffuse cirrhosis. Thus, the determination of tumor geography becomes less important than the discovery of cirrhosis in the nontumorous liver. An exception to the general proscription of resection in the Western cirrhotic is provided by the patient whose tumor ruptures and causes hemoperitoneum as a primary symptom. Urgent resection and debridement may be necessary to save the patient's life, although arterial ligation and embolization may provide alternatives for the wary clinician.

In the noncirrhotic patient, very large resections are possible for three reasons. First, the liver has an enormous functional reserve capacity. Second, the resection of more than 35 to 40 per cent of the liver stimulates that combination of hypertrophy and hyperplasia which we call regeneration (Chap. 3). Functional sufficiency is restored within a week or two after major resection and volume within a very few months. Third, as a large tumor fills one lobe, the other lobe gradually hypertrophies, so that even when a surgeon removes 75 to 80 per cent of the mass or weight of the liver, probably considerably less than half of the functioning parenchyma is removed. One should be extremely aggressive about resecting primary liver cancer in patients with noncirrhotic livers, particularly in children and in young adults with fibrolamellar carcinoma *if* the disease has not spread beyond Glisson's capsule. Extrahepatic spread precludes resection for cure (except in pediatric patients with embryonal tumors responsive to chemotherapy), but extrahepatic spread occurs late in many patients with hepatocellular carcinoma. Only 47 per cent of patients in one large series had extrahepatic spread at the time of their death and autopsy.[2] Direct invasion of contiguous structures such as diaphragm or colon by either primary or secondary liver cancer does not carry as poor a prognosis as embolic spread. Multivisceral resection may occasionally be indicated in these instances.

Modern imaging can determine *un*resectability in many patients and is probably better than the surgeon's eyes and hands in detecting spread into critical veins. Involvement of the portal vein bifurcation or the junction of the hepatic veins and the inferior vena cava by hepatocellular carcinoma, either within or without the vein lumen, precludes resection for cure. Size alone does not, particularly for primary cancer. Huge tumors can be resected safely if the vital confluences and bifurcations are spared. However, final decisions about resectability in apparently favorable cases are often best reserved for the operating room. With thorough inspection and palpation before and after appropriate dissection and mobilization, the geography of a tumor can be appreciated and the final decision can be made before incurring significant risk.[11] "Satellitosis," the congregation of several small nodules around a larger tumor mass, represents regurgitation into adjacent portal vein branches and should not preclude resection, but true multicentricity should probably contraindicate major resection for both primary and secondary disease.

OPERATIVE AND POSTOPERATIVE PROBLEMS

Death either during or after liver resection for tumor is unfortunately not uncommon. Table 46–1 illustrates a progressive decline in operative mortality rates, but 3 to 5 per cent of patients with secondary cancer still die after major liver resection. The figure is closer to 6 to 10 per cent for patients with primary cancer, who tend to have larger tumors. Table 46–2 lists causes of death. Failure to control hemorrhage on the operating table remains at the top of the list. Postoperative liver failure is largely a function of patient selection. It is due in a few instances to technical problems.

Postoperative liver failure is unusual after controlled resection of tumor from a noncirrhotic liver. The multiple metabolic problems described by the pioneering surgeons were (in retrospect) more closely related to the hypotension and hypothermia of bloody operations requiring multiple transfusions and to the postoperative sepsis that often accompanied resection by now outmoded techniques than it was to the loss of functioning parenchyma. Even the portal hypertension secondary to routing the total portal circulation through a small remnant of residual liver is transient. The reserve vascular capacity of this remarkable organ seems to parallel its functional reserve. Bile fistula, abdominal abscess, and upper gastrointestinal hemorrhage are rarely seen after controlled resection. The more common complications, such as atelectasis and wound infection, can be reduced by attention to detail. Pulmonary complications have been reduced by the ever-decreasing use of thoracic extension of an abdominal incision formerly used for almost all patients with bulky tumors. Thus, given a controlled gentle resection, the liver can tolerate removal of very large tumors. This brings us to the two key questions: (1) Do the results of resection justify assumption of the risk of operation? (2) How do survivors of resection fare when compared with similar patients treated by other modes of therapy? These two questions will be considered separately, first for primary liver cancer and then for secondary liver cancer.

PRIMARY LIVER CANCER

Table 46–3 lists rates of resectability for patients with primary liver cancer and illustrates an improving trend,

TABLE 46–1. OPERATIVE MORTALITY AFTER LIVER RESECTION FOR PRIMARY LIVER CANCER

Reference	Patients	Number/% of Deaths	Cirrhosis Present (%)
Asian			
Reports			
3	370	44/12	
4	88	14/16	51
5	301	56/19	79
6	181	16/9	70
7	165	33/25	85
8	274	17/62	
9	305	23/7.5	
10	109	6/5.5	64
Non-Asian			
Reports			
2	127	27/21	20
11	46	2/5	0
12	43	4/9	14

particularly in Asia. In the Liver Tumor Cancer Research Center at the Zhong Shan Hospital in Shanghai from 1961 through 1970, primary liver tumors were resectable in only 15.5 per cent of 387 patients whereas tumors were resectable in 36 per cent of 316 patients seen from 1977 to 1982.[15] Earlier recognition of disease and the evolution of safer operative techniques, allowing limited resection in cirrhotic patients, help to explain these gains made for Chinese and Japanese patients. The figures from Western centers may not be representative because of referral patterns that present only the most favorable cases to recognized centers for liver surgery.

Table 46–4 updates the results of resection in Western and Asian patients. The 35 to 40 per cent long-term survival in the West justifies an aggressive approach to primary liver tumor in noncirrhotic patients. Fibrolamellar carcinoma has not yet been reported from the East, but the collected review of Soreide and co-workers reemphasizes the good prognosis of this histologic variant in Western patients.[16] That this variant occurs more often in younger and often in female patients—that is, the same population at risk for benign solid liver tumors (focal nodular hyperplasia and liver cell adenoma)—is of considerable interest and probably is not coincidental. Five-year survival after liver resection for primary cancer usually means permanent cure for noncirrhotic patients, but whether this will be true for the cirrhotic patients remains to be seen. Although their original cancers may have been "cured," one would suspect that new cancers will develop with time in the cirrhotic patient.

The concept of subclinical cancer has resulted from the screening with alpha-fetoprotein of large high-risk populations.[15] Elevation of alpha-fetoprotein above 200 ng/ml is an indication for further evaluation of the patient. When resectable disease is found, conservative resections are based on segmental anatomy and the use of intraoperative ultrasonography. In patients with chronic active hepatitis-B infection and macronodular cirrhosis, operative mortality is markedly reduced, and long-term survival is increased when a limited resection can be performed.[15] Unfortunately, the use of alpha-fetoprotein as a screening test has not produced better results for resection in African patients, in whom the disease seems to be more aggressive, or in Western patients, in whom the disease is more often associated with alcoholism and a micronodular pattern of cirrhosis.

Table 46–5 lists survival in pediatric patients. Hepatoblastoma occurs in younger patients and has a better prognosis than hepatocellular carcinoma, probably because of its sensitivity to chemotherapeutic agents.

LIVER TRANSPLANTATION FOR PRIMARY LIVER CANCER (See Chap. 55)

Transplantation teams in Pittsburgh and Cambridge have accumulated enough experience with total hepatectomy and transplantation for primary liver cancer to allow some perspective. Starzl and his associates divide their experience into those patients who had primary liver cancer found incidentally in livers removed for some other condition and those patients for whom the hepatectomy was done for clinically evident massive involvement with primary liver cancer. In the first group, all 12 patients who survived the transplant operation are alive without evidence of disease from 4 months to 15 years after transplantation. In the second group with clinical cancer, 4 of 25 patients

TABLE 46–2. CAUSES OF OPERATIVE DEATHS AFTER LIVER RESECTION FOR NEOPLASIA

Reference	Death/Resection	Failure to Control Hemorrhage	Bile Duct Injury, Other Technical	Liver Failure, Postoperative	Upper Gastrointestinal Hemorrhage	Sepsis	Cardiopulmonary	Other
Foster and Berman (p + s) (1977)[2]	82/621	26	13	15	4	4	4	5 judgment error 3 air emboli; 2 recurrent cancer
Fortner et al. (p + s) (1978)[61]	10/108	2	2	0	1	0	1	4 coagulopathy + hepatic
Sorenson et al. (p + s) (1979)[59]	8/31	4	0	3	0	1	0	
Logan et al. (cm) (1982)[26]	1/19	0	0	0	1	0	0	
Adson et al. (p) (1981)[11]	3/66	3	0	0	0	0	0	
Adson et al. (cm) (1981)[11]	2/106	0	0	0	1	0	0	1 late death in 75-year-old with complicated course
Balasegaram (p + s) (1979)[4]	14/88	4	0	8	0	2	0	
Lee et al. (p) (1982)[7]	33/165	9	1	10	3	5	3	2 wound dehiscence
Mengchao et al. (p) (1980)[6]	16/181	2	0	9	0	1	0	4 coagulopathy
Bengmark et al. (p + s) (1982)[58]	3/21	3	0	0	0	0	0	all 3 in O.R.
Foster (p + s) (1988)[58a]	3/106	0	2	0	0	0	0	

Source: Data in this table were adapted from Foster JH. In: Decosse J, Sherlock P, eds. Clinical Management of Gastrointestinal Cancer. Martinus Nijhoff, 1984:93 (Table 6), with permission.[13]

p + s = primary and secondary neoplasms; cm = colorectal metastases only; p = primary neoplasms only.

with hepatocellular carcinoma are alive without disease at 5 to 45 months (3 of the 4 had fibrolamellar carcinoma). There were no survivors in ten patients transplanted for cholangiocarcinoma, and two patients have experienced long survival after total hepatectomy for primary sarcomas of the liver.[20]

Calne and his associates report 3 5-year survivors without evidence of disease in 31 patients transplanted for hepatocellular carcinoma. Most of those who died early succumbed to the complications of transplantation rather than cancer. Of 16 patients receiving transplantations for

cholangiocarcinoma, 12 died in the first year (2 with recurrence), 3 others had recurrences in the second year, and 1 patient is alive without evidence of recurrent cancer 1 year after transplantation.[21] The dedication, the persistence, and the skills required for these pioneering transplantation efforts can only be applauded. The work must continue and should become more encouraging as less morbid immunosuppressive regimens are developed, but for the present, liver transplantation for primary cancer cannot yet be recommended as an accepted form of therapy.

Non-operative therapy for primary liver cancer is re-

TABLE 46–3. RESECTABILITY RATES OF PATIENTS WITH PRIMARY LIVER CANCER

Reference	Patients with plc	Laparotomies for plc	Resections	Percentage Resectable	
				Total Patients	Patients with Laparotomy
56	3254	—	171	5.3	—
4	810	535	88	11	16
5	4031	1041	361	9	35
7	935	—	165	18	—
15	466 cc	—	115	25	—
	100 scc	90	60	60	67
57	187	—	118	63	—

Source: Adapted from Foster JH. Chirurg Gastroent Interdisz Gespr, 1987 (Table 2), with permission.[14]

plc = primary liver cancer; cc = clinical cancer; scc = subclinical cancer.

TABLE 46–4. SURVIVAL AFTER LIVER RESECTION FOR PRIMARY CANCER

Reference	Cases Resected	Operative Mortality (%)	Survival 3 Yrs (%)	Survival 5 Yrs (%)	Other
Western Experience					
1970 Foster (literature review)[60]	60	22		36*	
1977 Foster & Berman (national survey)[2]	127	21		30*	{36% in noncirrhotics { 0% in cirrhotics
1978 Fortner[61]	42	17		37†	
1981 Adson & Weiland[11]	43	5	65	36	
1983 Iwatsuki & Starzl[12]	43	9	56†	46†*	
1986 Soreide et al (fibrolamellar only)[16]	42	0		56	
Eastern Experience					
1970 Foster (literature review)[60]	236	24	—	6*	
1974 Yu & Tang (China)[62]	258	15	15.5		
1976 Ishikawa (Japan)[63]	297	22	8.4		
1979 Lin (Taiwan)[64]	132	11	18		
1980 Okuda (Japan)[5]	222	21.5	12		
1982 Lee (Hong Kong)[65]	165	20	20†		
1985 Tang (China)[15]					
Subclinical	60	2		73	
Clinical	25	6		16	
1986 Lee et al (Taiwan)[66]					
Subclinical	62	6	68		44 at 4 yrs
Clinical	47	4	32		8 at 4 yrs
1986 Nagasue et al (Japan)[57]	118	14.4	2 yr‡ 81	4 yr‡	81 noncirrhotic}
			55		35 cirrhotic }

Source: The data in this table are adapted from Foster JH. Chirurg Gastroent Interdisz Gespr, 1987 (Table 3), with permission.
*Operative survivors only.
†*Actuarial* survival.
‡Survival of 94 patients resected "for cure."

viewed in Chapter 45. The final report of a Hong Kong study is disappointing but illustrative of the usefulness of currently available techniques. One hundred sixty-six patients with hepatocellular carcinoma were prospectively randomized to receive (1) dearterialization, (2) hepatic artery ligation plus perfusion of the distal artery with chemotherapy, (3) hepatic artery ligation plus portal vein perfusion with chemotherapy, (4) external radiation, or (5) supportive care only. After 15 years of investigation, all of the patients have died. There were no differences in survival times among the treatment groups or between treated patients and those who received supportive care alone.[21a]

CONCLUSIONS AND RECOMMENDATIONS FOR THE TREATMENT OF PATIENTS WITH PRIMARY LIVER CANCER

At the present time, resection remains the only method for achieving cure for patients with hepatocellular carci-

TABLE 46–5. RESULTS OF RESECTION OF PRIMARY LIVER CANCER IN CHILDREN

Reference	Patients Resected	Survival
Exelby et al. 1975[17]	86 HB	50% at 3 yrs
	33 HCC	34% at 5 yrs
Foster & Berman 1977[2]	47 HB	47% at 5 yrs
	21 HCC	29% at 5 yrs
Randolph et al. 1978[18]	9 HB	5 alive (4 ned > 2 yrs)
	2 HCC	Both died
Okuda 1980[5]	40 HB	61.5% 5 yrs
Giacomantonio 1984[19]	22	12 alive, 6 > 5 yrs (all HB)

HB = hepatoblastoma; HCC = hepatocellular carcinoma; ned = no evidence of disease.

noma. No palliative benefit of resection has yet been demonstrated for patients with incurable disease. When resection is not possible, no treatment should be given to asymptomatic patients outside of an experimental protocol. The treatment of symptomatic patients remains in the realm of art. Supportive measures alone may provide more comfortable days at home than the use of more active treatment programs, which bring with them significant toxicity.

METASTATIC CANCER

RESECTION

The last decade has seen enormous strides in the accumulation of experience with liver resection for secondary liver tumors. Most of this experience is in patients with colorectal cancer. Adson has the largest experience,[22] and that together with a collected review[23] and a recent computerized survey by Hughes, Sugarbaker, and colleagues[24] provides useful answers to most of the questions about which patients with metastatic colorectal cancer will benefit from resection. Experience with other metastatic tumors is small, and the reports of resectional and other treatment are anecdotal.

Resection can be done safely by those with experience. Table 46–6 documents recent reports of operative mortality. Not enough patients have undergone liver transplantation for metastatic disease to justify definitive conclusions, but the dearth of experience testifies to the negative results of early attempts.

TABLE 46–6. OPERATIVE MORTALITY AFTER LIVER RESECTION FOR METASTATIC CANCER

Reference		Patients	Operative Mortality (%)
Foster & Berman	1977[2]	176	8
Wanebo et al	1978[25]	27	7
Logan et al	1982[26]	19	5
Fortner	1983[27]	65	7
Cady & McDermott	1984[28]	23	0
Butler et al	1986[29]	62	10
Iwatsuki et al	1986[30]	60	0
Ekberg et al	1986[31]	72	5.6
Adson	1987[22]	141	2.8

NONCOLORECTAL DISEASE

Table 46–7 summarizes survival of patients after liver resection for cancer metastatic from primary sites outside of the colon and rectum. Credit for long-term survival in patients with resected liver metastases from Wilms's tumors must be shared with chemotherapy and an aggressive approach to the resection of pulmonary (in addition to liver) metastases. The four five-year survivors after resection of liver deposits of melanoma, pancreatic cancer, and leiomyosarcoma are dead of recurrent cancer more than five years after liver resection, and thus natural history more than resection must be given credit. This collected experience is not sufficient to justify conclusions, but an occasional resection may be useful in a patient with a noncolorectal metastatic lesion in the liver if the tumor seems to be slow-growing, is unresponsive to other treatments, and the resection can be done safely.

COLORECTAL METASTASES

The liver is the most common site for metastasis of colorectal carcinoma.[49] Since most patients with such spread will die of their liver involvement,[49] it seems important to define the utility of resection in this group of patients. Table 46–8 reports survival in patients after resection of colorectal liver metastases. Five-year survival does not equate with cure, because 14 of 61 patients in one review[23] and one third of 5-year survivors in a collected series[24] eventually died of recurrent colorectal cancer. These figures must be compared with survival figures of patients without resection. Survival for 6 to 10 months after the diagnosis of liver metastasis has been used in the past as a standard

against which to measure the results of resectional and other therapy.[23] Adson's recent report of survival of 252 patients without resection (Fig. 46–1)[40] and the more selective statistics of Wood, Pettavel, Goslin, Finan, Wagner, and their associates are revealing (Table 46–9). Perhaps as many as 40 per cent of untreated patients with limited disease will survive two years after a diagnosis of liver metastasis. However, less than 1 per cent of patients will live five years.

How can we select the patient who will benefit from resection? The statistical analyses of Hughes and associates provide the clearest answer to date. They collected data on 859 patients from 24 institutions in the United States and Western Europe. All patients had survived liver resection for metastatic colorectal carcinoma. Table 46–10 documents the correlation of various factors with actuarial overall and disease-free survival. A patient with one or two resectable metastases from a Dukes's B primary cancer, with an interval between bowel and liver resections of more than one year and a resection margin in excess of 1 cm, had more than a 45 per cent chance of surviving five years after liver resection. Conversely, patients with three or more liver metastases from Dukes's C primary lesions whose liver metastases were discovered at the same time as the colon tumor or within one year did significantly less well after resection of the liver metastases.[24]

Although unsupported by data, the suggestion of Cady, Foster, and others to watch a patient with limited (resectable) colorectal liver metastasis for a few months after its discovery may have some merit.[28, 41] The patient with rapidly progressive disease may be spared a major operation, and the patient with indolent disease may still be "curable" if the observation period is not prolonged. Many patients have been followed with serial measurements of carcinoembryonic antigen (CEA) after bowel resection for colorectal cancer. If the CEA becomes elevated after an initial return to normal postcolectomy, will it accurately predict recurrence and can it provide a stimulus for re-operation, which might in turn provide an opportunity for "cure" of residual disease? The report of Martin and colleagues is more optimistic than any other in this regard. They found residual cancer in 95 per cent of 146 patients at CEA-directed relaparotomy. This residual disease was resectable in 81 patients. Liver resection was done in many patients, and 10 of 16 patients who can be evaluated have lived five years without evidence of recurrence after such a liver resection.[42]

Other reports of the results of CEA-directed "second-look" operations have not been as optimistic.[50–53] Resection

TABLE 46–7. SURVIVAL AFTER LIVER RESECTION FOR NONCOLORECTAL LIVER METASTASES

Primary Tumor	Operative Survivors	Survival		Died of Recurrence After 5 Years
		2 Yrs	5 Yrs	
Wilms's tumor	17	8/14	4/10	0
Melanoma	16	2/11	1/11	1
Leiomyosarcoma	13	4/9	1/9	1
Kidney	9	2/5	1/5	0
Pancreas	8	2/7	1/7	1 (islet cell)
Uterus and cervix	9	1/7	0/7	—
Stomach	10	1/8	1/8	0
Breast	6	0/3	0/2	—
Other sarcomas	5	1/3	1/3	1
Ovary	4	0/2	0/2	—
Unknown primary	4	0/3	0/3	—
Other*	9	2/4	0/2	—

Source: Adapted from Foster JH. In: DeCasse J, Sherlock P, eds. Clinical Management of Gastrointestinal Cancer. Martinus Nijhoff, 1984 (Table 10); Iwatsuki S, et al. Ann Surg 197:247, 1983, with permission.
*Includes 2 adrenal, 2 neuroblastoma, and 1 each lung, thyroid, paraganglionoma, pericytoma, and glucagonoma.

TABLE 46–8. SURVIVAL AFTER LIVER RESECTION FOR METASTATIC COLORECTAL CANCER

Reference		Patients	Survival (%)	
			2 Yrs	5 Yrs
Foster	1978[32]	259†	44	22
Ekberg et al.	1986[31]	72	30* (3 yrs)	16*
Iwatsuki et al.	1986[30]	60	72*	45*
Butler et al.	1986[29]	56†	50* (3 yrs)	34*
Hughes et al.	1987[24]	859†	—	33*
Adson	1987[22]	141	—	23

*Actuarial survival.
†Excludes operative deaths.
References 22, 29, and 31 are institutional; references 24 and 32 are collected series that may include cases from Iwatsuki, Butler, and Adson.

"for cure" was only possible in 10 to 25 per cent of patients. Long-term survival of this very small and selective group of patients has been fairly good.

NONRESECTIONAL THERAPY FOR PATIENTS WITH LIVER METASTASIS

This topic is a large one that is full of controversy. Only a short discussion will follow based upon the author's current personal opinions. Appropriate references are cited for further study.

CHEMOTHERAPY

No combination of chemotherapeutic agents given systemically has been shown to be better than 5-fluorouracil (5-FU) alone for patients with liver metastases from gastrointestinal carcinoma. Although 15 to 19 per cent of such patients will show a response to 5-FU, no survival benefit over untreated control patients has yet been demonstrated in spite of 25 years of experience.[54] Hepatic artery infusion for metastatic cancer was abandoned 20 years ago because of attendant morbidity and little demonstrable benefit. More recently, the development of a totally implantable infusion device and a better appreciation of the pharmacokinetics of various chemotherapeutic agents have prompted a renewal of interest in the use of 5-floxuridine

and other agents given by such a pump. Early reports of greater than 80 per cent response rates resulted in a large, uncontrolled experience that suggested less morbidity and probably increased benefit.[41] However, even these optimistic early reports showed no advantage to hepatic artery infusion for patients with extrahepatic disease, and this method of treatment was abandoned in that group of patients. Controlled trials were eventually set up and are on-going, but enough data have been accumulated to bring discouragement. Patients given systemic chemotherapy were compared with patients undergoing hepatic artery infusion. Although response rate was higher in the arterial infusion group, no significant survival advantage has yet been demonstrated. Toxicity was higher than anticipated in the hepatic artery infusion group and was sometimes reversible (hepatitis and gastritis), occasionally non-reversible (sclerosing cholangitis), and even fatal.[43-45] The responders lived 24 and 26 months in the most favorable reports, but this was not much different from the mean survival of untreated patients with limited disease previously reported by Wagner and co-workers.[40] Most would agree that hepatic artery infusion for patients with liver metastasis should be limited to patients on investigational protocols. Inclusion of untreated patients with similar performance status and tumor burden in these protocols would do much to clarify the place of hepatic artery infusion in the future.

RADIATION

Rapid growth, necrosis and hemorrhage, and invasion of the diaphragm may produce localized pain in a patient with bulky, unresectable liver metastasis. External beam radiation may be followed by pain relief, although survival will probably not be affected.[41] The response to radiation of patients with liver metastasis from radiosensitive tumors such as seminoma can be impressive, but unfortunately, patients with liver metastasis from the gastrointestinal tract, breast, lung, and prostate do not do as well.

The introduction of radiotagged microspheres via hepatic artery has also been attempted for patients with metastatic cancer, but no palliative or survival benefit has yet been shown in controlled investigations.[55]

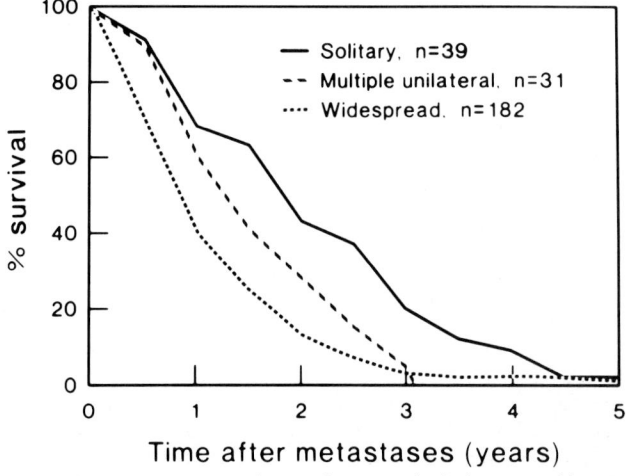
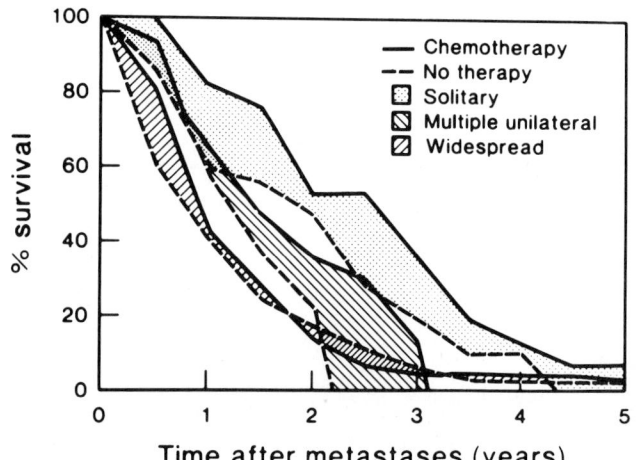

Figure 46–1. A, Survival rates of patients who had unresected hepatic metastases without evidence of other residual disease—classified with respect to extent and site of hepatic involvement. Three-year survival rates: solitary lesions 0.21; multiple unilateral 0.06; and widespread 0.04. Five-year survival rates: 0.03, 0.00, and 0.02, respectively. B. Survival rates of patients who had unresected hepatic metastases of varied extent who were and were not treated with chemotherapeutic agents. (Reproduced from Wagner JS, et al. Ann Surg 199:502, 1984, with permission.)

TABLE 46–9. SURVIVAL OF PATIENTS WITH LIVER METASTASES FROM COLORECTAL CANCER

Reference	Patients	Survival (%)				
		Mean (Mos)	1 Yr	2 Yrs	3 Yrs	5 Yrs
All Stages						
Pestana et al. 1964[33]	353	9				
Jaffe et al. 1968[34]	177	5				
Cady et al. 1970[35]	269	13	33	14	7	1
Staged Liver Involvement						
Wood et al. 1976[36]						
Solitary	15	16.7	60	—	—	1
Localized	11	10.6	27	—	—	0
Widespread	87	3.1	6	—	—	0
Pettavel et al. 1978[37]						
Minimal	12	21.5	100	—	—	—
Moderate	41	6.9	—	0	—	0
Widespread	30	1.4	0	—	—	—
Goslin et al. 1982[38]						
4 or more	87	10	—	—	—	0
Less than 4	38	24	—	—	—	0
Finan et al. 1985[39]						
Solitary	21	15.5	—	—	—	0
Multiple	65	8	—	—	—	0
Wagner et al. 1984[40]						
Solitary	39	21	>60	>40	>21	3
Widespread	182	9*	40*	12*	4	2

*Estimated.

HEPATIC ARTERY LIGATION

Metastatic tumors may shrink after hepatic artery ligation, but the response usually will be modest and temporary if it occurs at all.[41] Occasionally, a patient with debilitating symptoms from a hormone-producing tumor will find relief after arterial ligation or embolization (see the following section).

FUNCTIONING LIVER METASTASES FROM ENDOCRINE TUMORS

If there is a place for palliative (i.e., noncurative) liver resection for metastatic tumor, it is probably in the patient

TABLE 46–10. SURVIVAL AFTER LIVER RESECTION FOR METASTATIC COLORECTAL CANCER

Factor	5-Year Survival (%)*	
	Overall	Disease-Free
Number of Metastases		
1	37	25
2	37	25
≥3	18	7
Surgical Margin		
Positive or <1 cm	23	13
>1 cm	47	33
Stage of Primary Tumor		
Dukes's B	47	28
Dukes's C	23	18
Disease-Free Interval†		
<1 month	27	17
1 month to 1 year	31	22
1 year	42	26

Source: Adapted from Hughes KS, et al. Resection of the liver for colorectal carcinoma metastases: a multi-institutional study of indications for resection. Surgery 103:278, 1988.
Actuarial survival estimated by Kaplan-Meier method.
†Interval between bowel and liver resection.

who is disabled by symptoms caused by the hormones or other vasoactive substances released by a tumor metastasis in the liver. The carcinoid syndrome provides an excellent example. Long survival can be anticipated because of the slow growth rate of the primary tumor. More often than not, liver resection is not possible because of widespread disease, but when tumor geography allows safe resection of 95+ per cent of visible or palpable disease, palliation of hormone-induced symptoms will occur. Thirty-six of 37 patients who survived liver resection for carcinoid in a collected review were palliated. The only patient who was not benefited had resection of less than 50 per cent of the liver tumor deposits.[13] A rare patient with metastatic insulinoma or other limited, slow-growing endocrine tumor may also benefit from resection of hepatic deposits for control of symptoms caused by production of hormones.

McDermott and others have reported significant and prolonged palliation of a few patients with unresectable liver metastasis from carcinoid after hepatic artery ligation.[46, 47] The author's very limited experience with this situation has not been so fortunate.

CONCLUSIONS AND RECOMMENDATIONS FOR PATIENTS WITH METASTATIC LIVER CANCER

More accurate diagnosis and a better understanding of the natural history of liver metastasis have allowed recent clarification of the place of liver resection for metastatic tumors. Most patients with metastatic cancer in their livers will have involvement too extensive to allow resection, and many will have extrahepatic spread. Such patients, if asymptomatic, should probably not be treated off protocol unless they have a disease known to be sensitive to low-dose radiation or to chemotherapy and hormonal manipulation.

Liver resection should be limited to those patients with well-localized metastasis from colorectal carcinoma and perhaps an occasional patient with a slow-growing, bulky metastasis from some other site. The aim of liver resection for metastatic cancer is cure, not palliation, and prolonged survival will follow safe resection in 30 to 45 per cent of carefully selected patients with colorectal liver metastasis. Long and useful palliation without cure may occasionally be possible if the vast bulk of the hormone-producing liver metastasis from a slow-growing endocrine tumor is resected.

REFERENCES

1. Reed WP, Haney PJ, Elias EG, et al. Ethiodized oil emulsion enhanced computerized tomography in the preoperative assessment of metastases to the liver from the colon and rectum. Surg Gynecol Obstet 162:131, 1986.
2. Foster JH, Berman MM. Solid Liver Tumors, Vol 22 in Major Problems in Clinical Surgery series. Philadelphia, WB Saunders, 1977.
3. Shanghai Coordinating Group. Diagnosis and treatment of primary hepatocellular carcinoma in early stage. Chin Med J [Engl] 92:801, 1979.
4. Balasegaram M. Hepatic resection for malignant tumors. Surg Rounds p 14, Sept 1979.
5. Okuda K. Liver cancer study group of Japan: primary liver cancers in Japan. Cancer 45:2663, 1980.
6. Mengchao W, Han C, Xiaohua Z, et al. Primary hepatic carcinoma resection over 18 years. Chin Med J [Engl] 93:723, 1980.
7. Lee NW, Wong J, Ong GB. The surgical management of primary carcinoma of the liver. World J Surg 6:66, 1982.
8. Wu MC, Zhang XH, Chen H, et al. Experiences in hepatectomies of 467 cases. Chin J Digest [Chin] 2:190, 1982.
9. Tang ZY, Yu YQ, Zhou XD. The changing role of surgery in the treatment of primary liver cancer. Semin Surg Oncol 2:103, 1986.
10. Lee CS, Sung JL, Hwang LY, et al. Surgical treatment of 109 patients with symptomatic and asymptomatic hepatocellular carcinoma. Surgery 99:481, 1986.
11. Adson MA, Weiland LH. Resection of primary solid hepatic tumors. Am J Surg 141:18, 1981.
12. Iwatsuki S, Shaw BW, Starzl TE. Experience with 150 liver resections. Ann Surg 197:247, 1983.
13. Foster JH. Liver resection for malignant disease. In: Decosse J, Sherlock P, eds. Clinical Management of Gastrointestinal Cancer. Boston, Martinus Nijhoff, 1984:93.
14. Foster JH. Primary liver cancer. Chirurg Gastroent Interdisz Gespr 3:25, 1987.
15. Tang ZY, ed. Subclinical Hepatocellular Carcinoma. Heidelburg, Springer-Verlag, 1985.
16. Soreide O, Czerniak A, Bradpiece H, et al. Characteristics of fibrolamellar hepatocellular carcinoma. Am J Surg 151:518, 1986.
17. Exelby PR, Filler RM, Grosfeld JL. Liver tumors in children in particular reference to hepatoblastomas and hepatocellular carcinoma. American Academy of Pediatrics, Surgical Section Survey—1974. J Pediatr Surg 10:329, 1975.
18. Randolph JG, Altman RP, Arensman RM, et al. Liver resection in children with hepatic neoplasms. Ann Surg 187:599, 1978.
19. Giacomantonio M, Ein SH, Mancer K, et al. Thirty years of experience with pediatric primary malignant liver tumors. J Pediatr Surg 19:523, 1984.
20. Iwatsuki S, Gordon RD, Shaw BW Jr, et al. Role of liver transplantation in cancer therapy. Ann Surg 202:401, 1985.
21. Rolles K, Calne RY. Liver transplantation. In: Calne RY, ed. Transplantation Immunology. Clinical and Experimental. Oxford, Oxford University Press, 1984:436.
21a. Lai ECS, Choi TK, Tong SW, et al. Treatment of unresectable hepatocellular carcinoma: results of a randomized controlled trial. World J Surg 10:501, 1986.
22. Adson MA. Resection of liver metastases—when is it worthwhile? World J Surg 11:511, 1987
23. Foster JH, Lundy J. Liver metastases. Curr Probl Surg 18:161, 1981.
24. Hughes KS, Simon R, Songhorabodi S, et al. Resection of the liver for colorectal carcinoma metastases: a multi-institutional study of indications for resection. Surgery 103:278, 1988.
25. Wanebo HJ, Semoglou C, Attiyeh F, et al. Surgical management of patients with primary operable colorectal cancer and synchronous liver metastases. Am J Surg 135:81, 1978.
26. Logan SE, Meier SJ, Ramming KP, et al. Hepatic resection of metastatic colorectal carcinoma. Arch Surg 117:25, 1982.
27. Fortner JG, Silva JS, Golberg RB, et al. Multivariate analysis of a personal series of 247 consecutive patients with liver metastases from colorectal cancer. Ann Surg 199:306, 1984.
28. Cady B, McDermott WV. Major hepatic resection for metachronous metastases from colon cancer. Ann Surg 201:204, 1985.
29. Butler J, Attiyeh FF, Daly JM. Hepatic resection for metastases of the colon and rectum. Surg Gynecol Obstet 162:109, 1986.
30. Iwatsuki S, Esquivel CO, Gordon RD, et al. Liver resection for metastatic colorectal cancer. Surgery 100:804, 1986.
31. Ekberg H, Tranberg K-G, Andersson R, et al. Determinants of survival in liver resection for colorectal secondaries. Br J Surg 73:727, 1986.
32. Foster JH. Survival after liver resection for secondary tumors. Am J Surg 135:389, 1978.
33. Pestana C, Reitemeier RJ, Moertel CG, et al. The natural history of carcinoma of the colon and rectum. Am J Surg 108:826, 1964.
34. Jaffe BM, Donegan WL, Watson F, et al. Factors influencing survival in patients with untreated hepatic metastases. Surg Gynecol Obstet 127:1, 1968.
35. Cady B, Munson DO, Swinton NW. Survival of patients after colonic resection with simultaneous liver metastases. Surg Gynecol Obstet 131:697, 1970.
36. Wood CB, Gillis CR, Blumgart LH. A retrospective study of the natural history of patients with liver metastases from colorectal cancer. Clin Oncol 2:285, 1976.
37. Pettavel J, Morgenthaler F. Protracted arterial chemotherapy of liver tumors: an experience of 107 cases over a 12-year period. Prog Clin Cancer 7:217, 1978.
38. Goslin R, Steele R Jr, Zamcheck N. Factors influencing survival in patients with hepatic metastases from adenocarcinoma of the colon or rectum. Dis Colon Rectum 25:749, 1982.
39. Finan PJ, Marshall RJ, Cooper EH, et al. Factors affecting survival in patients presenting with synchronous hepatic metastases from colorectal cancer: a clinical and computer analysis. Br J Surg 72:373, 1985.
40. Wagner JS, Adson MA, Van Heerden JA, et al. The natural history of hepatic metastases from colorectal cancer. Ann Surg 199:502, 1984.
41. Foster JH. Treatment of metastatic disease of the liver: a skeptic's view. Semin Liver Dis 2:170, 1984.
42. Martin EW Jr, Minton JP, Carey LC. CEA-directed second-look surgery in the asymptomatic patient after primary resection of colorectal carcinoma. Ann Surg 202:310, 1985.
43. Kemeny MM, Goldberg D, Beatty JD, et al. Results of a prospective randomized trial of continuous regional chemotherapy and hepatic resection as treatment of hepatic metastases from colorectal primaries. Cancer 57:492, 1986.
44. Lewis BJ, Stagg RJ, Friedman MA, et al. Intra-arterial versus intravenous FUDR for colorectal cancer metastatic to the liver. A Northern California Oncology Group Study. In: Howell SB, ed. Intra-arterial and Intracavitary Cancer Chemotherapy. Boston, Martinus Nijhoff, 1984:77.
45. Kemeny N, Daly J, Chun H, et al. Randomized study of intrahepatic vs. systemic infusion of fluorodeoxyuridine in patients with liver metastases from colorectal carcinoma (preliminary results). In: Howell SB, ed. Intra-arterial and Intracavitary Cancer Chemotherapy. Boston, Martinus Nijhoff, 1984:85.
46. McDermott WV Jr, Paris AL, Clouse ME, et al. Dearterialization of the liver for metastatic cancer. Ann Surg 187:38, 1978.
47. Bengmark S, Ericsson M, Lunderquist A, et al. Temporary liver dearterialization in patients with metastatic carcinoid disease. World J Surg 6:46, 1982.
48. Kemeny MM, Sugarbaker PH, Smith TH, et al. A prospective analysis of laboratory tests and imaging studies to detect hepatic lesions. Ann Surg 195:163, 1982.
49. Edmondson HA, Peters RL. Neoplasms of the liver. In: Schiff L, Schiff EF, ed. Diseases of the Liver, 5th ed. Philadelphia, JB Lippincott, 1982.
50. Staab HJ, Anderer FA, Stumpf E, et al. Eighty-four potential second-look operations based on sequential carcinoembryonic antigen determinations and clinical investigations in patients with recurrent gastrointestinal cancer. Am J Surg 149:198, 1985.
51. Deveney KE, Way LW. Follow-up of patients with colorectal cancer. Am J Surg 148:717, 1984.
52. Wilking N, Petrelli NJ, Herrera L, et al. Abdominal exploration for suspected recurrent carcinoma of the colon and rectum based on elevated carcinoembryonic antigen alone or in combination with other diagnostic methods. Surg Gynecol Obstet 162:465, 1986.
53. Steele G Jr, Zamcheck N, Wilson R, et al. Results of CEA-initiated second-look surgery for recurrent colorectal cancer. Am J Surg 139:544, 1980.
54. Lokich JJ. Chemotherapy of liver cancer. In: Bottino JC, Opfell RW, Muggia FM, eds. Liver Cancer. Boston, Martinus Nijhoff, 1985.
55. Ensminger WD, Gyves JW. Pharmacologic studies of hepatic intra-arterial chemotherapy. In: Bottino JC, Opfell RW, Muggia FM, eds. Liver Cancer. Boston, Martinus Nijhoff, 1985.
56. Tang ZY, Yang BH. Primary liver cancer—clinical analysis of 3254 cases. Tumor Prevention Treatment Study (Chin) 2:207, 1974.
57. Nagasue N, Yukaya H, Ogawa Y, et al. Clinical experience with 118

hepatic resections for hepatocellular carcinoma. Surgery 99:694, 1986.
58. Bengmark S, Hafstrom L, Jeppsson B. Primary carcinoma of the liver: improvement in sight? World J Surg 6:54, 1982.
58a. Foster J. Personal observations. (unpublished.)
59. Sorenson TA, Aronsen KF, Aune S, et al. Results of hepatic lobectomy for primary epithelial cancer in 31 adults. Am J Surg 138:407, 1979.
60. Foster JH. Survival after liver resection for cancer. Cancer 26:493, 1970.
61. Fortner JG, Kim DK, MacLean BJ, et al. Major hepatic resection for neoplasia. Ann Surg 188:363, 1978.
62. Yu YQ, Tang ZY. Surgical resection of primary liver cancer—analysis of 258 cases. Tumor Prevention Treatment Study (China) 2:215, 1974.
63. Ishikawa K. Follow-up study of patients with primary liver cancer. Report 3. Acta Hepatol Jpn 17:460, 1976.
64. Lin TY. Resectional therapy for primary malignant tumors. Int Adv Surg Oncol 2:25, 1979.
65. Lee NW, Wong J, Ong GB. The surgical management of primary carcinoma of the liver. World J Surg 6:66, 1982.
66. Lee CS, Sung JL, Hwang LY, et al. Surgical treatment of 109 patients with symptomatic and asymptomatic hepatocellular carcinoma. Surgery 99:481, 1986.

IV E. Inherited Diseases of the Liver

47

Copper Metabolism, Wilson's Disease, and Hepatic Copper Toxicosis

John L. Gollan, M.D., Ph.D., F.R.A.C.P., F.R.C.P.

Copper is the prosthetic element in numerous metalloenzymes, and as such it is critical to a variety of mammalian functions, including mitochondrial energy generation, melanin formation, the scavenging of oxygen radicals, and the cross-linkage of collagen and elastin. The ubiquitous availability of copper in nature, and hence its relative excess in most diets, is reflected by the rarity of acquired copper deficiency in humans. Similarly, because of the efficiency of the physiologic mechanisms regulating copper balance, toxic accumulation of the metal is infrequent.

The liver plays a pivotal role in the maintenance of copper homeostasis. Following intestinal absorption, the metal is taken up by the liver, where it is stored, processed for excretion into bile, or incorporated into the plasma copper protein, ceruloplasmin. Derangements of human copper metabolism arise principally from genetic defects in these homeostatic mechanisms. In Wilson's disease (hepatolenticular degeneration), the liver is both the site of the inherited metabolic defect and the organ most frequently injured by the excessive tissue concentrations of copper. This chapter is introduced by a selective review of normal copper metabolism, with emphasis on the role of the liver, followed by a discussion of Wilson's disease and other hepatobiliary diseases associated with copper overload. For additional information, the reader is referred to comprehensive reviews on copper metabolism[1-14] and Wilson's disease,[15-28] and in particular the recent monograph by Scheinberg and Sternlieb.[29]

COPPER METABOLISM

TOTAL BODY AND HEPATIC COPPER

Although only a few determinations of total body copper have been made in humans,[4, 30, 31] values estimated for normal adults range between 50 and 150 mg. The most recent estimate of total body copper is approximately 100 mg for a 70-kg individual, of which about 8 mg (or 8 per cent) is found in the liver.[12] The highest concentrations of copper are found in liver, followed in decreasing order by brain, heart, and kidneys. Although the concentrations of copper in muscle and bone are low, these tissues contain about 50 per cent of total body copper because of their large mass.

The concentration of copper in fetal liver is considerably higher than that in adults (mean 32 μg/g dry weight, range 0 to 55 μg/g).[12] In the early phase of fetal development, almost all of the body copper is present in the liver, and most of this is contained in the hepatocyte lysosomes[32] in association with metallothionein.[33] Metallothionein (previously named mitochondrocuprein) is a cysteine-rich protein containing 4 per cent copper. The relative proportion of copper in the liver declines during fetal life, but at birth it still represents 50 to 60 per cent of total body copper.[12] During this period of transition in the newborn, copper appears to be irregularly distributed throughout the liver.[34] Thereafter, a rapid fall in hepatic copper concentration occurs during early infancy, apparently as a result of the combined influence of redistribution of hepatic copper to other organs, the postnatal growth spurt, and the relatively low copper content of human milk. By the age of 3 months, the concentration of hepatic copper is comparable to that of adults.[35]

DIETARY COPPER AND INTESTINAL ABSORPTION

The daily copper requirement for adults, estimated from copper balance studies (which neglect dermal loss), is 1.3 to 1.7 mg.[4, 36, 37] A daily intake of 2 to 5 mg is commonly quoted for the average North American diet, although amounts in excess of 10 mg or less than 1 mg[38] may not be unusual even with conventional diets. Oysters and other shellfish contain the highest concentrations of copper, followed in decreasing order by liver, nuts, chocolate, mushrooms, legumes, and cereals. The abundance of dietary copper relative to total body content is in contradistinction to the situation for iron—that is, a dietary supply of 15 mg daily in the face of a total body iron content of 3 to 5 g. Because the various nutrient solutions used in total parenteral nutrition are deficient in trace elements, including copper, it is recommended that a trace element preparation be administered routinely to all patients receiving parenteral nutrition.[39]

Dynamic studies with radiocopper indicate that 40 to 60 per cent of the average daily intake of dietary copper is absorbed.[40-42] The prompt appearance of radiocopper in blood following oral administration, and attainment of maximal radioactivity within one to two hours,[43-45] suggest that absorption of copper occurs principally in the upper gastrointestinal tract. Absorption of radiocopper is reduced in diffuse disease of the small intestine, such as celiac disease, scleroderma, or lymphosarcoma.[46] The availability of copper for absorption is influenced by the chemical form of ingested copper, the nature of other dietary components, and intraluminal factors.[10] The influence of these factors in humans has yet to be defined clearly, but extensive animal studies show that copper absorption is antagonized by the presence of other transition elements (e.g., cadmium, molybdenum and zinc),[47-49] ascorbic acid,[50] and anions such as sulfides, which form insoluble copper salts at alkaline pH.[51] The copper in raw meat is relatively unavailable for absorption,[52] whereas that in grassland herbage is absorbed readily by copper-deficient animals.[53] However, a decreased positive copper balance has been demonstrated in Wilson's disease patients fed a vegetarian diet,[54] and soybean proteins appear to affect adversely the utilization of copper.[55] These different effects of animal and vegetable protein on copper absorption probably reflect the formation of a variety of copper complexes, which may either facilitate or inhibit uptake.

It is unlikely that copper is absorbed in the ionic form because of the predilection of the metal to form complexes around neutral pH. Several lines of evidence suggest that the metal is absorbed as low–molecular weight, soluble complexes formed with both the products of food digestion and gastrointestinal secretions. Human saliva, gastric juice, and duodenal aspirate contain still unidentified low–molecular weight, copper-binding substances that prevent the formation and precipitation of cupric hydroxide at pH 8.[56, 57] Amino acids and oligopeptides, particularly those containing histidine, would appear to be the ligands responsible,[57] and indeed L-amino acids have been shown to facilitate the intestinal absorption of copper[58] and its uptake by a variety of tissues.[59, 60] The observation that amino acids and a small fraction of copper[61] are transported across the intestinal mucosa by energy-dependent processes has also led to the proposal that at least a portion of dietary copper is absorbed as copper–amino acid complexes.[10] It is apparent, however, that not all copper complexes formed by endogenous secretions facilitate absorption. Gallbladder bile contains a high–molecular weight substance that has a high binding affinity for copper and inhibits the intestinal uptake of radiolabeled copper in intact rats.[57] Thus, net uptake of ingested copper may reflect the differential binding of the metal in the gut lumen to both high– and low–molecular weight ligands present in the diet and the gastrointestinal secretions.[57]

The regulatory mechanisms, if any, that mediate the mucosal transport of copper have not been defined, although two distinct cytosolic copper-binding proteins have been demonstrated in rat duodenum and bovine duodenum.[48, 62] One fraction of copper is contained in a protein with the properties of the enzyme superoxide dismutase (see later) and the other in the sulfhydryl-rich protein metallothionein, which binds cadmium and zinc as well as copper by the formation of mercaptides. Moreover, the mucosal metallothionein content is increased by dietary zinc and cadmium,[63, 64] and since copper binds more tenaciously to metallothionein than either of these metals, the serosal transfer of copper is thereby impeded. Thus, it has been postulated that intestinal metallothionein may play a dual role in copper absorption,[10] first passively binding copper within the mucosal cell before it is complexed by amino acids for transport across the serosal surface and released into the portal circulation and second acting as a mucosal block to protect against absorption of toxic levels of copper. Although metallothionein and active transport of copper–amino acid complexes may influence copper absorption, there is no evidence that overall copper homeostasis, like that of iron, is regulated significantly at the level of the intestine.[65]

COPPER TRANSPORT IN BLOOD

Copper in whole blood is distributed in at least five different forms. In the red cell, more than half of the copper is associated with superoxide dismutase (formerly known as erythrocuprein), and the remaining fraction is found in a labile pool possibly complexed with amino acids.[66] The total copper content of erythrocytes remains relatively constant in the presence of either copper deficiency or copper excess, indicating that red cell copper is probably not the form in which the metal is transported to and from the tissues. In normal individuals, ceruloplasmin constitutes 90 to 95 per cent of the copper circulating in plasma, and the remaining portion is bound loosely to albumin, with a minor fraction bound to amino acids.

After absorption from the intestine or after intravenous administration, copper is bound to the nonceruloplasmin fraction[4, 67] (Fig. 47–1). This copper is cleared promptly by the liver (plasma $t_{1/2}$ in humans is about 10 minutes), where a highly efficient plasma membrane recognition system exists for albumin-bound copper. The hepatic uptake process exhibits saturation kinetics and competition by related substrates (e.g., zinc), which is indicative of facilitated transport.[68, 69] Studies with radiocopper indicate that within several hours, 60 to 90 per cent of the absorbed copper is deposited in the liver.[70] After about eight hours, hepatic radioactivity decreases as a portion of the copper is incorporated into ceruloplasmin and returned to the plasma.[60, 71]

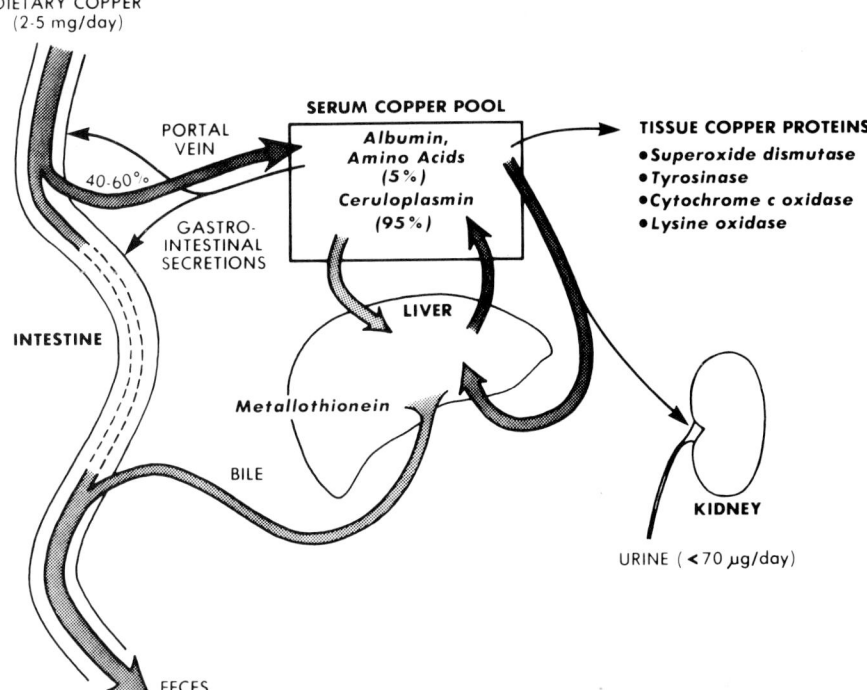

Figure 47–1. Absorption, excretion, and metabolic pathways of copper in normal adults.

It is generally considered that ceruloplasmin does not function as the immediate copper transport protein in blood, since copper incorporated into this molecule appears to be released only in the course of degradation of the protein.[72, 73]

Human, bovine, and rat serum albumins have a single and relatively specific high-affinity binding site for copper (dissociation constant $K_d = 7 \times 10^{-17}$ M). The theoretical copper-binding capacity of this site ($\sim 3,800$ μg/dl)[12] is virtually never exceeded even in pathologic situations. The binding site is located near the N-terminus of the albumin molecule. The imidazole nitrogen of the histidine in position 3 appears to be particularly important for binding, since dog albumin, which lacks this histidine residue, binds copper nonspecifically at multiple sites.[12] A small, highly labile, and functionally important ultrafilterable plasma fraction of nonceruloplasmin copper is accounted for by copper bound to amino acids.[74] Of the amino acids in human plasma, histidine has the highest affinity for copper ($K_d = 10^{-18}$ M for Cu(His)$_2$), followed by threonine, glutamine, and asparagine.[56] In addition, there is evidence for the existence of complexes with two amino acids (e.g., histidine-Cu-threonine) and ternary complexes with albumin (e.g., albumin-Cu-histidine).[75] Although characterization of these complexes has not been achieved in vivo, the following equilibria may pertain in the physiologic state:

$$Cu^{2+} + amino\ acid + albumin \rightleftharpoons Cu^{2+}\text{-amino acid}$$
$$+ albumin \rightleftharpoons albumin\text{-}Cu^{2+}\text{-amino acid} \qquad [1]$$
$$\rightleftharpoons albumin\text{-}Cu^{2+} + amino\ acid$$

The amino acid–bound copper complexes represent only a minor fraction of total plasma copper, but they probably are responsible for transport of the metal between blood and tissues[60] and across cell membranes. Rapid exchange of copper between high-affinity ligands (albumin, histidine, and amino acid complexes such as Gly-His-Lys),[76] which collectively account for ~ 6 per cent of plasma copper, is

believed to be important in the hepatic clearance of copper.[68, 77] The small amount of copper excreted in urine (less than 70 μg daily) probably emanates from the amino acid–bound plasma fraction or dissociation from the copper-albumin complex. Urinary copper of normal subjects does not reflect the dietary intake,[78] and contributes little to the maintenance of copper homeostasis except in abnormal states such as Wilson's disease.

HEPATIC COPPER PROTEINS

In the liver, as in other tissues, it is unlikely that free cupric ions exist in appreciable concentration. As outlined in Table 47–1, copper is found (1) in association with binding proteins (e.g., metallothionein, human liver copper protein, or L-6-D), in which form it presumably is in equilibrium with copper bound to other organic molecules such as amino acids, or (2) as a component of specific metalloenzymes (e.g., superoxide dismutase; cytochrome c oxidase; monoamine oxidase; and ceruloplasmin; and in extrahepatic tissues, tyrosinase and lysyl oxidase) in which the copper remains an integral part of the protein molecule throughout its biologic life. In normal adult human liver, about 80 per cent of the copper is present in the cytosolic proteins metallothionein, L-6-D, and superoxide dismutase (formerly known as hepatocuprein). In neonates, however, the bulk of the hepatic copper is located in lysosomes in the form of metallothionein[33] (or mitochondrocuprein, see Total Body and Hepatic Copper).

It has been suggested that the two low–molecular weight sulfhydryl-rich cytosolic proteins isolated from human liver, L-6-D[79] and metallothionein,[80, 81] are similar, if not identical.[10, 48] However, metallothionein contains only 0.1 per cent copper by weight in addition to as much as 7 per cent zinc and cadmium,[81] whereas L-6-D contains as much as 3 per cent copper and little zinc. The proteins apparently differ also with respect to their molecular

TABLE 47–1. COPPER PROTEINS IN HUMAN LIVER

Protein	Subcellular Location	Molecular Weight	Postulated Function(s)
L-6-D, or human liver copper protein	Cytosol	10,000	Storage? Donor for ceruloplasmin synthesis?
Metallothionein	Cytosol	6100	Storage? Detoxification? Donor for ceruloplasmin synthesis and biliary copper excretion?
Mitochondrocuprein (?metallothionein)	Lysosomes	Insoluble polymer	Storage? Detoxification?
Superoxide dismutase (hepatocuprein or cytocuprein)	Cytosol and mitochondrial intermembrane space	32,000	Prevents tissue injury by scavenging superoxide anion radicals
Cytochrome c oxidase	Mitochondrial inner membrane	290,000	Aerobic oxidation
Monoamine oxidase	Mitochondria	195,000	Oxidative deamination of catecholamines
Ceruloplasmin	Hepatic microsomes Plasma	132,000	Iron mobilization (ferroxidase activity); regulator of biogenic amine levels? Serum antioxidant

weights (Table 47–1) and cysteine contents; cysteine is far more abundant in metallothionein. Hence, the term *metallothionein*[12, 13] should be reserved at the present time for the protein that has been characterized by Vallee and his coinvestigators,[81–83] and is now known to bind zinc, cadmium, copper, mercury, and silver in increasing order of affinity.[84] Further studies are necessary to establish whether L-6-D in adult liver, mitochondrocuprein in fetal liver, and metallothionein are identical.

The physiologic role(s) of the low–molecular weight copper-binding protein(s) is uncertain, but it may be critical in the temporary storage and detoxification of copper, as a donor for the synthesis of ceruloplasmin or for excretion of copper into bile, or both. Following hepatic uptake from the plasma, copper is predominantly bound to cytosolic metallothionein,[85] although movement through this pool is relatively rapid. Thus, in rats, copper appears in the low–molecular weight proteins of liver within an hour of injection and continues to increase for as long as 12 hours.[12] Thereafter, copper levels in this pool decline exponentially, suggesting that the metal is either utilized rapidly for the synthesis of copper proteins (e.g., ceruloplasmin, superoxide dismutase) or excreted in bile. Distribution of copper between the temporary storage form bound to metallothionein and the two processing routes can change under different dietary conditions, by changes in circulating glucocorticoids or estrogens and in the presence of a variety of pathologic states.[10] Thus, the storage function of metallothionein and other low–molecular weight proteins in normal human liver appears to be adapted to relatively short-term needs, but with accumulation of copper such as occurs in the neonatal period, Wilson's disease, copper poisoning, and experimentally induced copper overload, the proportion of hepatic copper bound to these proteins increases greatly.[12] In these situations, the binding of copper by low–molecular weight proteins may render the metal less toxic, as is the case with other metallothionein-bound metals.[82] Finally, it has been shown that copper accumulates in the low–molecular weight fractions of rat liver cytosol after ligation of the bile duct,[86] suggesting that metallothionein may be involved in the excretion of biliary copper.

The enzyme *superoxide dismutase* (superoxide oxidoreductase) is believed to be present in all aerobic cells. In mammalian tissues, the highest activities are found in liver, kidney, and erythrocytes.[87, 88] The enzyme was isolated and characterized from red cells (erythrocuprein), liver (hepatocuprein), and brain (cerebrocuprein)[12, 89] and initially was thought to function in copper storage or transport. It now is established that all of these so-called cytocupreins[90] are cuprozinc enzymes with superoxide dismutase activity.[89, 91] Four different forms of superoxide dismutase have been found to date. The group containing copper and zinc is found in the cytosol and intermembrane space of mitochondria and is unrelated, except in its activity, to the other three, which contain manganese or iron. These enzymes catalyze the dismutation of the superoxide anion to form molecular oxygen and hydrogen peroxide as follows:

$$O_2^- + O_2^- + 2 H^+ \rightleftharpoons O_2 + H_2O_2 \qquad [2]$$

Superoxide dismutase may play a vital role in protecting the liver cell components from the damaging effects of the superoxide radical, which is a common intermediate of the reduction of oxygen (see also Chap. 30). Although the biosynthesis of cuprozinc superoxide dismutase occurs on free polysomes in the cytoplasm, metallothionein-copper does not appear to function as the precursor pool of copper for synthesis of the enzyme.[93]

Cytochrome c oxidase, a copper- and heme-containing lipoprotein found in the inner mitochondrial membrane, is the terminal oxidase in the electron transport chain.[94] The enzyme, which is composed of at least seven subunits[14] and contains two copper ions,[95] catalyzes the oxidation of reduced cytochrome c and the reduction of molecular oxygen to form oxidized cytochrome c and water.[96] Severe copper deficiency results in decreased cytochrome oxidase activity with an associated reduction in oxidative phosphorylation, although apoprotein molecules of the enzyme are present in copper-deficient cells.[12] Cytochrome c oxidase also appears essential for the normal mitochondrial uptake of iron and its incorporation into heme, since this process is defective in copper deficiency.[97]

The *monoamine oxidase* present in liver mitochondria catalyzes the oxidative deamination of a variety of monoamines, including epinephrine and serotonin, with stoichiometric formation of the corresponding aldehyde, ammonia, and hydrogen peroxide.[98] The enzyme contains four atoms of copper per molecule. *Tryptophan-2,3-dioxygenase* is a hemoprotein present in liver cytosol. It catalyzes the insertion of molecular oxygen into the pyrrole ring of L-tryptophan.[99] Despite the earlier belief that this enzyme was an authentic copper protein, recent studies with purified preparations have shown that the copper content is negligible,[100] and hence it is not a copper metalloenzyme.[101]

The blue copper-glycoprotein *ceruloplasmin* is synthesized almost exclusively in the liver prior to its appearance in the blood (Fig. 47–1).[73, 102, 103] It has been estimated that 0.5 to 1.0 mg of copper is incorporated into ceruloplasmin daily.[40, 73] Ceruloplasmin is predominantly a plasma protein that migrates electrophoretically as an alpha-2 globulin. Serum ceruloplasmin concentration is low in the human newborn[104] but increases to near adult levels during the first two years of life,[5] coincident with the postnatal decrease in hepatic copper concentration. The mean serum concentration of ceruloplasmin in adults is $\sim$ 30 mg/dl.[27, 28] Its copper comprises 95 per cent of the total serum content ($\sim$ 100 μg/dl). Ceruloplasmin is one of the so-called acute phase reactants (e.g., fibrinogen, haptoglobin);[105] its synthetic rate increases in response to inflammation. Plasma levels also reflect a wide range of humoral and hormonal influences.[10] In rats, adrenal insufficiency or hypothyroidism induces an increase in serum ceruloplasmin, and the rise can be prevented by administration of corticosteroids or thyroid hormone, respectively.[106] In all the mammalian species that have been examined,[10] estrogens increase serum ceruloplasmin concentrations, an effect that is probably the result of enhanced hepatic synthesis.[106] The effect of estrogens on serum ceruloplasmin (and hence serum copper) level is most apparent in women using oral contraceptives or during pregnancy.

Human ceruloplasmin is a globular glycoprotein consisting of a single polypeptide chain with 1046 amino acid residues, a molecular mass of 132 kd, and six to seven atoms of copper per molecule.[107, 108] Heterogeneity of the prosthetic carbohydrate groups appears to account for at least two different molecular forms in human serum.[109] Although copper is an integral part of the ceruloplasmin molecule, some of the metal can be removed in vitro by lowering the pH and by exposure to reducing agents. The blue color and enzymic activity of the molecule are lost in the resulting apoceruloplasmin but can be restored by the addition of cupric ions in vitro.[110] The functional relevance of this observation is uncertain, since the exchange of ceruloplasmin-copper has not been demonstrated directly in vivo.

The hepatic pathways for incorporation of copper into ceruloplasmin have been delineated only partially.[12] However, based on kinetic studies with radiocopper in isolated rat liver[111] and in humans,[112] the following model is proposed. The copper in ceruloplasmin and that excreted in bile are derived from separate intracellular compartments that do not exchange with one another. Radiocopper is apparently incorporated into ceruloplasmin by at least two pathways: a slow route that involves initial equilibration with a hepatic storage pool and a more rapid pathway that appears to bypass this pool.[112] The existence in vivo of these postulated compartments has not been established, and their relation to known organelles or copper-binding proteins in the hepatocyte is speculative. Moreover, it has been shown that copper recently transferred from albumin to the liver is utilized preferentially for incorporation into ceruloplasmin.[102, 113] Also, newly arrived hepatic radiocopper appears in high specific activity within microsomes, which it then leaves at about the same rate as it appears in ceruloplasmin.[102] The following sequence thus has been proposed for the synthesis of ceruloplasmin:[114] synthesis of the apoprotein (which proceeds at a steady rate, relatively independent of the presence of copper),[74] glycosylation, and insertion of copper in the hepatic microsomes.

The plasma disappearance of ceruloplasmin copper ($t_{1/2}$ $\sim$ 12 hours in the rat) is much slower than that of albumin-bound copper ($t_{1/2}$ $\sim$ 5 minutes), and the protein moiety of ceruloplasmin has the same rate of disappearance as its copper.[73, 115] Because ceruloplasmin copper is not readily exchangeable in vivo,[116] its distribution to various tissues, including liver, kidney, heart, and lung, appears to represent catabolism of the molecule rather than a true transport process. The catabolism of ceruloplasmin largely involves the liver,[117, 118] and uptake by the hepatocytes occurs via the proposed general mechanism for removal of glycoproteins from the circulation.[119] Removal of the terminal sialic acid group of ceruloplasmin results in hepatocyte uptake of the molecule, via the plasma membrane asialoglycoprotein receptor, and its transport to the lysosomes, where the copper is then removed and the protein is degraded. Indeed, desialation of ceruloplasmin with neuraminidase reduces the plasma half-time of asialoceruloplasmin to less than 0.5 hour.[119] It appears likely that liver endothelial cells take up circulating ceruloplasmin through a mechanism involving receptor-mediated endocytosis. Ceruloplasmin then is desialated and excreted, where it is recognized by the asialoglycoprotein receptor on the hepatocyte surface.[120]

The biologic role(s) of ceruloplasmin has not been clearly established, although it shows significant oxidase activity toward a variety of substrates.[121, 122] Ceruloplasmin functions as a ferroxidase by oxidizing ferrous to ferric iron and thus it may participate in iron mobilization from tissue iron-storage sites, including the liver, by controlling the rate of ferric iron uptake by the transport protein transferrin.[121] Consequently, copper deficiency results in low serum concentrations of ceruloplasmin and iron, reduced iron mobilization, and eventually, anemia in the presence of a high hepatic iron content. However, the ferroxidase activity of ceruloplasmin may not be essential for normal iron metabolism, since iron transport appears normal in patients with Wilson's disease, who have barely detectable serum levels of ceruloplasmin. Ceruloplasmin also catalyzes the oxidation of biogenic amines (e.g., epinephrine, 5-hydroxytryptamine, and dopamine), suggesting that it may influence circulating and tissue levels of biogenic amines and hence neurotransmitter activity in the central nervous system.[123, 124] A number of hallucinogenic drugs, tricyclic antidepressants,[125] and phenothiazine derivatives[126] influence the oxidase activity of ceruloplasmin. Despite these observations, the in vivo significance of the oxidase activity of ceruloplasmin toward natural substrates has yet to be determined.[122] It also has been suggested that ceruloplasmin may be a major antioxidant in serum, based on its ability to inhibit the auto-oxidation of lipids induced by ascorbic acid or inorganic iron.[127, 128] It also may serve as a circulating scavenger of superoxide anion radicals, mimicking the function of cytoplasmic superoxide dismutase.[129] Finally, there is evidence to suggest that ceruloplasmin may be required as a specific donor of copper for the biosynthesis of cytochrome *c* oxidase.[121]

BILIARY EXCRETION OF COPPER

The maintenance of copper balance depends primarily on the excretion of copper in bile. In healthy adults, mean biliary copper output determined by two different techniques was 1.2 to 1.7 mg/day,[130–131] compared with less than 0.07 mg/day in urine. Although other gastrointestinal secretions, such as saliva and gastric juice, contain much lower concentrations of copper than does bile,[132] when considered on the basis of their daily volumes, these secretions represent a significant pool of luminal copper. This may explain the observation that the amount of copper in the feces is more than can be accounted for by both biliary and unabsorbed dietary copper.[71] The importance of biliary excretion in copper homeostasis is illustrated by the excessive accumulation of hepatic copper that follows ligation of the bile duct in experimental animals[133, 134] or prolonged cholestasis associated with conditions such as primary biliary cirrhosis.[135, 136]

Little is known regarding the mechanisms or physiologic control of biliary excretion of copper. In rats, the concentration of copper in bile is decreased in late pregnancy and during the early postpartum period,[137] caused most likely by the diversion of a larger than normal proportion of hepatic copper to the synthesis of ceruloplasmin (which increases during pregnancy). The excretion of copper increases with the administered dose up to an apparent transport maximum and is strikingly dependent on body temperature, being 14 times greater at 40°C than at 30°C.[138] The major concentration gradient, however, is from plasma to liver, whereas the liver to bile gradient is relatively small.

Unfortunately, the immediate hepatic precursor pool(s) of biliary copper has not been defined, since this would appear to be the likely site for the defect underlying the abnormal biliary excretion of copper in Wilson's disease. On the basis of kinetic studies, it is apparent that the copper incorporated into ceruloplasmin and that excreted into bile are derived from different intracellular compartments.[111] The early appearance of albumin-bound radiocopper in the low–molecular weight proteins of hepatocyte cytosol (i.e., metallothionein)[139] and in bile[140] suggests that these proteins may represent at least one of the prebiliary copper compartments.[12] An alternative pathway for biliary copper excretion has been proposed by Sternlieb and coworkers;[141] these investigators administered ^{64}Cu orally to a healthy subject and a patient with Wilson's disease and found that specific activity of the copper in hepatic lysosomes was virtually identical to that in bile, suggesting that lysosomes might be the source of biliary copper. The wide variety of biliary components that have been claimed by different investigators to be the carrier of biliary copper suggests that there may be more than one prebiliary copper compartment. Indeed, in addition to copper arising from the catabolism of desialated ceruloplasmin in the lysosomal compartment (following receptor-mediated endocytosis), a small fraction of the desialated protein appears to be transported directly from the sinusoids to the bile canaliculi, either by a vesicular or paracellular pathway.[142]

In human bile, copper appears to be complexed to both low–molecular weight and macromolecular ligands.[143, 144] The low–molecular weight components predominate in hepatic bile, whereas the high–molecular weight species are found particularly in gallbladder bile.[143] In vitro simulation of gallbladder function by dialysis and concentration of hepatic bile produces a pattern of copper binding that resembles that of gallbladder bile,[57] suggesting that at least a portion of the low–molecular weight copper fraction undergoes reabsorption by the gallbladder. Whereas the low–molecular weight fraction probably represents copper bound to amino acids and small peptides,[145, 146] the nature of the macromolecular copper component(s) has yet to be determined. The trace amounts of copper excreted in bile as ceruloplasmin[142, 147] or its degradation products[142, 143] appear insufficient to account for the copper present in bile as a high–molecular weight complex. Similarly, binding to albumin or to other plasma proteins is unlikely to be responsible for this fraction of biliary copper.[148] Since most of the biliary copper migrates with the micellar fraction of bile on gel electrophoresis,[149, 150] it has been proposed that the high–molecular weight fraction actually reflects copper bound to bile acids, phospholipids, or conjugated bilirubin. However, the dissolution of micellar aggregates with acetone[57] or supramicellar concentrations of glycocholate[151] has no effect on the apparent molecular size, indicating that copper is not present in micellar form. Hence, the identity of the macromolecular copper complex in bile still eludes us. There is no evidence, however, to suggest that the copper overload in Wilson's disease is related to a qualitative defect in biliary copper.[141, 151]

Regardless of the form in which copper is complexed in bile, the intestinal reabsorption of biliary copper appears to be negligible,[57, 145, 152] and thus most of the copper excreted by this route will be eliminated in the feces. For example, in rats two hours after intraduodenal administration of human bile labeled in vivo with ^{64}Cu, only 4 per cent of the radioactivity was absorbed, compared with 13 per cent absorbed from a dose of [^{64}Cu] cupric acetate.[57] Also, in rats given intraduodenal doses of biliary copper collected from donor animals at various time intervals after radiocopper administration, the copper was absorbed more efficiently from bile collected during the early phase of radiocopper excretion than that obtained during the later time intervals.[145] These findings suggest that with increasing time after administration, the proportion of copper excreted in the form of low–molecular weight complexes decreases, and the proportion excreted in macromolecular form increases.

COPPER DEFICIENCY

Copper deficiency in humans is unusual, although both acquired and genetic forms are recognized. Both forms have features that resemble manifestations of spontaneous or experimental copper deficiency in animals, reflecting dysfunction of the central nervous system, hematopoietic system, bones, and connective tissue.[13, 153] Acquired copper deficiency is rare, but it has been reported to occur in severely malnourished infants,[154] particularly in premature babies, and in children or adults with malabsorption[155] or after extensive bowel operations[156] and has been associated with long-term, high-dose oral zinc therapy[157] and long-term total parenteral nutrition without copper supplementation.[158, 159] Because adequate methods for the assessment of total body copper are not widely accessible, the diagnosis of copper deficiency is made by the finding of very low serum concentrations of copper and ceruloplasmin in the clinical setting of a microcytic, hypochromic anemia, neutropenia, and osteoporosis or scurvy-like bone changes, all of which are reversed by the cautious administration of copper.[160, 161] Measurement of serum ceruloplasmin levels before and after copper repletion has been advocated as a method to detect mild copper deficiency.[160]

Menkes' syndrome (steely-hair disease), or trichopoliodystrophy,[162] is a rare, X-linked, inherited form of copper deficiency that appears six weeks to six months after birth and leads to death, usually by the age of 3 years, from progressive focal cerebral and cerebellar degeneration. The disorder is characterized by seizures, mental retardation, temperature instability, peculiar hair that has less crimp than normal and a steely texture (*pili torti*), presumably due to impaired disulfide bond formation, intimal abnormalities in arteries, and scorbutic bone changes.[25] Levels of serum copper and ceruloplasmin are markedly reduced, and hepatic copper concentration usually is decreased to the low-normal range.[163] Although hepatic cytochrome *c* oxidase levels are reduced and mitochondrial changes are observed occasionally on electron microscopy, the liver appears histologically normal.[13]

Findings in patients with Menkes' syndrome and in the mottled mouse (X-linked animal model) indicate defective placental transfer of copper in utero, and an even more marked defect in intestinal copper absorption after birth.[164, 165] Whereas the liver, plasma, brain, and most other organs show diminished copper concentrations, the primary defect produces abnormal accumulations of copper in the intestinal mucosa, kidney, placenta, and testis. The defective intestinal absorption of dietary copper (20 per cent of normal capacity) is probably the result of defective transport within the mucosal cell or across the serosal surface into the plasma.[164] It has been proposed that the basic defect in affected tissues of patients with Menkes' syndrome (e.g., intestinal mucosa) involves an increase in the affinity of metallothioneins for copper[166] or an apparent overproduction of this high-affinity ligand,[167] with impaired egress of copper from cells and hence accumulation of the metal. The observation that cultured fibroblasts[168] and lymphoblasts[167] from patients with Menkes' syndrome contain an abnormally high copper concentration supports the concept of a defect involving multiple cell types. Thus, overproduction of metallothionein in tissues other than the liver may explain the changes in copper metabolism observed in Menkes' disease. Since the X chromosome contains no metallothionein-related DNA sequences, the disorder cannot be due to mutations or amplification of the metallothionein genes themselves or of their cis-acting regulatory sequences.[169] Hence, the Menkes' mutation presumably affects human metallothionein gene expression through a trans-acting alteration in transcriptional regulation or indirectly by altering copper homeostasis. Attempted therapy with intravenous copper results in increased plasma copper and ceruloplasmin levels, but when brain disease is established, no sustained clinical improvement has been observed. The response appears more encouraging when therapy is initiated early and copper is administered intravenously in a slow-release form.[25, 170, 171]

Abnormalities in copper metabolism closely resembling those in Menkes' syndrome have been described in an X-linked, heritable connective tissue disorder, tentatively classified as type IX of the Ehlers-Danlos syndrome.[172, 173] Clinical features include bladder diverticula, inguinal hernias, slight skin laxity, and skeletal abnormalities, notably occipital horn-like exostoses. Lysyl oxidase activity is low in fibroblast cultures from both disorders, but arterial and neurologic changes are absent in type IX Ehlers-Danlos patients, and the disease is not lethal in childhood. Whether these two syndromes represent different degrees of severity of the same biochemical defect or distinct, albeit related, disorders has not been established.

EFFECTS OF EXCESSIVE HEPATIC COPPER

The biochemical and ultrastructural effects of hepatic copper toxicosis in humans and animals have been reviewed comprehensively by Sternlieb.[13, 174] Experimental studies in animals demonstrate that excess administered copper accumulates primarily in the liver. There is considerable species variation in hepatic storage capacities, as illustrated by the fact that the hepatic copper concentration in the normal dog is tenfold higher than that in humans,[175] and in certain specimens of Dominican toad *(Bufo marinus)* and mute swan *(Cygnus olor)*, which have black livers, the copper contents ($\leq$ 6 mg of copper/g of dry liver) are 50 to 100 times that of normal human liver.[13] Such species appear to have developed an efficient protective mechanism whereby excess copper is sequestered by lysosomes evident as numerous dense granules on microscopy),[174, 176, 177] apparently rendering the metal innocuous, since no hepatocyte injury is evident on light or electron microscopy. This mechanism is less apparent in humans and other animals such as sheep. For example, the chronic administration of copper to sheep leads to hepatic necrosis with release of hepatic copper to the circulation,[178] causing fatal hemolysis and renal insufficiency. This syndrome also is seen occasionally in patients with fulminant Wilson's disease.[179] Acute toxicity following accidental or suicidal ingestion of gram quantities of copper may occasionally result in hepatic necrosis and hemolysis, although the rapid onset of intense gastrointestinal irritation that follows ingestion, with vomiting and diarrhea, frequently protects patients from the more serious systemic injuries.[180–182]

Various mechanisms that remain poorly defined appear to be responsible for the subcellular injury of copper toxicosis, and virtually all components of the hepatocyte are susceptible to damage.[13, 174] The plasma membrane may be modified by the introduction of positive charges at normally uncharged or negatively charged sites, thus influencing membrane permeability and the diffusion of small molecules and ions. Such an effect has been shown in myocardial mitochondria, in which Cu^{2+} was presumed to have altered the protein component of the outer membrane or perturbed its relationship to membrane lipids.[183] This effect of copper on mitochondrial membranes may be responsible in part for the changes in hepatocyte mitochondria that are characteristic of the early stages of Wilson's disease.[16, 184]

Considering the high content of sulfhydryl groups in certain cytosolic proteins, Sternlieb has suggested that copper may promote the polymerization of metallothionein through S-Cu-S linkages formed by interactions with the abundant thiol groups.[13] In contrast, the binding of copper to sulfhydryl groups may interfere with the polymerization of tubulin[185] and may consequently affect microtubular functions such as protein and triglyceride secretion from the hepatocyte (steatosis with triglyceride inclusions is one of the earliest microscopic changes in Wilson's disease).[186, 187] Moreover, the action of copper on tubulin also may be related to the deposition of Mallory's hyalin, which is observed in the hepatocytes of some patients with advanced Wilson's disease, primary biliary cirrhosis, and Indian childhood cirrhosis (all conditions associated with excess of hepatic copper).[188] Other potentially damaging effects of copper may involve the depletion of glutathione reserves, the destabilization of nuclear DNA, the perturbation of lysosomal membranes with leakage of enzymes into the cytosol, and the stimulation of fibrinogenesis.[13, 174]

WILSON'S DISEASE (HEPATOLENTICULAR DEGENERATION)

In 1912, Kinnear Wilson collected six previously reported cases and contributed six additional cases to define the familial syndrome of progressive lenticular degeneration associated with cirrhosis of the liver.[189] Although Wilson's original clinical observations remain surprisingly valid, he failed to recognize the existence of the Kayser-Fleischer corneal ring, he did not appreciate that the disease was associated with abnormal copper metabolism, and he considered that the hepatic disease was not clinically significant. Since that time, considerable advances have been achieved in elucidating the biochemical and histologic features and in defining the natural history and therapy of the disease, although the underlying genetic defect in copper homeostasis has not yet been determined.

GENETICS

In his original monograph, Wilson considered that the familial incidence was attributable to environmental rather than to genetic factors. Almost a decade later, Hall reported that the disease was more frequent in siblings, in contradistinction to their parents, who rarely were affected.[190] In 1953, Bearn presented evidence for an autosomal recessive mode for inheritance,[191] and he later confirmed this view in an extended genetic analysis of 30 families.[192] Additional supportive studies subsequently have appeared from Japan,[193] England, and Taiwan.[17] The abnormal gene is distributed worldwide, and the disease has been found in virtually all races, including the Australian aborigine[194] and the South African black.[195]

The overall gene frequency, or heterozygote carrier rate, has been estimated as 1:200 to 1:400, which corresponds to a worldwide incidence of about five persons with Wilson's disease per million. However, recent estimates based on data from the United States,[29] Germany,[196] and Japan[197] suggest that prevalence of the disease may be as high as 1:30,000 in the general population. An increased rate of consanguinity, as occurs in certain isolated communities in Japan, Sardinia, and Israel, leads to a considerably higher incidence.[18] Since patients show a variety of clinical manifestations, including a juvenile hepatic form and a late-onset, predominantly neurologic form, it has been proposed that Wilson's disease may be genetically heterogeneous,[198] either with several allelomorphic forms at a single locus, or with multiple loci. However, different clinical forms of the disease are frequently evident in the same sibships, and hence this hypothesis requires further evaluation.

The abnormal gene responsible for the disease has been recently mapped, using conventional gene linkage analysis.[199] Twenty-seven autosomal markers were investigated for linkage in a large inbred kindred. Close linkage was found between the Wilson's disease gene and the esterase D locus on chromosome 13.[199, 200] The distance between the two loci was estimated as 6 to 7.5 centimorgans. On the basis of this finding, it should now be possible to proceed to cloning and characterization of the abnormal gene.

PATHOGENESIS

It is generally agreed that the clinical manifestations of Wilson's disease are the direct result of the excessive accumulation of tissue copper. Moreover, the apparent reversal of abnormal copper metabolism in patients following orthotopic liver transplantation strongly supports the concept that the primary defect is located in the liver.[201, 202]

The observations that serum ceruloplasmin levels are usually markedly reduced in Wilson's disease and that patients have profoundly diminished incorporation of radiocopper into ceruloplasmin (Fig. 47–2) relative to that in

healthy subjects and patients with other forms of liver disease has focused much attention on this protein and its potential role in disordered copper metabolism.[71, 112, 203–205] Although it is possible that the insertion of copper into ceruloplasmin is impaired in Wilson's disease, the primary defect does not appear to be directly related to this protein for the following reasons: (1) The gene for ceruloplasmin appears to be located on chromosome 3 in contrast to the gene for Wilson's disease, which is on chromosome 13. (2) Occasional patients (< 5 per cent) have serum ceruloplasmin concentrations within the normal range. (3) Heterozygous individuals may have greatly reduced ceruloplasmin levels, and yet they never develop toxic tissue levels of copper. (4) The serum ceruloplasmin concentration does not correlate with the clinical severity of the disease; in fact, in the course of long-term penicillamine therapy, ceruloplasmin levels frequently decline in association with a marked clinical improvement. (5) Intravenous administration of purified ceruloplasmin from normal subjects to patients with Wilson's disease does not appear to normalize copper metabolism.[206, 207] There is, in addition, no convincing evidence that ceruloplasmin participates in or exerts control over normal intestinal absorption or biliary excretion of copper, and thus the disturbance in ceruloplasmin synthesis appears likely to be secondary to the underlying metabolic defect.

Intuitively, the primary defect in Wilson's disease would seem to result in increased absorption of copper, decreased copper excretion, or both. In patients with Wilson's disease, the absorption of an oral dose of radiocopper commences as rapidly as it does in healthy subjects, but plasma radioactivity in patients attains a higher level and then declines more slowly.[43, 44, 51] These studies did not distinguish absorption from body retention of copper, but they were widely interpreted as reflecting overabsorption of the metal. However, studies employing dual isotope and

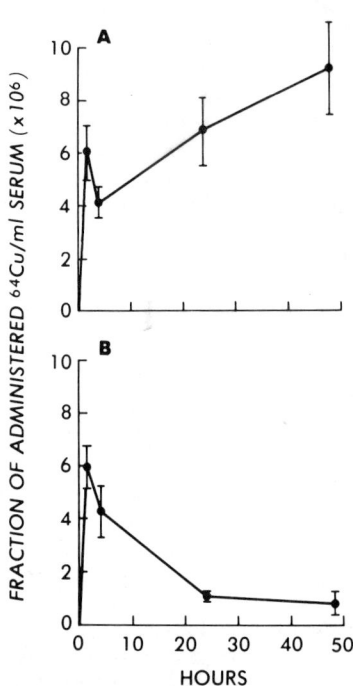

Figure 47–2. Serum ^{64}Cu concentrations (mean ± SE) after the ingestion of a 2-mg dose of radiocopper. A, Patients with miscellaneous liver diseases (non-Wilsonian); B, patients with Wilson's disease. (Modified with permission from Sternlieb I, Scheinberg IH. GASTROENTEROLOGY 77:138. Copyright 1978 by The American Gastroenterological Association.)

whole-body counting techniques have demonstrated that copper absorption varies considerably in normal individuals[41] and that absorption of copper in either homozygotes or heterozygotes for Wilson's disease does not differ from that of normal subjects or from that of cirrhotic patients.[42] Also, intestinal reabsorption of excreted biliary copper, which appears to be insignificant from normal bile,[143] does not appear to be enhanced in patients with Wilson's disease.[42]

It now is apparent that the diminished fecal excretion of copper in patients with Wilson's disease is caused by impairment of biliary excretion of the metal. In studies with intravenously administered ^{67}Cu ($t_{1/2}$ 61.9 hours, compared with the more commonly used ^{64}Cu, $t_{1/2}$ 12.6 hours), cumulative excretion, determined by fecal excretion and whole-body counting, ranged from 24 to 40 per cent in healthy subjects and from 4 to 13 per cent in patients with Wilson's disease.[208] Other investigators reported that whereas healthy subjects and cirrhotic patients excreted > 15 per cent (means 20 per cent and 23 per cent, respectively) of the dose, Wilson's disease patients generally excreted < 10 per cent (mean 5 per cent).[209] Diminished biliary copper excretion in Wilson's disease has been demonstrated by collections from the duodenum[208] (daily biliary copper 0.6 mg in Wilson's disease versus 1.2 mg in control subjects)[130] and common duct bile.[141] Radiocopper excretion recently has been measured in two patients after bile duct cannulation; very little of the injected copper was recovered in the bile of these patients, and there was no evidence of the marked secondary rise in the rate of excretion found after 12 hours in the controls.[210] It was concluded that the accumulation of tissue copper in Wilson's disease results from a defect in the bile secretory mechanism for the metal.

Several hypotheses recently have been advanced to explain the primary defect. The first suggests that the bile of patients with Wilson's disease is relatively deficient in a normal copper-binding component,[143] possibly the taurine conjugate of chenodeoxycholic acid,[149] and that this results in impaired biliary excretion of copper. Against this proposal is the observation that copper-binding proteins in the bile of patients with Wilson's disease appear to be normal qualitatively[141] and that no evidence of a primary disturbance in bile acid metabolism can be demonstrated.[211] According to the second hypothesis, Wilson's disease results from the synthesis of an abnormal hepatic copper-binding protein with an increased affinity for the metal.[212] This concept was revitalized by the report that hepatic metallothionein (see Hepatic Copper Proteins) isolated from the livers of two patients with Wilson's disease had a copper-binding constant four times that of the protein from two control subjects with biliary cirrhosis.[213] Because certain objections have been raised regarding the methods of data interpretation[214] and it is not conceptually easy to account for all of the observed abnormalities in Wilson's disease on the basis of an abnormal protein with high affinity for copper, further confirmation of this finding is still wanting.

The third and most tenable hypothesis, proposed by Sternlieb and colleagues,[141] holds that hepatic lysosomes participate in the intracellular processing and biliary excretion of copper. These investigators administered radiocopper to a patient with Wilson's disease and to one control subject prior to cholecystectomy and analyzed samples of bile and liver. The concentration of copper in the hepatic lysosomal fraction of the patient was about 40 times that of the control. Because of dilution of radiocopper by high concentrations of endogenous copper in the patient's lysosomes, the specific activity of copper in the lysosomal fraction was low in the patient. The specific activity of radiocopper in the patient's bile was low and differed from all specific activities in subcellular fractions examined except that of the lysosomes, to which it was virtually identical. These observations are compatible with the concept that a hepatic lysosomal defect in Wilson's disease interferes with the excretion of copper from lysosomes to bile and underlies the accumulation of excess hepatic copper in Wilson's disease.

The biochemical copper profile of the normal neonate is similar to that of patients with Wilson's disease (e.g., low serum copper and ceruloplasmin levels and high liver copper concentrations > 250 μg/g dry weight). Recently, it has been postulated that the repression of normal copper metabolism in the fetus and its induction within three months of birth are regulated by a controller gene. It is suggested, therefore, that Wilson's disease may result from a failure to switch from the positive copper balance of the fetus to the normal adult pattern, with concomitant activation of biliary excretion and export of ceruloplasmin from the liver, and that this may be caused by mutation of a controller rather than a structural gene.[215, 216]

Since further investigation is obviously needed to establish which of these theories is correct, recent interest has focused on copper toxicosis in Bedlington terriers, a potential animal model. In 1975, Hardy and associates[217] reported finding prominent dark cytoplasmic granules (lysosomes) in association with excessive amounts of hepatic copper and cirrhosis in two Bedlington terriers dying of liver failure. Subsequent studies have shown that many of the hepatic manifestations of Wilson's disease are shared by this canine disorder, although striking differences have been found with regard to other aspects.[13, 218–221] Both are inherited as an autosomal recessive trait, with normal intestinal absorption of copper but impaired biliary excretion of the metal.[222] In the Bedlington terrier, copper accumulates in hepatocellular lysosomes bound to metallothionein and forms the characteristic electron-dense granules,[223] which precede the development of hepatic injury. The appearance of chronic active hepatitis progressing to a mixed micronodular and macronodular cirrhosis is common in both diseases, and episodes of hemolysis occur in both. However, the pathologic effects in Bedlington terriers seem largely to be restricted to the liver, since neither the characteristic neurologic disturbances nor the Kayser-Fleischer rings of Wilson's disease are evident. Moreover, the liver differs histologically from the human condition in that the steatosis and the mitochondrial and peroxisomal changes that are characteristic of the early Wilsonian lesion are lacking,[16] and in the canine liver, copper is predominantly centrolobular in distribution, and Mallory bodies are absent. Finally, it is not possible to distinguish affected and nonaffected dogs on the basis of serum concentrations of ceruloplasmin,[218] in contradistinction to 95 per cent of Wilson's disease patients, in whom levels are reduced.[224]

CLINICAL MANIFESTATIONS

Although the accumulation of hepatic copper begins during infancy, clinical liver disease rarely appears before the age of 6 years. The age of symptomatic onset and the clinical pattern of disease vary considerably in different patients. During the early asymptomatic stages, minor histologic findings on liver biopsy may be the only evidence of disease apart from the primary biochemical abnormalities of copper metabolism. In a group of 151 asymptomatic patients, Sternlieb and Scheinberg found that 50 per cent had developed symptoms by age 15.[27] Thus, Wilson's disease occurs predominantly in older children, adolescents, and younger adults, although occasionally patients may remain in excellent health and their disease may be clinically undiagnosed until the sixth decade of life.[225, 226] In Sternlieb's series, the initial clinical manifestation was hepatic in 42 per cent, neurologic in 34 per cent, psychiatric in 10 per cent, hematologic or endocrinologic secondary to hepatic dysfunction in 12 per cent, and renal in 1 per cent. About 25 per cent of patients simultaneously developed two or more modes of onset. This pattern of disease resembles that observed in smaller series in the United States[23] and in other countries.[17, 227]

Hepatic

The manifestations of hepatic involvement tend to occur at a younger age than do those of the central nervous system disease and are nonspecific, mimicking the features of a variety of acute and chronic liver diseases, including acute and chronic hepatitis, fulminant hepatic failure, and cirrhosis. In the early asymptomatic phase of disease or in the presence of inactive cirrhosis, liver tests may be normal, or serum aspartate aminotransferase levels may be mildly elevated. Most commonly, the hepatic disease begins insidiously and pursues a chronic course progressively characterized by the onset of lassitude, fatigue, anorexia, jaundice, spider angiomas, splenomegaly, and hypersplenism, culminating in portal hypertension, ascites, variceal hemorrhage, and hepatic failure.

Patients with Wilson's disease frequently present with a shrunken or normal-sized liver and the features of postnecrotic *cirrhosis*; thus, progressive hepatic insufficiency, ascites, or bleeding esophageal varices may be a first and ominous manifestation of the disease.[16, 228] It is not unusual for Wilson's disease to be manifested with clinical, biochemical, and histologic characteristics similar to those of *chronic active hepatitis*.[16, 229–231] In a study of seven patients with histologic features of chronic hepatitis,[229] the diagnosis of Wilson's disease was made in one by the accidental finding of Kayser-Fleischer rings and in four others after neurologic features became manifest. In another series of 17 patients aged 7 to 21 years, with morphologic features indistinguishable from those of chronic active hepatitis, neurologic dysfunction was evident in 3 patients only, Kayser-Fleischer rings were absent in 8 patients, and serum ceruloplasmin was normal in 3 individuals with severe hepatic failure.[231] Nine of the patients with advanced liver disease died within two years of diagnosis, mostly from hepatic failure and despite the use of D-penicillamine. Although 10 to 30 per cent of patients with Wilson's disease may manifest features of chronic hepatitis, the disease represents an uncommon cause of HBsAg-negative chronic active hepatitis. Nevertheless, it is imperative that biochemical screening for Wilson's disease be undertaken in all patients under the age of 35 years who have clinical or histologic findings compatible with chronic active hepatitis (or other chronic parenchymal liver disease).

Occasionally, the disease may be manifested as *fulminant hepatic failure*,[179, 232–236] which is clinically indistinguishable from the viral syndrome of massive hepatic necrosis and usually terminates in death within days or weeks unless the resources for liver transplantation are available. Although it is critical to make a diagnosis of Wilson's disease in these patients for the purpose of family screening, treatment is generally unsuccessful, particularly when the disorder is associated with hemolysis and consequent renal insufficiency.[179, 235] Finally, cirrhosis and hemolysis, both of which are frequent manifestations of Wilson's disease, predispose to the development of *cholelithiasis*. Moreover, an increased incidence of mixed cholesterol gallstones has been reported in Wilson's disease;[237] hence, this possibility should be considered in the differential diagnosis of abdominal pain in such patients.

Neurologic

The neurologic manifestations commonly appear between the ages of 12 to 30 years[20] and almost invariably are accompanied by the presence of Kayser-Fleischer rings.[29, 238] Symptoms are subtle in the beginning and progress inexorably if patients are untreated. Early findings include incoordination (particularly involving fine movements), clumsiness, resting and intention tremors, dysarthria, excessive salivation, dysphagia, ataxia, and mask-like facies. Fortunately, the late manifestations of dystonia, spasticity, rigidity with development of flexion contractures, and grand mal seizures are now rare, as a result of earlier diagnosis and treatment. Deteriorating performance in school is a common initial complaint that apparently is not attributable to intellectual impairment. Electroencephalography is not helpful in diagnosis and reveals only nonspecific slow waves in patients with advanced neurologic or hepatic dysfunction.[239] The gross anatomic changes (degeneration and cavitation) that involve the putamen, globus pallidus, caudate nuclei, thalamus,[22, 29] and (less frequently) the brainstem and frontal cortex may be demonstrated at a relatively early stage by computed tomography.[240–241] However, the clinical neurologic status of patients with Wilson's disease is not reliably predicted by computed tomography[242, 243] or evoked potentials.[242] Magnetic resonance imaging appears to be more sensitive in defining structural changes in the cerebrum, cerebellum and brain stem, but is frequently normal in asymptomatic patients.[244] Liver function studies frequently are within normal limits during the neurologic stage of disease, although cirrhosis usually is present. Liver biopsy is not always necessary for diagnosis of neurologic Wilson's disease but provides information about the extent of liver injury.

Psychiatric

Psychiatric manifestations may be prominent, and affected individuals frequently are considered to have progressive psychiatric illness and are institutionalized before Wilson's disease is diagnosed. Patients, most commonly adolescents, may show behavioral changes that often are aggressive in nature, psychoneurosis, a manic-depressive or schizophrenic psychosis, or organic dementia.[20, 22, 29, 245] At least four symptom clusters can be identified—namely, affective, behavioral, schizophrenia-like, and cognitive.[247] These manifestations may reflect not only cerebral copper deposition but also the expressions of an individual frustrated by progressive, undiagnosed neurologic symptoms.[29] The psychologic stresses of the disease in this situation are reflected by the fact that therapy often results in only partial psychiatric recovery. Psychotherapy and the milder tranquilizing or antidepressant drugs are indicated when psychiatric disturbances are more than minimal, although specific therapy with D-penicillamine is still essential.

Ophthalmic

The *Kayser-Fleischer ring* is a golden-brown or greenish discoloration in the zone of Descemet's membrane in the limbic region of the cornea (Fig. 47–3). The array of colors and hues that can be seen is an optical phenomenon related to the distribution, density, and size of the copper granules.[248] The rings are usually complete and bilateral, but discoloration appears initially at the superior poles, followed by the inferior poles and the lateral regions. It has been postulated that this pattern of copper deposition is due to a relative stagnation of corneal solvent flow in the superior poles, allowing the precipitation of copper.[249] Moreover, the rings fade gradually over three to five years with adequate penicillamine treatment and disappear sequentially as a function of corneal solvent flow patterns, so that the superior corneal pole is the last region to be cleared. When not visible with the unaided eye, Kayser-Fleischer rings can be identified by slit-lamp ophthalmoscopy or gonioscopy. Using x-ray excitation spectrometry, it now is possible to quantitate and monitor the amount of copper in the cornea of affected patients.[250] The Kayser-Fleischer ring has been shown to consist of electron-dense granules, rich in copper and sulfur (suggesting that the

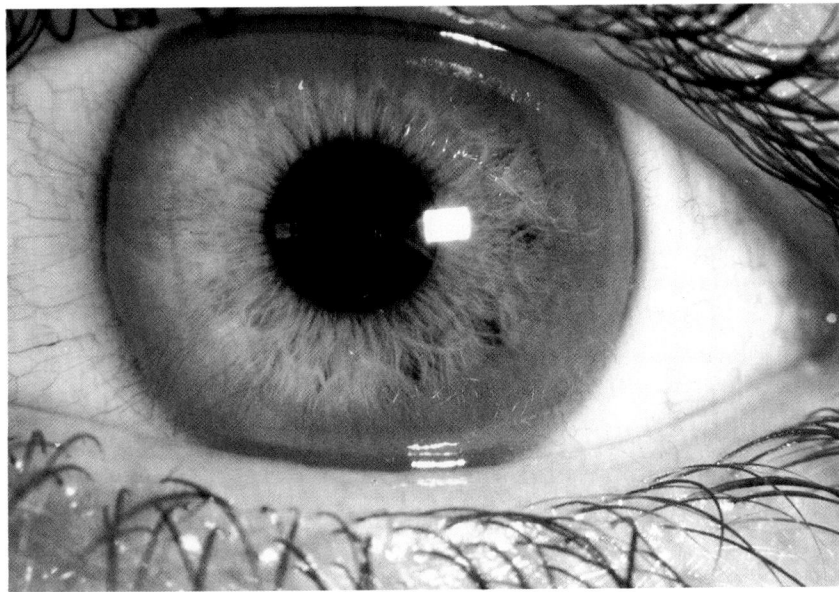

Fig. 47–3

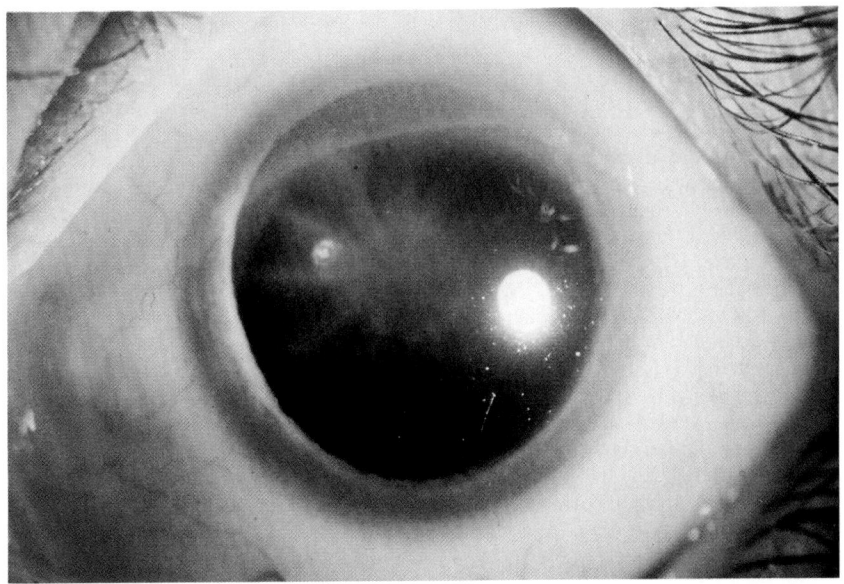

Fig. 47–4

Figure 47–3. Kayser-Fleischer ring. (Courtesy of Professor Dame S. Sherlock, London.)

Figure 47–4. Sunflower cataract. (Courtesy of I. Sternlieb, New York.)

metal may be bound to metallothionein), which are more numerous at the peripheral than in the central region of the cornea.[251] Interestingly, the central area of the cornea contains as much copper as the limbus, but the sulfur-containing moiety is present only in Descemet's membrane.[251]

Kayser-Fleischer rings are almost invariably present in patients with neurologic features but may be absent in asymptomatic children and patients who have hepatic disease, particularly those with chronic active hepatitis.[231] Although the Kayser-Fleischer ring is a useful diagnostic sign, it is no longer considered to be pathognomonic of Wilson's disease unless accompanied by neurologic manifestations. Pigmented corneal rings in the presence of chronic hepatobiliary disease have been associated with long-standing intrahepatic cholestasis of childhood,[252–254] partial biliary atresia,[255] primary biliary cirrhosis,[256] chronic active hepatitis with cirrhosis,[255–256] and cryptogenic cirrhosis.[255, 257] In all of these conditions, excessive deposition of copper in the liver and other organs probably is due to diminished biliary excretion of copper. However, these diseases can readily be distinguished from Wilson's disease by the clinical history, immunologic markers, serum level of ceruloplasmin, and radiocopper kinetics (Fig. 47–2).

Sunflower cataracts (Fig. 47–4, color plate, p. 1259) are a less frequent ocular manifestation of Wilson's disease that are found together with Kayser-Fleischer rings.[249, 258, 259] The cataract appears as a central green or golden disk in the anterior capsule of the lens, with radiating petals arising from the posterior capsule. Vision is unimpeded by the cataracts, and in general they tend to clear much more rapidly than do Kayser-Fleischer rings in response to penicillamine therapy.[249] Sunflower cataracts can be found in association with an intraocular copper-containing foreign body (chalcosis) and in this situation are often accompanied by Kayser-Fleischer rings.[260]

Hematologic

Acute intravascular hemolysis frequently complicates the course of Wilson's disease, and in at least 15 per cent of patients it may be the presenting feature.[261–264] Hemolysis usually is transient and self-limiting, preceding the onset of hepatic manifestations by several years. Since Kayser-Fleischer rings may be absent, the diagnosis should be excluded biochemically in all patients less than 20 years old who have Coombs-negative, nonspherocytic hemolytic anemia. Occasionally, acute hemolysis may manifest in association with acute hepatic failure; in this situation, death ensues within weeks from hepatic or renal failure.[179, 232, 234, 235] Although only a few instances of acute ongoing hemolysis have been studied, it is postulated that copper is released suddenly from the liver, increasing free plasma copper, which then is taken up by the red cells. This may lead to oxidative damage to red cell membranes and hemoglobin.[22, 262] Other investigators report that copper-induced oxidative stress is insufficient to explain the degree of hemolysis observed[265] and suggest that the primary toxic effect of copper is mediated by its oxidant action on membrane phospholipids.[266]

In patients with predominantly hepatic involvement, particularly acute hepatic failure or severe decompensated cirrhosis, defective synthesis of coagulation factors and qualitative platelet abnormalities may result in a bleeding tendency.[267] Cirrhosis with associated splenomegaly also is

thought to underlie the frequent finding of thrombocytopenia and leukopenia in the presenting laboratory data.[268]

Renal

A wide variety of defects in renal function have been found in association with Wilson's disease, including decreased glomerular filtration rate and renal plasma flow and renal tubular abnormalities.[22, 269–271] Proximal tubular dysfunction, presumably resulting from the toxic effect of copper on cellular function, is manifest most frequently as aminoaciduria, glucosuria, uricosuria (with an associated low serum uric acid concentration), hyperphosphaturia, and hypercalciuria. In addition, there is often proteinuria, involving low–molecular weight globulins, and peptiduria, consisting primarily of hydroxyproline-containing peptides derived from degradation of collagen.[272] Distal renal tubular acidosis, as reflected by the inability to acidify urine to a pH of less than 5.2 after ammonium chloride loading,[271, 273–275] appears to be of particular significance with regard to the development of renal stones, which occur in as many as 16 per cent of patients.[274] Penicillamine, which during the course of therapy produces a marked improvement in renal function,[271] occasionally may have serious adverse effects on the kidney, including nephrotic syndrome[29, 276] and a Goodpasture-like syndrome.[277]

Skeletal

Radiologic signs of skeletal involvement are common,[278–281] particularly those of bone demineralization.[19, 22, 29] Clinical symptoms are less evident, although patients often will admit to pain and stiffness in the knees, wrists, or other large joints.[280] Occasionally, skeletal complaints represent the first manifestation of the disease.[282] Radiologic changes include osteomalacia and rickets, osteoporosis, premature osteoarthrosis, spontaneous fractures, bone fragmentation near joints, subarticular cysts, osteochondritis desiccans, chondrocalcinosis, chondromalacia patellae, and premature degenerative arthritis of the knees and wrists. The pathogenesis of these osteoarticular lesions is unknown, and there is little evidence to indicate that copper toxicity is directly involved. Renal tubular abnormalities probably contribute to the changes (i.e., hypercalciuria and hyperphosphaturia), and other factors such as hepatic and neurologic dysfunction may also be involved.[22, 29] The increased urinary hydroxyproline excretion in patients does not appear to correlate with the severity of the skeletal lesions.[272]

Miscellaneous

Cardiac involvement has recently been recognized in Wilson's disease.[283, 284] Clinical manifestations include arrhythmias, cardiomyopathy, and autonomic dysfunction. In a group of 53 consecutive patients with a mean age of 21 years, electrocardiographic abnormalities were present in 34 per cent.[284] Although data are limited, the morphologic changes, which include variable degrees of interstitial and replacement fibrosis, small vessel sclerosis, focal inflammatory cell infiltration, and nodal degeneration,[285] appear to be proportional to the cardiac concentrations of copper.[29]

A variety of manifestations that arise secondary to hepatic dysfunction usually are corrected as the underlying liver disease abates with therapy. These include primary or secondary amenorrhea in women and delayed puberty and gynecomastia in boys.[27] Detailed hormonal analysis of four female patients suggests that the ovulatory disturbances (i.e., severe oligomenorrhea or amenorrhea) may be due to a primary disturbance of ovarian function.[285] Less frequent associations with Wilson's disease include parathyroid insufficiency,[286] glucose intolerance,[287] exocrine pancreatic insufficiency,[288] and abnormalities of humoral and cell-mediated immunity.[289] Blue lunulas of the fingernails are an unusual but characteristic finding.[290] Although an increase of fingertip whorls has been reported to be of diagnostic value,[291] these dermatoglyphic studies have not been confirmed by other investigators.[292]

NATURAL HISTORY

A theoretical concept of the natural history of Wilson's disease, which accounts for the diverse clinical presentations of the disorder,[29, 282, 293] has been conceived by Deiss and associates[15, 294] and modified by Dobyns and co-workers.[23] According to this concept, a modified version of which is shown in Figure 47–5, the natural history of the disease may be considered in four stages: stage I, the initial period of accumulation of copper by hepatic binding sites; stage II, the acute redistribution of copper within the liver and its release into the circulation; stage III, the chronic accumulation of copper in the brain and other extrahepatic tissues with progressive and eventually fatal disease unless copper balance is achieved by chelation therapy (stage IV).

During stage I, the patient remains asymptomatic, and copper accumulates diffusely in the cytosol of hepatocytes until all such hepatic binding sites have been saturated.[295] When the accumulation of copper reaches a critical level, some of the metal is redistributed from the cytosol to the lysosomes,[295] and a proportion is released into the blood (stage II). The phenomenon of redistribution of copper within hepatocytes is supported by morphologic studies[295] and that of hepatic copper release is consistent with the observation that the hepatic concentrations of copper in asymptomatic children are generally much higher than those in older symptomatic patients.[293] In most patients (~60 per cent) the process of hepatic redistribution and release occurs gradually, and the disease remains clinically inapparent during this stage. If, however, the hepatic release of copper is rapid, the abrupt rise in blood levels may be sufficient to cause hemolysis. Also, if the shift of copper from hepatocyte cytosol to lysosomes is rapid or erratic, hepatic necrosis or chronic active hepatitis with hepatic failure may ensue.

Those patients who become symptomatic in stage II may succumb as the result of hepatic failure or, rarely, hemolysis or may again become asymptomatic. During stage III, storage of copper in the lysosomes continues with associated development of hepatic fibrosis and cirrhosis, and extrahepatic accumulation of copper occurs in other tissues (e.g., brain, cornea, and kidneys). If the cirrhosis is inactive and progresses slowly and cerebral accumulation is slow, patients may remain asymptomatic for many years before finally manifesting hepatic or neurologic symptoms or both. If, on the other hand, hepatic injury proceeds rapidly, the manifestations of hepatic disease may merge imperceptibly with those of stage II. If the disease is diagnosed before progressive and fatal hepatic or neurologic disease supervenes, patients will achieve a state of copper balance after prolonged therapy (stage IV), and most will become asymptomatic, although some have residual evidence of portal hypertension or irreversible brain damage.

HEPATIC PATHOLOGY

Histologic changes usually are evident in biopsy samples of liver obtained from asymptomatic patients, even during the first decade of life.[29, 293] The earliest changes detectable on light microscopy are glycogen degeneration of nuclei in periportal hepatocytes[186, 296] and moderate fatty infiltration (Fig. 47–6).[187, 297] The lipid droplets, which are composed of triglycerides, progressively increase in number and size, so that the steatosis may resemble that induced by ethanol.[29] Coexistent with or preceding these changes, mitochondrial abnormalities may be apparent,[297] probably related pathogenetically to the steatosis. Hepatocyte mitochondria are heterogeneous in size and shape and have an increased matrix density, separation of the normally apposed inner and outer mitochondrial membranes, and widened intercristal spaces, and an array of vacuolated and crystalline inclusions or dense inclusions appear in the matrix (Fig. 47–7).[16, 228, 297, 298] Although these abnormalities may be seen individually in other pathologic conditions, the simultaneous occurrence of several in the same mitochondrion appears to be specific for young patients with Wilson's disease. In most patients, these mitochondrial features become less pronounced or disappear after several years of D-penicillamine therapy,[299] suggesting indirectly that the changes are a consequence of copper toxicity. Lipolysosomes, which are membrane-bound lipid droplets containing acid phosphatase activity, account for 1 to 2 per cent of the observed lipid droplets in the steatosis of Wilson's disease.[300] These lipid-containing lysosomes are nonspecific, however, since they have been observed in hepatocytes containing excess lipid as a consequence of a variety of other causes.[301] Ultrastructural changes also may be evident in peroxisomes (organelles also involved in lipid metabolism, as discussed in Chap. 5), which appear heterogeneous and contain a granular, flocculent, rather than homogeneous, matrix of varying electron density. These ultrastructural abnormalities, particularly the mitochondrial and fatty changes, regress as fibrosis and ultimately cirrhosis develop.[297] Except for an abundance of copper-rich lipofuscin granules in periportal hepatocytes, the electron microscopic appearances are usually normal in the later stages.[295] Occasionally, collagen fibrils or basement membrane material may be found in sinusoidal spaces[298] and abnormal separation of hepatocytes and pseudo-glandular formations are seen.[29]

The rate of progression of hepatic injury from fatty infiltration to cirrhosis varies considerably and occurs by one of two processes. Some patients develop changes indistinguishable from chronic active hepatitis arising from other causes (Figs. 47–8 and 47–9),[229–231] with mononuclear cell infiltrates, mostly lymphocytes and plasma cells, piecemeal necrosis extending beyond the limiting plate, parenchymal collapse, bridging hepatic necrosis, and fibrosis. This hepatic lesion may subside spontaneously and evolve into macronodular cirrhosis or may progress rapidly into a fulminant hepatitis, which responds poorly to treatment.[179, 232–236] The progression to cirrhosis may be accompanied by little parenchymal inflammatory infiltrate or by necrosis. In this situation, the histologic appearances are those of a macronodular or mixed micromacronodular cirrhosis,[303] with either wide or thin fibrous septa (containing predominantly types I and III collagen),[304] bile ductule prolifera-

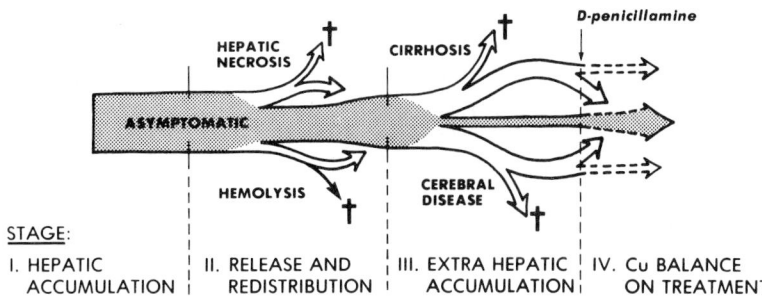

Figure 47–5. Natural history of Wilson's disease. (A conceptual scheme modified from Dobyns WB, et al. Mayo Clin Proc 54:35, 1979, with permission.)

tion, and variable septal round cell infiltration. At the periphery of nodules, hepatocytes frequently contain Mallory's cytoplasmic hyalin.[296, 303] All the changes of the precirrhotic stage, particularly excess cytoplasmic lipid and nuclei containing glycogen, also may be seen in the cirrhotic liver. In contradistinction to its high incidence in cirrhotic patients with hemochromatosis, hepatocellular carcinoma rarely complicates the course of Wilson's disease,[305–311] although in the latter, cirrhosis develops earlier and persists for many decades in treated patients. Since copper has been shown to protect against chemically induced hepatocellular carcinoma in rats, it has been suggested that the metal may exert a protective effect in patients with Wilson's disease.[308]

Despite consistently elevated hepatic copper levels in Wilson's disease, histochemical staining of this excess copper by rubeanic acid or rhodanine is negative in the majority of patients and therefore is of little value in diagnosis.[231, 293, 303] Moreover, orcein staining for copper-associated protein[312]

is negative in about half of the cases.[313] Copper-associated protein gives a granular stain with orcein and is an ill-defined entity that appears to be polymerized metallothionein sequestered in lysosomes.[295, 314–317] In contradistinction to Wilson's disease, other conditions in which hepatic copper is elevated (e.g., primary biliary cirrhosis, primary sclerosing cholangitis, biliary atresia, intrahepatic cholestasis of childhood, Indian childhood cirrhosis, and also in the newborn infant) are nearly always associated with stainable copper and the presence of copper-associated protein, particularly in periportal hepatocytes.[312, 313, 318–323] In seeking an explanation for these findings, two observations may be relevant: (1) in Wilson's disease with cirrhosis, copper is often localized in portal tracts and fibrous septa, whereas the regenerating nodules are almost devoid of copper;[303] and (2) diffusely distributed copper in the cytosol of younger patients with Wilson's disease[29, 305, 317] may be less readily apparent than the granular lysosomal staining that appears later in the course of the disease and is more typical

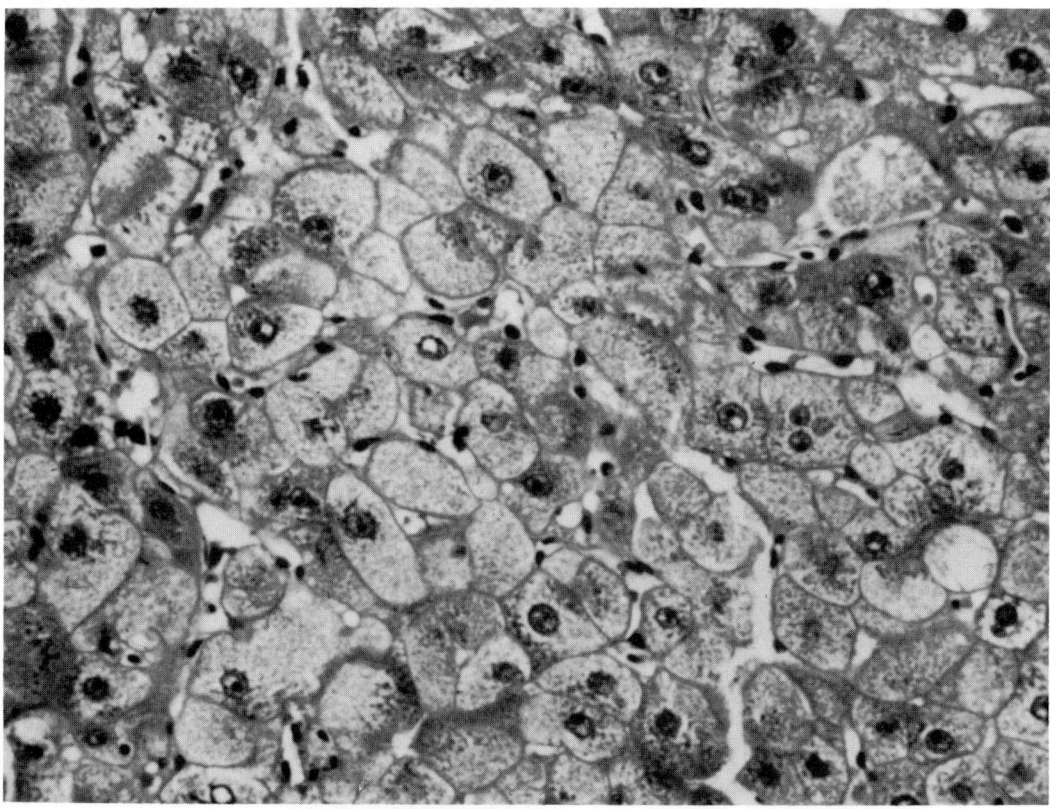

Figure 47–6. Light micrograph of a section of a liver biopsy obtained from an asymptomatic 14-year-old boy with a three-year history of persistently elevated serum aminotransferase levels. Serum ceruloplasmin concentration was 10.6 mg/100 ml and hepatic copper concentration 756 μg/g dry weight. There is fatty infiltration of pleomorphic hepatocytes, and glycogen vacuolation is present in some nuclei. Hematoxylin and eosin, × 300.

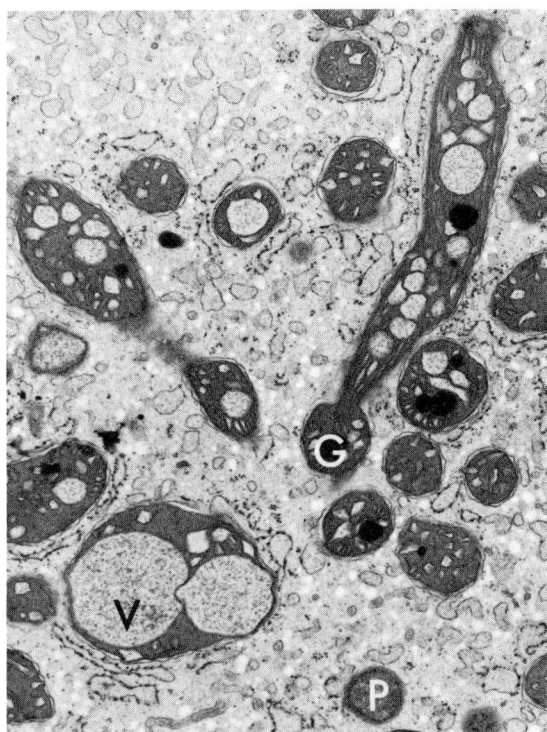

Figure 47–7. Striking pleomorphism of mitochondria that have abnormally arranged cristae, numerous large, electron-lucent vacuoles (V) with finely granular contents, and greatly enlarged mitochondrial granules (G). Mitochondrial crystals are also present, but are not apparent at this magnification. In this section, glycogen was extracted during processing, leaving blank spaces. Notice the granular matrix of the peroxisome (P). The specimen was obtained from a 24-year-old man with psychiatric, neurologic, and corneal signs of Wilson's disease. Fatty metamorphosis of hepatocytes was seen by light microscopy. Serum ceruloplasmin, 4.5 mg/dl; hepatic copper, 1055 μ/g dry weight (× 9250). (Reproduced from Sternlieb, I. In: Popper H, Schaffner F, eds. Progress in Liver Diseases, Vol. 4. Grune & Stratton, 1972:511, with permission.)

of other states in which hepatic copper is increased. Whether the production of copper-associated protein, which has been postulated to protect hepatocytes from the injurious effects of copper, is impaired in Wilson's disease[313] and whether metallothionein is involved in the basic defect in Wilson's disease remain intriguing but unanswered questions.[314, 317] Finally, copper-associated protein has been demonstrated in primary liver tumors,[323] including fibrolamellar liver cell carcinoma,[324] and may be helpful in distinguishing primary from metastatic tumors.

BIOCHEMICAL DIAGNOSIS

The great majority of patients with Wilson's disease have both Kayser-Fleischer rings (some of which may be apparent only on slit-lamp examination) and serum ceruloplasmin concentrations of less than 20 mg/dl. When corneal rings are absent or patients are asymptomatic, coexistence of a hepatic copper concentration of more than 250 μg/g dry weight and a low ceruloplasmin concentration is sufficient to establish the diagnosis.

Serum Ceruloplasmin

Measured by either the enzymatic or the immunochemical method, the normal serum concentration of this copper-

containing glycoprotein is 20 to 40 mg/dl. Although a decreased level of ceruloplasmin per se is not diagnostic of Wilson's disease, approximately 95 per cent of all patients and 85 per cent of individuals who have hepatic manifestations of the disease have concentrations of less than 20 mg/dl.[325] The molecular basis for the deficiency of ceruloplasmin in Wilson's disease is at least in part caused by a decrease in transcription (possibly translational or posttranslational) of the ceruloplasmin gene.[326] Hypoceruloplasminemia may arise as a transient consequence of nephrotic syndrome, protein-losing enteropathy, malabsorption, or severe malnutrition and, in these situations, should create no diagnostic difficulty.[22] Some confusion may however arise with regard to about 10 per cent of the heterozygous carriers of the Wilson's disease gene, in whom the disease never develops but whose low levels of ceruloplasmin are comparable to those found in patients (about one in 2000 persons in the general population).[293, 327] This problem may rarely be compounded in the heterozygote who fortuitously develops chronic active hepatitis or cirrhosis and who thus resembles the Wilson's disease homozygote clinically, biochemically, and histologically.[328] Sporadic reports suggest the existence of a benign entity distinct from Wilson's disease that is a hereditary form of hypoceruloplasminemia not associated with excessive copper binding.[329] Wilson's disease pedigrees in which quantitative discrepancies exist between plasma oxidase activity and plasma ceruloplasmin concentration determined by immunoassay have also been described.[330] An occasional diagnostic dilemma may arise in patients with fulminant hepatitis (non-Wilsonian), in whom hypoceruloplasminemia appears as a transitory response to the massive necrosis and diminished synthetic function of the liver.[331] Similarly, about 25 per cent of children with chronic active hepatitis have decreased serum concentrations of ceruloplasmin.[332] On the other hand, serum ceruloplasmin levels are virtually always normal or elevated in adults with chronic active hepatitis,[333, 334] and hence this is a useful screening test to differentiate Wilson's disease and chronic active hepatitis in adult patients. It thus is apparent that a diagnosis of Wilson's disease requires more than the mere demonstration of a reduced serum level of ceruloplasmin,[325] although such a finding in an asymptomatic individual with elevated serum transaminase levels is highly suggestive of the diagnosis.

Conversely, normal ceruloplasmin concentrations (usually 20 to 30 mg/dl) are found in as many as 15 per cent of patients with Wilson's disease who have severe chronic active liver disease.[231] These low-normal concentrations may reflect a temporary increase in the hepatic synthesis of ceruloplasmin (which is an acute-phase reactant) in response to the inflammatory process in the liver or an excess of circulating estrogens, or both.[335] In such patients, if the diagnosis remains in doubt or the severity of hepatic dysfunction contraindicates liver biopsy, a radiocopper loading test may be necessary to confirm the diagnosis of Wilson's disease.[205] The ceruloplasmin concentration usually subsides to the low level generally associated with Wilson's disease if the liver disease becomes less active,[294] and a further reduction frequently follows the initiation of D-penicillamine therapy.[27] Pregnancy or estrogen administration also may elevate serum ceruloplasmin levels in patients with Wilson's disease.[327, 335]

Nonceruloplasmin Serum Copper

In the healthy adult, the concentration of copper bound to serum albumin or amino acids (nonceruloplasmin cop-

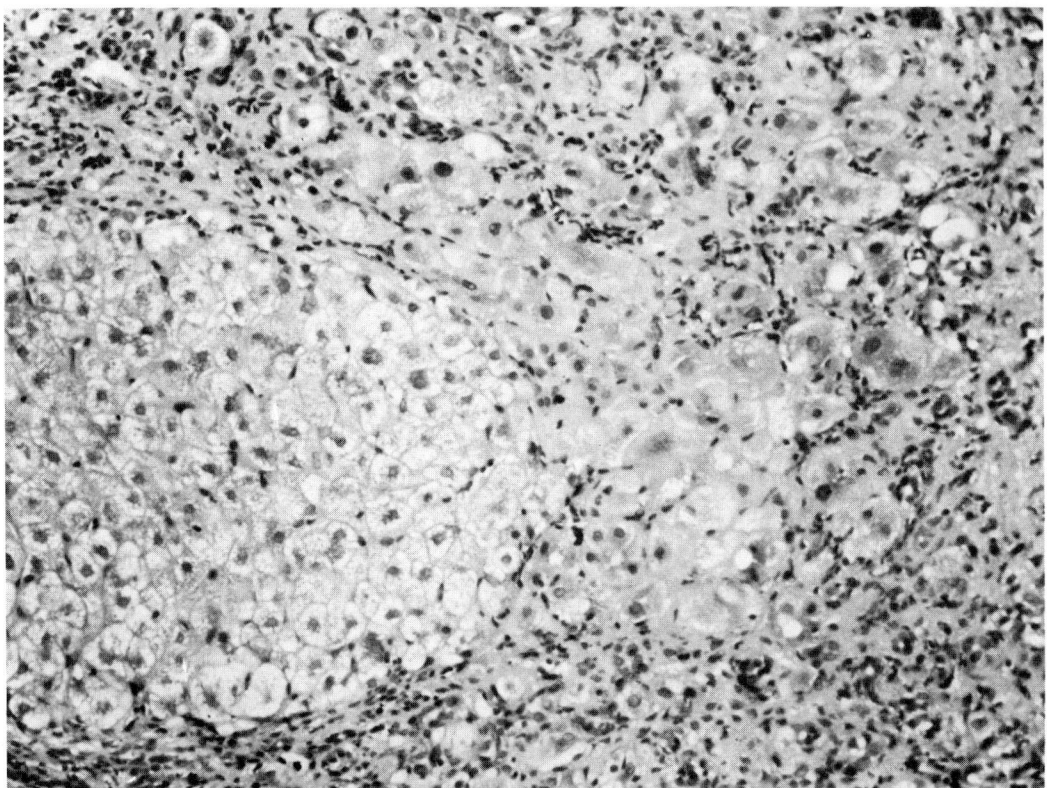

Figure 47–8. Light micrograph of a section of a liver biopsy obtained from a 15-year-old girl with Wilson's disease who presented with liver failure. The picture is one of chronic active hepatitis with cirrhosis and shows a regeneration nodule, isolation of small groups of ballooned liver cells, piecemeal necrosis, and marked infiltration with mononuclear inflammatory cells. Hematoxylin and eosin, × 185.

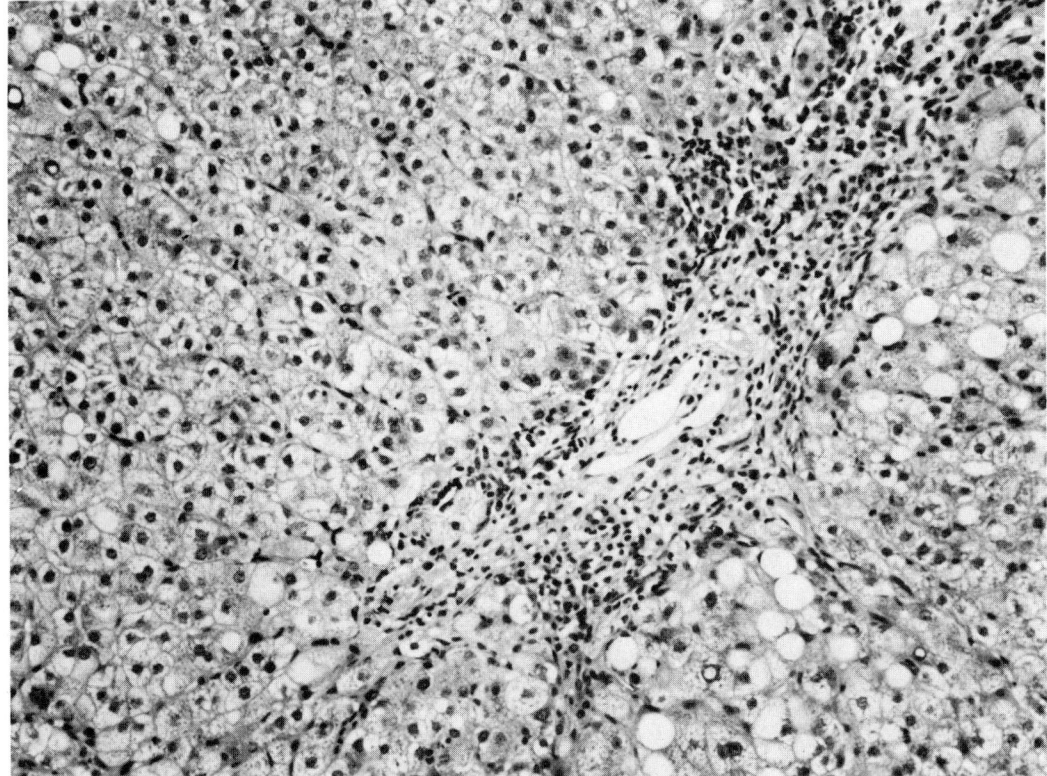

Figure 47–9. Light micrograph of a section of a liver biopsy obtained from an 18-year-old girl with neurologic abnormalities. The picture is that of a moderately active cirrhosis, showing a fibrous septum containing a few inflammatory cells but minimal piecemeal necrosis. Some hepatocytes contain fat, and occasional nuclei are vacuolated. Hematoxylin and eosin, × 185.

per) is 5 to 12 µg/dl.[336] Patients with untreated Wilson's disease have elevated concentrations, probably as a result of the passage of excessive hepatic copper to the circulation, that may be as high as 50 µg/dl.[51, 336] This increase in the nonceruloplasmin fraction usually is not sufficient to compensate for the reduced serum ceruloplasmin level in Wilson's disease, so that in most cases, total serum copper levels are below the normal range.[25, 51] Although heterozygotes and treated patients with Wilson's disease have normal serum levels of nonceruloplasmin copper, patients with a variety of parenchymal or cholestatic liver diseases have increased concentrations,[336] so that measurement of this fraction of serum copper has little diagnostic value.

Urinary Copper Excretion

Normal persons excrete less than 40 µg/24 hours of copper in the urine, most of which probably is derived from the readily filterable fraction of nonceruloplasmin copper in serum. Almost all patients with Wilson's disease who have progressed beyond stage I (see Fig. 47–3) or who are symptomatic excrete in excess of 100 µg/24 hours.[51] Occasionally, values as high as 1,000 µg or more/24 hours may be observed during stage II of the disease in association with hepatic necrosis, when hepatic copper stores suddenly are released into the circulation. Unfortunately, urinary copper levels are frequently elevated in patients with cirrhosis,[78, 337] chronic active hepatitis,[332, 333] and cholestasis, including primary biliary cirrhosis,[334, 337] and hence this measurement does not differentiate these entities from Wilson's disease. Administration of D-penicillamine to increase urinary copper excretion has not provided a more sensitive diagnostic index, since overlap is still evident in the ranges of copper excreted by patients with Wilson's disease, cholestasis, and chronic active hepatitis.[337, 338] Once the diagnosis is established, however, quantitative estimation of urinary copper provides a useful means of evaluating the response to D-penicillamine therapy and individualizing maintenance dosages.

Hepatic Copper Concentration

Normal hepatic copper concentrations are between 15 and 55 µg/g dry liver.[339] Various microanalytic techniques have been used to quantitate the copper content of biopsy samples,[13] including atomic absorption spectrophotometry, neutron activation analysis, and x-ray microanalysis.[340, 341] In order to obtain an accurate determination, it is crucial that the biopsy needle and container be free from contamination by copper and that an adequate-sized sample (a major portion of the biopsy core) be submitted for analysis. A disposable needle made entirely of steel or a Klatskin or a Menghini needle washed in EDTA and rinsed with demineralized water should be used, and the syringe should contain 5 per cent dextrose rather than saline.[29]

Hepatic copper concentrations are elevated in virtually all untreated patients with Wilson's disease to values of between 250 and 3000 µg/g of dry tissue.[293, 339] Values below 250 µg/g usually are attributable to the irregular distribution of copper in liver, particularly in the presence of cirrhosis, when small, fragmented biopsy samples are obtained. Heterozygous carriers of the Wilson's disease gene may have slightly elevated levels of hepatic copper (rarely, to 250 µg/g), but they do not develop signs of copper toxicosis.[293] As in patients with hepatic or neurologic dysfunction,

hepatic copper should be determined in asymptomatic individuals with family or clinical histories suggestive of Wilson's disease or in the presence of unexplained hypoceruloplasminemia.[293] The finding of a normal hepatic copper concentration excludes the diagnosis of untreated Wilson's disease. However, an elevated hepatic copper level per se does not establish the diagnosis of Wilson's disease, since concentrations higher than 250 µg/g may be found in primary biliary cirrhosis,[135, 334, 339, 341–346] primary sclerosing cholangitis, extrahepatic biliary obstruction[339] or atresia,[347] in intrahepatic cholestasis of childhood[348, 349] and other cholestatic syndromes,[252] in young patients with Indian childhood cirrhosis[188, 350–353] and in vineyard sprayers inhaling copper salts.[354] It is postulated that the excessive copper in these disorders may contribute to the hepatic injuries, although they each appear to have distinctive microscopic and histochemical features.[319, 341] Moreover, these patients are readily distinguished from those with Wilson's disease on the basis of history, physical findings, and liver tests. In the great majority of individuals with prolonged cholestatic disorders or chronic active hepatitis (in whom hepatic copper may be moderately elevated)[332, 333] serum ceruloplasmin concentrations are normal or increased.[333]

Histochemical stains such as rubeanic acid, rhodamine, and orcein are of little diagnostic value in Wilson's disease[231, 303] but may be useful in differentiation of cholestatic conditions.[312, 320] Computed tomography has little to offer in the diagnosis of Wilson's disease, since liver attenuation values are within the normal range, even in patients with a markedly elevated liver copper content.[355, 356] Similarly, nuclear magnetic resonance imaging is of no value in monitoring liver copper levels.[357]

Incorporation of Orally Administered Radiocopper into Ceruloplasmin

Occasionally, a diagnostic dilemma may arise in Wilson's disease patients who have normal ceruloplasmin concentrations or when liver biopsy is contraindicated, or in heterozygous carriers of the Wilson's disease gene, or patients with other forms of liver disease who have Kayser-Fleischer rings, elevated hepatic copper concentrations, or increased urinary copper excretion. A test of the incorporation of orally administered radiocopper (2 mg cupric acetate, containing 0.3 to 0.5 mCi ^{64}Cu mixed in fruit juice)[29] into ceruloplasmin, which simply requires measurement of serum radioactivity at 1, 2, 4, 24, and 48 hours, will generally resolve these problems.[70, 205] As shown in Figure 47–2, in healthy subjects or patients who have hepatic disorders that mimic Wilson's disease, the plasma concentrations of nonceruloplasmin radiocopper rise rapidly, are maximal within 1 to 2 hours, then fall and rise again over the ensuing 48 hours as radiocopper is incorporated into ceruloplasmin and released into the circulation.[67, 204, 205] On the contrary, patients who have Wilson's disease incorporate little or no radiocopper into newly synthesized ceruloplasmin;[205] the pattern of incorporation observed in heterozygotes is intermediate between that of Wilson's disease patients and that of healthy subjects.[45]

TREATMENT

Demonstration of the efficacy of D-penicillamine in 1956 by Walshe dramatically changed the picture of untreated Wilson's disease progressing relentlessly to death.[358]

An initial dose of 1 to 2 g daily of D-penicillamine generally results in complete reversal or alleviation of hepatic, neurologic, and psychiatric abnormalities.[15, 22, 27, 29, 359] The key to a successful outcome is early diagnosis and treatment, as reflected by the observation that clinical disease can be prevented indefinitely in asymptomatic patients, provided that they adhere to continuous maintenance therapy.[360, 361]

Chelation therapy with D-penicillamine produces an initial urinary copper excretion of 2 to 5 mg daily, although after several years of treatment, this decreases to 0.5 to 1.0 mg.[15] Although the drug's principal mode of action is generally ascribed to "de-coppering," it also may detoxify hepatic copper in the setting of markedly elevated tissue levels;[362] this may result from the formation of copper complexes with D-penicillamine and the induction of metallothionein synthesis by the drug,[363] both of which reduce unbound, toxic copper. Some patients respond dramatically within weeks of starting D-penicillamine therapy, whereas others may show no clinical improvement for many months or even have temporary deterioration of their neurologic status. In the latter situation, particularly when patients are in critical condition, the dose of D-penicillamine may be increased to as much as 4 g daily for short periods. After several years of therapy, when symptoms have largely resolved and a stable condition has been achieved, the dose of D-penicillamine may be reduced to 1.0 g daily. Thereafter, life-long therapy should be continued for all patients without interruption. In fact, noncompliance or discontinuation of D-penicillamine results in a high incidence of irreversible hepatic failure, which is often fatal (2½ years on average after cessation of therapy).[362, 364, 365] Abnormalities of liver tests may persist for a year or so after the initiation of treatment, but as they subside a corresponding abatement of the ultrastructural and histologic abnormalities is observed.[299, 366] The response to therapy of hepatic fibrosis and portal hypertension is less impressive.

Successful pregnancy is rare in untreated symptomatic Wilson's disease. However, in well-treated patients, pregnancy is not contraindicated, and continuation of D-penicillamine therapy (~1.0 g daily) protects the mother from relapse and does not appear to pose any risk to the fetus.[29, 367, 368] Although progressively more and more adverse effects of D-penicillamine have been recognized,[22, 27, 29, 369] serious complications in patients with Wilson's disease have been reported only infrequently. Up to 20 per cent of patients develop a hypersensitivity reaction in the second week of treatment, which usually is characterized by fever, pruritus, erythematous rash, malaise, and less often, by lymphadenopathy, leukopenia, or thrombocytopenia. These reactions subside if the drug is withdrawn, and the patient then can be desensitized by reinstituting D-penicillamine in slowly increasing doses with steroid coverage if necessary. Other occasional side effects, which are encountered usually after at least a year of therapy, include dysgeusia, desquamation and friability of the skin (penicillamine dermatopathy), elastosis perforans serpiginosa, aphthous mouth ulceration, nephrotic syndrome, and rarely, a Goodpasture-like syndrome, arthralgias and disseminated lupus erythematosus, myasthenia gravis, polymyositis, neuromyotonia, cholestasis, agranulocytosis, thrombocytopenia, red cell aplasia, aplastic anemia, and depression of serum IgA levels. Thus, in addition to occasional determinations of 24-hour urinary copper excretion, routine urinalysis and blood counts should be performed at regular intervals.

In the small proportion of patients who develop serious toxic reactions to D-penicillamine, an alternative chelating agent, triethylene tetramine dihydrochloride (trientine) appears to be effective.[365, 370, 371] Trientine is available as an "orphan drug" (as designated by the Food and Drug Administration) in the U.S., is administered orally in doses of 1 to 2 g daily, and is apparently free from adverse effects. Healthy infants have been born to women treated with trientine throughout pregnancy,[372] and the drug is successful in preventing the rapid clinical deterioration that frequently follows the discontinuation of D-penicillamine in Wilson's disease.[365] Unlike D-penicillamine, trientine causes the serum copper concentration to rise during cupruresis, suggesting that the two agents may mobilize copper from different copper pools.[370] Other highly promising compounds, such as 2,3,2-tetramine[373] and N,N'-bis-(2-aminoethyl)-1,3-propanediamine (APD),[374] which induce a greater cupruresis in copper-loaded rats than the aforementioned agents, may prove a useful adjunct to therapy if well tolerated by humans.

Dietary copper intake can be reduced by about one half to at least 1.5 mg per day by avoiding large quantities of foods that contain a high content of copper (e.g., shellfish, organ meats such as liver, nuts, mushrooms, cocoa, and legumes).[9] The use of domestic water softeners should also be avoided, since these may substantially increase the copper content of water.[9] The ubiquitous presence of copper in most foodstuffs makes severe dietary copper restriction impractical.[375] Potassium sulfide was previously advocated to reduce absorption of dietary copper during the first year of treatment, but because of the resulting unpleasant taste and disagreeable odor of hydrogen sulfide, few patients were able to tolerate this agent.

The use of zinc has been advocated to decrease copper absorption in patients with Wilson's disease who have been previously decoppered.[376-380] It has been reported that 50 mg elemental zinc, as sulphate or acetate, given three times daily between meals maintains neutral or negative copper balance.[379] It is postulated that zinc induces the synthesis of intestinal metallothionein, which in turn sequesters copper, so that it is unavailable for transfer into the portal circulation and is sloughed with intestinal cells into the lumen.[377] Although zinc inhibits the gastrointestinal absorption of copper, neutral copper balance does not necessarily imply that a significant decrease in the copper content of liver or brain will ensue or that the decoppered state will be sustained. Based on available data, zinc therapy thus should be reserved for those rare patients who exhibit intolerance to both D-penicillamine and trientine.[381] If, however, it can be shown that supplemental zinc acts synergistically with chelating agents, it may eventually find a role as adjunctive therapy with D-penicillamine in patients with symptomatic or progressive disease.[381]

Major surgery is tolerated poorly by patients who have Wilson's disease and hence should be undertaken only when absolutely essential and after thorough evaluation. Surgical decompression of portal hypertension should be reserved for those in whom recurrent variceal bleeding is uncontrollable by standard conservative measures, including endoscopic sclerotherapy (Chap. 23). Surgical intervention in such patients is frequently followed by the appearance or aggravation of neurologic symptoms and signs and, in many cases, death.[382] In situations where surgery is necessary because D-penicillamine may interfere with the cross-linking of collagen and wound healing, the dosage of the drug should be reduced for a week or two postoperatively.

Finally, orthotopic liver transplantation has been performed on numerous occasions in patients with potentially lethal hepatic injury caused by Wilson's disease.[383-386] The following patients should be considered as candidates for transplantation:[29, 387] (1) those with clinical features of acute fulminant hepatitis, with associated hemolysis and hypercupremia, either as the initial presentation or following the discontinuation of D-penicillamine[365] and (2) those who have decompensated cirrhosis with a progressive clinical course despite adequate chelation therapy for at least several months, together with general supportive measures (e.g., diuretics). The selection of patients for transplantation may be facilitated by determination of a prognostic index, which is based on the severity of abnormality of serum AST, bilirubin, and prothrombin time on admission, and appears to accurately predict a fatal or nonfatal outcome.[388] Liver transplantation as a last therapeutic resort may not only be life-saving in patients with hepatic decompensation but also may reverse the severe neurologic manifestations of Wilson's disease.[386] In two children with cirrhotic Wilson's disease who underwent hepatic transplantation,[383–384] both survived more than six years, during which time clinical signs abated, biochemical findings in serum and urine normalized, and the copper content of the grafted livers remained normal, reflecting the fact that the underlying metabolic defect in Wilson's disease resides in the liver.

REFERENCES

1. Scheinberg IH, Sternlieb I. Copper metabolism. Pharmacol Rev 12:355, 1960.
2. Adelstein SJ, Vallee BL. Copper metabolism in man. N Engl J Med 265:892, 1961.
3. Adelstein SJ, Vallee BL. Copper. In: Comar CL, Bronner F, eds. Mineral Metabolism. New York, Academic Press, 1962:371.
4. Cartwright GE, Wintrobe MM. Copper metabolism in normal subjects. Am J Clin Nutr 14:224, 1964.
5. Sass-Kortsak A. Copper metabolism. Adv Clin Chem 8:1, 1965.
6. Peisach JP, Aisen P, Blumberg WE. The Biochemistry of Copper. New York, Academic Press, 1966.
7. Schroeder HA, Nason AP, Tipton IH, et al. Essential trace elements in man: copper. J Chronic Dis 19:1007, 1966.
8. Dowdy RP. Copper metabolism. Am J Clin Nutr 22:887, 1969.
9. Underwood EJ. Trace Elements in Human and Animal Nutrition. New York, Academic Press, 1971:57.
10. Evans GW. Copper homeostasis in the mammalian system. Physiol Rev 53:535, 1973.
11. Frieden E, Hsieh HS. Ceruloplasmin: the copper transport protein with essential oxidase activity. Adv Enzymol 44:187, 1976.
12. Bloomer LC, Lee GR. Normal hepatic copper metabolism. In: Powell LW, ed. Metals and Liver. New York, Marcel Dekker, 1978:179.
13. Sternlieb I. Copper and the liver. Gastroenterology 78:1615, 1980.
14. Winge DR. Normal physiology of copper metabolism. Semin Liver Dis 4:239, 1984.
15. Deiss A, Lynch RE, Lee GR, et al. Long-term therapy of Wilson's disease. Ann Intern Med 75:57, 1971.
16. Sternlieb I. Evolution of the hepatic lesion in Wilson's disease (hepatolenticular degeneration). In: Popper H, Schaffner F, eds. Progress in Liver Diseases. Vol. 4. New York, Grune & Stratton, 1972:511.
17. Strickland GT, Frommer D, Leu M-L, et al. Wilson's disease in the United Kingdom and Taiwan. Q J Med 42:619, 1973.
18. Sternlieb I, Scheinberg IH. Wilson's disease. In: Schaffner F, Sherlock S, Leevy C, eds. The Liver and Its Diseases. New York, Intercontinental Press, 1974:328.
19. Strickland GT, Leu M-L. Wilson's disease. Clinical and laboratory manifestations in 40 patients. Medicine 54:113, 1975.
20. Cartwright GE. Diagnosis of treatable Wilson's disease. N Engl J Med 298:1347, 1978.
21. Werlin SL, Grand RJ, Perman JA, et al. Diagnostic dilemmas of Wilson's disease: diagnosis and treatment. Pediatrics 62:47, 1978.
22. Williams DM, Lee GR. Hepatolenticular degeneration (Wilson's disease). In: Powell LW, ed. Metals and the Liver. New York, Marcel Dekker, 1978:241.
23. Dobyns WB, Goldstein NP, Gordon H. Clinical spectrum of Wilson's disease (hepatolenticular degeneration). Mayo Clin Proc 54:35, 1979.
24. Walshe JM. Wilson's disease: questions and answers. In: Davidson CS, ed. Problems in Liver Diseases. New York, Stratton Intercontinental, 1979:220.
25. Danks DM. Hereditary disorders of copper metabolism in Wilson's disease and Menkes' disease. In: Stanbury JB, Wyngaarden JB, Fredrickson DS, et al., eds. The Metabolic Basis of Inherited Disease. New York, McGraw-Hill, 1983:1251.
26. Walshe JM. Copper: its role in the pathogenesis of liver disease. Semin Liver Dis 4:252, 1984.
27. Sternlieb I, Scheinberg IH. Wilson's disease. In: Wright R, Alberti KGM, Karran S, et al., eds. Liver and Biliary Disease. London, Baillière Tindall, 1985:949.
28. Walshe JM. The liver in Wilson's disease (hepatolenticular degeneration. In: Schiff L, ed. Diseases of the Liver. Philadelphia, JB Lippincott, 1987:1037.
29. Scheinberg IH, Sternlieb I. Wilson's Disease. In: Smith LH, ed. Major Problems in Internal Medicine Series. Philadelphia, WB Saunders, 1984.
30. Chou T-P, Adolph WH. Copper metabolism in man. Biochem J 29:476, 1935.
31. Tipton IH, Cook MJ. Trace elements in human tissue. Part II. Adult subjects from the United States. Health Physiol 9:103, 1963.
32. Porter H. Copper proteins in brain and liver in normal subjects and in cases of Wilson's disease. In: Bergsma D, Scheinberg IH, Sternlieb I, eds. Wilson's Disease. Birth Defects Original Article Series, Vol. 4. New York, National Foundation–March of Dimes, 1968:23.
33. Ryden L, Deutsch HF. Preparation and properties of the major copper-binding component in human fetal liver. J Biol Chem 253:519, 1978.
34. Faa G, Liguori C, Columbano A, et al. Uneven copper distribution in the human newborn liver. Hepatology 7:838, 1987.
35. Reed GB, Butt EM, Landing BH. Copper in childhood liver disease. A histologic, histochemical, and chemical survey. Arch Pathol 93:249, 1972.
36. Hartley TF, Dawson JB, Hodgkinson A. Simultaneous measurement of Na, K, Ca, Mg, Cu, and Zn balances in man. Clin Chim Acta 52:321, 1974.
37. Klevay LM, Sandstead H, Munoz J, et al. The copper requirement of healthy men. Am J Clin Nutr 31:711, 1978.
38. Klevay LM, Reck SJ, Barcome DF. Evidence of dietary copper and zinc deficiencies. JAMA 241:1916, 1979.
39. Shils ME, Burk AW, Greene HL, et al. Guidelines for essential trace element preparations for parenteral use. JAMA 241:2051, 1979.
40. Sternlieb I. Gastrointestinal copper absorption in man. Gastroenterology 52:1038, 1967.
41. Weber PM, O'Reilly S, Pollycove M, et al. Gastrointestinal absorption of copper: studies with ^{64}Cu, ^{95}Zr, a whole body counter and the scintillation camera. J Nucl Med 10:591, 1969.
42. Strickland GT, Beckner WM, Leu M-L. Absorption of copper in homozygotes and heterozygotes for Wilson's disease and controls: isotope tracer studies with ^{67}Cu and ^{64}Cu. Clin Sci 43:617, 1972.
43. Matthews WB. The absorption and excretion of radiocopper in hepatolenticular degeneration (Wilson's disease). J Neurol Neurosurg Psychiatr 17:242, 1954.
44. Bearn AG, Kunkel HG. Metabolic studies in Wilson's disease using Cu^{64}. J Lab Clin Med 45:623, 1955.
45. Sternlieb I, Morell AG, Bauer CD, et al. Detection of the heterozygous carrier of the Wilson's disease gene. J Clin Invest 40:707, 1961.
46. Sternlieb I, Janowitz HD. Absorption of copper in malabsorption syndromes. J Clin Invest 43:1049, 1964.
47. Van Campen DR, Scaife PU. Zinc interference with copper absorption in rats. J Nutr 91:473, 1967.
48. Evans GW, Majors PF, Cornatzer WE. Mechanisms for cadmium and zinc antagonism of copper metabolism. Biochem Biophys Res Commun 40:1142, 1970.
49. Fischer PWF, Giroux A, L'Abbe MR. The effect of dietary zinc on intestinal copper absorption. Am J Clin Nutr 34:1670, 1981.
50. Van Campen D, Gross E. Influence of ascorbic acid on the absorption of copper by rats. J Nutr 95:617, 1968.
51. Cartwright GE, Hodges RE, Gubler CJ, et al. Studies on copper metabolism. XIII. Hepatolenticular degeneration. J Clin Invest 33:1487, 1954.
52. Moore T, Constable BJ, Day KC, et al. Copper deficiency in rats fed upon raw meat. Br J Nutr 18:135, 1964.
53. Mills CF. The dietary availability of copper in the form of naturally occurring organic complexes. Biochem J 63:190, 1956.
54. Canelas HM, De Jorge FG, Tognola WA. Metabolic balances of copper in patients with hepatolenticular degeneration submitted to vegetarian and mixed diets. J Neurol Neurosurg Psychiatr 30:371, 1967.
55. Davis PN, Norris LC, Kratzer FH. Interference of soybean proteins with utilization of trace minerals. J Nutr 77:217, 1962.
56. Gollan JL, Davis PS, Deller DJ. A radiometric assay of copper binding in biological fluids and its application to alimentary secretions in normal subjects and Wilson's disease. Clin Chim Acta 31:197, 1971.

57. Gollan JL. Studies on the nature of complexes formed by copper with human alimentary secretions and their influence on copper absorption in the rat. Clin Sci Mol Med 49:237, 1975.

58. Kirchgessner M, Grassman E. The dynamics of copper absorption. In: Mills CF, ed. Trace Element Metabolism in Animals. Edinburgh, Churchill Livingstone, 1970:277.

59. Neumann PZ, Silverberg M. Active copper transport in mammalian tissues. A possible role in Wilson's disease. Nature 210:414, 1966.

60. Harris DIM, Sass-Kortsak A. The influence of amino acids on copper uptake by rat liver slices. J Clin Invest 46:659, 1967.

61. Crampton RF, Matthews DM, Poisner R. Observations on the mechanism of absorption of copper by the small intestine. J Physiol 178:111, 1965.

62. Evans GW, Cornatzer WE. Copper and zinc metalloproteins in the rat. Fed Proc 29:695, 1970.

63. Fischer PWF, Giroux A, L'Abbe MR. Effects of zinc on mucosal copper binding and on the kinetics of copper absorption. J Nutr 113:462, 1983.

64. DiSilvestro RA, Cousins RJ. Physiological ligands for copper and zinc. Annu Rev Nutr 3:261, 1983.

65. Marceau N, Aspin N, Sass-Kortak A. Absorption of copper[64] from gastrointestinal tract of rat. Am J Physiol 218:377, 1970.

66. Neumann PZ, Silverberg M. Metabolic pathways of red blood cell copper in normal humans and in Wilson's disease. Nature 213:775, 1967.

67. Bearn AG, Kunkel HG. Localization of Cu[64] in serum fractions following oral administration: an alteration in Wilson's disease. Proc Soc Exp Biol Med 85:44, 1954.

68. Schmitt RC, Darwish HM, Cheney JC, et al. Copper transport kinetics by isolated rat hepatocytes. Am J Physiol 244:G183, 1983.

69. Ettinger MJ, Darwish HM, Schmitt RD. Mechanism of copper transport from plasma to hepatocytes. Fed Proc 45:2800, 1986.

70. Sternlieb I, Scheinberg IH. Radiocopper in diagnosing liver disease. Semin Nucl Med 2:176, 1972.

71. Bush JA, Mahoney JP, Markowitz H, et al. Studies on copper metabolism. XVI. Radioactive copper studies in normal subjects and in patients with hepatolenticular degeneration. J Clin Invest 34:1766, 1955.

72. Scheinberg IH, Morell AG. Exchange of ceruloplasmin copper with ionic Cu[64] with reference to Wilson's disease. J Clin Invest 36:1193, 1957.

73. Sternlieb I, Morell AG, Tucker WD, et al. The incorporation of copper into ceruloplasmin in vivo: studies with copper[64] and copper[67]. J Clin Invest 40:1834, 1961.

74. Neumann PZ, Sass-Kortsak A. The state of copper in human serum. Evidence for an amino-acid bound fraction. J Clin Invest 46:646, 1967.

75. Lau S-J, Sarkar B. Ternary coordination complex between human serum albumin, copper (II) and L-histidine. J Biol Chem 246:5938, 1971.

76. Lau SJ, Sarkar B. The interaction of copper (II) and glycyl-L-histidyl-L-lysine, a growth modulating tripeptide from plasma. Biochem J 199:649, 1981.

77. Darwish HM, Cheney JC, Schmitt RC, et al. Mobilization of copper (II) from plasma components and mechanism of hepatic copper transport. Am J Physiol 246:G72, 1984.

78. Bearn AG, Kunkel HG. Abnormalities of copper metabolism in Wilson's disease and their relationship to the amino-aciduria. J Clin Invest 33:400, 1954.

79. Morell AG, Shapiro JR, Scheinberg IH. Copper-binding protein from human liver. In: Walshe JM, Cummings JN, eds. Wilson's Disease: Some Current Concepts. Springfield, Ill.: Charles C Thomas, 1961:36.

80. Porter H, Sweeney M, Porter EM. Human hepatocuprein: isolation of a copper protein from the subcellular soluble fraction of adult human liver. Arch Biochem Biophys 105:319, 1964.

81. Buhler RHO, Kagi JHR. Human hepatic metallothionein. Fed Eur Biochem Soc Lett 39:229, 1974.

82. Kagi JHR, Vallee BL. Metallothionein: a cadmium- and zinc-containing protein from equine renal cortex. J Biol Chem 235:3460, 1960.

83. Pulido P, Kagi JHR, Vallee BL. Isolation and some properties of human metallothionein. Biochemistry 5:1768, 1966.

84. Brady FO. The physiological function of metallothionein. Trends Biochem Sci 7:143, 1982.

85. Weiner AL, Cousins RJ. Copper accumulation and metabolism in primary monolayer cultures of rat liver parenchymal cells. Biochim Biophys Acta 629:113, 1980.

86. Worwood M, Taylor DM. Subcellular distribution of copper in rat liver after biliary obstruction. Biochem Med 3:105, 1969.

87. Beckman G, Lundgren E, Tarnvik A. Superoxide dismutase isoenzymes in different human tissues, their genetic control and intracellular localization. Hum Hered 23:338, 1973.

88. Hartz JW, Funakoshi S, Deutsch HF. The levels of superoxide dismutase and catalase in human tissues as determined immunochemically. Clin Chim Acta 46:125, 1973.

89. Fridovich I. Superoxide dismutases: studies of structure and mechanism. In: Yasunobu KT, Mower HF, Hayaishi O, eds. Iron and Copper Proteins. Advances in Experimental Medicine and Biology. Vol. 74. New York, Plenum Press, 1976:530.

90. Carrico RJ, Deutsch HF. Isolation of human hepatocuprein and cerebrocuprein. Their identity with erythrocuprein. J Biol Chem 244:6087, 1969.

91. McCord JM, Fridovich I. Superoxide dismutase. An enzymic function for erythrocuprein (hemocuprein). J Biol Chem 244:6049, 1969.

92. Fridovich I. Superoxide dismutases. Adv Enzymol 41:35, 1974.

93. Geller BL, Winge DR. Metal binding sites of rat liver Cu-thionein. Arch Biochem Biophys 213:109, 1982.

94. Wharton DC. Cytochrome oxidase. In: Eichhorn GL, ed. Inorganic Biochemistry. Vol. 2. New York, Elsevier, 1973:955.

95. Brunori M, Wilson MT. Cytochrome oxidase. Trends Biochem Sci 7:295, 1982.

96. Malmstrom BG. Cytochrome c oxidase: some current biochemical and biophysical problems. Q Rev Biophys 6:389, 1974.

97. Williams DM, Loukopoulos D, Lee GR, et al. Role of copper in mitochondrial iron metabolism. Blood 48:77, 1976.

98. Nostrand JF, Glantz MD. Purification and properties of human liver monamine oxidase. Arch Biochem Biophys 158:1, 1973.

99. Schultz G, Feigelson P. Purification and properties of rat liver tryptophan oxygenase. Biol Chem 247:5327, 1972.

100. Shimizu T, Nomiyama S, Hirata F, et al. Indoleamine 2,3-dioxygenase. Purification and some properties. J Biol Chem 253:4700, 1978.

101. Ishimura Y, Makino R, Ueno R, et al. Copper is not essential for the catalytic activity of L-tryptophan 2,3-dioxygenase. J Biol Chem 255:3835, 1980.

102. Sternlieb I, Morell AG, Scheinberg JH. The uniqueness of ceruloplasmin in the study of plasma protein synthesis. Trans Assoc Am Physicians 75:228, 1962.

103. Neifakh SA, Monakhov NK, Shaponshnikov AM, et al. Localization of ceruloplasmin synthesis in human and monkey liver cells and its copper regulation. Experientia 25:337, 1969.

104. Scheinberg IH, Cook CD, Murphy JA. The concentration of copper and ceruloplasmin in maternal and infant plasma at delivery. J Clin Invest 33:963, 1954.

105. Goldstein IM, Kaplan HB, Edelson HS, et al. Ceruloplasmin: an acute-phase reactant that scavenges oxygen-derived free radical. Ann NY Acad Sci 389:368, 1982.

106. Evans GW, Cornatzer NF, Cornatzer WE. Mechanism for hormone-induced alterations in serum ceruloplasmin. Am J Physiol 218:613, 1970.

107. Ryden L. Single-chain structure of human ceruloplasmin. Eur J Biochem 26:380, 1972.

108. Takahashi N, Ortel TL, Putnam FW. Single-chain structure of human ceruloplasmin: the complete amino acid sequence of the whole molecule. Proc Natl Acad Sci USA 81:390, 1984.

109. Ryden L. Human ceruloplasmin as a polymorphic glycoprotein: analysis by chromatography on hydroxyapatite. Int J Protein Res 3:131, 1971.

110. Morell AG, Scheinberg IH. Preparation of an apoprotein from ceruloplasmin by reversible dissociation of copper. Science 127:588, 1958.

111. Hazelrig JB, Owen CA, Ackerman E. A mathematical model for copper metabolism and its relation to Wilson's disease. Am J Physiol 211:1075, 1966.

112. Vierling JM, Shrager R, Rumble WF, et al. Incorporation of radiocopper into ceruloplasmin in normal subjects and in patients with primary biliary cirrhosis and Wilson's disease. Gastroenterology 74:652, 1978.

113. Gibbs K, Walshe JM. Studies with radioactive copper (^{64}Cu and [67]Cu); the incorporation of radioactive copper into ceruloplasmin in Wilson's disease and in primary biliary cirrhosis. Clin Sci 41:189, 1971.

114. Scheinberg IH, Morell AG. Ceruloplasmin. In: Eichhorn GL, ed. Inorganic Biochemistry. New York, Elsevier, 1973:306.

115. Marceau N, Aspin N. The association of the copper derived from ceruloplasmin with cytocuprein. Biochim Biophys Acta 328:351, 1973.

116. Marceau N, Aspin N. Distribution of ceruloplasmin-bound [[67]Cu] in the rat. Am J Physiol 222:106, 1972.

117. Waldman TA, Morell AG, Wochner RD. Measurement of gastrointestinal protein loss using ceruloplasmin labeled with [67]copper. J Clin Invest 46:10, 1967.

118. Gregoriadis G, Morell AG, Sternlieb I. Catabolism of desialylated ceruloplasmin in the liver. J Biol Chem 245:5833, 1970.

119. Ashwell G, Morell AG. The role of surface carbohydrates in the hepatic recognition of circulating glycoproteins. Adv Enzymol 4:99, 1974.

120. Irie S, Tavassoli M. Liver endothelium desialates ceruloplasmin. Biochem Biophys Res Commun 140:94, 1986.

121. Frieden E, Hsieh HS. The biological role of ceruloplasmin and its

122. Laurie SH, Mohammed ES. Ceruloplasmin: the enigmatic copper protein. Coord Chem Rev 33:279, 1980.

123. Barass BC, Coult DB, Pinder RM, et al. Substrate specificity of caeruloplasmin indoles and indole isosteres. Biochem Pharmacol 22:2891, 1973.

124. Barass BC, Coult DB, Rich P, et al. Substrate specificity of caeruloplasmin. Phenylalkylamine substrates. Biochem Pharmacol 23:47, 1974.

125. Barass BC, Coult DB. Effects of some centrally acting drugs on caeruloplasmin. In: Bradley PB, Brimblecombe RW, eds. Progress in Brain Research. Vol. 36. New York, Elsevier, 1972:97.

126. Lovstad RA. Interaction of phenothiazine derivatives with human ceruloplasmin. Biochem Pharmacol 23:1045, 1974.

127. Dormandy TL. Free-radical oxidation and antioxidants. Lancet 1:647, 1978.

128. Cranfield LM, Gollan JL, White AG, et al. Serum antioxidant activity in normal and abnormal subjects. Ann Clin Biochem 16:299, 1979.

129. Goldstein JM, Kaplan HB, Edelson HS, et al. Ceruloplasmin. A scavenger of superoxide anion radicals. J Biol Chem 254:4040, 1979.

130. Frommer DJ. Defective biliary excretion of copper in Wilson's disease. Gut 15:125, 1974.

131. Van Berge Henegouwen GP, Tangedahl TN, Hofmann AF, et al. Biliary secretion of copper in healthy man. Quantitation by an intestinal perfusion technique. Gastroenterology 72:1228, 1977.

132. Gollan JL, Davis PS, Deller DJ. Copper content of human alimentary secretions. Clin Biochem 4:42, 1971.

133. Worwood M, Taylor DM. Subcellular distribution of copper in rat liver after biliary obstruction. Biochem Med 3:105, 1969.

134. Owen CA. Copper metabolism after biliary fistula, obstruction or sham operation in rats. Mayo Clin Proc 50:412, 1975.

135. Fleming CR, Dickson ER, Baggenstoss AH, et al. Copper and primary biliary cirrhosis. Gastroenterology 67:1182, 1974.

136. Epstein O, Jain S, Lee RG, et al. D-Penicillamine treatment improves survival in primary biliary cirrhosis. Lancet 1:1275, 1981.

137. Terao T, Owen CA. Copper metabolism in pregnant and postpartum rat and pups. Am J Physiol 232:E172, 1977.

138. Klassen CD. Effect of alteration in body temperature on the biliary excretion of copper. Proc Soc Exp Biol Med 144:8, 1973.

139. Marceau N, Aspin N. The intracellular distribution of the radio-copper derived from ceruloplasmin and from albumin. Biochim Biophys Acta 293:338, 1973.

140. Terao T, Owen CA. Nature of copper compounds in liver supernate and bile of rats: studies with ^{67}Cu. Am J Physiol 224:682, 1973.

141. Sternlieb I, van den Hamer CJA, Morell AG, et al. Lysosomal defect of hepatic copper excretion in Wilson's disease. Gastroenterology 64:99, 1973.

142. Kressner MS, Stockert RJ, Morell AG, et al. Origins of biliary copper. Hepatology 4:867, 1984.

143. Gollan JL, Deller DJ. Studies on the nature and excretion of biliary copper in man. Clin Sci 44:9, 1973.

144. Bhargara MM, Samuels A, Chowdhury JR, et al. A novel, abundant protein in rat bile binds azo dye metabolites, copper, bilirubin and its glucuronides. Hepatology 2:721, 1982. (Abstract.)

145. Mistilis SP, Farrer PA. The absorption of biliary and non-biliary radiocopper in the rat. Scand J Gastroenterol 3:586, 1968.

146. Evans GW, Cornatzer WE. Biliary copper excretion in the rat. Proc Soc Exp Biol Med 136:719, 1971.

147. Aisen P, Morell AG, Alpert S, et al. Biliary excretion of ceruloplasmin copper. Nature 203:873, 1964.

148. Frommer D. The binding of copper by bile and serum. Clin Sci 41:485, 1971.

149. Lewis KO. The nature of the copper complexes in bile and their relationship to the absorption and excretion of copper in normal subjects and in Wilson's disease. Gut 14:221, 1973.

150. McCullars GM, O'Reilly S, Breman M. Pigment binding of copper in human bile. Clin Chim Acta 74:33, 1977.

151. Frommer DJ. Biliary copper excretion in man and the rat. Digestion 15:390, 1977.

152. Owen CA. Absorption and excretion of [Cu^{64}] labeled copper by the rat. Am J Physiol 207:1203, 1964.

153. O'Dell BL. Biochemistry of copper. Med Clin North Am 60:687, 1973.

154. Cordano A, Baertl JM, Graham GC. Copper deficiency in infancy. Pediatrics 34:324, 1964.

155. Cordano A, Graham GC. Copper deficiency complicating severe chronic intestinal malabsorption. Pediatrics 38:596, 1966.

156. Dunlap WM, James JC, Hume DM. Anemia and neutropenia caused by copper deficiency. Ann Intern Med 80:470, 1974.

157. Porter KG, McMaster D, Elmer ME, et al. Anemia and low serum copper during zinc therapy. Lancet 2:774, 1977.

158. Karpel JT, Peden VH. Copper deficiency in long-term total parenteral nutrition. Pediatrics 80:32, 1972.

159. McCarthy DM, May RJ, Maher M, et al. Trace metal and essential fatty acid deficiency during total parenteral nutrition. Digest Dis 23:1009, 1978.

160. Danks DM. Copper deficiency in humans. Ciba Found Symp 79:209, 1980.

161. Williams DM. Copper deficiency in humans. Semin Hematol 20:118, 1983.

162. Menkes JH, Alter M, Steigleder GK, et al. A sex-linked recessive disorder with retardation of growth, peculiar hair, and focal cerebral and cerebellar degeneration. Pediatrics 29:764, 1962.

163. French JH. X-chromosome linked copper malabsorption (X-cLCM). In: Vinken PJ, Bruyn GW, Klawans HL, eds. Handbook of Clinical Neurology. New York, Elsevier–North Holland Publishing Co, 1977:279.

164. Danks DM, Stevens BJ, Campbell PE, et al. Menkes kinky-hair syndrome. An inherited defect in the intestinal absorption of copper with widespread effects. Birth Defects Original Article Series, 10:132, 1974.

165. Camakaris J, Mann JR, Danks D. Copper metabolism in mottled mouse mutants. Copper concentrations in tissues during development. Biochem J 180:597, 1979.

166. Chan W-Y, Garnica AD, Rennert OM. Metal binding studies of metallothioneins in Menkes kinky-hair disease. Clin Chim Acta 88:221, 1978.

167. Riordan JR, Jolicoeur-Paquet L. Metallothionein accumulation may account for intracellular copper retention in Menkes' disease. J Biol Chem 257:4639, 1982.

168. Goka TJ, Stevenson RE, Hefferan PM, et al. Menkes disease: a biochemical abnormality in cultured human fibroblasts. Proc Natl Acad Sci USA 73:604, 1976.

169. Schmidt CJ, Hamer DH, McBride OW. Chromosomal location of human metallothionein genes: implications for Menkes' disease. Science 224:1104, 1984.

170. Grover WD, Scrutton MC. Copper infusion therapy in trichopoliodystrophy. J Pediatr 86:216, 1975.

171. Mann JR, Camakaris J, Danks DM, et al. Copper metabolism in mottled mouse mutants. Copper therapy of brindled (Mo^{br}) mice. Biochem J 180:605, 1979.

172. Kuivaniemi H, Peltonen L, Palotie A, et al. Abnormal copper metabolism and deficient lysyl oxidase activity in a hereditable connective tissue disorder. J Clin Invest 69:730, 1982.

173. Peltonen L, Kuivaniemi H, Palotie A, et al. Alterations in copper and collagen metabolism in the Menkes' syndrome and a new subtype of the Ehlers-Danlos syndrome. Biochemistry 22:6156, 1983.

174. Sternlieb I. Copper and liver injury. In: Brunner H, Thaler H, eds. Hepatology: A festschrift for Hans Popper. New York, Raven Press, 1985:243.

175. Twedt DC, Sternlieb I, Gilbertson SR. Clinical morphologic, and chemical studies on copper toxicosis of Bedlington terriers. J Am Vet Med Assoc 175:269, 1979.

176. Sternlieb I, Goldfischer S. Heavy metals and lysosomes. In: Dingle JT, Dean RT, eds. Lysosomes in Biology and Pathology. Vol. 5. New York, Elsevier, 1976:185.

177. Walshe JM. Copper: its role in the pathogenesis of liver disease. Semin Liver Dis 4:252, 1984.

178. Ishmael J, Gopinath C, Howell JM. Experimental chronic copper toxicity in sheep. Histological and histochemical changes during the development of lesions in the liver. Res Vet Sci 12:358, 1971.

179. Hamlyn AN, Gollan JL, Douglas AP, et al. Fulminant Wilson's disease with haemolysis and renal failure: copper studies and assessment of dialysis regimens. Br Med J 2:660, 1977.

180. Chowdhury AKR, Ghosh S, Debabrata P. Acute copper sulphate poisoning. J Indian Med Assoc 36:330, 1961.

181. Chultani HK, Gupta PS, Gulati S, et al. Acute copper sulfate poisoning. Am J Med 39:849, 1965.

182. Holtzman NA, Elliott DA, Heller RH. Copper intoxication. Report of a case with observations on ceruloplasmin. N Engl J Med 275:347, 1966.

183. Hwang KM, Scott KM, Brierley GP. Ion transport by heart mitochondria. The effects of Cu^{2+} on membrane permeability. Arch Biochem Biophys 150:746, 1972.

184. Sternlieb I. Mitochondrial and fatty changes in hepatocytes of patients with Wilson's disease. Gastroenterology 55:354, 1968.

185. Wallin M, Larsson H, Edstrom A. Tubulin sulfhydryl groups and polymerization in vitro. Effects of di- and trivalent cations. Exp Cell Res 107:219, 1977.

186. Schaffner F, Sternlieb I, Barka T, et al. Hepatocellular changes in Wilson's disease. Histochemical and electron microscopic studies. Am J Pathol 41:315, 1962.

187. Scheinberg IH, Sternlieb I. The liver in Wilson's disease. Gastroenterology 37:550, 1959.

188. Popper H, Goldfischer S, Sternlieb I, et al. Cytoplasmic copper and its toxic effects. Studies in Indian childhood cirrhosis. Lancet 1:1205, 1979.

189. Wilson SAK. Progressive lenticular degeneration: a familial nervous disease associated with cirrhosis of the liver. Brain 34:295, 1912.
190. Hall HC. La Degenerescence Hepato-lenticulaire; Maladie de Wilson Pseudo-sclerose. Paris, Masson, 1921:190.
191. Bearn AG. Genetic and biochemical aspects of Wilson's disease. Am J Med 15:442, 1953.
192. Bearn AG. Genetic analysis of 30 families with Wilson's disease (hepatolenticular degeneration). Ann Hum Genet 24:33, 1960.
193. Arima M, Sano I. Genetic studies of Wilson's disease in Japan. Birth Defects Original Article Series 4:54, 1968.
194. Gollan JL, Hicks EP, Gordon JV. Hepatolenticular degeneration (Wilson's disease) in an Australian aboriginal. Med J Aust 2:1197, 1970.
195. Van der Merwe C, Padayatchi P. Wilson se sikte in'n swart pasient. S Afr Med J 54:616, 1978.
196. Bachmann H, Lossner J, Gruss B, et al. Die Epidemiologie der Wilson schen Erkrankung in der DDR und die derzeitige Problematik einer populationgenetischen Bearbeitung. Psychiatr Neurol Med Psychol [Beih] 31:393, 1979.
197. Saito T. An assessment of efficiency in potential screening for Wilson's disease. J Epidemiol Community Health 35:274, 1981.
198. Cox DW, Fraser FC, Sass-Kortsak A. A genetic study of Wilson's disease; evidence for heterogeneity. Am J Hum Genet 24:646, 1972.
199. Frydman M, Bonné-Tamir B, Farrer LA, et al. Assignment of the gene for Wilson's disease to chromosome 13: linkage to the esterase D locus. Proc Natl Acad Sci USA 82:1819, 1985.
200. Bowcock AM, Farrer LA, Cavalli-Sforza LL, et al. Mapping the Wilson disease locus to a cluster of linked polymorphic markers on chromosome 13. Am J Hum Genet 41:27, 1987.
201. Dubois RS, Giles G, Rodgerson DO, et al. Orthotopic liver transplantation for Wilson's disease. Lancet 1:505, 1971.
202. Beart RW Jr, Putman CW, Porter KA, et al. Liver transplantation for Wilson's disease. Lancet 2:176, 1975.
203. Gibbs K, Walshe JM. Studies with radioactive copper (^{64}Cu and ^{67}Cu); the incorporation of radioactive copper into caeruloplasmin in Wilson's disease and in primary biliary cirrhosis. Clin Sci 41:189, 1971.
204. Sternlieb I, Scheinberg IH. Radiocopper in diagnosing liver disease. Semin Nucl Med 2:176, 1972.
205. Sternlieb I, Scheinberg IH. The role of radiocopper in the diagnosis of Wilson's disease. Gastroenterology 77:138, 1979.
206. Bickel H, Neale FC, Hall G. A clinical and biochemical study of hepatolenticular degeneration (Wilson's disease). Q J Med 26:527, 1957.
207. Scheinberg IH, Sternlieb I. The long-term management of hepatolenticular degeneration. Am J Med 29:316, 1960.
208. O'Reilly S, Weber PM, Oswald M, et al. Abnormalities of the physiology of copper in Wilson's disease. III. The excretion of copper. Arch Neurol 25:28, 1971.
209. Strickland GT, Beckner WM, Leu M-L, et al. Turnover studies in homozygotes and heterozygotes for Wilson's disease and controls: isotope tracer studies with ^{67}Cu. Clin Sci 43:605, 1972.
210. Gibbs K, Walshe JM. Biliary excretion of copper in Wilson's disease. Lancet 2:538, 1980.
211. Cowen AE, Korman MG, Hofmann AF, et al. Biliary bile acid composition in Wilson's disease. Mayo Clin Proc 50:229, 1975.
212. Uzman LL, Iber FL, Chalmers TC, et al. The mechanism of copper deposition in the liver in hepatolenticular degeneration (Wilson's disease). Am J Med Sci 231:511, 1956.
213. Evans GW, Dubois RS, Hambridge KM. Wilson's disease: identification of an abnormal copper-binding protein. Science 181:1175, 1973.
214. Scheinberg IH. Wilson's disease and copper-binding proteins. Science 185:1184, 1974.
215. Epstein O, Sherlock S. Is Wilson's disease caused by a controller gene mutation resulting in perpetuation of the fetal mode of copper metabolism into childhood? Lancet 1:303, 1981.
216. Srai SKS, Burroughs AK, Wood B, et al. The ontogeny of liver copper metabolism in the guinea pig: clues to the etiology of Wilson's disease. Hepatology 6:427, 1986.
217. Hardy R, Stevens J, Stowe C. Chronic progressive hepatitis in Bedlington terrier associated with elevated copper concentrations. Minn Vet 15:13, 1975.
218. Twedt DC, Sternlieb I, Gilbertson SR. Clinical, morphologic, and chemical studies on copper toxicosis of Bedlington terriers. J Am Vet Med Assoc 175:269, 1979.
219. Ludwig J, Owen CA, Barham SS, et al. The liver in the inherited copper disease of Bedlington terriers. Lab Invest 43:82, 1980.
220. Su L-C, Ravanshad S, Owen CA, et al. A comparison of copper-loading disease in Bedlington terriers and Wilson's disease in humans. Am J Physiol 243:G226, 1982.
221. Owen CA, Ludwig J. Inherited copper toxicosis in Bedlington terriers—Wilson's disease (hepatolenticular degeneration). Am J Pathol 106:432, 1982.
222. Su L-C, Owen CA, Zollman PE, et al. A defect of biliary excretion of copper in copper-laden Bedlington terriers. Am J Physiol 243:G231, 1982.
223. Johnson GF, Morrell AG, Stockert RJ, et al. Hepatic lysosomal copper protein in dogs with an inherited copper toxicosis. Hepatology 1:243, 1981.
224. Gibbs K, Walshe JM. A study of caeruloplasmin concentrations found in 75 patients with Wilson's disease, their kinships and various control groups. Q J Med 48:447, 1979.
225. Fitzgerald MA, Gross JB, Goldstein NP, et al. Wilson's disease (hepatolenticular degeneration) of late adult onset. Mayo Clin Proc 50:438, 1975.
226. Madden JW, Ironside JW, Triger DR, et al. An unusual case of Wilson's disease. Q J Med 55:63, 1985.
227. Walshe JM. Wilson's disease (hepatolenticular degeneration). In: Vinken PJ, Klaven HL (eds). Handbook of Clinical Neurology. Vol. 27. New York, American Elsevier Publishing Co. 1976:379.
228. Sternlieb I. The development of cirrhosis in Wilson's disease. Clin Gastroenterol 4:367, 1975.
229. Sternlieb I, Scheinberg IH. Chronic hepatitis as a first manifestation of Wilson's disease. Ann Intern Med 76:59, 1972.
230. Johnson RC, De Ford JW, Gebhart RJ. Chronic active hepatitis and cirrhosis in Wilson's disease. South Med J 70:753, 1977.
231. Scott J, Gollan JL, Samourian S, et al. Wilson's disease, presenting as chronic active hepatitis. Gastroenterology 74:645, 1978.
232. Roche-Sicot J, Benhamou J-P. Acute intravascular hemolysis and acute liver failure associated as a first manifestation of Wilson's disease. Ann Intern Med 86:301, 1977.
233. Adler R, Mahnovski V, Heuser ET, et al. Fulminant hepatitis. A presentation of Wilson's disease. Am J Dis Child 131:870, 1977.
234. Doering EJ, Savage RA, Dittner TE. Hemolysis, coagulation defects, and fulminant hepatic failure as a presentation of Wilson's disease. Am J Dis Child 133:440, 1979.
235. McCullough AJ, Fleming CR, Thistle JL, et al. Diagnosis of Wilson's disease presenting as fulminant hepatitis. Gastroenterology 84:161, 1983.
236. Hartleb M, Zahorska-Markiewicz B, Ciesielski A. Wilson's disease presenting in sisters as fulminant hepatitis with hemolytic episodes. Am J Gastroenterol 82:549, 1987.
237. Rosenfield N, Grand RJ, Watkins JB, et al. Cholelithiasis and Wilson disease. Pediatrics 92:210, 1978.
238. Ross ME, Jacobson IM, Dienstag JL, et al. Late onset Wilson's disease with neurological involvement in the absence of Kayser-Fleischer rings. Ann Neurol 17:411, 1985.
239. Westmoreland BF, Goldstein NP, Klaas DW. Wilson's disease. Electroencephalographic and evoked potential studies. Mayo Clin Proc 49:401, 1974.
240. Nelson RF, Guzman DA, Grahovac Z, et al. Computerized cranial tomography in Wilson's disease. Neurology 29:866, 1979.
241. Ropper AH, Hatten P, Davis KR. Computed tomography in Wilson disease: report of two cases. Ann Neurol 5:102, 1979.
242. Roach ES, Ford CS, Spudis EV, et al. Wilson's disease: evoked potentials and computed tomography. J Neurol 232:20, 1985.
243. Williams F, John B, Walshe JM. Wilson's disease. An analysis of the cranial computerized tomographic appearances found in 60 patients and the changes in response to treatment with chelating agents. Brain 104:42, 1981.
244. Starosta-Rubinstein S, Young AB, Kluin K, et al. Clinical assessment of 31 patients with Wilson's disease. Correlations with structural changes on magnetic resonance imaging. Arch Neurol 44:365, 1987.
245. Goldstein NP, Ewert JC, Randall RV, et al. Psychiatric aspects of Wilson's disease (hepatolenticular degeneration): results of psychometric tests during long term therapy. Am J Psychiatr 124:1555, 1968.
246. Scheinberg IH, Sternlieb I, Richman J. Psychiatric manifestations in patients with Wilson's disease. Birth Defects Original Article Series 4:85, 1968.
247. Dening TR. Psychiatric aspects of Wilson's disease. Br J Psychiatry 147:677, 1985.
248. Johnson BL. Ultrastructure of the Kayser-Fleischer ring. Am J Ophthalmol 76:455, 1973.
249. Wiebers DO, Hollenhorst RW, Goldstein NP. The ophthalmologic manifestations of Wilson's disease. Mayo Clin Proc 52:409, 1977.
250. Belkin M, Zeimer R, Chazek T, et al. Corneal copper quantitation in Wilson's disease. Metab Ophthalmol 2:389, 1978.
251. Johnson RE, Campbell RJ. Wilson's disease. Electron microscopic, X-ray energy spectroscopic, and atomic absorption spectroscopic studies of corneal copper deposition and distribution. Lab Invest 46:564, 1982.
252. Jones EA, Rabin L, Buckley CH, et al. Progressive intrahepatic cholestasis of infancy and childhood. A clinicopathological study of a patient surviving to the age of 18 years. Gastroenterology 71:675, 1976.

253. Kaplinsky C, Sternlieb I, Javitt N, et al. Familial cholestatic cirrhosis associated with Kayser-Fleischer rings. Pediatrics 65:782, 1980.
254. Dunn LL, Annable WL, Kliegman RM. Pigmented corneal rings in neonates with liver disease. J Pediatr 110:771, 1987.
255. Frommer D, Morris J, Sherlock S, et al. Kayser-Fleischer-like rings in patients without Wilson's disease. Gastroenterology 72:1331, 1977.
256. Fleming CR, Dickson ER, Wahner HW, et al. Pigmented corneal rings in non-Wilsonian liver disease. Ann Intern Med 86:285, 1977.
257. Rimola A, Bruguera M, Rodés J. Kayser-Fleischer-like ring in a cryptogenic cirrhosis. Arch Intern Med 138:1857, 1978.
258. Cairns JE, Williams HP, Walshe JM. "Sunflower cataract" in Wilson's disease. Br Med J 3:95, 1969.
259. Walshe JM. The eye in Wilson's disease. Birth Def 12:187, 1976.
260. Rosenthal AR, Marmor MF, Levenberger PL. Chalcosis: a study of natural history. Ophthalmology 86:1956, 1979.
261. McIntyre N, Clink HM, Levi AG, et al. Hemolytic anemia in Wilson's disease. N Engl J Med 276:439, 1967.
262. Deiss A, Lee GR, Cartwright GE. Hemolytic anemia in Wilson's disease. Ann Intern Med 73:413, 1970.
263. Czlonkowska A. A study of hemolysis in Wilson's disease. J Neurol Sci 16:303, 1972.
264. Iser JH, Stevens BJ, Stening GF, et al. Hemolytic anemia of Wilson's disease. Gastroenterology 67:290, 1974.
265. Meyer RJ, Zalusky R. The mechanisms of hemolysis in Wilson's disease: study of a case and review of the literature. Mt Sinai J Med 44:530, 1977.
266. Forman SJ, Kumar KS, Redeker AG, et al. Hemolytic anemia in Wilson's disease: clinical findings and biochemical mechanisms. Am J Hematol 9:269, 1980.
267. Owen CA Jr, Goldstein NP, Bowie EJ. Platelet function and coagulation in patients with Wilson's disease. Arch Intern Med 136:148, 1976.
268. Hoagland HC, Goldstein NP. Hematologic (cytopenic) manifestations of Wilson's disease (hepatolenticular degeneration). Mayo Clin Proc 53:498, 1978.
269. Uzman LL, Denny-Brown D. Amino-aciduria in hepatolenticular degeneration (Wilson's disease). Am J Med Sci 215:599, 1948.
270. Bearn AG, Tu TF, Gutman AB. Renal function in Wilson's disease. J Clin Invest 36:1107, 1957.
271. Leu M-L, Strickland GT, Gutman RA. Renal function in Wilson's disease: response to penicillamine therapy. Am J Med Sci 260:381, 1970.
272. Asatoor AM, Milne MD, Walshe JM. Urinary excretion of peptides and of hydroxyproline in Wilson's disease. Clin Sci Molec Med 51:369, 1976.
273. Fulop M, Sternlieb I, Scheinberg IH. Defective urinary acidification in Wilson's disease. Ann Intern Med 68:770, 1968.
274. Wiebers DO, Wilson DM, McLeod RA, et al. Renal stones in Wilson's disease. Am J Med 67:249, 1979.
275. Wilson DM, Goldstein NP. Bicarbonate excretion in Wilson's disease (hepatolenticular degeneration). Mayo Clin Proc 49:394, 1974.
276. Adams DA, Goldman R, Maxwell MH, et al. Nephrotic syndrome associated with penicillamine therapy of Wilson's disease. Am J Med 36:330, 1964.
277. Sternlieb I, Bennett B, Scheinberg IH. D-Penicillamine induced Goodpasture's syndrome in Wilson's disease. Ann Intern Med 82:673, 1975.
278. Mindelzun R, Elkin M, Scheinberg IH, et al. Skeletal changes in Wilson's disease: a radiological study. Radiology 94:127, 1970.
279. Feller ER, Schumacher HR. Osteoarticular changes in Wilson's disease. Arthritis Rheum 15:259, 1972.
280. Golding DN, Walshe JM. Arthropathy of Wilson's disease. Study of clinical and radiological features in 32 patients. Ann Rheum Dis 36:99, 1977.
281. Canelas HM, Carvalho N, Scaff M, et al. Osteoarthropathy of hepatolenticular degeneration. Acta Neurol Scand 57:481, 1978.
282. Walshe JM. Wilson's disease. The presenting symptoms. Arch Dis Child 37:253, 1962.
283. Factor SM, Cho S, Sternlieb I, et al. The cardiomyopathy of Wilson's disease. Myocardial alterations in nine cases. Virchows Arch [A], 397:301, 1982.
284. Kuan P. Cardiac Wilson's disease. Chest 91:579, 1987.
285. Kaushansky A, Frydman M, Kaufman H, et al. Endocrine studies of the ovulatory disturbances in Wilson's disease (hepatolenticular degeneration). Fertil Steril 47:270, 1987.
286. Carpenter TO, Carnes DL, Anast CS. Hypoparathyroidism in Wilson's disease. N Engl J Med 309:873, 1983.
287. Johansen K, Gregersen G. Glucose intolerance in Wilson's disease. Normalization after treatment with penicillamine. Arch Intern Med 129:587, 1972.
288. Lankisch G, Kaboth U, Koop H. Involvement of the exocrine pancreas in Wilson's disease? Klin Wochenschr 56:969, 1978.
289. Czlonkowska A, Milewski B. Immunological observations on patients with Wilson's disease. J Neurol Sci 29:411, 1976.
290. Bearn AG, McKusick VA. Azure lunale. An unusual change in the fingernails in two patients with hepatolenticular degeneration (Wilson's disease). JAMA, 166:304, 1958.
291. Hodges RE, Simon JR. Relationship between fingerprint patterns and Wilson's disease. J Lab Clin Med 60:629, 1962.
292. David TJ, Ajdukiewicz AB. Palmar dermatoglyphs in Wilson's disease. Br Med J 3:825, 1972.
293. Sternlieb I, Scheinberg IH. Prevention of Wilson's disease in asymptomatic patients. N Engl J Med 278:352, 1968.
294. Cartwright GE, Lee GR. The pathogenesis and evolution of Wilson's disease. Epatologia 20:51, 1974.
295. Goldfischer S, Sternlieb I. Changes in the distribution of hepatic copper in relation to the progression of Wilson's disease (hepatolenticular degeneration). Am J Pathol 53:883, 1968.
296. Anderson PJ, Popper H. Changes in hepatic structure in Wilson's disease. Am J Pathol 36:483, 1960.
297. Sternlieb I. Mitochondrial and fatty changes in hepatocytes of patients with Wilson's disease. Gastroenterology 55:354, 1968.
298. Sternlieb I. Characterization of the ultrastructural changes of hepatocytes in Wilson's disease. Birth Defects Original Article Series 4:92, 1968.
299. Sternlieb I, Feldman G. Effects of anticopper therapy on hepatocellular mitochondria in patients with Wilson's disease. An ultrastructural and stereological study. Gastroenterology 71:457, 1976.
300. Hayashi H, Sternlieb I. Lipolysosomes in human hepatocytes. Ultrastructural and cytochemical studies of patients with Wilson's disease. Lab Invest 33:1, 1975.
301. Hayashi H, Winship DH, Sternlieb I. Lipolysosomes in human liver: distribution in livers with fatty infiltration. Gastroenterology 73:651, 1977.
302. Sternlieb I, Quintana N. The peroxisomes of human hepatocytes. Lab Invest 36:140, 1977.
303. Stomeyer FW, Ishak HG. Histology of the liver in Wilson's disease. A study of 34 cases. Am J Clin Pathol 73:12, 1980.
304. Rojkind M, Giambrone MA, Biempica L. Collagen types in normal and cirrhotic liver. Gastroenterology 76:710, 1979.
305. Lygren T. Hepatolenticular degeneration (Wilson's disease) and juvenile cirrhosis in the same family. Lancet 1:275, 1959.
306. Kamakura K, Kimura S, Igarashi S, et al. A case of Wilson's disease with hepatoma. J Jpn Soc Intern Med 64:232, 1975.
307. Terao H, Itakura H, Nakata K, et al. An autopsy case of hepatocellular carcinoma in Wilson's disease. Acta Hepatol Jpn 23:439, 1982.
308. Wilkinson ML, Portmann B, Williams R. Wilson's disease and hepatocellular carcinoma: possible protective role of copper. Gut 24:767, 1983.
309. Buffet C, Servent L, Pelletier G, et al. Hepatocellular carcinoma in Wilson's disease. Gastroenterol Clin Biol 8:681, 1984.
310. Guan R, Oon CJ, Wong PK, et al. Primary hepatocellular carcinoma associated with Wilson's disease in a young woman. Postgrad Med J 61:357, 1985.
311. Madden JW, Ironside JW, Triger DR, et al. An unusual case of Wilson's disease. Q J Med 55:63, 1985.
312. Salaspuro M, Sipponen P. Demonstration of an intracellular copper-binding protein by orcein staining in long-standing cholestatic liver diseases. Gut 17:787, 1976.
313. Evans J, Newman SP, Sherlock S. Observations on copper-associated protein in childhood liver disease. Gut 21:970, 1980.
314. Editorial. Wilson's disease and copper-associated protein. Lancet 1:644, 1981.
315. Hanaichi T, Kidokoro R, Hayashi H, et al. Electron probe X-ray analysis on human hepatocellular lysosomes with copper deposits: copper binding to a thiol-protein in lysosomes. Lab Invest 51:592, 1984.
316. Lerch K, Johnson GF, Grushoff PS, et al. Canine hepatic lysosomal copper protein: identification as metallothionein. Arch Biochem Biophys 243:108, 1985.
317. Nartley NO, Frei JV, Cherian MG. Hepatic copper and metallothionein distribution in Wilson's disease (hepatolenticular degeneration). Lab Invest 57:397, 1987.
318. Jain S, Scheuer PJ, Archer B, et al. Histological demonstration of copper and copper-associated protein in chronic liver disease. J Clin Pathol 31:784, 1978.
319. Goldfischer S, Popper H, Sternlieb I. The significance of variations in the distribution of copper in liver disease. Am J Pathol 99:715, 1980.
320. Guarascio P, Yentis F, Cevikbas U. Value of copper-associated protein in diagnostic assessment of liver biopsy. J Clin Pathol 36:18, 1983.
321. Janssens AR, Van Noord MJ, Van Hoek CJ, et al. The lysosomal copper concentration in the liver in primary biliary cirrhosis. Liver 4:396, 1984.
322. Vaux DJT, Watt F, Grime GW, et al. Hepatic copper distribution in primary biliary cirrhosis shown by the scanning proton microprobe. J Clin Pathol 38:653, 1985.
323. Sumithram E, Looi LM. Copper-binding protein in liver cells. Hum Pathol 16:677, 1985.

324. Lefkowitch JH, Muschel R, Price JB, et al. Copper and copper-binding protein in fibrolamellar liver cell carcinoma. Cancer 51:97, 1983.
325. Sternlieb I. Diagnosis of Wilson's disease. Gastroenterology 74:787, 1978.
326. Czaja MJ, Weiner FR, Schwarzenberg SJ, et al. Molecular studies of ceruloplasmin deficiency in Wilson's disease. J Clin Invest 80:1200, 1987.
327. Cartwright GE, Markowitz H, Shields GS, et al. Studies on copper metabolism. XXIX. A critical analysis of serum copper in normal subjects, patients with Wilson's disease and relatives of patients with Wilson's disease. Am J Med 28:555, 1962.
328. Spechler SJ, Koff RS. Wilson's disease: diagnostic difficulties in the patients with chronic hepatitis and hypoceruloplasminemia. Gastroenterology 78:803, 1980.
329. Edwards CQ, Williams DM, Cartwright GE. Hereditary hypoceruloplasminemia. Clin Genet 15:311, 1979.
330. Gollan JL, Stocks J, Dormandy TL, et al. Reduced oxidase activity in the ceruloplasmin of two families with Wilson's disease. J Clin Pathol 30:81, 1977.
331. Walshe JM, Briggs J. Ceruloplasmin in liver disease. A diagnostic pitfall. Lancet 2:263, 1962.
332. Perman JA, Werlin SL, Grand RJ, et al. Laboratory measures of copper metabolism in the differentiation of chronic active hepatitis and Wilson's disease in children. J Pediatr 94:564, 1979.
333. LaRusso NF, Summerskill WHJ, McCall JT. Abnormalities of chemical tests for copper metabolism in chronic active liver disease: differentiation from Wilson's disease. Gastroenterology 70:653, 1976.
334. Ritland S, Steinnes E, Skrede S. Hepatic copper content, urinary copper excretion, and serum ceruloplasmin in liver disease. Scand J Gastroenterol 12:81, 1977.
335. German JL, Bearn AG. Effect of estrogen on copper metabolism in Wilson's disease. J Clin Invest 40:445, 1961.
336. Frommer DJ. Direct measurement of serum non-caeruloplasmin copper in liver disease. Clin Chim Acta 68:303, 1976.
337. Frommer DJ. Urinary copper excretion and hepatic copper concentrations in liver disease. Digestion 21:169, 1981.
338. Lynch RE, Lee GR, Cartwright GE. Penicillamine-induced cupriuria in normal subjects and in patients with active liver disease. Proc Soc Expl Biol Med 142:128, 1973.
339. Smallwood RA, Williams HA, Rosenoer VM, et al. Liver-copper levels in liver disease: studies using neutron activation analysis. Lancet 2:1310, 1968.
340. Wiesner RH, Barham SS, Dickson ER. X-ray microanalysis: a new technique to measure hepatic copper and iron in Wilson's disease and hemochromatosis. Gastroenterology 77:A47, 1979.
341. Humbert J, Aprahamian M, Stock C, et al. Copper accumulation in primary biliary cirrhosis. An electron and X-ray microanalytical study. Histochemistry 74:85, 1982.
342. Hunt AH, Parr RM, Taylor DM, et al. Relation between cirrhosis and trace metal content of liver with special reference to primary biliary cirrhosis and copper. Br Med J 2:1498, 1963.
343. Worwood M, Taylor DM, Hunt AH. Copper and manganese concentrations in biliary cirrhosis of liver. Br Med J 3:344, 1968.
344. Jain S, Scheuer PJ, Samourian S, et al. A controlled trial of D-penicillamine therapy in primary biliary cirrhosis. Lancet 1:831, 1977.
345. Benson GD. Hepatic copper accumulation in primary biliary cirrhosis. Yale J Biol Med 52:83, 1979.
346. Vierling JM. Copper metabolism in primary biliary cirrhosis. Semin Liver Dis 1:293, 1981.
347. Sternlieb I, Harris RC, Scheinberg JH. Le Cuivre dans la cirrhose biliaire de l'enfant. Rev Int Hepatol Paris 16:1105, 1966.
348. Evans J, Newman S, Sherlock S. Liver copper levels in intrahepatic cholestasis of childhood. Gastroenterology 75:875, 1978.
349. Evans J, Zerpa H, Nuttall L, et al. Copper chelation therapy in intrahepatic cholestasis of childhood. Gut 24:42, 1983.
350. Tanner MS, Portmann B, Mowat AP, et al. Increased hepatic copper concentration in Indian childhood cirrhosis. Lancet 1:1203, 1979.
351. Dung HS, Somasundarum S. Copper levels in Indian childhood cirrhosis. Lancet 2:246, 1979.
352. Klass HJ, Kelly JK, Warnes TW. Indian childhood cirrhosis in the United Kingdom. Gut 21:344, 1980.
353. Lefkowitch JH, Honing CL, King ME, et al. Hepatic copper overload and features of Indian childhood cirrhosis. N Engl J Med 307:271, 1982.
354. Pimental JC, Menzes AP. Liver granulomas in vineyard sprayer's lung: a new etiology of hepatic granulomatosis. Am Rev Respir Dis 111:189, 1975.
355. Smevik B, Ritland S, Nilsen T, et al. Liver attenuation values at computed tomography related to liver copper content. Scand J Gastroenterol 17:461, 1982.
356. Dixon AK, Walshe JM. Computed tomography of the liver in Wilson's disease. J Comput Assist Tomogr 8:46, 1984.
357. Lawler GA, Pennock JM, Steiner RE, et al. Nuclear magnetic resonance (NMR) imaging in Wilson's disease. J Comput Assist Tomogr 7:1, 1983.
358. Walshe JM. Penicillamine, a new oral therapy for Wilson's disease. Am J Med 21:487, 1956.
359. Sternlieb I, Scheinberg IH. Penicillamine therapy in hepatolenticular degeneration. JAMA 189:748, 1964.
360. Sternlieb I. Present status of diagnosis and prophylaxis of asymptomatic patients with Wilson's disease. In: Leevy CM, ed. Diseases of the Liver and Biliary Tract. Basel, S Karger, 1976:137.
361. Arima M. Takeshita K, Yoshino K, et al. Prognosis of Wilson's disease in childhood. Eur J Pediatr 126:147, 1977.
362. Scheinberg IH, Sternlieb I, Schilsky M, et al. Penicillamine may detoxify copper in Wilson's disease. Lancet 2:95, 1987.
363. Heilmaier HE, Jiang JL, Griem H, et al. D-penicillamine induces rat hepatic metallothionein. Toxicology 42:23, 1986.
364. Walshe JM, Dixon AK. Dangers of non-compliance in Wilson's disease. Lancet 1:845, 1986.
365. Scheinberg IH, Jaffe ME, Sternlieb I. The use of trientine in preventing the effects of interrupting penicillamine therapy in Wilson's disease. N Engl J Med 317:209, 1987.
366. Grand RJ, Vawter GF. Juvenile Wilson's disease: histologic and functional studies during penicillamine therapy. J Pediatr 87:1161, 1975.
367. Scheinberg IH, Sternlieb I. Pregnancy in penicillamine-treated patients with Wilson's disease. N Engl J Med 293:1300, 1975.
368. Walshe JM. Pregnancy in Wilson's disease. Q J Med 46:73, 1977.
369. Steen VD, Blair S, Medsger TA. The toxicity of D-penicillamine in systemic sclerosis. Ann Intern Med 104:699, 1986.
370. Walshe JM. Copper chelation in patients with Wilson's disease. A comparison of penicillamine and triethylene tetramine. Q J Med 62:441, 1973.
371. Walshe JM. Treatment of Wilson's disease with trientine (triethylene tetramine) dihydrochloride. Lancet 1:643, 1982.
372. Walshe JM. The management of pregnancy in Wilson's disease treated with trientine. Q J Med 58:81, 1986.
373. Borthwick TR, Benson GD, Schugar HJ. Copper chelating agents. A comparison of cupruretic responses to various tetramines and D-penicillamine. J Lab Clin Med 95:575, 1980.
374. May PM, Jones DC, Williams DR. Wilson's disease: an end to the search for new therapy? Lancet 1:1127, 1982.
375. Hook L, Brandt IK. Copper content of some low-copper foods. J Am Diet Assoc 49:202, 1966.
376. Hoogenraad TU, Koevoet R, de Ruyter Korvr EG. Oral zinc sulphate as long-term treatment in Wilson's disease (hepatolenticular degeneration). Eur J Neurol 18:205, 1979.
377. Brewer GJ, Hill GM, Prasad AS, et al. Oral zinc therapy for Wilson's disease. Ann Intern Med 99:314, 1983.
378. Van Caillie-Bertrand M, Degenhart HJ, Visser HKA, et al. Oral zinc sulphate for Wilson's disease. Arch Dis Child 60:656, 1985.
379. Hill GM, Brewer GJ, Prasad AS, et al. Treatment of Wilson's disease with zinc. 1. Oral zinc therapy regimens. Hepatology 7:522, 1987.
380. Hoogenraad TU, Van Hattum J, Van den Hamer CJA. Management of Wilson's disease with zinc sulphate. Experience in a series of 27 patients. J Neurol Sci 77:137, 1987.
381. Lipsky MA, Gollan JL. Treatment of Wilson's disease: In D-penicillamine we trust—What about zinc? Hepatology 7:593, 1987.
382. Sternlieb I, Scheinberg IH, Walshe JM. Bleeding oesophageal varices in patients with Wilson's disease. Lancet 1:638, 1970.
383. Beart RW, Putnam CW, Porter KA, et al. Liver transplantation for Wilson's disease. Lancet 2:176, 1975.
384. Starzl TE, Putnam CW, Koep L. Liver transplantation for inborn errors of metabolism. In: Bianchi L, Gerok W, Sickinger K, eds. Liver and Bile. Baltimore, University Park Press, 1977:343.
385. Rakela J, Kurtz SB, McCarthy JT, et al. Fulminant Wilson's disease treated with postdilution hemofiltration and orthotopic liver transplantation. Gastroenterology 90:2004, 1986.
386. Polson RJ, Rolles K, Calne RY, et al. Reversal of severe neurological manifestations of Wilson's disease following orthotopic liver transplantation. Q J Med 64:685, 1987.
387. Sternlieb I. Wilson's disease: indications for liver transplants. Hepatology 4:15S, 1984.
388. Nazer H, Ede RJ, Mowat AP, et al. Wilson's disease: clinical presentation and use of prognostic index. Gut 27:1377, 1986.

48

Hemochromatosis: Iron Metabolism and the Iron Overload Syndromes

Anthony S. Tavill, M.D., F.R.C.P. • *Bruce R. Bacon, M.D.*

HISTORY

The association of diabetes, cirrhosis of the liver, fibrosis of the pancreas, and pigmentation of the skin was first described by Trousseau in 1865.[1] Six years later Troisier reported a case of "pigment cirrhosis in sugar diabetes."[2] In 1889, Von Recklinghausen termed the association of these clinical features *hemochromatosis*, and although he established that the increased pigment in tissues was iron, he suspected that it originated from the blood.[3] Thereafter, the favored synonyms for this syndrome were bronze diabetes or pigment cirrhosis (French literature) and hemochromatosis (German literature), although it was not recognized at that time that they represented different stages of development of the same disease. Little new information was forthcoming on the natural history of hemochromatosis until Sheldon published his classic monograph in 1935.[4] With his detailed review of 311 published cases, he established for the first time a unifying concept of the multiple organ involvement of a single disease and offered evidence for its familial occurrence. On the basis of his family studies, he concluded that hemochromatosis was a hereditary disease resulting from an inborn error of metabolism. The genetic basis of the disease was initially questioned by Macdonald,[5] and it took another four decades after Sheldon's study for workers to establish firm phenotypic evidence for the genetic transmission of hemochromatosis based on the association between the histocompatibility antigen (HLA) alleles and predisposition to the disease.[6] Likewise, the association between excessive iron deposition and tissue damage has been supported conclusively in the clinical setting by careful evaluation of family members of affected individuals.[7, 8]

The term *hemochromatosis* is currently used to denote the pathologic deposition of excessive iron in the parenchymal cells of many organs, which leads to cell damage and functional insufficiency. *Hemosiderosis* is used virtually synonymously by pathologists to indicate excessive stainable iron in tissues, without regard to the specific target cell primarily involved or to the underlying pathogenesis of the iron deposition. When the condition is genetically determined by inappropriately high absorption of iron in the intestinal mucosa, it is termed *genetic* or *hereditary* (primary, idiopathic) *hemochromatosis*. Other conditions, many of disordered or ineffective erythropoiesis, lead to excessive iron absorption and tissue deposition. They have been termed *secondary iron overload*, because the increased absorption of intestinal iron is promoted by the underlying condition or by increased availability of intestinal iron.

Both genetic hemochromatosis and secondary iron overload have to be distinguished from parenteral iron overload, which leads to iron deposition initially confined to the reticuloendothelial system. When transfusion requirements are met in disorders of erythropoiesis, a combination of reticuloendothelial and parenchymal iron overload may coexist, and the total iron burden may be very large. Likewise, in transfusional hemosiderosis, late parenchymal iron overload has been explained as a spillover from the reticuloendothelial system. The degree of structural and functional damage to the organ parallels the extent of parenchymal cell involvement, regardless of the underlying cause.

Since methods are now available for the detection of genetic hemochromatosis in presymptomatic relatives of patients with the disease, the diagnosis can be applied legitimately to individuals in whom the toxic consequences of iron overload have not yet developed. It is no longer justified to confine the diagnosis only to those individuals who manifest the classic triad of cirrhosis, diabetes, and skin pigmentation. Rather, all those relatives who can be shown to share both haplotypes with a proven proband should be regarded as homozygous for genetic hemochromatosis. This concept has promoted the early diagnosis and treatment of the disease and undoubtedly has already led to increased survival and reduced morbidity.

CAUSES OF IRON OVERLOAD IN HUMANS

Although Sheldon postulated the hereditary basis for so-called idiopathic or primary hemochromatosis in 1935, the use of the older nomenclature has persisted until recently because of the lack of firm genetic markers of the disease. With the advent of detailed pedigree analyses combined with determination of HLA to assign significance to indirect markers of iron overload, idiopathic or primary hemochromatosis can be renamed, with confidence, genetic hemochromatosis. This is in contradistinction to the many causes of secondary iron overload, in which an identifiable underlying disorder leads to excessive accumulation of parenchymal iron, with the potential for pathologic and clinical consequences that are ultimately similar to those in the genetic form of the disease. The most important of these causes are listed in Table 48–1. In secondary iron overload, a combination of enhanced iron absorption and dietary or transfusional iron overload, or both, may be responsible for the accumulation of body iron stores that are comparable to those seen in genetic hemochromatosis. Particularly in situations of ineffective erythropoiesis, iron may accumulate very rapidly because of these combined factors, and patients may present with the consequences of

Part of the work reported was supported by grants RO1 DK31505 and R23 DK35469 from the National Institutes of Health.

1273

TABLE 48–1. CAUSES OF IRON OVERLOAD IN HUMANS

	Predominant Cellular Distribution in Liver	
	Early	Late
GENETIC HEMOCHROMATOSIS (hereditary, primary)	H	H, RE
SECONDARY IRON OVERLOAD Anemia due to ineffective erythropoiesis Thalassemia major Sideroblastic anemias	H	H, RE
Chronic liver disease Alcoholic cirrhosis Post-portacaval shunt	H, RE	H, RE
Increased oral intake of iron African dietary iron overload Medicinal iron ingestion	H, RE	H, RE
Other inherited or congenital defects Porphyria cutanea tarda Congenital atransferrinemia Neonatal iron overload (idiopathic perinatal hemochromatosis)	H	H, RE
PARENTERAL IRON LOADING Transfusional iron overload Excessive parenteral iron Associated with hemodialysis	RE	RE, H

H = hepatocellular; RE = reticuloendothelial.

iron toxicity many years earlier than is commonly seen in genetic hemochromatosis.[9, 10] Similarly, in African or Bantu hemochromatosis, the level of iron intake may regularly exceed 100 mg/day, and some of the largest iron stores have been reported in this condition.[11–14] In contrast, the iron burden observed in liver disease with secondary iron overload (whether acquired or caused by another associated genetic disorder, e.g., porphyria cutanea tarda) is considerably smaller and probably plays a minor role in the pathogenesis of the liver damage associated with these conditions.[7, 15–17] These diseases will be discussed in more detail later.

NORMAL IRON METABOLISM

To understand the altered iron metabolism seen in patients with hemochromatosis, it is necessary to describe briefly normal iron metabolism.

IRON DISTRIBUTION

The average total body iron of a normal 70-kg man is about 4 g, about 60 to 65 per cent of which is present as hemoglobin within circulating red blood cells. Myoglobin in skeletal muscle accounts for approximately 10 per cent, and about 5 per cent of body iron is present in tissues throughout the body in a variety of other heme-containing proteins (e.g., catalase, cytochromes), in enzymes with iron-sulfur complexes (primarily in mitochondria), and in iron-dependent enzymes (e.g., prolyl and lysyl hydroxylase, ribonucleotide reductase, and so on). The remaining 20 to 25 per cent (approximately 800 mg in men and 300 mg in women) is in the storage proteins ferritin and hemosiderin and is roughly divided equally between parenchymal cells of the liver, reticuloendothelial cells in the bone marrow

and spleen, and skeletal muscle. Only about 7 mg of iron is in transit in extracellular fluids (3.5 mg in plasma) bound to the iron transport protein transferrin.[18–20]

IRON ABSORPTION

About 1 to 2 mg of iron are absorbed by the duodenal mucosa each day from a normal Western diet containing 10 to 20 mg of iron. This absorbed iron balances the daily obligatory losses of iron from the body that occur mainly from exfoliated gastrointestinal mucosal cells. Smaller amounts also are lost via bile, urine, and skin. Iron balance is regulated normally through control of iron absorption; iron stores and iron absorption are reciprocally related so that as stores decline absorption increases. Increased erythropoietic activity also results in increased iron absorption. The regulation of iron absorption occurs in the proximal intestinal mucosa; however, the mechanism or mechanisms of regulation are poorly understood.[21] The amount and bioavailability (heme versus nonheme iron) of dietary iron,[22] the rate of plasma iron turnover,[23] gut motility, luminal factors such as acidity, and the presence of ascorbic acid, various amino acids and dietary components such as tannins and phytates all influence,[21, 22, 24] but do not regulate, iron absorption. Absorption of heme iron is largely independent of these factors, which exert a more profound influence on the absorption of nonheme iron.

Iron absorption by the enterocyte, with subsequent passage to the portal circulation, depends on cell uptake, intracellular transfer, cellular retention, and release to the portal circulation. Heme iron, which is present in meat in the form of hemoglobin, myoglobin, and heme enzymes, can enter the intestinal epithelial cell intact. Heme oxygenase removes iron from the protoporphyrin ring,[25] and iron is released either for incorporation into cellular ferritin or for transfer to the intravascular compartment in which it is bound to circulating transferrin.

Cell uptake of nonheme iron has been the subject of several recent studies by Simpson and colleagues,[26–28] in which differences between Fe^{2+} and Fe^{3+} iron uptake have been demonstrated using isolated brush border membrane vesicles from mouse duodenum. Absorption in this in vitro system has been compared with absorption of iron in mice in vivo and should provide a useful system for studying several aspects of intestinal iron uptake. An intracellular or transferrin-like protein, presumably derived from plasma,[29] may play a role in the intracellular transport of iron; however, it is unlikely that plasma transferrin is a major carrier of iron from the lumen of the intestine across the enterocyte and into the portal circulation.[30, 31] Recent immunocytochemical studies have demonstrated the presence of transferrin receptors (which are increased in iron deficiency but are normal in hemochromatosis) in the enterocyte basolateral (blood) membrane but not in the brush border (mucosal) membrane.[29, 32] Transferrin receptors are also present in colonic cells, so their relevance in iron absorption, if any, is unknown. Alternative carrier-mediated (protein or lipid, or both) transport mechanisms are currently being proposed and are under intensive investigation.[33, 34] Despite the recognition that iron absorption is affected by body iron stores and by the rate of erythropoiesis, little is known about how these factors influence the intestinal mucosa to regulate iron absorption. One hypothesis is that the donation of iron by transferrin to sites of use (bone marrow) or storage (liver, reticuloendothelial system) in some way immediately facilitates procurement of more iron from the enterocyte.[23, 24, 35] Alternatively, it has been proposed that the content of iron in macrophages in the lamina propria of the gut, mimicking the level of iron stores in the body, plays a regulatory role.[21]

HEPATIC IRON METABOLISM

The liver plays a central role in the maintenance of whole body iron homeostasis because of its dual role as the principal storage organ for iron and as the major site of synthesis of the iron transport protein transferrin (Fig. 48–1). Under normal circumstances, about one third of storage iron (ferritin and hemosiderin) in the body is found in the liver. Approximately 98 per cent of hepatic iron is found in hepatocytes, which compose 80 per cent of the total liver mass; the remaining 1.5 to 2 per cent of total liver iron is found in reticuloendothelial cells, endothelial cells, bile ductular cells, lipocytes, and fibroblasts.[36]

The majority of hepatocellular iron uptake is via receptor-mediated endocytosis of the ferric-transferrin moiety (see Chap. 7). The presence of transferrin receptors has been confirmed in studies using isolated hepatocytes in suspension, hepatocytes in cell culture, and the perfused liver. From studies of hepatocytes in suspension, it has been estimated that there are 31,000 to 162,000 specific saturable transferrin binding sites/cell with a high affinity for diferric transferrin.[19, 37–40] The transferrin–iron receptor complex enters the cell by endocytosis via clathrin-coated pits and vesicles, following which a nonlysosomal endocytic vesicle is formed. Iron is released from transferrin when the pH within the vesicle is lowered to 5.5 or less. Undegraded apotransferrin is then quickly recycled to the exterior of the cell, a process termed *diacytosis*. With exposure to the neutral pH of the cell surface, the apotransferrin is released from the receptor, which is recycled to be used in the next round of ferric-transferrin uptake. It has been estimated that the complete cycle of uptake, iron dissociation, and apotransferrin release takes less than 16 min.[19, 37, 41] At higher than normal levels of transferrin saturation (> 30 per cent), there is a nonsaturable, nonspecific mechanism of iron uptake that at one time was thought to be mediated by fluid-phase endocytosis.[42] Subsequent studies, however, have shown that both saturable and nonsaturable uptake of transferrin and iron appear to be associated with specific endocytosis and recycling of transferrin.[37]

Hepatocytes also have specific receptor-mediated mechanisms for the uptake of heme-hemopexin,[43] hemoglobin-haptoglobin,[44] and circulating ferritin.[45] In the normal situation (no intravascular hemolysis or tissue necrosis), the relative proportions that these forms of iron provide to the hepatocyte are probably quite small, and it is expected that transferrin-dependent uptake of iron represents the majority of hepatocellular iron uptake. In conditions of iron overload, iron in the circulation may be bound to protein other than transferrin.[46–48] Recent studies have demonstrated rapid uptake by the liver of this form of iron.[49–51]

Uptake of iron by reticuloendothelial cells is largely by phagocytosis of senescent red blood cells. Following phagocytosis, the cells are lysed within secondary lysosomes, and the hemoglobin is degraded with release of heme for additional degradation by microsomal heme oxygenase.[52] Reticuloendothelial cells are capable of incorporating small amounts of iron bound to transferrin, but they do not play a role in the uptake of iron from heme-hemopexin or hemoglobin-haptoglobin complexes.[53]

Once iron has entered the hepatocyte, it can be found in several biochemical forms: ferritin, hemosiderin, heme, and iron in the so-called intracellular transit pool or the low molecular weight chelate pool.[19, 37, 41, 54–56] Based on studies with experimental animals and human liver biopsy samples it has been estimated that in normal liver, approximately 50 to 60 per cent of liver iron is in ferritin, 15 to 20 per cent is in heme, 10 to 15 per cent is in hemosiderin, and the remaining 5 to 20 per cent is in the intracellular transit pool.[19, 41, 57–59] The measurement of the relative amounts of iron in these forms has been technically difficult because of lack of precision in distinguishing the various fractions of nonheme, nonferritin iron. Furthermore, once tissue has been homogenized and the cells disrupted, the original compartmentalization is altered and there is uncertainty about extrapolating the in vitro results to the situation in vivo. Iron released from transferrin and iron released intracellularly from the degradation of heme or hemoglobin enters the labile intracellular transit pool from which iron is then available for use by a number of cellular processes, including uptake by mitochondria for incorporation into heme and for synthesis of the iron-sulfur proteins and the various iron-dependent enzymes. The composition of the intracellular transit pool of iron has been poorly characterized; however, it has been proposed that guanosine triphosphate (GTP), adenosine triphosphate (ATP), adenosine diphosphate (ADP), pyrophosphates, 2,3-diphosphoglycerate, ascorbic acid, glutathione, cysteine, glucose, fructose, citrate, lactose, and riboflavin all may serve as chelators or transporters of intracellular iron.[54, 55] Based on the accumulated evidence, it seems reasonable to assume that such a labile intracellular pool of iron exists and functions as an expanding and contracting reservoir at the interface between the plasma membrane and sites of intracellular use or storage. Our current understanding of the intracellular movement of iron, however, is hampered by the inability to measure directly such a labile compartment and by the inability to reconcile the known kinetic and thermodynamic properties of intracellular iron with a specific role for several of the low molecular weight compounds listed previously.[55, 60]

Iron that enters the cell in excess of that needed for utilization (see earlier discussion) accumulates in the major storage forms of iron, ferritin, and hemosiderin. Morphologically, both ferritin and hemosiderin can be identified by routine transmission electron microscopy. In normal liver, crystalline ferritin can be seen predominantly in hepatocytes, with some in reticuloendothelial cells, whereas amorphous hemosiderin is identified predominantly in reticuloendothelial cells, with occasional deposits seen in hepatocytes.[61, 62] Ferritin is present largely in a free state in the cytosol, with some membrane-bound ferritin in secondary lysosomes, and smaller amounts in both the rough and smooth endoplasmic reticulum. Hemosiderin, however, is virtually always localized in secondary lysosomes and is electron dense without the crystalline pattern of ferritin. Morphologic identification of the other forms of intracellular iron is not possible; however, centrifugation studies show that the majority of heme iron is located within mitochondria and endoplasmic reticulum as cytochromes involved in electron transport and within the cytochrome P450 complex, respectively.

The ferritin protein shell, apoferritin, is composed of 24 subunits with a total molecular weight of approximately 450,000 daltons. The subunits enclose a spheric cavity in which variable amounts of iron (up to 4500 atoms of ferric iron) can be stored as hydrated ferric oxide. There are two

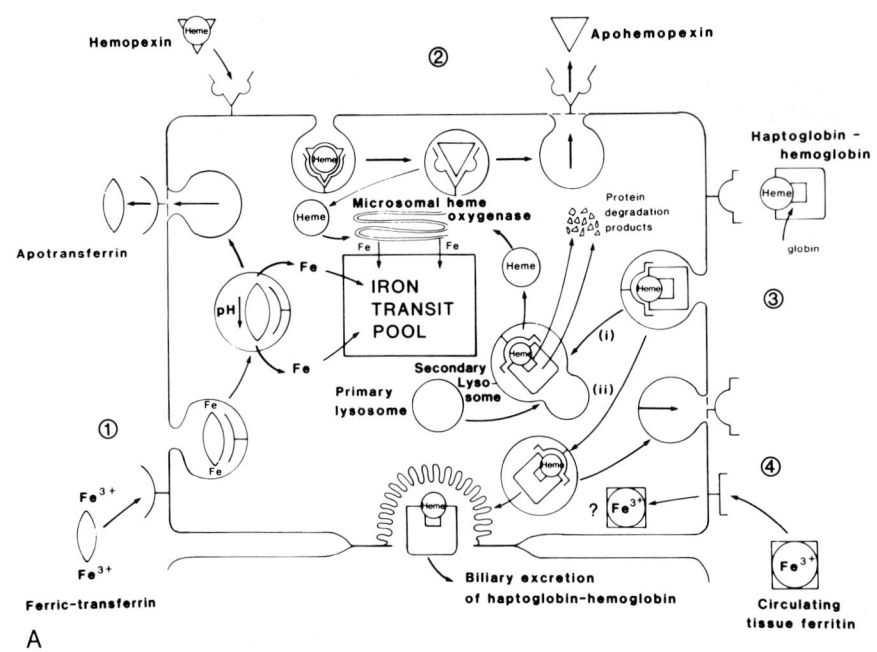

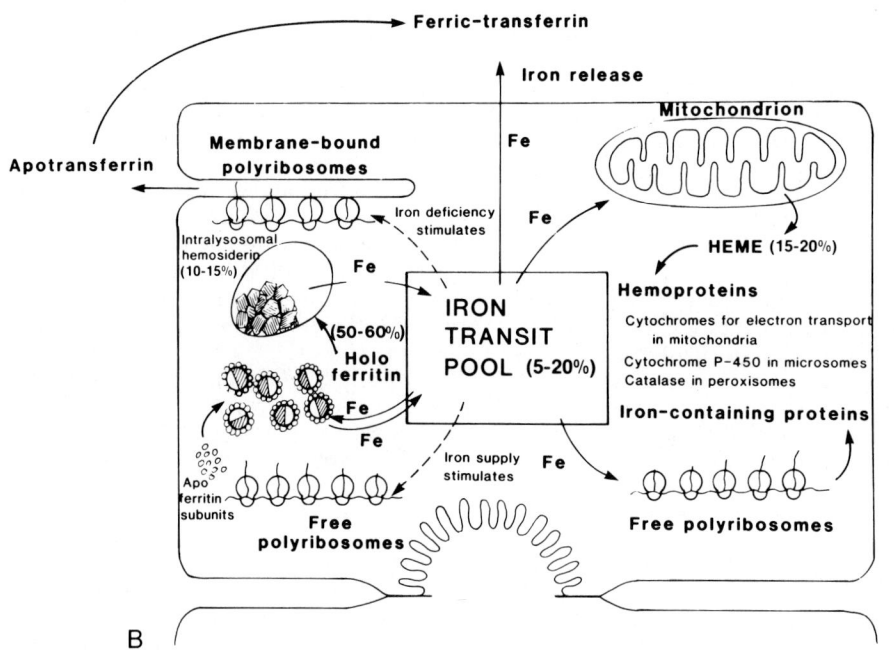

Figure 48–1. A, Schema of pathways of iron uptake by the hepatocyte. (*1*) Receptor-mediated binding and endocytosis of ferric-transferrin constitutes the major physiologic pathway for iron uptake. Critical reduction of pH within endosomes containing internalized ferric-transferrin releases iron to the iron transit pool and is followed by recycling of the receptor-transferrin complex and release of apotransferrin. (*2*) Uptake of heme-hemopexin also occurs by receptor-mediated endocytosis with release of heme to microsomal heme oxygenase and recycling of the receptor-apohemopexin complex. (*3,i*) Uptake of hemoglobin-haptoglobin is followed by fusion of the endocytotic vesicle with primary lysosomes to form secondary lysosomes. Heme is released to microsomal heme oxygenase, and globin and haptoglobin are degraded by lysosomal cathepsins. (*ii*) Alternatively, the hemoglobin-haptoglobin complex is excreted intact via a vesicular transport mechanism into the biliary canaliculus, with recycling of the receptor to the plasma membrane. (*4*) Uptake of circulating tissue ferritin, released by cell necrosis, can occur by receptor-mediated uptake. The subsequent fate of this ferritin iron is unknown. The iron transit pool is the postulated common recipient compartment for iron released from transferrin and degraded heme. **B, Schema of pathways of iron use, storage, and release by the hepatocyte.** The labile iron transit pool of low molecular weight chelates (5 to 20 per cent of the intracellular iron pool) is the presumed source of iron for incorporation into heme synthesized by mitochondria and a number of iron-containing or iron-requiring proteins synthesized on the rough endoplasmic reticulum. Heme iron constitutes 15 to 20 per cent of the total hepatocyte iron and is available as a prosthetic group for a variety of hemoproteins in mitochondria, microsomes, and peroxisomes. Iron available in excess of these requirements is incorporated into apoferritin for storage as holoferritin. Increased iron supply promotes formation of apoferritin and increased saturation of holoferritin, which at a critical level of iron overload leads to progressive formation of hemosiderin within secondary lysosomes. Under normal circumstances, ferritin and hemosiderin constitute about 50 to 60 per cent and 10 to 15 per cent of the total hepatic iron, respectively. In iron deficiency, depletion of ferritin iron and presumably also of transit iron stimulates the synthesis of apotransferrin.[339] Iron release is depicted to occur from the iron transit pool to transferrin. A variety of other chelators may accept iron released from the hepatocyte. (Modified from Bacon BR, Tavill AS. *Seminars in Liver Disease,* Volume 4, Number 3, New York, 1984, Thieme Medical Publishers, Inc. Reprinted with permission.)

types of ferritin subunits. The H subunits are heavier (molecular weight about 21,000 daltons) and more acidic and are found in greater proportion in heart and kidney. The L subunits are lighter (molecular weight approximately 19,000 daltons) and more basic and are found in greater proportion in liver and spleen.[19, 29, 63] Varying proportions of H and L subunits account for differences observed among isoferritins found in different organs, in neoplastic tissues, and at different degrees of iron loading. For example, in iron overload, the L subunit ferritins predominate in liver,[64, 65] whereas in certain types of cancer, H subunit ferritins are predominant.[66] With progressive iron uptake into hepatocytes, in excess of that needed for use, apoferritin synthesis is stimulated and ferric iron is incorporated into the crystalline core.

As levels of intracellular iron-loaded ferritin increase, ferritin is taken up by autophagic vacuoles, thus forming secondary lysosomes. Within the lysosomes, the protein component of ferritin is denatured and hydrolyzed by the lysosomal proteases, with the resultant formation of hemosiderin. Recent ultrastructural and biochemical studies support this scheme of hemosiderin formation.[41, 67–70] Hemosiderin remains relatively inert within secondary lysosomes. Despite the insolubility of hemosiderin, it is known from clinical studies of patients with iron overload that iron in hemosiderin can be mobilized.

Mechanisms of hepatocellular iron release are poorly understood. Under normal circumstances, hepatic iron efflux contributes less than 5 per cent to total plasma iron turnover.[71] However, when there is increased demand for iron (such as for erythropoiesis), the net mobilization of storage iron from both ferritin and hemosiderin is increased considerably. In experimental studies using the isolated perfused rat liver, the rate of iron efflux was inversely related to the time of prelabeling of the liver with radioactive iron so that the iron most recently taken up was the first to be released to circulating apotransferrin.[72] This observation supports the notion that the initial release of iron is from the intracellular transit pool; iron released subsequently is from the crystalline core of ferritin. Studies with perfused rat liver and with hepatocytes in suspension or culture have shown that iron efflux is directly proportional to apotransferrin concentration in either the perfusate or the incubation medium, with little or no release when circulating apotransferrin or other chelators are not present.[37, 72–74] Iron release from isolated hepatocytes was inversely related to oxygen tension,[74] which suggests that ferric iron must be reduced to ferrous iron as a requirement for release from storage sites such as ferritin. In addition, small amounts of iron are excreted in bile via lysosomal fusion at the canalicular membrane, with extrusion of lysosomal contents (iron and enzymes).[75] Manipulation of this mechanism with various drugs that affect lysosomal excretory pathways may be valuable in understanding the role of this form of iron excretion in both the normal situation and in states of iron overload.

PATHOGENETIC FACTORS IN IRON OVERLOAD

The expression of the metabolic defect in most forms of hemochromatosis is the inappropriate absorption of gastrointestinal iron, despite expanded stores. Plasma transferrin is saturated and the transferrin-bound iron is preferentially taken up by parenchymal cells, particularly those of the liver. There is progressive accumulation of storage iron, in the form of ferritin and hemosiderin, and associated cell injury.

GENETIC FACTORS

The mode of inheritance of genetic hemochromatosis has undergone considerable re-evaluation in recent years. It has been described variously as a dominant and a recessive disorder,[76] with earlier evidence offered by a number of workers pointing to each mode of inheritance. With the advent of HLA typing, it became apparent that patients with phenotypically characteristic hemochromatosis had a higher frequency of HLA-A3, and HLA-B14 antigens than did the control population.[77] This statistically significant association has been explained by the genetic linkage of the susceptibility locus for hemochromatosis to the major histocompatibility locus on chromosome 6.[6, 78–82] The demonstration of genetic linkage depends on evidence that the alleles for hemochromatosis susceptibility and HLA are preferentially transmitted together because their loci are physically close on the same chromosome.[83] Subsequent data point to a higher frequency of HLA-A3 in hemochromatosis than of the other associated antigens HLA-B7 and HLA-B14, suggesting that the hemochromatosis allele is located closer to the locus of HLA-A than to that of HLA-B.[80, 84, 85]

The term used to characterize the degree of linkage is the so-called *linkage disequilibrium*, which has been defined as the "non-random association of linked genes in the gametes of a population; the tendency for certain alleles of one locus to occur with certain alleles of another locus on the same chromosome with frequencies greater than that attributable to chance alone."[86] More precise genotypic evidence has been provided recently, which has helped to clarify current concepts on the location of the hemochromatosis allele. Simon and co-workers have compared 609 haplotypes carrying the hemochromatosis allele with 475 control haplotypes.[87] The strongest linkage disequilibria in hemochromatosis were for HLA-A3,B7 and HLA-A3,B14, both of which significantly exceeded those of controls. The observed frequency of the two haplotypes in hemochromatosis was 25 per cent for HLA-A3,B7 (compared with 6 per cent in controls) and 17.5 per cent for HLA-A3,B14 (compared with 1.6 per cent in controls). When these workers analyzed their data further to determine whether the HLA alleles A3, B7, and B14 each mark the hemochromatosis allele independently, it became apparent that only HLA-A3 was independently linked to the hemochromatosis locus. HLA-A3 occurred more frequently among all HLA-B7– or HLA-B14–negative haplotypes in hemochromatosis than in the control population. In contrast, without HLA-A3, HLA-B7 and HLA-B14 occurred no more frequently in hemochromatosis than in a control population. On the basis of these results, it is clear that the hemochromatosis allele is closer to locus A than to locus B. This information should prove to be valuable in the search for the genomic abnormality at a molecular level.[88]

The principal HLA markers of hemochromatosis, the haplotype HLA-A3,B7 is ubiquitous throughout the world, whereas HLA-A3,B14 has been found with increased frequency in Sweden, Great Britain, Ireland, Brittany, and Canada.[87] In this most recent study from Brittany, the overall frequency of HLA-A3 in the haplotypes carrying the hemochromatosis gene was 57.5 per cent, compared with a frequency among control haplotypes of 16 per cent. In a collective European series, HLA-A3 occurred in about

75 per cent of 384 patients with genetic hemochromatosis compared with 28 to 30 per cent of controls.[89, 90] Only about 30 per cent of all homozygous patients with hemochromatosis carry two HLA-A3 alleles; the remainder carry a single HLA-A3 allele, and homozygosity is defined in terms of the other shared haplotypes, namely, those of the B loci.[89] The gene frequencies estimated in two widely separated areas of the world, Utah in the United States and Brittany in France, are remarkably similar.[87, 91] The gene frequency in the respective populations is approximately 5 per cent. On the basis of the Hardy-Weinberg equation, this gives a heterozygote frequency of about 10.6 per cent and a homozygote frequency of about 0.3 per cent. The similarity of these gene frequencies in other areas of the world in which hemochromatosis is relatively more common, taken together with the observation that genetic hemochromatosis has been described only in white individuals, suggests that the gene arose by a unique mutation followed by chromosome recombinations, with subsequent spread of the gene by migration to certain areas of Europe, the United States, and Australia.[87]

Although it is accepted that the susceptibility allele for hemochromatosis cannot be detected reliably by any single phenotypic marker, it can be "fingerprinted" within a pedigree by determining the specific combination of antigenic alleles at the HLA-A and HLA-B loci, the HLA haplotype. In this way, haplotypes have been used to detect genotypes—those sharing both haplotypes with a proband being designated homozygotes—at maximum risk for the development of clinical disease. Likewise, a relative risk has been calculated for those individuals possessing particular alleles or haplotypes. For example, an individual with the HLA-A3 allele has a 5.3-fold enhanced risk of having hemochromatosis, whereas an individual with the haplotype HLA-A3, B14 has a 10.7-fold greater risk of having hemochromatosis than does a control population.[87] It should be emphasized that the absolute diagnostic value (see further on) of the HLA haplotype without pedigree information is small.

Since homozygotes show the highest levels of iron overload, as defined by hepatic iron concentrations,[7, 92] and heterozygotes show a variety of other phenotypic iron markers but do not have significant tissue iron overload,[92, 93] it is not entirely appropriate to speak in terms of dominant or recessive inheritance.[83] Autosomal recessive inheritance is not appropriate because heterozygotes have evidence of mild abnormalities in iron metabolism. However, if iron levels in tissue are used as a standard for the definition of the disease, it is clear that only homozygotes progress to fully developed tissue iron overload. An additional factor in the recessive versus dominant controversy is the relatively frequent opportunity for matings between homozygotes and heterozygotes. Since half the offspring of such matings will be homozygous for the hemochromatosis allele, the generation to generation appearance of the disease may give the false impression of autosomal dominant inheritance.

PATHOPHYSIOLOGY OF GENETIC HEMOCHROMATOSIS

A number of putative metabolic abnormalities have been suggested for the pathogenesis of iron overload in genetic hemochromatosis. The favored hypothesis is disordered regulation of intestinal iron absorption. Additional factors have been suggested, and the evidence for and against them will be summarized.

Intestinal Iron Absorption

In genetic hemochromatosis a relatively increased efficiency of absorption of iron by the intestinal mucosa results in a greater transfer of luminal iron to the circulation.[94-96] In vitro studies of duodenal biopsies from patients with genetic hemochromatosis have demonstrated that inappropriate transfer of iron occurs at normal luminal concentrations of iron.[97, 98] Patients with hemochromatosis show increased absorption of iron in spite of normal dietary intake and normal erythropoiesis.[99-103] There is inappropriately high absorption of iron in genetic hemochromatosis at all levels of body iron overload. Furthermore, relatives of symptomatic patients also demonstrate enhanced iron absorption, which is indicative of their heterozygous state.[104] The absorbed iron in patients with genetic hemochromatosis is bound to plasma transferrin, in which form it is delivered preferentially to parenchymal cells, particularly in the liver.[105] This is in marked contrast to the situation in normal individuals in whom a greater percentage of absorbed iron is directed to the erythropoietic tissues of the bone marrow.[106] The marked diversion of transferrin-bound iron to parenchymal cells in genetic hemochromatosis occurs even after phlebotomy therapy and in the face of iron deficiency.[107, 108] Mechanisms that have been suggested to explain the increased rate of transfer of dietary iron to the liver include putative intestinal luminal factors, failure of the reticuloendothelial system to process and retain iron adequately, abnormal transferrin function, and excessive avidity of parenchymal cells for iron. Earlier suggestions of a deficiency of a factor in gastric secretions (specifically a glycoprotein) in genetic hemochromatosis that inhibited iron absorption have not been borne out by later studies.[109-113]

Reticuloendothelial Function and Its Relationship to Iron Absorption. In genetic hemochromatosis the abnormal deposition of iron shows a predilection for parenchymal cells with a relative paucity of iron in the reticuloendothelial system and the mononuclear phagocytic cells of the bone marrow, leading to the suggestion that a failure to retain iron by reticuloendothelial cells could play a role in the pathogenesis of hemochromatosis.[114-117] Examination of the ability of human mononuclear phagocytic cells from patients with genetic hemochromatosis to store iron and to synthesize ferritin revealed no abnormality when compared with monocytes from normal subjects.[118-120] This seems to be the case whether uptake of iron is studied from a particulate source or from transferrin.[118, 120, 121] Although increased expression of transferrin receptor may occur in peripheral monocytes in hemochromatosis,[122] there is no reason to believe that there is an intrinsic abnormality in iron metabolism by the circulating monocytes in genetic hemochromatosis. However, it should be noted that iron-loaded macrophages can be observed randomly distributed in the lamina propria of the duodenal mucosa of patients with genetic hemochromatosis, in contrast to their normal predilection for the tips of the villi.[123] A relationship of this observation to the relative paucity of iron in the mucosal cells, and a role of the macrophage in abnormal iron absorption have yet to be elucidated.[124]

Transferrin Function and Its Relationship to Iron Absorption and Donation to Tissues. Although early experiments carried out in vitro and in vivo failed to reveal any abnormalitiy in transferrin function in genetic hemochromatosis,[125] later studies have continued to postulate a role for transferrin in normal and abnormal iron absorption. Although transferrin may have a function in the transfer of iron from the interior of the enterocyte to the plasma, this is by no means certain.[126, 127] Furthermore, brush border membranes do not bind transferrin and do not contain transferrin receptors.[29, 128] In all likelihood, the majority of transferrin found in mucosal extracts is derived from contamination of preparations with plasma. There is not enough transferrin present in the brush border of the enterocyte to mediate iron absorption or to play a significant role in the transport of iron from the lumen of the duodenum to the basolateral membrane of the mucosal cell.[31, 129–131] Finally, family studies have shown that the HLA-linked defect responsible for increased iron absorption in genetic hemochromatosis is not a consequence of an abnormality in the primary structure of transferrin.[125, 132] No linkage between the HLA loci and the transferrin loci could be demonstrated in this study, which is in keeping with the reported assignment of the transferrin locus to chromosome 3 (hemochromatosis locus on chromosome 6).[125]

Alternative views for the role of transferrin in the pathogenesis of hepatic iron overload have been based on the observation that if the glycan portion of transferrin is abnormal, there is excessive uptake of iron by the liver.[133] Although the sialic acid content of plasma transferrin is reduced in men who chronically consume more than 60 g of alcohol daily, the transferrin samples isolated from two patients with genetic hemochromatosis had normal electrophoretic patterns and contained normal amounts of sialic acid,[134] supporting the earlier data that all the major properties of transferrin are normal in genetic hemochromatosis.[125, 132, 135, 136]

Likewise, although earlier investigators suggested a reciprocity between cellular iron content and the expression of cell surface transferrin receptors,[137, 138] others have shown that an increase in plasma membrane receptors may be associated with enhanced iron uptake.[139, 139a] The regulatory signal for the suppression of transferrin receptor biosynthesis on K562 cells is the level of chelatable iron in the cells.[140] These findings have led to a search for abnormalities in transferrin receptor expression or function in hemochromatosis. No differences were found in the affinity for transferrin of receptors on fibroblasts or lymphocytes from individuals who were homozygous for hemochromatosis when compared with normal individuals.[141] However, a recent study using immunocytochemical localization of transferrin receptors in situ has shown that there is a greatly reduced number of transferrin receptors on the hepatocytes of untreated subjects with genetic hemochromatosis.[142, 142a] In light of the earlier work, this may be a function of down regulation, which occurred *after* the increase in iron stores. The suppression of transferrin receptor expression can therefore be regarded as a secondary consequence of excess iron storage.

Cellular Toxicity of Iron Overload

In genetic hemochromatosis, the liver is the major recipient of excess absorbed iron, and after several years of high tissue iron levels, fibrosis and, eventually, cirrhosis develop.[20, 143–146] Accordingly, despite the adverse effects of iron on many organs of the body, most of our understanding of the pathophysiologic effects of excess tissue iron is derived from clinical and experimental studies of the effects of iron on the liver. Clinical evidence for hepatotoxicity resulting from iron has been provided by studies of patients with genetic hemochromatosis,[7, 8, 147] African dietary iron overload,[148, 149] and secondary hemochromatosis due to β-

thalassemia,[150–153] in which correlation between hepatic iron concentration and the occurrence of liver damage has been demonstrated or in which therapeutic reduction of hepatic iron, either by phlebotomy or by chelation therapy, has resulted in clinical improvement. In both genetic hemochromatosis and African dietary iron overload, the hepatic iron concentration threshold for the development of hepatic fibrosis is about 4,000 to 5,000 μg Fe/g liver, wet weight (equivalent to about 22,000 μg/g dry weight).[7, 148, 154] In contrast, in patients with β-thalassemia who have not received chelation therapy, the threshold concentration for the development of fibrosis is nearly twice this level or about 9,000 to 10,000 μg Fe/g wet weight liver.[150, 151] This higher threshold in secondary iron overload may be related to the initial deposition of iron from transfused red blood cells in reticuloendothelial cells, the shorter duration of exposure of parenchymal cells to high concentrations of iron, a combination of these, or other unknown factors. Nonetheless, it appears from clinical studies that there is a relationship between both hepatic iron concentration and cellular distribution (parenchymal versus reticuloendothelial) and the development of iron-induced hepatotoxicity. Despite this convincing clinical evidence, the specific pathophysiologic mechanisms for hepatocyte injury and hepatic fibrosis in chronic iron overload are poorly understood.[155]

Several mechanisms whereby excess hepatic iron causes cellular injury with resultant fibrosis and cirrhosis have been proposed (Fig. 48–2). Iron-induced peroxidative injury to phospholipids of organelle membranes is a potentially unifying mechanism underlying the major theories of cellular injury in chronic iron overload. Early studies found increased susceptibility to lipid peroxidation in vitro in experimental iron overload. Wills,[156] using iron-loaded mice, found increased malondialdehyde production in hepatic microsomes that were incubated in vitro with ascorbate and an NADPH generating system. Heys and Dormandy found increased susceptibility to lipid peroxidation in vitro in iron-loaded spleens from patients with β-thalassemia.[157] Other investigators have measured ethane and pentane evolution in the breath as indicators of peroxidative breakdown of lipids in vivo following parenteral injections of iron salts or chelates;[158–160] however, in these experiments it was not possible to determine the specific sites (organ or organelle) of the increased lipid peroxidation. These studies and others have shown evidence of increased lipid peroxidation in iron overload.[161] However, until recently, evidence of any associated functional damage was lacking.

Peters and co-workers demonstrated that hemosiderin-laden secondary lysosomes isolated from liver biopsy spec-

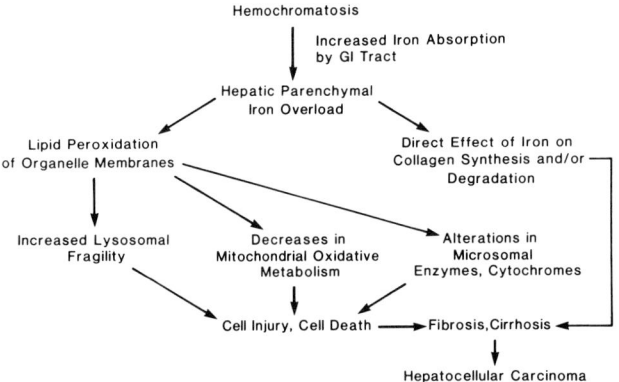

Figure 48–2. Proposed mechanisms for pathogenesis of cell injury and fibrosis and cirrhosis in hemochromatosis.

imens from patients with various types of iron overload have increased membrane fragility in vitro.[162] This increase in fragility correlated with the hemosiderin content in the liver, and it returned to normal in patients with hemochromatosis who were successfully treated with chronic phlebotomy therapy. Based on in vitro studies with normal lysosomes, increased membrane fragility can be caused by iron-induced peroxidative injury to lysosomal membranes.[163, 164] Furthermore, with the addition of ascorbate at a neutral pH, iron from ferritin or hemosiderin is available for initiation of the peroxidative reaction; however, at an intralysosomal pH of 5.5, iron is able to initiate peroxidation without the addition of exogenous reductants. The proposed mechanism whereby increased lysosomal fragility in iron overload could lead to cellular injury is that lysosomal rupture mediated by iron-induced lipid peroxidation causes leakage of hydrolytic lysosomal enzymes into the cytosol, resulting in damage to subcellular organelles and leading ultimately to injury and death of the cell.[165] It has not yet been demonstrated that the increased lysosomal fragility observed in vitro is directly related to increased lysosomal permeability in vivo. A recent study in iron-loaded thalassemia patients demonstrated a significant correlation between serum ferritin levels (representing tissue iron stores) and serum levels of N-acetyl-β-D-glucosaminidase,[166] (a lysosomal enzyme) supporting the hypothesis of increased lysosomal fragility causing liver injury in iron overload. Alternatively, cell damage (due to excess iron) could have resulted in cellular death by other mechanisms, without intracellular lysosomal rupture being a primary initiating event.

Iron-induced membrane lipid peroxidation of subcellular organelles other than lysosomes, such as mitochondria and microsomes, leading to functional insufficiency with subsequent cell injury and death is an alternative, though not mutually exclusive, theory. Recent experimental work using an animal model of dietary iron overload, in which hepatic iron deposition is quantitatively and qualitatively similar to that seen in human hemochromatosis, has found evidence of iron-induced lipid peroxidation (increased conjugated dienes) in vivo in hepatic mitochondria and microsomes.[167, 168] In subsequent studies, associated functional abnormalities in hepatic mitochondria showed a decrease in respiratory control caused by an irreversible inhibitory defect in electron transport.[169] Abnormalities in hepatic microsomal function included a reduction in the concentrations of cytochrome P450 and cytochrome b_5 and in aminopyrine demethylase activity.[170] Both lipid peroxidation and the associated organelle dysfunction were dependent on the degree of hepatic iron loading, and the iron concentration threshold was approximately 3000 μg/g wet weight.[167–170]

The biochemical form of intracellular iron responsible for initiating these hepatotoxic manifestations is unknown. In conditions of iron overload, the ability of the hepatocyte to maintain iron in the nontoxic, protein-bound ferric state may be exceeded, resulting either in small amounts of ferrous iron or in excessive amounts of low molecular weight chelated iron in the cytosol.[54] When cellular reductants (ascorbate, NADPH, O_2^-) are available, iron in the forms described or iron mobilized from ferritin may play a catalytic role in the initiation of peroxidative injury.[171–174] For example, ferrous iron (Fe^{2+}) can react with preformed lipid hydroperoxides (LOOH) to form alkoxyl radicals (LO•)

$$LOOH + Fe^{2+} \longrightarrow Fe^{3+} + OH^- + LO•$$

and ferric iron (Fe^{3+}) can similarly react with lipid hydroperoxides to form peroxyl radicals (LOO•)

$$LOOH + Fe^{3+} \longrightarrow Fe^{2+} + H^+ + LOO•$$

Both alkoxyl and peroxyl radicals can stimulate the chain reaction of lipid peroxidation by abstracting further hydrogen atoms.[161] Alternatively, it has been proposed that hydroxyl radicals (OH•) produced either by the Fenton reaction

$$Fe^{2+} + H_2O_2 \longrightarrow Fe^{3+} + OH• + OH^-$$

or by the iron-catalyzed Haber-Weiss reaction

$$Fe^{3+} \text{ complex} + O_2^- \longrightarrow Fe^{2+} \text{ complex} + O_2$$
$$Fe^{2+} \text{ complex} + H_2O_2 \longrightarrow Fe^{3+} \text{ complex} + OH• + OH^-$$

Net reaction:
$$O_2^- + H_2O_2 \xrightarrow[\text{catalyst}]{\text{Fe complex}} O_2 + OH• + OH^-$$

may be the radical species responsible for initiating the peroxidative reaction.[171, 172] Regardless of the initiating species, peroxidative decomposition of the polyunsaturated fatty acids of membrane phospholipids may result in specific abnormalities of organelle function.[175] Abnormalities in mitochondrial and microsomal function, along with the possible leakage of hydrolytic lysosomal enzymes from peroxidized lysosomal membranes, may provide sufficient organelle dysfunction to be deleterious to the maintenance of normal cell integrity. At the present time it is unknown whether any of these functional abnormalities in subcellular organelles (lysosomes, mitochondria, microsomes) are pathophysiologically significant in producing the chronic liver damage observed in the human conditions of iron overload. In the experimental model of dietary iron overload, however, lipid peroxidation and dysfunction occur earlier (2 to 5 months) and at lower levels of hepatic iron (3000 to 4000 μg/g wet weight) than the development of hepatic fibrosis (8 to 12 months and 8000 μg/g iron).[176] The experimental demonstration of fibrosis with long-term dietary iron loading suggests that the biochemical abnormalities described at lesser degrees of iron overload may be initiators of hepatic injury and fibrosis. Increased hepatic fibrosis in experimental iron overload was demonstrated in earlier studies in which massive amounts of parenteral iron chelates were administered over several years, but how these observations relate to genetic hemochromatosis is uncertain.[177–179]

Weintraub and co-workers propose that excess levels of iron in tissue are a direct stimulus to increased collagen biosynthesis, leading to the development of hepatic fibrosis in the absence of preceding iron-mediated cellular injury.[180] Ultrastructural evidence has been provided of increased collagen formation in thalassemia with iron overload without cellular injury.[181] Non–transferrin bound iron (plasma iron not in complex with transferrin) has been considered as potentially responsible for hepatic damage as well as for injury to other tissues.[46, 47, 182–184] None of these postulated mechanisms is mutually exclusive, and all may be operative concomitantly.

Role of Vitamin E. If lipid peroxidation is a likely mechanism of tissue injury in iron overload, it would be anticipated that α-tocopherol, an antioxidant, might be protective or perhaps be diminished (by increased "consumption") in patients with severe iron overload. Tissue and plasma levels of α-tocopherol (the major form of vitamin E) have not been determined in patients with genetic hemochromatosis. However, in thalassemia patients with secondary hemochromatosis, an inverse relationship between plasma levels of α-tocopherol and total body iron stores (determined by cumulative blood transfusions) has been demonstrated,[185] and tissue α-tocopherol levels were found to be decreased in spleens from iron-loaded thalassemia patients.[157] Additionally, Rachmilewitz and co-workers have found decreased plasma α-tocopherol levels associated with increased red blood cell lipid peroxidation in iron-loaded thalassemia patients.[186] In experimental studies, evidence of lipid peroxidation (increased exhaled ethane and pentane) has been found when iron was injected into vitamin E–deficient animals;[159] however, vitamin E supplementation has failed to reduce peroxidation in dietary iron overload.[187] At present, too little is known about the possible beneficial effects of vitamin E supplementation to use it therapeutically in patients with iron overload.

Role of Vitamin C. Abnormalities in ascorbic acid (vitamin C) metabolism have been described in patients with genetic hemochromatosis.[188] In African dietary iron overload, ascorbic acid deficiency occurs frequently, and frank scurvy may develop.[189] In the presence of heavy parenchymal iron deposition, there appears to be an acceleration in the catabolism of ascorbic acid in patients whose diets typically contain subnormal levels of vitamin C. Ascorbic acid deficiency is also seen occasionally in patients with transfusional iron overload.[190] Administration of ascorbic acid with deferoxamine enhances iron excretion.[191] Conversely, ascorbic acid deficiency diminishes the release of iron from reticuloendothelial cells.[192] There have been a few case reports of severe cardiac toxicity with death from cardiac failure when ascorbic acid has been administered to patients with transfusional iron overload.[193] It has been proposed that administration of ascorbic acid results in a redistribution of iron from reticuloendothelial cells to parenchymal cells and results in reduction of iron (Fe^{3+} to Fe^{2+}), leading to the formation of a potentially toxic form of iron in parenchymal cells.[194, 195] Thus in iron overload, marginal ascorbic acid deficiency may have beneficial protective effects, although efficacy of deferoxamine chelation therapy may be hindered.

PATHOLOGIC FINDINGS IN GENETIC HEMOCHROMATOSIS

The pathologic changes in the various affected organs reflect both the presence of excess storage iron and the secondary consequences of the prolonged presence of the excess iron. Since the primary metabolic abnormality in genetic hemochromatosis is thought to be present throughout life but does not produce clinical consequences until organ damage has occurred, there has been little opportunity for observation of pathologic manifestations in presymptomatic individuals. The concept of a threshold for organ damage encompasses both the level of accretion of iron in tissue and the duration of exposure to toxic levels of iron. Marked differences exist in the concentrations of iron in the various organs and in the relative abundance of iron in the different cell populations of each organ. Furthermore, there appear to be markedly different susceptibilities to tissue damage among the vulnerable organs that do not relate quantitatively to the concentration of iron in the organ. Finally, comparisons and contrasts need to be drawn with the pathologic changes in the various forms of secondary iron overload, in which both different cell distri-

bution and forms of excess iron stores may have a marked influence on the pathologic consequences of iron overload. When excessive alcohol intake accompanies iron overload, the pathologic features of iron storage disease may be significantly influenced, making the primary diagnosis sometimes difficult. For these reasons, we have chosen to review the pathologic changes in genetic hemochromatosis and then to compare and contrast them with the changes in various forms of secondary hemochromatosis and in alcoholic liver disease with iron overload.

HEPATIC PATHOLOGY

Liver iron levels are often 50 to 100 times the upper limit of normal by the time the patient with hemochromatosis first comes to the physician's attention (Fig. 48–3).[7] The most striking abnormality is the presence of hemosiderin granules (stained with Perls' Prussian blue) in the hepatocytes, often with a predominant pericanalicular distribution. The presence of excess ferritin iron is reflected by a diffuse bluish stain of the hepatocyte, which often is dwarfed by the dense staining of the granular hemosiderin. There is good correlation between the concentration of ferritin-hemosiderin clusters seen on electron microscopy and the degree of Perls' Prussian blue staining.[196] The progression of iron deposition from a completely normal state to uniform heavy deposition throughout all hepatocytes has been revealed by histopathologic studies of asymptomatic family members.[7, 196–199] Initial deposition is in the periphery of the lobule in the periportal region or zone 1 of Rappaport. Only with a progressive increase in the iron burden do the cells in the central areas of the lobule (zone 3) show equal degrees of iron staining. In contrast, the deposition of lipofuscin-like pigment seen in association with iron accumulation tends to be most abundant in centrilobular cells, again in a pericanalicular distribution within the cells.[196] In advanced hemochromatosis there is heavy iron deposition in bile ductular cells and Kupffer cells and in macrophages within fibrous tissue.[200] Associated pathologic changes of a nonspecific nature include steatosis and nuclear vacuolation, particularly in association with diabetes.

In symptomatic genetic hemochromatosis, fibrosis or cirrhosis is present almost invariably. Fibrous bands vary in width, beginning in a periportal distribution and surrounding partially preserved lobules or groups of lobules. In this regard, the distribution of fibrous tissue is similar to that seen in chronic partial biliary obstruction. The iron distribution in nodules is usually uniform within hepatocytes and spares the connective tissue. Only occasionally do nodules or areas of nodules seem to contain less iron than the surrounding parenchyma. This has suggested to some workers that nodules are formed predominantly by fibrous dissection of the parenchyma, rather than from regenerative foci of surviving cells.[200] This concept is at the root of a current controversy as to whether cirrhosis results from a primary stimulus to fibrosis or from a response to hepatocellular injury. Since evidence for ongoing hepatocellular necrosis is sparse, and the macrophages usually respond to the presence of dense aggregates of iron, the proponents of the fibrogenic theory seem to have this pathologic evidence in their favor. It should be noted that although an excellent correlation has been shown between the hepatic iron content and the presence of fibrosis and cirrhosis,[7] such a correlation has not been noted with the extent of stainable hepatic iron.[196] In particular, females with grade

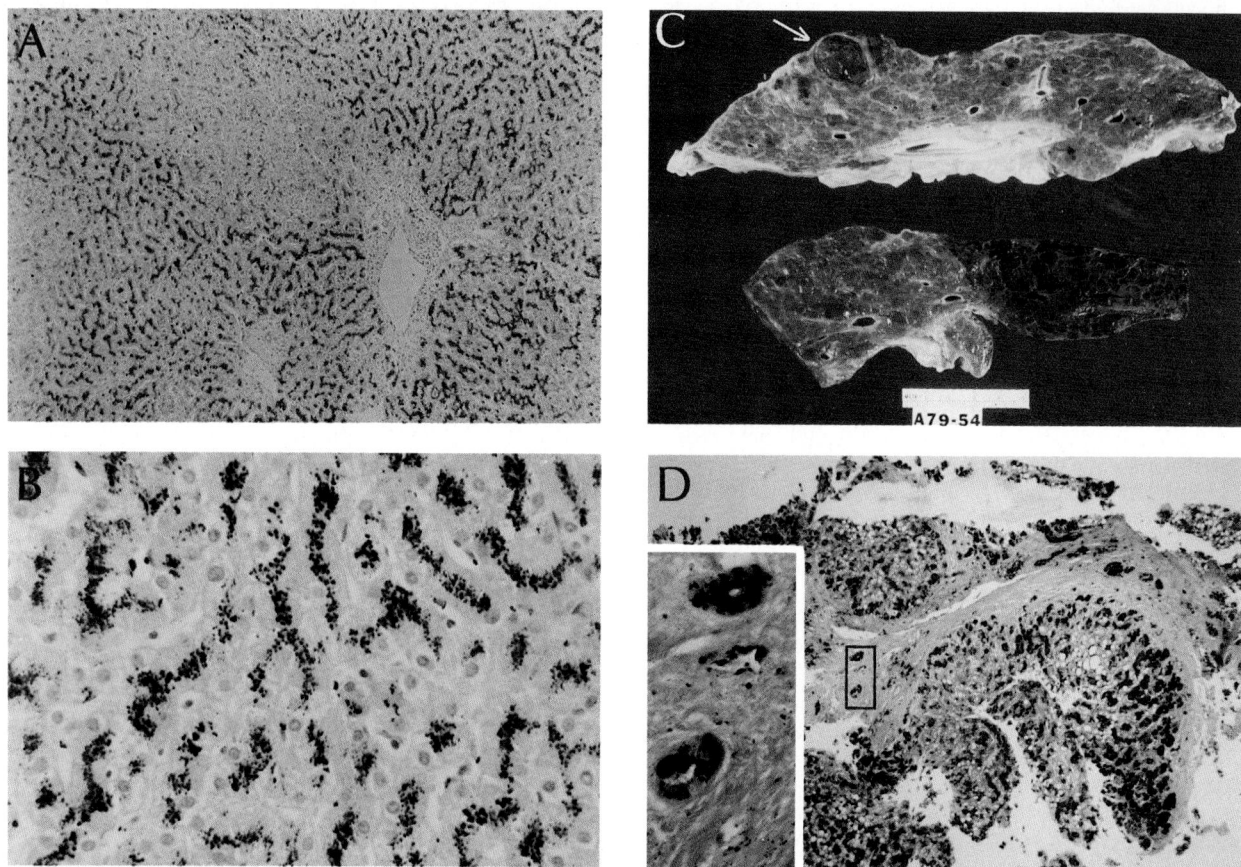

Figure 48–3. Hepatic pathologic features in genetic hemochromatosis. *A*, Precirrhotic, presymptomatic hemochromatosis in a 61-year-old woman who presented with hepatomegaly as the only physical finding. Perls' Prussian blue staining of liver tissue on light microscopy (magnification × 100) shows grade III deposition of iron, maximal in hepatocytes of zones 1 and 2 of Rappaport with relative sparing of zone 3 (pericentral). Hepatic iron concentration measured biochemically was 2470 μg/g wet tissue (upper 95 per cent confidence limit, 480 μg/g), equivalent to approximately 10,000 μg/g dry tissue. *B*, Higher magnification (× 500) of the same section shows predominant pericanalicular deposition of Perls' Prussian blue–positive granular hemosiderin. *C*, Gross autopsy specimen from a patient dying of cirrhotic hemochromatosis. The upper specimen shows cirrhosis and a small multicentric hepatocellular carcinoma (*arrow*). The lower specimen has been partially stained with potassium ferrocyanide (Perls' stain for ferric iron) and shows strong reactivity. *D*, Light microscopic appearance of the liver biopsy specimen from a patient with cirrhotic hemochromatosis (magnification × 150) showing an area of cirrhotic nodular regeneration, with intervening broad bands of fibrous tissue and no inflammatory infiltrate. The Perls' stain shows grade IV hemochromatosis with associated mild steatosis (the patient drank moderate amounts of alcohol). The magnified area (*inset*) demonstrates dense granular hemosiderin deposits in the bile duct epithelium.

IV iron staining may have relatively well-preserved hepatic histologic features without fibrosis or cirrhosis.[199]

At an ultrastructural level, there is evidence that both excessive quantities of crystalline ferritin and amorphous hemosiderin accumulate. In both experimental and clinical iron overload, increased cytosolic ferritin becomes membrane bound within so-called siderosomes. It is speculated that siderosome ferritin is a precursor of lysosomal ferritin that is then degraded to hemosiderin.[62, 68, 201–203] In the complex spectrum of advanced hemochromatosis or experimental iron overload, ferritin iron may be found free and membrane bound in siderosomes,[176, 179–181] whereas hemosiderin, which is by far the predominant form of storage iron in symptomatic patients,[204] is found largely within pericanalicular lysosomes.[162, 205]

CHANGES IN THE SPLEEN AND BONE MARROW

Even in the presence of massive hepatic iron overload, the amount of iron in the spleen and bone marrow is relatively low. In a semiquantitative analysis of the spleens of patients with symptomatic genetic hemochromatosis

there were only occasional fine granules of hemosiderin in some of the pulp macrophages,[206] with most of the iron confined to the capsule, trabeculae, and walls of blood vessels. Likewise, levels of iron in biopsy specimens of bone marrow from affected patients were not significantly elevated.[116]

CHANGES IN THE PANCREAS

Both the exocrine and endocrine secretory cells of the pancreas manifest excess iron storage. In symptomatic homozygotes, there is disorganization of acinar structure and fibrosis and a reduction in islet cells. Stainable iron is more prominent in acinar cells and fibrous tissue than in the islets of Langerhans, suggesting enhanced susceptibility of endocrine cells to the toxic effects of iron.[207]

CHANGES IN OTHER ENDOCRINE ORGANS

Hemosiderin deposits are present in cells of the thyroid acini, the zona glomerulosa of the adrenal cortex, the cells of the anterior pituitary (with the exception of the acidophil cells), and the parathyroid glands. In the testes, there is atrophy of the germinal epithelium in the presence of relatively low levels of iron.[207]

CHANGES IN THE SKIN

Most of the clinically visible pigmentation of the skin is due to melanin deposition in the basal layers of the epidermis. However, some of the grayish pigmentation is associated with hemosiderin deposition in the sweat glands, vascular endothelium, and connective tissue of the dermis, which may be particularly visible through the atrophic dermis and epidermis.[208]

CHANGES IN THE HEART

Most of the available information on cardiac pathology of iron overload has come from studies of patients with dyserythropoietic anemias, who had received a large number of blood transfusions over prolonged periods.[209] In individuals who have received more than 100 units of blood, hemosiderin deposits exist predominantly in ventricular myocardium, in the subepicardial regions, and in contractile cells more than in conducting tissues. Iron storage protein is visible in the perinuclear region of cardiomyocytes. These cells undergo degeneration and necrosis and replacement by fibrous tissue.

CHANGES IN THE JOINTS

There is heavy deposition of hemosiderin in the type B synovial lining cells (which undergo proliferation) and associated fibrosis. At an ultrastructural level, iron is confined to synthetic, fibrocytic cells and chondrocytes in contrast to the macrophages, which contain little iron. There are secondary degenerative changes in the chondrocytes and surrounding cartilage with associated calcification and subchondral cyst formation.[210-212]

COMPARISONS WITH SECONDARY HEMOCHROMATOSIS AND ALCOHOLIC LIVER DISEASE WITH IRON OVERLOAD

Although many of the causes of secondary hemochromatosis have in common with genetic hemochromatosis an increased delivery of transferrin-bound iron to parenchymal cells, there are valuable distinguishing features that reflect differences in pathogenesis, rates of accretion of storage iron, and the role of associated transfusional iron overload (see Table 48–1).

Since transfusional iron delivery is almost invariably associated with concomitant refractory anemia, the picture of iron overload is usually a mixed one, with increased iron in both parenchymal and reticuloendothelial cells. Most commonly, erythroid hyperplasia provides a major additional stimulus to dietary iron absorption and iron delivery to storage sites. This is not the case in hypoplastic anemias, in which iron overload is almost exclusively transfusional in origin. In the latter circumstances, iron-laden Kupffer cells predominate in the liver, and only later in the course of iron accumulation do parenchymal cells share in excessive storage.[213] Periportal fibrous tissue occurs very late,

and true cirrhosis is rare in this latter group of individuals. Another contrasting feature in transfusional hemosiderosis is the heavy deposition of iron in the macrophages of the spleen and bone marrow, emphasizing the important role of the reticuloendothelial system in processing the iron released from transfused red blood cells.

The situation in African (Bantu) hemochromatosis is more complex. Although evidence suggests that iron is particularly well absorbed from fermented maize cooked in iron pots, and the route of ingress of iron in this condition, like in genetic hemochromatosis, is via the alimentary tract, there are nevertheless marked differences in iron distribution. There is proportionately more iron in the spleen at all levels of hepatic iron overload than in genetic hemochromatosis.[13] The ratio of spleen to hepatic iron is approximately 2:1, and although concentrations of hepatic iron up to 6000 μg/g wet weight are seen by 40 to 50 years of age, the ratio between spleen and liver is maintained. Accumulation of iron in Kupffer cells and portal tract macrophages is prominent in comparison with parenchymal cells and bile ductular cells.[149] Nevertheless, the portal fibrosis and cirrhosis that develop are indistinguishable from the pattern in genetic hemochromatosis, except for the prominence of hemosiderin granules in the portal tracts and fibrous tissue. As in genetic hemochromatosis,[7] there is good correlation between the prevalence of fibrosis and cirrhosis and the concentration of hepatic iron in patients with African hemochromatosis.[13] At levels in excess of 5000 μg/g wet weight, more than 70 per cent of these individuals have established fibrosis or cirrhosis.[149]

The pathologic appearance of the liver may lead to confusion when alcoholism and iron overload coexist. The confusion arises as a result of the high prevalence of excessive alcohol intake in genetic hemochromatosis and the frequency of stainable iron in cirrhotic livers of alcoholics. Significant stainable iron was seen in 57 per cent of liver biopsy specimens from alcoholic patients.[214] Furthermore, the severity of the liver disease was not a factor in determining the overall prevalence of hemosiderosis, since it was present in 59 per cent of precirrhotic patients and in 55 per cent of cirrhotic patients. In this series of 157 patients, only 7 per cent showed grade III or grade IV iron deposition. In contrast, in the majority of alcoholic individuals with genetic hemochromatosis, the hepatic histopathologic appearance is indistinguishable from that of nonalcoholic genetic hemochromatosis.[200] However, in about 25 per cent of alcoholics with genetic hemochromatosis the histopathologic appearance was of micronodular alcoholic cirrhosis, in which the iron distribution in the nodules was very irregular. The authors concluded that both iron and alcohol were important for the pathogenesis of the liver lesions. It has been suggested by others that a predominantly centrilobular deposition of collagen and a relative paucity of iron in fibrous septa favor a primary alcoholic cause for cirrhosis.[215]

CLINICAL FEATURES OF GENETIC HEMOCHROMATOSIS

Sheldon's studies between 1927, when he published an original case report of a patient with hemochromatosis, and 1935, when his monograph was published,[4] enabled him to describe with lasting validity the constellation of clinical features in the fully established disease. He concluded that an iron burden of 25 to 50 g was required to establish symptomatic disease. In view of the age of onset at the time of diagnosis of the disease, he determined that the net rate of accretion was slow and probably averaged no more than 1.5 mg to 2.5 mg/day throughout life. Although the classic triad of hepatomegaly, diabetes mellitus, and skin pigmentation formed the common clinical denominator of disease in the majority of patients reviewed by Sheldon, data that were accumulated on patients and their families over the next 20 years (1935 to 1955) indicated that the triad had to be expanded to include a number of other clinical features, several of which could antedate the classic triad by many years. For an in-depth review of these features, the reader is referred to several important publications that document the phenotypic expression of the disease in large groups of patients observed firsthand over many years of detailed supervision.[8, 92, 144, 147, 199, 216–218]

It is important at the outset to recognize that since the advent of HLA typing for the identification of homozygous relatives of probands with symptomatic disease, the clinical picture of genetic hemochromatosis has taken on a much broader spectrum, ranging from totally asymptomatic individuals through the precirrhotic and prediabetic patients with early manifestations of the disease to those patients with fully established end-organ toxicity. Certain of the cited recent studies have included in their data features of such early disease and have provided much needed insights into the evolution of clinical manifestations as iron accumulates.[8, 92, 199, 218]

SEX, AGE OF ONSET, AND AGE OF PRESENTATION

The mean age at presentation with the first symptoms attributable to hemochromatosis is typically about 50 years.[144, 147, 199] However, the mean age at diagnosis is usually delayed four to five years because of failure to attribute the earliest symptoms and signs to hemochromatosis.[144] In a recent large study of 163 patients, the mean age and distribution by age were similar whether the patients were cirrhotic or noncirrhotic or diabetic or nondiabetic at the time of diagnosis.[8] In this study, the age at diagnosis was 46.2 ± 10.6 (mean ± SD) years with a range of 18 to 77 years. Of the 163 patients, 145 were men and 18 were women, a ratio of about 8:1, which is similar to results in other studies.[218] However, when investigations have been extended to include HLA typing, other homozygous family members have been discovered on the basis of haplotype alone. It is clear from this type of study that the frequency of the disorder in women is seriously underestimated when based solely on phenotypic expression.[93, 199] A ratio closer to 2:1 was reported by both the groups in Salt Lake City and in London, Ontario. Contrary to popular belief, when symptoms and signs were looked for in HLA-detected homozygotes, there was no significant difference in the ages of the affected men and women (57.3 years in men, 53.0 years in women).[199]

OVERVIEW OF CLINICAL FEATURES IN GENETIC HEMOCHROMATOSIS

It is of interest to compare the clinical features in three studies published in recent years (Table 48–2). One study selected 34 patients who presented to a single center over a 22-year period. Diagnosis was based on clinical and biochemical features.[144] The second study identified 35 homozygotes through pedigree studies, using a baseline of

14 symptomatic probands.[199] The third and most recent study endeavored to diagnose patients early through indirect and direct screening tests for iron overload.[8] The authors in the latter study identified and evaluated 163 patients, 51 of whom were shown to be in the precirrhotic phase of the disease and 74 of whom were nondiabetic.[8] This has allowed for comparison of the prevalence of the other features of genetic hemochromatosis, independent of the effects of liver disease. For example, several symptoms and signs were significantly more prevalent in patients with cirrhosis than in those who were noncirrhotic: weakness and lethargy, 88 and 73 per cent; abdominal pain, 67 and 39 per cent; loss of libido or potency in men, 43 and 25 per cent; hepatomegaly, 90 and 60 per cent; splenomegaly, 17 and 4 per cent; edema, 14 and 6 per cent; ascites, 9 and 0 per cent; and jaundice, 13 and 2 per cent. Other features such as arthralgias, skin pigmentation, and gynecomastia occurred with similar frequency in both cirrhotic and noncirrhotic patients. Overt diabetes mellitus (both non–insulin-dependent and insulin-dependent) was significantly more frequent in cirrhotic patients than in noncirrhotic patients (71 per cent versus 20 per cent). In the other two studies,[144, 199] there was a similar prevalence of the principal symptoms and signs in the probands as that observed in patients with established cirrhosis in the series reported by Niederau and co-workers.[8] This suggests strongly that probands in other reported series had advanced disease with already established irreversible cirrhosis. However, it is noteworthy that arthralgia figured prominently in the study that selected otherwise asymptomatic patients on HLA typing evidence alone,[199] and it usually antedated the diagnosis of hemochromatosis.

LIVER DISEASE

Hepatomegaly antedates the development of cirrhosis and may be related to the extent of iron overload. Its presence in 69 per cent of noncirrhotic patients with genetic hemochromatosis,[8] although significantly less than in patients with established cirrhosis (90 per cent), provides evidence that iron deposition per se plays a major factor in pathogenesis. Features of hepatocellular dysfunction and portal hypertension are observed most frequently when cirrhosis is established. Similarly, in the laboratory evaluation of hepatic dysfunction, those tests that most closely reflect hepatocyte function, such as serum albumin concentrations and prothrombin time, do not show abnormal results until cirrhosis is established.[8, 199] However, it is not uncommon to observe mild elevation (two- to fourfold) in the serum aminotransferase levels in the absence of cirrhosis.[199] These markers of hepatocellular necrosis usually return to normal with treatment, even though the cirrhosis itself is not reversible. As discussed earlier, other features such as loss of libido and potency, amenorrhea, the presence of gynecomastia, and diabetes are much less specific for the presence of cirrhosis. Rather, they reflect the independent effects of iron overload on endocrine tissues. The increased prevalence of some of these features in cirrhotic patients is a function of generalized tissue damage secondary to systemic iron overload.

A precise evaluation of the relationship between hepatic iron levels and the prevalence of cirrhosis or fibrosis in the liver has been made by Bassett and co-workers in Brisbane, Australia.[7] In 30 homozygous relatives of 17 probands with hemochromatosis, only those with hepatic iron levels in excess of 22,000 μg/g dry weight (equivalent

TABLE 48–2. PRINCIPAL CLINICAL FEATURES IN GENETIC HEMOCHROMATOSIS

Author	Niederau et al	Milder et al	Edwards et al
Reference	8	144	199
Number of Subjects	163*	34†	35*
Symptoms (%)			
Weakness, lethargy	83	73	20
Abdominal pain	58	50	23
Arthralgias	43	47	57
Loss of libido, impotence	38	56	29
Cardiac failure symptoms	15	35	0
Physical and Diagnostic Findings (%)			
Cirrhosis (biopsy)	69	94	57
Hepatomegaly	83	76	54
Splenomegaly	13	38	40
Loss of body hair	20	32	6
Gynecomastia	8	12	—
Testicular atrophy	—	50	14
Skin pigmentation	75	82	43
Clinical diabetes	55	53	6

*Patient selection occurred by both clinical features and family screening.
†Only symptomatic index cases were studied.

to about 4500 μg/g wet weight in their study) had fibrosis or cirrhosis on liver biopsy. Patients with cirrhosis tended to be older than the prefibrotic homozygotes (41.7 ± 10.5 years versus 26.5 ± 11.1 years, P <0.01). Furthermore, only in homozygotes was there an age-related rise in hepatic iron levels. This study was the first to provide clear evidence that a threshold exists in the liver for the development of fibrosis and cirrhosis. Confirmation has been provided by Niederau and co-workers,[8] who found in the course of phlebotomy therapy that those individuals whose cumulative iron stores were the greatest suffered more complications from cirrhosis and had the worst prognosis. Conversely, in the course of phlebotomy therapy, no patient whose initial liver biopsy revealed no cirrhosis showed cirrhosis in any subsequent biopsy specimen. In those patients with cirrhosis, the two major causes of death were the complications of chronic liver disease (19 per cent) and cancer of the liver (30 per cent). In about 70 per cent of the cirrhotic patients who expired, death occurred before iron depletion could be completed. Liver cancers developed more than 200-fold more frequently than expected in the general population. The tumors were confined to cirrhotic patients and occurred in those with the highest initial iron stores between 3 and 19 years after documentation of iron depletion. To date, no case of primary liver cancer in genetic hemochromatosis has developed without established cirrhosis being present. The majority of the cancers of the liver were primary hepatocellular carcinomata. A minority were carcinomata arising from intrahepatic bile ducts (19 per cent). It should be noted that in this large study the incidence of extrahepatic cancers was not excessive, in contradistinction to that reported in other studies.[147, 218]

Frequently there is associated unexplained epigastric or right upper quadrant pain, which is usually chronic but sometimes acute. In its acute form, it is severe and associated with circulatory shock.[219] A variety of explanations has been offered for this acute event, including bacterial peritonitis and gram-negative sepsis.[220]

DIABETES MELLITUS

Again, the recent large study of Niederau and co-workers provides an excellent source for data on the prevalence of diabetes mellitus.[8] In the cirrhotic group of subjects (n = 112), 79 individuals had overt diabetes. Of these subjects, 61 per cent were insulin-dependent, whereas the other 39 per cent were non–insulin-dependent. In contrast, in the noncirrhotic individuals (n = 51), only 10 were clinically diabetic, and of these individuals, 6 were non–insulin-dependent. Interestingly, in the remaining 74 patients without overt diabetes, there were 9 in the cirrhotic group and 14 in the noncirrhotic group with abnormal glucose tolerance test results. The overall prevalence of glucose intolerance (clinical and biochemical) was 79 per cent in the cirrhotic individuals and 33 per cent in the noncirrhotic individuals. Although this simply may reflect parallelism between selective islet cell damage and the liver damage in untreated hemochromatosis, it is also possible that it is partly a feature of the glucose intolerance of cirrhosis. Conversely, there is a higher prevalence of diabetes mellitus in the first-degree relatives of diabetic patients with genetic hemochromatosis than in those patients with hemochromatosis who do not have diabetes.[221] Although Sheldon reported that vascular complications of diabetes were rare in hemochromatosis,[4] it is probable that the prognosis was so limited by other complications of the disease that these complications had not yet had time to develop. In fact, as prognosis has improved, increased vascular complications (retinopathy, nephropathy, neuropathy, peripheral vascular disease) have been observed,[221] and in the case of retinopathy they occur with a frequency equal to that in other patients with longstanding diabetes without hemochromatosis.[222]

SKIN PIGMENTATION

Excessive skin pigmentation is detectable almost invariably, particularly in exposed areas. However, it frequently eludes the patient's own attention or the attention of relatives because of its insidious development. The frequency of skin pigmentation at the time of diagnosis (overall 75 per cent) is not significantly different in those with (79 per cent) or without (69 per cent) established cirrhosis.[8] The classic description of bronzed discoloration has to be modified in some cases in favor of a slate-gray pigmentation.[4] The former is caused by melanin pigmentation, whereas the latter is the result of iron deposition in the basal layers of epidermis and the lining cells of sweat glands. In advanced cases, pigmentation also involves the conjunctivae, lid margins, and the buccal mucosae.[208, 223]

CARDIAC MANIFESTATIONS

Cardiomyopathy, cardiac dysrhythmia, and heart failure are the most common causes of death in young patients with secondary hemochromatosis and associated transfusional iron overload.[224] The development of these complications carries a dire prediction of death within three months of onset.[225, 226] Iron deposits in secondary hemochromatosis favor the ventricles rather than the atria and contractile tissue rather than conducting tissue, resulting in cardiac failure rather than dysrhythmias.[227] Nevertheless, atrial tachyarrhythmias, ventricular ectopy, and tachycardia can aggravate the diminished systolic function produced by the iron-overload cardiomyopathy.[228] With the advent of effective phlebotomy therapy for genetic hemochromatosis, this complication has become relatively rare. Only 3 of 53 deaths in a recent series could be ascribed to cardiomyopathy.[8] However, even this low incidence was 300 times more frequent than expected in that population. Baseline noninvasive studies with M-mode echo have shown that ventricular enlargement principally results from increased wall thickness. Later cavity dilation occurs with the advent of congestive failure. Based on studies in fetal rat myocardial cells in culture,[229] it has been suggested that myocardial dysfunction is the consequence of iron-induced lipid peroxidation. Because of the sensitivity of myocardial tissue to iron-induced damage and the rapidity of fatal complications, the early detection of cardiac dysfunction is a clear indication for iron removal or detoxification.

ARTHROPATHY

The overall prevalence of the arthropathy of genetic hemochromatosis is difficult to assess. The frequency of arthralgias at the time of diagnosis varies between 43 per cent and 57 per cent in recent reports.[8, 199] The latter study included both probands and genotypic homozygotes discovered by HLA typing of first-degree relatives. Only 11 of the 20 patients complaining of arthralgias had objective physical signs of arthropathy. However, several of those without painful joints or abnormal physical signs had radiologic evidence of joint disease. The frequency of arthralgia in those with and without cirrhosis does not differ (44 per cent versus 41 per cent, respectively).[8] This supports the notion that arthralgia may be an important first symptom, and in some recently reported cases, arthritis may be the sole clinical manifestation of genetic hemochromatosis.[230]

The polyarthropathy of hemochromatosis tends to involve the metacarpophalangeal, proximal interphalangeal, knee, wrist, and vertebral joints. Although involvement is usually symmetric, it is occasionally unilateral.[217] Pain and stiffness usually precede objective evidence of enlargement, deformity, limitation of movement, and nodule formation, which are suggestive of osteoarthritis. Synovial thickening is not typically evident, and on radiologic evaluation several types of abnormalities can be detected. Characteristically, the arthropathy is manifested by subchondral cyst formation, osteopenia, squaring of the metacarpal joint heads, swelling of the metacarpophalangeal joints, and chondrocalcinosis.[199, 230, 231] The latter is present in about 50 per cent

of patients with arthropathy. Less typically, nonspecific radiologic evidence of degenerative joint disease is the only detectable radiologic abnormality.[199] Rarely, the arthritis progresses to devastating destruction of the smaller joints in spite of adequate iron removal. In other patients, episodes of acute inflammatory synovitis are superimposed on the more chronic changes. These episodes have been termed pseudogout and have been attributed to the precipitation of crystals of calcium pyrophosphate, possibly as a result of the inhibition of pyrophosphatase by iron deposited in synovial lining cells.[210, 212, 232, 233] Although the foregoing description has resulted from studies exclusively in genetic hemochromatosis, arthropathy has been described in a patient with secondary transfusional siderosis.[234]

OTHER ENDOCRINE ABNORMALITIES

In men with genetic hemochromatosis, loss of libido and impotence may occur relatively early in the course of the disease. Although these symptoms, accompanied by loss of secondary sexual characteristics and testicular atrophy, are often present with associated liver disease, they frequently antedate the development of cirrhosis. For example, loss of libido or potency was present in 43 per cent of cirrhotic patients and in 25 per cent of noncirrhotic patients ($P < 0.05$).[8] Interestingly, amenorrhea in women occurs with equal frequency whether established liver disease is present or not (18 per cent versus 29 per cent).[8] Gynecomastia is relatively less common in genetic hemochromatosis than in other causes of cirrhosis (only 9 per cent of patients with cirrhosis from hemochromatosis) and occurs in those without cirrhosis with equal frequency (7 per cent).[8] The majority of cases with gonadal failure have gonadotrophin insufficiency, with low levels of luteinizing hormone and follicle-stimulating hormone and diminished responsiveness to gonadotrophin-releasing hormone.[144, 199, 235–237] In contrast, pituitary-adrenal and pituitary-thyroid responsiveness is usually normal.[144, 199]

SUSCEPTIBILITY TO INFECTION

Although an increased susceptibility to infection in patients with iron overload has been postulated, the association remains to be proved conclusively. Nevertheless, reports continue to accumulate of unusual infections occurring in hemochromatosis. Yersinia enterocolitica septicemia and hepatic abscesses have been described in genetic hemochromatosis and in secondary iron overload due to β-thalassemia with and without liver disease.[238, 239] Other infections include those with Y. pseudotuberculosis,[240] Vibrio vulnificus,[241] and Listeria monocytogenes.[242] Based on both experimental and clinical observations, it has been suggested that increased bioavailability of iron predisposes the host to infection;[243, 244] the decrease in circulating apotransferrin leads to enhanced bacterial viability by making free iron available for bacterial growth and metabolism.[245–247] Alternatively, evidence has been presented to suggest that iron overload produces a defect in monocyte phagocytic capacity, which is reversed by phlebotomy.[242] In either event, the fundamental role of iron in bacterial metabolism and macrophage and neutrophil function in vivo requires further elucidation.

THE ASSOCIATION OF IRON OVERLOAD AND ALCOHOLIC LIVER DISEASE: THE PROBLEMS OF PATHOGENESIS AND DIAGNOSIS

The differentiation of the alcoholic patient with liver disease and associated hepatic iron overload from the patient with genetic hemochromatosis who ingests excessive quantities of alcohol is a frequent diagnostic problem. The problem is compounded by a number of factors: (1) the high prevalence of excessive alcohol ingestion in patients with genetic hemochromatosis (25 to 40 per cent),[217] (2) the presence of iron in a bioavailable form in certain alcoholic beverages,[248, 249] (3) the lack of correlation between stainable iron on liver biopsy specimens and the tissue iron concentration, and (4) the relatively low sensitivity and specificity of the indirect tests for assessment of iron overload in alcoholic patients.[250]

Although histologic siderosis is relatively more common in alcoholic patients, very few show grade III or IV Prussian blue stainable iron.[214] Furthermore, detailed evaluation of the body and liver iron stores of alcoholic patients in Sweden failed to reveal a significant increase in storage iron.[251, 252] In a follow-up study of 60 alcoholic patients and 25 patients with genetic hemochromatosis at the Royal Free Hospital in London,[15] 29 per cent of the alcoholic subjects had hepatic iron concentrations in excess of 1400 μg/g dry weight. In contrast, liver iron concentrations greater than 10,000 μg/g dry weight were found in all 15 patients with genetic hemochromatosis. In none of the alcoholic patients was the concentration this high. Thus, quantitative determination of hepatic iron clearly differentiated alcoholic patients with significant stainable iron from patients with genetic hemochromatosis. In the study by Bassett and co-workers from Brisbane, Australia, 30 homozygous relatives of patients with symptomatic genetic hemochromatosis were compared with 51 alcoholic patients with liver disease and 40 control subjects.[7] No patient with alcoholic liver disease had a liver iron concentration greater than 5000 μg/g dry weight. Although concentrations in presymptomatic homozygous genetic hemochromatosis were occasionally less than this level, no such individual manifested liver disease in the form of fibrosis or cirrhosis. Furthermore, there was no evidence for an age-related accumulation of hepatic iron in alcoholic liver disease. In contrast, alcoholic patients with gross hepatic iron overload probably have genetic hemochromatosis, as supported by estimation of total body iron stores and family studies.[253] A recent study from the Mayo Clinic has suggested that heavy deposition of iron should be regarded as evidence of genetic hemochromatosis, regardless of the degree of alcohol consumption.[254] However, it is also evident that excessive consumption of alcohol by individuals who are homozygous for hemochromatosis can accelerate the development of cirrhosis at levels of iron less than the toxic threshold.[7] Finally, HLA studies have shown that alcoholic patients with minor degrees of iron overload are not selectively heterozygous for the disease,[255] nor does heterozygosity predispose to any significant degree of hepatic iron accumulation.[92]

DIAGNOSIS OF HEMOCHROMATOSIS

The diagnosis of genetic hemochromatosis may be made in (1) symptomatic individuals with clinical features suggestive of the syndrome of iron overload, (2) asymptomatic relatives of patients with previously diagnosed genetic hemochromatosis (homozygotes detected by HLA-haplo-type sharing who have not yet accumulated sufficient iron to produce clinical evidence of toxic organ damage), and (3) asymptomatic individuals in whom suspicion of hemochromatosis has been raised by the serendipitous discovery of an abnormal indirect marker of iron overload. The latter group is particularly problematic because of the general lack of recognition that such indirect markers may be significant. Furthermore, because of the low specificity of many of these markers, there is a need to determine the cost-effectiveness of pursuing such clues by means of more specific and more invasive investigations. Nevertheless, there can be little doubt that with a gene frequency of approximately 5 per cent and a disease prevalence in the population of about 1 in 300, genetic hemochromatosis is currently underdiagnosed.

It has been shown by Bassett and co-workers that in genetic hemochromatosis the accretion of iron is a progressive, age-related phenomenon in which the critical factor in the onset of irreversible liver damage is the rate of iron accretion.[7] Since the excess iron burden accumulates at a maximum of about 1 g/year in men (less in women), and since it is unusual to see cirrhosis in individuals with iron stores of less than 20 g, an explanation is readily available for an inherited disease that does not manifest itself until the fourth decade of life. Therein lies the opportunity for prevention of organ damage, namely, the detection of phenotypic markers of iron overload before the toxic threshold has been reached. Clearly, there also remains the potential for early detection of homozygotes based on the degree of awareness of the significance of early clinical markers such as asymptomatic hepatomegaly with normal or minimally abnormal liver test results, loss of libido, and unexplained arthropathy with chondrocalcinosis (see earlier discussion). Similarly, appropriate investigation of asymptomatic individuals with positive serum markers of iron overload will yield a few with homozygous genetic hemochromatosis. Recent evidence from Germany has demonstrated that timely removal of iron by phlebotomy will produce a normal life expectancy in these individuals.[8] Therefore, it is generally agreed that all clues to the presence of iron overload should be pursued, and if they are proved to be in agreement, direct evidence of tissue damage should be sought and correlated with a specific measurement of the level of iron stores. To summarize, the minimum criteria for the diagnosis of genetic hemochromatosis include (1) increased iron stores with a predominantly parenchymal cell distribution, (2) no cause for secondary iron overload, and (3) a family history of iron overload.[143] In practice, however, there is frequently no family history of iron overload simply because of the lack of access to first-degree relatives.

DETECTION OF INCREASED IRON STORES

Available tests for the detection of increased iron stores can be stratified on the basis of ease of performance and degree of invasiveness. As the level of investigation escalates, so, for the most part, does the degree of invasiveness. However, there is a higher level of specificity and accuracy of diagnosis achieved by the more invasive tests.

Indirect Methods (Table 48–3)

The first line of investigation is the least costly,[256] and is usually used for screening. It consists of the determination

TABLE 48–3. EVALUATION OF INCREASED IRON STORES IN GENETIC HEMOCHROMATOSIS

Indirect Methods	Direct Methods
Serum iron concentration	Liver biopsy for stainable iron and quantitative iron concentration
Transferrin iron saturation	Measurement of physical properties of hepatic iron
Serum ferritin concentration	Computed tomography
	Magnetic susceptibility
	Magnetic resonance imaging
	Determination of iron removed by phlebotomy

of serum iron and transferrin concentrations, transferrin-iron saturation, and serum ferritin concentration. Since transferrin is the specific iron-binding protein of the circulating plasma, its concentration can be calculated from the iron-binding capacity and the known stoichiometry of iron and transferrin (2 atoms/mole at saturation). Normal values are shown in Table 48–4.[257] Unfortunately, false-positive elevations of serum iron occur commonly, for example, following ingestion of iron-containing multivitamin pills; in the presence of coincidental hepatocellular necrosis; in alcoholic patients, both with and without liver disease; and more confounding, also in individuals who are heterozygous for the hemochromatosis allele, but who have only minimally increased iron stores.[92, 93] The lack of sensitivity and specificity in the latter circumstance is particularly disconcerting. In a study of 242 relatives of 41 probands with genetic hemochromatosis, there was an unacceptably high frequency of false-positive and false-negative test results when serum iron was measured (10 and 24 per cent, respectively).[258] The transferrin saturation proved to be a much more sensitive test (92 to 100 per cent sensitive) in this study and others conducted on large pedigrees.[81, 258] However, because the transferrin concentration of plasma may vary independently of the level of the iron stores, it is not surprising that a false-positive elevation has been reported in as many as 24 per cent of asymptomatic relatives with normal iron stores.[259] This is particularly relevant when screening tests are used to detect genetic hemochromatosis in the very young relatives of symptomatic probands. In these circumstances, the predictive accuracy of serum iron and transferrin saturation is particularly low. In 34 homozygous relatives who were less than 35 years of age, all of whom had an elevated hepatic iron concentration, there was a sensitivity of only 82 per cent for serum iron and 85 per cent for transferrin saturation. Nevertheless, for practical purposes a transferrin saturation level of more than 62 per cent will identify 92 per cent of homozygous relatives and is a useful value for screening.[81] It should be borne in

TABLE 48–4. REPRESENTATIVE IRON STUDIES IN SYMPTOMATIC HEMOCHROMATOSIS*

Determination	Normal	Hemochromatosis
Serum iron (μg/dl)	50–150	180–300
Total iron binding capacity (μg/dl)	250–370	200–300
Transferrin saturation (%)	20–50	80–100
Serum ferritin (ng/ml)		
Men	20–300	500–6000
Women	15–250	
Hepatic iron concentration (μg/g, dry weight)	300–1800	10,000–30,000

*Source: Data from Bassett ML, et al. Hepatology 6:24, 1986; Chapman RW, et al. Dig Dis Sci 27:909, 1982; Powell LW, Halliday JW. Viewpoints Dig Dis 14:13, 1982; Worwood M. Clin Sci 70:215, 1986.

mind that the same group also reported a high frequency of elevated serum transferrin saturation in heterozygous relatives when no significantly increased iron stores existed.[92]

Because of its ease of performance, the serum ferritin determination is now included as a first-line investigation by most clinical laboratories. Its approximate cost at $31.50 makes it about two and one-half times as expensive as the serum iron and transferrin-iron saturation.[256] An increased serum ferritin level usually reflects an increase in total body iron. However, it fails to distinguish between parenchymal and reticuloendothelial iron, and it is not specific for iron overload. Furthermore, because tissue damage and inflammation can cause a nonspecific rise in serum ferritin, these are important limitations.[260]

The first demonstration of ferritin in human serum was regarded as a reflection of underlying hepatocellular necrosis.[261] However, with the development of a sensitive radioimmunoassay, others were able to show that it is present in normal serum, and that it is a marker of the amount of storage iron, levels being decreased in iron deficiency (<15 ng/ml) and elevated in iron overload (see Table 48–4).[257] Currently, a variety of assays are used (radioimmunoassay [RIA], immunoradiometric assay [IRMA], or enzyme-linked immunosorbent assay [ELISA]) to measure serum ferritin,[262–264] and a human liver ferritin standard is available as a reference agent for the assay.[265] In normal serum and that from patients with iron overload, serum ferritin is immunologically related to liver or spleen ferritin, reacting with antibodies to ferritins rich in light (L) subunits. However, it differs from tissue ferritin in that it is low in iron content (0.02 to 0.07 μg Fe/μg compared with >0.7 μg/μg of protein),[265] and it is glycosylated. The presence of the carbohydrate moiety on serum ferritin has suggested its origin as a specific secretory protein. In iron overload, the serum protein acquires an additional glycosylated subunit (the G subunit).[266] With hepatocellular necrosis, the direct release of tissue ferritin from damaged cells causes an increase in ferritin in serum, which is not glycosylated.[267, 268]

There is a wide range of normal values for serum ferritin in adults. Worwood quotes normal figures between 15 and 300 ng/ml, with men tending to have higher values than women.[265] Powell and Halliday give a narrower range with a lower upper limit of normal of 100 ng/ml.[257] Levels between 500 and 6000 ng/ml are seen in patients with iron overload. Studies of large numbers of families with genetic hemochromatosis in four countries have shown that the serum ferritin level correlates well with the size of the body iron stores and liver iron concentration.[89, 204, 250, 258, 259, 269, 270] However, it is realized that serum ferritin levels in precirrhotic young homozygotes with hemochromatosis may be normal despite significantly elevated liver iron levels and total body iron stores.[89, 204, 250, 259, 269, 271–274] In 34 homozygous relatives of 22 genetic hemochromatosis probands who were less than 35 years old at the time of study, there were 5 individuals with serum ferritin levels in the normal range (85 per cent sensitivity).[259] This can be compared with the 82 per cent sensitivity for transferrin iron saturation. However, only two individuals (aged 15 and 17 years) had both saturation and serum ferritin concentrations in the normal range. In this study the combined sensitivity of transferrin iron saturation and serum ferritin was 94 per cent. All 34 subjects had increased mobilizable iron, and it is noteworthy that although there was an excellent correlation between serum ferritin and mobilized body iron, there was also a progressive rise in serum ferritin with age. Those individuals with normal serum ferritin levels were younger (<20 years), and their mobilized iron was less than 5 g.

Finally, it should be re-emphasized that many conditions characterized by liver damage or inflammation, the presence of solid tumors, particularly with metastases, and lymphomas and leukemias can be associated with increased concentrations of serum ferritin.[265] For these reasons, specificity will always be limited. However, serum ferritin is a valuable screening tool for primary and secondary causes of iron overload. It is raised relatively early in the course of iron accretion, and usually long before the development of iron-induced damage to tissue. Furthermore, the combination of serum ferritin and transferrin saturation is highly sensitive and will detect the vast majority of asymptomatic individuals with homozygous genetic hemochromatosis. The serum ferritin level falls progressively during phlebotomy therapy, with an excellent correlation between its level and the amount of iron mobilized in an individual patient.[144] In contrast, the serum iron level does not fall until the excess stores have been completely mobilized, and the serum ferritin is reduced to less than 50 ng/ml.

Direct Methods (Table 48–3)

Although the serum ferritin determination gives an indication of the total iron stores, and a raised transferrin saturation points to their predominantly parenchymal location, a diagnosis of hemochromatosis requires direct documentation of excess iron in the liver. In addition, documentation of the extent of hepatic injury is helpful for management. There is no effective substitute for liver biopsy to achieve both these aims. The small core provided by percutaneous needle biopsy yields sufficient tissue for histopathologic evaluation and biochemical measurement of iron concentration. Perls' Prussian blue stain (potassium ferrocyanide for ferric iron) is used to identify and localize storage iron. A semiquantitative grading system (grades I to IV) has been established based on the extent of Prussian blue granule deposition.[196] This has been extended by Powell and Kerr so that stainable iron is represented as follows: grade IV, virtually 100 per cent of hepatocytes; grade III, 75 per cent; grade II, 50 per cent; and grade I, 25 per cent.[200] The latter approach seems logical in view of the initial periportal deposition of iron in genetic hemochromatosis, with subsequent involvement of the entire lobule as iron accretion progresses. Unfortunately, there is a poor correlation between stainable iron and direct chemical measurement of iron.[250, 269, 277] Grades I and II Prussian blue staining can be seen in normal liver,[275, 276] whereas grade III stainable iron is observed frequently in alcoholic cirrhosis, in which it correlates poorly with hepatic iron concentration.[15, 214] In genetic hemochromatosis there has been general disappointment with the histochemical grading of stainable iron. Although it is agreed that grade IV deposition indicates a heavy iron burden, grade III is much more difficult to interpret. However, staining for iron is used routinely as a screening test, and despite a significant number of false-positive results, it is useful in defining the cellular distribution of the iron.

The chemical determination of iron can be performed satisfactorily on formalin-fixed (but not embedded) tissue, untreated wet tissue, or on a lyophylized specimen. Current methods employ colorimetric or atomic absorption measurement of nonheme iron after appropriate washing and chemical digestion of the tissue. In practice, these methods give comparable results,[278] and the choice among them depends on the availability of atomic absorption spectrophotometry and the size of the available specimen. Graphite furnace atomic absorption spectrophotometry has an advantage when very small samples have to be processed. In our institution, the colorimetric method of Torrance and Bothwell has proved to be very reproducible, relatively simple, and inexpensive to perform.[217, 279] Normal concentrations of liver iron up to 1800 μg/g dry weight have been quoted,[7] with livers of patients with symptomatic hemochromatosis usually containing more than 10,000 μg/g.[7, 15] The livers of patients with established hepatic fibrosis and cirrhosis consistently have liver iron greater than 22,000 μg/g dry weight.[7] Patients with alcoholic liver disease and increased stainable iron fall in the range of 1400 to 5000 μg/g but never exceed 10,000 μg/g.[7, 15, 250] Those with hemochromatosis and cirrhosis who coincidentally drink excess amounts of alcohol fall in the range of 10,000 to 22,000 μg/g,[7] that is, less than the threshold level for fibrosis seen in uncomplicated genetic hemochromatosis. It should be emphasized that young, asymptomatic, precirrhotic homozygotes almost always have concentrations greater than the normal range, but since accretion is age related,[7] the actual level must be interpreted with the age of the subject in mind.

The hepatic iron concentration constitutes the "gold standard" by which iron overload is judged. The ultimate test of mobilizable iron is the amount removed by phlebotomy. Although this is to be regarded as a third-level investigation reserved for those individuals in whom biopsy is not possible, or when alternative noninvasive methods are not available for quantifying iron stores, it is the ultimate test of significant iron overload. Each unit of blood removed is equivalent to about 250 mg of iron, depending on the hematocrit value. Most individuals, including alcoholic persons with spurious indirect markers of iron overload, will become iron deficient after removal of more than 2 g of iron. Patients with symptomatic hemochromatosis will almost invariably require removal of at least 72 units of blood (equivalent to 15 to 20 g of iron) before becoming depleted of iron.

Alternative, noninvasive techniques have been sought for those individuals in whom liver biopsy is not possible. Such alternative techniques include (1) computed tomography (CT), (2) magnetic susceptibility measurement, and (3) magnetic resonance imaging (MRI). All exploit the physical properties of storage iron and depend on the calibration of that physical property against the hepatic iron concentration.

On CT scanning, the linear attenuation coefficient (CT number) is increased by iron because of its high relative electron density when compared with other cellular constituents.[280] In hemochromatosis, conventional single-energy CT scanning has not proved to be a very sensitive test for iron overload, although in one study it did appear to be more specific than the serum ferritin concentration.[281] In addition, it has been shown to correlate well with the hepatic iron concentration in patients with iron overload caused by thalassemia major.[282] Its sensitivity has been increased by the use of a dual-energy technique, which yielded an excellent positive correlation between the attenuation coefficient and the hepatic iron concentration in both the precirrhotic and cirrhotic stages of hemochromatosis.[283] However, this technique requires expensive nonstandard modifications of equipment and complicated calibration methodology.

The paramagnetic properties of ferritin and hemosiderin have been exploited for the measurement of hepatic iron stores.[284, 285] Noninvasive human determinations became possible with the development of the superconducting quantum interference device (SQUID). An induced magnetic field is amplified quantitatively by storage iron in the liver, and this enhancement can be measured sensitively and reproducibly by the magnetic susceptometer. With appropriate calibration, measurements made in humans with iron overload have shown excellent correlation over a 30-fold range of hepatic iron level, measured independently by a chemical method. Although an instrument is now available commercially, it is expensive and can be used only for the measurement of iron in the liver. As such, it will have limited applicability and will be affordable only in specialized referral centers.

MRI is currently being evaluated as a quantitative method for the assessment of hepatic iron concentration. Studies in experimental animals have shown decreased spin-echo image intensity in iron overload resulting from a marked decrease in the transverse (T2) relaxation time.[286] Use of tissue relaxation rates (1/T1 and 1/T2) and optimized spin-echo sequences have resulted in a reasonably accurate assessment of hepatic iron overload in patients with hemochromatosis. With further refinement, it is anticipated that MRI may provide an increasingly accurate noninvasive measurement of hepatic iron concentration; clinical studies are currently in progress in several centers.[287]

Before the current interest in physical methods for quantification of hepatic iron stores, the deferoxamine test was used as a marker of chelatable iron. Normal subjects excrete less than 1.5 mg of iron in the urine in the 24 hours following a dose of 0.5 g of deferoxamine intramuscularly. In hemochromatosis, the excretion is usually in excess of 3 mg. Unfortunately, the test is insensitive in presymptomatic genetic hemochromatosis, and like the serum ferritin and serum iron levels, the result can underestimate iron stores in the presence of ascorbic acid deficiency and overestimate them in a variety of conditions (inflammation, malignancy, liver disease) that are not in themselves associated with iron overload. It has therefore been largely discarded in favor of more direct methods.[288]

DIAGNOSIS OF THE PRESYMPTOMATIC GENETIC HOMOZYGOTE

In a genetic disease in which the presumed abnormality in iron absorption leads to a progressive accumulation of iron throughout life, there is clearly the opportunity to diagnose the disorder early based on its phenotypic expression (Table 48–5). As discussed earlier, there are biochemical forms of expression that antedate the development of irreversible tissue damage and that can be used to pre-empt the attainment of the toxic threshold of iron.[154] The first indication of risk is a family history of a first-degree relative with the disease. Current recommendations are for the genetic and biochemical screening of all first-degree relatives from the age of 10 years onward. HLA typing of such relatives indicates the extent of the risk. The likelihood of developing the disease is virtually nil for those relatives sharing neither HLA haplotype with the proband and

TABLE 48–5. DIAGNOSTIC SCREENING FOR PRESYMPTOMATIC HEMOCHROMATOSIS[87, 143]

Serum iron, transferrin saturation, and serum ferritin in all first-degree relatives of proband more than 10 years old
If any one is abnormal, liver biopsy is performed for stainable and biochemical iron and histopathologic features
HLA, A and B haplotypes: homozygote defined as sharing both with proband; yearly screening by indirect criteria is necessary

minimal for those sharing one haplotype, as the latter are presumed heterozygotes. The risk is very high in individuals with both haplotypes in common, that is, in presumed homozygotes.[90] Recent data have shown that when no other disease factors are present (for example, iron loss caused by chronic bleeding), all true homozygotes will inevitably manifest phenotypic features of hemochromatosis.[289] A rare exception to this rule is the misdiagnosis of the homozygous state because of chromosomal cross-over. For practical purposes, it is recommended that the combination of serum iron, transferrin saturation, and serum ferritin be used for phenotypic screening and HLA typing for genotypic screening.[143] In a homozygote with any abnormal biochemical marker, a liver biopsy should be performed to quantify the hepatic iron content, and phlebotomy should commence if the level is raised. In a homozygote with normal biochemical indices, the tests should be repeated annually. In a presumed heterozygote, the presence of an abnormality in the biochemical indices should not be cause for alarm. However, it is reasonable to repeat the tests annually. A transferrin saturation in excess of 62 per cent or a rising serum ferritin concentration should be an indication for a more direct quantification of hepatic iron. Hopefully, tests that are less invasive than liver biopsy will soon become generally available for the additional reassurance of these individuals and for the physicians taking care of them.

Abnormalities in Genetic Heterozygotes

Using the hepatic iron level as the reference standard for the diagnosis of iron overload, heterozygotes have been shown to have mean values that are significantly higher than those of controls (1880 µg/g compared with 800 µg/g) but that are significantly lower than the level seen in hemochromatosis homozygotes (16,700 µg/g).[7] However, unlike homozygotes, heterozygotes showed no progressive accretion of iron with age. In both these respects, hemochromatosis heterozygotes may be indistinguishable from patients with alcoholic liver disease; HLA typing of patients with alcoholic liver disease and minor degrees of iron overload provides no support for the concept of an enhanced incidence of liver damage in alcoholic patients who are heterozygous for hemochromatosis.[255]

With the knowledge that hepatic iron concentration tends to be slightly increased in most heterozygotes, it is not surprising that since the advent of HLA screening, virtually every study has shown a significant prevalence of positive indirect serum markers of iron overload in heterozygotes.[89, 92, 218, 259, 274, 290]

Value of HLA Typing

From what has been discussed, the value of HLA typing in diagnosis lies in defining the risk of the disease developing in a first-degree relative of a proband with genetic hemochromatosis, that is, the identification of homozygotes. By the same reasoning, HLA typing also permits reassurance of those relatives who show positive serum markers but who can be defined as risk-free heterozygotes or normal homozygotes because they share only one haplotype or no haplotypes, respectively, with the proband.[87]

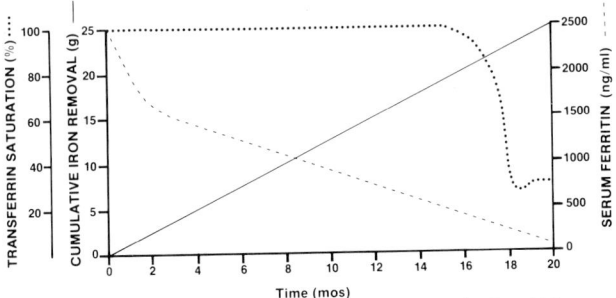

Figure 48–4. Response of indirect markers of iron overload to phlebotomy therapy. This figure illustrates the reciprocal relationship between the serum ferritin level and the removal of excess iron stores. The fall in transferrin iron saturation antedates the complete removal of storage iron (in this example, 25 g). At this time, a fall in the hematocrit value can be expected, indicating a relative iron deficiency.

TREATMENT AND PROGNOSIS OF HEMOCHROMATOSIS

Removal of iron by phlebotomy therapy is the mainstay of treatment in genetic hemochromatosis. Weekly or biweekly, if tolerated, removal of 500 ml of blood (equivalent to 250 mg of iron) should be continued until the storage pool of iron is depleted. In practice, this may take two to three years for those individuals with a very large iron burden (>30 g). In the study by Edwards and co-workers of 35 homozygotes,[199] the 20 treated men required an average of 68 phlebotomies removing 500 ml of blood to achieve depletion, whereas the 10 treated women required an average of 25 phlebotomies. Since the diagnosis can now be made in presymptomatic homozygotes, current recommendations are for the treatment of all individuals with genetic hemochromatosis who have evidence of iron overload based on quantitative determination of liver iron.[154]

The serum ferritin level can be expected to decline progressively during therapy,[144, 199] with the greatest fall/milligram of iron removed (1 ng/ml/2 mg of Fe) occurring during the early phlebotomies, and then slowing to about 1 ng/ml/4 mg of Fe after about 15 phlebotomies (Fig. 48–4). The serum iron level and the transferrin saturation can be expected to remain high until iron depletion has occurred. In practice, these determinations do not fall until the serum ferritin level falls to less than 30 to 50 ng/ml.[144, 199] At this point, the hematocrit also falls, which is an indication of the development of iron deficiency. The rate of phlebotomy can then be reduced to three to six/year to maintain the transferrin saturation at about 50 per cent. In presymptomatic patients without consistent abnormalities of all serum markers, it may be necessary to choose the one that most sensitively reflects the iron status in the individual case. In practice, it is not necessary to measure the serum ferritin level before every phlebotomy. Rather, the hematocrit, which should have returned to within 5 to 10 per cent of its baseline value, can be used as a suitable safeguard, with the serum iron level and transferrin saturation serving as markers of iron deficiency.

Several studies have evaluated the benefits of iron depletion by phlebotomy.[8, 144, 147] In the early years after recognition of the disease, the outcome was determined by the course of the diabetes mellitus. With the availability of insulin, the average life expectancy after diagnosis improved from two to about four years.[144] In the only recent study to evaluate outcome without removal of iron, the five-year survival rate was 18 per cent and the 10-year survival rate was 10 per cent.[147] In this study, in which cirrhosis was invariably present, the survival rate with phlebotomy improved to 66 per cent and 32 per cent at 5 and 10 years, respectively. Milder and co-workers give an overall survival rate of 70 per cent at 5 and 10 years after diagnosis in treated patients.[144] However, they point out that the prognosis is much worse when there is associated alcoholism. By the same reckoning, when there is no excessive alcohol ingestion, survival rates of 84 per cent at 5 to 10 years can be expected.

The critical role of the presence of diabetes mellitus and cirrhosis in prognosis has been evaluated by Niederau and co-workers (Table 48–6).[8] When there was no diabetes or cirrhosis, life expectancy of patients with genetic hemochromatosis was virtually identical to that expected of age and sex-matched controls. In the presence of established cirrhosis, 5- and 10-year survival rates were 90 and 70 per cent, respectively; with diabetes mellitus, survival rates of 90 and 63 per cent were observed at 5 and 10 years, respectively. Both complications significantly increased the mortality rate when compared with the control population. The major causative factor in determining the presence of these two major life-threatening complications was the size of the iron burden. Survival was normal in the 77 patients who were depleted of iron in 18 months by regular phlebotomy. In the 75 patients whose iron stores could not be depleted in 18 months, only 60 per cent were alive after ten years. The patients who died after achieving iron depletion had iron stores significantly larger than those who survived (32 g versus 21 g). Death rates from diabetes mellitus (an increase of 7-fold), cirrhosis (13-fold), primary liver cancer (220-fold), and cardiomyopathy (306-fold) were all significantly higher than those expected in a matched population. It is noteworthy that in 11 of the 13 patients who died from liver cancer, iron depletion had been achieved. However, all patients had established cirrhosis. The liver tumor developed 9.1 ± 4.5 years after iron depletion.

Although improvement in liver function and regression of hepatomegaly has been reported in about 50 per cent of patients treated by phlebotomy,[147] cirrhosis is not usually reversible.[8] However, there have been reports of regression of fibrosis and cirrhosis in association with iron removal.[291, 292] Although the possibility of sampling error was not ruled out by laparoscopic evaluation, the potential for reversibility has prevented an attitude of therapeutic nihilism in patients with established cirrhosis. This is supported by the improved survival rate of patients with cirrhosis treated by phlebotomy.[147] In contrast, less than one third of patients showed improvement in diabetes mellitus, as evidenced by unchanged insulin requirements.[147] It appears that insulin dependency resulting from pancreatic beta cell destruction is not reversible.[8] Pigmentation is improved by removal of iron, but hypogonadism and established arthropathy are

TABLE 48–6. CAUSES OF DEATH IN HEMOCHROMATOSIS

Cause of Death*	Mortality Ratio (Observed/ Expected)	Proportion of All Deaths (%)†
Cancer of liver	220	30
Cirrhosis	13	19
Diabetes mellitus	7	6
Cardiomyopathy	306	6

*Four causes of death among 53 patients who died in a series of 163 patients with genetic hemochromatosis were shown to be significantly higher than the expected rates in a normal population.[8]

†The remaining 39 per cent of deaths occurred from causes that did not occur significantly more frequently than in the control population.

not ameliorated. However, there is frequently relief of malaise, weakness, and lethargy, and of the common right upper quadrant pain occurring in patients with heavy hepatic iron deposits.

The single most common acute cause of death in primary and secondary iron overload is cardiomyopathy and cardiac dysrhythmia.[8, 144, 224] Heart disease due to iron overload is regarded as warranting accelerated removal of iron by a combination of phlebotomy and chelation therapy with deferoxamine B, a polyhydroxamic acid derivative produced by the soil fungus, *Streptomyces pilosus*.[152, 293] Although it has been shown that ascorbic acid treatment can serve to maximize the chelatable iron pool, caution has been expressed regarding the adjuvant use of ascorbic acid with iron mobilization therapy because of reported deterioration in cardiac function in association with administration of ascorbic acid.[193, 294]

Phlebotomy is the treatment of choice in genetic hemochromatosis because of the rapidity with which storage iron can be mobilized. It should be remembered that iron absorption from the gastrointestinal tract is promoted by therapeutic reduction of iron stores, increasing from 1 to 4 mg/day to 4 to 8 mg/day during phlebotomy.[100] This increase is equivalent to an extra unit of blood every two months. Phlebotomy has been used in various forms of secondary hemochromatosis, African hemochromatosis,[295] and porphyria cutanea tarda,[296] with evidence of clinical benefit. However, in a preliminary study, its use in patients with alcoholic liver disease and iron overload did not improve the outcome of the disease.[297] Although alcohol appears to have a synergistic effect in producing liver damage in genetic hemochromatosis,[7] the ill effects of smaller deposits (≤ 10 g total) of iron in patients with alcoholic liver disease could not be confirmed in this study.

Phlebotomy is not a feasible form of treatment in those forms of secondary hemochromatosis associated with anemia, in particular the thalassemia syndromes. It is in these diseases that considerable effort has been devoted to the development of suitable chelation therapy. Deferoxamine B, which was first introduced 25 years ago, is still the only iron-chelating agent that is clinically useful. It is effective when delivered parenterally, either by subcutaneous or intravenous infusion. Although three major studies have demonstrated the efficacy of deferoxamine in increasing life expectancy and arresting the development of hepatic fibrosis,[150, 298, 299] its use did not become widespread until it was shown that continuous infusions were superior to bolus injections in enhancing urinary iron excretion.[300] The infusions are administered five to six nights/week for 8 to 12 hours at a dose of 0.5 to 4.0 g, depending on the age and weight of the patient and the degree of iron loading. With increasing dosage, fecal iron excretion is progressively enhanced and may exceed urinary excretion.[301] Preliminary data in experimental rats supports the notion that the biliary route of iron excretion from the iron-overloaded liver may be preferentially enhanced under these circumstances.[302] It is generally recommended that ascorbic acid in a small dose (100 to 200 mg) be given *during* the deferoxamine infusion to enhance urinary excretion of iron.[293] This mode of administering ascorbic acid (i.e., small doses in the presence of a chelator) has not been associated with enhanced cardiac toxicity.

SECONDARY HEMOCHROMATOSIS

The foregoing account has been devoted largely to the clinical and pathologic consequences of iron overload in genetic hemochromatosis. The opportunity has been taken to compare and contrast the pathologic features of the various forms of secondary hemochromatosis (see Table 48–1). However, lifelong excessive gastrointestinal absorption of iron often compounded by the requirement for blood transfusions occurs in the dyserythropoietic anemias, in particular thalassemia major. The pattern of organ damage and the clinical consequences of that damage are indistinguishable from those occurring in genetic hemochromatosis.[224] Since the rate of iron accretion is so much more rapid in thalassemia, the major targets of damage—namely, the liver, the pancreas, and the heart—are vulnerable at a much earlier age than in genetic hemochromatosis, and the need for prophylactic therapy to prevent iron overload is therefore more urgent. Hence, an aggressive approach in the use of chelation therapy in young children has become the usual practice. It is relevant that in 15 nonthalassemic adults who were transfused with a mean of 120 units of blood, portal fibrosis was noted at a mean hepatic iron concentration of 22,000 μg/g,[303] which is in remarkably close agreement with that seen in genetic hemochromatosis.[7]

The common theme in the iron-loading anemias is refractory anemia, with hypercellular bone marrow and ineffective erythropoiesis. These anemias include thalassemia major, the sideroblastic anemias, pyruvate kinase deficiency, and a variety of other anemias characterized by defective incorporation of iron into hemoglobin. Although the parenchymal distribution of the iron overload is in keeping with enhanced iron absorption, the extent of iron overload cannot be related to the level of the anemia.[304] It has been postulated that either the extent of erythroid activity in some cases or a linkage to the hemochromatosis allele in others may be responsible for the variable degree of iron overload observed in dyserythropoietic anemias.[305] It has been argued that the prevalence of the hemochromatosis allele is relevant to the promotion of iron overload in very rare diseases, such as dyserythropoietic anemias, idiopathic refractory sideroblastic anemia, or porphyria cutanea tarda. Simon criticizes the evidence supporting such an association on the grounds that small sample sizes lead to lack of statistical significance.[305-307] Furthermore, he was unable to confirm an increased prevalence of HLA-A3 in 22 patients with idiopathic sideroblastic anemia in Brittany.[308] Likewise, he points out that it is very unlikely on genetic grounds that the prevalence of the hemochromatosis allele is greater in the various populations with secondary hemochromatosis than in the general population. In summary, in the study by Simon and co-workers there is no evidence linking the hemochromatosis gene to the pathogenesis of iron overload in idiopathic sideroblastic anemia,[308] porphyria cutanea tarda,[309] or alcoholic liver disease.[255]

PORPHYRIA CUTANEA TARDA

Porphyria cutanea tarda (see Chap. 14) is the most common form of hepatic porphyria. The liver is the site of the overproduction of porphyrins, which leads to the mutilating cutaneous manifestations of the disease.[296] The disease occurs in two forms: the more common sporadic porphyria cutanea tarda syndrome and the rarer familial form. In both forms, evidence has accumulated to suggest that excessive storage iron plays a central role in promoting the biochemical and clinical manifestations of porphyria cutanea tarda.

The classic sporadic porphyria cutanea tarda syndrome may represent an aberrant response to alcoholic liver disease with iron overload (~70 per cent of cases), African hemochromatosis, or estrogen-induced liver damage. Rare cases of toxic porphyria cutanea tarda are caused by exposure to the polyhalogenated hydrocarbon hexachlorobenzene. In sporadic porphyria cutanea tarda, it has been suggested that heterozygosity for genetic hemochromatosis may be responsible for the associated iron-overload and clinical expression of the disease.[309] Although evidence was presented for the over-representation of the HLA-A3 allele in the family of a proband with porphyria cutanea tarda, and in another group of 14 patients with porphyria cutanea tarda, all of whom were said to have excess hepatic iron stores,[310] no direct evidence was provided for the concurrence of the hemochromatosis allele with porphyria cutanea tarda in these individuals. Indeed, in a much larger study group, Beaumont and co-workers determined the HLA genotypes in 69 patients with porphyria cutanea tarda (42 sporadic and 27 familial).[311] The prevalence of the HLA-A3 haplotype (about 23 per cent) was similar in both groups and was no different from a control population. However, in an isolated patient with familial porphyria cutanea tarda who was HLA-A3 positive, it is possible that there was the coincidental presence of the hemochromatosis gene and the gene for porphyria cutanea tarda, the phenotypic expression of the former promoting expression of the latter. Adams and Powell conclude that the controversy will not be resolved until large numbers of pedigree studies of unselected patients with porphyria cutanea tarda, both familial and sporadic, are completed by several centers.[312] They emphasize that a final opinion on the role of the hemochromatosis allele in porphyria cutanea tarda will not be possible until the gene for genetic hemochromatosis has been identified and sequenced.

HEPATIC MANIFESTATIONS IN PORPHYRIA CUTANEA TARDA

No correlation between the porphyric activity and the extent of liver damage has been demonstrated. Liver damage usually has characteristics of alcohol damage, and cirrhosis is present in up to 30 per cent of patients. Other features of liver disease have been described, which may be more specific for porphyria cutanea tarda. Mild periportal hemosiderosis, focal lobular hepatocyte necrosis and steatosis, marked hepatocyte hyperplasia, and periductal lymphocytic aggregates, when observed together, have suggested that porphyrin deposition itself may be the basis for specific hepatotoxic manifestations.[296]

ROLE OF IRON IN PATHOGENESIS OF PORPHYRIA CUTANEA TARDA

About 75 per cent of patients with porphyria cutanea tarda have excessive hepatic iron on light microscopy that is distributed in both hepatocytes and Kupffer cells.[313] Hepatic iron also is increased based on biochemical analysis.[17] The degree of iron deposition usually is not severe and reflects total body iron stores of no more than 4 g (except in African hemochromatosis, in which stores are increased greatly). The role of this increased iron, and its interaction with the enzyme uroporphyrinogen decarboxylase, remains controversial. Some workers have suggested that iron may play a role in the inhibition of uroporphy-

rinogen decarboxylase,[314, 315] whereas others have not been able to demonstrate inhibition of this enzyme activity in vitro or in vivo in experimental iron overload.[316-318] In addition, removal of iron has not restored reduced hepatic enzyme activity in patients with porphyria cutanea tarda.[319] In contrast, a role for iron has been supported by reports documenting the beneficial effects of phlebotomy, and the deleterious effects of iron administration on the clinical manifestations of porphyria cutanea tarda.[320-323] It has been shown that the hepatic uroporphyrinogen decarboxylase activity may be restored to normal during remission.[324, 325] Furthermore, a distinction needs to be made between familial and sporadic porphyria cutanea tarda with regard to uroporphyrinogen decarboxylase activity and concentration. It is only in the former disease that an intrinsic deficiency of this enzyme has been demonstrated; this defect is inherited as an autosomal dominant trait.[326] It has been assumed that uroporphyrinogen decarboxylase deficiency in the liver leads to overproduction of uroporphyrin and thereby the clinical consequences of this illness. Iron may play a synergistic role in the inhibition of uroporphyrinogen decarboxylase. A more fundamental role has been postulated for an uncoupling of the cytochrome P450 reductase–cytochrome P_i450 system with the release of activated oxygen.[327-330] In the sporadic form of porphyria cutanea tarda, factors that rapidly induce this P450 system without providing a rapid turnover of porphyrinogen substrate can serve to initiate an attack of porphyria cutanea tarda. In these circumstances, the formation of an oxidant leads to oxidation of the porphyrinogen substrate to porphyrin, which together with the active oxidant inhibits uroporphyrinogen decarboxylase activity. Iron released from storage ferritin may serve to catalyze this free radical–induced toxic sequence.[171-174]

TREATMENT OF PORPHYRIA CUTANEA TARDA

Treatment, as for hemochromatosis, is the removal of iron by phlebotomy. Iron removal decreases the hepatic overproduction of porphyrins and leads to improvement of both the skin and hepatic abnormalities even without evidence of excessive iron in the liver. Removal of as little as 4 g of iron will produce remission of the porphyric symptoms.[320, 321] It remains to be demonstrated whether benefits for the associated liver disease also ensue. When alcohol is incriminated, only abstention offers an opportunity for potential reversal of hepatic damage.

NEONATAL IRON STORAGE DISEASE

During the past 30 years there have been several reports of infants dying during the perinatal period or in early infancy with documented hepatic iron overload and cirrhosis. There has been a recent epidemiologic review of 25 reported cases, and a detailed clinical and pathologic study of 5 cases.[331, 332] Other previous reports have documented individual cases in detail.[333, 334] In the study from Silver and co-workers,[332] the morphologic evaluation of tissue iron deposition was correlated with quantitative tissue iron measurements. Normal liver architecture was destroyed by diffuse fibrosis, and evidence of regeneration was found in the form of regeneration nodules, neocholangiolar proliferation, and multinucleated giant cells. Hepatic siderosis was graded III to IV+ and was always predominantly hepatocellular; extrahepatic siderosis was also seen in the parenchymal cells of several other organs, notably the exocrine pancreas and myocardium. Although hepatic iron concentrations were significantly higher than in control autopsies, the levels reported (mean, 622 µg/g) were well below the toxic range reported in adults with genetic hemochromatosis.[7] Nevertheless, the total hepatic iron stores were more than three times higher than in selected perinatal controls. The authors maintain that hepatic damage commenced between 16 and 30 weeks of gestation based on the liver weights and morphologic features at autopsy. Limited data are available on the maternal iron status. No excessive transferrin iron saturation or serum ferritin levels were noted in the mother of three affected infants, and although the HLA-A3 haplotype was present in both the mother and one of her affected infants, there was no way of knowing if the father was a heterozygote. Although it is conceivable that a fetus who is homozygous for hemochromatosis could have excessive transport of iron across the placenta, there has been no evidence for such a disordered mechanism in utero in the offspring of families known to carry the hemochromatosis allele. Current understanding of fetal iron metabolism during intrauterine development is limited to the concept that fetal iron is derived from maternal transferrin, which is bound by transferrin receptors on the trophoblastic brush border.[335–338] The mechanism for transport of iron across the trophoblast epithelium is not known. Until more detailed information is available on the possible pathophysiology of placental transport, and the structure and function of both maternal and fetal iron storage and transport mechanisms, the fundamental defect in the enigmatic condition of neonatal iron storage disease will remain elusive. On the basis of current information, it does seem, however, that the developing liver is vulnerable to iron toxicity at relatively low levels of iron in tissue.

SUMMARY AND FUTURE PERSPECTIVES

When Sheldon reviewed the literature on hemochromatosis available to him in 1935,[4] he concluded that the two principal features of tissue damage—cirrhosis and diabetes mellitus—evolved concurrently in the course of iron accumulation resulting from a common inherited pathogenetic mechanism. The data reviewed in this chapter support this concept. Since the previous edition of this book, the other major contributions to the literature have supported the notion that iron accumulation is progressive throughout the life of patients with genetic hemochromatosis, that a hepatic iron concentration threshold exists for the development of cirrhosis, and that the threshold may be preempted by timely initiation of phlebotomy therapy. Confirmation has been provided of the value of screening tests of iron overload in the homozygous relatives of patients with confirmed hemochromatosis and of the value of HLA haplotyping in the detection of those at risk for the disease. Careful observations of treated presymptomatic homozygotes will yield answers as to whether all phenotypic expression of the disease can be prevented.

Biochemical studies in humans and experimental animals have contributed new ideas about the putative pathways of iron-induced cytotoxicity, invoking recognized mechanisms of free radical–induced injury. Future work in these exciting areas of basic and applied toxicology should provide further insights into the molecular basis of membrane damage in iron overload. Other future developments that are awaited with interest relate to the exploitation of techniques of molecular genetics to locate and sequence the genome for hemochromatosis and to develop further the use of iron chelators that can be taken by mouth as an alternative to the tedium of repeated phlebotomy.

REFERENCES

1. Trousseau A. Glycosurie, diabète sucré. Clinique Médicale de l'Hotel-Dieu de Paris, 2nd ed., Vol. 2. Ballicre Paris, 1865:663.
2. Troisier M. Diabète sucré. Bull Soc Anat Paris 16:231, 1871.
3. Von Recklinghausen FD. Über Hämochromatose. Tagebl Versamml Natur Ärzte Heidelberg 62:324, 1889.
4. Sheldon JH. Haemochromatosis. London, Oxford University Press, 1935.
5. Macdonald RG. Hemochromatosis and Hemosiderosis. Springfield, IL, Charles C Thomas, 1964.
6. Simon M, Bourel M, Genetet B, et al. Idiopathic hemochromatosis: demonstration of recessive transmission and early detection by family HLA typing. N Engl J Med 297:1017, 1977.
7. Bassett ML, Halliday JW, Powell LW. Value of hepatic iron measurements in early hemochromatosis and determination of the critical iron level associated with fibrosis. Hepatology 6:24, 1986.
8. Niederau C, Fischer R, Sonnenberg A, et al. Survival and causes of death in cirrhotic and noncirrhotic patients with primary hemochromatosis. N Engl J Med 313:1256, 1985.
9. Modell CB. Transfusional haemochromatosis. In: Kief H, ed. Iron metabolism and its disorders. Amsterdam, Excerpta Medica, 1975:230.
10. Modell CB. Advances in the use of iron-chelating agents for the treatment of iron overoad. In: Brown EB, ed. Progress in Hematology, Vol 11. New York, Grune & Stratton, 1979:267.
11. Charlton RW, Bothwell TH, Seftel HC. Dietary iron overload. In: Callender ST, ed. Clin Haematol 2:383, 1973.
12. MacPhail AP, Simon MO, Torrance JD, et al. Changing patterns of dietary iron overload in black South Africans. Am J Clin Nutr 32:1272, 1979.
13. Bothwell TH, Bradlow BA. Siderosis in the Bantu. A combined histopathological and chemical study. Arch Pathol 70:279, 1960.
14. Isaacson C, Seftel H, Keeley KJ, et al. Siderosis in the Bantu. The relationship between iron overload and cirrhosis. J Lab Clin Med 58:845, 1961.
15. Chapman RW, Morgan MY, Laulicht M, et al. Hepatic iron stores and markers of iron overload in alcoholics and patients with idiopathic hemochromatosis. Dig Dis Sci 27:909, 1982.
16. Sauer GF, Funk DD. Iron overload in cutaneous porphyria. Arch Intern Med 124:190, 1969.
17. Lundvall O, Weinfeld A, Lundin P. Iron storage in porphyria cutanea tarda. Acta Med Scand 188:37, 1970.
18. Conrad ME, Barton JC. Factors affecting iron balance. Am J Hematol 10:199, 1981.
19. Bacon BR, Tavill AS. Role of the liver in normal iron metabolism. Semin Liver Dis 4:181, 1984.
20. Gordeuk VR, Bacon BR, Brittenham GM. Iron overload: causes and consequences. Ann Rev Nutr 7:485, 1987.
21. Refsum SB, Schreiner BB. Regulation of iron balance by absorption and excretion. A critical review and a new hypothesis. Scand J Gastroenterol 9:867, 1984.
22. Hallberg L. Bioavailability of dietary iron in man. Ann Rev Nutr 1:123, 1981.
23. Cavill I, Worwood M, Jacobs A. Internal regulation of iron absorption. Nature 256:328, 1975.
24. Charlton RW, Bothwell TH. Iron absorption. Ann Rev Med 34:55, 1983.
25. Weintraub LR, Weinstein MB, Huser H, et al. Absorption of hemoglobin iron: the role of a heme-splitting substance in the intestinal mucosa. J Clin Invest 47:531, 1968.
26. Simpson RJ, Peters, TJ. Fe^{2+} uptake by intestinal brush-border membrane vesicles from normal and hypoxic mice. Biochim Biophys Acta 814:381, 1985.
27. Simpson RJ, Peters TJ. pH-Sensitive transport of Fe^{2+} across purified brush-border membrane from mouse intestine. Biochim Biophys Acta 856:109, 1986.
28. Simpson RJ, Raja KB, Peters TJ. Fe^{2+} uptake by mouse intestinal mucosa in vivo and by isolated intestinal brush-border membrane vesicles. Biochim Biophys Acta 860:229, 1986.
29. Parmley RT, Barton JC, Conrad ME. Ultrastructural localization of transferrin, transferrin receptor and iron binding sites on human placental and duodenal microvilli. Br J Haematol 60:81, 1985.
30. Huebers HA, Huebers E, Csiba E, et al. The significance of transferrin for intestinal iron absorption. Blood 61:283, 1983.

31. Simpson RJ, Osterloh KRS, Raja KB, et al. Studies on the role of transferrin and endocytosis in the uptake of Fe^{3+} from Fe-nitrilotriacetate by mouse duodenum. Biochim Biophys Acta 884:166, 1986.

32. Banerjee D, Flanagan PR, Cluett J, et al. Transferrin receptors in the human gastrointestinal tract. Relationship to body iron stores. Gastroenterology 91:861, 1986.

33. Simpson RJ, Peters TJ. Iron-binding lipids of rabbit duodenal brush-border membrane. Biochim Biophys Acta 898:181, 1987.

34. Stremmel W, Lotz G, Niederau C, et al. Iron uptake by rat duodenal microvillous membrane vesicle: evidence for a carrier mediated transport system. Eur J Clin Invest 17:136, 1987.

35. Finch CA, Huebers H, Eng M, et al. Effect of transfused reticulocytes on iron exchange. Blood 59:364, 1982.

36. Van Wyk CP, Linder-Horowitz M, Munro HN. Effect of iron loading on non-heme iron compounds in different liver cell populations. J Biol Chem 246:1025, 1971.

37. Morgan EH, Baker E. Iron uptake and metabolism by hepatocytes. Fed Proc 45:2810, 1986.

38. Young SP, Aisen P. Transferrin receptors and the uptake and release of iron by isolated hepatocytes. Hepatology 1:114, 1981.

39. Cole ES, Glass J. Transferrin binding and iron uptake in mouse hepatocytes. Biochim Biophys Acta 762:102, 1983.

40. Morley CGD, Bezkorovainy A. The behavior of transferrin receptors in rat hepatocyte plasma membranes. Clin Physiol Biochem 1:318, 1983.

41. Crichton RR, Charloteaux-Wanters M. Iron transport and storage. Eur J Biochem 164:485, 1987.

42. Page MA, Baker E, Morgan EH. Transferrin and iron uptake by rat hepatocytes in culture. Am J Physiol 246:G26, 1984.

43. Smith A, Morgan WT. Hemopexin-mediated transport of heme into isolated rat hepatocytes. J Biol Chem 256:10902, 1981.

44. Kino K, Tsunoo H, Higa Y, et al. Hemoglobin-haptoglobin receptor in rat liver plasma membrane. J Biol Chem 255:9616, 1980.

45. Mack U, Powell LW, Halliday JS. Detection and isolation of a hepatic membrane receptor for ferritin. J Biol Chem 258:4672, 1983.

46. Hershko C, Graham G, Bates GW, et al. Nonspecific serum iron in thalassemia-abnormal serum iron fraction of potential toxicity. Br J Haematol 40:255, 1978.

47. Wang WC, Ahmet N, Hanna M. Non-transferrin-bound iron in long-term transfusion in children with congenital anemias. J Pediatr 108:552, 1986.

48. Gutteridge JMC, Rowley DA, Griffiths E, et al. Low-molecular-weight iron complexes and oxygen radical reactions in idiopathic haemochromatosis. Clin Sci 68:463, 1985.

49. Brissot P, Wright TC, Ma WL, et al. Efficient clearance of non-transferrin-bound iron by rat liver. Implications for hepatic iron loading in iron overload states. J Clin Invest 76:1463, 1985.

50. Graven CM, Alexander J, Eldridge M, et al. Tissue distribution and clearance kinetics of non-transferrin-bound iron in the hypotransferrinemic mouse: A rodent model for hemochromatosis. Proc Natl Acad Sci 84:3457, 1987.

51. Hershko C, Peto TEA. Annotation: non-transferrin plasma iron. Br J Haematol 66:149, 1987.

52. Tenhunen R. The enzymatic degradation of heme. Semin Hematol 9:19, 1972.

53. Deiss A. Iron metabolism in reticuloendothelial cells. Semin Hematol 20:81, 1983.

54. Jacobs A. Low molecular weight intracellular iron transport compounds. Blood 50:433, 1977.

55. Romslo I. Intracellular transport of iron. In: Jacobs A, Worwood M, eds. Iron in Biochemistry and Medicine II. London, Academic Press, 1980:325.

56. Morley CGD, Beskorovainy A. Identification of the iron chelate in hepatocyte cytosol. IRCS Med Sci 11:1106, 1983.

57. Selden C, Peters TJ. Separation and assay of iron proteins in needle biopsy specimens of human liver. Clin Chim Acta 98:47, 1979.

58. Zuyderhoudt FMJ, Hengeveld P, Van Gool J, et al. A method for measurement of liver iron fractions in needle biopsy specimens and some results in acute liver disease. Clin Chim Acta 86:313, 1978.

59. Mulligan M, Althaus B, Linder MC. Non-ferritin, non-heme iron pools in rat tissues. Int J Biochem 18:791, 1986.

60. Schneider W, Erni I. Chemistry of transit iron pools. In: Saltman P, Hegenauer J, eds. The Biochemistry and Physiology of Iron. New York, Elsevier-North Holland 1982:121.

61. Parmley RT, May ME, Spicer SS, et al. Ultrastructural distribution of inorganic iron in normal and iron-loaded hepatic cells. Lab Invest 44:475, 1981.

62. Richter GW. The iron-loaded cell—the cytopathology of iron storage. Am J Pathol 91:363, 1978.

63. Munro HN, Linder MC. Ferritin: structure, biosynthesis and role in iron metabolism. Physiol Rev 58:317, 1978.

64. Wagstaff M, Worwood M, Jacobs A. Iron and isoferritins in iron overload. Clin Sci 61:529, 1982.

65. Bomford A, Conlon-Hollingshead C, Munro HN. Adaptive responses of rat tissue isoferritins to iron administration. Changes in subunit synthesis, isoferritin abundance and capacity for iron storage. J Biol Chem 256:948, 1981.

66. Arosio P, Yokota M, Drysdale JW. Structural and immunological relationships of isoferritins in normal and malignant cells. Cancer Res 36:1735, 1976.

67. Wixom RL, Prutkin L, Munro HN. Hemosiderin: nature, formation and significance. Int Rev Exp Pathol 22:193, 1980.

68. Richter GW. Studies of iron overload. Rat liver siderosome ferritin. Lab Invest 50:26, 1984.

69. Weir MP, Gibson JF, Peters TJ. Biochemical studies on the isolation and characterization of human spleen haemosiderin. Biochem J 223:31, 1984.

70. Weir MP, Sharp GA, Peters TJ. Electron microscopic studies of human haemosiderin and ferritin. J Clin Pathol 38:915, 1985.

71. Cook JD, Hershko C, Finch CA. Storage iron kinetics. V. Iron exchange in the rat. Br J Haematol 25:695, 1973.

72. Baker E, Morton AG, Tavill AS. The regulation of iron release from the perfused rat liver. Br J Haematol 45:607, 1980.

73. Baker E, Vicary FR, Huehns ER. Iron release from hepatocytes. Br J Haematol 47:493, 1981.

74. Baker E, Page M, Morgan EH. Transferrin and iron release from hepatocytes in culture. Am J Physiol 248:G93, 1985.

75. LeSage GD, Kost LJ, Barham SS, et al. Biliary excretion of iron from hepatocyte lysosomes in the rat. A major excretory pathway in experimenal iron overload. J Clin Invest 77:90, 1986.

76. McKusick VA. Mendelian inheritance in man, 5th ed. Baltimore, Johns Hopkins University Press, 1978.

77. Simon M, Bourel M, Fauchet R, et al. Association of HLA-A3 and HLA-B14 antigens with idiopathic hemochromatosis. Gut 17:332, 1976.

78. Lipinski M, Hors J, Saleun JP, et al. Idiopathic hemochromatosis: linkage with HLA. Tissue Antigens 11:471, 1978.

79. Kravitz K, Skolnick M, Cannings C, et al. Genetic linkage between hereditary hemochromatosis and HLA. Am J Hum Genet 31:601, 1979.

80. Doran TJ, Bashir HV, Trejaut J, et al. Idiopathic haemochromatosis in the Australian population: HLA linkage and recessivity. Hum Immunol 2:191, 1981.

81. Dadone MM, Kushner JP, Edwards CQ, et al. Hereditary hemochromatosis: analysis of laboratory expression of the disease by genotype in 18 pedigrees. Am J Clin Pathol 78:196, 1982.

82. LaLouel JM, LeMignon L, Simon M, et al. A combined qualitative (disease) and quantitative (serum iron) genetic analysis of idiopathic hemochromatosis. Am J Hum Genet 37:700, 1985.

83. Kidd KR. Genetic linkage and hemochromatosis. N Engl J Med 301:209, 1979.

84. Saddi R, Muller JY, Pouliquen A, et al. HLA-A3,B7 linkage disequilibrium in hemochromatosis patients with or without insulin dependent diabetes. Tissue Antigens 17:473, 1981.

85. Simon M, Fauchet R, Hespel JP, et al. Idiopathic hemochromatosis and HLA. In: Farid N, ed. HLA in Endocrine and Metabolic Disorders. New York, Academic Press, 1981:291.

86. King RC, Stansfield WD, eds. Dictionary of Genetics, 3rd ed. New York, Oxford University Press, 1985:222.

87. Simon M, LeMignon L, Fauchet R, et al. A study of 609 HLA haplotypes marking the hemochromatosis gene (1) mapping of the gene near the HLA-A locus and characters required to define a heterozygous population and (2) hypothesis concerning the underlying cause of hemochromatosis-HLA association. Am J Hum Genet 41:89, 1987.

88. David V, Paul P, Simon M, et al. DNA polymorphism related to the idiopathic hemochromatosis gene: evidence in a recombinant family. Hum Genet 74:113, 1986.

89. Beaumont C, Simon M, Fauchet R, et al. Serum ferritin as a possible marker of the hemochromatosis allele. N Engl J Med 301:169, 1979.

90. Simon M, Alexandre J-L, Fauchet R, et al. The genetics of hemochromatosis. Prog Med Genet 4:135, 1980.

91. Edwards CQ, Skolnick MH, Kushner JP. Hereditary hemochromatosis: contributions of genetic analyses. Prog Hematol 12:43, 1981.

92. Cartwright GE, Edwards CQ, Kravitz K, et al. Hereditary hemochromatosis. Phenotypic expression of the disease. N Engl J Med 301:175, 1979.

93. Valberg LS, Lloyd DA, Ghent CN, et al. Clinical and biochemical expression of the abnormality in idiopathic hemochromatosis. Gastroenterology 79:884, 1980.

94. Boender CA, Verloop MC. Iron absorption, iron loss and iron retention in man: studies after oral administration of a tracer dose of $^{59}FeSO_4$ and $^{131}BaSO_4$. Br J Haematol 17:45, 1969.

95. Powell LW, Campbell CB, Wilson E. Intestinal mucosal uptake of iron and iron retention in idiopathic haemochromatosis as evidence for a mucosal abnormality. Gut 11:727, 1970.

96. Marx JJ. Mucosal uptake, mucosal transfer and retention of iron, measured by whole body counting. Scand J Haematol 23:293, 1979.

97. Cox TM, Peters TJ. Uptake of iron by duodenal biopsy specimens from patients with iron-deficiency anemia and primary haemochromatosis. Lancet 1:123, 1978.

98. Cox TM, Peters TJ. In vitro studies of duodenal iron uptake in patients with primary and secondary iron storage disease. Q J Med 49:249, 1980.

99. Chados RB, Ross JF, Apt L, et al. The absorption of food iron and inorganic iron by normal, iron-deficient and hemochromatotic subjects. J Clin Invest 36:314, 1957.

100. Smith PM, Godrey BE, Williams R. Iron absorption in idiopathic haemochromatosis and its measurement using a whole-body counter. Clin Sci 37:519, 1969.

101. Walters GO, Jacobs A, Worwood M, et al. Iron absorption in normal subjects and patients with idiopathic haemochromatosis: relationship with serum ferritin concentration. Gut 16:188, 1975.

102. Williams R, Manenti F, Williams HS, et al. Iron absorption in idiopathic haemochromatosis before, during and after venesection therapy. Br Med J 2:78, 1966.

103. Deller DJ. Iron-59 absorption measurements by whole body counting: studies in alcoholic cirrhosis, hemochromatosis and pancreatitis. Am J Dig Dis 10:249, 1965.

104. Williams R, Pitcher CS, Parsonson A, et al. Iron absorption in relatives of patients with idiopathic haemochromatosis. Lancet 1:1243, 1965.

105. Pollycove M, Mortimer R. The quantitative determination of iron kinetics and hemoglobin synthesis in human subjects. J Clin Invest 40:753, 1961.

106. Pollycove M. Iron overload syndromes. Clin Physiol Biochem 4:61, 1986.

107. Pollycove M, Fawwaz RA, Winchell HS. Transient hepatic deposition of iron in primary hemochromatosis with iron deficiency following venesection. J Nucl Med 12:28, 1971.

108. Batey R, Pettit JE, Nicholas AW, et al. Hepatic iron clearance from serum in treated hemochromatosis. Gastroenterology 7:856, 1978.

109. Davis PS, Luke CG, Deller DJ. Reduction of gastric iron-binding protein in haemochromatosis. A previously unrecognized metabolic defect. Lancet 2:1431, 1966.

110. Luke CG, Davis PS, Deller DJ. Gastric iron binding in haemochromatosis, secondary iron overload, cirrhosis and diabetes. Lancet 2:844, 1968.

111. Wynter CV, Williams R. Iron-binding properties of gastric juice in idiopathic haemochromatosis. Lancet 2:534, 1968.

112. Morgan OS, Gatenby PB, Weir DG, et al. Studies on an iron-binding component in human gastric juice. Lancet 1:861, 1969.

113. Powell LW, Wilson E. In vivo intestinal mucosal uptake of iron, body iron absorption and gastric juice iron-binding in idiopathic haemochromatosis. Aust Ann Med 19:226, 1970.

114. Valberg LS, Simon JB, Manley PN, et al. Distribution of storage iron as body iron stores expand in patients with hemochromatosis. J Lab Clin Med 86:479, 1975.

115. Ross CE, Muir WA, Alan BP, et al. Hemochromatosis. Pathophysiologic and genetic considerations. Am J Clin Pathol 63:179, 1975.

116. Brink B, Disler P, Lynch S, et al. Patterns of iron storage in dietary iron overload and idiopathic hemochromatosis. J Lab Clin Med 88:725, 1976.

117. Green R, Saab GA, Conjalka MS, et al. Monocyte ferritin levels disproportionately low in untreated hemochromatosis (Abstract). Blood (Suppl) 52(1):80, 1978.

118. Jacobs A, Summers MR. Iron uptake and ferritin synthesis by peripheral blood leucocytes in patients with primary idiopathic haemochromatosis. Br J Haematol 49:649, 1981.

119. Bassett ML, Halliday JW, Powell LW. Ferritin synthesis in peripheral blood monocytes in idiopathic hemochromatosis. J Lab Clin Med 100:137, 1982.

120. McLaren GD, Konijn AM, Bentley DP, et al. Iron uptake and ferritin synthesis by human peripheral blood monocytes incubated in vitro with a particulate suspension of radio iron. In: Saltman P, Hegenauer J, eds. The Biochemistry and Physiology of Iron. New York, Elsevier-North Holland, 1982:605.

121. Sizemore DJ, Bassett ML. Monocyte transferrin-iron uptake in hereditary hemochromatosis. Am J Hematol 16:347, 1984.

122. Björn-Rasmussen E, Hageman J, Van den Dungen P, et al. Transferrin receptors on circulating monocytes in hereditary hemochromatosis. Scand J Haematol 34:308, 1985.

123. Astaldi G, Meardi G, Lisino T. The iron content of jejunal mucosa obtained by Crosby's capsule in hemochromatosis and hemosiderosis. Blood 28:70, 1966.

124. Crosby WH. The control of iron balance by the intestinal mucosa. Blood 22:441, 1963.

125. Bothwell TH, Jacobs P, Torrance JD. Studies on the behavior of transferrin in idiopathic hemochromatosis. South African J Med Sci 27:35, 1962.

126. Levine PH, Levine AJ, Weintraub LR. The role of transferrin in the control of iron absorption: Studies at a cellular level. J Lab Clin Med 80:333, 1972.

127. Morgan EH. The role of plasma transferrin in iron absorption in the rat. Q J Exp Physiol 65:239, 1980.

128. Mazurier J, Montreuil J, Spik G. Visualization of lactotransferrin brush-border receptors by ligand-blotting. Biochem Biophys Acta 821:453, 1985.

129. Osterloh KRS, Simpson RJ, Peters TJ. The role of mucosal transferrin in intestinal iron absorption (annotation). Br J Haematol 65:1, 1987.

130. Schümann K, Schafer SG, Forth W. Iron absorption and biliary secretion of transferrin in rats. Res Exp Med 186:215, 1986.

131. Peters TJ, Simpson RJ, Snape SD. Significance of dietary residence time and luminal transferrin levels for a transferrin-mediated mechanisms of iron absorption in the mouse (Abstract). J Physiol 384:468, 1987.

132. Jenkins T, Bothwell TH, Maier G, et al. Is transferrin normal in idiopathic haemochromatosis? Br J Haematol 52:493, 1982.

133. Regoeczi E, Chindemi RA, Debanne MT. Transferrin glycans: a possible link between alcoholism and hepatic cirrhosis. Alcoholism: Clin Exp Res 8:287, 1984.

134. Tsau MF, Scheffel U. Transferrin sialic acid contents of patients with hereditary hemochromatosis. Am J Hematol 20:359, 1985.

135. Wheby MS, Balcerzak SP, Anderson P, et al. Clearance of iron from hemochromatotic and normal transferrin in vivo. Blood 24:765, 1964.

136. Cartei G, Causarano D, Naccarato R. Transferrin behavior in primary haemochromatosis. Experientia 31:373, 1975.

137. Ward JH, Kushner JP, Kaplan J. Regulation of HeLa cell transferrin receptors. J Biol Chem 257:10317, 1982.

138. Ward JH, Kushner JP, Kaplan J. Transferrin receptors of human fibroblasts, analysis of receptor properties and regulation. Biochem J 208:19, 1982.

139. Davis RJ, Corvera S, Czech MP. Insulin stimulates cellular iron uptake and causes the redistribution of intracellular transferrin receptors to the plasma membrane. J Biol Chem 261:8708, 1986.

139a. Bomford AB, Munro HN. Transferrin and its receptor: their roles in cell function. Hepatology 5:870, 1985.

140. Roualt T, Rao K, Harford J, et al. Hemin, chelatable iron, and the regulation of transferrin receptor biosynthesis. J Biol Chem 260:14862, 1985.

141. Ward JH, Kushner JP, Ray FA, et al. Transferrin receptor function in hereditary hemochromatosis. J Lab Clin Med 103:246, 1984.

142. Sciot R, Paterson AC, Van den Oord JJ, et al. Lack of hepatic transferrin receptor expression in hemochromatosis. Hepatology 7:831, 1987.

142a. Anderson GJ, Halliday JW, Powell LW. Transferrin receptors in hemochromatosis. Hepatology 7:967, 1987.

143. Powell LW, Bassett ML, Halliday JW. Hemochromatosis: 1980 update. Gastroenterology 78:374, 1980.

144. Milder MS, Cook JD, Sunday S, et al. Idiopathic hemochromatosis, an interim report. Medicine 59:39, 1980.

145. McLaren GD, Muir WA, Kellermeyer RW. Iron overload disorders. Natural history, pathogenesis, diagnosis and therapy. CRC Crit Rev Clin Lab Sci 19:205, 1983.

146. Bassett ML, Halliday JW, Powell LW. Genetic hemochromatosis. Semin Liver Dis 4:217, 1984.

147. Bomford A, Williams R. Long-term results of venesection therapy in idiopathic haemochromatosis. Q J Med 45:611, 1976.

148. Bothwell TH, Charlton RW. Historical overview of hemochromatosis. Ann NY Acad Sci 526:1, 1988.

149. Bothwell TH, Isaacson C. Siderosis in the Bantu. A comparison of the incidence in males and females. Br Med J 1:522, 1962.

150. Barry M, Flynn DM, Letsky EA, et al. Long-term chelation therapy in thalassemia major: effect on liver iron concentration, liver histology and clinical progress. Br Med J 2:16, 1974.

151. Risdon RA, Barry M, Flynn DM. Transfusional iron overload: the relationship between tissue iron concentration and hepatic fibrosis in thalassemia. J Pathol 116:83, 1975.

152. Cohen A, Martin M, Schwartz E. Depletion of excessive liver iron stores with desferrioxamine. Br J Haematol 58:369, 1984.

153. Cohen A, Witzleben C, Schwartz E. Treatment of iron overload. Semin Liver Dis 4:228, 1984.

154. Tavill AS, Bacon BR. Hemochromatosis: how much iron is too much? Hepatology 6:142, 1986.

155. Jacobs A. The pathology of iron overload. In: Jacobs A, Worwood MK, eds. Iron in biochemistry and medicine, II. London, Academic Press, 1980:427.

156. Wills ED. Effects of iron overload on lipid peroxide formation and oxidative demethylation by the liver endoplasmic reticulum. Biochem Pharmacol 21:239, 1972.

157. Heys AD, Dormandy TL. Lipid peroxidation in iron-overloaded spleens. Clin Sci 60:295, 1981.

158. Dillard CJ, Tappel AL. Volatile hydrocarbon and carbonyl products of lipid peroxidation: a comparison of pentane, ethane, hexane and acetone as in vivo indices. Lipids 14:989, 1979.

159. Dillard CJ, Downey JE, Tappel AL. Effect of antioxidants on lipid peroxidation in iron-loaded rats. Lipids 19:127, 1984.

160. Gavino VC, Dillard CJ, Tappel AL. Release of ethane and pentane from rat tissue slices: effect of vitamin E, halogenated hydrocarbons and iron overload. Arch Biochem Biophys 233:741, 1984.

161. Britton RS, Bacon BR, Recknagel RO. Lipid peroxidation and associated hepatic organelle dysfunction in iron overload. Chem Phys Lipids 45:207, 1987.

162. Selden C, Owen M, Hopkins JMP, et al. Studies on the concentration and intracellular localization of iron proteins in liver biopsy specimens from patients with iron overload with special reference to their role in lysosomal disruption. Br J Haematol 44:593, 1980.

163. Mak TI, Weglicki WB. Characterization of iron-mediated peroxidative injury in isolated hepatic lysosomes. J Clin Invest 75:58, 1985.

164. O'Connell MJ, Ward RJ, Baum H, et al. The role of iron in ferritin and haemosiderin-mediated lipid peroxidation in lysosomes. Biochem J 229:135, 1985.

165. Peters TJ, O'Connell MJ, Ward RJ. Role of free-radical mediated lipid peroxidation in the pathogenesis of hepatic damage by lysosomal disruption. In: Poli G, Cheesemen KH, Dianzani MU, et al., eds. Free Radicals in Liver Injury. Oxford, IRL Press, 1985:107.

166. Frigerio R, Mela Q, Passiu G, et al. Iron overload and lysosomal stability in β-thalassemia intermedia and trait: correlation between serum ferritin and serum N-acetyl-β-D-glucosaminidase levels. Scand J Haematol 33:252, 1984.

167. Bacon BR, Tavill AS, Brittenham GM, et al. Hepatic lipid peroxidation in vivo in rats with chronic iron overload. J Clin Invest 71:429, 1983.

168. Bacon BR, Brittenham GM, Tavill AS, et al. Hepatic lipid peroxidation in vivo in rats with chronic dietary iron overload is dependent on hepatic iron concentration. Trans Assoc Am Phys 96:146, 1983.

169. Bacon BR, Park CH, Brittenham GM, et al. Hepatic mitochondrial oxidative metabolism in rats with chronic dietary iron overload. Hepatology 5:789, 1985.

170. Bacon BR, Healey JF, Brittenham GM, et al. Hepatic microsomal function in rats with chronic dietary iron overload. Gastroenterology 90:1844, 1986.

171. Halliwell B, Gutteridge JMC. Oxygen toxicity, oxygen radicals, transition metals and disease. Biochem J 219:1, 1984.

172. Halliwell B, Gutteridge JMC. Oxygen free radicals and iron in relation to biology and medicine: some problems and concepts. Arch Biochem Biophys 2467:501, 1986.

173. Aust SD, Morehouse LA, Thomas CE. Role of metals in oxygen radical reactions. J Free Radical Biol Med 1:3, 1985.

174. Thomas CE, Morehouse LA, Aust SD. Ferritin and superoxide-dependent lipid peroxidation. J Biol Chem 260:3275, 1985.

175. Bacon BR, Tavill AS, Brittenham GM, et al. Hepatotoxicity of chronic iron overload. Role of lipid peroxidation. In: Poli G, Cheeseman KH, Dianzani MU, et al., eds. Free Radicals in Liver Injury. Oxford, IRL Press, 1985:49.

176. Park CH, Bacon BR, Brittenham GM, et al. Pathology of dietary carbonyl iron overload in rats. Lab Invest 57:555, 1987.

177. Lisboa PE. Experimental hepatic cirrhosis in dogs caused by chronic massive iron overload. Gut 12:363, 1971.

178. Brissot P, Campion JP, Guillouzo A, et al. Experimental hepatic iron overload in the baboon: results of a two-year study. Evolution of biological and morphological hepatic parameters of iron overload. Dig Dis Sci 28:616, 1983.

179. Iancu TC, Rabinowitz H, Brissot P, et al. Iron overload of the liver in the baboon: an ultrastructural study. J Hepatol 1:261, 1985.

180. Weintraub LR, Goral A, Grasso J, et al. Pathogenesis of hepatic fibrosis in experimental iron overload. Br J Haematol 59:321, 1985.

181. Iancu TC, Neustein HB, Landing BH. The liver in thalassaemia major: ultrastructural observations. In: Iron Metabolism, Ciba Foundation Symposium 51 (New Series). New York, Elsevier North-Holland, 1977:293.

182. Wheby MS. Liver damage in disorders of iron overload. A hypothesis. Arch Intern Med 144:621, 1984.

183. Aruoma OI, Bomford A, Polson RJ, et al. Nontransferrin-bound iron in plasma from hemochromatosis patients: effect of phlebotomy therapy. Blood 72:1416, 1988.

184. Gutteridge JMC, Rowley DA, Griffith E, et al. Low-molecular-weight iron complexes and oxygen radical reactions in idiopathic haemochromatosis. Clin Sci 68:463, 1985.

185. Miniero R, Piga A, Luzzatto L, et al. Vitamin E and β-thalassemia. Haematologica (Pavia) 68:562, 1983.

186. Rachmilewitz EA, Lubin BH, Shoret SB. Lipid membrane peroxidation in β-thalassemia major. Blood 47:495, 1976.

187. Bacon BR, Britton RS, O'Neill R. Effects of vitamin E deficiency on hepatic mitochondrial lipid peroxidation and oxidative metabolism in rats with chronic dietary iron overload. Hepatology 9:398, 1989.

188. Brissot P, Geugnier Y, Letreut A, et al. Ascorbic acid status in idiopathic hemochromatosis. Digestion 17:479, 1978.

189. Seftel HC, Malkin C, Schmaman A, et al. Osteoporosis, scurvy and siderosis in Johannesburg Bantu. Br Med J 1:642, 1966.

190. Cohen A, Cohen IJ, Schwarz E. Scurvy and altered iron stores in thalassemia major. N Engl J Med 304:158, 1981.

191. Hussain MAM, Flynn DM, Green N, et al. Effect of dose, time and ascorbate on iron excretion after subcutaneous desferrioxamine. Lancet 1:977, 1977.

192. Wapnick AA, Lynch SR, Charlton RW, et al. The effect of ascorbic acid deficiency on desferrioxamine-induced urinary iron excretion. Br J Haematol 17:563, 1969.

193. Nienhuis AW. Vitamin C and iron. N Engl J Med 304:170, 1981.

194. Roeser HP. The role of ascorbic acid in the turnover of storage iron. Semin Hematol 30:91, 1983.

195. Vender Weyden MB. Vitamin C, desferrioxamine and iron loading anemias. Aust NZ J Med 14:593, 1984.

196. Scheuer PJ, Williams R, Muir AR. Hepatic pathology in relatives of patients with haemochromatosis. J Pathol Bacteriol 84:53, 1962.

197. Brick IB. Liver histology in six asymptomatic siblings in a family with hemochromatosis; genetic implications. Gastroenterology 40:210, 1961.

198. Bothwell TH, Cohen I, Abrahams OL, et al. A familial study in idiopathic hemochromatosis. Am J Med 27:730, 1959.

199. Edwards CO, Cartwright GE, Skolnick MH, et al. Homozygosity for hemochromatosis: clinical manifestations. Ann Intern Med 93:519, 1980.

200. Powell LW, Kerr JFR. The pathology of the liver in hemochromatosis. Pathobiol Ann 5:317, 1975.

201. Trump BF, Valigorsky JM, Arstila AA, et al. The relationship of intracellular pathways of iron metabolism to cellular iron overload and iron storage diseases. Am J Pathol 72:295, 1973.

202. Hoy TG, Jacobs A. Ferritin polymers and the formation of haemosiderin. Br J Haematol 49:593, 1981.

203. Hoy TG, Jacobs A. Changes in the characteristics and distribution of ferritin in iron loaded cell cultures. Biochem J 193:87, 1981.

204. Beaumont C, Simon M, Smith PM, et al. Hepatic and serum ferritin concentration in patients with idiopathic hemochromatosis. Gastroenterology 79:877, 1980.

205. Seymour CA, Peters TJ. Organelle pathology in primary and secondary haemochromatosis with special reference to lysosomal changes. Br J Haematol 40:239, 1978.

206. Bothwell TH, Abrahams C, Bradlow BA, et al. Idiopathic and Bantu haemochromatosis: comparative histological study. Arch Pathol 79:163, 1965.

207. Jacobs A. Iron overload—clinical and pathologic aspects. Semin Hematol 14:89, 1977.

208. Chevrant-Breton J, Simon M, Bourel M, et al. Cutaneous manifestations of idiopathic hemochromatosis. A study of 100 cases. Arch Dermatol 113:161, 1977.

209. Buja LM, Roberts WC. Iron in the heart. Etiology and clinical significance. Am J Med 51:209, 1971.

210. Atkins CJ, McIvor J, Smith RM, et al. Chondrocalcinosis and arthropathy: studies in haemochromatosis and in idiopathic chondrocalcinosis. Q J Med 39:71, 1970.

211. Shumacher HR. Hemochromatosis and arthritis. Arthritis Rheum 7:41, 1964.

212. Schumacher HR. Articular cartilage in the degenerative arthropathy of hemochromatosis. Arthritis Rheum 25:1460, 1982.

213. Oliver RAM. Siderosis following transfusions of blood. J Pathol Bacteriol 77:171, 1959.

214. Jakobovits AW, Morgan MY, Sherlock S. Hepatic siderosis in alcoholics. Dig Dis Sci 24:305, 1979.

215. Kent G, Popper H. Liver biopsy in diagnosis of hemochromatosis. Am J Med 44:837, 1968.

216. Finch SC, Finch CA. Idiopathic hemochromatosis, an iron storage disease. Medicine 34:381, 1955.

217. Bothwell TH, Charlton RW, Cook JD, et al. Iron metabolism in man. Oxford, Blackwell Scientific, 1979.

218. Ammann RW, Müller E, Bansky J, et al. High incidence of extrahepatic carcinomas in idiopathic hemochromatosis. Scand J Gastroenterol 15:733, 1980.

219. Macsween RN. Acute abdominal crisis, circulatory collapse and sudden death in haemochromatosis. Q J Med 35:589, 1966.

220. Jones NL. Irreversible shock in haemochromatosis. Lancet 1:569, 1962.

221. Dymock IW, Cassar J, Pyke DA, et al. Observations on the pathogenesis, complications and treatment of diabetes in 115 cases of haemochromatosis. Am J Med 52:203, 1972.

222. Griffiths JD, Dymock IW, Davies EWG, et al. Occurrence and prevalence of diabetic retinopathy in hemochromatosis. Diabetes 20:766, 1971.

223. Davies G, Dymock IW, Harry J, et al. Deposition of melanin and iron

in ocular structures in haemochromatosis. Br J Ophthalmol 56:338, 1972.

224. Modell B, Berdoukas V. Death and survival. In: The Clinical Approach to Thalassemia. London, Grune & Stratton, 1984:151.

225. Engle MA. Cardiac involvement in Cooley's anemia. Ann NY Acad Sci 119:694, 1964.

226. Ehlers KH, Levin AR, Markenson AL, et al. Longitudinal study of cardiac function in thalassemia major. Ann NY Acad Sci 344:397, 1980.

227. Vigorita VJ, Hutchins GM. Cardiac conduction system in hemochromatosis: clinical and pathologic features of six patients. Am J Cardiol 44:418, 1979.

228. Candell-Riera J, Lu L, Seres L, et al. Cardiac hemochromatosis: beneficial effects of iron removal therapy. Am J Cardiol 52:824, 1983.

229. Link G, Pinson A, Hershko C. Heart cells in culture: a model of myocardial iron-overload and chelation. J Lab Clin Med 106:147, 1985.

230. Hamilton E, Williams R, Barlow KA, et al. The arthropathy of idiopathic haemochromatosis. Q J Med 37:171, 1968.

231. Askari AD, Muir WA, Rosner IA, et al. Arthritis of hemochromatosis. Clinical spectrum, relation to histocompatibility antigens and effectiveness of early phlebotomy. Am J Med 75:957, 1983.

232. Alexander GM, Dieppe PA, Doherty M, et al. Pyrophosphate arthropathy: a study of metabolic associations and laboratory data. Ann Rheum Dis 41:377, 1982.

233. Utsinger PD, Zvaifler NJ, Resnick D. Calcium pyrophosphate dihydrate deposition disease without chondrocalcinosis. J Rheumatol 2:258, 1975.

234. Abbott DF, Gresham GA. Arthropathy in transfusional siderosis. Br Med J 1:418, 1972.

235. Stocks AE, Martin FIR. Pituitary function in hemochromatosis. Am J Med 45:839, 1968.

236. Stocks AE, Powell LW. Pituitary function in idiopathic haemochromatosis and cirrhosis of the liver. Lancet 2:298, 1972.

237. Bezwoda WR, Bothwell TH, Van der Walt LA, et al. An investigation into gonadal function in patients with idiopathic haemochromatosis. Clin Endocrinol 6:377, 1977.

238. Capron JP, Capron-Chivrac D, Tosson H. Spontaneous Yersinia enterocolitica peritonitis in idiopathic hemochromatosis. Gastroenterology 87:1372, 1984.

239. Chiesa C, Pacifico L, Renzulli F, et al. Yersinia hepatic abscesses and iron overload. JAMA 257:3230, 1987.

240. Yamaschiro KW, Goldman RH, Harris DR, et al. Pasteurella pseudotuberculosis acute sepsis with survival. Arch Intern Med 128:605, 1971.

241. Blake PA, Merson MH, Weaver RE, et al. Disease caused by a marine vibrio. N Engl J Med 300:1, 1979.

242. Van Asbeck BS, Verbrugh HA, Van Oost BA, et al. Listeria monocytogenes meningitis and decreased phagocytosis associated with iron overload. Br Med J 284:542, 1982.

243. Weinberg ED. Iron withholding: a defense against infection and neoplasm. Physiol Rev 64:65, 1984.

244. Weinberg ED. Iron, infection and neoplasia. Clin Physiol Biochem 4:50, 1986.

245. Wright AC, Simpson LM, Oliver JD. Role of iron in the pathogenesis of Vibrio vulnificus infections. Infect Immunol 34:503, 1981.

246. Weinberg ED. Iron and susceptibility to infectious disease. Science 184:952, 1974.

247. Hegenauer J, Saltman P. Letter: Iron and susceptibility to infectious disease. Science 188:1038, 1975.

248. Perman G. Hemochromatosis and red wine. Acta Med Scand 182:281, 1967.

249. Barry M. Iron overload: clinical aspects, evaluation and treatment. Clin Haematol 2:405, 1973.

250. Brissot P, Bourel M, Henry D, et al. Assessment of liver iron content in 271 patients; a re-evaluation of direct and indirect methods. Gastroenterology 80:557, 1981.

251. Lundvall O, Weinfeld A, Lundin P. Iron stores in alcohol abusers. I. Liver iron. Acta Med Scand 185:259, 1969.

252. Lundvall O, Weinfeld A. Iron stores in alcohol abusers. II. As measured with the desferrioxamine test. Acta Med Scand 185:271, 1969.

253. Powell LW. The role of alcoholism in hepatic iron storage disease. Ann NY Acad Sci 252:124, 1975.

254. LeSage GD, Baldus WP, Fairbanks VF, et al. Hemochromatosis: genetic or alcohol-induced? Gastroenterology 84:1471, 1983.

255. Simon M, Bourel M, Genetet B, et al. Idiopathic hemochromatosis and iron overload in alcoholic liver disease: differentiation by HLA phenotype. Gastroenterology 73:655, 1977.

256. Charache S, Gittelsohn AM, Allen H, et al. Noninvasive assessment of tissue iron stores. Am J Clin Pathol 88:333, 1987.

257. Powell LW, Halliday JW. Iron metabolism, iron absorption and iron storage disorders. Viewpoints Dig Dis 14:13, 1982.

258. Halliday JW, Cowlishaw JL, Russo AM, et al. Serum ferritin in diagnosis of haemochromatosis—a study of 43 families. Lancet 2:621, 1977.

259. Bassett ML, Halliday JW, Ferris RA, et al. Diagnosis of hemochromatosis in young subjects: predictive accuracy of biochemical screening tests. Gastroenterology 87:628, 1984.

260. Finch CA. The detection of iron overload. N Engl J Med 307:1702, 1982.

261. Reissmann KR, Dietrich MR. On the presence of ferritin in the peripheral blood of patients with hepatocellular disease. J Clin Invest 35:588, 1956.

262. Addison GM, Beamish MR, Hales CN, et al. An immunoradiometric assay for ferritin in the serum of normal subjects and patients with iron deficiency and iron overload. J Clin Pathol 25:326, 1972.

263. Jacobs A, Miller F, Worwood M, et al. Ferritin in the serum of normal subjects and patients with iron deficiency and iron overload. Br Med J 4:206, 1972.

264. Walters GO, Miller FM, Worwood M. Serum ferritin concentration and iron stores in normal subjects. J Clin Pathol 26:770, 1973.

265. Worwood M. Editorial review: serum ferritin. Clin Sci 70:215, 1986.

266. Cragg SJ, Wagstaff M, Worwood M. Detection of a glycosylated subunit in human serum ferritin. Biochem J 199:565, 1981.

267. Prieto J, Barry M, Sherlock S. Serum ferritin in patients with iron overload and with acute and chronic liver diseases. Gastroenterology 68:525, 1975.

268. Worwood M, Cragg SJ, Wagstaff M, et al. Binding of human serum ferritin to concanavalin A. Clin Sci 56:83, 1979.

269. Edwards CQ, Carroll M, Bray P, et al. Hereditary hemochromatosis: diagnosis in siblings and children. N Engl J Med 297:7, 1977.

270. Batey RG, Hussein S, Sherlock S, et al. The role of serum ferritin in the management of idiopathic haemochromatosis. Scand J Gastroenterol 13:953, 1978.

271. Wands JR, Rowe JA, Mezey SE, et al. Normal serum ferritin concentrations in precirrhotic hemochromatosis. N Engl J Med 294:302, 1976.

272. Rowe JW, Wands JR, Mezey E, et al. Familial hemochromatosis: characteristics of the precirrhotic stage in a large kindred. Medicine (Baltimore) 56:197, 1977.

273. Feller ER, Pont A, Wands JR, et al. Familial hemochromatosis: physiological studies in the precirrhotic stage of the disease. N Engl J Med 296:1422, 1977.

274. Bassett ML, Powell LW, Halliday JM, et al. Early detection of idiopathic haemochromatosis: relative value of serum ferritin and HLA typing. Lancet 2:4, 1979.

275. Weinfeld A, Lundin P, Lundvall O. Significance for the diagnosis of iron overload of histochemical and chemical iron in the liver of normal subjects. J Clin Pathol 21:35, 1968.

276. Walker RJ, Miller JPG, Dymock IW, et al. Relationship of hepatic iron concentration to histochemical grading and total chelatable iron in conditions associated with iron overload. Gut 12:1011, 1971.

277. Barry M. Liver iron concentration, stainable iron and total body storage iron. Gut 15:411, 1974.

278. Kreeftenberg HG, Koopman BJ, Huizenga JR, et al. Measurement of iron in liver biopsies—a comparison of three analytical methods. Clin Chim Acta 144:255, 1984.

279. Torrance JD, Bothwell TH. A simple technique for measuring storage iron concentrations in formalinized liver samples. S Afr J Med Sci 33:9, 1968.

280. Mills SR, Doppman JL, Nienhuis AW. Computed tomography in the diagnosis of excessive iron storage of the liver. J Comp Asst Tomogr 1:101, 1977.

281. Howard JM, Ghent CN, Carey LS, et al. Diagnostic efficacy of hepatic computed tomography in the detection of body iron overload. Gastroenterology 84:209, 1983.

282. Houang MTW, Arozena X, Skalicka A, et al. Correlation between computed tomographic values and liver iron content in thalassemia major with iron overload. Lancet 1:1322, 1979.

283. Chapman RWG, Williams G, Bydder G, et al. Computed tomography for determining liver iron content in primary haemochromatosis. Br Med J 280:440, 1980.

284. Brittenham GM, Danish EH, Harris JW. Assessment of bone marrow and body iron stores: old techniques and new technologies. Semin Hematol 18:194, 1981.

285. Brittenham GM, Farrell DE, Harris JW, et al. Magnetic susceptibility measurement of human iron stores. N Engl J Med 307:1671, 1982.

286. Stark DD, Moseley ME, Bacon BR, et al. Magnetic resonance imaging and spectroscopy of hepatic iron overload. Radiology 154:137, 1985.

287. Stark DD. Liver. In: Stark DD, Bradley WG, eds. Magnetic Resonance Imaging, Chap. 38. St. Louis, CV Mosby Co, 1988:934.

288. Gollan JL. Diagnosis of hemochromatosis. Gastroenterology 84:418, 1983.

289. Powell LW, Axelson E, Bassett ML, et al. Do all homozygotes for

genetic hemochromatosis develop iron overload? (Abstr.) Hepatology 7:1051, 1987.

290. Bassett ML, Halliday JW, Powell LW. HLA typing in idiopathic hemochromatosis: distinction between homozygotes and heterozygotes with biochemical expression. Hepatology 1:120, 1981.

291. Weintraub LR, Conrad ME, Crosby WH. The treatment of hemochromatosis by phlebotomy. Med Clin North Am 50:1533, 1966.

292. Powell LW, Kerr JFR. Reversal of "cirrhosis" in idiopathic hemochromatosis following long-term intensive venesection therapy. Aust Ann Med 1:54, 1970.

293. Pippard MJ, Callender ST. The management of iron chelation therapy. Br J Haematol 54:503, 1983.

294. Nienhuis AW, Peterson DJ, Henry W. Evaluation of endocrine and cardiac function in patients with iron overload on chelation therapy. In: Zaino EC, Roberts RH, eds. Chelation Therapy in Chronic Iron Overload. Miami, Symposia Specialists, 1977:1.

295. Cliff JL, Speight ANP. Venesection in haemosiderosis. East Afr Med J 53:289, 1976.

296. Pimstone NR. Porphyria cutanea tarda. Semin Liver Dis 2:132, 1982.

297. Grace ND, Greenberg MS. Phlebotomy in the treatment of iron overload: a controlled trial (a preliminary report) (Abstr). Gastroenterology 60:744, 1971.

298. Modell B, Letsky EA, Flynn DM, et al. Survival and desferrioxamine in thalassaemia major. Br Med J 284:1081, 1982.

299. Hoffbrand AV, Gorman A, Laulicht M, et al. Improvement in iron status and liver function in patients with transfusional iron overload with long-term subcutaneous desferrioxamine. Lancet 1:947, 1979.

300. Propper RD, Shurin SB, Nathan DG. Reassessment of the use of desferrioxamine B in iron overload. N Engl J Med 294:1421, 1976.

301. Pippard MJ, Callender ST, Finch CA. Ferrioxamine excretion in iron-loaded man. Blood 60:288, 1982.

302. Wadiwala I, Tavill AS, Louis L, et al. Hepatobiliary iron excretion in dietary iron overload: preferential response to deferoxamine chelation (Abstr.). Hepatology 7:1107, 1987.

303. Schafer AI, Cheron RG, Dluhy R, et al. Clinical consequences of acquired transfusional iron overload in adults. N Engl J Med 304:319, 1981.

304. Weatherall DJ, Clegg JB. The Thalassaemia Syndromes, 3rd ed. Oxford, Blackwell Scientific, 1981.

305. Cartwright GE, Edwards CQ, Skolnick MH, et al. Association of HLA-linked hemochromatosis with idiopathic refractory sideroblastic anemia. J Clin Invest 65:989, 1980.

306. Simon M. Secondary iron overload and the hemochromatosis allele. Br J Haematol 60:1, 1985.

307. Fargion S, Piperno A, Panaiotopoulos N, et al. Iron overload in subjects with beta-thalassemia trait: role of idiopathic haemochromatosis gene. Br J Haematol 61:487, 1985.

308. Simon M, Beaumont C, Briere J, et al. Is the HLA-linked hemochromatosis allele implicated in idiopathic refractory sideroblastic anaemia? Br J Haematol 60:75, 1985.

309. Kushner JP, Edwards CQ, Dadone MM, et al. Heterozygosity for HLA-linked hemochromatosis as a likely cause of the hepatic siderosis associated with sporadic porphyria cutanea tarda. Gastroenterology 88:1232, 1985.

310. Kushner JP, Edwards CQ, Dadone MM, et al. HLA-linked hemochromatosis and sporadic porphyria cutanea tarda (letter). Gastroenterology 90:801, 1986.

311. Beaumont C, Fauchet R, Nhu Phung L, et al. Porphyria cutanea tarda and HLA-linked hemochromatosis: evidence against a systematic association. Gastroenterology 92:1833, 1987.

312. Adams PC, Powell LW. Porphyria cutanea tarda and HLA-linked hemochromatosis—all in the family? Gastroenterology 92:2033, 1987.

313. Grossman ME, Bickers DR, Poh-Fitzpatrick MB, et al. Porphyria cutanea tarda. Clinical and laboratory findings in 40 patients. Am J Med 67:277, 1979.

314. Mukerji SK, Pimstone NR, Burns M. Dual mechanism of inhibition of rat liver uroporphyrinogen decarboxylase activity by ferrous iron: its potential role in the genesis of porphyria cutanea tarda. Gastroenterology 87:1248, 1984.

315. Kushner JP, Steinmuller D, Lee GR. The role of iron in the pathogenesis of porphyria cutanea tarda II. Inhibition of uroporphyrinogen decarboxylase. J Clin Invest 56:661, 1975.

316. De Verneuil H, Sassa S, Kappas A. Effects of polychlorinated biphenyl compounds, 2,3,7,8-tetrachlorodibenzo-p-dioxin, phenobarbital and iron on uroporphyrinogen decarboxylase. Implications for the pathogenesis of porphyria. Biochem J 214:145, 1983.

317. Bonkovsky HL, Healey JF, Sinclair PR, et al. Iron and the liver: acute effects of iron-loading on hepatic heme synthesis of rats. Role of decreased activity of 5-amino-levulinate dehydrase. J Clin Invest 71:1175, 1983.

318. Bonkovsky HL, Healey JF, Lincoln B, et al. Hepatic heme synthesis in a new model of experimental hemochromatosis: studies in rats fed finely divided elemental iron. Hepatology 7:2295, 1987.

319. Felsher BF, Carpio NM, Engleking DW, et al. Decreased hepatic uroporphyrinogen decarboxylase activity in porphyria cutanea tarda. N Engl J Med 306:766, 1982.

320. Lundvall O. The effect of phlebotomy in porphyria cutanea tarda. Acta Med Scand 189:33, 1971.

321. Epstein JH, Redeker AG. Porphyria cutanea tarda: a study of the effect of phlebotomy. N Engl J Med 279:1301, 1968.

322. Lundvall O. The effect of replenishment of iron stores after phlebotomy therapy in porphyria cutanea tarda. Acta Med Scand 189:51, 1971.

323. Felsher BF, Jones ML, Redeker AG. Iron and hepatic uroporphyrin synthesis: relation in porphyria cutanea tarda. JAMA 226:663, 1973.

324. Elder GH, Tovey JA, Sheppard DM, et al. Immunoreactive uroporphyrinogen decarboxylase in porphyria cutanea tarda. Lancet 1:1301, 1983.

325. Elder GH, Urquhart AJ, DeSalamanca RE, et al. Immunoreactive uroporphyrin decarboxylase in the liver in porphyria cutanea tarda. Lancet 2:229, 1986.

326. Toback AC, Sassa S, Poh-Fitzpatrick MB, et al. Hepatoerythropoietic porphyria: clinical, biochemical and enzymatic studies in a three-generation family lineage. N Engl J Med 316:645, 1987.

327. Sinclair PR, Bement WJ, Bonkovsky HC, et al. Inhibition of uroporphyrinogen decarboxylase by halogenated biphenyls in chick hepatocyte cultures. Essential role for induction of cytochrome P-448. Biochem J 222:737, 1984.

328. Sinclair PR, Bement WJ, Bonkovsky HL, et al. Uroporphyrin accumulation produced by halogenated biphenyls in chick embryo hepatocytes. Revised of the accumulation by piperonyl butoxide. Biochem J 247:63, 1986.

329. Smith AG, Francis JE, Kay SJE, et al. Mechanistic studies of the inhibition of hepatic uroporphyrinogen decarboxylase in C57BL/10 mice by iron-hexachlorobenzene synergism. Biochem J 238:871, 1986.

330. Smith AG, Francis JE. Chemically-induced formation of an inhibitor of hepatic uroporphyrinogen decarboxylase in inbred mice with iron overload. Biochem J 246:221, 1987.

331. Knisely AS, Magid MS, Dische MR, et al. Neonatal hemochromatosis. Birth Defects 22:75, 1987.

332. Silver MM, Beverley DW, Valberg LS, et al. Perinatal hemochromatosis: clinical, morphologic, and quantitative iron studies. Am J Pathol 128:538, 1987.

333. Blisard KS, Bartow SA. Neonatal hemochromatosis. Hum Pathol 17:376, 1986.

334. Goldfischer S, Grotsky HW, Chang CH, et al. Idiopathic neonatal iron storage involving the liver, pancreas, heart, and endocrine and exocrine glands. Hepatology 1:58, 1981.

335. Faulk WP, Galbraith GMP. Trophoblast transferrin and transferrin receptors in the host-parasite relationship of human pregnancy. Proc R Soc Lond B 204:83, 1979.

336. Loh TT, Higuchi DA, Van Bockxmeer FM, et al. Transferrin receptors on the human placental microvillous membrane. J Clin Invest 65:1182, 1980.

337. Brown PJ, Molloy CM, Johnson PM. Transferrin receptor affinity and iron transport in the human placenta. Placenta 3:21, 1982.

338. Pearse BMF. Coated vesicles from human placenta carry ferritin, transferrin and immunoglobulin G. Proc Natl Acad Sci 79:451, 1982.

339. Morton AG, Tavill AS. The role of iron in the regulation of hepatic transferrin synthesis. Br J Haematol 36:383, 1977.

49

Inborn Errors of Metabolism That Lead to Permanent Liver Injury

Fayez K. Ghishan, M.D. • *Harry L. Greene, M.D.*

ABBREVIATIONS

ADP = adenosine diphosphate
ATP = adenosine triphosphate
BSP = sulfobromophthalein
FDPase = fructose-1,6-diphosphatase
GSD = glycogen storage disease
HFI = hereditary fructose intolerance
PAS = periodic acid–Schiff
P_i = inorganic phosphate
PRPP = phosphoribosyl pyrophosphate
THCA = $3\alpha,7\alpha,12\alpha$-trihydroxy-5β-cholestan-26-oic acid
TPN = total parenteral nutrition
UDP = uridine diphosphate

The liver is often affected by inborn errors of metabolism, but only a few of them injure it severly enough to cause permanent damage. The use of the Menghini needle for percutaneous liver biopsy has proved safe in infants and children, so histologic and biochemical evaluations of liver specimens from living patients has provided the means for major advances in the study of metabolic diseases during the last few years. Continued research in this area promises greater advances in diagnosis and treatment of metabolic illnesses as our understanding of the pathophysiology of such disorders improves. Table 49–1 lists the major metabolic diseases that involve the liver. Those marked with asterisks may lead to progressive disease and are discussed here or elsewhere in this book.

EVALUATION OF HEPATIC METABOLIC DISORDERS

The clinical history and physical examination are the first essentials in evaluating infants and children with metabolic liver disorders. Of particular importance is a family history of any metabolic liver disease. Symptoms that may be associated with metabolic liver disorders are usually nonspecific and include vomiting, diarrhea, jaundice, seizures, and abnormal urinary odor. Clinical findings include hepatosplenomegaly, hypotonicity or hypertonicity, coarse facial features, and respiratory distress. The physical examination should include adequate ophthalmologic examination by slit lamp for corneal, lenticular, and retinal alterations. Psychomotor evaluation to detect developmental delays is important in identifying those diseases that may involve the central nervous system. Initial laboratory screening tests such as analysis of the urine for reducing substances may help in early diagnosis of galactosemia. The peripheral blood smear may reveal vacuolation of the

TABLE 49–1. INBORN ERRORS OF METABOLISM RESULTING IN INJURY TO THE LIVER

Inborn errors of carbohydrate metabolism
　*Glycogen storage disease, types I–XII
　*Galactosemia
　*Fructose intolerance
　　Fructose-1-phosphate aldolase deficiency
　　Fructose-1,6-diphosphatase deficiency
Inborn errors of protein metabolism
　*Tyrosinemia
　Urea cycle enzymic defects
Inborn errors of lipid metabolism
　Gaucher's disease
　Niemann-Pick disease
　Gangliosidosis
　*Acid cholesterol ester hydrolase deficiency
　　Wolman's disease
　　Cholesterol ester storage disease
　Lipodystrophy
Inborn errors of mucopolysaccharide metabolism
Inborn errors of porphyrin metabolism
　*Protoporphyria (discussed in Chap. 14)
Inborn errors of bile acid metabolism
　*Byler's disease
　*Arteriohepatic dysplasia
　Benign recurrent cholestasis
　*Zellweger's syndrome
　*The THCA syndrome
Inborn error of copper metabolism
　*Wilson's disease (discussed in Chap. 47)
Unclassified
　*Alpha$_1$-antitrypsin deficiency
　*Cystic fibrosis

*Diseases that lead to progressive disease and are discussed in this chapter or other sections of this book.

lymphocytic cytoplasm, which signifies deposition of storage material. Skeletal x-rays may reveal changes consistent with certain storage diseases, as in the case of mucopolysaccharidosis. In general, storage diseases usually cause marked hepatomegaly. By contrast, disorders resulting in hepatocellular damage cause only modest hepatomegaly. Confirmatory tests depend on assays of appropriate enzymes in tissues such as leukocytes, skin fibroblasts, intestine, and liver.

DISORDERS OF CARBOHYDRATE METABOLISM

Inborn errors resulting from abnormal metabolism of lipids are mostly untreatable at present, and most of the errors in protein metabolism that respond to treatment require relatively stringent dietary restrictions. In contrast, most errors in carbohydrate metabolism, which respond favorably to treatment, do so with relatively modest dietary restrictions. Liver diseases that may occur in untreated patients with inborn errors of carbohydrate metabolism such as fructose intolerance and galactosemia are usually preventable. Although these particular conditions are relatively rare (about one in 30,000 live births for fructose intolerance and one in 20,000 live births for galactosemia), their combined incidence is similar to that of phenylketonuria (about one in 14,000 births in the United States). Considering the outcome in untreated patients and the simplicity of either measuring urinary reducing sugar or assaying the blood sample that is obtained to screen for phenylketonuria, it seems reasonable to implement the practice of routine screening of all newborn infants for both galactosemia and fructose intolerance.

Three inborn errors in carbohydrate metabolism that may result in permanent liver damage are disorders of fructose metabolism, disorders of galactose metabolism, and certain of the glycogen storage diseases (Fig. 49–1). These three abnormalities are discussed separately.

DISORDERS OF FRUCTOSE METABOLISM

Fructose Phosphate Aldolase Deficiency (Hereditary Fructose Intolerance) and Fructose-1,6-Diphosphatase Deficiency

Until the midfifties, the only identified defect in fructose metabolism was the benign disorder essential fructosuria, identified because of the large amounts of fructose in the urine following oral fructose ingestion.[1] It was recognized in 1956 that in some patients, ingestion of fructose was followed by vomiting, severe hypoglycemia, and liver disease.[2] A year later, this illness was characterized and named hereditary fructose intolerance (HFI).[3] A third disorder of fructose metabolism was identified in 1970. It was associated with fasting-induced as well as diet-induced hypoglycemia, but more strikingly, both fasting and dietary fructose caused lactic acidosis.[4] Each of these three disor-

ders is distinct from the others both clinically and biochemically. Essential fructosuria is due to deficient activity of hepatic fructokinase, HFI is due to deficiency of fructose-1-phosphate aldolase, and the third condition results from deficiency of fructose-1,6-diphosphatase (FDPase). Essential fructosuria does not cause liver injury. Patients with FDPase deficiency may show transient fatty infiltration of the liver. However, liver injury may be a permanent feature of HFI. For this reason, only HFI is discussed in detail.

Hereditary Fructose Intolerance

In 1957, Froesch and colleagues described the typical syndrome of HFI in two siblings and two relatives.[3] They recognized that the disorder, like essential fructosuria, was inherited and was associated with urinary excretion of fructose, but that it was due to a different enzymatic defect and had different prognostic implications.

Clinical Features

Patients with HFI may be extremely ill and may die after continuous exposure to fructose. However, affected patients are generally healthy and symptom-free so long as they do not ingest fructose or fructose-containing foods.[5, 6] For this reason symptoms do not arise until breast milk or cow's milk formulas are supplemented with fructose-containing foods. In fortunate cases, fructose is not introduced until after an affected infant is 5 to 6 months of age. By this time, the child is likely to associate nausea, vomiting, and symptoms of hypoglycemia with sweet-tasting food. In such cases, aversion to sweets is probably life-saving, and the diagnosis may go undetected until adulthood.[7] When this occurs, the diagnosis may be suspected on the basis of a careful history that recognizes the extreme aversion to dietary "sweets."

The largest single collection of patients consists of 55 patients diagnosed between 1961 and 1977 as having HFI.[8] Fifty of the patients had become symptomatic because of dietary fructose, and five cases were diagnosed shortly after

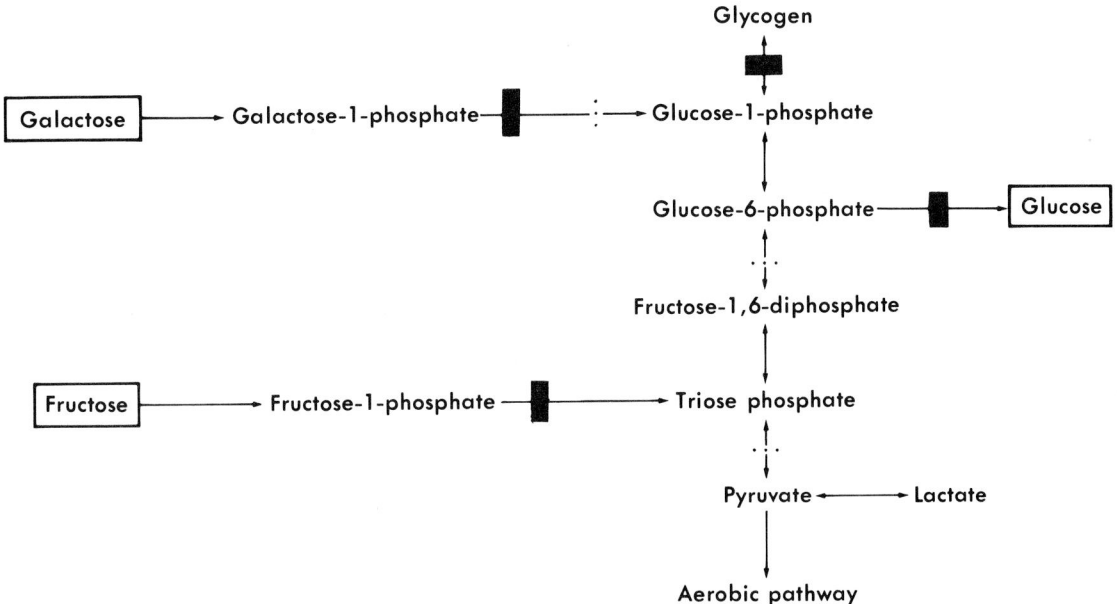

Figure 49–1. Metabolic relationship between disorders in glycogen, galactose, glucose, and fructose metabolism. Solid rectangle indicates site of metabolic block; . . . indicates omission in the metabolic sequence.

birth because an older sibling of each infant was known to have HFI. Fourteen patients received fructose in their first feedings, and symptoms usually appeared within a few days. The remaining patients received a fructose-free diet (breast milk or cow's milk formula). Their symptoms began immediately after introduction of dietary fructose or sucrose. Thirty-two (64 per cent) were diagnosed as having HFI at less than 6 months of age, 12 (24 per cent) between 6 and 12 months of age, and 6 (12 per cent) after 1 year of age.

The younger patients were usually admitted to the hospital on an emergency basis with acute liver impairment, sepsis, bleeding diathesis, shock, or dehydration. Patients less than 6 months old developed a triad of jaundice, edema, and bleeding tendency. Older patients were admitted more often because of liver enlargement or ascites or both.

Vomiting and hepatomegaly were observed in all patients. Half had anorexia, weight retardation, and bleeding tendency. About a third had jaundice, diarrhea, edema or ascites or both, and growth retardation. Thirteen of the 50 had developed an aversion to sweet foods. This aversion had developed as early as 3 months of age, and in 2 patients had resulted in continued breast-feeding until 9 months of age. Vomiting and diarrhea in the young children were sometimes severe enough to cause dehydration.

The laboratory findings were variable but liver function was severely deranged in the younger patients. Deficiency of clotting factors and elevated alanine aminotransferase (ALT) were present in all but one of the patients less than 6 months old. Two patients also had serum albumin levels of 2.8 g/dl. Fifteen patients had aminoaciduria; the predominant amino acids were tyrosine and methionine in 3 of the 15. All patients showed complete resolution of laboratory abnormalities in response to removal of fructose from the diet during a succeeding 2-week period.

Histologic abnormalities were found in the livers of all patients. Fibrosis without inflammation was present in either periportal or intralobular areas in most; all but three patients had some steatosis. These three patients were older

and had voluntarily restricted themselves to diets with small amounts of fructose.

Treatment of the symptomatic patients consisted of immediate cessation of fructose intake. Those with normal liver function were given fructose-free diets normal in protein content. Infants who had acute liver dysfunction were given intravenously a glucose-electrolyte mixture and were given exchange transfusion when there was a serious bleeding tendency. Thereafter, a fructose-free, low-protein diet was fed; when the liver dysfunction had been corrected, a diet normal in protein was begun.

Clinical and biochemical improvement was dramatic following exchange transfusion. Vomiting ceased immediately. The bleeding tendency disappeared in less than 24 hours, and renal tubular dysfunction disappeared within 3 days. All patients showed resolution of symptoms and normalization of laboratory findings within two weeks. Catch-up growth occurred within two to three years. The only persistent abnormality was hepatomegaly with steatosis, which was present from birth in the five patients restricted in dietary fructose.

Although there were no deaths in the series reported by Odievre and co-workers,[8] the continuous intake of fructose may cause death from hypoglycemic seizures or progressive liver failure and inanition. The second child of such a family may profit from experience with the first child by more rapid recognition of the illness.

With greater awareness, more cases of HFI in children are being diagnosed, and the condition is arrested by feeding fructose-restricted diets. One cautionary note relates to the fact that a number of proprietary milks, primarily the soy-based formulas, contain sucrose as a significant source of the carbohydrate calories. The remaining carbohydrate is usually a glucose oligosaccharide. Hypoglycemia and seizures may not be a problem in affected infants fed these formulas because the remaining carbohydrate is glucose. The liver disease may be progressive, however, and infants fed these formulas may simply fail to thrive or have hepatomegaly and vomiting or may progress to chronic liver failure and death. Acute liver failure from

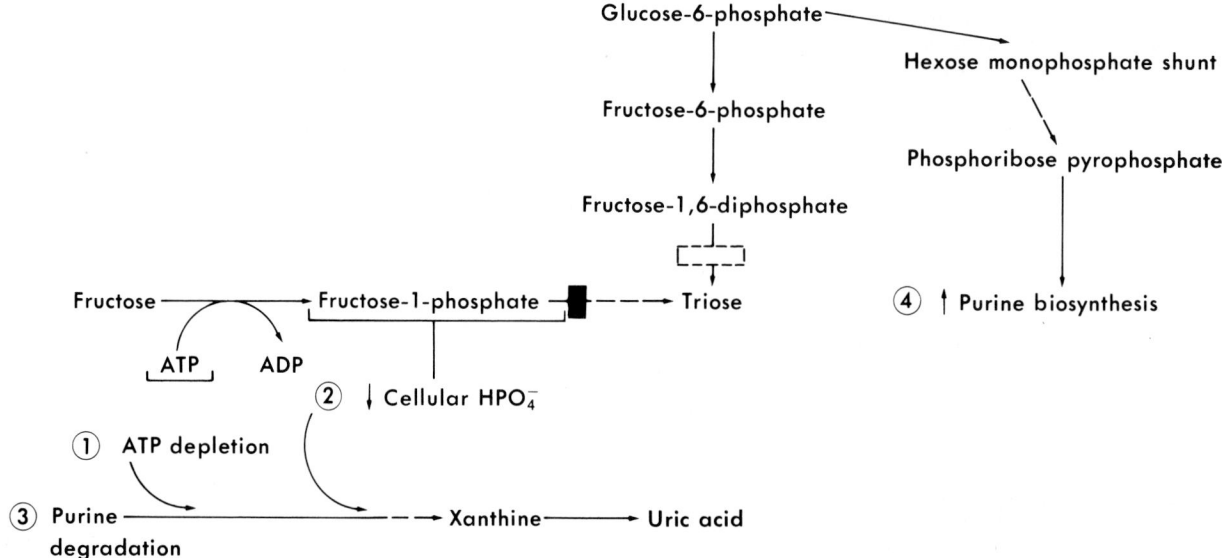

Figure 49–2. Mechanism of hyperuricemia and hypophosphatemia in hereditary fructose intolerance. Following fructose intake, there is rapid phosphorylation to fructose-1-phosphate, causing ATP depletion ① because of the aldolase block. The accumulated fructose-1-phosphate inhibits the aldolase step, preventing ATP generation from anaerobic glycolysis. Phosphate is not released from the sugar, causing depletion of intracellular phosphate ②. Low ATP and HOP_4^- levels favor degradation of preformed purines to uric acid ③. There is a compensatory increase in purine biosynthesis ④. Solid rectangle indicates site of metabolic block.

fructose intolerance is exceedingly unusual, and the absence of hepatomegaly in an infant who has severe liver disease and has reducing sugar in the urine should make one doubt the diagnosis of HFI. Although the disease has been identified for only 23 years, follow-up studies of infants and recognition of older patients with HFI indicate a normal life expectancy. Patients retain their sensitivity to dietary fructose as adults, but the hypoglycemic response to fructose may be somewhat more delayed in adults than in infants (45 to 60 minutes in infants; 60 to 90 minutes in adults).[6] The sensitivity to fructose may be life-threatening for adult patients. For example, patients with known HFI have been given sorbitol intravenously following surgery. Since sorbitol is metabolized to fructose, the patients died of complications from the sorbitol infusion.[9, 10]

Biochemical Characteristics

The clinical and biochemical abnormalities seen in patients with HFI result from deficient activity of hepatic fructose-1-phosphate aldolase. This enzyme is present normally in liver, renal tubular cells, and the intestinal mucosa.[11] It catalyzes the conversion of fructose-1-phosphate to D-glyceraldehyde and dihydroxyacetone phosphate (Reaction [1]).

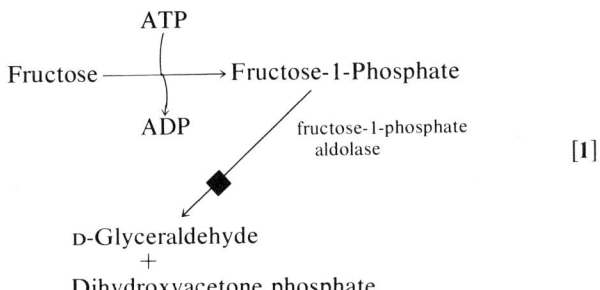

The metabolic consequences of this enzymatic deficiency are accumulation of large amounts of fructose-1-phosphate in the liver and depletion of inorganic phosphate (P_i) and adenosine triphosphate (ATP). The inability to metabolize fructose-1-phosphate in cells of affected patients leads to sequestration of large amounts of P_i. One of the many effects secondary to this is an inability to regenerate ATP, a process that depends on the presence of P_i. The clinical and laboratory features of HFI can be understood on the basis of this simple scheme (Fig. 49–2).

Patients with HFI have been shown to have levels of activity of fructose-1-phosphate aldolase ranging from 0 to 12 per cent of normal.[6, 12, 13] In addition, most patients have reduced levels of activity of hepatic fructose-1,6-diphosphate aldolase ranging from 25 to 85 per cent of normal.[12, 14] The differential between the activities of the two aldolase enzymes suggests that they are separate protein moieties. However, Gurtler and Leuthardt have crystallized human liver aldolase and have shown that both enzymatic activities

are attributable to a single liver aldolase.[15] In addition, slight alterations of the aldolase molecule, such as splitting off an end-terminal residue, may change the ratio of its affinity for fructose-1-phosphate or fructose-1,6-diphosphate.[16, 17]

Patients with HFI produce a protein that has the immunologic properties of fructose-1-phosphate aldolase but is biologically inactive.[18] On the basis of these findings, it seems probable that a mutation of the structural gene is responsible for the enzyme defect in HFI. More recent studies suggest that the mutation in HFI is not homogeneous.[19]

Accumulation of fructose-1-phosphate apparently causes the major manifestations of the disease through inhibition of other enzymatic reactions. Two metabolic pathways studied most extensively are gluconeogenesis and glycogenolysis (see also Chap. 4). Their inhibition by fructose-1-phosphate explains fructose-induced hypoglycemia. Concentrations of fructose-1-phosphate in excess of 10 mM completely inhibit fructose-1,6-diphosphate aldolase activity in vitro.[20] This finding suggests that fructose-1-phosphate inhibits gluconeogenesis at this enzymatic step. Inhibition at this site is further supported by the finding that fructose-induced hypoglycemia is not prevented by simultaneous infusions of gluconeogenic precursors such as dihydroxyacetone or glycerol. In addition, liver specimens from patients with HFI do not form glucose from ^{14}C-glycerol when fructose is present, whereas oxidation of ^{14}C-glycerol is apparently unaffected by fructose (Reaction [2]).[21]

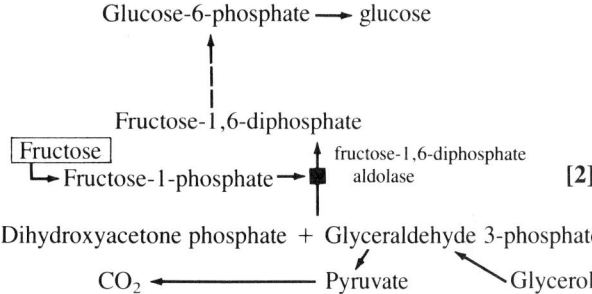

Patients with HFI apparently also have inhibition of glycogenolysis following fructose intake. This inhibition occurs above the level of phosphoglucomutase. In support of this, it was shown that when galactose is administered together with fructose, hypoglycemia is less pronounced and does not last as long as when fructose is given alone (Reaction [3]).[5] Thus, a defect in the phosphorylation of glycogen to glucose-1-phosphate is incriminated. Several studies of normal liver indicate that depletion of P_i as well as accumulation of fructose-1-phosphate may contribute to an almost complete failure of glycogen mobilization.[22–24] In addition, depletion of intracellular ATP levels may contribute to the lack of glycogen degradation to glucose-1-phosphate.[25–27]

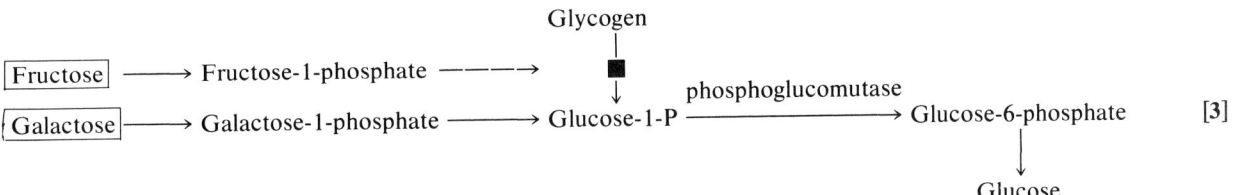

A variant of fructose intolerance has been described in which the red cell galactose-1-phosphate uridyl transferase activity was normal but galactose as well as fructose caused hypoglycemia.[28] The nature of this finding is unclear, since a reevaluation of these patients 12 years later showed normal blood glucose responses to fructose and galactose.[29]

Results of studies by Schwartz and colleagues suggest that newborn infants delivered at term have less capacity for fructose metabolism in the first few days of life as compared with later in life.[30] This is felt to be caused by the immaturity of the enzymes for handling fructose. In their studies, a rapid infusion of fructose caused a prompt but transient decrease in blood glucose and suppressed the glucagon-induced elevation of blood glucose. Although hepatic aldolase was not measured, the findings suggest that until further studies are completed, the use of fructose or sorbitol as a calorie source (as in total parenteral nutrition) for term infants in the first few days of life may not be justified. Enzymatic maturation may take longer in premature infants, although definitive studies have not been reported.

Laboratory Features

The primary laboratory features of HFI are fructose-induced hypoglycemia and hypophosphatemia, and/or chronic liver disease. In addition, serum and urinary urate levels may be increased.

Hypoglycemia. Hypoglycemia induced by dietary or intravenous fructose is a characteristic of the illness. The hypoglycemia is not due to an excess of circulating insulin.[20, 31] That sorbitol provokes hypoglycemia before substantial amounts of fructose are released into the circulation is evidence against a direct effect of fructose on blood glucose levels.[6] More likely, the adverse effects of fructose result from intracellular accumulation of a fructose metabolite, such as fructose-1-phosphate.[20, 32] The metabolite impairs both gluconeogenesis and glycogenolysis (Reactions [2] and [3]). Studies with ^{14}C-glucose indicate a complete cessation of hepatic glucose release following fructose infusion.[31] Also, glucagon does not increase blood glucose following fructose-induced hypoglycemia, even in the presence of normal to slightly elevated hepatic glycogen content.[33]

Hypophosphatemia. This is the second prominent feature of fructose-induced hypoglycemia. The reduction of inorganic phosphorus precedes that of glucose and may be the only abnormal finding when a small dose of fructose is administered.[6] Hypophosphatemia appears to be a consequence of binding and sequestration of phosphorus in the form of fructose-1-phosphate within the hepatocytes.[32, 34] The first step in fructose metabolism is phosphorylation by ATP. With large doses of fructose, ATP is depleted rapidly. With deficient activity of aldolase, as occurs in HFI, inorganic phosphate is not released back into the cell. To compensate, phosphate from the serum is sequestered by the liver, with a resulting reduction in available circulating phosphate levels.[6] Phosphorylation of fructose decreases intracellular phosphate in normal individuals, but the phosphate sequestered in normal liver is made available by further metabolism of fructose-1-phosphate. Thus, changes in serum levels of phosphate are extremely transient in the normal individual and depend upon the amount of fructose ingested.

Hepatic Enzyme Elevation. This appears to be the direct effect of increased hepatic fructose-1-phosphate levels. Within one and one half hours following a large dose of fructose, transaminase levels may increase more than twofold.[35] The mechanism of liver cell damage is not clear, but it may result from a combination of depletion of ATP and a direct toxic effect of elevated levels of the phosphorylated hexose.

Hyperuricemia and Increased Urate Excretion. These conditions appear to result from depletion of intracellular ATP and P_i. This depletion of ATP and P_i increases the rate of purine degradation to uric acid (Fig. 49–2).[25, 26]

Other laboratory findings are less consistent. Some patients show substantial decreases in serum potassium and increases in serum magnesium following fructose intake.[6, 33] Some have increases in serum lactate and pyruvate.[5, 6, 12] These changes appear to be related to the extent of liver damage and the severity of hypoglycemia. Granulocytosis may be seen with chronic fructose ingestion. A galactose infusion may relieve the hypoglycemia, but this also is an inconsistent finding. As blood glucose declines following fructose ingestion, insulin and insulin-like activity decrease. Levels of glucagon, epinephrine, and growth hormone increase. In response to these hormonal changes, the nonesterified fatty acids in plasma increase more than twofold, a response not seen in normal subjects.[5, 12, 36, 37]

Renal tubular acidosis and a Fanconi-like syndrome with renal tubular reabsorptive defects have been reported.[8, 38, 39] In one patient, renal tubular acidosis persisted despite restriction of dietary fructose.[8] The renal tubular acidosis is normalized in most patients as soon as fructose intake ceases.[40, 41] Fructose-1-phosphate aldolase normally is present in the renal tubules. It is absent in patients with HFI. Hence, the transient renal disturbance in affected patients may be due to accumulation of fructose-1-phosphate in renal tubular cells following fructose intake.[11]

Pathology

The changes in hepatic ultrastructure within one and one half to two hours after a single dose of fructose are "glycogen-associated membrane arrays" and cytolysosomes in various stages of development. These may represent lysosomes ingesting the accumulated fructose-1-phosphate in an attempt to get rid of it by acid hydrolysis. With chronic ingestion of fructose, the primary histologic changes are lipid accumulation and varying stages of hepatocellular necrosis and biliary duct proliferation. Liver disease may progress to cirrhosis with impairment of liver-dependent coagulation factors.[42]

In spite of extremely severe hepatic disease, the liver shows a remarkable ability to regenerate once dietary fructose is excluded. For example, a three-month-old child who had cirrhosis, hypoalbuminemia, hypoprothrombinemia, and ascites had normal liver function and disappearance of ascitic fluid after three weeks of a fructose-free diet. Except for slight fibrosis the hepatic architecture was normal three years later.[33]

The pathogenesis of acute and chronic liver cell injury following fructose intake has not been studied in detail. By analogy with galactosemia, a six-carbon sugar phosphorylated at carbon 1 may have a direct cytotoxic effect, whereas phosphorylation of the carbon 6 position apparently has no obvious toxicity. In addition, the severe alterations in energy metabolism may play a role in derangement of liver cell function and may thereby result in the pathologic changes seen following ingestion of dietary fructose. The reason for lipid accumulation is also unclear, but it may represent only general cellular dysfunction seen in a number of unrelated conditions.[5, 12, 37]

Although renal function may be severely impaired, there is little histologic change in the kidney other than some increase in medullary lipid.

The teeth of patients who have HFI are unusually free of caries. This has been taken to indicate that fructose and sucrose are important cariogenic substrates.[43]

In spite of the recurrent episodes of hypoglycemia and seizures that are common in undiagnosed cases, the brain is remarkably free of abnormalities. In contrast to patients with galactosemia who commonly show psychomotor retardation, HFI patients surviving even the most severe forms of liver disease appear to have normal intelligence after being given fructose-free diets.

Genetics

The genetic findings are compatible with an autosomal recessive trait. Levels of hepatic fructose-1-phosphate aldolase activity in five parents of patients with HFI were normal.[44] In addition, carriers usually metabolize substantial fructose loads without difficulty. This is in contradistinction to carriers of galactosemia, who metabolize galactose at slower rates than normal and who may develop lenticular opacification with chronic galactose ingestion.

Differential Diagnosis

During infancy, various conditions may be associated with hypoglycemia,[45, 46] but most of them are associated with fasting. Hypoglycemia following eating should be a clue to the possibility of HFI, particularly in the presence of urinary reducing sugar. Other diseases in which hypoglycemia follows ingestion of food are deficiency of fructose diphosphatase, galactosemia, and leucine intolerance. In addition, premature infants may have transient fructose intolerance due to immaturity of hepatic aldolase activity.[30] Some patients with Tay-Sachs disease have deficient levels of fructose-1-phosphate aldolase.[47, 48] Three such patients were given fructose loads, but did not develop hypoglycemia, hypophosphatemia, or the hypermagnesemia that is seen in patients with HFI. The relationship of the decreased enzymatic activity to the pathogenesis of Tay-Sachs disease is unknown, although measurement of fructose-1-phosphate aldolase activity has been used as a marker to detect the carrier state of Tay-Sachs disease.[48, 49]

The diagnosis of HFI can be made by an intravenous fructose tolerance test. The smallest dose that will produce the typical symptoms without causing nausea and vomiting is 0.25 g/kg body weight.[6] A dose of 0.25 g/kg body weight or 3 g/m^2 surface area is given as a single rapid injection. Marked, prolonged reductions of blood glucose and phosphate levels occur regularly with this dose. However, at least one infant with marked hepatomegaly and severely deranged hepatic function did not have the typical changes in blood glucose and phosphate until the intravenous dose was doubled. Thus, with severe liver disease, blood and urinary levels of fructose are inconsistently elevated with the lesser fructose load. The lower dose of fructose may be a valuable aid as an initial screen for HFI during use of an unrestricted diet, but a negative test, as described above, should not be used to rule out the diagnosis of HFI. Because the fructose load may cause symptomatic hypoglycemia, vomiting, and derangement of liver function, measurement of intestinal aldolase activity may be preferable in patients strongly suspected of having HFI.[50] The presumptive diagnosis made from tolerance tests should be confirmed by assay of enzyme activity in percutaneous liver biopsy specimens.

Treatment

A diet containing no fructose will alleviate all the symptoms and liver dysfunction associated with HFI.[3-7] It is important that the patient and the mother receive detailed dietary counseling concerning which foods contain fructose. Older children commonly may associate discomfort with specific foods and regularly avoid them. However, infants are completely dependent on dietary selections made by the parents.

The common practice of adding small amounts of sugar to processed foods demands almost constant attention to avoid substantial fructose intake. One patient with HFI who continued to consume small amounts of fructose had chronic slight elevations in aspartate amino transferase (AST) levels as well as hepatic fat accumulation. Because pharmacologic doses of folate are known to cause nonspecific increases in both aldolase activities, the patient was treated with 5 mg folate daily, with a resultant 53 per cent increase in hepatic fructose-1-phosphate aldolase activity. With no change in dietary intake there were decreases in AST and hepatic lipid contents. Tolerance tests however showed that folate treatment did not increase this patient's ability to handle a large dietary intake of fructose.[50]

Prognosis

Patients maintained on fructose-free diets have developed entirely normally, with normal life spans, although most continue to have slight hepatomegaly with hepatic steatosis.[8] Even infants with severely deranged liver function and substantial hepatic fibrosis can achieve remarkable recoveries once fructose is removed from their diets.

Fructose Diphosphatase Deficiency

In 1970, Baker and Winegrad described a patient who had a third type of genetic defect in fructose metabolism.[4] The predominant clinical findings were hepatomegaly and fasting-induced hypoglycemia with lactic acidosis. The patient was shown later to have deficient hepatic FDPase activity. Other cases with similar clinical and laboratory findings have been reported since.[51] The primary difference between patients with FDPase deficiency and patients with HFI is that fasting as well as dietary fructose induce symptoms in patients with deficiencies of FDPase. As a result, an occasional patient with FDPase deficiency has been diagnosed incorrectly as having type IB glycogen storage disease. Several patients have been found to have "partial" FDPase deficiencies. These patients do not have lactic acidosis but develop hypoglycemia during fasting or secondary to dietary intake of fructose or glycerol. One such patient had many of the characteristics of the syndrome "ketotic hypoglycemia."[52] Others have been erroneously diagnosed during infancy as having acute tyrosinosis. The deficiency of FDPase is inherited as an autosomal recessive trait.

DISORDERS OF GALACTOSE METABOLISM

In 1935, Mason and Turner provided the first detailed description of a patient intolerant of galactose.[53] Since then, numerous case reports have described the constellation of nutritional failure, liver disease, cataracts, and mental retardation that results from a deficiency of hepatic galactose-1-phosphate uridyl transferase activity.[54-56] There is evidence that this defect is due to a lack of synthesis of transferase protein rather than amino acid substitution.[57] Subsequently, Gitzelmann described the case of a 44-year-old patient with galactosuria and early onset cataracts.[58] Later reports indicated that this patient represented a second defect in galactose metabolism, which was found to be due to deficiency of galactokinase.[59, 60] Apparently this defect does not result in progressive liver disease and mental retardation. In 1972 Gitzelmann discovered a third type of galactosemia, caused by uridine diphosphate galactose-4-epimerase deficiency.[61] This condition has been considered benign inasmuch as the deficiency is limited to leukocytes and erythrocytes and the affected individuals show no other laboratory abnormalities or clinical abnormality.[62] More recently, generalized epimerase deficiency has been described.[63-67] These patients show signs and symptoms identical to those of transferase-deficiency galactosemia. Because each of these conditions results in milk-induced galactosemia but represents three distinct biochemical entities, it has been suggested that the term *galactosemia* be supplemented by the specific enzymatic defect, i.e., transferase-deficiency galactosemia, galactokinase-deficiency galactosemia, and epimerase-deficiency galactosemia.

Transferase-Deficiency Galactosemia

Human beings are capable of metabolizing large quantities of galactose, as demonstrated by the rapid elimination of galactose from blood.[68, 69] An elevation of the level of plasma glucose occurs shortly after galactose infusion as a result of conversion of galactose to glucose. Tracer studies indicate that as much as 50 per cent of galactose may be found in body glucose pools within 30 minutes of injection.[69] Under normal circumstances, plasma galactose is removed so rapidly by the liver that the rate of galactose clearance has been used as an index of hepatic blood flow[70] and liver function.[71] The removal mechanism is saturated at plasma levels of about 50 mg/dl, a level corresponding to the limits of the ability of galactokinase to phosphorylate the sugar.[72] With a load of galactose that increases blood levels by 30 to 40 mg/dl, urinary losses may be substantial, since the kidney threshold is at plasma levels of 10 to 20 mg/dl.[72]

Almost half of the calorie source in most mammalian milks is from hydrolysis of lactose to its two monosaccharides, glucose and galactose. Consequently, the series of enzymatic steps involved in conversion of galactose to glucose are most stressed during infancy. As a consequence,

enzymatic defects of this pathway are most likely to produce clinical signs and symptoms as well as marked elevations of blood and urinary galactose levels during this crucial period of development.

The first described defect resulting in galactosemia results from deficient activity of the enzyme required for the second of four steps in galactose metabolism (Fig. 49–3). The consequences of this defect are much more severe than are those of the other defects in galactose metabolism, galactokinase deficiency and uridine diphosphate (UDP)-galactose-4-epimerase deficiency.

Clinical Features

Since transferase-deficiency galactosemia was first described in 1935, numerous patients with the disorder have been followed for long periods. In 1970, Komrower and Lee reported the results of long-term follow-up of the 60 known cases of galactosemia in Great Britain.[73] More recently, long-term follow-up studies from 47 families have been reported from Los Angeles.[74]

The disease varies in severity. Some patients may present with an acute, fulminant illness after the first milk feedings or more commonly as a subacute illness with gastrointestinal symptoms (i.e., jaundice and failure to thrive). In milder cases, moderate intestinal upset following galactose ingestion may be the only manifestation. In severe cases, anorexia, abdominal distention, diarrhea, vomiting, and hypoglycemic attacks may be seen shortly after birth. The most common initial symptoms are failure to thrive and vomiting, usually starting within the first few days of milk ingestion. Table 49–2 lists the more common findings in 43 symptomatic patients.[74] Within the first week of life, hepatomegaly and jaundice are usually seen. In fact, prolonged obstructive jaundice in the neonate is a common presenting feature, and examination of urine for reducing sugar should be done in all cases of infants with clinical jaundice. The jaundice from intrinsic liver disease may be accentuated in some infants with galactosemia by severe hemolysis and erythroblastosis. With continued galactose ingestion, ascites may develop as early as two to five weeks after birth. Cataracts may be seen within a few days after birth; or, if the mother has consumed large amounts of milk late in gestation, they may be present at delivery. The cataracts, consisting of punctate lesions in the nucleus of the fetal lens, may be so small as to be seen only with slit-lamp examination. Retardation of mental development may be apparent after the first several months. A few patients homozygous for the disorder have been found to be entirely asymptomatic while ingesting milk. These patients, who are usually black, may be capable of metabolizing moderate amounts of galactose.[75]

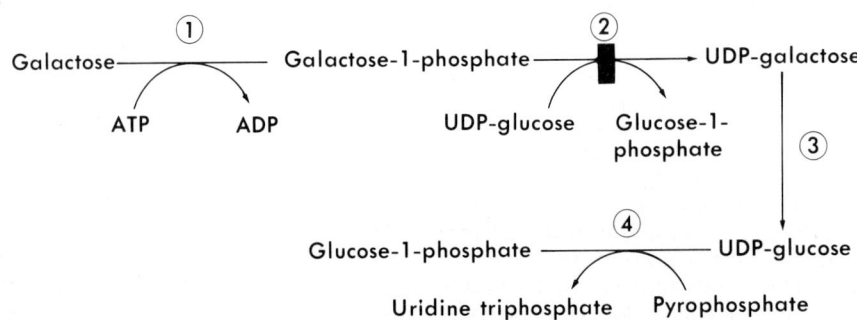

Figure 49–3. Reactions in the conversion of galactose to glucose. ① = galactokinase; ② = galactose-1-phosphate uridyltransferase; ③ = uridine diphosphate (UDP) galactose-4-epimerase; ④ = UDP glucose pyrophosphorylase.

TABLE 49–2. COMMON CLINICAL FINDINGS IN 43 SYMPTOMATIC GALACTOSEMIC PATIENTS

	Number of Patients	Per Cent Incidence
Anorexia and weight loss	23	53
Hepatomegaly	39	91
Jaundice	34	79
Ascites and/or edema	7	16
Vomiting	17	40
Abdominal distention	9	21
Cataracts	21	49
Infection	10	23
Sepsis	5	12

Source: Koch R, et al. In: Kelley VC, ed. Practice of Pediatrics. Harper & Row, 1979:4.

Since milk-substitute formulas have become easily accessible, infants who have recurrent vomiting and poor weight gains during the first few weeks of life are often given trials of one of the lactose-free formulas. An occasional infant with galactosemia may be unwittingly changed to such a formula with resulting improvement without any awareness of the child's underlying defect. In such instances, the patient may have the disease undetected until months or years later, when they may have motor retardation, hepatomegaly, and cataracts.[76]

An important clinical observation concerning galactosemia is that of Levy and associates, who showed the strong association between galactosemia and *Escherichia coli* sepsis.[77] In routine screening of more than 700,000 infants during a 12-year period, 8 infants with classic transferase-deficiency galactosemia were identified. Four of these infants had septicemia at the time galactosemia was detected (second week of life), and three of the four died. A review of results from eight other states that routinely screen newborns for galactosemia indicates that in screening more than 2.5 million newborns, 35 such patients were identified. Of the 35 patients, 10 are known to have had systemic infection, and 9 of the 10 died from bacteremia despite therapy. Infections usually seem to develop at the end of the first week or during the second week of life, and their incidence appears to correlate directly with continued intake of galactose. These findings suggest that infants with *E. coli* sepsis should be considered possibly galactosemic and that infants recently diagnosed as galactosemic should be considered possibly infected with *E. coli*.

With initiation of a galactose elimination diet, all acute manifestations of the disease usually improve within 72 hours, and hepatic dysfunction begins to normalize by one week. During the first year of life, small amounts of dietary galactose may cause symptoms; however, around puberty most patients show an improved tolerance to dietary galactose. To account for this improved tolerance, an alternative metabolic pathway for galactose has been postulated to develop around the time of puberty. This pathway is thought to bypass the deficient transferase step by forming UDP-galactose from the interaction of galactose-1-phosphate and uridine triphosphate (Fig. 49–4).[78] This reaction in liver and brain would reduce the concentration of galactose-1-phosphate to normal levels and would thus protect against the effects of the defective pathway. Although this hypothesis represents an attractive explanation for the increased ability to tolerate galactose later in life, tracer studies do not support an increased rate of galactose metabolism. A third pathway, involving the formation of xylulose, is unimportant in normal humans but may permit survival of some patients who continue to ingest galactose (Fig. 49–4).

Laboratory Findings

Routine laboratory findings may be varied but include elevated blood and urinary levels of galactose, hyperchloremic acidosis, albuminuria, aminoaciduria, hypoglycemia, and blood changes reflecting deranged liver function. Occasionally, infants may have severe and prolonged hypoglycemia. The galactosuria may be intermittent because of poor food intake or may disappear within three or four days of intravenous feeding. Thus, if the urine is not tested for reducing sugar during a period of galactosuria, the diagnosis may not be suspected. The finding of a urinary reducing substance that does not react with the glucose oxidase test should alert one to the possibility of galactosemia. This finding does not establish the diagnosis, since several other conditions such as fructosuria, lactosuria (from deficient intestinal lactase), and severe liver disease of any origin may impair the clearance of blood galactose and result in the presence of urinary reducing sugar that is not glucose.[76]

Biochemical Characteristics and Pathogenesis of Galactose Toxicity

The hepatic manifestations of transferase-deficiency galactosemia are due entirely to the abnormal metabolism of galactose, and patients never exposed to galactose should have no abnormality. Toxicity apparently results from accumulation of the metabolic products of galactose rather than from galactose itself. The two compounds that have been studied most extensively are galactose-1-phosphate and galactitol, the product of an alternate pathway (Fig. 49–5). The biochemical causes of toxicity in individual organs may differ, depending on the metabolic patterns and functions of the involved organs. For example, cataracts are apparently caused by galactitol accumulation, whereas this compound appears to have little, if any, relation to the renal abnormalities or hepatic dysfunction.

Hypoglycemia. Hypoglycemia that may occur following galactose ingestion is apparently caused by the inhibition of glucose release from glycogen. The mechanism responsible is postulated to be due to high levels of galactose-1-phosphate that interfere with phosphoglucomutase, the enzyme that catalyzes the conversion of glucose-1-phosphate to glucose-6-phosphate.[79] In addition, there is an inhibition of glucose formation through gluconeogenesis.[80] The galactose-1-phosphate may be toxic in other ways as well, although investigations aimed at answering this question depended primarily on changes induced in normal animals fed high-galactose diets and do not necessarily reflect the changes that occur in patients who have deficiencies of enzymatic activity.

The organs primarily involved in galactosemia are the lens of the eye, the liver, the brain, and the kidney. The mechanism whereby galactose feeding causes these pathologic changes is not understood for all tissues.

Lenticular Changes. Changes in the lens appear to result primarily from accumulation of galactitol. Van Heyningen showed galactitol accumulation, and Kinoshita and associates showed that an increase in galactitol concentration caused a concomitant increase in water content secondary to the oncotic pressure from the galactitol.[81-83] The poor diffusion of the alcohol from the lens makes this organ particularly susceptible. Reversing the osmotic effect of the galactitol accumulation with an osmotically balanced incubation medium prevents the lenticular opacification.[82] Many biochemical alterations occur concurrently in the lens as it

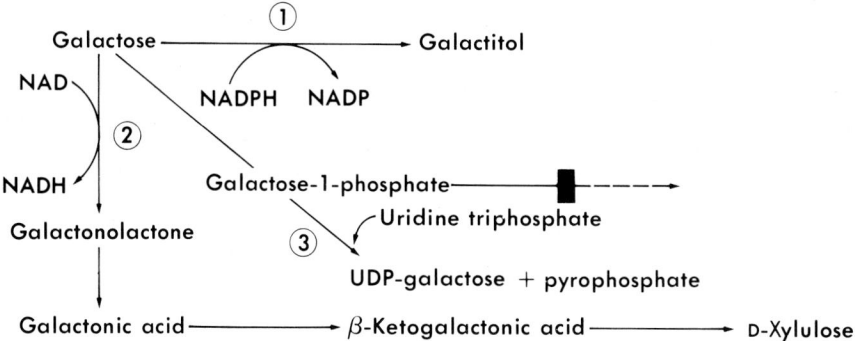

Figure 49–4. Alternate pathways of galactose metabolism. ① = aldose reductase or L-hexonate dehydrogenase; ② = galactose dehydrogenase; ③ = uridine diphosphate galactose pyrophosphorylase.

undergoes cataract formation. These include decreases in amino acid transport, protein synthesis, several enzymatic activities, and alteration of ion fluxes.[83–88] Glycolysis and respiration of the lens are reduced by about 30 per cent after about two days of galactose feeding and remain at this level until cataracts occur.[87] It is not surprising, then, that nutrient supplements can alter the rate of cataract formation in galactose-fed animals.[89] Thus, nutrient imbalances and alterations in lenticular water content from galactitol formation together are prime initiators of lenticular opacification. The causes of cellular damage in other organs are less clear.

Liver. Liver contents of both galactose-1-phosphate

and galactitol are elevated in patients fed galactose.[90, 91] However, the liver damage seen in patients with transferase deficiencies does not occur in normal animals fed high-galactose diets despite high hepatic levels of galactose-1-phosphate in the rat[92] and high hepatic galactitol levels in chicks.[93] In addition, patients with galactokinase deficiencies form large amounts of galactitol, but show no liver damage. This suggests that some other metabolite or metabolites may accumulate to act singly or in concert to cause cellular toxicity. In this respect, galactosamine, which was increased in the liver of one patient, is known to induce hepatocellular changes in animals.[93]

Kidneys. Kidneys of transferase-deficient patients de-

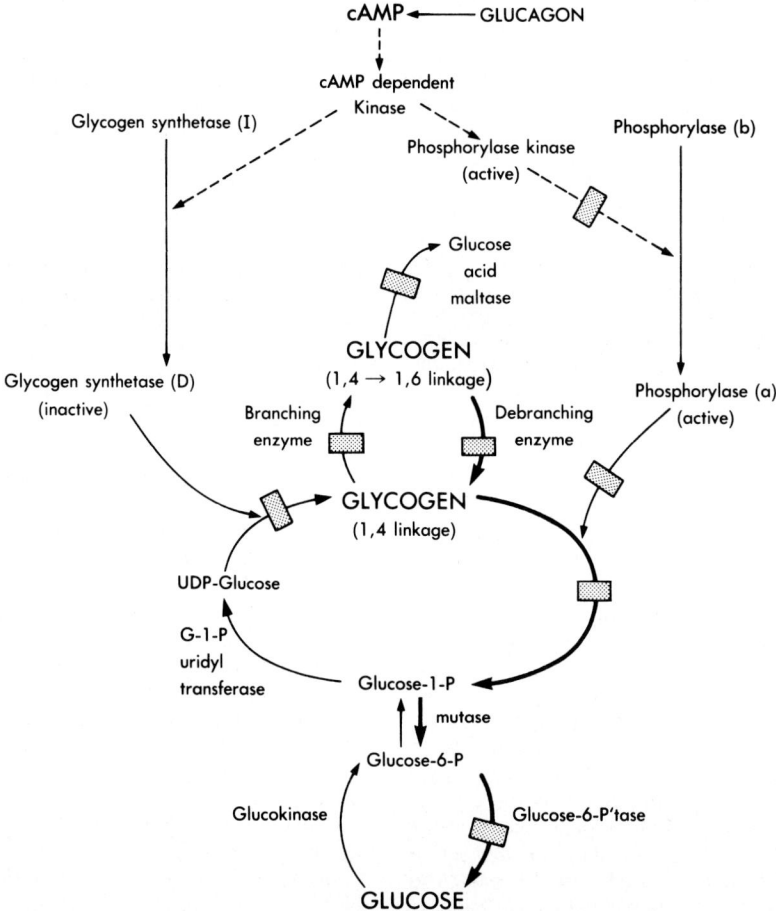

Figure 49–5. Pathway for glycogen synthesis and degradation to glucose. Broken lines indicate enzymic activation after glucagon stimulation; heavy arrows indicate glycogen degradation from glucagon infusion; and hatched boxes indicate points in the metabolic sequence where enzymic defects have been identified.

velop renal tubular dysfunction following galactose ingestion. They accumulate both galactose-1-phosphate and galactitol.[90, 91] However, accumulation of galactitol alone does not appear toxic, since patients with galactokinase deficiencies do not develop renal dysfunction but do excrete large amounts of galactitol. This suggests that the alcohol is not the primary renal insult in patients with transferase deficiency. Aminoaciduria can be induced in both normal man and rats by large amounts of galactose.[94, 95] This could be due to an accumulation of galactose-1-phosphate that secondarily impairs amino acid accumulation by the tubules.[96] If analogous to that in the human intestine, the inhibition is noncompetitive.[97]

Brain. Changes in the brains of patients with transferase-deficiency galactosemia may not be entirely reversible following galactose restriction. For this reason, substantial efforts have been made to delineate the pathogenesis of galactose-induced brain damage. In the brains of patients and those of rats fed galactose, galactitol accumulates in higher concentrations than in any other tissue except the lens.[92, 98] This suggests that galactitol accumulation may be important in the pathogenesis of the brain abnormality. However, in patients with galactokinase deficiencies galactitol accumulation does not appear to damage tissues other than the lens.

Studies in a chick brain showed that galactose administration diminished ATP, reduced brain glucose and glycolytic intermediates, redistributed hexokinase, enhanced fragility of neural lysosomes, and decreased fast axoplasmic transport.[99-103] The effects could be temporarily reversed by glucose.[104] Changes in the chick brain appear to be related to several factors such as hyperosmolality,[103] an alteration in energy metabolism,[100] abnormal serotonin levels,[105] and interference with active uptake of glucose into the neurons. Whether these changes in chicks are similar to galactose-induced abnormalities in patients with transferase deficiencies remains to be determined.

Although intestinal epithelium of the patient with galactosemia is also deficient in its activity of the transferase enzyme, this does not appear to alter intestinal transport of galactose. Many infants develop intestinal symptoms of vomiting and diarrhea following galactose ingestion, but it is unclear whether this is a direct effect on the intestine or secondary to the effects on the central nervous system.

Pathology

Early hepatic lesions, present in the first weeks of life, consist of cholestasis and diffuse fatty vacuolization with little or no inflammatory reaction. The fatty changes are extensive and generalized throughout the lobule. Later, disorganization of the liver cells with pseudoductular and pseudoglandular orientation occurs. This tendency toward pseudoglandular orientation of cells has been described as "characteristic" of galactosemia but is relatively nonspecific. As the disease progresses, delicate fibrosis appears, first in the periportal regions, eventually extending to bridge adjacent portal tracts. Regenerating nodules and hepatic fibrosis are late features that with continued galactose ingestion, progress to cirrhosis similar in many respects to the cirrhosis of ethanol abuse. Death usually occurs in the first year of life unless galactose intake is decreased or curtailed. Frank cellular necrosis is unusual but may occur with large amounts of dietary galactose. In spite of the severity of the hepatic lesion there is a remarkable lack of inflammatory infiltration.[106]

Except for cataract formation in the lens, the tissues show only minor changes. Kidneys show dilation of tubules at the corticomedullary junction. The spleen enlarges as a result of portal hypertension. Lesions in the brain are subtle, with minor loss of nerve cells and gliosis in the dentate nucleus and gliosis in the cerebral cortex and gray matter.[107]

Genetics

Investigations of red cell and leukocytic transferase activities in family members indicate that the disorder is transmitted as an autosomal recessive trait.[108] Heterozygotes have about 50 per cent of normal activity, and genotype detection is more accurate when the transferase:galactokinase ratio is determined.[109] Population studies indicate that the incidence of heterozygosity for galactosemia is between 0.9 and 1.25 per cent and that between 8 and 13 per cent carry the Duarte gene.[110] Incidences of transferase-deficiency galactosemia derived from large-scale screening in neonatal nurseries have been between 1:10,000 and 1:70,000 live births.[111, 112] At least one patient with transferase-deficiency galactosemia has delivered a normal heterozygous infant.[74]

Diagnostic Screening For Galactosemia

The rationale for genetic screening is threefold: (1) to detect disease at its incipient stage and thereby offset harmful expression of the mutant gene through appropriate medical treatment, (2) to identify a variant genotype for which reproductive options (family planning) may be provided, and (3) to identify gene frequency or biologic significance and natural history of variant phenotypes.

Various screening methods for galactosemia have been employed.[113] The original Guthrie test used filter paper blood samples from which a microbiologic assay detected elevated galactose levels. The newer Beutler test assays the erythrocyte transferase activity directly from dried filter paper, and the Paigen assay is an improved bacteriologic method that includes detection of elevated galactose and galactose-1-phosphate. Measurements of elevated galactose requires that the infant receive sufficient dietary galactose or a false negative test will result. Conversely, the normal enzyme may become inactive in a hot or humid climate, and a false positive (negative enzyme activity) may be reported.

The relatively common inaccuracies of the screening tests for galactosemia and the low prevalence of the illness, coupled with the observation that infants born into families without a known history of galactosemia may be affected at birth, has prompted some screening centers not to screen for galactosemia. For example, in Quebec the spaces on the blood sample filter paper assigned to galactosemia were given over to screening for congenital hypothyroidism with a striking increase in cost effectiveness.

In utero assay for galactosemia is indicated in pregnant women with a family history of galactosemia. Cultured fibroblasts from amniotic fluid can be assayed for transferase activity. Additionally, the technique of chorionic villus sampling has been used to detect galactosemia during the tenth week of gestation.[114]

Diagnosis

The presumptive diagnosis of galactosemia in an infant with vomiting and failure to thrive on milk feedings may be made by identification of a urinary reducing sugar that does not react with glucose oxidase reagents. It should be remembered that lactose, fructose, and pentose may give similar results, but if the formula is milk based and there is no other dietary sugar, galactosemia is the presumed diagnosis, and restriction of dietary galactose should be initiated immediately. Identification of the sugar can be made by paper or gas-liquid chromatography. Recently, paper impregnated with galactose oxidase has been introduced, which makes screening for galactosuria easier. Normal premature and some term infants may excrete as much as 60 mg/dl urinary galactose during the first week or two of life.

Unlike suspected fructose intolerance, which may be diagnosed by use of a fructose tolerance test, *demonstration of galactosuria or galactosemia by a galactose tolerance test should never be used.* Although not clearly documented, it has been suggested that a single large exposure to galactose may result in severe and prolonged hypoglycemia, with possible resulting brain damage. For this reason, the definitive diagnosis should be made on the basis of direct measurement of transferase activity and not by tolerance test.[74, 76]

The red cell UDP-glucose consumption test has been used extensively as an enzyme screening test for the past decade.[76, 111, 112, 115] It is based on the assay of UDP-glucose before and after incubation with galactose-1-phosphate and added red cell hemolysate as the enzyme source. Conversion of UDP-glucose to UDP-glucuronic acid by UDP-glucose dehydrogenase forms NAD from NADH, which is measured spectrophotometrically. With this procedure, a complete absence of red cell transferase activity is found in homozygous patients, and intermediate levels characterize heterozygous carriers. Infants identified as having 50 per cent of normal activity should have further tests to rule out other variants that may be homozygous at 50 per cent activity (see later).

With the advent of screening for galactosemia, multiple variants of this disease have become apparent, the variants being more prevalent than classic transferase-deficiency galactosemia.[116] There are three homozygotic types: (1) "Classic" galactosemia is autosomal recessive and there is no transferase activity in erythrocytes, fibroblasts, liver and presumably in any other tissue. In heterozygotic, unaffected carriers, activity is 50 per cent of normal. (2) The Duarte variant is the most common form of galactosemia and is detected only by enzyme screening, because these infants are asymptomatic. Red cell activity is 50 per cent of normal and on starch gel electrophoresis the enzyme migrates faster than normal. Red cells of patients who have this variant produce two distinct bands rather than the single normal band. In addition, red cells of a parent of a Duarte-homozygous patient have three bands for the variant enzyme. Homozygotic Duarte erythrocytes have 50 per cent of normal enzyme activity; heterozygous Duarte erythrocytes, 75 per cent. Ten to 15 per cent of the population may have Duarte-variant galactosemia. The Duarte gene is apparently allelic with the normal and galactosemic genes, since the most frequently detected abnormality on neonatal screening tests is the compound heterozygous state, consisting of classic galactosemia with the Duarte variant. Two protein bands are present on protein electrophoresis and erythrocyte transferase activity is 25 per cent. Although some of these infants appear asymptomatic at birth and remain so during infancy, others have systemic symptoms with metabolic manifestations of galactosemia. (3) In the "Negro" variant, erythrocytic transferase activity is absent, but 10 per cent of normal activity is present in liver and intestine. The Duarte and the Negro variants may be asymptomatic despite galactose ingestion, although patients with the variant may develop a galactose toxicity syndrome in the neonatal period.

In addition to the homozygotic variants, several heterozygotic variants have been identified: (1) An Indiana variant, in which erythrocytic transferase activity is approximately 35 per cent of normal and is highly unstable (mobility on starch gel electrophoresis is slower than normal), (2) a Rennes variant has about 7 to 10 per cent of normal transferase activity (this variant also travels more slowly than normal by electrophoresis), (3) the Los Angeles variant, which has erythrocytic transferase activity higher than normal (about 140%); this has been detected in six families. Electrophoretic mobility of this variant of the enzyme is similar to that of the Duarte variant. West German and Chicago variants have also been identified by screening procedures.

Treatment

Although the cause of the entire toxicity syndrome in transferase deficiency is uncertain, there is no disagreement that elimination of galactose intake will reverse the biochemical manifestations of transferase-deficiency galactosemia. Some patients seem to have increasing tolerance to galactose with advancing age; however, studies using ^{14}C-galactose do not support the clinical impression that alternate pathways of galactose metabolism develop at puberty,[74-76] nor is there any indication that any drug will increase galactose oxidation, although there are patients with variant forms of transferase deficiencies who can oxidize limited amounts of galactose.

The only acceptable treatment at present is the elimination of dietary galactose. Permissible diets are described in recent publications.[69, 74] Preparations employed in treating infants are Pregestimil, Nutramigen, and the soybean milk preparations. Both Pregestimil and Nutramigen are prepared from casein and may contain small amounts of lactose, but these do not appear to be sufficient to impair therapeutic efficacy. The soybean formulas contain small amounts of galactose in raffinose and stachyose, and other dietary constituents contain small amounts of galactosides, but these carbohydrates are not digested by human intestinal enzymes and should not affect the efficacy of treatment.[74] Because of the frequent addition of milk to a number of proprietary food items, strict attention must be given to the diet during and after weaning.

It is important to be aware that asymptomatic heterozygotic mothers may have elevated serum galactose levels following ingestion of diets high in milk. Infants delivered of such mothers may have the galactosemic syndrome at birth. For this reason, restriction of galactose during the pregnancies of women who have previously borne children with galactosemia is recommended.[74-76]

Prognosis

When untreated, galactosemia results in early deaths of many affected children and is attended by the prospect of mental retardation of those who survive. In a series of 43 galactosemic patients described by Koch and colleagues, there were 13 neonatal deaths.[74] The deaths, occurring at an average age of 6 weeks, were usually attributed to infection. Levy and co-workers noted that 9 of 35 patients died of *E. coli* infections and strongly recommended early cultures and institution of antibiotics effective against

E. coli in any case of an infant with galactosemia who appears ill.[77]

Treatment of the galactosemic patient with a galactose-free diet results in survival with reversal of the acute symptoms, normal growth, and complete recovery of liver function; however, the long-term outcome (particularly for intellectual development) is not entirely certain. Experience gained in the long-term follow-up of 59 patients in the Los Angeles area indicates that many patients have developed very well and have attained college-level educations.[74] Others who were equally well treated with galactose restriction have had various intellectual deficiencies. The causes of the variability in the responses to treatment need further exploration.

Hypergonadotrophic hypogonadism is another long-term disorder recently observed in galactosemic women.[117, 118] Although successful pregnancy is possible, 65 per cent of galactosemic women develop ovarian failure with atrophic gonads. The mechanism is felt to be related to excess galactose exposure during fetal and childhood development[119] or to galactose restriction and a specific galactose need during ovarian development. The male gonads, however, appear more resistant to the effects of galactosemia.[120]

While genetic and social factors may influence results of intelligence tests, such factors do not explain all the differences observed. Recent association of thyroid dysfunction with galactosemia may play some role in the outcome.[121, 122] A factor that definitely affects outcome is the age of the patient at diagnosis. Recent evidence supports the previous impression that a more favorable outcome can be expected when a patient is treated at an early age. For example, the mean IQ of 16 patients treated before 7 days of age was 99.5, whereas that of patients treated between 4 and 6 months of age was 62. It is generally desirable to institute treatment at the earliest possible age, and neonatal screening is an important step in this direction.

Although diagnosis and treatment at birth are desirable objectives, it is also possible that homozygotic galactosemic infants may have experienced unfavorable intrauterine exposure to galactose or its metabolites. Even with maternal dietary restriction of lactose during pregnancy, levels of erythrocytic galactose-1-phosphate in samples of cord blood from 12 homozygotic infants still averaged 11.3 mg/dl. Thus, it appears that the intrauterine environment is not ideal for the homozygotic galactosemic fetus.[74]

Galactokinase-Deficiency Galactosemia

Galactokinase deficiency is less common than classic transferase deficiency, with an incidence of about 1 in 10,000.[123] It does not result in progressive liver disease and mental retardation, but galactose exposure may result in cataract formation.[58–60] It is appropriate to compare this entity with transferase deficiency, since it affects the first reaction (kinase) and the transferase, the second reaction of the galactose pathway (see Fig. 49–3). Comparison of patients with these two defects and the defect involving the third reaction (epimerase) have helped to determine some of the mechanisms of toxicity in several organs, including the development of cataracts. With galactokinase deficiency, there is no accumulation of galactose-1-phosphate, no systemic manifestations, and no mental retardation. Cataract formation is related to synthesis of galactitol in the lens and osmotic disruption of lens fiber architecture, as discussed in the previous section. Maternal galactokinase

deficiency may result in fetal cataract formation.[123] Because of the potential for cataract formation, life-long elimination of galactose is suggested.

Uridine Diphosphate Galactose-4-epimerase–Deficiency Galactosemia

The galactose epimerase catalyzes the third reaction of galactose metabolism (see Fig. 49–3). Epimerase deficiency was discovered incidentally while screening for galactosemia and has an incidence of about 1 in 46,000 in Switzerland.[61] Patients have normal erythrocyte transferase activity but elevated levels of galactose-1-phosphate.[61, 62] This condition is apparently caused by a decreased stability of epimerase and leads to enzyme deficiency in those cells in which its turnover is slow or absent, such as erythrocytes.[124] It is therefore considered to be a benign illness inasmuch as the enzyme deficiency is limited to leukocytes and red blood cells. Affected persons have no symptoms. However, others have recently described patients with generalized epimerase deficiency.[63, 67] These patients have signs and symptoms identical to transferase-deficiency galactosemia. By contrast with transferase deficiency, in which uridine diphosphogalactose can be formed from uridine diphosphoglucose, one patient with epimerase deficiency was unable to synthesize the galactose precursor necessary for synthesis of glycoproteins and glycolipids. These glycosylated compounds are necessary for cell membrane integrity, especially in the central nervous system. Thus, in contrast to patients with transferase deficiency, the rare patient with systemic epimerase deficiency may require small quantities of galactose for normal growth and development. One patient with epimerase deficiency continued to show slightly elevated levels of galactose-1-phosphate in red cells even with dietary restriction of galactose. Appropriate treatment of this disorder therefore requires frequent monitoring of erythrocyte galactose-1-phosphate levels in order to best determine the optimal dietary level of galactose.

Glycogen Storage Diseases

Clinical and pathologic recognition of glycogen storage disease (GSD) affecting the liver and kidneys was described by von Gierke in 1929.[125] Three years later, Pompe recognized another type of glycogen storage disease that involved not only the liver and kidneys but most other organs as well.[126] In 1952, Cori and Cori showed that hepatic glucose-6-phosphatase activity was deficient in patients with von Gierke's disease.[127] This marked the beginning of a classification of glycogenoses by the types of enzymatic defects and the primary organs of involvement. In most types of GSD, the glycogen content of liver or muscle or both is excessive. In unusual cases, the glycogen content may be less than normal, the molecular structure of glycogen may be abnormal, or both may occur. In spite of differences in the specific enzymatic defects, most of the syndromes are not readily distinguishable on clinical grounds alone, and tissue analyses for glycogen content and enzymatic activity are necessary to confirm the diagnoses.[128, 129] Deficiencies of enzymes involving almost every step of glycogen synthesis and degradation have been identified. Their locations in the sequence of glycogen synthesis and degradation are illustrated in Figure 49–5.

Most enzymatic defects giving rise to hepatic glycogenosis involve the degradation of glycogen to glucose-6-

phosphate, or in rare instances, the synthesis of glycogen from glucose-6-phosphate.[128–131] On the other hand, patients with von Gierke's disease are deficient in the activity of glucose-6-phosphatase, a gluconeogenic enzyme. As a consequence of this enzymatic difference, many of the clinical and chemical features of von Gierke's disease, or type I glycogen storage disease (GSD-I), are unique among the glycogen storage diseases. For example, the tetrad of a bleeding tendency from thrombasthenia, urate stone formation from hyperuricemia, hyperlipidemia, and lactic acidosis accompanies GSD-I and is not part of the aberrations seen with other glycogenoses.

In spite of the number of enzymatic deficiencies leading to the glycogenoses, only types 0 (glycogen synthetase deficiency) and IV (α-1,4-glucan:α-1,4-glucan 6-glycosyl transferase deficiency) invariably lead to cirrhosis and liver failure. Patients who have type I (glucose-6-phosphatase deficiency) may develop benign hepatic adenomas and hepatic adenocarcinomas, and patients with Type III (amylo-1,6-glucosidase deficiency; debrancher enzyme deficiency) may develop hepatic fibrosis or cirrhosis. Since only a few patients have been reported with Type 0 GSD, only types I, III, and IV will be discussed in detail.

Type I Glycogenosis
(Glucose-6-phosphatase Deficiency)

Clinical Characteristics

This form of glycogenosis, the most commonly diagnosed type, represents about a fourth of all cases diagnosed. Type I GSD has been divided into types IA and IB, based on the finding that the IB patients have near normal in vitro activity of glucose-6-phosphatase but absent activity in vivo. Since both types have similar metabolic changes and respond similarly to treatment, a general discussion of type IA (designated GSD-I) is presented, followed by a brief discussion of type IB. The clinical picture is one of severe hepatomegaly, which may be apparent within the first two weeks of life. Profound hypoglycemia may develop shortly after birth or may not be prominent for several weeks, depending upon frequency of feeding, the presence of intercurrent infection, and the severity of the disease. Because glucose-6-phosphatase activity is also deficient in the kidney, patients have substantial enlargement of the kidneys. Serum transaminase levels may be slightly elevated, but become normal with effective treatment that maintains blood glucose between 75 and 110 mg/dl at all times. Neither the liver nor the kidneys show functional abnormalities other than the inability to release free glucose into the circulation. In this regard, patients who receive a renal transplant remain unable to maintain normal fasting blood glucose levels.[132] Consanguinity of parents is common, and the disease is transmitted as an autosomal recessive. During the past decade, major improvements in therapy have been documented.[133–136] The study of mechanisms whereby deficiencies of glucose-6-phosphatase activity can cause striking abnormalities in lipid, purine, and carbohydrate metabolism has been instrumental in these therapeutic advances. In order to place GSD-I in metabolic perspective, the mechanisms whereby this single enzyme deficiency can have such profound effects on other metabolic pathways are reviewed.

Biochemical Characteristics

Blood Glucose Changes. The most consistent and life-threatening feature of GSD-I is the low blood glucose levels that result from relatively short periods of fasting. Fasting for as short a time as two to four hours is almost always associated with decreases in blood glucose to less than 70 mg/dl, and it is not uncommon to observe six- to eight-hour fasting levels of 5 to 10 mg/dl. In normal individuals, blood glucose levels are maintained within a relatively narrow range by hepatotropic agents such as glucagon, which release glucose either from stored glycogen or by gluconeogenesis.[137] In GSD-I, degradation of glycogen can occur, or lactate or other gluconeogenic precursors can be converted to glucose-6-phosphate, but in the absence of glucose-6-phosphatase, glucose is not released, and blood glucose levels continue to decline. Blood hormone measurements indicate that during periods of hypoglycemia, insulin levels are appropriately low and glucagon levels are high.[129, 138] Following a glucose load, there is a substantial, although somewhat delayed, insulin release, with concomitant decreases in glucagon and alanine levels.[129, 133, 138] Thus, the hormonal response to changes in the blood glucose concentrations appears appropriate.

Lactic Acid Changes. Under normal circumstances, most circulating lactate is generated by muscle glycolysis during exercise. Removal and metabolism of this lactate is efficiently performed by the liver.[137] On the other hand, much of the circulating lactate in patients with GSD-I is generated by hepatic glycolysis.[139] This phenomenon apparently is the result of hepatic stimulation to release glucose from glycogen in combination with inefficient gluconeogenesis. Excess glucose-6-phosphate formed during glycogenolysis cannot be hydrolyzed to free glucose because of the lack of glucose-6-phosphatase activity. Instead, glucose-6-phosphate is diverted through the glycolytic pathway. This metabolic diversion appears to be the basis for enhancement of lactate formation, as illustrated in Figure 49–6.

Hyperlipidemia. Elevation of plasma lipids is a consistent and striking abnormality.[140, 141] Levels of triglyceride may reach 6000 mg/dl, with associated cholesterol levels of 400 to 600 mg/dl. Free fatty acid levels are also usually elevated. Around puberty, xanthomas can appear over extensor surfaces, but they may also appear in childhood, with involvement of the nasal septum. Those located on the septum may contribute to the frequency of prolonged nosebleeds seen in some patients.

As with lacticemia, elevated levels of triglyceride and cholesterol appear to be a consequence of increased rates of glycogenolysis and glycolysis. Observations by Sadeghi-Nejad and co-workers suggest that excess hepatic glycolysis increases hepatic nicotinamide-adenine dinucleotide (NADH), nicotinamide-adenine dinucleotide phosphate (NADPH), and acetyl coenzyme A (CoA), three compounds important in fatty acid and cholesterol synthesis.[139] Thus, increases in glycerol-3-phosphate and acetyl CoA generated by the glycolytic pathway, together with high levels of reduced cofactors, could sustain an increased rate of triglyceride and cholesterol synthesis.[142, 143] In addition to this apparent increased rate of lipid synthesis, an event concomitant with hypoglycemia is lipolysis from peripheral lipid stores. This further augments the tendency for hyperlipidemia and hepatic steatosis to occur by increasing circulating free fatty acids.[140–144]

Hyperuricemia. Although blood levels of uric acid and the tendency to develop gouty arthritis and nephropathy vary in different patients, those who survive puberty often have gouty complications.[145, 146]

Hyperuricemia was originally attributed to the increased levels of serum lactate and lipid, which competitively inhibit urate excretion.[141] However, the high level of

Type I glycogen storage disease

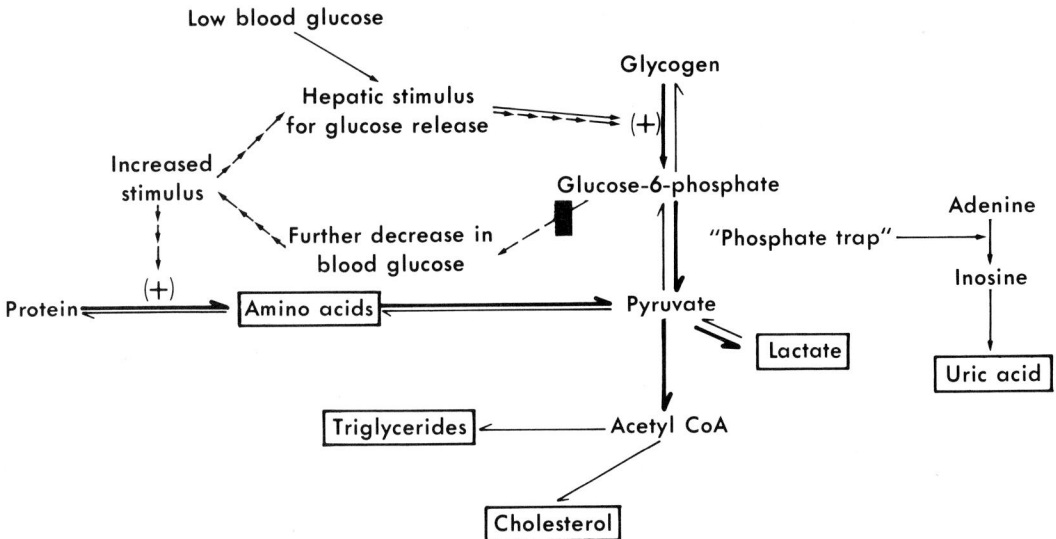

Figure 49–6. Biochemical basis for the primary laboratory findings in patients with glucose-6-phosphatase deficiency (indicated by the solid rectangle). The increased production of glucose-6-phosphate that results from continuous stimulation of glycogen breakdown apparently increases glycolysis, which in turn results in a net increase (indicated by dark arrows) in the production of lactate, triglyceride, cholesterol, and uric acid. Both glycogenolysis and gluconeogenesis are involved in the overproduction of substrate.

urate excretion together with the rate of incorporation of ^{14}C-L-glycine into plasma and urinary urate indicates that an increased rate of purine synthesis de novo is probably more important in the genesis of hyperuricemia than is a decrease in urate excretion.[147, 148] There are at least two mechanisms by which the rate of purine synthesis can be influenced: (1) alteration of the substrate (precursor) concentration (i.e., phosphoribosyl pyrophosphate [PRPP] and glutamine levels) and (2) alteration of the end product, or purine concentration (i.e., low intracellular purine levels increase purine synthesis).[149–151] In support of the former, two substrates, PRPP and glutamine, are necessary for the first committed reaction. This reaction transfers the amine from L-glutamine to PRPP to form 5-phosphoribosyl-1-amine and is apparently rate-limiting for the entire sequence of purine synthesis (Reaction [4]). Although tissue glutamate and glutamine levels have not been measured, blood levels of the two substrates obtained from hyperuricemic patients with GSD-I are three- to eightfold higher than are values obtained after urate is normalized by glucose infusion.[143] In addition to the possibility of increased availability of glutamine, the high levels of glucose-6-phosphate produced during periods of hypoglycemia and excessive glycogenolysis may increase synthesis of the second important substrate in purine synthesis, ribose-5-phosphate.[141, 145, 152] This suggests that an apparent increased availability of purine precursors, glutamine, and ribose-5-phosphate may cause a secondary increase in PRPP and thus increase the

rate of purine synthesis. Studies using human leukocytes indicate, however, that an increase in availability of glutamine and ribose-5-phosphate alone will not increase the generation of PRPP.[153] Assuming this is true in liver, the second mechanism, alteration of end-product concentration, should be more important in modulating the increased rate of purine synthesis in patients with GSD-I.

In support of the second mechanism for hyperuricemia, a decreased concentration of purine ribonucleotides would favor an increase in the rate of purine biosynthesis by releasing the glutamine pyrophosphate-ribose-phosphate amidotransferase from end-product inhibition.[154] Although hepatic nucleotide levels during hypoglycemic episodes have not been determined directly, indirect evidence suggests that in patients with GSD-I, hypoglycemia can reduce adenyl ribonucleotide levels. Such a conclusion is based on measured values of hepatic ATP before and after simulating the effects of hypoglycemia with intravenous glucagon administration.[155] Seven patients had threefold decreases in hepatic ATP levels with concomitant 1.3-fold decreases in ADP. Such a reduction in ATP has been shown to favor the rapid degradation of adenyl or guanyl ribonucleotides to xanthine and uric acid.[156, 157] The latter set of reactions is also favored by low intracellular phosphate levels, which apparently occur through "phosphate trapping" of the phosphorylated sugar. Normally, this accumulation of glucose-6-phosphate is prevented by the action of glucose-6-phosphatase.[156]

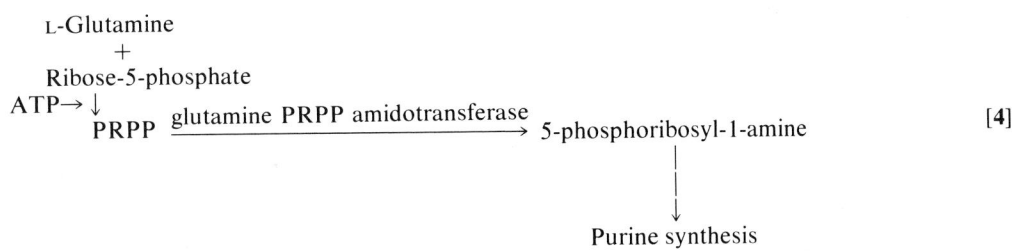

[4]

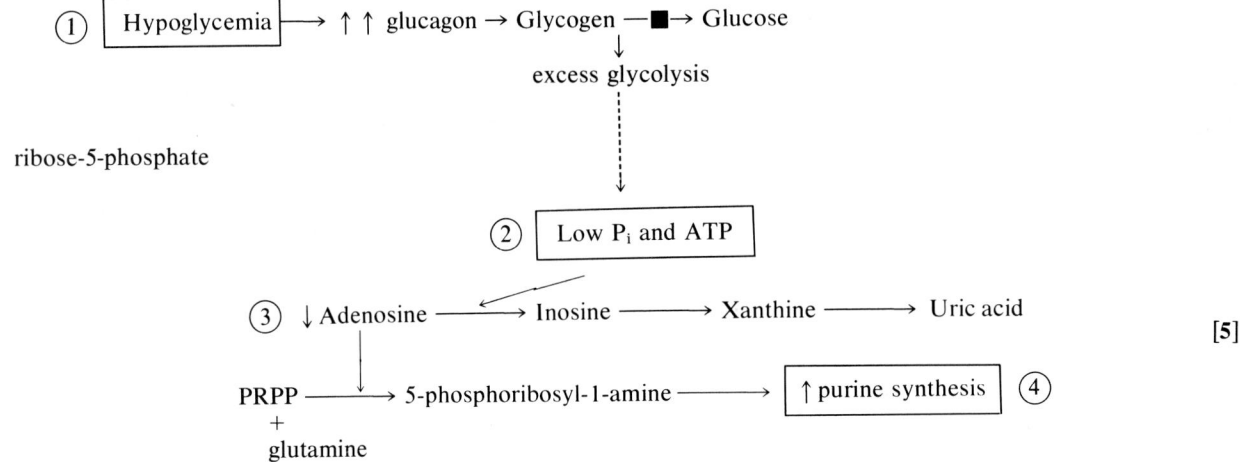

These observations suggest that the increase in urate production is secondary to recurrent episodes of hypoglycemia (Reaction [5]), which result in compensatory glucagon release. This hepatotropic agent stimulates glycogen degradation to glucose-6-phosphate. The absence of phosphatase activity results in a phosphate-trapping effect and lowering of ATP levels (Reaction [5]), which in turn promotes degradation of preformed purines to uric acid (Reaction [5]).[17, 157, 158] Finally, the decrease in end-product (purine) concentration promotes a high rate of purine biosynthesis (Reaction [5]).

Hypophosphatemia. Low serum phosphate levels are not an invariable finding, but are more likely to be present during periods of hypoglycemia and acidosis. It has been noted that a glucagon injection is followed by an acute decrease in serum phosphate that spontaneously reverts to the preinjection level within three hours. This suggests that cellular $[P_i]$ levels are rapidly depleted by the glucagon effects and that there is a compensatory shift of phosphate out of the circulating pool. A well-demonstrated corollary occurs after fructose ingestion in patients with hereditary fructose intolerance. This has been shown to result from phosphate trapping on the fructose moiety because of blockage of the aldolase step.[6, 17, 157, 158] As a result of the inability to release inorganic phosphate from the sugar, the liver cell must take up phosphorus from serum (Reaction [6]). For example, when 6.6 mmol of fructose are administered to an 8.8-kg infant, the fructose load exceeds the amount of inorganic phosphate mole per mole, in the entire extracellular fluid.[6]

A phenomenon analogous to that seen in hereditary fructose intolerance apparently occurs because of the phosphate trap created as a result of glucose-6-phosphatase deficiency. A relative metabolic block at the aldolase step would also be expected because of the progressive increase in NADH formed during the initial phase of the reaction cascade from glucose-6-phosphate to pyruvate. The demonstrated decrease in hepatic glycogen content by a mean of 2.3 per cent following a glucagon injection will provide a large amount of glucose-6-phosphate that cannot be hydrolyzed to release the bound inorganic phosphate[155] (Reaction [7]). The series of reactions (Reaction [7]) reflects the phosphate trapping by the accumulated sugars of the anaerobic pathway, thus causing an acute shift of circulating phosphate to the intracellular pool. As the phosphate is lost from the sugars, there will be a compensatory shift of phosphate back into the circulation.

Recurrent Fever. A few patients have recurrent fever in association with acidosis and hypoglycemia. In these patients, the fever can be reproduced by intravenous injection of glucagon if the patient is already slightly hypoglycemic (blood glucose 35 to 55 mg/dl) and acidotic (arterial blood pH 7.28 to 7.36). The febrile response begins 8 to 12 minutes following glucagon injection (0.1 mg/kg given over 3 minutes), and usually peaks 12 to 16 minutes later. If the low blood glucose level is corrected by intravenous administration of glucose and the acidosis is corrected by sodium bicarbonate, the temperature will usually return to normal within 45 minutes following glucagon infusion.

If the explanation for hypophosphatemia just postu-

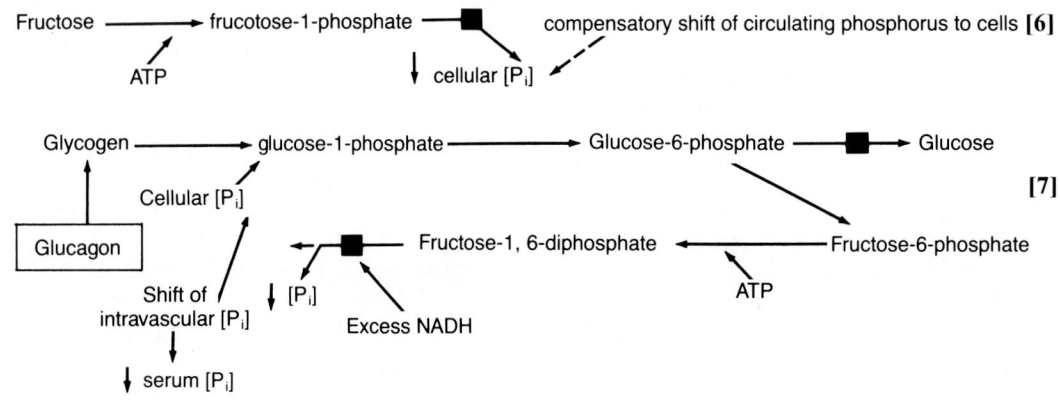

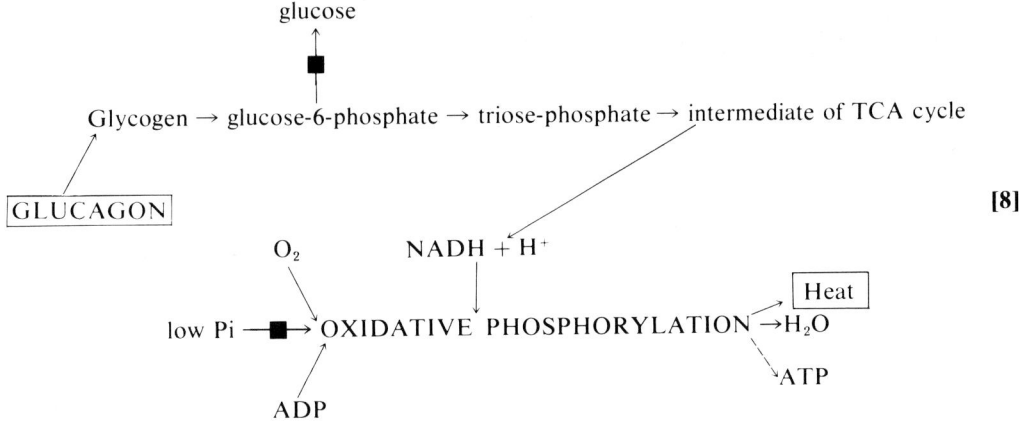

[8]

lated is correct, the febrile response may represent an uncoupling of oxidative phosphorylation secondary to lack of P_i. For example, the glucagon results in the excessive formation of glucose-6-phosphate from glycogen. Because of the glucose-6-phosphatase deficiency, a burst of glycolysis results in excess production of reduced cofactors, which normally produce high-energy phosphates. Because of low intracellular phosphate levels, oxidative phosphorylation, were it to occur, would have to be uncoupled, leading to production of heat rather than chemical energy in the form of ATP (Reaction [8]).

Platelet Dysfunction. Patients with GSD-I usually have prolonged bleeding times secondary to abnormal platelet aggregation. Corby and co-workers examined platelet function in 13 patients, each with deficient hepatic activity of one of the following enzymes: glucose-6-phosphatase, debrancher enzyme, phosphorylase, or phosphorylase kinase.[158] Only the seven patients with glucose-6-phosphatase deficiencies had abnormal platelet aggregation, and four of these also had abnormal platelet adhesiveness. The defect appears to be intrinsic, since crossover and resuspension studies using patient platelets in normal plasma and normal platelets in patient plasma did not alter in vitro platelet function. Two such patients had the ADP content of affected platelets measured, and in either instance it was normal. Nevertheless, the release of ADP from platelets in response to added collagen and epinephrine was markedly impaired. These observations suggest that the functional defect is an impairment of the ability of the platelet membrane to release ADP. Cooper has shown a similar defect in ADP release from platelets with elevated cholesterol content.[159] The elevated cholesterol content impaired fluidity of the membrane, causing secondary impairment of ADP and epinephrine-induced aggregation. Although platelet cholesterol levels of patients with GSD-I have not been measured, the elevated serum cholesterol content might reflect elevated platelet cholesterol content and therefore may contribute to the abnormality of platelet function in GSD-I patients. If this postulate is correct, then treatment that lowers blood and platelet cholesterol levels should also normalize platelet function. One of the author's patients recently was found to have abnormal platelet function but had normal serum cholesterol and triglyceride levels. This finding does not support the hypothesis.

Growth Impairment. Children who have GSD-I are of short stature but without disproportionate head sizes or limb or trunk lengths. The abdomen is usually massively enlarged as a result of hepatomegaly. Bones may be osteoporotic, and some patients have delayed bone age. The

mechanism leading to these changes is not clear. Growth hormone and thyroid hormone levels are normal or increased.[129, 133] Measurements of calorie-protein intake in three patients for two weeks indicated adequate caloric consumption. Recent observations suggest that chronic lactic acidosis and concomitant reversal of the insulin-glucagon ratio may be more important factors in preventing normal growth.

Hepatic Adenomas and Carcinomas. The development of adenomatous nodules within hepatic parenchyma was an infrequent finding until recently. Most patients with GSD-I who are more than 15 years old are now found to develop adenomas. This is at variance with the previously held view that they occur only infrequently. Adenomas develop in most patients during the second decade of life, but they may be seen in 3-year-old children. The nodules, which are best demonstrated by ultrasonography and radioisotopic scanning, show increased echodensity and decreased isotope uptake. At laparotomy, they appear as discrete, pale nodules that range in number from one to many and in size from 1 to 5 cm. A number of patients have been found to have solitary hepatocellular adenocarcinomas in individual nodules.[160–163] The mechanism causing the adenomas or their malignant degeneration is unknown, but treatment with portacaval shunting does not prevent their development. The authors now have two patients who had adenomas prior to nocturnal feedings, but after three years of treatment, nodules were no longer detectable by scanning (Fig. 49–7). A subsequent older patient (aged 16 years) developed adenomas during treatment with nocturnal feedings, that were later found to be inadequate to maintain blood glucose above 75 mg/dl. After readjustment of therapy, the nodules decreased in size but did not show complete resolution. This suggests that chronic stimulation of the liver by hepatotropic agents (glucagon and others) that increase blood glucose levels may be important in the genesis of the adenomas.

The tendency for adenoma formation and malignant transformation is highest in young adult patients and appears to be a consequence of supportive therapy which presently ensures survival into childhood and young adulthood. The mechanism leading to hepatic malignancy is unknown, although review of case histories suggests that the adenomatous cells rather than the nonadenomatous cells are transformed.[164] A similar progression has been observed in experimental hepatocarcinogenesis from exposure to N-nitrosomorpholine.[164] The progression from normal hepatocytes to malignancy appears to be as follows. First, multifocal areas of cells containing excessive glycogen

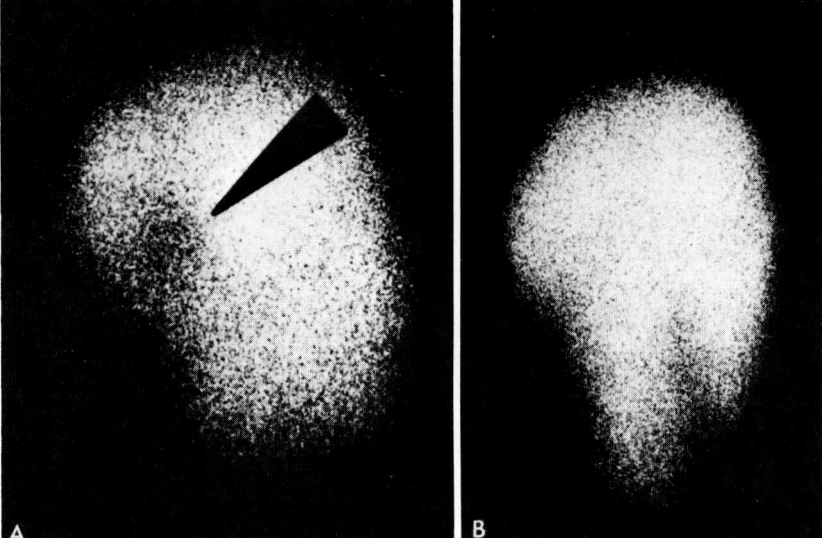

Figure 49–7. Technetium scan of the liver, showing regression of hepatic filling defect in response to dietary therapy. The arrow in *A* indicates a hepatic adenoma before therapy; *B* shows its disappearance, with reduction in the size of the liver, after four years of dietary therapy.

develop. The cells in these areas also show decreased glucose-6-phosphatase activity. Second, the focal cluster of cells develops a gradual reduction in glycogen content and a concomitant increase in ribosomes, reflected as basophilia by hematoxylin and eosin (H & E) staining. Finally, the foci enlarge and acquire the phenotypic markers of hepatocellular carcinoma. These experimental observations, coupled with the findings in patients with GSD-I, have led Bannasch and associates to postulate that the metabolic disturbance leading to hepatocellular glycogenesis is fixed at the genetic level in both the experimental animals and the patients and is causally related to the neoplastic transformation.[164]

Severity of Illness. In spite of the fact that there is no difference in activities of the phosphatase enzyme between patients, the expression of symptoms and of chemical anomalies vary substantially from one patient to another without detectable differences in management. Some patients may have only moderate abnormalities in blood chemistry and slightly decreased growth rates, whereas others may have marked alterations in blood lipids, require frequent hospitalizations for fever and lactic acidosis, or even die in infancy or early childhood.

In addition, there appears to be some abatement of hypoglycemia after patients have reached adulthood. In fact, a few patients who had had moderately severe symptoms during childhood improved so dramatically during adulthood that they were able to have successful pregnancies.[165–166]

Glucose Production. In 1967, Havel reported that two adult patients with GSD-I showed near normal basal rates of glucose production using ^{14}C-glucose as a marker.[167] This observation has been confirmed in patients of all ages by several investigators who used dideuteroglucose as the isotopic marker.[168–171] These studies indicate in addition several features of the illness that have important therapeutic implications. (1) Patients with GSD-I can release glucose into the circulation at close to normal basal rates. (2) Patients cannot increase glucose release during hypoglycemia or following a pharmacologic dose of glucagon; therefore, their basal rates of glucose production are also their maximal rates of production. (3) Maximal glucose production is variable between patients but is not related to residual activity of hepatic glucose-6-phosphatase. How-

ever, the tendency for fasting-induced hypoglycemia and severity of the clinical illness is directly related to maximal rates of glucose production. (4) Endogenous glucose production is not inhibited unless an exogenous source of glucose is provided at a rate of 8 mg/kg/minute, an amount that maintains blood glucose levels at about 90 mg/dl. (5) The improvement in ability to fast for a longer time period after the second decade of life appears to result from a decrease in glucose utilization rather than an increase in glucose production.

Diagnosis

Characteristically, these patients have no increase in blood glucose following administration of glucagon or epinephrine, and usually they show substantial decreases in blood glucose within 20 minutes following intravenous glucagon administration. As mentioned in the previous section, a major product of glycogenolysis is lactate rather than glucose. In some patients who are already slightly acidotic, glucagon stimulation may cause severe acidosis. Aside from the glucagon tolerance test, other tolerance tests have been used as an aid in diagnosing the type of glycogenosis. For example, neither galactose nor fructose is converted to free glucose in patients with GSD-I, and a tolerance test with either of these sugars results in a flat blood glucose curve. These tolerance tests have the advantage of avoiding liver biopsy. On the other hand, a substantial volume of blood is required to complete all the tolerance testing, and not infrequently, the results are inconclusive. For example, the authors have had several patients referred with erroneous diagnoses based on tolerance tests. Thus, for accurate diagnosis, the authors feel that measurement of hepatic enzyme activity is necessary. To provide a basis for some selectivity in the enzymatic analyses of biopsy specimens, the authors' practice is to determine serial blood glucose and lactate measurements during a 4- to 6-hour fast, followed by the maximum glucose response to glucagon before liver biopsy. For example, a rise in glucose of more than 30 mg/dl generally indicates a defect in phosphorylase kinase, which is not routinely measured from needle-biopsy material.

Before an effective form of treatment was available, the necessity for accurate diagnosis was less important than it is today. Because of the effectiveness of treatment of patients with glucose-6-phosphatase deficiency, the suspected diagnosis of glycogen storage disease should be confirmed by enzymatic assay of hepatic tissue. A diagnosis can be confirmed by examination of needle biopsy material, which avoids potential complications of surgery and general anesthesia.[172]

Pathology

In GSD-I the liver cells are distended with glycogen and often contain medium-sized to large lipid vacuoles. The lipid content in the liver of an untreated patient is substantially greater than that in the liver of a patient who has been treated, but in either instance, hepatic steatosis is a prominent morphologic feature. The liver cells are pale-staining and have prominent plasma membranes. Three notable features differentiate GSD-I from other glycogenoses: (1) the presence of substantial steatosis, (2) a lack of associated fibrosis, and (3) nuclear hyperglycogenosis. Nuclear glycogenosis is commonly seen in hepatocytes of normal children, but in GSD-I (and GSD-III), the nuclei are grotesquely enlarged—that is, hyperglycogenosis is present.

It is not possible to distinguish between normal and elevated levels of cytoplasmic glycogen in the liver in any of the forms of glycogenosis through the use of periodic acid-Schiff (PAS) stain.[173] Thus, to make a diagnosis of excessive glycogen content, a quantitative determination is necessary. It is also important to note that the livers of normal individuals and those of patients with glucose-6-phosphatase deficiencies can degrade glycogen. Thus, post-mortem analyses of surgical specimens that are not frozen promptly may give inappropriately low (e.g., "normal") levels.

Treatment

Patients with some glycogenoses—for example, those who have deficiencies of hepatic phosphorylase kinase activity and some patients with GSD-III (debrancher deficiency)—have excellent prognoses without specific treatment. In fact, with the exception of those who have defects in glycogen synthesis, generalized glycogenosis (acid maltase deficiency; GSD-II; Pompe's disease), or glucose-6-phosphatase deficiencies, most patients who have hepatic glycogenoses have favorable prognoses and are successfully managed with attention to frequencies of food intake. This, however, has not been true of most patients who have GSD-I.

Present recommendations for treatment of GSD-I stem primarily from the studies of Folkman and associates,[174] who first illustrated the reversal of most biochemical abnormalities after total parenteral nutrition (TPN). Their observation that both TPN and portacaval shunting[175, 176] delivered nutrients primarily into the systemic circulation suggested that hepatic exposure to nutrients was important in the pathogenesis of many biochemical abnormalities. Nevertheless, it was later demonstrated that the same beneficial effect seen with TPN or portacaval shunting could be achieved with an intragastric infusion of a nutrient solution similar in content to that used for TPN.[177] This suggested that bypassing the liver with nutrients was not the most important factor in reversing the abnormalities. The similarity in the three types of treatment (i.e., portacaval shunting, TPN, and continuous intragastric infusion of glucose) was that a hormonal stimulus to the liver to produce glucose was decreased or averted. Specifically, TPN and continuous intragastric feeding both prevented a hepatic stimulus for glucose release by maintaining blood glucose levels in the range of 90 to 150 mg/dl, whereas the portacaval shunt prevented such a stimulus by diverting pancreatic and enteric blood into systemic circulation. On this basis, the hypothesis for treatment illustrated in Figure 49–8 was formulated.

The hypothesis states that as blood glucose falls below a critical level, compensatory mechanisms cause glycogen degradation to glucose-6-phosphate. In the absence of glucose-6-phosphatase, glucose-6-phosphate is not hydrolyzed to release free glucose, and the hepatic stimulus for glycogenolysis results in formation of other intermediates such as lactate, triglycerides, and cholesterol. To interrupt the stimulus, treatment with an exogenous source of glucose would inhibit the release of hepatotropic stimuli and thus the excess glycogenolysis. If this postulate is correct, any method of treatment that maintains blood glucose above this critical level should also prevent or at least alleviate biochemical manifestations of the illness. In addition, the hypothesis suggests that diversion of portal vein blood flow should dilute hepatotropic agents in the systemic circulation. This dilution would result in less hepatic stimulation for glycogenolysis.

Theoretically, either portacaval shunting or continuous infusion of a high-glucose diet should be effective in reversing most manifestations of the illness, with the exception that portacaval shunting should have little or no beneficial effect on hypoglycemia. Thus, portacaval shunting is not recommended as a sole form of treatment for those patients who are expected to have frequent episodes of very low blood glucose levels or for small children, in whom shunts may be more likely to close spontaneously.

Although TPN and continuous intragastric infusion of glucose are effective treatment modalities for GSD-I, they are impractical on a long-term basis. A more practical method was devised to maintain blood glucose at physiologic concentrations or at levels that would prevent stimulation of excess glycogenolysis and glycolysis. This treatment consisted of a high-glucose diet given to simulate TPN. Thus, it was given enterally either by nasogastric tube or by gastrostomy during nighttime sleep, along with a high-starch diet, which was consumed at frequent intervals while the patient was awake. Such a regimen has successfully maintained a large number of patients relatively symptom-free for over ten years and has provided normal or near-normal growth and development.[178, 202]

More recently, Chen and colleagues have found that a number of patients can maintain normal blood glucose levels by taking cold, uncooked cornstarch (2 g/kg) at 6-hour intervals.[179] This regimen has been used by a number of patients to avoid the continuous nocturnal feedings. A number of the younger children have not been able to maintain normal glucose and lactate levels as well with the cornstarch regimen as they had with the continuous nocturnal feeding regimen.[180, 181] In the authors' experience, growth rates were less with the raw starch regimen than with continuous feedings, and one patient consumed such large quantities of cornstarch that protein intake was insufficient to maintain normal secretory proteins (albumin, transferrin, and retinol-binding protein). Thus, while the cornstarch feedings can be beneficial as a "time-release" form of glucose in some patients, a dose response to the starch preparation and careful monitoring of blood glucose levels should be carried out to ensure that treatment is appropriate for individual patients. The authors believe

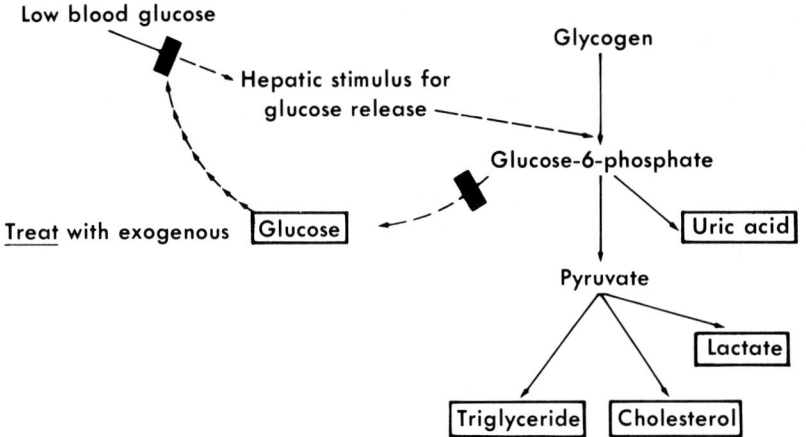

Figure 49–8. A biochemical basis for management of patients with glucose-6-phosphatase deficiency (indicated by solid rectangle). By preventing the decrease in blood glucose with an exogenous supply of glucose, excessive glycolysis and gluconeogenesis are prevented. This results in a net decrease in production of circulating triglyceride, cholesterol, lactate, and uric acid.

that many patients will require an intensive feeding regimen at least until they have stopped growing. This consists of high starch feedings at 2- to 3-hour intervals during the day, continuous nocturnal feeding of a complete, low lipid–containing (< 5 per cent calories) formula, and periodic monitoring to ensure normal blood glucose and lactate levels throughout the day and night. As the patients become fully grown and have a relatively lower requirement for glucose, the uncooked cornstarch regimen may allow discontinuation of the nighttime nasogastric feedings.

Prognosis

Until the use of nocturnal feedings, the first few years of life were usually marked by frequent hospitalizations for treatment of hypoglycemia and acidosis, with a high rate of death or permanent CNS impairment from recurrent and prolonged episodes of hypoglycemia. Patients who survived puberty appeared to have fewer problems than they had when younger. Patients with persistent hyperuricemia had gouty complications during the second and third decades of life and many patients had complications of hyperlipemia, with xanthomas, and with higher rates of cardiovascular disease and pancreatitis than those in the general population.[128–130, 137, 182] Recognition of hepatic adenomas has been relatively recent, and the incidence of complications from benign hepatic adenomas is unclear, although several patients have developed malignant hepatomas.[160, 162]

Long-term follow-up of the results of portacaval shunting or nocturnal feedings is not complete. Ten-year follow-up of patients treated with nocturnal feedings indicates that infants so treated have many fewer problems than they had prior to treatment, and that some patients with hepatic adenomas may show resolution after a few years of treatment. Too few patients have been followed into the third decade of life to permit conclusions, but early observations indicate that, for optimal treatment, the nocturnal feedings are necessary for most young patients, whereas raw cornstarch administration may suffice for older patients. On the other hand, patients generally have less tendency to hypoglycemia after the age of 20. A 22-year-old patient, severely affected at the age of 15 years, had been treated with nocturnal feedings for 6½ years, with complete resolution of all chemical manifestations of the illness except hypoglycemia (blood glucose 62 mg/dl) and lactate elevation (7 mEq/L) after a nine-hour fast. She was weaned off nocturnal feedings by gradually decreasing the hourly feeding over a period of a month. After 2½ years of no nocturnal

feedings, she continues to have completely normal blood chemistry results after an eight-hour fast. There is still no hepatic glucose-6-phosphatase activity, however.

So long as blood glucose is consistently maintained between 70 and 120 mg/dl, most children appear to lead fairly normal, healthy lives, with normal growth and development, although in at least one patient the disease has been unresponsive to this type of management.[183] A recent report indicates that a blood level of 90 mg/dl (achieved by a glucose infusion of 8 mg/kg minute) is necessary to completely inhibit endogenous glucose production. However, this dose provides additional calories, and unless the lower infusion rate does not correct the metabolic abnormalities, the greater tendency for obesity can be avoided by the lower rate of infusion.

Most recently, Chen and colleagues have observed that older patients (>18 yrs) with suboptimal treatment have a high incidence of progressive renal disease. The affected individuals show progressive glomerular sclerosis with proteinuria as an early manifestation.[183a] Although the cause of the lesion is unclear, it appears that the incidence is lowered by maintenance of good control of blood glucose and other blood abnormalities since none of the authors' nine patients ages 25 to 34 show renal abnormalities.

Glycogen Storage Disease Type IB

In 1968, Senior and Loridan described a patient with clinical and laboratory features identical to GSD-I except that no enzyme defect was identified from frozen liver.[164] Subsequently, a number of similar patients have been identified.[184–194] In addition to the hepatic abnormality, patients have repeated infections because of neutropenia and abnormal leukocyte migration,[188–192] and some show decreased neutrophil phagocytosis–stimulated oxygen consumption, decreased NBT reduction,[191] defective bactericidal activity, and defective hexose monophosphate shunt activity.[192] These patients have been diagnosed as having glycogen storage disease type IB. There has been little mention of a familial occurrence in the reports of GSD-IB. This is curious, since a number of patients with GSD-I have affected siblings. One of the author's patients with GSD-IB has seven unaffected siblings. The number of reported cases is small, however, and the mode of inheritance is presumed to be autosomal recessive.

The reason for the discrepancy between the in vitro and in vivo activity of glucose-6-phosphatase in patients with GSD-IB is not known. Steady-state kinetic measurements led Arion and associates to conclude that the normal microsomal glucose-6-phosphatase enzyme is a two-compartment system consisting of a specific glucose-6-phosphate carrier on the outer half (side) of the membrane of the endoplasmic reticulum and a catalytic phosphorylase component located on the inner half of the membrane.[193] Since disruption of isolated microsomes of patients with GSD-IB with cholate or freeze-thawing results in a marked increase in activity, the general assumption has been that the defect in GSD-IB is a deficiency of the translocase or carrier portion of the enzyme system,[185, 186, 193, 194] although the putative translocase has never been identified in microsomes from normal liver. Zakim and Edmonson, using methods to measure presteady-state kinetics,[195] have shown that the limiting step in the reaction is not glucose release from the enzyme but the release of phosphate. These findings in normal liver microsomes are similar in the liver of a patient with GSD-IB, although the presteady-state kinetics are blunted. These findings question the general concept of a translocase and suggest that patients with GSD-IB may have a configurational abnormality in the enzyme-membrane interaction which can be overcome by alteration of the membrane lipid rather than by an opening of the microsomal vescicle.[195, 196]

Treatment of GSD-IB is identical to that of GSD-IA with the possible exception that prophylactic antibiotics may improve the tendency for frequent infection.[188-192, 197] Improvement in neutrophil function with treatment has been reported by some investigators.[191, 192] However, the authors' experience was that the neutropenia and abnormal migration persisted even after three months of management that normalized all parameters of disease in the blood, and even after subsequent portacaval shunting.[197, 198] The lack of improvement in neutrophil function in some of the well-managed patients suggests that the defect in GSD-IB is intrinsic to both the liver and leukocytes. Since glucose-6-phosphatase is not known to have any importance for normal neutrophil function, the relationship between the hepatic enzyme defect and leukocyte dysfunction is not known.

Type III Glycogen Storage Disease (GSD-III) Amylo-1,6-Glucosidase (Debrancher) Deficiency

This glycogenosis accumulates a polysaccharide that has a structure of a limit dextrin produced by degradation of glycogen with phosphorylase and oligo 1,4-1,4 glucan-transferase but no debrancher activity (Reaction [9]).[199]

As depicted, the terminal α-1,4-glucosyl units are hydrolyzed by the combined activity of oligo 1,4-1,4 glucan-transferase and phosphorylase, but the inner branch points of α-1,6 linkages ($\boxed{G}$) are not hydrolyzed by debranching enzyme. Thus, the glycogen molecule is abnormal, with an excessive number of branch points (1,6 linkages). Depending upon the tissue(s) involved and enzymatic characteristics, subtypes of GSD-III have been described (i.e., GSD-IIIA, GSD-IIIB, and so on).

Clinical Characteristics

By physical examination alone, these patients cannot be readily distinguished from patients who have type I glycogenosis (GSD-I). Early in life, hepatomegaly and growth failure may be striking. However, a few patients may develop splenomegaly at 4 to 6 years of age.[200] These

patients usually have evidence of hepatic fibrosis but do not necessarily progress to cirrhosis and liver failure.

In addition to hepatic involvement, a number of patients with GSD-III have muscle weakness. Rapid walking and climbing result in increased weakness without cramps.[201] In some patients, there may be a progressive myopathy. Glycogen may also accumulate in the heart, and moderate cardiomegaly with nonspecific electrocardiographic changes is sometimes present.[202] However, congestive heart failure and cardiac arrhythmias are not reported. There is no renal enlargement in GSD-III, in contradistinction to GSD-I.

GLYCOGEN

G
|
G
|
G
|
$\boxed{G}$
|
G—G—G—G—G　G—G—G—G—G　　　　[9]
$\boxed{G}$　→ 1,6 link hydrolyzed normally by
G　　　debranching enzyme
|
G
|
G
|
G

The clinical course in GSD-III is generally much milder than that of GSD-I, in that severe hypoglycemia is not a problem except with prolonged fasting. Some patients have shown relative decreases in liver size around puberty,[199, 203] but rare patients have shown evidence of progressive fibrosis and liver failure.[128, 204, 205] The latter patients may have an additional phosphorylase or phosphorylase kinase deficiency.[128]

Biochemical Characteristics and Laboratory Findings

Lipid levels in plasma are variably elevated and to some extent appear to be related to the individual tendency toward fasting-induced hypoglycemia.[203] That is, the patients who develop lower glucose levels with six- to eight-hour fasts tend to have higher blood lipid levels. However, none of the patients approach the severe elevations of 4000 to 6000 mg/dl seen with GSD-I. Uric acid levels are generally normal, but rare patients reportedly have slight elevations. Serum transaminase levels are consistently moderately elevated (300 to 600 IU; normal <40 IU),[55] although some patients show elevations of 900 to 2000 IU.

Galactose and fructose are readily converted to glucose by these patients; similarly, protein and amino acid mixtures induce small and prolonged increases in blood glucose levels.[138, 203] Both glucagon and epinephrine increase blood glucose when given between one and one half and three hours following a meal but elicit little response after a 14-hour fast ("double glucagon tolerance test").[206] This result is interpreted to indicate available 1,4 glucosyl linkages that can be degraded by phosphorylase shortly after a meal. The glycogen in this case is degraded only until 1,6 linkages are encountered. Access to 1,4 linkages is blocked by terminal 1,6 glycosyl linkages that would be present after a prolonged fast, and these would prevent glucose increase after glucagon administration. Unfortunately, the glucose response to the double glucagon tolerance test is not a consistent finding, and it should not be used as a definitive diagnostic test. Since glucagon also stimulates gluconeogenesis, the inconsistency of the test results is possibly due to glucose formation via this pathway.

The liver content of glycogen is often markedly increased (to as much as 17.4 g/100 g tissue) in GSD-III.[199] By various techniques, the glycogen is found to have abnormally short outer branch points. Many patients also show some depression of glucose-6-phosphatase activity. Hug has found several patients with combined defects in phosphorylase and phosphorylase kinase. These patients are generally more severely affected and tend to develop cirrhosis.[128]

A series of techniques is available for measuring debrancher activity: (1) liberation of glucose from phosphorylase-treated limit dextrin, (2) incorporation of ^{14}C-glucose into glycogen, (3) 1,4 → 1,4 transfer of an oligoglucan (glucan transferase activity), and (4) hydrolysis of singly branched oligosaccharides. Using these various techniques, Hers and associates have identified a series of biochemical subtypes of GSD-III. These subtypes are also divided according to types of muscle glycogen.[199, 207, 208]

Pathology

The liver in GSD-III is very similar in appearance to that in GSD-I with two notable exceptions: (1) the presence of fibrous septa or frank cirrhosis and (2) the paucity of fat (Fig. 49–9). Until recently, there had been no demonstration of progression of the fibrosis to cirrhosis. Hug reports

that progression to cirrhosis is more likely to occur in patients who have combined enzymatic defects.[128, 208] The ultrastructural appearance of the liver is not distinguishable from that seen in GSD-I except that in GSD-III lipid vacuoles are small and are less frequent.[208]

If muscle is affected, excessive glycogen is readily demonstrable in ethanol-fixed specimens by the PAS method. Glycogen accumulates between intact myofibrils and in the subsarcolemmal position,[209] locations in which glycogen usually occurs but not in abundance. The diagnosis depends upon demonstration of deficient activity of amylo-1,6-glucosidase (debrancher enzyme).

Treatment

Treatment of this disorder remains investigative. It should be restricted to patients who have obvious muscle involvement, progressive fibrotic changes in the liver, or both. An accurate correlation between the type of glycogen accumulation and progression of liver disease, so that a clear-cut prognosis could be assigned to each patient, would be helpful in showing a positive therapeutic response.

Present investigative efforts combine the technique of nocturnal feedings with the known responses to protein and amino acids.[138, 203, 210] Slonim and coworkers have shown improved growth and increased muscle strength in a patient given a high-protein diet during the day and continuous nocturnal intragastric feedings of a high-protein liquid formula (Sustacal) at night.[211] More recently, Borowitz and Greene[212] have found that growth and transaminase and blood glucose levels were more positively influenced by a high starch diet with a standard (Recommended Dietary Allowance) protein intake. This therapy is therefore virtually identical to that for GSD-I. This circumstance is

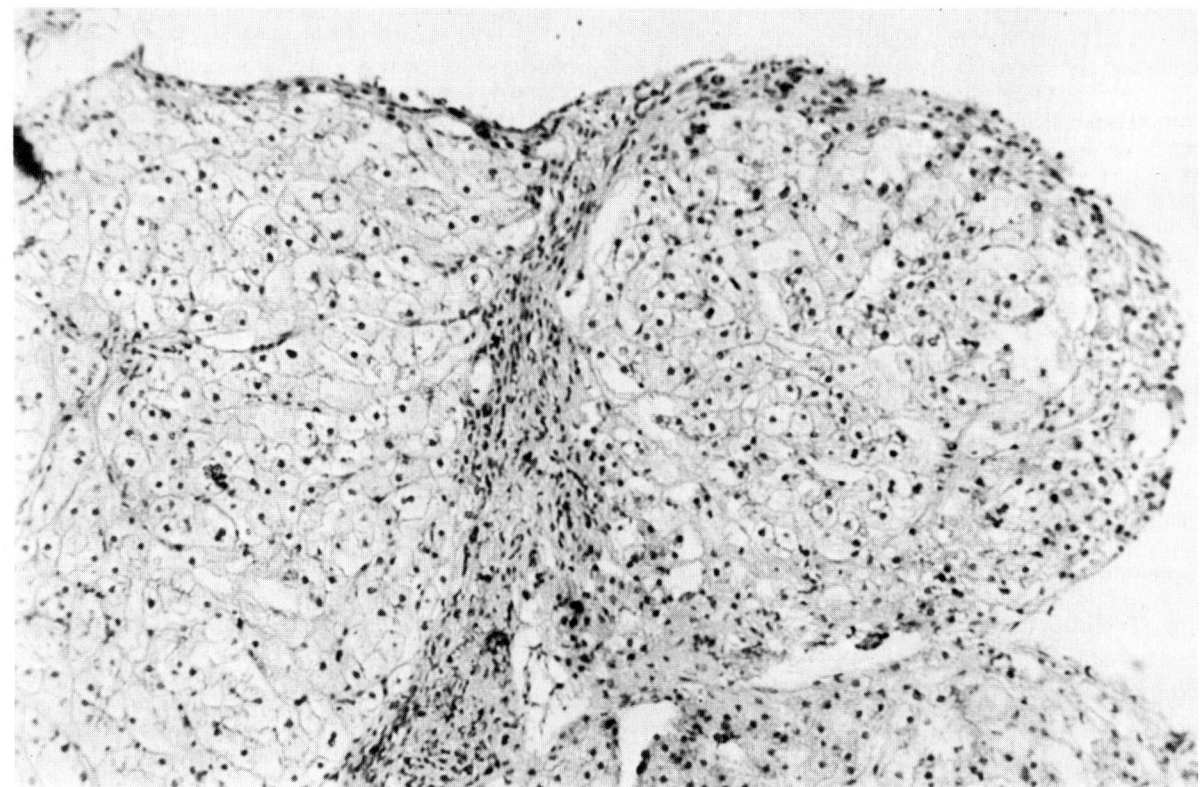

Figure 49–9. Percutaneous liver biopsy specimen from a patient with glycogen storage disease, type III, showing increased fibrosis. The hepatocytes do not contain fat deposition. × 80.

encouraging, but more extensive follow-up evaluation over a longer period of treatment is needed.

Type IV Glycogenosis (α-1,4 Glucan-6-Glycosyl Transferase Deficiency; GSD-IV)

Type IV glycogen storage disease, a rare form of glycogenosis, was first described clinically and pathologically in 1952 by Anderson.[213] Illingsworth and Cori showed that the glycogen possessed abnormally long outer and inner chains of glucose units.[214] Ten years later, Brown and Brown demonstrated the absence of branching enzyme activity in this disorder.[215] The few descriptions of the disorder (about 20 documented cases) have illustrated its unusual clinical, biochemical, and pathologic aspects.[216–222]

Clinical Characteristics

Infants are normal at birth and for some months thereafter. There is an insidious onset of symptoms during the first year of life. Symptoms may manifest as early as 3 months or as late as 15 months of age. The disorder is usually diagnosed because of hepatosplenomegaly, abdominal distention, signs and symptoms referable to hepatic dysfunction, nonspecific gastrointestinal symptoms, and failure to thrive. Muscle hypotonia and wasting may be present. Superficial veins over the distended abdomen are prominent as the disease progresses. Patients who live beyond infancy develop hepatic cirrhosis with accompanying portal hypertension, ascites, and esophageal varices. The terminal course is usually due to chronic hepatic failure and jaundice with bleeding esophageal varices, although a few patients develop cardiac failure, apparently from myofibrillar damage caused by polysaccharide deposits within myocardial cells. Intercurrent infection is a common terminal complication. The duration of survival after diagnosis is usually 2 to 37 months, although an occasional patient may survive 3 to 4 years.

Mental development is normal in some instances, although it is now clear that GSD-IV may involve the neuromuscular axis at all levels—skeletal muscle, peripheral nervous system, and central nervous system. The level and extent of the neuromuscular lesions appear to vary from patient to patient, and at least one patient showed signs of involvement of all levels simultaneously.[222]

A 59-year-old man was recently described with GSD type IV. The patient had deficient branching enzyme in skeletal muscle with normal muscle glycogen and low normal enzyme activity in leukocytes.[223] The man had a 30-year history of progressive, asymmetrical limb-girdle weakness and a vacuolar myopathy. The vacuoles contained glycogen, which was partially resistant to diastase. Ultrastructural changes resembled the amylopectin polysaccharide deposits seen in childhood GSD-IV. Three other adult patients have been reported with an amylopectin-like storage myopathy; two of these later developed involvement of the heart and brain, but none showed hepatic involvement.[224–226]

Approximately 50 per cent of infants with GSD-IV have signs suggestive of involvement of the neuromuscular system and abnormal deposits of polysaccharide in skeletal muscle.[227–230] The pathologic changes can occur in the absence of clinical changes.[230] Since the majority of these patients have not had comparative measurements of branching enzyme activity in fibroblasts, liver, muscle, and leukocytes, it is not possible to correlate apparent clinical

and pathologic findings with enzymatic changes. It has been suggested that there may be two branching enzymes acting at different sites[231, 232] and that the clinical expression of this disease depends on deficiency of organ-specific brancher isoenzymes.

The authors have had recent experience in managing two unusual patients with deficient branching enzyme measured in both the liver and skin fibroblasts (by Dr. Barbara Brown, St. Louis, Missouri). The first patient, a male, showed the usual progression to cirrhosis and liver failure by 18 months of age.[232a] At age 2 years, he underwent liver transplantation and standard treatment with immunosuppressants. He is presently 3 years posttransplant with normal liver function and shows no evidence of nerve, muscle, or cardiac abnormalities. Thus, in spite of the generalized nature of the defect, transplantation of a normal liver has not been associated with obvious progression in other organs. The second patient, a 6-year-old boy, was noted at 3 years of age to have hepatomegaly and chronically elevated serum transaminases.[232b] Open liver biopsy showed moderate, generalized micronodular fibrosis and typical PAS-positive, diastase-resistant deposits in about 25 per cent of the hepatocytes. Electronmicroscopy showed accumulation of Drochman fibrils characteristic of GSD-IV, but these fibrils were not present in all cells. During the succeeding three years, the boy showed normal growth and development with spontaneous normalization of liver tests. Liver biopsy at the age of 6 years showed minimal periportal fibrosis with no PAS-positive, diastase-resistant deposits present in any hepatocytes and normal-appearing glycogen by electron microscopic analysis. Assays of hepatocytes and skin fibroblasts showed no detectable branching enzyme activity. These two patients plus previous reports of GSD-IV indicate that branching enzyme deficiency may present in a variety of ways, the classic infantile variety primarily affecting the liver. As more patients have the opportunity for transplantation, it is anticipated that a more accurate classification system can be found for the various subgroups of this unusual disorder.

Laboratory Findings

Blood electrolytes are usually within normal limits except in patients with renal tubular defects, who have low bicarbonate concentrations. Serum transaminase and alkaline phosphatase levels are usually elevated to three to six times normal. Except with malnutrition, late in the disease, serum cholesterol is often slightly elevated. Until liver failure develops, serum albumin, globulin, bilirubin, and ammonia are normal. All liver tests become abnormal as liver failure becomes severe. Glucagon and epinephrine tolerance tests cause a positive glucose response, with levels of 15 to 23 mg/dl, the maximum response occurring about 30 minutes after hormone injection and two hours after a meal.[217] Both hormones may allow detection of urinary ketone bodies. Hypoglycemia is not a characteristic feature of the illness until terminal liver failure occurs. Chronic and severe acidosis may occur secondary to a renal tubular defect in hydrogen ion excretion.[218–220]

Oral glucose and fructose tolerance tests show no abnormality, and serum lactate and pyruvate levels are normal.[217]

Biochemical Characteristics

The stored polysaccharide in GSD-IV is a glucose polymer whose properties differ from those of normal mammalian glycogen. The normal level of liver glycogen in a child in the fed state is roughly 6 per cent of the hepatic wet weight.[233, 234] Normal glycogen has the following characteristics: (1) at least 36 per cent of the glucose units are susceptible to phosphorylase-catalyzed degradation, (2) chain lengths are 8 to 12 glycosyl units, (3) branch points (1,6 linkages) make up 8 per cent, and (4) the $KI:I_2$ absorption band is at 460 nm.[13]

Patients with GSD-IV usually have hepatic glycogen levels slightly lower than normal (3.5 to 5 per cent), although one patient had a level of 10.7 per cent.[235] Hepatic glycogen in these patients is unusually susceptible to phosphorylase-induced hydrolysis ($>$ 40 per cent phosphorylase degradation), suggesting that it has longer outer chain lengths and fewer branch points (about 6 per cent) than does normal glycogen. The polysaccharide is highly chromogenic, with a maximal $KI:I_2$ absorption band at about 525 nm.[235] About half the extracted polysaccharide may be insoluble and poorly characterized. Muscle glycogen appears normal; leukocytic glycogen is abnormal, as is brancher enzyme activity in these cells.

Although the deficiency of branching enzyme explains the formation of an amylopectin-like polysaccharide, it does not account for the presence of an appreciable proportion of branch points in the abnormal glycogen. Brown and Brown suggest that normal liver contains two enzymes with branching activities of different specificities, only one of which is measured by the methods used.[215] Another possibility is that the mutant gene in this disorder has produced a protein with substantially modified enzymatic specificity such that branching occurs mainly with long outer chains.[216]

The liver glycosyl deposits and myocardial deposits are felt to be biochemically the same, since they appear similar histochemically and are both resistant to digestion by α-amylase. This resistance to digestion by amylase is difficult to explain, because there is no other evidence for the existence of an α-amylase–resistant glycogen.

Pathology

Examination of the liver shows a uniform micronodular cirrhosis with broad bands of fibrous tissue extending around and into the lobules. Portal veins, lymphatic channels, and hepatic arteries are normal with slight portal biliary duct proliferation. Liver cell plates are distorted, and as the disease progresses, the lobules develop prominent sinusoidal channels with fibrous walls coursing between thick liver plates.

Pale amphophilic or basophilic deposits occur in liver cells, cardiac and skeletal muscle, and brain.[216, 219, 222] The deposits in cardiac muscle resemble "cardiac colloid" and those in brain resemble Lafora's bodies.[219, 222]

Liver cell nuclei are frequently eccentric in position. They appear (with H & E stain) to be displaced by pale, slightly eosinophilic or colorless inclusions deposited in the cytoplasm. This is the most striking and characteristic finding and is generally limited to the periphery of the lobule. The inclusions vary from hyaline to reticulate and are usually sharply demarcated from normal cytoplasm. Clear halos may surround the contents of the inclusions. In the late stages of the disease, nodular accumulations of a slightly different hyaline, fibrillar material are scattered throughout the hepatic lobules. This material is birefringent, appearing in polarized light as sheaths of crystals that cannot be easily distinguished from deposits that typify α_1-antitrypsin deficiency, except perhaps on the basis of their greater frequency and larger size in GSD-IV. In both

conditions, the peripheral lobular deposits are PAS-positive and diastase-resistant.[233]

Examination of myocardial tissue shows hypertrophied muscle fibers with large rectangular nuclei. Within the fibers, colorless discrete deposits similar to those in the liver are found. These deposits are uniformly distributed, with only a slight predilection for subendocardial regions. The epicardium and vessels are normal, without significant myocardial fibrosis, endocardial sclerosis, necrosis, or calcification.

PAS-positive material may be present within foamy macrophages of the spleen and lymph nodes, smooth muscle of the gastrointestinal tract and large blood vessels, and skeletal muscle around the larynx, diaphragm, tongue, and esophagus. Peripheral skeletal muscle is usually free of any abnormality except for scant amounts of abnormal polysaccharide.

Central nervous system abnormalities have been found in only 6 of 20 reported cases. In these instances, discrete, spherical PAS-positive globules were widely scattered throughout the neuraxis. They were usually most prominent in white matter and in subependymal and subapical regions but were also numerous in gray matter. Peripheral nerves also contain PAS-positive globules in the endoneurium. The PAS-positive deposits in neuronal tissue are also resistant to amylase digestion.[222]

Electronmicroscopic studies show a decrease in cytoplasmic organelles. The organelles are found in "tongues" of cytoplasm extending between large, irregular aggregates of low electron density. The contents of these aggregates are variable, and they contain two or three components: glycogen rosettes or the alpha particles of Drochman fibrils and granular material. Some areas, which contain primarily glycogen, frequently fail to stain well despite the use of lead citrate. The fibrils are straight or curved and are about 65 Å wide.[221]

Myocardial fibers are distended by zones of material with low electron density, similar to those seen in the liver. Unlike liver cells, cardiac cells rarely contain material thought to be glycogen.

Electron microscopic examination of skeletal muscle reveals granulofibrillar deposits similar to those in the viscera but less conspicuous; beta glycogen is more prominent in these deposits.

Ultrastructural studies of the central nervous system tissue show the presence of large numbers of globules with a granulofibrillar appearance and of medium electron density. In some deposits, the fibrils are oriented radially, and in others, they assume a whorled appearance. The material is mostly restricted to astrocytic processes. It is not found within neuronal perikaryons or processes.[217, 222]

Histochemical stains of the liver deposits indicate that the material is an abnormal glycogen with fewer branch points than usual. The deposits also have properties unusual for a glucose polymer: a positive colloidal iron stain and resistance to α-amylase digestion of conventional duration. Only pectinase was able to reduce the PAS and colloidal iron reactions significantly.

Genetics

Since a branching enzyme deficiency has been reported to occur in siblings, the condition is inherited, presumably as a recessive trait.[234] Although an autosomal inheritance is most likely, the preponderance of males reported suggests that X-linked inheritance cannot be ruled out. Most of the other glycogenoses are autosomal recessive. Examination of leukocytes from parents could not detect the heterozygotic state. Prenatal diagnosis is possible by enzymatic assay of fibroblasts from amniotic fluid cultures.

Treatment

Three types of treatment, without decided improvement, were used for one patient.[235] First, a high-protein, low-carbohydrate diet with corn oil added to the milk fat caused no change in weight gain or in the progression of cirrhosis. Second, with progression of the disease, treatment with purified α-glucosidase from *Aspergillus niger* was given for six days. This treatment resulted in a striking decrease in hepatic glycogen content, from 10 to 2 per cent. Although no unfavorable reaction occurred, liver size did not decrease. Glycogen content was maintained at 3 per cent by a third treatment, intramuscular injection of zinc-glucagon, 1 mg, three times a day for 24 days. Any positive effect of these treatments remains doubtful. On the other hand, the poor clinical results following the treatments might have been related to the advanced state of cirrhosis prior to their initiation.

Other than supportive nutritional management[232a] for terminal cirrhosis, no specific treatment appears to be beneficial. The finding that the Aspergillus extract caused a striking decrease in hepatic glycogen suggests that if the accumulation of abnormal glycogen is in some way hepatotoxic, this form of treatment might be studied in patients prior to the onset of severe cirrhosis.

INBORN ERRORS OF AMINO ACID METABOLISM

Hereditary tyrosinemia is the only inborn error of amino acid metabolism that results in permanent liver injury. This chapter summarizes the normal metabolic pathway of tyrosine, then discusses the disorders associated with abnormal tyrosine metabolism.

TYROSINE METABOLISM

The principal hepatic pathway for degradation of tyrosine is shown in Figure 49–10. These reactions normally catabolize 99 per cent of tyrosine. The steady-state plasma concentration of tyrosine is determined by two primary factors, (1) gastrointestinal uptake, which is regulated by an active transport system, and (2) the rate of production of tyrosine from phenylalanine and its subsequent catabolism to CO_2 and water. Most of the ingested phenylalanine is catabolized via tyrosine. The rate-limiting reaction in the tyrosine oxidation pathway is that catabolized by tyrosine transaminase (Fig. 49–10, Reaction [1]).[236, 237] Pyridoxal phosphate is the coenzyme. Tyrosine transaminase is found mainly in the cytosol of the liver. Its activity shows a circadian rhythm. Also, the activity of tyrosine transaminase is induced by various compounds, including corticosteroids.[238–240]

p-Hydroxyphenylpyruvic hydroxylase is the second enzyme involved in tyrosine catabolism. This enzyme is found in the cytosol of the human liver and kidney.[241, 242] It catalyzes the conversion of p-hydroxyphenylpyruvic acid to homogentisic acid (Fig. 49–10, Reaction [2]) and converts phenylpyruvic acid to p-hydroxyphenylacetic acid.[243] The enzyme requires a reducing agent. Ascorbic acid can serve both in vivo and in vitro in this capacity.[244] p-Hydroxyphenylpyruvic acid is not normally found in the urine. When its normal catabolism to homogentisic acid is blocked, the levels of both the α-keto acid and tyrosine in the plasma may be increased. At the same time, p-hydroxyphenyl lactic acid is formed through the action of lactic dehydrogenase. p-Hydroxyphenylacetic acid also can be formed from decarboxylation of p-hydroxyphenylpyruvic acid. Homogentisic acid oxidase catalyzes the conversion of homogentisic acid to maleylacetoacetic acid. This reaction also requires vitamin C for maximum activity in vivo. Fumaryl acetoacetase acts on maleylacetoacetic acid to yield fumaric acid and acetoacetic acid.

DISORDERS OF TYROSINE METABOLISM

Several conditions associated with abnormalities in tyrosine metabolism have been described; however, only hereditary tyrosinemia (hepatorenal type) is associated with permanent injury to the liver. Other abnormalities in tyrosine metabolism, summarized in Table 49–3, are discussed briefly.

TYROSINOSIS

The first known case of abnormal excretion of a tyrosine metabolite was described by Medes in 1927.[245] The patient, a 49-year-old Russian Jew who had myasthenia gravis, was found to have an unusual reducing substance in the urine. The reducing compound was later isolated and identified as p-hydroxyphenylpyruvic acid, the α-keto acid of tyrosine. The condition was named tyrosinosis by Medes.[246] When the patient was fasting, the urine contained 1.6 g p-hydroxyphenylpyruvic acid in a 24-hour period. This quantity was considered to represent endogenous production from the catabolism of endogenous protein.

TABLE 49–3. CONDITIONS ASSOCIATED WITH HYPERTYROSINEMIA

	Enzyme Deficiency	Clinical Features
Transitory tyrosinemia of the newborn	p-Hydroxyphenylpyruvic acid oxidase	None
Tyrosinosis (Medes' patient)	p-Hydroxyphenylpyruvic acid oxidase	None
Persistent tyrosinemia	Cytosol tyrosine transaminase in one case	Mental retardation Skin and eye lesions No hepatic or renal disease
Hereditary tyrosinemia (hepatorenal type)	Fumaryl acetoacetase	Cirrhosis, hepatomas Renal tubular defects
Hypertyrosinemia secondary to liver disease	Generalized partial defects of tyrosine transaminase, p-hydroxyphenylpyruvic acid oxidase and homogentisic acid oxidase	

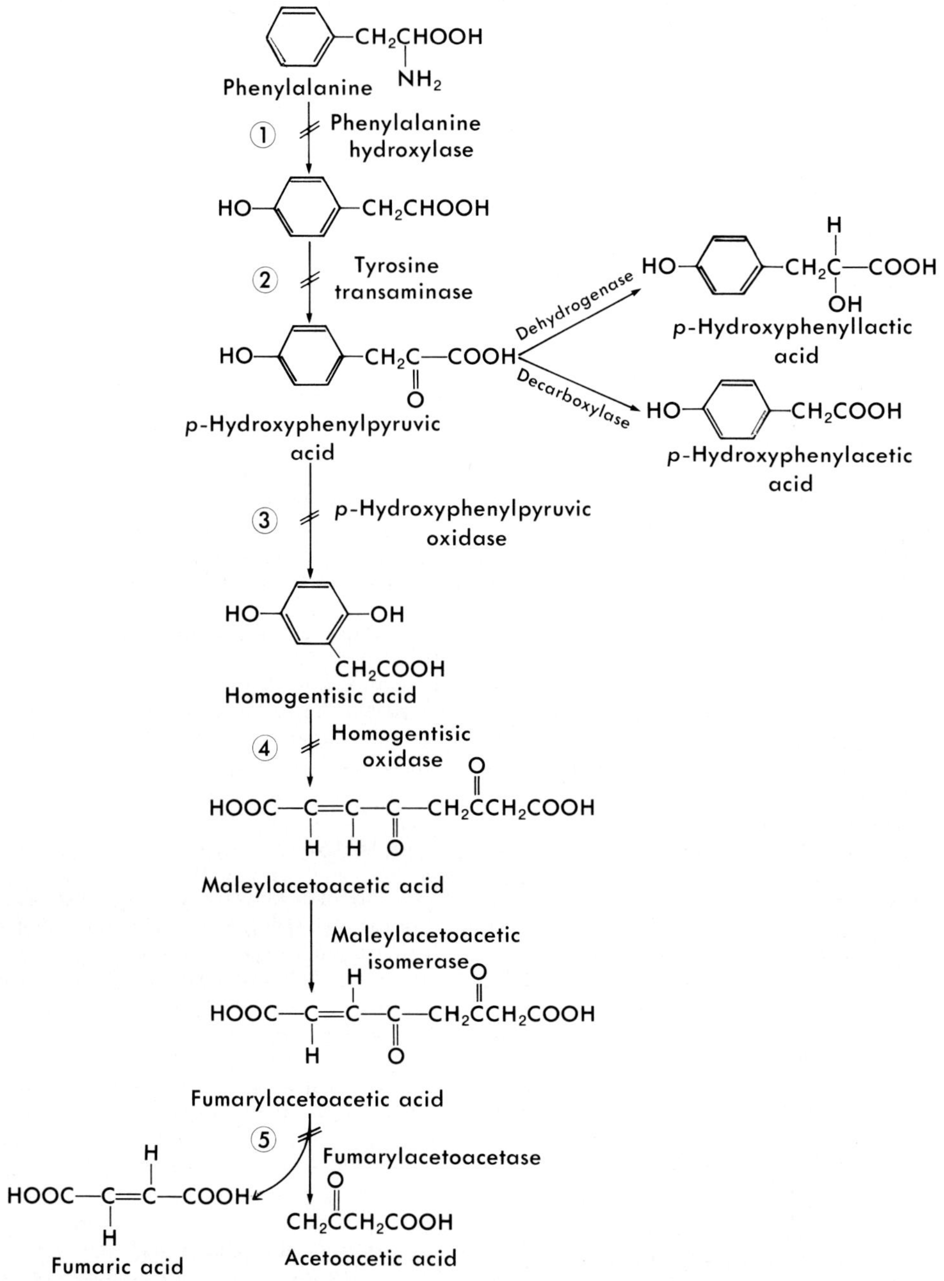

Figure 49–10. Metabolic pathway of phenylalanine and tyrosine. ⁄⁄ = block in the metabolic pathway; ① = block in phenylketonuria; ② = block in persistent hypertyrosinemia; ③ = block in Medes' tyrosinemia patient; ④ = block in alcaptonuria; ⑤ = ? block in hereditary tyrosinemia.

When the patient was fed a regular diet, the amount of urinary p-hydroxyphenylpyruvic acid doubled, and tyrosine also could be isolated from the urine. One of the interesting findings was that feeding large amounts of tyrosine also led to the excretion of 3,4-dihydroxyphenylalanine (dopa), a product of the minor pathway of tyrosine metabolism. Medes postulated a defect in the conversion of p-hydroxyphenylpyruvic acid to homogentisic acid. No other case of tyrosinosis has been described.

TRANSITORY TYROSINEMIA OF THE NEWBORN

This condition is seen in approximately 30 per cent of premature infants and as many as 10 per cent of full-term infants.[247–249] It is assumed that the hepatic enzymes catalyzing the early steps of tyrosine metabolism are not well developed in these infants.[250, 251] Administration of vitamin C, which is known to protect p-hydroxyphenylpyruvic oxidase from unphysiologic levels of its own substrate, will usually correct the transitory tyrosinemia.[252] The transitory tyrosinemia in infants usually disappears within a few weeks but occasionally persists for several months. A reduction in protein intake to 1.5 to 2 g/kg/day with administration of vitamin C should correct the condition. Although it is generally assumed that transitory tyrosinemia is harmless, this may not be true, since persistent hypertyrosinemia (see later) is regularly associated with mental retardation. There is a definite need for prospective studies of infants, specifically, premature infants with transitory hypertyrosinemia.

Persistent Hypertyrosinemia (Tyrosinemia II, Richner-Hanhart Syndrome)

Several patients have been described with persistent tyrosinemia without associated hepatic or renal disease.[253–258] The patients were reported to have cataracts, corneal ulcers, keratotic skin lesions, and neuropsychiatric abnormalities. Enzymatic studies were carried out in four patients. A total deficiency of cytosolic tyrosine transaminase was found in two;[255] however, the activity was only reduced in two others.[259] The keratotic lesions abated in response to low phenylalanine, low tyrosine diets in two cases.[257, 260] Large doses of vitamin C had no effect on the tyrosinemia in those patients.

HYPERTYROSINEMIA SECONDARY TO LIVER DISEASE

Patients with hepatic cirrhosis have a reduced capacity to metabolize tyrosine and other amino acids.[261] Cirrhotic patients have significantly increased fasting levels of plasma tyrosine and basal levels of p-hydroxyphenylpyruvic acid. They have impaired tolerance to oral loading doses of tyrosine, p-hydroxyphenylpyruvic acid, and homogentisic acid.[262] These findings suggest generalized partial defects in tyrosine transaminase, p-hydroxyphenylpyruvic acid oxidase, and homogentisic acid oxidase enzymes in patients with cirrhosis. Levels of tyrosine are also slightly elevated in other diseases, including cystic fibrosis,[263] hypoxemia with respiratory failure,[264] and rheumatoid arthritis.[265]

HEREDITARY TYROSINEMIA

In 1965, Baber reported the case of a 9-month-old infant with failure to thrive, abdominal distention, and diarrhea. The child was found to have cirrhosis of the liver, a renal tubular defect with gross aminoaciduria of a distinct type, and vitamin D–resistant rickets.[266]

In 1957 to 1959, Sakai and co-workers reported the case of another patient with a similar clinical picture and marked p-hydroxyphenyl lactic aciduria. They drew attention to the abnormal metabolism of tyrosine in this patient and named the condition atypical tyrosinosis.[267–269] Since then, many cases have been reported from Norway,[270] Canada,[271, 272] Sweden,[273] and the United States.[274, 275] Although a variety of names have been given to the disorder in these cases, hereditary tyrosinemia is generally accepted.

Clinical Features

Hereditary tyrosinemia may be either acute or chronic.[271, 276] Symptoms appear in the first month with acute disease, and the patient usually dies with hepatic failure within the first three to nine months.[271] In the chronic form of the disease, the symptoms appear later. The life spans of these patients are longer than those of patients who have the acute form.[271–276] Both forms can occur within the same family. The main symptoms are failure to thrive, vomiting, diarrhea, anorexia, hepatosplenomegaly, ascites, edema, jaundice, bruising, and rickets.[271] Some patients have slight mental deficiencies.

In the chronic form of the disease, hepatoma may develop.[277] A review of the literature by Weinberg in 1976 disclosed 16 cases of hepatoma in 43 patients surviving beyond 2 years of age. This incidence is higher than that seen in adults with macronodular cirrhosis.[277]

Laboratory Findings

Biochemical evidence of hepatocellular damage is found in elevated serum levels of AST and ALT. Total and direct bilirubin were elevated in 19 of 20 patients so tested.[271] However, total serum bilirubin levels were usually less than 10 mg/dl until the appearance of signs of liver failure, at which time they became markedly elevated. Synthetic function of the liver is also disturbed, as evidenced by low levels of serum albumin and vitamin K–dependent clotting factors. Hematologic studies show mild anemia, elevated reticulocyte counts, and normal serum iron levels. Bone marrow aspirates show erythroid hyperplasia. These findings suggest a hemolytic anemia, which may be related to an intracorpuscular defect secondary to abnormal accumulation of tyrosine metabolites.[278] In the chronic form of the disease, anemia, leukopenia, and thrombocytopenia are present secondary to hypersplenism.

A tendency to develop hypoglycemia has been found in association with hereditary tyrosinemia.[278, 279] Marked hyperplasia of the islets of Langerhans is a rather constant finding, but insulin levels are reported to be normal.[278] The responses to epinephrine and glucagon of two patients thus examined showed flat curves.[278] These findings suggest a disturbance in the release of glucose from glycogen; however, hepatic glycogen content and structure and glycogenolytic enzymes are normal. The glycolytic enzymes are also normal.

The laboratory findings related to the renal tubular defects include hyperphosphaturia, glucosuria, proteinuria, and gross aminoaciduria. Biochemical evidence of rickets secondary to hypophosphatemia is seen in almost all cases.[271] The urinary excretion of amino acids follows a distinctive pattern.[280] The aminoaciduria is more pronounced in the acute disease. The pattern of urinary excretion of tyrosine and phenolic acids (p-hydroxyphenyl lactic, p-hydroxyphenylpyruvic, and p-hydroxyphenylacetic acids) by tyrosinemic patients is similar to that described for premature infants with transitory tyrosinemia.[281]

Chromatography of the serum amino acids reveals slight hypertyrosinemia and, frequently, hypermethioninemia. Occasionally, other amino acids, including phenylalanine, are slightly elevated. Some of these results must be interpreted with caution, since liver damage may cause modest elevations of these amino acids.

In six patients with hereditary tyrosinemia, urinary δ-aminolevulinic acid levels were elevated to as much as a hundredfold above control values.[282] In two of these cases, attacks of abdominal pain and paresis of a peripheral type, resembling acute intermittent porphyria, prompted investigation for porphyrins. The amounts of porphobilinogen and porphyrins excreted were normal or slightly elevated, but δ-aminolevulinic acid levels were markedly elevated.[282] Similar abnormal pyrrole metabolism was found by Kang and Gaull in the case of a patient with hereditary tyrosinemia. δ-Aminolevulinic acid synthetase activity in liver tissue was increased.[275] It was believed that the abnormality of pyrrole metabolism is a secondary process related to induction of δ-aminolevulinic acid synthetase activity by one of the accumulated tyrosol metabolites. However, Lindblad and colleagues[283] and Melancon associates[284] have recently shown that the accumulation of succinyl acetoacetate inhibits porphobilinogen synthetase (δ-aminolevulinic acid dehydratase), leading to increased excretion of δ-aminolevulinic acid. This observation has been confirmed by Berger and co-workers.[285]

Biochemical Features

The clinical and biochemical improvements in the renal tubular condition and synthesis of proteins in the liver in response to introduction of a diet low in phenylalanine and tyrosine suggest that the aromatic amino acid derivatives exert a toxic effect on the kidney and liver. The failure to correct all the liver disease has been attributed to extensive, only partly reversible, pathologic changes.

Patients with hereditary tyrosinemia are reported to lack or to have markedly reduced activity of p-hydroxyphenylpyruvic acid oxidase in liver and kidneys.[286, 287] There is reason to question whether deficiency of this enzyme can account for the clinical manifestations in patients with hereditary tyrosinemia. Thus, activity of p-hydroxyphenylpyruvic acid oxidase is reduced in 30 per cent of premature infants, 10 per cent of full-term infants, and patients with persistent hypertyrosinemia (but these patients have no derangement of function of the liver or kidneys). Perry and colleagues induced experimental hypertyrosinemia in vitamin C–deficient newborn guinea pigs fed diets containing large amounts of tyrosine. There was no evidence of a liver or kidney disturbance.[288] Gaull and associates have therefore proposed that deficiency of p-hydroxyphenylpyruvic acid oxidase is not the primary defect in patients with hereditary tyrosinemia. These authors believe that there are deficiencies in methionine-activating enzyme and cystathionine synthetase in affected patients and that the signs and symptoms of the disease reflect these deficiencies.[289–290]

Feeding large amounts of methionine to guinea pigs in fact produced a syndrome similar to that seen in infants with hereditary tyrosinemia. The animals showed hyperty-

rosinemia, hypermethioninemia, generalized aminoaciduria, hypoglycemia, and pancreatic islet cell degeneration.[288] Hence, some metabolite of methionine may be the toxic factor responsible for the pathologic and biochemical changes seen in hereditary tyrosinemia. Some findings, however, do not support this idea. (1) Hypertyrosinemia usually precedes hypermethioninemia in infants with hereditary tyrosinemia. (2) Transient neonatal hypermethioninemia is an apparently benign condition unassociated with tyrosinemia. (3) Weanling rats fed high-methionine diets have increases of methionine, taurine, and alanine, but not tyrosine, in the serum.[291]

An apparently identical clinical and biochemical picture resembling hereditary tyrosinemia has occasionally been found in patients with hereditary fructosemia[292–294] but not in galactosemia, although severe liver damage is seen in both conditions. Plasma levels of tyrosine and methionine and the excretion of phenolic acid decreased markedly with the exclusion of fructose from the diets of patients with hereditary fructosemia.[293]

Recently, Lindblad and associates[283] reported increased excretion of succinyl acetone and succinyl acetoacetate in the urines of patients with hereditary tyrosinemia. These compounds presumably originate from maleylacetoacetate or fumarylacetoacetate, or both. Their accumulation indicates a block in metabolism of tyrosine at the fumarylacetoacetase reaction (see Fig. 49–10). These observations have been confirmed by Malancon and colleagues.[284] Since then, several groups have confirmed the defect in fumarylacetoacetase in liver tissues from patients with hereditary tyrosinemia.[295, 296, 297] Additionally, the activity of fumarylacetoacetase was found to be markedly decreased in patients with the acute form of hereditary tyrosinemia. It is reasonable to conclude that severe liver and kidney damage in hereditary tyrosinemia is secondary to accumulation of succinylacetone and succinylacetoacetate, which can bind to the SH group of proteins, thereby destroying their function. The liver and kidneys would be the organs affected principally by these metabolites, because these tissues are the only ones with p-hydroxyphenylpyruvate hydroxylase activity—that is, metabolism of tyrosine to potentially toxic metabolites depends on the presence of this enzyme. Of interest in this regard are the findings of Lindblad, indicating that patients with the more benign form of hereditary tyrosinemia have lower levels of activity of p-hydroxyphenylpyruvate hydroxylase in their livers than do patients who have more serious forms of the illness. The cause of the low activity of p-hydroxyphenylpyruvic hydroxylase in hereditary tyrosinemia remains to be determined. The possibility of a defect in a regulatory gene common to p-hydroxyphenylpyruvic hydroxylase and fumarylacetoacetase can be considered. Continued search for other possible biochemical defects that may be responsible for all the clinical and biochemical features is needed.

Pathology

The major pathologic findings are in the liver and kidneys.[238–300] Macroscopically, the liver is enlarged, firm, and nodular. The kidneys are enlarged, with poor architectural demarcations. Microscopically, the architecture of the liver is distorted by extensive fibrosis, with infiltration by lymphocytes and plasma cells in the portal areas. The liver cell cords have a pseudoglandular appearance. The hepatocytes show fatty metamorphosis, and some may undergo acidophilic degeneration and, occasionally, giant cell transformation. Glycogen is either lacking or markedly decreased.

Pancreatic islet cell hyperplasia has been found in the majority of cases.[298–300]

Genetics

Tyrosinemia has been found with increased frequency in French Canadians. Inheritance is autosomal recessive. The carrier rate in northeastern Quebec is 1:14, for an estimated frequency of 14.6 cases per 10,000 population.[301] An automated fluorometric test for hypertyrosinemia has been described.[302] In the province of Quebec, a neonatal screening program has been developed. The association of increased serum levels of alpha fetoprotein with hypertyrosinemia distinguishes patients with hereditary tyrosinemia from patients with transient hypertyrosinemia of the newborn.[303] Recently, prenatal diagnosis was accomplished by measurement of fumarylacetoacetase in cultured amniotic fluid cells.[304]

Treatment

A diet low in phenylalanine and tyrosine has been used in management of the acute and chronic forms of the disease by several groups of investigators.[270, 305–308] This diet decreases serum tyrosine. It increases serum phosphorus secondary to enhanced renal tubular reabsorption of phosphorus.[270] Similar beneficial effects on renal function are reflected by reductions of glycosuria, hyperaminoaciduria, and proteinuria. The effect of diet on hepatic dysfunction is uncertain. In only one acute case of tyrosinemia were reductions of fibrosis and infiltration of the liver by inflammatory cells found.[309] Other patients did not respond to the diet in this manner.[272, 307, 310] The available evidence suggests that a diet low in phenylalanine and tyrosine should be given to patients with the acute and chronic forms of the disease. Signs of deficiency of phenylalanine and tyrosine should be monitored in patients receiving this diet. The amounts of phenylalanine and tyrosine used in such diets are approximately 25 mg/kg/day of each; however, there is some variation in the optimal minimum requirements for individual patients.

In a recently reported case, dietary treatment returned the elevated levels of phenylalanine and tyrosine to normal in the serum of a patient with hereditary tyrosinemia. However, the patient continued to have hypermethioninemia and clinical evidence of liver disease. Strict control of his dietary intake of methionine, as well as phenylalanine and tyrosine, returned all serum amino acid levels to normal and eliminated the hepatic abnormalities.[311]

Large doses of vitamin D (10,000 to 15,000 U/day), together with dietary restrictions of phenylalanine and tyrosine, are necessary to correct the rickets of hereditary tyrosinemia.

Liver transplantation has been carried out in four patients with chronic hereditary tyrosinemia and hepatoma. All were reported to be alive and well three months to three years after transplantation. Therefore, this modality of therapy needs to be considered in patients who develop hepatoma as a complication from their chronic hereditary tyrosinemia.[312]

Prognosis

Patients who have acute hereditary tyrosinemia die in the first few months of life. Unfortunately, this is the commonest form of the disease.[271, 276] In patients with the chronic form, the disease progresses slowly, with the eventual development of cirrhosis. Hepatoma has been reported to occur in 37 per cent of patients with chronic hereditary tyrosinemia.[277]

INBORN ERRORS OF LIPID METABOLISM

INTRACELLULAR METABOLISM OF CHOLESTEROL

Metabolism of cholesterol and cholesterol esters has been studied primarily in cultured human fibroblasts (see Chap. 5). Study of patients with inborn errors of lipid metabolism has provided information that tends to support most of the general hypotheses developed from growing fibroblasts in cultures. A brief discussion of the origin, transport, and degradation of free cholesterol and cholesterol esters is included to provide a basis for understanding the metabolic consequences of a deficiency of lysosomal acid lipase.

Peripheral cells can synthesize free cholesterol and cholesterol esters, but they derive most cholesterol from exogenous sterols circulating in the serum as low-density lipoproteins. Intracellular levels of cholesterol are the primary regulators of the rate of synthesis of cholesterol and of uptake from low-density lipoproteins. The metabolism of cholesterol esters is illustrated schematically in Figure 49–11. The origin of lipoproteins enriched in cholesterol and cholesterol esters, which are the main sources of cholesterol for tissues, is discussed in Chapter 5.

As discussed in Chapter 5, the initial event in the intracellular metabolism of low-density lipoproteins (i.e., particles enriched in cholesterol esters) is binding to receptors on the cell surface. Low-density lipoprotein receptors bind only those human plasma lipoproteins that contain apolipoproteins B and E (e.g., low-density lipoprotein and very low-density lipoprotein). After low-density lipoprotein is bound to its specific receptor site, the lipoprotein remains metabolically inactive until the endosomes fuse with lysosomes (see Chap. 5). At this point, the protein component is hydrolyzed by lysosomal enzymes to products that consist mostly of free amino acids and small peptides (mol wt <1000). The cholesterol ester component of low-density lipoprotein is hydrolyzed by a lysosomal acid lipase. The liberated cholesterol is then available for metabolic utilization by the cell.[313] A consequence of the uptake and storage of low-density lipoprotein cholesterol is that the synthesis of cholesterol in nonhepatic tissues is maintained at a low level.

Patients with isolated deficiencies of acid hydrolase activity (Wolman's disease) should develop predictable changes in tissue lipids. For example, cholesterol ester as cholesterol linoleate should accumulate in lysosomes of affected individuals. This has been shown to occur.[314, 315] Because of a reduced rate of generation of free cholesterol within cells, there also should be decreased suppression of the activity of 3-hydroxy-3-methylglutaryl CoA reductase and reduced activation of endogenous cholesterol acyltransferase. (See Chap. 5 for details of these changes.) These two events will result in increased cholesterol synthesis by the cell and decreased cholesterol esterified with oleic acid, respectively. These abnormalities have been shown to occur

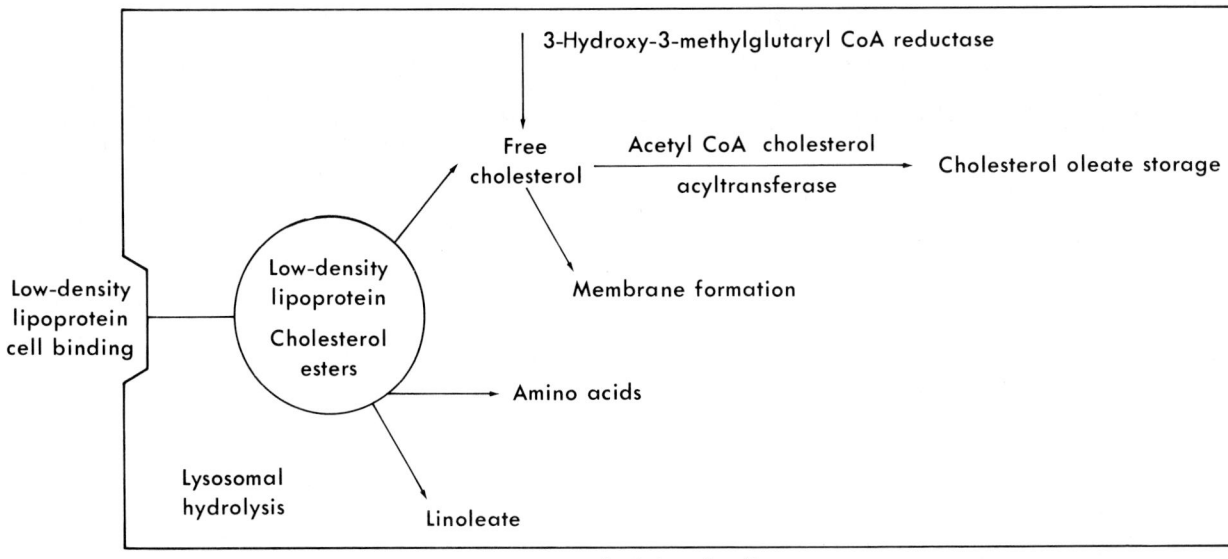

Figure 49–11. Metabolism of cholesterol esters.

in patients with cholesterol ester storage disease.[314, 315] However, patients with Wolman's disease have additional abnormalities such as accumulation of oxygenated steryl esters, which are difficult to explain solely on the basis of an isolated deficiency of acid hydrolase.[316] Similarly, patients with Wolman's disease have unexplained steatorrhea, which may be secondary to defects in the metabolism of bile acids.

WOLMAN'S DISEASE

Enzymatic Abnormalities

In 1965, Abramov, Schorr, and Wolman reported an infant who died at 2 months of age following a short illness characterized by abdominal distention, severe vomiting, diarrhea, hepatosplenomegaly, and radiographic evidence of calcification of the adrenal glands.[317] In 1961, Wolman and co-workers reported the cases of two siblings of their first patient who were found to have the same illness.[318] Accumulations of cholesterol esters and triglycerides were found in the liver, spleen, lymph nodes, and adrenal glands. The disorder was reported under the title *generalized xanthomatosis with calcified adrenals*.[318] In 1965, Crocker and associates described three patients with this disorder as having Wolman's disease; since then, the latter term has been widely accepted.[319] In 1969, Patrick and Lake confirmed that the accumulated cholesterol was esterified and demonstrated an acid hydrolase deficiency in the livers and spleens of those patients.[320] The activity of acid hydrolase was also deficient in cultured fibroblasts of patients with Wolman's disease.[321]

Deficiency of acid hydrolase or acid esterase manifests in two phenotypic forms. Wolman's disease represents the clinically acute and severe form. Affected patients die in the first year of life. Cholesterol ester storage disease represents a chronic form of deficiency of acid hydrolase. Patients who have this latter disorder do not have adrenal calcifications, and they live to adulthood.[314] Forty patients with Wolman's disease and more than 20 patients with cholesterol ester storage disease have been described so far.

Clinical Features

The majority of patients have similar clinical courses. Projectile vomiting, diarrhea, abdominal distention, and failure to thrive, the first noticeable symptoms, appear in about the second week of life.[317, 318] Some patients are jaundiced.[319, 322] Neurologic development of these infants is not normal. A decrease in activity may be noticed in the second month of life. It is not clear whether these symptoms are related to severe malnutrition or reflect neurologic defects. Konno and associates reported the case of an infant who had exaggerated tendon reflexes, ankle clonus, and opisthotonus.[322] Electroencephalography was reported to show no abnormality in this patient or several others.[315, 323] On physical examination the patient is usually slightly feverish, irritable, and wasted. Nonspecific skin eruptions may be observed. Abdominal distention with hepatosplenomegaly is seen in all patients; lymphadenopathy is detected in some. Subsequently progressive hepatosplenomegaly and abdominal distention, fever, and vomiting and diarrhea occur, persisting until the death of the patient, usually in the first six months of life.[317, 318]

Laboratory Findings

Anemia usually appears early in the course of the disease, and hemoglobin levels progressively decrease to as low as 5 g/dl. Peripheral blood lymphocytes show intracytoplasmic and intranuclear vacuolization.[319, 322, 324] Acanthocytosis was found in a Japanese infant.[322] Lipid-laden histiocytes or foam cells are seen in bone marrow aspirates and in the peripheral blood.[317]

Total serum bilirubin and the conjugated fraction are elevated in some patients.[318, 319, 322] Some have elevated serum levels of AST and ALT.[319, 322] Steatorrhea is present, evidenced by a high fecal fat content[319, 322, 323] and an abnormal ^{131}I-triolein absorption test.[323] The most consistent diagnostic finding, present in all reported cases of Wolman's disease, is calcification of the adrenal glands.[317, 318] The adrenal glands are symmetrically enlarged and show extensive punctate calcifications (Fig. 49–12).[317, 318] This is the only disease that causes such calcification of the adrenal

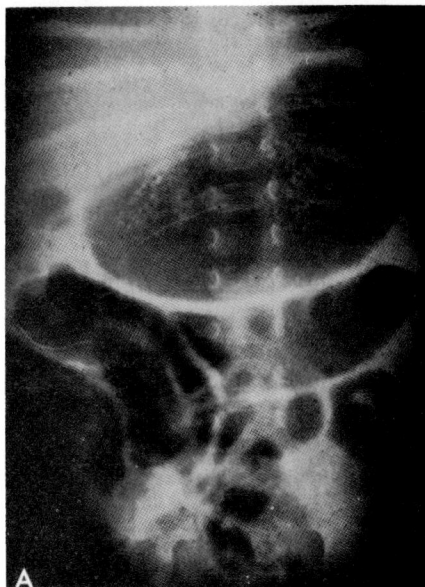
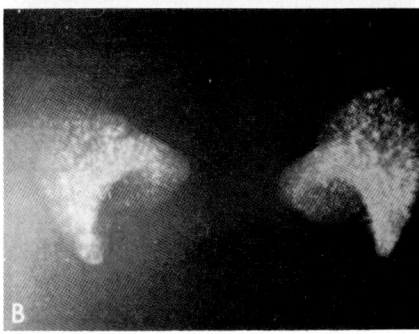

Figure 49–12. Radiograms showing the calcification of the enlarged adrenal glands in a patient with Wolman's disease. *A*, patient in the supine position; *B*, the adrenals after removal at autopsy. (Reproduced from Crocker AC, et al by permission of Pediatrics, Vol. 35, page 627, copyright 1965.)

glands. In all other conditions, the calcifications are scattered. In most patients, the responses of the adrenal glands to ACTH stimulation are depressed.

Plasma cholesterol and triglycerides are usually normal in patients with Wolman's disease.[318, 319, 322, 324, 325]

Triglycerides and very low-density lipoproteins were elevated in two patients.[324] It is expected that low-density lipoprotein levels should be high, because the acid hydrolase deficiency decreases cellular metabolism of low-density lipoproteins. Some patients, however, had hypolipoproteinemia.[323] The severe inanition and reduced production of lipoproteins by the liver probably offset the tendency towards hyperlipoproteinemia.

Biochemical Characteristics

Most of the enzymes that hydrolyze fatty acid esters are active at neutral or alkaline pH. Recently, an ester hydrolase active at acidic pH (4.0 to 5.6) has been found in lysosomes and cell membranes.[320] This enzyme requires no cofactors and utilizes triglycerides and cholesterol ester as substrates. Accumulation of cholesterol esters apparently results from the deficiency of cholesterol ester hydrolase activity.[326] Accumulations of triglycerides and other lipid products in large quantities are more difficult to explain. These biochemical abnormalities are discussed in more

detail in the section on cholesterol ester storage disease. Table 49–4 shows the results of analyses of lipids in various tissues in Wolman's disease.

The triglyceride content is severalfold greater in the liver and as much as 100-fold greater in the spleen of a patient with Wolman's disease than in comparable tissues of controls.[320] The total cholesterol in liver and spleen is elevated in every case of Wolman's disease. The majority of the increase is in the cholesterol ester fraction. Similar accumulations of triglycerides and cholesterol esters have been found in the bone marrow, thymus, and lymph nodes. Slight increases were also detected in the lungs and kidneys.[324] Cholesterol and triglyceride contents of the brain were reported to be elevated in some patients;[319, 324] however, they were normal in others.[322]

That severe malabsorption is seen in Wolman's disease but not in cholesterol ester storage disease could be explained by the differences in bile acid metabolism in these two diseases. Total serum bile acid levels were either normal or increased in patients with cholesterol ester storage disease.[315] Assmann and colleagues found oxygenated steryl esters in Wolman's disease but not in cholesterol ester storage disease. The accumulation of these oxygenated esters would suggest a defect in bile acid synthesis in Wolman's disease.[316] Boyd has suggested that cholesterol linoleate may be the precursor in 7α-hydroxycholesterol formation.[327] If the pathway from 7α-hydroxycholesterol to bile acids were blocked, an accumulation of oxygenated steryl ester would occur. These speculations await confirmation by the study of bile acid metabolism in Wolman's disease. Such a defect in bile acid synthesis in Wolman's disease would explain the steatorrhea.

Pathology

Liver. Enlargement of the liver is a constant finding. It is firm and appears yellow. The hepatic architecture is usually distorted. The hepatic parenchymal cells show marked steatosis. Sinusoids are plugged by swollen histiocytes with foamy, vacuolated cytoplasm. Kupffer cells are distended and vacuolated. The portal areas are enlarged, with increased fibrosis that extends to the periportal areas. The fibrosis may be extensive, and a classic picture of hepatic cirrhosis may be seen.[317, 318, 324, 325]

Electronmicroscopic examination of the liver shows that parenchymal organelles are distorted by the accumulation of large osmiophilic lipid droplets, which are identified as neutral lipids. These droplets are seen mostly in the lysosomes.[325] The smooth endoplasmic reticulum and rough endoplasmic reticulum appear distended, but are usually empty. The Kupffer cells are distended so as to almost obstruct the sinusoids.[325]

Spleen and Lymph Nodes. The spleen is greatly enlarged, is firm, and appears mottled with yellowish flecks. Microscopic section shows that the reticular cells are transformed into large foam cells. The lymphatic follicles are atrophied and compressed. The lymph nodes are enlarged, firm, and yellowish. Microscopically, the lymph nodes are similar to the spleen. The same changes are seen also in the bone marrow and thymus.[319, 324]

Intestines. The small intestine is usually thickened and has a yellowish serosal surface. The mucosa is greasy, yellowish, and granular. Microscopic sections show thick, flattened villi with numerous foamy, lipid-filled histiocytes in the lamina propria. Some of the foam cells extend into

TABLE 49–4. TISSUE LIPID ANALYSIS IN PATIENTS WITH WOLMAN'S DISEASE

	Triglyceride	Total Cholesterol	Free	Esterified	Reference
Liver, wet weight (mg/g)	137	97	38	59	322
	61	170	9	161	320
	44	32	14	18	316
Upper limit of normal	20	5	4	1	316
Spleen, wet weight (mg/g)	8	26	10	16	322
	99	35	8	27	320
	29	8	4	4	324
Upper limit of normal	1	5	4	<1	343, 344, 345

the muscularis mucosae. These changes are most evident in the proximal intestine or occasionally in the colon.[319, 324]

Adrenal Glands. Both glands are symmetrically enlarged, firm, and difficult to cut. The cortex on cut sections is yellowish. Medially, the tissue is whitish. Microscopic sections of the glands show preservation of the architecture of the cortex. Many of the cells are swollen and vacuolated and contain sudanophilic lipid.[324] Some of the foam cells are necrotic and appear as lipid cysts. Most of the calcium deposition occurs in a finely granular pattern; however, in some regions it may be condensed to form crystalline bumps.[324] There is extensive fibrosis in the inner cortical areas. The medullary cells are normal.

Electronmicroscopic sections show that the innermost part of the adrenal cortex is necrotic, with calcification. The histiocytes are filled with large amounts of both crystalline and droplet lipid. Histochemical analysis of the lipid indicates the presence of cholesterol esters and triglycerides.[324, 325]

Other Organs. The vascular endothelium shows lipid deposition, but frank atherosclerosis is not seen. Foam cells have been observed in the intestinal tissue and in the lungs, thyroid, testes, ovaries, leptomeninges, Purkinje cells, Auerbach's plexus, and Meissner's plexus.

Genetics

Wolman's disease is inherited as an autosomal recessive trait. Seven of the patients reported so far have been Jews of Iraqi or Iranian origin. The other patients have been reported from Japan, Western Europe, and North America. Young and Patrick reported that the enzyme acid hydrolase in the leukocytes of the parents and a sibling of one patient had half the normal activity.[324] Kyriakides and associates reported similar findings in skin fibroblasts from the parents of a patient.[321] A prenatal diagnosis using cultured amniotic fluid cells has been described.[328]

Differential Diagnosis

Calcifications of the adrenal glands, invariably present in Wolman's disease, can be seen in conditions such as Addison's disease, adrenal hemorrhage,[329] neuroblastoma, ganglioneuroma, adrenal cysts, pheochromocytoma, cortical carcinoma, and adrenal teratoma.[317, 329] However, the calcifications in Wolman's disease characteristically outline the shape of the adrenal gland. Niemann-Pick disease may result in gastrointestinal symptoms, hepatosplenomegaly, and failure to thrive in early infancy, but adrenal calcifications are absent. The definitive diagnosis of Wolman's disease depends on the clinical picture and assay of acid

hydrolase in cultured leukocytes or skin fibroblasts, using p-nitrophenyllaurate as a substrate.[330] Acid hydrolase activity that is less than 5 per cent of normal confirms the diagnosis.

Treatment and Prognosis

No specific therapy is available. Enzyme replacements have not been tried. The prognosis for a patient who has Wolman's disease is grave. All reported patients have died in the first few months of life.

CHOLESTEROL ESTER STORAGE DISEASE

Clinical Picture

In 1963, Fredrickson reported the first known case of hepatic cholesterol ester storage disease. The patient was a child with hepatomegaly and hyperlipidemia.[331] In 1967, Lageron and co-workers reported the case of a French adult with the same disease.[332, 333] In 1968, Schiff and associates reported the cases of a brother and sister with the disease. Mild cirrhosis was evident in liver biopsy specimens, along with marked increases in fat content. Four of five younger siblings were found to have hepatomegaly. Liver biopsy specimens from three of the siblings showed vacuoles in their hepatocytes similar to those seen in the hepatocytes of the original patients.[315] Partin and Schubert found deposits of cholesterol esters in the lamina propria and mucosal smooth muscle and vascular pericytes[334] in jejunal tissue samples from two of the severely affected children in the family described by Schiff.

The majority of patients come to medical attention early in childhood, but one patient sought treatment at the age of 23. Hepatomegaly has been present in all patients reported.[315, 331–340] In one patient, hepatomegaly was present at birth. Hepatomegaly is progressive; eventually, hepatic fibrosis develops. Splenomegaly was found in 54 per cent of patients. Esophageal varices secondary to portal hypertension were present in 27 per cent of the patients. One patient had recurrent episodes of abdominal pain without known cause.[333, 340] Two of the patients were reported to have had delays in sexual maturation.[336, 338]

Laboratory Findings

Results of liver tests are usually normal. Jaundice has not been found, except in two patients who may have developed hepatitis with lethal complications.[330, 337]

Schiff and colleagues studied the serum bile acid profiles of two patients and those of five siblings, both parents, an uncle, and a grandfather of these patients. Total serum bile acids were markedly elevated in one patient, and in all but three relatives. The ratio of cholic acid to chenodeoxycholic acid was decreased in duodenal bile obtained from one of the two patients.[315]

Plasma lipoprotein patterns show hypercholesterolemia and some hypertriglyceridemia. The majority of the patients have increased levels of low-density lipoprotein. Two patients had low levels of high-density lipoprotein.

Biochemical Characteristics

Results of lipid analyses of liver tissue obtained from three patients with cholesterol ester storage disease are shown in Table 49–5. The major abnormality was the marked increase in cholesterol esters. The fatty acid composition of the cholesterol esters showed a predominance of oleic and linoleic acids.[315, 321] The stored esters contained less than the expected amount of cholesterol linoleate.

Increased levels of low-density lipoproteins in serum are routinely found in cholesterol ester storage disease. The presence of atherosclerosis in two patients with cholesterol ester storage disease is of interest, since current speculation about the role of acid hydrolase in arterial intima predicts that accelerated atherosclerosis will be a consequence of the enzymatic deficiency.

The reason for the different clinical courses of Wolman's disease and cholesterol ester storage disease are unclear. It may be that there is a small but critical difference between the levels of residual acid hydrolase in the two groups of patients. A slightly greater deficiency of acid hydrolase in tissues has been recorded for patients with Wolman's disease.[335] Another possibility is that the two diseases are different at the levels of the enzymatic defects. For example, liver tissue from a patient with Wolman's disease did not hydrolyze DL-hexadecanyl-1,2-dioleate, whereas liver tissue from a patient with cholesterol ester storage disease hydrolyzed this substrate at a normal rate.[341] There could be isoforms of acid hydrolase with deficiency of different isoenzymes in Wolman's disease and cholesterol ester storage disease. Alternatively, it may be that the nature of the defect in a single type of acid hydrolase differs in these disorders.

More recently, Burton and co-workers reported that the intracellular acid hydrolase activity in cultured cells from Wolman's patients was 10 to 20 per cent of control hydrolytic activity, whereas cholesterol ester storage disease cells exhibited 30 to 45 per cent of control activity. These differences were found only when intracellular rather than cell lysate activity of the enzyme was measured.[342]

Pathology

The pathologic changes are secondary to the intralysosomal deposition of cholesterol esters and triglycerides.

Liver. Macroscopically, the liver is greatly enlarged and has an orange color. On microscopic examination, the hepatic parenchymal cells and Kupffer cells show deposition of lipid droplets (Fig. 49–13). In frozen sections, the lipid droplets in the hepatocytes are birefringent but not autofluorescent. Those in Kupffer cells are not birefringent but show yellow autofluorescence. The differences are thought to be due to peroxidation of the fatty acids of cholesterol esters in macrophages but not in parenchymal cells.

Electronmicroscopic studies show the lipid deposits to be limited by a single trilaminar membrane. The deposits in the hepatocytes are electron-lucent; however, those in the Kupffer cells are interspersed with electron-dense material.

In the majority of patients, dense bands of fibrous tissue extend through the liver, forming lobules of different sizes. Fibrosis may progress in some patients to give a classic picture of cirrhosis, with the development of portal hypertension and esophageal varices.[337]

Other Tissues. Partin and Schubert studied small intestinal biopsy specimens from two patients. The biopsy specimens had an orange tinge. In contradistinction to Tangier disease, which features storage of cholesterol esters, abnormal coloration of the colonic mucosa or the tonsils has not been found in cholesterol ester storage disease. Histologic sections of the small bowel show that the epithelial cells are normal; however, there were foam cells in the lacteal area and especially abundant in the villous tips. Free droplets of fat were present in the extracellular spaces of the lamina propria.[334]

Electronmicroscopic studies of small intestine show foam cells in clusters beneath the basement membrane of the epithelial cells surrounding the lacteals. The cytoplasm of the lacteal endothelium is distended by numerous large osmiophilic lipid vacuoles. Smooth muscle fiber cells, vascular pericytes, fibrocytes, and Schwann cells of nerve fibers contain lucent lipid droplets.

Deposits of lipids, similar to those seen in Wolman's disease, were found in other tissues. Although clinically there was no evidence of atherosclerosis in patients with cholesterol ester storage disease, two of three patients examined by necropsy had atherosclerosis.[337]

Genetics

Cholesterol ester storage disease is probably inherited as an autosomal recessive trait.[335] There is a preponderance of females among the patients reported. It is possible to detect heterozygotes by quantitation of acid hydrolase activity in leukocytes or cultured fibroblasts. Heterozygotes have 40 to 50 per cent of the reported normal enzymatic activity.[337] Prenatal diagnosis can be established utilizing cultured amniotic fluid cells.

Treatment and Prognosis

There is no specific therapy available for cholesterol ester storage disease. Enzyme replacements have not been

TABLE 49–5. LIPID CONCENTRATIONS IN LIVER TISSUE OF PATIENTS WITH CHOLESTEROL ESTER STORAGE DISEASE

	Total Lipids	Triglycerides	Total Cholesterol	Free	Esterified	Reference
Lipids, wet weight (mg/g)	280	64	121	9	187	344
	244	36	112	11	174	333
Upper limit of normal		19	4	3	1	345

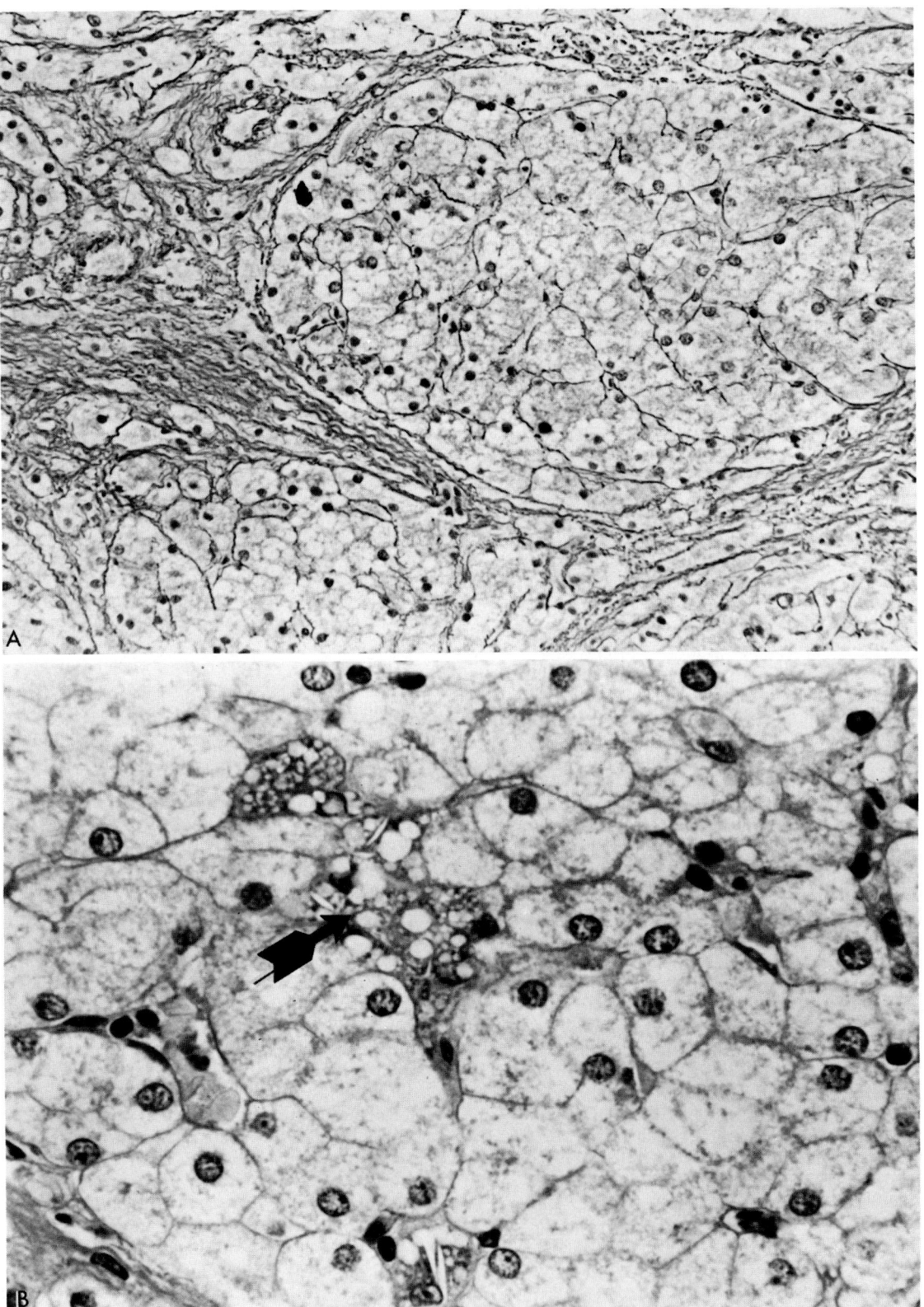

Figure 49–13. Biopsy specimens from a patient with cholesterol ester storage disease. *A,* liver, showing dense bands of connective tissue extending through the liver, forming nodules (Wilder's reticulum stain, × 200). *B,* the individual foam vacuoles of different sizes plus acinar clefts interpreted as cholesterol, indicated by arrow (Gomori's trichrome, × 500). *C,* the lamina propria of the small intestine, containing foam cells, indicated by arrow, in dense nodules distorting the involved villus (Gomori's trichrome, × 200). (Reproduced with permission from Beaudet AL, Ferry GD, Nichols BL, et al. J. Pediatr., 90:910, 1977, with permission.)

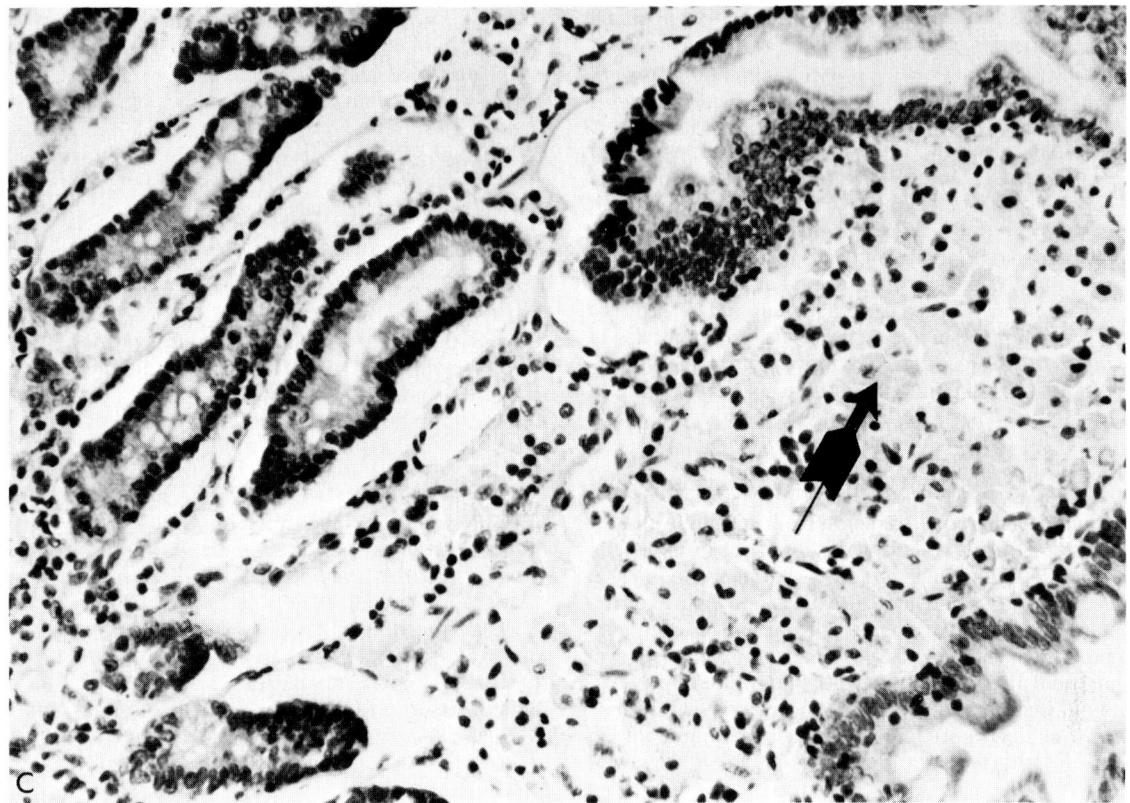

Figure 49–13 *Continued*

tried. Cholesterol ester storage disease is relatively benign. Death in childhood from hepatic complications has been reported.[337] Two patients died at 43 years of age.[332, 339]

INBORN ERRORS OF BILE ACID METABOLISM

Inborn errors of bile acid metabolism are a complex group of disorders, the biochemical characteristics of which need further investigation. With some of these disorders, the prognoses appear good, as for Summerskill's benign recurrent intrahepatic cholestasis. In the syndromes discussed here, hepatic cirrhosis has appeared either very early in life, as in Zellweger's syndrome, or after the first year of life, as in Byler's disease. Methods of therapy are limited. Phenobarbital and cholestyramine have been used to improve biliary flow but without effect on the progression of these diseases.

PROGRESSIVE INTRAHEPATIC CHOLESTASIS (Byler's Disease)

In 1965, Clayton and associates described a syndrome of progressive intrahepatic cholestasis in an extensive Amish kindred descended from Jacob Byler, who was born in the United States in 1799.[346] Six members of four interrelated, inbred Amish sibships were described in Clayton's original abstract.[346] The disease was characterized by onset of pruritus, jaundice, steatorrhea, and hepatosplenomegaly early in infancy. Four of the 6 patients died between 17 months and 8 years of age. Similar cases have been reported from France[347] and Japan.[348] Biochemically, all of Clayton's

patients had conjugated hyperbilirubinemia and elevated serum alkaline phosphatase with normal serum cholesterol. Two fathers in Clayton's pedigree had decreased maximum hepatic excretory rates (transport maximum: T_m) of sulfobromophthalein (BSP). The abnormalities in the two fathers and the pedigree pattern suggest an autosomal recessive inheritance. Clayton and colleagues suspected an error in bile acid metabolism in their patients.

Clinical Features

Progressive intrahepatic cholestasis usually manifests between the ages of 1 and 10 months.[348, 349] In four of the reported cases, onset of the disease occurred in the first week of life.[350] Pruritus and jaundice are the earliest symptoms. In infants, pruritus may be severe enough to interfere with sleep. The jaundice is usually accompanied by dark urine and pale stools that may become totally acholic. The stools are loose, foul-smelling, and greasy because of steatorrhea.[347–349, 351] The jaundice usually fluctuates. Recurrent cholestatic episodes alternate with periods of remission. The cholestatic episodes have been reported to be triggered by upper respiratory tract infections.[350] After several months, remissions are less frequent. Rickets is seen in some patients.[348] Most have growth retardation; developmental retardation was found in 30 per cent of the reported patients.[352] Bleeding episodes secondary to hypoprothrombinemia have been reported for approximately half the patients. Some patients have clubbing of the fingers.[352] Xanthomatosis of the skin does not occur. Hepatomegaly has been present in all patients reported so far, but splenomegaly has been found in only half of the patients. Liver enlargement persists during remissions, and with the progression of disease, the liver becomes hard, irregular, and nodular. The majority of patients die between the ages of 2 and 15 years, but occasionally a patient has survived until the age of 25 years.[350] Recently, Dahms reported the cases of twin brothers with Byler's disease, both of whom developed hepatocellular carcinomas. The two brothers died at 13 and 17 years of age of liver failure.[353]

Laboratory Findings

All reported patients have had elevations of total serum bilirubin. Levels of 40 to 50 mg/dl are not unusual during the cholestatic episodes.[352] The direct fraction is usually half of the total bilirubin.[347-351] The serum AST and ALT are elevated. Serum cholesterol is usually normal or low.[348] Prothrombin time and thromboplastin time are increased secondary to malabsorption of vitamin K. Malabsorption studies reveal severe steatorrhea, excretion of fat amounting to 50 to 80 per cent of intake.[347] T_m and storage capacity for BSP are both markedly reduced.[348] A parent heterozygotic for the trait is clinically normal but may have an abnormally decreased BSP T_m.[348]

Total serum bile acids have been elevated in the patients studied. Total bile acids in duodenal aspirates of one patient studied by Linarelli and associates were 0.07 to 0.5 mM, which is below the critical micellar concentration of 2 mM.[354, 355] The clearance of labeled cholic acid and chenodeoxycholic acid was normal at 20 minutes and slightly impaired at 60 minutes. The half-life of the labeled bile acid was prolonged. The major loss of the isotopes was in urine rather than feces.[355] Serum lithocholic acid was reported to be high in Linarelli's patient[355] and in two other patients;[356] however, other investigators did not confirm this observation.[357]

Radiographic examination of the biliary tree by operative cholangiography showed patency of the biliary tree in the patients studied. In the series reported from France, cholelithiasis and intrapancreatic calcification were found in some patients.[350]

The biochemical findings suggest a defect in the excretion of bile acids across the canalicular membrane of the liver cell, but the nature of the defect has yet to be determined.

Pathology

Light microscopy of liver biopsies early in the disease shows normal hepatic architecture. The hepatic lobules contain normal hepatocytes. Occasionally, the hepatic cells are arranged in tubular fashion. The portal areas contain normal bile ducts with minimal fibrosis. Moderate biliary duct proliferation is sometimes found;[350] however, other patients have decreased numbers of biliary ducts.[7] The striking feature of all liver biopsy specimens is the marked cholestasis in the parenchymal cells and in canaliculi, especially in the lumina of the tubular formations and around the veins.[355] As the disease progresses, the classic picture of biliary cirrhosis develops.[351]

Electronmicroscopic studies show markedly abnormal biliary duct canaliculi. The pericanalicular ectoplasm is greatly thickened, and the microvilli are swollen, fused, or blunted. The canalicular lumens are filled with coarsely particulate and amorphous granular material.[355]

Prognosis

Death usually occurs between the ages of 17 months and 8 years of hepatic complications such as liver failure, bleeding, and malnutrition. Occasionally, a patient has survived to 25 years of age.

Therapy

Methods of therapy are limited. Phenobarbital lowers the serum bilirubin levels and alleviates the pruritus even though it does not change serum levels of bile acid.[358] Cholestyramine, a resin exchanger, is ineffective. No therapy prevents the development of biliary cirrhosis. Alagille reported rapid relief of cholestasis in four patients in whom cholecystojejunostomy was performed; however, the long-term benefit from such a major surgical procedure is unknown.[347]

HEREDITARY LYMPHEDEMA WITH RECURRENT CHOLESTASIS (Norwegian Cholestasis; Aagenaes's Syndrome)

In 1968, Aagenaes and associates reported the cases of 16 patients from Norway in whom hereditary recurrent intrahepatic cholestasis appeared during the neonatal period.[359] In 1971, Sharp and Krivit reported two sisters of Norwegian extraction with a similar syndrome.[360] Consanguinity was present in six of the seven parental couples in the series reported by Aagenaes and co-workers, suggesting an autosomal recessive inheritance. In 1974, Aagenaes described two additional families with a similar syndrome.[361] All patients had early onset of intrahepatic cholestasis with elevated levels of total and direct serum bilirubin. Lymphedema of the lower extremities appeared late in childhood in all Aagenaes's patients. It appeared early and at the onset of cholestatic jaundice in the patients of Sharp and Krivit.

Clinical Features

All reported patients became jaundiced during the first month of life.[359-361] The jaundice lasted about one to six years, and during this period, the patients had severe pruritus. Growth retardation with complications of malabsorption such as rickets, anemia, and bleeding tendency was evident during the period of cholestasis. When the cholestasis resolved, catch-up growth occurred, so the patients' adult heights were normal. One or more further episodes of cholestasis have occurred in all adult patients. Lymphedema, once present, persists throughout life.

Laboratory Findings

Total serum bilirubin is elevated, with the direct fraction 50 to 80 per cent of the total. Especially during periods of cholestasis and in the first year of life, serum AST and ALT are increased.[359-361] Serum alkaline phosphatase is always increased. Results of the BSP excretion test are abnormal, with retention of 25 to 40 per cent at 45 minutes. Serum cholesterol and triglycerides are elevated. Lipoprotein electrophoresis shows increases in pre– beta and beta-lipoproteins. Protein electrophoresis shows elevation of the

α_2-globulin fraction with low serum albumin. Prothrombin time and thromboplastin time are elevated secondary to malabsorption of vitamin K. Fecal fat measurements show excretion of about 30 to 50 per cent of ingested fat. Fecal nitrogen excretion is normal.

Lymphangiography with visualization of the deep lymphatics was attempted in only one case. The lymphatics were found to be abnormally tortuous.[360] Injection of blue dye into the interdigital spaces in another patient resulted in a "chicken-wire" pattern, indicative of an absence of deep lymphatics.[360]

Pathology

Examination of liver biopsy specimens reveals intact architecture with marked bile stasis, giant cell transformation, and minimal hepatic cell necrosis. The portal areas show a slight increase in fibrosis, and in most instances, biliary ducts are difficult to find. In one patient, repeat liver biopsies at 10 years of age showed progression to cirrhosis.

Biochemical Characteristics

The elevated total serum bile acids and retention of BSP suggest deterioration of the excretory function of the liver. However, the nature of the defect is not known. The association of lymphedema of both lower extremities and cholestasis raises the possibility of abnormal lymphatic drainage from the liver. Aagenaes and colleagues injected colloidal gold into the liver capsule of one of their patients. Instead of normal excretion by lymphatic vessels, there was puddling of the isotope in the liver, which suggests a defect in the hepatic lymphatic system.[362] The close functional relationship between lymphatic and biliary drainage systems of the liver was shown experimentally in animals. Following experimental obstruction of the common bile duct, bilirubin and bile acids rapidly appeared in the lymphatic system prior to elevation in the serum.[363-366] Conversely, an increased biliary flow with increased excretion of bilirubin and bile acids occurred after interruption of the hepatic lymphatics in cats.[362] Thus, it is possible that abnormalities of the lymphatics of the liver contribute to the pathogenesis of this entity.

Prognosis

Initially, the syndrome was thought to carry a good prognosis;[360] however, a subsequent report indicated that one of the earlier reported patients had died of liver failure. As previously mentioned, in another patient, a repeat liver biopsy at 10 years of age showed evidence of cirrhosis.[361]

Therapy

No effective therapy is available. Cholestyramine has been used to alleviate pruritus during the cholestatic episodes. Because of the cholestasis, fat-soluble vitamins and fats in the form of medium-chain triglycerides should be given.

ARTERIOHEPATIC DYSPLASIA

Although reports of biliary duct hypoplasia and chronic liver disease appeared in the early 1950s,[367-369] it was not until 1973 that Watson and Miller described the cases of nine patients who had neonatal liver disease and familial pulmonary dysplasia.[370] A full description of the syndrome was provided by Alagille and co-workers. These authors emphasized the characteristic facial appearance and vertebral and cardiovascular anomalies.[371] The syndrome is probably not rare, since investigators were able to report groups of patients as large as 5,[372] 9,[370] and 15.[371]

Clinical Features

The major features of this syndrome are chronic liver disease, characteristic facies, cardiovascular and vertebral anomalies, and ophthalmologic abnormalities. Other abnormalities of the central nervous system and the renal and

TABLE 49–6. FINDINGS IN FIVE PATIENTS WITH ARTERIOHEPATIC DYSPLASIA*

	Patient				
	1	2	3	4	5
Liver					
Neonatal jaundice	+	+	+	−	+
Neonatal hypercholesterolemia	+	+	+	+	+
Paucity of intrahepatic bile ducts	+	+	+	+	+
Attenuated extrahepatic bile duct	−	−	+	−	−
Heart†					
Peripheral pulmonic stenosis	+	+	0	0	−
Pulmonic valvular stenosis	+	+	0	0	−
Ventricular septal defect	−	+	0	0	+
Murmur compatible with peripheral pulmonic stenosis	+	0	+	+	−
Eyes					
Posterior embryotoxon	+	+	+	+	+
Retinal pigmentary changes	+	−	+	+	+
High myopia	−	−	−	−	+
Posterior subcapsular cataracts	+	−	−	−	−
Strabismus	+	−	+	−	+
Bones					
Abnormal vertebrae	+	+	+	+	+
Lumbar spine					
Decreased interpedicular distance	+	+	+	+	+
Abnormal progression of interpedicular distance	+	0	+	−	+
Pointed anterior process C1	+	0	+	+	−
Short distal phalanges	+	0	+	+	+
Short ulnae	+	0	+	+	−
Central nervous system					
Absent reflexes	+	+	+	−	−
Poor school performance	+	0	+	+	+
Misdemeanors	+	0	+	+	+
Abnormal EEG	0	0	+	0	0
Kidneys					
Decreased creatinine clearance	+	−	−	+	0
Increased uric acid, increased blood urea nitrogen	+	−	−	+	−
Endocrine system					
Decreased thyroxine, EFT‡	+	−	−	−	−
Increased testosterone	+	0	0	0	+

Source: Riely CA, et al. Ann Intern Med 91:520, 1979, with permission.
*Key: + = tested and present; − = tested and not present; 0 = not tested or could not be evaluated.
†Cardiac catheterization was done in Patients 1, 2, and 5 only.
‡EFT = estimated free thyroxine.

endocrine systems have been described. Table 49–6 summarizes the findings in five cases reported by Riely and associates.[372]

Chronic Liver Disease

The syndrome is associated with cholestasis, which may develop during the neonatal period and usually becomes apparent in the first two years of life.[372–374] Pruritus develops early in infancy and persists despite the disappearance of jaundice. The liver is usually enlarged, firm, smooth, and nontender. The spleen may be enlarged even in the absence of portal hypertension.[375] The stools may be clay-colored and the urine dark yellow. Xanthomas may be seen on the extensor surfaces of the fingers and in creases of the palms, anal folds, and popliteal and vaginal areas. These xanthomas represent long-standing severe intrahepatic cholestasis. With the progression of the disease about the beginning of the second year of life, jaundice may subside or disappear, but cholestasis persists. The long-term outlook for the liver disease is usually benign, with only moderate portal fibrosis likely to occur even with long-standing cholestasis. Only 3 of 36 patients followed by the Alagille group developed hepatic cirrhosis.[375]

Characteristic Facies

The face is small with a prominent, broad forehead. The eyes are set widely and deeply (hypertelorism). The mandible is small and pointed, giving the appearance of a triangular face.[372, 373]

Cardiovascular Abnormalities

All patients have cardiac murmurs as infants. Most have peripheral pulmonary stenosis, which is usually mild and does not necessitate surgery.[376] Other cardiac lesions, including ventricular septal defects, coarctation of the aorta, and cyanotic heart disease, have also been reported.

Osseous Abnormalities

The hands show various degrees of shortening of the distal phalanges, stiffening, swelling, and limitation of motion at the proximal interphalangeal joints. Radiographs of the spine show either frank or incomplete butterfly vertebrae and decreased interpediculate distances in the lumbar spine.[372]

Ocular Findings

In each of the five recently reported cases, the patient has had a posterior embryotoxon visible to the unaided eye, by slit-lamp examination, or on gonioscopy. In addition, retinal pigmentary changes are usually found.

Other Abnormalities

Growth retardation, which decreased with age, was documented in the majority of cases of children. Slight to moderate mental retardation was documented in some of these cases.[371] Renal function is impaired, with hyperuricemia and decreased creatinine clearance in some patients.[372] Hypogonadism was suspected to be present in six male patients reported by Alagille and colleagues. Testicular biopsy showed no abnormality in two; in two others, fibrous tissue proliferation was present. In the other two, spermatogenic cells were almost completely lacking.[371]

Laboratory Findings

Total serum bilirubin is elevated during infancy, with levels between 4 and 14 mg/dl. The direct fraction is 30 to 50 per cent of the total. Serum bilirubin usually returns to normal after the second year of life.[371] Serum cholesterol levels may be as high as 200 mg/dl. Serum triglyceride levels range from 500 to 1000 mg/dl. Serum alkaline phosphatase and 5' nucleotidase levels are very high. Serum AST and ALT are slightly elevated. Despite the return of serum bilirubin to normal, biochemical evidence of severe cholestasis is usually found. Total serum bile acids have been markedly elevated in the patients so studied,[372, 374] with increases in both cholic acid and chenodeoxycholic acid. No major unidentified chromatographic peak was present in the serum or duodenal bile of the patients so studied.[372]

Retention of BSP at 45 minutes is abnormal; however, storage capacity for BSP is normal.[373] Prothrombin time and partial thromboplastin time are abnormal secondary to malabsorption of fats. Both values return to normal in response to intramuscular administration of vitamin K.

Pathology

Exploratory laparotomy of a patient who has arteriohepatic dysplasia will show uniformly patent extrahepatic biliary ducts. In the neonatal period, liver biopsy will show intact hepatic architecture, with marked cholestasis. The hepatocytes may be swollen, with balloon degeneration and minimal giant cell transformation. The most dramatic changes are in the portal areas, where a decrease in the number of biliary ducts is observed, with a slight increase in connective tissue. However, Ghishan and colleagues reported finding biliary duct proliferation in two patients with arteriohepatic dysplasia whose livers were biopsied when they were 5 and 49 days old, respectively. Subsequent liver biopsies, when the patients were 2 and 27 months old, respectively,[377] showed a paucity of biliary ducts in the portal areas. Biopsies of the livers of adult patients with arteriohepatic dysplasia have shown no biliary ducts in the portal areas, but no progression to cirrhosis.[372] However, 3 of 26 patients followed by the Alagille group developed hepatic cirrhosis.[375]

Genetics

The non–sex-linked vertical inheritance of arteriohepatic dysplasia, demonstrated by the father-to-son transmission reported by Riely and co-workers and the father-to-daughter transmission reported by Henriksen and associates,[374] supports the supposition that this syndrome is an autosomal dominant trait.

Biochemical Characteristics

Total serum bile acids are elevated in arteriohepatic dysplasia.[373, 374] Retention of BSP at 45 minutes is markedly increased, whereas the liver's ability to store BSP is normal.[372] A defect in bile acid formation or excretion with a subsequent diminution of bile flow, resulting in progressive atrophy of the intrahepatic biliary ducts, is a likely explanation for the clinical and pathologic picture of this syndrome. This hypothesis awaits confirmation.

Therapy

Phenobarbital and cholestyramine have not been shown to be effective in the treatment of arteriohepatic dysplasia; however, Alagille and colleagues reported alleviation of pruritus and reductions of serum cholesterol, triglyceride, and bilirubin levels in response to very high doses of cholestyramine—12 to 15 g/day.[371] Patients in whom the disorder was refractory to this regimen were subjected to cholecystojejunostomy.[375] Although their conditions improved clinically, follow-up data are insufficient to permit evaluation of the long-term effects of this major surgical procedure.

Prognosis

The long-term prognosis appears to be good. Three of Alagille's 26 patients developed cirrhosis,[372] but in all other reported cases the disease has followed a benign course, without progression to cirrhosis. The liver of a 27-year-old adult with arteriohepatic dysplasia was biopsied recently and found to show no evidence of cirrhosis, despite a complete lack of biliary ducts in the portal areas.

ZELLWEGER'S SYNDROME
(Cerebrohepatorenal Syndrome)

In 1964, Bowen and associates described an autosomal recessive disease occurring in two siblings. It was characterized by severe hypotonia, growth and mental retardation, renal cortical cysts, and hepatic dysfunction. Both patients died before the age of 5 months.[378] Patients with a similar clinical syndrome were described by Smith and co-workers[379] and by Passarge and McAdams.[380] In 1969, Opitz and colleagues described four new patients and identified the presence of iron deposition in the liver.[381] Since the original two were Professor Hans Zellweger's patients, his name was used by Opitz's group as an eponymic designation for this condition.[381] In 1972, Goldfischer and co-workers described mitochondrial abnormalities and lack of peroxisomes in electronmicroscopic studies of liver biopsy specimens from patients with Zellweger's syndrome.[382] In 1975, Danks and associates reported finding pipecolic acid in the urines of four patients.[383] In 1979, Hanson and colleagues described a defect in bile acid synthesis found in three patients with Zellweger's syndrome.[384]

Clinical Features

Severe hypotonia with simian creases is common, together with camptodactyly, which may involve several fingers. There may be some ulnar deviation of hands and fingers. Partial flexion of the knees with various degrees of equinovarus deformities of the feet are often seen. All patients have high foreheads with shallow supraorbital ridges and flat facies. Sucking and swallowing difficulties,

generalized seizures, and delays in developmental maturation are common. Patent ductus arteriosus and septal defects are present in approximately 40 per cent of the patients. Hepatomegaly is common; splenomegaly occasionally is found. Jaundice is evident in 30 to 50 per cent of the patients.[383]

Laboratory Findings

Hematologic investigations have shown elevated serum iron and nearly total saturation of the serum iron-binding protein in more than half the cases reported.[385] The true incidences of these abnormalities may be higher, as iron status has not been determined in many cases. Tissue concentrations of iron in the liver, spleen, kidneys, and lungs are increased. In one reported case, tissue iron in the liver was 50 mg/100 g wet weight (normal values for the same age group range from 7 to 21 mg/100 g). Ferrokinetic studies in this case demonstrated a rapid disappearance of iron and a markedly increased plasma iron turnover.[65] Fe incorporation into circulating red cells was significantly impaired, with abnormal accumulation of the radiolabeled iron in the liver. Intestinal absorption of iron was normal. Desferrioxamine induced a marked increase in urinary iron excretion. However, ferrokinetic studies of a second patient done by the same investigator showed no abnormality.[385]

Prothrombin time and thromboplastin time are usually prolonged, secondary to hepatic dysfunction. Serum AST and ALT are moderately elevated. Conjugated hyperbilirubinemia may be detected. Aminoaciduria was present in four cases.[383] Urinary excretion of pipecolic acid, a minor breakdown product of lysine, was found to be markedly increased in four cases of infants in which adequate qualitative tests were made.[383] Hanson and colleagues showed that three infants excreted excessive $3\alpha,7\alpha$-dihydroxy-5β-cholestan-26-oic acid (DHCA); $3\alpha,7\alpha,12\alpha$-trihydroxy-5β-cholestan-26-oic acid (THCA); and $3\alpha,7\alpha,12\alpha,24\xi$-tetrahydroxy-$5\beta$-cholestan-26-oic acid (varanic acid). These compounds are precursors of chenodeoxycholic acid and cholic acid that have undergone only partial side-chain oxidation.[384] These findings were confirmed recently in two other cases of Zellweger's syndrome.[386]

Radiographic studies of patients with Zellweger's syndrome reveal certain characteristic findings, mainly the presence of patches of calcification in cartilage. These have a dense cortex and a reticular central region and characteristically are present in the triradiate cartilage in the acetabulum, the patellae, the sternum, and the scapulae.[383, 387]

Pathology

Liver. Macroscopically, the liver appears grossly unremarkable. Histologic sections of biopsy and autopsy specimens of the liver show changes that may vary from minimal to severe diffuse fibrosis with cirrhosis.[383] The original patients were described as having biliary dysgenesis; however, recent reports show normal biliary ducts in the portal areas, with varying degrees of portal fibrosis. The hepatic lobules may contain foci of liver cell necrosis and loss. Prussian blue staining for iron shows a marked increase in iron deposition, mainly in the reticuloendothelial cells.[381] Some patients have minimal or no deposition of iron.[383, 388] There is no correlation between the extent of liver damage and iron deposition.[383] Electronmicroscopic studies show swollen hepatocytes filled with glycogen. The mitochondria are often extremely dense and reduced in number; their cristae are twisted and irregular, with dilation of the intracristate spaces. Typical arrays of rough endoplasmic reticulum are sparse. No peroxisomes can be found in the hepatocytes.[382]

Kidneys. Macroscopically, the surface is studded with small (< 3 mm in diameter) fluid-filled cysts. Microscopically, the cysts contain dysplastic glomerular and tubular elements and are lined by cuboidal or flattened epithelium. Cysts of glomerular origin and others that appear to be dilated tubular structures are also present. Ultrastructural studies demonstrate a lack of peroxisomes in the proximal tubules.[381, 382]

Central Nervous System. Severe cerebral gliosis, subependymal cyst formation, macrogyria, and polymicrogyria were noted. Myelinization was incomplete or lacking.[381] Prussian blue staining shows deposition of iron.[382] Ultrastructurally, the mitochondria of the cortical astrocytes are abnormally dense and often appear degenerate.[382]

Biochemical Features

The mitochondria in the livers, kidneys, and brains of patients with Zellweger's syndrome are structurally abnormal.[382] Functionally, oxygen consumption of mitochondrial fractions prepared from the livers and brains of two patients was diminished by 70 per cent. Addition of adenosine diphosphate (ADP) to the mitochondrial fractions failed to stimulate respiration, although this response was elicited in the control mitochondria.[382]

In vitro studies suggest that the formation of C24 bile acids (chenodeoxycholic acid and cholic acid) from cholesterol is defective in affected patients. It seems that mitochondrial defects are the cause of the abnormalities in bile acid synthesis (see Chap. 13). Since cholic acid and chenodeoxycholic acid are present in these patients, the defect in synthesis is not a complete one. It is possible that in Zellweger's syndrome, chenodeoxycholic and cholic acids are synthesized via an alternate pathway requiring only microsomal enzymes.[389, 390]

Prognosis

Patients who have Zellweger's syndrome die in the first year of life of malnutrition, liver failure, and intercurrent infections.[381, 383, 387] Desferrioxamine enhances urinary excretion of iron but unfortunately does not influence ultimate outcome.

Genetics

An autosomal recessive inheritance is suggested by family studies. A prenatal diagnosis based on detection of elevated levels of a very long-chain fatty acid, hexacosaenoic acid (C26:0) in cultured amniotic fluid cells has been described.[391] The impaired oxidation of very long-chain fatty acids is secondary to the absence of the peroxisomes seen in Zellweger's patients.

THE THCA SYNDROME

In 1972, Eyssen and co-workers reported the cases of two children with neonatal cholestatic liver disease and markedly elevated levels of THCA in the duodenal fluid. In normal individuals, THCA is not present in either serum or bile. The patients had other congenital abnormalities such as frontal bossing, epicanthal folds, and simian creases.[392] In 1975, Hanson and associates described two siblings with a rapidly progressive form of intrahepatic cholestasis that was associated with very high levels of THCA in bile and serum.[393] Hanson's patients differed from those described by Eyssen and colleagues in that no other congenital abnormality was present in the former group. However, all four patients had a paucity of bile ducts, and all died before the age of 2 years.

Clinical Features

The two patients reported by Eyssen's group had cholestatic jaundice at 2 to 3 months of age. Jaundice remitted in both between 4 and 5 months of age. The first patient died at the age of 8½ months of severe malnutrition.[392]

The two patients reported by Hanson's group had jaundice. Hepatosplenomegaly was present at birth in one and at 4 months of age in the other. Pruritus was not observed. Both patients failed to gain weight and died with progressive liver disease before the age of 2 years.[393]

Laboratory Findings

Both patients reported by Hanson and co-workers had elevated total and direct serum bilirubin. Serum alkaline phosphatase was markedly elevated; however, cholesterol and triglycerides were normal in one patient. Both patients had radiographic evidence of rickets. Results of bile acid analyses of the duodenal fluids of the patients of Eyssen and associates are shown in Table 49–7. In the two cases reported by Hanson, THCA amounted to 72 per cent and 65 per cent of total bile acids in the sera. Cholic acid was not detectable in the serum of the first patient and constituted only 6 per cent of serum bile acids in the second. Chenodeoxycholic acid amounted to 28 per cent and 22 per cent of the total bile acids, respectively. Normally, THCA is not detectable in human bile or serum.

Biochemical Features

All four patients had very high levels of THCA in their sera. The metabolism of THCA was studied in one patient after an intravenous injection of [³H]THCA, and the cause of the increase in THCA was found to be a metabolic defect in the conversion of THCA to cholic acid.[393]

Since varanic acid, a metabolite of THCA, could not be identified in the serum of either of the two patients reported by Hanson's group, it is reasonable to assume that the defect is due to a deficiency of the 24-hydroxylating enzyme system required to convert THCA to varanic acid.[393] The toxicity of THCA has not been investigated thoroughly, although Lee and Whitehouse demonstrated that THCA is a potent uncoupler of oxidative phosphorylation.[394] Thus, it is possible that the destruction of the intrahepatic biliary ducts might be due to an accumulation of THCA.

Pathology

Liver biopsy specimens show a paucity of ductular structures with an increase in connective tissue in the portal

TABLE 49-7. RESULTS OF DUODENAL BILE ACID ANALYSIS IN THCA SYNDROME*

	Age (Months)	Bile Salt Total Amount (mg/100 μl)	Relative Concentration (%)		
			Chenodeoxycholic Acid	Cholic Acid	THCA
Patient 1	4.5	26	23	58	19
Patient 2	3.5	61	18	37	45
Control 1	3	251	51	49	0
Control 2	4	424	39	61	0

*Patients of Eyssen H, et al. Biochim Biophys Acta 273:212, 1972.

areas. Subsequent liver biopsies show rapid progression to cirrhosis.

Prognosis

All four patients whose cases were reported died before the age of 2 years with hepatic cirrhosis.

Genetics

The disease appears to be inherited as an autosomal recessive trait.

Therapy

Cholestyramine therapy was not effective in preventing the development of hepatic cirrhosis.[393]

CYSTIC FIBROSIS

Cystic fibrosis is the commonest cause of chronic obstructive pulmonary disease and of pancreatic insufficiency in the first three decades of life in the United States. Today, as more patients with cystic fibrosis reach reproductive age, the hepatic complications of cystic fibrosis are encountered with increasing frequency. In her first study of cystic fibrosis of the pancreas, Anderson found three patients with hepatic cirrhosis already reported and added one of her own.[395] Farber provided an excellent description of an unfamiliar type of cirrhosis with gross lobulation of the liver, which he found in a few of his 87 patients with cystic fibrosis.[396] Early histologic changes in the liver included enlargement of the portal areas with biliary duct proliferation and accumulation of eosinophilic material within the lumens of the biliary ducts. The cirrhotic change was attributed to obstruction of the biliary ductules by inspissated secretions.[396] Bodian described focal cirrhotic lesions found in one fourth of 62 patients with cystic fibrosis examined at necropsy. These findings were present in virtually all patients more than 1 year of age. Bodian proposed the descriptive term *focal biliary cirrhosis*. This lesion had been asymptomatic in all of Bodian's patients.[397]

Craig and associates found 7 patients with cirrhosis of the liver among 150 patients with cystic fibrosis examined at necropsy. Microscopically, the authors found obstruction of biliary ductules by eosinophilic amorphous material surrounded by areas marked by fibrosis and biliary duct proliferation. The focal character of the extensive hepatic damage was stressed.[398]

di Sant'Agnese and Blanc described cystic fibrosis and multilobular hepatic cirrhosis in 7 patients 4 to 10 years old. To establish the evolution of the hepatic lesions, di Sant'Agnese and Blanc reviewed the autopsy material of 116 patients with cystic fibrosis. Of 25 patients who had cirrhotic lesions, 16 had single or multiple lesions of focal biliary cirrhosis. The changes were more extensive in nine. A multilobular biliary cirrhosis was found in six of these. Younger patients had focal biliary cirrhosis; older patients had multilobular cirrhosis.[399]

Clinical Features

Liver Disease in Infancy

Cystic fibrosis may manifest in the newborn period with obstructive jaundice.[400-406] In all of ten such infants, the onset of jaundice was before 3 weeks of age, and it occurred before 10 days of age in eight.[396] Jaundice persisted from 20 days to six months. Meconium ileus with or without small intestinal atresia or combined with volvulus was seen in approximately half of these patients.[401, 403, 404, 406] In three cases of patients subjected to laparotomy, accumulation of thick, viscid bile was thought to have caused extrahepatic obstruction.[404-406] Biliary duct proliferation without plugging by inspissated material was detected in the livers of five of nine patients with meconium ileus and intestinal atresia whose livers were examined. However, the authors do not rule out that the obstruction might have occurred in more central ducts.[401] Neonatal hepatitis with marked giant-cell transformation of the hepatocytes was documented in a 2-month-old cystic fibrosis patient with obstructive jaundice.[407] Some infants may make a complete recovery, and some may die from liver failure and other complications of cystic fibrosis. The diagnosis is suspected on the basis of a history of meconium ileus.

Liver Disease in Childhood and Adolescence

Symptomatic liver disease was seen in 2.2[408, 409] to 16 per cent[406] of patients with cystic fibrosis in two series. In the largest reported series, from Boston, 48 of 2500 patients with cystic fibrosis developed portal hypertension. The incidence of portal hypertension increases more than tenfold for patients who are adolescent or older.[410, 411] Interestingly, several members of the same family developed cirrhosis and its complications. A similar observation was reported by Stern and colleagues. Initial symptoms of hepatic complications begin between 9 and 19 years of age. Of 693 patients with cystic fibrosis seen over a period of 18 years, 15 developed clinical hepatic disease, an incidence of 2.2 per cent. In 13 of these 15 patients, all symptoms were related to portal hypertension, such as gastrointestinal bleeding or hypersplenism. Hepatocellular dysfunction was the principal feature in one of the remaining two cases, and massive hepatomegaly and failure to thrive were dominant in the other.[408] A similar experience was reported recently from Switzerland. Of 204 unselected patients with cystic fibrosis, 7 were found to have hepatic cirrhosis, an incidence of 3.4 per cent. Two of the seven patients came to medical attention because of hematemesis. The hepatic abnormality in the others was detected because of hepatosplenomegaly and failure to thrive.[412]

Documentation of mild hepatic involvement is often difficult, since clinical manifestations, including jaundice, may be lacking. Results of liver tests may be normal. The BSP excretion test may be of help in detecting early hepatic involvement.[413] The best early indication of hepatic involvement is an elevated level of the hepatic isoenzyme of alkaline phosphatase.[414, 415] Total serum alkaline phosphatase activity is not reliable in the evaluation of hepatic involvement in children with cystic fibrosis because age-related normal values for alkaline phosphatase are hard to establish. Also, puberty is often delayed in patients with cystic fibrosis, hence total alkaline phosphatase may appear to be normal in the presence of liver disease.[412]

It is important to emphasize that hepatic disease, including portal hypertension, may be present in patients with cystic fibrosis even when results of liver tests are normal or only slightly abnormal. In fact, the first manifestation of cystic fibrosis may be portal hypertension in a previously asymptomatic patient. Thus, children and young adults with unexplained portal hypertension or other hepatic abnormalities should be tested by pilocarpine iontophoresis and by chemical determination of the chloride level in sweat.

Gallbladder Disease

Clinical symptoms of cholelithiasis and cholecystitis have been found in some patients with cystic fibrosis. Microgallbladder has been reported to be present in approximately 15 per cent of cases and poor or nonvisualization of the gallbladder in another 25 per cent.[416] Gallbladder stones are found in as many as 8 per cent of patients.[417] The gallbladder disease in these patients may be related to occlusion of the cystic duct by precipitation of abnormal secretions and to abnormal biliary lipid composition.[418]

The pathogenesis of the increased incidence of gallbladder stones in cystic fibrosis was investigated by analysis of biliary lipid in 26 patients with cystic fibrosis, 7 children with cholelithiasis without cystic fibrosis, and 13 controls. For 14 patients with cystic fibrosis who had stopped taking pancreatic enzymes a week earlier, the molar percentage of lipid composition accounted for by cholesterol (mean ± SE 16.3 ± 2.9) and the saturation index (2.0 ± 0.3) were comparable with values obtained for the group with cholelithiasis but no cystic fibrosis. For 12 patients with cystic fibrosis taking pancreatic enzymes, the molar percentage of cholesterol (8.6 ± 1.7) and the saturation index (1.0 ± 0.1) did not differ from those of controls. Bile salt analysis revealed a striking preponderance of cholic acid over chenodeoxycholic acid, and the glycine:taurine ratio of conjugated bile acids was lower in enzyme-treated patients with cystic fibrosis than in those not currently receiving treatment. The high ratio of cholic acid to chenodeoxycholic acid is a well-known response to malabsorption of bile acids. The decrease of this ratio and the concomitant normalization of biliary lipids during treatment of patients with cystic fibrosis suggest that the lithogenic bile in cystic fibrosis is secondary to bile acid malabsorption.[418]

Biochemical Characteristics

Cystic fibrosis is related to an abnormality in secretions of the exocrine glands. These secretions contain high concentrations of sodium chloride. This abnormality is due to decreased chloride permeability in the ducts of sweat glands.[419–421] In addition, elevated concentrations of nucleotides, calcium, and various proteins have been described. A defect in alpha$_2$-macroglobulin–protease complex has been described. This defect may be caused by a lesser affinity for proteases, defective release of protease from alpha$_2$-macroglobulin–protease complex, or blockage of protease binding sites in cystic fibrosis alpha$_2$-macroglobulin.[422–427]

The biochemical characteristics of the liver disorder are not well understood. Intrahepatic obstruction by eosinophilic concentrations of mucus occurs early in the disease and has been proposed as the cause of cirrhosis in cystic fibrosis.[399] Shwachman found that cirrhosis did not develop in patients with cystic fibrosis who had pulmonary involvement without pancreatic involvement. Thus, defects in digestion and absorption appear to be prerequisites for liver disease, except possibly during the neonatal period.[425] Patients with cystic fibrosis and pancreatic insufficiency have markedly elevated fecal bile acid excretion compared with age-matched controls.[426]

Bile acid kinetics were investigated by double-isotope dilution technique in six children with previously untreated cystic fibrosis. All six children had pancreatic insufficiency. The bile acid pool sizes were small and turned over rapidly in untreated patients. When fat excretion was reduced by therapy, the turnover rate of the pool decreased, with twofold enlargement of the pool size. These findings suggest an interruption of enterohepatic circulation.[427] The pathophysiologic mechanism of the interruption of the enterohepatic circulation and its relation to hepatobiliary disease have not been defined.

Laboratory Findings

Sweat chlorides are elevated in all patients with cystic fibrosis. Total pancreatic exocrine dysfunction is found in 80 to 85 per cent of the patients. Five to ten per cent of the patients have partial insufficiency. The remainder have normal exocrine function. Steatorrhea and azotorrhea are the major consequences of the pancreatic insufficiency. Malabsorption of fat-soluble vitamins A, D, E, and K is the result of pancreatic insufficiency and the use of antibiotics, which alter the bacterial flora of the intestinal tract. Vitamin K deficiency may occur in the first year of life and produce overt hemorrhage.[428] Vitamin A levels are low in the serum but normal or elevated in the liver. There is probably a defect in the transport of vitamin A out of the liver.[429] Night blindness and benign increases in intracranial pressure secondary to low vitamin A levels in blood have been reported.[429, 430] Vitamin D is poorly absorbed; however, overt rickets is rare. Serum levels of 25-OH vitamin D are reported to be similar to values obtained for normal controls.[431] Two other studies demonstrated low serum levels of 25-OH vitamin D in four of 17 patients in one series[432] and in all 21 patients in another.[433] Differences in serum levels reflect different assays, and the times of the year during which the patients were studied, since 85 per cent of circulating 25-OH vitamin D is of endogenous origin.[431] When patients were studied in winter and early spring, values of serum 25-OH vitamin D were low;[433]

however, the other studies were conducted in the summer and early fall.[431, 433] These observations suggest a subtle deficiency of vitamin D in patients with cystic fibrosis deprived of sunlight and endogenous vitamin D production.

Liver tests usually show no abnormality. Conjugated hyperbilirubinemia and elevations of serum AST, ALT and alkaline phosphatase are seen in neonates with obstructive jaundice secondary to cystic fibrosis. Some infants with cystic fibrosis have hypoproteinemia and edema as a result of protein malabsorption, particularly infants who have been breast-fed or fed soybean-based formulas. Breast milk contains only 1.1 per cent protein; although adequate for normal infants, it is suboptimal for those who have cystic fibrosis. Soybean-based formula contains small amounts of antitryptic activity, which may potentiate the existing malabsorption.

The detection of mild liver involvement in cystic fibrosis is often difficult. The best early indication is elevated alkaline phosphatase of hepatic origin. Total serum alkaline phosphatase is not helpful (see the previous discussion). The kinetics of BSP excretion show a decrease in hepatic removal rate and biliary secretion and an increase in hepatic-to-plasma reflux as liver disease progresses.[413] In patients with cystic fibrosis and biliary cirrhosis, abnormal liver function and hematologic abnormalities or hypersplenism usually are detected. Abnormalities related to the gallbladder are seen in approximately 20 per cent of the patients. Oral cholecystography may result in nonvisualization of the gallbladder, or microgallbladder or cholesterol stones may be detected.[416]

Pathology

Focal biliary cirrhosis is found in approximately 25 per cent of patients with cystic fibrosis examined by necropsy.[399] Progression to a multilobular cirrhosis occurs in about 5 per cent of surviving children and adolescents.

Three histologic types of lesions were identified by Oppenheimer and Esterly[434] in young infants with cystic fibrosis.

1. Focal biliary cirrhosis, characterized by biliary duct proliferation, inspissated granular eosinophilic material filling the biliary ducts, chronic inflammatory infiltration, and variable degrees of fibrosis. The lesions are focal in distribution and vary in number and severity. The incidence of focal biliary cirrhosis increases with age.

2. Excess mucus in biliary duct radicles, or in the linings of epithelial cells with periportal changes. The distribution of the biliary mucus is variable and focal, but it is seen most often in the large intrahepatic ducts. Biliary duct proliferation and, less commonly, metaplasia of the ductal epithelium are seen. The periportal changes include edema and inflammatory infiltrate. This type of lesion is commonly seen in infants less than a year of age.

3. Periportal changes without biliary mucus. These changes are common in infants less than 3 months of age but are not seen in older children.

It appears that the periportal changes are nonspecific and transitory. The accumulation of biliary mucus appears to be related to cystic fibrosis, and since its frequency decreases with age, this indicates that biliary mucus is only one factor in the pathogenesis of focal biliary cirrhosis, which worsens with age and progresses to multilobular cirrhosis in only 5 per cent of the patients. Why such a small percentage of the patients progress to multilobular biliary cirrhosis remains uncertain. Shwachman noted a

familial tendency to develop hepatic complications.[425] Nutritional deficiencies and intercurrent infection do not explain the progression to multilobular cirrhosis. The relationship in cystic fibrosis between the abnormalities in bile salt metabolism and hepatobiliary disease awaits further investigation.

Hemosiderosis and fatty infiltration of the liver are two other pathologic features of the liver in cystic fibrosis. The increased intestinal absorption of iron that occurs in untreated patients with pancreatic insufficiency may produce hepatic hemosiderosis. The early institution of supplemental enzymes reduces the increased absorption of iron.[435] Hepatic infiltration with fat secondary to chronic malnutrition is frequently seen with cystic fibrosis.[425]

Genetics

Cystic fibrosis is inherited as an autosomal recessive trait.[436] The highest reported incidence of cystic fibrosis has been in Caucasians, primarily those of European origin. The incidence in the Caucasian population in the United States is approximately 1:2000.[437] The disease is less frequent in blacks and Asians.[438] No good incidence figures are available for nonwhites with the exception of Hawaiians, for whom the incidence has been reported to be 1:90,000.[439]

Recently, prenatal diagnosis was accomplished using a DNA probe (DOCRl-917) that detects restriction fragment length polymorphisms following DNA digestion with Hind III and Hinc II. The location of this probe was shown to be about 15 centimorgan from the cystic fibrosis locus.[440] The DOCRI-917 locus was mapped to chromosome 7. Other DNA markers such as met oncogene and PJ3.11, which are known to be on chromosome 7, are also close to the cystic fibrosis locus and have been used recently by Beaudet and co-workers for prenatal diagnosis.[441]

Therapy

Hepatic complications of cystic fibrosis that need treatment include those of newborns with obstructive jaundice and those of patients first seen for treatment as adolescents with multilobular biliary cirrhosis and portal hypertension. Jaundiced neonates may escape severe hepatic involvement later. Drugs that stimulate bile flow are not helpful. Flushing of the extrahepatic biliary tree with normal saline has been successful in two cases.[404, 406] In some cases, spontaneous relief of the jaundice has occurred without treatment.[406] The decision to perform portal-systemic shunting in an older patient with portal hypertension depends largely on pulmonary status. Patients who have severe pulmonary disease are poor candidates for surgery. The long-term survival of these patients is poor, and the complication rate for such a major operation is very high. Those patients who have had single episodes of hemorrhaging or have esophageal varices with good pulmonary function are considered candidates for the shunting procedure.[410, 411]

REFERENCES

1. Sachs B, Sternfeld L, Kraus G. Essential fructosuria: its pathophysiology. Am J Dis Child 63:252, 1974.
2. Chalmers RA, Pratt RTC. Idiosyncrasy to fructose. Lancet 2:340, 1956.

3. Froesch ER, Prader A, Labhart A, et al. Die hereditäre Fructose intoleranz, ein bisher nicht bekannte kongenitale Stoff wechselstorung, Schweiz Med Wochenschr 87:1168, 1957.
4. Baker L, Winegrad AI. Fasting hypoglycemia and metabolic acidosis associated with deficiency of hepatic fructose-1,6-diphosphatase activity. Lancet 2:13, 1970.
5. Cornblath M, Rosenthal IM, Reisner SH, et al. Hereditary fructose intolerance. N Engl J Med 269:1271, 1963.
6. Froesch ER, Wolf HP, Baitsch H, et al. Hereditary fructose intolerance: an inborn defect of hepatic fructose-1-phosphate splitting aldolase. Am J Med 34:151, 1963.
7. Swales JD, Smith ADM. Adult fructose intolerance. Q J Med 35:455, 1966.
8. Odievre M, Gentil C, Gautier M, et al. Hereditary fructose intolerance in childhood. Am J Dis Child 132:605, 1978.
9. Mass RE, Smith WR, Welsh JR. The association of hereditary fructose intolerance and renal tubular acidosis. Am J Med Sci 251:516, 1966.
10. Schulte MJ, Widukind L. Fatal sorbitol infusion in a patient with fructose-sorbitol intolerance. Lancet 2:188, 1977.
11. Morris RC Jr, Ueki I, Loh D, et al. Absence of renal fructose-1-phosphate aldolase activity in hereditary fructose intolerance. Nature 214:920, 1967.
12. Perheentupa JE, Pitkanen E, Nikkila EA, et al. Hereditary fructose intolerance: a clinical study of four cases. Ann Paediatr Fenn 8:221, 1962.
13. Shapira F, Dreyfus JC. L'Aldolase hépatique dans intolerance au fructose. Rev Fr Etud Clin Biol 12:486, 1967.
14. Hers HG, Joassin G. Anomalie de l'aldolase hépatique dans l'intolérance au fructose. Enzymol Biol Clin 1:4, 1961.
15. Gurtler B, Leuthardt F. Ueber die Heterogeniatat der Aldolase. Helv Chim Acta 53:654, 1970.
16. Rutter JW, Richards OC, Woodfin BM. Comparative studies of liver and muscle aldolase. I. Effects of carboxypeptidase on catalytic activity. J Biol Chem 236:3193, 1961.
17. Drechler JE, Boyer PD, Kowalesky AG. The catalytic activity of carboxypeptidase-degraded aldolase. J Biol Chem 234:2627, 1959.
18. Nordmann Y, Shapira F, Dreyfus JC. A structurally modified aldolase in fructose intolerance: immunologic and kinetic evidence. Biochem Biophys Res Commun 31:884, 1968.
19. Gitzelmann R, Steinmann B, Bally C, et al. Antibody activation of mutant human fructose-diphosphate aldolase B in liver extracts of patients with hereditary fructose intolerance. Biochem Biophys Res Commun 59:1270, 1974.
20. Froesch ER, Prader A, Wolf HP, et al. Die hereditäre Fructose intoleranz. Helv Paediat Acta 14:99, 1959.
21. Froesch ER. Essential fructosuria, hereditary fructose intolerance, and fructose-1,6-diphosphatase deficiency. In: Stanbury JB, Wyngaarden JB, Fredrickson DS, eds. The Metabolic Basis of Inherited Disease, 4th ed. New York, McGraw-Hill, 1978:131.
22. van Den Berg G, Hue L, Hers HG. Effect of administration of fructose on glycolytic action of glucagon. An investigation of the pathogeny of hereditary fructose intolerance. Biochem J 134:637, 1973.
23. Kaufmann U, Froesch ER. Inhibition of phosphorylase-a by fructose-1-phosphate, α-glycerophosphate and fructose-1,6-diphosphate: Explanation for fructose-induced hypoglycemia and fructose-1,6-diphosphatase deficiency. Eur J Clin Invest 3:407, 1973.
24. Thurston JH, Jones EM, Hauhart RE. Decrease and inhibition of liver glycogenphosphorylase after fructose. An experimental model for the study of hereditary fructose intolerance. Diabetes 23:597, 1974.
25. Woods HF, Eggleston LV, Krebs HA. The cause of hepatic accumulation of fructose-1-phosphate on fructose loading. Biochem J 119:501, 1970.
26. Raivio KO, Kekomaki MP, Maenpaa PH. Depletion of liver adenine nucleotides induced by D-fructose: dose dependency and specificity of the fructose effect. Biochem Pharmacol 18:2615, 1969.
27. Levine B, Snodgrass GJAI, Oberholzer VG, et al. Fructosemia: observations on seven cases. Am J Med 45:826, 1968.
28. Dormandy TL, Porter RJ. Familial fructose and galactose intolerance. Lancet 1:1189, 1961.
29. Turner RC, Spathis GS, Nabarro JDN, et al. Familial fructose and galactose intolerance. Lancet 2:872, 1972.
30. Schwartz R, Gamsu H, Mulligan PB, et al. Transient intolerance to exogenous fructose in the newborn. J Clin Invest 43:333, 1964.
31. Dubois R, Loeb H, Ooms HA, et al. Etude d'un cas d'hypoglycémie fonctionell par intolérance au fructose. Helv Paediat Acta 16:90, 1961.
32. Milhaud G. Téchnique nouvelle de misc en evidence d'erreurs congénitales du métabolism chez l'homme. Argent Bras Endocr 13:49, 1964.
33. Levin B, Oberholzer VG, Snodgrass GJAI, et al. Fructosemia: an inborn error of fructose metabolism. Arch Dis Child 38:220, 1963.
34. Lelong M, Alagille D, Gentil C, et al. Cirrhose hépatique et tubulopathie par absence congénitale de l'aldolase hépatique: intolérance héréditaire au fructose. Bull Soc Med Hop (Paris) 113:58, 1962.

35. Leven B, Snodgrass GJAI, Oberholzer VG, et al. Fructosemia: observation of seven cases. Am J Med 45:826, 1968.
36. Gentil C, Colin J, Valette AM, et al. Investigation of carbohydrate metabolism in hereditary intolerance to fructose: attempt at interpretation of hypoglycemia. Rev F Etud Clin Biol 9:596, 1964.
37. Nikkila EA, Perheentupa J. Non-esterified fatty acids and fatty liver in hereditary fructose intolerance. Lancet 2:1280, 1962.
38. Morris RC. Fructose-induced disruption of renal acidification in patients with hereditary fructose intolerance. J Clin Invest 44:1076, 1965.
39. Morris RC. Evidence for an acidification defect of the proximal renal tubule in experimental and clinical renal disease. J Clin Invest 45:1048, 1966.
40. Morris RC Jr. An experimental renal acidification defect in patients with hereditary fructose intolerance. I. Its resemblance to renal tubular acidosis. J Clin Invest 47:1389, 1968.
41. Morris RC Jr. An experimental renal acidification defect in patients with hereditary fructose intolerance. II. Its distinction from classical renal tubular acidosis: Its resemblance to the renal acidification defect associated with the Fanconi syndrome of children with cystinosis. J Clin Invest 47:1648, 1968.
42. Phillips MJ, Path MC, Little JA, et al. Subcellular pathology of hereditary fructose intolerance. Am J Med 44:910, 1968.
43. Marthaler TM, Froesch ER. Hereditary fructose intolerance: dental status of eight patients. Br Dent J 132:597, 1967.
44. Raivio K, Perheentupa J, Nikkila EA. Aldolase activities in the liver of patients with hereditary fructose intolerance. Clin Chim Acta 17:275, 1967.
45. Cornblath M, Schwartz R. Carbohydrate Metabolism in the Neonate. Philadelphia, WB Saunders 1966.
46. Greenberg RE, Christiansen O. The critically ill child: hypoglycemia. Pediatrics 46:915, 1970.
47. Aronson SM, Perle G, Saifer A, et al. Biochemical identification of the carrier state in Tay-Sachs disease. Proc Soc Exp Biol Med 64:4, 1962.
48. Schneck LG, Perle G, Volk BW. Fructose intolerance in Tay-Sachs disease. Pediatrics 36:273, 1965.
49. Volk BD, Aronson SM, Saifer A. Fructose-1-phosphate aldolase deficiency in Tay-Sachs disease. Am J Med 36:481, 1964.
50. Greene HL, Stifel FB, Herman RH. Hereditary fructose intolerance: treatment with pharmacologic doses of folic acid. Clin Res 20:274, 1972.
51. Melancon SB, Khachadurian AK, Nadler HL. Metabolic and biochemical studies in fructose-1,6-diphosphatase deficiency. J Pediatr 82:650, 1973.
52. Greene HL, Stifel FB, Herman RH. "Ketotic hypoglycemia" due to fructose diphosphatase deficiency and treatment with folic acid. Am J Dis Child 124:415, 1972.
53. Mason HH, Turner ME. Chronic galactosemia. Am J Dis Child 50:359, 1935.
54. Komrower GM, Schwarz V, Holzel A, et al. A clinical and biochemical study of galactosemia. Arch Dis Child 31:254, 1956.
55. Isselbacher KJ, Anderson EP, Kurahashi K, et al. Congenital galactosemia, a single enzymatic block in galactose metabolism. Science 123:635, 1956.
56. Donnell GN, Bergren WR, Cleland RS. Galactosemia. Pediatr Clin North Am 7:315, 1960.
57. Anderson MW, Williams VP, Helmer GR Jr, et al. Transferase-deficiency galactosemia: evidence for the lack of a transferase protein in galactosemic red cells. Arch Biochem Biophys 222:326, 1983.
58. Gitzelmann R. Hereditary galactokinase deficiency, a newly recognized cause of juvenile cataracts. Pediatr Res 1:14, 1967.
59. Chacko CM, McCrone L, Nadler HL. A study of galactokinase and glucose-4-epimerase from normal and galactosemic skin fibroblasts. Biochim Biophys Acta 284:552, 1972.
60. Dahlqvist A, Gamstrup I, Madsden H. A patient with hereditary galactokinase deficiency. Acta Pediatr Scand 29:669, 1970.
61. Gitzelmann R. Deficiency of uridine diphosphate galactose-4-epimerase in blood cells of an apparently healthy infant. Helv Paediat Acta 27:125, 1972.
62. Gitzelmann R, Steinmann B, Mitchell B. Uridine diphosphate galactose-4-epimerase deficiency. IV. Report of eight cases in three families. Helv Paediat Acta 31:44, 1976.
63. Holton JB, Gillett MG, MacFaul R, et al. Galactosemia: a new variant due to uridine diphosphate galactose-4-epimerase deficiency. Arch Dis Child 56:885, 1981.
64. Henderson MJ, Holton JB, MacFaul R. Further observations in a case of uridine diphosphate galactose-4-epimerase deficiency with a severe clinical presentation. J Inherited Metab Dis 6:17, 1983.
65. Marchese N, Borrore C. Galactosemia caused by generalized uridine diphosphate galactose-4-epimerase deficiency. J Pediatr 103:927, 1983.
66. Bowling FG, Fraser DK, Clague AE, et al. A case of uridine diphos-

phate galactose-4-epimerase deficiency detected by neonatal screening for galactosemia. Med J Aust 144:150, 1986.

67. Garibaldi LR, Canine S, Supert-Furga A, et al. Galactosemia caused by generalized uridine diphosphate galactosemia-4-epimerase deficiency. J Pediatr 103:927, 1983.

68. Stenstam T. Peroral and intravenous galactose tests: comparative study of their significance in different conditions. Acta Med Scand Suppl 177, 1946.

69. Segal S, Blair A. Some observations on the metabolism of D-galactose in normal man. J Clin Invest 40:2016, 1961.

70. Tygstrup N, Winkler K. Galactose blood clearance as a measure of hepatic blood flow. Clin Sci 17:1, 1958.

71. Colcher H, Patek AJ, Kendall FE. Galactose disappearance from the blood stream: calculation of a galactose removal constraint and its application as a test of liver function. J Clin Invest 25:768, 1946.

72. Tygstrup N. Determination of the hepatic elimination capacity (Lm) of galactose by single injection. Scand J Clin Lab Invest 18:suppl 92, 118, 1966.

73. Komrower GM, Lee DH. Long-term follow-up of galactosemia. Arch Dis Child 45:367, 1970.

74. Koch R, Donnell GN, Fishler K, et al. Galactosemia, In: Kelley VC, ed. Practice of Pediatrics. Hagerstown, Md, Harper and Row, 1979:14.

75. Segal S, Blair A, Roth H. The metabolism of galactose by patients with congenital galactosemia. Am J Med 38:62, 1965.

76. Segal S. Disorders of galactose metabolism. In: Stanbury JB, Wyngaarden JB, Fredrickson DS, eds. The Metabolic Basis of Inherited Disease. New York, McGraw-Hill, 1978:164.

77. Levy HL, Sepe SJ, Shih VE, et al. Sepsis due to Escherichia coli in neonates with galactosemia. N Engl J Med 297:823, 1977.

78. Segal S, Cuatrecasas P. The oxidation of ^{14}C galactose by patients with congenital galactosemia. Evidence for a direct oxidative pathway. Am J Med 44:340, 1968.

79. Sidbury JB Jr. The role of galactose-1-phosphate in the pathogenesis of galactosemia, In: Gardner LE, ed. Molecular Genetics and Human Disease. Springfield, Ill.: Charles C Thomas, 1960:61.

80. Tada K. Glycogenesis and glycolysis in the liver from congenital galactosemia. Tohoku J Exp Med 82:168, 1964.

81. van Heyningen R. Formation of polyols by the lens of the rat with "sugar" cataracts. Nature 184:194, 1959.

82. Kinoshita JH, Dvornik D, Krami M, et al. The effect of aldose reductase inhibition on the galactose exposed rabbit lens. Biochim Biophys Acta 158:472, 1968.

83. Kinoshita JH, Barber GW, Merola LO, et al. Changes in levels of free amino acids and myo-inositol in the galactose-exposed lens. Invest Ophthalmol 8:625, 1969.

84. Dische Z, Zelmenis G, Youlous J. Studies on protein and protein synthesis—during the development of galactose cataract. Am J Ophthalmol 44:332, 1957.

85. Sippel TO. Enzymes of carbohydrate metabolism in developing galactose cataracts of rats. Invest Ophthalmol 6:59, 1967.

86. Korc I. Biochemical studies on cataracts in galactose fed rats. Arch Biochem 94:196, 1961.

87. Sippel TO. Energy metabolism in the lens during development of galactose cataract in rats. Invest Ophthalmol 5:576, 1966.

88. Kinoshita JH, Merola LO, Tung B. Changes in cation permeability in the galactose-exposed rabbit lens. Exp Eye Res 7:80, 1968.

89. Heffley JD, Williams RJ. The nutritional teamwork approach. Prevention and regression of cataracts in rats. Proc Natl Acad Sci USA 71:4164, 1974.

90. Schwarz V. The value of galactose phosphate determination in the treatment of galactosemia. Arch Dis Child 35:428, 1960.

91. Quan-Ma R, Wells H, Wells W, et al. Galactitol in the tissues of a galactosemic child. Am J Dis Child 112:477, 1966.

92. Quan-Ma R, Wells W. The distribution of galactitol in tissues of rats fed galactose. Biochem Biophys Res Commun 20:486, 1965.

93. Keppler D, Decker K. Studies on the mechanisms of galactosamine hepatitis. Eur J Biochem 10:219, 1969.

94. Fox M, Thier S, Rosenberg L, et al. Impaired renal tubular function induced by sugar infusion in man. J Clin Endocrinol 24:1318, 1964.

95. Rosenberg L, Weinberg A, Segal S. The effect of high galactose diets on urinary excretion of amino acids in the rat. Biochim Biophys Acta 48:500, 1961.

96. Their S, Fox M, Rosenberg L, et al. Hexose inhibition of amino acid uptake in the rat kidney cortex slice. Biochim Biophys Acta 93:106, 1964.

97. Saunders S, Isselbacher KJ. Inhibition of intestinal amino acid transport by hexoses. Biochim Biophys Acta 102:397, 1965.

98. Wells W, Pittman T, Wells H, et al. The isolation and identification of galactitol from the brains of galactosemia patients. J Biol Chem 240:1002, 1965.

99. Wells HJ, Gordon M, Segal S. Galactose toxicity in the chick: oxidation of radioactive galactose. Biochim Biophys Acta 222:327, 1970.

100. Granett SE, Kozak LP, McIntyre JP, et al. Studies on cerebral energy metabolism during the course of galactose neurotoxicity in chicks. J Neurochem 19:1659, 1972.

101. Knull HR, Lobert PF, Wells WW. Galactose neurotoxicity in chicks. Effects on fast axoplasmic transport. Brain Res 79:524, 1974.

102. Malone J, Wells H, Segal S. Decreased uptake of glucose by brain of the galactose toxic chick. Brain Res 43:700, 1972.

103. Malone JI, Wells HJ, Segal S. Galactose toxicity in the chick: hyperosmolality. Science 174:952, 1971.

104. Knull HR, Wells WW. Recovery from galactose-induced neurotoxicity in the chick by the administration of glucose. J Neurochem 20:415, 1973.

105. Wooly DW, Gommi BW. Serotonin receptors. IV. Specific deficiency of receptors in galactose toxicity and its possible relationship to the idiocy of galactosemia. Proc Natl Acad Sci USA 52:14, 1964.

106. Robbins SL, Cotran RS. Diseases of infancy and childhood, In: Robbins SL, Cotran RS, eds. Pathologic Basis of Disease. 2nd ed. Philadelphia, WB Saunders, 1979:582.

107. Smetana HF, Olen E. Hereditary galactose disease. Am J Clin Pathol 38:3, 1962.

108. Walker FA, Hsia DYY, Slatis HM, et al. Galactosemia: a study of 27 kindreds in North America. Ann Hum Genet 25:287, 1962.

109. Kirkman HN, Bynum E. Enzymatic evidence of a galactosemic trait in parents and galactosemic children. Ann Hum Genet 23:117, 1959.

110. Mellman WJ, Tedesco TA, Feige P. Estimation of the gene frequency of the Duarte variant of galactose-1-phosphate uridyl transferase. Ann Hum Genet 32:1, 1968.

111. Brandt MJ. Frequency of heterozygotes for hereditary galactosemia in a normal population. Acta Genet (Basel) 17:289, 1967.

112. Tedesco TA, Miller KL, Rawnsley BE, et al. Human erythrocyte galactokinase and galactose-1-phosphate uridyltransferase: a population survey. Am J Hum Genet 27:737, 1975.

113. Scriver CR. Population screening: report of a workshop. Prog Clin Biol Res 163B:89, 1985.

114. Kleijer WJ, Janse HC, van Diggelen OP, et al. First trimester diagnosis of galactosemia. Lancet 1(8583):748, 1986.

115. Anderson EP, Kalckar HM, Kurahashi K, et al. A specific enzymatic assay for the diagnosis of congenital galactosemia. J Lab Clin Med 50:569, 1957.

116. Kliegman RM, Sparks JM. Perinatal galactose metabolism. J Pediatr 107:831, 1985.

117. Kaufman F, Kogut M, Donnell G, et al. Hypergonadotropic hypogonadism in female patients with galactosemia. N Engl J Med 304:994, 1981.

118. Steinmann B, Grizelmann R, Zachmann M. Hypogonadism and galactosemia. N Engl J Med 304:995, 1981.

119. Chen YT, Mattison DR, Feigenbaum L, et al. Reduction in oocyte number following prenatal exposure to a diet high in galactose. Science 214:1145, 1981.

120. Chen YT, Mattison DR, Bercu BB, et al. Resistance of the male gonad to a high galactose diet. Pediatr Res 18:345, 1984.

121. Campbell S, Kulin HE. Transient thyroid-binding globulin deficiency with classic galactosemia. J Pediatr 105:335, 1984.

122. Holtzman NA. Pitfalls of newborn screening (with special attention to hypothyroidism): When will we ever learn? Birth Defects 19:111, 1983.

123. Segal S. Disorders of galactose metabolism. In: Stanbury J, Wyngaarden J, Fredrickson D, et al, eds. The Metabolic Basis of Inherited Disease, 5th ed. New York McGraw-Hill, 1983:167.

124. Gitzelmann R, Haigis E. Appearance of active UPD-galactose-4-epimerase in cells cultured from epimerase-deficient persons. J Inherited Metab Dis 1:41, 1978.

125. von Gierke E. Hepato-nephromegalia glykogenia (Glykogenspeicherkrankheiten Leber und Nieren). Beitr Pathol Anat 82:497, 1929.

126. Pompe JC. Over idiopatische hypertrophie van het hart. Ned Tijdschr Geneeskd 76:304, 1932.

127. Cori GT, Cori DF. Glucose-6-phosphatase of the liver in glycogen storage disease. J Biol Chem 199:661, 1952.

128. Hug G. Glycogen storage disease. Birth Defects 12:145, 1976.

129. Howell RR. The glycogen storage diseases. In: Stanbury JB, Wyngaarden JB, Fredrickson DS, eds. The Metabolic Basis of Inherited Disease, 4th ed. New York McGraw-Hill, 1977:137.

130. Senior B. The glycogenoses. Clin Perinatol 3:79, 1976.

131. Tarui S, Okuno G, Ikuka Y, et al. Phosphofructokinase deficiency in skeletal muscle: a new type of glycogenosis. Biochem Biophys Res Commun 19:517, 1965.

132. Emmett M, Narins RG. Renal transplantation in type I glycogenosis: failure to improve glucose metabolism. JAMA 239:1642, 1964.

133. Greene HL, Slonim AE, O'Neill JA Jr, et al. Continuous nocturnal intragastric feeding for management of type I glycogen storage disease. N Engl J Med 294:423, 1976.

134. Roe TF, Kogu MD. Chronic effects of oral glucose alimentation and portacaval shunt in patients with glycogen storage disease type I. Pediatr Res 10:414, 1976. (Abstract.)

135. Baker L, Mills JL. Long-term treatment of glycogen storage disease type I: clinical improvement but persistent abnormalities of lactate and triglyceride concentration. Pediatr Res 12:502, 1978. (Abstract.)

136. Crigler JR Jr, Folkman J. Glycogen storage disease: new approaches to therapy. In: Porter R, Whelan J, eds. Hepatotrophic Factors. Amsterdam, Ciba Foundation Symposium, 1978:331.

137. Coleman JE. Metabolic interrelationships between carbohydrates, lipids, and proteins. In: Bondy PK, Rosenberg LE, eds. Diseases of Metabolism, 7th ed. Philadelphia WB Saunders, 1974:107.

138. Slonim AE, Lacy WW, Terry AB, et al. Nocturnal intragastric therapy in type I glycogen storage disease: effect on hormonal and amino acid metabolism. Metabolism 28:707, 1979.

139. Sadeghi-Nejad A, Presente E, Binkiewiez A, et al. Studies in type I glycogenosis of the liver. The genesis and deposition of lactate. J Pediatr 85:49, 1974.

140. Jakovcic S, Khachadurian AK, Hsia DYY. The hyperlipidemia in glycogen storage disease. J Lab Clin Med 68:769, 1966.

141. Howell RR, Ashton DM, Wyngaarden JB. Glucose-6-phosphatase deficiency glycogen storage disease. Studies on the interrelationships of carbohydrate, lipid and purine abnormalities. Pediatrics 29:553, 1962.

142. Ockerman PA. Glucose, glycerol and free fatty acids in glycogen storage disease type I blood levels in the fasting and nonfasting state: effect of glucose and adrenalin administration. Clin Chim Acta 12:370, 1965.

143. Forget PP. Fernandes J, Begemann PH. Triglyceride clearing in glycogen storage disease. Pediatr Res 8:114, 1974.

144. Hulsmann WD, Eijenboom WHM, Koster JF, et al. Glucose-6-phosphatase deficiency and hyperlipaemia. Clin Chim Acta 30:775, 1970.

145. Fine RN, Strauss J, Connel GN. Hyperuricemia in glycogen storage disease type I. Am J Dis Child 112:572, 1966.

146. Howell RR. The interrelationship of glycogen storage disease and gout. Arthritis Rheum 8:780, 1965.

147. Alepa FP, Howell RR, Klineberg JR, et al. Relationships between glycogen storage disease and tophaceous gout. Am J Med 42:58, 1967.

148. Jakovcic S, Sorensen LB. Studies of uric acid metabolism in glycogen storage disease associated with gouty arthritis. Arthritis Rheum 10:129, 1967.

149. Henderson JF, Khoo KY. Synthesis of 5-phosphoribosyl-1-pyrophosphate from glucose in Ehrlich ascites tumor cells in vitro. J Biol Chem 240:2349, 1965.

150. Greene ML, Seegmiller JE. Elevated erythrocyte phosphoribosylpyrophosphate in x-linked uric aciduria: importance of PRPP concentration in regulation of human purine biosynthesis. J Clin Invest 48:32a, 1969.

151. Raivio KO, Seegmiller JE. Role of glutamine in purine synthesis and in guanine nucleotide formation in normal fibroblasts and in fibroblasts deficient in hypoxanthine phosphoribosyltransferase activity. Biochim Biophys Acta 299:282, 1973.

152. Howell RR. Hyperuricemia in childhood. Fed Proc 27:1078, 1968.

153. Brosh S, Boer P, Jupfer J, et al. De novo synthesis of purine nucleotides in human peripheral blood leukocytes: excessive activity of the pathway in hypoxanthine-guanine phosphoribosyltransferase deficiency. J Clin Invest 58:289, 1976.

154. Holmes EW, McDonald JA, McCord JM, et al. Human glutamine phosphoribosyl-pyrophosphate amidotransferase: kinetic and regulatory properties. J Biol Chem 248:143, 1973.

155. Greene HL, Wilson FA, Hefferan P, et al. ATP depletion a possible role in the pathogenesis of hyperuricemia in glycogen storage disease type I. J Clin Invest 62:321, 1978.

156. Bode JC, Zelder O, Rumpelt HJ, et al. Depletion of liver adenosine phosphates and metabolic effects of intravenous infusion of fructose or sorbitol in man and in the rat. Eur J Clin Invest 3:436, 1973.

157. Roe TF, Kogut MD. The pathogenesis of hyperuricemia in glycogen storage disease type I. Pediatr Res 11:664, 1977.

158. Corby DG, Putnam CW, Greene HL. Impaired platelet function in glucose-6-phosphate deficiency. J Pediatr 85:71, 1974.

159. Cooper RA. Abnormalities of cell-membrane fluidity in the pathogenesis of disease. N Engl J Med 297:371, 1977.

160. Howell RR, Stevenson RE, Ben-Menachem Y, et al. Hepatic adenomata with type I glycogen-storage disease. JAMA 236:1481, 1976.

161. Roe TF, Kogut MD, Buckingham BA, et al. Hepatic tumors in glycogen-storage disease type I. Pediatr Res 13:931, 1979.

162. Levine G, Mierau G, Favara BE. Hepatic glycogenosis, renal glomerular cysts and hepatocarcinoma. Am J Pathol 82:PPC-37, 1976.

163. Maruyama Y, Kida E, Takagi M. An autopsy case of glycogen storage disease in female adults. J Osaka Med College 25:207, 1962.

164. Bannasch P, Hacker HJ, Klimek, Mayer D. Hepatocellular glycogenosis and related pattern of enzymatic changes during hepatocarcinogenesis. Adv Enzyme Regul 22:97, 1983.

165. Sidbury JB. The genetics of the glycogen storage diseases. Progr Med Genet 4:32, 1965.

166. Farber M, Knuppel RA, Binkiewicz A, et al. Pregnancy and von Gierke's disease. Obstet Gynecol 47:226, 1976.

167. Havel RJ, Blasse EO, Williams HE, et al. Splanchnic metabolism in von Gierke's disease (glycogenosis type I). Tran Assoc Am Physicians 82:302, 1969.

168. Tsalikian E, Simmons P, Gerich JE, et al. Glucose production and utilization in children with glycogen storage disease type I. Am J Physiol 247:E513, 1984.

169. Kalhan SC, Gilfillan C, Tserng K-Y, et al. Glucose production in type I glycogen storage disease. J Pediatr 101:159, 1982.

170. Powell RC, Wentworth SM, Brandt IK. Endogenous glucose production of type I glycogen storage disease. Metabolism 30:443, 1981.

171. Schwenk WF, Haymond MW. Optimal rate of enteral glucose administration in children with glycogen storage disease type I. N Engl J Med 314:682, 1986.

172. Edelstein G, Hirschman CA. Hyperthermia and ketoacidosis during anesthesia in a child with glycogen storage disease. Anesthesiology 52:90, 1980.

173. McAdams AJ, Hug G, Bove KE. Glycogen storage disease types I to X. Criteria for morphologic diagnosis. Hum Pathol 5:463, 1974.

174. Folkman J, Philippart A, Tze WJ, et al. Portacaval shunt for glycogen storage disease: value of prolonged intravenous hyperalimentation before surgery. Surgery 72:306, 1972.

175. Starzl TE, Marchioro TL, Secton AW, et al. The effect of portacaval transposition on carbohydrate metabolism: experimental and clinical observations. Surgery 57:687, 1965.

176. Riddell RG, Davies RP, Clark AD. Portacaval transposition in the treatment of glycogen storage disease. Lancet 2:1205, 1966.

177. Burr IM, O'Neill JA, Karzon DT, et al. Comparison of the effects of total parenteral nutrition, continuous intragastric feeding, and portacaval shunt on a patient with type I glycogen storage disease. J Pediatr 85:792, 1974.

178. Greene HL, Slonim AE, Burr IM. Type I glycogen storage disease: advances in treatment. Adv Pediatr 26:63, 1979.

179. Chen YT, Cornblath M, Sidbury JB. Cornstarch therapy in type I glycogen storage disease. N Engl J Med 310:171, 1984.

180. Collins JE, Leonard JV. The dietary management of inborn errors of metabolism. Hum Nutr Appl Nutr 39:255, 1985.

181. Leonard JV, Dunger DB. Hypoglycemia complicating feeding regimens for glycogen storage disease. Lancet 2:1203, 1978.

182. Greene HL, Slonim AE, Burr IM, et al. Type I glycogen storage disease: five years of management with nocturnal intragastric feeding. J Pediatr 96:590, 1980.

183. Michels VV, Beaudet AL, Pott VE, et al. Glycogen storage disease: long-term follow-up of nocturnal intragastric feeding. Clin Genet 17:220, 1980.

183a. Chen Y-T, Coleman RA, Sheinman JI, et al. Renal disease in type I glycogen storage disease. N Engl J Med 318:7, 1988.

184. Senior B, Loridan L. Studies of liver glycogenosis with particular reference to the metabolism of intravenously administered glycerol. N Engl J Med 279:958, 1968.

185. Bialek DS, Sharp HL, Kane WJ, et al. Latency of glucose-6-phophatase in type IB glycogen storage disease. J Pediatr 91:938, 1977. (Abstract.)

186. Harisawa K, Igarashi Y, Otomo H, et al. A new variant of glycogen storage disease type I, probably due to a defect in the glucose-6-phosphatase transport system. Biochem Biophys Res Commun 83:1360, 1978.

187. Lange AJ, Arion WJ, Beautet AL. Type Ib glycogen storage disease is caused by a defect in the glucose-6-phosphate translocase of the microsomal glucose-6-phosphatase system. J Biol Chem 255:8381, 1980.

188. Anderson DC, Mace ML, Brinkley BR, et al. Recurrent infection in glycogenosis type IB: abnormal neutrophil motility related to impaired redistribution of adhesion sites. J Infect Dis 143:447, 1981.

189. Beaudet AL, Anderson DC, Michels VV, et al. Neutropenia and impaired neutrophil migration in type Ib glycogen storage disease. J Pediatr 97:906, 1980.

190. Heyne K, Gahr M. Phagocytatic extra-respiration: differences between cases of glycogenosis type Ia and Ib. Eur J Pediatr 133:186, 1980.

191. Seger R, Steinmann B, Tiefenauer L, et al. Glycogenosis Ib: neutrophil microbicidal defects due to impaired monophosphate shunt. Pediatr Res 18:297, 1984.

192. Arion WJ, Wallen BK, Lange AJ, et al. On the involvement of a glucose-6-phosphate transport system in the function of microsomal glucose-6-phosphatase. Mol Cell Biochem 6:75, 1975.

193. Skaug WA, Warford LL, Figueroa JM, et al. Glycogenosis type IB: Possible membrane transport defect. South Med J 74:761, 1981.

194. Lange AJ, Arion WJ, Beaudet L. Type Ib glycogen storage disease is caused by a defect in the glucose-6-phosphatase system. J Biol Chem 255:8381, 1980.

195. Zakim D, Edmonson DE. The role of the membrane in regulation of activity of microsomal glucose-6-phosphatase. J Biol Chem 257:1145, 1982.

196. Greene HL, Zakim D, Edmonson D. Measurement of hepatic steady state and pre-steady state kinetic of glucose-6-phosphatase in a patient with type Ib glycogen storage disease. Pediatr Res 1986.

197. Ambruso DR, McCabe ERB, Anderson D, et al. Infectious and bleeding complications in patients with glycogenosis type Ib. Am J Dis Child 139:691, 1985.

198. Corbeel L, Boogaerts M, Van den Berghe G, et al. Clinical and biochemical findings before and after portal-caval shunt in a girl with type Ib glycogen storage disease. Pediatr Res 15:58, 1981.

199. Brown B, Brown DH. The glycogen storage diseases: types I, III, IV, V, VII, and unclassified glycogenoses. In: Whelan WJ, ed. Carbohydrate Metabolism and its Disorders, Vol. 2 New York, Academic Press, 1968:123.

200. Brandt IK, DeLuca VA Jr. Type III glycogenosis: a family with an unusual tissue distribution of the enzyme lesion. Am J Med 40:779, 1966.

201. Murase T, Ikeda H, Muro T, et al. Myopathy associated with type III glycogenosis. J Neurol Sci 20:287, 1973.

202. Levin S, Moses SW, Chayoth R, et al. Glycogen storage diseases in Israel. Isr J Med Sci 3:397, 1967.

203. Van Creveld S, Huijing F. Glycogen storage disease. Am J Med 38:554, 1965.

204. Starzl TE, Putnam CW, Porter KA, et al. Portal diversion for the treatment of glycogen storage disease in humans. Ann Surg 178:525, 1973.

205. Alagille D, Odievre M. Inborn errors of metabolism. In: Alagille D, Odievre M, eds. Liver and Biliary Tract Disease in Children. New York, John Wiley & Sons, 1979:217.

206. Hug G, Krill CE Jr, Perrin EV, et al. Cori's disease (amylo-1,6-glucosidase deficiency). N Engl J Med 268:113, 1963.

207. Hers HG. Amylo-1,6-glucosidase activity in tissues of children with glycogen storage disease. Biochem J 76:69, 1960.

208. van Hoof F, Hers HG. The subgroups of type III glycogenosis. Eur J Biochem 2:265, 1967.

209. McAdams AJ, Hug G, Bove KE. Glycogen storage disease, types I to X. Criteria for morphologic diagnosis. Hum Pathol 5:463, 1974.

210. Garancis JS, Panares RR, Good TA, et al. Type III glycogenosis: a biochemical and electron microscopic study. Lab Invest 22:468, 1970.

211. Slonim AE, Terry AB, Moran R, et al. Differing food consumption for nocturnal intragastric therapy in types I and III glycogen storage disease. Pediatr Res 12:512/894, 1978. (Abstract.)

212. Borowitz SM, Greene HL. Cornstarch therapy in a patient with type III glycogen storage disease. J Pediatr Gastroenterol Nutr 6:631, 1987.

213. Anderson DH. Studies on glycogen disease with report of a case in which the glycogen was abnormal. In: Ajjar VA, ed. Carbohydrate Metabolism. Baltimore, Johns Hopkins Press, 1952:28.

214. Illingworth B, Cori GT. Structure of glycogens and amylopectins. III. Normal and abnormal human glycogen. J Biol Chem 199:653, 1952.

215. Brown BI, Brown D. Lack of an α-1,4-glucan:α-1,4 glucan 6-glycosyl transferase in a case of type IV glycogenosis. Proc Nat Acad Sci USA 56:725, 1966.

216. Reed GB Jr, Dixon JFP, Neustein HB, et al. Type IV glycogenosis. Patient with absence of a branching enzyme α-1,4-glucan:α-1,4-glucan 6-glycosyl transferase. Lab Invest 19:546, 1968.

217. Levin B, Burgess EA, Mortimer PE. Glycogen storage disease type IV, amylopectinosis. Arch Dis Child 43:548, 1968.

218. Motoi J, Sonobe H, Ogawa K. Two autopsy cases of glycogen storage disease—cirrhotic type. Acta Pathol Jpn 23:211, 1973.

219. Brass K. Zur histologischen diagnose der glykogenose type IV (Amylopektinose). A Kinkerheilk 117:187, 1974.

220. Ishihara T, Uchino F, Adachi H. Type IV glycogenosis: a study of two cases. Acta Pathol Jpn 25:613, 1975.

221. Bannayan GA, Dean WJ, Howell RR. Type IV glycogen storage disease. Am J Clin Pathol 66:702, 1976.

222. McMaster KR, Powers JM, Hennigar GR Jr, et al. Nervous system involvement in type IV glycogenosis. Arch Pathol Lab Med 103:105, 1979.

223. Ferguson IT, Mahon M, Cumming WJK. An adult case of Anderson's disease—Type IV glycogenosis. J Neurol Sci 60:337, 1983.

224. Holmes JM, Houghton CR, Woolf AL. A myopathy presenting in adult life with features suggestive of glycogen storage disease. J Neurol Neurosurg Psychiatr 23:302, 1960.

225. Torvik A, Dietrichson P, Svaar H, et al. Myopathy with tremor and dementia—a metabolic disorder? Case report with post-mortem study. J Neurol Sci 21:181, 1974.

226. Pelissier JF, DeBarsy T, Bille J, et al. Polysaccharide (amylopectin-like) storage myopathy—histochemical, ultrastructural and biochemical studies. Acta Neuropathol (Suppl) 7:292, 1970.

227. Schochet SS, McCormick WF, Zellweger H. Type IV glycogenosis (amylopectinosis)—light and electron microscopic observations. Arch Pathol 90:354, 1970.

228. Howell RR, Kaback MM, Brown BI. Type IV glycogen storage disease—branching enzyme deficiency in skin fibroblasts and possible heterozygote detection. J Pediatr 78:638, 1971.

229. McMaster KR, Powers JM, Hennigan GR, et al. Nervous system involvement in type IV glycogenosis. Arch Pathol Lab Med 103:105, 1979.

230. Ishihara TF, Uchino H, Adachi M, et al. Type IV glycogenosis—a study of 2 cases. Acta Path Jpn 25:613, 1975.

231. Brown BI, Brown DH. Lack of α-1,4 glucan-α-1,4 glucan 6 glucosyl transferase in a case of type IV glycogenosis. Proc Natl Acad Sci 56:725, 1966.

232. Reed GB, Dixon JFP, Neustein HB, et al. Type IV glycogenosis—patient with absence of a branching enzyme α-1,4 glucan-α-1,4 glucan 6-glucosyltransferase. Lab Invest 19:546, 1968.

232a. Greene HL, Ghishan FK, Brown B, et al. Hypoglycemia in type IV glycogenosis: hepatic improvement in patients treated to normalize blood glucose concentrations. J Pediatr 112:55, 1988.

232b. Greene HL, Brown B, McClanathan DI. A new variant of type IV glycogenosis: deficiency of branching enzyme activity without apparent progressive liver disease. Hepatology 8:302, 1988.

233. Hers HG. Glycogen storage disease. In: Levine R, Luft R, eds. Advances in Metabolic Disorders Vol 1. New York, Academic Press, 1964:1.

234. Ockerman PA. Glycogen storage disease in Sweden. Acta Paediatr Scand, Suppl 160, 1965.

235. Fernandes J, Huijing F. Branching enzyme deficiency glycogenosis: studies in therapy. Arch Dis Child 43:347, 1968.

236. Lin ECC, Knox WE. Specificity of the adaptive response of tyrosine-α-ketoglutarate transaminase in the rat. J Biol Chem 233:1186, 1958.

237. La Du BN, Zannoni VG, Laster L, et al. The nature of the defect in tyrosine metabolism in alcaptonuria. J Biol Chem 230:251, 1958.

238. Shambaugh GE, Warner DA, Biesel WR. Hormonal factors altering rhythmicity of tyrosine-α-ketoglutarate transaminase in rat liver. Endocrinology 81:811, 1967.

239. Gelehrter TD, Tomkins GM. Control of tyrosine aminotransferase synthesis in tissue culture by a factor in serum. Proc Natl Acad Sci USA 64:723, 1969.

240. Granner D, Chase LR, Auerbach GD, et al. Tyrosine aminotransferase: enzyme induction independent of adenosine 3,5'-monophosphate. Science 162:1018, 1968.

241. Goswami MND, Knox WE. Developmental changes of p-hydroxyphenylpyruvate oxidase activity in mammalian liver. Biochim Biophys Acta 50:35, 1961.

242. Fellman JH, Fujita TS, Roth ES. Assay, properties and tissue distribution of p-hydroxyphenylpyruvate hydroxylase. Biochim Biophys Acta 284:90, 1972.

243. Taniguchi K, Armstrong MD. The enzymatic formation of α-hydroxyphenylacetic acid. J Biol Chem 238:4091, 1963.

244. Goswami MND, Knox WE. An evaluation of the role of ascorbic acid in the regulation of tyrosine metabolism. J Chronic Dis 16:363, 1963.

245. Medes G, Berglund H, Lohmann A. An unknown reducing urinary substance in myasthenia gravis. Proc Soc Exp Biol Med 25:210, 1927.

246. Medes G. A new error of tyrosine metabolism: tyrosinosis. The intermediary metabolism of tyrosine and phenylalanine. Biochem J 26:917, 1932.

247. Mathews J, Partington MW. The plasma tyrosine levels of premature babies. Arch Dis Child 39:371, 1964.

248. Avery ME, Clow CI, Menkes JH, et al. Treatment tyrosinemia of the newborn: dietary and clinical aspects. Pediatrics 39:371, 1964.

249. Levy HI, Shih VE, Madigan PM, et al. Transient tyrosinemia in full-term infants. JAMA 209:249, 1969.

250. Constantsas NS, Nicolopoulos DA, Agathopoulos AS, et al. Properties and developmental changes of human hepatic and pyruvate enzymes. Biochim Biophys Acta 192:545, 1969.

251. Rizzardini M, Abeliuk P. Tyrosinemia and tyrosyluria in low birth-weight infants. A new criterion to assess maturity at birth. Am J Dis Child 121:182, 1971.

252. Bakker HD, Wadman SK, Van Sprang FJ, et al. Tyrosinemia and tyrosyluria in healthy prematures. Time courses not vitamin C-dependent. Clin Chim Acta 6:73, 1975.

253. Wadman SK, Van Sprang FJ, Mass JW, et al. An exceptional case of tyrosinosis. J Ment Defic Res 12:269, 1968.

254. Holston JL Jr, Levy HL, Tomlin GA, et al. Tyrosinosis: a patient without liver or renal disease but with mental retardation. Pediatr Res 48:393, 1971.

255. Kennaway NG, Buist NRM. Metabolic studies in a patient with hepatic cytosol tyrosine aminotransferase deficiency. Pediatr Res 5:287, 1971.

256. Zaleski WA, Hill A. Tyrosinosis: a new variant. Can Med Assoc J 108:477, 1973.
257. Goldsmith LA, Kang E, Bienfang DC, et al. Tyrosinemia with plantar and palmar keratosis and keratitis. J Pediatr 83:798, 1973.
258. Louis WJ, Pitt DD, Davies H. Biochemical studies in a patient with tyrosinosis. Aust NZ J Med 4:281, 1974.
259. Goldsmith LA, Thorpe JM, Roe CR. Hepatic enzymes of tyrosine metabolism in tyrosinemia II. J Invest Dematol 73:530, 1979.
260. Zaleski WA, Hill A, Kushniruk W. Skin lesions in tyrosinosis. Response to dietary treatment. Br J Dermatol 88:335, 1973.
261. Levine RJ, Conn HO. Tyrosine metabolism in patients with liver disease. J Clin Invest 46:2012, 1967.
262. Norlinger BM, Fulenwider JT, Ivey GL, et al. Tyrosine metabolism in cirrhosis. J Lab Clin Med 94:833, 1979.
263. Van Der Heiden C, Wauters EAK, Ketting D, et al. Gas chromatographic analysis of urinary tyrosine and phenylalanine metabolites in patients with gastrointestinal disorders. Clin Chim Acta 34:289, 1971.
264. Newberry PD, Rohrer JW, Cherian G, et al. Degree and duration of hypoxia needed to produce tyrosyluria. Lancet 1:750, 1972.
265. Kallimaki JL, Lehtonen A, Seppala P. Oral tyrosine tolerance test in rheumatoid arthritis. Ann Rheum Dis 25:469, 1966.
266. Baber MA. A case of congenital cirrhosis of the liver with renal tubular defects akin to those in the Fanconi syndrome. Arch Dis Child 31:335, 1956.
267. Sakai K, Kitagawa T. An atypical case of tyrosinosis. I. Clinical and laboratory findings. Jikeikai Med J 4:1, 1957.
268. Sakai K, Kitagawa T. An atypical case of tyrosinosis, II. A research on the metabolic block. Jikeikai Med J 4:11, 1957.
269. Sakai K, Kitagawa T. An atypical case of tyrosinosis. III. The outcome of the patient. Pathological and biochemical observations on the organ tissues. Jikeikai Med J 6:15, 1959.
270. Halvorsen S, Gjessing LR. Studies on tyrosinosis: 1, effect of low-tyrosine and low-phenylalanine diet. Br Med J 2:1171, 1964.
271. Larochelle J, Mortezai A, Belanger M, et al. Experience with 37 infants with tyrosinemia. Can Med Assoc J 97:1051, 1967.
272. Scriver CR, Larochelle J, Silverberg M. Hereditary tyrosinemia and tyrosyluria in a French Canadian geographic isolate. Am J Dis Child 113:41, 1967.
273. Gentz J, Jagenburg R, Zetterstrom R. Tyrosinemia: an inborn error of tyrosine metabolism with cirrhosis of the liver and multiple renal tubular defects (de Toni-Debre-Fanconi syndrome). J Pediatr 660:670, 1965.
274. Kogut MD, Shaw KN, Donnell GN. Tyrosinosis. Am J Dis Child 113:47, 1967.
275. Kang ES, Gerald PS. Hereditary tyrosinemia and abnormal pyrrole metabolism. J Pediatr 77:397, 1970.
276. Halvorsen S, Pande H, Løken AC, et al. Tyrosinosis: a study of 6 cases. Arch Dis Child 41:238, 1966.
277. Weinburg AG, Mize CE, Worthen HG. The occurrence of hepatoma in the chronic form of hereditary tyrosinemia. J Pediatr 88:434, 1976.
278. Sass-kortsak A, Ficici S, Paunier L, et al. Secondary metabolic derangements in patients with tyrosyluria. Can Med Assoc J 97:1079, 1967.
279. Scriver CR, Silverberg M, Clow CL. Hereditary tyrosinemia and tyrosyluria: clinical report of four patients. Canad Med Assoc J 97:1047, 1967.
280. La Du BN, Gjessing LR. Tyrosinosis and tyrosinemia. In: Stanbury JB, Wyngaarden JB, Fredrickson DS, eds. The Metabolic Basis of Inherited Disease, 4th ed. New York, McGraw-Hill, 1978:256.
281. Coward RF, Smith P. Urinary excretion of 4-hydroxyphenyllactic acids and related compounds in man, including a screening test for tyrosyluria. Biochem Med 2:216, 1968.
282. Gentz J, Johansson S, Lindblad B, et al. Excretion of δ-aminolevulinic acid in hereditary tyrosinemia. Clin Chim Acta 23:257, 1969.
283. Lindblad B, Lindstedt S, Steen G. On the enzymic defects in hereditary tyrosinemia. Proc Natl Acad Sci USA 74:4641, 1977.
284. Melancon SB, Gagne R, Grenier A, et al. Deficiency of fumarylacetoacetase in the acute form of hereditary tyrosinemia with reference to prenatal diagnosis. In: Fisher MM, Roy CC, eds. Pediatric Liver Disease. New York, Plenum Press, 1983:223.
285. Berger R, Van Farssen H, Smith GPA. Biochemical studies on the enzymatic deficiencies in hereditary tyrosinemia. Clin Chim Acta 134:129, 1983.
286. Taniguchi K, Gjessing LR. Studies on tyrosinosis: 2, activity of the transaminase, parahydroxyphenylpyruvate oxidase, and homogentisic acid oxidase. Br Med J 1:969, 1965.
287. Gentz J, Lindblad B. p-Hydroxyphenylpyruvate hydroxylase activity in fine-needle aspiration liver biopsies in hereditary tyrosinemia. Scand J Clin Lab Invest 29:115, 1972.
288. Perry TL, Hardwick DF, Hansen S, et al. Methionine induction of experimental tyrosinaemia. J Ment Defic Res 11:246, 1967.
289. Gaull GE, Rassin DK, Solomon GE, et al. Biochemical observations on so-called hereditary tyrosinemia. Pediatr Res 4:337, 1970.
290. Gaull GE, Rassin DK, Sturman JA. Significance of hypermethioninaemia in acute tyrosmosis. Lancet 1:1318, 1968.
291. Daniel RG, Waisman HA. The influence of excess methionine on the free amino acids of brain and liver of the weanling rat. J Neurochem 16:787, 1969.
292. Lindemann R, Gjessing LR, Merton B, et al. Fructosaemia/"acute-tyrosinosis." Lancet 1:891, 1969.
293. Grant DB, Alexander FW, Seakins JWT. Abnormal tyrosine metabolism in hereditary fructose intolerance. Acta Paediatr Scand 59:432, 1970.
294. Bakker HD, De Bree PK, Ketting D, et al. Fructose-1,6-diphosphatase deficiency: another enzyme defect which can present itself with the clinical features of "tyrosinosis." Clin Chim Acta 55:41, 1974.
295. Berger R, Smith GPA, Stoker-deVries SA, et al. Deficiency of fumarylacetoacetate in a patient with hereditary tyrosinemia. Clin Chim Acta 114:37, 1981.
296. Kviltingen EA, Jellum E, Stokke O. Assay of fumarylacetoacetate fumarylhydroxylase in human liver–deficient activity in a case of hereditary tyrosinemia. Clin Chim Acta 115:311, 1981.
297. Furukawa N, Kinugasa A, Seo T, et al. Enzyme defect in a case of tyrosinemia type I acute form. Pediatr Res 18:463, 1984.
298. Prive L. Pathological findings in patients with tyrosinemia. Can Med Assoc J 97:1054, 1967.
299. Partington MW, Haust MD. A patient with tyrosinemia and hypermethioninemia. Can Med Assoc J 97:1059, 1967.
300. Perry TL. Tyrosinemia associated with hypermethioninemia and islet cell hyperplasia. Can Med Assoc J 97:1067, 1967.
301. Bergeron P, LaBerge C, Grenier A. Hereditary tyrosinemia in the province of Quebec. Prevalence at birth and geographic distribution. Clin Genet 5:157, 1974.
302. Grenier A, Laberge C. A modified automated fluorometric method for tyrosine determination in blood spotted on paper. A mass screening procedure for tyrosinemia. Clin Chim Acta 57:71, 1974.
303. Grenier A, Belanger L, Laberge G. Alpha-1-fetoprotein measurement. Clin Chem 22:1011, 1976.
304. Kvittingen EA, Steinmann B, Gitzelmann R, et al. Prenatal diagnosis of hereditary tyrosinemia by determination of fumarylacetoacetase in cultured amniotic fluid cells. Pediatr Res 19:334, 1985.
305. Gentz J, Lindblad B, Lindstedt S, et al. Dietary treatment in tyrosinemia (tyrosinosis) with a note on the possible recognition of a carrier state. Am J Dis Child 113:31, 1967.
306. Halvorsen S. Dietary treatment of tyrosinosis. Am J Dis Child 113:38, 1967.
307. Sass-Kortsak A, Ficici S, Paunier L, et al. Observations on treatment in patients with tyrosyluria. Can Med Assoc J 97:1089, 1967.
308. Kogut MS, Shaw KN, Donnell GN. Tyrosinosis. Am J Dis Child 113:54, 1976.
309. Tada K, Wada Y, Yazaki N, et al. Dietary treatment of infantile tyrosinemia. Tohoku J Exp Med 95:337, 1968.
310. Bodegard G, Gentz J, Lindblad B, et al. Hereditary tyrosinemia. III. On the differential diagnosis and the lack of effect of early dietary treatment. Acta Paediatr Scand 58:37, 1969.
311. Michals K, Matalon R, Wong PWK. Dietary treatment of tyrosinemia type I. J Am Diet Assoc 73:507, 1978.
312. Starzl TE, Zitelli BJ, Shavv B Jr, et al. Changing concepts: liver replacement for hereditary tyrosinemia and hepatoma. J Pediatr 106:604, 1985.
313. Goldstein JD, Dana SE, Faust JR, et al. Role of lysosomal acid lipase in the metabolism of plasma low density lipoprotein: observations in cultured fibroblasts from a patient with cholesteryl ester storage disease. J Biol Chem 250:8487, 1975.
314. Sloan HR, Fredrickson DS. Enzyme deficiency in cholesteryl ester storage disease. J Clin Invest 51:1923, 1972.
315. Schiff L, Schubert WK, McAdams AJ, et al. Hepatic cholesterol ester storage disease, a familial disorder. I. Clinical aspects. Am J Med 44:538, 1968.
316. Assmann G, Fredrickson DS, Sloan HR, et al. Accumulation of oxygenated steryl esters in Wolman's disease. J Lipid Res 16:28, 1975.
317. Abramov S, Schorr S, Wolman M. Generalized xanthomatosis with calcified adrenals. J Dis Child 91:282, 1956.
318. Wolman M, Sterk VV, Gatt S, et al. Primary familial xanthomatosis with involvement and calcification of the adrenals. Report of two more cases in siblings of a previously described infant. Pediatrics 28:742, 1961.
319. Crocker AC, Vawter GF, Neuhauser EBD, et al. Wolman's disease: three new patients with a recently described lipidosis. Pediatrics 35:627, 1965.
320. Patrick AD, Lake BD. Deficiency of an acid lipase in Wolman's disease. Nature 222:1067, 1969.
321. Kyriakides EC, Paul B, Balint JA. Lipid accumulation and acid lipase deficiency in fibroblasts from a family with Wolman's disease, and their apparent correction in vitro. J Lab Clin Med 80:810, 1972.
322. Konno T, Fujii M. Wolman's disease: the first case in Japan. Tohoku J Exp Med 90:375, 1966.

323. Eto Y, Kitagawa T. Wolman's disease with hypolipoproteinemia and acanthocytosis: clinical and biochemical observations. J Pediatr 77:862, 1970.

324. Marshall WC, Ockenden BG, Fosbrooke AS, et al. Wolman's disease: a rare lipidosis with adrenal calcification. Arch Dis Child 44:331, 1969.

325. Lough J, Fawcett J, Wiegensberg B. Wolman's disease. An electron microscopic, histochemical and biochemical study. Arch Pathol 89:103, 1970.

326. Young EP, Patrick ND. Deficiency of acid esterase activity in Wolman's disease. Arch Dis Child 45:664, 1970.

327. Boyd GS. Effect of linoleate and estrogen on cholesterol metabolism. Fed Proc (Suppl 11) 21:86, 1962.

328. Coates PM, Cortner J. Acid lipase in cultured amniotic fluid cells. Implications for the prenatal diagnosis of Wolman's disease. Pediatr Res 12:450, 1978.

329. Meyers MA. Diseases of the Adrenal Glands in Radiologic Diagnosis. Springfield, Ill. Charles C Thomas, 1963.

330. Beaudei AL, Lipson MH, Ferry GD, et al. Acid lipase in cultured fibroblasts. Cholesterol ester storage disease. J Lab Clin Med 84:54, 1974.

331. Fredrickson DS. Newly recognized disorders of cholesterol metabolism. Ann Intern Med 58:718, 1963.

332. Largeron A, Caroli J, Stralin H, et al. Polycorie cholésterolique de l'adulte. I. Etude clinique, électronique, histochimique. Presse Med (Paris) 75:2785, 1967.

333. Infante R, Polonovski J, Caroli J. Polycorie cholésterolique de l'adulte. II. Etude biochimique. Presse Med (Paris) 75:2829, 1967.

334. Partin JC, Schubert WK. Small intestinal mucosa in cholesterol ester storage disease: a light and electron microscope study. Gastroenterology 57:524, 1969.

335. Sloan HR, Fredrickson DS. Enzyme deficiency in cholesterol ester storage disease. J Clin Invest 51:1923, 1973.

336. Burke JA, Schubert WK. Deficient activity of hepatic acid lipase in cholesterol ester storage disease. Science 176:309, 1972.

337. Beaudet AL, Ferry GD, Nichols BL Jr, et al. Cholesterol ester storage disease: clinical, biochemical, and pathological studies. J Pediatr 90:910, 1977.

338. Wolf H, Hug G, Michaelis R, et al. Seltene angeborene Erkraukung mit Cholesterinester Speicherung in der Leber. Helv Paediat Acta 29:195, 1974.

339. Lageron A, Lichtenstein H, Bodin F, et al. Polycorie cholesterolique de l'adulte: à propos d'une nouvelle observation. Nouv Presse Med 3:1233, 1974.

340. Lageron A, Lichtenstein H, Bodin F, et al. Polycorie cholesterolique de l'adulte: aspects cliniques et histochimiques. Med Chir Dig 4:9, 1975.

341. Fredrickson DS, Sloan HF, Ferrans VJ, et al. Cholesterol ester storage disease: a most unusual manifestation of deficiency of two lysosomal enzyme activity. Trans Assoc Am Physicians 85:109, 1972.

342. Burton BK, Remy WT, Rayman L. Cholesterol ester and triglyceride metabolism in intact fibroblasts from patients with Wolman's disease and cholesterol ester storage disease. Pediatr Res 18:1242, 1984.

343. Suomi WD, Agranoff BW. Lipids of the spleen in Gaucher's disease. J Lipid Res 6:211, 1965.

344. Fredrickson DS, Ferrans VJ. Acid cholesterol ester hydrolase deficiency. In: Stanbury JB, Wyngaarden JB, Fredrickson DS, eds. The Metabolic Basis of Inherited Disease, 4th ed. New York, McGraw-Hill, 1978:678.

345. Kwiterovich PO, Sloan HR, Fredrickson DS. Glycolipids and other lipid constituents of normal human liver. J Lipid Res 11:322, 1970.

346. Clayton RJ, Iber FL, Ruebner BH, et al. Byler's disease: fatal familial intrahepatic cholestasis in an Amish kindred. J Pediatr 67:1025, 1965. (Abstract.)

347. Hirooka M, Ohno T. A case of familial intrahepatic cholestasis. Tohoku J Exp Med 94:293, 1968.

348. Clayton RJ, Iber FL, Ruebner BH, et al. Byler disease: fatal familial intrahepatic cholestasis in an Amish kindred. Am J Dis Child 117:112, 1969.

349. Gray OP, Saunders RA. Familial intrahepatic cholestatic jaundice in infancy. Arch Dis Child 41:320, 1966.

350. Alagille D, Odievre M. Liver and Biliary Tract Disease in Children. New York, John Wiley & Sons, 1978.

351. Odievre M, Gautier M, Hadchouel M, et al. Severe familial intrahepatic cholestasis. Arch Dis Child 48:806, 1973.

352. Ballow M, Margolis CZ, Schachtel B, et al. Progressive familial intrahepatic cholestasis. Pediatrics 51:998, 1973.

353. Dahms BB. Hepatoma in familial cholestatic cirrhosis of childhood: its occurrence in twin brothers. Arch Pathol Lab Med 103:30, 1979.

354. Watkins JB, Perman JA. Bile acid metabolism in infants and children. Clin Gastroenterol 6: no 1, 1977.

355. Linarelli LG, Williams CN, Phillips MJ. Byler's disease: fatal intrahepatic cholestasis. J Pediatr 81:484, 1972.

356. Williams CN, Kaye R, Baker L, Progressive familial cholestatic cirrhosis and bile acid metabolism. J Pediatr 81:493, 1972.

357. Banfield WJ, Thaler MM, Alagille D, et al. Bile acid concentration in Byler's disease. Gastroenterology 67:779, 1974.

358. Ghent CH, Bloomer JR, Hsia AE. Efficacy and safety of long term phenobarbital therapy in familial cholestasis. J Pediatr 93:127, 1978.

359. Aagenaes Ø, Van Der Hagen CB, Refsum S. Hereditary recurrent intrahepatic cholestasis from birth. Arch Dis Child 43:646, 1968.

360. Sharp HL, Krivit W. Hereditary lymphedema and obstructive jaundice. J Pediatr 78:491, 1971.

361. Aagenaes Ø. Hereditary recurrent cholestasis with lymphoedema—two new families. Acta Paediatr Scand 63:465, 1974.

362. Aagenaes Ø, Cudeman B, Sigstad H, et al. Clinical and experimental relationships between cholestasis and abnormal hepatic lymphatics. Pediatr Res 4:377, 1970.

363. Bloom W. The role of the lymphatics in the absorption of bile pigment from the liver in early obstructive jaundice. Bull Johns Hopkins Hosp 34:316, 1923.

364. Shafiroff BG, Doubilet H, Ruggiero W. Bilirubin resorption in obstructive jaundice. Proc Soc Exp Biol Med 42:203, 1939.

365. Cain JC, Grindlay JH, Bollman JL, et al. Lymph from liver and thoracic duct. Surg Gynecol Obstet 85:559, 1947.

366. Friedman M, Byers SO, Omoto C. Some characteristics of hepatic lymphs in the intact rat. Am J Physiol 184:11, 1956.

367. Ahrens EH Jr, Harris RC, MacMahon HE. Atresia of the intrahepatic bile ducts. Pediatrics 8:628, 1951.

368. MacMahon HE, Thannhauser SJ. Congenital dysplasia of the interlobular bile ducts with extensive skin xanthomata: congenital acholangic biliary cirrhosis. Gastroenterology, 21:488, 1952.

369. Haas L, Dobbs RH. Congenital absence of the intrahepatic bile ducts. Arch Dis Child 33:396, 1958.

370. Watson GH, Miller V. Arteriohepatic dysplasia: familial pulmonary arterial stenosis with neonatal liver disease. Arch Dis Child 48:459, 1973.

371. Alagille D, Odievre M, Gautier M, et al. Hepatic ductular hypoplasia associated with characteristic facies, vertebral malformations, retarded physical, mental, and sexual development, and cardiac murmur. J Pediatr 86:63, 1975.

372. Riely CA, Cotlier E, Jensen PS, et al. Arteriohepatic dysplasia: a benign syndrome of intrahepatic cholestasis with multiple organ involvement. Ann Intern Med 91:520, 1979.

373. Riely CA, LaBrecque DR, Ghent C, et al. A father and son with cholestasis and peripheral pulmonic stenosis. J Pediatr 92:406, 1978.

374. Henriksen NT, Langmark F, Sörland SJ, et al. Hereditary cholestasis combined with peripheral pulmonary stenosis and other anomalies. Acta Paediatr Scand 66:7, 1977.

375. Alagille D, Odievre M. Liver and Biliary Tract Disease in Children. New York, John Wiley & Sons, 1979.

376. Greenwood RD, Rosenthal A, Crocker AC, et al. Syndrome of intrahepatic biliary dysgenesis and cardiovascular malformations. Pediatrics 58:243, 1976.

377. Ghishan FK, LaBreque DR, Mitros F, et al. The evolving course of infantile obstructive cholangiopathy. J Pediatr 97:27, 1980.

378. Bowen P, Lee CSN, Zellweger H, et al. A familial syndrome of multiple congenital defects. Bull Johns Hopkins Hosp 114:402, 1964.

379. Smith DW, Opitz JM, Inhorn SL. A syndrome of multiple developmental defects including polycystic kidneys and intrahepatic biliary dysgenesis in two siblings. J Pediatr 67:617, 1965.

380. Passarge E, McAdams AJ. Cerebro-hepatorenal syndrome. J Pediatr 71:691, 1967.

381. Opitz JM, ZuRhein GM, Vitale L, et al. The Zellweger syndrome (cerebro-hepato-renal syndrome). Birth Defects. Original Article series, Vol. 5, 1968.

382. Goldfischer S, Moore CL, Johnson AD, et al. Peroxisomal and mitochondrial defects in the cerebro-hepato-renal syndrome. Science 182:62, 1972.

383. Danks DM, Tippett P, Adams C, et al. Cerebro-hepato-renal syndrome of Zellweger: a report of eight cases with comments upon the incidence, the liver lesion and a fault in pipecolic acid metabolism. J Pediatr 86:382, 1975.

384. Hanson RF, Szczepanik-Vanleeuwen P, Williams GC, et al. Defects of bile acid synthesis in Zellweger's syndrome. Science 203:1107, 1979.

385. O'Brien RT. Iron overload. Pediatrics Semin Hematol 115:122, 1977.

386. Monnens L, Bakkeren J, Parmentier G, et al. Disturbances in bile acid metabolism of infants with the Zellweger (cerebro-hepato-renal) syndrome. Eur J Pediatr 133:31, 1980.

387. Williams JP, Secrist L, Fowler GW, et al. Roentgenographic features of the cerebrohepatorenal syndrome of Zellweger. Am J Roentgenol Radium Ther Nucl Med 115:607, 1972.

388. Patton RG, Christie DL, Smith DW, et al. Cerebro-hepato-renal

syndrome of Zellweger: two patients with islet cell hyperplasia, hypoglycemia, and thymic anomalies, and comments on iron metabolism. Am J Dis Child 124:840, 1972.

389. Setoguchi T, Salen G, Tint GS, et al. A biochemical abnormality in cerebrotendinous xanthomatosis: impairment of bile acid biosynthesis associated with incomplete degradation of the cholesterol side chain. J Clin Invest 53:1393, 1974.

390. Salen G, Shefer S, Setoguchi T, et al. Bile alcohol metabolism in man: conversion of 5β-cholestane-3α, 7α, 12α, 25-tetrol to cholic acid. J Clin Invest 56:226, 1975.

391. Maser AE, Singh I, Broum FR, et al. The cerebro-hepato-renal (Zellweger) syndrome. Increased levels and impaired degradation of very long-chain fatty acids and their use in prenatal diagnosis. N Engl J Med 310:1141, 1984.

392. Eyssen H, Parmentier G, Compernolle F, et al. Trihydroxycoprostanic acid in the duodenal fluid of two children with intrahepatic bile duct anomalies. Biochim Biophys Acta 273:212, 1972.

393. Hanson RF, Isenberg JN, Williams GC, et al. The metabolism of 3α, 7α, 12α-trihydroxy-5β cholestan-26-oic acid in two siblings with cholestasis due to intrahepatic bile duct anomalies. J Clin Invest 56:577, 1975.

394. Lee MJ, Whitehouse MW. Inhibition of electron transport and coupled phosphorylation in liver mitochondria by cholenic (bile acids) and their conjugates. Biochim Biophys Acta 100:317, 1965.

395. Anderson DH. Cystic fibrosis of the pancreas and its relation to celiac disease. Am J Dis Child 56:344, 1938.

396. Farber S. Pancreatic function and disease in early life. V. Pathologic changes associated with pancreatic insufficiency in early life. Arch Pathol 37:238, 1944.

397. Bodian M, ed. Fibrocystic Disease of the Pancreas. London, Heinemann, 1952.

398. Craig JM, Gellis SS, Hsia DY. Cirrhosis of the liver in infants and children. Am J Dis Child 90:299, 1955.

399. di Sant'Agnese PA, Blanc WA. A distinctive type of biliary cirrhosis of the liver associated with cystic fibrosis of the pancreas. Pediatrics 18:387, 1956.

400. Gatzimos CD, Jowitt RH. Jaundice in mucoviscidosis. Am J Dis Child 89:182, 1955.

401. Bernstein J, Vawter G, Harris GBC, et al. The occurrence of intestinal atresia in newborns with meconium ileus. Am J Dis Child 99:804, 1960.

402. Sheir KJ, Horn RC Jr. The pathology of liver cirrhosis in patients with cystic fibrosis of the pancreas. Can Med Assoc J 89:645, 1963.

403. Talamo RC, Hendren WH. Prolonged obstructive jaundice. Am J Dis Child 115:74, 1968.

404. Kulczycki LL. Editorial note. In: Quarterly Annotated References to Cystic Fibrosis. Volume 6, New York, National Cystic Fibrosis Research Foundation, 1967:2.

405. Bachand JP. Un cas insuité de mucoviscidose: atteinte hépatique néonatale. Laval Med 38:371, 1967.

406. Valman HB, France NE, Wallis PG. Prolonged neonatal jaundice in cystic fibrosis. Arch Dis Child 46:805, 1971.

407. Rosenstein BJ, Oppenheimer EH. Prolonged obstructive jaundice and giant cell hepatitis in an infant with cystic fibrosis of pancreas. J Pediatr 91:1022, 1977.

408. Stern RC, Stevens DP, Boat TF, et al. Symptomatic hepatic disease in cystic fibrosis: incidence, course, and outcome of portal systemic shunting. Gastroenterology 70:645, 1976.

409. Feigelson J, Pecau Y, Cathelineau L, et al. Additional data on hepatic function tests in cystic fibrosis. Acta Paediatr Scand 64:337, 1975.

410. Tyson KRT, Schuster SR, Shwachman H. Portal hypertension in cystic fibrosis. J Pediatr Surg 3:271, 1968.

411. Schuster SR, Shwachman H, Toyama WM, et al. The management of portal hypertension in cystic fibrosis. J Pediatr Surg 12:201, 1977.

412. Schwarz HP, Kraemer R, Thurnheer U, et al. Liver involvement in cystic fibrosis. A report of 9 cases. Helv Paediat Acta 33:351, 1978.

413. Lebenthal E, Jacobson M, Kevy S, et al. Predictive value of BSP kinetics for early liver involvement in cystic fibrosis. Gastroenterology A-30:807, 1974.

414. Boat TF, Doershuk CF, Stern RC, et al. Serum alkaline phosphatase in cystic fibrosis. Interpretation of elevated values based on electrophoretic analysis. Clin Pediatr 13:505, 1974.

415. Kattwinkel J, Taussig LM, Statland BE, et al. The effects of age on alkaline phosphatase and other serologic liver function tests in normal subjects and patients with cystic fibrosis. J Pediatr 82:234, 1973.

416. Rovsing H, Sloth K. Micro-gallbladder and biliary calculi in mucoviscidosis. Acta Radiol 14:588, 1973.

417. Warwick WT, L'heurex PR, Sharp HL, et al. Gallstones in cystic fibrosis. Proceedings of VII International Cystic Fibrosis Congress, 1976:100.

418. Roy CC, Weber AM, Morin CL, et al. Abnormal biliary lipid composition in cystic fibrosis. Effect of pancreatic enzymes. N Engl J Med 297:1301, 1977.

419. Quinton PM. Chloride impermeability in cystic fibrosis. Nature 301:421, 1983.

420. Frizzell RA, Rechkemmer G, Shoemaker RL. Altered regulation of airway epithelial cell chloride channels in cystic fibrosis. Science 233:558, 1986.

421. Quinton PM. Missing Cl conductance in cystic fibrosis. Am J Physiol 251:C649, 1986.

422. Rao GJS, Nadler HL. Deficiency of trypsin-like activity in saliva of patients with cystic fibrosis. J Pediatr 80:573, 1972.

423. Wilson GB, Fudenberg HH. Studies on cystic fibrosis using isoelectric focusing. II. Demonstration of deficient proteolytic cleavage of α_2-macroglobulin in cystic fibrosis plasma. Pediatr Res 10:87, 1976.

424. Shapira E, Rao GJS, Wessel HU, et al. Absence of an α_2-macroglobulin-protease complex in cystic fibrosis. Pediatr Res 10:812, 1976.

425. Shwachman H. Gastrointestinal manifestation of cystic fibrosis. Pediatr Clin North Am 22:787, 1975.

426. Weber AM, Roy CC, Chartrand L, et al. Relationship between bile acid malabsorption and pancreatic insufficiency in cystic fibrosis. Gut 17:295, 1976.

427. Watkins JB, Tercyak S, Klein PD. Bile salt kinetics in cystic fibrosis: influence of pancreatic enzyme replacement. Gastroenterology 73:1023, 1977.

428. Walters TJ, Koch HF. Hemorrhagic diathesis and cystic fibrosis in infancy. Am J Dis Child 124:641, 1972.

429. Underwood BA, Denning CR. Blood and liver concentrations of vitamins A and E in children with cystic fibrosis of the pancreas. Pediatr Res 6:26, 1972.

430. Keating J, Feigin RD. Increased intracranial pressure associated with probable vitamin A deficiency in cystic fibrosis. Pediatrics 41:46, 1970.

431. Weisman Y, Reiter E, Stern RC, et al. Serum concentrations of 25-hydroxyvitamin D and in patients with cystic fibrosis. J Pediatr 95:416, 1979.

432. Hubbard VS, Farrell PM, di Sant'Agnese PA. 25-Hydroxycholecalciferol levels in patients with cystic fibrosis. J Pediatr 94:84, 1979.

433. Hahn TJ, Squires AE, Halstead LR, et al. Reduced serum 25-hydroxyvitamin D concentration and disordered mineral metabolism in patients with cystic fibrosis. J Pediatr 94:38, 1979.

434. Oppenheimer EH, Esterly TR. Hepatic changes in young infants with cystic fibrosis: possible relation to focal biliary cirrhosis. J Pediatr 86:683, 1975.

435. Caplan A, Gross S. Hematologic and serologic studies in cystic fibrosis. J Pediatr 73:540, 1968.

436. Danks DM, Allan J, Anderson CM. A genetic study of fibrocystic disease of the pancreas. Ann Hum Genet 28:323, 1965.

437. Merritt AD, Hanna BL, Todd CW, et al. The incidence and mode of inheritance of cystic fibrosis. J Lab Clin Med 60:998, 1962.

438. Oppenheimer EH, Esterly JR. Cystic fibrosis in non-Caucasian patients. Pediatrics 42:547, 1968.

439. Wright SW, Morton NE. Genetic studies on cystic fibrosis in Hawaii. Am J Hum Genet 20:157, 1968.

440. Tsui LC, Buchwald M, Barker D, et al. Cystic fibrosis locus defined by a genetically linked polymorphic DNA marker. Science 230:1054, 1985.

441. Beaudet AL, Rosenbloom C, Spece JE, et al. Linkage of cystic fibrosis and the met oncogene. Pediatr Res 20:470A, 1986.

50

Alpha₁-Antitrypsin Deficiency

Fayez K. Ghishan, M.D. • Harry L. Greene, M.D.

ABBREVIATIONS

PAS = periodic acid–Schiff
Pi = protease inhibitor

In 1963, Laurell and Eriksson discovered a genetically determined deficiency in a major serum protease inhibitor, α_1-antitrypsin. This deficiency was associated with the early onset of emphysema in adults.[1] In 1969, Sharp and coworkers reported the association of α_1-antitrypsin deficiency and hepatic cirrhosis in children.[2] Since then, several reports from different parts of the world have included histories of neonatal hepatitis.[2] Soon it became apparent from several published reports that approximately 15 to 30 per cent of neonates with conjugated hyperbilirubinemia have α_1-antitrypsin deficiencies.[3, 4]

CHARACTERISTICS OF α_1-ANTITRYPSIN

α_1-Antitrypsin derived its name from its identification as α_1 globulin and from the original method used for measuring its activity. α_1-Antitrypsin is a glycoprotein synthesized in the liver. It has a relatively short half-life of four to five days.[5] Ninety per cent of the serum's ability to inhibit trypsin is due to this glycoprotein, which also inhibits chymotrypsin, pancreatic elastase, skin collagenase, renin, urokinase, Hageman-factor cofactor, and the neutral proteases of polymorphonuclear leukocytes.[6] α_1-Antitrypsin is present in tears, duodenal fluid, saliva, nasal secretions, cerebrospinal fluid, pulmonary secretions, and mother's milk. Its level in normal amniotic fluid is approximately 10 per cent of the normal serum level. Inflammation, neoplastic disease, pregnancy, or estrogen therapy increases the serum level of α_1-antitrypsin two- to threefold. Such a stimulus has little inductive effect, however, in a patient deficient in α_1-antitrypsin.[6]

MEASUREMENT AND TYPING OF PROTEASE INHIBITOR *(Pi)*

Approximately 2 mg α_1-antitrypsin are present in 1 ml serum. α_1-Antitrypsin function can be quantitated by measuring the ability of serum samples to inhibit the action of trypsin.[7]

The production of antiserum to the α_1-globulin fraction has made possible the use of radial immunodiffusion plates for measuring the concentration of this protein. In general, the results of this inhibitor function correlate well with the electroimmunodiffusion assay.[8] Protein electrophoresis on starch gel has contributed greatly to our understanding of

variations in α_1-antitrypsin.[9] α_1-Globulins appear in this system as a series of characteristic bands of variable intensity. A system of labeling based on the letters of the alphabet has been adopted. Faster-moving protein complexes are identified by earlier letters in the alphabet, and the slowest-moving protein is labeled Z. The system itself is titled *Pi* (protease inhibitor). The technique of isoelectric focusing on polyacrylamide gel has considerably improved the separation of the protein bands.[10]

Fagerhol and Laurell have demonstrated that the serum α_1-antitrypsin is inherited via a series of codominant alleles that appear to control the electrophoretic mobility of the α_1-antitrypsin.[11, 12] There are at least 26 different alleles for this gene.[12] Each person inherits a maximum of two different alleles. Different allelic forms of α_1-antitrypsin have different capacities for inhibiting trypsin. The activities of different phenotypes are listed in Table 50–1. The P and S alleles have 12.5 and 30 per cent activity of α_1-antitrypsin. Thus, a PiPS individual—that is, a person found to have protease inhibitor (Pi) PS—would have 42.5 per cent of maximum activity of α_1-antitrypsin. Children and adults who have hepatic cirrhosis secondary to deficiencies of α_1-antitrypsin are PiZZ. The association of hepatic cirrhosis with heterozygotic expressions such as PiSZ or PiFZ is uncertain, because only a few reports of such associations have been published.

PATHOPHYSIOLOGIC BASIS OF THE DEFECT

Microscopic examinations of livers from patients who are PiZZ almost uniformly disclose globules of an amorphous material within the hepatocytes, particularly in the periportal area.[13] These globules, which enlarge as the infant matures, are most easily discerned by positive PAS staining, after treatment of the liver biopsy specimen with diastase. These globules are also detected in the livers of patients who are PiZZ but have no liver disease and in those of healthy heterozygotes.

TABLE 50–1. RELATIONSHIP BETWEEN Pi PHENOTYPES AND SERUM CONCENTRATIONS OF α_1-ANTITRYPSIN

Phenotype	Serum Concentration (%)
MM	100
MZ	60
SS	60
FZ	60
M—	50
PS	40
SZ	42.5
ZZ	15
Z—	10
—	0

1349

A basic difference between PiZ and PiM molecules has been demonstrated by peptide mapping. A glutamic acid in a peptide fragment from normal α_1-antitrypsin is replaced by a lysine in the abnormal form.[14, 15] Recently, α_1-antitrypsin was isolated from the liver of a patient with PiZZ. The differences between the carbohydrate contents of the ZZ and MM phenotypes are shown in Table 50–2. Notice the absences of galactose and sialic acid, the decreased amount of hexosamine, and the twofold increase in mannose in the ZZ compared with the MM phenotype.[16]

The polypeptide portion and core carbohydrates of glycoproteins are assembled in the rough endoplasmic reticulum and Golgi apparatus, respectively. The transfer of the core carbohydrate to the protein portion of a glycoprotein takes place only in the rough endoplasmic reticulum. Further, glycoproteins do not leave the rough endoplasmic reticulum until this process is completed. Defective glycosylation hence can interfere with the excretion of glycoproteins from the rough endoplasmic reticulum of liver to the extracellular space.[16]

In contradistinction to the abnormalities in the carbohydrate content of α_1-antitrypsin deposits in liver with the ZZ phenotype, α_1-antitrypsin in the sera of PiZZ patients has the same carbohydrate composition as in persons of the MM phenotype.[17] Thus, it is possible that some molecules are fully glycosylated and subsequently leave the rough endoplasmic reticulum. The deposition of α_1-antitrypsin globules in the liver is also present in the heterozygote. The few reported patients with no detectable α_1-antitrypsin globules in their sera, phenotype Pi null, had no deposition of α_1-antitrypsin globules in their livers. Why only 15 to 30 per cent of infants who are phenotype ZZ develop cholestatic jaundice and only a minority have hepatic cirrhosis in childhood and adulthood is not known. Possibly other factors act in concert with the circulating α_1-antitrypsin deficiency or with the deposition of α_1-antitrypsin in the liver to produce the hepatic changes. Certainly the etiologic puzzle of liver disease with PiZZ needs further study.

MOLECULAR BASIS OF THE DEFECT IN α_1-ANTITRYPSIN DEFICIENCY

Recent advances in DNA technology allowed a new way to study the molecular defect in α_1-antitrypsin. As indicated previously, the basis of the defect in the PiZZ type of α_1-antitrypsin deficiency is the substitution of lysine for glutamic acid at position 52 from the carboxyl terminus in the Z type protein. Complementary DNA clones from baboon and humans have demonstrated that mature α_1-antitrypsin is composed of 394 amino acids.[18]

Sequencing of human cDNA indicated that the codon for the glutamic acid residue at position 342 of the protein

TABLE 50–2. CARBOHYDRATE ANALYSIS OF α_1-ANTITRYPSIN LIVER PREPARATION

Carbohydrate	Residues per Mole	
	MM Phenotype	ZZ Phenotype
Galactose	8.1	<0.1
Mannose	12.0	21.2
N-Acetylglucosamine	8.9	3.9
Sialic acid	6.3	<0.1
Hexosamine	12.6	5.6

Source: Adapted from Herez A, et al. Science 201:1229, 1978, with permission.

is GAG. It is believed that the α_1-antitrypsin deficiency is caused by a point mutation involving the G to A position—that is, nucleic acid GAG in the M type is changed to AAG in the Z type. This mutation occurs in exon V region of the human α_1-antitrypsin gene. The structure of the gene has been established by electron microscopy of hybrid molecules formed between the cloned chromosomal DNA and baboon α_1-antitrypsin mRNA. The chromosomal α_1-antitrypsin gene contains five exon coding regions and four introns that do not code for protein sequence. The molecular defect in the S type of protein appears to be a substitution of glutamic acid by valine.[19] In the null type (absence of detectable serum levels of α_1-antitrypsin), however, the defect appears to be an inability of the gene to direct the synthesis of a detectable mRNA transcript.[20]

Genetics

The most common allele is PiM, which has a frequency distribution of 0.86 to 0.99, depending on the population studied.[21] In Americans, the frequency is about 0.95, with a frequency of 0.98 in blacks.[22] The next two most common alleles in the United States are PiS at 0.03 and PiZ at 0.01. Blacks have lower frequencies of these alleles.[21, 22] In Sweden, the frequency of PiZ is 0.026.[23] Calculations from allelic frequencies predict that in the United States PiZZ will occur in about one in 3630 subjects and PiSZ in one in 830.

Levels of circulating α_1-antitrypsin are unreliable in identification of the heterozygous state. Thus, members of families containing a patient with PiZZ should be phenotyped.[24] Prenatal diagnosis is now available to detect the ZZ α_1-antitrypsin deficiency. The Z mutation, like many single-base substitutions, does not occur within a restriction recognition site; however, it can be detected by using a mutation-specific oligonucleotide. This method has been successfully used to detect the ZZ type, using amniotic cells.[25, 26]

Clinical Features

Although α_1-antitrypsin deficiency was originally described in association with pulmonary emphysema in early adulthood,[1] this chapter discusses only the hepatic manifestations. Extrahepatic manifestations, such as pancreatic fibrosis[27] and membranoproliferative glomerulonephritis,[28] are not dealt with here.

Liver Disease in Children

The association of PiZZ and neonatal cholestasis is now well established.[3] Early reports indicated that by the second decade of life most patients had developed overt cirrhosis and that the clinical outlook for these patients was grave.[13] Recent reports have not substantiated this outlook.[29, 30]

In a recent prospective study of 200,000 Swedish newborns, 125 were found to have the phenotype PiZZ. Eleven per cent of these infants developed neonatal cholestatic jaundice. At 2 years of age only 3 of them had cirrhosis. About 50 per cent of the asymptomatic PiZZ subjects had occasional elevations of ALT. In 15 per cent, the level of ALT was probably permanently elevated. In the same study, 48 infants with the phenotype PiSZ were identified. None of these infants had significant liver disease, and only two had elevated ALT levels.[23, 29] In screening 107,038 newborns in the United States, 21 infants were found to have the phenotype PiZZ. Of the 18 infants followed, only one had neonatal cholestatic jaundice. Five had hepatomegaly, biochemical abnormalities, or both. At 3 to 6 years of age, none of the children had evidence of hepatic cirrhosis.[30]

In contrast, a recent report suggests that infants with PiZZ who present with neonatal cholestasis are more likely to develop serious liver disease in the future compared with those without a history of neonatal cholestasis.[31a]

The cholestatic jaundice may appear during the first week of life. Acholic stools and dark urine may be seen. On physical examination, hepatomegaly is usually detected. The biochemical signs of obstructive jaundice are found. The jaundice usually disappears during the second to fourth months of life.[29] Histologic studies of liver biopsies from those infants with cholestatic jaundice may be helpful in predicting the course of liver disease. Details of such histologic studies of livers of infants with cholestatic jaundice are provided in the section describing the pathology of α₁-antitrypsin deficiency. Hepatic cirrhosis may develop during the second year of life or later in childhood.[29, 31] The long-term consequences of the PiZZ phenotype in patients without neonatal cholestatic jaundice remain to be determined by following such infants to adulthood.

Liver Disease in Adults

Ganrot and co-workers initially reported two cases of cirrhosis and one case of primary hepatic carcinoma in adults with the PiZZ phenotype.[32] Subsequently, several case reports of hepatic cirrhosis in adults with the PiZZ phenotype were published.[33, 34] One study of 13 autopsied patients from Sweden revealed cirrhosis or hepatic fibrosis in 8, 3 of whom also had hepatomas.[35] However, the patients were selected from an unspecified number of autopsies. In another study, 9 patients with hepatic cirrhosis were discovered among a group of 200 adult patients who had the PiZZ phenotype. None of these patients had a history of neonatal cholestasis. Most of these patients experienced the fairly acute onset of portal hypertension without prior histories of alcoholic liver disease. Coma or bleeding from varices or both was the commonest cause of death.[35] Emphysema was common in this group. It is estimated that the risk of developing hepatic cirrhosis in adults with α₁-antitrypsin deficiency is about 10 per cent.[35] Recently Eriksson and colleagues assessed the risk of developing liver cirrhosis and primary liver cancer in a retrospective study based on 17 autopsied cases of α₁-antitrypsin deficiency identified in the city of Malmö, Sweden during the period 1963 to 1982. Each autopsied case was matched with four controls selected from the same autopsy register. The results indicated a strong relation between α₁-antitrypsin deficiency and cirrhosis and primary liver cancer. However, when the data were analyzed according to sex, these associations were significant only for male patients. This study suggests clearly that male patients are at higher risk for the development of cirrhosis and hepatoma with α₁-antitrypsin deficiency. The reason for male selectivity is not clear; however, it could be secondary to a small sample size or to a true lower risk for women.[36]

The relationship between cirrhosis and partial deficiency or heterozygotic phenotypes of α₁-antitrypsin is not well defined.

Campra and associates reported a case of a patient with adult-onset cirrhosis associated with the phenotype PiSZ.[37] Similar case reports followed, with an association between FZ and MZ phenotypes and hepatic cirrhosis.[38, 39] However, in a recent prospective study, the heterozygous state occurred with approximately equal frequencies in patients with and those without hepatobiliary disease.[40] A more recent study showed an increased prevalence of phenotype MZ in patients with cryptogenic cirrhosis and with non-B chronic active hepatitis.[42] The possibility remains that patients with partially deficient states are at greater risk for the development of chronic liver disease when exposed to certain unspecified stimuli. This possibility needs to be explored by long-term prospective follow-up studies of patients with heterozygous phenotypes who do not have liver disease.

Cirrhotic patients with α₁-antitrypsin deficiencies have an exceedingly high incidence of hepatomas. Thus, Eriksson found six hepatomas in the nine cirrhotic adults who were phenotypically PiZZ. Four of these tumors were hepatocellular carcinomas and two were cholangiocarcinomas. The hepatoma cells did not contain α₁-antitrypsin globules.[35]

Pathology

Sharp found distinctive, sharply defined, round-to-oval deposits 1 to 40 μm in diameter in the periportal hepatocytes of individuals who were PiZZ, regardless of whether they had liver disease or not.[13] These globules, which enlarge with increasing age, become increasingly easy to detect as the infant matures. They are seen with hematoxylin-eosin staining as slightly eosinophilic deposits in the cytoplasm of the hepatocytes. They are discerned most easily by positive PAS staining after diastase treatment (Figs. 50–1 and 50–2).

Immunofluorescent and immunocytochemical studies have shown that the inclusions consist of material antigenically related to α₁-antitrypsin. These globules have also been observed in heterozygous individuals.[6] There appears to be no definite relationship between the intensity and extent of involvement with the globules and the occurrence of liver disease.[6] However, the absence of liver disease in the few Pi-null individuals who have no deposits of these globules suggests that the deposits may have a role in the pathogenesis of liver disease.[41–43]

Hepatic stenosis has been a nonspecific finding in some patients with α₁-antitrypsin deficiencies.[3]

Electron microscopy shows the hepatocyte to contain characteristic amorphous deposits primarily within dilated rough endoplasmic reticulum,[6, 16] although one study demonstrated the deposits to be in the smooth endoplasmic reticulum.[43] Such deposits were not present in Golgi apparatus. The amounts of material in the deposits vary from one patient to another, and they are not limited to the hepatocytes but may also be seen in biliary duct cells. Glycogen, clear vacuoles, and heterogeneous electron-dense bodies (lipofuscin) may be seen in the cytoplasm of the hepatocytes.[43] Bile stasis may be present in some hepatocytes.

In neonates of the PiZZ phenotype with cholestatic jaundice secondary to α₁-antitrypsin deficiencies, three morphologic patterns of hepatic alterations can be distinguished:[44]

1. Hepatocellular damage. Features in this group include giant cell transformation and relatively little infiltration with chronic inflammatory cells. The bile ducts are normal, with either no or minimal fibrosis. Bile stasis is present; however, bile plugs are not seen in the portal area.

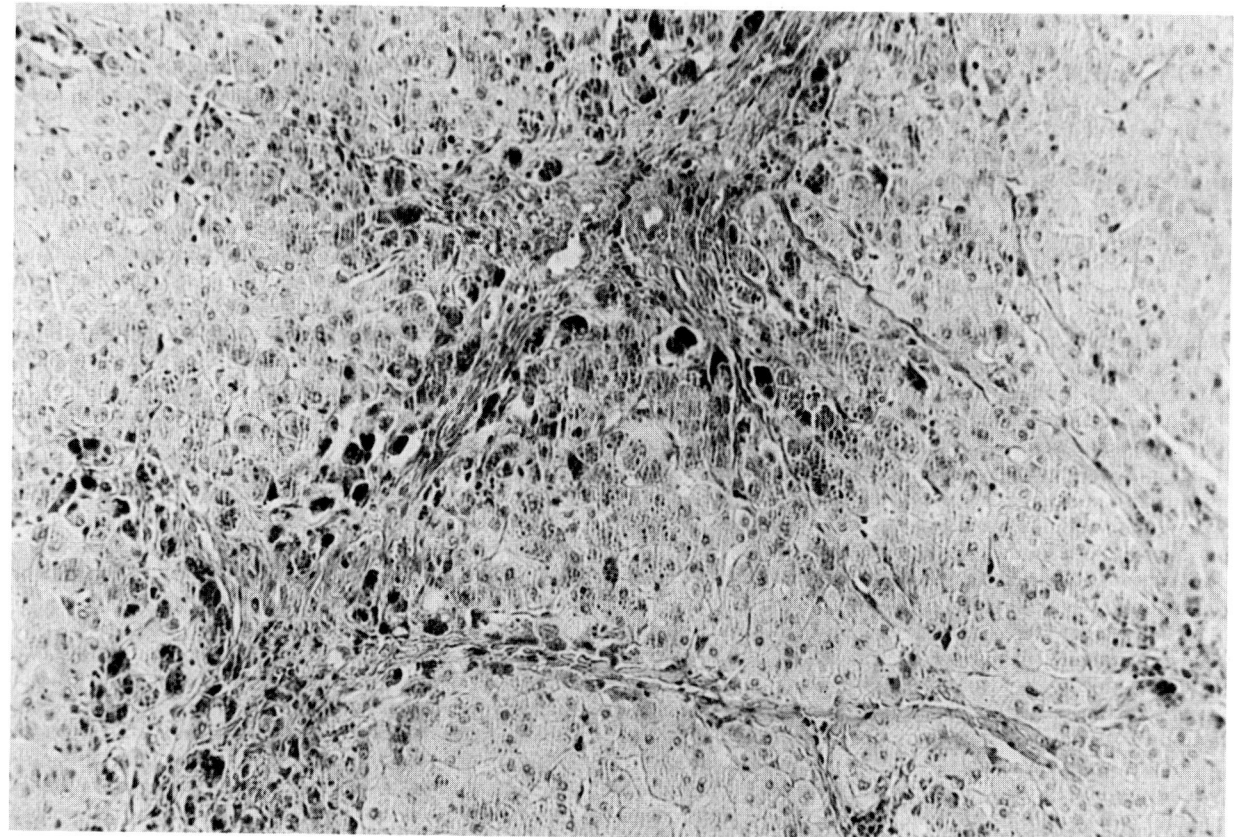

Figure 50–1. Wedge biopsy of the liver, showing cirrhosis. The hepatocytes contain deposits of typical α_1-antitrypsin. PAS staining with diastase, $\times$ 80.

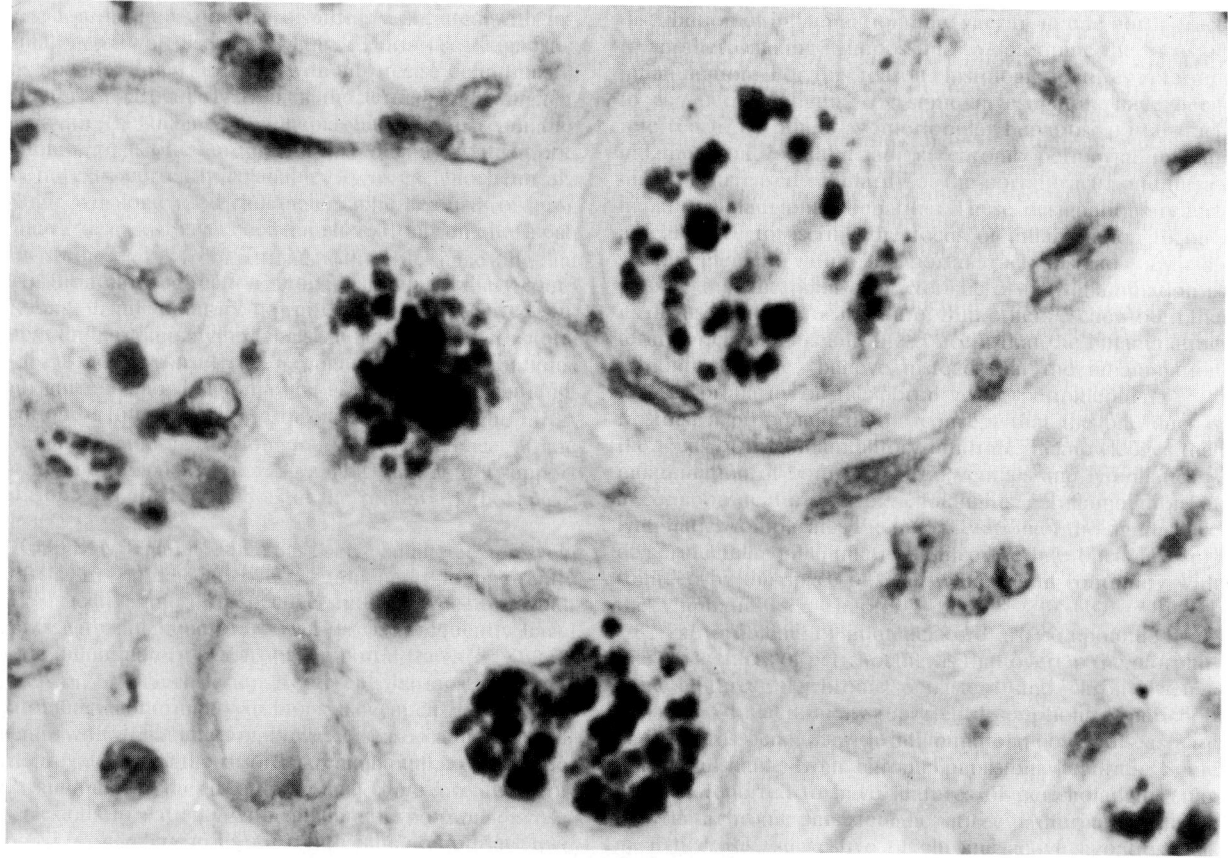

Figure 50–2. Hepatocytes containing deposits of α_1-antitrypsin. PAS staining with diastase, $\times$ 400.

TABLE 50–3. METABOLIC LIVER DISEASES THAT LEAD TO PERMANENT INJURY

Inborn Errors of Metabolism	Enzyme Deficiency	Common Clinical Manifestations	Laboratory Data	Treatment
A. Carbohydrate metabolism				
1. Hereditary fructose intolerance	Fructose-1-phosphate aldolase	Vomiting, jaundice, hepatomegaly	↓ Glucose, ↓ PO_4, ↑ uric acid, ↑ SGOT, renal tubular dysfunction	Fructose-free, sucrose-free diet
2. Galactosemia	Galactose-1-phosphate uridyl transferase	Vomiting, jaundice, hepatomegaly, failure to thrive	↓ Glucose, reducing substances in the urine, abnormal liver function tests, renal tubular dysfunction	Lactose-free diet
3. Glycogen storage disease, Type I	Glucose-6-phosphatase	Hepatomegaly, growth failure	Hypoglycemia, hyperlipemia, acidosis, ↑ uric acid	Nocturnal nasogastric feedings
4. Glycogen storage disease, Type III	Amylo-1,6-glucosidase (debrancher enzyme)	Hepatomegaly, growth failure, muscle weakness	Hypoglycemia, hyperlipemia	Frequent feedings of high-protein diet
5. Glycogen storage disease, Type IV	α-1,4-Glucan 6-glycosyl transferase (brancher)	Vomiting, diarrhea, failure to thrive, hepatosplenomegaly	Abnormal liver function tests, acidosis	Frequent feedings of high-protein diet
B. Protein metabolism				
1. Hereditary tyrosinemia	Fumaryl acetoacetase	Failure to thrive, jaundice, hepatosplenomegaly, rickets	Abnormal liver function tests, renal tubular dysfunction	Low-phenylalanine, low-tyrosine diet
C. Lipid metabolism				
1. Wolman's disease	Acid lipase	Vomiting, diarrhea, hepatosplenomegaly, failure to thrive	Symmetrical calcification of adrenals, anemia, vacuolation of lymphocytes, deposition of triglycerides and cholesterol ester in various organs	None
2. Cholesterol ester	Acid lipase	Hepatosplenomegaly	Deposition of triglyceride and cholesterol ester in various organs, portal hypertension	None
D. Bile acid metabolism				
1. Byler's disease	Not known, ? ↓ excretion of bile acids across canalicular membrane	Pruritus, jaundice, steatorrhea, hepatosplenomegaly	↑ Bilirubin, ↑ alkaline phosphatase	? Phenobarbital and ? cholestyramine
2. Arteriohepatic dysplasia	Not known, ? ↓ bile acid formation or excretion	Characteristic facies, pulmonary stenosis, vertebral anomalies, posterior embryotoxon, pruritus, jaundice, hepatomegaly	↑ Bilirubin, ↑ cholesterol, ↑ alkaline phosphatase, ↑ bile acids	? Phenobarbital and ? cholestyramine
3. Zellweger's syndrome	Defect in bile acid formation	Characteristic facies, hypotonia, jaundice, hepatomegaly	↑ Precursors of cholic and chenodeoxycholic acid, ↑ serum iron	None
4. Hereditary lymphedema with recurrent cholestasis	? Impaired bile acid secretion ? Abnormalities of liver lymphatics	Pruritus, jaundice, lymphedema of the lower extremities	↑ Bilirubin, ↑ cholesterol, ↑ alkaline phosphatase, abnormal lymphangiograms	? Phenobarbital and ? cholestyramine
5. THCA (3α,7α,12α-trihydroxy-5β-cholestan-26-oic acid) syndrome	Block in conversion of ? THCA → variant acid	Jaundice, hepatosplenomegaly	↑ THCA in serum and bile	? Phenobarbital and ? cholestyramine
E. Unclassified				
1. Alpha-1-antitrypsin deficiency	Not known	Neonatal cholestatic jaundice, hepatomegaly, portal hypertension	↓ Serum alpha-1-antitrypsin phenotype→PiZZ	None medically; liver transplant
2. Cystic fibrosis	Not known, ? alpha-2-macroglobulin defect	Pancreatic insufficiency, pulmonary infection, neonatal cholestatic jaundice, hepatomegaly, portal hypertension	↑ Sweat Cl, steatorrhea, possibly abnormal liver function tests	No specific therapy

2. Portal fibrosis with biliary duct proliferation. Extensive portal fibrosis, sometimes sufficiently advanced to give a picture of cirrhosis, is usually seen. Marked ductular proliferation is present, and bile plugs are occasionally seen in the ducts. In five such infants, jaundice disappeared before the age of 6 months, but the liver and spleen became progressively larger and harder. Portal hypertension was later found in two of these infants. Four of the five infants underwent exploratory surgery for presumed extrahepatic biliary atresia. A normal, patent extrahepatic biliary tree was found in each.

3. Ductular hypoplasia. The hepatic architecture is intact, with minimal hepatocellular damage. The portal areas show minimal fibrosis, but there is a marked diminution of the number of biliary ducts. In one such infant, no biliary duct could be detected in 11 portal areas. Bile stasis, randomly distributed in the hepatic lobules, is always present. The clinical course in these infants is one of continued jaundice with pruritus and high levels of serum cholesterol.

This classification may be useful in predicting the course of liver disease, but exceptions to these categories will occur. Longer follow-up is necessary to determine the long-term outcome in infants with neonatal cholestatic jaundice secondary to severe α_1-antitrypsin deficiency.

Therapy

Exciting progress has been made during the last few years in the area of genetic engineering. This research could potentially be used to devise therapies for α_1-antitrypsin deficiency. It is conceivable that the Z gene could be manipulated to produce α_1-antitrypsin. Other areas of current research involve development of α_1-antitrypsin products to replace the missing inhibitor. Two products are under investigation; one product is derived from recombinant DNA methods and the other from a blood fraction.[47]

Currently, liver transplantation is the only available form of therapy for patients of phenotype PiZZ who have end-stage hepatic cirrhosis. Hood and co-workers reported the results of liver transplantation in seven patients.[45] The type of α_1-antitrypsin in the serum after transplantation was the same as the donor phenotype in every recipient. Three of the seven patients are alive and well after 13, 21, and 36 months. The other patients died 12 to 28 months after transplantation. It remains to be seen whether patients treated by liver transplantation are immune to the development of other complications of the disease, such as pulmonary disease.

SUMMARY

Various metabolic disorders may permanently injure the liver. Most such disorders carry enzymatic defects that have been identified; others remain speculative. Most of the diseases that are associated with enzymatic defects in carbohydrate metabolism are treatable, with good to excellent results. However, most defects in lipid and bile acid metabolism are poorly responsive to dietary or drug therapy. Table 50–3 summarizes the disorders discussed in Chapters 49 and 50.

REFERENCES

1. Laurell CB, Eriksson S. The electrophoretic alpha-1-globulin pattern of serum in alpha-1-antitrypsin deficiency. Scand J Clin Lab Invest 15:132, 1963.
2. Sharp HL, Bridges RA, Krivit W, et al. Cirrhosis associated with alpha-1-antitrypsin deficiency: a previously unrecognized inherited disorder. J Lab Clin Med 73:934, 1969.
3. Porter CA, Mowat AP, Cook PJK, et al. α_1-Antitrypsin deficiency and neonatal hepatitis. Br Med J 3:435, 1972.
4. Mowat AP, Psacharopoulos HT, Williams R. Extrahepatic biliary atresia versus neonatal hepatitis. Arch Dis Child 51:763, 1976.
5. Makino S, Reed CE. Distribution and elimination of exogenous alpha-1-antitrypsin. J Lab Clin Med 75:742, 1970.
6. Sharp HL. The current status of α-1-antitrypsin, a protease inhibitor, in gastrointestinal disease. Gastroenterology, 70:611, 1976.
7. Statement of methods for selecting alpha-1-antitrypsin abnormalities. In: Mittman C, ed. Pulmonary Emphysema and Proteolysis. New York, Academic Press, 1972:141.
8. Talamo RC, Langley CE, Hyslop JR. A comparison of functional and immunochemical measurement of serum alpha-1-antitrypsin. In: Mittman C, ed. Pulmonary Emphysema and Proteolysis. New York, Academic Press, 1972:167.
9. Fagerhol MK. Quantitative studies on the inherited variants of serum alpha-1-antitrypsin. Scand J Clin Lab Invest 23:97, 1967.
10. Allen RC, Harley RA, Talamo RC. A new method for determination of α_1 AT phenotypes using isoelectric focusing on polyacrylamide gel slabs. Am J Clin Pathol 62:732, 1974.
11. Fagerhol MK, Laurell CB. The polymorphism of "prealbumins" and alpha-1-antitrypsin in human sera. Clin Chim Acta 16:199, 1967.
12. Fagerhol MK. Pi typing techniques. In: Peters H, ed. Twenty-second Colloquium on Peptides of Biological Fluids. Amsterdam, Elsevier, 1975:493.
13. Sharp HL. Alpha-1-antitrypsin deficiency. Hosp Prac 6:83, 1971.
14. Jeppson JO. Amino acid substitution Glu→LYS in α_1-antitrypsin PiZ. FEBS Lett 65:195, 1976.
15. Yoshida A, Lieberman J, Giadulis L, et al. Molecular abnormality of human alpha-1-antitrypsin variant (PiZZ) associated with plasma activity deficiency. Proc Natl Acad Sci USA 73:1324, 1976.
16. Hercz A, Katona E, Cutz E, et al. α_1-Antitrypsin: the presence of excess mannose in the Z variant isolated from liver. Science 201:1229, 1978.
17. Hercz A, Barton M. The purification and properties of human antitrypsin variant Z. Eur J Biochem 74:603, 1977.
18. Kyrachi K, Chandra T, Friezneo SJ, et al. Cloning and sequence of cDNA coding for alpha-1-antitrypsin. Proc Natl Acad Sci USA 78:6826, 1981.
19. Long G, Chandra T, Woo S, et al. Complete sequence of cDNA for human alpha-1-antitrypsin and the gene for the S variant. Biochemistry 23:4878, 1984.
20. Garver RI, Mornex JF, Nukiwa T, et al. Alpha-1-antitrypsin deficiency and emphysema caused by homozygous inheritance of non-expressing alpha-1-antitrypsin genes. N Engl J Med 314:762, 1986.
21. Kueppers F. Alpha-1-antitrypsin: physiology, genetics and pathology. Hum Genet 11:177, 1971.
22. Pierce JA, Eradio B, Dew TA. Antitrypsin phenotypes in St. Louis. JAMA 231:609, 1975.
23. Sverger T. Liver disease in alpha₁-antitrypsin deficiency detected by screening of 200,000 infants. N Engl J Med 294:1316, 1976.
24. Talamo RC, Langley CE, Levine BW, et al. Genetic vs. quantitative analysis of serum alpha₁ antitrypsin. N Engl J Med 287:1067, 1972.
25. Kidd V, Wallace RB, Itakura K, et al. Alpha-1-antitrypsin deficiency detection by direct analysis of the mutation in the gene. Nature 304:230, 1983.
26. Kidd V, Golbus MS, Wallace RB, et al. Prenatal diagnosis of alpha-1-antitrypsin deficiency by direct analysis of the mutation site in the gene. N Engl J Med 310:639, 1984.
27. Freeman HJ, Weinstein WM, Shnitka TK, et al. Alpha-1-antitrypsin deficiency and pancreatic fibrosis. Ann Intern Med 85:73, 1976.
28. Moroz SP, Cutz E, Balfe JW, et al. Membranoproliferative glomerulonephritis in childhood cirrhosis associated with alpha-1-antitrypsin deficiency. Pediatrics 57:232, 1976.
29. Sveger T. α_1-antitrypsin deficiency in early childhood. Pediatrics 62:22, 1978.
30. O'Brien ML, Buist NRM, Murphey H. Neonatal screening for alpha-1-antitrypsin deficiency. J Pediatr 92:1006, 1978.
31. Odievre M, Martin JP, Hadchouel M, et al. Alpha₁-antitrypsin deficiency and liver disease in children: phenotypes, manifestations, and prognosis. Pediatrics 57:226, 1976.
31a. Ghishan FK, Greene HL. Liver disease in children with PiZZ α_1-antitrypsin deficiency. Hepatology 8:307, 1988.
32. Ganrot PO, Laurell CB, Eriksson S. Obstructive lung disease and trypsin inhibitors in α_1-antitrypsin deficiency. Scand J Clin Lab Invest 19:205, 1967.
33. Ishak KG, Jenas EH, Marshall ML, et al. Cirrhosis of the liver associated with alpha-1-antitrypsin deficiency. Arch Pathol 94:445, 1972.
34. Berg NO, Eriksson S. Liver disease in adults with alpha-1-antitrypsin deficiency. N Engl J Med 287:1264, 1972.

35. Eriksson S, Hagerstrand I. Cirrhosis and malignant hepatoma in α_1-antitrypsin deficiency. Acta Med Scand 195:451, 1974.
36. Eriksson S, Carlson J, Velez R. Risk of cirrhosis and primary liver cancer in alpha-1-antitrypsin deficiency. N Engl J Med 314:736, 1986.
37. Campra JL, Craig JP, Peters RL, et al. Cirrhosis associated with partial deficiency of alpha-1-antitrypsin in adults. Ann Intern Med 78:233, 1973.
38. Brand B, Bezahler GH, Gould R. Cirrhosis and heterozygous FZ alpha-1-antitrypsin deficiency in an adult. Case report and review of the literature. Gastroenterology 66:264, 1974.
39. Rawlings W, Moss J, Cooper HS, et al. Hepatocellular carcinoma and partial deficiency of alpha-1-antitrypsin (MZ). Ann Intern Med 81:771, 1974.
40. Fisher RL, Taylor L, Sherlock S. α_1-Antitrypsin deficiency in liver disease: the extent of the problem. Gastroenterology 71:646, 1976.
41. Talamo RC, Langley CE, Reed CE, et al. α_1-Antitrypsin deficiency: a variant with no detectable α_1-antitrypsin. Science 181:70, 1973.
42. Martin JP. Further examples confirming the existence of Pi null (Pi-). Pathol Biol 23:521, 1975.
43. Yunis EJ, Agostini RM, Glen RH. Fine structural observations of the liver in α-1-antitrypsin deficiency. Am J Pathol 82:265, 1976.
44. Hadchouel M, Goutier M. Histopathologic study of the liver in the early cholestatic phase of alpha-1-antitrypsin deficiency. J Pediatr 89:211, 1976.
45. Hood JM, Koep LJ, Peters RL, et al. Liver transplantation for advanced liver disease with alpha-1-antitrypsin deficiency. N Engl J Med 302:272, 1980.
46. Hodges JR, Millwand-Sadler GH, Barbatis C, et al. Heterozygous MZ alpha$_1$-antitrypsin deficiency in adults with chronic active hepatitis and cryptogenic cirrhosis. N Engl J Med 304:557, 1981.
47. Cohen A. Unraveling the mysteries of alpha-1-antitrypsin deficiency. N Engl J Med 314:778, 1986.

51

Cholestatic Syndromes of Infancy and Childhood

Valeer J. Desmet, M.D., Ph.D.
Francesco Callea, M.D., Ph.D.

ABBREVIATION

EHBDA = extrahepatic bile duct atresia

EXTRAHEPATIC CHOLESTASIS

Various diseases of the extrahepatic bile ducts may cause obstruction to bile flow and cholestasis in neonates and children. By far the most frequent condition in this group is extrahepatic bile duct atresia (EHBDA). Because of its relative frequency, its differential diagnostic problems, and the extensive studies devoted to this condition in the last 25 years, EHBDA is the main subject of this chapter.

ATRESIA OF EXTRAHEPATIC BILE DUCTS

Historic Overview

Atresia of the extrahepatic bile ducts is defined as the lack of a lumen in part or all of the extrahepatic biliary tract, causing complete obstruction to bile flow.[1] This definition is biased by the precision (or lack of precision) of the investigative method used, that is, palpation or macroscopic inspection, or both, of transected (whether or not obliterated) ducts, inspection of the ducts through surgical microscopes, operative cholangiography, or microscopic examination of specimens. The reliability of these various investigative approaches differs. In the previous century, observations of EHBDA were made by inspecting with the naked eye the bile ducts at autopsy. By definition, this represented investigation in the end stage of the disease. It is extremely important to study the early stages of the disease, which became feasible only in recent times.

The earliest observations of EHBDA were made around the middle of the nineteenth century.[2-4] Quite early in the course of study, controversy arose about the etiology and pathogenesis of this disease, which was considered to result from either a lack of development (agenesis) or antenatal infection.[5]

Thomson,[6-8] who published one of the first major reviews of EHBDA (49 patients), concluded that it represented a progressive inflammatory lesion of bile ducts, whatever the cause. Other early investigators also adhered to the idea of a descending cholangitis instead of a malformation.[9] Congenital syphilis, fetal peritonitis, and erythroblastosis fetalis were considered to be causes for this acquired condition.[10] By contrast, several authors favored the concept of a developmental anomaly.[11, 12] Controversy over whether the etiology and pathogenesis was developmental or caused by an infection still persists, although the classically invoked infectious agents have been replaced by a virus that remains to be identified.[13] Surgical treatment of EHBDA was first discussed by Holmes in 1916;[11] he predicted that a conventional biliary-enteric anastomosis might be feasible in the 16 per cent of patients with dilated, bile-containing proximal segments of extrahepatic ducts. This correctable group of patients was separated from the majority, in whom the entire extrahepatic biliary tract was obliterated. Successful surgery was first reported by Ladd in 1928.[14] One of his early patients was reported to be doing well 37 years later.[15] However, few reports of survival were published in the next four decades; Bill counted only 52 reported successes after operations for biliary atresia performed between 1927 and 1970,[16] and most of them had a limited period of follow-up.

In early clinical reports, EHBDA frequently was confused with inspissated bile syndrome (see further on),[17] neonatal hepatitis (see further on), and choledochal cyst. (see Chap. 52).

In the 1940s, curative surgery in the newborn was confined almost exclusively to patients with the inspissated bile syndrome.[18] Obstruction in these patients was thought to be a consequence of thick, tenacious bile that required operative irrigation of the extrahepatic bile ducts. This indication for surgery disappeared when it was demonstrated that the vast majority of these patients had a primary hepatic parenchymal disorder associated with massive hemolysis due to Rh or ABO incompatibility or acute dehydration. Cholestasis resolved in most patients without surgical intervention.[19]

In 1953, Gross documented that EHBDA was the most common condition causing obstructive jaundice in the first months of life,[20] and that most patients had the noncorrectable type of lesion. Early death was an inevitable consequence in these patients.

The uselessness of surgery in inspissated bile syndrome and the inability of surgery to correct the lesion in the vast majority of patients with true EHBDA led to delaying operation for jaundice in the newborn in the 1950s and 1960s. Even infants with remediable lesions were operated on so late that irreversible liver damage had already occurred.[18] This tragedy led Clatworthy and McDonald to advocate brief diagnostic laparotomy and operative cholangiography in the first months of life in all infants with inexplicable jaundice.[21]

In the meantime, advances had been made in the distinction of several types of nonobstructive forms of neonatal jaundice and cholestasis of the newborn. It appeared that operation could be harmful in infants with neonatal hepatitis.[22-24] Since the diagnosis of biliary atresia versus neonatal hepatitis could not be established in most infants during the early months of life, it was recommended that operation be postponed until the patient was four months old.[23] The price for avoiding operation in patients with neonatal hepatitis would be paid by those infants with remediable causes of obstructive jaundice.[18] The surgeon's case for early operation was further inhibited by several reports describing spontaneous cure of biliary atresia.[18] Operative cholangiography was not performed in many of these patients, however, casting doubt on the accuracy of the original diagnosis of biliary atresia. The rather mystic belief that a totally fibrotic extrahepatic duct system might subsequently become patent persisted, nevertheless, because of claims that the development of the bile ducts proceeded for some time after birth.[25] The surgical pessimism in that period produced the feeling that EHBDA represented one of the darkest chapters in pediatric surgery.[26]

A new era in the study and therapy of EHBDA was inaugurated by a new surgical management of this disease, which was developed in Japan. In 1957, Dr. Morio Kasai performed exploratory surgery on an infant and found no patent extrahepatic ducts. He made a shallow exploration into the porta hepatis, just anterior to the portal vein, and found a small amount of bile seepage. He then anastomosed a segment of small bowel to the liver capsule around the raw opening into the liver. A good flow of bile developed in this baby, and the patient remained well for more than 17 years.[27] An account of this surgical approach—hepatic portoenterostomy, or the Kasai operation—was published in Japanese in 1959,[28] in German in 1963,[29] and in the English literature in 1968.[30] Although it originally met with skepticism,[31, 32] hepatic portoenterostomy and its subsequent modifications have become the treatment of choice for noncorrectable EHBDA. In more recent years, liver transplantation is emerging as an alternative treatment.

The Kasai operation has made the noncorrectable lesions correctable, so confusion may arise about the term *noncorrectable*. In the post-Kasai period, truly uncorrectable biliary atresia means a patient with late, severe cirrhosis.[33]

The work of Kasai and his colleagues introduced two new concepts into the pathologic study of biliary atresia.[34] First, they showed that intrahepatic bile ducts were patent from the interlobular ducts of the liver to the porta hepatis in nearly all patients during the first two or three months after birth. Interlobular bile ducts appeared to be destroyed rapidly and their number decreased progressively after two months of age. This explained why surgery was most effective for patients younger than ten weeks of age, which made early and rapid investigation mandatory. Second, the radical approach of portoenterostomy with resection of the obliterated extrahepatic ducts provided unique specimens not hitherto available. Histopathologic study of these fibrous remnants (discussed further on) confirmed the concept that EHBDA represents an ongoing inflammatory process leading to progressive destruction of the extrahepatic bile ducts.[35, 36] It soon appeared also that the intrahepatic bile ducts participated in the dynamic inflammatory process and were subject to progressive destruction.[16, 37, 38]

Increased experience worldwide with hepatic portoenterostomy has revealed that the intrahepatic component of duct inflammation and destruction is of great importance in determining the prognosis, even in patients with good bile flow soon after surgery (see Liver Lesions After Portoenterostomy). Hepatic portoenterostomy, including all subsequent variations and technical improvements in the operation, is not tantamount to cure.[39-40] A significant number of patients still show abnormalities on liver tests and signs of portal hypertension may develop.[39]

This then is the present state of a disease described for the first time more than 150 years ago. Results today are encouraging but not ideal because the cause or causes of EHBDA are unknown, diagnosis is difficult, and only a minority of infants are truly cured by radical surgery.[41] It looks as if a completely satisfactory solution will not be reached without an understanding of the fundamental causes and pathogeneses involved.[41, 42] What is really known today about EHBDA is that whatever its cause, it is a progressive inflammatory lesion of the bile ducts, which as mentioned was the proposal of Thomson almost a century ago.[6-8]

Incidence of Extrahepatic Bile Duct Atresia

The incidence of biliary atresia was reported in 1963 to be 1/25,000;[43] but in recent studies a frequency of 1/10,000 to 13,000 live births is mentioned.[34, 40, 44] The incidence is similar in studies from Japan,[45] North America,[46] and the United Kingdom.[47] The suggestion that the Chinese population has a significantly higher incidence was not confirmed in the Chinese population of San Francisco.[45, 48] EHBDA occurs more frequently in girls than in boys.[49-53] Only a few familial cases have been noted.[35, 54–57] Since no specific mode of inheritance for repeated occurrences is evident, genetic counseling is of uncertain value, except for families with more than one affected child, in which the future risk of recurrence is not likely to be less than 20 per cent.[58, 59]

At present, EHBDA is considered to be an acquired rather than a genetic disorder.[13, 35] In this respect, the following observations are of interest: Neonatal hepatitis and biliary atresia occur in subsequent members of the same sibship.[60, 61] There are reports of progression from neonatal hepatitis to biliary atresia in the same infant,[62, 63] and EHBDA has occurred in only one of two histocompatibility locus antigen (HLA)-identical twins.[64, 65] The existence of EHBDA with other disorders is reported occasionally, for example, the heterozygous state of galactosemia,[66] α_1-antitrypsin deficiency,[67–69] and small-bowel atresia.[70] Such cases apparently represent fortuitous and unusual associations of different pathogenic processes.

EHBDA is often associated with a number of malformations, some of them constituting the polysplenia syndrome.[71–75] This comprises multiple spleens, venous anomalies (partial lack of the inferior vena cava with azygos drainage, preduodenal portal vein, bilateral superior vena cava), dextro- or levocardia, cardiac anomalies, tendency to levoisomerism, and inversion of abdominal viscera. Associated malformations of this type are reported in 11 per cent of patients with EHBDA.[40, 75, 76] Besides their importance with respect to surgical techniques, these associated malformations suggest that the causal agent responsible for EHBDA may be operative relatively early during intrauterine development.

Pathologic Features of Extrahepatic Bile Duct Atresia

Pathologic Features of the Extrahepatic Bile Ducts

Macroscopic Lesions. EHBDA occurs in various anatomic variants.

As early as 1916, Holmes described 116 different configurations of the extrahepatic biliary system and, since then, an equal number of different types have been reported. The variations range from total absence of the system at one extreme, to complete normality at the other, with presence, or absence, or stenosis, or patency of all or any parts in between. Because of this extreme variation, comparison of the effects of the disease in different patients and consideration of its causes solely on the basis of the anatomy of the extrahepatic biliary tree proves to be impossible.[77]

However, it appeared useful to distinguish between correctable and noncorrectable types.[11] Correctable variants of EHBDA correspond to patients in whom only limited segments of the extrahepatic bile ducts have interrupted permeability; the obliterated segment can be resected and the preserved proximal parts of the extrahepatic system can be reimplanted in the duodenum.[40] Kasai proposed a classification of the numerous observed anatomic variants.[78] The main anatomic groups with the types I, II, and III according to Kasai are represented in Figure 51–1. Type I corresponds to atresia of the common bile duct, whereas the more proximal extrahepatic bile duct segments are intact. Type IIa represents obliteration in the common hepatic duct with or without atresia of its main branches; the common bile duct, the cystic duct, and the gallbladder are normal. Reanastomosis in this type of EHBDA is

performed through cystically dilated ducts near the porta hepatis. Type IIb also belongs to the correctable category, although all main branches of the extrahepatic system of bile ducts (common duct, hepatic ducts, and cystic ducts) are obliterated or missing. Reanastomosis with the duodenum is possible through cystically dilated ducts in the hilum. Recently, however, the value of this type of corrective surgery was questioned.[79] Unfortunately, the correctable types I, IIa, and IIb represent less than 10 per cent of all patients with EHBDA;[79] 90 per cent or more of patients cannot be helped by the reanastomoses mentioned. They belong to Kasai's type III category, which represents noncorrectable biliary atresia, that is, the lack of or atresia of common, hepatic, and cystic ducts. There are no cystically dilated hilar ducts that can be used for anastomosis in these patients. Often one notes the presence of a peculiar prehilar fibrous cone. The gallbladder is involved in the atretic process in about 80 per cent of patients.[80]

Kasai revolutionized the surgical treatment of biliary atresia by introducing the portojejunostomy procedure,[30] which includes en bloc resection of the entire extrahepatic biliary tree, including the gallbladder and the fibrous cone at the hilum. The operation and its subsequent modifications are discussed on page 1375.

Microscopic Lesions. Numerous studies have been performed on the histopathologic characteristics of fibrous remnants of the resected extrahepatic biliary tree.[36, 37, 40, 42, 75, 78, 81–95] The authors of these studies have focused their interest on (1) the topography and the nature of the lesions observed in the extrahepatic duct remnants and (2) the correlation between the numbers and sizes of identifiable duct structures at the porta hepatis and the success of increased bile flow after hepatic portoenterostomy.

TOPOGRAPHY AND TYPES OF LESIONS. The histologic procedure usually followed includes serial sectioning of the formalin-fixed extrahepatic fibrous remnant in 2- to 3-mm thick slices, which are embedded in paraffin for preparation of microscopic slides. A constant finding is complete fibrous obliteration of at least a segment of the extrahepatic biliary tree, confirming the diagnosis of EHBDA at the microscopic level. Usually, however, only a segment is reduced to a fibrous cord, whereas the remaining parts reveal remnants of lumina and inflammatory changes to a variable extent. The variable histologic appearance is categorized usually into three or four types.[84–86, 92] One type of histologic picture (type I according to Gautier and co-workers and type III according to Miyano and co-workers and Chandra and Altman)[84, 86, 92] corresponds to the lack of any lumen lined by biliary epithelium (Fig. 51–2). The bile duct segment is replaced by a fibrous cord, often with concentric arrangement of collagen bundles and without inflammatory infiltration.[40, 81] A second type of appearance (type II according to Gautier and co-workers and Miyano and co-workers) represents lumina lined by cuboidal epithelia (Fig. 51–3).[84, 92] The lumina may be distributed randomly or grouped in clusters at the periphery of the section. Some lumina are surrounded by concentric rings of dense connective tissue. Periluminal inflammatory cells are usually found, and signs of necrosis and sloughing of epithelial cells are frequently observed. Bile plugs may be present in the lumina. A third pattern (type III according to Gautier and colleagues) is characterized by a central structure that unquestionably corresponds to an altered bile duct (Fig. 51–4).[84] In some specimens, the structure contains a loose network of connective tissue without visible epithelium. In a larger proportion of specimens, the lumen is filled either with cellular debris and macrophages containing bile or

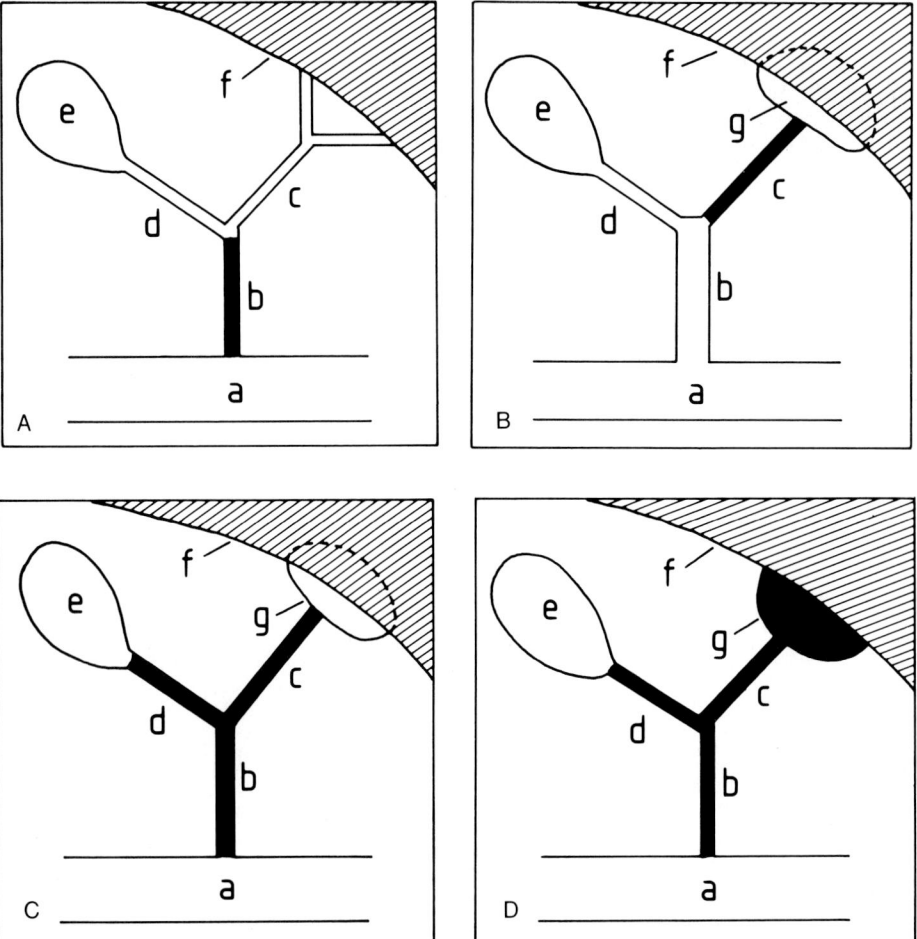

Figure 51–1. Anatomic types of EHBDA according to Kasai. *A,* EHBDA, type I. Correctable form of atresia. The common bile duct is partially or completely occluded or is reduced to a fibrous cord. *B,* EHBDA, type IIa. Correctable form of atresia. Obliteration of common hepatic duct. The common bile duct and cystic duct are patent, and the gallbladder is intact. Presence of cystically dilated bile ducts at the porta hepatis. *C,* EHBDA, type IIb. Correctable form of atresia. Obliteration of common bile duct and hepatic and cystic ducts. Gallbladder is not involved. Presence of cystically dilated bile ducts at the porta hepatis. *D,* EHBDA, type III. Noncorrectable form of atresia. Obliteration of common, hepatic, and cystic ducts. No anastomosable ducts at the porta hepatis. Presence of a prehilar fibrous cone. a = duodenum, b = common bile duct, c = common hepatic duct, d = cystic duct, e = gallbladder, f = liver, g = cystically dilated ducts at porta hepatis. (Modified after Schweizer P, Müller G. Cholestase-syndrome in Neugeborenen- und Sauglingsalter. Stuttgart, Hippokrates Verlag, 1984.)

with a biliary concrement. In other instances, the lumen appears free but narrowed by surrounding inflammatory tissue; in three quarters of such specimens the epithelial lining is columnar, but it incompletely lines the perimeter of the lumen. Smaller epithelial structures may be seen at the peripheral part of the section and are similar to type II lesions. This type III lesion roughly corresponds to what is termed type I by Miyano and co-workers,[84, 92] who further

subdivided the specimens into type Ia (luminal diameter more than 300 μ) and type Ib (luminal diameter between 100 μ and 300 μ) and to type I by Chandra and Altman (luminal diameter more than 150 μ).[86]

All investigators agree that the variable histologic

[Figure 51-2 image]

Figure 51–2. EHBDA. Fibrous remnant, Gautier type I. The extrahepatic bile duct has disappeared and is replaced by dense fibrous connective tissue (hematoxylin and eosin, × 64).

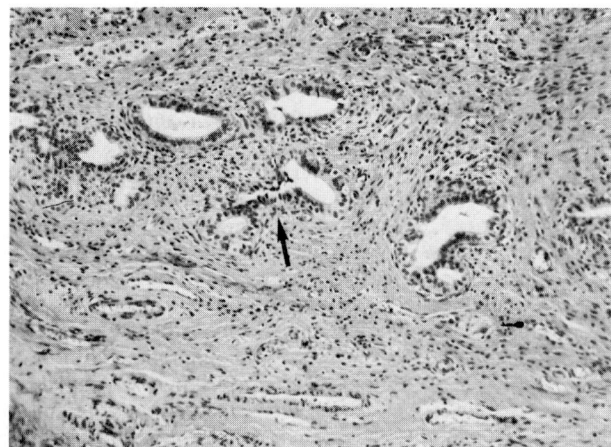

Figure 51–3. EHBDA. Fibrous remnant, Gautier type II. A cluster of small epithelium-lined tubes lies embedded in connective tissue, characterized by inflammatory cell infiltration and beginning fibrosis. Note degenerative changes (e.g., nuclear pycnosis) (*arrow*) in part of the lining epithelial cells (hematoxylin and eosin, × 128).

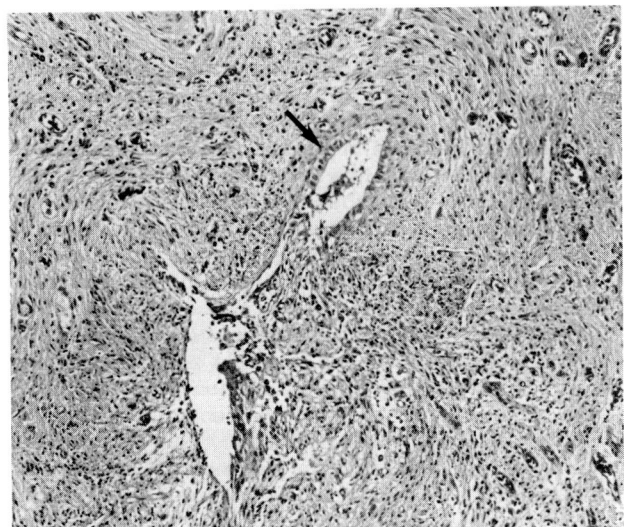

Figure 51–4. EHBDA. Fibrous remnant, Gautier type III. Most of the lining bile duct epithelium is destroyed; some segments remain (arrow). A lumen can still be recognized, surrounded by granulation-like tissue rich in fibroblasts and inflammatory cells (hematoxylin and eosin, × 160).

appearance reflects a dynamic process of progressive inflammatory destruction of the extrahepatic bile ducts. The earliest stage corresponds to periductal inflammation with necrosis and sloughing of the epithelial lining, followed by progressive periductal fibrosis and narrowing of the lumen (Fig. 51–5). The end stage is a complete fibrous scar of a destroyed epithelium-lined tube that remains identifiable as a fibrous cord in which the collagen texture is more dense than the surrounding connective tissue of the hepatoduodenal ligament and in which the collagen bundles may display a concentric arrangement. The most advanced stage of complete obliteration is frequently seen at the distal end of the common hepatic duct,[40, 83, 84, 92] whereas the more proximal segments and the prehepatic fibrous cone often show the early stages of inflammatory destruction. This has led to the hypothesis that the lesion represents an ascending, progressive inflammatory process.[83]

An important observation is that the degree of fibrous obliteration of the extrahepatic ducts increases with the increasing age of the patient, in parallel with increasing fibrosis in the liver.[92] Of equal interest is the finding that

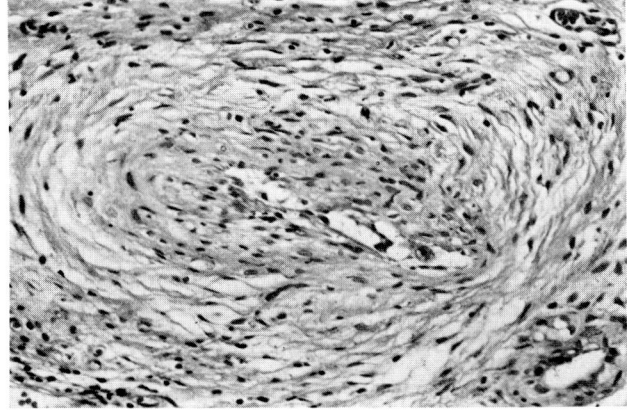

Figure 51–5. EHBDA. Fibrous remnant. Transitional stage between Gautier type III and type I. The epithelial lining of the duct has virtually disappeared. A slit-like lumen is still discernible, surrounded by concentric fibrosis. Collapse of the lumen and further fibrosis would lead to formation of a fibrous cord (hematoxylin and eosin, × 40).

epithelial necrobiosis and inflammatory infiltration may be observed distal to regions of complete obstruction, indicating that these changes are not secondary to occlusion of bile ducts.[37]

CORRELATION BETWEEN NUMBER AND SIZE OF BILE DUCTS NEAR THE PORTA HEPATIS AND POST-OPERATIVE DRAINAGE OF BILE. The rationale of hepatic portoenterostomy lies in establishing continuity between the bile ducts near the porta hepatis and the intestinal lumen. Theoretically, successful restoration of bile flow is expected in patients with patent biliary structures near the porta hepatis. Postoperative bile flow would be expected to be greatest in patients with biliary structures having the largest diameters or in patients with the greatest numbers of such structures, or both. Investigations by Kasai and co-workers and Kimura indicated that a satisfactory postoperative flow of bile is obtained only when the diameter of the patent ducts near the porta hepatis is at least 200 μ.[78, 88] Suruga and colleagues concluded that duct lumina of 100 μ diameter were sufficient for assuring adequate flow of bile.[96] Some authors recommend intraoperative confirmation by frozen section of the presence of microscopically patent ducts at the level of anastomosis in portoenterostomy.[97, 98] However, in the studies mentioned, the correlation between the presence of patent ducts and postoperative flow of bile was not 100 per cent. Furthermore, other authors reported no correlation between postoperative drainage of bile and the number or size of bile ducts at the porta hepatis.[84, 89, 93] Gautier and associates found,[84] for example, that 6 of 13 patients with no demonstrable bile ducts at the porta hepatis had an adequate bile flow postoperatively. Later studies have applied a sophisticated computer analysis of the size of bile ducts.[90] From these data, no correlation is seen between the degree of postoperative drainage of bile and the number of ducts or the area of the largest bile ducts, but the total area of all bile duct structures (about 100,000 μ²) was significantly larger in patients with adequate postoperative drainage versus those with poor postoperative drainage (about 30,000 μ²; p <0.05). More effective bile flow was evident in patients with more than 50,000 μ² total area of bile ducts, as compared with those with less than 50,000 μ² total area. In four patients, however, there was good postoperative flow of bile despite a small total area for bile ducts at the porta hepatis. Moreover, in all studies bile failed to drain after operation in a significant number of infants with presumably favorable histologic findings. In view of these inconsistencies, further analysis was carried out by Ohi and associates.[95] These authors concluded that distinction should be made among different types of biliary structures at the porta hepatis, that is, among bile ducts, collecting ducts of biliary (periductal) glands, and biliary glands themselves. Only bile ducts, and not collecting ducts and glands, communicate with the intrahepatic biliary system and assure drainage of bile after hepatic portoenterostomy.

Matsukawa concluded from three-dimensional histometry of bile ducts in the porta hepatis that the sites of obstruction may be located very close to the liver tissue and that interruptions of bile duct continuity are found at any level of the fibrous, scarred tissue cone.[91] This finding suggests a preponderant importance of the bile duct configuration high up in the porta hepatis. Finally, it was concluded in a recent study that the size of the bile ducts at the porta hepatis does not have much influence on operative results.[99, 100]

Although refinement in recognition and measurement of bile ducts draining at the porta hepatis might help to assure a better predictive value of operative intervention, the results already mentioned still do not explain the occurrence of adequate bile flow in patients without recognizable epithelial structures. These puzzling cases raise the question of how bile is drained when there is no duct continuity and point to alternative pathways like lymphatic drainage of bile constituents.[101] The concept of lymphatic drainage forms the basis for some modifications of the Kasai procedure (omentopexy).[40]

Pathologic Features of the Liver and Intrahepatic Bile Ducts in Extrahepatic Bile Duct Atresia

In discussing the changes observed in the liver and intrahepatic bile ducts in EHBDA, it is useful to distinguish between (1) pure EHBDA, (2) EHBDA associated with hypoplasia of intrahepatic bile ducts, and (3) EHBDA associated with hyperplasia of intrahepatic bile ducts.

Pure Extrahepatic Bile Duct Atresia

INTERPRETATION OF HISTOLOGIC CHANGES. There has been much discussion about the value of liver biopsy in the diagnosis of EHBDA. Although some early studies emphasized the usefulness of liver histopathologic features,[77, 102] other authors pointed out the lack of reliability of the histopathologic diagnosis, especially on needle biopsy specimens. From a questionnaire sent to several authorities, Brent obtained divergent opinions about the usefulness of liver biopsy.[35] In 1967, Hays and associates reported the diagnostic accuracy of percutaneous (needle) liver biopsy to be approximately the same as for operative (open) liver biopsy, with a failure rate of 33 per cent. Similar figures were given by Landing.[13, 104] Alagille and associates found that needle biopsy yielded a firm diagnosis in only one third of cases and a strongly suggestive diagnosis in another third.[105] Surgical liver biopsy was diagnostic in 58 per cent of cases and was strongly suggestive in nearly all the remaining cases, with a failure rate of 10 per cent. Eliot and associates found that results from needle biopsies correlated fairly well with those from surgical biopsies and concluded that needle biopsy was of great value but could not be used as the sole diagnostic procedure.[106] In more recent years, the diagnostic accuracy of liver biopsy is reported to be up to 90 per cent and even 95 per cent.[40, 107–110]

The improvement in accuracy of histopathologic interpretation of liver biopsy specimens in the diagnosis of EHBDA seems to be due to attributing less importance to parenchymal giant cells and more attention to changes in the portal tracts, including interlobular bile duct damage, and above all, to awareness that the histopathologic changes (including the diagnostic features) are profoundly influenced by the age of the patient. The most important message for the histopathologist is that he or she is studying a snapshot of a dynamic process.

EHBDA is a cause of extrahepatic cholestasis that brings about a series of changes in the liver, the most characteristic of which are those observed in the portal tracts.[111] Basically, the neonatal liver reacts to extrahepatic cholestasis in much the same way as does the adult liver, except for a more fetal type of ductular reaction and an accelerated progression of the lesions. This is reflected in the development of fully established and irreversible biliary cirrhosis in less than two months.

The following description of histologic abnormalities of the liver and intrahepatic bile ducts, observed in preoperative biopsy specimens and in follow-up specimens after hepatic portoenterostomy (the latter is discussed on page 1378) is based on reports from the literature and on microscopic study of patients observed personally, the majority being patients from Italy under the care of Professor Guido Caccia (Brescia).

The *interpretation* of the histopathologic findings may appear somewhat at variance with classic descriptions reported in the literature on this subject up to now. This interpretation is based on some new aspects of the histopathologic characteristics of cholestasis in general (e.g., cholate stasis without bilirubinostasis), on some new insights into so-called ductular proliferation, and on renewed interest in the embryologic development of intrahepatic bile ducts (e.g., ductal plates and ductal plate malformation). Hence we place emphasis on features not commonly discussed in the pertinent literature. We recognize that some of these interpretations are subject to debate, but hopefully they will stimulate further progress in understanding the course of events in EHBDA.

The interpretation of the histopathologic changes described in this chapter relies on the following six concepts, which are not commonly treated in the pediatric literature of the last 25 years: (1) the embryologic development of the intrahepatic bile ducts, (2) the long time it takes for development of the intrahepatic biliary tree throughout fetal life, (3) the apparent fetal type of ductular reaction in early neonatal life in patients with EHBDA, (4) the concept of ductular metaplasia of hepatocytes in acinar zone I in longstanding cholestasis, (5) the diagnostic value of cholate stasis besides bilirubinostasis, (6) the diagnostic usefulness of better visualization of ducts and ductules and signs of cholestasis in histologic sections of liver.

Embryologic Development of Intrahepatic Bile Ducts. The intrahepatic bile ducts are derived by transformation from primitive precursors of parenchymal cells. With few exceptions, most embryologic studies describe the early formation of intrahepatic ducts by transformation of primitive parenchymal cells around the branches of the ingrowing portal vein, which is surrounded by a sheet of mesenchyme.[112] First a layer of primitive hepatocytes in direct contact with the mesenchymal sheet converts into biliary types of cells (Fig. 51–6). This is followed by a similar conversion of a second discontinuous layer of cells, resulting in the formation of a partly double epithelial cylinder surrounding the portal vein and its accompanying mesenchyme. There is a slit between the two epithelial layers. This primitive bile duct thus assumes the shape of a cylinder, with a cylindric slit-like lumen that is lined on both sides by a biliary type of epithelium. The primitive bile duct with cylindric configuration, located around the primitive portal tract, is termed the *ductal plate*.[113] Very soon, and even before completion of the biliary transformation of the outer epithelial layer, some parts of the slit-like lumen dilate (Fig. 51–7). Most of the cylindric structure disappears at the same time in relation to ingrowth of mesenchyme. This remodeling of the ductal plate results in an anastomosing system of tube-shaped ducts, located within the portal connective tissue. Derangement in, or arrest of, remodeling results in total or partial persistence of the ductal plate, that is, an excess of primitive embryologic structures, appearing as hyperplasia of bile ducts with unusual, curved, and often concentric patterns.[114]

Development of Intrahepatic Bile Ducts Throughout Fetal Life. Intrahepatic bile ducts begin their development at the hilum of the liver in the early embryonic stage and proceed toward the periphery throughout fetal life.[77] Distinction should be made between *differentiation* of the intrahepatic bile duct cells from hepatocytes and *growth* of both hepatocytes and bile duct structures. Differentiation

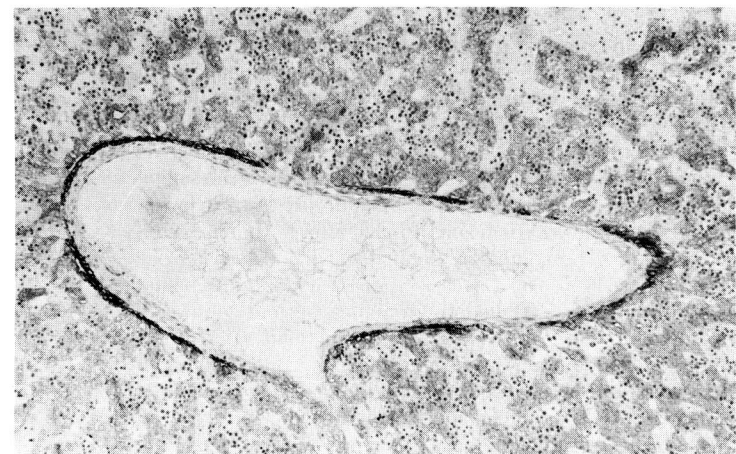

Figure 51–6. Immunoperoxidase stain for cytokeratins 8, 18, and 19 on liver section from an 11-week-old human fetus. This antibody stains cytokeratins in hepatocytes and bile duct structures. A large portal vein is shown, surrounded by a narrow sleeve of mesenchyme. The cell layer in contact with the mesenchyme shows an enhanced expression of cytokeratins, which appear only weakly stained in parenchymal cells. The strongly stained cell layer represents an early ductal plate. (Immunoperoxidase with anticytokeratin CAM 5.2 [Becton-Dickinson]. Counterstained with hematoxylin, × 160.)

of the bile duct system requires more than differentiation of bile duct cells from hepatocytes. The primitive cylindric ductal plate is gradually remodeled into an anastomosing system of tubes. The remodeling of ductal plates occurs over a long period, starting with the early ductal plates near the hilum of the liver and continuing until the end of fetal life as more peripheral plates are formed around the terminal ramifications of the portal vein (Fig. 51–8).[115] Occasional reports in the literature mention the possibility of postnatal maturation of the intrahepatic system of bile ductals in infants initially shown to have a paucity of intrahepatic bile ducts.[40, 116–120]

Postnatal Persistence of the Fetal Type of Duct Formation. The entire complex system for intrahepatic bile duct development, that is, the formation of ductal plates and their remodeling, is potentially susceptible to the action of disturbing factors or influences over a long period. The observation of ductal plates in liver specimens from infants with EHBDA thus suggests an antenatal interference with intrahepatic maturation of bile ducts.

Examination of liver specimens from three- to five-month-old infants with EHBDA suggests that formation of ductal plates continues after birth. This may be due either to retardation in the maturation process of the liver as a whole or to persistence after birth of a fetal type of ductular reaction in response to obstruction in cases of EHBDA. Adequate remodeling of ductal plates appears to be disturbed in EHBDA in view of the frequency with which ductal plates continue to be found after birth (see page 1368).

Ductular Proliferation Corresponding to Ductular Transformation of Hepatocytes. Any form of extrahepatic cholestasis elicits an intrahepatic ductular reaction. There is an increase in the number of the smallest branches of the intrahepatic biliary tree.[111] A significant portion of the increased number of ductular structures does not result from multiplication of pre-existing ductules but from ductular metaplasia of hepatocytes in acinar zone I (periportal).[112, 114, 121] This is especially true in cholestasis of long duration. It is associated with or is caused by a change in the composition of the biomatrix of connective tissue surrounding hepatocytes.[122, 123] In cholestatic conditions in older

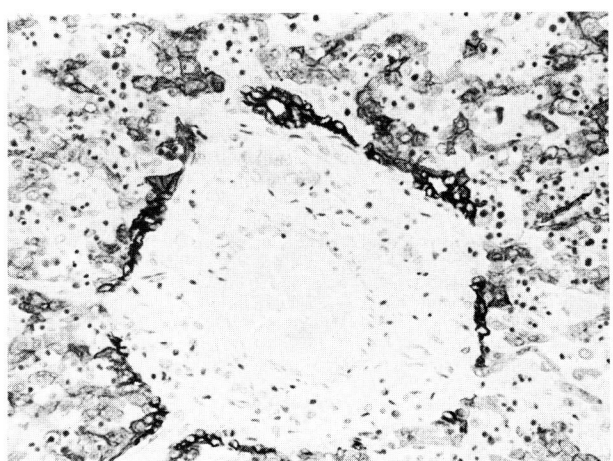

Figure 51–7. Immunoperoxidase stain for cytokeratins 8, 18, and 19 on a liver section from 16 week-old-human fetus. This antibody stains cytokeratins in hepatocytes and bile ducts. The picture shows a portal vein with surrounding mesenchyme (portal tract), encircled by a partly double layer of cells with more marked cytokeratin expression (ductal plate). In two places, the double epithelial layer molds around a lumen, leading to the primitive form of individualized bile ducts, still located at the periphery of the portal tract. This represents an early stage of remodeling of the ductal plate. (Immunoperoxidase with anticytokeratin CAM 5.2 [Becton-Dickinson]. Counterstained with hematoxylin, × 400.)

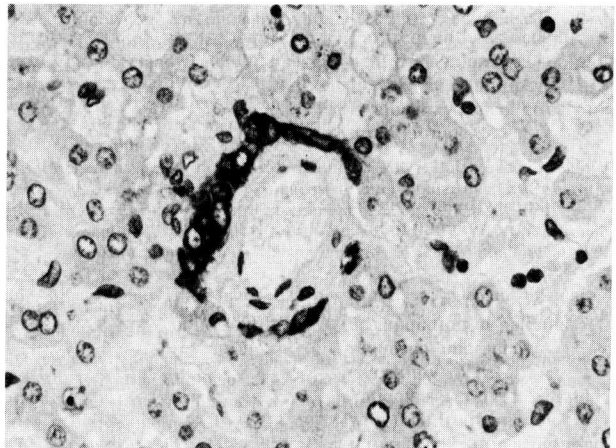

Figure 51–8. Immunoperoxidase stain for epidermal type of keratin on a liver section from a neonate (day 1). Only bile duct epithelium shows positive staining. The parenchymal cells stain negative. At birth, some bile ducts still appear as cylindric structures surrounding smaller (more peripheral) portal tracts. Such ductal plate configuration represents an immature state of bile duct development. (Immunoperoxidase with rabbit polyclonal antihuman cytokeratin [Dako Corporation, Santa Barbara, CA]. Counterstained with hematoxylin, × 640.)

infants and adults, the population of ductular cells derived from cholangiocytic metaplasia of hepatocytes assumes the appearance previously described as atypical ductular proliferation.[124] These newly formed ductules are not arranged in concentric ductal plates, but they basically retain the labyrinthic anastomosing pattern of the hepatocellular muralia system.[112] This pattern has been beautifully illustrated in some three-dimensional reconstruction studies.[125] It thus appears that ductular reaction in the younger infant follows a fetal pattern with renewed formation of ductal plates. With increasing age, the ductular reaction to obstruction corresponds to a more adult pattern of so-called ductular proliferation, which includes ductular metaplasia of hepatocytes.

Cholate Stasis and Bilirubinostasis. In conventional terminology, histologic cholestasis corresponds to accumulation of bilirubin pigment, most characteristically in the form of intercellular bile plugs.[126] Javitt has insisted that a cholestatic condition is better reflected by a rise in serum bile salt levels than by increased concentrations of conjugated bilirubin in the serum.[127] Thus, cholestasis may exist without clinical jaundice and in the presence of normal levels of bilirubin in serum. The same principle applies to the recognition of histologic cholestasis. Especially in cases of low-grade cholestasis (e.g., in patients with longstanding but incomplete obstruction of the biliary passages), the liver parenchyma may show changes reflecting cholestasis without accumulation of bile pigment. Hence, it seems useful to distinguish between bilirubinostasis and cholate stasis.[124, 128] In several examples of slowly progressive, smoldering cholestasis—as in primary biliary cirrhosis, primary sclerosing cholangitis, and in follow-up specimens from patients after successful portoenterostomy for EHBDA—cholate stasis is a more reliable indicator of a cholestatic state than is bilirubinostasis.

Cholate stasis refers to a microscopic change in hepatocytes in acinar zone I (periportal). The parenchymal cells appear swollen, with coarsely granular cytoplasm, often associated with intercellular edema, and there is increased fibrosis and infiltration with inflammatory cells, including polymorphs. With time, the cells show gradual accumulation of copper (best demonstrated with the rhodamine stain) and of metallothionein or copper-binding protein (demonstrable with Shikata's orcein stain). In severe degrees of cholate stasis, the altered cells may reflect disturbances in their cytoskeleton by the appearance of Mallory bodies.[124, 128] Further parenchymal features of cholestasis that are not necessarily accompanied by bilirubinostasis are so-called feathery degeneration and cholestatic liver-cell rosettes.[129] In summary, ductular reaction, cholate stasis, and cholestatic liver-cell rosettes are more reliable histologic markers of a low-grade, smoldering cholestatic state than is the microscopically visible accumulation of bile pigment (bilirubinostasis).

Histologic Visualization of Intrahepatic Bile Ducts. The microscopic identification of intrahepatic bile ducts may be difficult in altered portal tracts with dense inflammatory infiltration. This difficulty is even greater in the case of small ducts, as in liver biopsy specimens from infants and in specimens with damaged, involuted, or disappearing ducts. Histologic analysis of tissue sections from livers with disease of intrahepatic bile ducts is facilitated by staining techniques that enhance the contrast in visualization of bile duct structures. Several special techniques can be used for this purpose.[112] A good and reliable method is the immunohistochemical demonstration, with the use of specific antibodies, of subtypes of intermediate filaments that are specific for bile-duct types of cells. Adequate results are obtained with rabbit polyclonal antibodies raised against the epidermal type of keratin (Fig. 51–9).[112, 128, 130-132] Immunohistochemical staining for tissue polypeptide antigen (TPA) gives similar results.[133, 134] Besides being useful for better visualization of bile ducts, these techniques are useful for revealing mild cholestatic changes in liver parenchymal cells in acinar zone I (see Figs. 51–11, 51–28, 51–31, 51–33, 51–36 and 51–39).[128]

OPTIMAL TIME FOR DIAGNOSTIC LIVER BIOPSY. Even if ductular reaction is accepted as a most reliable but not a pathognomonic criterion in diagnosing extrahepatic obstruction in liver tissue specimens,[108] it should be realized that this alteration takes some time to develop. This explains why some authors recommend postponing liver biopsy until the end of the sixth postnatal week in order to assure an optimal chance for confident diagnosis of EHBDA.[40] However, our own experience, as well as that of others, indicates that there is a broad variability in the extent of liver alteration and ductular reaction in patients of the same age, that diagnostic histologic features may be observed in some infants at a younger age than six weeks (i.e., four weeks), and that in some early severe cases the lesions may be far advanced and close to biliary cirrhosis at the age of four to six weeks as we observed in ten patients from a personal series of 41 cases.[18]

If one accepts that surgical correction should be performed as early as possible, in any case before the liver is severely affected by advanced fibrosis or biliary cirrhosis, it may be unwise to postpone diagnostic liver biopsy until the end of the sixth week of life. Furthermore, it is reasonable to accept the fact that the speed of progress of the disease varies in individual patients, as it has been shown to vary according to the sex of the patient.[53] Moreover, in some patients, the pathologic jaundice appears only after the first postnatal month, entailing a similar delay in the development of diagnostic features in the liver. Hence, it appears that the optimal time for diagnostic liver biopsy depends to a large extent on clinical judgement and the experience of the pediatrician or pediatric surgeon. A liver biopsy that is obtained too early in the course of the disease may be nondiagnostic, necessitating a second, later biopsy.[135]

HISTOPATHOLOGIC FEATURES. It may be of interest to distinguish between classic or typical cases to which most

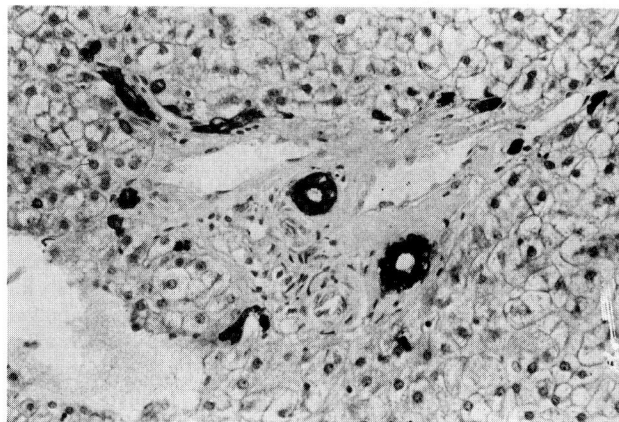

Figure 51–9. Portal tract in normal human adult liver. Immunoperoxidase stain with polyclonal anticytokeratin. Only bile ducts in the portal tract and small ductules at the portal-parenchymal interphase show strong positive staining. (Immunoperoxidase stain with polyclonal rabbit antikeratin, wide spectrum screening [Dako Corporation, Santa Barbara, CA]. Counterstained with hematoxylin, × 400.)

descriptions in published reports correspond and a group of early severe cases, which display somewhat aberrant features in the interlobular bile ducts. The latter group corresponds to what was described as "association between EHBDA and hyperplasia of intrahepatic bile ducts,"[40] and is discussed later (see page 1368).

Liver specimens with classic features of EHBDA show histologic alterations that change in the course of the disease, allowing some chronologic staging of the lesions in successive periods.[40] As emphasized before, the timing of the stages may be only approximate. The earliest stage (from about one to four weeks) is characterized by nonspecific features of bilirubinostasis, consisting of granules of bile pigment in hepatocytes and intercellular bile plugs.[40] A few hepatocytes may show degeneration and necrosis. Parenchymal giant cells may be seen, but usually in small numbers and without striking hydropic change. There is no inflammatory infiltration in either the parenchyma or the portal tracts. The amount of bilirubin in Kupffer cells increases with the duration of cholestasis. Foci of extramedullary hematopoiesis may persist to a variable extent. The histopathologic features in this early period do not allow for a firm diagnosis.

In the second stage of the disease, from about four to seven weeks,[40] the portal tracts show changes that are characteristic for extrahepatic obstruction of the bile duct. They consist of rounding of the portal tract, edema, dilation of lymph vessels, and ductular proliferation (Figs. 51–10, 51–11, 51–12). The increase in ductules occurs typically at the periphery of the portal tracts, so-called marginal bile duct proliferation.[136] The ductular reaction becomes associated with an inflammatory infiltration, including lymphocytes and polymorphonuclear leukocytes. The density of the inflammatory infiltrate is variable. The ductular reaction in the periphery of the portal tracts creates a diffuse borderline between portal connective tissue and periportal parenchyma (acinar zone I). This stage is considered diagnostic of EHBDA and explains the recommendation by some to postpone diagnostic liver biopsy until the sixth week of life.[40]

Most authors agree on the diagnostic usefulness of so-called marginal bile duct proliferation. Also, in older studies, ductular proliferation was considered the most reliable histologic change.[10, 35, 105, 108, 137, 138] It was recognized, however, that ductular proliferation takes some time to reach full development.[105, 138–140]

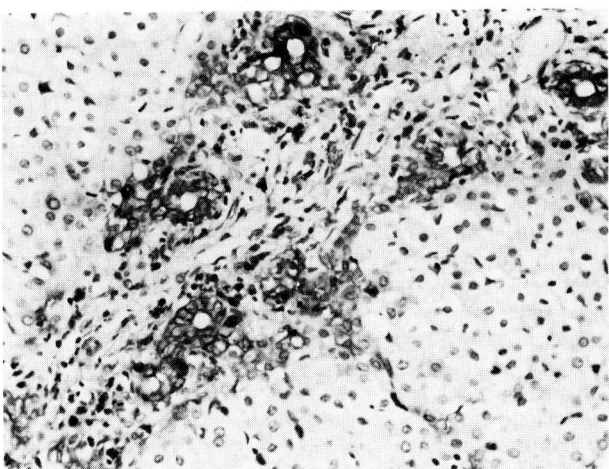

Figure 51–11. EHBDA in infant aged 60 days. Immunoperoxidase stain for epidermal type keratin. The figure shows part of a portal tract; it contains several strongly positive-staining bile ducts, some of them in close connection with periportal parenchyma. The most peripheral hepatocytes show mild keratin staining, indicating a phenotypic shift toward bile duct type cells (ductular metaplasia of hepatocytes). (Immunoperoxidase with rabbit polyclonal antihuman cytokeratin [Dako Corporation, Santa Barbara, CA]. Counterstained with hematoxylin, × 400.)

Equally important, from a diagnostic point of view, are the lesions of the portal bile ducts, which can be summarized as inflammatory destruction. The ducts show permeation by inflammatory cells, disruption of their basement membranes, and epithelial abnormalities that include increased acidophilia, vacuolization, flattening, and shedding or necrosis of the epithelium (Figs. 51–12 and 51–13). The ductal inflammatory lesions bear striking resemblance to those observed in the extrahepatic bile duct remnants, and they are responsible for the progressive disappearance of intrahepatic bile duct segments. An occasional portal tract may display bile ducts, usually of small size, in ductal plate configuration.

During a subsequent third stage (from seven to eight weeks),[40] portal and periportal fibrosis develops, associated with periportal extension of the ductular reaction. The density of the inflammatory infiltrate may decrease, and portal edema and lymphangiectasis become less prominent.

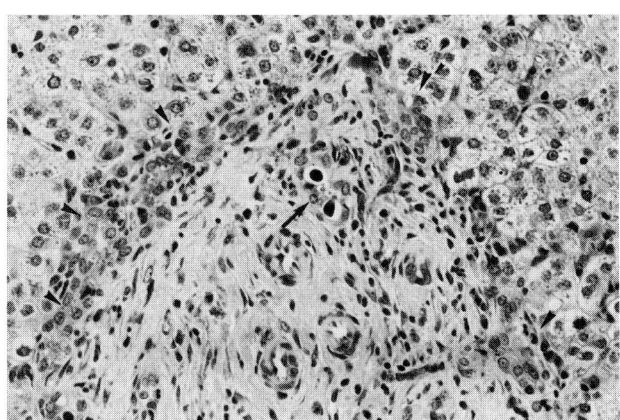

Figure 51–10. EHBDA in infant aged 43 days. The portal tract shows mild mononuclear cell infiltration. The bile duct contains bile concrements (arrow). Immediately surrounding the bile duct, an early stage of ductular reaction (mainly ductular metaplasia of hepatocytes) is seen (arrowheads) (hematoxylin and eosin, × 400.)

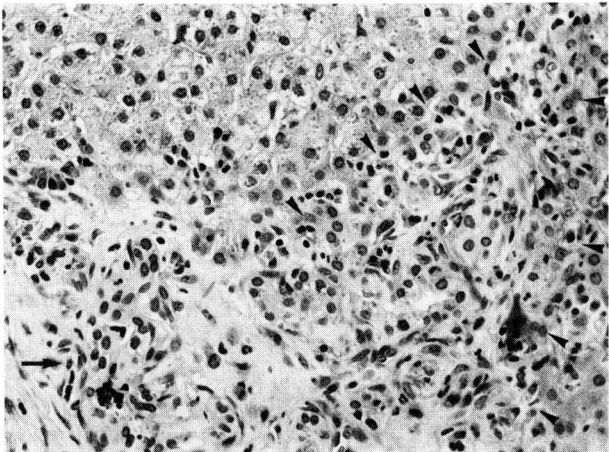

Figure 51–12. EHBDA in infant aged 30 days. The figure shows part of a portal tract (lower left). It contains bile ducts, some of them with damaged epithelial lining and bile concrements in the lumen (arrow). A wedge-shaped area of ductular proliferation, with admixed inflammatory cells and collagen fibers, extends into the parenchyma (arrowheads) (hematoxylin and eosin, × 400).

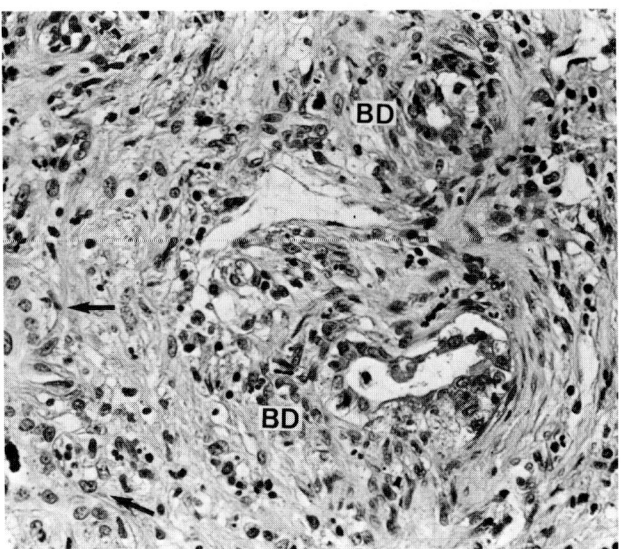

Figure 51–13. EHBDA in infant aged eight weeks. Portal tract with two bile ducts (*BD*), which show swelling, vacuolization, attenuation, and sloughing of their lining epithelial cells. There is mild inflammatory infiltration. Ductular proliferation occurs at the margin of the portal tract (*arrows*) (hematoxylin and eosin, × 400).

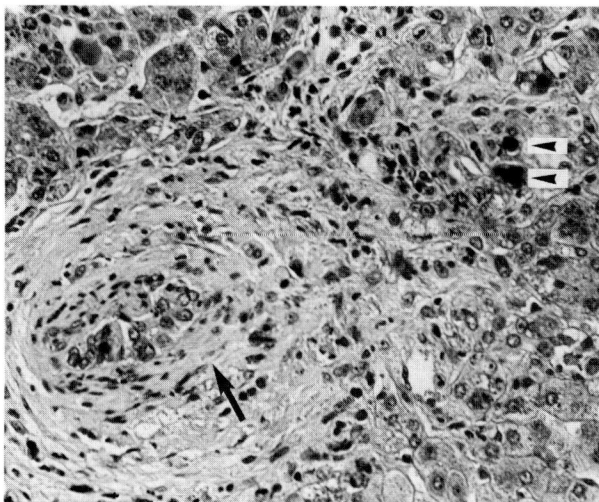

Figure 51–15. EHBDA in infant aged eight weeks. The portal tract contains a bile duct with degenerating epithelial lining, encircled by beginning concentric periduct fibrosis (*arrow*). Bile plugs are seen in the periportal parenchyma (*arrowheads*) (hematoxylin and eosin, × 400).

Bile concrements appear in the lumina of some of the ductular segments, which is typical in EHBDA.[40, 80, 109] The ductules often show signs of biliary reabsorption as vacuolization, lipofuscin and bilirubin pigment (Fig. 51–14),[128, 141] and reduplication of the basement membranes on electron microscopic examination.[126, 142] The parenchymal changes by themselves remain nondiagnostic. The extent and topography of bilirubinostasis is variable; coarse bile plugs are scattered throughout the parenchyma and some hepatocytes show feathery degeneration. Damage to liver cells and necrosis of single cells seem to depend on the degree of bile stasis. There is no appreciable intralobular inflammation. Pigmented macrophages tend to cluster in periportal regions.

After about the tenth week,[40] the periportal fibrosis gradually extends into the surrounding parenchyma, whereas the density of the inflammatory infiltration tends to decrease. Also, the number of ductular structures seems to decrease, and the remaining ductules often show dilation of the lumen and bile concrements. The interlobular bile ducts display fibrous cholangitis, with irregular narrowing of their lumina, thickening of their basement membranes, and development of concentric periductal fibrosis. The strangulated ducts show progressive atrophy of the epithelial lining (Figs. 51–15 and 51–16). The progressing periportal fibrosis causes linkage of adjacent portal tracts, reaching the stage of biliary fibrosis but not yet fully developed biliary cirrhosis.[143] The liver lesions at this time are advanced beyond the optimal stage for successful hepatic portoenterostomy, and they indicate a high-risk patient with regard to successful postoperative drainage of bile.

The fifth and final stage (beyond 12 weeks) corresponds to further progression to secondary biliary cirrhosis,[40] characterized by nodular regeneration of the parenchyma and perinodular septal fibrosis (Fig. 51–17). Admittedly, the distinction between biliary fibrosis and biliary cirrhosis is not a clear one, especially when judged on needle-biopsy

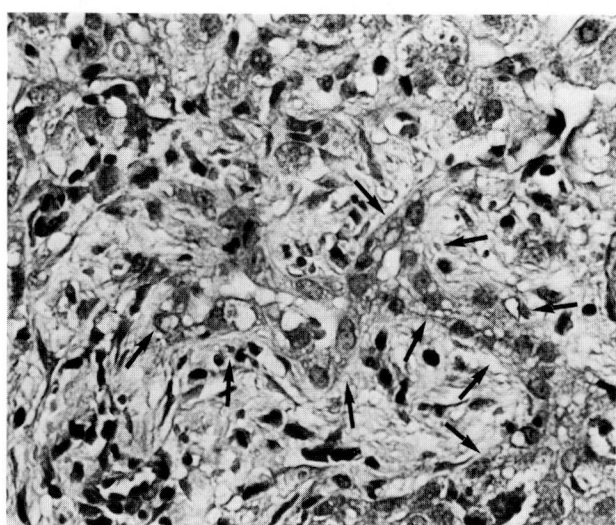

Figure 51–14. EHBDA in infant aged 56 days. Edge of an edematous portal tract containing an anastomosing ductular network. The ductular lining cells show striking vacuolation (*arrows*) (hematoxylin and eosin, × 640).

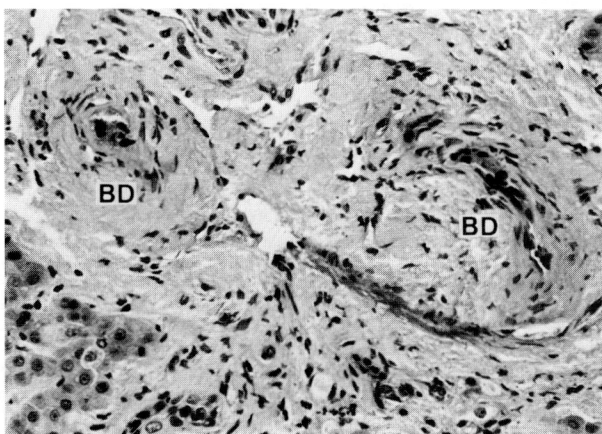

Figure 51–16. EHBDA in infant aged six months. Portal tract with two bile ducts (*BD*) in advanced stage of destruction: some atrophic lining cells with nuclear pyknosis remain. The ducts are surrounded by broad layers of dense collagen (fibrous obliterating cholangitis) (hematoxylin and eosin, × 400).

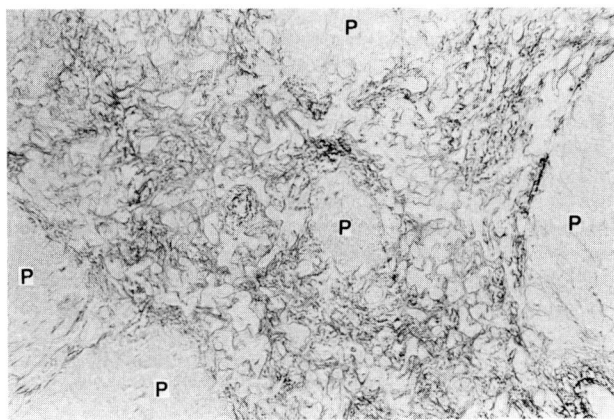

Figure 51–17. EHBDA in infant aged 10 months. Stage of biliary cirrhosis. The figure shows extensive fibrosis and an increase in ductules between the nodular parenchymal areas (P) (Shikata's orcein stain, × 160).

specimens. This uncertainty accounts for the controversy concerning the reversibility of biliary cirrhosis.[143] The finding of biliary cirrhosis (the fifth stage of disease) on liver biopsy specimens is a contraindication for corrective surgery.[40]

Several authors have specifically emphasized the alterations that can be observed at the level of the interlobular bile ducts in the central part of the portal tracts.[37, 82, 144] These changes consist of a spectrum of lesions of the bile duct lining cells, including intracellular vacuoles, flattening and condensation of cells with pyknotic nuclei, and necrosis of bile duct cells, as well as mitosis of these cells. Similar lesions of the lining epithelium of bile ducts were observed in larger intrahepatic ducts at the porta hepatis.[37, 42] Based on the distribution of these changes in the original specimens and their persistence after corrective surgery, it was believed that they were not secondary to distal obstruction alone and that they apparently represented an intrahepatic component of the basic disease process affecting the extrahepatic ducts.[37]

Ongoing damage to the bile ducts leads to progressive disappearance of the interlobular bile ducts.[39, 87] EHBDA thus represents a "disappearing bile duct disease."[145, 146] The lack of interlobular bile ducts in late stages of EHBDA probably results from various causes: damage from distal extrahepatic obstruction,[143] strangulation by progressive fibrosis,[87] ischemia due to compression of the peribiliary capillary plexus by portal fibrosis,[129] and, perhaps most importantly, from a relentless progression of the primary process of the sclerosing cholangitis that affects the extrahepatic ducts.[27, 37, 147–150] This topic is relevant for the discussion of liver lesions in follow-up biopsies after hepatic portoenterostomy (see page 1378).

Lesions of the intrahepatic bile ducts can be recognized by radiographic studies that demonstrate hypoplasia of the intrahepatic biliary tree.[18, 79, 151–153]

Not only is progression of EHBDA associated with the disappearance of intrahepatic bile ducts, but the branches of the portal vein often appear strikingly hypoplastic in the sclerosing portal tracts.[154] In later biopsy specimens from patients with EHBDA, one may observe fusion between large preterminal portal tracts, resulting in enlarged fibrous areas. There is an apparent lack of the finer ramifications of portal tracts. This picture suggests a lack of continued outgrowth of terminal ramifications of the portal tracts and the vessels they contain. Such apparently stunted growth of portal tracts may be part of the previously mentioned

retardation in growth and differentiation of intrahepatic bile ducts, and it may also be responsible for the hypoplastic pattern of the portal vein.[154]

Studies by Landing and co-workers have disclosed a particular time course for the intrahepatic lesions in untreated or unsuccessfully treated EHBDA.[155] Their data show an early phase of rapid proliferation of bile ductules, peaking at 205 days, followed by rapid regression to approximately 400 days. There is a slower progressive loss of intrahepatic ducts thereafter. The connective tissue in the portal tracts increases on a slower course and continues to increase after maximum regression of ducts is reached, indicating a dissociation between the ductular reaction and fibrosis in EHBDA. It was also found that boys with EHBDA show a statistically significant longer survival than girls.[53] Girls show a greater degree of proliferation of intrahepatic ductules in the early phase (<200 days) and greater regression of ducts and more rapid development of fibrosis than do boys between 200 and 400 days. The more stormy progression of the disease in girls may be significant from a pathogenetic point of view (see page 1372).

HISTOLOGIC DIFFERENTIAL DIAGNOSIS OF EXTRAHEPATIC BILE DUCT ATRESIA

Histologic Differential Diagnosis Between Extrahepatic Bile Duct Atresia and Neonatal Hepatitis. The histopathologic features of neonatal hepatitis are described on page 1386. The criteria for differentiating neonatal hepatitis from EHBDA follow: more pronounced parenchymal changes, focal necrosis, often more numerous parenchymal giant cells with a hydropic change (ballooning) of their cytoplasm, intralobular inflammatory infiltration, less conspicuous changes in the portal tracts with virtually no ductular proliferation. The histopathologic diagnosis remains in doubt in a small percentage of patients with EHBDA (5 to 7 per cent). The problematic biopsy specimens are those in which ductular proliferation is not prominent, and parenchymal damage, in the form of giant cell transformation with ballooning and focal necrosis, is pronounced. If this histologic appearance is present and other investigations are also inconclusive, it is still advisable to proceed to exploratory laparotomy. This is true despite published warnings that surgery may be harmful to patients with neonatal hepatitis.[23] Several surveys have demonstrated that limited surgery is tolerated well and has no negative effect on prognosis in this condition.[51, 78, 88, 156].

Histologic Differential Diagnosis Between Extrahepatic Bile Duct Atresia and Other Syndromes of Neonatal Cholestasis. A great number of entities must be considered in the differential diagnosis of neonatal cholestasis (Table 51–1).[157] From the point of view of histopathologic differentiation, however, only a few metabolic disorders have to be considered, and they include galactosemia, fructose intolerance, and α1-antitrypsin deficiency (see Chaps. 49 and 50). The other cholestatic syndromes reveal characteristic findings on liver biopsy or can be diagnosed by other means.

Galactosemia and α1-antitrypsin deficiency represent abnormalities that manifest clinically in the same age group as does EHBDA. In both conditions, the early stage is characterized by ductular proliferation in the portal tracts, albeit to a lesser extent than in EHBDA. Galactosemia is characterized further by severe histologic cholestasis, with bile plugs in pseudoglandular arrangements of hepatocytes and a constant fatty change.[120, 158] Fructose intolerance causes a somewhat similar picture, usually with less ductular proliferation and minor cholestasis. Furthermore, most often it causes clinical symptoms at a later age, beyond the third month of life. α1-Antitrypsin deficiency can be rec-

TABLE 51–1. NEONATAL CHOLESTASIS—PROPOSED CLASSIFICATION OF RECOGNIZED DISEASE ENTITIES*

I. Extrahepatic disorders
   A. Biliary atresia
   B. Biliary hypoplasia
   C. Bile duct stenosis
   D. Anomalies of choledochal-pancreatico-ductal junction
   E. Spontaneous perforation of bile duct
   F. Mass (neoplasia, stone)
   G. Bile-mucous plug
II. Intrahepatic disorders
   A. Idiopathic
      1. Idiopathic neonatal hepatitis
      2. Intrahepatic cholestasis, persistent
         a. Arteriohepatic dysplasia (Alagille's syndrome)
         b. Byler disease (severe intrahepatic cholestasis with progressive hepatocellular disease)
         c. Trihydroxycoprostanic acidemia (defective bile acid metabolism and cholestasis)
         d. Zellweger's syndrome (cerebrohepatorenal syndrome)
         e. Nonsyndromic paucity of intrahepatic ducts (apparent absence of bile ductules)
      3. Intrahepatic cholestasis, recurrent (syndromic?)
         a. Familial benign recurrent cholestasis
         b. Hereditary cholestasis with lymphedema (Aagenaes)
   B. Anatomic
      1. Congenital hepatic fibrosis or infantile polycystic disease
      2. Caroli's disease (cystic dilation of intrahepatic ducts)
   C. Metabolic disorders
      1. Disorders of amino acid metabolism
         a. Tyrosinemia
      2. Disorders of lipid metabolism
         a. Wolman's disease
         b. Niemann-Pick disease
         c. Gaucher's disease
      3. Disorders of carbohydrate metabolism
         a. Galactosemia
         b. Fructosemia
         c. Glycogenosis IV

   4. Metabolic disease in which the defect is uncharacterized
      a. α_1-antitrypsin deficiency
      b. Cystic fibrosis
      c. Idiopathic hypopituitarism
      d. Hypothyroidism
      e. Neonatal iron storage disease
      f. Infantile copper overload
      g. Multiple acyl-CoA dehydrogenation deficiency (glutaric acid type II)
      h. Familial erythrophagocytic lymphohistiocytosis
   D. Hepatitis
      1. Infectious
         a. Cytomegalovirus
         b. Hepatitis B virus (non-A, non-B virus?)
         c. Rubella virus
         d. Reovirus type 3
         e. Herpesvirus
         f. Varicella virus
         g. Coxsackievirus
         h. ECHO virus
         i. Toxoplasmosis
         j. Syphilis
         k. Tuberculosis
         l. Listeriosis
      2. Toxic
         a. Cholestasis associated with parenteral nutrition
         b. Sepsis with possible endotoxemia (urinary tract infection, gastroenteritis)
   E. Genetic or chromosomal
      1. Trisomy E
      2. Down's syndrome
      3. Donahue's syndrome (leprechaunism)
   F. Miscellaneous
      1. Histiocytosis X
      2. Shock or hypoperfusion
      3. Intestinal obstruction
      4. Polysplenia syndrome

*Source: Reprinted by permission from Balistreri, W. F.: *Seminars in Liver Disease* Volume 7, Thieme Medical Publishers, New York, 1987.

ognized by the characteristic, periodic acid-Schiff (PAS)-positive, diastase-resistant globular inclusions in periportal hepatocytes. They can be identified more specifically by means of immunohistochemical methods (immunofluorescence, immunoperoxidase), even on paraffin-embedded tissue.[159, 160]

Extrahepatic Bile Duct Atresia Associated with Hypoplasia of Intrahepatic Bile Ducts. Atresia of the intrahepatic bile ducts is usually not complete but consists of a reduced ratio in the number of interlobular bile ducts to the number of portal tracts. This explains why the term *intrahepatic biliary atresia* is replaced by the terms *intrahepatic bile duct hypoplasia* and *paucity of intrahepatic bile ducts*.[117, 161, 162] Hypoplasia of intrahepatic bile ducts may be an isolated defect or may be associated with other extrahepatic anomalies.[109] The latter variety corresponds to arteriohepatic dysplasia or Alagille's syndrome and the cerebrohepatorenal or Zellweger's syndrome (see Chap. 49).[163–168] An isolated or nonsyndromatic paucity of interlobular bile ducts occurs in patients with congenital rubella, α_1-antitrypsin deficiency, trihydroxy coprostanic acidemia, Down's syndrome, cystic fibrosis, choledochal cyst, hypopituitarism, Ivemark's syndrome, and lymphedema, and furthermore in patients with no apparent associated disorders (idiopathic forms).[169, 170]

A sound morphologic diagnosis of hypoplasia of the interlobular bile ducts rests on a sufficient biopsy specimen

and morphometric evaluation of bile ducts. Alagille and co-workers recommend a surgical biopsy of the liver.[80, 163] Others feel that a simple percutaneous needle biopsy may be adequate.[40, 171] Between 6 and 20 portal tracts should be present.[40] Hypoplasia of intrahepatic bile ducts is diagnosed if the ratio of interlobular bile ducts to the number of portal areas is less than 0.5, whereas in normal children this ratio lies between 0.9 and 1.8.[163, 164, 172] Schweizer and Müller consider hypoplasia to be definitely proved only when less than two of at least ten portal tracts display an interlobular bile duct.[40] The portal areas without bile ducts usually appear hypoplastic as a whole. Furthermore, it has been shown that the total number of portal tracts/mm^2 of tissue is reduced in patients with hypoplasia in comparison with normal controls.[173] During the last five years, however, this histologic picture of bland, ductless, and somewhat hypoplastic portal areas with a paucity of interlobular bile ducts has been questioned, as will be discussed further.

Cases of combined EHBDA and hypoplasia of interlobular bile ducts have been described repeatedly.[10, 118, 120, 138, 165, 174] Schweizer and Müller noted such association in more than 10 per cent of their patients with EHBDA (8 of 69 infants).[40] Liver biopsy in such patients reveals the typical portal reaction to EHBDA (edema, ductular proliferation) in those portal areas with an interlobular bile duct, at least when the biopsy is performed during the diagnostic phase of EHBDA. In contrast, the portal areas that are devoid of an interlobular bile duct (50 to 80 per cent of all portal tracts) show no reaction at all. This histologic picture with both variants of portal tracts is considered diagnostic for combined EHBDA and hypoplasia of interlobular bile ducts.[40, 118, 120] Since small-needle biopsies may contain only portal tracts lacking an interlobular duct, only hypoplasia of interlobular bile ducts may be diagnosed despite the presence of associated EHBDA. Interestingly, it seems as if the lack of interlobular bile ducts in the portal tracts prevents the development of ductular proliferation in response to extraheptic obstruction.[118, 120, 138]

It appears from results of several studies that the interlobular bile ducts are not congenitally lacking in patients with syndromatic paucity of intrahepatic bile ducts (Alagille's syndrome). During the first few weeks of life, interlobular bile ducts can be demonstrated in the portal areas of liver biopsy specimens from such patients, but their number gradually diminishes over the course of time.[169, 171, 175-180] The gradual disappearance of portal bile ducts appears to be due to destructive inflammation. There is infiltration with mononuclear leukocytes, and the epithelial lining cells of the bile ducts show desquamation and necrobiosis. Gradually, the lumen is obliterated by connective tissue, with fading of the inflammatory component.[169, 175, 181-183] The number of interlobular bile ducts decreases with aging of the patient. There is no characteristic age at which bile ducts disappear completely.[175] Some studies document a virtual lack of interlobular ducts during the first four weeks of life,[171, 184] whereas in another study of five children, paucity of interlobular ducts was established after three months of age.[169] It would appear therefore that the histopathologic picture, described earlier as typical for combined EHBDA and hypoplasia of intrahepatic bile ducts, applies only for patients in whom destruction of interlobular ducts is far enough advanced to reach the stage of paucity. This age may be around three months or even younger.[169, 171, 184] Hence, the histopathologist cannot rely on a lack of portal ducts to diagnose hypoplasia or paucity of ducts in earlier stages of Alagille's syndrome.

Whether ductular proliferation in the margin of portal areas carrying a duct remains a valid criterion for diagnosis of EHBDA in association with hypoplasia of intrahepatic ducts appears to be a difficult question. According to some authors,[171, 178, 185-187] there may be ductular proliferation during the phase of inflammatory destruction of ducts in cases of Alagille's syndrome without associated EHBDA. Possibly, all patients with Alagille's syndrome would show an initial proliferation of bile ducts if biopsy was performed early enough.[171] Other authors insist, however, that ductular proliferation is lacking in the destructive phase that leads to a paucity of bile ducts and that the ductular proliferation observed occasionally is secondary to cholangitis.[169, 180]

Ductular proliferation must be evaluated carefully in the diagnosis of EHBDA. In 158 cases with adequate clinical follow-up, liver biopsy has been diagnostic in approximately 95 per cent. Errors stemmed most often from "over-reading" mild or moderate degrees of bile duct hyperplasia in hepatitis and interpreting the lesion as extrahepatic obstruction.[107, 108]

LaBrecque and co-workers state that one should rely on the extrahepatic manifestations (characteristic facies, vertebral abnormalities, heart murmur, posterior embryotoxon) for the diagnosis of Alagille's syndrome. It should be realized that not all features are present in every patient.[164] Confirmation of the diagnosis can usually be obtained by a simple percutaneous liver biopsy, which reveals a paucity of intrahepatic ducts. On occasion, the

initial biopsy may reveal an increase in ducts, suggesting extrahepatic obstruction and a diagnosis of EHBDA. In such cases, exploratory laparotomy may be necessary to confirm patency of the extrahepatic ducts. Patients with extrahepatic biliary atresia have been reported to have also some of the typical features of Alagille's syndrome.[163, 165, 188]

In the nonsyndromatic type of paucity of intrahepatic bile ducts, biopsy specimens show decreased numbers of interlobular ducts from the first three months of life, and evidence is found of inflammatory destruction of remaining ducts. The picture is characterized further by mild periportal fibrosis.[170] In one study two patients were mentioned with ductular proliferation in portal tracts. This lesion was found to be due to cholangitis in one patient (aged six weeks), and EHBDA developed in another infant (aged two weeks).[170] In the English literature, two further patients have been reported with EHBDA in association with paucity of intrahepatic ducts of the nonsyndromatic type on initial biopsy.[107, 178] Repeat biopsy performed three weeks later in one of these patients showed development of ductular proliferation,[178] which led to the correct diagnosis of associated EHBDA. Apparently, the first biopsy (at four weeks of age) was performed too early for ductular proliferation to have developed; the second biopsy (at seven weeks of age) was performed in a more diagnostic phase according to Schweizer and Müller.[40]

The recent reports on paucity of intrahepatic bile ducts, emphasizing that intrahepatic bile ducts may be present but subject to subsequent inflammatory destruction as seen in early liver biopsy specimens from such patients, render the histopathologic diagnosis of associated EHBDA more complicated. Several other observations confuse the issue. EHBDA itself leads to inflammatory destruction of intrahepatic bile ducts, resulting in paucity of bile ducts. Conversely, the disease in Alagille's syndrome need not be limited to the liver and intrahepatic bile ducts but may also affect the major extrahepatic ducts.[165] A newly described form of sclerosing cholangitis with neonatal onset, leading to disappearance of intrahepatic bile ducts, may result from the same type of bile duct injury as EHBDA, representing a "near-miss" biliary atresia.[189] The main message for the histopathologist from this confusion is that he or she should remain conscious of the evolving nature of the lesions in these obstructive cholangiopathies and realize that histologic recognition of combined intrahepatic paucity and EHBDA in biopsy specimens may be difficult early in life. Interpretation of liver biopsy specimens from such patients requires close collaboration with the clinician.

A further area of controversy with regard to the combination of EHBDA and hypoplasia of intrahepatic bile ducts concerns the nature of the lesion of extrahepatic bile ducts—whether it represents atresia or hypoplasia. Schweizer and Müller mention a 10 per cent incidence of associated intrahepatic paucity of ducts (unspecified how many syndromatic and nonsyndromatic types) in patients with verified true EHBDA based on operative cholangiograms and microscopic studies of excised fibrous remnants.[40]

The New York group reported five children with Alagille's syndrome.[169, 180] Three of these patients had a lesion of the common hepatic duct that was considered hypoplastic not atretic. Hypoplasia was defined as a narrow but patent lumen on microscopic examination (not complete obliteration). Alagille mentions five patients with extrahepatic manifestations of Alagille's syndrome and intraoperative cholangiograms suggesting atresia of proximal extrahepatic ducts.[190] These patients reportedly had patent but hypoplastic extrahepatic bile ducts on histologic examination of excised tissue. The infant described by Kocoshis and co-workers had clinical stigmata of Alagille's syndrome and apparently diffuse EHBDA.[188] Re-examination of the excised fibrous duct remnants led to the conclusion that this child had severe extrahepatic hypoplasia rather than atresia.[180]

American authors recommend avoiding reconstructive surgery and hepatoportoenterostomy in infants with Alagille's syndrome and associated hypoplasia of the extrahepatic bile ducts in order to avoid the debilitating effects of cholangitis related to a hepatoportoenterostomy.[171, 180] In contrast, German authors recommend hepatoportoenterostomy in patients with combined EHBDA and hypoplasia of intrahepatic bile ducts.[40] This opinion is based on the recognition that the evolution to secondary biliary cirrhosis resulting from EHBDA is slower in patients with both EHBDA and paucity of intrahepatic ducts than in patients with isolated EHBDA. This apparently is so because there is no ductular proliferation in patients with paucity of intrahepatic, interlobular bile ducts. Ductular proliferation may be regarded as the pacemaker for the development of secondary biliary cirrhosis.[143] On reviewing the course of 80 patients with Alagille's syndrome,[164] it was noted that the 11 children in whom surgery was performed early because of mistaken diagnosis (EHBDA) or for tentative therapy (cholecystostomy or cholecystojejunostomy) did not have a worse long-term prognosis.

An intriguing finding in patients with Alagille's syndrome and hypoplasia of the common hepatic duct was that changes in bile ducts in the porta hepatis were indistinguishable from those seen in fibrous remnants in EHBDA. Structures of the Gautier types II and III were found.[84, 169] The authors' interpretation was that it remained unclear whether these findings reflected hypoplasia of the extrahepatic biliary tree or focal atresia. This finding raises the suspicion, however, that Alagille's syndrome, like EHBDA, represents a sclerosing cholangitis, which may affect the entire biliary tract—extrahepatically as well as intrahepatically.[165] It also raises the intriguing question about a possible common or related pathogenesis in EHBDA and syndromatic paucity of intrahepatic bile ducts.

Extrahepatic Bile Duct Atresia Associated with Hyperplasia of the Intrahepatic Bile Ducts (Early Severe Forms). Congenital hyperplasia of the intrahepatic bile ducts is known in the English literature as congenital hepatic fibrosis,[191] in the German literature as cholangiodysplastische Pseudo-Zirrhose and "cholangiodysplasia of the hyperplastic type,"[40, 192] and in the French literature as fibroangiodénomatose.[193-195]

The basic lesion of the intrahepatic bile ducts in this entity corresponds to a lack of resorption and remodeling of the excess epithelial structure that is formed in the first embryonic stage of intrahepatic development of bile ducts, that is, the so-called ductal plate.[113] Lack of remodeling into mature bile ducts with persistence of the original embryonic ductal plate structure is termed the *ductal plate malformation*.[196] The bile ducts appear hyperplastic in this condition.

The ductal plate malformation constitutes the basic lesion of congenital hepatic fibrosis, infantile polycystic disease, von Meyenburg complexes, Ivemark's syndrome, Meckel's syndrome, and Caroli's disease.[114, 131] However, ductal plate malformation of the intrahepatic bile ducts may also be associated with EHBDA.[114, 129, 131] In the German literature, this was described recently as "association between EHBDA and cholangiodysplasia of the hyperplastic type" (so-called cholangiodysplastische Pseudo-Zir-

rhose) in 7 of 69 patients with EHBDA (incidence of 10 per cent).[40]

The histologic picture seen on preoperative liver biopsy specimens showed a combination of intrahepatic bile duct hyperplasia (ductal plate malformation) and the typical features of EHBDA—edema, inflammatory infiltrate, and marginal ductular proliferation. In two of these patients, biopsies were performed 10 and 12 months after successful hepatoportoenterostomy. Interestingly, these biopsy specimens showed regression of the portal alterations caused by EHBDA but persistence of the lesion representing intrahepatic bile duct hyperplasia (or ductal plate malformation) apparently identical to congenital hepatic fibrosis.[40] Similar congenital hepatic fibrosis–like patterns were observed by us in 5 of 16 "cured" patients followed-up for four to seven years after successful portoenterostomy (see page 1378) and at the time of Kasai's operation in 10 patients of a series of 41 personally studied patients.[497]

The age of these ten patients at the time of surgical intervention ranged from 30 to 70 days. In all cases, even in the youngest at four weeks of age, histologic features revealed already advanced biliary fibrosis, with serpiginous fibrous bands connecting portal tracts (Fig. 51–18). These patients thus can be considered early severe cases. As a rule, such specimens show no extramedullary hematopoiesis or parenchymal giant cell transformation. The original portal tracts are enlarged and are characterized by excess numbers of branches of the hepatic artery and a relatively small sized portal vein or veins (Fig. 51–19). The portal bile ducts display a peculiar pattern, composed of curved segments of variable length surrounding the portal vessels, assuming the basic configuration of an embryonic ductal plate. In several instances, the portal vessels are surrounded by two and even three concentric structures, corresponding to interrupted and partially remodeled ductal plates (Fig. 51–20). This observation suggests that repetitive formation of ductal plates may occur in successive waves during the first few weeks of life in patients with early severe EHBDA. These ductal plates represent an embryonic type of excess of duct structures, recognized as duct hyperplasia. Several enla.ged portal areas seem to correspond to fused clusters of smaller portal tracts, since multiple aggregates of complex ductal plates surrounding arterial sprouts may be observed in the same large mesenchymal area (Figs. 51–21 and 51–22). Apparently such histologic features result from sectioning through abnormally branching portal tracts: instead of growing by regular tree-like branching, resulting

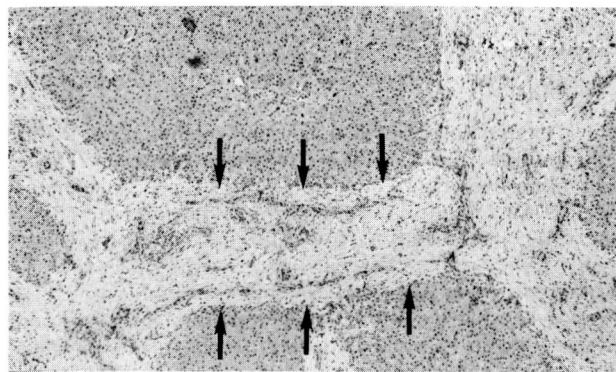

Figure 51–18. EHBDA in infant aged 30 days. Disturbed liver architecture by fusion between large portal areas. The latter contain several bile ducts. Some of these appear in ductal plate configuration (*arrows*). This degree of fibrosis at the age of 30 days represents early, severe EHBDA. Note the resemblance to congenital hepatic fibrosis (hematoxylin and eosin, × 64).

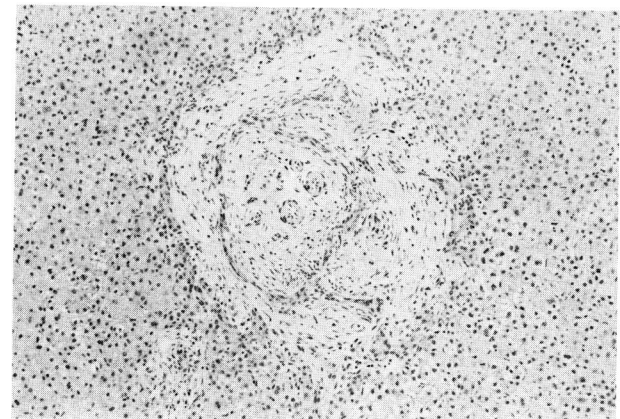

Figure 51–19. EHBDA in infant aged 43 days. Portal tract with bile ducts in ductal plate configuration. Some segments of the ductal plate show epithelial irregularities and involution. A mild ductular reaction occurs at the interphase between portal tract and parenchyma. Note prominent arteries and poorly developed portal vein in the portal tract (hematoxylin and eosin, × 160).

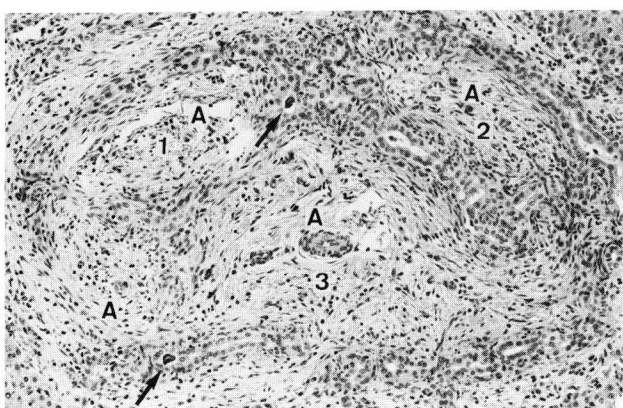

Figure 51–22. EHBDA in infant aged 30 days. Large portal tract with numerous abnormal bile duct segments. In analogy with Figure 51–21, this appearance suggests a fusion between adjacent ductal plates (their presumed centers numbered 1, 2, and 3). Note the presence of arterial branches (A) but poor development (or lack) of portal vein. Bile concrements are present in some parts of the ductal plates (arrows) (hematoxylin and eosin, × 160).

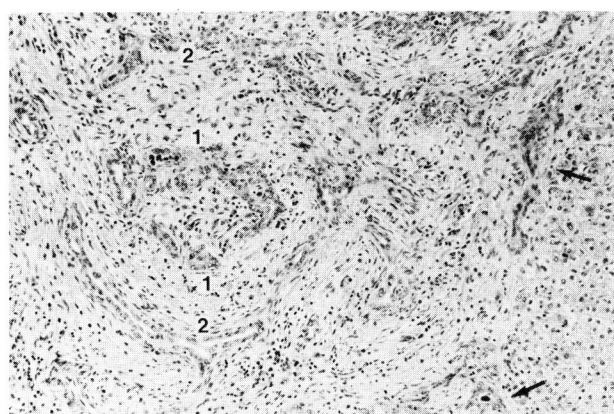

Figure 51–20. EHBDA in infant aged 48 days. Enlarged portal tract with moderately dense inflammatory infiltration. Two concentric rings of bile ducts in ductal plate configuration can be recognized (1,2). Ductular proliferation occurs at the portal-parenchymal interface (arrows) (hematoxylin and eosin, × 160).

in individualized portal tracts separated by intervening parenchyma, the portal tracts give rise to multiple sprouts of smaller portal twigs that remain in close proximity. Such features may indicate a stunted growth of portal tracts, presumably caused by inadequate development (hypoplasia) of the branches of the portal vein. This finding would correlate with the observation that portal pressure is often increased at the time of corrective surgery.[198] The immature ducts with ductal plate configuration appear to be subjected to the same fate as their normal or mature counterparts in untreated or progressive EHBDA. They show variable degrees of necrobiosis in their lining cells and become subject to progressive atrophy and fibrous obliteration (Figs. 51–23 through 51–26).

In summary, the natural course of EHBDA follows a comparable course in both classic and early severe cases. In both instances, progression of the disease is accompanied by variably progressive destruction of intrahepatic segments of bile ducts, either normally shaped, mature ducts in classic cases or immature types of ducts with ductal plate configuration in early severe cases. Table 51–2 compares the histologic features of classic and early severe EHBDA. Reduplication of ductal plates followed by variable degrees of destruction of ducts results in a varying degree of duct

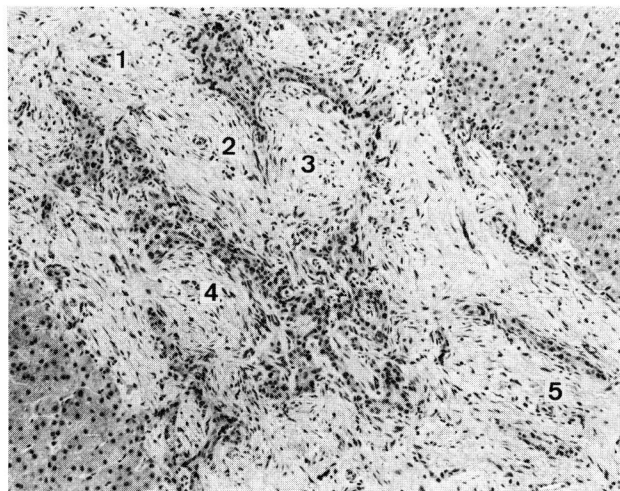

Figure 51–21. EHBDA in infant aged 30 days. Large fibrous area containing numerous irregular bile duct segments. This appearance suggests a close approximation of several portal tracts centered by vessels (1,2,3,4,5) with surrounding incomplete ductal plates (hematoxylin and eosin, × 160).

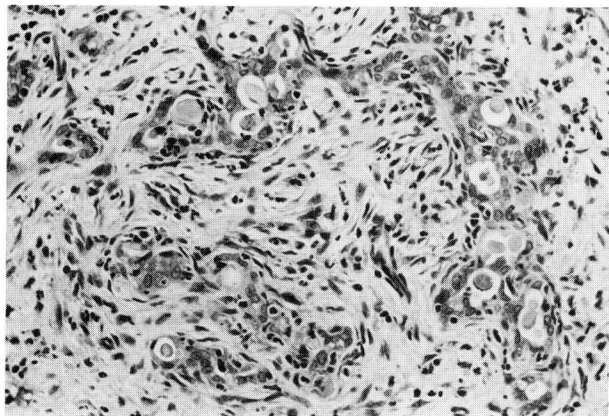

Figure 51–23. EHBDA in infant aged 55 days. Detail of portal tract with moderately dense inflammatory infiltration. Bile duct segments (in ductal plate configuration) show irregular dilation of their lumen with bile concrements and interepithelial inflammatory infiltration (hematoxylin and eosin, × 400).

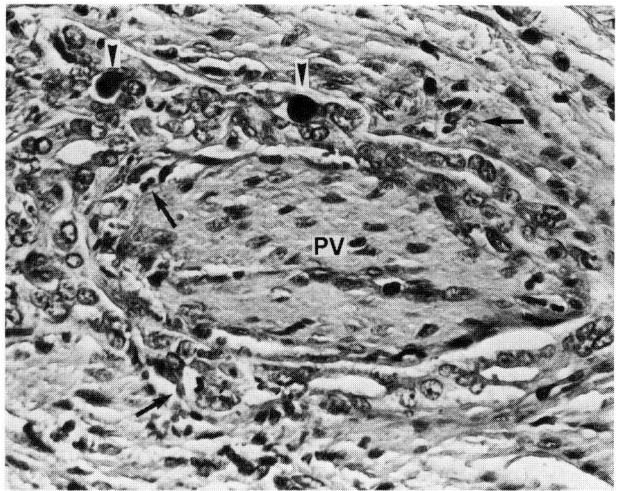

Figure 51–24. EHDBA in infant aged eight weeks. Detail of portal tract with bile duct in ductal plate configuration. Collapsed portal vein in the central connective tissue area (*PV*). The bile duct epithelium shows degenerative changes like anisocytosis and vacuolization. A few polymorphonuclear leukocytes infiltrate near the bile duct structure (*arrows*). Occasional bile concrements are found in the lumen of the ductal plate (*arrowheads*) (hematoxylin and eosin, × 640).

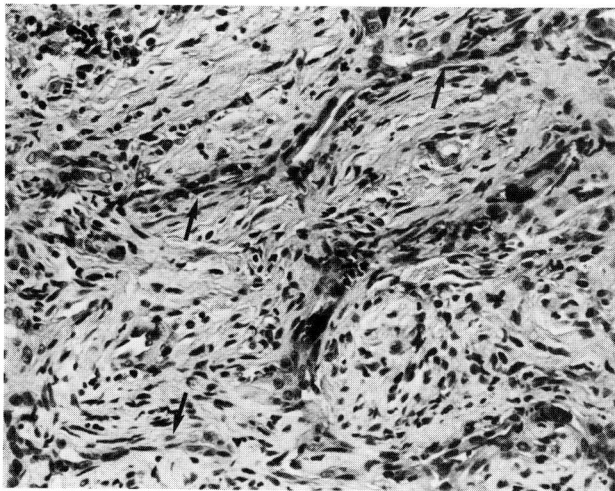

Figure 51–26. EHBDA in infant aged four and one-half months. Necroinflammatory ductal plate. Detail from enlarged portal tract containing bile duct structures in ductal plate configuration. The epithelial lining cells show marked degenerative changes: cellular shrinkage and nuclear pyknosis and extreme flattening in some segments (*arrows*). The surrounding portal connective tissue is highly cellular with moderately dense inflammatory infiltration (hematoxylin and eosin, × 400).

hyperplasia and resemblance to the pattern of congenital hepatic fibrosis. The hypothesis can be proposed that the duct patterns peculiar to early severe cases are responsible for the later development of a congenital hepatic fibrosis–like pattern—especially when intrahepatic duct destruction is slowed down by relief of the extrahepatic component of obstruction after successful portoenterostomy (see page 1378). The histologic features and clinical course of early severe forms of EHBDA strongly support the concept of an antenatal start of the basic disease process of EHBDA; the latter apparently interferes with the normal maturation and remodeling of the embryonic ductal plates and the normal development of portal vein branches.

Etiology and Pathogenesis of Extrahepatic Bile Duct Atresia

Pathogenesis

EHBDA has been considered a congenital anomaly because of failure of recanalization of the bile duct that

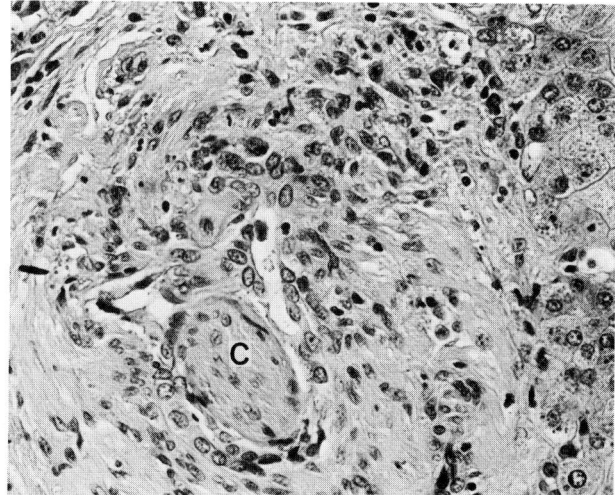

Figure 51–25. EHBDA in infant aged eight weeks. Portal tract containing bile duct in ductal plate configuration with central connective tissue in core (*C*). The lining epithelial cells display pronounced degenerative changes: anisocytosis, atrophy, vacuolization, and pyknosis of nuclei; the epithelium tends to lift from the mesenchyme (hematoxylin and eosin, × 400).

was thought to be occluded by proliferated epithelial cells early in fetal life.[12] The other prevailing concept has been that EHBDA represents a progressive destruction of developed extrahepatic and even intrahepatic bile ducts by an inflammatory process of unspecified nature.[6-8] Blanc emphasized that EHBDA was a condition acquired in utero.[35] He based his conviction on the arguments that (1) there was little in traditional embryology to support the hypothesis of the segmental lack of formation of bile ducts; (2) EHBDA is observed rarely in stillborn infants or in autopsies performed on premature infants in the neonatal period; (3) inflammation and progressive obliteration of extrahepatic ducts were observed in surgical specimens from the hilum of the liver taken from areas in which no ducts were grossly visible; (4) when sections of the liver hilum were taken at autopsy, cord-like fibrous remnants of bile ducts were found, indicating that epithelium had been present and then had disappeared, possibly as a result of some late fetal or neonatal injury; and (5) the disappearance of the lumen of a duct might result from inflammation. Brent added two further factors to Blanc's ideas: (1) there is inconstant documentation for clay-colored stools early in the disease in patients who eventually had EHBDA, and (2) just as intestinal atresia seldom is reported by experimental teratologists, extrahepatic biliary atresia is also a rarity.[35] A further argument in favor of an acquired disease is the discordance of EHBDA in monozygotic twins.[64, 65] Landing proposed the concept of infantile obstructive cholangiopathy based on the histopathologic similarity of the

TABLE 51–2. MAIN HISTOLOGIC FEATURES IN CLASSIC AND EARLY SEVERE FORMS OF EHBDA

	Classic EHBDA	Early Severe EHBDA
Onset of the basic disease process	Neonatal-postnatal	Fetal-antenatal
Bile duct configuration	Tubular ducts	Ductal plates (even multiple concentric ductal plates)
Extramedullary hematopoiesis	Present	None
Parenchymal giant cells	Present	None

liver lesions in patients with neonatal hepatitis, EHBDA, and choledochal cyst.[13, 145] According to this concept, EHBDA is the result of a cholangiopathic process that starts in postnatal life in most cases. The cholangiopathy is due to an inflammatory process, which affects and destroys the liver parenchymal cells as well as the bile duct epithelium, the latter resulting in obliteration of the bile duct lumina. According to the predominance of parenchymal or duct lesions, the disease corresponds to either neonatal hepatitis or EHBDA. The etiology of the parenchymal and duct inflammatory lesions was presumed to be of viral origin. Parenchymal giant cells were considered the morphologic hallmark of a specific disease process. Although the concept of infantile obstructive cholangiopathy had great impact in the subsequent literature on the subject, it should be realized that it represents a hypothesis. Its main merit is in stimulating thought about EHBDA as an acquired, progressive, and destructive process. Additional support for this idea was found in resected specimens of remnants of bile ducts, which became available after the introduction of hepatic portoenterostomy as a surgical treatment of EHBDA. At present, some of the facets of the hypothesis of infantile obstructive cholangiopathy are hardly tenable, and others remain unconfirmed.

The similarity in the histopathologic appearance of the liver in neonatal hepatitis and EHBDA could still be stressed at a time when liver biopsy could not achieve distinction between these two entities in at least 30 per cent of cases.[13, 145] Currently, however, EHBDA is recognizable by liver histopathologic features in 90 to 95 per cent of cases,[40] it is difficult to accept a common etiology for diseases with recognizably different histopathologic lesions.[179] One no longer can consider parenchymal giant cells as the morphologic hallmark of a distinct disease process. It is clear that parenchymal giant cell transformation is observed in neonatal liver diseases of diverse causes.[199]

The hypothesis of a viral etiology, more specifically a viral infection with variable impact on parenchymal cells as well as bile duct cells, remains unrefuted but equally unproved. Somewhat disturbing for the concept of EHBDA as a postnatally acquired disorder is the observation that up to 30 per cent of patients have associated malformations.[40, 76] Reports on the familial occurrence of EHBDA are also disturbing.[54, 56–58] Schweizer and Müller presented a new theory on the pathogenesis of EHBDA,[40] which takes into account most of the observed facts and available information. They propose to distinguish between two types of EHBDA, a fetal-embryonic form and a pre-, peri-, or postnatal acquired form of the disease.

It is proposed that the fetal-embryonic form is characterized clinically by the early onset of jaundice. Without a jaundice-free interval, the physiologic jaundice of the newborn turns into a pathologic, conjugated hyperbilirubinemia in the second or third week of life. The level of conjugated bilirubin in serum starts to rise progressively. An analysis of the clinical records from ten hospitals of 342 children with EHBDA indicates that this type of clinical course is observed in 34 per cent of patients.[40] This putative pathogenetic type of EHBDA is characterized morphologically by complete lack of epithelial bile duct remnants in the hepatoduodenal ligament. In their own four patients with this type of disease, Schweizer and Müller found associated malformations of malrotation in all four patients and ectopic pancreas in the hepatoduodenal ligament in one patient.[40] This constellation of findings has been taken as evidence that the atresia of bile ducts started in the

embryonic or fetal period. The bile duct was missing at the time of birth either because it had not been formed or because it became obliterated completely in the embryonic or fetal period. These patients have a poor prognosis. Postoperative bile flow was not obtained after hepatoportoenterostomy in any of them.

The prenatal, perinatal, or postnatal form of EHBDA is characterized clinically by a shorter or longer jaundice-free period following the physiologic jaundice of the newborn. The jaundice-free period often lasts only a few days; in some cases, however, it may be as long as several weeks. As a rule, the pathologic jaundice develops after a latent period in the third to fifth weeks of life. From a study of 342 children with EHBDA observed in ten different hospitals,[40] it appeared that 66 per cent had had a jaundice-free period with a mean duration of six days. Bile duct remnants were demonstrated regularly in the hepatoduodenal ligament of these patients, in the form of segments with epithelium-lined lumina or epithelial clusters. Associated malformations could not be demonstrated in any of the patients with this form of EHBDA. The constellation of findings in this group suggests that the bile duct was present at birth but that it became obliterated subsequently as an acquired disease. The prognosis in these children is better than in children with the former type of disease. Adequate postoperative flow of bile was achieved in 12 of 16 of these patients.

The ideas of Schweizer and Müller concerning different types of EHBDA is supported by a series of observations. Schweizer and Müller treated a patient with atretic hepatic ducts with hepatoportocholecystostomy, since the common bile duct was shown to be patent.[40] Postoperatively, stools became green, and the serum level of conjugated bilirubin dropped from 12.4 mg/dl to 5.2 mg/dl. Three weeks later, the patient became more jaundiced and passed acholic stools. At a second operation, a complete and microscopically verified occlusion of the cystic and common bile ducts was demonstrated. Thus the obliterative process was progressive and led to complete atresia of the common bile duct over five weeks in this patient. A similar observation was reported by Holder.[200]

The development of pathologic jaundice following a jaundice-free period after the physiologic neonatal jaundice indicates that the obliteration of the extrahepatic duct system occurred only after birth. The experimental findings of Holder and Ashcraft support this view.[201] These authors produced bile duct occlusion experimentally in rabbit fetuses and observed that animals born with occluded bile ducts were jaundiced at birth.

The presence of normal-colored meconium in the majority of cases of atresia also may be considered an argument in favor of the pre- or perinatally acquired nature of EHBDA and against the dysembryonic hypothesis.[182]

In their microscopic study of resected bile duct remnants, Schweizer and Müller often found epithelium-lined luminal segments and epithelial clusters in children operated on in the sixth to eighth weeks of life, whereas no epithelial remnants and only completely obliterated fibrous scars were found in patients operated on later than the 12th week of life. Furthermore, several investigators have reported that bile duct remnants with microscopic lumina are demonstrable in the connective tissue of the porta hepatis in the early stages of EHBDA.[78, 86, 151, 202–209] These remnants become obliterated and usually are no longer demonstrable after the 12th week of life.

Etiology

The etiology of EHBDA remains unknown. The inflammatory destruction of the bile duct could be of infectious, ischemic, or toxic origin.

Infectious Etiology. Since the beginning of this century,[9] the hypothesis has been formulated that EHBDA is the result of an infectious hepatitis resulting in destructive cholangitis. Reports were published of families in which one or more of the siblings succumbed to neonatal hepatitis, and the others died of EHBDA.[60, 61, 210] Some reports mentioned cases of neonatal hepatitis that subsequently evolved to EHBDA.[62, 63] A single report of an association with *Listeria monocytogenes* was published.[211] Cytomegalovirus infection was considered as a possible cause of EHBDA,[212] with subsequent negation,[213] repeated reconsideration,[214, 215] but overall failure to establish a relationship.[40, 42, 216] A similar lack of relationship applies for neonatal herpes simplex infection, and for viral hepatitis type A and type B.[217–220] An association between EHBDA and the non-A, non-B hepatitis virus cannot be investigated adequately for lack of reliable serologic tests and confident morphologic identification of this virus.[221–223]

Infection with the Epstein-Barr virus has been noted in an occasional child with EHBDA.[224] In recent years, interest arose in infection by reovirus type III because of similarities between the lesions of bile ducts caused by this virus in mice and those of human EHBDA.[225] A higher incidence of reovirus III antibodies was detected in patients with EHBDA than in controls;[226, 227] reovirus III immunoreactivity was demonstrated in inflammatory and necrotizing remnants of ducts in a patient with EHBDA,[228, 229] and reovirus III antibody titers were found to be elevated in an infant rhesus monkey with EHBDA.[230] Furthermore, the incidence of serum antibodies to reovirus type III in infants with idiopathic neonatal hepatitis was similar to that of patients with EHBDA.[231, 232] Other groups could not confirm these results,[233, 234] which may result from variation in methods or to different causes of EHBDA in various parts of the world.[235] In conclusion, the proof of a viral cause of EHBDA is still under debate. At present, reovirus type III is the best supported candidate.[236]

Ischemic Etiology. An ischemic cause for EHBDA has been suggested repeatedly. It has been proposed that EHBDA could be related to insufficient vascularization of the biliary tree caused by lack of development of some anastomotic loops or their terminal branches in an anatomic region without vessels of its own.[83] Fibrous obliteration of the common duct could be produced experimentally by inducing ischemia of bile ducts.[237] Experimental atresia of bile ducts was induced in fetal rabbits and sheep by ligation of the hepatic artery or its branches.[238, 239] Definite proof for an ischemic origin in human EHBDA, however, is lacking.[83]

Exogenous Toxic Origin. An association of EHBDA with amphetamine ingestion by pregnant mothers was mentioned,[240] but no causative link could be demonstrated with teratogenic drugs or ionizing radiation.[34, 35] Some epidemiologic studies on EHBDA have revealed a time-space clustering that is compatible with an exogenous toxic origin of the disease.[241]

Endogenous Toxic Origin. Irritation of the bile passages by pathologic bile salts has been proposed.[242] It is of interest that unusual bile acids have been demonstrated in the fetus and newborn infant, as compared with adults, and that the number of bile acids in fetuses and newborns is closer to 40 compared with the 4 bile acids present in adults.[243, 244] Javitt identified a patient with neonatal cholestasis who failed to convert 3β-hydroxy-5-cholenoic acid to chenodeoxycholic acid,[245] raising the possibility that the lack of a C-24-7alpha-hydroxylase is the metabolic basis of persistent cholestasis in some neonates. Abnormal 27-carbon bile acids have been shown to accumulate in bile, serum, and urine of children with paucity of intrahepatic bile ducts.[246, 247] Unusual bile acids, including large amounts of 3β-hydroxy-cholenoic acid, were detected in the sera of children with Alagille's syndrome.[248] Biliary injury resembling that observed in EHBDA has been reproduced by administration of certain bile acids (lithocholic acid, chenodeoxycholic acid) to newborn animals or to their mothers in late pregnancy.[41, 249, 250]

There is a preponderance of EBHDA in girls.[49, 50] And as mentioned already, girls show a greater degree of ductular proliferation than do boys in the early phase of EHBDA, as well as more rapid development of fibrosis.[53] Relevant reported biochemical differences between the sexes that may merit investigation in this regard include the rate of processing of xenobiotics in the hepatocyte's endoplasmic reticulum and differences in the patterns of excretion of bile acids.[251, 252]

Reflux of Pancreatic Juice in the Biliary Tree. A further possible cause of EHBDA is reflux of pancreatic juice into the biliary duct system. This could be favored by abnormal anatomic relationships between the common bile duct and the pancreatic duct in the region of the ampulla of Vater. A high incidence of a congenitally abnormal junction of the common bile duct and pancreatic duct, that is, a long common channel and poorly developed musculature of the sphincter of Oddi, was found in autopsies of patients with EHBDA.[252–255] Reflux of pancreatic juice may cause tryptic digestion of the lining of the bile duct, leading to weakening of the wall and eventually choledochal cyst or repetitive cholangitis with progressive stenosing fibrosis.

Angiofibromatosis. Histologic examination of fibrous remnants of extrahepatic bile ducts and fibrous plaques near the porta hepatis often reveals impressive numbers of blood vessels, which may be arranged in nodular areas with concentric fibrosis, giving the impression of an angiofibromatosis.[40, 81, 85] The suggestion has been made that these vascular anomalies might be causally related to EHBDA.[40]

Experimental Extrahepatic Bile Duct Atresia

Experimental induction of EHBDA has been attempted by several means. Induction of ischemia of the bile ducts in fetal animals was alluded to previously, and as mentioned, it is hypothesized that some cases of biliary atresia and neonatal hepatitis are initiated by an adverse effect of unsaturated monohydroxy bile acids on the fetal and infantile hepatobiliary system.[250] Intravenous injection of lithocholic acid into preterm rabbits produced obstruction within the biliary tract of newborn rabbits. Obstruction was found in the gallbladder in 2 of 16 rabbits born to mothers given lithocholic acid. No instances of obstruction were observed in 28 controls.[41]

A study on fascioliasis showed that a possible mechanism for the enlargement of the common bile duct by the parasite *Fasciola hepatica* was excess L-proline secreted by this parasite.[256] This suggested that L-proline might be a specific growth factor for bile duct epithelium. Intra-abdominal infusion of L-proline in mice led to bile duct enlargement;[257] this finding led the authors to suggest that bile duct hypoplasia and atresia may result from a defect in proline metabolism and that proline administration might possibly be therapeutic during the early phase of EHBDA.[257]

Phenylene-1,4-diisothiocyanate is an antihelminthic drug that produces inflammatory changes in the hepatobiliary system of rats.[258] It has been used in experiments set up to simulate EHBDA.[259] Rats given the drug after birth showed dilation of the extrahepatic bile ducts with inflammation. Animals receiving the drug during the fetal period or just after birth showed stenotic or atretic extrahepatic bile ducts caused by thickening and fibrosis of the wall. The results of this experimental model suggest that the differences in the pathologic features in infantile obstructive cholangiopathy (biliary atresia, neonatal hepatitis, and bile duct dilation) may be the result of variation in the developmental stage in which the pathogenic process is acting. When studying clinical cases of EHBDA, these authors came to the conclusion that the correctable type of EHBDA may be due to the impact of the pathogenic process in later developmental stages than is the case in the noncorrectable type of EHBDA.[259]

Other authors used chemicals that are known to produce intrahepatic ductular proliferation, for example, the aromatic amine p, p¹-diaminodiphenylmethane. This toxin was responsible for so-called Epping jaundice (see Chap. 32).[260] When administered to pregnant rats, this toxin produced ductular proliferation in the mothers but only parenchymal steatosis in the fetal livers.[261]

A number of investigators have studied the physiologic involution and atresia of the bile ducts in the lamprey during metamorphosis as an animal model of human EHBDA.[262-265] The most interesting aspects of this work concern the mechanism of bile duct involution and the adaptation of the liver and the organism to survival without a draining biliary system. An analogous problem of ductless livers is encountered in syndromic paucity of intrahepatic bile ducts (Alagille's syndrome) and in several long-term survivors of hepatic portoenterostomy (see p. 1378).

Clinical Features—Diagnostic Work-up

The goals of diagnostic investigation in infants with protracted hyperbilirubinemia are to define specific treatable entities and to identify the infant who may benefit from surgical treatment. Prompt identification of cholestasis is imperative because this condition is never benign in contrast to unconjugated hyperbilirubinemia.[50] The pathophysiologic characteristics and the clinical and biochemical features of cholestasis are considered in Chapter 12.

Clinical Features

Unfortunately, there is no pathognomonic clinical symptom of extrahepatic biliary atresia, since intrahepatic and extrahepatic forms of cholestasis share numerous clinical and biochemical features. Nevertheless, clinical features may aid in the discrimination between EHBDA and the numerous other causes of cholestasis in early childhood mentioned in Table 51–1.

EHBDA occurs more frequently in girls, usually of normal birthweight, whereas neonatal hepatitis appears to be more common in boys (up to 70 per cent of cases).[266] Familial cases are rare in EHBDA, whereas a familial incidence is noted in 15 to 20 per cent of patients with neonatal hepatitis. Associated polysplenia syndrome pleads in favor of EHBDA.[72]

In EHBDA the stools are consistently acholic, whereas incompletely or intermittently decolored stools indicate incomplete cholestasis of the intrahepatic type. However, intrahepatic cholestasis may also be severe and complete, causing a total lack of bile pigment in stools. In neonatal hepatitis, the pathologic jaundice follows the physiologic hyperbilirubinemia without interval and is already observed in the second week of life. In EHBDA, the neonatal physiologic jaundice also persists in 34 per cent of cases; in contrast, in 66 per cent of patients, an intercalated jaundice-free period of about two weeks occurs between the physiologic jaundice and the appearance of pathologic icterus.[40] Hepatomegaly is often palpable in the first or second week in neonatal hepatitis, whereas liver enlargement becomes detectable usually in the third or fourth week of life in EHBDA.

Pathologic jaundice (indicating cholestasis) should be considered present in a patient with hyperbilirubinemia if the conjugated (direct reacting) fraction composes more than approximately 20 per cent of the total.[50] In EHBDA, direct-reacting bilirubinemia shows a more progressive rise than in neonatal hepatitis. Serum enzymes are not very helpful in discrimination. In the first three months of life, neonatal hepatitis may cause higher elevations of aspartate aminotransferase (AST) and alanine aminotransferase (ALT), whereas γ-glutamyl transpeptidase levels are more abnormal in cases of EHBDA.

Different scoring systems based on clinical and laboratory data have been developed in attempts to better differentiate EHBDA from neonatal hepatitis.[267-269] According to Alagille,[109] clinical features and laboratory data allow a differentiation between EHBDA and neonatal hepatitis in 83 per cent of cases before the age of three months. The following features occur significantly more frequently in infants with neonatal hepatitis than in those with EHBDA: male gender (66 per cent versus 45 per cent), low birthweight (mean 2680 g versus 3230 g), other congenital anomalies (32 per cent versus 17 per cent), onset of jaundice (mean 23 days versus 11 days of age), onset of acholic stools (mean 30 days versus 16 days), white stools during the first ten days after admission (26 per cent versus 79 per cent), and enlarged liver with a firm or hard consistency (53 per cent versus 87 per cent). Other studies confirm the helpful discriminating value of clinical symptoms.[40]

Further Investigation in the Infant with Protracted Conjugated Hyperbilirubinemia

Further investigations in the diagnostic work-up for differentiating extrahepatic from intrahepatic cholestasis are in two general categories: (1) those that measure hepatobiliary secretion, providing information about the patency of the biliary system, and (2) those that attempt to establish a definite diagnosis.

A series of additional investigations have been introduced for differentiating extrahepatic from intrahepatic cholestasis and, hence, for checking the patency of extrahepatic bile ducts. The discriminating value of such tests was evaluated recently.[270]

Alpha Fetoprotein. Zeltzer and co-workers suggested that quantitative estimation of serum alpha fetoprotein (AFP) was of value in distinguishing EHBDA from neonatal hepatitis.[271] The mean serum concentration of AFP in neonatal hepatitis is significantly higher than the mean concentration in infants with EHBDA. Using a sensitive radioimmunoassay method, a peak serum AFP level of greater than 40 μg/ml was diagnostic of neonatal hepatitis. This conclusion was confirmed in later studies that emphasized the diagnostic value of serum AFP levels during the first three months of life.[272] However, in the majority of patients with hepatobiliary disease, there is considerable overlap among the various groups, so discrimination was not possible routinely.

Bile Acids. The serum values of bile acids in infants with biliary atresia or neonatal hepatitis are not increased sufficiently to differentiate these infants from those who are normal (with physiologic cholestasis of the newborn) or to segregate patients according to specific liver disease.[252] Javitt and colleagues proposed that the ratio of chenodeoxycholic acid to cholic acid in serum might help to identify patients with EHBDA, particularly after administration of cholestyramine.[252] Although results of other studies failed to substantiate this observation,[273] the test is still used for differential diagnosis.[40]

Lipoprotein X. Most forms of cholestasis are accompanied by the appearance of an abnormal lipoprotein (lipoprotein X [LPX]) in the serum (see Chap. 5). Cholestyramine-induced stimulation of bile flow decreases the concentration of LPX in serum more in patients with intrahepatic cholestasis than in infants with EHBDA. Poley and co-workers thus recommend the quantitative determination of LPX in serum before and after a ten-day course of cholestyramine as a simple and reproducible screening test for EHBDA.[274] Others use a three-day course of cholestyramine.[40] EHBDA can be diagnosed only if the value of LPX decreases less than 35 per cent. It is agreed that the lack of LPX in the serum excludes EHBDA.[40, 274] Combined testing of LPX and γ-glutamyl transpeptidase, proposed by some to differentiate between EHBDA and intrahepatic cholestasis,[275] is still under debate.[276, 277]

Vitamin E Absorption Test. Decreased serum levels of vitamin E and an increase in peroxide-induced hemolysis were demonstrated in infants with obstructive jaundice. Although the clinical usefulness of an oral vitamin E tolerance test remains to be clarified, it may be used in conjunction with serum levels of vitamin E to assess the need for parenteral vitamin E supplementation.[278] It is not expected to be particularly helpful in the differential diagnosis of cholestasis.[270]

Riboflavin Absorption Test. Children with biliary obstruction have some impairment in the intestinal absorption of the water-soluble vitamin riboflavin, resulting either from alteration in its enterohepatic circulation or from a still unproven role for bile acids in the absorptive process.[279] This test has not gained wide use in the diagnosis of cholestatic syndromes.

Duodenal Intubation for Bilirubin Content. Greene and co-workers recommended 24-hour collection and visual examination of duodenal fluid as an easy, inexpensive, noninvasive, and rapid method for determining complete cholestasis.[280] They concluded that no laboratory measurements are necessary to detect the typically yellow bilirubin pigment and that quantitation is not necessary to differentiate between the presence or lack of bilirubin pigment. In case of a doubtful result, Schweizer and Müller recommend repeating the test after intravenous injection of cholecystokinin.[40] A positive result excludes EHBDA. A negative result allows no discrimination, since intrahepatic cholestasis also may cause complete lack of bile flow into the intestine.

Other authors find that the bilirubin coloration of intestinal secretions is not reliable because it may be secondary to jaundice, with transmucosal leakage of bilirubin, rather than to true bile flow.[281] The use of qualitative thin-layer chromatography to detect differences in bile acid excretion into the duodenum has been helpful in some cases.[282]

Endoscopic Retrograde Cholangiopancreatography. This procedure has been performed successfully and without complication in very few patients with EHBDA.[283, 284] Considerable skill and expertise are required on the part of the endoscopist, and even then serious complications like sepsis, pancreatitis, cholangitis, and rupture of the duodenum occur.[40, 270] Also, the risk of general anesthesia must be calculated. With further technical refinement (i.e., development of instruments designed specifically for pediatric use), this procedure may gain broader applicability.[285-287]

Percutaneous Transhepatic Cholangiography. Percutaneous transhepatic cholangiography (PTC) (see Chaps. 26 and 60) in infants is a feasible procedure and may be easier to perform than endoscopic retrograde cholangiopancreatography (ERCP).[288] Demonstration of the intrahepatic bile ducts is possible in 40 to 45 per cent of cases. Visualization of a patent biliary tract with antegrade flow of contrast medium into the duodenum negates the need for laparotomy.[270]

Laparoscopy. Application of laparoscopy in neonatal cholestatic jaundice has not found wide acceptance, although diagnoses of EHBDA, choledochal cyst, and neonatal hepatitis have been established by laparoscopy.[289] Schweizer and Müller,[40] while admitting the efficacy of laparoscopy, doubt its necessity. Other procedures allow one to diagnose EHBDA with such a high degree of certainty that they can be the basis for deciding on surgical intervention. Laparoscopy has no advantage over a small laparotomy. Both require narcosis and an invasive procedure. However, when EHBDA is confirmed at exploratory laparotomy, the surgeon can proceed by enlarging the incision and performing corrective surgery.

If noninvasive methods do not provide sufficient data for deciding on a laparotomy, percutaneous needle liver biopsy is indicated. Liver biopsy is a less invasive procedure than laparoscopy, needs no general anesthesia, and allows for the diagnosis of EHBDA in 90 to 95 per cent of patients.[40]

Excretion of Rose Bengal Sodium Iodine-131. Rose bengal sodium ^{131}I has been used to assess the patency of bile ducts in infants with cholestatic jaundice.[290] After intravenous injection of 0.5 to 1.0 μCi of rose bengal sodium ^{131}I, the stools are collected over a 72-hour period, and the excreted fraction of ^{131}I is measured. Since rose bengal is excreted with bile, 5 to 10 per cent, at most, of the injected radioactivity is detected in the stools in patients with extrahepatic biliary obstruction. Isotope in stool in these instances is derived from metabolism of the parent compound. If fecal excretion of isotope is less than 10 per cent, one cannot differentiate between EHBDA and intrahepatic cholestasis. In the instance of dubious results, the test can be repeated after a five-day course of cholestyramine or phenobarbital to stimulate bile flow. Biliary excretion of ^{131}I usually increases to greater than 10 per cent in patients with intrahepatic cholestasis but remains less than 10 per cent in patients with EHBDA.[40] Recently, the accuracy of the test was reported to be 91 per cent, with a specificity of 88 per cent.[291] Other authors consider rose bengal scanning to be of only historic interest.[292]

Hepatobiliary Scintigraphy. Major disadvantages of rose bengal sodium ^{131}I for hepatobiliary imaging include the high radiation dose resulting from beta emission, the long half-life of the isotope (eight days), the poor resolution of the images, and a false-positive rate of 20 per cent.[293, 294] The development of technetium 99m (^{99m}Tc)-labeled hepatobiliary imaging agents, particularly of an iminodiacetic acid analog (^{99m}Tc-IDA) is a major advance in imaging of the biliary system. Hepatobiliary scintigraphy with derivatives of ^{99m}Tc-IDA is recommended as a reliable test for differentiating EHBDA from other causes of neonatal jaundice, provided (1) the patient is pretreated with phenobarbital and (2) both hepatic uptake and excretion of tracer are taken into consideration in the interpretation of the scan.[293] Recent studies continue to emphasize the diagnostic utility of hepatobiliary scintigraphy in conjunction with clinical data (birthweight).[295, 296] Septo-optic dysplasia, an unusual clinical syndrome associated with intrahepatic cholestasis, should be recognized to avoid false-positive results.[297]

Ultrasonography. The value of ultrasonography was enhanced by the development of high resolution gray-scale recording and real-time imaging techniques. This safe, simple, and noninvasive procedure should be performed in all infants with cholestatic jaundice.[270] It permits rapid detection of a choledochal cyst,[298] and it is important in identifying associated abnormalities that have an impact on surgical procedures.[299, 300] A recent study indicates that ultrasonographic demonstration of a decrease in gallbladder size following feeding virtually eliminates the possibility of EHBDA.[301] One case has been reported of antenatal sonographic diagnosis of EHBDA.[302]

Liver Histologic Features. As described on page 1357, histopathologic examination of a liver biopsy specimen can provide valuable assistance in determining whether exploratory laparotomy is indicated. Several authors consider the liver histopathologic features the most reliable evidence for EHBDA.[50, 107-109, 303-305]

A liver biopsy specimen can be obtained in most patients by using the Menghini technique of percutaneous aspiration with local anesthesia.[50, 305] Since not all portal tracts may show ductular reaction to the same extent, the biopsy specimen should consist of at least five portal tracts.[40] As mentioned on page 1360, some authors recommend postponing liver biopsy until the sixth week of life in order to give ductular proliferation a chance to develop to a recognizable extent.[40] As discussed before, it appears that the time of onset or the rate of progression of this lesion, or both, varies in different patients.

Diagnostic Work-up

The first goal in the management of the newborn infant with jaundice is prompt identification of cholestasis and early differentiation from physiologic jaundice or jaundice induced by breast milk. The next goal is early recognition of specific, treatable primary causes of cholestasis.[50] The need for early surgical correction in patients with EHBDA leaves the pediatrician with a short time for diagnostic evaluation.

The clinical findings usually allow the experienced pediatrician or surgeon to recognize EHBDA in a number of patients.[109]

A series of additional investigations serve to confirm the diagnosis or to identify other causes of neonatal cholestasis, or both. Table 51-3 represents an example of a recommended staged evaluation of the infant with suspected cholestasis.[157] Similar diagnostic protocols have been published by other authors.[135, 306] Whichever plan of investigation is chosen, the emphasis must be on early diagnosis, as surgical results are related to the age of the infant at operation.[34]

TABLE 51-3. STAGED EVALUATION OF THE INFANT WITH SUSPECTED CHOLESTASIS*

Clinical evaluation (history, physical examination)
Fractionated serum bilirubin or serum bile acid determination
Stool color
Index of hepatic synthetic function (prothrombin time)
Viral and bacterial cultures (blood, urine, spinal fluid)
Viral serology (HBsAg, TORCH) and VDRL titers
Alpha$_1$-antitrypsin phenotype
Thyroxine and thyroid-stimulating hormone
Sweat chloride
Metabolic screen (urine or serum amino acids, urine-reducing substances)
Ultrasonography
Hepatobiliary scintigraphy or duodenal intubation for bilirubin content
Liver biopsy

*Source: Reprinted by permission from Balistreri, W. F.: *Seminars in Liver Disease*, Volume 7, Thieme Medical Publishers, New York, 1987.

Treatment of Extrahepatic Bile Duct Atresia

The prognosis of untreated EHBDA is very poor. Adelman performed a baseline study for comparison with the results of hepatic portoenterostomy.[307] Follow-up information was obtained for 89 infants who underwent surgical exploration without corrective reconstruction for biliary atresia. The rate of apparent cure was 1.1 per cent. The average age at death was 12 months (ranging from 2 months to 4 years). The mean age was 10 months. These findings correlate with previous data,[308] which defined the life span of patients with EHBDA who did not undergo corrective surgery at one to two years.

Hepatic Portoenterostomy

Numerous operative techniques have been applied in order to re-establish drainage of bile in uncorrectable types of EHBDA.[40] Attempts were made to assure drainage through a parenchymal wound by resection of the left lobe of the liver,[309-311] by resection of the quadrate lobe,[312] or by wedge resection of the quadrate lobe.[313] Some surgical techniques included implantation of biliary stents in the liver.[314-316] Other operative procedures attempted to divert bile into hepatic lymph by drainage of the thoracic duct either externally or into the esophagus.[317-320] Alternative methods for lymphatic drainage of bile included connecting lymph nodes of the hepatoduodenal ligament with the intestine.[321] None of these methods was successful because of scarring of parenchymal wounds and obliteration of stents and lymphatic anastomoses.[40] As mentioned in the beginning of this chapter, the hepatic portoenterostomy or Kasai procedure revolutionized the treatment of EHBDA.[30]

The rationale of hepatic portoenterostomy is the presence of patent ducts at the porta hepatis, at least in the early stages of EHBDA. A transection is made in the parenchyma above the fibrous cone of obliterated proximal ducts, and the exposed area of crude liver surface is anastomosed to the intestine (Fig. 51-27). Kasai's unorthodox approach was met with skepticism by surgeons and pediatricians in North America,[31, 202, 322] but nevertheless acquired broad application.[32, 38, 151, 292, 323, 324] It was recognized at an international meeting in 1977 as the standard procedure for treatment of EHBDA and is even recommended now for so-called correctable EHBDA.[79, 325]

One of the frequent and sometimes fatal complications in patients with successful portoenterostomy and adequate drainage of bile is recurrent cholangitis, especially in the

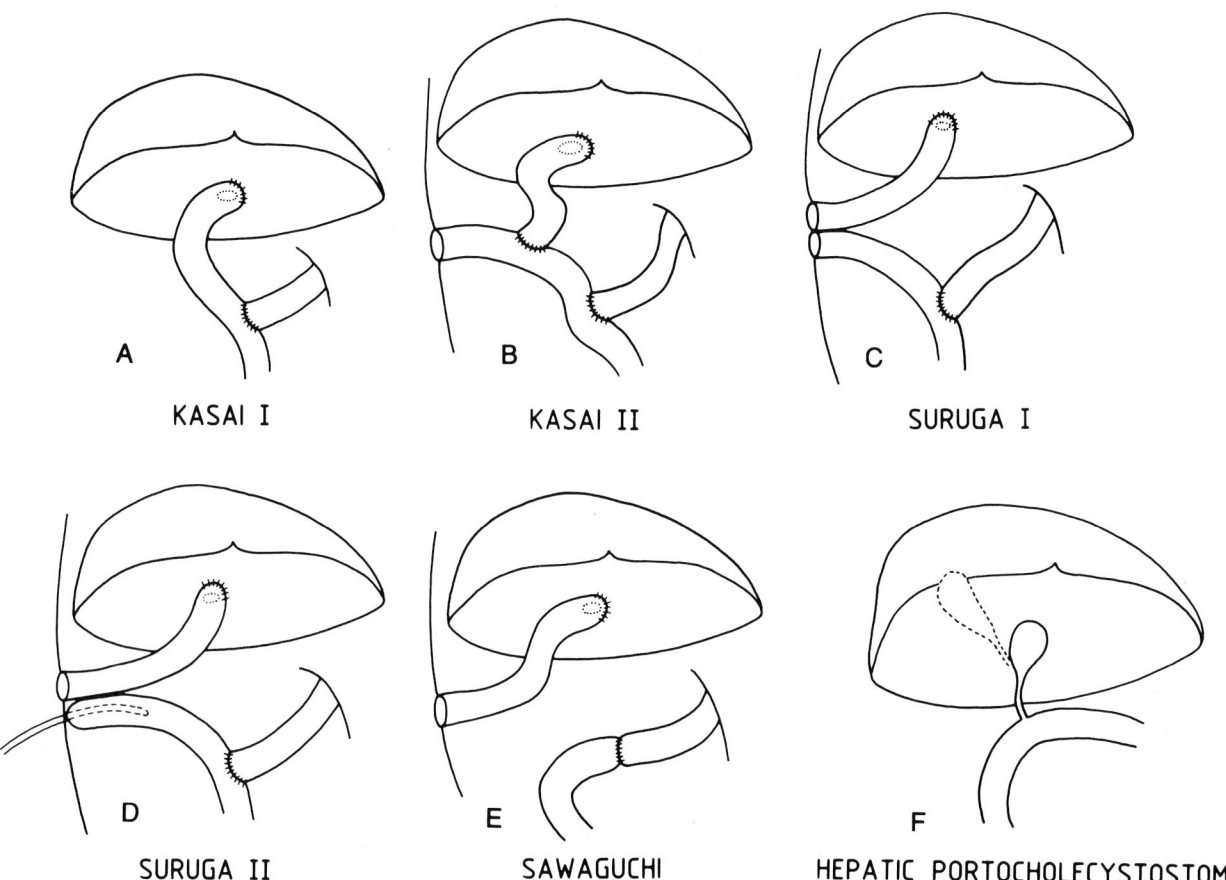

KASAI I   **KASAI II**   **SURUGA I**

SURUGA II   **SAWAGUCHI**   **HEPATIC PORTOCHOLECYSTOSTOMY**

Figure 51–27. The most common surgical procedures used for EHBDA. *A*, Kasai I: the original hepatic portoenterostomy. *B*, Kasai II: double Roux-en-Y hepatic portoenterostomy. *C*, Suruga I: double barrelled hepatic portoenterostomy *D*, Suruga II: refinement of Suruga I procedure to include subcutaneous enterostomy for the distal jejunal limb with the insertion of a jejunal tube. *E*, Sawaguchi: hepatic portojejunostomy with external stoma (requires hospitalization until second operation, substitution of fluid and electrolytes, and reinfusion of bile through gastric intubation). *F*, Hepatic portocholecystostomy.

first two years after operation, with a reported incidence of about 40 per cent.[34, 324] The etiology and pathogenesis of postoperative cholangitis is not entirely clear. It is thought to be due to reflux of intestinal contents from the draining intestinal loop toward the porta hepatis. This has led to several modifications of the original Kasai procedure with construction of external venting conduits. A full discussion of the technical aspects of the various surgical procedures is beyond the scope of this chapter. The most frequently applied techniques (Fig. 51–27) are the Kasai I, the Kasai II,[78] the Suruga I,[326] the Suruga II,[327] and the Sawaguchi procedures and the use of a cutaneous double-barreled enterostomy constructed by the Mikulicz technique.[38, 328, 329] The usefulness of external diversion of bile for preventing the development of cholangitis after portoenterostomy remains a matter of debate.[330] Conversely, in the belief that postoperative cholangitis is not of ascending origin, some surgeons have recommended lymphatic drainage by omentopexy.[40, 76, 331]

Specific modifications of the Kasai operation include the use of microsurgery,[100] extended dissection into the porta hepatis and the use of an intussuscepted ileocolic conduit,[332, 333] or special techniques for revision of the portoenterostomy in case of inadequate bile flow.[334] Recently, there has been a return to the original Kasai procedure in order to avoid complicating the technical performance of liver transplantation at a later date in case of failure of the portoenterostomy.[330, 335]

Hepatic portocholecystostomy (Fig. 51–27) is the method of choice in the approximately 25 per cent of patients with obstruction of the common hepatic duct but with a patent cystic duct, gallbladder, and common bile duct. This type of anastomosis, using biliary conduits for re-establishing continuity, has the advantage of preventing the complications of cholangitis.[336]

The important factors contributing to optimal operative results include (1) an early operation, preferably within 60 days after birth; (2) a precise dissection and adequate transection of the porta hepatis; (3) prevention of postoperative cholangitis; (4) reoperation in indicated cases; and (5) the experience of the surgeon. The earliest reported operation was performed at 76 hours after birth.[302] When the operation is carried out by 60 days of age, excretion of bile is obtained in 82 per cent of the patients. The ability to achieve good postoperative bile flow decreases with the advancing age of the patient. Active bile flow is obtained in only 40 per cent of patients who are older than 90 days at the time of surgery.[337]

A large series of reports has been published on the postoperative complications and their treatment and the overall long-term results.[98–100, 150, 152, 197, 266, 332–334, 336–356] Some of the long-term results of corrective surgery in larger series of patients with EHBDA are summarized in Table 51–4.

Over the years, the results of portoenterostomy have improved gradually. The group of Kasai reported that they performed corrective surgery on 214 patients in the 31-year period from 1953 through 1983.[348] The disease was treated successfully in only 14 per cent of 96 patients in the first 18

TABLE 51–4. LONG-TERM FOLLOW-UP AFTER CORRECTIVE SURGERY FOR EHBDA
(SUMMARY OF SOME LARGER PUBLISHED SERIES)

Authors	Number of Patients Operated on	Duration of Follow-up	Surviving Patients (%)	(Number)	Portal Hypertension (%)
Alagille et al.[39]	121	>5 years	36.6	(44)	52
Kitamura et al.[341]	144	>5 years	26.4	(38)	48.6 (Esophageal varices in 17 patients)
Kobayashi et al.[344]	132	>5 years	29.5	(39)	46 (16 patients of 35 studied)
Altmann and Levy[306]	100	1–9 years	54		
Caccia et al.[342]	90	2–10 years	40.3	(39)	51
Schweizer[355]	Review of 683 patients	>5 years (214 patients)	21	(45)	
Ohi et al.[348]	214	>5 years	33	(70)	>⅓ of patients examined

years of this period. In the next seven years (1971 to 1977), jaundice cleared in 55 per cent of 65 patients, of which 29 patients (45 per cent) were alive without jaundice at the time of reporting (1985). In the last six years, the jaundice cleared in 66 per cent of 53 patients, and 53 per cent of patients were free of jaundice at the time of reporting (1985). It is estimated on the basis of recent operative results that 66 to 80 per cent of patients with EHBDA can be cured if an adequate corrective operation is carried out before 60 days of age and postoperative cholangitis is prevented.[352, 355] Encouraging short-term and long-term results (more than 90 per cent success rate) were reported with a modified Sawaguchi procedure.[351]

Although the hepatic portoenterostomy has improved the outcome of patients with EHBDA, it has provided a population with unique health problems, including recurrent cholangitis, nutritional and growth deficiencies, delayed development, portal hypertension, osteomalacia and osteoporosis, and social and psychiatric difficulties.[357] These complications usually respond to aggressive medical therapy and support, which are detailed in recent reviews.[50, 358] However, even successful portoenterostomy is not tantamount to cure.[39, 292] It appears particularly difficult to determine fully and accurately the ultimate outcome in patients with EHBDA because the short-term or midterm cure does not clearly reflect the eventual prognosis of EHBDA. These difficulties are reflected in the various terms used by pediatric surgeons, such as *cure expected* or *no jaundice* or *more than five years survival*.[100] Perhaps the most disappointing aspect of the hepatic portoenterostomy is the failure of hepatic parenchymal disease to resolve in many patients. It is the exceptional patient who shows histologic improvement after operation.[18, 40] Even in patients with correctable EHBDA, that is, those with patency of the proximal extrahepatic bile ducts, there is a mortality rate of 14.6 per cent in patients in whom there was complete success in establishing drainage of bile. Thus re-establishment of bile flow does not equate with cure in EHBDA.[49] The histopathologic features of hepatic parenchymal disease after hepatoportoenterostomy are discussed further on.

Liver Transplantation

Human orthotopic liver transplantation was pioneered by Starzl in 1963.[359] Early pediatric cases included patients with extrahepatic biliary atresia and concomitant hepatocellular carcinoma.[360] Metabolic liver diseases and biliary atresia were the major indications for liver transplantation in the pediatric age group, and results of liver transplantation have always been better in children than in adults.[361, 362] However, even after so-called successful trans-

plantation, the quality of life often was degraded by the side effects of high-dose steroid therapy, for example, cushingoid facies, growth retardation, and osteoporosis. Despite the continued efforts over the last 20 years to improve the survival and the quality of life after organ transplantation, real progress came only after the discovery and clinical use since 1980 of cyclosporine.[363, 364]

In pediatric liver transplantation, the one-year survival rate improved from 40 to 70 per cent with cyclosporine and low-dose steroid therapy.[365] Infectious complications became less frequent and more treatable than was true with conventional immunosuppression therapy.[363] Virtually all survivors are clinically well and living at home, but medical and psychologic problems remain in several patients.[366] Specific aspects of patient selection, treatment, and complications are discussed in a separate chapter on liver transplantation (see Chap. 55).

A number of centers in the world have started hepatic transplantation programs,[362] and results continue to be promising.[365, 367–370] Several authors consider hepatic portoenterostomy to be the treatment of choice for patients with EHBDA.[40, 351, 355] Even in less successful cases, this procedure may allow survival of the patient until a more appropriate age for liver transplantation is reached. However, the observation of more than minor complications in many patients with long-term follow-up after successful portoenterostomy, and the improvement of the results of liver transplantation in the cyclosporine era, may change the choice of preferential treatment in the years to come, although a shortage of donor livers will impose restrictions. Successful liver transplantation represents a more complete treatment of EHBDA, since it not only assures re-establishment of bilioenteric continuity but also replaces a diseased organ with a healthy one. One of the major complications of liver transplantation is transplant rejection, which may cause destruction and disappearance of intrahepatic bile ducts.[371–374]

Liver Alterations After Hepatic Portoenterostomy

There is no doubt that some patients with EHBDA are cured by hepatic portoenterostomy. Kasai's patient with the longest survival is older than 25 years of age and is well. However, real cure seems to be limited to a minority of patients who undergo surgery. Most reports on long-term follow-up mention some abnormalities in liver enzymes and serum bile salt levels, as well as hepatomegaly, splenomegaly, and often portal hypertension, occasionally with severe bleeding from esophageal varices.[18, 34, 39, 150, 292, 339, 340, 342, 343, 345, 349, 375–381]

The time of appearance of complications like cirrhosis and portal hypertension is variable in different patients. In surgical reports, the complication of cirrhosis with portal hypertension is usually ascribed to the occurrence of repetitive episodes of cholangitis. However, there is a growing probability that the more serious long-term hepatic complications after portoenterostomy reflect the relentless, slow progression of the intrahepatic component of the basic disease process of EHBDA. As formulated by Landing in 1974,[13] EHBDA indeed represents a progressive inflammatory destruction of the entire biliary tree—intrahepatic as well as extrahepatic. The inflammatory destructive process may resolve at any stage and at any level,[13] which probably accounts for some reported instances of spontaneous cure in EHBDA.[18] Hepatic portoenterostomy seems to exert a beneficial effect on the progression of the intrahepatic lesion, not so much by arresting the basic disease process as by eliminating the superimposed obstruction caused by progressive obliteration of the extrahepatic bile ducts. This relief of obstruction saves the patient from rapid deterioration to the stage of secondary biliary cirrhosis and is responsible for the increased survival of patients whose prognosis is extremely poor without treatment.[307] However, the basic inflammatory process affecting the intrahepatic branches of the biliary system continues to operate in many patients, albeit at variable speed, similar to destruction of intrahepatic bile ducts in adults with primary biliary cirrhosis or primary sclerosing cholangitis. One report cites a patient who had end-stage cirrhosis at the age of 33 years after a portoenterostomy was performed in infancy.[382] The following section summarizes the major histologic findings in follow-up studies after hepatic portoenterostomy and ends with an attempt at interpretation of the lesions observed.

Description of Histologic Findings

Development of Bile Duct Cysts and Bile Duct Dilation Mostly After Unsuccessful Portoenterostomy. In patients with inadequate postoperative flow of bile or attacks of cholangitis, the development of large bile duct cysts has been demonstrated, possibly as a result of the operative procedure.[206, 383, 384] Dilation of intrahepatic bile ducts was observed in a postmortem study of patients who died after a portoenterostomy with an unsuccessful postoperative course.[385] The pathogenesis of development of intrahepatic bile duct dilation and cyst formation remains unclear. The possibility of associated Caroli's disease should be considered.[300, 351]

Improvement in the Histologic Appearance of the Liver After Successful Portoenterostomy. In several reports on histologic studies of liver specimens from patients followed-up after hepatic portoenterostomy,[377, 386, 387] an improvement in the hepatic histologic alterations was observed in some patients. Such improvement included a decrease in parenchymal and ductular cholestasis, in ballooning and damage of liver cells, in the degree of infiltration by inflammatory cells, and in periportal fibrosis.

Progressive Liver Damage Observed in Long-term Follow-up After Successful Portoenterostomy. Successful portoenterostomy in this context implies adequate postoperative flow of bile, disappearance of jaundice, and a patient in generally good condition. These patients may have episodes of cholangitis, especially during the first postoperative year, and portal hypertension develops later in a substantial number of these patients. In addition, a variety of histologic abnormalities have been observed in several

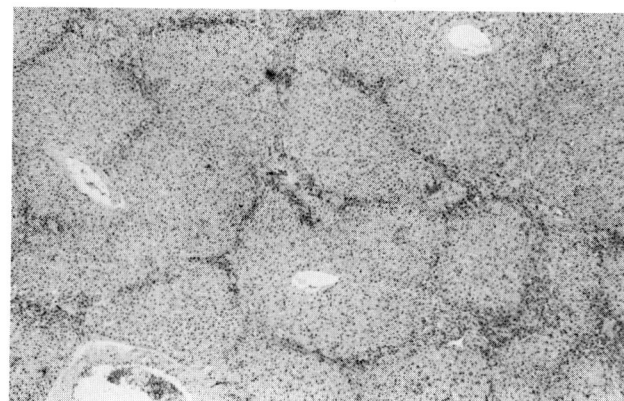

Figure 51–28. EHBDA. Follow-up liver biopsy four and a half years after successful portoenterostomy (no jaundice). The overall liver architecture is preserved, but the lobules are accentuated by delicate fibrous extensions between adjacent portal tracts, simulating the normal appearance of pig's liver (hematoxylin and eosin, × 64).

studies of such patients who were followed for five years and longer.[150, 197, 343, 386, 388]

MILD PERIPORTAL FIBROSIS. In some patients, only mild periportal fibrosis is observed, with virtual lack of inflammatory infiltration (Fig. 51–28). The lobular parenchyma appears normal. This pattern was observed in 4 of a series of 16 studied cases.[197] In some cases, however, careful analysis often reveals a number of additional abnormalities. Many portal tracts are large and densely collagenized. The histologic appearance leaves the impression that a number of smaller terminal portal tracts are missing. An occasional portal tract lacks an identifiable interlobular duct (Fig. 51–29). The interlobular ducts may be ensheathed in a hyaline layer, which is not identical to the laminated concentric periduct fibrosis of classic chronic cholangitis. On PAS-diastase stained sections, the basement membrane of the ducts is more prominent than normal. A few small foci of small ductules usually are found close to or even inside the lobular parenchyma. Almost invariably, one finds some periductular edema and an occasional neutrophilic polymorph, indicating a minimal degree of cholangiolitis.

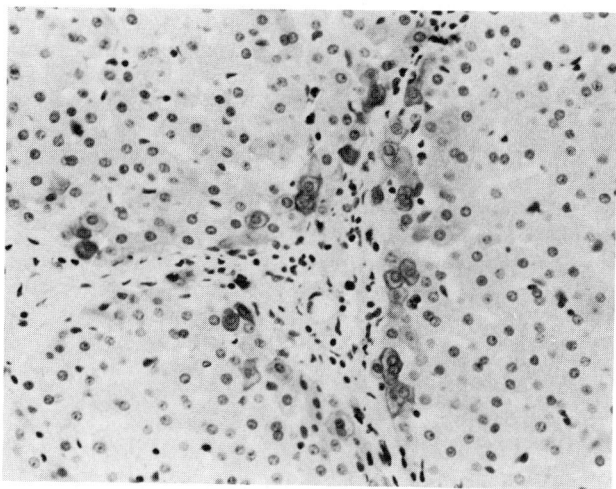

Figure 51–29. EHBDA. Follow-up liver biopsy four and a half years after successful portoenterostomy. Same patient as in Figure 51–28. An occasional portal tract is found in which an interlobular bile duct is missing. The parenchymal cells adjacent to the portal tract show positive staining for bile duct–type cytokeratins, indicating a mild, smoldering cholestasis. (Immunoperoxidase staining with rabbit polyclonal antihuman cytokeratin [Dako Corporation, Santa Barbara, CA]. Counterstained with hematoxylin, × 400.)

Rhodamine staining for copper usually yields negative results. On preparations immunostained for an epidermal type of keratin or TPA, the foci of ductular proliferation are revealed to a better extent. Moreover, the periportal hepatocytes (acinar zone I) stain positive for keratin or TPA, indicating an early stage of biliary metaplasia and revealing a state of latent cholestasis (Fig. 51–29).[128, 130] Such histologic features are observed in patients who are cured clinically. They have normal levels of bilirubin in sera but often have a mild rise in alkaline phosphatase levels.

When the periportal fibrosis is somewhat more pronounced, the lobular pattern of the liver is accentuated, and the histologic appearance at first glance reminds one of the normal histologic appearance of the pig liver.

CONGENITAL HEPATIC FIBROSIS–LIKE PATTERN. In clinically cured cases, without jaundice or overt cholestasis, the liver histologic appearance may resemble that of so-called congenital hepatic fibrosis (Fig. 51–30). This pattern was observed in 5 of 16 cases studied.[197] The congenital hepatic fibrosis–like histologic appearance is characterized by large portal tracts with dense collagenized stroma and periportal fibrosis. The portal areas of connective tissue contain an increased number of bile ducts, occasionally showing curved shapes and even typical circular or nearly circular patterns of ductal plates (Figs. 51–31 and 51–32). Closer analysis reveals features that are not typical of the classic descriptions of congenital hepatic fibrosis. Several segments of bile ducts show necrobiosis of lining cells, with acidophilic condensation of cytoplasm and pyknosis of nuclei. This lesion may affect a few single cells scattered in the section, or the epithelial damage with "melting down" of the bile duct lining may be extensive. Several segments of bile duct are surrounded by thick, hyaline, collagenous sheets (Fig. 51–33). Minute foci of intralobular ductules, which are often, but not necessarily, at the periphery of the parenchyma, reveal discrete signs of cholangiolitis. Rhodamine staining for copper yields negative results or minimal positivity. Immunostaining for keratin or TPA emphasizes the duct hyperplasia and shows to better advantage the foci of ductular reaction, but also reveals the keratin positivity of periportal hepatocytes (Fig. 51–34). A striking feature often noted in such cases is the hypoplastic size of portal vein branches in the portal tracts. Medial smooth muscle cells develop in the wall of the portal vein branches, correlating with the degree of portal hypertension.[389] A decrease in the

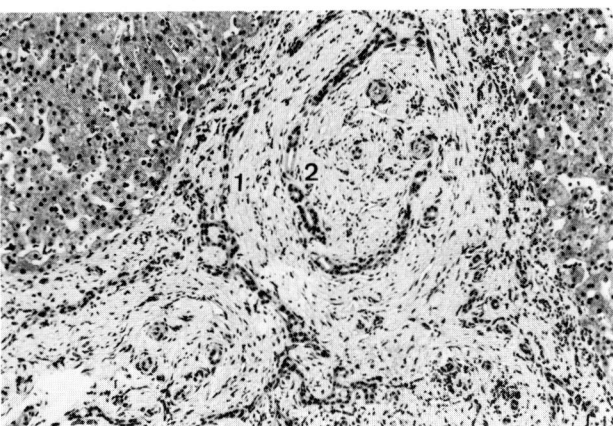

Figure 51–31. EHBDA. Follow-up liver biopsy four years after successful portoenterostomy in same patient as in Figure 51–30. Congenital hepatic fibrosis–like appearance. The ducts in the portal tracts and connecting septa often appear in ductal plate configuration. Double concentric ductal plates are often found (1,2). Compare with ductal plate duplication in early stages (see Figure 51–20) (hematoxylin and eosin, × 160).

caliber of the main portal vein also was recently observed by abdominal sonography in patients with poor hepatobiliary function.[390]

All patients showing a congenital hepatic fibrosis–like picture on follow-up biopsy specimens showed ductal plate malformation of the intrahepatic bile ducts at the time of portoenterostomy.

SECONDARY BILIARY FIBROSIS AND CIRRHOSIS. In a proportion of clinically cured cases, histologic study of late follow-up biopsy specimens reveals extensive fibrosis, with numerous portal-portal connective tissue septa. In some patients, the picture is that of secondary biliary cirrhosis. The borderline between biliary fibrosis and biliary cirrhosis is unclear, since longstanding cholestasis leads to increasing fibrosis with predominant localization in zone I. Only in later stages does further development of portal-central septa occur, realizing the complete picture of true biliary cirrhosis.[143] Reports in the literature do not always distinguish between advanced biliary fibrosis and secondary biliary cirrhosis.[343, 391] For this reason, and because of the admitted difficulty in making this distinction clearly on small speci-

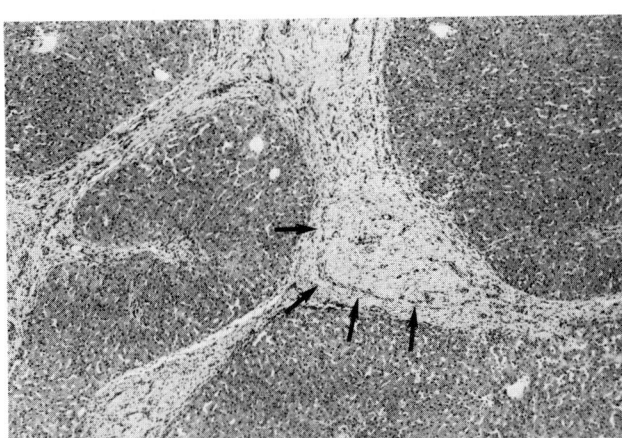

Figure 51–30. EHBDA. Follow-up liver biopsy four years after successful portoenterostomy (no jaundice). The overall histologic pattern corresponds to that of congenital hepatic fibrosis. Portal tracts are connected by broad connective tissue bands, containing numerous bile ducts. Some bile ducts appear in ductal plate configuration (*arrows*). See also Figure 51–31 (hematoxylin and eosin, × 64).

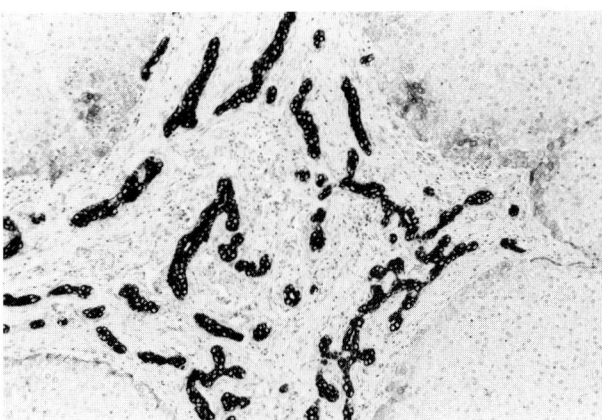

Figure 51–32. EHBDA. Follow-up liver biopsy four and a half years after successful portoenterostomy (no jaundice). Congenital hepatic fibrosis–like pattern. Immunostaining for bile duct cell markers (TPA) reveals better the numerous bile duct structures, their similarity to ductal plates, and sometimes double concentric layering. Periportal hepatocytes show weakly positive staining, indicating chronic, mild cholestasis. See also Figure 51–34. (Immunoperoxidase staining for tissue polypeptide antigen (TPA). Counterstained with hematoxylin, × 160.)

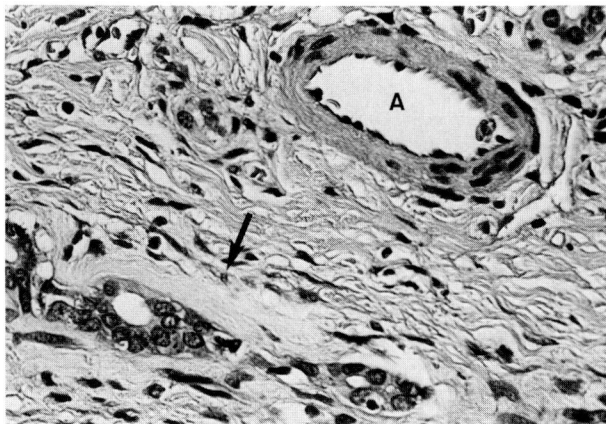

Figure 51–33. EHBDA. Follow-up liver biopsy four years after successful portoenterostomy (no jaundice) in same patient as in Figures 51–30 and 51–31. Congenital hepatic fibrosis–like appearance. This higher magnification shows that some of the bile duct segments are encased by broad sheets of fibrillar fibrosis (sclerosing cholangitis) (arrow) hematoxylin and eosin, × 640; A = hepatic artery.

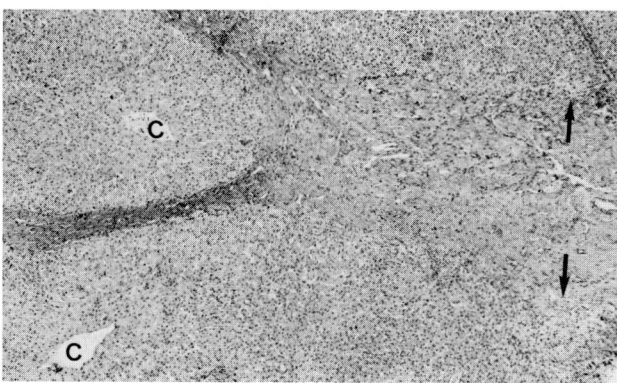

Figure 51–35. EHBDA. Follow-up liver biopsy four years after successful portoenterostomy (no jaundice). Acholangic biliary fibrosis. Broad fibrous septa connect adjacent portal tracts. The basic lobular architecture is preserved: parenchymal lobules are centered by draining veins (C). There is total lack of bile ducts inside portal tracts and septa. Occasional foci of ductular proliferation occur at the connective tissue—parenchymal interphase (arrows), indicating a very mild cholestatic state. Compare with Figures 51–36 and 51–37 (hematoxylin and eosin, × 64).

mens of tissue, advanced biliary fibrosis and biliary cirrhosis are treated together. An additional reason for emphasizing this problem is to warn the reader against accepting too easily the concept of reversibility of true biliary cirrhosis, an impression that may arise from occasional reports.[392, 393]

In patients with advanced biliary fibrosis, the basic pattern of connective tissue is similar to that described in the congenital hepatic fibrosis–like pattern. There is predominance of connective tissue septa from portal area to portal area (Fig. 51–35). The parenchyma appears as garland-shaped masses between these septa. The portal vein branches in the portal tracts appear hypoplastic. There may be an increased number of dilated lymphatic channels.[388] They are recognizable by positive staining with Ulex Europeus lectin and the negativity for factor VIII–related antigen of their lining endothelium.[197] Lymphocytic infiltration may be present, especially in the periphery of the portal tracts; however, usually it does not infiltrate the parenchyma (lack of or only little piecemeal necrosis). A striking feature is the lack of interlobular bile ducts (Fig. 51–35). This stage corresponds to acholangic biliary fibrosis or cirrhosis, or both. This pattern was observed in 2 of a

series of 16 personally studied patients.[197] Several small foci of cholangiolitis can be found in the form of small clusters of ductules near to or even inside the parenchyma, associated with some interstitial edema and a rare neutrophilic polymorph (Fig. 51–36). In some cases, the loss of ducts is not total. An occasional portal tract still contains an interlobular bile duct, showing signs of involution and necrobiosis of its lining cells. Such ducts may have normal tubular shape or may exhibit a ductal plate configuration. Occasionally the involuting duct is surrounded by lymphocytes (lymphocytic cholangitis).[394, 395] This pattern of paucity of ducts was observed in 5 of 16 personally studied patients.[197]

The presence of some remaining ducts or ductal plates represents a pattern that is intermediate between the picture described as congenital hepatic fibrosis–like and the pattern classified as acholangic biliary fibrosis or cirrhosis, or both. Even in instances of a total lack of interlobular bile ducts, there is no bilirubinostasis either in the parenchyma or in the occasional remaining ducts or ductules.

Rhodamine staining for copper may be negative, or may show some accumulation of copper in peripheral hepatocytes, especially in specimens with complete loss of

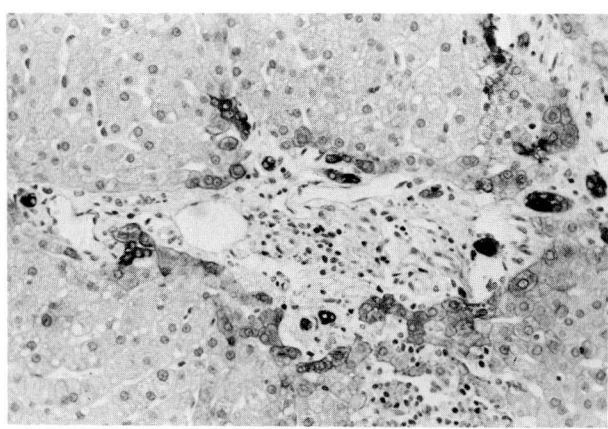

Figure 51–34. EHBDA. Follow-up liver biopsy four years after successful portoenterostomy (no jaundice) in same patient as in Figures 51–30 and 51–31. Immunostaining for bile duct cell markers reveals positive reaction in periportal hepatocytes and ductules, suggesting an early stage of ductular metaplasia of zone 1 hepatocytes. This finding indicates mild, smoldering cholestasis. (Immunostaining for TPA. Counterstained with hematoxylin, × 400.)

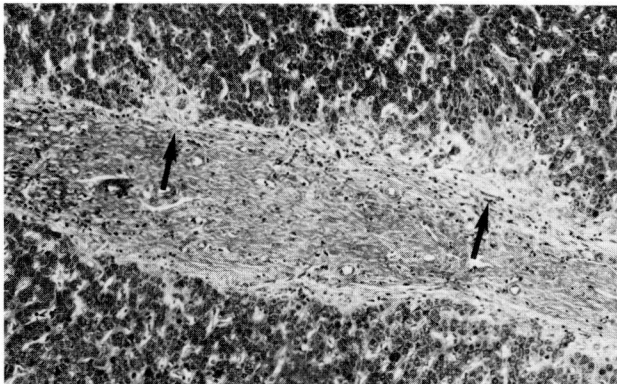

Figure 51–36. EHBDA. Follow-up liver biopsy four years after successful portoenterostomy (no jaundice). Acholangic biliary fibrosis. Detail of fibrous septum linking portal tracts. There are no bile ducts inside the portal tract and septum. Higher magnification and use of trichrome stain reveal to a better extent small foci of ductular proliferation at the septal-parenchymal interface (arrows). Compare with Figures 51–35 and 51–37. These alterations indicate a mild, smoldering cholestatic state (Masson's trichrome stain, × 160).

ducts. Immunostaining for the epidermal type of keratin or for TPA emphasizes the decreased number of ducts, reveals the foci of ductular proliferation much better than routinely stained histologic sections, and shows positive keratin staining of peripheral hepatocytes and of cholestatic liver cell rosettes (Fig. 51–37). The latter feature, together with the foci of cholangiolitis, attests to the existence of a mild, smoldering state of cholestasis.

LIVER LESIONS OBSERVED NEAR THE TIME OF CLINICAL DETERIORATION IN PATIENTS WITH LONG-TERM CLINICAL CURE. Some patients remain jaundice-free for years after successful portoenterostomy. In some, jaundice reappears after four to seven years. Biopsies performed at this time show active biliary disease superimposed on one of the patterns described on page 1378. There is seldom periportal fibrosis, more often a congenital hepatic fibrosis–like pattern or a biliary fibrosis-cirrhosis pattern. In a series of 21 personally studied patients with long-term follow-up (four to seven years), 16 patients were jaundice-free.[197] However, five other patients showed clinical signs of deterioration with appearance of jaundice. The follow-up liver specimens of these children showed lesions of acholangic biliary fibrosis or cirrhosis, or both, displaying the active features described further on.[197]

Besides the features described on page 1378, these specimens are characterized by a diffuse borderline between the area of connective tissue and the remaining parenchyma. The irregularity in outline is caused by so-called biliary piecemeal necrosis (Figs. 51–38, 51–39, 51–40).[124, 128, 396]

The peripheral parenchymal cells are dissociated by interstitial edema and infiltration with inflammatory cells, including mononuclear and polymorphonuclear leukocytes.

The dissociated liver cell plates may show features of ductular metaplasia or cholate stasis, or both (Figs. 51–40 and 51–41).

Bilirubinostasis is found in the parenchyma, usually as intercellular plugs of bile and bilirubin staining of hypertrophic Kupffer cells and macrophages. Some foci of parenchymal cells show features of feathery degeneration.[124]

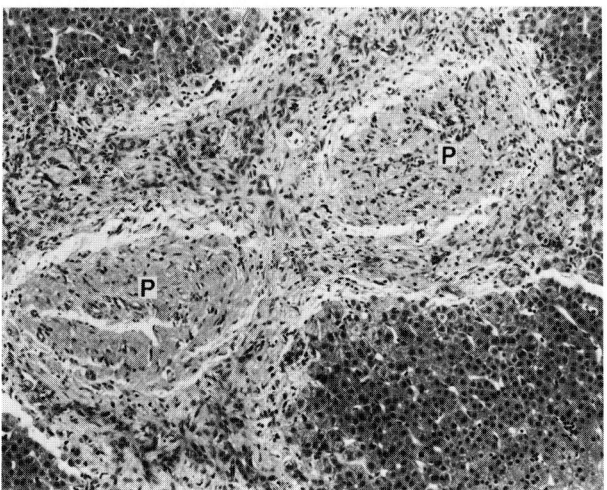

Figure 51–38. EHBDA. Follow-up liver biopsy five years after portoenterostomy. The patient was free of jaundice for five years but recently a rise of bilirubin in serum developed. The figure shows two interconnected portal tracts (P) composed of dense fibrous tissue without interlobular ducts. They are surrounded by a layer of loose connective tissue carrying numerous ductules. The connective tissue–parenchymal interface is irregular because of edema, ductular proliferation, and inflammatory infiltration (so-called biliary piecemeal necrosis). This alteration indicates active biliary disease with progressive cholestatic changes (hematoxylin and eosin, × 160).

Cholestatic liver cell rosettes are present to a variable extent.[128] The concurrent presence of these features indicates active (instead of slowly smoldering) biliary disease, with more severe degrees of progressive cholestatic lesions.

The portal tracts may still contain an involuting bile duct in tubular or ductal plate configuration, showing atrophy and epithelial involution and occasionally lymphocytic infiltration (lymphocytic cholangitis).[394, 395] Examples may be found of lymphoid aggregates only, possibly at the site of a pre-existing but now vanished duct.

Interpretation of Histologic Findings

In patients with an unsuccessful postoperative course, the liver lesions correspond to those of the underlying liver

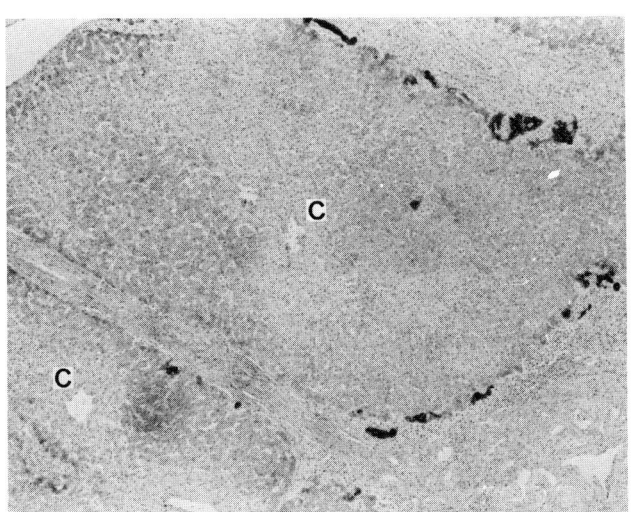

Figure 51–37. EHBDA. Follow-up liver biopsy four years after successful portoenterostomy (no jaundice). Acholangic biliary fibrosis. Fibrosis septa connect adjacent portal tracts; parenchymal lobules carry central draining veins (C). There are no interlobular ducts inside portal tracts and septa. Foci of ductular proliferation at the connective tissue–parenchymal interface are better revealed by positive staining for bile duct cell markers. Compare with Figures 51–35 and 51–36. (Immunostaining for TPA. Counterstained with hematoxylin, × 64.)

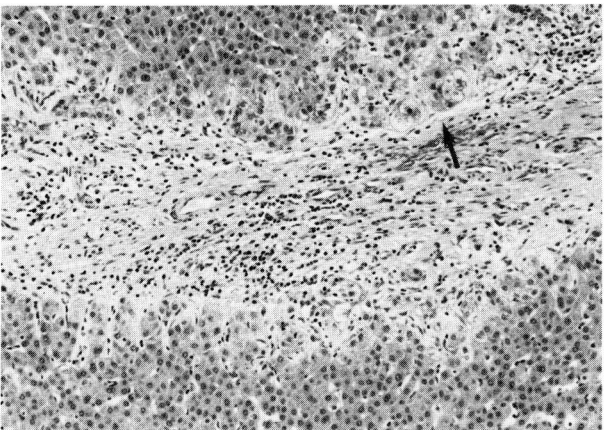

Figure 51–39. EHBDA. Follow-up liver biopsy five years after portoenterostomy. The patient was free of jaundice for five years, but recently a rise of bilirubin in serum developed. Same patient as in Figure 51–38. The figure shows a fibrous septum with moderately dense lymphocytic infiltration. There are no interlobular bile ducts. The septal-parenchymal interface is irregular because of edema, ductular proliferation, and inflammatory infiltration (biliary piecemeal necrosis). Several periseptal hepatocytes appear swollen and coarsely granular (so-called cholate stasis) (arrow). These features indicate active biliary disease with progressive cholestatic changes (hematoxylin and eosin, × 160).

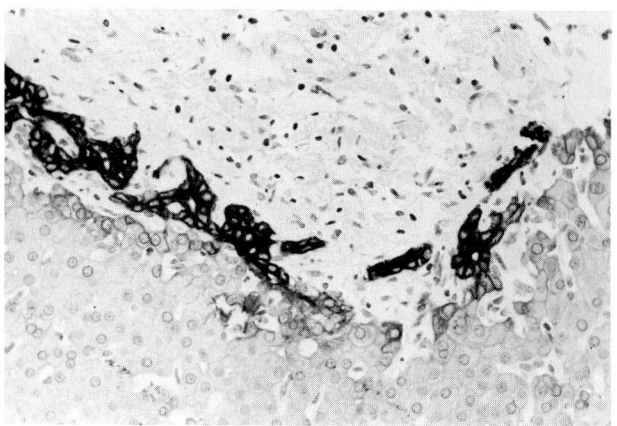

Figure 51–40. EHBDA. Follow-up liver biopsy five years after portoenterostomy. The patient was free of jaundice for five years, but recently a rise of bilirubin in serum developed. Same patient as in Figures 51–38 and 51–39. Detail of septal-parenchymal interface. Immunostaining for bile duct cell markers reveals better the ductular reaction and the moderately positive staining of periseptal hepatocytes. Positive staining is most marked in the periphery of these hepatocytes. (Immunostaining for TPA. Counterstained with haematoxylin, × 400.)

disease, possibly aggravated by postoperative complications of ischemia, renewed obstruction, and especially acute cholangitis.

In patients with a successful postoperative course, the variety of liver lesions observed allows the formulation of the following hypothesis. The core of the hypothesis is not new and refers to EHBDA as a progressive destructive inflammation of intrahepatic and extrahepatic bile ducts.[13, 37] The hypothesis further implies that the underlying basic disease process continues at its own pace and during its own and individually determined period of time in spite of successful surgery. The effect of portoenterostomy has been to relieve the patient of extrahepatic obstruction and its own disastrous effects, but it leaves the patient with the intrinsic intrahepatic disease of bile ducts (the basic disease process).[37] Apparently, the basic disease process may resolve spontaneously, resulting in a patient with complete clinical and histologic normalization. There is not much histologic documentation of this course of events. In some patients, the intrahepatic disease of bile ducts, with its accompanying inflammation and fibrosis, continues for a while, resulting in some periportal fibrotic scarring before

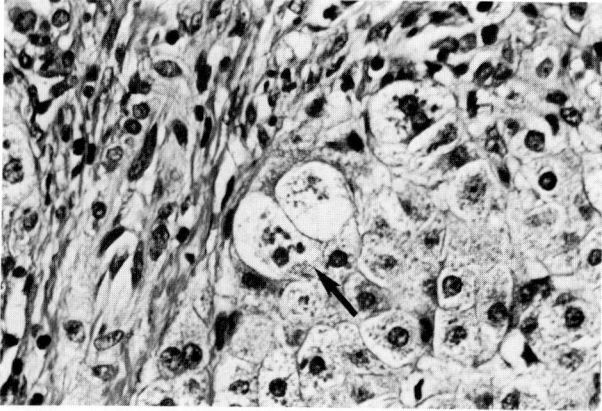

Figure 51–41. EHBDA. Follow-up biopsy four years after portoenterostomy. The patient was free of jaundice for nearly four years, but recently a rise of bilirubin in serum developed. Detail of septal-parenchymal interphase, with features of cholate stasis in periseptal hepatocytes: they appear swollen and coarsely granular and occasionally contain Mallory bodies (arrow) (hematoxylin and eosin, × 640).

it finally heals. This course of events would apply for those patients who remain clinically well and biochemically normal but in whom some mild and functionally insignificant periportal fibrosis is found. The only sequel is that the normal human histologic pattern of the liver has come closer to that of the pig liver (Fig. 51–28).

As described in Pathologic Features of the Liver in Extrahepatic Bile Duct Atresia, several cases are characterized by a particular type of ductular reaction in the form of ductal plate formation, and even repetitive ductal plate formation, resulting in often incomplete concentric rings of bile duct structures (early severe EHBDA).

When after successful portoenterostomy, the basic disease process causing intrahepatic bile duct destruction stops in an early phase, the liver is left in a state characterized by an excess of immature types of bile duct structures. The bile duct destruction stops, but the remodeling of the ductal plate is deranged. This bile duct hyperplasia, together with the increase in portal and periportal connective tissue accompanying the later waves of ductal plates, creates the histologic appearance described as congenital hepatic fibrosis–like. It is intriguing to speculate whether natural congenital hepatic fibrosis (see Chap. 52) is not brought about by a comparable process of excess stimulation of ductal plate formation with arrest of the normal remodeling process. In this view, congenital hepatic fibrosis would represent a fetal type of biliary fibrosis. It is equally intriguing to speculate whether the congenital hepatic fibrosis–like pattern in EHBDA may not be responsible for the development of portal hypertension in the same way that natural congenital hepatic fibrosis does. Development of portal hypertension, followed by the complications of esophageal varices and variceal hemorrhage, is now recognized universally as a late complication of successful hepatic portoenterostomy,[148, 339, 349, 376, 397, 398] although spontaneous alleviation of portal hypertension has been observed in some patients.[339, 379, 399]

It looks as if the arrest in remodeling of the ductal plate may be complete or variably incomplete. Complete arrest of remodeling would result in a congenital hepatic fibrosis–like pattern with ductal plate configurations in numerous portal areas. Partial remodeling would result in a congenital hepatic fibrosis–like pattern with ductal plates or ductal plate remnants in some portal tracts and normally shaped (remodeled) ducts in other portal areas. The variability in degree of ductal plate formation, and the variability in degree of remodeling (or arrest of the latter) might explain the variability in the time-dependent development of portal hypertension. The mechanism of development of portal hypertension in congenital hepatic fibrosis is not established, but presumed mechanisms include the sometimes documented hypoplasia of interlobular branches of the portal vein and the excess fibrous connective tissue in and around the portal tracts.[154] Whatever the mechanism of development of portal hypertension, it may be the only complication in patients who undergo surgery. The liver parenchyma is normal, and since progressive destruction of the intrahepatic bile ducts stops, there is no perpetuation of the state of smoldering cholestasis. Liver test results are normal. The abnormally shaped intrahepatic bile ducts seem to assure adequate drainage of the bile produced by the liver. In several patients, however, continued low-grade destruction of intrahepatic bile ducts (in excess numbers and in ductal plate configuration) continues to occur.

This is reflected in the histologic picture described: a congenital hepatic fibrosis–like pattern, but with superimposed signs of smoldering cholestasis. This low-grade destructive cholangitis may lead, over months and years, to progressive disappearance of intrahepatic bile ducts of whatever shape, mature and immature, resulting in ductless portal tracts expanded by increasing amounts of connective tissue and periportal fibrosis. This gradually leads to the secondary biliary fibrosis and cirrhosis with virtually complete lack of ducts. The patient may still be free of jaundice. However, the cholestasis will be reflected in raised serum levels of alkaline phosphatase, γ-glutamyl transpeptidase, cholesterol, and bile salts.[280] It is not clear how the liver manages to get rid of bile pigments. The suggestion has been made that drainage occurs through hepatic lymph vessels when no intrahepatic bile ducts are present.[400] The finding of excess numbers of dilated lymphatics is of interest in this respect.[197] This stage may be characterized by portal hypertension due to hypoplasia of intrahepatic portal vein branches, extensive portal and periportal fibrosis, and nodular cirrhotic transformation of the liver architecture.

In some patients, a long-term state of clinical cure may deteriorate with reappearance of jaundice. This may be due to clinical episodes of cholangitis, as often reported in the surgical literature. However, some authors state that there is no correlation between development of biliary cirrhosis in their patients and the presence or lack of repeated episodes of cholangitis.[343] The reason for this deterioration is not clear. It might be late occlusion of the anastomosis at the porta hepatis or late-stage obliteration of the larger intrahepatic draining ducts caused by the basic disease process; it may be a block in lymphatic drainage by slow, progressive fibrosis; or it may be a change in metabolic pathways inside the liver cells. Whatever the mechanism, the clinical deterioration is accompanied, and even preceded by, histologic changes of active biliary disease as described previously.

Finally, the nonhomogeneous spread of lesions observed in follow-up biopsy specimens from patients after portoenterostomy should be stressed.[388, 401] An unequal distribution of the lesions is not surprising in progressive and destructive intrahepatic bile duct disease in view of what is known from experience in adults with primary biliary cirrhosis and sclerosing cholangitis. The lack of homogeneity of lesions throughout the liver, however, causes problems for adequate assessment in liver specimens of restricted size like those obtained by percutaneous needle biopsy. This explains why some authors recommend surgical biopsy in order to assure a more representative tissue sample.[39, 343]

For the sake of completeness, it should be mentioned that other mechanisms have been proposed to explain the progression of lesions—for example, immunologic mechanisms and an autonomic fibromatosis of certain fibroblast clones resulting in progressive fibrosis.[402, 403] At present, it is not clear whether these mechanisms should be considered alternatives or integral parts of the basic disease process in the hypothesis described earlier.

In conclusion, the histologic studies of liver specimens obtained from patients after long-term follow-up for hepatic portoenterostomy allow the conclusion that the basic disease process of the intrahepatic bile ducts continues to run its natural course. This has been proposed on several occasions.[18, 34, 37, 39] The advantage of portoenterostomy is in the relief of the extrahepatic bile duct occlusion, which itself is the result of the extrahepatic component of the basic process of sclerosing cholangitis. After re-establishment of bilioenteric continuity, the intrahepatic bile duct disease may heal spontaneously or may progress at faster or slower rates.

The pathologic mechanisms result in progressive obliteration and disappearance of intrahepatic bile ducts accompanied by increasing periportal fibrosis, resulting in the end stage of biliary fibrosis or cirrhosis, or both. The histologic pattern of changes is modulated by the extent to which ductal plate formation and derangement in remodeling of ductal plates has occurred. Presumably this depends largely on an earlier antenatal onset of disease and persistence of a fetal type of ductular reaction to obstruction during the first two months of life.

BILE DUCT HYPOPLASIA

Bile duct hypoplasia is a lesion characterized by an exceptionally small but grossly visible and radiographically patent extrahepatic biliary duct system.[18, 36, 109] The diagnosis is almost always made at exploratory laparotomy for jaundice in infancy. Bile duct hypoplasia is not a specific disease entity but a manifestation of a variety of hepatobiliary disorders. It may be associated with atresia of extrahepatic ducts and with intrahepatic cholestasis of any cause (see Table 51–1).[109] Bile duct hypoplasia may represent an intermediate stage in the development of EHBDA. Infants have been observed in whom hypoplasia of extrahepatic ducts progressed to total obliteration.[103, 200, 404] There is also evidence that the obliterating disease that leads to bile duct hypoplasia may stabilize at this stage or may even improve. Resolution of jaundice has occurred spontaneously in patients with hypoplastic extrahepatic bile ducts who underwent operation in infancy,[20, 405] but the extent of improvement, if any, of the hypoplastic bile duct system was not substantiated. In patients with persistence of bile duct hypoplasia, liver cirrhosis is slowly progressive.[406] This slow development of cirrhosis is comparable to the progressive biliary disease that develops in adults with narrowed extrahepatic ducts.[407] A case history has been reported with the documented sequence of choledochal cyst to biliary hypoplasia to biliary atresia.[404] Narrowing and other duct irregularities have been demonstrated by cholangiography in patients suffering from neonatal hepatitis.[103]

Small extrahepatic bile ducts have been demonstrated by operative cholangiography in patients with the homozygous form of α₁-antitrypsin deficiency.[408–410] The hypoplasia of the extrahepatic bile ducts in this setting may represent a form of disuse atrophy caused by decreased bile flow as a result of intrahepatic cholestasis.[103] A similar hypothesis might apply to hypoplasia of the extrahepatic bile duct associated with hypoplasia of intrahepatic ducts as documented in some patients with Alagille's syndrome.[165, 169, 190, 411, 412] However, as mentioned previously, histologic study of the extrahepatic bile ducts in some of these patients revealed inflammatory and epithelial degenerative lesions, which were indistinguishable from those observed in fibrous remnants from patients with EHBDA.[169]

Treatment of bile duct hypoplasia depends on the primary hepatobiliary disorder. Bile duct hypoplasia secondary to low flow states (e.g., neonatal hepatitis, α₁-antitrypsin deficiency) cannot be improved by surgery. Patients in whom hypoplastic extrahepatic bile ducts appear to progress to total biliary obstruction should be considered for hepatic portoenterostomy after an observation period of six weeks.[18]

SPONTANEOUS PERFORATION OF THE COMMON BILE DUCT

Spontaneous perforation of the common bile duct is a highly specific clinical entity in infancy and should always be considered in an infant in whom jaundice develops after an anicteric period of good health.[18, 323] It is a rare condition; some 50 cases have been reported since the first description in 1932.[413] The cause is unknown. In a majority of patients, the perforation occurs at the union of the cystic and common ducts. This suggests a developmental weakness at this site,[414] but a viral infection has also been suggested as a cause for this disease.[415]

Clinical signs of the disease commonly are noted between one week and two months after birth, although instances of later onset have been reported.[323] The clinical presentation may be one of an intra-abdominal catastrophe. Usually, however, fluctuating jaundice, acholic stools, and dark urine slowly develop in these patients. Symptoms may be so mild that the development of an inguinal or umbilical hernia secondary to ascites may be the first sign of illness.[416] In some cases, general symptoms of weight loss, irritability, and vomiting may be noted before jaundice.

On clinical examination, one notes abdominal distention from bile ascites and sometimes bile staining of the umbilicus or scrotum caused by bile tracking along patent hernial sacs.[323] Signs of peritonitis and pyrexia usually are lacking. Laboratory investigation reveals a moderate rise in serum levels of bilirubin; liver enzyme tests give normal results, a feature that differentiates this condition from EHBDA. Definitive preoperative diagnosis can be made by abdominal paracentesis yielding fluid with a high concentration of bilirubin.[417] Intravenous cholangiography demonstrates a leak in the extrahepatic bile ducts. Scanning with rose bengal sodium ^{131}I or other isotopes indicates free isotope in the peritoneal cavity.[18, 323] Treatment is surgical. The type of operation performed depends to some extent on the findings at operation.[18, 323, 418–420]

BILE PLUG SYNDROME AND INSPISSATED BILE SYNDROME

The terms *bile plug syndrome* and *inspissated bile syndrome* are often used interchangeably,[18, 323] although Bernstein and co-workers stated explicitly that obstruction of the common duct by a plug of secretions and bile is to be differentiated from the so-called inspissated bile syndrome.[421]

The term inspissated bile syndrome was derived in the nineteenth century and used by surgeons to indicate patients with prolonged jaundice in whom the surgeon found normal extrahepatic bile ducts containing inspissated bile at exploration for presumed EHBDA.[17, 35] This concept was later extended in pediatric practice to include patients with apparent obstructive jaundice in early infancy in whom jaundice cleared spontaneously after several weeks.[19, 120, 422] The majority of these infants have massive hemolytic jaundice caused by Rh and ABO blood group incompatibility.[19, 422] From a questionnaire sent to 12 leading pediatricians in 1962,[35] it appeared that the inspissated bile syndrome in its extended meaning was not considered a disease entity and was felt to represent "a pigment of our imagination." The histologic features of bile plugs in the parenchyma are the result rather than the cause of cholestasis and are caused by bilirubin overload of the liver and by dehydration. Since hemolytic disease of the newborn caused by blood group incompatibility is treated more adequately by exchange transfusion, this form of neonatal cholestasis has become infrequent.[40, 118]

The bile plug syndrome represents a form of extrahepatic cholestasis in which obstruction is caused by inspissated concrements of secretions and bile in the common bile duct.[421] Usually the syndrome occurs in patients with hemolytic disease.[40] Clinically, bile plug syndrome cannot be differentiated from EHBDA; the diagnosis is made at exploratory laparotomy. The inspissated material can be removed by simple irrigation of the biliary tree.[423] On occasion, inspissation may proceed to the point of production of stones, necessitating manual removal of the calculi.[18, 323]

BILE DUCT STENOSIS

A rare cause of extrahepatic obstruction in children beyond the neonatal age is a localized narrowing of the distal part of the common bile duct.[80] In three such cases, the proximal segments of the duct were dilated, and they contained small biliary concrements that had accumulated near the narrowed part. The condition was cured by simple choledochotomy and cleaning of the duct. Mention is made of two cases of post-traumatic stricture of the common bile duct, possibly caused by previous blunt abdominal trauma, and of two patients with partial stenosis of the confluence of the hepatic ducts without evidence of antecedent trauma.[80]

DUPLICATION OF THE BILIARY TREE

Duplication of the biliary tree is a condition of exceptional rarity according to authors with vast experience.[80, 424, 425] The etiology is probably identical to that of intestinal duplication. Clinical symptoms include abdominal pain and recurring intestinal obstruction. The cholestasis may be anicteric or icteric. A hard mass of variable size may be palpated in the right hypochondrium. Usually, the diagnosis is made during surgical intervention for presumed cholangitis or choledochal cyst.

GALLSTONES

Gallstone formation can occur in premature infants treated with parenteral nutrition and furosemide.[426] Gallstones in children are rare and usually appear in the period before puberty. In contrast with adult gallstone disease, there is no female predominance.[80] Possible causes include chronic hemolysis, mucoviscidosis, and bile duct malformations. Ethnic, genetic, and familial factors may predispose to gallstone disease.[80]

BILE DUCT TUMORS

Tumors of the extrahepatic bile ducts are extremely rare in children. The tumors correspond to embryonal rhabdomyosarcoma.[427, 428] The clinical symptoms are those of complete cholestasis with progressive onset; an abdominal mass may be palpable. Operative cholangiography reveals the obstruction, which is often near the ampullary region.[80] Treatment consists of surgical excision. The prognosis is poor: 24 of 25 infants died within 16 months.[428]

EXTRAMURAL COMPRESSION OF THE COMMON BILE DUCT

Occasionally, extrahepatic cholestasis in a child is caused by extrinsic compression of the common bile duct.

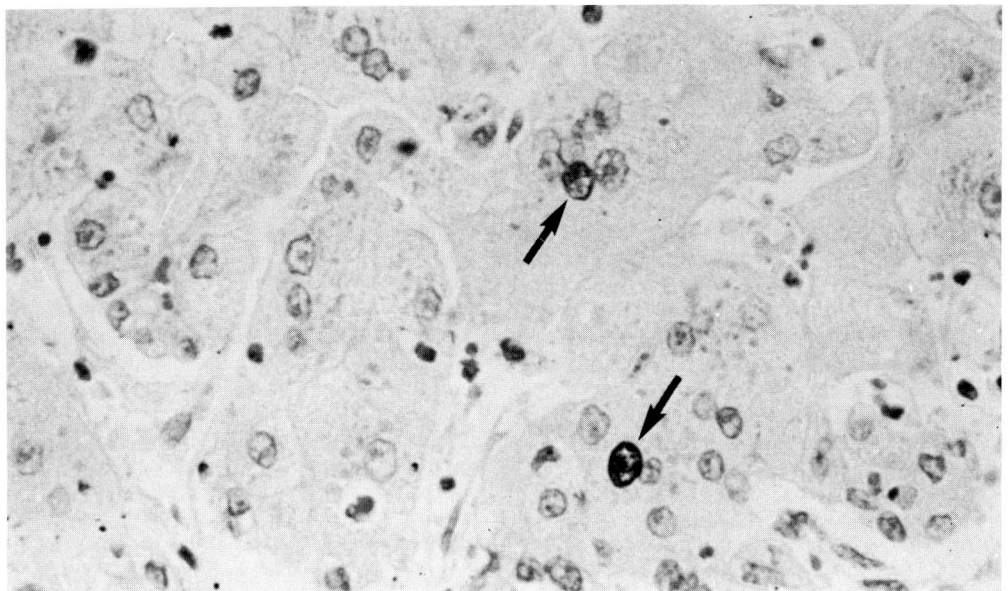

Figure 51–42. Fatal acute viral hepatitis type B in ten-month-old child. Liver biopsy showed multilobular and bridging hepatic necrosis (not shown). The surviving parenchyma is characterized by parenchymal giant cell transformation. Some of the nuclei in the multinucleated giant cells contain hepatitis B core antigen (HBcAg) (*arrows*). (Immunoperoxidase stain for HBcAg. Counterstained with hematoxylin, × 640.)

A case has been reported of bile duct obstruction by peritoneal bands, and cure was effected by simple division of the constricting bands.[429] Other causes include malignant tumors of lymph nodes near the porta hepatis (Hodgkin's and non-Hodgkin's lymphomas) and benign lesions like chronic pancreatitis and post-traumatic cyst of the pancreas.[80] Both benign and malignant tumors of the pancreas or duodenum have been reported as causes of obstructive jaundice in infants (duodenal fibrosarcoma and carcinoma and hemangioendothelioma of the pancreas).[323]

PRIMARY SCLEROSING CHOLANGITIS

Primary sclerosing cholangitis is characterized by chronic inflammatory constriction of the intra- and extrahepatic biliary tree often associated with ulcerative colitis in adults (see Chap. 43).[131, 395] Until recently, the condition was thought to be rare in children. The few cases reported can be separated in several groups:[189] those with sclerosing cholangitis that is somewhat similar to that reported in adults,[430, 431] sclerosing cholangitis associated with immunodeficiency syndrome,[432–434] sclerosing cholangitis associated with histiocytosis X,[435] and retroperitoneal fibrosis.[80, 436, 437]

Recent studies show that primary sclerosing cholangitis in children may have a higher incidence than would appear from the literature; in 1987 two series of 13 and 8 patients were reported.[438, 439] Sixteen of these 21 children also suffered from chronic inflammatory bowel disease. An increased awareness of primary sclerosing cholangitis by pediatricians and pathologists, together with the more widespread use of ERCP, should clarify the true incidence of primary sclerosing cholangitis in children.

An apparently new subgroup of patients with sclerosing cholangitis of childhood was recently identified.[189] This report described eight children with cholestasis from the first week of life, followed by early cirrhosis and portal hypertension; percutaneous cholecystography (at age eight months to nine years) disclosed rarefaction of segmental branches, stenosis, and focal dilation of the intrahepatic bile ducts. The extrahepatic bile ducts were involved in six patients. The authors suggest that this form of primary sclerosing cholangitis with neonatal onset starts before birth and may result from the same type of bile duct injury as does EHBDA but without the same extent of damage to the extrahepatic bile ducts, resulting in "near-miss" EHBDA.[189]

CONGENITAL DILATION OF THE INTRAHEPATIC BILE DUCTS (CAROLI'S DISEASE) AND CHOLEDOCHAL CYST

These conditions are described in Chapter 52.

INTRAHEPATIC CHOLESTASIS

Intrahepatic cholestasis comprises all forms of bile secretory failure of the liver in which the pathogenetic mechanisms are operative within the anatomic confines of the organ. This group of diseases can be further divided into two broad categories: (1) those conditions in which the primary lesion is confined to the intrahepatic bile ducts (e.g., paucity of intrahepatic bile ducts) and (2) the diseases that apparently correspond to a primary disturbance of the liver parenchymal cells.[111]

In the neonate and young child, the latter group of diseases has often been designated with the vague terms *neonatal giant cell hepatitis* or *neonatal hepatitis*. The following discussion is devoted to this apparently multifactorial category of neonatal hepatitis.

NEONATAL HEPATITIS

History and Terminology

In 1952, Craig and Landing described a "form of hepatitis in the neonatal period simulating biliary atresia."[440]

The disease presented clinically as obstructive jaundice that was indistinguishable from EHBDA and was histologically characterized by parenchymal giant cell transformation. A normal, patent biliary tree was present on abdominal exploration or at postmortem examination. The histopathologic picture was interpreted as "active hepatitis having the characteristics of viral hepatitis." At that time, there were no serologic tests available for viral hepatitis A or B, and the viral etiology remained unproved. In the meantime, it has become clear that viral hepatitis in the neonate may present a histologic picture with or without parenchymal giant cells (Fig. 51–42).[40, 118] In this respect, the original authors were right in stating that "perhaps we have overemphasized the diagnostic importance of the multinucleate giant cell in this group of cases."[440]

According to the experience of French pediatric hepatologists,[109] neonatal hepatitis or intrahepatic cholestasis was almost as frequent (49.3 per cent) as extrahepatic bile duct abnormalities (51.7 per cent). The incidence of neonatal hepatitis in southeastern England was found to be 1/2500 live births.[441]

Failure to identify a specific viral infection in the majority of cases and the clinical similarity to EHBDA has led to the use of terms like *neonatal hepatitis syndrome*,[442] *infantile obstructive cholangiopathy*,[13] and *cryptogenic infantile cholestasis type I*.[322] As can be deduced from Table 51–1, the list of specific causes of prolonged, conjugated hyperbilirubinemia in the neonatal age is long and diverse. The early detection of specific infectious diseases, intoxications, and disorders of amino acid, lipid, and carbohydrate metabolism is important, because in many instances, cholestasis attributable to these factors is treatable and reversible. A similar clinical picture of obstructive jaundice may be seen in homozygous α_1-antitrypsin deficiency and in cystic fibrosis. Endocrine disorders (hypopituitarism and hypothyroidism) may also be associated with cholestasis.[50, 443] For clinical and therapeutic purposes, then, the terms *neonatal hepatitis syndrome* and *infantile obstructive cholangiopathy* are no longer adequate, because these terms have various connotations and remain too vague.[40, 50, 80, 444]

Distinction between extrahepatic and intrahepatic cholestasis, and subdivision of the latter into extralobular and intralobular cholestasis, may be more adequate.[111] In the group with intralobular (or parenchymal) cholestasis, the disease process is thought to focus on the hepatocyte and not, or only secondarily, on intrahepatic and extrahepatic segments of the biliary tree.[109] Intralobular cholestasis may be due to infectious, metabolic, toxic, and unknown causes.

In the infectious category, distinction should be made between hepatitis in a neonate and idiopathic neonatal hepatitis.[50] Hepatitis in a neonate refers to infection with a specific, identified virus, such as hepatitis B or cytomegalovirus (Fig. 51–42). These cases represent only a minority (about 10 per cent) of cases with neonatal hepatitis syndrome.[322] However, idiopathic neonatal hepatitis remains a form of cholestasis of undetermined cause. This explains why some authors prefer to drop the term *hepatitis* altogether and to use the more objective, nonprejudiced term *cholestasis*.[80] Just as α_1-antitrypsin deficiency, which was formerly included in the idiopathic category, has now become clearly separable as a delineated subcategory, new developments in the future may identify further subcategories in the presumably multifactorial group now indicated with the terms *idiopathic neonatal hepatitis* or *idiopathic* or *cryptogenic neonatal cholestasis*.

Since most of the conditions listed in Table 51–1 are treated in other chapters, a detailed discussion of the various causes and diagnostic investigations of the neonatal hepatitis syndrome is not given here. The further discussion is limited to the histopathologic features and overall prognosis of idiopathic neonatal hepatitis or idiopathic neonatal cholestasis.

Ever since the recognition of neonatal cholestasis with patent extrahepatic bile ducts, the main challenge for the clinician and the histopathologist has been to differentiate between EHBDA or other anatomic forms of obstruction (e.g., choledochal cyst) on the one hand and neonatal hepatitis without mechanical occlusion of the drainage system on the other. The reasons are the importance of early identification of patients who can be treated by surgery and the concern of avoiding unnecessary and potentially harmful laparotomy in infants with diseased livers.

From a study by Thaler and Gellis,[23] it appeared that surgical exploration of the bile ducts had a harmful effect on the prognosis of patients with neonatal hepatitis. In contrast, Lawson and Boggs concluded from their studies that exploratory laparotomy, without biliary duct exploration, need not alter the future course of infants with neonatal hepatitis when they lack a positive family history.[445] They suggested that familial forms of neonatal hepatitis syndrome caused the apparent poor prognosis in their total operative series and that early laparotomy may be safe and useful not only in establishing diagnosis but also in salvaging a number of infants with surgically correctable biliary atresia. In spite of further warning,[322] the conclusions from the Lawson and Boggs study were mainly emphasized by pediatric surgeons who insist on early settling of the diagnostic differentiation from EHBDA.[18, 337] In a follow-up study from France it was noted that progression to cirrhosis was mainly observed in patients who had undergone surgery,[446] but the authors remarked that the potentially adverse role of laparotomy must be judged with respect to the severity of the liver disease. The majority of their patients who were subjected to surgery had permanently pale stools, hard livers, and histologic features suggesting mechanical bile duct obstruction. Such findings correlate with another study in which poor prognosis was mainly observed in patients with neonatal hepatitis mimicking biliary atresia, that is, severe forms with complete cholestasis.[447] Notwithstanding some controversy about the strategies of diagnostic work-up, no one will doubt the principle that unnecessary surgery should be avoided as much as possible. Clinical features may be helpful in distinguishing neonatal hepatitis from EHBDA. These features were mentioned on page 1373. Liver biopsy may be helpful in discriminating between neonatal hepatitis and EHBDA.

Histopathologic Features

In general, the histologic liver alterations in neonatal hepatitis are more prominent in the parenchyma than in the portal tracts (Fig. 51–43).[139, 448] Usually there is more extensive parenchymal giant cell transformation than in patients with EHBDA; giant cells are larger, appear more hydropic or ballooned, and often show degenerative features. Necrosis of parenchymal giant cells may be associated with infiltration by neutrophils;[120] on occasion, this feature has to be differentiated from so-called surgical necrosis in surgically resected wedge biopsy specimens.[449]

One study has drawn attention to the occurrence of a peculiar large type of cell with strongly eosinophilic cytoplasm and a bizarrely shaped, homogeneously staining

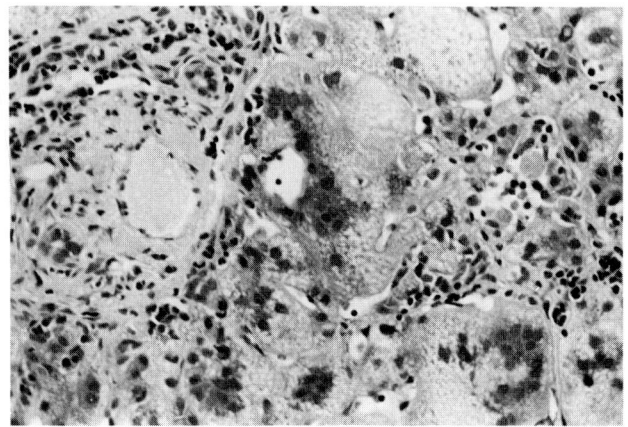

Figure 51–43. Neonatal giant cell hepatitis in infant aged eight weeks. The portal tract (*upper left*) shows mild mononuclear cell infiltration; the interlobular bile duct appears normal; and there is no ductular proliferation. The lobular parenchyma shows parenchymal giant cell transformation, focal necrosis, and mononuclear cell infiltration (hematoxylin and eosin, × 512).

nucleus.[450] It is difficult to differentiate these cells from megakaryocytes, and their nature remains unclear. Foci of extramedullary hematopoiesis are found more often in neonatal hepatitis than in EHBDA, but they do not represent a differentiating feature. Hemosiderin deposition in parenchymal cells and Kupffer cells is more conspicuous in neonatal hepatitis than in EHBDA.[139] Intralobular inflammation and Kupffer cell hyperplasia is usually more striking in neonatal hepatitis, whereas portal and periportal inflammation predominates in EHBDA.[139, 448] Bilirubinostasis (histologic cholestasis) is variable but may be marked, with pigment granules in parenchymal cells and Kupffer cells and variably sized intercellular plugs of bile. Bile concrements in portal ductules may be seen on occasion but are found more often in EHBDA.[139] Ductular proliferation at the periphery of portal tracts may be observed in some cases, but it never reaches the extent found in EHBDA. However, the finding of mild ductular proliferation may be misleading.[139] The fibrosis is more intralobular in neonatal hepatitis, in contrast to the more periportal predominance of fibrosis in EHBDA.[132, 158]

Liver Parenchymal Giant Cells

The multinucleated giant cells in neonatal hepatitis are of parenchymal nature, according to their position in liver cell plates and light microscopic and ultrastructural features. The number of nuclei in parenchymal giant cells is variable, as is the location of the nuclei inside the cytoplasmic mass, either central or peripheral. On hematoxylin and eosin–stained sections, the cytoplasm is pale staining, possibly because of glycogen and also because of a hydropic change in several instances. Giant cells often contain brownish pigment granules, which correspond to bilirubin, lipofuscin, or hemosiderin, or a combination of these pigments. Histochemical characteristics of parenchymal giant cells include intense PAS-staining caused by glycogen (diastase-digestible), intense staining for glucose-6-phosphatase, succinic dehydrogenase and nicotinamide adenine dinucleotide (NAD) and nicotinamide adenine dinucleotide phosphate (NADP) diaphorases,[451] numerous acid phosphatase-positive inclusions, and increased staining for nonspecific alkaline phosphatase at the sinusoidal border.[452]

Electron microscopic study of parenchymal giant cells

reveals well-preserved organelles: normal nuclei, mitochondria, endoplasmic reticulum, and plasma membrane. Apparently, the organelles for energy provision and protein synthesis are normal. An increased number of vacuoles and autophagosomes (cytolysosomes) indicates degenerative changes or increased turnover of organelles, whereas the large number of nuclei can be considered a sign of regeneration.[452] Bile canaliculi can be demonstrated in giant cells;[453] the sinusoidal microvilli are shortened and reduced in number.[452]

Giant cells seem to be deficient in bile secretion, as is seen from the accumulation of bilirubin deposits in their cytoplasm and the delayed excretion of rose bengal sodium ^{131}I.[451] The formation of giant cells has been a matter of debate. Some authors considered parenchymal giant cells to be the result of faulty development of hepatocytes with aplasia of intercellular canaliculi, possibly on a hereditary basis.[454] Others considered the possibility that these multinucleated cells arose by nuclear multiplication not followed by cell division, resulting in multinucleated plasmodial cells.[455, 456] Circumstantial evidence suggests that parenchymal giant cells may represent syncytial masses formed by fusion of several mononuclear hepatocytes. Possibly the cell fusion occurs in liver cell plates with pseudoglandular arrangement.[132, 440, 451]

The problem of the spontaneous disappearance of giant cells is similarly unresolved. Serial biopsy specimens from infants with giant cell transformation suggest that giant cells possess a limited life span of only a few months (from two or three months to six months).[118, 120, 451] Their disappearance after several months generally parallels recovery from cholestasis.[451] The biologic significance of parenchymal giant cells remains unsolved. It has been suggested that parenchymal giant cells are not a nonspecific type of reaction to injury but that they represent a morphologic marker of infantile obstructive cholangiopathy.[13] However, parenchymal giant cells may occur in virtually all liver disorders of early infancy.[451] Thus, the mere presence or lack of parenchymal giant cells is of relatively limited diagnostic value. A list of neonatal diseases associated with hepatocellular giant cell transformation is given in Table 51–5.[451] It thus may be concluded that parenchymal giant cell transformation represents a nonspecific reaction of the infant's hepatocytes to various types of injury.[139] Parenchymal giant cell transformation is more age-specific than disease-specific. Even this statement may not be taken too strictly, since parenchymal giant cells have also been observed in adult liver disease, like viral hepatitis and drug-induced liver disease.[457–459] Experimentally, parenchymal giant cell transformation has been induced in the liver by administration of *Escherichia coli* endotoxin to rabbits and rats and aflatoxin B$_1$ to marmosets.[460–463]

Prognosis of Neonatal Hepatitis

A few studies have reported on the follow-up of patients with neonatal hepatitis. The outcome is highly variable.[50, 441, 446, 447, 464] In general, the outcome is better in sporadic cases without known associated factors, whereas the prognosis is poor in familial cases and in patients with associated conditions like α_1-antitrypsin deficiency. For example, of the sporadic cases reported by Danks and coworkers,[447] approximately 60 per cent of the patients recovered, 10 per cent had persisting inflammation or fibrosis, 2 per cent had cirrhosis, and 30 per cent died. The outcome was worse in familial cases: 30 per cent of the patients

TABLE 51–5. CONDITIONS ASSOCIATED WITH GIANT CELL TRANSFORMATION*

Mechanical Obstruction	Nonobstructive Disease
Extrahepatic biliary atresia	*Diseases of established nature*
	Hepatitis B
Choledochal cysts	Rubella
	Cytomegalovirus
Intrahepatic biliary atresia	Herpes simplex
	Coxsackievirus
	Toxoplasmosis
	Congenital syphilis
	Escherichia coli pyelonephritis
	α_1-antitrypsin deficiency
	Cystic fibrosis
	Galactosemia
	Myeloproliferative disorder
	Niemann-Pick disease
	Gaucher's disease
	Down's syndrome
	17–18 trisomy
	Mucolipidosis
	Turner's syndrome
	Indian childhood cirrhosis
	ABO and Rh incompatibility
	Spherocytosis
	Anomalous pulmonary venous return to portal vein
	Endocardial cushion defect
	Neonatal hepatic necrosis
	Arnold-Chiari malformation
	Diseases of unestablished nature
	Primary giant cell transformation or neonatal hepatitis

Source: Modified from Ruebner B, Thaler M. In: Javitt NB, ed. Neonatal Hepatitis and Biliary Atresia. US Department of Health, Education, and Welfare, DHEW Publication No. (NIH) 79–1296, 1979:2990.

recovered, chronic liver disease with cirrhosis developed in 10 per cent, and 60 per cent died.

Adverse effects of diagnostic laparotomy are not universally recognized,[23, 445, 447] but it may be that the patients with the most severe disease causing complete cholestasis and carrying the worst prognosis are the first candidates for diagnostic laparotomy in case of uncertainty after noninvasive investigation.[446]

REFERENCES

1. Danks DM, Campbell PE, Clarke M, et al. Extrahepatic biliary atresia. The frequency of potentially operable cases. Am J Dis Child 128:684, 1974.
2. Donop CF. De ictero specialisme neonatorum. Inaug. Diss., Berlin, 1852. Cited by Schweizer, P, Müller, G. Gallengangsatresie. Cholestasesyndrome in Neugeborenen-und Säuglingsalter. Stuttgart, Hippokrates Verlag, 1984.
3. Heschl J. Vollständiger Defekt der Gallenwege beobachtet bei einem 7 Monate alt verstorbenen weiblichen Kinde. Wien Med Wochenschr 15:493, 1865.
4. Legg JW. Congenital deficiency of the common bile duct, the cystic and hepatic ducts ending in a blind sac; cirrhosis of the liver. Trans Pathol Soc Lond 27:178, 1875/76.
5. Lomer R. Ueber einen Fall von congenitaler partieller Obliteration der Gallengänge. Arch Pathol Anat Physiol und Klin. Medizin 99:130, 1885.
6. Thomson J. On congenital obliteration of the bile ducts. Edinburgh Med J 37:523, 1891.
7. Thomson J. On congenital obliteration of the bile ducts. Edinburgh Med J 37:604, 1892.
8. Thomson J. On congenital obliteration of the bile ducts. Edinburgh Med J 37:724, 1892.
9. Rolleston HD, Hayne LB. A case of congenital hepatic cirrhosis with obliterative cholangitis (congenital obliteration of the bile ducts). Br Med J 1:758, 1901.
10. Moore TC. Congenital atresia of the extrahepatic bile ducts. Surg Gynecol Obstet 96:215, 1953.
11. Holmes JB. Congenital obliteration of the bile ducts. Diagnosis and suggestions for treatment. Am J Dis Child 11:405, 1916.
12. Ylppö A. Zwei Fälle von kongenitalem Gallengangverschlusz: Fett- und Bilirubin- Stoffwechselversuche bei einem derselbe. Z Kinderheilk 9:319, 1913.
13. Landing BH. Considerations on the pathogenesis of neonatal hepatitis, biliary atresia and choledochal cyst. The concept of infantile obstructive cholangiopathy. Prog Pediatr Surg 6:113, 1974.
14. Ladd WE. Congenital atresia and stenosis of the bile duct. JAMA 91:1082, 1928.
15. Lou MA, Schmutzer KJ, Regan JF. Congenital extrahepatic biliary atresia. Arch Surg 105:771, 1972.
16. Bill AH. World progress in surgery. Biliary atresia—introduction. World J Surg 2:557, 1978.
17. Ladd WE. Congenital obstruction of bile ducts. Ann Surg 102:742, 1935.
18. Lilly JR, Altman RP. The biliary tree. In: Ravitch MM, Welch KJ, Benson CD, et al, eds. Pediatric Surgery, 3rd ed. Chicago, Year Book Medical, 1979:827.
19. Dunn PM. Obstructive jaundice and haemolytic disease of the newborn. Arch Dis Child 38:54, 1963.
20. Gross RE. The Surgery of Infancy and Childhood. Philadelphia, WB Saunders Co, 1953.
21. Clatworthy HW Jr, McDonald VG Jr. The diagnostic laparotomy in obstructive jaundice in infants. Surg Clin North Am 36:1545, 1956.
22. Thaler MM, Gellis SS. Studies in neonatal hepatitis and biliary atresia. Am J Dis Child 116:257, 1968.
23. Thaler MM, Gellis SS. Studies in neonatal hepatitis and biliary atresia. II. The effect of diagnostic laparotomy on long-term prognosis of neonatal hepatitis. Am J Dis Child 116:262, 1968.
24. Thaler MM, Gellis SS. Studies in neonatal hepatitis and biliary atresia. III. Progression and regression in cirrhosis in biliary atresia. Am J Dis Child 116:271, 1968.
25. Carlson E. Salvage of the "noncorrectable" case of congenital biliary atresia. Arch Surg 81:893, 1960.
26. Herzog B. Zur Gallengangatresie. Helv Chir Acta 35:515, 1968.
27. Bill AH, Brennom WS, Huseby TL. Biliary atresia: new concepts of pathology, diagnosis and management. Arch Surg 109:367, 1974.
28. Kasai M, Suzuki S. A new operation for "non-correctable" biliary atresia: hepatic portoenterostomy. Shujitsu, 13:733, 1959.
29. Kasai M, Kimura S, Wagatsuma M, et al. Die chirurgischen Behandlungen der angeborenen Miszbildungen des Gallenganges. Therapiewoche 13:710, 1963.
30. Kasai M, Kimura S, Asakura S, et al. Surgical treatment of biliary atresia. J Pediatr Surg 3:665, 1968.
31. Campbell DP, Poley JR, Bhatia M, et al. Hepatic portoenterostomy—is it indicated in the treatment of biliary atresia? J Pediatr Surg 9:329, 1974.
32. Lilly JR. The Japanese operation for biliary atresia: remedy or mischief? Pediatrics 55:12, 1975.
33. Gans SL. Editorial: Correctable or not correctable: biliary atresia. J Pediatr Surg 18:107, 1983.
34. Howard ER. Extrahepatic biliary atresia—a review of current management. Br J Surg 70:193, 1983.
35. Brent RL. Persistent jaundice in infancy. J Pediatr 61:111, 1962.
36. Witzleben CL. The pathogenesis of biliary atresia. In: Javitt NB, ed. Neonatal Hepatitis and Biliary Atresia. U.S. Department of Health, Education and Welfare, DHEW Publication No (NIH) 79–1296, 1979:339.
37. Haas JE. Bile duct and liver pathology in biliary atresia. World J Surg 2:561, 1978.
38. Lilly J, Altman RP, Schroter G, et al. Surgery of biliary atresia. Current Status. Am J Dis Child 129:1429, 1975.
39. Alagille D, Valayer J, Odièvre M, et al. Long-term follow-up in children operated on by corrective surgery for extrahepatic biliary atresia. In: Kasai M, ed. Biliary Atresia and its Related Disorders. Amsterdam, Excerpta Medica, 1983:233.
40. Schweizer P, Müller G. Gallengangsatresie. Cholestase-syndrome in Neugeborenen- und Säuglingsalter. Stuttgart, Hippokrates Verlag, 1984.
41. Jenner RE. New perspectives on biliary atresia. Ann R Coll Surg Engl 60:367, 1978.
42. Witzleben CL, Buck BE, Schnaufer L, et al. Studies on the pathogenesis of biliary atresia. Lab Invest 38:525, 1978.
43. Danks D, Bodian M. A genetic study of neonatal obstructive jaundice. Arch Dis Child 38:378, 1963.
44. Tunte W. Zur Häufigkeit der angeborenen Gallengangsatresie. Z Kinderheilk 102:275, 1968.
45. Shim KT, Kasai M, Spence MA. Race and biliary atresia. In: Kasai M, Shiraki K, eds. Cholestasis in Infancy. Tokyo, University of Tokyo Press, 1980:5.

46. Silverman A, Roy CC, Cozzetto FJ. Pediatric clinical gastroenterology. St. Louis, CV Mosby, 1971:293.
47. Psacharopoulos HT, Howard ER, Portmann B, et al. Extrahepatic biliary atresia: preoperative assessment and surgical results in 47 consecutive cases. Arch Dis Child 55:851, 1980.
48. Thaler MM. Discussion: epidemiological studies in biliary atresia. In: Kasai M, Shiraki K, eds. Cholestasis in Infancy. Tokyo, University of Tokyo Press, 1980:24.
49. Lilly JR, Stellin G, Pau CML, et al. Historical background of the biliary atresia registry. In: Daum F, ed. Extrahepatic Biliary Atresia. New York, Marcel Dekker, 1983:73.
50. Balistreri WF. Neonatal cholestasis. J Pediatr 106:171, 1985.
51. Balistreri WF, Schubert WK. Liver disease in infancy and childhood. In: Schiff L, Schiff ER, eds. Diseases of the Liver, 5th ed. Philadelphia, JB Lippincott, 1982:1265.
52. Brough AJ, Bernstein J. Liver biopsy in the diagnosis of infantile obstructive jaundice. Pediatrics 43:519, 1969.
53. Wells TR, Ramicone E, Landing BH, et al. Preferentially longer survival of males than of females with untreated extrahepatic biliary atresia: correlations with time course of intrahepatic lesions and suggestion of possible ethnic influences. Pediatr Pathol 4:321, 1985.
54. Krauss AN. Familial extrahepatic biliary atresia. J Pediatr 65:933, 1964.
55. Lutz-Richner AR, Landolt RF. Familiäre Gallengangsmissbildungen mit tubulärer Niereninsuffizienz. Helv Paediat Acta 28:1, 1973.
56. Mowat AP, Psacharopoulos HT, Williams R. Extrahepatic biliary atresia versus neonatal hepatitis. Review of 137 prospectively investigated infants. Arch Dis Child 51:763, 1976.
57. Whitten WW, Adie GC. Congenital biliary atresia. J Pediatr 10:539, 1952.
58. Nevin NL, Bell M, Frazer MJL, et al. Congenital extrahepatic biliary atresia in two brothers. J Med Genet 6:379, 1969.
59. Sommer AM, Moody PE, Reiner CB. Familial extrahepatic biliary atresia, report of a case situation. Clin Pediatr 15:627, 1976.
60. Scott RB, Wilkins W, Kessler A. Viral hepatitis in early infancy. Report of three fatal cases in siblings simulating biliary atresia. Pediatrics 13:447, 1954.
61. Petermann MG. Neonatal hepatitis in siblings. J Pediatr 50:315, 1957.
62. Willnow U. Zur Klinik, Morphologie und Pathogenese der mit Riesenzellbildung einhergehenden connatalen Lebererkrankungen. Arch Kinderheilkd 182:153, 1971.
63. McDonald PJ, Stehman FB, Stewart DR. Infantile obstructive cholangiopathy. Am J Dis Child 133:518, 1979.
64. Hyams JS, Glaser JH, Leichtner AM, et al. Discordance for biliary atresia in two sets of monozygotic twins. J Pediatr 107:420, 1985.
65. Moore TC, Hyman PE. Extrahepatic biliary atresia in one human leucocyte antigen identical twin. Pediatrics 76:604, 1985.
66. Robertson AF. Case report: the coincidence of biliary atresia and the heterozygous state of galactosemia. Pediatrics 35:1008, 1965.
67. Nord KS, Saad S, Yoshi VV, et al. Concurrence of alpha-1-antitrypsin deficiency and biliary atresia. J Pediatr 111:416, 1987.
68. Fos E, Arcas R, Cabre J, et al. Deficit de alfa-1-antripsina y atresia de vias biliares. An Esp Pediatr One 25:467, 1986.
69. Christen H, Bau J, Halsband H. Hereditary alpha-1-antitrypsin deficiency associated with congenital extrahepatic bile duct hypoplasia. Klin Wochenschr 53:90, 1975.
70. Lecoultre C, Fête R, Cvendet A, et al. An unusual association of small bowel atresia and biliary atresia: a case report. J Pediatr Surg 18:136, 1983.
71. Dimmick JE, Bove KE, McAdams J. Extrahepatic biliary atresia and the polysplenia syndrome. J Pediatr 86:644, 1975.
72. Chandra RS. Biliary atresia and other structural anomalies in congenital polysplenia syndrome. J Pediatr 85:649, 1974.
73. Lilly JR, Chandra RS. Surgical hazards of co-existing anomalies in biliary atresia. Surg Gynecol Obstet 139:49, 1974.
74. Rumler W. Ueber die kongenitale Gallenwegsatresie: zum familiären Vorkommen und zur Genese dieser Fehlbildung. Arch Kinderheilk 164:238, 1961.
75. Choulot JJ, Gautier M, Eliot N, Odièvre M. Les malformations associées à l'atrésie des voies biliaires extrahépatiques. Arch Fr Pediatr 36:19, 1979.
76. Rickham PP, Hirsig J. Biliary atresia: recent advances in aetiology, diagnosis and treatment. Z Kinderchir Grenzgeb 26:114, 1979.
77. Stowens D. Congenital biliary atresia. Ann NY Acad Sci 11:337, 1963.
78. Kasai M. Treatment of biliary atresia with special reference to hepatic porto-enterostomy and its modifications. In: Bill AH, Kasai M, eds. Prog Pediatr Surg. 6:5, 1974.
79. Lilly JR, Hall RJ, Vasquez-Estevez J, et al. The surgery of "correctable" biliary atresia. J Pediatr Surg 22:522, 1987.
80. Alagille D, Odièvre M. Liver and biliary tract disease in children. New York, Wiley-Flammarion, 1979.
81. Alagille D, Gautier M. Anatomy II: anatomic data of the biliary system with respect to extrahepatic biliary atresia. In: Bianchi L, Gerok W, Sickinger K, eds. Liver and Bile. Baltimore, University Press, 1977:33.
82. Bill AH, Haas JE, Foster GL. Biliary atresia: histopathologic observations and reflections upon its natural history. J Pediatr Surg 12:977, 1977.
83. Gautier M. L'atrésie des voies biliaires extrahépatiques: hypothèse étiologique basée sur l'étude histologique de 130 reliquats fibreux. Arch Fr Pediatr (Suppl)36:3, 1979.
84. Gautier M, Jehan P, Odièvre M. Histologic study of biliary fibrous remnants in 48 cases of extra-hepatic biliary atresia: correlation with postoperative bile flow restoration. J Pediatr 89:704, 1976.
85. Gautier M, Elliot N. Extrahepatic biliary atresia. Morphological study of 98 biliary remnants. Arch Pathol Lab Med 105:397, 1981.
86. Chandra RS, Altman RP. Ductal remnants in extrahepatic biliary atresia. A histopathological study with clinical correlations. J Pediatr 93:196, 1978.
87. Kasai M. Intra- and extrahepatic bile ducts in biliary atresia. In: Javitt NB, ed. Neonatal Hepatitis and Biliary Atresia. U.S. Department of Health, Education and Welfare. DHEW Publication No (NIH) 79–1296, 1979:351.
88. Kimura S. The early diagnosis of biliary atresia. Prog Pediatr Surg 6:91, 1974.
89. Lawrence D, Howard ER, Tsannatos C, et al. Hepatic portoenterostomy for biliary atresia; a comparative study of histology and prognosis after surgery. Arch Dis Child 56:460, 1981.
90. Matsuo S, Ikeda K, Yakabe S, et al. Histologic study of the remnant of porta hepatitis in patients with extrahepatic biliary atresia—a computed picture analysis of 30 cases. Z Kinderchir 39:46, 1984.
91. Matsukawa Y. Three-dimensional histometry of bile ducts in the porta hepatis tissue in cases of biliary atresia. Arch Jpn Chir 53:47, 1984.
92. Miyano T, Suruga K, Tsuchiya H, et al. A histopathological study of the remnant of extrahepatic bile duct in so-called uncorrectable biliary atresia. J Pediatr Surg 12:19, 1977.
93. Mustard R Jr, Shandling B, Gillam J. The Kasai operation (hepatic portoenterostomy) for biliary atesia—experience with 20 cases. J Pediatr Surg 14:511, 1979.
94. Ohi R, Okamoto A, Kasai M. Morphologic studies of extrahepatic bile ducts in biliary atresia. In: Kasai M, Shiraki K, eds. Cholestasis in Infancy. Tokyo, University of Tokyo Press, 1980:157.
95. Ohi R, Shikes RH, Stelling GP, et al. In biliary atresia duct histology correlates with bile flow. J Pediatr Surg 19:467, 1984.
96. Suruga K, Miyano T, Kimura K, et al. Reoperation in the treatment of biliary atresia. J Pediatr Surg 17:1, 1982.
97. Altman RP. Biliary atresia: a surgical-histopathologic correlation. In: Javitt NB, ed. Neonatal Hepatitis and Biliary Atresia. U.S. Department of Health, Education and Welfare DHEW Publications No (NIH) 79–1296, 1979:391.
98. Altman RP. The portoenterostomy procedure for biliary atresia: a five year experience. Ann Surg 188:357, 1978.
99. Suruga K, Miyano T, Arai T, et al. A study of patients with long-term bile flow after hepatic portoenterostomy for biliary atresia. J Pediatr Surg 20:252, 1985.
100. Suruga K, Miyano T, Arai T, et al. A study on hepatic portoenterostomy for the treatment of atresia of the biliary tract. Surg Gynecol Obstet 159:53, 1984.
101. Schweizer P, Flach A. Lympho-digestive Gallendrainage an der Leberpforte bei extrahepatischer Gallengangsatresie. Tierexperimentelle Studie Zschr Kinderchir 18:271, 1976.
102. Stowens D. Congenital biliary atresia. Am J Gastroenterol 32:577, 1959.
103. Hays DM, Woolley MM, Snyder WH, et al. Diagnosis of biliary atresia: relative accuracy of percutaneous liver biopsy, open liver biopsy and operative cholangiography. J Pediatr 71:598, 1967.
104. Landing BH. Protracted obstructive jaundice in infancy. In: Becker FF, ed. The Liver, Normal and Abnormal Functions. Part B. New York, Marcel Dekker, 1975:821.
105. Alagille D, Gautier M, Habib E-C, et al. Les données de la biopsie hépatique pré- et peroperatoire au cours des cholostases prolongées du nourrisson. Etude de 128 observations. Arch Fr Pediatr 26:283, 1969.
106. Eliot N, Hadchouel M, Gautier M, et al. Valeur de la biopsie hépatique à l'aiguille et de la biopsie chirurgicale dans le diagnostic des cholestases néonatales. Gastroenterol Clin Biol 2:1025, 1978.
107. Brough HJ, Bernstein J. Conjugated hyperbilirubinemia in early infancy. A reassessment of liver biopsy. Hum Pathol 5:507, 1974.
108. Brough AJ, Bernstein J. Morphologic approach to the evaluation of infantile conjugated hyperbilirubinemia. In: Javitt NB, ed. Neonatal Hepatitis and Biliary Atresia. U.S. Department of Health, Education and Welfare. DHEW Publication No (NIH) 79–1296, 1979:381.
109. Alagille D. Cholestasis in the first three months of life. In: Popper H, Schaffner F, eds. Progress in Liver Diseases., Vol VI. New York, Grune & Stratton, 1979:471.

110. Manolaki AG, Larcher VF, Mowat AP, et al. The prelaparotomy diagnosis of extrahepatic biliary atresia. Arch Dis Child 58:591, 1983.

111. Desmet VJ. Cholestasis: extrahepatic obstruction and secondary biliary cirrhosis. In: MacSween RNM, Anthony PP, Scheuer PJ, eds. Pathology of the Liver, 2nd ed. Edinburgh, Churchill Livingstone, 1987:364.

112. Desmet VJ. Modulation of bile duct epithelium. In: Reutter W, Popper H, Arias IM, et al., eds. Modulation of Liver Cell Expression. Lancaster, MTP Press, 1987:195.

113. Hammar JA. Ueber die erste Entstehung der nicht kapillaren intrahepatischen Gallengänge beim Menschen. Z Mikrosk Anat Forsch 5:59, 1926.

114. Desmet VJ. Intrahepatic bile ducts under the lens. J Hepatol 1:545, 1985.

115. Van Eyken P, Sciot R, Desmet VJ. Intrahepatic bile duct development in the rat: a cytokeratin-immunohistochemical study. Lab Invest 59:52, 1988.

116. Lüders D. Hypoplasie der intrahepatischen Gallengänge mit gutartigem Verlauf. Monatsschr Kinderheilkd 121:717, 1973.

117. Gherardi GJ, MacMahon HE. Hypoplasia of terminal bile ducts. Am J Dis Child 120:151, 1970.

118. Roschlau G. Leberbiopsie im Kindesalter. VEB Gustav Fischer Verlag, Jena, 1978.

119. Sacher M, Paky F, Stoegmann W, et al. Passagere Hypoplasien der intrahepatischen Gallengänge. Klinische und morphologische Beobachtungen. Monatschr Kinderheilkd 133:840, 1985.

120. Thaler H. Leberkrankheiten. Histologie, Pathophysiologie, Klinik. Berlin, Springer-Verlag, 1982:214.

121. Nakanuma Y, Ohta G. Immunohistochemical study on bile ductular proliferation in various hepatobiliary diseases. Liver 6:205, 1986.

122. Hahn EG, Kirchner J, Schuppan D. Perisinusoidal fibrogenesis and ductular metaplasia of hepatocytes in focal nodular hyperplasia of the liver. J Hepatol 5:S32, 1987.

123. Schulz R, Schuppan D, Hahn EG. Connective tissue and ductular metaplasia of hepatocytes. In: Wolff JR, Sievers J, Berry M, eds. Mesenchymal-epithelial Interactions in Neural Development. Nato ASI Series, Vol. H5. Berlin-Heidelberg, Springer-Verlag, 1987:119.

124. Bianchi L. Liver biopsy interpretation in hepatitis. Part I. Presentation of critical morphologic features used in diagnosis (Glossary). Pathol Res Pract 178:2, 1983.

125. Chiba T. Reconstruction of intrahepatic bile ducts in congenital biliary atresia. Tohoku J Exp Med 115:99, 1975.

126. Desmet VJ. Morphologic and histochemical aspects of cholestasis. In: Popper H, Schaffner F, eds. Progress in Liver Diseases, Vol IV. New York, Grune & Stratton, 1972:97.

127. Javitt NB. Bile salts and liver disease in childhood. Postgrad Med J 50:354, 1974.

128. Desmet VJ. Current problems in diagnosis of biliary disease and cholestasis. Semin Liver Dis 6:233, 1986.

129. International Group. Histopathology of the intrahepatic biliary tree. Liver 3:161, 1983.

130. Butron Vila M, Haot J, Desmet VJ. Cholestatic features in focal nodular hyperplasia of the liver. Liver 4:387, 1984.

131. Desmet VJ. Cholangiopathies: past, present and future. Semin Liver Dis 7:67, 1987.

132. Van Eyken P, Sciot R, Van Damme B, et al. Keratin immunohistochemistry in normal human liver. Cytokeratin pattern of hepatocytes, bile ducts and acinar gradient. Virchows Arch A 412:63, 1987.

133. Nathrath WBJ, Heidenkummer P, Björklund V, et al. Distribution of tissue polypeptide antigen (TPA) in normal human tissue. Immunological study on unfixed, methanol, ethanol and formalin fixed tissue. J Histochem Cytochem 33:99, 1985.

134. Burt AD, Stewart JA, Aitchison M, et al. Expression of tissue polypeptide antigen (TPA) in fetal and adult liver: changes in liver disease. J Clin Pathol 40:719, 1987.

135. Ferry GD, Selby ML, Udall J, et al. Guide to early diagnosis of biliary obstruction in infancy. Clin Pediatr 24:305, 1985.

136. Matzen P, Junge J, Christoffersen P, et al. Reproducibility and accuracy of liver biopsy findings suggestive of an obstructive cause of jaundice. In: Brunner H, Thaler H, eds. Hepatology, a Festschrift for Hans Popper. New York, Raven Press, 1985:285.

137. Kasai M, Yakovac W, Koop EC. Liver in congenital biliary atresia and neonatal hepatitis. A histopathologic study. Arch Pathol 74:152, 1962.

138. Gathmann HA, Osswald P, Müller G. Differentialdiagnose und Verlaufsbeobachtungen bei Säuglingen und Kleinkindern mit längerdauernder Cholestase. Z Kinderheilk 120:259, 1975.

139. Ruebner BH, Miyai K. The pathology of neonatal hepatitis and biliary atresia with particular reference to hemopoiesis and hemosiderin deposition. Ann NY Acad Sci 111:375, 1963.

140. Lorenz G. Histomorphologische Leberveränderungen bei extrahepa-

141. Hollander M, Schaffner F. Electron microscopic studies in biliary atresia. Am J Dis Child 16:57, 1968.

142. Sasaki H, Schaffner F, Popper H. Bile ductules in cholestasis. Morphologic evidence for secretion and absorption in man. Lab Invest 16:84, 1967.

143. Desmet VJ. Cirrhosis: aetiology and pathogenesis: cholestasis. In: Boyer JL, Bianchi L, eds. Liver Cirrhosis. Lancaster, MTP Press, 1987:101.

144. Ito I, Nagaya M, Niinomi N, et al. Intrahepatic bile ducts in biliary atresia. In: Ohi R, ed. Biliary Atresia. Tokyo, Professional Postgraduate Services, 1987:62.

145. Landing BH, Wells TR, Reed GB, et al. Diseases of the bile ducts in children. In: Gall EA, Mostofi FK, eds. The Liver. Baltimore, Williams & Wilkins, 1973:480.

146. Sherlock S. The syndrome of disappearing intrahepatic bile ducts. Lancet 2:493, 1987.

147. Ohi R, Endo N, Kasai M. Histopathological studies of the liver in biliary atresia—further observations. In: Kasai M, ed. Biliary Atresia and its Related Disorders. Amsterdam, Excerpta Medica, 1983:71.

148. Howard ER, Driver M, McClement J, et al. Prolonged survival after operation for extrahepatic biliary atresia. In: Kasai M, ed. Biliary Atresia and its Related Disorders. Amsterdam, Excerpta Medica, 1983:167.

149. Ito T, Horisawa M, Ando H. Intrahepatic bile ducts in biliary atresia—a possible factor determining the prognosis. J Pediatr Surg 18:124, 1983.

150. Altman RP, Chandra R, Lilly J. Ongoing cirrhosis after successful porticoenterostomy in infants with biliary atresia. J Pediatr Surg 10:685, 1975.

151. Lilly JR, Altman P. Hepatic portoenterostomy (the Kasai operation) for biliary atresia. Surgery 78:76, 1975.

152. Odièvre M, Valayer J, Razemon-Pinta M, et al. Hepatic portoenterostomy or cholecystostomy in the treatment of extrahepatic biliary atresia. J Pediatr 88:774, 1976.

153. Lilly JR, Karrer FM. Contemporary surgery of biliary atresia. Pediatr Clin North Am 32:1233, 1985.

154. Ohuchi N, Ohi R, Takahashi T, et al. Postoperative changes in intrahepatic portal veins in biliary atresia. A 3-D reconstruction study. J Pediatr Surg 21:10, 1986.

155. Landing BH, Wells TR, Ramicone E. Time course of the intrahepatic lesion of extrahepatic biliary atresia. A morphometric study. Pediatr Pathol 4:309, 1985.

156. Kasai M, Suzuki H, Ohashi E, et al. Technique and results of operative management of biliary atresia. World J Surg 2:571, 1978.

157. Balistreri WF. Foreword. Neonatal cholestasis: lessons from the past, issues for the future. Semin Liver Dis 7:61, 1987.

158. Scheuer PJ. Liver Biopsy Interpretation, 3rd ed. London, Bailliere Tindall, 1980.

159. Ray MB, Desmet VJ. Immunofluorescent detection of alpha-1-antitrypsin in paraffin embedded liver tissue. J Clin Pathol 28:717, 1975.

160. Callea F, Fevery J, De Groote J, et al. Detection of PiZ phenotype individuals by alpha-1-antitrypsin (AAT) immunohistochemistry in paraffin-embedded liver tissue specimens. J Hepatol 2:389, 1986.

161. Ahrens EH Jr, Harris RC, MacMahon HE. Atresia of the intrahepatic bile ducts. Pediatrics 8:628, 1951.

162. Sharp HL, Carey JB, White JG, et al. Cholestyramine therapy in patients with a paucity of intrahepatic bile ducts. J Pediatr 71:723, 1967.

163. Alagille D, Odièvre M, Gautier M, et al. Hepatic ductular hypoplasia associated with characteristic facies, vertebral malformations, retarded physical, mental and sexual development and cardiac murmur. J Pediatr 86:63, 1975.

164. Alagille D, Estrada A, Hadchouel M, et al. Syndromatic paucity of interlobular bile ducts (Alagille syndrome or arteriohepatic dysplasia): review of 80 cases. J Pediatr 110:195, 1987.

165. Riely CA. Familial intrahepatic cholestatic syndromes. Semin Liver Dis 7:119, 1987.

166. Perrault G. Paucity of interlobular bile ducts: getting to know it better. Dig Dis Sci 26:481, 1981.

167. Kelley RI. Review: the cerebrohepatorenal syndrome of Zellweger; morphologic and metabolic aspects. Am J Med Genet 16:503, 1983.

168. Eyssen H, Eggermont E, Van Eldere J, et al. Bile acid abnormalities and the diagnosis of cerebro-hepato-renal syndrome (Zellweger syndrome). Acta Paediatr Scand 74:539, 1985.

169. Kahn EI, Daum F, Markowitz J, et al. Arteriohepatic dysplasia. II. Hepatobiliary morphology. Hepatology 3:77, 1983.

170. Kahn E, Daum F, Markowitz J, et al. Nonsyndromatic paucity of interlobular bile ducts: light and electron microscopic evaluation

of sequential liver biopsies in early childhood. Hepatology 6:890, 1986.

171. LaBrecque DR, Mitros FA, Nathan RJ, et al. Four generations of arteriohepatic dysplasia. Hepatology 2:467, 1982.

172. Alagille D, Odièvre M, Hadchouel M. Paucity of interlobular bile ducts: recent concepts. In: Kasai M, ed. Biliary Atresia and its Related Disorders. Amsterdam, Excerpta Medica, 1983:59.

173. Hadchouel M, Hugon RN, Gautier M. Reduced ratio of portal tracts to paucity of intrahepatic bile ducts. Arch Pathol Lab Med 102:402, 1978.

174. Alagille D, Le Tan Vinh: L'absence congénitale des voies biliaires intrahépatiques. Rev Medicochir Mal Foie 37:57, 1962.

175. Dahms BB, Petrelli M, Wyllie R, et al. Arteriohepatic dysplasia in infancy and childhood—a longitudinal study of six patients. Hepatology 2:350, 1982.

176. Berman MD, Ishak KG, Schaefer EJ, et al. Syndromatic hepatic ductular-hypoplasia (arteriohepatic dysplasia). Dig Dis Sci 26:485, 1981.

177. Heathcote J, Deodhar KP, Scheuer P, et al. Intrahepatic cholestasis in childhood. N Engl J Med 295:801, 1976.

178. Ghishan FK, Labrecque DR, Mitros FA, et al. The evolving nature of infantile obstructive cholangiopathy. J Pediatr 97:27, 1980.

179. Danks DM, Campbell PE, Jack I, et al. Studies on the aetiology of neonatal hepatitis and biliary atresia. Arch Dis Child 52:360, 1977.

180. Markowitz J, Daum F, Kahn EI, et al. Arteriohepatic dysplasia. I. Pitfalls in diagnosis and management. Hepatology 3:74, 1983.

181. Pilloud P. Un cas de syndrome de MacMahon-Thannhauser congénital: modalité pathogénique particulière de l'agénésie biliaire intrahépatique. Helv Paediatr Acta 21:327, 1966.

182. Perez-Soler A. The inflammatory and atresia-inducing disease of the liver and bile ducts. Monographs in Paediatrics, Vol. 8. Basel, S Karger, 1976.

183. Odawara M, Partin JC, Schubert WK. Intrahepatic biliary atresia: ultrastructural study of three cases (Abstr). Gastroenterology 60:179, 1971.

184. Valencia-Mayoral P, Weber J, Cutz E, et al. Possible defect in the bile secretory apparatus in arteriohepatic dysplasia (Alagille's syndrome): a review with observations on the ultrastructure of the liver. Hepatology 4:691, 1984.

185. Riely CA, LaBrecque DR, Ghent C, et al. A father and son with cholestasis and peripheral pulmonic stenosis. A distinct form of intrahepatic cholestasis. J Pediatr 92:406, 1978.

186. Riely CA, Cotlier E, Jensen PS, et al. Arteriohepatic dysplasia: a benign syndrome of intrahepatic cholestasis with multiple organ involvement. Ann Intern Med 91:520, 1979.

187. Novotny NM, Zetterman RK, Antonson DL, et al. Variation in liver histology in Alagille's syndrome. Am J Gastroenterol 75:449, 1981.

188. Kocoshis SA, Cottrill CM, O'Connor WN, et al. Congenital heart disease, butterfly vertebrae and intrahepatic biliary atresia: a variant of arteriohepatic dysplasia? J Pediatr 99:436, 1981.

189. Amedee-Manesme O, Bernard O, Brunelle F, et al. Sclerosing cholangitis with neonatal onset. J Pediatr 111:225, 1987.

190. Alagille D. Intrahepatic neonatal cholestasis. In: Javitt NB, ed. Neonatal Hepatitis and Biliary Atresia. US Department of Health, Education and Welfare, DHEW Publication No (NIH) 79–1296, 1979:177.

191. Kerr DNS, Harrison CV, Sherlock S, et al. Congenital hepatic fibrosis. Q J Med 30:91, 1961.

192. Fink U. Ueber intrahepatische Gallengangshyperplasien und Komplikationen. Zentralbl Allg Pathol 93:497, 1955.

193. Kerneis JP, Ferron A de, Gordeef A, et al. La fibro-angio-adénomatose du foie avec hypertension portale. II. Anatomie pathologique. Physiopathologie. Nosologie. Presse Med. 69:1406, 1961.

194. Ferron A de, Gordeef A, Ferron C de, et al. La fibro-angio-adénomatose du foie avec hypertension potale. I. Clinique. Radiologie. Traitement. Presse Med 69:1147, 1961.

195. Caroli J, Corcos V. Maladies des voies biliaires intrahépatiques segmentaires. Paris, Masson, 1964:59.

196. Jörgensen MJ. The ductal plate malformation. Acta Pathol Microbiol Scand (Suppl) 257:1, 1977.

197. Callea F, Facchetti F, Lucini L, et al. Liver morphology in anicteric patients at long-term follow-up after Kasai operation: a study of 16 cases. In: Ohi R, ed. Biliary Atresia. Tokyo, Professional Postgraduate Services, 1987:304.

198. Valayer J. Hepatic porto-enterostomy: surgical problems and results. In: Berenberg SR, ed. Liver Disease in Infancy and Childhood. The Hague, Martinus Nijhoff Medical Division, 1976.

199. Montgomery CK, Ruebner BH. Neonatal hepatocellular giant cell transformation. A review. In: Rosenberg HS, Bolande RP, eds. Perspectives in Pediatric Pathology, Vol. 3. Chicago, Year Book Medical Publishers, 1976:85.

200. Holder TM. Atresia of the extrahepatic bile duct. Am J Surg 107:458, 1964.

201. Holder TM, Ashcraft KW. The effect of bile duct ligation and inflammation in the fetus. J Pediatr Surg 2:35, 1967.

202. Koop CE. Biliary atresia and the Kasai operation. Pediatrics 55:9, 1975.

203. Koop CE. Progressive extrahepatic biliary obstruction of the newborn. J Pediatr Surg 10:169, 1975.

204. Chiba T. Histopathological studies on the prognosis of biliary atresia. Tohoku J Exp Med 122:249, 1977.

205. Kimura K, Tsugawa C, Kubo M, et al. Technical aspects of hepatic portal dissection in biliary atresia. J Pediatr Surg 14:27, 1979.

206. Fonkalsrud EW, Arima E. Bile lakes in congenital biliary atresia. Surgery 77:384, 1975.

207. Scotto JM, Stralin HG. Congenital extrahepatic biliary atresia. Arch Pathol Lab Med 101:416, 1977.

208. Schweizer P. Die Cholestase im Kindesalter aus chirurgischer Sicht. Monatsschr Kinderheilkd 128:292, 1980.

209. Suruga K, Kono S, Miyano T, et al. Treatment of biliary atresia: microsurgery for hepatic portoenterostomy. Surgery 80:558, 1976.

210. Suda J, Nakajima S, Okaniwa M, et al. Neonatal hepatitis and extrahepatic biliary atresia in the same sibship. Tohuku J Exp Med 133:445, 1981.

211. Becroft DM. Biliary atresia associated with prenatal infection by *Listeria monocytogenes*. Arch Dis Child 47:656, 1972.

212. Oppenheimer EH, Esterly JR. Cytomegalovirus infection: a possible cause of biliary atresia. Am J Pathol 71:2a, 1973.

213. Le Tan Vinh, Tran Van Duc, Thieffry St, et al. Association de malformation congénitale et de cytomégalie: étude de 18 observations anatomo-cliniques. Nouvelle Presse Med 2:1411, 1973.

214. Lang DJ, Marshall WC, Pincott JR, et al. Cytomegalovirus: association with neonatal hepatitis and biliary atresia. In: Javitt NB, ed. Neonatal Hepatitis and Biliary Atresia. US Department of Health, Education and Welfare. DHEW Publication No (NIH) 79–1296, 1979:33.

215. Finegold MJ, Carpenter RJ. Obliterative cholangitis due to cytomegalovirus: a possible precursor of paucity of intrahepatic bile ducts. Hum Pathol 13:662, 1982.

216. Numazaki Y, Oshima T, Tanaka A, et al. Neonatal liver disease and cytomegalovirus infection. In: Kasai M, Shiraki K, eds. Cholestasis in Infancy. Tokyo, University of Tokyo Press, 1980:61.

217. Nahmias AJ, Visintine AM. Liver involvement in neonatal herpes simplex virus infection. In: Javitt NB, ed. Neonatal Hepatitis and Biliary Atresia. US Department of Health, Education and Welfare. DHEW Publication No (NIH) 79–1296:47.

218. Szmuness W, Stevens CE. Epidemiology of viral hepatitis A and B with particular reference to children. In: Javitt NB, ed. Neonatal Hepatitis and Biliary Atresia. US Department of Health, Education and Welfare, DHEW Publication No (NIH) 79–1296, 1979:59.

219. Shiraki K, Sakurai M, Yoshihara N, et al. Vertical transmission of HB virus and neonatal hepatitis. In: Kasai M, Shiraki K, eds. Cholestasis in Infancy. Tokyo, University of Tokyo Press, 1980:67.

220. Balistreri WF, Tabor E, Gerety RJ. Negative serology for hepatitis A and B viruses in 18 cases of neonatal cholestasis. Pediatrics 66:270, 1980.

221. De Vos R, Vanstapel MJ, Desmyter J, et al. Are nuclear particles specific for non-A, non-B hepatitis? Hepatology 3:532, 1983.

222. Desmet VJ, De Vos R. Ultrastructural findings in non-A, non-B viral hepatitis. In: Brunner H, Thaler H, eds. Hepatology, a Festschrift for Hans Popper. New York, Raven Press, 1985:159.

223. Spichtin HP, Gudat F, Berthold H, et al. Nuclear particles of non-A, non-B type in healthy volunteers and patients with hepatitis B. Hepatology 4:510, 1984.

224. Weaver LT, Nelson R, Bell TM. The association of extrahepatic bile duct atresia and neonatal Epstein-Barr virus infection. Acta Paediatr Scand 73:155, 1984.

225. Bangaru B, Morecki R, Glaser J, et al. Comparative studies of biliary atresia in the human newborn and reovirus-induced cholangitis in weanling mice. Lab Invest 43:456, 1980.

226. Morecki R, Glaser J, Cho S, et al. Biliary atresia and reovirus type 3 infection. N Engl J Med 307:481, 1982.

227. Glaser JH, Balistreri WF, Morecki R. Role of reovirus type 3 in persistent infantile cholestasis. J Pediatr 105:912, 1984.

228. Morecki R, Glaser JH, Johnson AB, et al. Detection of reovirus type 3 in the porta hepatis of an infant with extrahepatic biliary atresia: ultrastructural and immunocytochemical study. Hepatology 4:1137, 1984.

229. Morecki R, Glaser JH, Horwitz MS. Etiology of biliary atresia: the role of reo 3 virus. In: Daum F, ed. Extrahepatic Biliary Atresia. New York, Marcel Dekker, 1983:1.

230. Cornelius CE, Rosenberg DP. Animal model of human disease. Neonatal biliary atresia. Am J Pathol 118:168, 1985.

231. Morecki R, Glaser J. Pathogenesis of extrahepatic biliary atresia and reovirus type 3 infection. In: Kasai M, ed. Biliary Atresia and its Related Disorders. Amsterdam, Excerpta Medica, 1983:20.

232. Glaser J, Morecki R, Balistreri WF, et al. Neonatal obstructive cholangiopathy and reovirus type 3 infection (Abstr). Hepatology 2:719, 1982.

233. Dussaix E, Hadchouel M, Tardieu M, et al. Biliary atresia and reovirus type 3 infection. N Engl J Med 310:658, 1984.
234. Brown W, Sokol RJ, Levin M, et al. An immunological search for evidence that infection with reovirus 3 causes extrahepatic biliary atresia or neo-natal hepatitis. Gastroenterology 92:1721, 1987.
235. Morecki R, Glaser JH, Cho S, et al. Biliary atresia and reovirus type 3 infection (letter). N Engl J Med 310:1610, 1984.
236. Glaser JH, Morecki R. Reovirus type 3 and neonatal cholestasis. Semin Liver Dis 7:100, 1987.
237. Schweizer P. Modell einer extrahepatischen Gallengangsatresie. Z Kinderchir 15:90, 1974.
238. Morgan WW Jr, Rosenkrantz JB, Hill RB Jr. Hepatic arterial interruption in the fetus. An attempt to simulate biliary atresia. J Pediatr Surg 1:342, 1966.
239. Pickett LK, Briggs HC. Biliary obstruction secondary to hepatic vascular ligation in fetal sheep. J Pediatr Surg 4:95, 1969.
240. Levin JN. Amphetamine ingestion with biliary atresia. J Pediatr 79:130, 1971.
241. Strickland AD, Shannon K. Studies in the etiology of extrahepatic biliary atresia: time-space clustering. J Pediatr 100:749, 1985.
242. Harris RC, Anderson DH. Intrahepatic bile duct atresia. Am J Dis Child 100:783, 1960.
243. Lester R, Pyrek J St, Little JM, et al. Diversity of bile acids in the fetus and newborn infant. J Pediatr Gastroenterol Nutr 2:355, 1983.
244. Colombo C, Zuliani G, Ronchi M, et al. Biliary bile acid composition of the human fetus in early gestation. Pediatr Res 21:197, 1987.
245. Javitt NB. Neonatal cholestasis: identification of a metabolic error in bile acid synthesis. In: Ohi R, ed. Biliary Atresia. Tokyo, Professional Postgraduate Services, 1987:30.
246. Hanson RF, Isenberg JN, Williams GC, et al. The metabolism of 3alpha, 7alpha, 12alpha-trihydroxy-5beta-cholestan-26-oic acid in two siblings with cholestasis due to intrahepatic bile duct anomalies. J Clin Invest 56:577, 1975.
247. Eyssen H, Parmentier G, Compernolle F, et al. Trihydroxy-coprostanic acid in the duodenal fluid of two children with intrahepatic bile duct anomalies. Biochim Biophys Acta 273:212, 1972.
248. Hernanz A, Codoceo R, Jara P, et al. Unusual serum bile acid pattern in children with the syndrome of hepatic ductular hypoplasia. Clin Chim Acta 145:289, 1985.
249. McSherry CK, Morrissey KP, Swarm RL, et al. Chenodeoxycholic acid-induced liver injury in pregnant and neonatal baboons. Ann Surg 184:490, 1976.
250. Jenner RE, Howard ER. Unsaturated monohydroxy bile acids as a cause of idiopathic obstructive cholangiopathy. Lancet 2:1073, 1975.
251. Theron CN, Neethling AC, Taljaard JJF. Sex-dependent differences in phenobarbitone-induced oestradiol-2 hydroxylase activity in rat liver. S Afr Med J 60:279, 1981.
252. Javitt NB, Keating JP, Grand RJ, et al. Serum bile acid patterns in neonatal hepatitis and extrahepatic biliary atresia. J Pediatr 90:736, 1977.
253. Miyano T, Suruga K, Kimura K, et al. A histopathologic study of the region of the ampulla of Vater in congenital biliary atresia. Jpn J Surg 10:34, 1980.
254. Miyano T, Suruga K, Suda K. Abnormal choledocho-pancreaticoductal junction related to etiology of infantile obstructive jaundice diseases. J Pediatr Surg 14:16, 1979.
255. Suda K, Miyano T, Hashimoto K. The choledocho-pancreatico-ductal junction in obstructive jaundice diseases. Acta Pathol Jpn 30:187, 1980.
256. Isseroff H, Sawma JT, Reino D. Fascioliasis: role of proline in bile duct hyperplasia. Science 198:1157, 1977.
257. Vacanti JP, Folkman J. Bile duct enlargement by infusion of L-proline: potential significance in biliary atresia. J Pediatr Surg 14:814, 1979.
258. Selye H, Szabo S. Experimental production of cholangitis by 1,4-phenylenediisothiocyanate. Arch Pathol 94:486, 1972.
259. Ogawa T, Suruga K, Kojima Y, et al. Experimental study of the pathogenesis of infantile obstructive cholangiopathy and its clinical evaluation. J Pediatr Surg 18:131, 1983.
260. Kopelman H, Robertson MH, Sanders PG, et al. The Epping jaundice. Br Med J 1:514, 1966.
261. Bourdelat D, Moulinoux JP, Chambon Y, et al. Prolifération ductulaire biliaire intrahépatique chez la ratte gestante traitée par le 4,4' diaminodiphenylmethane (4,4 DDPM). Bull Assoc Anat (Nancy) 67:375, 1983.
262. De Vos R, De Wolf-Peeters C, Desmet V. A morphologic and histochemical study of biliary atresia in lamprey liver. Z Zellforsch 136:85, 1973.
263. Sidon EW, Youson JH. Morphological changes in the liver of the sea lamprey, Petromyzon marinus L., during metamorphosis: I. Atresia of the bile ducts. J Morphol 177:109, 1983.
264. Sidon EW, Youson JH. Relocalization of membrane enzymes accompanies biliary atresia in lamprey liver. Cell Tissue Res 236:81, 1984.
265. Youson JH, Sidon EW. Lamprey biliary atresia—first model system for the human condition. Experientia 34:1084, 1978.
266. Hays DM, Kimura K. Biliary atresia: the Japanese experience. Cambridge, MA, Harvard University Press, 1980.
267. Chiba T, Kasai M. Differentiation of biliary atresia from neonatal hepatitis by routine clinical examinations. Tohoku J Exp Med 115:327, 1975.
268. Shiraki K, Okaniwa M, Landing BH. Cholestatic syndromes of infancy and childhood. In: Zakim D, Boyer TD, eds. Hepatology. A Textbook of Liver Disease. Philadelphia, WB Saunders, 1982:1176.
269. Sakurai M, Shiraki K. Quantitative diagnosis of biliary atresia and neonatal hepatitis. In: Kasai M, Shiraki K, eds. Cholestasis in Infancy. Tokyo, University of Tokyo Press, 1980:293.
270. Sunaryo FP, Watkins JB. Evaluation of diagnostic techniques for extrahepatic biliary atresia. In: Daum F, ed. Extrahepatic Biliary Atresia. New York, Marcel Dekker, 1983:11.
271. Zeltzer PM, Neerhout RC, Fonkalsrud EW, et al. Differentiation between neonatal hepatitis and biliary atresia by measuring serum alpha-fetoprotein. Lancet 1:373, 1974.
272. Andres JM, Lilly JR, Altman RP, et al. Alpha-1-fetoprotein in neonatal hepatobiliary disease. J Pediatr 91:217, 1977.
273. Manthorpe D, Mowat AP. Serum bile acids in the neonatal hepatitis syndrome. In: Alagille D, ed. Liver Diseases in Children (Hepatologie Infantile). Paris, Editions INSERM, 1976:57.
274. Poley JR, Alaupovic P, Knight-Gibson C, et al. The quantitative determination of serum lipoprotein-X and apolipoproteins in infants with cholestatic liver and biliary tract disease. In: Daum F, ed. Extrahepatic Biliary Atresia. New York, Marcel Dekker, 1983:33.
275. Tazawa Y, Yamada M, Nakagawa M, et al. Significance of serum lipoprotein-X and gammaglutamyltranspeptidase in the diagnosis of biliary atresia. A preliminary study in 27 cholestatic young infants. Eur J Pediatr 145:54, 1986.
276. Fung KP. Lipoprotein-X and diagnosis of biliary atresia (letter). Eur J Pediatr 146:312, 1987.
277. Deutsch J, Kurz R, Mueller WD, et al. Lipoprotein X, gamma-glutamyltranspeptidase and biliary atresia (letter). Eur J Pediatr 146:313, 1987.
278. Melhorn DK, Gross S, Izant RJ. The red cell hydrogen peroxide hemolysis test and vitamin E absorption in the differential diagnosis of jaundice in infancy. J Pediatr 81:1082, 1972.
279. Jusko WJ, Levy G, Yaffe SJ, et al. Riboflavin absorption in children with biliary obstruction. Am J Dis Child 121:48, 1971.
280. Greene HL, Helinek GL, Moran R, et al. A diagnostic approach to prolonged obstructive jaundice by 24-hour collection of duodenal fluid. J Pediatr 95:412, 1979.
281. Hashimoto S, Tsugawa C, Kimura K, et al. Naso-duodenal tube insertion technique for rapid diagnosis of congenital biliary atresia. J Jpn Soc Pediatr Surg 14:889, 1978.
282. Yamashiro Y, Robinson PG, Lari J, et al. Duodenal bile acids in diagnosis of congenital biliary atresia. J Pediatr Surg 18:278, 1983.
283. Lebwohl O, Waye JD. Endoscopic retrograde cholangio-pancreatography in the diagnosis of extrahepatic biliary atresia. Am J Dis Child 133:647, 1979.
284. Waye JD. Endoscopic retrograde cholangiopancreatography in the infant. Am J Gastroenterol 65:461, 1976.
285. Allendorph M, Werlin SL, Geenen JE, et al. Endoscopic retrograde cholangiopancreatography in children. J Pediatr 110:206, 1987.
286. Guelrud M, Jean D, Torres P, et al. Endoscopic cholangiopancreatography in the infant: evaluation of a new prototype pediatric duodenoscope. Gastrointest Endosc 33:4, 1987.
287. Takahashi H, Kuriyama Y, Maie M, et al. ERCP in jaundiced infants. In: Ohi R, ed. Biliary Atresia. Tokyo, Professional Postgraduate Services, 1987:110.
288. Howard ER, Nunnerley HB. Percutaneous cholangiography in prolonged jaundice of childhood. J R Soc Med 72:495, 1979.
289. Leape LL, Ramenofsky ML. Laparoscopy in infants and children. J Pediatr Surg 12:929, 1977.
290. White WE, Welsh JS, Darrow DC, et al. Pediatric application of the radioiodine (I-131) Rose Bengal method in hepatic and biliary system disease. Pediatrics 32:239, 1963.
291. Antico VF, Denhartog P, Ash JM, et al. The I-131 Rose Bengal excretion test is not dead. Clin Nucl Med 10:171, 1985.
292. Ryckman FC, Noseworthy J. Neonatal cholestatic conditions requiring surgical reconstruction. Semin Liver Dis 7:134, 1987.
293. Majd M. Radionuclide studies in the evaluation of neonatal jaundice. In: Daum F, ed. Extrahepatic Biliary Atresia. New York, Marcel Dekker, 1983:23.
294. Majd M, Reba R, Altman R. Hepatobiliary scintigraphy with 99m technetium PIPIDA in the evaluation of neonatal jaundice. Pediatrics 67:140, 1981.
295. Verreault J, Danais S, Blanchard H, et al. Scintigraphie hepato-biliaire au disida-99mTc et cholangiopathies obstructives infantiles. Chir Pediatr 28:1, 1987.

296. Spivak W, Sarkar S, Winter D, et al. Diagnostic utility of hepatobiliary scintigraphy with 99m TC-DISIDA in neonatal cholestasis. J Pediatr 110:855, 1987.
297. Kumura D, Miller JH, Sinatra FR. Septo-optic dysplasia: recognition of causes of false-positive hepatobiliary scintigraphy in neonatal jaundice. J Nucl Med 28:966, 1987.
298. Han BK, Babcock DS, Gelfand MH. Choledochal cyst with bile duct dilatation: sonography and 99m Tc-IDA cholescintigraphy. Am J Roentgenol 136:1075, 1981.
299. Abramson SJ, Berdon WE, Altman RP, et al. Biliary atresia and noncardiac polysplenic syndrome: US and surgical considerations. Radiology 163:377, 1987.
300. Marchal GI, Desmet VJ, Proesmans WC, et al. Caroli disease: high-frequency U.S. and pathologic findings. Radiology 158:507, 1986.
301. Green D, Carroll BA. Ultrasonography in the jaundiced infant. J Ultrasound Med 5:323, 1986.
302. Greenholz SK, Lilly JR, Shikes RH, et al. Biliary atresia in the newborn. J Pediatr Surg 21:1147, 1986.
303. Balistreri WF. Neonatal cholestasis. In: Lebenthal E, ed. Textbook of Gastroenterology and Nutrition in Infancy. New York, Raven Press, 1981:1081.
304. Mowat AP. Liver Disorders in Children. London, Butterworths, 1979.
305. Mowat AP. Paediatric liver disease: medical aspects. In: Wright R, Millward-Sadler GH, Alberti KGMM, et al., eds. Liver and Biliary Disease, 2nd ed. London, Philadelphia, Baillière Tindall, WB Saunders, 1985:1201.
306. Altman RP, Levy J. Biliary atresia. Pediatr Ann 14:481, 1985.
307. Adelman S. Prognosis of uncorrected biliary atresia: an update. J Pediatr Surg 13:389, 1978.
308. Hays DM, Snyder WH. Life-span in untreated biliary atresia. Surgery 54:373, 1963.
309. Longmire WP Jr, Sanford MC. Intrahepatic-cholangiojejunostomy with partial hepatectomy for biliary atresia. Surgery 24:264, 1948.
310. Krumhaar D, Hecker W, Joppich J, et al. Analyse von 49 Gallenweg-serkrankungen im Kindesalter. Arch Kinderheilkd 182:47, 1970.
311. Suruga K, Yamazaki Z, Iwai S, et al. The surgery of infantile obstructive jaundice. Arch Dis Child 40:158, 1965.
312. Hasse W. Studien über die intrahepatische Gefäsztopographie des Frischgeborenen und Säuglings. Erg Chir Orthop 48:1, 1966.
313. Nixon HH. Leberchirurgie im Säuglings- und Kindesalter. Z Kinderchir 1:83, 1964.
314. Sterling JA, Lowenburg AH. Observations of infants with hepatic duct atresia and use of artificial duct prothesis. Pediatr Clin North Am 9:485, 1962.
315. Aterman K, Lav H, Gillis DA. The response of the liver to implantation of artificial bile ducts. J Pediatr Surg 6:413, 1971.
316. Shimura H, Nakamura Y, Sakai M. Indication of surgical treatment for biliary atresia. Shujitsu 17:872, 1963.
317. Absolon KB, Rikkers H, Aust JB. Thoracic duct lymph drainage in congenital biliary atresia. Surg Gynecol Obstet 120:123, 1965.
318. Hasse W, Waldschmidt J, Grohne H, et al. Experimental studies on thoracic duct anastomosis with the esophagus in dogs. J Pediatr Surg 2:553, 1967.
319. Suruga K, Nagashima N, Hirai Y, et al. A clinical and pathological study of congenital biliary atresia. J Pediatr Surg 2:558, 1967.
320. Williams LF, Dooling JA. Thoracic duct–esophagus anastomosis for relief of congenital biliary atresia. Surg Forum 14:189, 1963.
321. Fonkalsrud EW, Kitawaga S, Longmire WP Jr. Hepatic lymphatic drainage to the jejunum for congenital biliary atresia. Am J Surg 112:188, 1966.
322. Thaler MM. Cryptogenic liver disease in young infants. In: Popper H, Schaffner F, eds. Progress in Liver Diseases, Vol. 5. New York, Grune & Stratton, 1976:476.
323. Howard ER. Paediatric liver disease: surgical aspects. In: Wright R, Millward-Sadler GH, Alberti KGMM, et al., eds. Liver and Biliary Disease, 2nd ed. London, Philadelphia, Baillière Tindall, WB Saunders, 1985:1219.
324. Ohi R, Chiba T, Ohkochi N, et al. The present status of surgical treatment for biliary atresia: report of the questionnaire for the main institutions in Japan. In: Ohi R, ed. Biliary Atresia. Tokyo, Professional Postgraduate Services, 1987:125.
325. Javitt NB. Neonatal hepatitis and biliary atresia. (An International Workshop, March 1977). US Department of Health, Education and Welfare. DHEW Publication Np (NIH) 79–1296, 1978.
326. Suruga K. Congenital biliary atresia—surgical treatment of congenital biliary atresia. Shujutsu 24:543, 1970.
327. Suruga K, Miyano T, Kitahara T, et al. Treatment of biliary atresia: a study of our operative results. J Pediatr Surg 16:621, 1981.
328. Sawaguchi S, Akiyama Y, Saeki M, et al. The treatment of congenital biliary atresia with special reference to hepatic portoenteroanastomosis. Tokyo, Fifth Annual Meeting of the Pacific Association of Pediatric Surgeons, 1972.
329. Lilly JR, Hitch DC. Postoperative ascending cholangitis following portoenterostomy for biliary atresia: measures for control. World J Surg 2:581, 1978.

330. Burnweit CA, Coln D. Influence of diversion on the development of cholangitis after hepatoportoenterostomy for biliary atresia. J Pediatr Surg 21:1143, 1986.
331. Hirsig J, Rickham PP, Briner J. The importance of hepatic lymph drainage in experimental biliary atresia. Effect of omentopexy on preventation of cholangitis. J Pediatr Surg 14:142, 1979.
332. Ito T, Nagaya M, Ando H, et al. Modified hepatic portal enterostomy for biliary atresia. Z Kinderchir 39:242, 1984.
333. Endo M, Katsumata K, Yokoyama J, et al. Extended dissection of the porta hepatis and creation of an intussuscepted ileocolic conduit for biliary atresia. J Pediatr Surg 18:784, 1983.
334. Hata Y, Uchino J, Kasai Y. Revision of porto-enterostomy in congenital biliary atresia. J Pediatr Surg 20:217, 1985.
335. Shim WKT, JIN-ZHE Z. Antirefluxing roux-en-Y biliary drainage valve for hepatic portoenterostomy: animal experiments and clinical experience. J Pediatr Surg 20:689, 1985.
336. Matory YL, Miyano T, Suruga K. Hepaticportoenterostomy as surgical therapy for biliary atresia. Surg Gynecol Obstet 161:541, 1985.
337. Kasai M. Hepatic portoenterostomy for the so-called "noncorrectable" type of biliary atresia. In: Daum F, ed. Extrahepatic Biliary Atresia. New York, Marcel Dekker, 1983:79.
338. Kobayashi A, Utsunomiya T, Kawai S, et al. Congenital biliary atresia. Am J Dis Child 130:830, 1976.
339. Odièvre M. Long-term results of surgical treatment of biliary atresia. World J Surg 2:589, 1978.
340. Hays DM, Kimura K. Biliary atresia: new concepts of management. Curr Probl Surg 18:546, 1981.
341. Kitamura T, Sawaguchi S, Akiyama H, et al. Langzeitresultate nach Operation der angeborenen Gallengansatresie bei 144 eigenen Fällen. Z Kinderchir 31:239, 1980.
342. Caccia G, Dessanti A, Alberti D. Clinical results in 90 patients with biliary atresia: 2–10 years. In: Ohi R, ed. Biliary Atresia. Tokyo, Professional Postgraduate Services, 1987:281.
343. Gautier M, Valayer J, Odièvre M, et al. Histologic liver evaluation 5 years after surgery for extrahepatic biliary atresia: a study of 20 cases. J Pediatr Surg 19:263, 1984.
344. Kobayashi A, Itabashi F, Ohbe Y. Long-term prognosis in biliary atresia after hepatic portoenterostomy: analysis of 35 patients who survived beyond 5 years of age. J Pediatr 105:243, 1984.
345. Ohi R, Mochizuki I, Komatsu K, et al. Portal hypertension after successful hepatic portoenterostomy in biliary atresia. J Pediatr Surg 21:271, 1986.
346. Altman RP. Long-term results after the Kasai procedure. In: Daum F, ed. Extrahepatic Biliary Atresia. New York, Marcel Dekker, 1983:91.
347. Howard ER, Driver M, McClement J, et al. Biliary atresia: the results of surgery in 88 consecutive cases. In: Daum F, ed. Extrahepatic Biliary Atresia. New York, Marcel Dekker, 1983:99.
348. Ohi R, Hanamatsu M, Mochizuki I, et al. Progress in the treatment of biliary atresia. World J Surg 9:285, 1985.
349. Valayer J. Biliary atresia and portal hypertension. In: Daum F, ed. Extrahepatic Biliary Atresia. New York, Marcel Dekker, 1983:105.
350. Canty TG, Self TW, Collins DL, et al. Recent experience with a modified Sawaguchi procedure for biliary atresia. J Pediatr Surg 20:211, 1985.
351. Canty TG Sr. Encouraging results with a modified Sawaguchi hepato-portoenterostomy for biliary atresia. Am J Surg 154:19, 1987.
352. Kasai M. Advances in treatment of biliary atresia. Jpn J Surg 13:265, 1983.
353. Kasai M, Ohi R, Chiba T. Long-term survivors after surgery for biliary atresia. In: Ohi R, ed. Biliary Atresia. Tokyo, Professional Postgraduate Services, 1987:277.
354. McClement JW, Howard ER, Mowat AP. Results of surgical treatment for extrahepatic biliary atresia in United Kingdom 1980–2. Br Med J 290:345, 1984.
355. Schweizer P. Langzeitergebnisse in der Behandlung der extrahepatischen Gallengangsatresie. Z Kinderchir 40:263, 1985.
356. Schweizer P. Treatment of extrahepatic bile duct atresia: results and long term prognosis after hepatic portoenterostomy. Pediatr Surg Int 1:30, 1986.
357. Barkin RM, Lilly JR. Biliary atresia and the Kasai operation: continuing care. J Pediatr 96:1015, 1980.
358. Balistreri WF. Clinical aspects. In: Ishak KG, ed. Hepatopathology 1985. AASLD Postgraduate Course 1985. American Association for the Study of Liver Diseases, Chicago, 1985:69.
359. Starzl TE, Marchioro TL, von Kaulla KN, et al. Homotransplantation of the liver in humans. Surg Gynecol Obstet 117:659, 1963.
360. Van Wijk J, Halgrimson CG, Giles G, et al. Liver transplantation in biliary atresia with concomitant hepatoma. S Afr Med J 46:885, 1972.
361. Starzl T, Iwatsuki S, Van Thiel D, et al. Evolution of liver transplantation. Hepatology 2:614, 1982.
362. Krom RAF. Liver transplantation (1963–1983): a review of results of

the centers Pittsburgh, Cambridge, Hannover, Groningen, Innsbruck and Paris. In: Gips CH, Krom RAF, eds. Progress in Liver Transplantation. Dordrecht, Martinus Nijhoff, 1985:3.

363. Iwatsuki S, Starzl TE, Shaw BW Jr, et al. Pediatric liver transplantation. In: Gips, CH, Krom RAF, eds. Progress in Liver Transplantation. Dordrecht, Martinus Nijhoff, 1985:196.

364. Starzl TE. Liver transplantation for biliary atresia. In: Daum F, ed. Extrahepatic Biliary Atresia. New York, Marcel Dekker, 1983:111.

365. Iwatsuki S. Liver transplantation for children with biliary atresia. In: Ohi R, ed. Biliary Atresia. Tokyo, Professional Postgraduate Services, 1987:315.

366. Gartner JC, Zitelli BJ, Malatack JT, et al. Orthotopic liver transplantation in children: two-year experience with 47 patients. Pediatrics 74:140, 1984.

367. Ascher NL, Najarian JS. Hepatic transplantation and biliary atresia: early experience in eight patients. World J Surg 8:57, 1984.

368. Gips CH, Krom RAF. Progress in Liver Transplantation. Dordrecht, Martinus Nijhoff, 1985.

369. Otte J-B, De Hemptinne B, De Ville de Goyet J, et al. Liver transplantation in children. In: Ohi R, ed. Biliary Atresia. Tokyo, Professional Postgraduate Services, 1987:320.

370. Bismuth H, Castaing D, Ericzon BG, et al. Hepatic transplantation in Europe. First report of the European liver transplant registry. Lancet 2:674, 1987.

371. Fennell RH, Vierling JM. Electron microscopy of rejected human liver allografts. Hepatology 5:1083, 1985.

372. Sharp HL, Snover DC, Burke BA, et al. The role of clinical evaluation in graft rejection following liver transplantation. In: Daum F, ed. Extrahepatic Biliary Atresia. New York, Marcel Dekker, 1983:119.

373. Ludwig J, Wiesner RH, Batts KP, et al. The acute vanishing bile duct syndrome (acute irreversible rejection) after orthotopic liver transplantation. Hepatology 7:476, 1987.

374. Snover DC, Freese DK, Sharp HL, et al. Liver allograft rejection. An analysis of the use of biopsy in determining outcome of rejection. Am J Surg Pathol 11:1, 1987.

375. Alagille D. Extrahepatic biliary atresia. Hepatology (Suppl) 4(1):7S, 1984.

376. Miyata M, Satani M, Ueda T, et al. Long-term results of hepatic portoenterostomy for biliary atresia; special reference to postoperative portal hypertension. Surgery 76:234, 1974.

377. Kasai M, Watanabe I, Ohi R. Follow-up studies of long-term survivors after hepatic portoenterostomy for "non correctable" biliary atresia. J Pediatr Surg 10:173, 1975.

378. Kasai M, Okamoto A, Ohi R, et al. Changes of portal vein pressure and intrahepatic blood vessels after surgery for biliary atresia. J Pediatr Surg 10:152, 1981.

379. Lilly JR, Stellin G. Variceal hemorrhage in biliary atresia. J Pediatr Surg 19:476, 1984.

380. Sondheimer JW, Shandling B, Weber JL, et al. Hepatic function following portoenterostomy for extrahepatic biliary atresia. Can Med Assoc J 118:255, 1978.

381. Howard ER, Mowat AP. Hepatobiliary disorders in infancy: hepatitis, extrahepatic biliary atresia; intrahepatic biliary hypoplasia. In: Thomas HC, MacSween RNM, eds. Recent Advances in Hepatology. Edinburgh, Churchill Livingstone, 1983:153.

382. Bussutil RW. Discussion on paper by Canty TG. Am J Surg 154:25, 1987.

383. Werlin SL, Sty JR, Starshak RJ, et al. Intrahepatic biliary tract abnormalities in children with corrected extrahepatic biliary atresia. J Pediatr Gastroenterol Nutr 4:537, 1985.

384. Saito S, Nishina T, Tsuchida Y. Intrahepatic cysts in biliary atresia after successful hepatoportoenterostomy. Arch Dis Child 59:274, 1984.

385. Gautier M, Moitier G, Odièvre M. "Uncorrectable" extrahepatic biliary atresia. Relationship between intrahepatic bile duct pattern and surgery. J Pediatr Surg 15:129, 1980.

386. Watanabe I, Ohi R, Okamoto A, et al. Postoperative changes in the histologic picture of the liver in biliary atresia. In: Kasai M, Shiraki K, eds. Cholestasis in Infancy. Tokyo, University of Tokyo Press, 1980:381.

387. Dessanti A, Ohi R, Hanamatsu M, et al. Short term histological liver changes in extrahepatic biliary atresia with good postoperative bile drainage. Arch Dis Child 60:739, 1985.

388. Hadchouel M, Gautier M, Valayer J, et al. Histopathology of the liver five years after successful surgery for extrahepatic biliary atresia. In: Daum F, ed. Extrahepatic Biliary Atresia. New York, Marcel Dekker, 1983:65.

389. Nio M, Takahashi T, Ohi R. Changes of intrahepatic portal veins in biliary atresia: formation and development of medial smooth muscles correlated with portal hypertension. In: Ohi R, ed. Biliary Atresia. Tokyo, Professional Postgraduate Services, 1987:243.

390. Hernandez-Cano AM, Geis JR, Rumack CH, et al. Portal vein dynamics in biliary atresia. J Pediatr Surg 22:519, 1987.

391. Weinbren K, Hadjis NS, Blumgart LH. Structural aspects of the liver in patients with biliary disease and portal hypertension. J Clin Pathol 38:1013, 1985.

392. Bunton GL, Cameron R. Regeneration of liver after biliary cirrhosis. Ann NY Acad Sci 111:412, 1963.

393. Yeong ML, Nicholson GI, Lee SP. Regression of biliary cirrhosis following choledochal cyst drainage. Gastroenterology 82:332, 1985.

394. Ludwig J, Czaja AJ, Dickson ER, et al. Manifestations of nonsuppurative cholangitis in chronic hepatobiliary diseases: morphologic spectrum, clinical correlations and terminology. Liver 4:105, 1984.

395. Ludwig J. New concepts in biliary cirrhosis. Semin Liver Dis 7:293, 1987.

396. Popper H. Changing concepts of the evolution of chronic hepatitis and the role of piecemeal necrosis. Hepatology 3:758, 1983.

397. Akiyama H, Saeki M, Ogata T. Portal hypertension after successful surgery for biliary atresia. In: Kasai M, ed. Biliary Atresia and its Related Disorders. Amsterdam, Excerpta Medica, 1967:276.

398. Okamoto E, Toyosaka A, Okasora T. Surgical treatment of portal hypertension in biliary atresia. In: Kasai M, ed. Biliary Atresia and its Related Disorders. Amsterdam, Excerpta Medica, 1983:283.

399. Kasai M, Okamoto A, Ohi R, et al. Changes of portal vein pressure and intrahepatic blood vessels after surgery for biliary atresia. J Pediatr Surg 16:152, 1981.

400. Mallet-Guy D, Michoulier J, Beau S. Experimental studies on liver lymph flow: conditions affecting bilio-lymphatic transfer. In: Taylor W, ed. The Biliary System. Philadelphia, FA Davis, 1965:69.

401. Kimura S, Togon H, Sakai K. Histological studies of the liver in long-term survivors. In: Ohi R, ed. Biliary Atresia. Tokyo, Professional Postgraduate Services, 1987:299.

402. Larcher VF, Vegnente A, Psacharopoulos HT, et al. Immune responses in patients with obstructive jaundice in infancy. Acta Paediatr Scand 72:59, 1983.

403. De Freitas LAR, Chevallier M, Louis D, Grimaud J-A. Human extrahepatic biliary atresia: portal connective tissue activation related to ductular proliferation. Liver 6:253, 1986.

404. Lilly JR. The surgery of biliary hypoplasia. J Pediatr Surg 11:815, 1976.

405. Longmire WP. Congenital biliary hypoplasia. Ann Surg 159:335, 1964.

406. Krant SM, Swenson O. Biliary duct hypoplasia. J Pediatr Surg 8:301, 1973.

407. Afroudakis A, Kaplowitz N. Liver histopathology in chronic common bile duct stenosis due to chronic alcoholic pancreatitis. Hepatology 1:65, 1981.

408. Altman RP, Chandra R. Biliary hypoplasia as a consequence of alpha-1-antitrypsin deficiency. Surg Forum 27:377, 1976.

409. Odièvre M, Martin JP, Hadchouel M, et al. Alpha-1-antitrypsin deficiency and liver disease in children: phenotypes, manifestations and prognosis. Pediatrics 57:226, 1976.

410. Porter CA, Mowat AP, Cook PJL, et al. Alpha-1-antitrypsin deficiency and neonatal hepatitis. Br Med J 3:435, 1972.

411. Gorelick FS, Dobbins JW, Burrell M, et al. Biliary tract abnormalities in patients with arteriohepatic dysplasia. Dig Dis Sci 27:815, 1982.

412. Morelli A, Pelli MA, Vedovelli A, et al. Endoscopic retrograde cholangiopancreatography study in Alagille's syndrome: first report. Am J Gastroenterol 78:241, 1983.

413. Dijkstra CH. Galuitstorting in de buikholte bij een zuigeling. Maandschr Kindergeneesk 1:409, 1932.

414. Johnston JH. Spontaneous perforation of the common bile ducts in infancy. Br J Surg 48:532, 1961.

415. Moore TC. Massive bile peritonitis in infancy due to spontaneous bile duct perforation with portal vein occlusion. J Pediatr Surg 10:537, 1975.

416. Caulfield E. Bile peritonitis in infancy. Am J Dis Child 52:1348, 1936.

417. Prevot J, Babut JM. Spontaneous perforations of the biliary tract in infancy. Prog Pediatr Surg 3:187, 1971.

418. Howard ER, Johnston DI, Mowat AP. Spontaneous perforation of common bile duct in infants. Arch Dis Child 51:883, 1976.

419. Lilly JR, Weintraub WH, Altman RP. Spontaneous perforation of the extrahepatic bile ducts and bile peritonitis in infancy. Surgery 75:664, 1974.

420. Dunn DC, Lees VC. Spontaneous perforation of the common bile duct in infancy. Br J Surg 73:929, 1986.

421. Bernstein J, Braylan R, Brough AJ. Bile plug syndrome: a correctable cause of obstructive jaundice in infants. Pediatrics 43:273, 1969.

422. Hsia DYY, Patterson P, Allen FH, et al. Prolonged obstructive jaundice in infancy. Pediatrics 10:243, 1952.

423. Rickham PP, Lee EYC. Neonatal jaundice: surgical aspects. Clin Pediatr 3:197, 1964.

424. Akers DR, Favara BE, Franciosi RA, et al. Duplications of the alimentary tract: report of three unusual cases associated with bile and pancreatic ducts. Surgery 71:817, 1972.

425. Wrenn EL Jr, Favara BE. Duodenal duplication (or pancreatic bladder) presenting as double gallbladder. Surgery 69:858, 1971.

426. Whittington PF, Black DD. Cholelithiasis in premature infants treated with parenteral nutrition and furosemide. J Pediatr 97:647, 1980.
427. Taira Y, Nakayama I, Moriuchi A, et al. Sarcoma botryoides arising from the biliary tract of children—a case report with review of the literature. Acta Pathol Jpn 26:709, 1976.
428. Akers DR, Needham ME. Sarcoma botryoides (Rhabdomyosarcoma) of the bile ducts with survival. J Pediatr Surg 6:474, 1971.
429. Nixon HH. Paediatric liver disease: surgical aspects. In: Wright R, Alberti KGMM, Karran S, et al., eds. Liver and Biliary Disease, 1st ed. London, WB Saunders, 1979:962.
430. Werlin SL, Glicklich M, Jona J, et al. Sclerosing cholangitis in childhood. J Pediatr 96:433, 1980.
431. Spivak W, Grand RJ, Eraklis A. A case of primary sclerosing cholangitis in childhood. Gastroenterology 82:129, 1982.
432. Naveh Y, Mendelsohn M, Spira G, et al. Primary sclerosing cholangitis associated with immunodeficiency. Am J Dis Child 137:114, 1983.
433. Descos B, Brunelle F, Fischer A, et al. Sclerosing cholangitis in children with immunodeficiency (Abstr). Pediatr Res 18:1059, 1984.
434. Record CO, Shilkin KB, Eddleston ALWF, et al. Intrahepatic sclerosing cholangitis associated with a familial immunodeficiency syndrome. Lancet 2:18, 1973.
435. Leblanc A, Hadchouel M, Jehan P, et al. Obstructive jaundice in children with histiocytosis X. Gastroenterology 80:134, 1981.
436. Hellstrom HR, Perez-Stable EC. Retroperitoneal fibrosis with disseminated vasculitis and intrahepatic sclerosing cholangitis. Am J Med 40:184, 1986.
437. Alpert LI, Jindrak K. Idiopathic retroperitoneal fibrosis and sclerosing cholangitis associated with a reticulum cell sarcoma. Gastroenterology 62:111, 1972.
438. El-Shabrawi M, Wilkinson ML, Portmann B, et al. Primary sclerosing cholangitis in childhood. Gastroenterology 92:1226, 1987.
439. Classen M, Götze H, Richter H-J, et al. Primary sclerosing cholangitis in children. J Pediatr Gastroenterol Nutr 6:197, 1987.
440. Craig JM, Landing BH. Form of hepatitis in neonatal period simulating biliary atresia. Arch Pathol 54:321, 1952.
441. Dick MC, Mowat AP. Hepatitis syndrome in infany—an epidemiological survey with 10 year follow up. Arch Dis Child 60:512, 1985.
442. Chandra RK. The neonatal hepatitis syndrome. Trop Gastroenterol 2:94, 1981.
443. Felber S, Sinatra F. Systemic disorders associated with neonatal cholestasis. Semin Liver Dis 7:108, 1987.
444. Alagille D. Closing remarks. In: Kasai M, ed. Biliary Atresia and its Related Disorders. Amsterdam, Excerpta Medica, 1983:301.
445. Lawson EE, Boggs JD. Long-term follow-up of neonatal hepatitis: safety and value of surgical exploration. Pediatrics 53:650, 1974.
446. Odièvre M, Hadchouel M, Landrieu P, et al. Long-term prognosis for infants with intrahepatic cholestasis and patent extrahepatic biliary tract. Arch Dis Child 56:373, 1981.
447. Danks DM, Campbell PE, Smith AL, et al. Prognosis of babies with neonatal hepatitis. Arch Dis Child 52:368, 1977.
448. Ruebner B. The pathology of neonatal hepatitis. Am J Pathol 36:151, 1960.
449. Christoffersen P, Poulsen H, Skeie E. Focal liver cell necroses accompanied by infiltration of granulocytes arising during operation. Acta Hepato-Splenolog (Stuttgart) 17:240, 1970.
450. Kadas I. Neonatal hepatitis: histological and differential diagnostic aspects. Acta Morphol Acad Sci Hung 24:223, 1976.
451. Ruebner B, Thaler MM. Giant-cell transformation in infantile liver disease. In: Javitt NB, ed. Neonatal Hepatitis and Biliary Atresia. US Department of Health, Education and Welfare, DHEW Publication No. (NIH) 79–1296, 1979:299.
452. Schaffner F, Popper H. Morphologic studies in neonatal hepatitis with emphasis on giant cells. Ann NY Acad Sci 111:358, 1963.
453. Czenkar B. Pathologie der Riesenzellenhepatitis von Neugeborenen und Säuglingen. Virchows. Arch Pathol Anat 331:696, 1958.
454. Smetana HF, Edlow JB, Glunz PR. Neonatal Jaundice. A critical review of persistent obstructive jaundice in infancy. Arch Pathol 80:553, 1965.
455. Dible JH, Hunt WE, Pugh VW, et al. Foetal and neonatal hepatitis and its sequelae. J Pathol Bacteriol 67:195, 1954.
456. Oledzka-Slotwinska H, Desmet V. Morphologic and cytochemical study on neonatal liver "giant" cell transformation. Exp Mol. Pathol 10:162, 1969.
457. Schmid M, Pirovino M, Altorfer J, et al. Acute hepatitis non-A, non-B; are there any specific light microscopic features? Liver 2:61, 1982.
458. Thaler H. Post-infantile giant cell hepatitis. Liver 2:393, 1982.
459. Pessayre D, Degos F, Feldmann G, et al. Chronic active hepatitis and giant multinucleated hepatocytes in adults treated with clometacin. Digestion 22:66, 1981.
460. Campbell LV Jr, Gilbert EF. Experimental giant-cell transformation in the liver induced by E. coli endotoxin. Am J Pathol 51:855, 1967.
461. Andres JM, Walker WA. Effect of Escherichia coli endotoxin on the developing rat liver. I. Giant cell induction and disruption in protein metabolism. Pediatr Res 13:1290, 1979.
462. Andres JM, Darby BR, Walker WA. The effect of E. coli endotoxin on the developing rat liver. II. Immunohistochemical localization of alpha-fetoprotein in rat liver multinucleated giant cells. Pediatr Res 17:1017, 1983.
463. Svoboda DJ, Reddy JK, Liu C. Multinucleate giant cells in livers of marmosets given aflatoxin B1. Arch Pathol 91:452, 1971.
464. Deutsch J, Smith AL, Danks DM, et al. Long-term prognosis for babies with neonatal liver disease. Arch Dis Child 60:447, 1985.

52

Cystic Diseases of the Liver

Camillus L. Witzleben, M.D.

ABBREVIATIONS

DPM = ductal plate malformation
CHF = congenital hepatic fibrosis
APCD = adult polycystic disease (dominantly inherited polycystic disease)
IPCD = infantile polycystic disease (recessively inherited polycystic disease)

We define a cyst in this chapter as a tissue-enclosed space that is abnormal in location or size. The space, or cyst, may contain only air, or it may be filled wholly or partially with liquid or solids. So defined, a cyst may be a normal structure that has become dilated, for example, a biliary duct, or it may be an abnormal structure with a discrete wall. The latter can be fibrous or composed of a variety of tissues, including those in which it has formed. Abscesses, which would be a variety of cyst as defined here, are not discussed in this chapter (see Chaps. 39 and 40). Table 52–1 presents a proposed classification of hepatic cysts. It includes several types (e.g., parasitic, neoplastic) that are discussed more extensively in Chapters 39 and 45.

The classification in Table 52–1 differs somewhat from those usually presented. In the author's opinion, most

TABLE 52–1. PROPOSED CLASSIFICATION OF HEPATIC CYSTS

Parasitic
Nonparasitic
A. Solitary (sporadic; occasionally multiple, possibly multiple origins)
B. Polycystic (heritable; ductal origin; multiple; lesions in other viscera)
   1. Noncommunicating ductal cysts
      a. Adult polycystic disease (APCD)*
   2. Communicating ductal cysts with DPM
      a. CHF
      b. IPCD
      c. Malformation syndromes
         (1) Meckel-Gruber syndrome
         (2) Other (Ivemark's syndrome and so on)
      d. CHF—nephronophthisis†
   3. Communicating ductal cysts without DPM (simple Caroli's disease)‡
C. Systemic biliary dilation (not heritable, no DPM, no lesions in other viscera)
   1. With choledochal cyst
   2. Without choledochal cyst
D. Other
   1. Traumatic
   2. Infarcts
   3. Duodenal duplication
   4. Neoplastic
      a. Cystadenoma and cystadenocarcinoma
      b. Mesenchymal hamartoma
      c. Giant cavernous hemangioma
      d. Teratoma
      e. Other
   5. Peliosis

*Some percentage of cases have DPM (see text).
†May be unrelated to polycystic disease (see text).
‡Caroli's disease is rare, if it occurs at all (see text).
The author feels the distinctions between solitary and polycystic (as defined here) and between communicating and noncommunicating are more significant in pathogenetic terms, and more legitimately applied, than the usual distinction between congenital and acquired.

classifications of hepatic cysts make capricious (and in some respects clinically insignificant) distinctions between congenital and acquired cysts, and use the terms *Caroli's disease* and *polycystic disease* in an imprecise way. In the text of this chapter we discuss in detail the definitions employed in the classification contained in Table 52–1.

SOLITARY CYSTS

Solitary cysts have no consistent association with cysts in other viscera. They do not have an obvious vascular or lymphatic origin nor are they components or complications of a discernible tumor. Finally, they are unassociated with a history of trauma. Not all so-called solitary cysts are truly solitary, however, as will be discussed later. Also, there is enough variation among the cysts included in this group to leave open the possibility that there are a variety of origins and types of solitary cysts. On occasion solitary cysts are congenital, in the sense of being present at birth. They are not hereditary, however. Whether or not *all* solitary cysts deserve to be considered congenital (as indicated in some classifications) is uncertain. A few of the reported cases of solitary cysts (especially when multiple) may have been unrecognized examples of one of the polycystic diseases.

The origins of the cysts included in the group of solitary cysts are not known. The age range of the patients and the variability in the types of lining cells, as well as the numbers and sizes of the cysts, raise the possibility that more than

one type of cystic disease is represented in this group. There is no convincing evidence for teratomatous origin or for other neoplastic origin (e.g., cystadenoma). The typical lack of bile argues against a duct retention origin in most cases. Possibly, some solitary cysts that lack an epithelial lining have a traumatic origin. The frequent presence of columnar epithelium in solitary cysts suggests that many are of ductal origin, but the precise genesis is unclear.

Solitary cysts are uncommon, although increasing numbers of cases are being discovered with the increased use of hepatic sonography. Nevertheless, the incidence in the population at large has not been defined. Henson and co-workers found only 38 cases in a 47-year period at the Mayo Clinic.[1] The ratio of symptomatic to asymptomatic solitary cysts was approximately 1:2 in this series.[1] Thus, the majority of solitary cysts are asymptomatic.

Solitary cysts have been reported to occur at all ages—from before birth to the ninth decade of life,[2, 3] but symptomatic solitary cysts occur predominantly in the fourth and fifth decades of life. In adults there is a clear predominance in women, perhaps in the range of 4:1.[4] This is less well established in children.[5]

Increased abdominal girth is perhaps the most common presenting complaint or finding in patients with solitary cysts. This is nearly always accompanied by a palpable, but poorly delineated, abdominal mass in the right upper quadrant. Patients also may complain of fullness, flatulence, diarrhea, vomiting, or pain. Nausea, weakness, dysphagia, and weight loss have been reported. Pain, when present, can be either dull, with some aggravation resulting from changes in position, or sharp and intermittent.[1] The latter seems to correlate with pathologic evidence of hemorrhage into the cyst and may be accompanied by chills and fever.[1] Other complications include inflammation, with or without infection, and perforation, which may occur either spontaneously or following trauma.[2] Laboratory findings are typically normal when infection is not present. Occasionally, however, the pressure of a large cyst, usually against the extrahepatic biliary system, causes obstructive jaundice.

The diaphragm may be elevated on the right side, and a mass or density may be evident in the right upper quadrant. Calcification occurs but much less frequently than in hydatid cysts. Other abdominal viscera may be displaced. Sonography is accurate in evaluating hepatic cystic masses (Fig. 52–1), and in selected cases it may be combined with needle aspiration, culture, and microscopic examination of the aspirate.[6] The fluid in a typical solitary cyst is sterile, clear, and cytologically negative. Occasionally, however, there may be bleeding into the cyst, or it may communicate with the biliary system. Hydatid disease should be ruled out before aspirating the cyst or cysts (see Chap. 39).[6] Scans may be useful in determining the size, number, and location of cysts and, if appropriate, can be combined with excretory radiography (Fig. 52–1). As mentioned, so-called solitary cysts are not always solitary; not uncommonly three or four cysts may be present close to one another. There may be multiple cysts throughout one lobe or, on occasion, there may be cysts in both lobes.[4] In all cases of cysts of the liver, but particularly in cases of multiple cysts, a careful search should be made for cysts or other abnormalities in the other viscera, especially the kidneys. This search must include a careful family history. Extrahepatic cysts, a positive family history, or the presence of the ductal plate malformation (dpm) suggests that the patient has one of the polycystic diseases (see further on).

Solitary cysts involve the right lobe of the liver more frequently than the left. The most common locus is on the

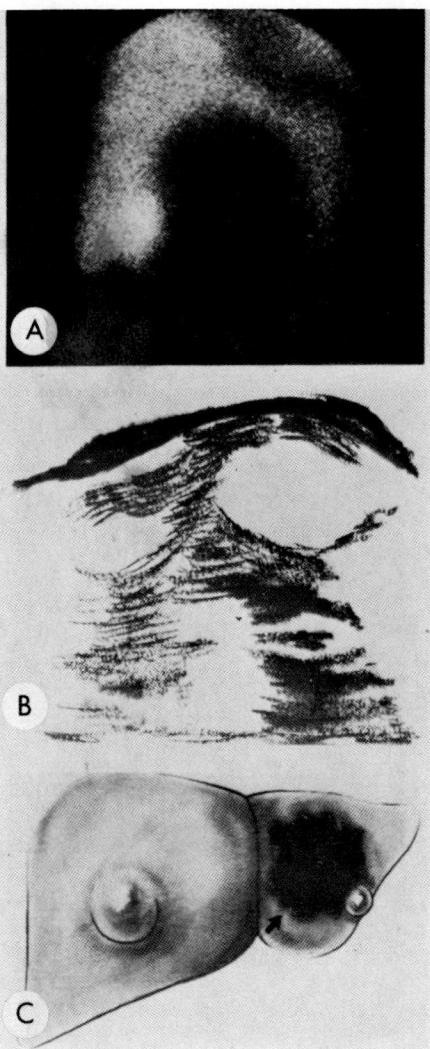

Figure 52–1. Two solitary cysts demonstrated by scan (A) and ultrasonography (B) and as seen at operation (drawing; C). (Hadad AR, et al. Am J Surg 134:739, 1977, with permission.)

anterior-inferior surface. Solitary cysts (Fig. 52–2) may be completely intrahepatic or pedunculated. They can vary in diameter from a few millimeters to many centimeters. One of the largest reported cysts contained 17 l of fluid.[2] In general, the cysts in symptomatic cases are larger than those in asymptomatic cases.[1]

The external surface of the cyst is smooth and usually translucent; the wall thickness is usually 1 cm or less. Although they are usually unilocular, solitary, multilocular cysts have been described (Fig. 52–2). The lining is usually described as smooth. The contents vary from pale yellow, serous fluid through viscid material to semisolid, brownish black material. Among the contents that have been identified are blood, mucin, cellular debris, albumin, cholesterol, and rarely, bile. The pH is said to be alkaline.[2, 4] Usually there are no connections with the biliary system, vasculature, or lymphatics. Connections with the biliary system may be present, however, in rare cases.

Microscopically, the cyst wall is said to have three layers. The outermost layer consists of moderately dense fibrous tissue with abundant blood vessels, biliary ducts, and hepatic parenchymal cells; occasionally, muscle cells may be present.[7] The middle layer consists of dense fibrous tissue of variable vascularity. The inner layer consists of less dense fibrous tissue. Often, but not always, it has an epithelial lining. A number of lining epithelia have been described. A single layer of columnar epithelium is most common. Ciliated columnar epithelium has been observed,[1] and in at least one case stratified squamous epithelium was present.[1] Some of the contents of the cyst may adhere to the inner layer. Inflammation can be present in any of the layers; when present, it is usually modest in amount and generally is interpreted as a secondary phenomenon. Carcinoma has been observed rarely to arise in a solitary cyst.[8] Benign common duct tumors have been associated sufficiently often that this additional lesion should be considered, especially in jaundiced patients.[9]

In considering the treatment of solitary cysts, the essentially benign character of these lesions must be kept in mind. The advisability of aspirating asymptomatic cysts with a typical sonographic appearance is debatable; and aspiration is generally ineffective as therapy.[10] Surgical treatment is indicated, however, when symptoms and complications develop, such as pain, weight loss, jaundice, infection, hemorrhage into the cyst, rupture of the cyst, torsion and strangulation of a pedunculated cyst, or malignancy. The appropriate surgical procedure depends on a number of factors, including the overall condition of the patient. Removing fluid too rapidly from a large cyst has resulted in death.[3] External drainage of infected cysts has been recommended, although prolonged sinus formation may develop following external drainage.[3] Excision should be carried out whenever possible. If excision is not feasible, subtotal resection is recommended, with removal of at least a third of the cyst wall to allow drainage into the peritoneal cavity. This procedure should not be performed, however, when there is bile drainage into the cyst. Some authors suggest, in fact,[11] that radiopaque material be injected intraoperatively to rule out communication of the cyst with the biliary tree. If the cyst or cysts are multilocular, establishment of drainage requires extensive removal of the septa. The wall of the cyst should be examined grossly and microscopically as extensively as possible, in order to diagnose rare instances of malignancy. If the cyst cannot be excised completely and the wall is uniform, random sections may be taken. Focal areas of abnormality should be sampled if present. If the cyst contains bile, or if bile radicles can be observed to enter the cyst, peritoneal drainage is contraindicated. Cystojejunostomy is recommended in this instance.[12] The use of currently available sclerosing agents seems ill-advised.

The prognosis for patients with solitary cysts is generally excellent if ill-advised surgical procedures and complications of surgery are avoided. So far as we can determine, only one patient who was not treated surgically has died with apparent cyst-related problems.[1] This patient had prolonged diarrhea and vomiting and may have died from inadequate replacement therapy. Despite the occasional occurrence of hemorrhage into a cyst, there is no report of a fatality from this complication.

TRAUMATIC CYSTS

Traumatic cysts are uncommon.[13] They probably are sequelae to intrahepatic hemorrhage. The blood is resorbed, and bile leaks into the space.[13] Presumably because of this pathogenesis, traumatic or post-traumatic cysts often do not manifest for some time after the initial trauma.

The symptoms and signs of a traumatic cyst may include abdominal distention, pain, and anorexia. On oc-

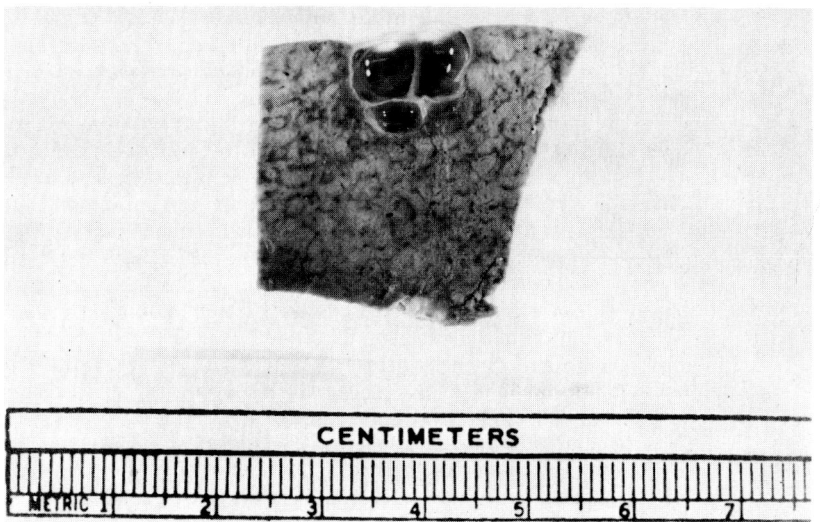

Figure 52–2. Gross photograph of asymptomatic solitary cyst found incidentally at autopsy. The cyst is multilocular and cyst walls are translucent.

casion, obstructive jaundice may be present.[13] Perforation and its symptoms may lead to recognition of such cysts. Rarely, the cyst becomes infected secondarily, and the patient has signs of infection.[13] A history of trauma usually can be obtained because the initiating trauma often is severe. Also, a history of trauma usually is the basis for concluding that the cyst is post-traumatic.

An abdominal mass often is palpable. Serum bilirubin levels may be elevated. Routine x-ray films may show elevation of the diaphragm or displacement of other abdominal viscera. Post-traumatic cysts occur predominantly in the right lobe of the liver and vary considerably in size. They may contain as much as several liters of fluid. As indicated already, most of these cysts are filled with bile unless they are infected, in which case they contain pus. The wall of the cyst is composed of fibrous tissue with variable amounts of inflammation, which is typically chronic. An epithelial lining is not present. A variety of surgical treatments have been employed with success, including incision and packing, incision and drainage, and partial excision and marsupialization to the abdominal wall. Simple drainage seems to be adequate treatment in most cases.[13]

CYSTS SECONDARY TO INFARCTION

It has been recognized recently that cysts can develop following apparently focal arterial insufficiency of the liver. Clinically, this is a rare occurrence. In one patient in whom hepatic cysts were observed to develop on the basis of vascular insufficiency,[14] the cysts were apparently asymptomatic. They were discovered during a computed tomographic (CT) scan and were found to be avascular on angiography. Microscopically, the cysts had fibrous walls, were lined by endothelium, and contained bile. There was exuberant formation of biliary ducts in the area adjacent to the cyst. Similar lesions have been created in monkeys by introducing emboli into the hepatic arterial tree.[14] Cysts that are secondary to infarction may become infected.[14]

The experimentally induced cystic lesions are presumed to develop secondary to focal hepatic infarction. They contain bile and therefore seem to connect with the bile ducts. However, they lack an epithelial lining and thus do *not* appear to us to be identical with those in Caroli's

disease. The role of vascular lesions in the genesis of hepatic cysts of undetermined origin, for example, bile-containing solitary cysts, remains to be elucidated.

DUODENAL DUPLICATION

Duodenal duplication is an uncommon anomaly of the gastrointestinal tract. Imamoglu and Walt described an extraordinary case in which such a duplication, which had luminal continuity with the normal duodenum, lay within the liver.[15] The patient had a five-year history of recurrent epigastric distress. The duplication, identified by barium examination of the upper gastrointestinal tract, was found at laparotomy to be located within the liver as a large cystic mass. External drainage failed to reduce its size. At a second operation, a loop of jejunum was anastomosed to the cyst wall at the hepatic surface by a Roux-en-Y anastomosis. This appeared to be successful. So far as we are aware, this was a unique occurrence.

CYSTS ASSOCIATED WITH NEOPLASMS

Virtually any hepatic neoplasm, whether primary or metastatic, can be cystic, at least by virtue of the occurrence of central necrosis. Other tumors involving the liver may be cystic on the basis of their fundamental structure. We limit this discussion to primary hepatic tumors for which a cystic component is a frequent or constant feature that is not related to central necrosis.

CYSTADENOMA AND CYSTADENOCARCINOMA

Cystadenomata and cystadenocarcinomata are among the most consistently cystic tumors involving the liver. Cystadenomata may involve either the liver or the extrahepatic biliary tree (including the gallbladder), the former predominantly. By contrast, cystadenocarcinomata have been seen thus far only within the liver.[16] Cystadenomata are more common in females than in males. Approximately two-thirds occur when the patient is 40 years old or older. They are extremely rare in children.[16, 17] The most common presenting symptoms of cystadenomata are right upper quadrant or epigastric pain, increasing abdominal girth, and a palpable abdominal mass.[16, 17] Less commonly, biliary obstruction may be a presenting complaint. On occasion, the obstruction may be episodic. In one patient, the tumor was discovered following perforation into the peritoneal cavity. Rarely, the tumor is found incidentally during abdominal surgery or at autopsy.[16] Plain x-ray films of the abdomen may reveal distortion of the stomach, colon, right hemidiaphragm, kidney, or ureter. Occasionally, the wall of the cyst may be calcified.[18] Hepatic scans reveal a filling defect, and ultrasonography typically shows a cystic lesion that is thick-walled and septated and has mural nodules. The definitive diagnosis is made only at operation. The lesions most frequently involve the right lobe only but may involve the left lobe or both lobes. In one case, there was a concomitant pancreatic cystadenoma.[18]

Cystadenomata vary markedly in size, ranging from 1.5 to 15 cm in diameter, and weighing as much as 6000 g.[16, 17] Grossly, the lesions usually have a smooth external surface and characteristically are multilocular, although rarely they may be unilocular. The contents are liquid and variable in appearance and composition. Cholesterol crystals or bile may be present.[16] The lining of the cyst may be smooth or rough, and papillary projections may be evident. Microscopically, the cystadenomata are lined by mucus-secreting cuboidal or columnar epithelium, often in papillary folds. Ultrastructural studies may reveal absorptive and argentaffin cells as well as mucus-secreting cells.[19] Ulcerations may be present. The stroma immediately beneath the epithelium is typically quite cellular, resembling ovary, but may be simply fibrotic. Wheeler and Edmondson have suggested that cysts with a cellular stroma (mesenchyme) are an entity that is distinct from those without and that they occur predominantly in females and have a low incidence of malignancy (see further on).[20] A few smooth muscle fibers, as well as inflammatory cells, may be present in the wall, and lipofuscin-laden macrophages are common. The outer layers of the wall may contain arteries, veins, nerve fibers, and bile ducts. On occasion, apparent bile duct hamartomata (von Meyenburg complexes) may be adjacent.

The histologic features of the tumor and its occurrence both in liver and in the extrahepatic tree indicate that it is derived from the biliary ducts. In one case, the tumor was seen to arise in a large bile duct. Bile is present in some of these tumors, and in one case an aberrant duct connected the tumor to the extrahepatic biliary system.[16]

Treatment of these tumors is surgical. Because of the thick capsule, the lesions often can be excised. If the tumor is sufficiently large, lobectomy may be indicated. Because of the apparent potential for malignant transformation of cystadenomata (see further on), less definitive procedures, such as drainage or marsupialization, should be considered only if excision is contraindicated in an individual case. Recurrence is uncommon, but it has been reported to occur in those tumors involving the extrahepatic biliary tree.[16]

The cystadenocarcinomata are said to arise by malignant change in cystadenomata. The malignant change may be focal.[16] Wheeler and Edmonson argue, as mentioned already, that most cystadenocarcinomata do not arise from the group of cystadenomata with cellular stroma.[20] Cystadenocarcinomata are less common than are cystadenomata. Up to 1986, there have been 64 cystadenomata and 27 cystadenocarcinomata reported.[21] As previously mentioned, cystadenocarcinomata have not been reported to arise in the extrahepatic biliary tree. Female predominance may be less marked than with cystadenoma.[16] The tumor has been

seen as early as the third decade of life. When there is no spread, the gross features are those of cystadenoma. The tumor is an adenocarcinoma and may involve the entire lining or may be focal. The lesion is capable of extrahepatic spread and distant metastasis, but it can be cured by complete excision. It may be biologically less aggressive than cholangiocarcinoma.[16] The effect of nonsurgical therapy for the tumor is unknown.

MESENCHYMAL HAMARTOMA

So-called mesenchymal hamartomata are uncommon primary hepatic neoplasms in children, usually occurring before the age of one year. On occasion they may be predominantly cystic.[22-24] They have a predilection for occurrence in males.

Characteristically, the tumor presents as a painless abdominal mass. Routine x-ray films show no distinctive features. Calcification is typically lacking. Imaging techniques reveal a multiloculated mass with variation in the size of septae and cystic spaces.[25] Angiography may reveal hypovascular or avascular foci, which probably represent the cystic areas of the tumor. More than half of the tumors occur in the right lobe, but a small proportion may involve both lobes. The tumors usually are quite large at the time of diagnosis—some have exceeded 1000 g in weight. Their gross appearances vary considerably. They are typically solitary. Such a tumor may be nearly solid, with only scattered small cystic areas. It may consist of a large number of cysts or may be predominantly cystic. Typically, the cysts contain gelatinous or mucoid material, and their lining is smooth. The tissue intervening between the cystic structures is solid but gelatinous. Histologically (Fig. 52–3), the lesions are heterogeneous, with clusters of normal-appearing hepatocytes entrapped in a poorly cellular mesenchyme that contains variable numbers of lymphatic-like spaces. Typically, the latter are the cysts, but dilated biliary lined channels may be present or even predominate.[24, 26] Bands of collagen may be present in the mesenchyme, and clusters of bile ducts are typically scattered throughout. Islands of hematopoiesis and scattered blood vessels are common features. No significant atypical features are present in any of the elements. Electron microscopic studies indicate a derivation from both mesenchyme and bile ducts.[27] The lesions show no predisposition to malignant transformation, and resection is curative. Because of their basically benign nature, radical surgery probably is inappropriate.

CAVERNOUS HEMANGIOMATA

Hemangiomata of the liver are essentially of two types, hemangioendotheliomata and cavernous hemangiomata. The former are seen principally in childhood, usually in the first year of life.[22] They tend to be solid, or at least relatively so. The cavernous hemangiomata, which are the more common of the two, are more consistently cystic.

Cavernous hemangiomata are the most common benign hepatic tumors in all age groups.[28] They have no significant capacity for invasion of tissue and none for metastasis. Probably fewer than 20 per cent become symptomatic.[28] By convention, lesions more than 4 cm in diameter have been designated giant cavernous hemangiomata.[29, 30] In one series of 122 cases, 49 of these tumors were giant, and of them, 40 per cent were symptomatic.[31] It appears from autopsy series that the incidence in males

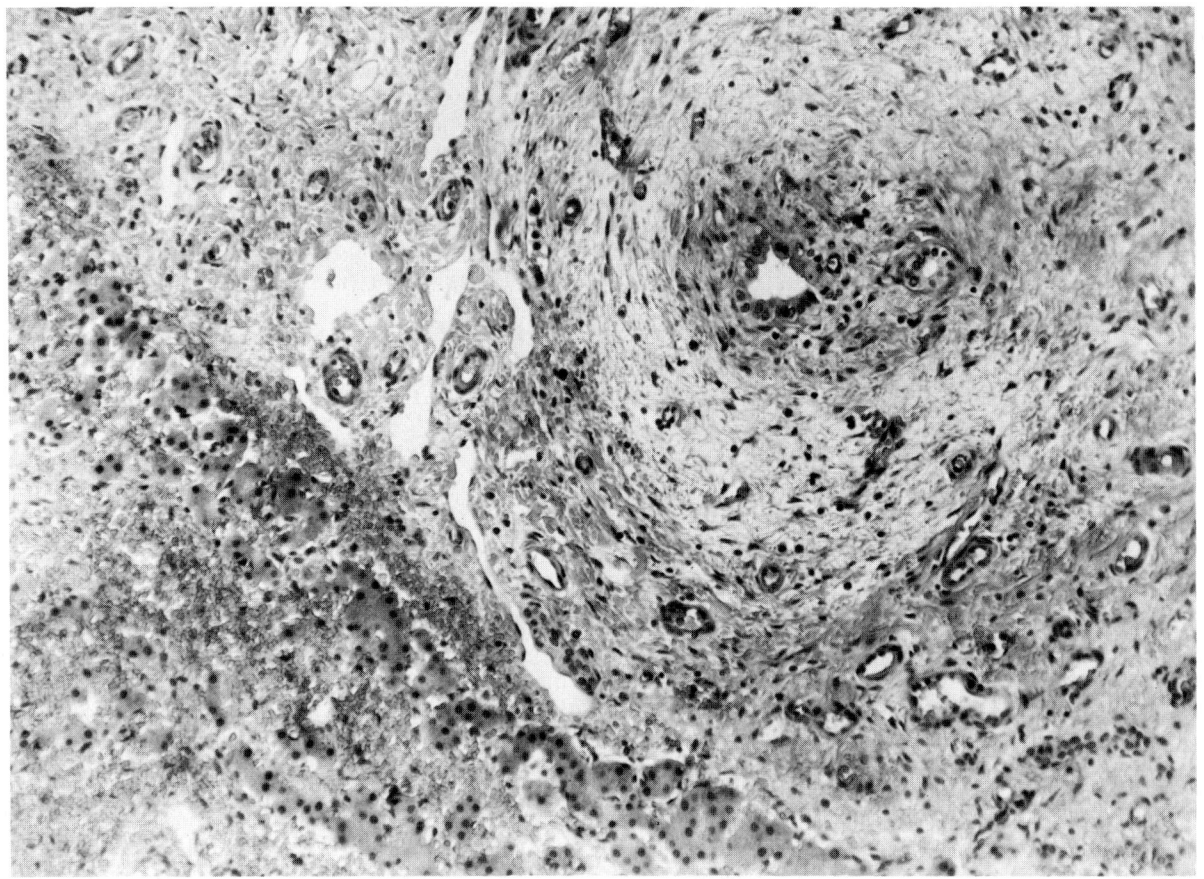

Figure 52–3. Light micrograph of a mesenchymal hamartoma, illustrating several duct elements in the mesenchyme (*upper right*), lymphatic-like spaces (*center*), and adjacent entrapped hepatocytes (*lower left*) (hematoxylin and eosin, × 10).

and females is approximately equal, but surgical series (which deal largely with symptomatic patients) have had a striking female predominance. Generally speaking, symptoms from these tumors become more common with increasing age. There is reason to suspect that hormones, especially estrogenic ones, enhance their growth, an effect that probably increases the probability of symptoms. Symptoms may arise from the effects of a mass in the abdomen and may include fullness, belching, weight loss, abdominal distention, vomiting, and pain. Anemia (caused by sequestration of the red blood cells in the tumor), hemorrhage (caused by extensive clotting within the tumor), or rupture of the tumor may also occur. Rupture usually is secondary to blunt abdominal trauma, but it may follow either percutaneous or operative attempts at biopsy. It also may develop spontaneously.

An upper abdominal mass may be palpable. Routine x-ray films of the abdomen can show elevation of the diaphragm. Calcification of the tumor or phleboliths may be evident. Scans or ultrasonography will show a defect. The most valuable diagnostic test, however, is angiography, which shows distinctive features in typical cases. The angiographic features include large feeding vessels displaced and curled at the margins of the lesions, varix-like spaces that fill rapidly and remain opacified throughout the examination, and a tendency for the vascular spaces to be arranged in rings or to be C-shaped.[28, 32]

The tumors are usually single. There appears to be a slight predilection for occurrence in the right lobe. In approximately 20 per cent of patients with giant hemangio-

mata, both lobes are involved.[30] Reported tumors cover a great range of sizes, from a few millimeters to 45 cm in diameter.[29] A few have been pedunculated.[28] Typically, they are reddish-blue or purple, cystic, and quite clearly vascular. Some may appear solid. The cut surfaces are honeycombed, with varying degrees of fibrosis, thrombosis, and calcification. Microscopically, the lesions consist of large, dilated, blood-filled channels lined by epithelium. A variable inflammatory reaction is present in the underlying fibromuscular wall. Thrombosis and calcification are common. Biopsy of hepatic hemangiomata is contraindicated.

Unless symptomatic, it appears that there is minimal risk to management by observation.[31] If treatment is necessary, the treatment of choice is surgical. The precise procedure depends on the size of the tumor, the number of lesions, and the general condition of the patient. Because of the possibility of rupture, the operating room staff must be prepared to provide clotting factors or large amounts of blood, or both, rapidly. The lesions should be removed by a wedge resection through normal liver or, if necessary and feasible, by lobectomy. Lesser procedures are likely to result in significant hemorrhage, and even operative biopsy and aspiration have precipitated life-threatening hemorrhage.[29] Rarely, when a tumor is unresectable, it may be possible to selectively ligate the arteries supplying it.[30] More commonly, irradiation is employed in these circumstances. Administration of steroids is associated with shrinkage of the lesion in some cases in children. The extent of an inoperable tumor can be delineated by placing clips along its margins during laparotomy. Irradiation does not eradicate the tumor,[29] but it may relieve symptoms. Rupture of the tumor, either pre- or intraoperatively, is associated with a high mortality rate, but when there is no rupture, mortality is very low and the prognosis is good.

TERATOMATA

Primary hepatic teratomata are rare, with roughly a dozen cases reported to date.[33–35] These tumors occur predominantly in children and, like teratomata elsewhere, they may have a significant cystic component. The great majority are seen within the first year of life. One patient was anencephalic and another had trisomy 13.[35] The symptoms are those of an enlarging hepatic mass. Routine x-ray films may show calcification, representing either teeth or bits of bone arising as components of the tumor. Angiograms and scans of the liver show an avascular defect within it. The majority of reported tumors have been in the right lobe of the liver. Characteristically, the tumor has both solid and cystic regions. Such tumors are relatively large; lobectomy may be necessary for excision. Histologically, the features are typical of a teratoma, with well-differentiated tissues (some of which may be immature) derived from multiple germ layers. The cystic areas contain keratinized debris with strands of hair. The cystic structures are a component of the tumor and are not related to the biliary duct system. In several of the reported cases, the tumors have had histologically malignant areas, one in the form of squamous cell carcinoma and the other in the form of hepatoblastoma. Pulmonary metastases developed in both of these patients. All but three of the nine patients with malignant changes in the tumor died, with or without resection of the tumor. Nevertheless, resection appears to be the treatment of choice. Subsequent therapy, if any, would depend on the presence and character of any malignant element.

OTHER CYSTIC NEOPLASMS

A single case of a malignant cystic hepatic neoplasm, possibly of mesothelial origin, has been reported in a six-month-old girl.[36]

PELIOSIS HEPATIS

Peliosis hepatis is characterized by the presence in the liver of blood-filled cavities, which may or may not be lined with sinusoidal cells. The individual cysts or cavities usually do not exceed several centimeters in diameter. The lesions may be diffuse or focal. The gross appearance of angiectatic lesions on the cut surface of the liver is distinctive. The lesions are not always limited to the liver and have been found (usually but not invariably in patients with liver lesions) in spleen, bone marrow, lung, pleura, kidney, and gut.[37, 38] There may be slight fibrosis of the walls of the cavities, and there may or may not be associated hepatocellular necrosis. The cysts are typically continuous with adjacent, more normal sinusoids, and they sometimes can be seen in continuity with hepatic venous tributaries. A distinction between phlebectatic and parenchymal types has been made,[39] with attendant pathogenetic implications, but the merit and applicability of this distinction is uncertain.

The lesion is usually diagnosed by gross or microscopic examination, but wedged hepatic venography has been reported to reveal quite specific findings.[40] When suspected,

it can be diagnosed by percutaneous biopsy.[41–44] Significant bleeding following biopsy seems to be uncommon.[41]

No consistent hepatic functional abnormalities are found, but in steroid-associated cases (see further on), there may be hepatic failure or rupture and peritoneal hemorrhage.[41]

Primarily associated in the past with wasting diseases, such as tuberculosis, malignancy, and chronic suppurative infection, peliosis hepatis is seen most commonly now in association with the administration of anabolic steroids and in a variety of clinical disorders.[41, 42, 45] It can be seen in a variety of experimental situations and as a naturally occurring disease in animals.[46]

The pathogenesis of peliosis hepatis remains obscure. Among suggested possibilities are necrosis of parenchyma with secondary vascular dilation, congenital weakness of vessel walls, angiitis, vascular (venous) obstruction with secondary dilation, and injury to endothelial cells. Certainly, more than one of these factors could operate to give a common morphologic end result. Recent ultrastructural studies,[46, 47] and the occurrence of a similar lesion in multiple organs in individual patients, suggest, however, that injury to endothelium may be the primary causative basis in many cases. Since the lesion usually is found incidentally and may be diffuse, surgical therapy is not considered. There are instances of regression of the disease following withdrawal of steroids.[41–43]

POLYCYSTIC LIVER DISEASE

The major uncertainties or controversies in the classification of hepatic cysts exist in the area of so-called polycystic diseases. We use the term *polycystic disease* to designate heritable disorders in which there is actual or potential cystic dilation of elements of the bile ducts *and* actual or potential development of renal lesions, especially cysts of tubular origin. There is current controversy over how many different disorders are encompassed in such a definition. Resolution of this controversy is of importance because of the prognostic implications in a given affected family and because the answer will define the number of pathogenetic mechanisms that will have to be delineated.

There is general agreement that polycystic disease so defined can be divided into at least two major groups. The first is a dominantly inherited condition, often called adult polycystic disease (APCD), in which the cysts of evident bile duct origin *do not* ordinarily communicate with the rest of the biliary system (noncommunicating). The second group comprises an undetermined number of recessively inherited disorders in which the cysts communicate with the bilary system (communicating). A major area of controversy centers around how many entities are included in the latter group. In addition, recent observations indicate that some of the hepatic morphologic features of the dominantly and recessively inherited groups may not be separated as clearly as thought previously (see further on).

A number of terms recur in the literature on polycystic disease. Some of these are used, whether accurately or inaccurately, as synonyms for all or specific polycystic diseases; others are used to describe certain features of these disorders. Among such terms are ductal plate malformation, fibropolycystic disease, biliary fibroadenomatosis, fibrocystic disease, congenital hepatic fibrosis (CHF), infantile polycystic disease (IPCD), and Caroli's disease. It is worthwhile to discuss several of these (ductal plate malformation and Caroli's disease) as a prelude to the discussion of the various specific polycystic diseases.

DUCTAL PLATE MALFORMATION

The term *ductal plate malformation* (DPM) is used to designate a distinctive lesion of the portal tract that is seen in a number of seemingly distinct polycystic disorders.

Typically, DPM consists of a nonreactive increase in the number of bile ducts in the portal areas together with an increase in fibrous tissue (Fig. 52–4). The bile ducts have unusual, distinctive profiles in two-dimensional views on routine sections. The bile ducts in some patients appear normal, but this is not a typical feature. The abnormalities of the portal tracts occur without inflammation or abnormalities of the hepatocytes. Bile often is present in the abnormal ducts. It appears that this lesion represents a developmental anomaly rather than a reactive lesion, that is, the lesion reflects an arrest of development or a failure during embryogenesis of "remodeling" of the intrahepatic biliary tree.[48, 49] Evidence has recently been presented suggesting that in at least some cases the fibrosis progresses to create parenchymal nodularity. The implications of this observation are uncertain, but they may challenge the morphometric observations of Landing.[50] DPM usually is present diffusely in portal tracts throughout the liver, but it may be limited in distribution.

DPM is seen in a number of polycystic conditions that are inherited recessively. There are a variety of associated abnormalities in the other viscera in these diseases. Among these diseases there is considerable controversy as to whether DPM and IPCD (Table 52–1) can be separated.

Landing introduced a new element in both the concept

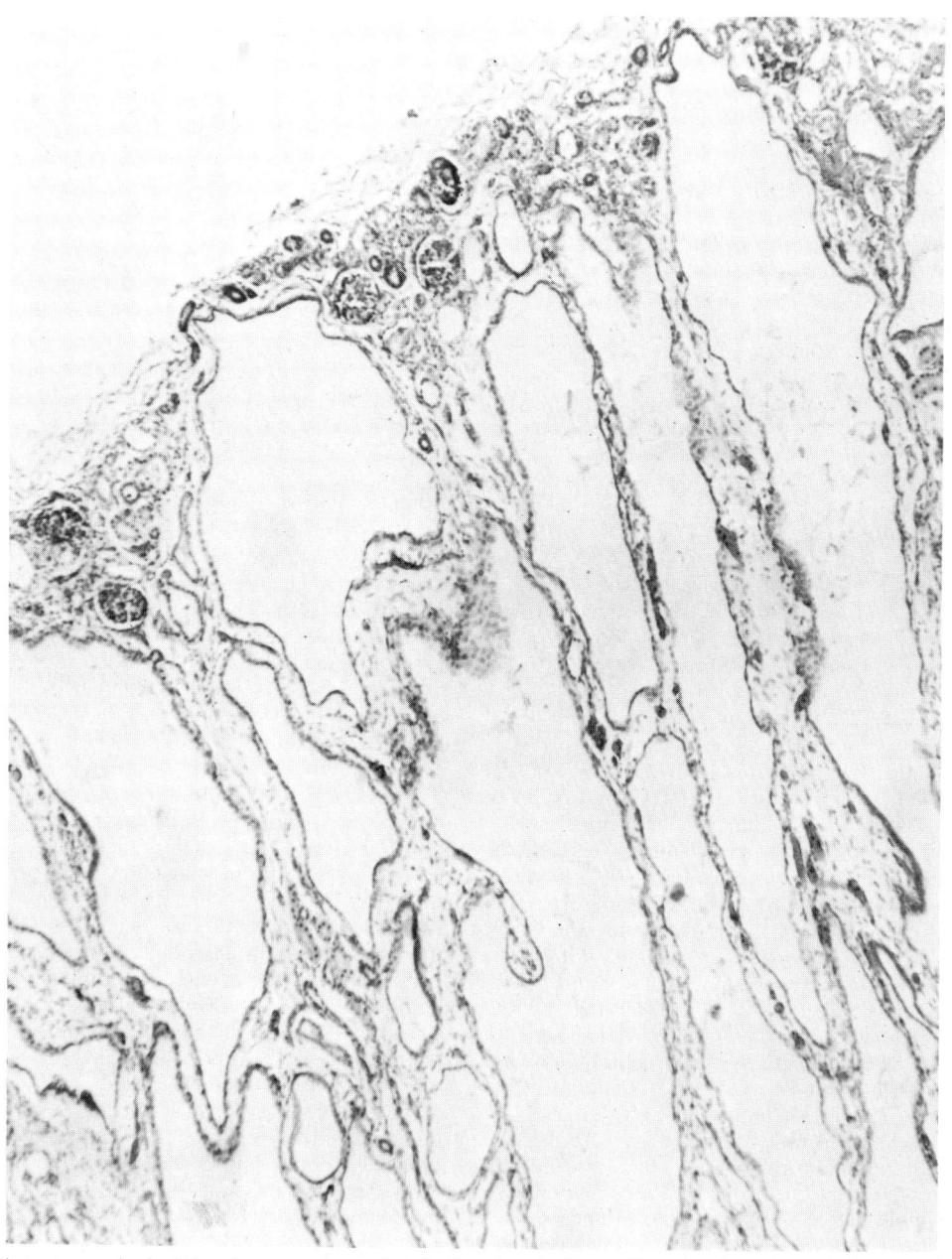

Figure 52–4. Photomicrograph of a kidney from a newborn with infantile polycystic disease, illustrating the typical radially oriented cysts. The cortical surface is at the top of the field (hematoxylin and eosin, × 4).

of DPM and the argument over the distinctiveness of CHF and IPCD and other polycystic disorders that are inherited recessively. He and his colleagues analyzed morphometric measurements of the portal tracts in these various conditions.[50] Their analyses showed that the lesions in each of the various conditions studied were distinctive in morphometric terms. Of particular importance was the observation that was made in several patients in whom multiple biopsies were performed over time—that is, that the morphometric parameters did not change with age within a given condition. This finding suggests that the differences between IPCD and CHF are not explained by the different ages at which these two conditions usually are diagnosed. Bernstein and co-workers[50a] have however presented evidence that in at least some patients there is a progression of the DPM lesion. It would be vital to determine whether such progression was a primary phenomenon or instead an inconstant result of complications (e.g., cholangitis). Landing and his co-workers further concluded that the multiple subdivisions of IPCD proposed by Blyth and Ockenden are not meaningful, a conclusion that was also reached by Gang and Herrin.[51, 52]

Other observers,[53, 54] nevertheless, appear to hold that the apparent similarity of the hepatic lesions (and the fact that the renal lesions of IPCD tend to evolve with time) indicate that these two disorders are only differing clinical presentations of the same disorder.[55] Landing has presented recent morphometric data from the renal lesions that indicate the two disorders are separable.[56] For the convenience of discussion, the two conditions are treated as separate entities in this chapter, recognizing that the issue is a matter of reasonable debate.

CAROLI'S DISEASE

The term *Caroli's disease* has come to be used by some authors for essentially all conditions in which there is nonobstructive dilation of the biliary tree, extending even to those entities not included in our definition of polycystic disease (i.e., cases without heritability, DPM, and renal lesions) for example, choledochal cyst. Other authors seem to use it for all polycystic diseases.[57] It is our opinion that either use is indiscriminate and serves only to confuse the classification of hepatic cystic disease. It is pertinent to review Caroli's observations.[58] He described two forms of congenital dilation of the segmental intrahepatic biliary tree. One of them (the simple type) was characterized by ectasia of hepatic bile ducts without the presence of other histologic abnormalities (i.e., no DPM) and without the presence of portal hypertension or hepatosplenomegaly. The other form (the periportal fibrosis–associated type) was characterized by lesions in the portal tract, conforming to what we now know as DPM, and the frequent presence of hepatosplenomegaly, hypersplenism, esophageal varices, and gastrointestinal hemorrhages. Both forms could be seen in the same family. Renal disease was associated with both forms. The renal disease was different from that seen in polycystic liver disease (presumably meaning APCD), and almost always involved infantile medullary spongiosis with dilation of the collecting ducts. The periportal fibrosis–associated type conforms quite obviously to polycystic diseases that are inherited recessively, as we have defined them (most probably CHF and IPCD). The current counterpart of the simple type is unclear. In fact, since Caroli's reports, few patients with the simple type have been described. We want to emphasize that the liver lesion in this form of the disease, that is, ectasia of bile ducts without DPM, resembles that seen with choledochal cysts (see further on).

In view of the lack of specificity with which the term *Caroli's disease* is used, we believe, as previously stated, that use of the term serves only to propagate confusion. We encourage the use of newer and potentially more discriminating terminology when discussing the various diseases in which there is a tendency for dilation of the biliary duct system. We have included the term *Caroli's disease* in Table 52–1 to describe only those patients with *inherited* cysts of bile ducts *without* DPM but *with* renal cysts and noted that patients of this sort have been described almost exclusively by Caroli.

NONCOMMUNICATING (DOMINANT) POLYCYSTIC DISEASE (APCD)

Reviews of multiple, nonparasitic cysts of the liver represent collections of a number of discrete entities, probably including multiple solitary cysts, choledochal cysts, and both recessively (communicating) and dominantly (noncommunicating) inherited cystic diseases of the liver. Such series also include a number of patients with noncommunicating multiple cysts and *no* apparent renal disease. The latter patients may have had multiple solitary cysts, or renal disease in these patients may have been overlooked. Alternatively, these patients may have had a purely hepatic type of polycystic disease, that is, multiple noncommunicating cysts of bile ducts. This latter entity has been postulated on the basis of a large series of autopsies.[59] Conversely, the data supporting the existence of this entity lack family histories. The heritability of such an entity, if it exists at all, is thus unclear. Because of this and other apparent uncertainties, we will not deal with it. Our focus instead is on the well-known noncommunicating and dominantly inherited polycystic disease commonly called APCD.

APCD is the most common heritable renal disorder. Its frequency is estimated to be 1 in 1500 to 1 in 5000 in the general population. It affects approximately 500,000 people in the United States.[60] The disease is inherited in an autosomal dominant manner with high penetrance. Although beyond the scope of this presentation, it is of note that molecular genetics studies have identified the locus of the critical gene and provided a marker for this disorder. These same approaches have generated debate about the possible heterogeneity of APCD.[60a, 60b] The peak incidence is in adult life (>40 years of age), but it is also recognized in children, usually in infancy.[61, 62] In studying a population of patients with autosomal dominant polycystic disease of the kidney, using sophisticated imaging techniques, Milutinovic and co-workers found recognizable hepatic cysts in 29 per cent of 158 patients.[63] A few relatives of such patients may have had hepatic cysts *only*, demonstrable by imaging techniques (see earlier discussion).[64] In an autopsy series of patients with APCD, hepatic cysts were found in 17 of 19 patients.[65]

There is considerable variation in the size of the liver in patients with APCD; it may remain the same size for many years and then become enlarged. It is believed that there is a slow but definite progression of liver disease in these patients.[66] Thus, infants with APCD rarely have recognizable cysts of the liver, and the diagnosis of cysts in the liver increases with age.[63] Tests of liver function usually are nearly normal, even with increasing liver size.[66] On occasion, however, slight elevations of indirect bilirubin or slight retention of sulfobromophthalein may be present. Rarely, large cysts cause mechanical obstruction of the biliary system.

The liver cysts are lined by biliary epithelium. Usually they are diffuse, but they may be localized.[65] The cysts, as noted, usually do not communicate with the biliary system and do not contain bile. Occasionally, however, they may rupture into adjacent bile ducts.[65] In a detailed autopsy study, Grunfeld and co-workers found two additional lesions of bile ducts in 60 per cent of the patients.[65] They were the so-called von Meyenburg complexes (which typically do not communicate with the biliary system) and fibroadenomatosis or DPM. The latter, at least by simple light microscopy, was identical with the lesions of DPM seen in patients with IPCD and CHF. Heretofore, only rare cases have been reported as demonstrating the coexistence of APCD and CHF.[67] The finding that both communicating (DPM) and noncommunicating lesions of bile ducts coexist relatively commonly in patients with autosomal dominant renal disease is quite surprising and interesting. The precise significance of this observation for our understanding of the pathogenesis and classification of the polycystic disease is as yet unclear. It could indicate that there is a pathogenetic continuum among the various disorders. Despite the apparent histologic overlap, it still seems valid to separate APCD from the recessively inherited communicating types of polycystic diseases because of (1) the predominance of one type of lesion of the bile ducts (i.e., communicating or noncommunicating) over the other in the different diseases, (2) the differing pattern of inheritance (dominant versus recessive), and (3) the frequently different symptoms and complications of the hepatic component of each disorder.

Approximately 5 per cent of patients with APCD have cysts in other viscera, including pancreas, spleen, uterus, ovaries, and seminal vesicles. These patients also have an increased incidence of berry aneurysms. The latter may rupture on occasion and may be the basis of a major complication of the disease.

The hepatic lesions in APCD generally have been thought to be insignificant clinically. Some of the small number of symptomatic cases reported previously may have been examples of CHF rather than APCD (or combinations of the two). Nevertheless, as more patients with APCD have survived for longer periods, it has become clear there is a significant incidence of liver disease associated with APCD. In the most thorough analysis of this issue, 10.5 per cent of the deaths in patients with APCD were considered to result from hepatic complications. There were, in addition, a number of surviving patients with significant, associated liver disease.[65] The complications included infection of cysts (caused by rupture into adjacent bile ducts?), cholangiocarcinoma, and portal hypertension. Analysis of the last-mentioned complication is obscured by the occurrence of posthepatic cirrhosis and chronic hepatitis in these patients, and by the possible confusion of some cases of CHF or long-surviving patients with IPCD, or both, with cases of APCD (a distinction now potentially made more difficult in histologic terms by the finding of DPM in APCD).

Symptoms may develop in a few patients from direct pressure effects of the cysts, and the symptoms may include obstructive jaundice or severe pain.[68] Such patients may benefit from unroofing of as many cysts as possible, with drainage into the peritoneal cavity.[68] Some patients with portal hypertension may benefit from portacaval shunting.

PATHOPHYSIOLOGIC CORRELATES OF DPM

In addition to its significance as an aid in morphologic diagnosis, DPM is important in that it is associated frequently with portal hypertension. This association is most prominent in patients diagnosed clinically as having CHF. Portal hypertension also occurs, however, in other possibly different polycystic conditions, such as IPCD. The basis for the association of the lesion of the portal tract with portal hypertension is not clear. The two most likely possibilities are an alteration of venous resistance resulting from the fibrosis of the portal tracts or a primary but associated abnormality of the intrahepatic portal veins. An early observation of a reduced number of branches of intrahepatic portal veins in CHF has not been corroborated.[69] Clinically, it often appears that the portal hypertension develops over time, suggesting that it may be associated with a change in the amount or character of the portal fibrosis, a phenomenon that has previously been discussed. In terms of the role of a primary associated abnormality of radicles of the portal vein, a duplication of these intrahepatic radicles was found in a high percentage of a small number of cases in which it was sought.[54, 70] There also appears to be a strong (but not invariable) association of portal hypertension with the presence of this duplication.[54]

THE DISEASE OF CONGENITAL HEPATIC FIBROSIS

In 1961, Kerr and colleagues described a group of their own patients and those from the literature with a common disorder for which they coined the name congenital hepatic fibrosis.[69] Affected patients had (1) portal hypertension without hepatic parenchymal disease or obstruction of the main portal vein, (2) a common lesion of the portal tract consisting of increased numbers of bile ducts of unusual profiles and a bland fibrosis (DPM), and (3) a paucity of portal vein radicles in the portal tracts. Cystic disease of the kidney was common. The condition appeared to be inherited as an autosomal recessive trait. Subsequent studies have confirmed the observations of Kerr and co-workers, except for the finding of a paucity of portal veins at the level of the portal tracts. As previously alluded to, however, the passage of time has given rise to the question of whether or not CHF is distinct from IPCD or simply a different presentation of the same disorder.

There is a considerable range of clinical presentations in patients with CHF. Most patients first come to attention because of portal hypertension in the first several decades of life. Ascites is rare. Some patients present with cholangitis (see further on) and rarely with hepatic encephalopathy.[71] Still other cases of CHF are discovered only incidentally at autopsy (latent CHF).[72]

Visceral abnormalities, in addition to those in liver and kidney, seen in single patients or small groups of patients with CHF include emphysema, cerebellar hemangioma, enlargement and deformity of the gallbladder, berry aneurysms, congenital heart disease, and intestinal lymphangiectasia or protein-losing enteropathy, or both.[72–76] Which of these conditions are coincidental is as yet unclear.

The renal lesions may be so minimal as to be discernible only at autopsy, but in some cases they are or become sufficiently severe to cause hypertension and azotemia and, occasionally, frank renal failure.[54, 55] Anatomically, the lesions are initially and primarily medullary, with dilation of collecting ducts and distal tubules.[56, 77] Later, cortical cysts develop. According to Landing and colleagues, both the extent of initial medullary involvement and the time-dependent variation in the ratio of cystic changes in cortical to medullary areas differ in CHF and IPCD.[56]

DPM is a characteristic of CHF, but on occasion it may be confined to one, or a segment of one, lobe.[78-80] The lesion is not always equally prominent in all involved portal tracts, so needle biopsy may be unreliable for making the diagnosis. Furthermore, in a few cases the extent of changes in bile ducts has been quite minimal.[81] In some patients, profiles of the bile ducts are normal. In terms of hepatic cysts, Jorgensen found an increase in the average diameter of bile ducts in patients with CHF as compared with controls.[48] The incidence of formation of gross cysts, however, is not established, nor is it clear whether or not the incidence of such cysts increases with age. Bouquien and co-workers found formation of cysts in each of five patients studied by cholangiography or injection studies at operation or necropsy.[82] Alvarez and colleagues found it in 12 of 17 children.[54] Dilation of the common duct (choledochal cyst) may be present and may exist with or be independent of dilation of intrahepatic ducts. Dilation of bile ducts becomes clinically significant when it is associated with either cholangitis or malignant transformation (see further on). Although the intrahepatic dilation, when present, tends to be diffuse, occasionally only a single lobe may be involved.[83] In one case, a blind but bile-containing dilated duct was observed.[69]

Cholangitis is a significant, although uncommon, complication of CHF. As noted, it may be the presenting symptom of the disorder.[84] When it occurs, dilation of the intrahepatic ducts is typically present. Murray-Lyon reported five cases and collected reports of others from the literature.[85] Most, but not all, of the patients had associated portal hypertension, and a considerable number had renal cysts, as seen on biopsy results or x-ray films. A number also had cystic dilation of the common duct or gallbladder, or both. The ages of these patients ranged from 1 month to 36 years. Calculi may form in the dilated ducts and may complicate the management of patients with pre-existing cholangitis, or perhaps initiate cholangitis and mandate surgery. The genesis of the cholangitis in patients in whom this complication develops is not clear. Possibly, operative cholangiography or biliary tract surgery initiates the process in some patients. Perhaps it tends to occur in patients with the most marked dilation of intrahepatic ducts and bile stasis, with or without calculi. In general, patients in whom cholangitis develops have poor prognoses.[85] Biliary tract surgery or operative cholangiography, or both, may contribute to the poor prognosis.[85] Because of the potentially deleterious effects of operative cholangiography and surgery on the biliary tract, it is suggested that conservative treatment be used as long as possible for all patients with CHF, including those with fever. Chenodeoxycholic acid should be used to prevent formation of calculi.[86] However, the potential for the development of malignancy (discussed later), together with the possibility of resecting localized duct dilations, as a prophylaxis against development of stones and cholecystitis, may constitute reasons for an aggressive approach to the management of selected patients with CHF.

When there is no cholangitis or malignancy, the major problem in management of patients with CHF is bleeding esophageal varices. Considerable initial success has been achieved in relieving portal hypertension in both children and adults by portal-systemic shunting. However, the long-term results need evaluation.[87]

An uncommon, although significant, complication in CHF is the development of malignancy. Only a few such cases have been reported.[88] Cholangiocarcinoma has been the most common tumor observed.[88] Ages at tumor development are variable. The tumor is also seen in association with choledochal cysts, or with cystic dilation of intrahepatic biliary ducts when DPM is not present. It is not clear whether dilation of ducts has always been present in patients with CHF with tumors of the bile ducts.

THE LESION OF CONGENITAL HEPATIC FIBROSIS AND NEPHRONOPHTHISIS

In a small number of patients, severe progressive renal disease has been accompanied by a hepatic lesion bearing a resemblance to DPM.[89, 90] The condition is included in this chapter because of the combination of heritability and the simultaneous presence of renal disease and a DPM-like lesion, but hepatic cysts are not a feature in these patients. Several of the patients have had retinal degeneration and cerebellar hypoplasia. The condition bears some similarities to retinal-renal dystrophy, but in the latter there is no associated liver lesion. In all patients reported there with the combination of a DPM-like lesion and severe progressive renal disease, the disease has been detected before the patient reached 20 years of age. Most of the patients were frankly uremic by this age. The condition is familial.

The pathologic features of the renal disease are different from those of typical IPCD and CHF. The renal histopathologic features include interstitial fibrosis and inflammation, tubular atrophy and cyst formation, and glomerular sclerosis. This histologic picture most closely resembles so-called nephronophthisis, but this is a descriptive impression only. The renal disease may not be similar pathogenetically to the more common juvenile nephronophthisis of Fanconi. The first observed abnormality of renal function is a concentrating defect.

The hepatic lesion, although generically consistent with DPM, is nevertheless somewhat atypical. The bile ducts rarely show unusual profiles, and in a few instances inflammation has been present. In one case, the portal lesion showed a quite marked change with time. Morphometric studies by Landing and co-workers show that the lesion of the portal tracts in these patients is different from IPCD and CHF.[50, 56] Hepatomegaly is the most common initial sign of the disease, yet abnormalities of liver function are scant. Splenomegaly is common, but complications of portal hypertension have not been reported.

CYSTIC DISEASE OF THE LIVER IN INFANTILE POLYCYSTIC DISEASE

IPCD (Potter's type I cystic renal disease) is an autosomal recessive disorder characterized by a combination of hepatic and renal diseases. The lesion in the liver is DPM. The lesion in the kidney consists of cysts of the collecting ducts. As noted earlier, there is disagreement over whether or not the disease is truly distinct from CHF. In the typical case, the affected infant has bilateral masses in the flanks at birth and survives only a few days, weeks, or months. A few patients, apparently those with less extensive renal disease, survive for prolonged periods.[55, 77] Although it has been suggested that the disease follows the same clinical course in all affected members of a single family, it now appears that this may not be true.[51, 52] This must be taken into account in genetic counseling.

The kidneys in a typical case present a distinct gross appearance of massive enlargement and radially oriented, minute cysts. This appearance correlates well with the microscopic features (Fig. 52–4). There is dilation of the collecting ducts.[77] Any intervening nephrons are normal, and there is no dysplasia. Renal fibrosis is scant or lacking, but fibrosis may increase with increasing survival. With advancing age there is also a tendency for the cysts to decrease in number, to lose their obvious radial orientation, and to become rounded.[55] It may be difficult to make the diagnosis in such instances without knowledge of the hepatic morphologic appearance and family history. Landing and co-workers have emphasized the morphometric differences between the renal lesions of IPCD and those of CHF.[50, 56]

The hepatic lesion is relatively uniform in appearance. Grossly recognizable cysts are present only rarely in the newborn;[91] gross cysts are uncommon even in older patients. At the microscopic level, the hepatic lesion is characterized by increased fibrous tissue in portal tracts and increased numbers of biliary ducts. The ducts often have unusual shapes (Fig. 52–5). They do not appear to be proliferating actively. There is no obstruction in the biliary tract and no parenchymal disease. An occasional patient may have only an inconspicuous increase in the number of bile ducts.[55] Reconstruction (stereologic) studies suggest that the ducts communicate both proximally and distally with the remainder of the biliary drainage system. The precise incidence of portal hypertension in IPCD is unclear, although it appears to be less than that in CHF. At least some of this apparent difference in the frequencies of portal hypertension reflects

that children with IPCD often die in infancy; the incidence of portal hypertension in IPCD may prove to be substantial in children with long survival times. It has been observed that there is a substantial correlation between the presence of portal hypertension and the presence of duplicated intrahepatic portal vein radicles in patients with IPCD-CHF.[70] There may be some evolution of the hepatic lesion with age, as indicated by the descriptions of Blyth and Ockenden,[51] which suggests that grossly recognizable hepatic cysts may become more frequent with age.

Deaths of patients with IPCD are often assumed to result from renal failure. Moreover, mortality seems to correlate with the extent of renal abnormality. It has been suggested, however, that the immediate cause of neonatal death usually is pulmonary disease.[55] In patients who survive the neonatal period, hypertension currently seems to be the principal factor determining survival.[55] Renal function abnormalities are nonspecific and include a decreased glomerular filtration rate, a decreased ability to concentrate urine, and defective acidification.[77] Portacaval shunting in those patients with clinically important portal hypertension results in significant improvement, at least in the short term.[55] Renal transplantation may be indicated on occasion. Occasional patients with IPCD may have pancreatic fibrosis with duct dilation or proliferation, or both.[55]

CHOLEDOCHAL CYST (CONGENITAL CYSTIC DILATION OF THE COMMON BILE DUCT)

Choledochal cysts are associated commonly with dilation of the intrahepatic bile ducts, and for this reason it is

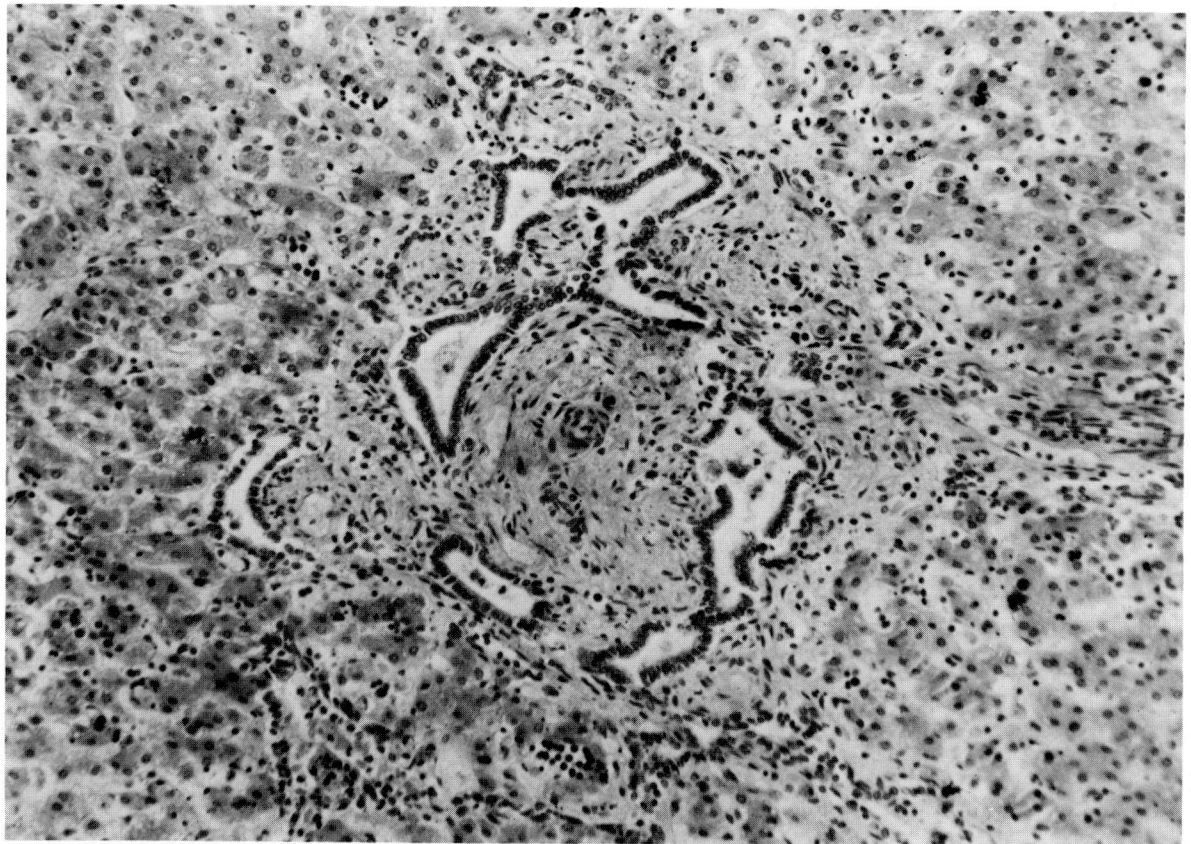

Figure 52–5. Photomicrograph of the portal tract from a newborn with infantile polycystic disease, illustrating congenital hepatic fibrosis lesion. Fibrous tissue and bile ducts are increased. The ducts are slightly dilated and of unusual shapes (hematoxylin and eosin, × 10).

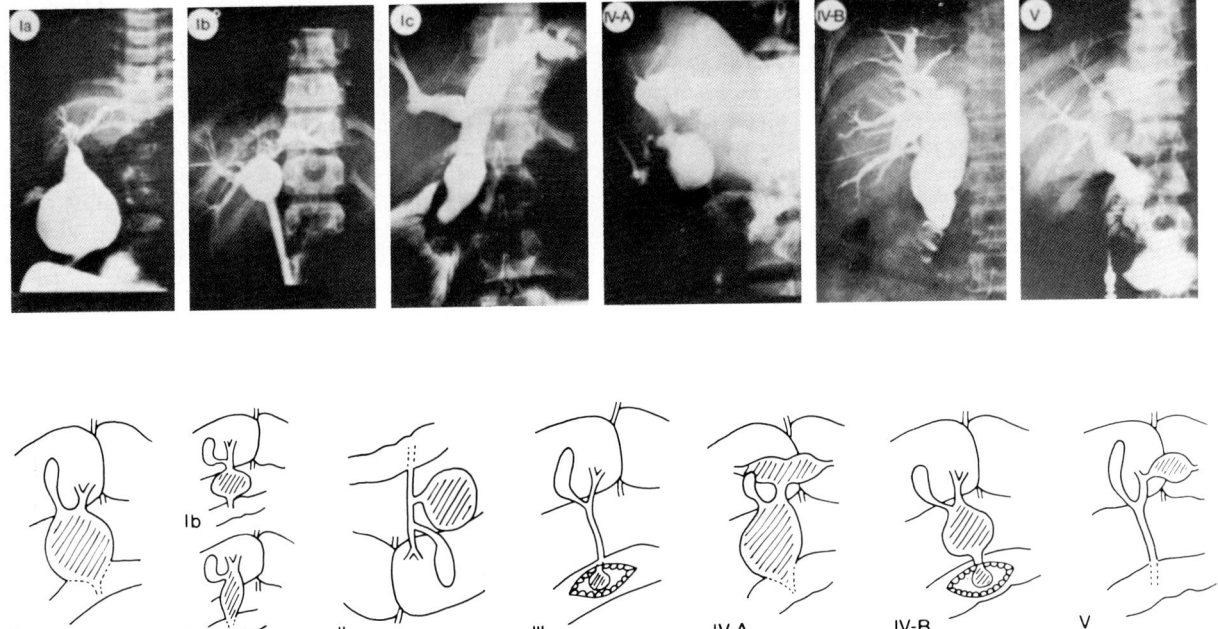

Figure 52–6. *Top,* Operative cholangiograms of congenital biliary duct cysts as classified by Todani and co-workers: (*left to right*) *Ia,* common type; *Ib,* segmental dilatation; *Ic,* diffuse dilatation; *II,* diverticulum; *III,* choledochocoele; *IV-A,* multiple cyst (intra- and extrahepatic); *IV-B,* multiple cyst (extrahepatic); *V,* intrahepatic. *Bottom,* Diagrams of the various types of communicating cysts. This classification emphasizes the frequent co-existence of intra- and extrahepatic duct dilation. (Reproduced from Todani T, et al. Am J Surg 134:263, 1977, with permission.)

appropriate to discuss them in this chapter (Fig. 52–6). The combination of intra- and extrahepatic cysts is similar to that seen in at least one of the polycystic diseases—CHF, but choledochal cysts differ significantly from the polycystic diseases because they are not heritable, are not associated with DPM, and are not associated ordinarily with lesions in other organs.

Choledochal cysts are more common in Japan than in western countries,[92] and Japanese workers deserve the credit for emphasizing that choledochal cysts are associated frequently with dilation of intrahepatic ducts as shared elements of a systemic dilatory change (Fig. 52–6).[93, 94] As noted previously, this does *not* connote the presence of polycystic disease as we have defined it, and in fact CHF may be unusual in Japan.[95]

Choledochal cysts, with the exception of one variety (see further on), are more common in females. They may present at any age. They have been demonstrated in utero and have been observed to develop in adult life.[96] Approximately 60 per cent present before the age of 10 years. Although they are often said to be congenital lesions, it is probably more consistent to say that affected patients have a congenital *propensity* for the development of cysts. Todani and co-workers have defined a subgroup of patients in whom the cysts are cylindric or diffuse.[97, 98] Such cases lack a female predominance and differ from other cases of choledochal cysts in a number of respects.[97, 98] Other workers have suggested that patients in the pediatric age group can be divided into several different groups.[99] It is important, therefore, to keep in mind that several conditions, differing in origin and possibly in other aspects as well, may be included in the broad classification of choledochal cysts without DPM.

The clinical manifestations of choledochal cysts are quite variable.[100, 101] Epigastric pain is the most common symptom. Fever and jaundice are the next most common findings in patients with choledochal cysts and intrahepatic

duct dilation. In the latter group, abdominal masses are relatively uncommon when compared with patients with only choledochal dilation.[100] The classic triad of pain, jaundice, and an abdominal mass is present in no more than one quarter of patients.[102] Symptoms may develop, regress, and recur in a repetitive fashion.[99]

When the diagnosis is suspected, ultrasonography is the initial study of choice.[103, 104] Combination with TcIDA cholescintigraphy or transhepatic cholangiography should allow delineation of both intra- and extrahepatic dilation.[103, 104] The anatomy must be thoroughly understood before instituting definitive therapy because the pancreatic duct may drain into the cyst.[104, 105]

The pathogenesis of choledochal cyst is a matter of debate and speculation. Suggested possibilities include congenital weakness of the wall, a primary abnormality of the mucosa, and congenital obstruction.[105] As already noted, it is by no means clear that all cases have the same pathogenesis. The possible role of pancreatic reflux, associated with an abnormal junction of the pancreatic and common bile ducts, has been much discussed. There is a high incidence, but not an invariable occurrence, of such an abnormality, as well as a high incidence of stenosis of the bile duct of variable severity.[98, 106]

Histologically, the cysts have a fibrous wall, typically with absent or mild inflammation (the inflammation is chronic). Most often, there is no epithelial lining. When this lining is present, its appearance varies from flattened to typically biliary.

As mentioned, intrahepatic dilation of bile ducts has often been demonstrated in association with choledochal cysts. The reported incidence varies widely from country to country. Todani found such dilation in somewhat less than 30 per cent of his patients.[100] It is present less commonly in young children than in older patients.[100] It is sufficiently common that it should always be sought in patients with choledochal cyst. It is diffuse in two thirds of affected patients and may involve only the left lobe of the liver, but it seldom involves only the right lobe.[97, 100] The intrahepatic dilation of bile ducts, when associated with the cylindric type of choledochal cyst, tends to regress after excision of the choledochal cyst.[97, 98] Dilation of the pancreatic duct is seen with some frequency in patients with choledochal cyst.[107, 108]

Complications, other than obstruction, include stone formation (which occurs in approximately 8 per cent of patients),[102] cholangitis, carcinoma and, rarely, perforation. Perforation is particularly likely to occur when the junction of the bile duct and the pancreatic duct allows free egress of pancreatic secretions into the common duct.[98] Carcinoma is said to develop in 2 to 8 per cent of cases.[101, 102, 109] These figures were derived in large part before the widespread use of excisional therapy, which may reduce the incidence of malignancy substantially. It is unlikely to eliminate it entirely, however, since carcinomata have developed after excision of cysts.[104, 110] The incidence of carcinoma increases with age.[111] The tumors may arise in various parts of the pancreaticobiliary system, including liver, gallbladder, intrahepatic ducts, pancreatic ducts, and pancreas. The usual type is adenocarcinoma, but squamous carcinoma, adenoacanthoma, and undifferentiated carcinoma have been seen.[107] The outcome in patients in whom malignancy develops is very poor.

It is now generally agreed that choledochal cysts require surgical treatment. The procedure of choice is excision of the cyst.[93, 104, 112] This procedure minimizes, but does not completely eliminate, cholangitis and also presumably reduces the incidence of subsequent development of carcinoma. Todani has suggested that patients with normal junctions between the bile duct and pancreatic duct may require only an adequate transduodenal sphincteroplasty.[98] Cholecystectomy is usually done at the same time. Most American surgeons seem to favor Roux-en-Y choledochojejunostomy for restoring biliary-enteric continuity. Todani has also used hepaticoduodenostomy.[97] A wide anastomosis is important for minimizing cholangitis. In situations in which cyst excision is not feasible, either because of the local anatomy or the elderly status of the patient, Roux-en-Y jejunal loop drainage with a large anastomosis may be the operation of choice. In patients with associated dilation of intrahepatic ducts, partial hepatic resection may be appropriate, but only if the dilated ducts are localized to a single lobe.[97, 113]

MALFORMATION SYNDROMES

It is not definitely known whether ductal cysts in all the various malformation syndromes are communicating or not. Many of the patients die so early in life that cholangiography is not carried out. Also, reconstruction studies in these conditions are rare. The author has chosen, however, to classify these cysts as communicating because the associated liver lesion usually appears to be DPM. Additional studies are needed to determine whether, or in which conditions, this is appropriate.

MECKEL-GRUBER SYNDROME (DYSENCEPHALIA SPLANCHNOCYSTICA)

This syndrome is inherited as a recessive trait. It is characterized by the presence of many malformations, with death usually occurring perinatally or in early infancy.[114–117]

The classic triad of findings in the syndrome—postaxial polydactyly, occipital encephalocele, and cystic kidneys—is not always present. The range of abnormalities that may be present makes diagnosis occasionally difficult or uncertain. A variety of central nervous system lesions may be present. The renal lesion appears to be cystic dysplasia. The range of abnormalities raises the possibility that certain other reported malformation constellations,[118] which include DPM, central nervous system lesions, and renal abnormalities, but are not typically included as examples of the Meckel-Gruber syndrome, *may* be variants.

Although DPM was recognized in some patients in early reports, recent studies have suggested it is nearly always present.[119, 120] In some patients dilation of intrahepatic bile ducts results in gross cysts.[115] Some reconstruction studies and occasional reports have suggested that the morphologic features in these patients were similar to IPCD.[121, 122] Other reconstruction studies suggest that the lesions differ in the two conditions.[123] Landing and coworkers determined by morphometric analysis that the lesion of portal tracts in the Meckel-Gruber syndrome was more fibrotic than that in either CHF or IPCD.[50] The latter authors emphasized a fibrous sheath around intratubular canals of Hering. Rarely, pancreatic cysts may be present.[114]

JEUNE'S SYNDROME (THORACIC ASPHYXIATING DYSTROPHY)

Jeune's syndrome is an autosomal recessive form of dwarfism characterized by an extremely constricted thorax, shortened limbs, abnormalities of the pelvis, and cystic disease of the kidneys. There is also apparently a relatively high incidence of hepatic lesions, characterized by portal fibrosis and large numbers of bile ducts.[124–126] As far as we know, gross cysts have not been described. Histologically, the hepatic lesions are at least compatible with DPM. Landing has observed that the morphometric features are generally similar to those in CHF but that the portal tracts are smaller.[50] Bernstein observed microcysts of the pancreas in several cases.[122] The kidney disease is characterized by the development of progressive renal insufficiency. The pathophysiologic features of the liver disease have not been defined.

ELLIS–VAN CREVELD SYNDROME

It is interesting that in a single case of Ellis–van Creveld syndrome (chondroectodermal dysplasia), portal fibrosis, an increase in the number of bile ducts, and cystic dysplasia of the kidneys were found.[127]

IVEMARK'S SYNDROME

So-called Ivemark's syndrome was described as a familial dysplasia of kidneys, liver, and pancreas.[128] The liver lesions appear to have been consistent with DPM. Only rare instances of the complete syndrome have been reported.[129] Apparent forme frustes without liver disease are seen somewhat more frequently.[130] A case with similar lesions was reported with trisomy C.[131]

OTHER CONDITIONS

Potter, in her discussion of renal cysts,[132] noted that some patients with her type III cystic kidneys have associated liver lesions, and a few of these patients may have pancreatic cysts and fibrosis as well. No familial occurrence was described. In an illustrated case, the picture and accompanying description indicate that the hepatic lesions consisted of minimal proliferation of connective tissue and a very slight increase in biliary ducts.[132] Such lesions, as we have indicated, might be considered examples of DPM, as broadly interpreted. Potter states that the hepatic lesions seen in association with type III kidneys can "ordinarily be easily distinguished from those found in type I (IPCD)." Classification of these cases of Potter with combined liver and pancreatic lesions and type III kidneys is further complicated by the facts that type III kidneys are not confined to a single genetic entity and Potter does not use dysplasia as a diagnostic designation. Landing has pointed out that hepatic lesions of a possibly similar nature may occur in the vaginal atresia syndromes and in tuberous sclerosis,[50] but little information is available on this point. In one case of the trisomy E syndrome, a fibrocystic liver was observed.[133]

REFERENCES

1. Henson SW Jr, Gray HK, Dockerty MB. Benign tumors of the liver. III. Solitary cysts. Surg Gynecol Obstet 103:607, 1956.
2. Flagg RS, Robinson DW. Solitary nonparasitic hepatic cysts. Arch Surg 95:964, 1967.
3. Stoesser AV, Wangensteen OH. Solitary nonparasitic cysts of the liver. Am J Dis Child 38:241, 1929.
4. Caplan LH, Simon M. Nonparasitic cysts of the liver. Am J Roentgenol 96:421, 1966.
5. Desser P, Smith S. Nonparasitic liver cysts in children. J Pediatr 49:297, 1956.
6. Roemer C, Ferrucci J, Mueller P, et al. Hepatic cysts: diagnosis and therapy by sonographic needle aspiration. Arch J Radiol 136:1065, 1981.
7. Rosch J, Mayer BS, Campbell JR, et al. "Vascular" benign liver cyst in children: report of two cases. Radiology 126:747, 1978.
8. Bloustein PA. Association of carcinoma with congenital cystic conditions of the liver and bile ducts. Am J Gastroenterol 67:40, 1977.
9. Saini S, Ferrucci J, Mueller PR, et al. Percutaneous aspiration of hepatic cysts done to provide definitive therapy. Am J Radiol 141:559, 1983.
10. Austin E, Mitchell G, Oliphant M, et al. Solitary hepatic duct polyp: a heretofore unheralded association. Surgery 89:359, 1981.
11. Lambruschi PG, Rudolf LE. Massive unifocal cyst of the liver in a drug abuser. Ann Surg 189:39, 1979.
12. Longmire WP Jr, Sergio AM, Gordon HE. Congenital cystic disease of the liver and biliary system. Ann Surg 174:711, 1971.
13. Henson SW Jr, Hallenbeck GA, Gray HK, et al. Benign tumors of the liver. V. Traumatic cysts. Surg Gynecol Obstet 104:302, 1957.
14. Doppman JL, Dunnick NR, Girton RT, et al. Bile duct cysts secondary to liver infarcts: report of a case and experimental production by small vessel hepatic artery occlusion. Radiology 130:1, 1979.
15. Imamoglu KH, Walt AJ. Duplication of the duodenum extending into the liver. Am J Surg 133:628, 1977.
16. Ishak KG, Willis GW, Cummins SD, et al. Biliary cystadenoma and cystadenocarcinoma. Report of 14 cases and review of the literature. Cancer 39:322, 1977.
17. Marsh JL, Dahms B, Longmire WP. Cystadenoma and cystadenocarcinoma of the biliary system. Arch Surg 109:41, 1974.
18. Keech M. Cystadenomas of the pancreas and intrahepatic bile ducts. Gastroenterology 19:568, 1951.
19. Devine P, Ucci A. Biliary cystadenocarcinoma arising in a congenital cyst. Hum Pathol 16:92, 1985.
20. Wheeler D, Edmondson H. Cystadenoma with mesenchymal stroma (CMS) in the liver and bile ducts. Cancer 56:1434, 1985.
21. Marcial M, Hauser S, Cibas E, et al. Intrahepatic biliary cystadenoma. Dig Dis Sci 31:884, 1986.
22. Dehner L. Hepatic tumors in the pediatric age group. In: Rosenberg H, Bolande R, eds. Perspectives in Pediatric Pathology, Vol 4. Chicago, Yearbook Medical, 1978.
23. Ishak R. Primary hepatic tumors in childhood. Prog Liver Dis 5:636, 1976.
24. Stocker T, Ishak K. Mesenchymal hamartoma of the liver: report of 30 cases and review of the literature. Pediatr Pathol 1:245, 1983.
25. Ros P, Goodman A, Ishak K, et al. Mesenchymal hamartoma of the liver: radiologic-pathologic correlation. Radiology 158:629, 1986.
26. Witzleben CL. Unpublished observations.
27. Dehner L, Ewing S, Sumner H. Infantile mesenchymal hamartoma of the liver. Histologic and ultrastructural observations. Arch Pathol 99:379, 1975.
28. Ishak KG, Rabin L. Benign tumors of the liver. Med Clin North Am 59:995, 1975.
29. Adam YG, Huvos AG, Fortner JG. Giant hemangiomas of the liver. Ann Surg 172:239, 1970.
30. Hirner A, Haring R. Giant cavernous hemangiomas of the liver. Case report and review of the literature. Langenbeck's Arch Chir 364:25, 1978.
31. Trastek V, van Heerden J, Sheedy P, et al. Cavernous hemangiomas of the liver: resect or observe. Am J Surg 145:49, 1983.
32. Olmsted WW, Stocker JT. RPC from the AFIP. Diag Radiol 117:59, 1975.
33. Watanabe I, Kasai M, Suzuki S. True teratoma of the liver—report of a case and review of the literature. Acta Hepatogastroenterol 25:40, 1978.
34. Witte D, Kissane J, Askin F. Hepatic teratomas in children. Pediatr Pathol 1:81, 1983.
35. Robinson R, Nelson L. Hepatic teratoma in an anencephalic fetus. Arch Pathol Lab Med 110:655, 1986.
36. DeStephano D, Wesley J, Heidelberger K, et al. Primitive cystic hepatic neoplasm of infancy with mesothelial differentiation. Pediatr Pathol 4:291, 1985.
37. Ichijima K, Kobashi Y, Yamabe H, et al. Peliosis hepatis. An unusual case involving multiple organs. Acta Pathol Jpn 30:109, 1980.
38. Warfel K, Ellis G. Peliosis of the spleen. Arch Pathol Lab Med 106:99, 1982.
39. Yanoff M, Rawson A. Peliosis hepatis: an anatomic study with demonstration of two varieties. Arch Pathol 77:159, 1964.
40. Lyon J, Bookstein J, Cartwright CA, et al. Peliosis hepatis: Diagnosis by magnification wedged hepatic venography. Radiology 150:647, 1984.
41. Nadell J, Kosek J. Peliosis hepatis: twelve cases associated with oral androgen therapy. Arch Pathol Lab Med 101:405, 1977.
42. Bagheri A, Boyer J. Peliosis hepatis associated with androgenic-anabolic steroid therapy: a severe form of hepatic injury. Ann Intern Med 81:610, 1974.
43. Poulsen H, Winkler K. Liver disease with periportal sinusoidal dilatation. Digestion 8:441, 1973.
44. Ross R, Kovacs K, Horvath E. Ultrastructure of peliosis hepatis in percutaneous biopsy. Pathol Eur 7:273, 1972.
45. Ishak K. Hepatic lesions caused by anabolic and contraceptive steroids. Semin Liver Dis 1:116, 1981.
46. Lee K. Peliosis hepatis–like lesion in aging rats. Vet Pathol 20:410, 1983.
47. Zafrani E, Cazier A, Baudelot A-M, et al. Ultrastructural lesions of the liver in human peliosis. Am J Pathol 114:349, 1984.
48. Jorgensen M. The ductal plate malformation. Acta Pathol Microbiol Scand A (Suppl) 257, 1977.
49. Desmet V. Cholangiopathies: past, present and future, State of the Art Lecture. Chicago, American Association for the Study of Liver Diseases, 1985.
50. Landing BH, Wells TR, Claireaux AE. Morphometric analysis of liver lesions in cystic diseases of childhood. Hum Pathol (Suppl)11:549, 1980.
50a. Bernstein J, Stickler GB, Neel IV. Congenital hepatic fibrosis: evolving morphology. APMCS Suppl 4:1726, 1988.
51. Blyth H, Ockenden BG. Polycystic disease of kidneys and liver presenting in childhood. J Med Genet 8:257, 1971.
52. Gang D, Herrin J. Infantile polycystic disease of the liver and kidneys. Clin Nephrol 25:28, 1986.
53. Sherlock S. Cysts and congenital biliary abnormalities. In: Sherlock S, ed. Diseases of the Liver and Biliary System. Oxford, Alden Press, 1981:406.
54. Alvarez E, Bernard O, Brunelle F, et al. Congenital hepatic fibrosis in children. J Pediatr 99:370, 1981.
55. Lieberman E, Madrigal-Salinas L, Gwin JL, et al. Infantile polycystic disease of the kidneys and liver: clinical, pathological and radiological correlations and comparisons with congenital hepatic fibrosis. Medicine 50:277, 1971.
56. Landing B, Wells T, Helczynski L. Some problems in the meanings of terms, as exemplified by tubulointerstitial and medullary cystic diseases of the kidneys (cystic diseases of liver and kidneys). In: Rosenberg H, Bernstein J, eds. Perspectives in Pediatric Pathology. Vol. 12. Basel, S. Karger, 1988:20.
57. Marchal GJ, Desmet VJ, Proesmans WC, et al. Caroli disease: high frequency US and pathologic findings. Radiology 158:507, 1986.
58. Caroli S. Diseases of the intrahepatic biliary tree. Clin Gastroenterol 2:147, 1973.
59. Karhunen P, Tenhu M. Adult polycystic liver and kidney diseases are separate entities. Clin Genet 30:29, 1986.

60. Grantham J. Clinical aspects of adult and infantile polycystic kidney disease. Contr Nephrol 48:178, 1985.
60a. Reeders ST, Breuning H, Davies KE, et al. A highly polymorphic DNA marker linked to adult polycystic disease on chromosome 16. Nature 317:542, 1985.
60b. Romeo G, Devoto M, Costa G, et al. A second genetic locus for autosomal dominant polycystic kidney disease. Lancet 2:8, 1988.
61. Kaplan BS, Rabin I, Drummond KN. Autosomal dominant polycystic renal disease in children. J Pediatr 90:782, 1977.
62. Shokeir MHK. Expression of "adult" polycystic renal disease in the fetus and newborn. Clin Genet 14:61, 1978.
63. Milutinovic J, Fialkow PJ, Rudd TG, et al. Liver cysts in patients with autosomal dominant polycystic kidney disease. Am J Med 68:741, 1980.
64. Levine E, Cook L, Grantham J. Liver cysts in autosomal dominant polycystic kidney disease: clinical and computed tomographic study. Am J Radiol 145:229, 1985.
65. Grunfeld J-P, Albouze G, Junger P, et al. Liver changes and complications in adult polycystic kidney disease. Adv Nephrol 14:1, 1985.
66. Comfort MW, Gray HK, Dahlin DC, et al. Polycystic disease of the liver: a study of 24 cases. Gastroenterology 20:60, 1952.
67. Manes JC, Kissane JM, Valdes AJ. Congenital hepatic fibrosis, liver cell carcinoma, and adult polycystic kidneys. Cancer 39:2619, 1977.
68. Lin T-Y, Chen C-C, Wang S-M. Treatment of nonparasitic cystic disease of the liver: a new approach to therapy with polycystic liver. Ann Surg 168:921, 1968.
69. Kerr DNS, Harrison CV, Sherlock S, et al. Congenital hepatic fibrosis. Q J Med 30:91, 1961.
70. Odievre M, Chaumont P, Montague J, et al. Anomalies of the intrahepatic portal venous system in congenital hepatic fibrosis. Radiology 122:427, 1977.
71. Richard-Molard B, Couzigou P, Julien J, et al. Fibrose hepatique congenitale tardivement revelee par une encephalopathie hepatique. Gastroenterol Clin Biol 9:449, 1985.
72. Fauvert R, Benhamou J. Congenital hepatic fibrosis. In: Schaffner F, Sherlock S, Leery C, eds. The Liver and its Diseases. New York, Intercontinental Medical Book Corp. 1974:283.
73. Williams R, Scheuer PJ, Heard BE. Congenital hepatic fibrosis with an unusual pulmonary lesion. J Clin Pathol 17:135, 1964.
74. Naveh Y, Roguin N, Ludatscher R, et al. Congenital hepatic fibrosis with congenital heart disease. Gut 21:799, 1980.
75. Pelletier V, Galenao N, Brouchu P, et al. Secretory diarrhea with protein-losing enteropathy, enterocolitis cystic superficialis, intestinal lymphangiectasis and congenital hepatic fibrosis: a new syndrome. J Pediatr 108:61, 1986.
76. Pedersen P, Tygstrup I. Congenital hepatic fibrosis combined with protein-losing enteropathy and recurrent thrombosis. Acta Paediatr Scand 69:571, 1980.
77. Anand SK, Chan JC, Lieberman E. Polycystic disease and hepatic fibrosis in children: renal function studies. Am J Dis Child 130:810, 1975.
78. Hauser R, Alexander R. Localized congenital hepatic fibrosis presenting as an abdominal mass. Hum Pathol 5:473, 1978.
79. Faivre J, Richir C, Deraud C. Agenesis of the left hepatic lobe, persistent ascites. Cruveilhier-Baumgarten's disease. Arch Mal Appar Dig 57:359, 1968.
80. Leong A. Segmental biliary ectasia and congenital hepatic fibrosis in a patient with chromosomal abnormality. Pathology 12:275, 1980.
81. Parker RGF. Fibrosis of the liver as a congenital anomaly. J Pathol Bacteriol 71:359, 1956.
82. Bouquien H, Delumeau G, Lenne Y, et al. Cited by Murray-Lyon IM, Shilkin KB, Laws JW, et al. Non-obstructive dilatation of the intrahepatic biliary tree with cholangitis. Q J Med 41:477, 1972.
83. Vic-Dupont, Mignot J, Halle B. Cited by Murray-Lyon IM, Shilkin KB, Laws JW, et al. Non-obstructive dilatation of the intrahepatic biliary tree with cholangitis. Q J Med 41:477, 1972.
84. Alvarez F, Hadchoel M, Bernard O. Latent chronic cholangitis in congenital hepatic fibrosis. Eur J Pediatr 139:203, 1982.
85. Murray-Lyon IM, Shilkin KB, Laws JW, et al. Non-obstructive dilatation of the intrahepatic biliary tree with cholangitis. Q J Med 41:477, 1972.
86. Howlett SA, Shulman ST, Ayoub EM, et al. Cholangitis complicating congenital hepatic fibrosis. Case report. Dig Dis 20:790, 1975.
87. Kerr DNS, Okonkwo S, Choa RG. Congenital hepatic fibrosis: the long-term prognosis. Gut 19:514, 1978.
88. Daroca PJ, Tuthill R, Reed RJ. Cholangiocarcinoma arising in congenital hepatic fibrosis. Arch Pathol 99:592, 1975.
89. Boichis H, Passwell J, David R, et al. Congenital hepatic fibrosis and nephronophthisis: a family study. Q J Med 42:221, 1973.
90. Witzleben CL, Sharp A. "Nephronophthisis-congenital hepatic fibrosis." An additional hepatorenal disorder. Hum Pathol 13:728, 1982.
91. Bernstein J. Cystic diseases of the liver in infancy. In: Javitt NP, ed. Neonatal Hepatitis and Biliary Atresia. Bethesda, MD, Public Health Service, DHEW publication NIH #79-1296, 1979.

92. Hays DM, Goodman GN, Snyder WH, et al. Congenital cystic dilatation of the common bile duct. Arch Surg 98:457, 1969.
93. Saito S, Tsuchida Y, Hashizume K, et al. Congenital cystic dilatation of the biliary ducts: surgical procedures and long-term results. Z Kinderchir 19:49, 1976.
94. Todani T, Watanabe Y, Narusue M, et al. Congenital bile duct cysts. Classification, operative procedures, and review of thirty-seven cases including cancer arising from choledochal cyst. Am J Surg 134:263, 1977.
95. Nonomura A, Ohta G, Yoshida K, et al. Congenital hepatic fibrosis. A case report with study of three dimensional reconstruction of serial sections of the liver. Acta Pathol Jpn 28:949, 1978.
96. Wideman MA, Tan A, Martinez CJ. Fetal sonography and neonatal scintigraphy of a choledochal cyst. J Nucl Med 86:893, 1985.
97. Todani T, Watanabe Y, Fujii T, et al. Congenital choledochal cyst with intrahepatic involvement. Arch Surg 119:1038, 1984.
98. Todani T, Watanabe Y, Fujii T, et al. Cylindrical dilatation of the choledochus: a special type of congenital bile duct dilatation. Surgery 98:964, 1985.
99. Barlow B, Tabor E, Blanc WA, et al. Choledochal cyst: a review of 19 cases. J Pediatr 89:934, 1976.
100. Todani T, Naruse M, Watanabe Y, et al. Management of congenital choledocal cyst with intrahepatic involvement. Ann Surg 187:272, 1978.
101. Flanigan DP. Biliary cysts. Ann Surg 177:705, 1973.
102. Yamaguchi M. Congenital choledochal cyst. Analysis of 1433 patients in the Japanese literature. Am J Surg 140:653, 1980.
103. Han BK, Babcock D, Gelfand M. Choledochal cyst with bile duct dilatation: sonography and ^{99}mTcIDA cholescintigraphy. Am J Radiol 136:1075, 1981.
104. Takiff H, Stone M, Fonkalsrud E. Choledochal cysts: results of primary surgery and need for reoperation in young patients. Am J Surg 150:141, 1985.
105. Spitz L. Choledochal cyst. Surg Gynecol Obstet 147:444, 1978.
106. Babbitt D, Starsuk R, Clemett A. Choledochal cyst: a concept of etiology. Am J Radiol 119:57, 1973.
107. Rattner D, Schapiro RH, Warshaw AL. Abnormalities of the pancreatic and biliary ducts in adult patients with choledochal cyst. Arch Surg 118:1068, 1983.
108. Uno J, Sakoda K, Akita M. Surgical aspects of cystic dilatation of the bile duct. Ann Surg 195:203, 1982.
109. Todani T, Tabuchi K, Watanabe Y, et al. Carcinoma arising in the wall of congenital bile duct cysts. Cancer 44:1134, 1979.
110. Gallagher P, Millis R, Mitchinson M. Congenital dilatation of the intrahepatic ducts with cholangiocarcinoma. J Clin Pathol 25:804, 1972.
111. Vogles C, Smadja C, Shands W, et al. Carcinoma in choledochal cysts. Age-related incidence. Arch Surg 118:986, 1983.
112. Deziel D, Rossi R, Munson L, et al. Management of bile duct cyst in adults. Arch Surg 121:410, 1986.
113. Lorenzo Z, Seed R, Beal J. Congenital dilatation of the biliary tract. Am J Surg 121:510, 1971.
114. Opitz JM, Howe JJ. The Meckel syndrome (dysencephalia splanchnocystica, the Gruber syndrome). Birth Defects 5:167, 1969.
115. Fried K, Liban E, Lurie M, et al. Polycystic kidneys associated with malformations of the brain, polydactyly, and other birth defects in newborn sibs. A lethal syndrome showing the autosomal-recessive pattern of inheritance. J Med Genet 8:285, 1971.
116. Mecke S, Passarge E. Encephalocele, polycystic kidneys, and polydactyly as an autosomal recessive trait simulating certain other disorders: the Meckel syndrome. Ann Genet 14:97, 1971.
117. Hsia YE, Bratu M, Herbordt A. Genetics of the Meckel syndrome (dysencephalia splanchnocystica). Pediatrics 48:237, 1971.
118. Miranda D, Schinella RA, Finegold MJ. Familial renal dysplasia. Microdissection studies with associated central nervous system and hepatic malformations. Arch Pathol 93:483, 1972.
119. Rapola J, Salonen R. Visceral anomalies in the Meckel syndrome. Teratology 31:193, 1985.
120. Salonen R. The Meckel syndrome: clinicopathological findings in 67 patients. Am J Med Genet 18:671, 1984.
121. Jorgensen M. A case of abnormal intrahepatic bile duct arrangement submitted to three dimensional reconstruction. Acta Pathol Microbiol Scand A 79:303, 1971.
122. Bernstein J, Brough J, McAdams AJ. The renal lesion in syndromes of multiple congenital malformations. Cerebrohepatorenal syndrome; Jeune asphyxiating thoracic dystrophy; tuberous sclerosis; Meckel syndrome. Birth Defects 10:35, 1974.
123. Adams CM, Danks DM, Campbell PE. Comments upon the classification of infantile polycystic diseases of the liver and kidney based upon three-dimensional reconstruction of the liver. J Med Genet 11:234, 1974.
124. Shokeir MHK, Houston CS, Awen CF. Asphyxiating thoracic chondrodystrophy. Association with renal disease and evidence of possible heterozygous expression. J Med Genet 8:107, 1971.

125. Edelson PJ, Spackham TJ, Belliveau RE, et al. A renal lesion in asphyxiating thoracic dysplasia. Birth Defects 10:51, 1971.
126. Cremin BJ. Infantile thoracic dystrophy. Br J Radiol 43:199, 1970.
127. Bohm N, Fukuda M, Staudt R, et al. Chondroectodermal dysplasia (Ellis–Van Creveld syndrome) with dysplasia of renal medulla and bile ducts. Histopathology 2:267, 1978.
128. Ivemark BI, Oldfelt V, Zetterstrom R. Familial dysplasia of kidneys, liver and pancreas. A probably genetically determined syndrome. Acta Pediatr 48:1, 1959.
129. Strayer DS, Kissane J. Dysplasia of the kidneys, liver and pancreas: report of a variant of Ivemark's syndrome. Hum Pathol 10:228, 1978.
130. Yeoh G, Bannatyne P, Russel P, et al. Combined renal and pancreatic dysplasia in the newborn. Pathology 17:653, 1985.
131. Blair JD. Trisomy C and cystic dysplasia of kidneys, liver and pancreas. Birth Defects 12:139, 1976.
132. Potter E. Normal and Abnormal Development of the Kidney. Chicago, Yearbook Medical, 1972.
133. Butler LJ, Snodgrass GJA, France NE, et al. E (16–18) trisomy syndrome: analysis of 13 cases. Arch Dis Child 40:600, 1965.

IV F. Special Topics

53

The Liver in Systemic Conditions

John P. Cello, M.D. • *James H. Grendell, M.D.*

ABBREVIATIONS

AST = serum aspartate aminotransferase
ALT = serum alanine aminotransferase
SLE = systemic lupus erythematosus
HBV = hepatitis B virus
HBsAg = hepatitis B surface antigen
CMV = cytomegalovirus
HSV = herpes simplex virus
MAI = mycobacterium avium–intracellulare
HIV = human immunodeficiency virus

As the body's largest parenchymal organ, receiving one fourth of the resting cardiac output and accounting for almost one fifth of the total resting oxygen consumption, the liver invariably is involved as an incidental target organ in a vast array of systemic conditions. The liver may occasionally be so severely compromised by such conditions as to threaten survival. This chapter surveys primarily nonhepatic conditions that are associated on occasion with substantial hepatic disease. The list of the conditions reviewed is by no means exhaustive but rather is illustrative of the liver's vulnerability in a number of systemic diseases.

AMYLOIDOSIS

Hepatic involvement in patients with systemic amyloidosis is quite common; however, significant hepatic disease is rare in these patients.

NATURE OF AMYLOID

Amyloid appears as a uniform, homogeneous, amorphous protein when viewed by light microscopy. It stains pale pink with hematoxylin and eosin (Fig. 53–1). Methyl violet and crystal violet stain amyloid metachromatically. Characteristically, a unique green birefringence, specific for amyloid, is visible on polarized light microscopy of tissue stained with Congo red. Electron microscopy demonstrates rigid, nonbranching fibrils, 50 to 150Å in width.

Solubilization and isolation of amyloid proteins require alkali degradation of the amyloid fibrils in tissue.[1] Gel filtration of degraded tissue fibrils of amyloid leads to isolation of at least two types of protein components, indicating that the amyloid found in different patients with amyloidosis is not a homogeneous protein. One of the proteins found in amyloid deposits in tissue is related to fragments of immunoglobulin light chains. The other has some homology with specific serum proteins. Fragments of the immunoglobulin light chains are the major components of the amyloid in a majority of patients with *primary* amyloidosis or amyloidosis resulting from multiple myeloma.[2] Both κ and λ light chain fragments are seen, but the κ type of light chain predominates. These fragments of immunoglobulin light chains have molecular weights ranging from 8000 to 25,000.[3] The light chain immunoglobulin fragments are similar to the Bence Jones protein isolated in the serum and urine of many patients with myeloma. The majority of patients with *primary* amyloidosis or amyloidosis in association with myeloma, but not those with other forms of amyloidosis, have detectable Bence Jones protein in their urines.

The second type of protein fragment, variously called amyloid protein A (AA), amyloid subunit, or amyloid fibrillar protein, can sometimes be isolated by gel filtration of the alkali-degraded fibrils, most commonly from patients with the so-called secondary form of the disease.[4] This protein is unrelated to the immunoglobulins but is similar to serum amyloid A protein, high-density apolipoprotein with a molecular weight of 100,000. Serum amyloid A protein is an acute-phase reactant that may undergo proteolytic cleavage by macrophage or polymorpholeukocyte proteinases to form amyloid A protein, which is deposited in tissue.[5,6]

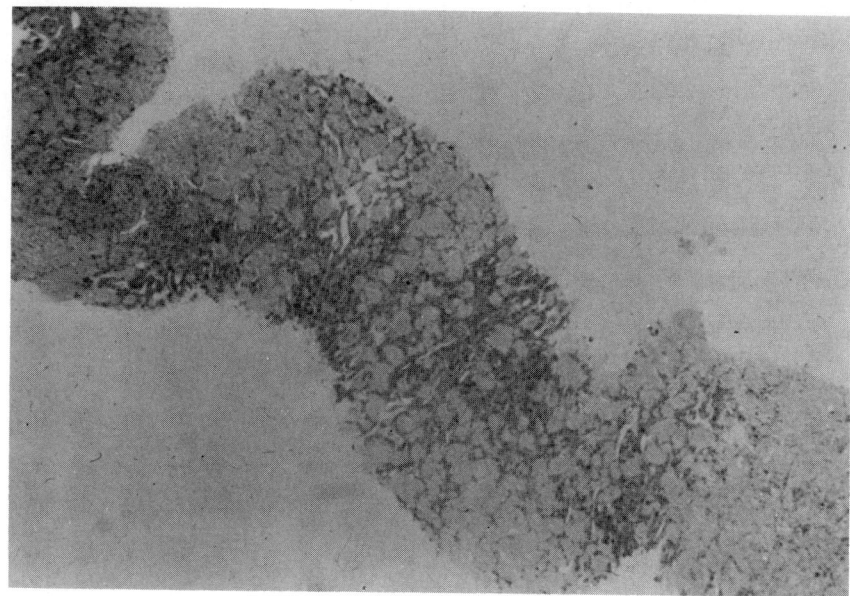

Figure 53–1. Amyloidosis of the liver. Hematoxylin and eosin. Extensive panlobular deposition of the pale pink–staining amyloid is evident on low-power microscopy in this tissue section from a patient with amyloidosis secondary to tuberculosis.

CLASSIFICATION OF AMYLOIDOSIS

No universally satisfactory classification system exists for amyloidosis. Classification may be done on the basis of (1) apparent pathogenesis; (2) major protein components in tissue, serum, or urine; or (3) clinical pattern of disease.[7, 8] The *pathogenetic* classification is most often employed (Table 53–1).[7] Approximately one fourth of all patients with amyloidosis have multiple myeloma. In these patients, the amyloid fibrils are composed of fragments of immunoglobulin light chains (so-called AL amyloid). The disease states most commonly associated with secondary amyloidosis (representing only 8 per cent of patients with systemic amyloidosis) include rheumatoid arthritis, osteomyelitis, tuberculosis, lepromatous leprosy, and Hodgkin's disease or other lymphomas. The amyloid fibrils of these patients are derived from nonimmunoglobulin proteins, largely amyloid A protein. The amyloid from patients with chronic inflammatory status is therefore termed amyloid AA. The majority of patients with systemic amyloidosis, however, do not have myeloma, chronic suppurative disease, or lymphoma and are said to have primary amyloidosis. Plasma cell malignancies are not found in these patients, but Bence Jones protein is frequently present. The amyloid fibrils in tissue deposits of patients with primary amyloidosis are composed of fragments of immunoglobulin light chains. Localized amyloidosis (about 9 per cent of all cases of amyloidosis) is encountered selectively in the bladder, lungs, skin, larynx, central nervous system, pancreas, heart, or hip joints. The local deposition of amyloid in these patients is not related, however, to the amyloid-like substance commonly found in the organs of elderly patients. Patients who have familial amyloidosis make up a small proportion of all amyloidosis patients seen in Western society. Aside from the test for Bence Jones protein in serum or urine, tests for amyloid protein A, serum amyloid A–related protein, and other protein units of amyloid are largely unavailable for routine clinical use.

A new classification system that is based on the apparent *pattern of organ involvement* has been suggested by Isobe and Osserman (Table 53–2).[8] Disease classified as pattern I appears to involve predominantly the heart, tongue, and gastrointestinal tract. Paraprotein M components are identifiable in all patients who have this pattern. A few patients with amyloidosis have the disease limited to the liver, spleen, kidneys, and adrenals. This pattern of organ involvement is classified as pattern II. Half the patients with pattern II have paraproteins. Many patients have mixed patterns I and II. These patients may have generalized organ involvement, but a substantial number of them have localized patterns of amyloid distribution in association with M proteins. The clinical usefulness of the Isobe-Osserman system of amyloid classification has yet to be demonstrated, and it is not widely used.

TABLE 53–1. DISTRIBUTION OF PATIENTS WITH AMYLOIDOSIS BY TYPE

	Patients	
	No.	*%*
Primary amyloidosis (AL)	132	56
Amyloidosis with myeloma (AL)	61	26
Secondary amyloidosis (AA)*	19	8
Localized amyloidosis	22	9
Familial amyloidosis (AF)	2	1
Total	236	100

Source: Adapted from Kyle RA, Bayrd ED. Medicine 54:271, © by Williams & Wilkins, 1975, with permission.

*AL, AA, and AF refer to the type of amyloid fibril present in these patients.

PATHOLOGY OF HEPATIC AMYLOIDOSIS

Gross inspection of the liver from a patient with hepatic amyloidosis reveals a large, smooth organ, pale brown in color. The consistency is quite firm.[9, 10] Occasionally, the liver may feel hard and have a yellow, waxy appearance. Although quite commonly it is modestly enlarged, the liver may on occasion weigh as much as 5 kg. Some of the hepatomegaly encountered at autopsy may be related to the congestive heart failure seen in many patients dying with systemic amyloidosis. The liver may occasionally be nodular, but cirrhosis resulting from amyloid alone is not encountered on either gross or microscopic examination.

Microscopic examination of the involved liver reveals

TABLE 53–2. CLINICAL PATTERNS OF AMYLOIDOSIS

	Distribution	No. of Patients	Patients with M-Paraprotein Detected	
			No.	%
Pattern I	Heart, tongue, GI tract	50	50	100
Pattern II	Liver, spleen, kidney, adrenals	17	9	53
Mixed patterns I and II	Patterns I and II combined	30	26	87
Localized pattern	Isolated organs*	3	3	100
Total		100	88	88

Source: Adapted from information appearing in NEJM, Isobe T, Osserman EF. N Engl J Med 290:473, 1974, with permission.
*Bladder, lung, skin, larynx, pancreas, etc.

three basic patterns of amyloid: intralobular, periportal and perivascular, and a mixture of these types.[9, 10] The space of Disse and the sinusoids are involved extensively in the *intralobular* type of hepatic amyloidosis. The amyloid may compress and distort the normal cell cords, leaving little of the normal parenchyma of the liver. Sparing of the central venous area may be seen occasionally in what is otherwise extensive intralobular amyloid infiltration. This intralobular involvement is found in approximately one fourth of patients with hepatic amyloidosis. *Periportal and vascular involvement* is seen in more than 40 per cent of patients with hepatic amyloidosis (Figs. 53–1, 53–2, and 53–3). The parenchyma of the liver may be spared in these patients, with little infiltration of amyloid into the sinusoids or the space of Disse. A *mixed pattern* with diffuse vascular and intralobular involvement together is encountered in approximately 20 per cent of patients with hepatic amyloidosis. Patients with predominantly portal and periportal involvement generally have less hepatosplenomegaly as compared with patients with extensive intralobular amyloid. Massive hepatosplenomegaly, ascites, and jaundice are seen far more commonly in patients with extensive intralobular involvement of the liver by amyloid. This extensive intralobular hepatic amyloidosis also is associated frequently with amyloid involvement of the heart and kidneys.

CLINICAL PRESENTATIONS OF SYSTEMIC AND HEPATIC AMYLOIDOSIS

Fatigue and weakness (54 per cent), weight loss (45 per cent), dyspnea on exertion (33 per cent), and edema (41 per cent) are the most common presenting symptoms reported by patients with systemic amyloidosis.[7, 9] On occasion, the presenting symptoms may be related to specific organ involvement, such as the carpal tunnel syndrome, nephrotic syndrome, congestive heart failure, malabsorption, peripheral neuropathy, or orthostatic hypotension. Brawny waxy skin lesions or macroglossia are diagnostic findings for amyloidosis. Intracutaneous hemorrhage due to amyloid involvement of the vessels of the skin may be seen occasionally.[11, 12] Few if any symptoms suggest significant liver disease. Hepatomegaly is found in 50 per cent of patients with systemic amyloidosis. Splenomegaly is less common (8 per cent of patients). Jaundice rarely is encountered upon initial examination.

The symptoms that predominate in patients with histologically proven hepatic amyloidosis are nonspecific: weight loss (24 per cent), peripheral edema (41 per cent), and weakness (Table 53–3).[7, 9] Hepatomegaly is found in only 60 per cent of patients with biopsy-proven hepatic amyloidosis. On occasion, however, the liver may become

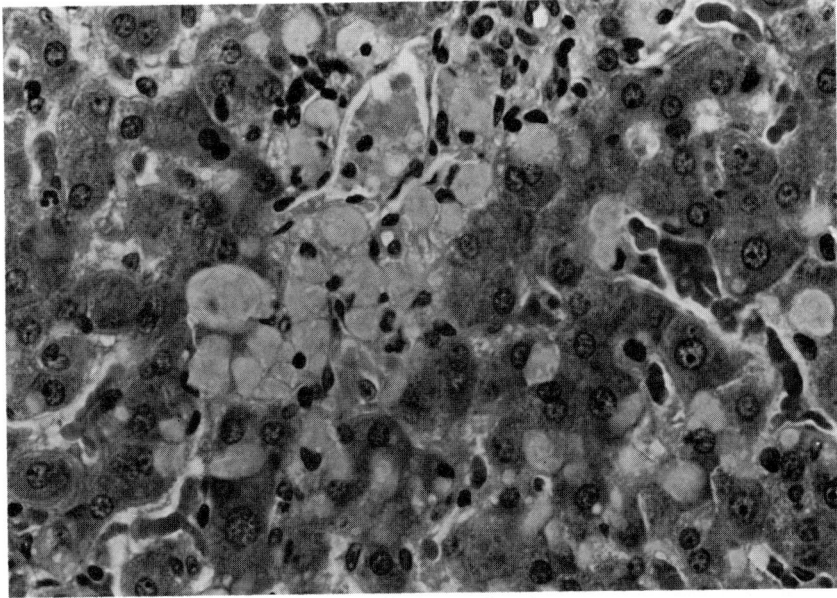

Figure 53–2. Amyloidosis. Hematoxylin and eosin. Focal amyloid deposits are readily recognizable by their apparently amorphous, pale pink nature. Deposition has occurred predominantly around a central vein in this liver from a patient with Hodgkin's disease.

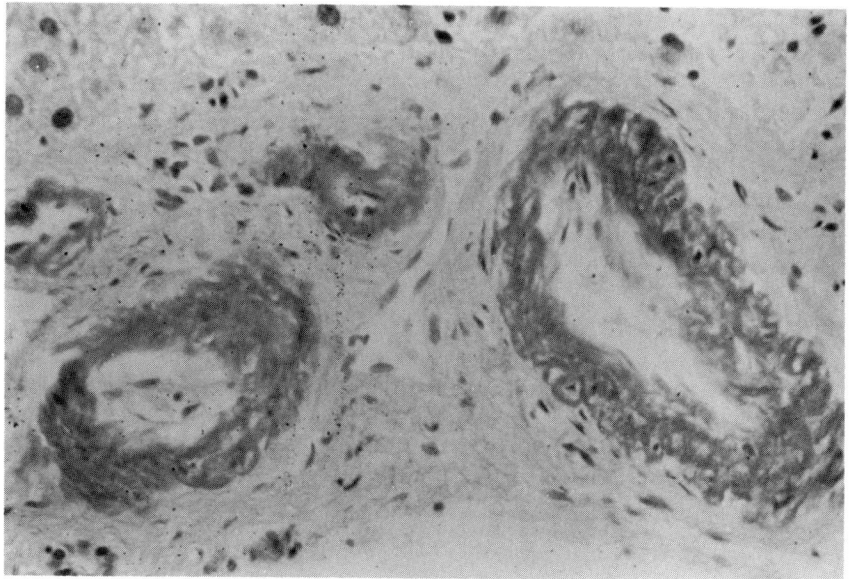

Figure 53–3. Amyloidosis. Hematoxylin and eosin. Extensive amyloid infiltration is limited to the media and adventitia of large vessels, with sparing of adjacent parenchyma.

massively enlarged, with diffuse amyloid infiltration. Splenomegaly (18 per cent) and ascites (19 per cent) may be found in association with hepatic amyloidosis.[7, 9, 10]

LABORATORY DIAGNOSIS—LIVER TESTS IN HEPATIC AMYLOIDOSIS

No specific noninvasive test is available that can firmly establish the diagnosis of hepatic amyloidosis. However, the presence of substantial hepatomegaly in a patient with myeloma or a chronic suppurative process should suggest hepatic amyloidosis. A paucity of significant chemical abnormalities will be encountered on routine blood testing of most patients with hepatic amyloidosis.[9, 10]

Retention of sulfobromophthalein is often cited as the most sensitive indicator of hepatic amyloidosis, since it is abnormally increased in 75 per cent of patients.[9, 10] Serum alkaline phosphatase activity is elevated in 60 per cent of patients with hepatic amyloidosis. The increase is rarely greater than twice the upper limit of normal. Leucine aminopeptidase and 5'-nucleotidase also may be increased.

Hyperbilirubinemia (bilirubin >1 mg/dl) is found in 20 per cent of patients with hepatic amyloidosis, but jaundice is unusual even in those patients who have massive hepatomegaly. On the other hand, severe intrahepatic cholestasis may be seen occasionally, and serum levels of bilirubin in such patients have been as high as 40 mg/dl.[13–15] Patients

TABLE 53–3. CLINICAL FEATURES IN 68 PATIENTS WITH AMYLOIDOSIS WITH BIOPSY-PROVEN HEPATIC INVOLVEMENT

Feature	Patients	
	No.	%
Weight loss	16	24
Edema	28	41
Jaundice	5	7
Ascites	13	19
Hepatomegaly	42	62
Splenomegaly	12	18

Source: Adapted from Levine RA. Am J Med 33:349, 1962; Levy M, et al. Digestion 10:40, 1974; with permission.

with hepatic amyloidosis and cholestasis invariably will have alkaline phosphatase elevations to as much as 30 times normal, hypercholesterolemia, and marked hepatomegaly.

Serum levels of transaminases usually are normal. Altered serum levels of albumin and globulin are encountered in only a minority of patients.

Abnormalities of coagulation are common among patients with amyloidosis, with an elevated prothrombin time the most frequently encountered abnormality.[16] Less commonly noted are prolonged partial thromboplastin time and thrombin time. On rare occasions, patients who have hepatic amyloidosis may have reduced coagulation factors. An isolated, selective deficiency of Factor X may be seen in systemic amyloidosis.[17, 18] This Factor X deficiency may be related to the affinity of Factor X for amyloid deposits. Coincidental deficiencies of both Factor IX and Factor X have been found in patients with systemic amyloidosis. These deficiencies of clotting factors are associated with abnormal prothrombin and partial thromboplastin times. Splenic sequestration of these clotting factors has been suggested in one case report of a patient in whom splenectomy was associated with a prompt and lasting reversal of abnormalities in prothrombin time and serum levels of Factor IX and Factor X.[18] Primary fibrinolysis and disseminated intravascular coagulation have also been found in association with systemic amyloidosis.[19]

Radionuclide liver-spleen scans of patients who have hepatic amyloidosis generally show enlarged livers with slightly decreased but homogeneous hepatic uptake of the radionuclide, although patchy uptake may occasionally be seen. Asymmetric hepatic uptake of the radionuclide has been associated in a number of patients with asymmetric deposition of amyloid, confirmed by liver biopsies obtained at surgery or laparoscopy.[20] The right lobe appears to be involved more commonly when involvement is asymmetric. Gallium citrate uptake may also be decreased in livers with extensive amyloid involvement; the decreased uptake of gallium citrate matches areas of decreased uptake by technetium sulfur colloid.[21] Extensive hepatic uptake of technetium-labeled diphosphonate has been reported to occur in patients with hepatic amyloidosis.[22] This bone-seeking radionuclide normally is taken up only minimally by the liver. The explanation for this unusual hepatic uptake of technetium diphosphonate is uncertain, but abnormal articular uptake may also be seen in patients with localized amyloid deposits in the hip or shoulder.

DIAGNOSIS OF SYSTEMIC AMYLOIDOSIS

Amyloid involvement of any organ can be demonstrated by histologic examination of tissue stained with methyl violet, crystal violet, or Congo red.[23, 24] It is rarely necessary to confirm infiltration of the liver by amyloid in patients with systemic amyloidosis. Sigmoidoscopic rectal valve biopsies provide the most convenient and safest means of demonstrating systemic amyloidosis. These biopsies are positive in more than 80 per cent of patients.[7] Skin biopsies also have been demonstrated to be positive in 80 per cent of patients.[23] Likewise, biopsies of the small bowel and gingiva are positive in more than three fourths of patients with systemic amyloidosis. The liver is involved in 50 per cent of patients with systemic amyloidosis. Significant clinical liver disease secondary to amyloid involvement is uncommon. Hence, there is no clinical imperative to confirm the presence of hepatic involvement.

Deaths from hemorrhage following percutaneous hepatic biopsies have been reported. These deaths, from fracture of liver extensively infiltrated with amyloid, have been the basis of recommendations that liver biopsies not be performed in patients suspected of having hepatic amyloidosis. In a series of one hundred patients with amyloidosis, eight had significant bleeding following diagnostic or therapeutic procedures.[16] Although an elevated prothrombin time was more commonly noted among the 41 amyloid patients with bleeding problems (including petechiae, gastrointestinal hemorrhage, and postprocedure bleeding), no coagulation test could have predicted postprocedure bleeding in these patients. All eight patients with postprocedure hemorrhage did however have a history of other bleeding episodes such as petechiae, gastrointestinal bleeding, hematuria, or hemoptysis.[16] Although it is considered unnecessary to perform a percutaneous needle biopsy of the liver of a patient who has confirmed systemic amyloidosis merely to diagnose hepatic involvement, the performance of liver biopsy in patients with suspected but not confirmed amyloidosis is not contraindicated if clotting tests and platelet counts are within acceptable limits and the patient has no history of a bleeding diathesis.

MEDICAL THERAPY AND OUTCOME

The clinical course of patients with systemic amyloidosis even with extensive hepatic infiltration is not determined by the extent of hepatic involvement.[7] Hepatic failure and other complications of extensive hepatic involvement are rare. The most common causes of death of patients with systemic amyloidosis are related to the involvement of other vital organs. Congestive heart failure is responsible for death in 30 per cent of cases. The underlying myeloma is responsible for death in an additional 30 per cent. The remainder of patients with extensive systemic amyloidosis die from progressive renal failure. Death related to amyloidosis of the liver has not been reported.

There is no specific medical therapy for systemic amyloidosis.[7] Chemotherapy for amyloidosis has been largely unsuccessful. Treatment with several courses of melphalan and prednisone has stabilized or partially reversed the amyloidosis in a few patients with primary amyloidosis.[25]

One patient with primary (AL) amyloidosis and massive hepatomegaly treated with monthly courses of melphalan and prednisone responded dramatically.[26] When treatment was continued for 35 months and the patient followed for a total of 93 months, histologic, biochemical, and clinical regression was documented. Remissions may be seen in amyloidosis associated with multiple myeloma upon successful chemotherapy of the myelomatosis. The progression of secondary amyloidosis may cease with successful eradication of the chronic inflammatory process in patients with Crohn's disease, tuberculosis, or leprosy.[27] Dramatic reversals of systemic amyloidosis due to familial Mediterranean fever have been reported. In four patients, three of whom had amyloidosis related to familial Mediterranean fever and one due to primary amyloidosis, treatment with colchicine was associated with marked decreases in proteinuria accompanied by improvements of renal function.[28] Among 1070 Israeli patients with familial Mediterranean fever treated prospectively with 1 to 2 mg per day of colchicine, prevention or stabilization of renal disease was documented.[29] Only 2 of 906 (0.2 per cent) medication-compliant patients developed progressive renal disease, whereas 16 of 54 (30 per cent) of noncompliant patients suffered progressive renal disease. Unfortunately, all patients who initially had significant renal disease, manifested by frank nephrosis or uremia, deteriorated despite colchicine therapy. Overall, colchicine treatment was effective only when given prior to the development of significant proteinuria. The mechanism of colchicine reversal in amyloidosis associated with familial Mediterranean fever is unknown, but it may be related to some direct or indirect inhibitory effect of colchicine on leukocyte function or serum amyloid A protein secretion. Experimentally, colchicine protects mice from the amyloidogenic stimulus of intravenous casein.

No specific therapy is necessary with respect to hepatic involvement in most patients with amyloidosis, since significant hepatic dysfunction is uncommon. However, in the management of those patients who have extensive prolonged cholestasis, some attention should be directed towards the replacement of fat-soluble vitamins. Intense pruritus may respond to cholestyramine. Experimental chemotherapy with prednisone and melphalan (see the preceding) should be reserved for patients with severe liver disease, and therapy should be administered only in a controlled clinical environment. The outcome of systemic amyloidosis is determined by the extent, severity, and progression of the renal and cardiac disease.

LIVER DYSFUNCTION IN HEART DISEASE

CONGESTIVE HEART FAILURE

Congestion of the liver (occasionally termed congestive hepatopathy) has been recognized for many years as a complication of severe chronic or acute congestive heart failure. Hepatic congestion has been found in all forms of heart disease, both acquired and congenital. In one large series of 175 patients with severe right-sided congestive heart failure and hepatic dysfunction, 33 per cent had arteriosclerotic cardiovascular disease (Table 53–4).[30] Twenty per cent had hypertensive cardiovascular disease, and 30 per cent had rheumatic valvular heart disease. Cor pulmonale accounted for an additional 6 per cent of patients with severe, right-sided congestive heart failure. Constrictive pericarditis was observed in only 4 per cent of patients who had right-sided congestive heart failure and hepato-

TABLE 53–4. CONGESTION OF THE LIVER IN RIGHT-SIDED HEART FAILURE

	Patients with Congested Livers			
	No.	*% of Total*	*No. with Acute Disease*	*No. with Chronic Disease*
Coronary artery disease	58	33.1	34	24
Hypertension	38	21.7	29	9
Rheumatic valve disease	56	32.0	33	23
Cor pulmonale	10	5.7	5	5
Congenital disease	3	1.7	1	2
Constrictive pericarditis	7	4.0	1	6
Scleroderma	1	0.6	1	0
Syphilis	1	0.6	1	0
Ball valve thrombus	1	0.6	1	0
TOTAL	175	100.0	106	69

Source: Adapted from Richman SM, et al. Am J Med 30:211, 1961, with permission.

megaly. Smaller numbers of patients had congenital heart disease, scleroderma, syphilitic heart disease, and complications associated with prosthetic valves. The most severe hepatic congestion occurred in patients who had rheumatic mitral stenosis with tricuspid insufficiency.

The pathogenesis of the hepatic dysfunction found in association with severe congestive heart failure has been the subject of much speculation.[31–39] Several factors have been postulated to be in part or entirely responsible for the hepatic dysfunction. These include (1) decreased hepatic blood flow with reduction of the oxygen supply to the liver and (2) increased hepatic venous pressure, producing central venous and sinusoidal stasis. The importance of either of these components in the alteration of hepatic function in patients with congestive heart failure has not been established. For example, although severe decreases in total hepatic blood flow are associated with hypoxic damage to the liver, the oxygen utilization by the liver remains fairly constant over a wide range of cardiac output.[40, 41] Experimentally, acute elevation of the hepatic venous pressure produces proportionate centrolobular damage, but hepatic dysfunction in congestive heart failure does not correlate precisely with the right atrial pressure.[33]

CLINICAL MANIFESTATIONS OF RIGHT VENTRICULAR FAILURE

In the majority of patients with congestive heart failure and severe passive congestion of the liver, the clinical picture is dominated by the signs and symptoms of the severe heart failure rather than those of liver disease (Table 53–5).[30, 34] A mild aching discomfort in the right upper quadrant may be reported by patients with acute passive congestion of the liver. Clinical jaundice is encountered in approximately 10 to 20 per cent of patients who have passive congestion of the liver.[34] Physical examination usu-

ally reveals signs of congestive heart failure, including distended jugular veins and hepatojugular reflux. Hepatomegaly is to be expected in the majority of patients with significant right-sided congestive heart failure. On occasion, the hepatomegaly can be massive. In 50 per cent of patients with both acute and chronic right-sided congestive heart failure, the liver extends 5 cm or more below the right costal margin.[30] As fibrosis develops during the course of severe hepatic congestion, the liver can decrease in size to near normal dimensions. With substantial tricuspid insufficiency, a pulsatile liver may be found. Ascites and peripheral edema may be present in 15 per cent of patients with severe congestive heart failure. Ascites is usually a sign of chronic right-sided congestive heart failure rather than a manifestation of cirrhosis. Splenomegaly occurs in one fourth of patients with acute or chronic right-sided congestive heart failure.

LABORATORY EVALUATION OF THE LIVER IN CONGESTIVE HEART FAILURE (Table 53–6)

There is no absolute correlation between the clinical severity of passive congestion of the liver and abnormalities of liver tests. In general, however, patients who have the highest right atrial pressures and the most profound clinical manifestations of congestive heart failure have the most dramatic alterations of tests of hepatocellular function.[33, 36] Retention of sulfobromophthalein had been felt for many years to be the most sensitive index of liver disease in patients with congestion of the liver, in that sulfobromophthalein retention is increased in more than 80 per cent of patients who have confirmed passive congestion of the liver.[30, 37, 38] In some cases, this may be the only abnormal test. Elevations of the serum bilirubin will be encountered in 25 to 75 per cent of patients with congestive heart failure. The bilirubin elevations, like sulfobromophthalein reten-

TABLE 53–5. SYMPTOMS AND SIGNS OF CONGESTED LIVERS IN 175 PATIENTS WITH RIGHT-SIDED HEART FAILURE

	% of Patients with Acute Heart Failure	% of Patients with Chronic Heart Failure
Any hepatomegaly (>11 cm)	99	95
Marked hepatomegaly*	57	49
Peripheral edema	77	71
Pleural effusion	25	17
Splenomegaly	20	22
Ascites	7	20

Source: Adapted from Richman SM, et al. Am J Med 30:211, 1961, with permission.
*Liver palpable to 5 cm below the right costal margin.

TABLE 53–6. TESTS OF HEPATOCELLULAR FUNCTION OF 175 PATIENTS WITH RIGHT-SIDED HEART FAILURE

Index of Liver Function	Acute Congestive Heart Failure		Chronic Congestive Heart Failure	
	No. Patients Tested	*Percentage Abnormal*	*No. Patients Tested*	*Per Cent Abnormal*
Bilirubin	86	37	57	21
BSP retention	71	87	55	71
Alkaline phosphatase	80	10	55	9
Aspartate aminotransferase (AST; SGOT)	67	48	37	5
Alanine aminotransferase (ALT; SGPT)	53	15	29	3
Globulins	100	60	67	37
Prothrombin time	68	84	43	74
Albumin	100	32	67	27
Cholesterol	87	49	60	42

Source: Adapted from Richman SM. Am J Med 30:211, 1961, with permission.

tion, correlate only weakly with right atrial pressure.[33] Hyperbilirubinemia of dramatic proportions is more commonly manifest during acute right-sided congestive heart failure than during chronic passive congestion of the liver. The hyperbilirubinemia appears to be related to actual hepatocellular dysfunction itself, with little contribution from increased pigment production, although the latter point is debated.[33, 34] Approximately 50 to 60 per cent of the increased bilirubin in patients with congestive heart failure is in the indirect-reacting fraction or largely unconjugated bilirubin. Serum alkaline phosphatase is usually within normal limits or at most twice the upper limit of normal. A normal serum alkaline phosphatase level is particularly helpful in supporting the clinical diagnosis of hepatic congestion, since most other hepatic diseases are associated with substantial abnormalities of alkaline phosphatase. Elevations of serum aspartate aminotransferase (AST) and alanine aminotransferase (ALT), on the other hand, are encountered in 5 to 50 per cent of patients with congestive heart failure.[30, 33, 34] Increases in the serum aminotransferases may be seen in both acute and chronic right-sided congestive heart failure, although the most dramatic elevations invariably are encountered in patients with *acute* worsening of already severe congestive heart failure. On the other hand, abnormal aminotransferase levels are found in only 5 per cent of patients with *chronic* right-sided congestive heart failure. The elevations of the aminotransferases in the latter patients are usually less than four or five times the upper limits of normal, whereas higher levels (more than ten times the upper limits of normal) are found in patients who have acute passive congestion of the liver. The AST elevation, however, reverses rapidly within a few days of circulatory improvement. The ALT level may be less impressively elevated than the AST in passive congestion of the liver. Some of the disproportionate elevation of AST over ALT may well be due to concomitant rhabdomyolysis, and simultaneous measurement of creatine phosphokinase (CPK) isoenzyme levels in serum are helpful in diagnosing the muscular injury. Modest elevations of serum globulins and decreases in serum albumin may be found in association with both acute and chronic right-sided congestive heart failure. The prothrombin time commonly is prolonged (70 to 80 per cent of patients) with passive congestion of the liver and usually is unresponsive to parenteral administration of vitamin K. The prothrombin time returns to normal slowly with clinical abatement of the congestive heart failure. Other abnormal liver tests, particularly the serum transaminases, rapidly return toward normal after substantial alleviation of congestive heart failure. However, sulfobromophthalein retention will remain abnormal for one to two weeks following clinical improvement. Similarly, hypoprothrombinemia may not be reversed until several weeks following clinical improvement.[30]

There is no biochemical means to distinguish a congested noncirrhotic liver from one with cardiac cirrhosis. Cardiac cirrhosis also is rare, probably because most patients who have severe passive congestion die of their underlying cardiovascular disease long before cirrhosis develops. The diagnosis of cardiac cirrhosis should be considered, however, in four clinical situations: (1) severe rheumatic heart disease, especially mitral stenosis; (2) chronic constrictive pericarditis; (3) prolonged or recurrent severe congestive heart failure; (4) clinically severe passive congestion of the liver with a small liver, ascites, and splenomegaly.[34] In addition, the absence of hepatic pulsations in a patient who has well-documented tricuspid insufficiency should alert one to the possibility of cardiac cirrhosis.

PATHOLOGY OF THE LIVER IN CONGESTIVE HEART FAILURE

Grossly, the liver appears large and purple, with blunted edges (Fig. 53–4).[33, 34] It is not uncommon for the liver to shrink appreciably soon after death and to appear much smaller on postmortem examination compared with the last clinical examination. Cut section of the liver in

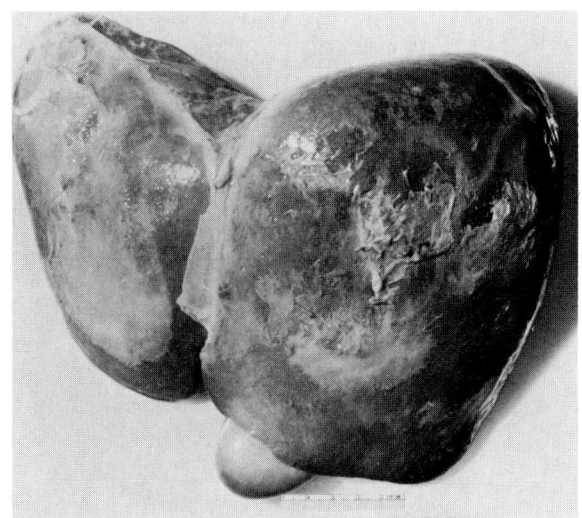

Figure 53–4. Liver in congestive failure. Gross specimen from a woman who died with acute cor pulmonale. The liver is large, with a mottled purple color. See Figures 53–5, 53–6, and 53–7 for microscopic views of this specimen.

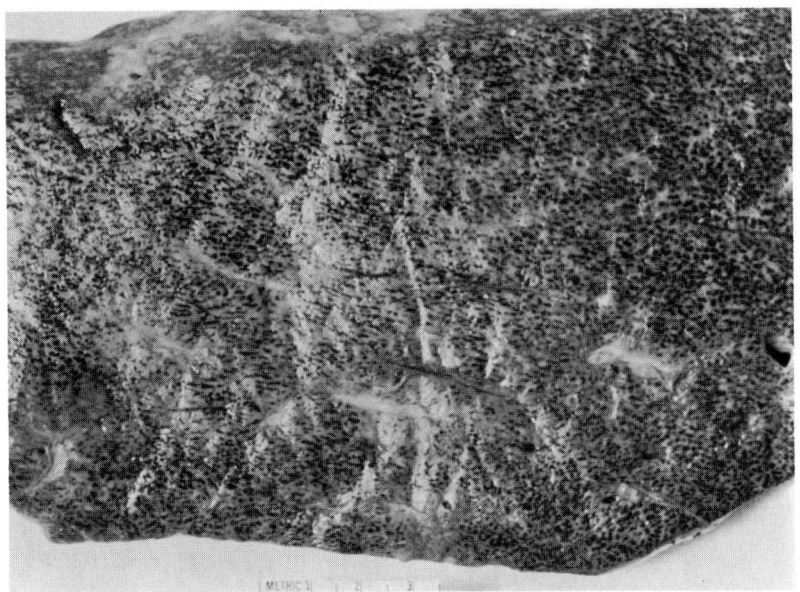

Figure 53–5. Liver in congestive failure. The cut surface shows bright red hemorrhagic areas adjacent to more normal-appearing parenchyma.

severe passive congestion has a "nutmeg" appearance (i.e., similar to the cross-section of a whole nutmeg kernel). There are reddish, hemorrhagic areas in sharp contrast to pale areas (Figs. 53–5 and 53–6). The lighter regions are more normal-appearing portal and periportal areas of the lobule; the reddish areas are hemorrhagic centrolobular zones. There is no absolute correlation between the severity of clinical congestive heart failure and the extent of hepatocellular necrosis determined microscopically.[33, 34]

The earliest and mildest histopathologic changes encountered in the congested liver are limited to the central lobular area. Early in congestive heart failure, the central veins become engorged and dilated. Sinusoids adjacent to the central vein also are dilated for variable distances toward the portal areas. The centrolobular hepatocytes are compressed, distorted, and atrophied in severe passive congestion. Dropout of liver cells, granular changes in the cytoplasm, and pyknotic nuclei with fragmentation may be found. With severe congestive heart failure, necrosis is accompanied by an increase in a brownish pigment in the cells, usually in the center of the lobule. This brown pigment, neither iron nor hemofuscin, is stained green with methylene blue and appears to be related to bile. The congestive and degenerative changes are invariably more severe in the portion of the lobule immediately adjacent to the dilated central veins (Fig. 53–7). As the congestive heart failure worsens, the changes in the parenchyma surrounding the central veins seem to spread toward the portal areas. In the most severe forms of passive congestion of the liver, only a small zone of normal-appearing parenchyma will remain in the periportal area. The reticulin network of the liver generally is maintained; however, with prolongation of severe passive congestion, the reticulin network may collapse around the central veins, and fine bands of fibrous tissue and collapsed reticulin will be seen extending from central vein to central vein (Fig. 53–8). This fibrous bridging of adjacent central veins, called reverse lobulation, is a feature unique to cardiac cirrhosis.

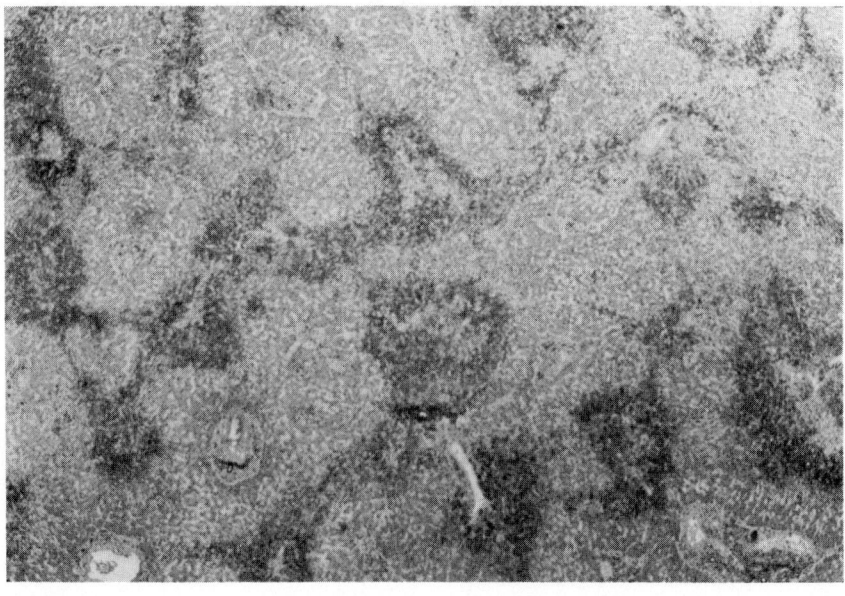

Figure 53–6. Liver in congestive failure. Hematoxylin and eosin. Low-power microscopic view of the liver shown in Figures 53–4 and 53–5. A confluence of centrolobular hemorrhagic necrosis is evident, with relative sparing of the periportal regions. Little inflammation is visible.

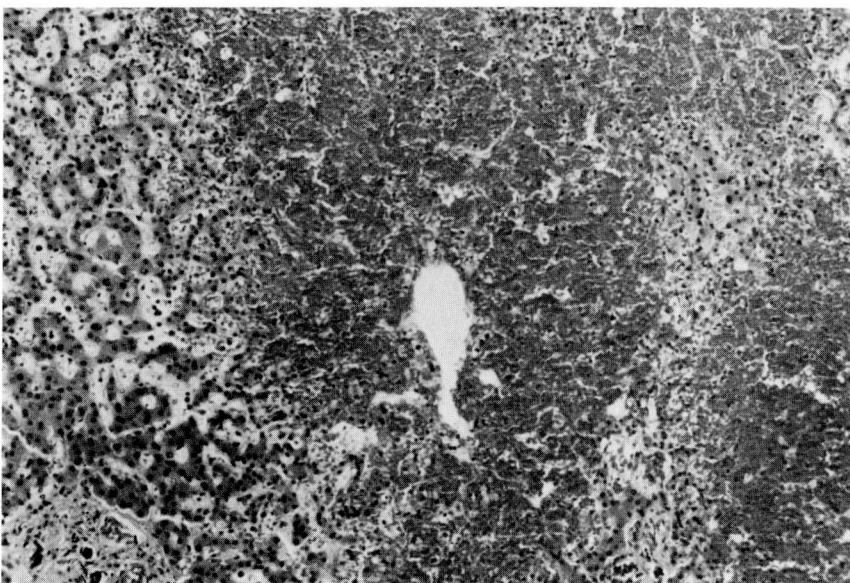

Figure 53–7. Liver in congestive heart failure. Hematoxylin and eosin. High-power microscopic view of the liver in Figure 53–6. A large central vein is surrounded by an extensive zone of hemorrhagic necrosis. At the right lower portion of the field, a periportal region is relatively spared of congestion.

Cardiac cirrhosis on liver biopsy may show only a small residual zone of normal-appearing parenchyma next to portal areas (Fig. 53–9). Extensive nodular regeneration of the liver in patients with cardiac cirrhosis is rare, since many patients with severe passive congestion of the liver die early in the course of their illness from the cardiovascular disease.

Midzonal hepatic necrosis has also been noted in patients with antecedent shock.[42] In 214 patients with centrolobular necrosis, De la Monte and co-workers reported 18 (8 per cent) with midzonal necrosis as well. No clinical features distinguished these patients with midzonal necrosis from those with centrolobular necrosis alone. This histologic pattern, usually seen only in yellow fever and experimental furosemide toxicity, is associated with the selective necrosis of hepatocytes in midzonal regions, the regeneration of hepatocytes in centrolobular areas following centrolobular necrosis, or both (Fig. 53–10).

DIAGNOSIS, THERAPY, AND OUTCOME

Severe passive congestion of the liver is suggested first by the presence of severe congestive heart failure in a patient with a large, somewhat tender liver. Findings of modest increases in serum bilirubin and aminotransferase levels and an elevated prothrombin time with no significant alteration of the serum alkaline phosphatase suggest the diagnosis of passive congestion of the liver. Substantial and rapid improvements in liver tests concomitant with improvement in circulatory status further support the clinical diagnosis of a congested liver. Diagnosis can be made firmly only by histologic examination of the liver. In theory, however, an elevated venous pressure enhances the risk of bleeding after percutaneous liver biopsy.[34] In the management of patients with severe congestive heart failure and abnormal liver tests, liver biopsy can and should be postponed until the congestive heart failure abates. If, however,

Figure 53–8. Liver in long-standing congestive failure. Hematoxylin and eosin. A broad band of fibrous tissue, representing both newly deposited collagen and reticulin collapse, is visible across the lower half of the field.

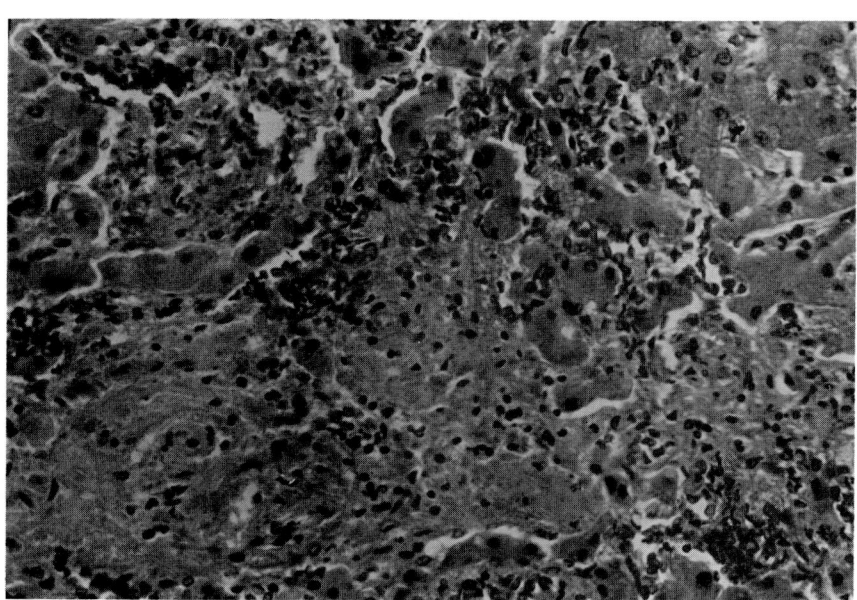

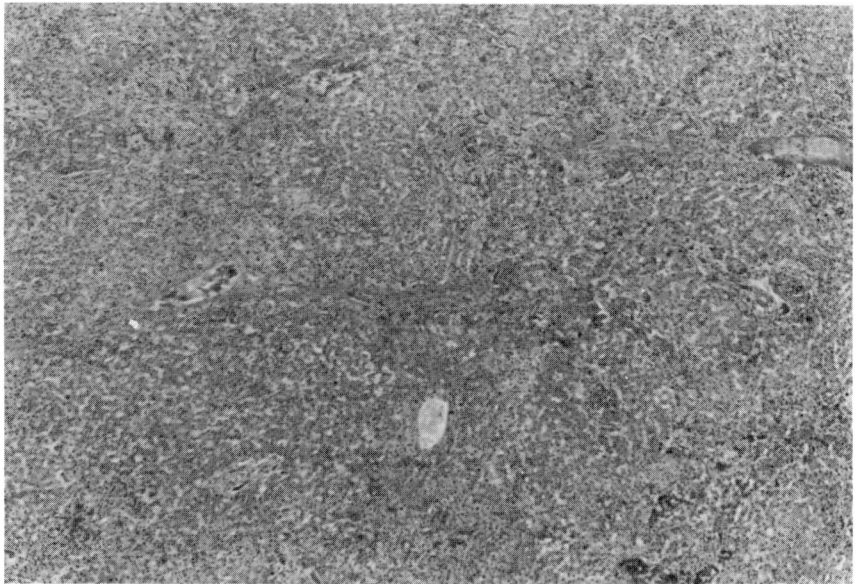

Figure 53–9. Cardiac cirrhosis. Hematoxylin and eosin. Narrow bands of fibrous scarring can be seen throughout the entire liver. Bridging fibrosis from central vein to central vein may produce a "reverse lobulation" of the hepatic architecture.

a tissue diagnosis is imperative in order to establish the nature of underlying liver disease, liver biopsy can be performed with the Menghini technique, provided coagulation indices, including prothrombin time and platelet count, are within acceptable limits.

Therapy should be directed at correcting or alleviating the congestive heart failure through the administration of digoxin, diuretics, or afterload-reducing agents. On occa-

sion, however, hepatocellular dysfunction itself may contribute to patient morbidity. Rarely, for example, patients who have severe passive congestion of the liver have profound hypoglycemia and mental confusion.[43] In most such patients the alteration of mental function is more likely to be a manifestation of decreasing cardiac output than of hepatic dysfunction.

Cardiac cirrhosis in and of itself does not lead to the

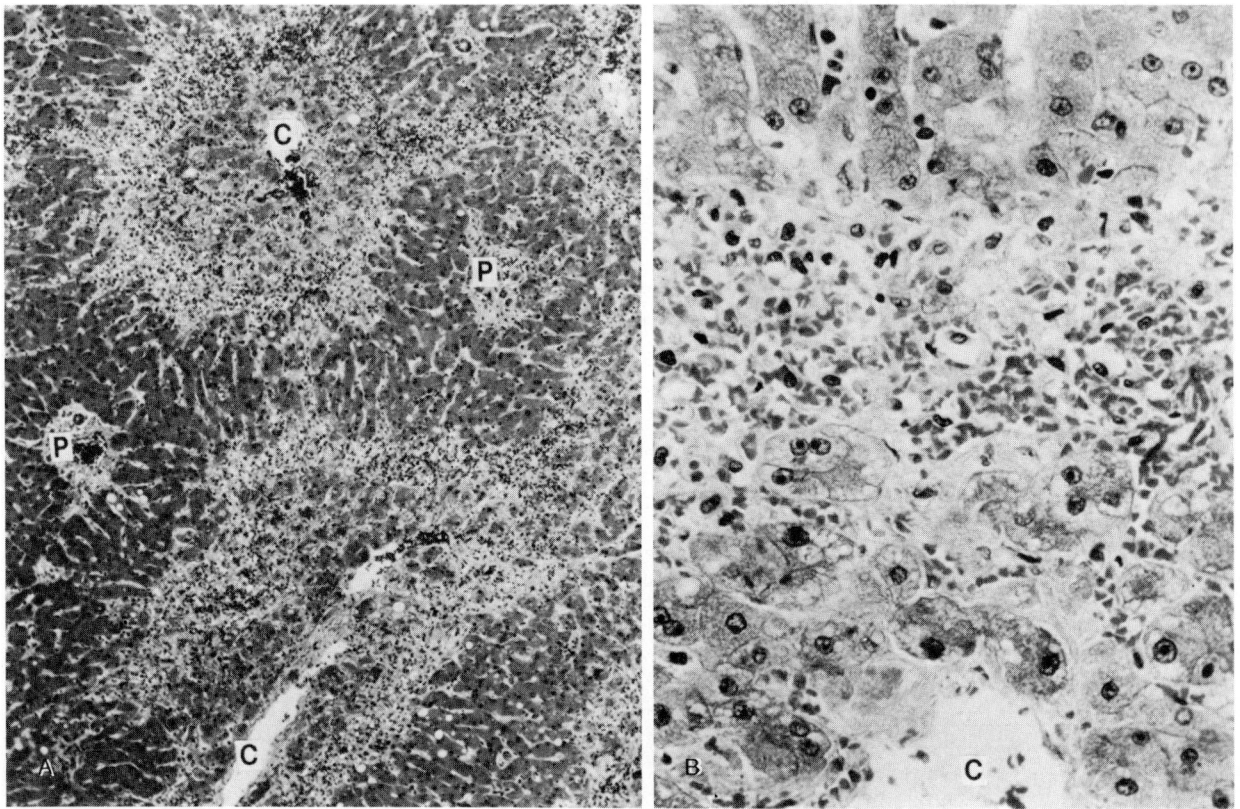

Figure 53–10. A, Two hepatic lobules with midzonal necrosis, seven days' survival after an episode of hypotension. The parenchyma around the central veins (C) and around the portal area (P) is spared (× 60). B, Portion of the lobule in the upper part of A. The central vein is below (C), and the region of midzonal necrosis extends across the middle of the field (× 320). (Reprinted with permission from Dela Monte SM, et al. Gastroenterology 86:627. (Copyright 1984 by The American Gastroenterological Association.)

development of either severe portal hypertension or bleeding from gastroesophageal varices, but splenomegaly and ascites may be encountered. Other stigmata of chronic liver disease, such as palmar erythema, spider angiomas, or caput medusae, are rare in patients with cardiac cirrhosis of the liver. In general, therefore, there appears to be no enhanced morbidity or mortality from the development of cardiac cirrhosis. Clinical improvement of cardiac function such as the dramatic reversal encountered following prosthetic valve placement, relief of constrictive pericarditis, or correction of a congenital anomaly, will lead to substantial and even dramatic improvement in hepatocellular tests.

LEFT VENTRICULAR FAILURE

Patients with acute left ventricular failure with or without chronic passive congestion of the liver may experience the abrupt onset of centrolobular necrosis of the liver.[35, 39, 44–47] This so-called "shock liver" or "ischemic hepatitis" most commonly is associated with an acute myocardial infarction and cardiogenic shock. However, significant centrolobular necrosis of the liver occurs in patients who have decompensated mitral valve disease, subacute bacterial endocarditis, the abrupt onset of atrial fibrillation with decreasing left ventricular output, and other cardiac diseases. The incidence of shock liver among patients with acute myocardial infarction is less than 1 per cent. Only two cases of centrolobular necrosis of the liver were seen in more than 300 patients treated for acute myocardial infarction between 1964 and 1976 in Copenhagen hospitals.[39] Since many patients with cardiogenic shock and the associated shock liver have both acute right and left ventricular failure, the factors responsible for the hepatocellular necrosis cannot be distinguished accurately. However, a sizeable proportion of patients with biopsy-proven centrolobular necrosis have few clinical findings suggestive of right ventricular failure—that is, no engorged jugular veins or palpable hepatomegaly. Substantial hepatocellular abnormalities also may be seen in patients without pre-existing liver disease following hemorrhagic shock and trauma. The incidence of acute hepatic necrosis in this situation is surprisingly low, with only 12 of 500 patients who had sustained life-threatening trauma and hypotension developing hyperbilirubinemia and abnormal serum aminotransferases.[35]

Physical findings are dominated by the elements of shock. Laboratory evaluation reveals dramatic increases in serum AST and ALT. Serum CPK is normal in shock liver unless accompanied by myocardial infarction or rhabdomyolysis. Prolongation of the prothrombin time may occur abruptly, together with a slow, steady increase in serum bilirubin. As with acute right-sided heart failure, dramatic improvements in the serum aminotransferases may be seen with improvement in cardiovascular status. Gradual improvements in the prothrombin time and bilirubin are to be anticipated with improvement in cardiac output. Histologic examination of the liver of a patient with acute left ventricular failure shows centrolobular necrosis, hemorrhage, and sinusoidal dilatation with bile stasis. Diffuse hepatic parenchymal calcification has been reported in one patient who survived for two years following an episode of ischemic hepatitis while uremic.[48] Calcium was noted on electron microscopy within mitochondria of hepatocytes in areas of degeneration. Preexisting right ventricular failure from either valvular or ischemic heart disease may predispose to ischemic hepatitis. Shock liver may be confused on biochemical testing but rarely on a clinical basis with acute viral hepatitis. The elevations of AST and ALT, however, return more rapidly toward normal in shock liver than with acute viral hepatitis. The reductions in aminotransferase levels may be quite dramatic with abrupt improvements in cardiac function.[44]

Infrequently, patients who have clinically inapparent left ventricular failure may develop biochemical abnormalities suggestive of acute viral hepatitis.[45–47] Although the majority of patients who have hepatic dysfunction associated with cardiac failure, especially those with shock liver, have definite physical and radiographic findings suggestive of cardiac dysfunction, in some patients abnormal liver tests will be the first sign of left ventricular failure. This unusual presentation of ischemic hepatic dysfunction has been reported to occur in patients with myocardial infarction, subacute bacterial endocarditis, and rheumatic valvular heart disease (particularly mitral regurgitation with a new onset of acute atrial fibrillation). On rare occasions, pain in the right upper quadrant, nausea, vomiting, and jaundice may be found in these patients without any symptom suggestive of congestive heart failure. In some of these patients, no physical findings of severe left or right ventricular failure can be detected clinically. Histologic examination of the liver of a patient who has this syndrome of ischemic hepatitis masking as viral hepatitis will establish the correct diagnosis. In the few cases reported, clinical alleviation of previously inapparent left ventricular dysfunction has produced dramatic improvements in liver tests.

CONGENITAL HEART DISEASE

Hepatic abnormalities also are encountered in children with congenital heart disease.[38] In approximately 20 per cent of patients dying with congenital heart disease at less than 1 month of age, postmortem examinations show histologic abnormalities of the livers. The hepatic abnormalities are similar to those found in adults with congestive heart failure except that subcapsular hemorrhage may be seen as an additional feature in infants. On occasion, midzonal hepatic necrosis rather than the more common centrolobular necrosis may be demonstrated in infants with congenital heart disease. Moreover, asymmetric lobar involvement has been found in children, with the left hepatic lobe more likely to be involved than the right. The clinical presentations of these infants invariably are related to their congenital heart disease. On occasion, however, hemorrhage from various sites may be a problem in children with severe hepatic dysfunction because of prolongation of their prothrombin and partial thromboplastin times. As in adults, there is failure to respond to parenteral administration of vitamin K.

Among 65 infants, children, and young adults (mean age ± SD 6.7 ± 1.2 years) with hemodynamic abnormalities (54, or 83 per cent, with congenital heart disease), the most striking abnormalities in hepatic biochemical tests were noted among patients with low cardiac outputs.[49] Those patients with cardiac outputs less than half normal (1.9 ± 0.4 L/min/m versus 4.0 ± 0.2 L/min/m) had the most striking abnormalities in prothrombin times, partial thromboplastin times, serum transaminases, and bilirubin (Table 53–7). Whereas significant elevations in serum transaminases and bilirubin were likewise noted in patients with both hypoxemia and systemic venous congestion, less impressive alterations in biochemical tests were noted among patients with hypoxemia alone or systemic venous conges-

TABLE 53–7. ABNORMAL LABORATORY TESTS IN INFANTS, CHILDREN, AND YOUNG ADULTS WITH CARDIAC DISEASE

	Number with Abnormal Results				
Laboratory Test	*1* *Mild* *(N=17)*	*2* *Hypoxemia* *(N=17)*	*3* *SVC* *(N=12)*	*4* *Hypoxemia* *and SVC* *(N=12)*	*5* *Low CO* *(N=7)*
Prothrombin time	0	4	4	7	7
Partial thromboplastin time	0	6	3	7	7
AST	1	10	8	8	6
Total bilirubin	0	2	0	8	7
Total protein	0	3	6	8	7

Source: Adapted from Mace S, et al. Am J Dis Child 139:60. Copyright 1985, American Medical Association.
SVC = systemic venous congestion; CO = cardiac output.

tion alone. Patients with acute cardiac failure tended to have the higher serum transaminase levels and more abnormal tests of coagulation, whereas those with chronic congestive failure had the higher serum bilirubin values.

Although a wide variety of congenital heart diseases have been associated with hepatic necrosis, disproportionate numbers of patients with hepatocellular necrosis have either hypoplastic left heart syndrome or infantile coarctation of the aorta. Thirty-eight per cent of patients dying from these conditions are found to have hepatic necrosis, as compared with 5 per cent of patients dying with other congenital heart lesions. In addition to reduced systemic blood flows, left-to-right shunts and marked elevations of right ventricular pressures are also encountered in these children. In addition to the problems of clotting defects in children with congenital heart disease and hepatic dysfunction, profound, irreversible hypoglycemia may be encountered rarely.

THE NEPHROGENIC HEPATIC DYSFUNCTION SYNDROME

BACKGROUND

Stauffer, in 1961, described abnormalities in hepatocellular function in five patients with renal cell carcinomas.[50] These patients with confirmed hypernephroma had a number of abnormalities in hepatocellular function as their sole initial manifestations of the renal cell tumors. Elevations of serum alkaline phosphatase and thymol turbidity as well as prothrombin times and sulfobromophthalein retention were found. Affected patients also had increases in α_2-globulin and decreased serum albumin. Hepatomegaly was common. Since this initial report, a number of additional patients with abnormal hepatocellular function secondary to a variety of nonmetastatic malignancies of the kidney have been described.[51–56] The nephrogenic hepatic dysfunction syndrome is a term that must however be reserved for patients proven to have no hepatic metastases from the underlying renal malignancy. Thus, before this diagnosis can be applied to any individual patient, adequate documentation of the absence of hepatic metastases must be provided by biopsy, surgical exploration, or angiographic study of the liver and long-term clinical follow-up. This syndrome must also be differentiated from the uncommon situation wherein a patient with solitary or multiple hepatic metastases from renal cell carcinoma undergoes spontaneous remission following removal of the primary cancer.[57] The elevation of the serum alkaline phosphatase so characteristically seen in patients with nephrogenic hepatic dysfunction syndrome has been regarded by some as reflect-

ing an isoenzyme of tumor origin.[53] Although metabolites from the tumor might be responsible for abnormal hepatic function and histologic characteristics, the injection of extracts of hypernephroma tissue into experimental animals has failed to produce liver cell injury histologically or biochemically equivalent to nephrogenic hepatic dysfunction syndrome.[51]

CLINICAL MANIFESTATIONS (Table 53–8)

Patients who have hypernephroma often have abnormal tests of hepatocellular function. In one study, 45 per cent of patients with hypernephroma had abnormal results of at least three of five tests of hepatic function (sulfobromophthalein, prothrombin time, globulins, bilirubin, and alkaline phosphatase).[51] It is doubtful that such a high percentage of patients with hypernephroma truly have nephrogenic hepatic dysfunction syndrome. Although many reports of such cases have detailed the features of a paraneoplastic syndrome, there has not been sufficient follow-up of the majority of these patients. There are, however, 30 patients with well-documented nephrogenic hepatic dysfunction syndrome in whom the absence of hepatic metastases was proved by extensive investigation and long-term clinical follow-up. The majority of these

TABLE 53–8. FEATURES OF NEPHROGENIC HEPATIC DYSFUNCTION SYNDROME IN 29 PATIENTS

	Patients	
	No.	*%*
Clinical features		
Fever	23/27	85
Weight loss	23/23	100
Abdominal mass	10/25	40
Hepatomegaly	18/27	67
Splenomegaly	11/23	48
Abnormal laboratory tests		
Hematocrit <35%	11/15	73
WBC >10,000/mm³	8/21	38
Platelets >350,000/mm³	13/21	62
BUN >25 mg/dl	5/15	33
Bilirubin >1 mg/dl	2/20	10
Aspartate aminotransferase (AST) >40 IU/l	3/14	21
Elevated alkaline phosphatase	24/27	90
Prothrombin time elevation	18/23	77
Sulfobromophthalein (BSP) >8% in 45 min	18/18	100
Albumin <3.5 g/dl	18/22	82
Globulins >4.1 g/dl	12/22	55

Source: Adapted from Strickland RC, Schenker S. Dig Dis 22:49, 1977, with permission.

patients with nephrogenic hepatic dysfunction syndrome had renal cell carcinomas. However, two patients with reversible hepatic dysfunction had xanthogranulomatous pyelonephritis. Moreover, there have been isolated reports of reversible hepatic dysfunction coexisting with sarcoma and primary carcinoma of the gastrointestinal tract.[55]

The most common clinical features of proven nephrogenic hepatic dysfunction syndrome include fever (85 per cent of patients), weight loss (100 per cent), a palpable abdominal mass (40 per cent), hepatomegaly (77 per cent), and splenomegaly (45 per cent). The systemic symptoms of low-grade fever with temperatures occasionally as high as 102° F and weight loss may persist for many months prior to the diagnosis of the renal cell carcinoma. Most of these patients will be found to have hematuria and a palpable mass in the region of one or both kidneys, with obvious malignancy demonstrable on intravenous pyelography. Nevertheless, some of these renal tumors will remain undiagnosed for appreciable periods of time following the onset of nephrogenic hepatic dysfunction syndrome. Thrombocytosis, with platelet counts greater than 350,000/mm³, has been found in 60 per cent of these patients. Decreased hematocrits and hemoglobin levels with leukocytosis and elevations of blood urea nitrogen (BUN) are present in more than one third of patients with this syndrome. Although liver test abnormalities are characteristic of nephrogenic hepatic dysfunction syndrome, they are usually only minimal.[51-55] In patients with well-documented nephrogenic hepatic dysfunction syndrome, sulfobromophthalein retention has been increased universally. Serum alkaline phosphatase is elevated in more than 90 per cent of patients with this syndrome, with serum levels as high as five times the upper limits of normal. Similar increases have been reported in the serum levels of γ-glutamyl transpeptidase and 5'-nucleotidase. Alterations in serum proteins are commonly encountered, with 80 per cent of patients found to have albumin levels of less than 3.5 g/dl. Fifty per cent of patients with nephrogenic hepatic dysfunction syndrome are found to have elevated serum globulins, especially the α_2-fraction. Significant hyperbilirubinemia and elevations of serum aminotransferases rarely are encountered; however, prolonged prothrombin times have been reported. The erythrocyte sedimentation rate may be increased profoundly to as much as 100 mm/hr (Westergren method).

Many patients with nephrogenic hepatic dysfunction syndrome had substantial improvements in hepatocellular tests as well as alleviation of symptoms following the successful removal of the primary renal malignancy.[53-55] The clinical features of malaise, fever, and weight loss likewise may revert to normal. The resolution of symptoms and abnormalities of liver function may occur within one to two months following successful surgery. In some patients, recurrence of malignancy in the renal bed has been associated with a recrudescence of the preoperative abnormalities of hepatocellular tests.[51]

HEPATIC HISTOLOGY

The histologic characteristics of the liver in nephrogenic hepatic dysfunction syndrome are nondiagnostic.[51, 53] The majority of patients have proliferation of Kupffer cells, which occasionally form small intrasinusoidal clusters and small nodules. On occasion, there may be focal hepatocytolysis and an increase in periportal mononuclear cells. Special histochemical stains have been reported to show increased canalicular staining for alkaline phosphatase in the centrolobular area.[53]

LYMPHOMA (HODGKIN'S AND NON-HODGKIN'S)

The liver has an extensive reticuloendothelial system and hence can be involved in generalized lymphomas of the Hodgkin's and non-Hodgkin's varieties. In addition to distinct nodular or diffuse lymphomatous infiltration of the liver, nonspecific histologic abnormalities such as steatosis, granulomas, or hemosiderosis may be encountered on biopsy of the liver of an affected patient. Because of differences in extent of involvement and pathologic findings in patients with Hodgkin's disease and non-Hodgkin's lymphomas, these two conditions are considered separately.

HODGKIN'S DISEASE (Table 53–9)

Malignant infiltration of the liver is uncommon in patients with Hodgkin's disease (Fig. 53–11). Malignant histiocytes, Reed-Sternberg cells, or both were encountered in livers of only 8 of 103 untreated patients with Hodgkin's disease undergoing laparotomy.[58, 59] Other nonspecific histologic abnormalities, however, were found in the livers of these patients.[60] For example, 10 per cent had hepatic granulomas.[58, 59] These were largely periportal and noncaseating and were rarely associated with malignant histiocytes or Reed-Sternberg cells. In addition, nonspecific lymphocytic infiltration of the portal areas with generalized increases in mononuclear cells, benign histiocytes, and eosinophils is seen in the liver biopsy specimens of as many as 30 per cent of patients with documented Hodgkin's disease, even though frank malignant infiltration of the liver is uncommon at the time of diagnostic staging.

On occasion, gross inspection of the liver of a patient with Hodgkin's disease demonstrates small nodules (1 to 2 mm) on the hepatic surface. Sometimes, larger confluent tumor masses are seen. Histologically, portal areas are enlarged as a result of infiltration of histiocytes and mononuclear cells. Reed-Sternberg cells may be difficult to find. In the livers of some patients, especially those who have lymphocyte-depleted Hodgkin's disease, definite invasion of the portal vein may be encountered. A replacement of the adjacent parenchyma of the liver by malignant histiocytes may lead to the finding of confluent tumor masses on

TABLE 53–9. HEPATIC PATHOLOGY IN HODGKIN'S DISEASE

	Untreated* (n = 103)		Treated† (n = 25)	
	No.	%	No.	%
Hodgkin's disease‡	8	7.7	2	8
Granulomas (no Hodgkin's disease)	8	7.7	1	4
Hepatitis	0		2	8
Lymphocytes in portal area	33	32.0	6	24
Hemosiderosis (no Hodgkin's disease)	5	4.9	4	16
Steatosis	11	10.7	4	16

Source: Adapted from Abt AB, et al. Cancer 33:1564, 1974, with permission.

*Includes 9 patients with stage I, 40 patients with stage II, 45 patients with stage III, and 9 patients with stage IV disease.

†Of these 25 patients, 17 were treated with radiation therapy and chemotherapy, 4 with chemotherapy alone, and 4 with radiation therapy alone.

‡Six biopsy specimens contained Reed-Sternberg cells.

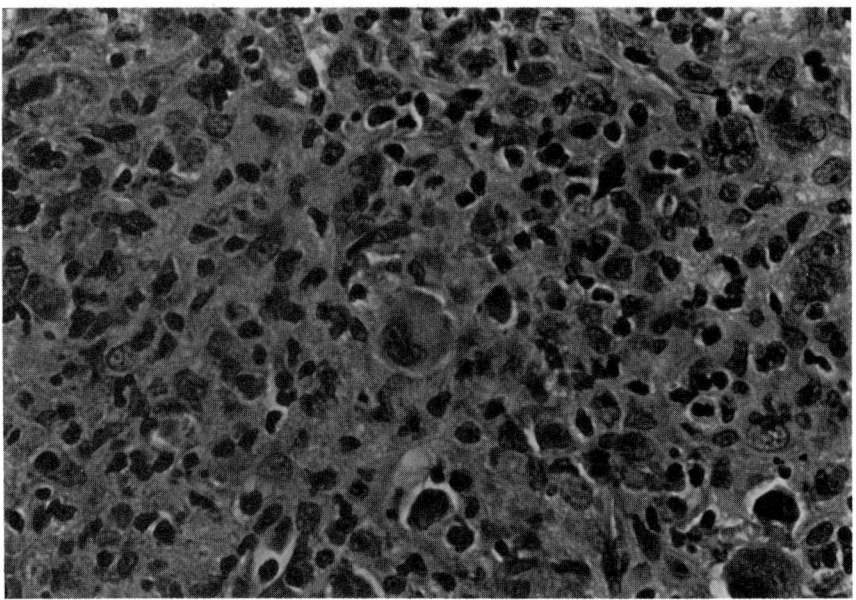

Figure 53–11. Hodgkin's disease in the liver. Hematoxylin and eosin. Malignant histiocytes and lymphocytes are readily identifiable in this portal area. Several large histiocytes have "owl-eye" nuclei and are Reed-Sternberg cells.

gross and microscopic examination. Rarely, focal hepatocellular necrosis and bile stasis may be present. Prominent portal fibrosis can be seen in the livers of patients with either nodular sclerosing or lymphocyte-depleted Hodgkin's disease.

Hodgkin's disease involving extrahepatic bile ducts and lymph nodes in the porta hepatis has been reported. Involvement of the extrahepatic bile ducts or gallbladder with Hodgkin's disease is invariably accompanied by hepatic involvement as well.[61]

The most commonly abnormal liver test in patients with Hodgkin's disease is an elevated serum alkaline phosphatase.[62, 63] Progressive increases in the proportions of patients who have elevated alkaline phosphatase levels occur with the advancing stages of the disease. Forty-one per cent of patients with Hodgkin's disease admitted to the Massachusetts General Hospital for staging were found on routine testing to have elevations of serum alkaline phosphatase.[62] In this group of patients, however, only 14 per cent of those subsequently confirmed to have stage I or stage II Hodgkin's disease were found to have elevations of serum alkaline phosphatase. Sixty-five per cent of the patients with stage III disease and 81 per cent with stage IV disease had elevated serum alkaline phosphatase levels. Moreover, alkaline phosphatase elevations were more common in patients with fever. Surprisingly, a low incidence of elevations of serum alkaline phosphatase was found in patients who had pruritus. Alkaline phosphatase elevations are generally between one and one half and two times the upper limits of normal. On occasion, pronounced alkaline phosphatase elevations to as much as five times the upper limit of normal have been reported to occur in patients with Hodgkin's disease of the liver. In an investigation of the sources of the elevated alkaline phosphatase levels in 31 patients, 23 were found to have increases in the liver fraction alone.[62] Three patients had normal livers but had increased levels of liver and bone alkaline phosphatase. The remaining three patients had elevated serum alkaline phosphatase levels, but determination of the contribution from liver or bone was not possible. Elevated levels of 5′-nucleotidase were found in 9 of 31 patients, and sulfobromophthalein retention was prolonged in 6 of 15 patients so

tested. The elevations in serum of liver alkaline phosphatase do not necessarily imply hepatic infiltration with Hodgkin's disease—that is, stage IV disease.

The source of the elevated serum alkaline phosphatase levels in patients with Hodgkin's disease has been the subject of much debate. There are no data to suggest that this increased serum alkaline phosphatase is a tumor isoenzyme. Moreover, the correlation of elevated serum alkaline phosphatase levels with fever may suggest a nonspecific, acute-phase type of reaction of the liver. One investigation of pathogenesis of severe intrahepatic cholestasis in a Hodgkin's disease patient failed to demonstrate abnormal estrogen, cortisol, follicle-stimulating hormone or adrenocorticotropic hormone levels. Moreover, no increase in serum lipoprotein X could be shown (see Chap. 5).[64] On occasion, intrahepatic or extrahepatic cholestasis with intense hyperbilirubinemia may be encountered.[63] The other tests of hepatocellular function are rarely increased in patients with Hodgkin's disease, aside from prolongation of the prothrombin times in those patients who have severe cholestasis resulting from extrahepatic obstruction of the biliary tree.

Liver involvement is infrequently encountered in clinical stage I or II Hodgkin's disease patients undergoing laparotomy, having been noted in only 10 of 255 patients (4 per cent) staged at the University of Alabama.[65] The presence of abdominal Hodgkin's disease correlated with symptoms, histologic type (nodular sclerosing < lymphocyte-predominant < mixed cellularity < lymphocyte-depleted), and sex (females < males). The lowest risk of abdominal disease was observed among females with nodular sclerosing (6 per cent) or lymphocyte-predominant (8 per cent) histology, whereas men with multiple systemic complaints and either mixed-cellularity (85 per cent) or lymphocyte-depleted (93 per cent) histology had the highest risk.[65] Among 135 patients with initially negative laparotomies, subsequent hepatic involvement was rare.

Since the diagnosis of hepatic infiltration with Hodgkin's lymphoma defines a patient as having stage IV disease, the documentation of hepatic involvement has important therapeutic implications. Elevated serum alkaline phosphatase levels cannot be taken as evidence of hepatic involvement with the tumor. Radionuclide scanning of the liver is too insensitive and nonspecific to be of clinical benefit in most cases of Hodgkin's disease.[66] False-positive tests demonstrating hepatomegaly or even focal defects of the liver are common. The liver biopsy is the only reasonable means of demonstrating infiltration of the liver by tumor. Percutaneous liver biopsy will fail to detect involvement of the liver, however, in a substantial number of patients.[67, 68] Laparoscopic biopsy of the liver does improve the diagnostic yield in patients with Hodgkin's disease, because multiple biopsies can be taken from both hepatic lobes and any visible superficial nodules can be biopsied. In general, six specimens obtained by laparoscopically directed liver biopsy, three from each lobe, appear equivalent to a similar number of specimens taken directly from the liver at laparotomy.[67] Thus, for purposes of excluding hepatic infiltration with Hodgkin's disease, the laparoscopic biopsy of the liver enhances the yield of percutaneous biopsy and appears equivalent to biopsies obtained at laparotomy.[67, 68]

NON-HODGKIN'S LYMPHOMA INVOLVING THE LIVER (Table 53–10)

Lymphomatous infiltration of the liver is encountered commonly in non-Hodgkin's lymphoma. In one series of 82 patients with non-Hodgkin's lymphoma, 11 of 40 (23 per cent) patients with lymphocytic lymphoma and 10 of 42 (24 per cent) patients with histiocytic lymphoma had lymphomatous infiltration of the liver on percutaneous biopsy.[60] Hepatic infiltration is thus significantly more frequent in patients who have non-Hodgkin's lymphoma compared with those with Hodgkin's lymphoma. On occasion, a primary hepatic lymphoma without generalized lymphoma may be encountered.[69] Only 29 well-documented cases of primary hepatic lymphoma have been reported.[69, 70, 71] Most (22 of 29 patients) were in middle-aged men (mean 51.9 years) with hepatomegaly. A single hypoechoic area may be noted on ultrasonography or a large space-occupying, low-attenuation area may be seen on computed tomography. The most common histologic type of primary hepatic lymphoma is diffuse large cell lymphoma (formerly called diffuse histiocytic lymphoma) of B cell origin. Ultrastructurally, lymphoma cells contain cleaved-to-round nuclei with finely dispersed chromatin and nucleoli of increased size.[71] In many adult patients, the lymphoma remains confined to the liver without involvement of spleen, lymph nodes, or bone marrow. This tendency to remain confined to the liver helps to explain the reports of long-term survival following hepatic resective surgery alone.[71] The liver and spleen generally are involved together in patients with systemic non-Hodgkin's lymphoma. The liver may be markedly enlarged with diffuse lymphomatous involvement, and on microscopic examination, large lymphoblasts or atypical histiocytes may be seen in the periportal regions (Figs. 53–12 to 53–14). On occasion, malignant histiocytes or lymphocytes will be found in the sinusoids or the parenchyma of the liver. Various additional, nonspecific findings may be found in association with non-Hodgkin's lymphoma. Chronic persistent hepatitis, chronic active hepatitis, steatosis, and hemosiderosis may be encountered upon occasion.[60]

Liver tests show moderate increases of serum alkaline phosphatase, with other test results being normal. On occasion, however, hepatic infiltration may produce profound intrahepatic cholestasis and jaundice. For staging purposes, the laparoscopically directed liver biopsy significantly enhances diagnostic yield, compared with percutaneous biopsy.[67, 72] However, unlike the staging situation in patients with Hodgkin's disease, in which the laparoscopic liver biopsy results appear equivalent to those from laparotomy, a substantial number of false-negative results of laparoscopic liver biopsy have been reported for patients with non-Hodgkin's lymphoma of the liver.[67] Thus, biopsy at laparotomy is superior to both percutaneous and laparoscopic liver biopsies in patients with non-Hodgkin's lymphoma. In addition to detecting histologic patterns of disease on liver biopsy sections, immunotyping of lymphoid malignancies is now possible using specific monoclonal antibodies and tissue obtained by percutaneous, laparoscopic, or operative means.[73] Special care is needed to block nonspecific hepatic staining caused by endogenous hepatic parenchymal cell biotin. Specimens for immunotyping must not however be placed in routine formalin fixative.

LIVER INVOLVEMENT IN MULTIPLE MYELOMA

Hepatic biochemical test abnormalities and altered hepatic histology may be seen in patients with multiple myeloma.[74] In one study, 48 per cent of myeloma patients for whom hepatic histology was available had infiltration of the liver by malignant plasma cells.[74] The infiltration is usually diffuse in nature, although nodular involvement may be seen. Most patients with diffuse infiltrates have hepatomegaly, and it may recede with successful chemotherapy. It is important to remember that hepatomegaly may likewise be due to amyloidosis or myeloid metaplasia. Extrahepatic cholestasis is less common in patients with multiple myeloma compared with patients with lymphoma.

SICKLE CELL ANEMIA

James B. Herrick, in 1910, first reported the clinical findings and morphologic characteristics of the red blood cells of a patient with sickle cell anemia. In the first patients described, jaundice, fever, chills, and pain in the right upper quadrant were observed. Thus, hepatic dysfunction in sickle cell anemia was recognized as a component of the disease from the beginning.[75] A variety of hepatic disorders may be seen in patients with sickle cell anemia, ranging from acute viral hepatitis to hepatic crises to severe intrahepatic cholestasis and cholelithiasis with common duct stones. In one series of 88 patients with sickle cell anemia admitted to the University of Alabama Hospital over a ten-year period, hepatitis was diagnosed by liver biopsy or by finding hepatitis B surface antigen in five patients.[76] Cho-

TABLE 53–10. HEPATIC PATHOLOGY IN NON-HODGKIN'S LYMPHOMAS

	Patients with Lymphocytic Lymphoma		Patients with Histiocytic Lymphoma	
	No.	%	No.	%
Lymphoma	11	22.5	10	23.8
Chronic persistent hepatitis	6	15	10	23.8
Chronic active hepatitis	2	5	1	2.4
Steatosis	3	7.5	3	7.1
Hemosiderosis	2	5	1	2.4
Normal	16	40	17	40.5
TOTAL	40		42	

Source: Adapted from Roth A, et al. Tumori 64:45, 1978, with permission.

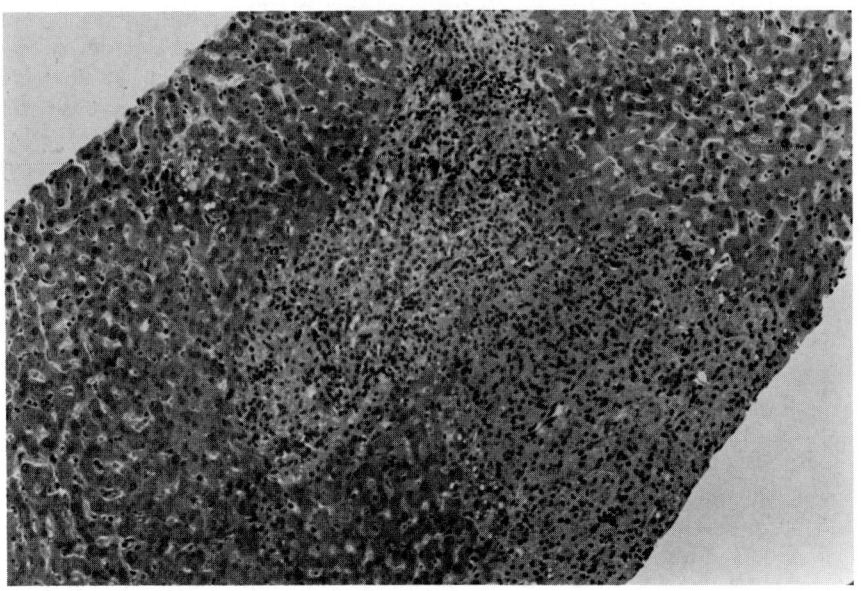

Figure 53–12. Lymphosarcoma of the liver. Hematoxylin and eosin. Low-power light microscopic view. A large area surrounding the portal zone contains a homogeneous population of malignant histiocytes.

lelithiasis, choledocholithiasis, or both were documented in 11 patients. A crisis involving intense pain in the right upper quadrant and cholestasis was encountered in nine patients. In other studies, cirrhosis of the liver is found at autopsy in approximately 20 per cent of patients with sickle cell disease. Whereas some patients have severe antecedent congestive heart failure or excess iron stores on histochemical staining, the majority have no clear-cut etiology for the cirrhosis.[77–79]

Acute viral hepatitis associated with the repeated blood transfusions can be expected in patients with sickle cell anemia. The clinical and laboratory features of acute viral hepatitis in patients with sickle cell anemia are identical with those of such patients without sickle cell anemia except that jaundice may be much greater in the former. However, confusion may occur in differentiating acute viral hepatitis from hepatic crises and the intrahepatic cholestasis that may be encountered in patients with sickle cell anemia. Acute hepatic failure has been reported in sickle cell disease

patients.[77] This rare complication is associated with a dramatic prolongation of the prothrombin time and extreme hyperbilirubinemia but transaminases less than ten times upper limit of normal. Most patients who develop acute hepatic failure die from the disease. A possible relationship between zinc deficiency and hepatic encephalopathy in sickle cell disease patients has been suggested; occasional dramatic reversals in weight loss and encephalopathy have been reported with zinc replacement.[77]

The incidences of cholelithiasis established by radiography, surgery, autopsy, or all three have been variably estimated from 7 to 37 per cent.[76, 80, 81] In 825 patients seen for sickle cell disease at Duke University over an 18-year period, 20 patients had extrahepatic biliary tract disease.[80] Thirteen patients had radiopaque gallstones, and four were documented to have common bile duct stones. Eighteen of 20 patients had signs and symptoms of chronic cholecystitis, and one had acute cholecystitis. Calculous disease in patients with sickle cell anemia may be manifested earlier in

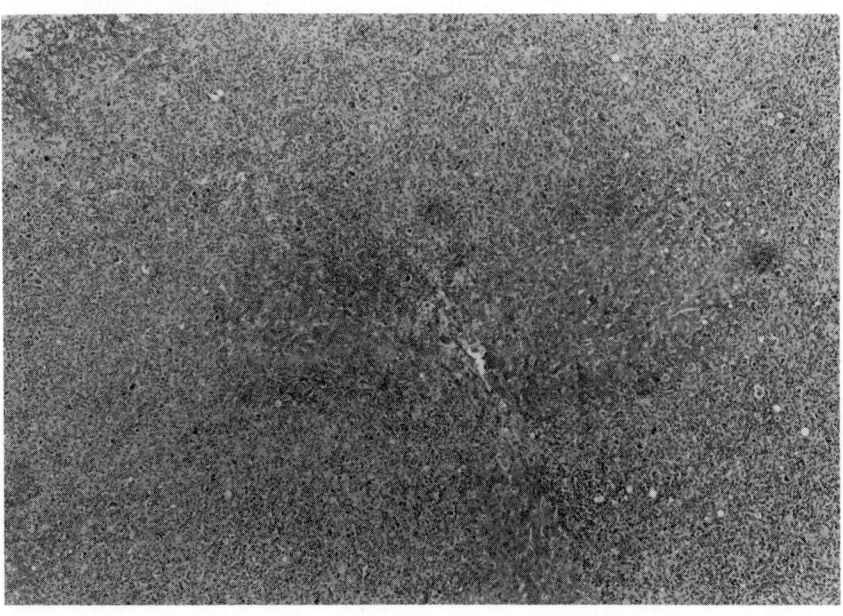

Figure 53–13. Lymphosarcoma of the liver. Hematoxylin and eosin. Low-power light microscopic view. The entire parenchyma of the liver except for a small region in the center of the field is replaced by a malignant lymphosarcoma infiltrate.

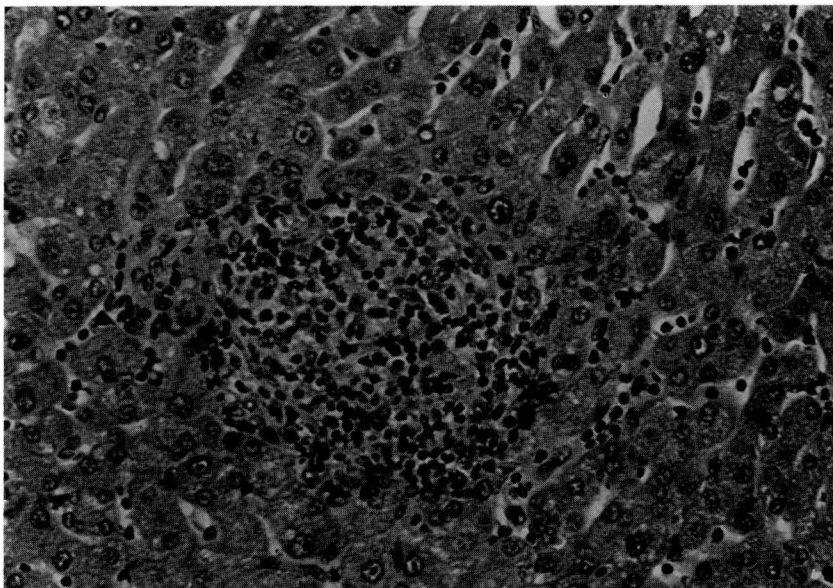

Figure 53–14. Mixed lymphoma of the liver. Hematoxylin and eosin. High-power light microscopic view. An nodular focus of mature and immature mononuclear cells is visible in the center of the field.

life compared with the general population.[81] The stones encountered are invariably small, multifaceted pigment stones resulting from the excessive hemolysis and enhanced pigment load. Gallstone disease in the teenage years has been reported, but in the vast majority of patients, the onset of cholelithiasis occurs in the 20s and 30s. The clinical picture of cholelithiasis in patients with sickle cell disease may be difficult to differentiate from an acute hepatic crisis with intense intrahepatic cholestasis.[75, 77, 80–84] Intravenous cholangiography and oral cholecystography cannot be done in the vast majority of such patients because of the significant hyperbilirubinemia. Noninvasive imaging techniques such as ultrasonography and computed axial tomography are useful for demonstrating biliary tract disease. In addition, acute obstruction of the cystic duct may be diagnosed by technetium radionuclide scanning. Confirmation of obstructed extrahepatic bile ducts, cystic duct obstruction, or both may be obtained by transhepatic cholangiography or endoscopic retrograde cholangiopancreatography when necessary. Although not indicated in sickle cell disease patients with incidental asymptomatic gallstones, elective cholecystectomy is recommended for patients with gallstones in whom there is difficulty in differentiating cholecystitis from abdominal sickle cell crisis.[77] Care must be taken in preparing these patients for elective surgery, with particular attention paid to preoperative exchange transfusion and hydration and oxygenation during surgery.

A unique clinical disorder, hepatic sickle crisis or sickle "hepatopathy," may be encountered in patients with sickle cell anemia. This disorder is characterized by intense pain in the right upper quadrant, fever, leukocytosis, jaundice, and tender hepatomegaly.[74, 82, 83] The clinical presentation thus may mimic that of acute cholangitis. Laboratory tests of patients with the hepatic crisis of sickle cell anemia show that bilirubin is elevated to levels ranging from 2 to 20 mg/dl (with half or more being the direct-reacting fraction). On occasion, patients with sickle cell hepatic crises have bilirubin levels as high as 45 to 100 mg/dl. Alkaline phosphatase usually is elevated only moderately, in the range of two to three times the upper limits of normal. Leukocytosis can be present, with leukocyte counts as high as 20,000/mm³. The prothrombin time usually is normal, but

on occasion may be prolonged. Aminotransferase levels range from moderately elevated to 10 to 15 times the upper limits of normal. Moderate increases in gamma-globulins can be detected on protein electrophoresis. In many instances, the hepatic crisis is accompanied by crises of pain in the kidneys and joints. On other occasions, however, the entire clinical picture of sickle cell crisis will be limited to hepatic manifestations.

Biopsy of the liver of a patient with the hepatic crises of sickle cell disease shows sinusoids filled with Kupffer cells laden with engulfed red blood cells. Sludging of erythrocytes in hepatic sinusoids should however not be overinterpreted to mean sickle hepatic crisis, since these changes are almost invariably seen in the livers of sickle cell patients, regardless of clinical features and laboratory results.[79] In fact, the formalin fixative commonly employed in processing liver tissue will artifactually increase sickling. Additional histologic features, such as coagulative necrosis, distorted hepatocytes, or acidophil bodies, are required to support the diagnosis of sickle hepatic crisis. These changes are most prominent in the centrolobular areas, where hyaline fibrin–like thrombi in the sinusoids may also be encountered. Increased iron stores will be evident in most patients, with iron found in both reticuloendothelial cells and hepatocytes. On electron microscopy, Kupffer cells are hypertrophied, and the hepatocytes may have a washed-out appearance, with a marked decrease in glycogen stores together with changes in smooth and rough endoplasmic reticulum. Repeat biopsies obtained shortly after the resolution of the hepatic crisis reveal that the histologic changes reverse rapidly.

The clinical course of a patient who has intense intrahepatic cholestasis and sickle cell anemia is dramatic. One usually sees impressive and dramatic symptomatic improvement together with substantial decreases in AST, hepatomegaly, and leukocytosis after a few days of therapy consisting of bedrest, hydration, and analgesics. The hyperbilirubinemia however, may persist for several days to several weeks with only gradual resolution. Since this syndrome of intense intrahepatic cholestasis in the hepatic crisis of sickle cell anemia may be indistinguishable from acute cholangitis, careful evaluation of the patient together with a combination of invasive and noninvasive abdominal imaging techniques must be done.

A rare benign form of extreme hyperbilirubinemia may occasionally be seen in children with sickle cell anemia.[85, 86] Bilirubin elevations to levels greater than 20 mg/dl (with more than 50 per cent direct-reacting) are unaccompanied by severe pain, fever, or generalized sickle cell crisis. Moreover, there is no dramatic change in hematocrit or reticulocyte count suggestive of significant hemolytic crisis. The clinical course is uneventful, with the hyperbilirubinemia resolving over a several weeks' course without permanent sequelae. The existence of this unusually high but benign hyperbilirubinemia contradicts the alleged grave prognosis of elevations of bilirubin (to more than 20 mg/dl) in patients with sickle cell disease. The cause of this hyperbilirubinemia is unknown, but it probably is not the result of bile duct obstruction or sickle crisis. Altered hepatic conjugation of bilirubin cannot be demonstrated. In fact, uridine diphosphate-glucuronyltransferase activity is substantially higher in jaundiced sickle cell patients than in non-jaundiced controls.[87]

NUTRITION AND LIVER DISEASE

JEJUNOILEAL BYPASS AND LIVER DISEASE

Morbid obesity is a serious health and emotional problem in the Western world. Numerous approaches have been employed to help these patients lose weight. One of the most effective is the jejunoileal bypass operation, in which a large portion of the absorptive small bowel is bypassed, causing severe malabsorption and thus weight loss. Although this type of operation, because of potentially severe complications, has been largely abandoned in favor of other surgical techniques (e.g., gastroplasty), there remains a substantial number of patients who still have a jejunoileal bypass anastomosis in place.

Pathogenesis

Although a variety of theories have been proposed to explain the liver disease that develops in patients following jejunoileal bypass operations, the cause remains unknown. Release of bacterial toxins or toxic bile acids (e.g., lithocholic acid) has been proposed as a possible mediator of liver damage.[88] This is supported by a clinical study showing prevention or reversal of hepatic steatosis following intestinal bypass in patients treated with metronidazole[89] and by animal studies showing a reduction in liver injury following jejunoileal bypass in rats undergoing removal of the defunctionalized loop[90] and a decrease in hepatic steatosis and cellular necrosis in dogs treated with tetracycline following small-intestine bypass.[91]

A variety of nutritional theories have also been proposed. Liver disease usually begins to develop soon after performance of the bypass, during the period of maximum weight loss, when fat from adipose tissue is being rapidly mobilized and levels of essential serum amino acids fall.[92] However, patients undergoing rapid weight loss caused by fasting or following gastroplasty do not suffer similar liver injury. Also, improvement in nutrition through use of parenteral hyperalimentation has yielded mixed results when used in patients with liver disease following jejunoileal bypass.[93–96]

Pathology

Morbidly obese individuals frequently have abnormal livers (Table 53–11). The most frequent finding is steatosis (28 to 88 per cent of patients).[97–99] A much smaller number of obese patients have hepatic fibrosis and lesions similar to those of alcoholic hepatitis.[99] Jejunoileal bypass has been shown to cause a worsening of hepatic lesions in some patients and to cause the de novo appearance of serious hepatic abnormalities in others (Table 53–11).[100, 101] Histologic abnormalities include worsening of steatosis, inflammation of both the hepatic lobule and portal areas, granuloma formation, portal fibrosis, and cirrhosis.[102] Within 5 to 7 years after jejunoileal bypass, cirrhosis is observed in 5 to 10 per cent of patients.[98–100] A normal preoperative biopsy does not preclude the development of liver disease, and there is no correlation between the postoperative hepatic abnormality and rate of weight loss,[100] although the pathologic changes appear to be most severe during the period of rapid weight loss, after which they typically stabilize or abate. However, in some patients hepatic inflammation and fibrosis persist.[100] The hepatic pathology that develops following jejunoileal bypass is very similar to that seen in patients with alcoholic liver disease;[96, 102] similarly, perivenular fibrosis on liver biopsy is believed to be a marker for progression to cirrhosis both in alcoholic liver disease and following a jejunoileal bypass.

Clinical Features

Liver disease following jejunoileal bypass for morbid obesity may range from only a slight abnormality in hepatic tests to asymptomatic hepatic fibrosis or cirrhosis to jaundice and liver failure. Abnormal hepatic tests, including elevations of alkaline phosphatase and AST, decreases in serum albumin, or increased retention of sulfobromophthalein, are common in the first 12 months following bypass surgery.[102–104] The failure of these tests to improve after three months is suggestive of a serious hepatic lesion.[104]

Hepatic failure is reported to develop in 2.2 to 6 per cent of patients following jejunoileal bypass and usually occurs in the first 12 to 18 months.[99, 102–104] Hepatic failure is more frequent in females. Anorexia, weakness, abdominal pain, nausea, and vomiting are frequent complaints. Within 3 to 14 months of the bypass procedure, jaundice is noted. Hepatomegaly, splenomegaly, ascites, and spider angiomas may also be present. Bilirubin levels initially are increased slightly; however, with worsening of the liver disease, values may exceed 30 mg/dl. The AST activity is increased two- to tenfold, whereas ALT activity is normal or nearly so. Prolongation of the prothrombin time and

TABLE 53–11. PREOPERATIVE AND POSTOPERATIVE FINDINGS IN LIVER BIOPSY SPECIMENS FROM PATIENTS UNDERGOING JEJUNOILEAL BYPASS

	Patients Studied Preoperatively		Patients Studied Postoperatively	
	No.	%	No.	%
Normal	59	62.1	13	13.7
Steatosis	18	18.9	36	37.9
Alcoholic hepatitis	14	14.7	28	29.5
Fibrosis	4	4.2	18	18.9
TOTAL	95		95	

Source: Adapted from Nasrallah SM, et al. Ann Surg. 192:726, 1980.

hypoalbuminemia are commonly present. Leukocytosis with white blood cell counts as high as 35,000/mm³ may be present.[102-104] Liver biopsy shows hepatic steatosis and alcoholic hepatitis.

Cirrhosis has been observed to develop in 5 to 9 per cent of patients followed by serial liver biopsy for up to 7 years.[97, 99] It may follow recovery from an episode of hepatic failure. However, the development of cirrhosis more commonly is insidious, with minimal associated clinical findings.[102] In several series, significant "precirrhotic" histologic changes (hepatic fibrosis and histologic features similar to alcoholic hepatitis) were found in about 50 per cent of postbypass patients.[97, 103] Occasional deaths caused by cirrhosis and liver failure have been reported as long as 7 to 10 years following jejunoileal bypass.

Prognosis and Treatment

Patients who have slight and transient abnormalities in hepatic function early in the postoperative period appear to have an excellent short-term prognosis.[104] The long-term prognosis for this group of patients remains undefined. The onset of icterus (bilirubin exceeding 2.5 mg/dl) or prolongation of the prothrombin time by more than 3 seconds is a poor prognostic sign. In addition, failure of hepatic tests to improve with time are indicative of worsening liver disease.[104] Fatality rates following the onset of icterus are reported to be 17 to 100 per cent.[102] Death may occur despite takedown of the shunt or the use of hyperalimentation.

The management of these patients is complicated by two factors. First, the pathogenesis of the disease is poorly understood, so that specific therapies have not been developed. Second, patients frequently are reluctant to have the shunt taken down, as they fear regaining the lost weight.

The onset of icterus is indicative of a severe hepatic lesion and is a strong indication for restoring intestinal continuity. Some patients have died following takedown of the jejunoileal bypass; however, most were severely ill and poor operative risks.[102, 104] Earlier reoperation may have improved survival in these latter patients. Improvement in cirrhosis has also been reported to occur following restoration of intestinal continuity.[105] Intravenous hyperalimentation may improve both hepatic function and histologic integrity of the liver in some patients with severe postbypass liver disease.[93, 94] A therapeutic role for metronidazole in this condition has been proposed but its efficacy has not been established.[89] Failure to improve with medical management or relapse of liver disease following initial improvement is an indication for prompt reversal of the jejunoileal bypass. Patient compliance with a high-protein, low-carbohydrate, low-fat, and no-alcohol diet has been claimed to reduce the frequency of severe postbypass liver problems, but this has not been investigated in a controlled trial.[99]

A difficult management problem is posed by patients who have normal or only slightly abnormal hepatic tests. Biochemical tests of hepatic function are poor indicators of the severity of the hepatic lesions that develop following jejunoileal bypass. Because of this, liver biopsy is frequently performed a year after the operation. Many of these patients will have serious histologic lesions, thus forcing a decision as to whether or not the jejunoileal bypass should be taken down. The presence of an alcoholic hepatitis–like lesion or increasing hepatic fibrosis is a strong indication for restoring intestinal continuity. If a decision not to reoperate is made, liver biopsy should be performed on these patients at six-month to yearly intervals.

HEPATIC DYSFUNCTION DURING TOTAL PARENTERAL NUTRITION

Paradoxically, total parenteral nutrition, which may be beneficial in patients with hepatic damage following jejunoileal bypass, is itself associated with liver disease. Clinically, this dysfunction may result in abnormal hepatic tests and, occasionally, in hepatomegaly and jaundice. On liver biopsy, varying degrees of steatosis and intrahepatic cholestasis may be seen.[106-108] Often it is not clear to what extent other factors, such as previous liver disease, alcoholism, anesthesia, hypoperfusion, sepsis, malnutrition, and drugs, may be contributing to the liver dysfunction.

Pathogenesis

The pathogenesis of the liver injury that develops in patients receiving total parenteral nutrition is not known, although several mechanisms have been postulated. These include an increased rate of hepatic lipid synthesis caused by glucose overload and hyperinsulinemia,[106] decreased elimination of excess fat from the liver secondary to essential fatty acid or carnitine deficiency,[107] free radical generation due to a deficiency in vitamin E and selenium,[109] or an imbalance between conjugated and unconjugated bile acids, perhaps resulting from bacterial overgrowth in the intestine.[110]

Pathology

Histologically, the most common findings are varying degrees of fatty metamorphosis and intrahepatic cholestasis. There also may be bile duct proliferation, bile plugs within canaliculi, centrolobular cholestasis, and pigment accumulation within hepatocytes. These changes are evident after about three weeks of total parenteral nutrition. Thereafter, periportal inflammation may be found. In an occasional patient, some periportal fibrosis also is present.[106, 107] Rarely, the lesion progresses to cirrhosis with liver failure and death.[111] Periportal copper deposition also has been described.[112]

Clinical Findings

In adults, the first liver test abnormalities usually observed are elevations of the serum alkaline phosphatase, transaminases, and γ-glutamyl transpeptidase following the first week of treatment.[108, 113] In infants, increased serum bilirubin is more frequently seen early on,[108] whereas in adults increases in serum bilirubin and lactate dehydrogenase may be observed later in the illness.[114] These biochemical changes usually normalize spontaneously but occasionally may persist or worsen.[112, 115]

Management

Decreasing the amount of glucose in total parenteral nutrition solutions or institution of an oral or enteral diet usually leads to improvements in hepatic tests and morphology.[108]

COLLAGEN VASCULAR DISEASE AND THE LIVER

Striking hepatic damage is uncommon in the so-called collagen vascular diseases. Although advanced liver disease is rare, hepatic dysfunction is not uncommon. This discussion of hepatic involvement in collagen vascular diseases encompasses systemic lupus erythematosus (SLE), rheumatoid arthritis, Sjögren's syndrome, disseminated systemic sclerosis (scleroderma), dermatomyositis, and polymyalgia rheumatica (PR).

SYSTEMIC LUPUS ERYTHEMATOSUS

Clinical liver disease is unusual in SLE. About one third of patients, however, have slight hepatomegaly. Whether hepatic enlargement is related to the duration or severity of illness or (in part) to adrenocorticosteroid therapy, is unclear. There is no characteristic histologic lesion present in the liver of patients with SLE. The term *lupoid hepatitis* is used to describe the hepatic lesion of patients with chronic active hepatitis and a positive LE cell test (see Chap. 38).[116, 117] Lupoid hepatitis does not occur with increased frequency in patients with SLE.

A variety of histologic lesions have been observed on liver biopsy in patients with SLE, including cholestasis with prominent bile plugs, steatosis, acute or chronic hepatitis, granulomatous hepatitis, and cirrhosis.[118] Elevations in serum AST, ALT, and alkaline phosphatase are common and tend to reflect more closely the level of activity of the patient's SLE rather than hepatic histologic abnormalities. Involvement of the thyroid gland appears to occur more frequently in SLE patients with liver disease.[118]

Some of the liver injury found in patients with SLE may be the result of use of aspirin. Prolonged and high-dose use of salicylates by some patients has resulted in hepatic dysfunction and in rare instances, in clinical liver disease. This is true for patients with SLE and other rheumatologic diseases (see Chap. 31).[119–121] The pathologic picture of salicylate toxicity is striking. There may be diffuse hepatocyte injury, poor definition of the limiting plate, early stellate fibrosis, chronic portal inflammation with plasma cells predominating, and some lymphoid follicles in portal areas.[119] An occasional patient may show histologic changes of a more acute injury that are distinguishable from those of viral hepatitis. In contradistinction to viral hepatitis, there is no lobular disarray; ballooning of injured cells is localized to the centrolobular areas, acidophilic bodies are more numerous and scattered, and there is only moderate portal inflammation.[119] The serum AST and ALT levels are frequently increased in patients with aspirin hepatotoxicity. Occasionally, serum alkaline phosphatase is elevated, but elevation of bilirubin is rare.

Aspirin appears to be a direct hepatotoxin, as the hepatic damage is related to the amount of aspirin taken. Toxicity occurs most frequently in patients whose serum salicylate levels exceed 20 mg/dl. After withdrawal of the drug, liver tests improve before salicylate levels return to normal. These patients do not have classic aspirin sensitivity—that is, they lack rash, urticaria, bronchospasm, fever, eosinophilia, and nasal polyps. The clinical and histologic abnormalities are completely reversible after withdrawal of the drug.

It is important to withdraw salicylates in the management of patients with collagen vascular diseases who have signs or symptoms or laboratory or histologic evidence of hepatitis. Only in this way can the occasional patient with aspirin-induced hepatic injury, who may be erroneously diagnosed as having chronic active hepatitis, be accurately identified.

RHEUMATOID ARTHRITIS

Rheumatoid arthritis may be associated with hepatic dysfunction. Liver disease is found most commonly in patients who have Sjögren's syndrome or Felty's syndrome.[121–123] Patients who have rheumatoid arthritis may also develop hepatic dysfunction while taking salicylates (see the preceding section).[120]

Some patients with long-standing rheumatoid arthritis develop splenomegaly and neutropenia (Felty's syndrome). In this syndrome, mild hepatomegaly is common, and elevations of the serum transaminases and alkaline phosphatase are seen in about 25 per cent of patients.[123] Nodular regenerative hyperplasia of the liver has been described in Felty's syndrome and rarely in other patients with rheumatoid arthritis.[122–124] Histologically, there may be mild portal fibrosis and infiltration of portal areas with lymphocytes and plasma cells. Obliteration of the portal venules that produce atrophy and formation of regenerative nodules may result in portal hypertension, ascites, and gastrointestinal hemorrhage.[122–124] The pathogenesis of the hepatic injury has not been established but has been proposed to arise from immune complex–mediated venular injury.[124]

SJÖGREN'S SYNDROME

Sjögren's syndrome consists of keratoconjunctivitis sicca, xerostomia, and swelling of the salivary glands. Other clinical features include Raynaud's phenomenon, achlorhydria, alopecia, splenomegaly, and leukopenia. The sera of these patients frequently contain antinuclear factors, complement-fixing or precipitating antibodies to a wide variety of tissues and organs, and other laboratory evidence of defects in the immune system. These patients have a high incidence of allergy to intradermal antigens, including tuberculin. Achlorhydria and high titers of parietal cell antibodies and antithyroid antibodies also are present, with or without autoimmune thyroiditis.[125]

Ten per cent of patients who have Sjögren's syndrome and 42 per cent of those who have Sjögren's syndrome and rheumatoid arthritis have antimitochondrial antibodies and either clinical or biochemical evidence of liver disease.[126, 127] The abnormalities of liver function in Sjögren's syndrome with or without rheumatoid arthritis include elevations of alkaline phosphatase, AST, and ALT. Increase in sulfobromophthalein retention has also been reported. Positive titers for antimitochondrial antibodies are usually accompanied by histologic abnormalities consistent with primary biliary cirrhosis (see Chap. 44).[121, 128]

DISSEMINATED SYSTEMIC SCLEROSIS (Scleroderma)

The association of liver disease and scleroderma has been reported. Reynolds and associates described six female patients with scleroderma who had Raynaud's phenomenon, calcinosis cutis, and telangiectasia (CRST syndrome).[129] The telangiectasias resembled those of Rendu-Osler-Weber syndrome. They were located on the finger pads and lips and occasionally in the mucosa of the upper gastrointestinal tract. These patients uniformly have antimitochondrial antibodies in their sera and frequently have positive titers for antinuclear antibodies as well as rheumatoid factor. On liver biopsy, they appear to have primary biliary cirrhosis (see Chap. 44).

POLYMYALGIA RHEUMATICA

Abnormalities of liver tests, including increases of alkaline phosphatase, serum globulins, and aminotransferases, have been found in patients with polymyalgia rheumatica and giant cell arteritis.[130] Liver biopsy of these patients may show focal hepatocellular necrosis, portal inflammation, and isolated small epithelioid granulomas.[131] Granulomas in the liver in polymyalgia rheumatica have been reported both with and without documented evidence of giant cell arteritis involving the temporal artery. An increased incidence of hepatitis B antibody in the sera of the patients with polymyalgia rheumatica has been reported but not confirmed. Tests for HbsAg have been negative (see Chap. 37). No evidence of vasculitis has been found in the livers of these patients. The liver disease in polymyalgia rheumatica appears to be entirely benign, especially when the patient is adequately treated with corticosteroids.[130, 131]

RENAL TRANSPLANTATION AND LIVER DISEASE

Patients undergoing hemodialysis and then renal transplantation are at risk for developing hepatic dysfunction and clinical liver disease. The basis for the hepatic damage in most instances appears to be infectious. An extremely small proportion of cases may be attributable to treatment with drugs, particularly either α-methyldopa or azathioprine.

The infectious agents thought to be responsible for post-transplantation hepatic dysfunction are hepatitis B virus (HBV) and non-A, non-B hepatitis viruses, cytomegalovirus (CMV), herpes simplex virus (HSV), and in rare instances, certain fungi and parasites.[132]

The overall reported incidences of abnormal liver tests in patients 2 to 54 months after renal transplantation vary from 6 to 60 per cent, the average being about 15 per cent. In the majority of patients, the abnormalities appear within three months. Clinically, those patients with liver dysfunction after renal transplantation cover a wide range. A small group is made up of those with recognizable acute hepatitis, the majority of whom recover completely. Patients in another, larger, group have persistently abnormal liver tests, with a few progressing to cirrhosis. A few patients move from acute to chronic hepatitis; however, the majority who develop chronic disease have an insidious onset of their liver disease. Fortunately, only 15 per cent of those with liver test abnormalities develop clinically evident liver disease.

ACUTE VIRAL HEPATITIS IN POST-TRANSPLANTATION PATIENTS

Acute viral hepatitis is reported to occur in about 4.5 per cent of those patients who have had renal transplants. The occurrence of acute hepatitis in post-transplantation patients is related both to the number of transfusions and to the duration of hemodialysis.[132–134] Viral hepatitis is defined in this situation by a threefold or greater increase in AST or by the development of circulating HBsAg. Hepatitis B is not the major cause of hepatic dysfunction in this group, however, as it is present in only about 15 per cent of patients with postoperative hepatic dysfunction 1 to 30 months after surgery.[132] The overall mortality of acute viral hepatitis in these patients is 1 per cent or less, and fatal cases are presumably caused by CMV, HSV, and non-A, non-B hepatitis as often as by hepatitis B virus.

CHRONIC LIVER DISEASE AFTER TRANSPLANTATION

Chronic hepatic disease is due to hepatitis B virus in a minority of cases. Many cases are probably caused by other viral agents such as non-A, non-B hepatitis viruses, CMV, or HSV. Liver biopsy in these patients reveals chronic persistent or chronic active hepatitis with or without cirrhosis. In some series, 50 per cent of patients have developed cirrhosis.[132–134]

CYTOMEGALOVIRUS HEPATITIS

The exact importance of CMV in causing hepatic dysfunction in post-transplantation patients is unknown. The difficulty in assessing its role lies in the fact that CMV is ubiquitous in this group of individuals. Seroconversion is found in 75 to 90 per cent of patients who have undergone transplantation. Strict diagnosis should depend on the isolation of the organism from tissue.[132, 134] Some investigators believe that CMV is a major cause of hepatic dysfunction in this group of patients.[134] The source of the CMV infection appears to be the blood transfused during hemodialysis or transplantation. The development of infection in the recipient correlates well with the presence of a significant CMV antibody titer in the donor. Also, there may be reactivation of endogenous infection, since infection rates are influenced by the seropositivity of the patient prior to transplantation.

There are several clinical pictures of hepatitis caused by CMV in the post-transplantation patient. There is an acute illness, usually ushered in by fever with temperatures of 40°C or more, often with chills, followed by a course clinically indistinguishable from that of viral hepatitis. These patients have significant rises in antibody titers to CMV, and the organism is frequently cultured from the urine and in a few cases is isolated from hepatic tissue. The higher the titer of complement-fixing antibodies in a patient, the more likely it is that he or she will develop hepatitis. Thus, a four- to eightfold rise in the titer is associated with a 67 per cent incidence of acute hepatitis, and a greater than eightfold rise is associated with hepatitis incidence of 100 per cent. Although most of these patients do not have severe illness or in many cases noticeable clinical symptoms, they nonetheless have abnormalities of liver function that can persist.[132, 134] Recovery is usually the rule although, rarely, the disease can be fatal. A second group of patients suffers from a more indolent and chronic form of hepatitis.

TABLE 53–12. HEPATIC HISTOLOGY IN BIOPSY OR AUTOPSY SPECIMENS FROM PATIENTS WITH AIDS

Finding	Biopsy (% of total) (n = 26)	Autopsy (% of total) (n = 59)	Combined (% of total) (n = 85)
Normal	1 (3.8)	9 (15.3)	10 (11.8)
Steatosis	10 (38.5)	26 (44.1)	36 (42.4)
Portal inflammation	14 (53.8)	16 (27.1)	30 (35.3)
Congestion	1 (3.8)	18 (30.5)	19 (22.4)
Granulomata	10 (38.5)	2 (3.4)	12 (14.1)
Focal necrosis	5 (19.2)	5 (8.5)	10 (11.8)
Fibrosis/cirrhosis	4 (15.4)	4 (6.8)	8 (4.7)
Bile stasis	2 (7.7)	3 (5.1)	5 (5.9)
Kupffer cell hyperplasia	3 (11.5)	3 (5.1)	6 (7.1)
Piecemeal necrosis	2 (7.7)	1 (1.7)	3 (1.2)

Source: Adapted from Schneiderman DJ, et al. Hepatology 7:925, 1987, © by Am. Assoc. for the Study of Liver Diseases.

In view of the ubiquity of CMV in post-transplantation patients, judgment as to the role of CMV in the pathogenesis of cirrhosis in these patients must be reserved.[134]

HERPES SIMPLEX VIRUS

The incidence of HSV infection in post-transplantation patients is extremely low. Unfortunately, however, such an infection may be virulent. One report described four patients who died of disseminated HSV infections after renal transplantation.[135] On the other hand, recovery was complete in 17 patients reported from another medical center.[136] It is of interest that the patients in the group that had completely benign courses had no detectable antibodies before transplantation. The virulence of the infection, like that of the HSV infections in patients with thymic dysplasia, Hodgkin's disease, burns, steroid-treated pemphigus, or asthma, may be related to the extent of immunosuppression of the patient.

DRUGS AND POST-TRANSPLANTATION HEPATIC DYSFUNCTION

It has long been appreciated that immunosuppressants, particularly azathioprine, cause hepatic dysfunction in patients with leukemia. The role of azathioprine in post-transplantation liver disease is uncertain. For example, increased ALT levels and the severity of liver damage cannot be related to dosages of the drug taken by patients. In a series of 196 patients treated with azathioprine, 13 per cent showed evidence of hepatic dysfunction.[137] No correlation between the liver damage and the dosage of azathioprine could be discovered. It did not seem to matter whether the patient also was a carrier of hepatitis B. Cessation of drug therapy had no effect on the course of the illness. In five patients, the liver disease diminished despite continued use of azathioprine.

OTHER COMPLICATIONS

Malignancy and veno-occlusive disease are other complications that have been reported to occur in patients following renal transplantation. The incidence of malignancy is about one hundredfold greater than that in an age-matched population. Most of the tumors are mesenchymal; only one case of hepatocellular carcinoma has been reported.[132] Very rarely, a patient may develop veno-occlusive disease while receiving immunosuppressive drugs (see Chap. 23).

THE LIVER AND BILIARY TRACT IN THE ACQUIRED IMMUNE DEFICIENCY SYNDROME (AIDS)

The liver is frequently involved in AIDS, although hepatic abnormalities are only rarely a major contributor to morbidity or mortality. Hepatomegaly and elevated serum transaminases and alkaline phosphatase are common.[138, 139] Elevations in serum bilirubin are infrequently seen, however.

HISTOLOGIC ABNORMALITIES ON LIVER BIOPSY OR AT AUTOPSY

A variety of histologic abnormalities (Table 53–12) have been described in liver biopsy and autopsy material obtained from patients with AIDS.[138–146] The most common findings, such as macrovesicular steatosis and portal inflam-

TABLE 53–13. SPECIFIC AIDS-RELATED DIAGNOSES MADE FROM BIOPSY OR AUTOPSY SPECIMENS FROM PATIENTS WITH AIDS

Finding	Biopsy (% of total) (n = 26)	Autopsy (% of total) (n = 59)	Combined (% of total) (n = 85)
No pathogens	15 (57.7)	34 (57.6)	49 (57.6)
MAI	8 (30.8)	6 (10.2)	14 (16.5)
KS	0 (0.0)	11 (18.6)	11 (12.9)
CMV	2 (7.7)	6 (10.2)	8 (9.4)
Lymphoma	2 (7.7)	2 (3.4)	4 (4.7)
Cryptococcus	0 (0.0)	2 (3.4)	2 (2.4)
Histoplasma	0 (0.0)	1 (1.7)	1 (1.2)
Coccidioides	0 (0.0)	1 (1.7)	1 (1.2)

Source: Adapted from Schneiderman DJ, et al. Hepatology 7:925, 1987, © by Am. Assoc. for the Study of Liver Diseases.
MAI = mycobacterium avium–intracellulare; KS = Kaposi's sarcoma; CMV = cytomegalovirus.

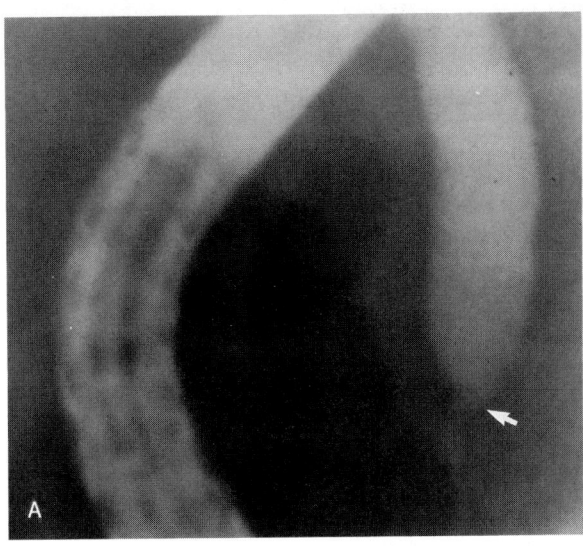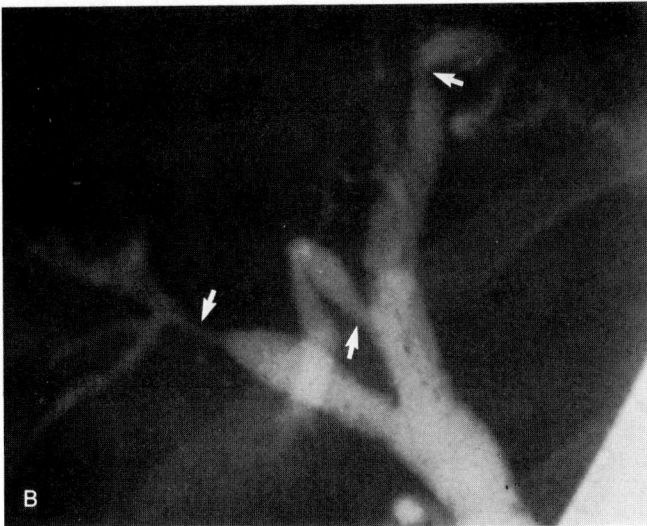

Figure 53–15. Typical bile duct abnormalities in patients with acquired immunodeficiency syndrome identified by endoscopic retrograde cholangiography. A, Dilated common bile duct with a short stricture consistent with papillary stenosis (arrow) in the most distal duct. B, Multiple strictures, consistent with sclerosing cholangitis, in the intrahepatic ducts (arrows).

mation, are nonspecific. Granulomas have frequently been observed and are most commonly associated with mycobacterial infection, usually *Mycobacterium avium–intracellulare*.[138, 139, 145, 146] Although this organism can usually be identified histologically by special techniques, cultures of liver tissue may at times be positive in the absence of histologically identifiable organisms.[139, 146] A variety of other specific AIDS-related diagnoses (Table 53–13) can be made by examination of liver tissue obtained by biopsy or at autopsy, including lymphoma, Kaposi's sarcoma, and infections with CMV, *Cryptococcus, Histoplasma,* and *Coccidioides* organisms.[138–146] However, these diagnoses will frequently have been made prior to liver biopsy, by other means,[139] or they involve diseases for which there is no effective therapy. Thus, in many patients with AIDS, the information obtained through liver biopsy rarely affects therapeutic decisions or leads to improved survival.[138] For this reason, it has been proposed that liver biopsy be reserved for those with unexplained fever and an elevated serum alkaline phosphatase and for those with focal mass lesions in the liver identified by sonography or computed tomography.[139]

HEPATITIS B VIRUS INFECTION IN AIDS

From 75 to 95 per cent of patients with AIDS have serologic evidence of active or previous infection with the HBV.[138, 139, 145] This range is slightly higher than the 50 to 75 per cent observed in studies of homosexual men performed at sexually transmitted disease clinics in the United States without regard to AIDS status.[147] Conversely, it has been reported that almost one third of homosexual males who tested positive for HBsAg had antibodies to the human immunodeficiency virus (HIV).[148] Coexisting infection with HBV and HIV appears to increase HBV replication and may extend the period of active viral replication or even lead to reactivation of HBV infection.[148, 149] This may increase the potential for transmission of HBV by these doubly infected patients. Interestingly, HIV infection appears to diminish the inflammatory component of chronic HBV infection, perhaps by reducing the immunologic response.[148, 149]

ABNORMALITIES OF THE BILE DUCTS IN AIDS

Strictures of the bile ducts have been reported in patients with AIDS.[150, 151] These may involve only the most distal portion of the common duct (papillary stenosis) or more commonly, may diffusely affect both the intrahepatic and extrahepatic ducts (sclerosing cholangitis). Patients usually present with epigastric or right upper quadrant abdominal pain and may give a history of nausea and vomiting, fever, and rigors. Bacterial cholangitis has been reported. Serum alkaline phosphatase levels have uniformly been elevated two- to more than tenfold above normal values, with less striking aminotransferase elevations. Serum bilirubin is frequently normal, although mild elevations (2 to 3 mg/dl) have been observed.[150, 151]

Although abdominal sonography and computed tomography will frequently identify biliary abnormalities in patients with AIDS, endoscopic retrograde cholangiopancreatography (ERCP) most clearly demonstrates the abnormalities.[152] Although one patient has been reported with isolated papillary stenosis and common duct dilation,[151, 152] typically there are focal areas of dilation mixed with areas of irregularity and stricturing of the intrahepatic and extrahepatic bile ducts (Fig. 53–15).

The cause of these bile duct abnormalities in AIDS patients has not yet been determined with certainty. However, it is likely that they are the result of opportunistic infections, and both cytomegalovirus and *Cryptosporidium* organisms have been observed on biopsies of the ampulla of Vater or bile ducts.[151, 152] Surgical T-tube drainage and sphincteroplasty[150] and endoscopic sphincterotomy[151, 152] have been employed in an attempt to treat this disorder. The experience with surgical approaches has been too limited to allow for any firm conclusions as to their efficacy but has not resulted in substantial, lasting improvement.[150] Endoscopic sphincterotomy has resulted in a decrease in abdominal pain in most patients but did not consistently prevent recurrent cholangitis or decrease bile duct dilation or serum alkaline phosphatase levels.[151, 152] The diffuse involvement of the bile ducts seen in most patients appears to limit the effectiveness of both surgical and endoscopic forms of therapy.

TABLE 53–14. FEATURES OF ADULT REYE'S SYNDROME

Viral Illness	ASA	AST	PT	Bilirubin	Ammonia	Died*
6/7‡	5/6	<36† 270–1500	≥2 sec 6/7	<2 mg/dl 6/7	<60 µg/dl† 136–381	2/7

Source: Adapted from information appearing in NEJM, Isobe T, Osserman EF. N Engl J Med 290:473, 1974.
*One patient suffered serious permanent neurologic injury.
†Upper limit of normal.
‡5 had influenza A or B, 1 had varicella.

REYE'S SYNDROME

In 1963 Reye and co-workers described an illness in children that was marked by encephalopathy and fatty infiltration of the liver.[153] The illness typically follows an episode of influenza or varicella and begins with the onset of pernicious nausea and vomiting. In early stages of illness, the patients are awake and alert but irritable. Patients may develop only a mild encephalopathy (lethargy or disorientation without coma), or there may be progressive deterioration of their mental state leading to deep coma (decerebrate rigidity or flaccidity) and death from cerebral edema. Blood ammonia levels may be normal in patients who are mildly encephalopathic, but levels become abnormal as the coma worsens and tend to be highest in those with the worst encephalopathy. The liver may be enlarged, and there is evidence of hepatic injury at the earliest stages of the disease. Serum levels of the aminotransferases (AST and ALT) are increased, as is the prothrombin time. The serum bilirubin, however, is normal or only mildly increased.[153–157] If a liver biopsy is performed, the hepatocytes are swollen and contain microvesicular droplets of fat that is similar in appearance to that found in fatty liver of pregnancy, Jamaican vomiting, valproic acid toxicity and a number of inherited disorders of fatty acid metabolism. Liver cell necrosis and portal inflammation are absent or minimally present.[158] To fulfill the Centers for Disease Control criteria for the diagnosis of Reye's syndrome, the patient must have (1) acute noninflammatory encephalopathy clinically documented by an alteration in consciousness and if available, cerebrospinal fluid containing less than 8 leukocytes/mm³; (2) hepatopathy documented by liver biopsy or autopsy or a threefold or greater rise of AST, ALT, or serum ammonia; (3) no more reasonable explanation for the cerebral or hepatic abnormalities.[159]

Although Reye's syndrome is most common in children, well-described cases in adults have been reported by a number of authors.[160–162] The findings from a group of seven adult patients with Reye's syndrome are shown in Table 53–14. The illness in adults is quite similar to that in children in that it is preceded by a viral illness and aspirin use is common. The severity of biochemical abnormalities also are similar, and the mortality (28 per cent) in this small series is not different from that seen with children (Fig. 53–16). Treatment of a patient with Reye's syndrome is similar to that given to any patient with acute hepatic failure of any etiology and is detailed in Chapter 17.

Reye's syndrome is principally a disease of children. In 1985, 91 cases of Reye's syndrome were reported to the Centers for Disease Control, with 53 per cent aged less than 4, 20 per cent 5 to 9, 19 per cent 10 to 14, 15 per cent 15 to 19, and 3 per cent more than 20 years.[163] Since 1980, the incidence of Reye's syndrome in the population of the United States has dropped dramatically (Fig. 53–16). The peak incidence of Reye's syndrome occurred in 1980 with 0.88 cases per 100,000 population less than 18 years of age. In 1986, this incidence had fallen to 0.16 cases per 100,000 population.[164] The most dramatic fall has been observed in the 0 to 9 years age group.[163] The reasons for this decline are unclear, but it is associated with a decrease in the use of aspirin for treatment of respiratory tract diseases in this same population.[165, 166] Although this would seem to suggest a causal association between aspirin usage and Reye's syndrome (see later), after an epidemic of Reye's syndrome in New Zealand in the late 1950s and early 1960s, the disease has virtually disappeared from that country for unexplained reasons.[155] A similar event may be occurring in the United States.

The pathogenesis of Reye's syndrome is not understood. The current state of our understanding has recently been reviewed,[155] and the focus of interest is on alterations in the mitochondria and their metabolism of fatty acids. The mitochondria of the liver in a patient with Reye's syndrome are abnormal both functionally and morphologically. They are enlarged, with disrupted cristae and reduced numbers of dense bodies.[167] Reductions in mitochondrial enzymes involved in synthesis of urea and citric acid cycle have been reported.[168–170] In addition, there are increased levels of dicarboxylic acids in the urines of patients with Reye's syndrome, suggesting decreased β-oxidation of fatty acids in the mitochondria (see Chap. 4).[155] Unfortunately, it is unclear what leads to these alterations in mitochondrial function and how these alterations affect the clinical presentation of the disease. For example, in the brain, mitochondrial enzyme activities are not reduced in patients with Reye's syndrome.[155]

Recently, there has been a great deal of interest in the role of salicylates in the pathogenesis of Reye's syndrome. Based on a number of epidemiologic studies, there appears to be an association between Reye's syndrome and recent use of aspirin.[171–173] The calculated odds ratio of developing Reye's syndrome after aspirin exposure and an appropriate viral illness was calculated to be 16:1.[173] The mechanism whereby aspirin may contribute to the development of Reye's syndrome is unclear, and patients can develop the syndrome in the absence of ingestion of aspirin. Despite a

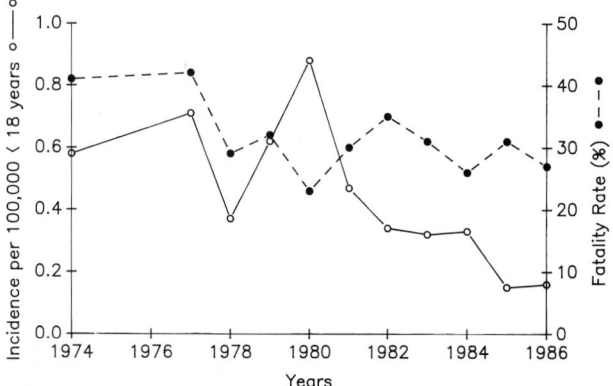

Figure 53–16. Yearly incidence of Reye's syndrome and associated case: fatality ratio (mortality) reported to the Centers for Disease Control. Incidence is per 100,000 population less than 18 years of age. (Data is from MMWR 36:689, 1987.)

lack of understanding of how aspirin may contribute to the development of Reye's syndrome, the epidemiologic evidence of an association is compelling enough to restrict the use of salicylates in children during periods of influenza activity or in the presence of varicella. Although adults with Reye's syndrome also frequently had taken salicylates, there is inadequate data to determine whether this also contributed to the appearance of Reye's syndrome in these older patients. With the decreasing incidence of Reye's syndrome in the United States and, secondarily, decline in an awareness of this rare disease, the physician will have to remain alert to the possibility of Reye's syndrome in both children and adults with vomiting and mild changes in sensorium following a viral illness. Only by maintaining this awareness can the patient with Reye's syndrome be diagnosed early and appropriate therapy be undertaken.[174, 175]

REFERENCES

1. Cornwell GG, Husby G, Westermark P, et al. Identification and characterization of different amyloid fibril proteins in tissue sections. Scand J Immunol 6:1071, 1977.
2. Husby G, Natvig JB, Michaelsen TE. Unique amyloid protein subunit common to different types of amyloid fibril. Nature 244:326, 1973.
3. Franklin EC. The complexity of amyloid (editorial). N Engl J Med 290:512, 1974.
4. Husby G, Sletten K, Michaelsen TE, et al. Amyloid fibril protein subunit, Protein A': distribution in tissue and serum in different clinical types of amyloidosis including that associated with myelomatosis and Waldenstrom's macroglobulinemia. Scand J Immunol 2:395, 1973.
5. Rosenthal CJ, Franklin EC. Variation with age and disease of an amyloid A protein-related serum component. J Clin Invest 55:746, 1975.
6. DeBeer FC, Mallya RK, Fagan EA, et al. Serum amyloid-A protein concentration in inflammatory diseases and its relationship to the incidence of reactive systemic amyloidosis. Lancet 2:231, 1982.
7. Kyle RA, Bayrd ED. Amyloidosis: review of 236 cases. Medicine 54:271, 1975.
8. Isobe T, Osserman EF. Patterns of amyloidosis and their association with plasma-cell dyscrasia, monoclonal immunoglobulins and Bence-Jones proteins. N Engl J Med 290:473, 1974.
9. Levine RA. Amyloid disease of the liver. Am J Med 33:349, 1962.
10. Gange RW. Systemic amyloidosis. Proc R Soc Med 69:231, 1976.
11. Rubinow A, Cohen AS. Skin involvement in generalized amyloidosis. Ann Intern Med 88:781, 1978.
12. Levy M, Polliack A, Lender M, et al. The liver in amyloidosis. Digestion 10:40, 1974.
13. Rubinow A, Koff RS, Cohen AS. Severe intrahepatic cholestasis in primary amyloidosis. Am J Med 64:937, 1978.
14. Mir-Madjlessi SH, Farmer RG, Hawk WA. Cholestatic jaundice associated with primary amyloidosis. Cleveland Clin Q 39:167, 1972.
15. Levy M, Fryd CH, Eliakim M. Intrahepatic obstructive jaundice due to amyloidosis of the liver. Gastroenterology, 61:234, 1971.
16. Yood RA, Skinner M, Rubinow A, et al. Bleeding manifestations in 100 patients with amyloidosis. JAMA 249:1322, 1983.
17. Westermark P, Stenkvist B. A new method for the diagnosis of systemic amyloidosis. Arch Intern Med 132:522, 1973.
18. Pasternack A. Fine-needle aspiration biopsy of spleen in diagnosis of generalized amyloidosis. Br Med J 2:20, 1974.
19. McPherson RA, Onstad JW, Ugoretz RS, et al. Coagulopathy in amyloidosis: combined deficiency of factors IX and X. Am J Hematol 3:225, 1977.
20. Greipp PR, Kyle RA, Bowie EJW. Factor X deficiency in primary amyloidosis. N Engl J Med 301:1050, 1979.
21. Redleaf PD, Davis RB, Kucinski C, et al. Amyloidosis with an unusual bleeding diathesis. Ann Intern Med 58:347, 1963.
22. Suzuki K, Okuda K, Yoshida T, et al. False-positive liver scan in a patient with hepatic amyloidosis: case report. J Nucl Med 17:31, 1976.
23. Goergen TG, Taylor A, Alazraki N. Lack of gallium uptake in primary hepatic amyloidosis. Am J Roentgenol 126:1246, 1976.
24. Vanek JA, Cook SA, Bukowski RM. Hepatic uptake of Tc-99m-labeled diphosphonate in amyloidosis; case report. J Nucl Med 18:1086, 1977.
25. Bradstock K, Clancy R, Uther J, et al. The successful treatment of
26. Gertz MA, Kyle RA. Response of primary hepatic amyloidosis to melphalan and prednisone: a case report and review of the literature. Mayo Clin Proc 61:218, 1986.
27. Fausa O, Nygaard K, Elgjo K. Amyloidosis and Crohn's disease. Scand J Gastroenterol 12:657, 1977.
28. Ravid M, Robson M, Kedar I. Prolonged colchicine treatment in four patients with amyloidosis. Ann Intern Med 87:568, 1977.
29. Zemer D, Pras M, Sohar E, et al. Colchicine in the prevention and treatment of the amyloidosis of familial Mediterranean fever. N Engl J Med 314:1001, 1986.
30. Bradley SE. The circulation and the liver. Gastroenterology 44:403, 1963.
31. Tygstrup N. Aspects of hepatic hypoxia: observations on the isolated perfused pig liver. Bull NY Acad Med 51:551, 1975.
32. Richman SM, Delman AJ, Grob D. Alterations in indices of liver function in congestive heart failure with particular reference to serum enzymes. Am J Med 30:211, 1961.
33. Sherlock S. The liver in heart failure. Br Heart J 13:273, 1952.
34. Dunn GD, Hayes P, Breen KS, et al. The liver in congestive heart failure: a review. Am J Med Sci 265:174, 1973.
35. Nunes G, Blaisdell FW, Margaretten W. Mechanism of hepatic dysfunction following shock and trauma. Arch Surg 100:546, 1970.
36. Losowsky MS, Ikram H, Snow HM, et al. Liver function in advanced heart disease. Br Heart J 27:578, 1965.
37. Semb BKH, Halvorsen SF, Fossdal JE, et al. Visceral ischemia following coeliac and superior mesenteric artery occlusion. Acta Chir Scand 143:185, 1977.
38. Weinberg AG, Bolande RP. The liver in congenital heart disease. Am J Dis Child 119:390, 1970.
39. Birgens HS, Henriksen S, Matzen P, et al. The shock liver. Acta Med Scand 204:417, 1978.
40. Ware AJ. The liver when the heart fails (editorial). Gastroenterology 74:627, 1978.
41. Myers JD, Hickam JB. An estimation of the hepatic blood flow and splanchnic oxygen consumption in heart failure. J Clin Invest 27:620, 1948.
42. De la Monte SM, Arcidi JM, Moore GM, et al. Midzonal necrosis as a pattern of hepatocellular injury after shock. Gastroenterology 86:627, 1984.
43. Kisloff B, Schaffer G. Fulminant hepatic failure secondary to congestive heart failure. Dig Dis Sci 21:859, 1976.
44. Bynum TE, Boitnott JK, Maddrey WC. Ischemic hepatitis. Dig Dis Sci 24:129, 1979.
45. Logan RG, Mowry FM, Judge RD. Cardiac failure simulating viral hepatitis. Ann Intern Med 56:784, 1962.
46. Cohen JA, Kaplan MM. Left-sided heart failure presenting as hepatitis. Gastroenterology 74:583, 1978.
47. Field RS, Meyer GW. Hepatic dysfunction in congestive heart failure simulating hepatitis. South Med J 71:221, 1978.
48. Shibuya A, Unuma T, Sugimoto T, et al. Diffuse hepatic calcification as a sequela to shock liver. Gastroenterology 89:196, 1985.
49. Mace S, Borkat G, Liebman J. Hepatic dysfunction and cardiovascular abnormalities: occurrence in infants, children, and young adults. Am J Dis Child 139:60, 1985.
50. Stauffer MH. Nephrogenic hepatosplenomegaly (abstr). Gastroenterology 40:694, 1961.
51. Utz DC, Warren MM, Gregg JA, et al. Reversible hepatic dysfunction associated with hypernephroma. Mayo Clin Proc 45:161, 1970.
52. Ramos CV, Taylor HB. Hepatic dysfunction associated with renal carcinoma. Cancer 29:1287, 1972.
53. Axelsson U, Hagerstrand I, Zettervall O. Unusual pattern of hepatic alkaline phosphatase activity and renal carcinoma. Acta Med Scand 195:223, 1974.
54. Jacobi GH, Phillipp T. Stauffer's syndrome—diagnostic help in hypernephroma. Clin Nephrol 4:113, 1975.
55. Strickland RC, Schenker S. The nephrogenic hepatic dysfunction syndrome: a review. Dig Dis 22:49, 1977.
56. Madayag MA, Bosniak MA, Kinkhabwala M, et al. Hemangiomas of the liver in patients with renal cell carcinoma. Radiology 126:391, 1978.
57. Deweerd JH, Hawthorne J, Adson MA. Regression of renal cell hepatic metastasis following removal of primary lesions. J Urol 117:790, 1977.
58. Abt AB, Kirschner RH, Belliveau RF, et al. Hepatic pathology associated with Hodgkin's disease. Cancer 33:1564, 1974.
59. Kadin ME, Donaldson SS, Dorfman RF. Isolated granulomas in Hodgkin's disease. N Engl J Med 283:859, 1970.
60. Roth A, Kolaric K, Dominis M. Histologic and cytologic liver changes in 120 patients with malignant lymphomas. Tumori 64:45, 1978.
61. Davey FR, Doyle WF. Hepatic alterations in Hodgkin's disease. NY State J Med 73:1981, 1973.
62. Aisenberg AC, Kaplan MM, Rieder SV, et al. Serum alkaline phosphatase at the onset of Hodgkin's disease. Cancer 26:318, 1970.

63. Meinders LE, Werre JM, Brandt KH, et al. Intrahepatic cholestasis in Hodgkin's disease. Neth J Med 19:287, 1976.
64. Piken EP, Abraham GE, Hepner GW. Investigation of a patient with Hodgkin's disease and cholestasis. Gastroenterology 77:145, 1979.
65. Trotter MC, Cloud GA, Davis M, et al. Predicting the risk of abdominal disease in Hodgkin's lymphoma. Ann Surg 201:465, 1985.
66. Harris JM, Tang DB, Weltz MD. Diagnostic tests and Hodgkin's disease. Cancer 41:2388, 1978.
67. Bagley CM, Thomas LB, Johnson RE, et al. Diagnosis of liver involvement by lymphoma: results in 96 consecutive peritoneoscopies. Cancer 31:840, 1973.
68. Coleman M, Lightdale CJ, Vinciguerra VP, et al. Peritoneoscopy in Hodgkin's disease. JAMA 236:2634, 1976.
69. Chambers TJ, O'Donoghue DP, Stansfeld AG. A case of primary lymphoma of the liver. J Clin Pathol 29:967, 1976.
70. Ryoo JW, Manaligod JR, Walker MJ. Primary lymphoma of the liver. J Clin Gastroenterol 8:308, 1986.
71. Osborne BM, Butler JJ, Guarda LA. Primary lymphoma of the liver. Cancer 56:2902, 1985.
72. Kolaric K, Roth A, Dominis M, et al. The diagnostic value of percutaneous liver biopsy in patients with non-Hodgkin's lymphoma—a preliminary report. Acta Hepatogastroenterol 24:440, 1977.
73. Verdi CJ, Grogan TM, Protell R, et al. Liver biopsy immunotyping to characterize lymphoid malignancies. Hepatology 6:6, 1986.
74. Perez-Soler R, Estebon R, Allende E, et al. Liver involvement in multiple myeloma. Am J Hematol 20:25, 1985.
75. Rosenblate HJ, Eisenstein R, Holmes AW. The liver in sickle cell anemia. Arch Pathol 90:235, 1970.
76. Sheehy TW. Sickle cell hepatopathy. South Med J 70:533, 1977.
77. Schubert TT. Hepatobiliary system in sickle cell disease. Gastroenterology 90:2013, 1986.
78. Johnson CS, Omata M, Tong MJ, et al. Liver involvement in sickle cell disease. Medicine 64:349, 1985.
79. Omata M, Johnson CS, Tong M, et al. Pathological spectrum of liver diseases in sickle cell disease. Dig Dis Sci 31:247, 1986.
80. Flyè MW, Silver D. Biliary tract disorders and sickle cell disease. Surgery 72:361, 1972.
81. Solanki DL, McCurdy PR. Cholelithiasis in sickle cell anemia: a case for elective cholecystectomy. Am J Med Sci 277:319, 1979.
82. Klion FM, Weiner MJ, Schaffner F. Cholestasis in sickle cell anemia. Am J Med 37:829, 1964.
83. Owen DM, Aldridge JE, Thompson RB. An unusual hepatic sequela of sickle cell anemia: a report of five cases. Am J Med Sci 249:175, 1965.
84. Green TW, Conley CL, Berthrong M. The liver in sickle cell anemia. Johns Hopkins Med J 92:127, 1953.
85. Buchanan GR, Glader BE. Benign course of extreme hyperbilirubinemia in sickle cell anemia: analysis of six cases. J Pediatr 91:21, 1977.
86. Krishnamurthy M, Elguezabal A, Lee CK, et al. Bland cholestasis—unusual hepatic sequela in sickle cell anemia. Postgrad Med 64:215, 1978.
87. Maddrey WC, Cukier SO, Maglalang AC, et al. Hepatic bilirubin UDP-glucuronyltransferase in patients with sickle cell anemia. Gastroenterology 74:193, 1978.
88. O'Leary JP, Maher JW, Hollenbeck JI, et al. Pathogenesis of hepatic failure after obesity bypass. Surg Forum 15:256, 1974.
89. Drenick EJ, Fisler J, Johnson D. Hepatic steatosis after intestinal bypass—prevention and reversal by metronidazole irrespective of protein-calorie malnutrition. Gastroenterology 82:535, 1982.
90. Vanderhoof JA, Tuma DJ, Sorrell MF. Role of defunctionalized bowel in jejunoileal bypass–induced liver disease in rats. Dig Dis Sci 24:916, 1979.
91. Hollenbeck JI, O'Leary JP, Maher JW, et al. An etiologic basis for fatty liver after jejunoileal bypass. J Surg Res 18:83, 1975.
92. Moxley R, Pozeksky T, Lockwood DH. Protein nutrition and liver disease after jejunoileal bypass for morbid obesity. N Engl J Med 290:921, 1974.
93. Ames F, Copeland E, Leeb D, et al. Liver dysfunction following small-bowel bypass for morbid obesity. N Engl J Med 290:921, 1974.
94. Baker AL, Elson CO, Gaspan J, et al. Liver failure with steatonecrosis after jejunoileal bypass. Arch Intern Med 139:289, 1979.
95. Brown R, O'Leary J, Woodward E. Hepatic effects of jejunoileal bypass for morbid obesity. Am J Surg 127:53, 1974.
96. Peters R, Gay T, Reynolds TB. Post–jejunoileal-bypass hepatic disease. Am J Clin Pathol 63:318, 1975.
97. Kaminski DL, Hermann VM, Martin S. Late effects of jejunoileal bypass operations on hepatic inflammation, fibrosis, and lipid content. Hepatogastroenterology 32:159, 1985.
98. Galdmbos JT, Wills CE. Relationship between 505 paired liver tests and biopsies in 242 obese patients. Gastroenterology 74:1191, 1978.
99. Baddeley RM. An epilogue to jejunoileal bypass. World J Surg 9:842, 1985.
100. Nasrallah SM, Wills CE, Galambos JT. Liver injury following jejunoileal bypass. Are there markers? Ann Surg 192:726, 1980.
101. Montorsi W, Doldi SB, Klinger R, et al. Surgical therapy for morbid obesity. Int Surg 71:84, 1986.
102. Peters RL. Hepatic morphologic changes after jejunoileal bypass. In: Popper H, Schaffner F, eds. Progress in Liver Diseases, Vol 6. New York, Grune & Stratton, 1979:518.
103. Halverson J, Wise L, Wazna M, et al. Jejunoileal bypass for morbid obesity: a critical appraisal. Am J Med 64:461, 1978.
104. Weismann RE, Johnson RE. Fatal hepatic failure after jejunoileal bypass: clinical and laboratory evidence of prognostic significance. Am J Surg 134:253, 1977.
105. Soyer MT, Ceballos R, Aldrete JS. Reversibility of severe hepatic damage caused by jejunoileal bypass after re-establishment of normal continuity. Surgery 79:601, 1976.
106. Sheldon GF, Petersen SR, Sanders R. Hepatic dysfunction during hyperalimentation. Arch Surg 113:504, 1978.
107. Lindon KD, Fleming CR, Abrams A, et al. Liver function values in adults receiving total parenteral nutrition. JAMA 241:2398, 1973.
108. Bower RH. Hepatic complications of parenteral nutrition. Semin Liver Dis 3:216, 1983.
109. Nanji AA. The pathogenesis of cholestasis in parenteral nutrition. (Letter.) J Parenter Enter Nutr 9:524, 1985.
110. Giner M, Curtas S. Adverse metabolic consequences of nutritional support: macronutrients. Surg Clin N Amer 66:1025, 1986.
111. Postuma R, Trevenes CL. Liver disease in infants receiving total parenteral nutrition. Pediatrics 63:110, 1979.
112. Bowyer BA, Fleming CR, Ludwig J, et al. Does long-term home parenteral nutrition in adult patients cause chronic liver disease? J Parenter Enter Nutr 9:11, 1985.
113. Nanji AA, Anderson FH. Sensitivity and specificity of liver function tests in the detection of parenteral nutrition-associated cholestasis. J Parenter Enter Nutr 9:307, 1985.
114. Grant JP, Cox CE, Kleinman LM, et al. Serum hepatic enzyme and bilirubin elevations during parenteral nutrition. Surg Gynecol Obstet 145:573, 1977.
115. Craig RM, Neuman T, Jeejeebhoy KN, et al. Severe hepatocellular reaction resembling alcoholic hepatitis with cirrhosis after massive small-bowel resection and prolonged total parenteral nutrition. Gastroenterology 79:131, 1980.
116. Harvey AMG, Shulman LE, Tumulty PA, et al. Systemic lupus erythematosus: review of the literature and analysis of 138 cases. Medicine (Baltimore) 33:291, 1954.
117. MacKay IR, Taft LI, Cowling DC. Lupoid hepatitis and the hepatic lesions of systemic lupus erythematosus. Lancet 1:65, 1969.
118. Runyon BA, LaBrecque DR, Anuras S. The spectrum of liver disease in systemic lupus erythematosus. Report of 33 histologically proved cases and review of the literature. Am J Med 69:187, 1980.
119. Seaman WE, Ishak KG, Plotz PH. Aspirin-induced hepatotoxicity in patients with systemic lupus erythematosus. Ann Intern Med 80:1, 1974.
120. Rich RR, Johnson JS. Salicylate hepatotoxicity in patients with juvenile rheumatoid arthritis. Arthritis Rheum 16:1, 1973.
121. Whaley K, Williamson J, Dick WC, et al. Liver disease in Sjögren's syndrome and rheumatoid arthritis. Lancet 1:861, 1970.
122. Blendis LM, Parkinson ML, Shelkin KB, et al. Nodular regenerative hyperplasia of the liver in Felty's syndrome. Q J Med 43:252, 1974.
123. Thorne C, Urowitz MD, Wanless I, et al. Liver disease in Felty's syndrome. Am J Med 73:35, 1982.
124. Wanless IR, Godwin TA, Allen F, et al. Nodular regenerative hyperplasia of the liver in hematologic disorders: a possible response to obliterative portal venulopathy. Medicine (Baltimore) 59:367, 1980.
125. Vanselow NA, Dodson VN, Angell DC. A clinical study of Sjögren's syndrome. Ann Intern Med 58:124, 1963.
126. Whaley K, Goudie RB, Dick WC, et al. Liver disease in Sjögren's syndrome and rheumatoid arthritis. Lancet 1:861, 1970.
127. Webb J, Whaley K, MacSween RNM, et al. Liver disease in rheumatoid arthritis and Sjögren's syndrome: prospective study using biochemical and serological markers of hepatic dysfunction. Ann Rheum Dis 34:70, 1975.
128. Doniach D, Walker JG. A limited concept of autoimmune hepatitis. Lancet 1:813, 1969.
129. Reynolds TB, Denison EK, Frankl HD. Primary biliary cirrhosis with scleroderma, Raynaud's phenomenon and telangiectasia. Am J Med 50:302, 1971.
130. Dickson ER, Maldonado JE, Sheps SG, Cain JA Jr. Systemic giant-cell arteritis with polymyalgia rheumatica. JAMA 224:1496, 1973.
131. Litvack KD, Bohan A, Silverman L. Granulomatous liver disease and giant cell arteritis. Case report and literature review. J Rheumatol 4:307, 1977.

132. Sopko J, Anuras S. Liver disease in renal transplant recipients. Am J Med 64:139, 1978.
133. Anuras S, Piros J, Bonney WW, et al. Liver disease in renal transplant recipients. Arch Intern Med 137:42, 1977.
134. Ware AJ, Luby SP, Eigenbrodt EH, et al. Spectrum of liver disease in renal transplant recipients. Gastroenterology 68:755, 1975.
135. Montgomerie JZ, Becroft DM, Croxson MD, et al. Herpes simplex virus infection after renal transplantation. Lancet 2:867, 1969.
136. Pien FD, Smith TF, Adenson CF, et al. Herpes viruses in renal transplant patients. Transplantation 16:489, 1973.
137. Ireland P, Rashid A, Von Lechtenberg F, et al. Liver disease in kidney transplant patients receiving azathioprine. Arch Intern Med 132:29, 1973.
138. Gordon SC, Reddy KR, Gould EE, et al. The spectrum of liver disease in the acquired immunodeficiency syndrome. J Hepatol 2:475, 1986.
139. Schneiderman DJ, Arenson DM, Cello JP, et al. Hepatic disease in patients with the acquired immune deficiency syndrome (AIDS). Hepatology 7:925, 1987.
140. Mobley K, Rotterdam HZ, Lerner CW, et al. Autopsy findings in the acquired immune deficiency syndrome. Pathology 20:45, 1985.
141. Glasgow BJ, Anders K, Layfield LJ, et al. Clinical and pathologic findings of the liver in the acquired immune deficiency syndrome (AIDS). Am J Clin Pathol 83:582, 1985.
142. Guarda LA, Luna MA, Smith JL, et al. Acquired immune deficiency syndrome: post-mortem findings. Am J Clin Pathol 81:549, 1984.
143. Welch K, Finkbeiner W, Alpers CE, et al. Autopsy findings in the acquired immune deficiency syndrome. JAMA 252:1152, 1984.
144. Reichert CM, O'Leary TJ, Levens DL, et al. Autopsy pathology in the acquired immune deficiency syndrome. Am J Pathol 112:357, 1983.
145. Lebovics E, Thung SN, Schaffner F, Radensky PW. The liver in the acquired immunodeficiency syndrome: a clinical and histologic study. Hepatology 5:293, 1985.
146. Orenstein MS, Tavitian A, Yonk B, et al. Granulomatous involvement of the liver in patients with AIDS. Gut 26:1220, 1985.
147. Schreder MT, Thompson SE, Hadler SC, et al. Hepatitis B in homosexual men: prevalence of infection and factors related to transmission. J Infect Dis 146:7, 1982.
148. Krogsgaard K, Lindhardt BO, Nielsen JO, et al. The influence of HTLV-III infection on the natural history of hepatitis B virus infection in male homosexual HbsAg carriers. Hepatology 7:37, 1987.
149. Perrillo RP, Regenstein FG, Roodman ST. Chronic hepatitis B in asymptomatic homosexual men with antibody to the human immunodeficiency virus. Ann Intern Med 105:382, 1986.
150. Margulis SJ, Honig CL, Soave R, et al. Biliary tract obstruction in the acquired immunodeficiency syndrome. Ann Intern Med 105:207, 1986.
151. Schneiderman DJ, Cello JP, Laing FC. Papillary stenosis and sclerosing cholangitis in the acquired immunodeficiency syndrome. Ann Intern Med 106:546, 1987.
152. Dolmatch BL, Laing FC, Federle MP, et al. AIDS-related cholangitis: radiographic findings in nine patients. Radiology 163:313, 1987.
153. Reye RDK, Morgan G, Baral J. Encephalopathy and fatty degenera-

154. DeVivo DC. Reye syndrome. Neurol Clin North Am 3:95, 1985.
155. Heubi JE, Partin JC, Partin JS, et al. Reye's syndrome: current concepts. Hepatology 7:155, 1987.
156. Schubert WK, Partin JC, Partin JS. Encephalopathy and fatty liver (Reye's syndrome). In: Popper H, Schaffner FF, eds. Progress in Liver Disease, Vol 4. New York, Grune & Stratton, 1972:489.
157. Bove KE. Reye's syndrome. In: Zakim D, Boyer TD, eds. Hepatology: A Textbook of Liver Disease, 1st ed. Philadelphia, WB Saunders, 1982:1212.
158. Bove KE, McAdams AJ, Partin JC, et al. The hepatic lesion in Reye's syndrome. Gastroenterology 69:685, 1975.
159. Sullivan-Boligai JZ, Corey L. Epidemiology of Reye syndrome. Epidemiol Rev 3:1, 1981.
160. Meythaler MM, Varma RR. Reye's syndrome in adults. Arch Intern Med 147:61, 1987.
161. Peters LJ, Wiener GJ, Gilliam J, et al. Reye's syndrome in adults. Arch Intern Med 146:2401, 1986.
162. Kirkpatrick DB, Ottoson C, Bateman LL. Reye's syndrome in an adult patient. West J Med 144:223, 1986.
163. Reye Syndrome—United States, 1985. MMWR 35:66, 1986.
164. Reye Syndrome Surveillance—United States, 1986. MMWR 36:689, 1987.
165. Barrett MJ, Hurwitz ES, Schonberger LB, et al. Changing epidemiology of Reye syndrome in the United States. Pediatrics 77:598, 1986.
166. Arrowsmith JB, Kennedy DL, Kuritsky JN, et al. National patterns of aspirin use and Reye syndrome reporting. United States, 1980 to 1985. Pediatrics 79:858, 1987.
167. Partin JC, Schubert WK, Partin JS. Mitochondrial ultrastructure in Reye's syndrome (encephalopathy and fatty degeneration of the viscera). N Engl J Med 285:1339, 1971.
168. Brown RE, Forman DT. The biochemistry of Reye's syndrome. Crit Rev Clin Lab Sci 17:247, 1982.
169. Brown T, Hug G, Lansky L, et al. Transiently reduced activity of carbamyl phosphate synthetase and ornithine transcarbamylase in liver of children with Reye's syndrome. N Engl J Med 294:861, 1976.
170. Mitchell RA, Ram ML, Arcinue EL, et al. Comparison of cytosolic and mitochondrial enzyme alterations in Reye's syndrome. Pediatr Res 14:1216, 1980.
171. Starko KM, Ray CG, Dominquez LB, et al. Reye's syndrome and salicylate use. Pediatrics 66:859, 1980.
172. Waldman RJ, Hall WN, McGee H, et al. Aspirin as a risk factor in Reye's syndrome. JAMA 247:3089, 1980.
173. Hurwitz ES, Barrett MJ, Bregman D, et al. Public health service study on Reye's syndrome and medications. N Engl J Med 313:849, 1985.
174. Dezateux CA, Helms RD, Matthew DJ. Recognition and early management of Reye's syndrome. Arch Dis Child 61:647, 1986.
175. Heubi JE, Daugherty CC, Partin JS, et al. Grade I Reye's syndrome—outcome and predictors of progression to deeper coma grades. N Engl J Med 311:1539, 1984.

tion of the viscera, a disease entity in childhood. Lancet 2:749, 1963.

54

The Liver in Pregnancy

Rebecca W. Van Dyke, M.D.

DEFINITIONS

AFLP = Acute fatty liver of pregnancy
BSP = Bromsulphalein (sulfobromophthalein sodium)
GGTP = Gamma glutamyl transferase
HELLP syndrome = *H*emolysis, *E*levated *L*iver enzymes, and *L*ow *P*latelet count
IHCP = Intrahepatic cholestasis of pregnancy

The pregnant state is associated with physiologic changes in hepatic function that may cause uncertainty about the presence or absence of liver disease. In addition, common disorders of the liver may present with unusual features during pregnancy. Finally, several types of liver disease are unique to pregnancy. The aspects of liver function and liver disease during pregnancy discussed in this chapter include (1) normal changes in hepatic function during pregnancy, (2) unusual aspects of common liver disorders, (3) liver disorders related to pregnancy, and (4) liver disorders unique to pregnancy.

NORMAL PHYSIOLOGIC CHANGES IN LIVER ANATOMY AND FUNCTION DURING PREGNANCY

ANATOMY AND HISTOLOGY

Liver size and gross appearance do not change during normal pregnancy.[1, 2] Subtle changes in histologic appearance may be seen but are nonspecific in nature. These include (1) increased variability in the size and shape of hepatocytes,[3, 4] (2) granularity of the cytoplasm,[3] (3) more frequent cytoplasmic fat vacuoles in centrilobular hepatocytes,[4] and (4) hypertrophy of the Kupffer cells.[5] Hepatocytes during normal pregnancy also exhibit proliferation of the smooth and rough endoplasmic reticulum; enlarged, rod-shaped, and giant mitochondria with paracrystalline inclusions; and increased numbers of peroxisomes.[6, 7] Many of these changes also are seen in women taking oral contraceptives.[8–10]

LIVER BLOOD FLOW

Blood volume increases by 40 to 50 per cent during pregnancy,[11–13] and there is an increase in cardiac stroke volume and output and a decrease in peripheral resistance.[11] Hepatic blood flow, measured as clearance of BSP (Bromsulphalein [sulfobromophthalein sodium]) or ^{125}I-denatured albumin, is unaltered during pregnancy.[14, 15] Therefore, hepatic blood flow in late pregnancy amounts to a smaller fraction of cardiac output.[14]

CHANGES IN LIVER FUNCTION

Plasma Proteins

Levels of serum albumin in pregnancy are 10 to 60 per cent below those in nonpregnant women, reflecting the increase in plasma volume in pregnancy.[16–20] In addition, synthesis of albumin may be impaired during pregnancy. Levels of albumin and synthesis of albumin also decrease in women taking oral contraceptives.[20, 21] Similarly, plasma levels of antithrombin III and haptoglobin fall during pregnancy or during use of oral contraceptives. These decreases are attributed to decreased hepatic synthesis of these proteins.[20, 22] Plasma concentrations of other serum proteins (e.g., ceruloplasmin, fibrinogen, thyroxine-binding globulin, corticosteroid-binding globulin, transferrin, and other α_1-, α_2-, and β-globulins) and presumably hepatic synthesis are increased in pregnant women[17, 20, 23] and in women receiving oral contraceptives.[17, 22] Prothrombin times, however, are normal during pregnancy.[24]

Plasma Lipids

Increases in peripheral lipolysis of triglycerides, flux of free fatty acids through the liver, hepatic synthesis of triglycerides, hepatic synthesis and secretion of very low–density (VLDL), high-density (HDL), and low-density lipoproteins (LDL) occur during pregnancy.[17, 25–27] These changes are reflected by progressive increases in plasma triglycerides (up to 300 per cent), cholesterol (25–60 per cent), and phospholipids.[19, 25, 26] The increased fat in liver biopsies of some pregnant women may be due to these changes in triglyceride and lipoprotein metabolism. The concentration of cholesterol in bile also is increased during pregnancy or during the use of oral contraceptives.[28]

Drug Metabolism

17-Ethynyl estrogens decrease cytochrome P-450 activity, probably via suicide inactivation of the enzyme.[29] Pharmacokinetic studies suggest impaired metabolism of promazine, pethidine, and cortisol in pregnant women[30, 31] and depressed antipyrine metabolism in women receiving oral contraceptives.[32–34] Estrogens and pregnancy also are associated with decreased hepatic activity of glucuronosyltransferase in rats.[35] In contrast, progestational agents induce hepatic mixed function oxidase activity in animals[36] and oral contraceptives increase clearance of morphine in humans.[37] Thus, pregnancy and oral contraceptives appear to alter drug metabolism, but the effects on any one drug are not readily predictable. The clinical significance of such changes in humans remains unclear.

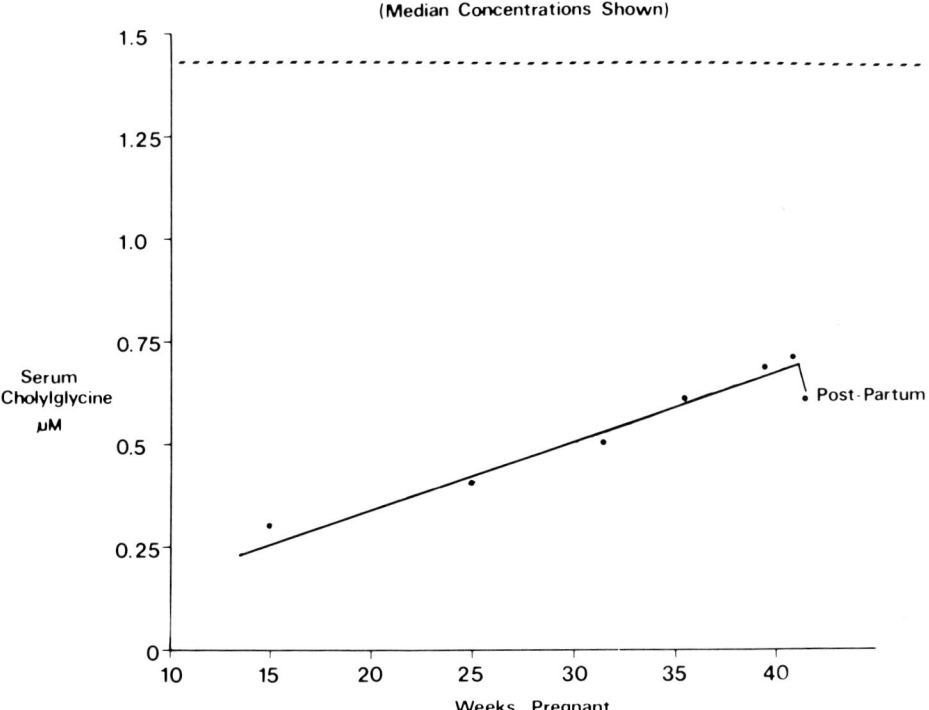

Figure 54–1. Median fasting serum cholylglycine levels measured in 297 normal pregnant women. (Reprinted with permission from Lunzer M, et al. Gastroenterology 91:825. Copyright 1986 by the American Gastroenterological Association.)

Bile Formation

Organic anion transport, including bilirubin,[38–40] and formation of bile are impaired during pregnancy and by administration of estrogens or oral contraceptives. Close to term, many pregnant women exhibit plasma levels of bilirubin that are at the upper limit of the normal range,[41–44] but not generally above it. Retention of the organic anion BSP in plasma increases progressively during pregnancy. Retention of BSP is increased two- to threefold in the third trimester of pregnancy, compared with values measured early in pregnancy or 6 to 16 weeks postpartum,[42, 45] al-though BSP concentration in plasma at 45 minutes generally remains within the broad range of normal values.[2, 42, 45] Hepatic storage capacity (S) for BSP is increased by 22 per cent, and biliary transport maximum (Tm) is decreased by 27 to 70 per cent in late pregnancy.[2, 42] Conjugation of BSP with glutathione appears unaffected in pregnancy suggesting that the transport defect is at the canalicular membrane.[2, 42] Women receiving estrogens or oral contraceptives exhibit similar changes in BSP metabolism.[46, 47]

Concentrations of bile salts in blood are within the normal range in most pregnant women, but concentrations of glycocholate, taurocholate, and chenodeoxycholate may

TABLE 54–1. LIVER TESTS DURING PREGNANCY

Test	Change During Pregnancy	Physiology
Serum bilirubin	None to slight increase	Mild impairment of bilirubin transport with decreased hepatic clearance
Serum bile acids	Progressive increase in serum levels during pregnancy to 200–300% of nonpregnant values	Impaired hepatic transport and/or biliary secretion
Sulfobromophthalein (BSP)	Progressive increase in plasma retention 45 min after administration and decrease in plasma clearance	Slightly increased storage capacity to 122% of nonpregnant values Decrease in biliary transport maximum (T_m) to 27–70% of non-pregnant values
Alkaline phosphatase	Progressive increase in serum activity to 1.5–2 times nonpregnant values	Release of placental alkaline phosphatase
Leucine aminopeptidase	Progressive increase in serum activity	Release of placental enzyme
Gamma glutamyl transpeptidase	Serum activity normal or low	Impaired release, particularly in disease states
Aminotransferases (AST/ALT)	No change	—
Serum albumin	Decreased levels	Hemodilution; possible decrease in synthesis
Prothrombin time	No change	—

rise progressively until term and may exceed levels measured early in pregnancy by two- to threefold (Fig. 54–1).[44, 48–50] These changes in transport of three different organic anions imply that bile formation is impaired during pregnancy or during estrogen administration. This hypothesis is supported by extensive studies in animals[51] (see Chap. 12).

LIVER TESTS (Table 54–1)

During normal pregnancy, alkaline phosphatase activity rises progressively, particularly during the last four months (Fig. 54–2). At term, 42 to 77 per cent of women exhibit alkaline phosphatase activities above the upper limit of normal.[19, 41–43] Values rarely exceed two times the upper limit of normal.[19, 24, 26, 41] The origin of the elevated plasma alkaline phosphatase activity during pregnancy is the placenta, not the liver.[52–55] Plasma leucine aminopeptidase activity also rises during pregnancy[56] (see Fig. 54–2). As with the increase in alkaline phosphatase, this is due to release of a placental enzyme. 5-Nucleotidase is reported either to increase during pregnancy or not to change.[56, 57]

Plasma levels of gamma glutamyl transferase (GGTP) activity may fall slightly during pregnancy[56, 58] (see Fig. 54–2). Levels of GGTP are inappropriately low in women with

viral hepatitis who are either late in pregnancy or taking oral contraceptives.[59] Serum aminotransferase activities (AST/ALT) remain within the normal range during pregnancy.[24, 26, 42] Thus, these latter enzymes are useful tests for identifying hepatocellular damage during pregnancy.

SKIN CHANGES

Several cutaneous vascular changes, commonly associated with chronic liver disease, appear frequently during pregnancy. Vascular spiders in pregnancy, which were first reported in 1914,[60] generally begin as a pale area of skin. A small, central red spot develops subsequently, followed by branching radicles and surrounding erythema.[61] The distribution of spiders is on the face, neck, anterior chest, lower arms, and dorsum of the hand. Bean and colleagues[61] observed vascular spiders in 67 per cent of 484 Caucasian women and 14 per cent of 749 black women at term. In contrast, spiders were seen in only 12 per cent of nonpregnant Caucasian women. Spiders appeared beginning in the second month of pregnancy, with the peak incidence at term. The spiders disappear in 75 per cent of affected women by seven weeks postpartum. A few women, particularly those with frequent pregnancies, exhibit vascular spiders indefinitely.

Palmar erythema is observed during pregnancy in 63 per cent of Caucasian women and 39 per cent of black women,[61] beginning in the second month and increasing in incidence to a peak at term. By seven weeks postpartum, only 9 per cent of Caucasian women and 4 per cent of black women continue to exhibit palmar erythema.

COINCIDENT OCCURENCE OF LIVER DISEASE AND PREGNANCY

This section is a brief review of the manifestations of a group of fairly common liver diseases in the pregnant woman. The reader is referred to Chapters 13, 37, 38, 44, and 47 for complete discussions of these disorders.

ACUTE VIRAL HEPATITIS

In 17 reviews of jaundice during pregnancy, hepatitis, presumably viral in etiology, accounted for 40 per cent of 654 cases of clinical jaundice.[24, 41, 62] The true incidence of clinical and subclinical viral hepatitis in pregnancy is not known; however, from 1970 to 1974 at Parkland Hospital in Dallas, an incidence of 1 in 700 deliveries was noted.[63] The data in Table 54–2 indicate the important features of the disease for mother and fetus.

Maternal Features

The clinical manifestations of acute viral hepatitis in pregnant women do not differ from those noted in nonpregnant women and in men. Laboratory data also are similar to values in nonpregnant individuals. In developed countries, maternal mortality from fulminant hepatitis and liver failure is low. In contrast, in India and the Middle East, pregnant women appear to manifest more severe disease (see Table 54–2). The reasons for these differences in mortality are not clear, although nutritional and viral

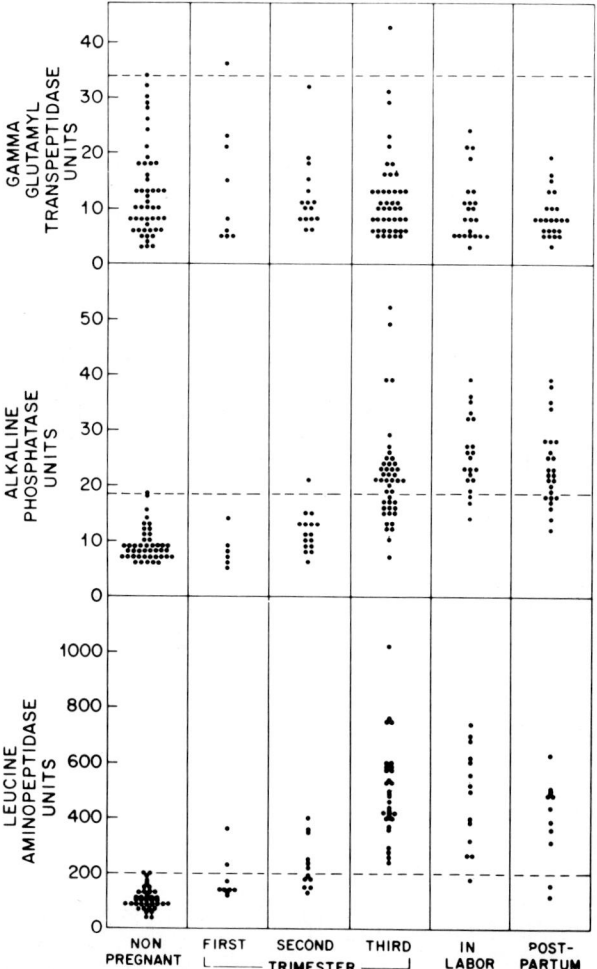

Figure 54–2. Serum activities of three enzymes in normal nonpregnant women and in women in various stages of pregnancy. The broken lines indicate the highest value obtained for each enzyme in nonpregnant women. (Reprinted with permission from The American College of Obstetricians and Gynecologists. Obstetrics and Gynecology, vol. 43, 1974, p. 745.)

TABLE 54–2. ACUTE VIRAL HEPATITIS IN PREGNANCY

Features	Observations
Incidence	0.026–1.2% of gestations
Number of patients	1346
Time of onset (trimester)	
I	13.9%
II	33.5%
III	52.6%
Etiology	4 series: epidemics of non-A, non-B hepatitis
	1 series: epidemic of hepatitis A
	5 series: 11–78% hepatitis B
Fulminant hepatic failure	31.4% (range 0–60%)
Maternal mortality	21.4% (range 0–54%)
	1.2% in the United States, Australia, Israel
	27.0% in India, Middle East
Premature birth	24.6% (range 8.3–54%)
Fetal/neonatal death	29.4% (range 4–89%)
	8.1% in the United States, Australia, Israel
	48.4% in India, Middle East

Source: Data derived from references 64–81.

factors (such as epidemics of non-A, non-B hepatitis[76, 78]) may be important.

Vertical Transmission

In all geographic locations, the fetus is at substantial risk of acquiring acute B-type viral hepatitis from the mother, by a mode of transmission termed vertical transmission.[82] Vertical transmission of hepatitis B is discussed in further detail in Chapters 35 and 37. Vertical transmission of non-A, non-B hepatitis may also occur,[81] and one report documents vertical transmission of delta hepatitis.[83] Vertical transmission of hepatitis A has not been reported.[81] Maternal-fetal transmission most often occurs at the time of delivery; therefore, there is a great risk of transmission when women develop viral hepatitis in the third trimester of pregnancy or when women are chronic carriers of the hepatitis B virus, particularly if they are also positive for HBeAg.[81, 84–87] Immunoprophylaxis with hepatitis B immune globulin and vaccine, administered at the time of birth, is highly effective in preventing vertical transmission of hepatitis B infection to the newborn.[88–92]

ALCOHOL-RELATED LIVER DISEASE

The unique aspect of alcohol ingestion during pregnancy is fetal involvement and the fetal alcohol syndrome. This syndrome generally includes facial abnormalities, congenital malformations, growth retardation, and central nervous system dysfunction. Liver dysfunction also has been found in some affected infants.[93–95] In five infants, hepatomegaly and elevated serum levels of transaminases and alkaline phosphatase were noted. Liver histology was abnormal in all cases, with varying degrees of fatty infiltration, centrizonal hepatocyte degeneration, perivenular sclerosis, portal and perisinusoidal fibrosis, and proliferation of bile ducts. One affected child exhibited cirrhosis and esophageal varices by 8 years of age.[95]

CHRONIC LIVER DISEASE

Fertility appears to be decreased in women with significant liver dysfunction[96] (see Chap. 19). Infertility, which may be reversed by immunosuppressive therapy, may be a presenting symptom in some women with chronic active hepatitis. Women with chronic alcoholic liver disease often exhibit severe and irreversible gonadal failure, amenorrhea, and infertility and rarely become pregnant (see Chap. 19).

Chronic Hepatitis

Seven women with stable, probably autoimmune, chronic persistent hepatitis were followed for three to eight years.[97] During that period all seven women had normal menstrual periods, four had documented normal basal temperature charts, and all seven became pregnant at least once. Pregnancy had no discernable adverse effect on the liver. The pregnancies all resulted in normal, full-term deliveries.

Women with autoimmune chronic active hepatitis treated with immunosuppressive therapy are surviving for increasing periods of time. Some have become pregnant. In general, women with chronic active hepatitis who are receiving immunosuppressive therapy tolerate pregnancy fairly well.[96, 98–101] However, modest deteriorations in liver tests, particularly serum bilirubin and alkaline phosphatase, occur. These changes usually return after delivery to the patient's previous baseline values and most likely represent the imposed cholestatic effects of pregnancy. Two women experienced an exacerbation of disease during pregnancy, which responded to increased doses of corticosteroids; two other women who were not on immunosuppressive therapy developed liver failure and died. Since no controlled studies have been reported, it is not known whether the adverse outcomes in these four women represent an adverse effect of pregnancy per se on their liver disease. The outcome for the fetus appears to be worse than that for the mother. Seven spontaneous abortions and seven perinatal deaths were reported in 42 pregnancies in women with chronic active hepatitis.[96, 98–101] The infants born alive were apparently healthy and did well. With use of immunosuppressive therapy, it appears that women with autoimmune chronic active hepatitis can conceive and deliver healthy children with relative safety and can survive for a considerable period thereafter.

Only two instances of pregnancy in women with chronic active hepatitis and cirrhosis due to hepatitis B have been reported.[102] Both women experienced progressive liver failure during pregnancy and died. One baby was born alive, although premature; the other died in utero.

Cirrhosis

Women with cirrhosis can and do become pregnant, although pregnancy in these women is uncommon. Reports have been published of at least 144 pregnancies in 115 women with cirrhosis of varying etiology.[98, 103–113] Evaluating the actual risk of hepatic complications during pregnancy is difficult, however; only one study identified a potential control group of nonpregnant, cirrhotic women.[103] Similarly, few authors have compared rates of obstetric complications in women with cirrhosis with rates in women without liver disease.

During the course of pregnancy, liver tests (most

commonly serum bilirubin and alkaline phosphatase activity) were reported to deteriorate in 30 to 40 per cent of cirrhotic women,[98, 104–106] but in two thirds of these patients, postpartum tests returned to baseline values. Much of this apparent deterioration could reflect the natural cholestatic effect of pregnancy.

Maternal morbidity and mortality is high during pregnancy in cirrhotic patients (10.5 per cent mortality in the 115 reported cases). Development of jaundice, ascites, hepatic encephalopathy, and postpartum hemorrhage are common (Table 54–3). Maternal deaths are due primarily to gastrointestinal hemorrhage from varices. Liver failure accounts for many of the remaining deaths (see Table 54–3), but the morbidity and mortality from cirrhosis during pregnancy may not differ greatly from the natural history of cirrhosis in these women. For example, Borhanmanesh and Hagighi[103] noted (over a 40-month period), two deaths among 9 pregnant cirrhotic women and three deaths among 12 age-matched, nonpregnant, cirrhotic women.

Bleeding from eophageal varices occurs in 18 to 32 per cent of pregnant women with cirrhosis, but can occur in up to 50 per cent of those women known to have portal hypertension.[106] Patients with a past history of variceal bleeding may or may not bleed again during pregnancy.[106, 110–112] Variceal bleeding can be prevented by a portosystemic shunt.[106, 110–112] Therapeutic portocaval shunts have been performed successfully during pregnancy with survival of all ten mothers and eight of ten babies.[104–106, 110–113] Sclerotherapy would seem to be a reasonable alternative to emergency or elective portosystemic shunting in the treatment of variceal bleeding during pregnancy. Prophylactic elective portosystemic shunts do not seem to be justified, particularly in light of the widespread availability of sclerotherapy. Finally, although elective delivery by cesarean section has been recommended to avoid the strain of labor and risk of precipitating variceal hemorrhage, there is no evidence that vaginal deliveries precipitate hemorrhage.[106]

As outlined in Table 54–3, the rates of spontaneous abortion, premature birth, and perinatal death are all greater than expected in women with cirrhosis. Infants born alive, however, generally are normal and do well. Fetal distress and perinatal mortality may be due, in part, to hepatic decompensation of the mother with its attendant metabolic abnormalities. Maternal hyperbilirubinemia is one possible toxic factor, and conceivably could cause kernicterus in utero. Two well-documented cases of severe maternal hyperbilirubinemia (16 and 33 mg/dl) have been reported,[114, 115] in which the infants were born severely jaundiced due to maternal-to-infant placental transfer of unconjugated bilirubin. Both infants exhibited fetal distress in utero, required multiple exchange transfusions after birth, and experienced many complications during the first few days of life. One infant exhibited neurologic signs of kernicterus.[114] Both infants improved with therapy and on follow-up appeared to have normal neurologic function. It would seem prudent to monitor closely the fetuses of cirrhotic women and to consider early delivery when fetal distress and/or severe maternal hyperbilirubinemia is detected.

Wilson's Disease

Chelation therapy has allowed patients with Wilson's disease to survive in good health into and through the reproductive years. Many such patients become pregnant and bear children (see Chap. 47). Amenorrhea, infertility, and spontaneous abortions are common in symptomatic, untreated women, due in part to high tissue copper levels as well as to the effects of liver dysfunction; however, therapy restores fertility and allows a normal reproductive life.[116–118] Some women with Wilson's disease, although satisfactorily treated with chelators, have liver disease, including cirrhosis, that antedates initiation of therapy. These women have increased fetal and maternal morbidity and mortality.

In both normal women and those with Wilson's disease, concentrations of copper and ceruloplasmin in serum and urine increase during pregnancy or with the use of estrogens.[23, 117–121] In women with Wilson's disease, concentrations of ceruloplasmin and copper in sera may double by the third trimester of pregnancy. The former may increase into the low-normal range. Nevertheless, discontinuing therapy with D-penicillamine in nine pregnant women was associated with symptomatic exacerbation of disease activity in three women.[116, 122] D-Penicillamine is potentially teratogenic, however. Fatal connective tissue defects have been observed in two infants born to women receiving large doses of the drug (0.9–2 g/day) for cystinuria and rheumatoid arthritis.[123, 124] One infant, born to a women with Wilson's disease who received 1.5 grams of D-penicillamine per day throughout her pregnancy exhibited cutis laxa at birth but appeared to be normal by 2 months of age.[125] For comparision, 65 normal infants have been born to women with Wilson's disease, most of whom received D-penicillamine throughout pregnancy.[116, 117, 121, 122, 126, 127] It is recommended that treatment with D-penicillamine be continued throughout pregnancy but at relatively low doses (0.25–0.5 g/day).[116, 122, 127, 128] Also, because of the antipyridoxine effects of D-penicillamine, oral supplementation with pyridoxine is recommended. Trientine (triethylene tetramine dihydrochloride) is an alternative to treatment with D-penicillamine.[118, 129] This drug has been used in seven women during 11 pregnancies; it appears to be effective, safe, and well tolerated.[118]

Dubin-Johnson Syndrome

Pregnancy or use of oral contraceptives in women with the Dubin-Johnson syndrome (see Chap. 11) causes a reversible 2- to 2.5-fold increase in plasma concentrations

TABLE 54–3. PREGNANCY AND CIRRHOSIS

Features	Shunted (29 Women)	Unshunted (83 Women)
Variceal hemorrhage	0	18–32%
Maternal death	3.5%	13.1%
Gastrointestinal hemorrhage	0	40–70%
Liver failure	100%	20–25%
Other	0	10–35%
Complication		
Jaundice	NA	26.5%
Ascites	NA	16.2%
Hepatic encephalopathy	NA	4.4%
Spontaneous abortions	2.8%	17.2%
Premature births	NA	20.7%
Perinatal deaths	16.7%	20.3%
Postpartum hemorrhage	24.1%	5.9%

Source: Data compiled from references 98, 103–105, 109–113.
NA = data not available.

of bilirubin.[130-132] Plasma concentrations of bile acids remain normal.[130] Affected women may be deeply jaundiced during pregnancy, but pruritus and other signs of generalized cholestasis are not seen. The transient exacerbation or unmasking of the Dubin-Johnson syndrome during pregnancy is related presumably to the cholestatic effects of estrogens superimposed on a liver with markedly impaired capacity for canalicular excretion of conjugated bilirubin.

LIVER DISORDERS PROBABLY RELATED TO PREGNANCY

BILIARY TRACT ABNORMALITIES

Gallstone Formation

Women develop cholesterol gallstones and clinical symptoms related to gallstones more frequently than do men[133, 134] (see Chaps. 13 and 57). The increased incidence of gallstone formation begins at puberty and tapers off after menopause, suggesting that sex hormones may be important etiologic factors.

Compared with men, women exhibit increased saturation of bile with cholesterol and have a smaller pool of bile acids[133] (see Chap. 13). Use of oral contraceptives[22, 133, 135-137] or pregnancy[138] increases the concentration and total output of cholesterol in hepatic and gallbladder bile. The total amount of bile acids is increased during pregnancy, but there is also increased sequestration of the bile acid pool in the intestine. As a result, there is little change, or even a decrease, in the bile acids secreted into bile, and the enterohepatic cycling of bile acids is decreased in pregnancy, as is the proportion of chenodeoxycholic acid relative to cholic acid. These changes all predispose to precipitation of cholesterol in bile. In addition, pregnancy and oral contraceptives increase the residual volume and the volume during fasting of the gallbladder, but the contractility[137-140] and the rate of emptying[139, 140] of the gallbladder are markedly reduced.

In spite of these changes in bile and gallbladder function, autopsy studies fail to show an increased prevalence of gallstones in women who have been pregnant, compared with those who have not.[134] On the other hand, a 2- to 2.5-fold increase in symptomatic gallbladder disease due to cholesterol gallstones has been reported in women taking oral contraceptives for up to 11 years, in postmenopausal women receiving estrogens, and in men treated with diethylstilbestrol for prostatic cancer.[141-144] Much of the increase in clinical symptoms seen in these studies is within the first one to two years of therapy, suggesting that exogenous estrogens accelerate development of symptoms in patients with pre-existing gallstones.[141-144]

Analysis of a series of young women who underwent cholecystectomy for symptomatic cholesterol gallstones suggests that pregnancy may similarly promote symptomatic gallbladder disease. Of the 300 women whose records were reviewed, 219 had at least one pregnancy; 89 noted the onset of symptoms during pregnancy; and 90 noted the onset of symptoms less than one year after a pregnancy.[145]

Biliary Tract Disease

Acute cholecystitis is the second most common cause of nonobstetric surgery during pregnancy, accounting for one to eight cases per 10,000 pregnancies.[146-148] Further-

more, common duct stones are a common cause of jaundice during pregnancy.[24] Diagnosis of biliary tract disease, with modern ultrasound, is straightforward;[148-151] ^{99}Tc-HIDA and other nuclear medicine scans are probably best avoided during pregnancy.

Therapy for symptomatic biliary tract disease during pregnancy is generally conservative. Many patients with biliary colic and/or acute cholecystitis respond to general medical management. Frequently, surgery can be postponed until after delivery.[148] Patients with recurrent symptoms or common bile duct obstruction may require surgery during pregnancy. This can be accomplished with relatively little maternal or fetal mortality.[146-148, 152, 153] Most surgeons advocate delaying surgery until the second trimester or until after delivery but do not hesitate to operate because of intractable symptoms or clinical deterioration.[146-148, 152-155]

HEPATIC NEOPLASMS

The liver is an estrogen-responsive organ that contains estrogen receptors.[156] Estrogens, either endogenous or exogenous, are thought to be responsible for several vascular and neoplastic changes in the liver. These include dilatation of the sinusoids, focal nodular hyperplasia, hepatocellular adenoma, and possibly some cases of hepatocellular carcinoma[157, 158] (see Chap. 45). Strong but circumstantial epidemiologic evidence links these processes to use of oral contraceptives; the association between pregnancy and these abnormalities is based on case reports and by analogy to the effects of oral contraceptives.

Dilatation of Hepatic Sinusoids

This lesion, with associated hepatomegaly and abdominal pain, has been reported in a few women receiving oral contraceptives. It has been noted in livers that contained oral contraceptive–associated adenomas.[157, 159-162] Improvement follows discontinuance of oral contraceptives. The prognosis is benign.[159, 160, 162]

Focal Nodular Hyperplasia

Focal nodular hyperplasia is a benign lesion that is often found incidentally and consists of normal liver elements disposed around a central stellate scar. The lesion occurs almost exclusively in women[163, 164] (see Chap. 45). An association with the use of oral contraceptives has been suggested.[163, 165-168] Since lesions may increase in size during pregnancy, surgery should be considered prophylactically in women with estrogen-responsive lesions who desire to bear children.[168]

Hepatocellular Adenomas

These adenomas are benign hepatocellular tumors linked causally to estrogens and the use of oral contraceptives[163, 165, 166, 169-172] (see Chap. 45). It is not clear whether estrogens actually initiate the adenomas, but they promote growth[173] and the development of serious complications and clinical symptoms such as a mass lesion, abdominal pain, acute hemorrhage, necrosis, and rupture.[174] Many adenomas regress after removal of estrogens.[175, 176] Pregnancy has not been associated with an increased incidence of hepatocellular adenomas, but pregnancy is associated with growth of adenomas, development of symptoms (nausea, vomiting, right upper-quadrant pain), and a propensity to rupture.[170, 177-180] Surgical excision, which is usually well tolerated, should be considered for large, symptomatic tumors, for those that do not shrink after oral contraceptive use has been discontinued, and for tumors in women who desire to bear children.[181, 182]

BUDD-CHIARI SYNDROME

Budd-Chiari syndrome (see Chap. 23) associated with use of oral contraceptives was noted as early as 1966, and the association has been well documented.[183-194] Development of hepatic vein thrombosis is attributed to an oral contraceptive–induced increase in clotting factors plus a generalized propensity for venous thrombosis.[183, 195, 196] Budd-Chiari syndrome associated with pregnancy is much less common. Twenty-five cases have been reported.[195-203] The predisposing factors for hepatic vein occlusion are thought to be the estrogen-related increases in clotting factors associated with a decrease in the activity of plasma antithrombin III (see Chap. 22). In some women, hepatic vein occlusion is associated with widespread venous thrombosis and may represent local propagation of clot originating in the iliac veins and inferior vena cava. Another syndrome that clinically resembles the Budd-Chiari syndrome, hepatic veno-occlusive disease, has been reported in three women post partum[204] and in one woman receiving an oral progestational agent for contraceptive purposes.[205] Clinical symptoms of the Budd-Chiari syndrome frequently begin post partum or immediately after an abortion rather than during the pregnancy itself. The general clinical features, diagnostic evaluation, and treatment are discussed in Chapter 23.[206]

LIVER DISORDERS UNIQUE TO PREGNANCY

Four unique syndromes of liver dysfunction have been identified during pregnancy: hepatic involvement in hyperemesis gravidarum, intrahepatic cholestasis of pregnancy, acute fatty liver of pregnancy, and pre-eclampsia/eclampsia-related liver disease.

HEPATIC INVOLVEMENT IN HYPEREMESIS GRAVIDARUM

Hyperemesis gravidarum is not a liver disese, but liver dysfunction occurs in severely affected patients. For example, among women requiring hospitalization for dehydration and weight loss, liver dysfunction and jaundice were noted in 13 to 33 per cent and 10 to 13 per cent, respectively.[24, 206]

Liver dysfunction usually presents in the first trimester, within one to three weeks after the onset of severe vomiting. Jaundice, dark urine, and occasionally pruritus are the major hepatic manifestations.[24, 41, 206-209] Mild hyperbilirubinemia is the laboratory abnormality (mean value 1.7 mg/dl) noted most frequently. Moderate increases in serum transaminases (two to three times normal) occur in slightly more than half of the patients. Alkaline phosphatase activities are elevated in a minority of patients. Excretion of BSP, which is a sensitive indicator of hepatic capacity for organic anion transport, is markedly impaired in women with liver

dysfunction and hyperemesis, compared with control, pregnant women.[207] Autopsy specimens from 19 women who died of hyperemesis (6 of whom were jaundiced), exhibited excess pigment in centrilobular areas, but no necrosis. Moderate deposits of fat in large vacuoles, usually in centrilobular heptocytes, were seen in 12 patients.[210] Cholestasis has been seen in liver biopsies from some affected women,[208] but most biopsies are normal.[206] The etiology of hepatic dysfunction is unknown but may be related to dehydration and malnutrition.[211, 212] Hepatic dysfunction in hyperemesis gravidarum is a relatively benign process with little clinical consequence. Women who have died of hyperemesis in the past did so from starvation and dehydration, not from liver failure. If vomiting is controlled, the hepatic dysfunction rapidly resolves, usually within a few days, although it may recur in subsequent pregnancies.[24, 41, 206, 208, 209]

INTRAHEPATIC CHOLESTASIS OF PREGNANCY

Intrahepatic cholestasis of pregnancy (IHCP) is a relatively benign cholestatic disorder that generally commences late in pregnancy, disappears abruptly after delivery, and frequently recurs with subsequent pregnancies. The main clinical manifestations are pruritus and jaundice. The term pruritus gravidarum is frequently applied to women with pruritus and biochemical cholestasis, whereas the terms cholestatic jaundice of pregnancy or cholestasis of pregnancy are often applied to those women who also develop clinically apparent jaundice.

Incidence

IHCP is recognized in less than 1 per cent of pregnancies in the United States and Europe. The disorder appears to be more frequent in Scandinavia and Chile, being reported in 1 to 6 per cent of all pregnancies in these countries.[213-229] It accounts for 20 to 50 per cent of all causes of jaundice in pregnancy in series reported from Scandinavia;[24, 41, 213] however, the overall incidence appears to have decreased in the past two decades.[224, 228]

Etiology

The etiology and pathogenesis of IHCP remain poorly defined, but both genetic and hormonal factors appear to be important. The best hypothesis is that IHCP reflects a heritable sensitivity to the cholestatic effects of estrogens. Heritable factors are suggested, as IHCP frequently affects female relatives of index cases,[216, 222, 224, 229] and pedigree studies have demonstrated IHCP in up to three generations of women in some families, suggesting dominant transmission of the trait.[225, 230, 231] IHCP also has been observed in nine women in a large family; four other members exhibited familial benign recurrent intrahepatic cholestasis.[232] The clinical features of IHCP closely resemble the cholestasis and jaundice that develop in some women receiving estrogens or oral contraceptives,[233-235] and the two disorders frequently overlap. Thus, as many as 50 per cent of women who experienced IHCP develop pruritus and cholestasis when using oral contraceptives.[217, 236, 237] IHCP and/or estrogen-related cholestasis also occur frequently in both mothers and sisters of women who develop cholestasis while using oral contraceptives. In one well-controlled study of

TABLE 54–4. INTRAHEPATIC CHOLESTASIS OF PREGNANCY: CLINICAL FEATURES

Incidence in Pregnancy	United States and Europe: 0.04–0.6% Scandinavia: 1–3% Chile: 4.7–6.1%
Age	Any
Parity	Any
Onset	70% third trimester 30% before third trimester
Onset of pruritus	Average, 28–30 weeks; range, 7–40 weeks
Onset of jaundice	1–4 weeks later
Recurrence in subsequent pregnancies	58% (average of 10 series)

Signs and symptoms
  Pruritus
  Jaundice
  Nausea, vomiting
  Abdominal pain
	
	100%
	25%
	5–75%
	9–24%

Physical findings
  Skin excoriations
  Jaundice
  Hepatomegaly
	
	Common
	25%
	Rare

Source: Data derived from references 213–229, 240.

129 women who developed jaundice after receiving oral contraceptives and of 129 matched controls, IHCP was reported as having occurred in 14% of the mothers of jaundiced patients but only in 2% of mothers of the controls, and in 15 per cent versus 1 per cent of the subjects' sisters. Fourteen per cent of patients' sisters, but none of the control subjects' sisters, developed cholestasis while receiving oral contraceptives.[238] Additionally, ethinyl estradiol impairs BSP excretion in both men and women, although the effect is much more marked both in women with a history of IHCP and in women and men with a family history of this disorder.[239]

Clinical Features

The clinical and laboratory features of IHCP are summarized in Tables 54–4 and 54–5 and in Figure 54–3. Lipoprotein X (see Chap. 5) may be present in plasma,[229] and gallbladder size and residual volume are often increased.[245, 246, 257] Serum transaminase activities in a few patients with IHCP will overlap with those typical of hepatocellular disorders such as acute viral hepatitis. Serologic tests for hepatitis viruses A and B, and the clinical course of the disease, particularly after delivery, may be helpful in the differential diagnosis. Liver biopsy is generally unnecessary for diagnosis. Liver failure and hepatic encephalopathy are not reported in IHCP. The appearance of these abnormalities indicates another etiology for the liver disease.

The pruritus can be disabling and, in exceptional cases, can be so severe as to mandate termination of pregnancy. Thirty-four cases of severe postpartum hemorrhage have been reported in women with IHCP. Although it is not clear whether vitamin K deficiency was responsible for this manifestation, patients should be treated with vitamin K if the prothrombin time is abnormal.

Pathology

The histopathology of IHCP is shown in Figure 54–4. Typical findings include centrilobular cholestasis, canaliculi containing bile plugs, and bile pigment in hepatocytes.[24, 247] Cholestasis may be patchy and subtle. Inflammation and hepatocellular necrosis usually are absent. Portal tracts and interlobular bile ducts are normal. Electron microscopic examination shows dilated bile canaliculi with loss of microvilli and occasional abnormal mitochondria.[247, 248] All histologic changes disappear after delivery and after resolution of clinical symptoms.[24, 247]

Natural History and Prognosis

The cholestasis of IHCP generally progresses until the time of delivery or termination of pregnancy. The severity of cholestasis and of laboratory abnormalities can be quite variable, both during one pregnancy and between different pregnancies.[221] For example, serum transaminase activities and even bilirubin concentrations may fluctuate and even temporarily normalize as pregnancy progresses.[221] Pruritus, however, rarely improves before delivery. After delivery, pruritus quickly disappears, often within 24 to 48 hours. Biochemical abnormalities and histologic findings resolve over the following weeks to months.[42] Long-term follow-up (up to 15 years) of women with IHCP has been achieved in Sweden.[41, 249] Other than a significantly higher incidence (i.e., 1.4- to 2.3-fold that of matched controls) of cholelithiasis and gallbladder disease, the prognosis for these women is excellent.[215, 229, 249]

The prognosis for the fetus is not as benign as for the mother. Earlier series document high rates of premature labor and neonatal death (11 per cent).[49, 213–229, 240, 250, 251] Fetal monitoring has documented high rates of fetal distress during labor (19 to 60 per cent) (the cause of which is unknown) and meconium staining at birth (35 per cent).[227, 244, 250] The latter is attributed by some authors to a stimulant effect of bile salts on fetal colonic muscle. Several recent controlled series from Sweden and Finland fail to confirm statistically significant differences in fetal mortality. When these studies are combined, however, there appears to be a trend toward increased fetal deaths (1.7 per cent mortality in 359 infants born to women with IHCP, compared with 0.77 per cent mortality in 390 infants born to unaffected women).[42, 49, 215, 216, 242] These findings have prompted a number of experienced physicians routinely to monitor patients closely during the third trimester and to opt for early delivery if any signs of fetal distress are found.[216, 220, 222, 225]

Therapy

Pruritus may respond to oral cholestyramine.[252–254] A few patients also are reported to have responded to phenobarbital.[253] Hypnotics may be helpful, as nocturnal pruritus can be the most distressing symptom. Vitamin K administration, especially near term, is reasonable, particularly for women with jaundice or prolonged cholestasis.

A new therapeutic agent, S-adenosyl-L-methionine, has been tried in a few women. This agent, which methylates phospholipids, appears to antagonize some of the cholestatic effects of estrogens in humans[255] and animals.[256] In a small, randomized clinical trial, pruritus and biochemical tests improved significantly in six women with IHCP who received large intravenous doses of S-adenosyl-L-me-

TABLE 54–5. INTRAHEPATIC CHOLESTASIS OF PREGNANCY: LABORATORY FINDINGS

Test	No. of Patients	% of Women With Abnormal Values	Average Value Reported	Range of Values Reported	Normal Values*
Bilirubin	558	25	1.0 (all patients) 2.9 (jaundiced patients)	0.4–8.4	≤ 1.1 mg/dL
Alkaline phosphatase	575	70	146 ± 66 (2.4-fold upper limit of nl)	nl–750 (up to 12.5-fold upper limit of nl)	≤ 60 KU/L
AST	409	60	119 ± 51	nl–736	≤ 40 IU/L
ALT	321	55	131 ± 96	nl–1030	≤ 40 IU/L
Serum bile salts	128	90	47 μM	nl–430 μM	≤ 6.5 μM
Serum cholic acid	64	70	17 μM	nl–109 μM	≤ 1.5 μM
BSP retention at 45 min	77	97–100	23%	10–33%	≤ 12%
Prothrombin time	128	16†	—	—	—
Fecal fat					
Patients with jaundice	12	—	14.0	2–31	≤ 7 g/24 hr
Patients with pruritus	11	—	4.0	1–10	≤ 7 g/24 hr

Source: Data derived from references 49, 213–229, 232–235.
*For non-pregnant individuals.
†All corrected with vitamin K.
nl = Normal; AST = aspartate aminotransferase; ALT = alanine aminotransferase; BSP = Bromsulphalein (sulfobromophthalein sodium).

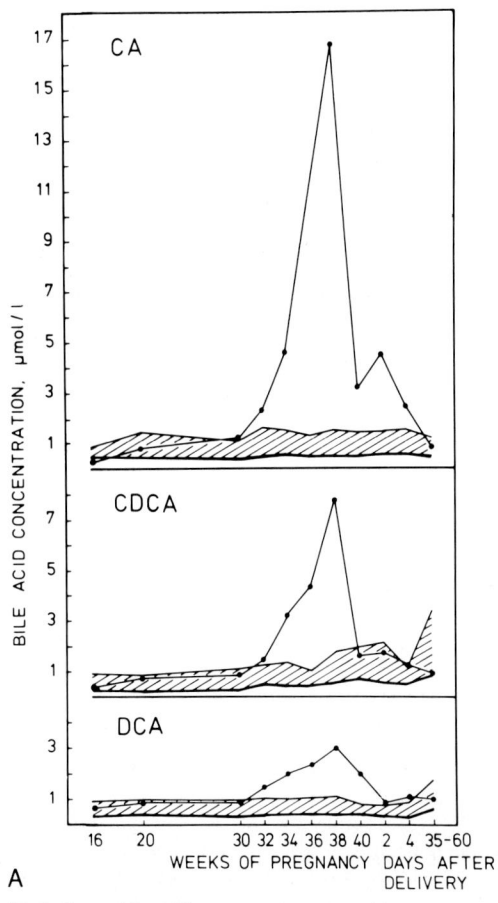

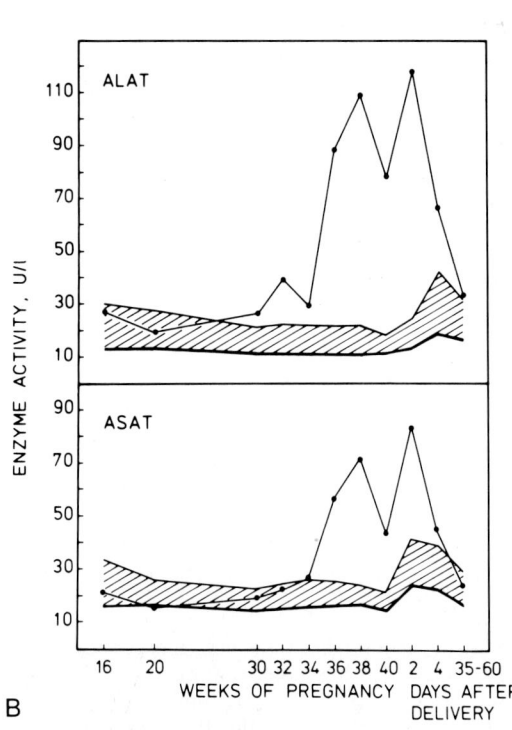

Figure 54–3. Serum bile acid concentrations (A) and liver tests (B), during pregnancy in control women (shaded areas; mean ± 2 S.D.) and in eight women who developed intrahepatic cholestasis of pregnancy (dotted line; mean values). CA = cholic acid; CDCA = chenodeoxycholic acid; DCA = oxycholic acid; ALAT = alanine aminotransferase; ASAT = aspartate aminotransferase. (Reprinted with permission from The American College of Obstetricians and Gynecologists. Obstetrics and Gynecology, vol. 61, 1983, p. 581.)

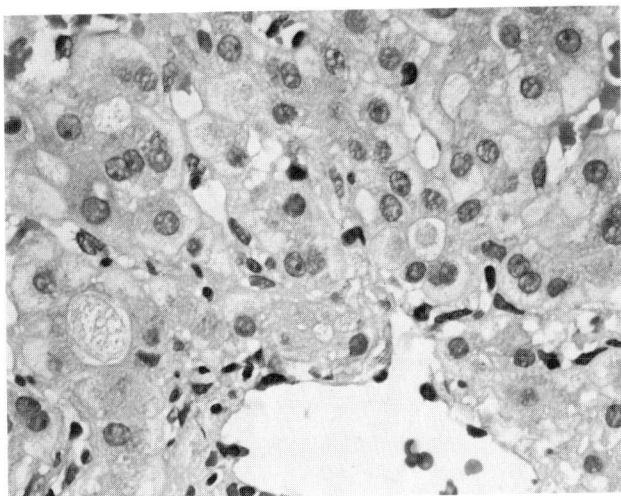

Figure 54–4. Intrahepatic cholestasis of pregnancy. Micrograph shows canalicular bile plugs, well-preserved hepatocytes, and a terminal hepatic venule at the bottom of the field. Hematoxylin and eosin, ×630. (Reproduced from Rolfes DB, Ishak KG. Histopathology 10:555, 1986, with permission of Blackwell Scientific Publications Limited.)

thionine for up to three weeks, compared with values in 12 other women given lower doses or placebo.[257] A preliminary report by the same investigators suggests that oral administration of S-adenosyl-L-methionine prevented the development of hepatic biochemical abnormalities in four women with a history of IHCP who were challenged with oral estrogen administration.[258] The greatest concern about this new therapy is the effect of S-adenosyl-L-methionine on the fetus.

ACUTE FATTY LIVER OF PREGNANCY

Acute fatty liver of pregnancy (AFLP) is a rare and frequently fatal, idiopathic disorder that appears exclusively during the third trimester of pregnancy.[259, 260] Its principal and distinctive histologic feature is infiltration of centrilobular hepatocytes with microvesicular fat (Fig. 54–5). This histology is strikingly similar to that in Reye's syndrome, Jamaican vomiting sickness, valproic acid hepatotoxicity, tetracycline hepatotoxicity, and medium- and long-chain acyl CoA dehydrogenase deficiency.[261–267] This group of disorders collectively has been termed the hepatic microvesicular steatoses,[261–267] and they share many clinical and laboratory features.

Estimates of incidence are poor, but values of one case per million deliveries are quoted frequently. Less than 200 total cases have been reported.[268–300] Instances of mild disease are now being identified more frequently, however, and AFLP may occur more commonly than has been appreciated. The most accurate figures for incidence probably derive from the Los Angeles County–USC Medical Center where, over a 10-year period, AFLP was identified in 1 per 13,000 deliveries[268] (Table 54–6). AFLP accounts for 16 to 43 per cent of the incidence of severe liver disease during pregnancy and consequently, for a large percentage of maternal deaths from liver disease.[269, 301] Although it can occur with any pregnancy, it is more common in primagravidas, in women with twin pregnancies, and in those with a male fetus (Table 54–6).

Etiology

The underlying cause of AFLP is unknown, but a metabolic abnormality seems most likely. It is clearly neither infectious nor inherited and does not recur in subsequent pregnancies. The characteristic lesion is infiltration of hepatocytes with microvesicular fat, in conjunction with pleomorphic, and abnormal mitochondria. These findings suggest an important (although not necessarily etiologic) abnormality in lipid metabolism or in mitochondrial function. In AFLP, hepatic fat constitutes 10 to 20 per cent of liver weight, is principally triglycerides and free fatty acids[270–272] and exists in small non–membrane-bound cytoplasmic droplets. These findings suggest that fatty acid oxidation, triglyceride synthesis, and/or lipoprotein synthesis and secretion are impaired. Triglycerides are relatively innocuous compounds, even when present in large concentrations, but free fatty acids are not. Fatty acids are known to interfere with mitochondrial function, to disrupt membranes, and to affect protein synthesis. Careful analysis of hepatic lipid content has been performed in only one case of AFLP, and extraordinary, levels of free fatty acids were found.[270] It is possible that abnormalities in fatty acid oxidation and/or triglyceride synthesis, in conjunction with the large hepatic fluxes of fatty acids that occur in pregnancy, lead to an increase in hepatic content of free fatty acids that in turn causes widespread metabolic dysfunction. On the other hand, tetracycline, which interferes with ribosome function and impairs protein synthesis, causes fatty liver and hepatic toxicity that has several clinical and laboratory features in common with AFLP. Thus, a primary disorder of protein synthesis is a potential cause of AFLP.

Specific abnormalities in mitochondrial function or in urea cycle enzymes have been proposed as pathogenic factors in AFLP by analogy to Reye's syndrome and to the congenital deficiencies of urea cycle enzymes (see Chap. 16). Transient defects in ornithine transcarbamylase (OTC) activity were identified in liver tissue from two women with AFLP;[274] however, in two other patients, hepatic activity of OTC was normal.[303] Arginosuccinate lyase activity, however, was low in one of the latter two patients.[303] These observations are perhaps more consistent with generalized mitochondrial dysfunction as a secondary phenomenon than as a primary specific abnormality.

Clinical Features

The clinical features of acute fatty liver of pregnancy are summarized in Tables 54–6 and 54–7. Illness begins in the third trimester, usually around 35 weeks of gestation, although onset of illness as early as 26 weeks and as late as the immediate postpartum period have been reported. The early manifestations are nonspecific. Nausea, fatigue, malaise, vomiting, and abdominal distress (right upper-quadrant or epigastric pain that may resemble reflux esophagitis) are the most common symptoms. Fever, headache, diarrhea, back pain suggestive of pancreatitis, and myalgias are reported in some patients. Clinical signs of liver dysfunction and even frank liver failure, such as jaundice, hepatic encephalopathy, or bleeding ensue one to two weeks later.

Physical findings often are minimal. Early on, right upper-quadrant tenderness may be the only abnormality found. The liver generally is small and not palpable. As the disease progresses, jaundice, changes in mental status, edema, and ascites may appear. Hypertension and proteinuria, the hallmarks of pre-eclampsia, are seen in 21 per

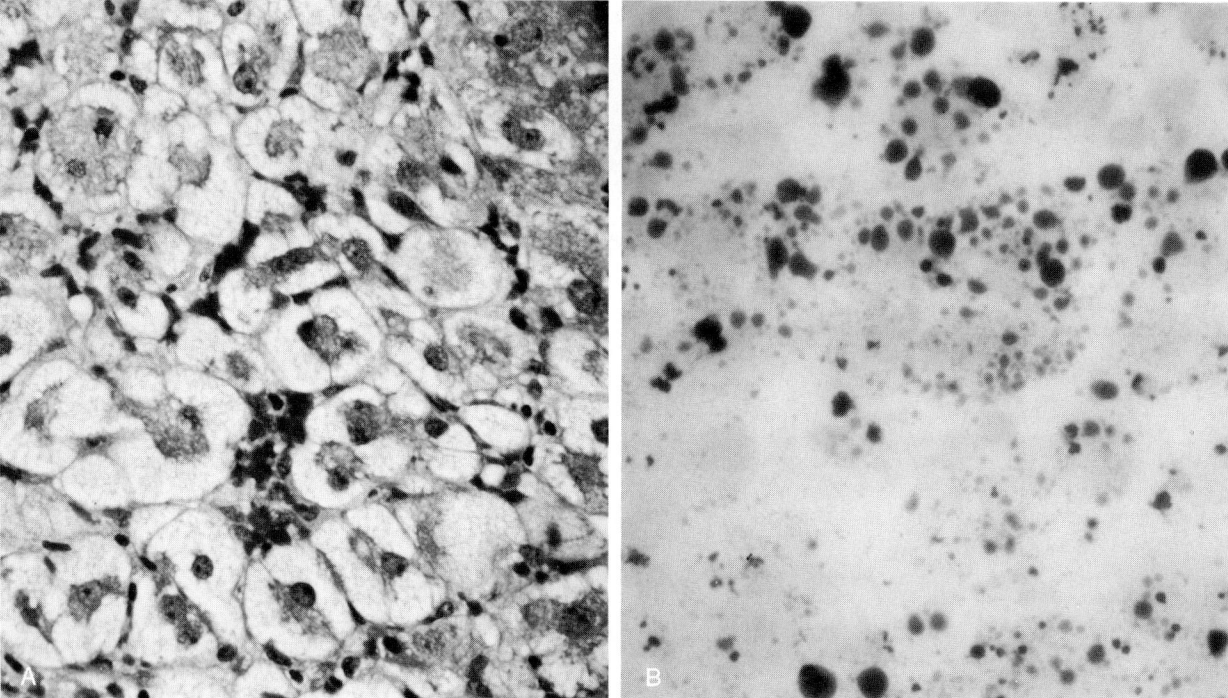

Figure 54–5. Acute fatty liver of pregnancy. Micrographs demonstrate microvesicular fatty infiltration. *A,* Hematoxylin and eosin; *B,* Oil red O stain.

cent of patients. This is a two- to fourfold greater incidence than is seen in normal pregnancy.[304]

Acute fatty liver of pregnancy is associated with a number of abnormal laboratory findings (Table 54–8). The blood smear frequently contains nucleated red blood cells and in those patients with disseminated intravascular coagulation (DIC), fragmented erythrocytes, and Burr cells. Leukocytosis virtually is universal, even in women with no evidence of infection. Coagulation disorders, including thrombocytopenia, decreased clotting factors, and frank DIC are common. (The decrease in clotting factors probably represents both impaired hepatic synthesis and accelerated consumption.) The inciting trigger for DIC is not known, although a marked decrease in plasma antithrombin III activity, noted in all of seven women tested,[294-296] may be one factor.[294]

Liver test abnormalities include hyperbilirubinemia, increases in alkaline phosphatase activity, and modest elevations of serum transaminase activities (usually ≤ 300 IU/L). A few patients with otherwise typical AFLP, exhibit

markedly elevated serum transaminase values. The generally modest abnormalities of liver tests can be misleading, as they do not reflect accurately the severe degree of liver dysfunction in these patients. For example, many patients may have hypoglycemia, impaired synthesis of clotting factors, and hepatic encephalopathy. Hypoglycemia occurs in fact in as many as 25 per cent of patients. It should be looked for initially and blood glucose levels need to be monitored frequently until liver failure resolves.

Renal dysfunction and elevation of BUN and creatinine occur in many patients with AFLP. Most patients suffer only mild renal dysfunction, but frank renal failure does occur and may require dialysis. The cause(s) of renal failure are not clearly defined. A characteristic laboratory abnormality, often seen early in the course of AFLP, is a marked

TABLE 54–6. ACUTE FATTY LIVER OF PREGNANCY: FEATURES AND PRESENTATION IN 111 CASES

Feature	Average Frequency *(Range of Values Reported)*
Incidence	1/13,000 deliveries
Age	27 years (18–38)
Primagravidas	42%
Twin gestations	13%
Male fetus	76%
Recurrences	0/19
Onset	35 weeks (26–40)
Hypertension or proteinuria	37%
Pre-eclampsia (hypertension, proteinuria, and edema)	21%

Source: Data derived from references 268–293, 295, 300, 315.

TABLE 54–7. ACUTE FATTY LIVER OF PREGNANCY: SIGNS AND SYMPTOMS

	No. of Patients*	Frequency (%)
Feature		
Nausea, vomiting	107	84
Abdominal pain, epigastric distress	111	62
Encephalopathy	105	72
Jaundice	111	98
Edema	96	39
Hypoglycemia	111	25
Ascites	30	50
Extrahepatic Manifestations		
Gastrointestinal hemorrhage	86	42
Coagulopathy (DIC)	64	56
Renal impairment	70	76
Pancreatitis	33	27

Source: Data derived from references 268–293, 295, 300, 315.
*For whom data is available.
DIC = disseminated intravascular coagulation.

TABLE 54–8. ACUTE FATTY LIVER OF PREGNANCY: LABORATORY ABNORMALITIES

Laboratory Test	No. of Patients	Frequency of Abnormal Results (%)	Abnormal Values	
			Average	Range
RBC smear	38	50*		
WBC count	100	97	—	12,000–46,000
Platelet count	90	86	—	5,000–121,000
Prothrombin time	92	92	22 sec	normal to 24 sec prolonged
Antithrombin III level	7	100†	—	—
Bilirubin	111	98	15 mg%	1.8–36 mg%
Alkaline phosphatase	83	100	4.4-fold upper limit of nl	up to 10-fold upper limit of nl
AST (nl ≤ 40)	72	100	258 IU/L	87–1300
ALT (nl ≤ 40)	50	98	228 IU/L	44–800
Serum uric acid	32	81	—	up to 18.5 mg%
Serum creatinine	68	75	3.0 mg/dL	up to 6.6 mg/dL

Source: Data derived from references 268–293, 295, 300, 315.
*Nucleated RBCs seen frequently; RBC fragments in those with disseminated intravascular coagulation (DIC).
†All 7 patients exhibited DIC.
RBC = red blood cell; WBC = white blood cell; nl = normal; AST = aspartate aminotransferase; ALT = alanine aminotransferase.

increase in the level of uric acid in serum. This occurs prior to the onset of frank renal insufficiency, suggesting a defect in renal tubular function.

Imaging studies of the liver, using ultrasound or computed tomography (CT), may suggest the presence of a fatty liver. Ultrasound, however, is not particularly sensitive.[297, 298] CT scans may be more useful than sonography in detecting fatty liver,[305] although only two cases have been reported in which it was used.[297, 299]

Pathology

The histologic appearance of AFLP is well described.[259, 268, 272, 274, 275, 292, 293] At the light microscopic level, lobular architecture is intact but the lobules are swollen, with compression of the sinusoids. As mentioned previously, centrilobular fatty infiltration of hepatocytes with microvesicular fat is the key feature of AFLP (see Fig. 54–5). However, in an occasional patient, diffuse cytoplasmic ballooning or large fat vacuoles, reminiscent of those seen in alcoholic steatosis, is observed.[292] Fat deposits are always located in the centrilobular area (zone 3) with a more variable involvement of zones 1 and 2. The fat is readily appreciated when fat stains such as oil red 0 are used on frozen sections of tissue (see Fig. 54–5). The lesion frequently is missed if routinely fixed tissue is examined, because the fat is removed during fixation. In addition to fatty metamorphosis, centrilobular cholestasis, as indicated by bile canalicular plugs and bile-stained hepatocytes, frequently is seen. Biopsies in a few patients also exhibit bile duct proliferation and acute cholangiolitis.[292]

Although widespread hepatic necrosis is virtually never seen, subtle signs are evident of hepatocyte necrosis and hepatocytolysis. Other clues suggesting that substantial loss of hepatocytes has occurred include the small size of livers at autopsy,[259, 292] close apposition of portal tracts and central veins, prominent lipid- and lipofuscin-laden Kupffer cells, occasional acidophilic bodies, and numerous mitotic figures.[292] Confluent centrizonal coagulative necrosis is seen in occasional patients who experience preterminal shock and is most likely a superimposed lesion of hepatic ischemia.[292]

Like hepatocyte necrosis, inflammation is subtle and may be absent. Most commonly, a few inflammatory cells, predominantly mononuclear cells and lymphocytes, are scattered throughout the lobule. Up to 25 per cent of

biopsies may exhibit substantial infiltration by lymphocytes and plasma cells in the lobule and/or portal tracts. The histological picture in these patients can resemble acute viral hepatitis, particularly if fat stains are not performed on frozen tissue. Other nonspecific findings include glycogen depletion, extramedullary hematopoiesis in up to 75 per cent of cases, absence of sinusoidal fibrin deposits, and rarely, central vein phlebitis.[292]

At the electron microscopic level, the swollen hepatocytes contain numerous small, non–membrane-bound cytoplasmic lipid droplets.[274, 285, 292, 303] Fat has also been reported in lysosomes,[306] rough and smooth endoplasmic reticulum, and the Golgi apparatus.[307] Glycogen depletion, proliferation of smooth endoplasmic reticulum, and a remarkable absence of lipoproteins in the Golgi apparatus also are seen.[274, 285, 292, 306] Mitochondria are large, pleomorphic, and ameboid-shaped and contain lamellar crystalline inclusions. Most,[274, 285, 292, 306] but not all,[307] investigators feel that these mitochondrial lesions are distinct from those seen in Reye's syndrome, a disease in which dilated mitochondria with rarefaction and flocculation of the matrix are characteristic. Bile canaliculi are dilated with loss of microvilli. Precipitated material is seen in canalicular lumens as well as in intracellular pericanalicular vesicles.

Other organs also may be involved. Fatty metamorphosis of pancreatic acinar cells and renal tubular epithelia is well described.[272, 293, 300] This involvement may account for the clinical findings of pancreatitis and renal insufficiency in some patients. The exact frequency with which other organs undergo fatty metamorphosis is not known.

Differential Diagnosis

The principal liver diseases that may be confused with AFLP are acute viral hepatitis, pre-eclampsia–related liver disease, and tetracycline-induced fatty liver.[308] The clinical presentation of all four diseases can be similar, but laboratory tests are helpful in distinguishing them. Diagnosis of AFLP is based on compatible clinical and laboratory abnormalities in a woman in the third trimester of pregnancy, in conjunction with a liver biopsy (including fat stains on frozen tissue) showing microvesicular fat. In contrast to AFLP, acute viral hepatitis may present at any time during pregnancy. A history of exposure to an individual with hepatitis is often obtained and serologic tests for hepatitis viruses A and B may be positive. Serum transaminase values tend to be much higher in acute viral hepatitis than in AFLP, and DIC is uncommon in the former disease. Pre-eclampsia–related liver disease always is associated with hypertension and proteinuria, whereas pre-eclampsia is often absent in fatty liver of pregnancy. Pre-eclampsia–related liver disease exhibits a greater degree of hematologic abnormalities and of hepatocellular necrosis than does AFLP. Indeed, in severe cases, liver infarction and hemorrhage frequently are seen in the former condition.

Tetracycline, particularly when administered in high doses and/or to patients with impaired renal function, can cause a syndrome that is virtually identical to AFLP.[267, 273, 302, 309–313] In the past, the two disorders were often lumped together, because high-dose intravenous tetracycline was used frequently to treat urinary tract infections and pyelonephritis in pregnant women.[267] Tetracycline-induced fatty liver has virtually disappeared; however, one recent case possibly related to chronic use of tetracycline for treatment of acne has been reported.[312]

Natural History and Prognosis

All the complications of fulminant hepatic failure (see Chap. 17) can occur in AFLP, including cerebral edema, gastrointestinal hemorrhage, renal failure, and infection. Patients usually die of one of these complications. Once liver dysfunction becomes evident, spontaneous labor or fetal death in utero commonly ensues. Delivery is often complicated by severe postpartum hemorrhage. After delivery, liver function improves. If patients do not die in the interim secondary to the complications of liver failure, signs and symptoms gradually resolve over the next few weeks. Long-term follow-up studies show that liver function returns to normal. All histologic abnormalities resolve without any evidence of chronic liver disease.[276, 278]

Overall outcome, as reported in the literature, is summarized in Table 54–9. Both maternal and fetal mortality is high (about 50 per cent). The high rate of fetal mortality is related to rapid maternal decompensation, premature delivery, and maternal DIC, with fibrin deposition in the placenta leading to placental infarcts and insufficiency and fetal asphyxia.[313] Improved survival of both mothers and infants has been reported in more recent series, in which prompt delivery (as soon as the diagnosis of AFLP is made) was undertaken, along with improved medical treatment for fulminant liver failure and for premature infants.

AFLP seems to be a sporadic disease. At least 14 women who survived the disorder have become pregnant

TABLE 54–9. ACUTE FATTY LIVER OF PREGNANCY: OUTCOME

Maternal Mortality

All reports*	49% (54/111 reported cases)
Recent series†	22% (10/45 cases)
Recent reports in which delivery was initiated promptly‡	15% (6/40 cases)

Infant Mortality

All reports*	49% (63/129 reported cases)
Recent series†	42% (22/53 cases)
Recent reports in which delivery was initiated promptly‡	36% (14/38 cases)

*Data derived from references 268, 293, 295, 300, 315.
†Data derived from references 268, 285, 288–291.
‡Data derived from references 268, 285, 288–291, 298, 300.

again (10 months to 7 years later), four of them twice. In all 14 women, the disease did not recur.[268, 269, 281, 290, 314, 315]

Therapy

There is no specific therapy for AFLP. Many investigators advocate a policy of prompt termination of pregnancy as soon as the diagnosis is made.[260] Although the true utility of this treatment will probably never be tested in controlled clinical trials, it is a reasonable recommendation. Since AFLP usually presents late in pregnancy and affected infants often die in utero with little warning, immediate delivery would be expected to improve fetal survival as well.

LIVER DISEASE RELATED TO PREGNANCY-INDUCED HYPERTENSION (TOXEMIA) AND PRE-ECLAMPSIA/ECLAMPSIA

Hypertension is a common complication of late pregnancy, arising de novo or, less commonly, superimposed on pre-existing hypertension. The term pre-eclampsia is applied to concomitant development of proteinuria and edema, whereas further progression to seizures heralds the onset of true eclampsia.[316, 317] Although pre-eclampsia and eclampsia are not primarily liver diseases, any organ system can be involved in the disease process, and a substantial fraction of affected women manifest some degree of liver damage. This ranges from mild hepatocellular necrosis to hepatic rupture. Since liver involvement is similar in pre-eclampsia and eclampsia, the former term will be used in most of this discussion.

Pre-eclampsia

Incidence

Pre-eclampsia develops in 5 to 10 per cent of all pregnancies. Frequency is greatest in young primagravidas[318–320] and extraordinarily high in women with the lupus anticoagulant.[321] The disorder can be mild or can progress rapidly to seizures and eclampsia, associated with renal failure, coagulopathy, microangiopathic hemolytic anemia, and widespread patchy ischemic necrosis of many tissues. Eclampsia has a high mortality rate, accounting for about 8 per cent of all maternal deaths[322] and 3 to 21 deaths per 100,000 pregnancies.[320, 322]

Pathophysiology

The pathophysiology underlying pregnancy-induced hypertension, pre-eclampsia, and eclampsia is not understood; however, it is clear that the vasculature of affected women exhibits an exquisite sensitivity to endogenous pressors and to catecholamines. This is in marked contrast to the decreased sensitivity to these agents seen in unaffected pregnant women.[316–318] Plasma levels of pressors such as angiotensin and vasopressin are within normal limits, but these levels would be considered high in light of the elevated blood pressure.[318] Patients exhibit a decrease in plasma levels of prostaglandins of the E and I series, which could be an important factor in triggering vasospasm and hypertension. Contraction of plasma volume and hemoconcentration appear early and may contribute to initiation of hypertension. Associated renal findings include intense arteriolar vasospasm and swelling of mesangial and epithelial cells in the renal glomerulus. Related to these abnormalities, patients develop decreased glomerular filtration rate, impaired natriuresis, and edema. The intense vasospasm is thought to cause damage to the vascular endothelium resulting in platelet deposition, thrombocytopenia, and fibrin deposition.[316] In many patients, deposition of fibrin thrombi and platelet aggregation are thought to lead to further ischemia and infarction, to microangiopathic hemolytic anemia, and, in some cases, to disseminated intravascular coagulopathy.

Clinical Findings

Pregnancy-induced hypertension usually is present for weeks prior to development of clinical symptoms; however, seizures, renal failure, and organ ischemia may appear without warning and are unrelated to the severity of the previous hypertension and proteinuria.[318]

HEPATIC INVOLVEMENT

Most women with pre-eclampsia exhibit no clinical or laboratory evidence of liver disease.[42, 323, 324] The liver is involved, however, in at least 10 per cent of women with pre-eclampsia.[24, 319, 325–327] Conversely, pre-eclampsia accounts for about 5 per cent of cases of jaundice in pregnancy. Liver involvement is more common in severe eclampsia, constituting the primary cause of death in 15 to 21 per cent of fatal cases.[320, 322] Over 70 per cent of women dying of pre-eclampsia/eclampsia show histologic evidence at autopsy of some degree of liver involvement.[320]

The hepatic lesion of pre-eclampsia (discussed later in more detail) is a combination of hemorrhage and patchy hepatocellular necrosis of various severity (Fig. 54–6). Two syndromes have been described and they will be discussed in more detail. One is a moderately severe disorder of patchy hepatocyte necrosis associated with thrombocytopenia, termed the HELLP syndrome. The second is acute liver hemorrhage and rupture, a rare but often fatal event.

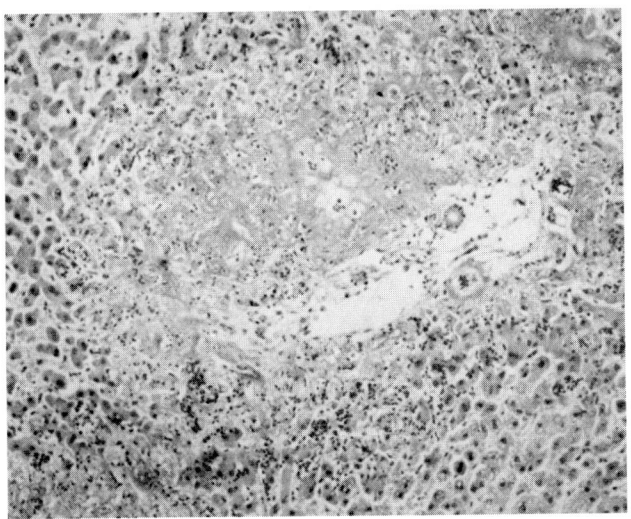

Figure 54–6. Micrograph of liver in eclampsia, showing periportal hemorrhage and patchy necrosis. Hematoxylin and eosin. (Courtesy of Dr. L. Ferrell.)

Hepatic Pathology

Liver biopsies in many women with pre-eclampsia are normal or exhibit only slight anisocytosis and anisonucleosis, hyperplasia of Kupffer cells, and occasional yellow pigment in hepatocytes.[4, 5, 328] In four series of 84 women with pre-eclampsia, all of whom underwent liver biopsy, hepatic histology was essentially normal in 70, whereas in 14 patients small scattered areas of necrosis were seen.[4, 5, 328, 329] Increased serum transaminase activities were noted in 60 per cent of the 84 women, suggesting that elevated transaminase values frequently indicate an insignificant degree of liver damage. Hepatic abnormalities are found more frequently in women with eclampsia. Six of 20 unselected patients undergoing liver biopsy[4, 5] and 65 to 72 per cent of unselected autopsy specimens of women dying of eclampsia exhibited focal hepatic necrosis.[320, 330]

The characteristic hepatic lesion of pre-eclampsia has three main features: (1) diffuse deposition of fibrin along the sinusoids and occasionally in portal tract capillaries, hepatic arterioles, and portal veins;[329] (2) periportal and portal tract hemorrhage;[4, 5, 330] and (3) ischemic necrosis, usually focal but occasionally confluent[4, 5, 328–320] (see Fig. 54–6). In cases with severe liver necrosis, diffuse blotchy areas of hemorrhage and necrosis are visible grossly both within the parenchyma of the liver and in subcapsular locations. Large hematomas may form beneath the capsule and these may rupture, resulting in exsanguination.

HELLP Syndrome

The HELLP syndrome was defined by Louis Weinstein in 1982, based on 29 patients observed within 30 months at the University of Arizona.[331] Although patients with the characteristics of this syndrome were reported as early as 1954, the name was coined by Weinstein from the characteristic laboratory features of Hemolysis, Elevated Liver enzymes and Low Platelet count. Patients with this syndrome probably represent the middle of the spectrum of liver involvement in pre-eclampsia (and eclampsia). The HELLP syndrome has been reported to occur in about 10 per cent of all women with pre-eclampsia.[325–327] An identical syndrome has been reported in a few women without clinically apparent pre-eclampsia; however, liver biopsies in most of these patients showed lesions characteristic of pre-eclampsia.[332]

Clinical features, summarized in Table 54–10,[325–327, 331–343] do not differ greatly from findings in many women with pre-eclampsia who do not manifest liver involvement. The syndrome is defined by its characteristic laboratory abnormalities, summarized in Table 54–11. Hemolysis (due to microangiopathic hemolytic anemia[343, 344]), thrombocytopenia, and increased serum transaminase activity are essentially universal features. Onset of these abnormalities may be sudden and without warning. Evidence of true disseminated intravascular coagulopathy is much less common. Although hepatocyte necrosis is present in all patients, the degree to which overall liver function is impaired may be difficult to assess. For example, hyperbilirubinemia, present in 42 per cent of reported cases, is probably due to a combination of hemolysis and liver dysfunction, whereas elevated values for the prothrombin time probably reflect a combination of decreased synthesis and increased peripheral consumption. Renal dysfunction also is virtually universal in women with the HELLP syndrome. It is not known whether the incidence and extent of renal impairment in women with this syndrome differ from those in other women with pre-eclampsia.

TABLE 54–10. THE HELLP SYNDROME: CLINICAL FEATURES

Feature	Average Value (Range)
No. of patients	293
Age	24 years (14–40)
Gestational duration	33.3 weeks (23–40)
Primiparas	56%
Frequency among all women with pre-eclampsia	10% (9–12%)
Hypertension*	92%
Proteinuria*	83%
Nausea, vomiting	36%
Epigastric/right upper-quadrant pain*	81%
Headache*	57%
Edema*	61%
Hepatic tenderness	100%
Ascites (often identified only at cesarean section)	65%

Source: Data compiled from references 325–327, 331–343. All but three cases (ref. 333) were reported after 1974.

*Signs and symptoms that are also commonly seen in women with pre-eclampsia who do not manifest the characteristic laboratory abnormalities of the HELLP syndrome.

A general outline for the treatment of the HELLP syndrome includes diagnosis and close monitoring of the mother's platelet count and serum transaminase activity, treatment of hypertension with MgSO$_4$ and other antihypertensive agents as needed, volume expansion, fetal monitoring and assessment of fetal lung maturity. If the fetal lungs are mature, or if fetal distress is apparent, or if maternal clinical or laboratory features deteriorate, immediate delivery is undertaken, usually by cesarean section. If the fetal lungs are immature and the fetus and mother are stable, administration of steroids (to hasten lung maturation) and close observation for a few days prior to delivery may be warranted.[316, 317, 325, 343] Platelet transfusions and steroids (to reverse the thrombocytopenia) have been given to some women without clear-cut beneficial results.[327, 339, 340]

Retardation of intrauterine growth and sudden fetal death are common in pregnancies complicated by pre-eclampsia and the HELLP syndrome.[345] Since the disorder generally appears late in pregnancy, the chances of fetal survival are better with prompt delivery. Prompt delivery also is indicated because the HELLP syndrome may worsen precipitously.

Maternal mortality in patients with this syndrome is low (2.4 per cent of 293 reported cases), possibly because most patients are delivered promptly; however, a causal relationship between early delivery and decreased maternal mortality has never been proven. Liver necrosis generally heals rapidly, with little evidence of fibrosis or of chronic liver disease. Fetal mortality is high, due primarily to placental insufficiency and fetal hypoxia. Some[345] but not all[346] investigators feel that infants born to women with the HELLP syndrome may exhibit transient thrombocytopenia and/or neutropenia and have recommended delivery by cesarean section to reduce the risk of intracranial hemorrhage during labor.

A few women develop pre-eclampsia in more than one pregnancy and are therefore at risk of recurrence of the HELLP syndrome. However, only one instance of recurrence of the HELLP syndrome has been reported.[327]

Hepatic Hemorrhage and/or Rupture

Hepatic rupture in pregnancy was first described by Abercrombie in 1844.[347] More than 60 cases (94 per cent associated with pre-eclampsia or eclampsia) have been reported since 1969.[319, 320, 347–372] Hepatic hemorrhage and/or rupture is probably due to confluent hepatic necrosis from pre-eclampsia. It is reported to occur in between 1 and 77 of every 100,000 deliveries and in 1 to 2 per cent of women with pre-eclampsia.[319, 320, 352] The highest figures are derived from a study in which abdominal CT scans were used to identify contained hepatic hematomas in women with few symptoms other than right upper quadrant abdominal pain.[319]

Hemorrhage occurs late in pregnancy or up to 48 hours post partum. Clinical or histologic features of pre-eclampsia are found in 92 per cent of patients. Information about laboratory abnormalities in reported cases is limited, but many patients would satisfy the criteria for the HELLP syndrome. Hepatic hemorrhage and rupture are heralded by the sudden onset of right upper-quadrant pain. Hepatic tenderness, diffuse abdominal pain, peritoneal findings, and chest and shoulder pain are noted in some patients. Shock ensues in over half of the patients. Shock may develop within a few hours of the onset of pain or be delayed for up to 48 hours. Anemia or a rapid drop in hematocrit is noted in many patients. These signs and symptoms are not diagnostic and are similar to those seen in a variety of intra-abdominal catastrophes, including rupture of a hepatic

TABLE 54–11. THE HELLP SYNDROME: LABORATORY ABNORMALITIES

Test	% of Patients with Abnormal Values	Average Value	Range of Values
Abnormal RBC morphology*	89.5	—	—
Thrombocytopenia	95	—	12,000–100,000
Fibrinogen	16	Decreased	—
Fibrin degradation products	42	Increased	—
Prothrombin time	13	Increased	—
Partial thromboplastin time	13	Increased	—
Serum bilirubin	42	—	1.4–19 mg/dL
AST (nl ≤ 40)	99	434 IU/L	nl–2300 IU/L
ALT (nl ≤ 40)	100	239 IU/L	49–702 IU/L
Impaired renal function (increased BUN and creatinine)	50–100	—	—
Creatinine clearance (120–150 ml/min is normal in pregnant women)	90–100	55 ml/min	0–138 ml/min

Source: Data represents reports on 293 cases and is derived from references 325–327, 331–344.

*RBC fragments, schistocytes, spherocytes; signs of microangiopathic hemolytic anemia.

RBC = red blood cell; AST = aspartate aminotransferase; ALT = alanine aminotransferase; nl = normal; BUN = blood urea nitrogen.

adenoma, abruptio placentae, perforated viscus, and intestinal infarction.

Diagnosis is based on clinical suspicion and visualization of the liver, either radiologically or at laparotomy. Currently, abdominal CT scans (Fig. 54–7) are the most sensitive and specific way to detect hepatic hemorrhage and/or rupture.[319, 360, 364, 374] Liver/spleen scans and angiograms also are useful. Ultrasound is easy to perform, but nonspecific findings and false-negative studies are frequent.[319, 360, 366, 370] Paracentesis can be useful in confirming intra-abdominal hemorrhage but does not clarify the site of bleeding and will be negative in patients with contained hematomas. Magnetic resonance imaging (MRI) scans, which do not expose the fetus to radiation (adverse effects of magnets and radiowaves are not known), display chronic hematomas[374] but are less accurate than CT scans in detecting acute hemorrhage.

Survival of a patient with an untreated, ruptured subcapsular hematoma has never been reported. In contrast, hemorrhage into a contained hematoma may resolve with medical support.[319, 352, 363] Treatment of hepatic hemorrhage and rupture requires rapid diagnosis and intensive therapy by a multidisciplinary team.[375, 376] The most important factors in ensuring maternal survival are identification of the disorder before irreversible shock occurs, rigorous hemodynamic support with large volume transfusions of blood and platelets (transfusion of over 20 units of blood is not uncommon), and, if rupture of Glisson's capsule has occurred (or is suspected), emergency laparotomy.

At surgery, hematomas are drained and hemostasis attempted with packing, sutures and/or lobectomy. Angiographic embolization has been attempted in four cases[361, 367, 368] and was successful in two.[367, 368] Obviously, one can expect this therapy to work only in patients with rupture limited to one portion of the liver. Reports describe successful arrest of hemorrhage with ligation of the hepatic artery; however, three of four patients later succumbed to liver failure associated with extensive ischemic necrosis.[362, 366, 368] Apparently the liver cannot survive the combination of ischemia due to pre-eclampsia and ligation of the hepatic artery.[362]

Women with contained hepatic hematomas, diagnosed by radiologic procedures, may do well without surgery if they receive adequate hemodynamic support and are followed closely.[319] Exploratory laparotomy should be undertaken, however, if there is any suspicion of free rupture into the peritoneum.

Overall maternal and fetal mortality is high, approximately 49 per cent and 59 per cent, respectively. Mortality is lower in women with contained hematomas and in those who undergo prompt laparotomy. In patients who survive, hematomas gradually resolve, and subsequent successful pregnancy has been reported.[371] Healing can be documented by serial CT scans.[319, 360, 364, 367] Recurrences have not been reported.

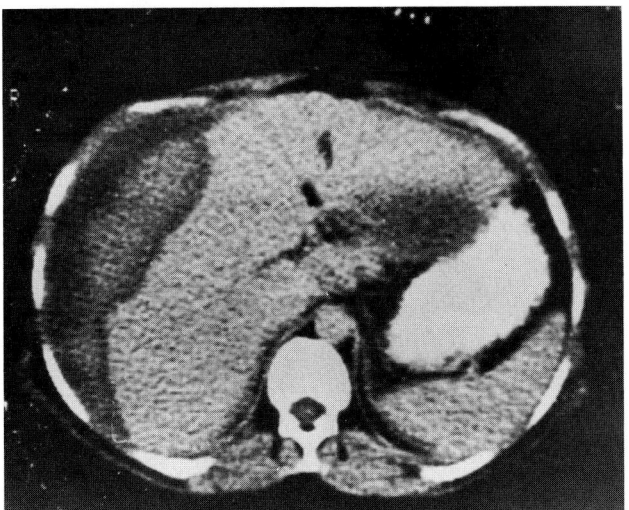

Figure 54–7. Abdominal CT scan, showing a subcapsular hematoma along the right margin of the liver. (Reprinted by permission of the New England Journal of Medicine from Manas KJ, et al. N Engl J Med 312:424, 1985.)

REFERENCES

1. Sheehan HL. Jaundice in pregnancy. Am J Obstet Gynecol 81:427, 1961.
2. Combes B, Shibata H, Adams R, et al. Alterations in sulfobromophthalein sodium–removal mechanisms from blood during normal pregnancy. J Clin Invest 42:1431, 1963.
3. Nixon WCW, Egeli ES, Laqueur W, et al. Icterus in pregnancy. J Obstet Gynaecol Br Emp 54:642, 1947.
4. Ingerslev M, Teilum G. Biopsy studies on the liver in pregnancy I, II, III. Acta Obstet Gynecol 25:339, 352, 361, 1945/46.
5. Antia FP, Bharadwaj TP, Watsa MC, et al. Liver in normal pregnancy, pre-eclampsia, and eclampsia. Lancet 2:776, 1958.
6. Gonzalez-Angulo A, Aznar-Ramos R, Marquez-Monter H, et al. Ultrastructure of liver cells in women under steroid therapy. I. Normal pregnancy and trophoblastic growths. Acta Endocrinol 65:193, 1970.
7. Perez V, Gorodisch S, Casavilla F, et al. Ultrastructure of human liver at the end of normal pregnancy. Am J Obstet Gynecol 110:428, 1971.
8. Larsson-Cohn U, Stenram U. Liver ultrastructure and function in icteric and non-icteric women using oral contraceptive agents. Acta Med Scand 181:257, 1967.
9. Martinez-Manautou J, Aznar-Ramos R, Bautista-O'Farrill J, et al. The ultrastructure of liver cells in women under steroid therapy. II. Contraceptive therapy. Acta Endocrinol 65:207, 1970.
10. Perez V, Gorodisch S, de Martire J, et al. Oral contraceptives: long-term use produces fine structural changes in liver mitochondria. Science 165:805, 1969.
11. Rovinsky JJ, Jaffin H. Cardiovascular hemodynamics in pregnancy. Am J Obstet Gynecol 95:787, 1966.
12. Pritchard JA. Changes in the blood volume during pregnancy and delivery. Anesthesiology 26:393, 1965.
13. Lund CJ, Donovan JC. Blood volume during pregnancy. Am J Obstet Gynecol 98:393, 1967.
14. Munnell EW, Taylor HC Jr. Liver blood flow in pregnancy—hepatic vein catheterization. J Clin Invest 26:952, 1947.
15. Laakso L, Ruotsalainen P, Punnonen R, et al. Hepatic blood flow during late pregnancy. Acta Obstet Gynecol Scand 50:175, 1971.
16. Iber FL. Jaundice in pregnancy—a review. Am J Obstet Gynecol 91:721, 1965.
17. Song CS, Rifkind AB, Gillette PN, et al. Hormones and the liver. The effects of estrogens, progestins, and pregnancy on hepatic function. Am J Obstet Gynecol 105:813, 1969.
18. Adlercreutz H, Tenhunen R. Some aspects of the interaction between natural and synthetic female sex hormones and the liver. Am J Med 49:630, 1970.
19. McNair RD, Jaynes RV. Alterations in liver function during normal pregnancy. Am J Obstet Gynecol 80:500, 1960.
20. Ramcharan S, Sponzilli EE, Wingerd JC. Serum protein fractions. Effects of oral contraceptives and pregnancy. Obstet Gynecol 48:211, 1976.
21. Honger PE, Rossing N. Albumin metabolism and oral contraception. Clin Sci 36:41, 1969.
22. Shaaban MM, Hammad WA, Fathalla MF, et al. Effects of oral contraception on liver function tests and serum proteins in women with past viral hepatitis. Contraception 26:65, 1982.
23. Burrows S, Pekala B. Serum copper and ceruloplasmin in pregnancy. Am J Obstet Gynecol 109:907, 1971.
24. Haemmerli R. Jaundice during pregnancy with special emphasis on recurrent jaundice during pregnancy and its differential diagnosis. Acta Med Scand 179(Suppl 444):1, 1966.
25. Svanborg A, Vikrot O. Plasma lipid fractions, including individual phospholipids, at various stages of pregnancy. Acta Med Scand 178:615, 1965.

26. Knopp RH, Warth MR, Carrol CJ. Lipid metabolism in pregnancy. I. Changes in lipoprotein triglyceride and cholesterol in normal pregnancy and the effects of diabetes mellitus. J Reprod Med 10:95, 1973.

27. Novikoff PM. Intracellular organelles and lipoprotein metabolism in normal and fatty livers. In: Arias IM, Popper H, Schachter D, et al, eds. The Liver: Biology and Pathobiology. New York: Raven Press, 1982:143.

28. Bennion LJ, Ginsberg RL, Garnick MB, et al. Effects of oral contraceptives on the gallbladder bile of normal women. N Engl J Med 294:189, 1976.

29. Schmid SE, Au WYW, Hill DE, et al. Cytochrome P-450–dependent oxidation of the 17α-ethinyl group of synthetic steroids. D-Homoannulation or enzyme inactivation. Drug Metab Dispos 11:531, 1983.

30. Crawford JS, Rudofsky S. Some alterations in the pattern of drug metabolism associated with pregnancy, oral contraceptives, and the newly born. Br J Anaesth 38:446, 1966.

31. Vore M, Bauer J, Pascucci V. The effect of pregnancy on the metabolism of [^{14}C]phenytoin in the isolated perfused rat liver. J Pharmacol Exp Ther 206:439, 1978.

32. Homeida M, Halliwell M, Branch RA. Effects of an oral contraceptive on hepatic size and antipyrine metabolism in premenopausal women. Clin Pharmacol Ther 24:228, 1978.

33. Carter DE, Goldman JM, Bressler R, et al. Effect of oral contraceptives on drug metabolism. Clin Pharmacol Ther 15:22, 1973.

34. O'Malley K, Stevenson IH, Crooks J. Impairment of human drug metabolism by oral contraceptive steroids. Clin Pharmacol Ther 13:552, 1972.

35. Brock WJ, Vore M. Hepatic morphine and estrone glucuronyltransferase activity and morphine biliary excretion in the isolated perfused rat liver. Drug Metab Dispos 10:336, 1982.

36. Vore M, Montgomery C. The effect of estradiol-17β treatment on the metabolism and biliary excretion of phenytoin in the isolated perfused rat liver and in vivo. J Pharmacol Exp Ther 215:71, 1980.

37. Watson KJR, Ghabrial H, Mashford ML, et al. The oral contraceptive pill increases morphine clearance but does not increase hepatic blood flow. Gastroenterology 90:1779, 1986 (Abstract).

38. Schreiber AJ, Simon FR. Estrogen-induced cholestasis: Clues to pathogenesis and treatment. Hepatology 3:607, 1983.

39. Soffer LJ. Bilirubin excretion as a test for liver function during normal pregnancy. Bull Johns Hopkins Hosp 52:365, 1933.

40. Sullivan CF, Tew WP, Watson EM. The bilirubin excretion test of liver function in pregnancy. J Obstet Gynaecol Br Emp 41:347, 1934.

41. Thorling L. Jaundice in pregnancy. A clinical study. Acta Med Scand 151(Suppl. 302):1, 1955.

42. Ylostalo P. Liver function in hepatosis of pregnancy and pre-eclampsia with special reference to modified bromsulphthalein tests. Acta Obstet Gynecol Scand 49(Suppl 4):4, 1970.

43. Kessler WB, Andros GJ. Hepatic function during pregnancy and puerperium. Obstet Gynecol 23:372, 1964.

44. Järnfelt-Samsioe A, Eriksson B, Waldenström J, et al. Serum bile acids, gamma-glutamyltransferase and routine liver function tests in emetic and nonemetic pregnancies. Gynecol Obstet Invest 21:169, 1986.

45. Simcock MJ, Forster FMC. Pregnancy is cholestatic. Med J Aust 2:971, 1967.

46. Mueller MN, Kappas A. Estrogen pharmacology. I. The influence of estradiol and estriol on hepatic disposal of sulfobromophthalein (BSP) in man. J Clin Invest 43:1905, 1964.

47. Kleiner GJ, Kresch L, Arias IM. Studies of hepatic excretory function. II. The effect of norethynodrel and mestranol on bromsulfalein sodium metabolism in women of childbearing age. N Engl J Med 273:420, 1965.

48. Fulton HC, Douglas JG, Hutchon DJR, et al. Is normal pregnancy cholestatic? Clin Chim Acta 130:171, 1983.

49. Heikkinen J. Serum bile acids in the early diagnosis of intrahepatic cholestasis of pregnancy. Obstet Gynecol 61:581, 1983.

50. Lunzer M, Barnes P, Byth K, et al. Serum bile acid concentrations during pregnancy and their relationship to obstetric cholestasis. Gastroenterology 91:825, 1986.

51. Kern F. Effect of estrogens on the liver. Gastroenterology 75:512, 1978.

52. Romslo I, Sagen N, Haram K. Serum alkaline phosphatase in pregnancy. Acta Obstet Gynecol Scand 54:437, 1975.

53. Sammour MB, Ramadan MA, Khalil FK, et al. Serum and placental lactic dehydrogenase and alkaline phosphatase isoenzymes in normal pregnancy and in pre-eclampsia. Acta Obstet Gynecol Scand 54:393, 1975.

54. Sussman HH, Bowman M, Lewis JL. Placental alkaline phosphatase in maternal serum during normal and abnormal pregnancy. Nature 218:359, 1968.

55. Birkett DJ, Done J, Neale FC, et al. Serum alkaline phosphatase in pregnancy: an immunological study. Br Med J 1:1210, 1966.

56. Walker FB, Hoblit DL, Cunningham FG, et al. Gamma glutamyl transpeptidase in normal pregnancy. Obstet Gynecol 43:745, 1974.

57. Seitanidis B, Moss DW. Serum alkaline phosphatase and 5'-nucleotidase levels during normal pregnancy. Clin Chim Acta 25:183, 1969.

58. Rosalki SB, Rau D, Lehmann D, et al. Determination of serum γ-glutamyl transpeptidase activity and its clinical applications. Ann Clin Biochem 7:143, 1970.

59. Combes B, Shore GM, Cunningham FG, et al. Serum γ-glutamyl transpeptidase activity in viral hepatitis: suppression in pregnancy and by birth control pills. Gastroenterology 72:271, 1977.

60. Bean WB. The cutaneous arterial spider: a survey. Medicine 24:243, 1945.

61. Bean WB, Cogswell R, Dexter M. Vascular changes of the skin in pregnancy. Surg Obstet Gynecol 88:739, 1949.

62. Friedlaender P, Osler M. Icterus and pregnancy. Am J Obstet Gynecol 97:894, 1967.

63. Hieber JP, Dalton D, Shorey J, et al. Hepatitis and pregnancy. J Pediatr 91:545, 1977.

64. Cahill KM. Hepatitis in pregnancy. Surg Gynecol Obstet 114:545, 1962.

65. Adams RH, Combes B. Viral hepatitis during pregnancy. JAMA 192:195, 1965.

66. Parker MLM: Infectious hepatitis in pregnancy. Med J Aust 2:967, 1967.

67. Bennett NM, Forbes JA, Lucas CR, et al. Infective hepatitis and pregnancy: analysis of liver function test results. Med J Aust 2:974, 1967.

68. Rao AVN, Devi CS, Savithri P, et al. Infectious hepatitis in pregnancy and puerperium—a study of 60 cases. Indian J Med Sci 23:471, 1969.

69. D'Cruz IA, Balani SG, Iyer LS. Infectious hepatitis and pregnancy. J Am Coll Obstet Gynecol 31:449, 1968.

70. Gelpi AP. Fatal hepatitis in Saudi Arabian women. Am J Gastroenterol 53:41, 1970.

71. Borhanmanesh F, Haghighi P, Hekmat K, et al. Viral hepatitis during pregnancy. Severity and effect on gestation. Gastroenterology 64:304, 1973.

72. Christie AB, Allam AA, Aref MKJ, et al. Pregnancy hepatitis in Libya. Lancet 2:827, 1976.

73. Adams WH, Shrestha SM, Adams DG. Coagulation studies of viral hepatitis occurring during pregnancy. Am J Med Sci 272:139, 1976.

74. Gelpi AP. Viral hepatitis complicating pregnancy: mortality trends in Saudi Arabia. Int J Gynecol Obstet 17:73, 1979.

75. Singh DS, Balasubramaniam M, Krishnaswami S, et al. Viral hepatitis during pregnancy. J Indian Med Assoc 73:90, 1979.

76. Khuroo MS, Teli MR, Skidmore S. Incidence and severity of viral hepatitis in pregnancy. Am J Med 70:252, 1981.

77. Mallia CP, Nancekivell AF. Fulminant virus hepatitis in late pregnancy. Ann Trop Med Parasitol 76:143, 1982.

78. Mandal D, Chowdhury NNR. Viral hepatitis in pregnancy. J Indian Med Assoc 79:96, 1982.

79. Shalev I, Bassan HM: Viral hepatitis during pregnancy in Israel. Br J Gynaecol Obstet 20:73, 1982.

80. Pain GC, Chakraborty AK, Choudhury NR. Outbreak of non-A non-B type viral hepatitis in a Calcutta slum. J Indian Med Assoc 80:125, 1983.

81. Tong MJ, Thursby M, Rakela J, et al. Studies on the maternal-infant transmission of the viruses which cause acute hepatitis. Gastroenterology 80:999, 1981.

82. Snydman DR. Hepatitis in pregnancy. N Engl J Med 313:1398, 1985.

83. Zanetti AR, Ferroni P, Magliano EM, et al. Perinatal transmission of the hepatitis B virus and of the HBV-associated delta agent from mothers to offspring in northern Italy. J Med Virol 9:139, 1982.

84. Gerety RJ, Schweitzer IL. Viral hepatitis type B during pregnancy, the neonatal period, and infancy. J Pediatr 90:368, 1977.

85. Tong MJ, McPeak CM, Thursby MW, et al. Failure of immune serum globulin to prevent hepatitis B virus infection in infants born to HBsAg-positive mothers. Gastroenterology 76:535, 1979.

86. Lee AKY, Ip HMH, Wong VCW. Mechanisms of maternal-fetal transmission of hepatitis B virus. J Infect Dis 138:668, 1978.

87. Stevens CE, Neurath RA, Beasley RP, et al. HBeAg and anti-HBe detection by radioimmunoassay: correlation with vertical transmission of hepatitis B virus in Taiwan. J Med Virol 3:237, 1979.

88. Beasley RP, Hwang L-Y, Lin C-C, et al. Hepatocellular carcinoma and hepatitis B virus. Lancet 2:1129, 1981.

89. Nair PV, Weissman JY, Tong MJ, et al. Efficacy of hepatitis B immune globulin in prevention of perinatal transmission of the hepatitis B virus. Gastroenterology 87:293, 1984.

90. Beasley RP, Hwang L-Y, Lee G C-Y, et al. Prevention of perinatally transmitted hepatitis B virus infections with hepatitis B immune globulin and hepatitis B vaccine. Lancet 2:1099, 1983.

91. Beasley RP, Hwang L-Y, Stevens CE, et al. Efficacy of hepatitis B immune globulin for prevention of perinatal transmission of the hepatitis B virus carrier state: final report of a randomized double-bind, placebo-controlled trial. Hepatology 3:135, 1983.

92. Stevens CE, Toy PT, Tong MJ, et al. Perinatal hepatitis B virus transmission in the United States. Prevention by passive-active immunization. JAMA 253:1740, 1985.

93. Lefkowitch JH, Rushton AR, Feng-Chen K-C. Hepatic fibrosis in fetal alcohol syndrome. Gastroenterology 85:951, 1983.

94. Møller J, Brandt NJ, Tygstrup I. Hepatic dysfunction in patient with fetal alcohol syndrome. Lancet 1:605, 1979.

95. Habbick BF, Casey R, Zaleski WA, et al. Liver abnormalities in three patients with fetal alcohol syndrome. Lancet 1:580, 1979.

96. Steven MM, Buckley JD, Mackay IR. Pregnancy in chronic active hepatitis. Q J Med 48:519, 1979.

97. Infeld DS, Borkowf HI, Varma RR. Chronic-persistent hepatitis and pregnancy. Gastroenterology 77:524, 1979.

98. Whelton MJ, Sherlock S. Pregnancy in patients with hepatic cirrhosis. Lancet 2:995, 1968.

99. Joske RA, Pawsey HK, Martin JD. Chronic active liver disease and successful pregnancy. Lancet 2:712, 1963.

100. Choudhury KL, Chogtu L. Chronic active hepatitis and pregnancy. J Indian Med Assoc 63:196, 1974.

101. Powell D. Pregnancy in active chronic hepatitis on immunosuppressive therapy. Postgrad Med J 45:292, 1969.

102. Schweitzer IL, Peters RL. Pregnancy in hepatitis B antigen positive cirrhosis. Obstet Gynecol 48 (Suppl 1):53S, 1976.

103. Borhanmanesh F, Haghighi P. Pregnancy in patients with cirrhosis of the liver. Obstet Gynecol 36:315, 1970.

104. Schreyer P, Caspi E, El-Hindi JM, et al. Cirrhosis—pregnancy and delivery: a review. Obstet Gynecol Surv 37:304, 1982.

105. Cheng Y-S. Pregnancy in liver cirrhosis and/or portal hypertension. Am J Obstet Gynecol 128:812, 1977.

106. Britton RC. Pregnancy and esophageal varices. Am J Surg 143:421, 1982.

107. Moore RM, Hughes PK. Cirrhosis of the liver in pregnancy. Obstet Gynecol 15:753, 1960.

108. Varma RR, Michelsohn NH, Borkowf HI, et al. Pregnancy in cirrhotic and noncirrhotic portal hypertension. Obstet Gynecol 50:217, 1977.

109. Niven P, Williams D, Zeegen P. Pregnancy following the surgical treatment of portal hypertension. Am J Obstet Gynecol 110:1100, 1971.

110. Salam AA, Warren WD. Distal splenorenal shunt for the treatment of variceal bleeding during pregnancy. Arch Surg 105:643, 1972.

111. Chattopadhyay TK, Kapoor VK, Iyer KS, et al. Successful splenorenal shunt performed during pregnancy. Jpn J Surg 14:405, 1984.

112. Brown HJ. Splenorenal shunt during pregnancy. Am Surg 37:441, 1971.

113. Krol-Van Straaten J, De Maat CEM. Successful pregnancies in cirrhosis of the liver before and after portacaval anastomosis. Neth J Med 27:14, 1984.

114. Waffarn F, Carlisle S, Pena I, et al. Fetal exposure to maternal hyperbilirubinemia. Am J Dis Child 136:416, 1982.

115. Cotton DB, Brock BJ, Schifrin BS. Cirrhosis and fetal hyperbilirubinemia. Obstet Gynecol 57 (Suppl):25S, 1981.

116. Scheinberg IH, Sternlieb I. Pregnancy in penicillamine-treated patients with Wilson's disease. N Engl J Med 293:1300, 1975.

117. Toaff R, Toaff ME, Peyser MR, et al. Hepatolenticular degeneration (Wilson's disease) and pregnancy. Obstet Gynecol Surv 32:497, 1977.

118. Walshe JM. The management of pregnancy in Wilson's disease treated with trientine. Q J Med 58:81, 1986.

119. German JL III, Bearn AG. Effect of estrogens on copper metabolism in Wilson's disease. J Clin Invest 40:445, 1961.

120. Dreifuss FE, McKinney WM. Wilson's disease (hepatolenticular degeneration) and pregnancy. JAMA 195:960, 1966.

121. Biller J, Swiontoniowski M, Brazis PW. Successful pregnancy in Wilson's disease: a case report and review of the literature. Eur Neurol 24:306, 1985.

122. Marecek Z, Graf M. Pregnancy in penicillamine-treated patients with Wilson's disease. N Engl J Med 295:841, 1976.

123. Mjølnerød OK, Dommerud SA, Rasmussen K, et al. Congenital connective-tissue defect probably due to D-penicillamine treatment in pregnancy. Lancet 1:673, 1971.

124. Solomon L, Abrams G, Dinner M, et al. Neonatal abnormalities associated with D-penicillamine treatment during pregnancy. N Engl J Med 296:54, 1977 (Letter).

125. Linares A, Zarranz JJ, Rodriguez-Alarcon J, et al. Reversible cutis laxa due to maternal D-penicillamine treatment. Lancet 2:43, 1979 (Letter).

126. Morimoto I, Minomiya H, Komatsu K, et al. Pregnancy and penicillamine treatment in a patient with Wilson's disease. Jpn J Med 25:59, 1986.

127. Walshe JM. Pregnancy in Wilson's disease. Q J Med 46:73, 1977.

128. Endres W. D-Penicillamine in pregnancy—to ban or not to ban? Klin Wochenschr 59:535, 1981.

129. Walshe JM. Treatment of Wilson's disease with trientine (triethylene tetramine) dihydrochloride. Lancet 1:643, 1982.

130. Cohen L, Lewis C, Arias IM. Pregnancy, oral contraceptives, and chronic familial jaundice with predominantly conjugated hyperbilirubinemia (Dubin-Johnson syndrome). Gastroenterology 62:1182, 1972.

131. Di Zoglio JD, Cardillo E. The Dubin-Johnson syndrome and pregnancy. Obstet Gynecol 42:560, 1973.

132. Shani M, Seligsohn U, Gilon E, et al. Dubin-Johnson syndrome in Israel. Q J Med 39:549, 1970.

133. Bennion LJ, Grundy SM. Risk factors for the development of cholelithiasis in man. N Engl J Med 299:1221, 1978.

134. Thistle JL. Gallstones in women. Med Clin North Am 58:811, 1974.

135. Pertsemlidis D, Panveliwalla D, Ahrens EH. Effects of clofibrate and of an estrogen-progestin combination on fasting biliary lipids and cholic acid kinetics in man. Gastroenterology 66:565, 1974.

136. Bennion LJ, Mott DM, Howard BV. Oral contraceptives raise the cholesterol saturation of bile by increasing biliary cholesterol secretion. Metabolism 29:18, 1980.

137. Kern F, Everson GT, DeMark B. Biliary lipids, bile acids, and gallbladder function in the human female: effects of contraceptive steroids. J Lab Clin Med 99:798, 1982.

138. Kern F, Everson GT, DeMark B, et al. Biliary lipids, bile acids, and gallbladder function in the human female. Effects of pregnancy and the ovulatory cycle. J Clin Invest 68:1229, 1981.

139. Braverman DZ, Johnson ML, Kern F Jr. Effects of pregnancy and contraceptive steroids on gallbladder function. N Engl J Med 302:362, 1980.

140. Everson RB, Byar DP, Bischoff AJ. Estrogen predisposes to cholecystectomy but not to stones. Gastroenterology 82:4, 1982.

141. Wingrave SJ, Kay CR. Oral contraceptives and gallbladder disease. Royal College of General Practitioners oral contraception study. Lancet 2:957, 1982.

142. Oral contraceptives and venous thromboembolic disease, surgically confirmed gallbladder disease, and breast tumors. Report from the Boston Collaborative Drug Surveillance Programme. Lancet 2:7817, 1973.

143. Surgically confirmed gallbladder disease, venous thromboembolism, and breast tumors in relation to postmenopausal estrogen therapy. Report from the Boston Collaborative Drug Surveillance Program. N Engl J Med 290:15, 1974.

144. Everson GT, McKinley C, Lawson M. Gallbladder function in the human female: Effect of the ovulatory cycle, pregnancy, and contraceptive steroids. Gastroenterology 82:711, 1982.

145. Glenn F, McSherry CK. Gallstones and pregnancy among 300 young women treated by cholecystectomy. Surg Gynecol Obstet 127:1067, 1968.

146. Friley MD, Douglas G. Acute cholecystitis in pregnancy and the puerperium. Am Surg 38:314, 1972.

147. Hill LM, Johnson CE, Lee RA, et al. Cholecytectomy in pregnancy. Obstet Gynecol 46:291, 1975.

148. Landers D, Carmona R, Crombleholme W, et al. Acute cholecystitis in pregnancy. Obstet Gynecol 69:131, 1987.

149. Bartoli E, Calonaci N, Nenci R. Ultrasonography of the gallbladder in pregnancy. Gastrointest Radiol 9:35, 1984.

150. Williamson SL, Williamson MR. Cholecystosonography in pregnancy. J Ultrasound Med 3:329, 1984.

151. Mintz MC, Grumbach K, Arger PH, et al. Sonographic evaluation of bile duct size during pregnancy. Am J Radiol 145:575, 1985.

152. Printen KJ, Ott RA. Cholecystectomy during pregnancy. Am Surg 44:432, 1978.

153. Hiatt JR, Hiatt JCG, Williams RA. Biliary disease in pregnancy: strategy for surgical management. Am J Surg 151:263, 1986.

154. Simon JA. Biliary tract disease and related surgical disorders during pregnancy. Clin Obstet Gynecol 26:810, 1983.

155. Griffen WO Jr, Dilts PV Jr, Roddick JW Jr. Non-obstetrical surgery during pregnancy. In: Ravitsh MM, Ellison EH, Julian OC, et al., eds. Current Problems in Surgery. Chicago, Year Book Medical Pub., Nov 1969:1.

156. Porter LE, Elm MS, Van Thiel DH, et al. Characterization and quantitation of human hepatic estrogen receptor. Gastroenterology 84:704, 1983.

157. Ishak KG. Hepatic lesions caused by anabolic and contraceptive steroids. Semin Liver Dis 1:116, 1981.

158. Christopherson WM, Mays ET, Barrows GH. Liver oncogenesis and steroids. In: Ariel IM, ed. Progress in Clinical Cancer, Vol. III. New York, Grune & Stratton, 1978:153.

159. Winkler K, Poulsen H. Liver disease with periportal sinusoidal dilata-

tion. A possible complication to contraceptive steroids. Scand J Gastroent 10:699, 1975.

160. Spellberg MA, Mirro J, and Chowdhury L. Hepatic sinusoidal dilatation related to oral contraceptives. Am J Gastroenterol 72:218, 1979.

161. Thung SN, Gerber MA. Precursor stage of hepatocellular neoplasm following long exposure to orally administered contraceptives. Hum Pathol 12:472, 1981.

162. Dienstag JL. Case records of the Massachusetts General Hospital. N Engl J Med 307:934, 1982.

163. Kerlin P, Davis GL, McGill DB, et al. Hepatic adenoma and focal nodular hyperplasia: clinical, pathologic, and radiologic features. Gastroenterology 84:994, 1983.

164. Knowles DM II, Casarella WJ, Johnson PM, et al. The clinical, radiologic, and pathologic characterization of benign hepatic neoplasms. Medicine 57:223, 1978.

165. Klatskin G. Hepatic tumors: Possible relationship to use of oral contraceptives. Gastroenterology 73:386, 1977.

166. Fechner RE. Benign hepatic lesions and orally administered contraceptives. Hum Pathol 8:255, 1977.

167. Stauffer JQ, Lapinski MW, Honold DJ, et al. Focal nodular hyperplasia of the liver and intrahepatic hemorrhage in young women on oral contraceptives. Ann Intern Med 83:301, 1975.

168. Scott LD, Katz AR, Duke JH, et al. Oral contraceptives, pregnancy, and focal nodular hyperplasia of the liver. JAMA 251:1461, 1984.

169. Baum JK, Holtz F, Bookstein JJ, et al. Possible association between benign hepatomas and oral contraceptives. Lancet 2:926, 1973.

170. Rooks JB, Ory HW, Ishak KG, et al. Epidemiology of hepatocellular adenoma. JAMA 242:644, 1979.

171. Edmondson HA, Henderson B, Benton B. Liver-cell adenomas associated with use of oral contraceptives. N Engl J Med 294:470, 1976.

172. Nissen ED, Kent DR, Nissen SE, et al. Association of liver tumors with oral contraceptives. Obstet Gynecol 48:49, 1976.

173. Wanless IR, Medline A. Role of estrogens as promoters of hepatic neoplasia. Lab Invest 46:313, 1982.

174. Guzman IJ, Gold JH, Rosai J, et al. Benign hepatocellular tumors. Surgery 82:495, 1977.

175. Edmondson HA, Reynolds TB, Henderson B, et al. Regression of liver cell adenomas associated with oral contraceptives. Ann Intern Med 86:180, 1977.

176. Bühler H, Pirovino M, Akovbiantz A, et al. Regression of liver cell adenoma. Gastroenterology 82:775, 1982.

177. Hayes D, Lamki H, Hunter IWE. Hepatic-cell adenoma presenting with intraperitoneal haemorrhage in the puerperium. Br Med J 3:1394, 1977.

178. Kent DR, Nissen ED, Nissen SE, et al. Maternal death resulting from rupture of liver adenoma associated with oral contraceptives. Obstet Gynecol 50 (Suppl.):5S, 1977.

179. Kent DR, Nissen ED, Nissen SE, et al. Effect of pregnancy on liver tumor associated with oral contraceptives. Obstet Gynecol 51:148, 1978.

180. Kent DR, Nissen ED, Nissen SE. Liver tumors and oral contraceptives. Int J Gynaecol Obstet 15:137, 1977.

181. Check JH, King LC, Rakoff AE. Uncomplicated pregnancy following oral contraceptive–induced liver hepatoma. Obstet Gynecol 52 (Suppl.):28S, 1978.

182. Malt RA. Surgery for hepatic neoplasms. N Engl J Med 313:1591, 1985.

183. Irey NS, Manion WC, Taylor HB. Vascular lesions in women taking oral contraceptives. Arch Pathol 89:1, 1970.

184. Ecker JA, McKittrick JE, Failing RM. Thrombosis of the hepatic veins. Am J Gastroenterol 45:429, 1966.

185. Sterup K, Mosbech J. Budd-Chiari syndrome after taking oral contraceptives. Br Med J 4:660, 1967.

186. Somayaji BM, Eeles GH, Paton A, et al. Budd-Chiari syndrome after oral contraceptives. Br Med J 1:53, 1968.

187. Rothwell-Jackson RL. Budd-Chiari syndrome after oral contraceptives. Br Med J 1:252, 1968.

188. Grayson MJ, Reilly MCT. Budd-Chiari syndrome after oral contraceptives. Br Med J 1:512, 1968.

189. Hoyumpa AM, Schiff L, Helfman EL. Budd-Chiari syndrome in women taking oral contraceptives. Am J Med 50:137, 1971.

190. Frederick WC, Howard RG, Spatola S. Spontaneous rupture of the liver in patient using contraceptive pills. Arch Surg 108:93, 1974.

191. Alpert LI. Veno-occlusive disease of the liver associated with oral contraceptives: case report and review of the literature. Human Pathol 7:709, 1976.

192. Wu S-M, Spurny OM, Klotz AP. Budd-Chiari syndrome after taking oral contraceptives. A case report and review of 14 cases. Dig Dis 22:623, 1977.

193. Powell-Jackson PR, Melia W, Canalese J, et al. Budd-Chiari syndrome: clinical patterns and therapy. Q J Med 51:79, 1982.

194. Lewis JH, Tice HL, Zimmerman HJ. Budd-Chiari syndrome associated with oral contraceptive steroids. Review of treatment of 47 cases. Dig Dis Sci 28:673, 1983.

195. Van Steenbergen W, Beyls J, Vermylen J, et al. "Lupus" anticoagulant and thrombosis of the hepatic veins (Budd-Chiari syndrome). J Hepatol 3:87, 1986.

196. Mackworth-Young CG, Melia WM, Harris EN, et al. The Budd-Chiari syndrome. Possible pathogenetic role for anti-phospholipid antibodies. J Hepatol 3:83, 1986.

197. Krass IM: Chiari's syndrome. Report of a case following pregnancy. J Obstet Gynaecol Brit Emp 64:715, 1957.

198. Hancock KW: The Budd-Chiari syndrome in pregnancy. J Obstet Gynaecol Br Cwlth 75:746, 1968.

199. Oettinger M, Levy N, Lewy Z, et al. The Budd-Chiari syndrome in pregnancy. J Obstet Gynaecol Br Cwlth 77:174, 1970.

200. Rosenthal T, Shani M, Deutsch V, et al. The Budd-Chiari syndrome after pregnancy. Am J Obstet Gynecol 113:789, 1972.

201. Khuroo MS, Datta DV. Budd-Chiari syndrome following pregnancy. Report of 16 cases, with roentgenologic, hemodynamic and histologic studies of the hepatic outflow tract. Am J Med 68:113, 1980.

202. Artigas JMG, Estabanez, Faure MRA. Pregnancy and the Budd-Chiari syndrome. Dig Dis Sci 27:89, 1982.

203. Covillo FV, Nyong AO, Axelrod JL. Budd-Chiari syndrome following pregnancy. Mo Med 81:356, 1984.

204. Hodkinson HJ, McKibbin JK, Tim JO, et al. Postpartum veno-occlusive disease treated with ascitic fluid reinfusion. S Afr Med J 54:366, 1978.

205. Girardin M-FS-M, Zafrani ES, Prigent A, et al. Unilobular small hepatic vein obstruction: possible role of progestogen given as oral contraceptive. Gastroenterology 84:630, 1983.

206. Adams RH, Gordon J, Combes B. Hyperemesis gravidarum. I. Evidence of hepatic dysfunction. Obstet Gynecol 31:659, 1968.

207. Combes B, Adams RH, Gordon J, et al. Hyperemesis gravidarum. II. Alterations in sulfobromophthalein sodium–removal mechanisms from blood. Obstet Gynecol 31:665, 1968.

208. Larrey D, Rueff B, Feldmann G, et al. Recurrent jaundice caused by recurrent hyperemesis gravidarum. Gut 25:1414, 1984.

209. Chatwani A, Schwartz R. A severe case of hyperemesis gravidarum. Am J Obstet Gynecol 143:964, 1982.

210. Sheehan HL. The pathology of hyperemesis and vomiting of late pregnancy. J Obstet Gynaecol Br Emp 46:685, 1939.

211. Verdy M. BSP retention during total fasting. Metabolism 15:769, 1966.

212. Webber BL, Freiman I. The liver in kwashiorkor. Arch Pathol 98:400, 1974.

213. Haemmerli UP, Wyss HI. Recurrent intrahepatic cholestasis of pregnancy. Report of six cases, and review of the literature. Medicine 46:299, 1967.

214. Rencoret R, Aste H. Jaundice during pregnancy. Med J Aust 1:167, 1973.

215. Johnson P, Samsioe G, Gustafson A. Studies in cholestasis of pregnancy. I. Clinical aspects and liver function tests. Acta Obstet Gynecol Scand 54:77, 1975.

216. Ylöstalo P, Ylikorkala O. Hepatosis of pregnancy. A clinical study of 107 patients. Ann Chir Gynaecol Fenniae 64:128, 1975.

217. Medline A, Ptak T, Gryfe A, et al. Pruritus of pregnancy and jaundice induced by oral contraceptives. Am J Gastroenterol 65:156, 1976.

218. Wilson BRI, Haverkamp AD. Cholestatic jaundice of pregnancy: New perspectives. Obstet Gynecol 54:650, 1979.

219. Johnston WG, Baskett TF. Obstetric cholestasis. Am J Obstet Gynecol 133:299, 1979.

220. Reyes H, Radrigan ME, Gonzalez MC, et al. Steatorrhea in patients with intrahepatic cholestasis of pregnancy. Gastroenterology 93:584, 1987.

221. Reyes H, Gonzalez MC, Ribalta J, et al. Colestasia intrahepatica de la embarazada: variabilidad clinica y bioquimica. Rev Med Chile 110:631, 1982.

222. Shaw D, Frohlich J, Witmann BAK, et al. A prospective study of 18 patients with cholestasis of pregnancy. Am J Obstet Gynecol 142:621, 1982.

223. Zhong-da Q, Qi-nan W, Yue-han L, et al. Intrahepatic cholestasis of pregnancy. Chung Hua I Hsueh Tsa Chih 96:902, 1983.

224. Berg B, Helm G, Petersohn L, et al. Cholestasis of pregnancy. Acta Obstet Gynecol Scand 65:107, 1986.

225. Reyes H. The enigma of intrahepatic cholestasis of pregnancy: lessons from Chile. Hepatology 2:87, 1982.

226. Reyes H, Gonzalez MC, Ribalta J, et al. Prevalence of intrahepatic cholestasis of pregnancy in Chile. Ann Intern Med 88:487, 1978.

227. Reyes H, Taboada G, Ribalta J. Prevalence of intrahepatic cholestasis of pregnancy in La Paz, Bolivia. J Chronic Dis 32:499, 1979.

228. Glasinovic JC, Marinovic I, Vela P. The changing scene of cholestasis of pregnancy in Chile. An epidemiological study. Hepatology 6:1161, 1986 (Abstract).

229. Furhoff A-K. Itching in pregnancy. Acta Med Scand 196:403, 1974.
230. Reyes H, Ribalta J, Gonzalez-Ceron M. Idiopathic cholestasis of pregnancy in a large kindred. Gut 17:709, 1976.
231. Holzbach RT, Sivak DA, Braun WE. Familial recurrent intrahepatic cholestasis of pregnancy: A genetic study providing evidence for transmission of a sex-limited, dominant trait. Gastroenterology 85:175, 1983.
232. De Pagter AGF, van Berge Henegouwen GP, ten Bokkel Huinink JA, et al. Familial benign recurrent intrahepatic cholestasis. Gastroenterology 71:202, 1976.
233. Cullberg G, Lundström R, Stenram U. Jaundice during treatment with an oral contraceptive, lyndiol. Br Med J 1:695, 1965.
234. Eisalo A, Jarvinen PA, Luukkainen T. Hepatic impairment during the intake of contraceptive pills: clinical trial with postmenopausal women. Br Med J 2:426, 1964.
235. Thulin KE, Nermark J. Seven cases of jaundice in women taking an oral contraceptive, anovlar. Br Med J 1:684, 1966.
236. Kreek MJ, Weser E, Sleisenger MH, et al. Idiopathic cholestasis of pregnancy. N Engl J Med 277:1391, 1967.
237. Kreek MJ, Sleisenger MH, Jeffries GH. Recurrent cholestatic jaundice of pregnancy with demonstrated estrogen sensitivity. Am J Med 43:795, 1967.
238. Dalen E, Westerholm B. Occurrence of hepatic impairment in women jaundiced by oral contraceptives and in their mothers and sisters. Acta Med Scand 195:459, 1974.
239. Reyes H, Ribalta J, Gonzalez C, et al. Sulfobromophthalein clearance tests before and after ethinyl estradiol administration, in women and men with familial history of intrahepatic cholestasis of pregnancy. Gastroenterology 81:226, 1981.
240. Misra PS, Evanov FA, Wessely Z, et al. Idiopathic intrahepatic cholestasis of pregnancy. Am J Gastroenterol 73:54, 1980.
241. Laatikainen TJ. Fetal bile acid levels in pregnancies complicated by maternal intrahepatic cholestasis. Am J Obstet Gynecol 122:852, 1975.
242. Laatikainen T, Ikonen E. Serum bile acids in cholestasis of pregnancy. Obstet Gynecol 50:313, 1977.
243. Heikkinen J, Mäentausta O, Ylöstalo P, et al. Changes in serum bile acid concentrations during normal pregnancy, in patients with intrahepatic cholestasis of pregnancy and in pregnant women with itching. Br J Obstet Gynaecol 88:240, 1981.
244. Laatinainen T, Tulenheimo A. Maternal serum bile acid levels and fetal distress in cholestasis of pregnancy. Int J Gynaecol Obstet 22:91, 1984.
245. Ylöstalo P, Kirkinen P, Keikkinen J, et al. Gallbladder volume and serum bile acids in cholestasis of pregnancy. Br J Obstet Gynaecol 89:59, 1982.
246. Kirkinen P, Ylöstalo P, Heikkinen J, et al. Gallbladder function and maternal bile acids in intrahepatic cholestasis of pregnancy. Eur J Obstet Gynecol Reprod Biol 18:29, 1984.
247. Adlercreutz H, Svanborg A, Ånberg Å. Recurrent jaundice in pregnancy. I. A clinical and ultrastructural study. Am J Med 42:335, 1967.
248. Van Haelst U, Bergstein N. Electron microscopic study of the liver in so-called idiopathic jaundice of late pregnancy. Pathol Eur 5:198, 1970.
249. Furhoff A-K, Hellström K. Jaundice in Pregnancy. A follow-up study of the series of women originally reported by L. Thorling. II. Present health of the women. Acta Med Scand 196:181, 1974.
250. Laatikainen T, Ikonen E. Fetal prognosis in obstetric hepatosis. Ann Chir Gynaecol Fenniae 64:155, 1975.
251. Reid R, Ivey KJ, Rencoret RH, et al. Fetal complications of obstetric cholestasis. Br Med J 1:870, 1976.
252. Engström J, Hellström K, Posse N, et al. Recurrent cholestasis of pregnancy. Acta Obstet Gynecol Scand 49:29, 1970.
253. Heikkinen J, Mäentausta O, Ylöstalo P, et al. Serum bile acid levels in intrahepatic cholestasis of pregnancy during treatment with phenobarbital or cholestyramine. Eur J Obstet Gynec Reprod Biol 14:153, 1982.
254. Laatikainen T. Effect of cholestyramine and phenobarbital on pruritus and serum bile acid levels in cholestasis of pregnancy. Am J Obstet Gynecol 132:501, 1978.
255. Di Padova C, Tritapepe R, Cammareri G, et al. S-adenosyl-L-methionine antagonizes ethynylestradiol-induced bile cholesterol supersaturation in humans without modifying the estrogen plasma kinetics. Gastroenterology 82:223, 1982.
256. Stramentinoli G, di Padova C, Gualano M, et al. Ethynylestradiol-induced impairment of bile secretion in the rat: Protective effects of S-adenosyl-L-methionine and its implication in estrogen metabolism. Gastroenterology 80:154, 1981.
257. Frezza M, Pozzato G, Chiesa L, et al. Reversal of intrahepatic cholestasis of pregnancy in women after high dose S-adenosyl-L-methionine administration. Hepatology 4:274, 1984.
258. Frezza M, Tritapepe R, Di Padova C. S-adenosylmethionine and hepatobiliary function in women with previous intrahepatic cholestasis of pregnancy. Hepatology 6:1144, 1986 (Abstract).
259. Sheehan HL. The pathology of acute yellow atrophy and delayed chloroform poisoning. J Obstet Gynaecol Br Emp 47:40, 1940.
260. Kaplan MM. Acute fatty liver of pregnancy. N Engl J Med 313:367, 1985.
261. Sherlock S. Acute fatty liver of pregnancy and the microvesicular fat diseases. Gut 24:265, 1983.
262. Partin JC, Schubert WK, Partin JS. Mitochondrial ultrastructure in Reye's syndrome (encephalopathy and fatty degeneration of the viscera). N Engl J Med 285:1339, 1971.
263. Bourgeois C, Olson L, Comer D, et al. Encephalopathy and fatty degeneration of the viscera: A clinicopathologic analysis of 40 cases. Am J Clin Pathol 56:558, 1971.
264. Heubi JE, Partin JC, Partin JS, et al. Reye's syndrome: Current concepts. Hepatology 7:155, 1987.
265. Treem WR, Witzleben CA, Piccoli DA, et al. Medium-chain and long-chain acyl CoA dehydrogenase deficiency: Clinical, pathologic and ultrastructural differentiation from Reye's syndrome. Hepatology 6:1270, 1986.
266. Mock DM. Fatty acids and Reye's syndrome. Hepatology 6:1414, 1986.
267. Combes B, Whalley PJ, Adams RH. Tetracycline and the liver. In: Popper H, Schaffner F, eds. Progress in Liver Diseases, Vol. IV. New York, Grune & Stratton, 1972:589.
268. Pockros PJ, Peters RL, Reynolds TB. Idiopathic fatty liver of pregnancy: findings in ten cases. Medicine 63:1, 1984.
269. Davies MH, Wilkinson SP, Hanid MA, et al. Acute liver disease with encephalopathy and renal failure in late pregnancy and early puerperium: a study of fourteen patients. Br J Obstet Gynaecol 87:1005, 1980.
270. Eisele JW, Barker EA, Smuckler EA. Lipid content in the liver of fatty metamorphosis of pregnancy. Am J Pathol 81:545, 1975.
271. Kahil ME, Fred HL, Brown H, et al. Acute fatty liver of pregnancy. Arch Intern Med 113:63, 1964.
272. Ober WB, LeCompte PM. Acute fatty metamorphosis of the liver associated with pregnancy. Am J Med 19:743, 1955.
273. Kunelis CT, Peters JL, Edmondson HA. Fatty liver of pregnancy and its relationship to tetracycline therapy. Am J Med 38:359, 1965.
274. Weber FL Jr, Snodgrass PJ, Powell DE, et al. Abnormalities of hepatic mitochondrial urea-cycle enzyme activities and hepatic ultrastructure in acute fatty liver of pregnancy. J Lab Clin Med 94:27, 1979.
275. Duma J, Dowling EA, Alexander HC, et al. Acute fatty liver of pregnancy. Ann Intern Med 63:851, 1965.
276. Joske RA, McCully DJ, Mastaglia FL. Acute fatty liver of pregnancy. Gut 9:489, 1968.
277. Breen KJ, Perkins KW, Mistilis SP, et al. Idiopathic acute fatty liver of pregnancy. Gut 11:822, 1970.
278. Hatfield AK, Stein JH, Greenberger NJ, et al. Idiopathic acute fatty liver of pregnancy. Dig Dis Sci 17:167, 1972.
279. Holzbach RT. Acute fatty liver of pregnancy with disseminated intravascular coagulation. Obstet Gynecol 43:740, 1974.
280. Cano RI, Delman MR, Pitchumoni CS, et al. Acute fatty liver of pregnancy. JAMA 231:159, 1975.
281. MacKenna J, Pupkin M, Crenshaw C Jr, et al. Acute fatty metamorphosis of the liver. Am J Obstet Gynecol 127:400, 1977.
282. Moldin P, Johansson O. Acute fatty liver of pregnancy with disseminated intravascular coagulation. Acta Obstet Gynecol Scand 57:179, 1978.
283. Varner M, Rinderknecht NK. Acute fatty metamorphosis of pregnancy. J Reprod Med 24:177, 1980.
284. Koff RS. Weekly clinicopathological exercises. N Engl J Med 304:216, 1981.
285. Burroughs AK, Seong NH, Dojcinov DM, et al. Idiopathic acute fatty liver of pregnancy in 12 patients. Q J Med 51:481, 1982.
286. Korula J, Malatjalian DA, Badley BWD. Acute fatty liver of pregnancy. Can Med Assoc J 127:575, 1982.
287. Cheng CY. Acute fatty liver of pregnancy—survival despite associated severe preeclampsia, coma and coagulopathy. Aust NZ J Obstet Gynecol 23:120, 1983.
288. Bernuau J, Degott C, Nouel O, et al. Non-fatal acute fatty liver of pregnancy. Gut 24:340, 1983.
289. Hague WM, Fenton DW, Duncan SLB, et al. Acute fatty liver of pregnancy. J R Soc Med 76:652, 1983.
290. Ebert EC, Sun EA, Wright SH, et al. Does early diagnosis and delivery in acute fatty liver of pregnancy lead to improvement in maternal and infant survival? Dig Dis Sci 29:453, 1984.
291. Hou SH, Levin S, Ahola S, et al. Acute fatty liver of pregnancy. Dig Dis Sci 29:449, 1984.
292. Rolfes DB, Ishak KG. Acute fatty liver of pregnancy: A clinicopathologic study of 35 cases. Hepatology 5:1149, 1985.
293. Czernobilsky B, Bergnes MA. Acute fatty metamorphosis of the liver in pregnancy with associated liver cell necrosis. Obstet Gynecol 26:792, 1965.
294. Liebman HA, McGehee WG, Patch MJ, et al. Severe depression of

antithrombin III associated with disseminated intravascular coagulation in women with fatty liver of pregnancy. Ann Intern Med 98:330, 1983.

295. Laursen B, Frost L, Mortensen JZ, et al. Acute fatty liver of pregnancy with complicating disseminated intravascular coagulation. Acta Obstet Gynecol Scand 62:403, 1983.

296. Mosvold J, Abildgaard U, Jenssen H, et al. Low antithrombin III in acute hepatic failure at term. Scand J Haematol 29:48, 1982.

297. Shimizu M, Okumura M, Yuh K, et al. Ultrasonically undetectable fatty liver in acute fatty liver of pregnancy and Reye's syndrome. J Clin Ultrasound 13:679, 1985.

298. Campillo B, Bernuau J, Witz M-O, et al. Ultrasonography in acute fatty liver of pregnancy. Ann Intern Med 105:383, 1986.

299. McKee CM, Weir PE, Foster JH, et al. Acute fatty liver of pregnancy and diagnosis by computed tomography. Br Med J 292:291, 1986.

300. Slater DN, Hague WM. Renal morphological changes in idiopathic acute fatty liver of pregnancy. Histopathology 8:567, 1984.

301. Sheehan HL. Jaundice in pregnancy. Am J Obstet Gynecol 81:427, 1961.

302. Whalley PJ, Adams RH, Combes B. Tetracycline toxicity in pregnancy. JAMA 189:357, 1964.

303. Maier J, Daugherty CC, Hug G, et al. Hepatic mitochondrial enzymes and ultrastructural abnormalities in acute fatty liver of pregnancy (AFLP). Gastroenterology 82:1123, 1982 (Abstract).

304. Riely CA, Latham PS, Romero R, Duffy TP. Acute fatty liver of pregnancy: a reassessment based on observations in nine patients. Ann Intern Med 106:703, 1987.

305. Bydder GM, Kreel L, Chapman RWG, et al. Accuracy of computed tomography in diagnosis of fatty liver. Br Med J 281:1042, 1980.

306. Malatjalian DA, Badley BWD. Acute fatty liver of pregnancy. Light and electron microscopic studies. Gastroenterology 84:1384, 1983 (Abstract).

307. Bertram PD, Anderson GD, Kelly S, et al. Ultrastructural alterations in acute fatty liver of pregnancy: similarity to Reye's syndrome. Gastroenterology 74:1008, 1978 (Abstract).

308. Riely CA. Acute fatty liver of pregnancy—1984. Dig Dis Sci 29:456, 1984.

309. Schultz JC, Adamson JS Jr, Workman WW, et al. Fatal liver disease after intravenous administration of tetracycline in high dosage. N Engl J Med 269:999, 1963.

310. Horwitz ST, Marymont JH Jr. Fatal liver disease during pregnancy associated with tetracycline therapy. Obstet Gynecol 23:826, 1964.

311. Schiffer MA. Fatty liver associated with administration of tetracycline in pregnant and nonpregnant women. Am J Obstet Gynecol 96:326, 1966.

312. Wenk RE, Gebhardt FC, Bhagavan BS, et al. Tetracycline-associated fatty liver of pregnancy, including possible pregnancy risk after chronic dermatologic use of tetracycline. J Reprod Med 26:135, 1981.

313. Moise KJ Jr, Shah DM. Acute fatty liver of pregnancy: etiology of fetal distress and fetal wastage. Obstet Gynecol 69:482, 1987.

314. Breen KJ, Perkins KW, Schenker S, et al. Uncomplicated subsequent pregnancy after idiopathic fatty liver of pregnancy. Obstet Gynecol 40:831, 1972.

315. Sakamoto S, Tsuji Y, Koga S, et al. Idiopathic fatty liver of pregnancy with a subsequent uncomplicated pregnancy and a progressive increase in serum cholinesterase activity during the third trimester. A case report. Hepatogastroenterology 33:9, 1986.

316. DeVoe SJ, O'Shaughnessy R. Clinical manifestations and diagnosis of pregnancy-induced hypertension. Clin Obstet Gynecol 27:836, 1984.

317. Cunningham FG, Pritchard JA. How should hypertension during pregnancy be managed? Med Clin North Am 68:505, 1984.

318. Lindheimer MD, Katz AI. Hypertension in pregnancy. N Engl J Med 313:675, 1985.

319. Manas KJ, Welsh JD, Rankin RA, et al. Hepatic hemorrhage without rupture in preeclampsia. N Engl J Med 312:424, 1985.

320. Villegas H, Azuela JC, Maqueo M. Spontaneous rupture of liver in toxemia of pregnancy. Int J Gynecol Obstet 8:836, 1970.

321. Branch DW, Scott JR, Kochenour NK, et al. Obstetric complications associated with the lupus anticoagulant. N Engl J Med 313:1322, 1985.

322. Hibbard LT. Maternal mortality due to acute toxemia. Obstet Gynecol 42:263, 1973.

323. Sibai BM, Anderson GD, McCubbin JH. Eclampsia. II. Clinical significance of laboratory findings. Obstet Gynecol 59:153, 1982.

324. Rosing U, Kallner A. Serum cholic and chenodeoxycholic acids during pregnancy and puerperium in normal and pre-eclamptic women. Acta Obstet Gynecol Scand 65:11, 1986.

325. MacKenna J, Dover NL, Brame RG. Preeclampsia associated with hemolysis, elevated liver enzymes, and low platelets—an obstetric emergency? Obstet Gynecol 62:751, 1983.

326. Beller FK, Dame WR, Ebert C. Pregnancy-induced hypertension complicated by thrombocytopenia, haemolysis and elevated liver

enzymes (HELLP) syndrome. Renal biopsies and outcome. Aust NZ J Obstet Gynaecol 25:83, 1985.

327. Sibai BM, Taslimi MM, El-Nazer A, et al. Maternal-perinatal outcome associated with the syndrome of hemolysis, elevated liver enzymes, and low platelets in severe preeclampsia-eclampsia. Am J Obstet Gynecol 155:501, 1986.

328. Maqueo M, Ayala LC, Cervantes L. Nutritional status and liver function in toxemia of pregnancy. Obstet Gynecol 23:222, 1964.

329. Arias F, Mancilla-Jimenez R. Hepatic fibrinogen deposits in pre-eclampsia. N Engl J Med 295:578, 1976.

330. Sheehan HL, Lynch JB. Pathology of Toxaemia of Pregnancy. Edinburgh, Churchill Livingstone, 1973:328.

331. Weinstein L. Syndrome of hemolysis, elevated liver enzymes, and low platelet count: A severe consequence of hypertension in pregnancy. Am J Obstet Gynecol 142:159, 1982.

332. Aarnoudse JG, Houthoff HJ, Weits J, et al. A syndrome of liver damage and intravascular coagulation in the last trimester of normotensive pregnancy. A clinical and histopathological study. Br J Obstet Gynaecol 93:145, 1986.

333. Pritchard JA, Weisman R Jr, Ratnoff OD, et al. Intravascular hemolysis, thrombocytopenia and other hematologic abnormalities associated with severe toxemia of pregnancy. N Engl J Med 250:89, 1954.

334. Killam AP, Dillard SH Jr, Patton RC, et al. Pregnancy-induced hypertension complicated by acute liver disease and disseminated intravascular coagulation. Am J Obstet Gynecol 123:823, 1975.

335. Goodlin RC. Severe pre-eclampsia: Another great imitator. Am J Obstet Gynecol 125:747, 1976.

336. Long RG, Scheuer PJ, Sherlock S. Pre-eclampsia presenting with deep jaundice. J Clin Pathol 30:212, 1977.

337. Goodlin RC, Cotton DB, Haesslein HC. Severe edema-proteinuria-hypertension gestosis. Am J Obstet Gynecol 132:595, 1978.

338. Goodlin RC, Holt D. Impending gestosis. Obstet Gynecol 58:743, 1981.

339. Schwartz ML, Brenner WE. Pregnancy-induced hypertension presenting with life-threatening thrombocytopenia. Am J Obstet Gynecol 146:756, 1983.

340. Thiagarajah S, Bourgeois FJ, Harbert GM Jr, et al. Thrombocytopenia in preeclampsia: Associated abnormalities and management principles. Am J Obstet Gynecol 150:1, 1984.

341. Bertakis KD, Hufford DB. Hemolysis, elevated liver enzymes and low platelet count. West J Med 144:81, 1986.

342. Clark SL, Phelan JR, Allen SH, et al. Antepartum reversal of hematologic abnormalities associated with the HELLP syndrome. J Reprod Med 31:70, 1986.

343. Weinstein L. Preeclampsia/eclampsia with hemolysis, elevated liver enzymes, and thrombocytopenia. Obstet Gynecol 66:657, 1985.

344. Cunningham FG, Lowe T, Guss S, et al. Erythrocyte morphology in women with severe preeclampsia and eclampsia. Am J Obstet Gynecol 153:358, 1985.

345. Brazy JE, Grimm JK, Little VA. Neonatal manifestations of severe maternal hypertension occurring before the thirty-sixth week of pregnancy. J Pediatr 100:265, 1982.

346. Pritchard JA, Cunningham FG, Pritchard SA, et al. How often does maternal preeclampsia-eclampsia incite thrombocytopenia in the fetus? Obstet Gynecol 69:292, 1987.

347. Bis KA, Waxman B. Rupture of the liver associated with pregnancy: A review of the literature and report of 2 cases. Obstet Gynecol Survey 31:763, 1976.

348. Barry AP, Meagher DJ. Rupture of the liver complicating pregnancy. Obstet Gynecol 23:381, 1964.

349. Castaneda H, Garcia-Romero H, Canto M. Hepatic hemorrhage in toxemia of pregnancy. Am J Obstet Gynecol 107:578, 1970.

350. Severino LJ, Freedman WL, Maheshkumar AP. Spontaneous subcapsular hematoma of liver during pregnancy. NY State J Med 70:2818, 1970.

351. Portnuff J, Ballon S. Hepatic rupture in pregnancy. Am J Obstet Gynecol 114:1102, 1972.

352. Hibbard LT. Spontaneous rupture of the liver in pregnancy: A report of eight cases. Am J Obstet Gynecol 126:334, 1976.

353. Jewett JF. Eclampsia and rupture of the liver. N Engl J Med 297:1009, 1977.

354. Nelson EW, Archibald L, Albo D Jr. Spontaneous hepatic rupture in pregnancy. Am J Surg 134:817, 1977.

355. Sommer DG, Greenway GD, Bookstein JJ, et al. Hepatic rupture with toxemia of pregnancy: Angiographic diagnosis. Am J Roentgenol 132:455, 1979.

356. Golan A, White RG. Spontaneous rupture of the liver associated with pregnancy. S Afr Med J 56:133, 1979.

357. Westergaard L. Spontaneous rupture of the liver in pregnancy. Acta Obstet Gynecol Scand 59:559, 1980.

358. Roopnarinesingh S, Jankey N, Gopeesingh T. Rupture of the liver as a complication of pre-eclampsia: Case report and review of the literature. Int Surg 66:169, 1981.

359. Henny CP, Lim TE, Brummelkamp WH, et al. Spontaneous rupture of Glisson's capsule during pregnancy. An acute surgical emergency. Neth J Surg 34:72, 1982.
360. Lubbe WF, Walkom P, Alexander CJ. Hepatic and splenic haemorrhage as a complication of toxaemia of pregnancy in a patient with circulating lupus anticoagulant. NZ Med J 95:842, 1982.
361. Herbert WNP, Brenner WE. Improving survival with liver rupture complicating pregnancy. Am J Obstet Gynecol 142:530, 1982.
362. Aziz S, Merrell RC, Collins JA. Spontaneous hepatic hemorrhage during pregnancy. Am J Surg 146:680, 1983.
363. Sloan DA, Schlegel DM. Spontaneous hepatic rupture associated with pregnancy. Contemporary Surg 24:39, 1984.
364. Ekberg H, Leyon J, Jeppsson B, et al. Hepatic rupture secondary to pre-eclampsia—Report of a case treated conservatively. Ann Chir Gynaecol 73:350, 1984.
365. Greca FH, Coelho JCU, Filho ODB, et al. Ultrasonographic diagnosis of spontaneous rupture of the liver in pregnancy. J Clin Ultrasound 12:515, 1984.
366. Gonzalez GD, Rubel HR, Giep NN, et al. Spontaneous hepatic rupture in pregnancy: Management with hepatic artery ligation. South Med J 77:242, 1984.
367. Loevinger EH, Vujic I, Lee WM, et al. Hepatic rupture associated with pregnancy: Treatment with transcatheter embolotherapy. Obstet Gynecol 65:281, 1985.
368. Wagner WH, Lundell CJ, Donovan AJ. Percutaneous angiographic embolization for hepatic arterial hemorrhage. Arch Surg 120:1241, 1985.
369. Stalter KD, Sterling WA Jr. Hepatic subcapsular hemorrhage associated with pregnancy. Surgery 98:112, 1985.
370. Winer-Muram HT, Muram D, Salazar J, et al. Hepatic rupture in preeclampsia: The role of diagnostic imaging. J Can Assoc Radiol 36:34, 1985.
371. Sakala EP, Moore WD. Successful term delivery after previous pregnancy with ruptured liver. Obstet Gynecol 68:124, 1986.
372. Heller TD, Goldfarb JP. Spontaneous rupture of the liver during pregnancy. NY State J Med 86:314, 1986.
373. Dammann HG, Hagemann J, Runge M, Klöppel G. In vivo diagnosis of massive heptic infarction by computed tomography. Dig Dis Sci 27:73, 1982.
374. Wilcox DM, Weinreb JC, Lesh P. MR imaging of a hemorrhagic hepatic cyst in a patient with polycystic liver disease. J Comput Assist Tomogr J Comput Assist Tomogr 9:183, 1985.
375. Henny CP, Lim AE, Brummelkamp WH, et al. A review of the importance of acute multidisciplinary treatment following spontaneous rupture of the liver capsule during pregnancy. Surg Gynecol Obstet 156:593, 1983.
376. Herbert WNP. Hepatic rupture and pregnancy. NY State J Med 86:286, 1986.

55

Liver Transplantation

Neville R. Pimstone, M.D. • Leonard I. Goldstein, M.D.
Richard Ward, M.D. • Boris H. Ruebner, M.D.

Liver transplantation is now a recognized therapeutic option for patients with progressive, irreversible liver disease, acute or chronic, or life-threatening hepatic metabolic disturbances, in whom conventional forms of medical therapy offer no prospect for prolonged survival. In the mid-1950s and early 1960s, pioneering research in animals by Welch and colleagues laid the groundwork for development of techniques for heterotopic homotransplantation (i.e., the insertion of an extra liver at an ectopic site) and orthotopic homotransplantation (i.e., the removal of the host liver and replacement with an allograft).[1-5]

The first successful orthotopic liver transplantations in humans were reported by Starzl's group in 1963.[6] The initial track record was dismal, with seven consecutive failures in three institutions leading to a moratorium on clinical trials. However, coincident with improving technique and with the introduction of cyclosporine as a potent antirejection drug in 1979,[7] the overall six-month to one-year actuarial survival of patients since 1980 has significantly improved (Figs. 55–1 and 55–2)[8-18, 101, 107] from 30 to 45 per cent to as high as 70 to 80 per cent. With improved survival, liver transplantation has become accepted as a proven therapy rather than an experimental advance in the treatment of liver diseases. This trend gained impetus following a Na-

tional Institutes of Health (NIH) Consensus Development Conference on Liver Transplantation in June 1983, which concluded that liver transplantation "is a therapeutic modality for end-stage liver disease that deserves broad application." At the time of the consensus, 540 liver transplantations had been performed in humans. Since 1983, the number of centers performing liver transplantation has

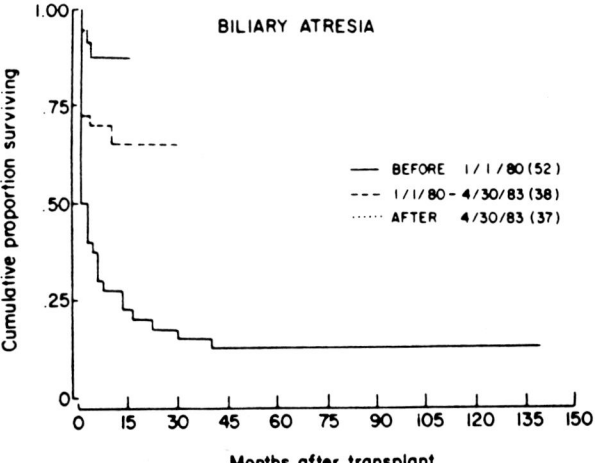

Figure 55–1. Actuarial survival of 127 patients who received liver transplants for biliary atresia as of August 1984. (From Scharschmidt BF. In: Thomas HC, Jones EA, eds. Recent Advances in Hepatology. Churchill Livingstone, 1986:175, with permission.)

This chapter was supported in part by National Institutes of Health Grant 2 R01 Dk30094.

We would like to thank Anthony H. Haulk, M.D., UC Davis, Division of Gastroenterology, for his help in preparing the liver histopathology photomicrographs for this chapter.

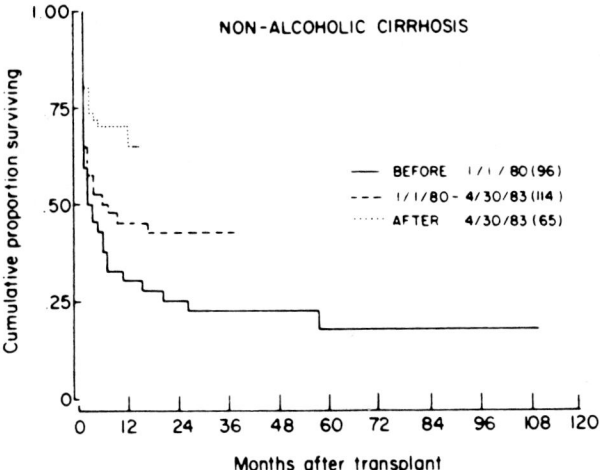

Figure 55–2. Actuarial survival of 275 patients who received liver transplants for nonalcoholic cirrhosis as of August 1984. (From Scharschmidt BF. In: Thomas HC, Jones EA, eds. Recent Advances in Hepatology. Churchill Livingstone, 1986:175, with permission.)

mushroomed to 32 currently in Europe, involving over 1200 patients per year,[114] and approximately 40 in the United States, performing approximately 1000 transplantations per year. Based on demographic studies, Dr. Starzl (personal communication) predicts 30 to 40 new adult and pediatric patients per million population per year to be acceptable candidates. The present concern now is the availability of donor organs for eligible recipients.

This chapter attempts to evaluate liver transplantation through the eyes of the hepatologist, focusing mainly on candidacy of prospective recipients and evaluation of liver dysfunction posttransplantation.

INDICATIONS FOR TRANSPLANTATION

The University of California at Davis criteria for transplantation follow closely the guidelines of the NIH Consensus Statement concerning patients for whom transplantation of the liver should be considered appropriate therapy. There are five main groups as listed in Table 55–1.

CHRONIC END-STAGE LIVER DISEASE

There are many causes of chronic liver injury of more than six months' duration that may lead to progressive liver failure, that grossly impairs the quality of life, or limits life expectancy. Seven categories are enumerated in Table 55–2. The choice of liver transplantation is predicated on the knowledge that other therapies are ineffective or unlikely to improve survival or decrease morbidity.

Causes

Viral Hepatitis

Chronic viral hepatitis may result from hepatitis B virus (HBV) with or without coinfection with hepatitis delta

virus (HDV) or from non-A, non-B hepatitis virus. There is no evidence that corticosteroid or immunosuppressant therapy has any beneficial effect on the natural course of the disease, and it may indeed be detrimental.[19, 20] The use of interferons may be effective in eliminating the virus and retarding disease progression in chronic hepatitis B.[21] Controlled prospective studies both in the United States and Europe have demonstrated parenteral alpha interferon given over a 3- to 6-month period to have a positive serologic, histologic, and clinical response in 25 to 45 per cent of patients,[22–25] but it currently is unclear what the long-term prognosis is for the patients who responded to treatment. Because interferons both inhibit viral replication and stimulate immunity, the beneficial effects may be associated with increased hepatic necrosis. Thus, in candidates with chronic hepatitis and cirrhosis with impaired reserve, interferon therapy might precipitate a significant clinical deterioration that could have a negative impact on the timing of transplant surgery.

Liver transplantation for end-stage HBV chronic hepatitis and cirrhosis is immediately successful in restoring liver function. Unfortunately, regardless of the e antigen status of the patient, recurrence of HBV infection in the liver allograft not only is almost invariable, but the liver disease may be more aggressive than the original illness.[26, 105, 118] Of 26 patients studied in Pittsburgh, 46 per cent of this group had antibodies for HDV. The expression of viral disease after transplantation ranged from acute hepatitis to cirrhosis with the development of hepatocellular carcinoma (HCC) and was dramatically compressed in time in that the spectrum of illness described was observed in less than a year following transplantation (Van Thiel, personal communication). This contrasts with the 30- to 40-year time period required for similar disease expression in individuals who are not immunosuppressed or transplanted. By contrast, in the UCLA experience with 15 patients with hepatitis B, only 1 patient has developed serious chronic hepatitis B over a 4-year period of observation.

Two other potentially HBV-related events occur posttransplantation. One has been a high incidence of postoperative pancreatic inflammatory disease. This might represent a trophism of the HB virus for pancreatic tissue. The second is the development of bone marrow hypoplasia or aplasia of one or more of stem cell lines (Van Thiel, personal communication). For liver transplantation to have a place in the treatment of chronic liver failure secondary to HBV infection, effective elimination of the virus or prevention of its replication needs to be achieved. Recurrence of allograft viral reinfection is not prevented by hepatitis B immunoglobulin and hepatitis vaccination perisurgery and postsurgery. Interferon therapy may prevent

TABLE 55–1. INDICATIONS FOR LIVER TRANSPLANTATION

Chronic end-stage liver disease
Fulminant and subfulminant hepatic failure
Primary hepatic cancer?
Metabolic liver disease
Failure of previous liver transplant

TABLE 55–2. CAUSES OF CHRONIC END-STAGE LIVER DISEASE

Viral hepatitis
Autoimmune lupoid hepatitis
Congenital errors of metabolism
Wilson's disease
α_1-Antitrypsin deficiency
Hemochromatosis
Protoporphyria
Biliary cirrhosis
Primary
Secondary, e.g., to sclerosing cholangitis, neonatal biliary atresia, neonatal bile duct paucity
Budd-Chiari syndrome without coagulopathy
Cryptogenic chronic active hepatitis and cirrhosis
Selected alcoholic liver injury

reinfection but on the other hand, may enhance the rejection process. Studies are currently in progress at Pittsburgh to evaluate these possibilities.[98]

Chronic non-A, non-B hepatitis resulting from as yet unidentified viral agents usually is transmitted by blood or blood products. An estimated 10 to 25 per cent of infected patients ultimately develop cirrhosis (see Chap. 37). As with HBV infection, non-A, non-B hepatitis does not respond to prednisone therapy or acyclovir[27] but may be responsive to the antiviral effects of the interferons.[28-30] In a pilot study reported by Hoofnagle and co-workers,[28] parenteral alpha interferon administered to patients with chronic non-A, non-B hepatitis resulted in biochemical and histologic improvement in eight of ten patients sustained on low doses of interferon (1 million units three times weekly). Similar data have been obtained from studies in England[29] and with beta interferon in Japan.[30] However, as with HBV, it is unclear whether there is a significant improvement in the prognosis of these patients.

The prognosis following liver transplantation for end-stage cirrhosis following non-A, non-B hepatitis is more promising than in HBV-related disease. Although acute liver injury ascribed to non-A, non-B hepatitis may recur post-transplantation, chronic non-A, non-B hepatitis has not yet been observed. Thus, the role of alpha interferon as adjuvant therapy to liver transplantation may be difficult to assess in a disease in which no viral markers are available to identify reinfection of the allograft.

Autoimmune Lupoid Hepatitis (See Chap. 38)

Autoimmune lupoid chronic hepatitis most commonly afflicts young women between 15 and 25 years of age, with a second age prevalence peak postmenopause. Frequently, there is multisystem involvement, and in 70 per cent of patients, antinuclear and smooth muscle antibodies are present. The hepatic histologic lesions generally are more severe than in chronic viral hepatitis, and prospective controlled trials of prednisolone therapy are undoubtedly beneficial in prolonging life to a mean of 12.2 years, with a five-year survival of 85 per cent, compared with 40 per cent in the untreated group.[31] When end-stage liver disease supervenes, the likelihood of resident opportunistic infections, particularly fungal infections, is high, because patients have been on chronic immunosuppressive therapy. These need to be sought prior to transplant surgery.

Congenital Errors of Metabolism

Liver disease resulting from congenital metabolic errors is addressed by other authors in this textbook. Wilson's disease (see Chap. 47) is effectively treated by copper chelation with drugs such as D-penicillamine. Candidates for liver transplantation include those patients presenting with fulminant hepatitis or cirrhosis with severe hepatic decompensation unresponsive to medical therapy. Very few patients will fall within this latter group. Of interest, in one patient receiving liver transplantation for Wilson's disease, liver copper was normal several years after surgery, suggesting reversal of the metabolic defect responsible for the disease.[32] α_1-Antitrypsin deficiency (see Chap. 50) is far more common in whites of European ancestry and its prevalence is high, particularly in Southern England. After successful transplantation, the protease inhibitor status is reversed and depressed serum α_1-antitrypsin levels return to normal.[33-35] Hemochromatosis (see Chap. 48) as a cause of cirrhosis is prevented or controllable by treatment mo-

dalities that diminish iron overload (e.g., phlebotomy therapy) and rarely is detected so late in the course of disease that liver transplantation is indicated. Protoporphyria (see Chap. 14) is a rare autosomal dominant disorder of heme biosynthesis, secondary to decreased mitochondrial ferrochelatase activity. Expression of this metabolic defect by the bone marrow results in increased circulating plasma protoporphyrin, which is cleared almost exclusively by the liver. Hepatobiliary disorders in protoporphyria are characterized by hepatic accumulation of protoporphyrin.[36-40] Hepatic injury may range from mild focal necrosis to cirrhosis. When jaundice supervenes in cirrhotic individuals in whom there is no extrahepatic obstruction (e.g., the latter from protoporphyrin gallstones), death is inevitable, usually within six months. In this clinical situation, liver transplantation is the only option.

Biliary Cirrhosis (See Chaps. 43 and 44)

In adults in the Pittsburgh experience,[44] chronic cholestatic disorders with cirrhosis account for 38 per cent of all patients requiring liver transplantation. Primary biliary cirrhosis and biliary cirrhosis secondary to sclerosing cholangitis are the most common chronic cholestatic liver disorders in adults assessed for liver transplantation. These two conditions typify the importance of clinical and biochemical assessment of end-stage liver disease in determining the timing for liver transplantation. Roll and colleagues reviewed the prognostic importance of clinical and histologic features in primary biliary cirrhosis.[41] A computer model could not predict a 50 per cent mortality in a time period of less than five years. Neuberger and associates, using age, serum bilirubin, serum albumin, and histologic evidence of cirrhosis, central cholestasis, or both, were able to estimate prognosis in terms of months in patients with primary biliary cirrhosis.[91] The latter model has not been universally adopted and currently the usual criteria for end-stage liver disease are used to determine which patients with biliary cirrhosis are candidates for transplantation.[41-43] Other factors that may influence the decision process include intractable pruritus or progressive osteoporosis with bone pain and recurrent bone fractures.

Pediatric causes of biliary cirrhosis secondary to chronic cholestatic states are well summarized by Alagille.[45, 46] Extrahepatic atresia (see Chap. 51), characterized by a partial or total absence of patent bile ducts between the porta hepatis and duodenum, is by far the most common indication for liver transplantation in children. The illness becomes manifest in the neonate and is marked by increasingly severe cholestasis during the first three months of life. Unless treated, the disorder is universally fatal. The relentless course of the disease has been influenced by the performance of the Kasai procedure—that is, hepatic portoenterostomy. In those in whom liver surgery can be performed (surgery is precluded in many because of associated anomalies), approximately 40 per cent will require liver transplantation. This is usually performed when the liver weight is approximately seven kilograms or greater (i.e., at the age of 1 to 2 years). Of the 60 per cent with apparently successful surgical restoration of bile flow, approximately 30 per cent will develop postsurgical cholestasis and cholangitis, which will ultimately lead to the need for liver transplantation. Of the remaining 30 per cent, most will develop cirrhosis and portal hypertension; approximately 5 per cent of these will require liver transplantation between the ages of 5 and 10 years for persistent or recurrent cholestasis. Thus, 75 per cent of children with the diagnosis of biliary atresia will ultimately require a hepatic allograft. Fortunately, children appear to tolerate transplant surgery better than adults, and in most series,[13, 14] the survival in children (~ 80 to 85 per cent ≥ three years) is about 10 per cent greater than that in adults.

Budd-Chiari Syndrome (See Chap. 23)

Budd-Chiari syndrome without coagulopathy and in the absence of myeloproliferative disorders is an indication for transplantation when there is progressive liver failure. If the underlying cause of hepatic vein thrombosis can be elucidated—i.e., polycythemia rubra vera, oral contraceptives, inferior vena cava web syndrome, the coagulopathy of primary liver cancer, renal cell carcinoma, and so forth—and treated, then the disease may improve without further therapy. If liver failure is progressive, especially in situations in which the phlebitis extends to the lobular veins, the prognosis is very poor in that most patients will die within months to three years of diagnosis.[47-50] A side-to-side portacaval shunt is effective in decompressing the congested liver in some patients,[47] and currently it is unclear which patients are better managed by a shunt and which by transplantation.

Cryptogenic Cirrhosis

This is a heterogeneous group of patients with cirrhosis in whom no defined inciting agent can be identified. It is likely that many patients with cryptogenic cirrhosis have non-A, non-B hepatitis and simply had no clinically identifiable symptoms with the acute infection. Likewise, in women with cryptogenic cirrhosis, the disease may be the end-stage of seronegative chronic autoimmune hepatitis. There are no special features of this subset with regard to liver transplantation.

Selected Alcoholic Liver Injury

A gray area exists in the selection of patients who abuse alcohol or drugs. Approximately 10 per cent of the adult population in the United States is alcoholic, and alcoholic liver disease is a major cause of cirrhosis in this country. Whereas transplantation of these patients is restricted to a select few who have been rehabilitated successfully, active alcoholism does not preclude other major surgery such as coronary artery bypass, portacaval shunt surgery for variceal hemorrhage, and major pancreatic surgery. The relative contraindication of alcohol abuse remains an area in which acceptance in a program requires active involvement of social workers, psychiatrists, and other professionals to assess the potential pre- and postoperative responses to counseling and rehabilitation.

Criteria for Chronic End-Stage Liver Disease

The criteria for liver transplant in patients with advanced chronic disease are enumerated in Table 55–3. The key question is what constitutes end-stage liver disease. With recently published data of greater than 70 per cent, one-year survival in adults and a greater than 80 per cent one-year survival in children, hepatologists are adopting a bolder approach in selecting candidates with an estimated survival of about 12 months.[107] Yet the decision is a demanding one, because to advise liver transplantation, one is advising a form of therapy with a one-year mortality of

TABLE 55–3. CRITERIA FOR END-STAGE LIVER DISEASE

Failure of excretion
  Rising bilirubin, e.g., 1 mg every one to two months or a total bilirubin or more than 15 mg/dl
Diminished liver protein synthetic function
  Prothrombin time that is uncorrectable following parenteral vitamin K and is increasing steadily or is greater than control by 5 seconds
  Diminished and decreasing serum albumin of 3.0 g/dl or less
Diminished renal function secondary to liver disease
  Refractory ascites with urine sodium less than 10 mEq per day
  Hepatorenal syndrome
Hepatic encephalopathy (needs to be of sufficient clinical severity to prevent the individual from functioning at normal level despite full medical therapy with lactulose with or without neomycin on a protein-restricted diet)
Subjective criteria that make quality of life intolerable (i.e., uncorrectable intense pruritus, intense fatigue)

between 20 and 30 per cent. On the other hand, a wait-and-see policy may allow for rapid disease progression such that the patient will die awaiting a donor organ; or at the time of surgery, the recipient's health will be so compromised that the perioperative mortality may be prohibitive. Thus, the ideal window is that period in which the patient *begins to show* progressive deterioration but at the stage when the general health will permit successful major surgery. Optimal management of potential candidates requires close cooperation between the referring physician and the transplant unit such that the referring physician has confidence that the candidate will not be operated on too early and the transplant team similarly knows that it will not be called upon to perform miracles in moribund patients.[114] Important prognostic indicators of a good response are reasonable nutrition, lack of coagulopathy, and no previous history of biliary tract or portal vein surgery. In the typical patient, a progressively rising bilirubin, increasing prothrombin time, refractory ascites, and recurrent hepatic encephalopathy in the absence of acute reversible hepatocellular injury are reliable indicators of impending death.[92] In many cirrhotics with such a picture, especially those with severe jaundice, visualization of the biliary tree for silent stones may be indicated to rule out potentially reversible extrahepatic obstruction. Also, pigment loading of the liver (i.e., from hemolysis or extravasated blood), especially in the presence of renal impairment, may complicate assessment of hepatic excretory function.

Complications of portal hypertension—that is, esophageal varices—do not usually constitute indications for transplantation. They can be treated by other means (e.g., endoscopic sclerosis of varices or portal systemic shunt surgery in a location where liver transplant can be performed should liver failure supervene postsurgery). Whereas portacaval shunt and biliary surgery increase the technical difficulties of transplantation and should be avoided if possible, the modern technical expertise is such that these are now relative rather than absolute contraindications. In fact, Warren or mesocaval shunt surgery, by decreasing collaterals, may facilitate the removal of the liver from the recipient and not deprive the allograft of blood flow should transplantation become necessary.

Fulminant and Subfulminant Hepatic Failure (See Chap. 17)

Fulminant hepatic failure is defined as the occurrence of severe impairment of liver function progressing to encephalopathy, stage III or IV, within eight weeks of onset of illness when there is no preexisting chronic liver disease.[110] Subfulminant hepatic failure refers to progressive irreversible liver failure 8 to 26 weeks following the onset of symptoms, also in patients without a previous history of antecedent liver disease. Both forms of disease carry a grave prognosis.[57, 59, 111] In fulminant hepatic failure from a variety of causes, the mortality rate is greater than 70 per cent when stage IV hepatic encephalopathy supervenes.[55–57, 90, 117] The mortality within subsets varies. Fulminant non-A, non-B hepatitis appears to have the worst prognosis, whereas in patients with stage IV hepatic encephalopathy secondary to acetaminophen-induced hepatic necrosis, there is approximately 50 per cent survival (15 of 32 cases).[111] The success of liver transplantation in this situation is hampered first because of the rapid rate of disease progression and second because of the development of irreversible brain damage from cerebral edema. The logistics of organ procurement, coupled with the difficulty in assessing cerebral function, makes this subset a difficult group to treat. In contrast, in subfulminant hepatic failure progressing beyond six weeks of the onset of the illness, transplantation can be performed in a more elective fashion.

The first successful transplant for fulminant hepatic failure was reported by the University of California at Davis group in 1985 in a 3-year-old girl with acute toxic liver necrosis secondary to *Amanita phalloides* poisoning.[93] Since that report, over 60 cases of orthotopic liver transplantation for fulminant hepatic failure have been reported.[59, 112, 115–117, 119–123] The survival rate is between 60 and 70 per cent. Two of the largest studies are briefly described.[59, 112] In one series,[123] 17 of 23 patients with fulminant hepatic failure survived 2 to 15 months following liver transplant, two dying from poor allograft function, one from complications postsurgery, two from decerebration during or immediately after surgery, and one from transmitted acute infection with the human immunodeficiency virus. The overall antecedent mortality figure in the same institution for similar disease was 85 per cent. The causes of liver damage were diverse—viral, drug-induced, or unknown. The Pittsburgh experience has been reviewed in three reports.[58, 59, 120] In one report,[59] there was an 80 per cent mortality in those receiving supportive therapy alone as opposed to a 45 per cent mortality in those in whom orthotopic liver transplantation had been performed. The spectrum of primary liver disease causing liver failure included viral hepatitis, Wilson's disease, and drug toxicity. Sixteen patients had fulminant hepatic failure, of whom six received transplantation, three surviving. Residual central nervous system damage was not commented on. Of the ten who did not receive liver transplantation, three survived, and seven died awaiting a donor organ. In the subfulminant hepatic failure group, 13 patients were evaluated, of whom 7 received transplantation and 4 survived. Of the six patients not transplanted, all died. Of interest is that one patient with fulminant hepatitis B became hepatitis B surface antibody–positive postoperatively, underscoring the proposed hyperimmune response to viral infection as a contributing factor to liver failure.

It is still too early to conclude that liver transplantation is the best approach for treating patients with fulminant hepatic failure, a condition in which spontaneous recovery can occur and for which other heroic measures, such as charcoal and other resin hemoperfusion, total–body exchange transfusion, temporary liver support, and steroids,[60–63] which were initially thought to be effective have not stood the test of randomized prospective studies. Time and analysis of data

from multiple centers will ultimately determine the efficacy of transplantation in acute liver failure. The small series just reviewed suggests that survival in patients with subfulminant hepatic failure will be improved by timely transplantation.

PRIMARY LIVER CANCER (See Chap. 45)

Hepatocellular carcinoma, the most common primary hepatic malignant neoplasm, has an aggressively lethal course. The median survival of 600 consecutive patients with primary liver cancer was only 1.6 months from the time of diagnosis.[51] When stratified for the extent of disease, those patients with surgically resectable tumors lived significantly longer than nonsurgical patients with comparable disease, the median survival for the two groups being 19.6 months and 2.8 months, respectively.

In one series, 40 patients had orthotopic liver transplantation for primary liver cancer or intrahepatic cholangiocarcinoma.[52] Of this group, 60 per cent had no recurrence of disease with a follow-up period of more than one year in 22 of 24 patients. Four patients survived beyond five years. Of the 40 per cent with recurrence of disease, 13 of 16 survived beyond one year. Limitations of the study include a short follow-up for tumor recurrence and absence of histologic subtyping of the hepatocellular carcinoma. The latter is important, as fibrolamellar hepatoma has a far more indolent course and may recur many years following resection. Tumor recurrence was universal in the eight patients with extrahepatic bile duct cancer (the "Klatskin tumor").

The experience in the United States with orthotopic liver transplantation as a treatment modality for hepatocellular carcinoma is less encouraging.[53, 54] Between 1963 and 1987, Starzl's group has evaluated liver transplantation in 81 patients, of whom 21 had incidental hepatic malignancy diagnosed either at the time of surgery or on subsequent pathologic examinations.[53, 54] These were patients in whom liver transplantation was performed for end-stage liver disease. Sixty patients underwent transplantation as a potential curative treatment for hepatic malignancy when conventional subtotal resection was not possible. With regard to both categories, 23 patients were operated in the pre-cyclosporine era, and 58 patients received the surgery after 1980. The one-year survival in patients with incidental tumor approximated 90 per cent as opposed to 70 per cent in the elective category. Recurrence of tumor in the incidental group was not observed. By three years, only 30 per cent of patients who originally harbored conventionally unresectable tumor were still alive, and tumor recurrence exceeded 90 per cent. The survival was similar, regardless of the type of immunosuppression used (i.e., cyclosporine did not influence the outcome).

In the category of 60 patients with primary hepatic malignancy that was not resectable, 37 had primary hepatocellular carcinoma, of whom 9 had the fibrolamellar variant. The projected five-year survival in nonfibrolamellar and fibrolamellar hepatocellular carcinoma was 29 per cent, with similar frequency of recurrence in the two groups. However, whereas in the fibrolamellar subtype, tumor recurrence occurred late (i.e., about three years posttransplant) with a subsequently indolent course, in nonfibrolamellar hepatocellular carcinoma, malignancy usually was noted in the allograft or as metastases within the first year posttransplant and was much more aggressive in its behavior. Recurrence of bile duct cancer was invariable in ten patients with the Klatskin tumor, and all ten patients expired during the four-year follow-up period.

In summary, the place of liver transplantation in the treatment of primary liver cancer is still an open question. Adjuvant radiation or chemotherapy protocols in association with transplantation have not been assessed. The United States data strongly suggest that there is recurrence in more than 90 per cent of patients one to three years postsurgery regardless of the histologic subtype. At the present time, transplantation for nonresectable hepatic malignancy appears to be palliative at best, whereas a primary tumor discovered incidentally at the time of transplantation does not adversely impact the long-term survival of the patient.

METABOLIC LIVER DISEASE

Orthotopic liver transplantation has been considered for two categories of metabolic disease of the liver: in the first subset there is associated life-threatening liver injury, and in the second there is no hepatic injury, but the adverse effects of the metabolic disease can be reversed by liver transplantation. In the first category, Wilson's disease, hemochromatosis, α_1-antitrypsin deficiency, tyrosinemia, glycogen storage diseases types 1 and 4, and protoporphyria all can result in progressive fulminant, subfulminant, or chronic liver failure. Successful liver transplantation normalizes liver function and in some patients may additionally cure the metabolic disorder responsible for the original liver injury—as in, tyrosinemia or α_1-antitrypsin deficiency.[44, 63]

Metabolic diseases of the liver such as hemophilia, urea cycle enzyme deficiencies, phenylketonuria, hyperlipoproteinemia type 2, and Crigler-Najjar syndrome are examples of metabolic disorders that may be life-threatening and reversible by liver transplantation. The Crigler-Najjar syndrome (see Chap. 11) was first reported in 1952,[64] and to date there are approximately 100 reported cases.[65] The type 1 syndrome is inherited as an autosomal recessive disorder and beyond the first week of life the unconjugated hyperbilirubinemia is severe enough to cause kernicterus and death, usually by the age of 15 months. Only three reported cases have survived into the teen-age years before developing progressive neurologic deterioration.[66, 67] Given this poor prognosis, liver transplantation is the only hope for survival. Liver transplantation should also be considered for children with type 2 hyperlipoproteinemia and for patients where a deficiency of urea cycle enzymes leads to recurrent encephalopathy, severely impairing the quality of life. In both of these two situations, transplantation should be performed before there is permanent damage to other organs. Patients with hemophilia have been transplanted because of the development of HBV or non-A, non-B hepatitis that progressed to cirrhosis. Following successful liver transplantation, not only was the hepatic failure cured but also the underlying hemophilia. Reversal of severe neurologic manifestations of Wilson's disease following orthotopic liver transplantation was reported from the King's College Hospital group.[124] One patient was a bedridden akinetic rigid individual who recovered to a state of minimal neurologic disability within four months of transplant surgery and required no further copper chelation treatment. The second patient recovered rapidly, suggesting that the new liver was highly efficient in mobilizing extrahepatic tissue copper. Reversal or prevention of progression of nonhepatic disease in α_1-antitrypsin deficiency awaits

further study, but of interest is the report that in 11 patients receiving orthotopic liver transplantation for liver failure, within 3 days postsurgery α_1-antitrypsin activity was already present in the serum of the recipient, and subsequently, the retransplanted liver continued to synthesize α_1-antitrypsin of the donor phenotype.[125]

In summary, liver transplantation emerges as one of the most exciting new approaches for the treatment of incapacitating or potentially lethal metabolic disorders in which the metabolic lesion is limited to or expressed by the hepatocytes.

FAILURE OF PREVIOUS LIVER TRANSPLANTATION

There are multiple causes of posttransplantation liver dysfunction (see the section on allograft dysfunction), of which primary nonfunction, immunologic rejection, and technical difficulties relating to the surgery can result in need for retransplantation.[68] Allograft rejection is the most common cause of life-threatening dysfunction and calls for intensive antirejection therapy. Failure or restriction of such therapy, caused by existing bacterial, viral, or fungal infections, constitutes the major indication for retransplantation.

Ischemic liver injury, which occurs either during harvesting, in the course of transplantation or postsurgery from hepatic artery thrombosis, is another important cause of allograft dysfunction. In harvesting-related injury,[69] progressive liver failure with elevation of bilirubin and serum transaminases occurs shortly after transplantation, and in most situations, retransplantation is the only hope for survival. Hepatic artery thrombosis when suspected by Doppler ultrasound should be confirmed by selective angiography, and the extent of ischemic necrosis needs to be assessed by liver biopsy. Retransplantation will be predicated by the clinical and biochemical indicators of progressive liver failure.

In the Pittsburgh experience,[68] the need for retransplantation has arisen in about 20 to 25 per cent of liver recipients. Since 1980, of 69 reported retransplants, 60 were for second and nine were for third episodes of allograft dysfunction. The most common indications for retransplantation were rejection (57 per cent), followed by primary nonfunction (22 per cent), with technical failure accounting for an almost equivalent percentage. In the last group, this was far more common in children (32 per cent) than in adults (8 per cent). In this report, the overall survival in patients retransplanted approached 50 per cent at one year and beyond. Although survival after retransplantation is similar regardless of the initial disease, the one-year survival rate for ischemic injury during harvesting of the donor liver is only 20 per cent, compared with 60 per cent for chronic rejection or arterial thrombosis.[69] Liver retransplantation overall improves (compared with patients receiving a single transplant) the actuarial five-year survival by approximately 15 per cent. In general, the retransplant procedure is technically easy, with far less blood loss than the initial operation, and should be considered before serious clinical deterioration compromises the chance of success.

Summary

The determining factor regarding candidacy of a prospective liver recipient is a balance in the risk-benefit ratio in which the benefit to the patient and to society is positive in the final evaluation. Initial candidacy is determined by a hepatologist, who weighs the morbidity and mortality of liver transplantation against state-of-the-art new modalities evolving to reverse progressive liver failure. Ultimately, the evaluation requires input from many clinical experts from multiple clinical and paramedical disciplines—that is, the personnel that constitute the liver transplant team. In the total evaluation process, the absolute and relative contraindications outlined in Table 55–4 need to be determined. Age above 60 years has been listed as a relative contraindication. Starzl compared the outlook of 363 adult transplant patients who were less than 50 years of age with 92 patients who were between the ages of 50 and 77.[126] Although actuarial survival was slightly more favorable among the young recipients, the difference was not statistically significant. These statistics may relax age criteria in the assessment of transplant candidacy. Whatever the age of the candidate, all require rigorous work-up, which *includes a check of portal vein* patency by Doppler ultrasound and a subspecialty evaluation of the cardiopulmonary, renal, and psychosocial status of the patient. In primary malignant disease of the liver, angiography will be required to determine resectability of the tumor. In the final analysis, the best treatment for the patient is the one that is least invasive.

TRANSPLANT SURGERY

This is a major endeavor for both the transplant center and the team that calls for a commitment from all parties involved. The basic requirements have been reviewed recently by Klintmalm and colleagues.[70, 101] These include qualified surgeons capable of and willing to perform the procedure; hepatologists who have a good working relationship with the operating surgeons; an active renal dialysis program; adequate intensive care and operating room facilities with staff capable of accommodating the transplant surgery; an active infectious disease program capable of recognizing unusual viral, fungal, and protozoal infections; a blood bank that can provide the necessary blood products on demand, often with little advance warning; a pathologist with special interest in liver and transplant histopathology; a psychiatric and social service to support patients and their

TABLE 55–4. CONTRAINDICATIONS FOR ORTHOTOPIC LIVER TRANSPLANTATION

Absolute Contraindications
Advanced cardiopulmonary diseases, including severe arteriovenous shunting, renal failure, or life-limiting disorders of any other organ system that are not correctable by liver transplantation
Active infection outside the hepatobiliary system (includes HIV positivity)
Inability to accept the procedure, understand its nature, and cooperate in the medical care required following transplantation
Portal vein thrombosis
Primary malignant disease outside the hepatobiliary system
Active alcohol and/or substance abuse and dependency
Option of alternative effective medical or surgical therapy
Weight of infant less than 7 kg
Relative Contraindications
Age over 60 years
Alcoholic liver disease
Previous biliary or portacaval shunt surgery
Metastatic hepatobiliary malignancy
HbsAg-positive or HBeAg-positive state

families; a broad-based community support program that includes housing for patients and their families; and an adequate staff, including transplant co-ordinators, transplant fellows, laboratory support, and enough persons in each group to prevent "burn out." The last is particularly important, as success in transplantation requires obsessive and demandingly meticulous attention to detail 24 hours per day, 365 days a year. This in effect requires at least two experts in each area committed to all levels of patient care.

Once the potential candidate is identified, the patient's name is entered into the United Network for Organ Sharing (UNOS) computer list. Other factors entered are the blood type,[106] the patient's size and weight, and potential transplant center. Finally, the clinical status of the recipient is entered in order to prioritize the need for donor organs.

DONOR LIVER PROCUREMENT

Donors are persons who are brain dead and are hemodynamically stable. They should have normal liver function and no evidence of cancer, liver trauma, HIV infection, or hepatitis, and they should be less than 50 years of age. When the donor is identified, the potential recipient should be alerted by pager to come to the Transplant Surgery Center.

An absolute prerequisite for successful surgery is prompt functioning of the donor organ. The requirements are more stringent than in renal transplantation. First, there is no dialysis equivalent in allograft failure. Second, the metabolically active liver needs to be grafted within 8 to 10 hours of harvesting to maintain function, compared to kidney transplantation in which viability can be maintained for as much as 48 hours or more. Third, size matching is important so that blood vessel size is comparable and the surgeon can comfortably close the abdomen following transplant surgery.[73] This is a problem, particularly in children. Preliminary reports from France[74] and Chicago[75] suggest that transplantation of a single lobe of adult liver to children may be a feasible alternative to procuring a pediatric donor organ.

The techniques for the standard donor operation are well reviewed in the literature[71, 72] and require that the donor liver be carefully dissected, maintaining as much of the biliary and vascular components as possible (Fig. 55–3).[71, 72] The harvesting should be so planned that immediate perfusion via the portal vein with a cold isotonic solution in situ will ensure rapid core cooling. Final preservation is obtained by perfusing both the liver and the kidneys in situ with an intracellular electrolyte solution (Collins') to wash all blood out prior to removal and packaging. Several organs may be procured from a single donor.[72]

ALLOGRAFT REPLACEMENT

The technical aspects of allograft replacement have been described in detail elsewhere.[13, 71] Only the principles are summarized in this chapter. The abdomen is entered by a bilateral subcostal incision with midline extensions to the xiphoid in adults. In 1984, the development of venovenous bypass without systemic anticoagulation was a major technical advance and is used almost routinely in adults and in some children.[76–79] The bypass (Fig. 55–4) is performed using a closed circuit apparatus that does not require heparinization. Its purpose is to maintain normal hemody-

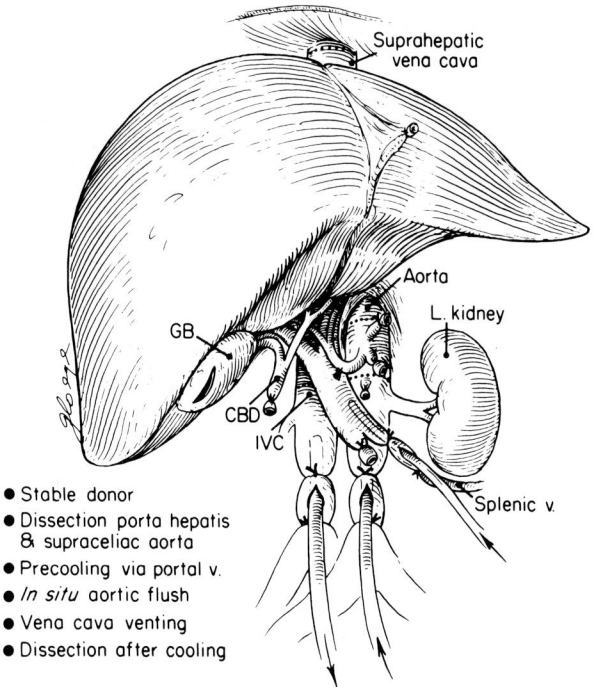

- Stable donor
- Dissection porta hepatis
  & supraceliac aorta
- Precooling via portal v.
- *In situ* aortic flush
- Vena cava venting
- Dissection after cooling

Figure 55–3. Preparation for harvesting of the donor liver. (From Busuttil RW, et al. Ann Surg 206:387, 1987, with permission.)

namic physiology during the critical anhepatic phase of orthotopic transplantation of the liver by diverting the inferior vena cava and portal circulation to the heart. Without it, when the inferior vena cava is cross-clamped at the diaphragm, there is a sudden decrease in both central

venous return and pulmonary arterial wedge pressures, resulting in a reduction of cardiac output. When the portal vein also is clamped, there is a marked increase in the hydrostatic pressure both in the portal and systemic venous beds, causing pooling of blood in the splanchnic area. This may increase transfusion requirements to maintain pressure during surgery and also intraoperative ischemic damage to kidney, bowel, and pancreas. Postsurgical fluid redistribution may result in fluid overload. The veno-venous bypass uses a femoral and portal venous return channel and repumps the blood via the axillary-jugular vein back to the heart. This permits decompression of the portal venous circulation and reduces the vascular engorgement, which in turn permits more easy dissection of the liver with minimal blood loss.

In the anhepatic phase, no hepatic disposition of citrate can occur, which may be a problem with the transfusion of citrated blood. To pre-empt precipitous falls in blood calcium levels, frequent monitoring of ionized calcium during surgery is necessary to permit therapeutic maintenance of serum calcium levels.[80]

Vascular anastomoses are performed in the following order: suprahepatic inferior vena cava (IVC), infrahepatic IVC, portal vein, and hepatic artery (Fig. 55–5). Following vascular anastomoses, biliary reconstruction is performed to restore the patency of the biliary tract (Fig. 55–6). At the present time, only graft duct to recipient duct reconstruction with a stent or a choledochojejunostomy to a jejunal Roux limb is recommended.[13, 71] There is a critical need for hemostasis postsurgery. This should be meticulously performed prior to closing of the abdomen. The usual blood transfusion requirement should be less than 20 units.

After surgery, the patients are followed in an intensive care unit for an average of about ten days. The early postoperative care has recently been reviewed by Grenvik and Gordon, who address the immediate immunosuppression regimen, pulmonary, cardiovascular, hepatic, renal, metabolic, bleeding, coagulation, and infection complica-

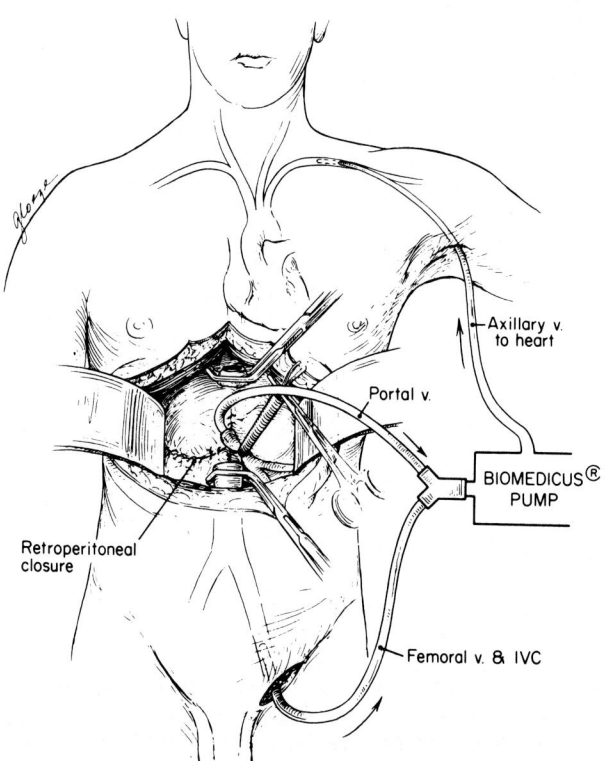

Figure 55–4. Veno-venous bypass for circulatory support during the anhepatic phase. (From Busuttil RW, et al. Ann Surg 206:387, 1987, with permission.)

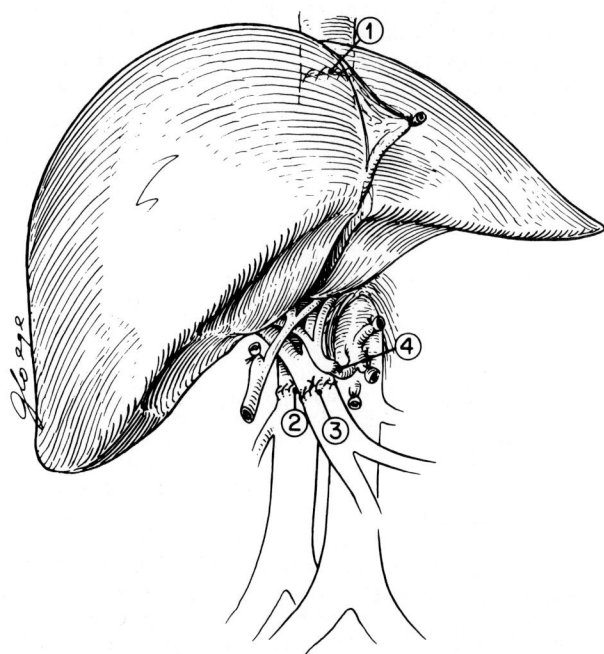

Figure 55–5. Order of vascular anastomoses. (From Busuttil RW, et al. Ann Surg 206:387, 1987, with permission.)

DONOR LIVER

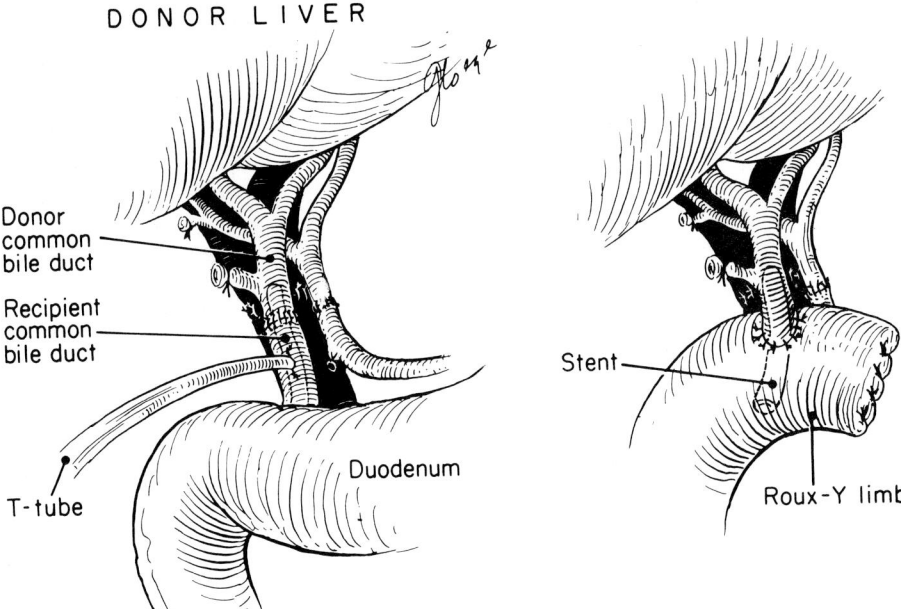

Donor common bile duct

Recipient common bile duct

T-tube

Duodenum

Stent

Roux-Y limb

Figure 55–6. Biliary reconstruction by choledochocholedochostomy with T-tube stent (left) or Roux-Y choledochojejunostomy with indwelling straight stent. (From Busuttil RW, et al. Ann Surg 206:387, 1987, with permission.)

tions as well as postoperative nutrition and pain control.[81] Immunosuppression postsurgery usually involves the use of cyclosporin A and steroids. An acceptable regimen would include 1 g methylprednisolone given intravenously in the operating room as well as 2 mg/kg cyclosporin A intravenously after revascularization of the allograft. In patients with renal failure, a monoclonal antibody to T lymphocytes (e.g., OKT3) is administered both preoperatively and postoperatively.[82] Perioperative antibiotics are continued for three days. The goals of postoperative care and criteria for discharge are to control rejection, to maintain multiorgan function, to contain infection, to clamp the T tubes so that oral cyclosporin A can be absorbed (this fat-soluble drug requires bile acids for absorption), and to achieve adequate oral nutrition.

Nonhepatic complications will be reviewed briefly.[81, 83] Right-sided pleural effusions are common and should be treated aggressively to pre-empt infection. Hypertension frequently occurs in the early postoperative period, requiring treatment, for example, with intravenous medication such as hydralazine. Renal function may be perturbed at the time of surgery because of diminished renal blood flow in end-stage liver disease, especially in patients with refractory ascites or hepatorenal syndrome. Cholestasis presurgery may render the renal tubules susceptible to acute injury following shock or sepsis during or following transplantation. Aminoglycoside antibiotics and immunosuppressant drugs such as cyclosporin A are nephrotoxic and can initiate or potentiate the renal dysfunction frequently seen in the postoperative period.

The immunocompromised patient is particularly susceptible to infections. Bacterial infections can affect the wound, lung, urinary tract, and operative sites, including liver and biliary tree. About 50 per cent of infections occur within the first month of transplantation. Frequent surveillance of all available body fluids and secretions is required, and blood cultures may be positive even in asymptomatic patients. When necessary, antibiotics should be used primarily against gram-positive and gram-negative organisms, and scrupulous aseptic technique must be followed in the care of these patients. Bacterial products such as endotoxin

may cause cholestasis, which may mimic rejection and result in inappropriate usage of immunosuppression.[84] Common bacterial isolates are staphylococcal, streptococcal, including enterococcus, enteric organisms, *Pseudomonas, Serratia,* and *Legionella* organisms. Viral infections such as cytomegalovirus (either reactivation or primary infection) and other members of the herpesvirus group, including herpes simplex I and II, herpes zoster, varicella, and the Epstein-Barr virus, cause significant morbidity and mortality.[84, 85] Recurrence of the primary hepatic infection (i.e., hepatitis B or hepatitis non-A, non-B) may also complicate the picture. Cytomegalovirus infection in conjunction with immunosuppressive therapy predisposes to the development of other opportunistic infections, including those with fungi, viruses, and bacteria. When the liver is involved (e.g., by cytomegalovirus or herpesvirus), this may cause enzyme abnormalities often attributed to rejection.[86, 87] Cyclosporin is less prone to be complicated by infectious complications than are high dose steroids and azathioprine. Fungal infections are common. Most liver transplant recipients become colonized or infected or both by yeasts. *Candida* is most common, but other infections include *Aspergillus,*[88] *Mucor,* and *Cryptococcus* organisms.[83]

Adverse drug effects of immunosuppressants also are common. With cyclosporin A, these include hypertension, nephrotoxicity, glucose tolerance, seizures, gingival hypertrophy, and hirsutism. Steroids can cause hyperglycemia, hyperlipidemia, osteopenia, hypercatabolic state, impaired wound healing, and mood change. Azathioprine may lead to bone marrow suppression. Monoclonal antibodies to T-lymphocytes–OKT3, for example, can cause fever, serum sickness, and pulmonary edema.

The neurologic complications following orthotopic liver transplantation have recently been reviewed,[127, 128] and in one study,[127] 17 of 52 patients exhibited cerebral dysfunction. In both studies, the clinical syndromes range from confusion to coma, cortical blindness, quadriplegia, and epilepsy. The causes were diverse and represented air embolism, cerebral hemorrhage secondary to coagulopathy, cerebral infarction as a result of perioperative hypotension, opportunistic infection of the brain, central pontine myelinosis, and drug-induced, predominantly cyclosporin A-related seizures. Complications following cyclosporin A appear to have occurred more frequently after intravenous administration and when blood cholesterol levels were low.[128] Hypocalcemia and hypomagnesemia increase; the neurotoxicity of cyclosporin A. Of therapeutic importance is the fact that while Dilantin controls seizures, the concomitant induction of hepatic microsomal enzymes accelerates cyclosporin A metabolism, thereby increasing the dose required to maintain therapeutic blood levels.

The diversity of complications in the postoperative period underscores the need for the critical care team to obtain appropriate consultation from transplant-oriented experts in infectious diseases, nephrology, and pulmonary medicine. After surgery, the hepatologist/gastroenterologist is primarily involved in the evaluation of hepatic dysfunction, and for this reason, the post-transplantation causes, histopathology, and management of allograft injury are discussed separately.

HEPATIC ALLOGRAFT DYSFUNCTION

Table 55–5 outlines the causes of hepatic dysfunction following liver transplantation. The cause of liver dysfunction may be difficult to identify as so many of the clinical and biochemical features are nonspecific (i.e., fever, jaundice, increased liver parenchymal and bile duct enzymes, and so forth).[103] In the course of evaluation, titers of antibodies to viral infection, biliary ultrasound, or T-tube cholangiogram and arterial ultrasound with angiography are frequently used to identify infection or assess patency of bile ducts and hepatic artery. Liver biopsy and cultures of biopsy tissue may be necessary to evaluate histopathology and allograft infection. Some transplant centers advocate biopsy of all patients in order to better interpret biopsies taken during allograft dysfunction. Liver biopsies in allograft dysfunction should be performed early in the work-up, before treatment for rejection.[102] This makes interpretation easier. Repeat biopsies are facilitated by a surgical facial window left post-transplant.[12] Even following full evaluation, Williams and co-workers have reported a self-limited, nonspecific "cholestasis syndrome" in 23 of 53 episodes of allograft dysfunction after liver transplantation for which no specific cause could be identified.[12]

HARVESTING-INDUCED INJURY

Allograft dysfunction may occur shortly after surgery as a result of ischemic injury incurred during harvesting. This may result from an unstable donor who is hypotensive and on vasopressors, inadequate perfusion and preservation, prolonged cold ischemia, or prolonged warm ischemia.[69] Clinically, there is little difficulty in making the diagnosis. It is manifest by initial nonfunction of the graft, which is marked by diminished bile flow and failure to

TABLE 55–5. ETIOLOGY OF HEPATIC DYSFUNCTION POSTTRANSPLANTATION

Harvesting-induced injury
Vascular thrombosis
Rejection
Infection
Bile duct complications
Drug-induced hepatic injury
Hemolysis

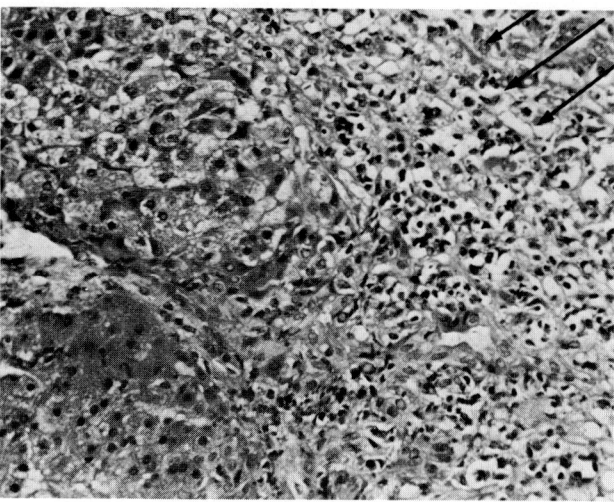

Figure 55–7. Ischemic necrosis 24 hours post-transplantation. Section shows a hepatic lobule with extensive necrosis (see arrows), predominantly centrilobular. Viable hepatocytes are seen surrounding a portal triad. Acute inflammatory cells are present at the interface between the necrotic and viable areas. H & E × 250.

reverse coagulopathy even following large volumes of fresh blood products. After surgery, there is an immediate progressive elevation of bilirubin; serum transaminases are usually 10 to 20 times greater than normal, and patients exhibit coagulopathy, hypoglycemia, renal failure, and varying degrees of encephalopathy. Liver biopsy clearly distinguishes harvesting-related injury (Fig. 55–7) from that of acute rejection (Figs. 55–8 and 55–9). Mild to moderate vascular injury may be limited to peripheral and subcapsular areas, and liver function may recover. Extensive ischemic damage and necrosis can only be treated by retransplantation. The one-year survival rate of retransplantation for ischemic injury is only 20 per cent, compared with 60 per cent for chronic rejection or arterial thrombosis.[69]

VASCULAR THROMBOSIS

The incidence of thrombosis of the hepatic artery as a cause of graft dysfunction is approximately 1.5 per cent in

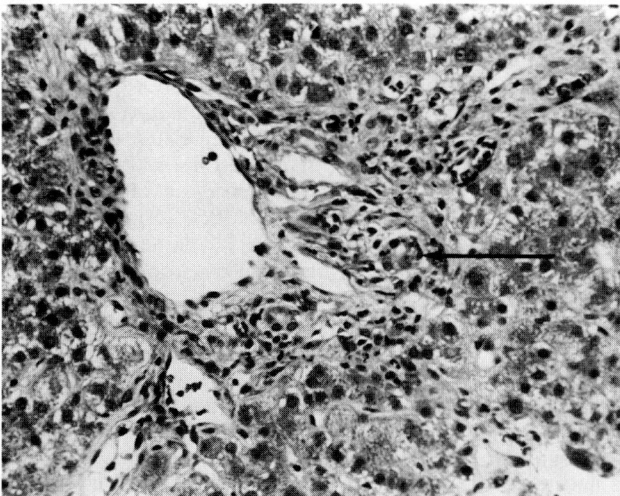

Figure 55–8. Rejection cholangitis. Note the marked portal inflammation composed of round cells with some polymorphs. Some of these inflammatory cells have penetrated the interlobular bile ducts (arrow), which show degenerative changes. H & E × 250.

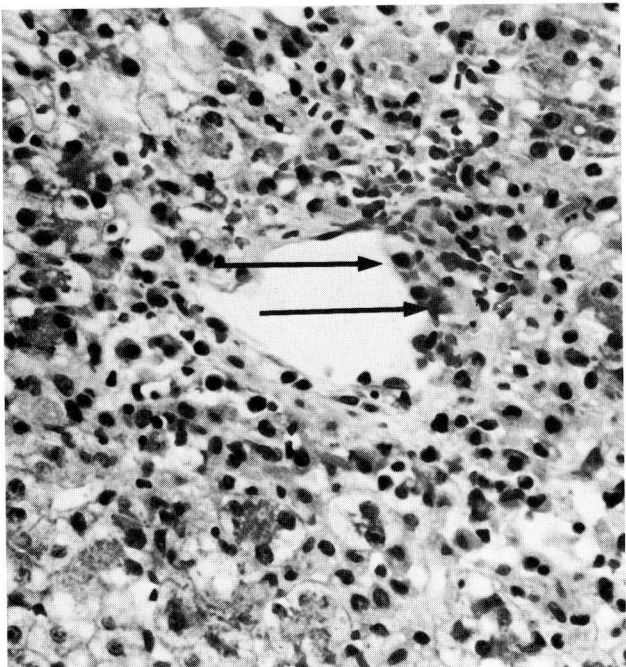

Figure 55–9. Endotheliitis caused by acute rejection. Central vein is surrounded by acute and chronic inflammatory cells. In addition, inflammatory cells are attached to the luminal endothelium (see arrows). H & E × 250.

adults and 11.8 per cent in children.[69] Extensive hepatic necrosis in this setting is the second most common indication for retransplantation in the pediatric population, although occasional patients will survive with a graft perfused solely by the portal vein. The clinical illness is milder than that of harvesting-induced injury, with fever, shaking chills, and moderate elevation of the transaminases after initial restoration of liver function. If thrombosis is partial, there may be regional necrosis of the liver, which increases the risk of abscess formation. These abscesses are best detected by liver imaging. Bile duct necrosis with leakage and bile peritonitis may further complicate the clinical spectrum. In the work-up of liver dysfunction, the use of a Doppler ultrasonography is helpful in determining the patency of the hepatic artery and portal vein. Thrombosis, when suspected, can be confirmed by selective angiography. Occasionally, subcapsular hepatic necrosis in liver transplant allografts can occur in postsurgical shock without occlusions in the extrahepatic arteries or the portal or hepatic veins.[104]

LIVER REJECTION AND ITS TREATMENT

Classically, rejection is classified as acute when it occurs three days to two months after transplantation and as chronic when it occurs more than two months following transplantation. However, because there are many examples of clinical and histologic acute rejection that have become manifest many months after transplantation, we prefer using histologic criteria for classification.

The liver appears to be relatively resistent to hyperacute rejection, and the first evidence of acute rejection rarely occurs before the fourth or fifth postoperative day. Clinically, the patient feels poorly, often has a low-grade fever, and complains of anorexia, abdominal discomfort, back pain, or respiratory distress.[83] On physical examina-

tion, the liver homograft is usually enlarged, but regardless of the amount of histologic inflammation, tenderness may be absent owing to denervation of the donor liver. Biochemically, serum transaminases, bilirubin, γ-glutamyl transpeptidase (GGT), and alkaline phosphatase levels are raised. A prolonged prothrombin time indicates serious liver injury.

Clinically, rejection should be suspected when liver dysfunction is unassociated with extrahepatic biliary obstruction, hepatic artery occlusion, or mass lesions in the liver on liver imaging, the last suggesting infarction or abscess formation. The reason for an aggressive approach in procuring allograft biopsies is the nonspecificity of the clinical illness and of the biochemical parameters of liver injury, which may be identical in rejection and in systemic or hepatic infection.[105] Thus, immunosuppression appropriate for rejection would aggravate bacterial, viral, or fungal infection. This underscores the need for rational therapy predicated on an adequate data base.

The histopathologic hallmarks of allograft rejection—that is, nonsuppurative cholangitis (Fig. 55–8) and endotheliitis (Fig. 55–9)—probably reflect the strong expression of histocompatibility antigens (HLA) in endothelial cells and bile duct epithelial cells.[102] Rejection cholangitis is of greater prognostic significance and may lead to destruction and complete loss of small bile ducts—the so-called vanishing bile duct syndrome[94]—whereas endotheliitis is generally of more diagnostic significance. Histologically, rejection cholangitis is characterized by evidence of bile duct damage with epithelial anisonucleosis and cytoplasmic vacuolation associated with a mixed or predominantly mononuclear portal infiltrate (Fig. 55–8). Endotheliitis is characterized by the attachment of lymphocytes (immunocytes) to the endothelium of the portal and terminal hepatic veins (i.e., the central vein) (Fig. 55–9). Acute cellular rejection is potentially reversible. A fibrotic process with obliteration of bile ducts (the vanishing bile duct syndrome)[94] and fibrosis of blood vessels with or without xanthomatous changes in the intima characterizes rejection that has progressed to an irreversible stage and will not respond to therapy. This constitutes chronic, irreversible rejection. Clinically, signs of impending acute vanishing bile duct syndrome include high fever and increasing jaundice with marked elevation of serum bilirubin and alkaline phosphatase levels that persist despite antirejection treatment.[13, 94] The pathogenesis of the syndrome is unclear. Bile duct epithelium is rich in HLA class I antigens. In one study, in 62 patients undergoing orthotopic liver transplantation, it was observed that a complete mismatch for class I antigens was more common in those patients with the vanishing bile duct syndrome than in those with normal graft function.[129] Conversely, a mismatch for HLA class II antigens was less common in those with the syndrome.

Response to antirejection therapy in a person with appropriate histopathology and symptoms (i.e., an improvement in the clinical, biochemical, and morphologic findings) strongly supports the diagnosis of rejection. However, absence of a response, or a response of only one or two manifestations—for instance, clinical and biochemical—does not rule out the presence of rejection. The mainstay of the treatment of rejection is cyclosporin A. This drug has selectivity for suppression of alloimmunity rather than of nonspecific host resistance, thereby achieving an improved therapeutic index for clinical transplantation. Cyclosporin A is a lipophilic undecapeptide extracted from the soil fungus *Tolypocladium inflatum* (Gams) and purified chromatographically. Its immunosuppressive effect is due to its relatively selective action on T, rather than B, lymphocytes.[95] Because cyclosporin A does not inhibit production of antibody against lipopolysaccharide antigens in nude mice, T-cell independent B-cell responses are intact. Moreover, its effects on polymorphonuclear leukocytes, macrophages/monocytes, and natural killer cells are only modest. The action of cyclosporin A on its target, T-cell lymphocytes, is reversible, and discontinuance of the drug leads to resumption of the immune response. Thus, the drug does not deplete T-cell precursors. The dose of cyclosporin A should be monitored by blood levels, preferably using high-pressure liquid chromatography, which selectively detects cyclosporin A in the presence of its metabolites. The optimal plasma level should range between 200 and 300 ng/ml.

Immunosuppressive agents used in conjunction with cyclosporin A include azathioprine, prednisone, and antibodies to lymphocytes. Azathioprine, an imidazole derivative of 6-mercaptopurine, has a lower therapeutic index than cyclosporin A. It competitively inhibits critical enzymes in the nucleic acid synthetic pathway and causes more myelosuppression than inhibition of lymphocyte proliferation. It can also cause liver injury. Prednisone has well-known widespread metabolic side effects and exhibits a broader immunosuppressive effect. In more serious rejection situations, polyclonal antibodies (e.g., antilymphocyte globulin) or specific monoclonal antibodies to T cells (e.g., OKT3) may be used.[96, 101]

First used for acute renal allograft rejection,[130] OKT3 has now been applied in hepatic allograft rejection. Twenty-four of 25 patients with acute hepatic allograft rejection resistant to steroids, antilymphocytic globulin therapy, or both responded to anti-OKT3, the response being complete in 14 and partial in 10.[82] With a mean follow-up of 18.2 months, allograft salvage rate has been 90 per cent and patient survival 88 per cent. When rejection recurred, these subsequent episodes usually responded to steroid therapy. In another study,[131] 52 patients required anti-OKT3 therapy for resistant rejection. A survival of 77 per cent was recorded in this subset, in which the mean follow-up period was 12.2 months. Evidence for reversal of rejection was not obvious for three to four days, and continued improvement thereafter was a general rule. A newer agent, FK-506, a macrolide extracted from the fermentation broth of *Streptomyces tsukubaensis*, inhibits production of T-cell lymphokines such as interleukin 2 in vitro at 110-fold lower concentrations than that of cyclosporin.[132] Its usefulness awaits further study.

When there is a probable liver rejection episode in a patient on combination immunosuppressive therapy, the usual first-line approach is to give a steroid bolus intravenously and then to taper rapidly. When rejection cholangitis is treated successfully, the inflammation recedes and the ducts remain undamaged. Sometimes periductal fibrosis may develop in this situation. When treatment failure occurs, duct destruction progresses as a consequence of rejection. It is characterized by degenerative changes such as cytoplasmic vacuolation; pyknosis of ductal epithelial cells; infiltration of the ductal wall by inflammatory cells, including immunocytes and neutrophils; and damage to the basement membrane. This last feature appears to be a sign of irreversibility. The loss of small bile ducts with the accompanying loss of antigenic stimulation leads to disappearance of inflammatory cells in the affected areas, a "burnt-out" portal tract,[97] and the development of fibrosis of the biliary type. If the steroid boluses do not reverse the process, then a once-only trial with antilymphocyte globulin

or anti-OKT3 is indicated. If the liver lesion does not regress, retransplantation may be the only option available.

LIVER INFECTION

Abnormalities of liver function as a response to systemic or intra-abdominal infections have already been alluded to. Direct infections of the liver include cholangitis; liver abscess (e.g., following ischemic necrosis); and those relating to transfusions, opportunistic organisms, or reinfection of the donor liver with the agent that caused the original liver disease. In patients with HBV infection, the inevitability and seriousness of recurrence of the viral disease has already been discussed in this chapter, and recurrence is unrelated to the e antigen status. Non-A, non-B hepatitis, either from recurrence of the original infection or as an acquired new infection after liver transplantation is more difficult to diagnose in the recipient liver because of the absence of specific serologic markers. Allograft dysfunction caused by hepatitis is characterized by a predominantly lobular injury (Fig. 55–10) rather than the predominantly portal reaction seen in rejection.

The second group of infections relate to those transmitted by transfused blood. These include HBV infection, non-A, non-B hepatitis, and HIV and CMV infections. The last can occur either as a primary infection or reactivation. The usual incubation period posttransfusion for CMV infection is three to six weeks. Both primary and reactivation infections in immunocompromised patients are associated with prolonged excretion of the virus at high titers in urine and in saliva. In some patients, the main presenting features of symptomatic infection are malaise, fever, and tiredness with atypical mononuclear cells in the peripheral blood. Epstein-Barr viral titers are negative. Liver tests are modestly abnormal. Histologic examination of liver biopsy material shows intranuclear and cytoplasmic inclusions in hepatocytes and bile duct cells (Fig. 55–11). Other changes include neutrophilic envelopment of hepatocytes containing inclusion bodies and focal areas of lymphocytic inflammation that resemble granulomas. There have been case

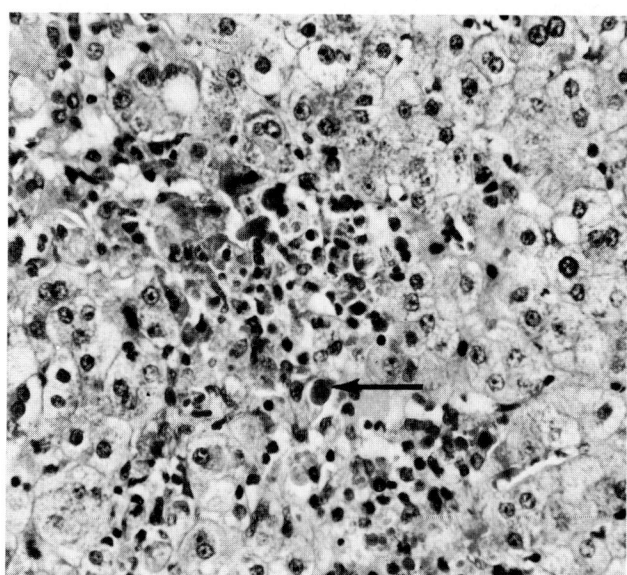

Figure 55–10. Viral hepatitis post-transplantation for presumed non-A, non-B cirrhosis. This section shows an area of focal necrosis with a chronic inflammatory cell infiltrate and an acidophilic body (arrow). Ballooning degeneration is seen in surrounding hepatocytes. H & E × 250.

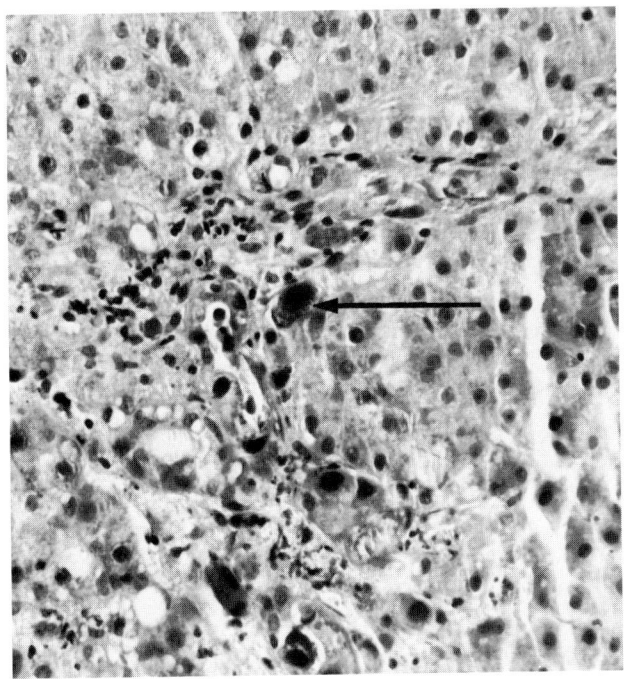

Figure 55–11. Cytomegaloviral (CMV) hepatitis post-transplantation. This section shows a portal bile duct with surrounding acute and chronic inflammation. CMV inclusions are seen in hepatocytes and in bile duct cells. The arrow points to a representative cell with intranuclear and cytoplasmic inclusions. H & E × 250.

reports of acute, fatal massive hepatic necrosis that appears to be related to CMV infection.[98]

Opportunistic infections of the liver can occur in any immunodeficiency state. These infections include fungal, protozoal, mycobacterial, and atypical presentations of viral illnesses.[83] Hepatic dysfunction manifested biochemically by increased levels of bilirubin, transaminase, and alkaline phosphatase may be due primarily to the effects of these infections or to the hepatotoxicity of the therapeutic agents used in their treatment.

BILE DUCT COMPLICATIONS

Complications of bile duct anastomosis in liver transplantation have been minimized by the standardization of reconstructive techniques that includes an understanding of and technical attention to the donor ductal system.[99] Nevertheless, bile leaks and biliary obstruction are still important causes of hepatic dysfunction.[69] Bile duct disruption may occur within ten days of surgery and is manifest with bile appearing in the abdominal drains. An internal bile leak frequently causes acute peritonitis with mild elevation of bilirubin and liver parenchymal enzymes. Stenotic obstruction of the bile duct is a late complication and when unrecognized, may mimic graft rejection, leading to inappropriate use of immunosuppressive agents. Acute bacterial cholangitis may also occur. The latter type of patient may be toxic and febrile and exhibit positive blood cultures. In the evaluation of graft dysfunction, a T-tube cholangiogram, radionuclide biliary scans, and ultrasonograms are useful in detecting bile duct complications for which endoscopic or surgical repair is indicated.

DRUG-INDUCED HEPATIC INJURY

Multisystem dysfunctions are common after liver transplantation, and the polypharmacy required to combat these disorders is frequently associated with adverse drug reactions, which include hepatic toxicity. In this section, the focus is on the hepatotoxic effects of immunosuppressive agents used to control rejection. The main culprits are cyclosporin A and azathioprine. Azathioprine causes a cholestatic liver injury with hepatocellular necrosis. Cyclosporin A also has been associated with chemical liver injury. The histopathology of the last lesion has not been clearly defined. Whereas perioperative hepatic ischemia may render the liver more susceptible to cyclosporin A–induced injury, this phenomenon has also been well described after renal transplantation. Patients with hepatotoxicity are more likely to have other adverse side effects of cyclosporin A, including nephrotoxicity and neuroectodermal toxicity. In a recent and comprehensive study on the hepatobiliary and pancreatic complications of cyclosporin A therapy in 466 renal transplant recipients, Lorber and associates identified 228 of 466 patients (49 per cent) with at least one hepatotoxic episode, half of which occurred during the first month of therapy.[100]

The biochemical profile of cyclosporin A hepatotoxicity is nonspecific and includes hyperbilirubinemia, increases in parenchymal enzymes, lactic dehydrogenase, and alkaline phosphatase.[100] Cholestasis also has been implicated as an early manifestation of liver injury. The best treatment for presumed cyclosporin A hepatotoxicity is to reduce the dose so that trough plasma levels, measured by high-performance liquid chromatography, are at the lower level of the therapeutic range, which for plasma is 200 to 300 ng/ml. Lowering the dose reversed hepatotoxicity in 81 per cent of cases.[100] Pancreatic abnormalities also have been observed. In one series, of the 228 patients with cyclosporin A–induced hepatotoxicity,[100] asymptomatic hyperamylasemia was noted in 12 (5.3 per cent) as opposed to 5 of the 238 patients without liver dysfunction. In the former group, three patients had acute pancreatitis; and three, pancreatic abscesses. Thus, a total prevalence of 4.9 per cent, or 23 of 446 patients, on cyclosporin A and prednisone had pancreatic abnormalities.

HEMOLYSIS

Graft dysfunction, whether subclinical or overt, decreases the capacity of the liver to eliminate bilirubin. Pigment loading in this situation, whether from intravascular hemolysis or from the breakdown of extravasated blood, frequently raises serum bilirubin levels. The prognostic importance of this is far less ominous than when increases in bilirubin are due to intrinsic hepatocellular injury or biliary tract disease. Intravascular hemolysis has been observed in approximately 17 per cent of patients receiving ABO unmatched transfusions.[69] Also, liver grafts from donors having an ABO subtype different from that of the recipient can produce antirecipient ABO antibodies. These antibodies have been detected within three weeks of transplantation and may persist one to two months afterward.[106]

REFLECTIONS ON THE PAST AND THE FUTURE

Long-term success after orthotopic liver transplantation has continued to improve since 1980, with a current one-year survival rate close to 80 per cent in children, which is about 10 per cent more than in adults (see Figs.

55–1 and 55–2). This may relate either to the inherent ability of children to respond better to major surgery or to the nature of the underlying pediatric liver disease. For example, children with biliary atresia are known to be prospective candidates for liver transplantation when the diagnosis is first made, especially if the porto-enterostomy (the Kasai operation) is unsuccessful. This provides opportunity for the transplant surgeon to optimize replacement with an allograft when the condition of the recipient is still excellent nutritionally and with regard to cardiopulmonary and renal function.

In contrast, the timing of transplant surgery in adults with chronic liver disease whose clinical status is deteriorating is much more critical. Most centers have reported patients who either died before an appropriate liver was obtained or who, while awaiting a donor organ, deteriorated to the point at which their clinical state was too poor to tolerate major surgery. This may have accounted for earlier reports of better survival in indolent chronic cholestatic cirrhotic disorders such as primary biliary cirrhosis. However, in more recent reports the one-year survival in children and adults is similar as is that of patients in different categories of liver disease, including seriously ill recipients.

Why is there continued improvement in survival over the past 2 to 3 years? The answer is both speculative and multifactorial.

In 1979, Calne and his associates reported prolonged renal graft survival using cyclosporin A in immunosuppressive regimen.[7] Since 1980, cyclosporin A and prednisone have been fairly standard immunosuppressive agents in liver transplantation. Cyclosporin A, because of its greater specificity as an antirejection drug, has been cited as a major reason for improved results;[14] however, this conclusion has been questioned by Scharschmidt.[18] In the latter analysis of 540 patients receiving liver allografts from four different centers, he observed that overall survival in the post-1980 era (50 per cent) was significantly better than the 29 per cent reported pre-1980 ($P < 0.001$). However, when he compared the results in the post-1980 period and separated the patients into two groups that either received cyclosporin A or alternative antirejection drugs, no significant difference between the two groups was observed ($P < 0.39$). However, interpretation of this data is complicated by the routine use of cyclosporin A in one major center as opposed to its nonuse in another.

Technical improvements in transplant surgery have played a major role in the improvement in long-term survival. One such technical development was the introduction of the veno-venous bypass, to maintain hemodynamic stability during the anhepatic phase of transplant surgery as well as to decompress the portal circulation before dissecting out the diseased liver. Other technical advances relate to better understanding of bile duct reconstruction, biliary epithelial preservation during harvesting, and improved techniques at biliary reanastomosis—all of which have led to a diminished incidence of postsurgical biliary leakage and fistula formation.

The indications for retransplantation have been clearly defined, and overall, this has resulted in an approximately 15 per cent increase in one-year survival. The procurement of donor livers requires sophisticated communication between harvesting and transplant centers, and this is far more efficient than in the pre-1980 days of liver transplantation.

The inappropriate use of immunosuppression not only increases prevalence of infection but also modifies expression of disease, delaying diagnosis and appropriate therapy. Improvement in this area includes better detection of existing infection in the prospective recipients, particularly in patients on steroids for autoimmune lupoid hepatitis, the histopathologic monitoring of allograft injury to permit titration of antirejection therapy to the lowest dose necessary to combat allograft rejection, and the experience of infectious disease teams in caring for immunocompromised patients with early diagnosis and appropriate treatment of atypical infections.

For whatever reason, there has clearly been an improvement in the benefit-risk ratio of orthotopic liver transplantation, which in turn has influenced the hepatologist to refer patients for transplant surgery earlier in the course of the disease. This cycle of increased confidence leading to better candidacy coupled with the improved total management of the patient should result in an even greater success rate in future years.

Liver diseases, both acute and chronic, that lead to death are relatively common in both children and adults. The prevalence rates based on demographic studies approximates 20 to 40 per million per year. Thus, in California, one might anticipate between 500 and 1000 transplant cases per year. An average large center should probably deal with 50 to 150 cases per year, suggesting that California might be able to sustain 5 to 10 transplant centers. The age range for transplantation is increasing as transplant centers report better results for patients aged 60 years and older. This will clearly enlarge the prospective liver recipient population. The costs and benefits of liver transplantation have recently been reviewed. The overall cost of transplantation has been estimated to lie between $50,000 and $250,000 per patient for the first year, including pre- and post-surgery expenses.[133] This encompasses the mean cost at the University of California, Los Angeles, which approximates $175,000 for adults and $125,000 for children. Williams and colleagues stratified the hospital costs (professional fees excluded) according to the recipients' health status at the time of transplantation.[113] At the University of Tennessee, the expenses for group I (ambulatory) patients averaged $57,404. In group II, patients that required inpatient care, the cost was marginally higher ($59,171), whereas for those recipients with renal failure or constant encephalopathy or who were confined to intensive care units (ICU) at the time of transplantation, the costs averaged $137,028.

Van Thiel and colleagues analyzed transplantation costs and benefits at the University of Pittsburgh but chose not to give a dollar amount because fee for service rendered varies so much from center to center, particularly worldwide.[108] They addressed the program developmental cost in hiring extra personnel and in expanding hospital facilities. They assessed the cost factors related to ICU days and non-ICU days as well as blood production requirements and pre- and postoperative laboratory costs. The costwise benefits of liver transplantation were difficult to assess. The authors state their "gut feeling" that "transplantation might convert a health care consumer into a health care premium payer."[108] Also addressed is the cost of caring for patients with advanced liver disease, especially if one considers multiple admissions for recurrent complications. Thus, the earlier that candidacy is established, the better will be the overall cost saving. Philosophically, Van Thiel and colleagues indicate that dollar figures cannot be equated to broader benefits of transplantation-related research in which the beneficiaries are not only the hepatologist, surgeon, radiologist, and immunologist but health care in general. McMahon indicates in his critique that the Pittsburgh study is neither a cost-benefit nor a cost-effective analytic study in the strict sense.[109] The questions raised in this commentary are philosophic: "Do the benefits justify the cost? We live at a time of increasing concern about the costs of medical care. Liver transplantation is both high-cost and life-saving for a small number of patients." Society, he claims, is concerned that the few patients who do benefit from liver transplantation may siphon off a disproportional amount of resources from other patients also in the need of health care. The author also addresses the inherent systematic bias to underestimate costs and to assess benefits that is caused by a conflict of interest when those directly engaged in a line of research are asked to evaluate its worth. However, he concurs that the "bottom line" is repugnance for a decision to withhold effective intervention based solely on economic grounds. As Bismuth has emphasized,[114] with the pressure of demands of motivated patients and informed doctors, it will be difficult not to offer the patients with potentially fatal liver disease the only curative therapeutic option, namely liver transplantation.

A key message is the need for liver transplant programs to be prospectively evaluated at a national level. In the United States, the National Institutes of Health are closely monitoring transplant centers by formulating and analyzing a wide variety of questions regarding candidacy, rejection, cost, and so forth. The purpose is to promote growth in a controlled and orderly manner. The rigorous policies of insurance companies in funding only centers with established successful track records or the potential to achieve this will tend to retard unrestrained growth. This is essential for the most effective implementation of a new and important therapeutic modality in liver disease.

Major advances have been made since the first edition of this textbook was published. We have attempted to present an overview of the state of the art that is clearly optimistic with regard to end-stage liver disease, subfulminant hepatic failure, and metabolic liver disease. By the time the next edition of this book is published, liver transplantation may well be a routine procedure performed at a much reduced cost. As the spectrum of indications increases and the age for recipients expands, the supply of donor organs may become rate limiting, and the philosophical aspects of who will and who will not receive a transplant may well be the main theme for future authors.

REFERENCES

1. Welch CS. A note on transplantation of the whole liver in dogs. Transplant Bull 2:54, 1955.
2. Goodrich EO, Welch HF, Nelson JA, et al. Homotransplantation of the canine liver. Surgery 39:244, 1956.
3. Sicular A, Paronetto F, Kark AE, et al. Rejection of the homotransplanted dog liver in the absence of hepatic insufficiency. Proc Soc Exp Biol Med 112:760, 1963.
4. Starzl TE, Marchioro TL, Huntley RT, et al. Experimental and clinical homotransplantation of the liver. Ann NY Acad Sci 120:739, 1964.
5. Starzl TE, Marchioro TL, Rowlands DT, et al. Immunosuppression after experimental and clinical homotransplantation of the liver. Ann Surg 160:411, 1964.
6. Starzl TE, Marchioro TL, von Kaulla K, et al. Homotransplantation of the liver in humans. Surg Gynecol Obstet 117:659, 1963.
7. Calne RY, Rolles K, White DG, et al. Cyclosporin A initially as the only immunosuppressant in 34 recipients of cadaveric organs: 32 kidneys, 2 pancreases, and 2 livers. Lancet 2:1033, 1979.
8. McMaster P, Jurewicz WA, Gunson BK, et al. The current state of liver and pancreas transplantation. Scand Gastroenter 117:69, 1985.
9. Starzl TE, Punam CW, Hansbrough JF, et al. Biliary complications after liver transplantation: with special reference to the biliary cast syndrome and techniques of secondary duct repair. Surgery 81:212, 1977.
10. Rolles K, Williams R, Neuberger J, et al. The Cambridge and King's College Hospital experience of liver transplantation, 1968–1983. Hepatology 4:50S, 1984.
11. Starzl TE, Shunzaburo I, Shaw BW, et al. Analysis of liver transplantation. Hepatology 4:47S, 1984.
12. Williams JR, Vera SR, Peters TG, et al. Survival following hepatic transplantation in the cyclosporine era. Am Surg 52:291, 1986.
13. Busuttil RW, Colonna JO, Hiatti JR, et al. The first 100 liver transplants at UCLA. Ann Surg 206:387, 1987.
14. Starzl TE, Iwatsuki S, Shaw BW, et al. Immunosuppression and other nonsurgical factors in the improved results of liver transplantation. Semin Liver Dis 5:334, 1985.
15. Williams R, Calne RY, Rolles K, et al. Current results with orthotopic liver grafting in Cambridge/King's College Hospital series. Br Med J 290:49, 1985.
16. Krom RAF. Liver transplantation at the Mayo Clinic. Mayo Clin Proc 61:278, 1986.
17. Wall WJ, Duff JH, Ghent CN, et al. Liver transplantation: the initial experience of a Canadian Centre. Can J Surg 28:286, 1985.
18. Scharschmidt BF. Human liver transplantation: analysis of data on 540 patients from four centers. Hepatology 4:95S, 1984.
19. Lam KC, Lai CL, Ng RP, et al. Deleterious effect of prednisolone in HBsAg-positive chronic active hepatitis. N Engl J Med 304:380, 1981.
20. A trial group of European Association for the Study of the Liver. Steroids in chronic B-hepatitis. A randomized, double-blind, multinational trial on the effect of low-dose, long-term treatment on survival. Liver 6:227, 1986.
21. Peters MG, Davis GL, Dooley JG, et al. The interferon system in acute and chronic viral hepatitis. In: Popper H, Schaffner F, eds. Progress in Liver Diseases, Vol 8. Orlando, Fla.: Grune & Stratton, 1986:453.
22. Dusheiko G, Di Bisceglie A, Boyer A, et al. Recombinant leukocyte interferon treatment of chronic hepatitis B. Hepatology 5:556, 1985.
23. Hoofnagle JH, Peters MG, Mullen KD, et al. Randomized, controlled trial of a four-month course of human alpha interferon in chronic type B hepatitis. Hepatology 5:1033, 1985. (Abstract.)
24. Perrillo R, Regenstein F, Peters M, et al. Prednisone withdrawal followed by alpha interferon in the treatment of chronic hepatitis B. Hepatology 6:1129, 1986. (Abstract.)
25. Alexander GJM, Brahm J, Fagan EA, et al. Loss of HBsAg with interferon therapy in chronic hepatitis B virus infection. Lancet 1:66, 1987.
26. Demetris AJ, Jaffe R, Sheahan DG, et al. Recurrent hepatitis B in liver allograft recipients: differentiation between viral hepatitis B and rejection. Am J Pathol 125:161, 1986.
27. Pappas SC, Hoofnagle JH, Young N, et al. Treatment of chronic non-A, non-B hepatitis with acyclovir; pilot studies. J Med Virol 15:1, 1985.
28. Hoofnagle JH, Mullen KM, Jones DB, et al. Pilot study of recombinant human alpha interferon in chronic non-A, non-B hepatitis. N Engl J Med 315:1575, 1986.
29. Thomson BJ, Doran M, Lever AMI, et al. Alpha-interferon therapy for non-A, non-B hepatitis transmitted by gammaglobulin replacement therapy. Lancet 1:539, 1987.
30. Nagashina H, Arima T, Suzuki H, et al. Treatment of chronic non-A, non-B hepatitis with human interferon-beta. J Med Virol 21:128A, 1987. (Abstract.)
31. Kirk AP, Jain S, Pocock S, et al. Late results of the Royal Free Hospital prospective controlled trial of prednisolone therapy in hepatitis B surface antigen–negative chronic active hepatitis. Gut 21:78, 1980.
32. Groth CG, Dubois RS, Corman J, et al. Metabolic effects of hepatic replacement in Wilson's disease. Transplant Proc 5:928, 1973.
33. Starzl TE, Iwatsuki S, Van Thiel DH, et al. Evolution of liver transplantation. Hepatology 2:614, 1982.
34. Putnam CW, Porter KA, Peters RL, et al. Liver replacement for alpha-1-antitrypsin deficiency. Surgery 81:258, 1977.
35. Hood JM, Koep LJ, Peters RL, et al. Liver transplantation for advanced liver disease with alpha-1-antitrypsin deficiency. N Engl J Med 302:272, 1980.
36. Barnes HD, Hurworth E, Millar JHD. Erythropoietic porphyrin hepatitis. J Clin Pathol 21:157, 1968.
37. Bloomer JR, Phillips MJ, Davidson DL, et al. Hepatic disease in erythropoietic protoporphyria. Am J Med 58:869, 1975.
38. Lamon JM, Poh-Fitzpatrick MB, Lamola AA, et al. Hepatic protoporphyrin production in human protoporphyria. Effects of intravenous hematin and analysis of erythrocyte protoporphyrin distribution. Gastroenterology 779:115, 1980.
39. Pimstone NR, Webber BL, Blekkenhorst GH, et al. The hepatic lesion in protoporphyria (PP): preliminary studies of haem metabolism, liver structure and ultrastructure. Ann Clin Res 8:122–132, 1976.

40. Pimstone NR. The hepatic aspects of the porphyrias. In: Read AE, ed. Modern Trends in Gastroenterology, Vol. 5. London, Butterworths, 1975:373.

41. Roll J, Boyer JL, Barry D, et al. The prognostic importance of clinical and histologic features in asymptomatic and symptomatic primary biliary cirrhosis. N Engl J Med 308:1, 1983.

42. Kaplan MM. Primary biliary cirrhosis. N Engl J Med 316:521, 1987.

43. Beswick DR, Boyer JL. Primary biliary cirrhosis. Hepatology 4:29S, 1984.

44. Maddrey WC, Van Thiel DH. Liver transplantation: an overview. Hepatology 8:948, 1988.

45. Alagille D. Liver transplantation in children—indications in cholestasis states. Transplant Proc 19:3242, 1987.

46. Alagille D. Extrahepatic biliary atresia. Hepatology 4:7S, 1984.

47. Mitchell MC, Boitnott JK, Kauman S, et al. Budd-Chiari syndrome: etiology, diagnosis and management. Medicine 61:199, 1982.

48. Parker RGF. Occlusion of the hepatic veins in man. Medicine 38:369, 1959.

49. Clain DJ, Freston J, Krell K, et al. Clinical diagnosis of the Budd-Chiari syndrome. Am J Med 43:544, 1967.

50. Tavill AS, Wood EJ, Krell L, et al. The Budd-Chiari syndrome: correlation between hepatic scintigraphy and the clinical, radiological, and pathological findings in nineteen cases of hepatic venous outflow obstruction. Gastroenterology 68:509, 1975.

51. Okuda K, Obata H, Mahakima Y, et al. Prognosis of primary hepatocellular carcinoma. Hepatology 4:3S, 1984.

52. Rolles K, Williams R, Neuberger J, et al. The Cambridge and King's College Hospital experience of liver transplantation, 1968–1983. Hepatology 4:50, 1984.

53. Iwatsuki S, Starzl TE. Liver transplantation in the treatment of liver cancer. New York, Marcel Dekker, Inc., 1986:477.

54. Iwatsuki S, Gordon RD, Shaw BW, et al. Role of liver transplantation in cancer therapy. Ann Surg 202:401, 1985.

55. EASL Study Group. Randomized trial of steroid therapy in acute liver failure. Gut 20:20, 1979.

56. Ring-Larsen H, Palazzo V. Renal failure in fulminant hepatic failure and terminal cirrhosis. Gut 22:585, 1981.

57. Williams R, Gimson AES. An assessment of orthotopic liver transplantation in acute liver failure. Hepatology 4:33S, 1984.

58. Iwatsuki S, Esquivel CO, Gordon RD, et al. Liver transplantation for fulminant hepatic failure. Semin Liver Dis 5:325, 1985.

59. Peleman RR, Gavaler JS, Van Thiel DH, et al. Orthotopic liver transplantation for acute and subacute hepatic failure in adults. Hepatology 7:484, 1987.

60. Burnell JM, Dawborn JK, Epstein RB, et al. Acute hepatic coma treated by cross-circulation or exchange transfusion. N Engl J Med 276:935, 1967.

61. Abouna G, Ameniya H, Fisher L, et al. Hepatic support by intermittent liver perfusion and exchange blood transfusions. Transplant Proc 3:1589, 1971.

62. Gazzard BG, Weston MJ, Murray-Lyon IM, et al. Charcoal hemoperfusion in the treatment of fulminant hepatic failure. Lancet 1:1307, 1974.

63. Shade RR. The changing indications for liver transplantation. Transplant Proc 19:2–6, 1987.

64. Magnus IA, Jarret A, Prankerd TAJ, et al. Erythropoietic protoporphyria: a new porphyria with solar urticaria due to protoporphyrinaemia. Lancet 2:448, 1961.

65. Bloomer JR, Sharp HL. The liver in Crigler-Najjar syndrome, protoporphyria, and other metabolic disorders. Hepatology 4:18S, 1984.

66. Wolkoff AW, Chowdhury JR, Gartner LA, et al. Crigler-Najjar syndrome (type I) in an adult male. Gastroenterology 76:840, 1979.

67. Blaschke TF, Berk PD, Scharschmidt BF, et al. Crigler-Najjar syndrome: an unusual course with development of neurologic damage at age eighteen. Pediatr Res 8:573, 1974.

68. Shaw BW, Gordon RD, Iwatsuki S, et al. Retransplantation of the liver. Semin Liver Dis 5:394, 1985.

69. Esquivel CO, Jaffe R, Gordon RD, et al. Liver rejection and its differentiation from other causes of graft dysfunction. Semin Liver Dis 5:369, 1985.

70. Klintmalm G, Moore AE. Organization of a new liver transplant center. Semin Liver Dis 5:412, 1985.

71. Starzl TE, Iwatsuki S, Esquivel CO, et al. Refinements in the surgical technique of liver transplantation. Semin Liver Dis 5:349, 1985.

72. Starzl TE, Hakala TR, Shaw BW, et al. A flexible procedure for multiple cadaveric organ procurement. Surg Gynecol Obstet 158:223, 1984.

73. Kam I, Lynch S, Svanas G, et al. Evidence that host size determines liver size: studies in dogs receiving orthotopic liver transplants. Hepatology 7:362, 1987.

74. Bismuth H, Samuel D, Gugenheim J, et al. Emergency liver transplantation for fulminant hepatitis. Ann Intern Med 107:337, 1987.

75. Broelsch C, Emond J, Thistlewaite R, et al. Liver transplantation with reduced-size donor organs. Transplantation 45:519, 1988.

76. Griffith BP, Shaw BW, Hardesty RL, et al. Veno-venous bypass without systemic anticoagulation for human liver transplantation. Surg Gynecol Obstet 160:270, 1985.

77. Shaw BW, Martin DJ, Marquez JM, et al. Venous bypass in clinical liver transplantation. Ann Surg 200:524, 1984.

78. Shaw BW. Some further notes on venous bypass for orthotopic transplantation of the liver. Transplant Proc 4:13–16, 1987.

79. Shaw BW, Martin DJ, Marquez JM, et al. Advantages of venous bypass during orthotopic transplantation of the liver. Semin Liver Dis 5:344, 1985.

80. Kost GJ, Jammal MA, Ward RE, et al. Monitoring of ionized calcium during human hepatic transplantation. Am J Clin Pathol 86:61, 1983.

81. Grenvik A, Gordon R. Postoperative care and problems in liver transplantation. Transplant Proc (Suppl. 3) 19:26, 1987.

82. Colonna J, Goldstein L, Brems J, et al. A prospective study on the use of monoclonal anti-T3-cell antibody (OKT3) to treat steroid resistant liver transplant rejection. Arch Surg 122:1120, 1987.

83. Busuttil RW, Goldstein LI, Danovitch GM, et al. Liver transplantation today. Ann Intern Med 104:377, 1986.

84. Ho M, Wajszczuk CP, Hardy A, et al. Infections in kidney, heart and liver transplant recipients on cyclosporine. Transplant Proc 31:62, 1983.

85. Dhein B, Bartell L, Ferguson RM. Infectious complications and lymphomas in cyclosporine patients. Transplant Proc 15:3162, 1983.

86. Betts RF, Hanshaw JB. Cytomegalovirus (CMV) in the compromised host(s). Annu Rev Med 28:1037, 1977.

87. Hirsch MS, Schooley RT. Drug therapy: treatment of herpes virus infections. N Engl J Med 309:1034, 1983.

88. Walsh TJ, Hamilton SR. Disseminated aspergillosis complicating hepatic failure. Arch Intern Med 143:1189, 1983.

89. Ruebner BH, Paul MP, Pimstone N, et al. Histopathology of early and late human allograft rejection. Hepatology 7:203, 1987.

90. Tygstrup N, Ranek L. Assessment of prognosis in fulminant hepatic failure. Semin Liver Dis 6:129, 1986.

91. Neuberger J, Altman DG, Christensen E, et al. Use of a prognostic index in evaluation of liver transplantation for primary biliary cirrhosis. Transplantation 41:713, 1986.

92. Zitelli BJ, Malatack JJ, Gartner JC, et al. Evaluation of the pediatric patient for liver transplantation. Pediatrics 78:559, 1986.

93. Woodle ES, Moody RR, Cox KL, et al. Orthotopic liver transplantation in a patient with Amanita poisoning. JAMA 253:69, 1985.

94. Ludwig J, Wiesner RH, Batts KP, et al. The acute vanishing bile duct syndrome (acute irreversible rejection) after orthotopic liver transplantation. Hepatology 7:476, 1987.

95. Borel JF, Feurer C, Gubler HU, et al. Biological effects of cyclosporin A: a new antilymphocytic agent. Agents Actions 6:468, 1976.

96. Casimi AB, Chos I, Delmonico FL, et al. A randomized clinical trial comparing OKT3 and steroids for treatment of hepatic allograft rejection. Transplantation 43:91, 1987.

97. Ludwig J. New concepts in biliary cirrhosis. Semin Liver Dis 7:293, 1987.

98. Yoo Y, Whiteside TL, Chen K, et al. The effect of human alpha interferon (IFN$_a$) on lymphocyte subpopulations and HLA-DR expression in liver tissue of hepatitis B virus (HBV)–positive subjects. Gastroenterology 94:A607, 1988.

99. Starzl TE, Putnam CW, Hansbrough JR, et al. Biliary complications after liver transplantation: with special reference to the biliary cast syndrome and techniques of secondary duct repair. Surgery 81:212, 1977.

100. Lorber MI, Van Buren CT, Flechner SM, et al. Hepatobiliary and pancreatic complications of cyclosporine therapy in 466 renal transplant recipients. Transplantation 43:35, 1987.

101. Jenkins RL. The Boston Center for Liver Transplantation (BCLT). Arch Surg 121:424, 1986.

102. Snover DC, Freese DK, Sharp HL, et al. Liver allograft rejection: an analysis of the use of biopsy in determining outcome of rejection. Am J Surg Pathol 11:1, 1987.

103. Frei JV. Workshop on the pathology of liver transplantation: a summary. Transplant Proc 18 [Suppl 4]:167, 1986.

104. Russo PA, Yunis EJ. Subcapsular hepatic necrosis in orthotopic liver allografts. Hepatology 6:708, 1986.

105. Demetris AJ, Jaffe R, Sheahan DG, et al. Recurrent hepatitis B in liver allograft recipients: differentiation between viral hepatitis B and rejection. Am J Pathol 125:161, 1986.

106. Ramsey G, Nusbacher J, Starzl TE, et al. Isohemagglutinins of graft origin after ABO-unmatched liver transplantation. N Engl J Med 311:1167, 1984.

107. Scharschmidt BF. Human liver transplantation: an analysis of 819 patients from eight centers. In Thomas HC, Jones EA, eds. Recent Advances in Hepatology. New York, Churchill Livingstone, 1986:175.

108. Van Thiel DH, Tarter R, Gavaler JD, et al. Liver transplantation in

adults. An analysis of costs and benefits at the University of Pittsburgh. Gastroenterology 90:211, 1986.
109. McMahon LF. Costs of liver transplantation: primum non obfuscare. Hepatology 6:1436, 1986.
110. Trey C, Davidson C. The management of fulminant hepatic failure. In: Popper H, Schaffner F, eds. Progress in Liver Disease, Vol 3. New York, Grune & Stratton, 1970:282–298.
111. O'Grady JG, Gimson AES, O'Brien CJ, et al. Controlled trials of charcoal hemoperfusion and prognostic factors in fulminant hepatic failure. Gastroenterology 94:1186, 1988.
112. Brems JJ, Hiatt JR, Ramming KP, et al. Fulminant hepatic failure: the role of liver transplantation as primary therapy. Am J Surg 205:415, 1987.
113. Williams JW, Vera SR, Peters TG, et al. Prediction of complications and costs of hepatic transplantation. Hepatology 5:1040.
114. Bismuth H, Castaing D, Ericzon BG, et al. Hepatic transplantation in Europe. Lancet 674, 1987.
115. Wall WJ, Duff JH, Ghent CN, et al. Liver transplantation: the initial experience of a Canadian Centre. Can J Surg 28:286, 1985.
116. Adams DH, Kirley RM, McMaster P, et al. Fulminant hepatic failure treated by hepatic transplantation. Lancet 2:1037, 1986.
117. Sokol RJ, Francis PD, Gold SH, et al. Orthotopic liver transplantation for acute fulminant Wilson's disease. J Pediatr 107:549, 1985.
118. Rizzetto M, Macagno S, Chiaberge E, et al. Liver transplantation in hepatitis delta virus disease. Lancet 469, 1987.
119. Ringe B, Pichlmayr R, Lauchart W, et al. Indications and results for fulminant hepatitis. Transplant Proc 18:86, 1986.
120. Van Thiel DH. Liver transplantation. Pediatr Ann 14:475, 1985.
121. O'Grady JG, Williams R. Transplantation in fulminant hepatic failure. Lancet 2:1227, 1986.
122. Rokela J, Kurtz SB, Ascher NL, et al. Fulminant Wilson's disease treated with postdilution hemofiltration and orthotopic liver transplantation. Gastroenterology 90:2004, 1986.
123. Bismuth H, Samuel D, Gugenheim J, et al. Emergency liver transplantation for fulminant hepatitis. Ann Intern Med 107:337, 1987.
124. Polson RJ, Rolles K, Calne RY, et al. Reversal of severe neurological manifestations of Wilson's disease following orthotopic liver transplantation. Q J Medicine 244:685, 1987.
125. Van Furth R, Kramps JA, Van der Putten ABMM, et al. Change in α_1-antitrypsin phenotype after orthotopic liver transplant. Clin Exp Immunol 66:669, 1986.
126. Starzl TE, Todo S, Gordon R, et al. Liver transplantation in older patients. N Engl J Med 316:484, 1987.
127. Adams DH, Ponsford S, Gunson B, et al. Neurological complications following liver transplantation. Lancet 949:951, 1987.
128. De Groon PC, Aksamit AJ, Rakela J, et al. Central nervous system toxicity after liver transplantation. N Engl J Med 317:861, 1987.
129. Donaldson PT, Alexander GJM, O'Grady J, et al. Evidence for an immune response to HLA class I antigens in the vanishing–bile duct syndrome after liver transplantation. Lancet 8:945, 1987.
130. Cosimi AB, Burton RC, Colvin RB, et al. Treatment of acute renal allograft rejection with OKT3 monoclonal antibody. Transplantation 32:535, 1981.
131. Fung JJ, Demetris AJ, Porter KA, et al. Use of OKT3 with cyclosporin and steroids for reversal of acute kidney and liver allograft rejection. Nephron 46:19, 1987.
132. Iwasaki Y, Starzl TE, Makowka L, et al. FK-506, a potential breakthrough in immunosuppression. Transplant Proc 10:19, 1987.
133. Luebs HW. Cost considerations. Semin Liver Dis 5:402, 1985.

56

Liver Trauma

James H. Foster, M.D.

INTRODUCTION

The liver is a large, blood-filled, soft, friable, and partially fixed organ that takes up much of the center of the trunk. Although protected by overlying ribs, its central location makes it particularly vulnerable to homicidal attacks and to compression by steering wheels. Two sets of inflow vessels (hepatic artery and portal vein) and two sets of outflow vessels (hepatic veins and bile ducts) take up much of the volume of the liver. The walls of these vessels are delicate and fragile as they pass through liver parenchyma. Liver injury, which is common throughout the United States, is more likely to be due to penetrating knife and gunshot wounds than to blunt traumas in our central cities; however, in the suburbs and more rural areas, blunt trauma from automobile injuries or athletic accidents is the usual cause of injury. Most liver injuries occur in young people without other major illnesses. This is fortunate indeed, because survival depends at least as much on normal hemostatic mechanisms and the ability to heal a wound as it does on adequate medical care. However, every hospital that cares for trauma patients must be prepared to deal with major liver injuries because massive hemorrhage will not wait for transfer.

This chapter deals only briefly with iatrogenic liver trauma, including that produced by closed chest massage. Transhepatic cholangiography, needle biopsy, selective angiography, and operative liver retraction during procedures for extrahepatic disease may produce life-threatening complications including bile leak, hemorrhage, subcapsular hematoma, arteriovenous or arteriobiliary fistulae, and even delayed rupture. These complications are also discussed elsewhere in this volume, and the reader is referred to those chapters for more thorough coverage.

There are no longer many major controversies among surgeons who work at trauma centers that handle liver injuries frequently. The arguments about diagnostic tests, caval shunts, hepatic artery ligation, major resection, packing, and nonoperative management, which raged in the last decade or two, have largely been resolved by the lessons of increasing experience matured by careful analysis of data from several centers. The contributions from Detroit Receiving Hospital,[1] Bellevue Hospital Center,[2] Ben Taub Hospital,[3] Parkland Hospital,[4] Denver General Hospital,[5] Charity Hospital,[6] and Sydney, Australia,[7] have been particularly useful. Walt's recent review of this subject is encyclopedic.[8] The middle ground seems to have won out over the advocates of either extreme as these important issues have been resolved.

The immediate risk of patients with liver trauma is hemorrhage. Bile leakage, devitalized tissue, and sepsis threaten at a later time. Delayed rupture and hemobilia, although very rare, may occur weeks after injury.[9] Metabolic failure after liver trauma is seldom seen unless the liver has been devascularized or unless there was a pre-existing diffuse liver disease.

Overall mortality has changed very little and remains about 10 to 15 per cent. Table 56–1 summarizes mortality rates from different mechanisms of injury. Half of the deaths are due to associated injuries, often intracranial. Bleeding in most patients with liver injuries stops spontaneously; when this does not occur, sophisticated and rapid judgments about operative care are needed. About half of the patients who make it to major trauma centers, and who eventually die of their liver injury, die in the operating room of uncontrolled hemorrhage—a dramatic testimony to the fact that the difficulties of vascular repair in this vascular and friable organ tax the technical skills of even the most experienced trauma surgeons. Thus, efficiency in diagnosis and proficiency in liver surgery and vascular control are critical in these desperate circumstances, which fortunately involve less than 10 per cent of patients with liver injury.

We shall consider diagnosis and resuscitation together because these two measures are usually carried out simultaneously. Care of the unusual patient with more severe problems will be emphasized.

DIAGNOSIS AND RESUSCITATION

The priorities of management of a trauma patient have been inscribed in stone, and rightly so. Only after an adequate airway and sufficient respiration have been ensured should one look for signs of liver injury. A penetrating wound of the central trunk usually is obvious; however, when signs of hypovolemia are present without obvious external blood loss or skin penetration, one should look very carefully for minor bruises or for tenderness over the lower ribs and upper abdomen. Rapid deceleration behind a steering wheel or any other mechanism for crushing the sternum and lower rib cage against the vertebral column (including closed chest massage) may produce compression and laceration of the center of the liver or shearing injury to the junction of the fixed portion of the liver (inferior vena cava) and the mobile portion. Hypovolemia requires resuscitation before further diagnostic steps. If rapid volume replacement fails to restore stability and no cause other than abdominal bleeding is obvious, or if signs point obviously to an upper abdominal injury, the patient needs an emergency operation. If questions remain, peritoneal lavage usually will resolve them. Patients with shotgun blasts and high-velocity gunshot wounds in the vicinity of the liver almost always need exploration, even if hemodynamically stable. If a patient with blunt trauma is hemodynamically stable, evaluation of the rest of the body should be carried out expeditiously and priorities assigned. Only hemorrhage is an immediate risk to life following liver injury. The diagnosis of continuing hemorrhage depends upon signs of hypovolemia. For management decisions, localization of the source of hemorrhage (if no external bleeding is obvious) needs only an answer to the question, "Is it retroperitoneal, intraperitoneal, or thoracic?"

Rapid deterioration after a period of apparent stability is not uncommon. Restoration of normal volume and central venous pressure may restart venous hemorrhage, vasospasm may relax, or platelet plugs may come undone if not supported and reinforced by solid fibrin clot. Although many concerns are raised about delayed rupture (i.e., significant bleeding occurring several days after injury), it is quite rare in my own experience and in reports by those with much larger experience.

The patient with massive hemorrhage needs immediate laparotomy. The patient with persistent hypovolemia of undetermined source needs diagnostic peritoneal lavage. But what does the stable patient with historic or physical evidence suggesting possible liver injury need in the way of a diagnostic work-up? Radionuclide scans (^{99m}technetium pertechnetate) have been much used in the past for both spleen and liver injuries, and angiography continues to have advocates in this setting. Neither of these techniques, however, has proved to be as valuable as ultrasonography and/or computed tomography (CT). If available, a CT scan will detect most significant liver injuries, collections of blood or other fluid in the peritoneal cavity, and injuries to adjacent structures such as the pancreas, spleen, and kidney.[21] Ultrasonography is perhaps almost as effective in diagnosing subcapsular hematoma or major liver laceration and often will provide a cheaper and equally effective way to follow the evolution of a liver lesion discovered by either sonography or CT.

With the availability of ultrasound and CT, liver trauma is being diagnosed more often, and abnormal images have been found in many patients without clinical signs of liver injury. A few years ago, operation was recommended for all patients with subcapsular or central hematomas or other major radiographic abnormalities,[10] but additional experience has led to more confidence in a nonoperative approach in some asymptomatic patients. Hematomas in patients without clinical signs are seldom of clinical significance. Then why look for them in the absence of clinical signs of hepatic injury? A case for not looking can be made, particularly in this age of cost-consciousness; but perhaps a stronger case can be made for a diagnostic evaluation. Thus, appreciation of a liver injury should

TABLE 56–1. MORTALITY OF LIVER INJURIES IN 1974–1976 AND 1980–1983 (WAYNE STATE UNIVERSITY)*

Agent	(1974–1976)		(1980–1983)	
	No. of Patients	Deaths	No. of Patients	Deaths
Gunshot wound	186	28 (15.1%)	87	8 (9%)
Stabs	91	1 (1.1%)	80	4 (5%)
Blunt	40	8 (20.0%)	17	5 (29%)
Shotgun	13	3 (23.1%)	3	1 (33%)
Iatrogenic	1	0	1	0
Total	331	40 (12.1%)	188	18 (9.6%)

Source: Reproduced from Walt AJ: Liver Injuries. In: Bengmark S, Blungart LH, eds. Liver Surgery. London, Churchill Livingstone, 1986:130, with permission.

*Note: Mortality in 1961–1968 was 10.5% (46/436); in 1969–1973 it was 14.6% (93/637).

prompt closer observation, longer hospitalization, serial imaging, and restricted post-hospital activity.

Should a patient with a large but non-expanding subcapsular hematoma of the liver stay in bed, and if so, for how long? When can this patient play football again? No general answers that will apply to all cases can be given, but the "natural history" of a subcapsular hematoma is less dangerous than we supposed a decade ago.[17, 18] Expansion with or without rupture usually occurs, if at all, soon after injury. It is difficult for this author to see how bed rest will splint the injury when every breath moves the liver up and down several centimeters. Activities that increase central venous pressure should probably be proscribed for seven to ten days, and violent physical activity for several weeks, but these recommendations are based on what seems reasonable and not scientific evidence.

Few laboratory tests affect management decisions for patients with liver trauma. An initial hematocrit level, if high, should not be reassuring in the face of signs of hypovolemia, and a low initial hematocrit level probably relates to resuscitation rather than to the degree of injury. However, serial hematocrit determinations may be useful in following a patient with suspected or documented injury. Coagulation abnormalities that would contraindicate elective operation should not deter an attempt to control massive hemorrhage by laparotomy after trauma. Various enzyme tests may or may not be abnormal and may reflect soft tissue injury other than that to liver, but they seldom contribute to a decision about operation.

Peritoneal lavage should *not* be done in many patients with liver injury and probably has been overused as a result of the very commendable campaign by the American College of Surgeons to establish protocols for patients with major injury. When a patient has obvious signs of continuing intra-abdominal hemorrhage, further confirmation is not needed before operation. Patients with multiple injuries who have no signs of vascular instability often have been subjected to unnecessary laparotomy because of positive peritoneal lavage findings. Volume replacement is often pushed when lavage is positive and may be detrimental to a patient with an intracranial injury. A patient with active intra-abdominal bleeding needs laparotomy, whereas a patient with intraperitoneal blood may not. It is common to find no active bleeding at the time of operation even after a positive tap has led to laparotomy. Peritoneal lavage, however, may be of critical importance in the unconscious patient and in the patient with signs of hypovolemia without an obvious source of bleeding.

Resuscitation of patients with liver injury initially means volume replacement. Balanced electrolyte solutions should be used with close monitoring of blood pressure, pulse, and urine output. Blood (preferably fresh whole blood), should be given as soon as possible if more than 2 liters of crystalloid are needed to restore vital signs to an acceptable range. Fresh frozen plasma should accompany packed red blood cells if more than a few units are necessary.

There is a delicate balance between the benefits of a delay to allow resuscitation and a safer operation and the adverse consequences of such a delay, which might allow further deterioration of the patient. In general, continued or worsening signs of hypovolemia after 2 to 3 liters of rapid infusion of crystalloid indicate that operation should be done immediately. In most such instances, it is better to attempt resuscitation in the operating room than in the emergency room. Many have advocated emergency room thoracotomy with placement of a clamp across the descend-

ing aorta in these desperate situations.[22, 23] Although the suggestion is reasonable, the results of such attempts have been dismal.

OPERATIVE MANAGEMENT

The gradual evolution of principles of operative management for patients with liver trauma has confirmed the wisdom of some of the lessons of World War II and the Korean conflict, so well summarized by Madding and Kennedy.[10] Operative management depends on a thorough knowledge of anatomy and considerable experience in applying this knowledge. Textbooks show the hepatic veins clearly, but often they are hard to find within the liver. This chapter will not stress anatomic detail or operative technique but will attempt to summarize current thinking about various options.

Table 56–2 shows the distribution of severity of injury at laparotomy. Fortunately, in most cases only simple techniques are needed to secure hemostasis and drainage. For more difficult problems, one could generalize by saying that the use of mattress sutures, major resection, intracaval shunting devices, and hepatic artery ligation has decreased in recent years,[5, 11, 12] whereas such "old-fashioned" measures as direct suture control of bleeding vessels, inflow occlusion, and even packing have made a comeback.[5, 13–15] An important principle of operative management cannot be restated too strongly: when the abdomen is open, hemorrhage must be arrested immediately. Attempts at definitive control must be delayed until the patient has been resuscitated, blood volume has been restored, and sufficient exposure and technical assistance are at hand. Transient control of a posterior venous injury is afforded by tamponading the liver up against the diaphragm and vertebral column. Hilar clamping and/or packing will slow or stop most other types of bleeding. Peeking or pecking is contraindicated until the patient is hemodynamically stable.

The source of bleeding from a deep laceration or a stellate fracture can be difficult to visualize. Superficial closure of such fractures often results in the formation of central hematomas, continued bleeding, and late complications such as abscess or hematobilia (hemobilia). Mattress sutures decrease hemorrhage but leave devitalized tissue and pose risk of injury to vital ducts and vessels. As we have learned the techniques of elective liver resection, we have gained confidence in our ability to enlarge a laceration

TABLE 56–2. METHODS OF TREATMENT OF LIVER INJURIES IN 1968–1976 AND 1980–1983 (WAYNE STATE UNIVERSITY)

Procedure	1968–1976 No. of Patients	1980–1983 No. of Patients
Laparotomy alone	492 (50.8%)	123 (67.5%)
Suture	367 (37.9%)	40 (21.3%)
Debridement	46 (4.8%)	5 (2.7%)
Hemihepatectomy	25 (2.6%)	5 (2.7%)
Hepatic artery ligation	14 (1.4%)	3 (1.6%)
Inferior vena cava cannulation	8 (0.8%)	2 (1.0%)
Packs	3 (0.3%)	6 (3.2%)
Death at operation or details unavailable	13 (1.4%)	4 (2.1%)
Total	968 (100%)	188 (100%)

Source: Reproduced from Walt AJ: Liver Injuries. In: Bengmark S, Blungart LH, eds. Liver Surgery. London, Churchill Livingstone, 1986:130, with permission.

by blunt technique to allow direct control of bleeding vessels. Experience shows that inflow occlusion (the Pringle maneuver) for periods of up to 60 minutes may be tolerated better than frequent declamping and reclamping every 10 to 15 minutes.[2] Whether hypothermia (by cooling the splanchnic viscera) or steroids protect against anoxic injury under these circumstances remains unproven.

Posterior tears of the major veins may not be obvious until the lobe is lifted up at exploration, when rapid loss of enormous amounts of blood may occur. The liver in this case must be replaced rapidly and tamponaded while proximal and distal control of the inferior vena cava is secured. This can be done through an abdominal incision in most children and in some adults by incising the diaphragm into the pericardium anterior to the caval hiatus; however, in adults, thoracic extension of the incision (usually by median sternotomy) is usually required. The Heaney maneuver (clamping of the aorta below the diaphragm) is no longer used by most experts in liver trauma, even in these desperate circumstances.

Resection of parenchyma for trauma is now largely limited to two circumstances. First, when fragments of liver are clearly devitalized, they should be debrided, usually by finger fracture technique. Most of the torn vessels will have stopped bleeding before the surgeon gets there, and it will be necessary to clamp only a few vessels. The second circumstance occurs when lobectomy (usually right lobectomy) is required to gain control of bleeding from the junction of the inferior vena cava and the major hepatic veins. Rapid blunt transection of the central plane has proved to be of more use than intracaval shunts in this most lethal of liver injuries.[11]

Hepatic artery ligation may be useful occasionally but will not stop bleeding from portal or hepatic veins. Most arterial bleeding will stop spontaneously, and much of the rest can be handled by direct control of the bleeding vessel. In the rare instance of continued definite arterial bleeding, whenever the hilar clamp is removed and direct control is not possible, the hilar branch should be tied as distally as possible. The risk of ischemic necrosis is small in patients with an uninjured portal venous system and in those in whom shock is transient.[8]

Packing seldom will be necessary at an experienced center, but it may be life-saving. Perihepatic compression, usually by mutiple laparotomy pads, will tamponade liver surfaces together to control hemorrhage long enough to allow correction of a coagulopathy or transfer to another hospital.[13–15] The packing should not be placed within a laceration or posteriorly to control major venous hemorrhage and should be removed in the operating room within 48 hours after placement to reduce the possibility of sepsis. The omentum can be used as a "plug" for an oozing laceration. At the end of a difficult repair, perhaps necessitating many units of transfused blood, diffuse oozing representative of a clotting abnormality may occur. It is sometimes the better part of wisdom to oppose raw liver surfaces either to omentum or other adjacent viscera and to close the abdomen than to persist in efforts to achieve absolute hemostasis.

The multiple soft drains advocated in the past have largely been replaced by closed suction drains. Routine biliary drainage has been shown to be unhelpful and perhaps harmful.[24] It is now used only to protect a biliary suture line.

POSTOPERATIVE PROBLEMS

The profound metabolic problems described by the pioneers after elective liver operation (injury) correlate better with the hypotension, hypothermia, multiple transfusions, and other challenges of major hemorrhage than with the liver injury itself. The liver quickly regains its metabolic capabilities if injury does not continue (e.g., sepsis, adult respiratory distress syndrome, devitalized tissue). Jaundice more often is caused by the excessive prehepatic load of multiple transfusions than by hepatocellular dysfunction. In this case, it should clear rapidly. Persistent hyperbilirubinemia means bile duct injury until proved otherwise. (The general problem of postoperative cholestasis is discussed in Chapter 34.) Serum albumin often drops dramatically after major liver resection, probably as a result of excessive loss from raw surfaces, but quickly returns toward normal without exogenous replacement in most patients.

Bile leakage often is seen and can be directed to the outside by proper placement of suction drains. It usually stops within a few days if there is no distal obstruction of the ducts. Persistent fistula means distal blockage or sequestration of a viable portion of liver. With adequate drainage, investigation of these possibilities can and should be delayed.

Localized sepsis usually is a sequela of devitalized tissue or fluid collection. Operative technique can reduce its incidence, and placement of percutaneous catheters under radiologic control can often reduce the morbidity of an established abscess.

NONOPERATIVE MANAGEMENT

In the past, the demonstration or even suspicion of liver injury prompted emergency laparotomy. As experience accumulated, it became apparent that bleeding often had stopped before the surgeon entered the abdomen, and that little was accomplished by operation except to rule out more severe injury. As our interest in splenic salvage has increased (secondary to improved knowledge of the spleen's immunologic function), more traumatized spleens are left in place, with or without laparotomy. The predicted dire consequences of this approach have not occurred. A selective approach analogous to that for patients with demonstrated splenic injury has evolved for stable patients with liver injuries, particularly in children.

A decade ago, surgical exploration was mandatory for all patients with penetrating wounds of the liver. More recently, patients with knife wounds and certain low-velocity bullet wounds have been treated selectively,[16] although there are those who continue to doubt the wisdom of this policy.

After blunt injury, in the patient with significant bleeding from a liver laceration, there are usually sufficient findings on physical examination to prompt exploration. In contrast, many patients with subscapular hematomas, even when the lesion is huge, may have no complaints or positive physical signs. Occult liver injuries usually are detected by radiologic imaging done because of a history of trauma that suggests upper abdominal injury or because of a decreasing hematocrit level.[21] Ultrasonography and CT (Fig. 56–1) have replaced nuclide scintigraphy in most institutions because they provide more accurate information. Ultrasound is particularly useful in serial examinations.

The key to nonoperative management of a patient with a liver injury is close observation. Clinical signs rather than radiologic findings should determine a change in treatment. Two other factors have also contributed to a trend toward nonoperative management in the stable patient. First, we

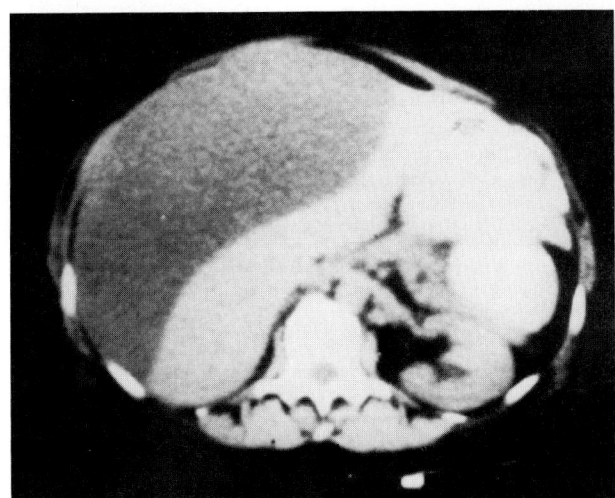

Figure 56–1. Computed tomography (CT) scan of the liver showing a large hematoma. The scan was made four days after blunt trauma suffered by a 35-year-old woman. She had no abdominal symptoms and recovered uneventfully from multiple extremity fractures without abdominal complaints. Four weeks later, CT showed marked reduction in the size of the hematoma.

have more reported experience with the method, and both early and late results suggest a natural history more benign than might have been predicted.[17, 18] Second, when operation is undertaken for subcapsular hematoma, what should the surgeon do? Should he leave undisturbed a stable lesion? Should he risk major hemorrhage by opening the capsule to attempt specific vascular control? Will he introduce contamination into a previously sterile field? These questions remain unanswered, but they correctly imply that there are risks as well as benefits in exploration.

The consequences of missing a major venous injury may be lethal. Exsanguination may occur quickly when volume is restored. Nevertheless, the operative mortality rate for repair of these lesions remains very high. If a nonoperative approach is chosen, one must prepare for the worst eventuality. Sufficient blood for transfusion must be at hand, and monitoring must be frequent and thorough. How long should this vigil continue? Again, no definite answer can be given, but experience suggests that most trouble will occur in the first 48 to 72 hours after injury.

If clinical signs of recurrent hemorrhage occur, there are those who would advocate arteriography and embolization.[25] I have no personal experience with this and would be hesitant to recommend it until more experience accumulates.

LIVER TRAUMA IN CHILDREN

The trend to nonoperative management has been led by surgeons caring for children. The experience in Cincinnati is representative.[19] Of 53 patients with liver injury, 4 had emergency laparotomy for exsanguinating bleeding; 2 of these patients died from hepatic vein injuries, and 2 survived right lobectomy. The other 49 patients were not operated upon acutely, and only 4 developed complications. One patient had hemobilia, which resolved without operation. Three patients required late debridement, drainage, and/or repair. No unoperated patient developed late hemorrhage or sepsis, and 51 patients survived without problems related to their liver injury. The authors appropriately credit these results to modern radiologic imaging and careful monitoring.

When a child is operated on, the serious lesions are more likely to be hepatic vein/inferior vena caval tears.[20] Their management is less likely to require thoracic extension of the incision. Both of these situations are probably related to the markedly increased mobility of the liver and the flexibility of the rib cage in children.

IATROGENIC INJURY

Liver laceration due to closed chest massage is probably more common than we realize and, if circumstances allow, should be managed using the same guidelines and principles as other types of liver injury. The unusual circumstances of fatty or cirrhotic liver in an alcoholic patient who suffers arrest due to exsanguinating upper gastrointestinal hemorrhage has compounded the problem of liver repair in more than one instance in this author's experience.

Bile leakage after needle puncture necessitates biliary decompression if there is any element of obstruction. Without obstruction, most cases will resolve quickly. Significant intraperitoneal hemorrhage after diagnostic needle biopsy should rarely occur if the indications and contraindications for biopsy are observed carefully. Needle biopsy should not be performed on lesions known to be hypervascular (e.g., hemangioma, focal nodular hyperplasia, liver cell adenoma, some primary cancers) unless the biopsy findings critically alter a major management decision. Hemangiomas can be diagnosed by ultrasonography, CT, angiography, or tagged red blood cell scans sufficiently accurately to allow observation without biopsy confirmation. More tissue than can be provided by a needle is necessary for histologic diagnosis of liver cell adenoma and focal nodular hyperplasia, and the geography of a tumor and the condition of the nontumorous liver may contribute more to a decision about tumor resection than does tumor histology in many patients.

If hemorrhage occurs after needle biopsy in a patient without a coagulation abnormality, operative correction should be undertaken if more than two or three units of blood are required or if the patient is exsanguinating. Coagulopathies should be corrected if possible before laparotomy.

Operative trauma to the liver usually occurs because of too vigorous retraction or capsular avulsion while the surgeon is dissecting adhesions from old disease or previous operation. Although initial bleeding may be alarming, a few moments of gentle compression will solve most of these problems—illustrating again the enormous hemostatic ability of the raw liver surface in an otherwise healthy patient.

CONCLUSIONS

Liver trauma is common, and the principles of its management should be known by most physicians and surgeons. Blunt trauma predominates in suburban and rural areas, whereas penetrating trauma is most common in our inner cities.

The management of a patient with liver trauma requires critical judgment based largely on clinical factors. Modern imaging has allowed a greater appreciation of the nature and extent of blunt injuries and, together with increasing experience, has allowed a selective approach to operative correction. Although a patient with major liver injury can tax the facilities and faculties of the most modern hospital, the tools and principles needed to treat the patient are relatively simple and straightforward.

REFERENCES

1. Walt AJ. Liver injuries. In: Bengmark S, Blumgart LH, eds. Liver Surgery. London, Churchill Livingstone, 1986:130.
2. Pachter HL, Spencer FC, Hofstetter SR, et al. Experience with the finger-fracture technique to achieve intrahepatic hemostasis in seventy-five patients with severe liver injuries. Ann Surg 197:771, 1983.
3. Feliciano DV, Jordan GL, Bitondo CG, et al. Management of 1000 consecutive cases of hepatic trauma (1979–1984). Ann Surg 204:438, 1986.
4. Trunkey DD, Shires GT, McClelland R. Management of liver trauma in 811 consecutive patients. Ann Surg 179:722, 1974.
5. Moore FA, Moore EE, Seagraves A. Nonresectional management of major hepatic trauma. An evolving concept. Am J Surg 150:725, 1985.
6. Levin A, Gover P, Nance FC, et al. Surgical restraint in the management of hepatic injury: a review of Charity Hospital experience. J Trauma 18:399, 1978.
7. Little JM, Fleischer G. Liver injuries in Sydney: a 20-year experience. Aust NZ J Surg 50:495, 1980.
8. Walt AJ. Trauma to the liver. In: Moody FG, Carey LC, Jones RS, et al., eds. Surgical Treatment of Digestive Disease. Chicago, Year Book Medical Publishers, 1986:397.
9. Sandbloom P, Saegesser F, Mirkovitch V. Hepatic hemobilia: hemorrhage from the intrahepatic biliary tract. A review. World J Surg 8:41, 1984.
10. Madding GF, Kennedy PA. Trauma to the Liver, 2nd ed. Philadelphia, WB Saunders, 1971.
11. Pachter HL, Spencer FC, Hofstetter SR, et al. The management of juxta-hepatic venous injuries without an atriocaval shunt: preliminary clinical observations. Surgery 99:569, 1986.
12. Flint LM, Polk HC. Selective hepatic artery ligation: limitations and failures. J Trauma 19:319, 1979.
13. Calne RY, McMaster P, Pentlow BD. The treatment of major liver trauma by primary packing with transfer of the patient for definitive treatment. Br J Surg 66:338, 1979.
14. Feliciano DV, Mattox KL, Jordan GL Jr. Intra-abdominal packing for control of hepatic hemorrhage, a reappraisal. J Trauma 21:285, 1981.
15. Svoboda JA, Peter ET, Dang CF, et al. Severe liver trauma in the face of coagulopathy: the case for temporary packing and early re-exploration. Am J Surg 144:717, 1982.
16. Demetriades D, Rabinowitz B, Sofianos C. Non-operative management of penetrating liver injuries: a prospective study. Br J Surg 73:736, 1986.
17. Lambeth W, Rubin BE. Nonoperative management of intrahepatic hemorrhage and hematoma following blunt trauma. Surg Gynecol Obstet 148:507, 1979.
18. Cheatham JE Jr, Smith EI, Tunell WP, et al. Nonoperative management of subcapsular hematomas of the liver. Am J Surg 140:852, 1980.
19. Oldham KT, Guice KS, Ryckman F, et al. Blunt liver injury in childhood: evolution of therapy and current perspective. Surgery 100:542, 1986.
20. Coln D, Crighton J, Schorn L. Successful management of hepatic vein injury from blunt trauma in children. Am J Surg 140:858, 1980.
21. Moon KL, Federle MP. Computed tomography in hepatic trauma. Am J Roentgenol 141:309, 1983.
22. Ledgerwood AM, Kazmers M, Lucas CE, et al. The role of thoracic aortic occlusion for massive hemoperitoneum. J Trauma 16:610, 1976.
23. Cogbill TH, Moore EE, Millikan JS, et al. Rationale for selective application of emergency department thoracotomy in trauma. J Trauma 23:453, 1983.
24. Lucas CE, Walt AJ. Analysis of randomized biliary drainage for liver trauma in 189 patients. J Trauma 12:925, 1922.
25. Rubin RE, Katzan BT. Selective hepatic artery embolization to control massive hepatic hemorrhage after trauma. Am J Roentgenol 129:253, 1977.

IV G.   Diseases of the Biliary Tree

57

Pathogenesis and Dissolution of Gallstones

Douglas M. Heuman, M.D. • *Edward W. Moore, M.D.*
Z. Reno Vlahcevic, M.D.

DEFINITIONS

CDCA = chenodeoxycholic acid
UDCA = ursodeoxycholic acid
MTBE = methyl tert-butyl ether
kd = kilodalton
HMG CoA reductase =
   3-hydroxy-3-methylglutaryl coenzyme A reductase

INTRODUCTION

Gallstones represent a failure to maintain certain biliary solutes, principally cholesterol and calcium salts, in a solubilized state or, as Walter Cannon[1] might have put it, a failure to maintain the "homeostasis" of bile.[2] In the past decade, an explosion of new information has produced a radical departure from previous concepts and beliefs. Indeed, the pendulum has swung almost 180 degrees from its position just 15 years ago.

The modern age of gallstone research, which we will call the "thermodynamic age," began with the now-classic studies of Small and colleagues,[3–7] which placed cholesterol solubility on a seemingly firm physicochemical footing. Phase diagrams were created, later revised by Carey and Small[8] and tabulated by Carey,[9] that quantitatively described cholesterol solubility in micellar systems containing bile salts, phospholipid, and cholesterol. This work was a great stimulus to gallstone research and provided a physicochemical basis for the use of oral bile salts as bile desaturating agents for treatment of cholesterol stones. In

This work was supported by the Veterans Administration, by NIH grants AM 07417, AM 18887, DK 32130, DK 39913, and DK 38030 and by a grant from the A. D. Williams Foundation.

this phase of the understanding of gallstone disease, it was widely believed that the insights derived from the thermodynamic approach would eventually lead to a solution of the gallstone problem.

In the subsequent decade it was generally held that gallstones result primarily from defects in hepatic secretion of biliary lipids (i.e., that gallstones are primarily a "liver disease"). Thus, in 1974, Swell et al.[10] wrote: ". . . it has now become quite clear that the gallbladder per se is not responsible for the formation of stones . . . . The mounting evidence indicates that cholelithiasis may be yet another liver disease characterized by a defect in the mechanism synthesizing and/or transporting the biliary lipids." This view largely ignored the fact that most gallstones form in the gallbladder. Indeed, one of the most striking features of gallstones is their propensity to form in the gallbladder, as opposed to the hepatic or common ducts. This, in itself, suggests that the gallbladder may play an important role in gallstone formation. In the 1980s it has become increasingly clear that this is indeed the case; alterations in gallbladder mucosal and motor function are now key areas of gallstone research.

This is not to say that the role of the liver in the production of cholesterol stones is of minor importance; rather, it means that the problem is far more complicated than previously appreciated. Thus, for cholesterol stones, the production of bile supersaturated with cholesterol and subsequent precipitation of cholesterol from solution involve multiple factors[11-16] that are incompletely understood.[8, 17, 18] From thermodynamic (phase diagram) considerations alone it is not possible to predict who will or will not develop gallstones. On one side of the coin, bile supersaturated with cholesterol is common in subjects without stones,[8, 19-22] whereas on the other, crystals of cholesterol monohydrate have been observed in sludge-containing bile samples[23] and in model solutions of bile[24] with cholesterol saturation indices of less than one. The problem is not simply one of proper calculation of saturation indices. It has required a fresh reappraisal of the entire problem of cholesterol supersaturation and nucleation in bile.

In order for cholesterol nucleation and crystal growth to occur, bile must be supersaturated with cholesterol. But supersaturated where? Evidence from animal models indicates that cholesterol nucleation occurs in the mucus gel that overlies the gallbladder epithelium. The conditions in this phase may be quite different from those in the bulk phase of bile, from which saturation indices are calculated. At present, information on the microenvironment in the mucus gel is insufficient to permit quantitative assessment of these differences. We do know that gels tend to lower the activation energies needed for nucleation[25] and have other properties that may favor nucleation.[18, 26] In addition, there is now convincing evidence that cholesterol nucleation occurs by, or results from, the aggregation of phospholipid-cholesterol vesicles. The importance of nonmicellar transporters of cholesterol in bile has been recognized only recently; the partitioning of cholesterol between micelles and vesicles is a dynamic and complex process.[17, 27, 28] Therefore, calculation of cholesterol saturation in bile from data obtained in micellar systems alone does not, and probably cannot, provide an accurate assessment of the true solubility of cholesterol at the locus of nucleation.

It is not possible, in this brief space, to give a comprehensive survey of all facets of gallstone pathogenesis. The problems encompass a wide range of knowledge, from intracellular biochemical/biophysical processes and mem-

brane transport to geologic processes and marine biology. The study of gallstone pathogenesis involves the physical chemistry of solutions, gels, and surfaces. Bile, a multiphase system and the "mother liquor" of gallstones, is surely one of the most complex fluids in all biology. We will concentrate therefore on those areas that have received the greatest attention in the past decade and that hold promise of eventually leading to an understanding of gallstone pathogenesis.

An overview of the pathogenesis of gallstones is depicted in the Venn diagram shown in Figure 57–1. We suggest that all factors in gallstone pathogenesis can be discussed in terms of three general categories: (1) *thermodynamics,* (2) *kinetics,* and (3) *time.* While each circle in the diagram could be subdivided into several others, the simplicity of the illustration serves to focus our attention on these three distinct principles:

1. Thermodynamics: Unless a solution is saturated with some solute, the formation of crystalline precipitates is thermodynamically impossible. In bile the thermodynamic areas of primary concern are the *solubility of cholesterol and calcium salts.* Since the solubilities of cholesterol and calcium involve different factors, they will be considered separately.

2. Kinetics: The fact that an event *can* occur does not mean that it *will* occur. Many events that are thermodynamically favored occur at negligible rates. With regard to gallstone formation, the kinetic factors of concern are *nucleation* and *crystal growth.* In this global category we include all nucleating and anti-nucleating factors in bile for both cholesterol and calcium. At present, it is not known whether these factors are different for cholesterol and calcium.

3. Time: This refers to residence time of a quantum of bile in a specific region of the biliary tract. Although, strictly speaking, time is a subset of kinetics, it is convenient to consider it separately. The time factor is of particular importance for nucleation from metastable (supersaturated) solutions. In more familiar terms, we use time to refer to the effects of *bile stasis,* particularly in the gallbladder.

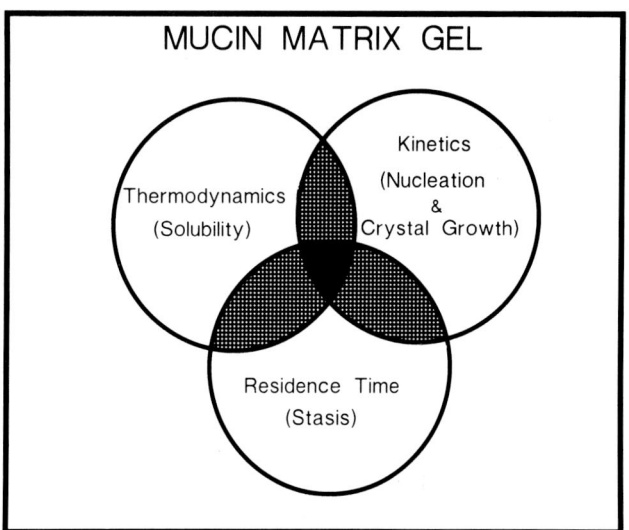

Figure 57–1. Venn diagram illustrating the concept that pathogenesis of gallstones involves multiple simultaneous defects in three broad areas—thermodynamics, kinetics, and time—and that the events of gallstone formation occur in the environment of a mucin gel.

GALLSTONE STRUCTURE AND COMPOSITION

Much progress has been made recently in defining the composition and structure of gallstones, using a wide variety of chemical, physical, and optical techniques. These include scanning electron microscopy,[29-36] infrared spectroscopy,[30, 32, 37-48] x-ray diffraction,[32, 33, 38, 48-57] polarized light microscopy,[33, 53, 58] nuclear magnetic resonance,[59] column and gas chromatography,[60] mass spectroscopy,[47] plasma O_2 and argon ion-etching,[34] electron probe microanalysis,[34, 40, 47, 61-63] and energy-dispersive elemental analysis (energy-dispersive x-ray analysis).[29, 30, 32, 34, 36, 61]

Classic teaching holds that there are two types of gallstones, based on chemical composition: "cholesterol" stones and "pigment" stones. Pigment stones are further subdivided into black pigment stones (found in the setting of chronic hemolysis) and brown pigment stones (associated with chronic biliary infection). In addition, many stones having features of both cholesterol and pigment types are classified in a "mixed" category. While such a classification has clinical usefulness, particularly in decisions regarding therapy, it has been of only limited value as a framework for understanding gallstone pathogenesis.

We believe that it may be useful to consider all gallstones as *a spectrum of calcium-containing rocks*. The reasons for this are as follows. It has been recognized for over 60 years that cholesterol stones contain visible pigment[64] in their central regions. The preponderance of data now strongly indicate that all cholesterol stones contain pigment[30, 31, 37, 40, 51, 65-67] and calcium[29, 36, 37, 40, 68] in their central nidus and that the pigment exists as one or more forms of calcium bilirubinate. The bilirubin is unconjugated.[69] The actual form of calcium bilirubinate varies from stone to stone.[70] Attempts have been made to define the type of salt by x-ray diffraction and by infrared spectroscopy, but the two methods do not always give similar results.[37, 38] Bilirubin may be divalent, or it may be monovalent if one of the two carboxyl groups is ionized. By x-ray diffraction and infrared spectroscopy, the predominant form is the "acid salt," which has the formula $Ca(HB^-)_2$ and is most easily envisioned as a salt of one Ca^{2+} ion and two bilirubin anions, each with one carboxyl group internally hydrogen-bonded. The dianionic salt is detectable by infrared spectroscopy and may be present as neutral salt (CaB) or as an intermediate salt having the formula $Ca_2(HB^-)_2B^{2-}$. The latter compound has been prepared synthetically.[38] Also, using scanning electron microscopy and energy-dispersive x-ray fluorescence, Pitchumoni et al.[36] have found striking calcium peaks in the central cloudy matrix of all cholesterol stones examined. This cloudy matrix, which probably represents mucin glycoproteins,[71] is believed to represent the nidus around which the stone forms.

All *pigment stones* are composed of the calcium salts of one or more of four anions:[72] (1) bilirubinate, (2) carbonate, (3) phosphate, and (4) long-chain fatty acids, mainly palmitate.[73, 74] These have been termed "calcium-sensitive" anions, meaning that their calcium salts are poorly soluble and prone to precipitate.[70] In both black pigment and brown, "earthy" stones, the calcium appears to be randomly distributed throughout the stone.[40, 68] Malet et al.,[30] using infrared spectroscopy, have found calcium bilirubinate, calcium carbonate, and calcium phosphate in the central nidus region of black pigment stones, and the presence of a mucin glycoprotein matrix in this type of stone has been demonstrated by Lamont et al.[75] Similar studies of the central regions of brown pigment stones are

needed, but it appears that all pigment stones, like all cholesterol stones, contain calcium, pigment, and glycoproteins in their central nidus.

Thus, at one end of the spectrum of calcium-containing rocks, there are so-called "pure" cholesterol stones, which actually contain calcium and pigment in their central region. At the other end of the spectrum are black pigment stones, containing calcium along with polymerized bilirubin and related pigments[41, 43, 44, 47, 63, 76, 77] throughout the stone. In between these two extremes are variable mixtures of cholesterol, calcium, and matrix protein. It is apparent therefore that any general theory of the pathogenesis of gallstones, including both cholesterol and pigment stones, must account for the universal presence of calcium, pigment, and matrix protein in the central nidus of the stone.

GALLSTONE PRECURSORS

ANIMAL MODELS

The cut surface of a gallstone, like the rings of a tree, provides a record of events occurring over time; the earliest events are recorded near the center. Events at the surface of a gallstone (reflecting the composition of bile at the time of gallstone removal) may have little relation to the state of affairs in bile at the time when stone formation began (often years previously). From ^{14}C-dating studies, human gallstones have been estimated to grow at the rate of 1 to 2 mm per year.[78] It is apparent, therefore, that if we are to understand gallstone pathogenesis, heavy reliance must be placed on animal models in which events during the first hours and days of gallstone formation can be studied.

Numerous animal models have been used for study of both cholesterol and pigment stones, as reviewed by Gurll and DenBesten,[79] and more recently by Rege and Nahrwold.[80] These include hamster,[81-86] rat,[87, 88] rabbit,[89-95] pig,[96] guinea pig,[97-101] mouse,[102-107] squirrel monkey,[108] dog,[109, 110] prairie dog,[111-116] and Richardson ground squirrel.[116-118] Many of the principles discussed in subsequent sections are based on findings in these animal models. Although it probably would be risky to place too much trust in any particular animal model as being representative of human gallstone formation, similar findings in several models or species would lend credence to the potential relevance of the finding to humans.

BILIARY SLUDGE

The term "sludge" refers to a mixture of cholesterol liquid crystals, cholesterol monohydrate crystals, and calcium bilirubinate granules in a mucin gel matrix.[119-121] It produces a low-amplitude echo pattern by ultrasonography, layers in the dependent part of the gallbladder, and does not produce post-acoustic shadowing.[122] Pigment granules and cholesterol crystals are the source of the acoustic echoes.[123]

Prospective studies of gallstone formation in man indicate that sludge is universally present before gallstone formation.[124-126] This supports the concept that mucus hypersecretion precedes stone development in humans, as noted in experimental animals. A macromolecular complex of mucin and bilirubin is present in the central organic matrix of cholesterol gallstones; the composition of this material appears to be similar to that of biliary sludge.[119, 127] These observations strongly suggest that nucleation of cholesterol and calcium occurs in the mucus gel near the epithelial surface, rather than in the bulk aqueous phase of bile.[18, 128]

Experimentally, pigment sludge has been produced in dogs following cystic duct ligation,[23] in prairie dogs fed a high-carbohydrate diet,[129] in pigs receiving total parenteral nutrition (TPN),[96] and in the Richardson ground squirrel fed a high-cholesterol diet.[118] The last of these studies have provided insight into some of the initial events leading to gallstone formation: within 12 hours after initiation of the diet, the cholesterol saturation index began to rise, followed (within 18 hours) by accumulation of mucus on the epithelial surface of the gallbladder. Cholesterol crystals appeared at 24 hours, which formed aggregates of parallel crystals at about 2 weeks. These aggregates then formed larger clusters that grew to visible stones up to 1 mm in diameter by 10 weeks. In a short time frame, these events followed a previously proposed sequence for forming cholesterol gallstones in humans: supersaturation, nucleation, crystal deposition, and stone growth.[130, 131] There is now little doubt that the mucus gel is the site in which nucleation occurs and stones develop.

MUCUS

Chemistry and Physiology

Current knowledge of the chemistry of mucin and physiology of mucin secretion by the gallbladder has been summarized by Lamont et al.[132, 133] (see also refs. 134–140). Briefly, the word "mucus" refers to the slimy secretion of various epithelial membranes, which is composed of water, inorganic salts, and proteins, including immunoglobulins. "Mucin" refers to a high molecular weight ($>2 \times 10^6$ daltons) polymeric glycoprotein that imparts viscoelastic properties to the secretion. There are also smaller mucin glycoproteins in bile that have not been well characterized. As a group, all the mucin glycoproteins are characterized by having their sugar (glycan) chain linked covalently to the polypeptide core via O-glycosidic bonds to serine and/or threonine. The composition of mucins from various mammalian organs and species appears to vary only slightly and consists of about 75 per cent carbohydrates, 20 per cent peptide core, and 5 per cent bound counterions and H_2O.[132]

The structure of the mucin molecule has been likened to a "bottle brush," in which the unbranched polypeptide core is the central backbone, and the radially arranged oligosaccharide side chains are the bristles of the brush.[138] In dilute aqueous solutions, mucin exists mainly as monomers (500 kd). Pearson et al. have proposed that both gastric mucin[141] and gallbladder mucin[142] contain a covalently linked protein (70 kd) that cross-links mucin monomers by disulfide bonds to form polymeric mucin molecules. With increasing concentration, these polymers aggregate to form a gel, with marked increase in viscosity.

Mucin is a major secretory product of the gallbladder epithelial cell and appears to be secreted by a process of exocytosis, following fusion of intracellular secretory granules with the apical membrane.[143] Lee[144] has suggested that secretion of mucin by the gallbladder is a merocrine process, analogous to the exocytosis of zymogen granules by pancreatic acinar cells. Following translocation across the membrane, the mucin gel ("gel" phase) adheres to the luminal face of the membrane; as distance from the membrane increases, an increasing proportion of the glycoprotein is present as monomers, the more soluble, or "sol," phase.[132]

The mucin gel is believed to constitute an important part of the unstirred layer (diffusion-resistance barrier) that separates the cell membrane from the bulk solution of bile.[145–149]

In the fasting state, there is a low level of mucin secretion by the gallbladder.[145] Rapid release follows endogenous[150] or exogenous[143] stimulation with cholecystokinin (CCK). In the past decade, several studies have suggested an important role for prostaglandins as stimulants of mucin secretion. Lee et al.[112] have shown that hypersecretion of mucin in the prairie dog model is blocked by aspirin. Lamont and coworkers[145] found that arachidonic acid stimulates mucin secretion by explants of prairie dog gallbladder, an effect that is blocked by indomethacin. In explants of guinea pig gallbladder, Moore and colleagues[151] showed that arachidonate-stimulated mucin secretion and release of prostaglandin F_1 was inhibited by hydrocortisone, an inhibitor of phospholipase A_2. In cholesterol-fed prairie dogs, LaMorte et al.[152] noted increased synthesis of prostaglandins prior to the development of cholesterol stones. In contrast, cholesterol-fed guinea pigs developed hemolysis and pigment stones, with no increase in synthesis of prostaglandins.

At present, it is not known whether these findings apply to humans. Cantafora et al.[153] have reported a higher percentage of arachidonic acid esterified to the sn-2 position of biliary lecithin in patients with cholesterol gallstones than in patients without stones. Interestingly, Ahlberg and coworkers[154] have noted a decrease in the percentage of arachidonate in biliary lecithins during chenodeoxycholate administration. Important areas for future study[18] include (1) the role of prostaglandins in mucus hypersecretion and (2) the possibility that hydrolysis of biliary arachidonyl lecithins in the gallbladder lumen serves as a stimulus for prostaglandin synthesis.

Role of Mucus in Gallstone Formation

The importance of mucus in the pathogenesis of gallstones appears to have been recognized since antiquity. In 1932, Weiser and Gray[155] wrote: "Hippocrates and Galen attributed gallstones and other concretions to an accumulation of mucus which clings to the organ and serves as a nucleus for stones which subsequently formed." In 1856, Meckel von Helmsbach[156] wrote: "Two basic factors underlie the formation of every true gall or urinary stone; first, the presence of an organic substance, mucus, in which there may be deposition of salts; second, a suitable urinary or gall fluid to serve as the mother liquor for these sediments."

In 1953, Kleeberg[157, 158] succeeded in making concretions in vitro using gelatin, potassium dichromate, NaCl, and AgCl, in which there was rhythmic precipitation (Liesegang rings[159]) and deposition of gel giving a laminated appearance similar to that often seen in human pigment stones.[50, 61, 160] In 1963, Womack et al.,[58] using histochemical techniques, showed that mucus plays a dominant role as a scaffolding protein in gallstone formation. Subsequently, Bouchier and colleagues[161] reported that human gallbladder bile from patients with stones contained increased hexosamine and was more viscous than normal bile; these findings have been confirmed in other studies.[162, 163]

In 1969, Freston et al.,[89] using the dihydrocholesterol-fed rabbit model of cholesterol stones, showed that mucus hypersecretion *precedes* the development of gallstones, and these workers concluded that the stimulus for this secretion appears to be present in bile. Womack,[65] using a hamster model, confirmed in 1971 the presence of mucus hypersecretion prior to stone development and noted the presence of mucopolysaccharides in cholesterol stones. Maki[162] simultaneously reported the presence of sulfated glycoproteins in human pigment stones. In 1981, Lee and associates confirmed Freston's observations in the rabbit and in three additional models of gallstones: Lincomycin-treated guinea pigs,[164] mice fed cholesterol–cholic acid,[165] and cholesterol-fed prairie dogs.[112] In the last-mentioned work, which may prove to be a landmark paper, it was found that mucus hypersecretion preceded the development of cholesterol crystals and that mucus hypersecretion, cholesterol nucleation, and gallstone formation were all abolished by administration of aspirin. Mucus hypersecretion in the prairie dog model has been observed in several other studies[152, 166, 167] in the nb/nb mouse hemolytic model of pigment stones,[168] and in the canine model of pigment stones.[110]

It is clear that mucus plays an important role in gallstone formation. Glycoproteins are a major component of both human cholesterol and pigment stones[75, 127, 162, 163, 169] and are amply present in bile.[170] Mucus serves as a matrix gel in which nucleation reactions occur and serves as a scaffolding protein in subsequent stone growth. The possible role of mucin as a nucleating protein is considered below (see Nucleation and Crystal Growth).

CALCIUM

OVERVIEW

A major advance in the past decade has been the evolution of the field of biliary calcium and the application of electrochemical techniques[171, 172] for the study of free ionized calcium (Ca^{2+}) in bile and model bile systems. Calcium is one of the most abundant and important cations in the human body, serving two general types of functions, as a structural (cross-linking) component and as a messenger agent (i.e., information transfer).[173] It is known to be a factor of importance in several aspects of gallstone formation. Thus, calcium salts are structural components of gallstones: (1) Calcium, as the salt of one or more "calcium-sensitive"anions, is the major inorganic component of all pigment stones; (2) calcium bilirubinates (and often carbonates) are major constituents of biliary sludge and of the central nidus region of all cholesterol stones; (3) calcium salts may serve as a nucleus or "seed" for cholesterol nucleation and crystal growth;[32, 40, 62, 70, 130, 174–176] and (4) calcium salts, particularly $CaCO_3$, often form a rim or shell on the surface of cholesterol stones that reduces or prevents dissolution by oral bile salts.[33, 177–181]

Free Ca^{2+} also has a variety of effects that may be of importance in the events leading to gallstone formation. Free Ca^{2+} (1) promotes fusion of phospholipid-cholesterol vesicles,[182, 183] (2) promotes cholesterol phase transitions,[184] (3) promotes cholesterol crystal growth by roughly fourfold,[24, 185] (4) increases solubility of intestinal mucus,[136] (5) promotes tissue activity of phospholipase A_2 and may thus be involved in prostaglandin synthesis from arachidonyl lecithins,[18] (6) binds to intestinal mucus,[186] (7) decreases bile salt solubility,[187] (8) binds to both monomeric[70, 175, 188–193] and micellar[70, 174, 175, 188–192, 194–196] bile salts, (9) enters into all calcium solubility relations in bile,[70] and (10) appears to lower the critical micellar concentration of certain bile salts such as glycocholate,[70] thus decreasing its own high-affinity binding to bile salt monomers. Space does not permit detailed comment on all of these factors; some will be noted below in relation to nucleation and theories of pathogenesis.

PHYSICOCHEMICAL STATE OF CALCIUM IN BILE

Free Ca^{2+} interacts with many components of bile; the major ones are shown in Figure 57–2. The central and critical species is free Ca^{2+} (for a consideration of the relationships between activities and concentrations, see refs. 70, 172, 197–202). The concentration of free Ca^{2+} (abbreviated $[Ca^{2+}]$) is about 1.15 mM in normal human plasma[203] and 1.22 mM in canine plasma. In humans[204, 205] and dogs[206–208] both the concentration of free ionized calcium and the total calcium concentration increase linearly with increasing bile salt concentration. Both $[Ca^{2+}]$ and total calcium concentration in gallbladder bile are therefore much higher than in common duct bile. Thus, concentrations of these components are linearly related to one another in humans[205, 209] and dogs.[206]

The difference between total calcium and free calcium concentrations in a given sample of bile represents calcium bound to the various anionic species shown in Figure 57–2. In both humans and dogs, only about 30 per cent of the total calcium exists as the free ion, in both common duct and gallbladder bile. The major buffers for Ca^{2+}, particularly in gallbladder bile, are bile salts. This involves both high-affinity binding of Ca^{2+} to premicellar (presumably monomeric) bile salts[70, 175, 188–193] and low-affinity binding to bile salt micelles.[70, 174, 175, 188–196] In common duct bile, calcium complexation with HCO_3^- and CO_3^{2-} ions,[210] and with bilirubin diglucuronide (BG_2)[211] are also quantitatively important. Complexation with phosphate is not important, owing to the low concentrations of inorganic phosphate in bile (approximately 0.35 mM in common duct and 0.6 mM in gallbladder bile).[212]

Recently, it has been shown that if all of the known calcium complexes in bile are summated with free Ca^{2+} to give a predicted total calcium, the resulting value is about 10 per cent less than that actually observed.[208] This difference most likely represents Ca^{2+} bound to mucin glycoproteins. Forstner[186] has found that intestinal mucin binds calcium with an affinity of about 0.02 mmoles per gram (at 1 mM Ca^{2+} in 0.14 M NaCl). Interestingly, this is virtually identical to Ca^{2+}-binding to human crystalline albumin[213] and to albumin in human plasma.[214] We know of no studies of binding of Ca^{2+} to gallbladder mucin, but it is likely to be similar to that of intestinal mucin. Work is currently in progress to develop a quantitative thermodynamic model

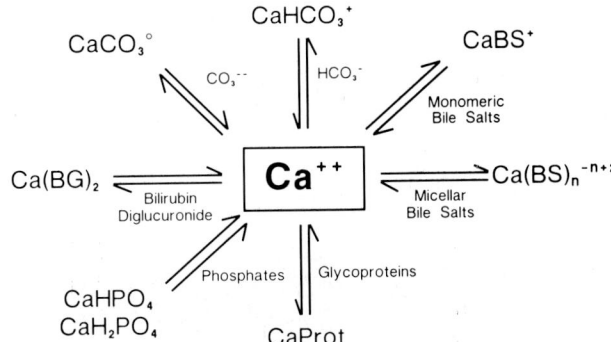

Figure 57–2. Interactions of free Ca^{2+} with multiple anionic ligands in bile to form soluble calcium complexes. The sum of all species represents total calcium concentration. In both humans and dogs, free Ca^{2+} accounts for only about 30 per cent of the total calcium concentration in bile.

of biliary calcium, similar to that recently reported for calcium in pancreatic juice.[215]

ENTRY OF CALCIUM INTO BILE

If therapeutic modulation of biliary free Ca^{2+} concentration is to be achieved for treatment and possible prevention of calcium-containing gallstones, knowledge of the mechanism(s) of calcium entry into bile is essential. In 1984, Cummings and Hofmann[216] found a strong parallel relation between total calcium outputs and bile salt outputs in canine bile upon infusion of a variety of bile salts. Results were believed to be compatible with passive entry of Ca^{2+} into bile, but no definitive conclusions could be made because free Ca^{2+} was not measured. Subsequent studies in guinea pigs,[217] dogs,[218] and humans[219] have shown clearly that free Ca^{2+} enters bile by passive convection and diffusion throughout the biliary tract, so that Ca^{2+} entry is tightly linked to bile flow. In all three species, plots of calcium outputs versus bile flow yield intercepts at or near the origin. Thus, any measure that increases bile flow will increase calcium output but may or may not affect the concentration of free Ca^{2+}, depending on Gibbs-Donnan effects (see section on Regulation of Ionized Calcium in Bile).

The passive distribution of free Ca^{2+} between bile and plasma has important implications for its possible therapeutic reduction in bile. Calcium will always be present in bile, and there appear to be no cellular secretory mechanisms for calcium to serve as targets for pharmacologic inhibitors. Possible therapeutic reduction of biliary Ca^{2+} must be accomplished therefore by chelation within the lumen of the biliary tract. Such chelation would shift the equilibrium only temporarily, however, owing to passive re-entry of Ca^{2+}, as noted above. No such agents for oral use are currently available; their synthesis is an important area for future research.

SOLUBILITY OF CALCIUM IN BILE

The solubility of calcium salts, like that of cholesterol, is a critical factor in gallstone pathogenesis. As recently noted,[70] calcium precipitation occurs only if the solubility product (K'sp) of one or more of four calcium salts is exceeded; that is, if

$[Ca^{2+}]\cdot[bilirubin] > K'sp$ for calcium bilirubinate,
$[Ca^{2+}]\cdot[CO_3^{2-}] > K'sp$ for calcium carbonate,
$[Ca^{2+}]\cdot[phosphate] > K'sp$ for calcium phosphate, or
$[Ca^{2+}]\cdot[palmitate] > K'sp$ for calcium palmitate

In bile, the pathways leading to precipitation of calcium salts could include

1. Increase in $[Ca^{2+}]$,
2. Increase in $[anion^-]$, or
3. Both of these

It is apparent that the concentration (or activity) of free Ca^{2+} is critical for all calcium solubility relationships. Any measure that will reduce free $[Ca^{2+}]$ in bile will correspondingly reduce the likelihood of calcium precipitation.

In "pigment" gallstones, $CaCO_3$ exists as one or more of three polymorphs: calcite, aragonite, and vaterite.[220] Vaterite, which is uncommon in nature (found in shells of

certain mollusks), often predominates. The reason for this is not clear but may be related to pH at the locus of crystallization. There appear to have been no studies of vaterite solubility under physiologic conditions. However, K'sp for calcite has recently been determined with the Ca^{2+} electrode: 3.76×10^{-8} M at 37°C.[221] Aragonite appears to be slightly more soluble than calcite.[222]

Using K'sp for calcite as reference for $CaCO_3$ solubility in bile, it has been shown that canine common duct bile, but not gallbladder bile, is markedly supersaturated with $CaCO_3$,[223, 224] as shown in Figure 57–3. Human common duct bile is also supersaturated.[225] Similar degrees of supersaturation have been observed in canine pancreatic juice;[226] however, the dog does not spontaneously develop either gallstones or pancreatic stones. *These findings indicate that kinetic (nucleating/anti-nucleating) factors are of critical importance in calcium precipitation in bile.* Indeed, saturation indices for $CaCO_3$ as high as 75 have been produced by the addition of calcium to canine bile without evidence of precipitation.[227] Such high degrees of metastability almost certainly reflect the presence of proteins in bile that inhibit calcium nucleation.

The profound (> 200-fold) decrease in the ion-product $[Ca^{2+}]\cdot[CO_3^{2-}]$ in gallbladder bile seen in Figure 57–3 is due entirely to acidification of gallbladder contents, with a marked decrease in the concentration of CO_3^{2-}. (As noted above, free $[Ca^{2+}]$ actually increases with increasing concentration of bile.) Such beneficial effects of acidification by the gallbladder also apply to the solubility of calcium bilirubinate and probably also to calcium phosphate and palmitate (although these have not been quantified). Ostrow et al.[228] have recently shown that the monoanion of bilirubin predominates (>90 per cent) at the pH of bile. Preliminary studies of the solubility of calcium bilirubinates by Ostrow and Celic[229] indicate that the degree of saturation with these salts is also strongly pH-dependent, so that gallbladder bile having a normal bilirubin concentration would be super-saturated with $Ca(HB)_2$ above a pH of approximately 6.8. Clearly, acidification of bile by the gallbladder greatly decreases the saturation (increases the solubility) of both $CaCO_3$ and calcium bilirubinate.

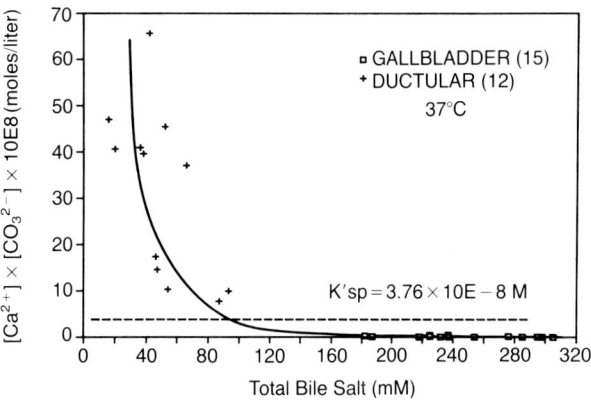

Figure 57–3. Observed ion product $[Ca^{2+}]\cdot[CO_3^{2-}]$ in bile from the canine common bile duct or gallbladder. The dashed line represents the solubility product constant (K'$_{sp}$) for calcite (3.76×10^{-8} M). Note that all common bile duct samples were supersaturated, whereas all gallbladder bile samples were markedly unsaturated. The gallbladder reduced the ion product by an average of >200-fold via acidification of bile, which led to a marked reduction in carbonate ion concentration. (Reproduced from Rege RV, Moore EM. *The Journal of Clinical Investigation*, 1986, 77:21, by copyright permission of the American Society for Clinical Investigation.)

REGULATION OF IONIZED CALCIUM IN BILE

Perhaps the most important advances in the field of biliary calcium has been the realization that (1) bile salts, at the pH of bile, are impermeant anions that generate powerful Gibbs-Donnan forces in the biliary lumen;[230] (2) these forces dictate that the concentrations (activities) of all freely permeable cations will be higher in bile than in plasma; and (3) Ca^{2+} is a permeable cation and thus is subject to these forces. At equilibrium, the relation between bile/plasma activity ratios for permeant cations and anions is given by the Gibbs-Donnan ratio (g):

$$g = \frac{[Na^+]_B}{[Na^+]_P} = \frac{[K^+]_B}{[K^+]_P} = \frac{[Cl^-]_P}{[Cl^-]_B} = \frac{([Ca^{2+}]_B)^{1/2}}{([Ca^{2+}]_P)^{1/2}} \quad [1]$$

where B and P refer to bile and plasma, respectively.

Using equilibrium dialysis of taurocholate, one finds, as expected from theory, that g_{Ca++} is linearly related to the concentration of bile salt anion (BS^-):[230]

$$g = 1 + 0.0025 [BS^-] \quad [2]$$

so that, for a univalent ion such as K^+,

$$[K^+]_B = (g_{K+}) \cdot [K^+]_P \quad [3a]$$

$$[K^+]_B = (1 + 0.0025[BS]) \cdot [K^+]_P \quad [3b]$$

and for Ca^{2+},

$$[Ca^{2+}]_B = (g^2_{Ca2+} \cdot [Ca^{2+}]_P \quad [4a]$$

$$[Ca^{2+}]_B = (1 + 0.0025[BS])^2 \cdot [Ca^{2+}]_P \quad [4b]$$

From Equations 2 and 4, it is apparent that free $[Ca^{2+}]$ in bile will depend on the ambient concentration of bile salt. At plasma $[Ca^{2+}] = 1.15$ mM and $[BS^-] = 30$ mM (as in the common bile duct), predicted biliary $[Ca^{2+}]$ is 1.33 mM; at 300 mM $[BS^-]$ (i.e., maximally concentrated gallbladder bile), predicted $[Ca^{2+}]$ is 3.52 mM.

Close relationships between the observed $[Ca^{2+}]$ and that predicted by the Gibbs-Donnan effect have been found in rabbit gallbladder bile[231] and in canine common duct and gallbladder bile.[207] Similarly, close relationships have been found for the distribution of K^+ in rabbit gallbladder bile[232] and in canine common duct and gallbladder bile.[233]

One may conclude from these studies of calcium entry and distribution that Ca^{2+} enters bile primarily by passive *convection* in the osmotic water flux from plasma to bile, in response to canalicular secretion of bile salt. Ca^{2+} entry probably occurs across paracellular aqueous channels, the importance of which has been noted by Boyer.[234] This convective entry accounts for the close relationships noted by Cummings and Hofmann[216] between calcium output and bile salt output. In addition, $[Ca^{2+}]$ in bile rises above plasma levels in transit through the biliary ductules by *diffusion* from plasma. At low rates of bile flow, observed $[Ca^{2+}]$ levels in canine common duct bile are those predicted from equilibrium Gibbs-Donnan relationships (see Equation 4). At high flow rates, there is insufficient residence time for diffusional equilibrium to be obtained, so that $[Ca^{2+}]$ in duct bile rises only slightly above corresponding plasma values. This points up the importance of the third circle in the Venn diagram shown in Figure 57–1. The concept of residence time in bile ducts and gallbladder is a key to understanding Ca^{2+} concentrations (activities) and therefore calcium solubility in bile.

Bile salts have both "black hat" and "white hat" effects on calcium solubility. First, they induce Ca^{2+} entry into bile by virtue of their osmosity;[235] then they promptly bind it to both bile salt monomers and micelles. This binding reduces free $[Ca^{2+}]$ and increases calcium solubility. However, the reduction in $[Ca^{2+}]$ increases the plasma-to-bile gradient, favoring further diffusion of Ca^{2+} into bile, as dictated by Gibbs-Donnan forces. This diffusion, by increasing $[Ca^{2+}]$, again reduces calcium solubility.

SUMMARY

The findings presented above have important implications in the pathogenesis of "pigment" gallstones. Free $[Ca^{2+}]$ in bile is dependent on, or related to, (1) bile salt–induced Gibbs-Donnan forces, (2) plasma $[Ca^{2+}]$ (see Equation 4), and (3) residence time. It follows that

1. Any factor that increases the concentration of bile salt, such as the concentration of bile by the gallbladder, will increase free $[Ca^{2+}]$ in bile and thus, at a given concentration of anion, will increase the likelihood of calcium precipitation.

2. Any factor that increases plasma free $[Ca^{2+}]$ will tend to be amplified by the g^2 term in the Gibbs-Donnan equation (Equation 4). This may be related to the apparent increased incidence of gallstones in patients with hyperparathyroidism.[236-239]

3. Any factor that increases residence time in the bile ducts (cholestasis) or gallbladder (stasis) will increase the time available for Gibbs-Donnan diffusional forces to operate across the epithelium. With sufficient time, biliary $[Ca^{2+}]$ will rise until a Gibbs-Donnan equilibrium state is achieved across the epithelium. These Gibbs-Donnan forces are substantial and increase the likelihood of calcium precipitation.

In preliminary studies of normocalcemic patients (13 control patients without stones and 40 patients with stones [14 cholesterol, 19 mixed, and 7 black pigment]), there were no significant differences in $[Ca^{2+}]$ concentrations in bile between patients with and without gallstones or between patients with different types of stones.[205] For all 53 patients, $[Ca^{2+}]$ was linearly related to [BS]: $[Ca^{2+}] = 1.05 + 0.0033$ [BS], as shown in Figure 57–3. Thus, in normocalcemic patients (the vast majority of gallstone patients), pigment gallstones do not appear to represent an abnormality in biliary $[Ca^{2+}]$. Rather, they appear to result from increases in biliary anions, (i.e., in the [anion⁻] term in the ion-product relations noted above). Thus, unconjugated bilirubin increases in bile if the bilirubin load increases, as in sickle cell anemia[240-244] and spherocytosis,[245] or if there is excessive deconjugation of bilirubin,[246] as by bacteria.[247-250] Calcium phosphates and calcium salts of long-chain fatty acids such as palmitate may result from excessive hydrolysis of biliary lecithins by bacterial phospholipases.[251] Similarly, $CaCO_3$ precipitates do not appear to reflect an increase in $[Ca^{2+}]$, but rather an increase in $[CO_3^{2+}]$, as occurs with defective acidification of gallbladder bile (discussed below).

In principle, it should be possible to temporarily reduce the ion-product for all calcium salts to below saturation (K'sp) by chelation of Ca^{2+} in bile. If calcium precipitation is thus rendered impossible, nucleating and anti-nucleating factors will become of little or no consequence. If safe, effective methods for chelation of Ca^{2+} in bile can be

CHOLESTEROL

OVERVIEW

The connection between cholesterol and gallstones dates back over two centuries. Indeed, the name "cholesterol" reflects the fact that this omnipresent component of animal cell membranes was first discovered in gallstones.[252] In the mid-1700s, the French investigator Poulletier de la Salle noted that an alcohol extract of gallstones contained a novel, waxy substance. De Fourcroy[253] in 1789 confirmed and was the first to publish this finding. This substance initially was thought to be identical to spermacetine, a wax found in the heads of sperm whales; however, Chevreul[254, 255] found that the new substance had a much higher melting point than spermacetine or other known waxes. He named the new substance cholesterine, from the Greek words meaning "bile solid." With the demonstration in the late nineteenth century that cholesterine was actually a secondary alcohol,[256, 257] the name was modified to cholesterol.

Cholesterol (cholest-5-ene-3β-ol) is a planar hydrocarbon found throughout the animal kingdom. It is derived from acetate via a series of steps involving synthesis and polymerization of the basic building block, isopentenyl pyrophosphate (see also Chap. 5). It is characterized structurally by (1) a linked series of four hydrocarbon rings (the cyclophenopentophenanthrene nucleus) that is entirely saturated except for a single double bond in the 5 position, (2) a single hydroxyl group in the 3β position, (3) β-oriented methyl groups in the 13 and 10 positions (carbons 18 and 19, respectively), and (4) a branched, saturated 8-carbon side chain attached in the 17β position (carbons 20–27). Most tissues in the human body have the capacity to synthesize cholesterol.[258] The principal role of cholesterol appears to be stabilization of membranes.[259] Cholesterol also serves as a chemical precursor of bile acids and steroid hormones (see Chap. 13).

In the nomenclature of Small,[260] cholesterol is classified as an insoluble, non-swelling amphiphile. Its solubility in water is very low, on the order of 3×10^{-8} M at room temperature.[261, 262] However, cholesterol is not entirely non-polar; the 3β hydroxyl group renders the molecule slightly amphiphilic. Because of this, cholesterol at an air-water or lipid-water interface forms a stable, spreading monolayer,[260] much as do phospholipids. Its hydroxyl group interacts with the aqueous phase and its non-polar ring and side chain project away from the interface. Cholesterol in membranes has a similar orientation. Cholesterol is both more water-soluble and more weakly amphiphilic than membrane phospholipids, which may account for the relatively rapid exchange of free cholesterol between membranes and other aqueous carriers such as vesicles and micelles, as well as the relative rapidity with which cholesterol "flip-flops" across a membrane bilayer.[263] When a fatty acyl group is esterified to the 3β hydroxyl group to form a cholesterol ester, amphiphilicity is lost. Cholesterol esters are therefore entirely non-polar, like triglycerides. Cholesterol esters are not found in bile.

PHYSICOCHEMICAL STATES OF CHOLESTEROL IN MODEL SOLUTIONS AND BILE

In aqueous systems, the hydroxyl group of cholesterol associates with a molecule of water to form a stable monohydrate. Cholesterol precipitates from aqueous solution as the crystalline monohydrate.[261] Cholesterol monohydrate crystals have a characteristic structure[264] that is easily recognized by microscopic examination. The microscopic finding of cholesterol monohydrate crystals in bile almost invariably accompanies cholesterol gallstone disease,[265] and formation of these crystals is believed to represent an obligatory step in the formation of cholesterol gallstones.[266]

Cholesterol is present in human gallbladder bile at concentrations on the order of 10 to 20 mM, about one million times its solubility as monomers in water; yet crystals of cholesterol monohydrate are absent from normal bile. Thus, some carrier for cholesterol must be present in bile to prevent it from precipitating. From the first, attention was focused on the two other principal lipid components of bile—bile salts and phosphatidylcholine (lecithin)—as the carriers for cholesterol.

The modern era of cholesterol gallstone science began with the studies of Small, Bourges, and Dervichian in the mid-1960s. Although previous investigators[267–269] had shown that bile salts could solubilize cholesterol and that the addition of lecithin to bile salts markedly increased the micellar solubility of cholesterol, these authors were the first to conduct comprehensive quantitative studies of the interactions of cholesterol, lecithin, and bile salts in aqueous media. Their findings, presented in a series of classic papers,[3–6] laid the groundwork for our current understanding of the complex physical chemistry of biliary lipids. These authors found that bile salts are freely soluble in water at pH 10 to concentrations greater than 1 M (this is not true, however, of monohydroxy bile salts such as lithocholate[13]). Bile salts in excess of the critical micellar concentration (around 5 mM) form micelles. In a system containing high concentrations of bile salts with cholesterol, 20 to 130 molecules of bile salts are required to solubilize one molecule of cholesterol.[270] At a bile salt concentration of 100 mM, comparable to that of gallbladder bile, cholesterol solubility is about 2 mM (five- to tenfold less than the cholesterol concentrations actually found in bile, but five orders of magnitude greater than the solubility of cholesterol in water).[3]

Lecithin is highly insoluble in water. When water is added to lecithin, one observes spontaneous formation of "paracrystalline" lipid bilayers that, depending on the mechanical conditions of formation, may be multilamellar or unilamellar, sheets (membranes) or spheres (vesicles).[271] This arrangement, which has properties of both fluidity and structure, is called a liquid crystalline state; it is further distinguished from other possible liquid crystalline states as the Lα phase.[272] This is the characteristic physicochemical state of cell membrane phospholipids.

When cholesterol is added to a phospholipid bilayer, it nests between the phospholipid acyl chains with its polar hydroxyl group toward the lipid-water interface (possibly interacting via hydrogen bonds with the carbonyl oxygens of the fatty acyl groups).[273] Incorporation of cholesterol has three important effects on a phospholipid bilayer:[274] (1) it reduces the random mobility of the phospholipid acyl chains, thereby reducing membrane fluidity; (2) it prevents orderly packing of the phospholipid acyl chains and thus dramatically lowers or eliminates the tendency of membranes to gel or "freeze" at low temperature; and (3) it causes tighter packing of the phospholipid molecules, leading to "condensation" of the bilayer.

Cholesterol added to lecithin in water is incorporated into bilayers up to a cholesterol:lecithin equilibrium ratio of 1:1 (mole:mole).[4] Although under certain conditions lecithin membranes can be enriched with cholesterol up to a 2:1 cholesterol:lecithin mole ratio,[275] the excess cholesterol eventually must precipitate as crystalline cholesterol monohydrate. Lipid bilayers containing cholesterol in their smallest and simplest form are unilamellar vesicles; these eventually will aggregate to form multilamellar vesicles, globules that are grossly visible by light microscopy and exhibit characteristic "Maltese cross" birefringence under polarized light.[276] The ternary system of bile salt–lecithin–water behaves differently. At low bile salt concentrations, lecithin forms bilayers. As the bile salt:lecithin ratio increases above about 1:2, these bilayers completely dissolve to form micelles. The structure of the bile salt–phospholipid mixed micelle is believed to consist of a small, disc-shaped phospholipid bilayer surrounded by a rim of bile salt and also incorporating some bile salts into the bilayer in the form of reverse micelles. When all four components are combined by adding cholesterol to a bile salt–lecithin–water system containing greater than 75 per cent water, a system is created in which micelles, liquid crystalline bilayers, and cholesterol monohydrate crystals each may be present, depending on the proportions of the four components.[5-7] In the region corresponding to the normal composition of human gallbladder bile (assuming 90 per cent water), only a single phase is found—the micellar phase. At slightly higher concentrations of cholesterol, however, two separate phases—micelles and solid cholesterol monohydrate crystals—may coexist. In more dilute or bile salt–poor systems, formation of micelles is impaired, and phospholipid and cholesterol instead form liquid crystalline bilayers; if cholesterol is present in excess, then cholesterol monohydrate crystals may coexist with lamellar liquid crystals.

Admirand and Small[7] found in 1968 that the lipid composition of gallbladder bile of patients with cholesterol gallstones invariably exceeded the limits of micellar cholesterol solubility as defined by the quaternary phase diagram (Fig. 57–4). In contrast, the lipid composition of gallbladder bile from normal controls was found to fall within the zone in which only a single micellar phase was expected. Thus differences in biliary content of the three principal lipids appeared to be both necessary and sufficient to account for gallstone formation.

Several quantitative indices subsequently were developed to express the degree of cholesterol saturation of bile.[277-280] The most widely accepted is the cholesterol saturation index of Carey and associates,[8, 9, 281] based on extensive studies with model solutions of bile salts, lecithin, and cholesterol. The cholesterol saturation index is defined as the ratio of the actual amount of cholesterol present in a sample to the amount of micellar cholesterol that can be solubilized at equilibrium in a model solution containing the same ratio of bile salts to lecithin and the same total lipid concentration. In the model of Admirand and Small,[7] a cholesterol saturation index greater than 1 (100 per cent) is a prerequisite for gallstone formation.

REGULATION OF BILIARY CHOLESTEROL SATURATION

Soon after the landmark publications of Small and associates, several groups[282-284] reported that the lipid composition of gallbladder bile both in normal individuals and in patients with gallstones was essentially identical to that of hepatic bile; only the water content was different. Thus it was concluded that supersaturation of gallbladder bile was caused by the liver's excretion of excessive cholesterol relative to bile acids and phospholipids. This finding has led to the strong bias throughout much of the past two decades that cholesterol gallstones are the physical manifestation of an underlying metabolic liver disorder, and much subsequent work has focused on regulation of biliary cholesterol secretion and the nature of the abnormality in cholesterol gallstone disease.

In general, bile supersaturated with cholesterol could result from either deficiency in secretion of bile salts and/or phospholipids or disproportionately increased secretion of cholesterol. It is known that secretion of bile salts stimulates secretion of cholesterol and phospholipid into bile.[19, 285-290] However, the relationship is not linear. As secretion of bile salts increases, the rate of secretion of cholesterol plateaus and the cholesterol:bile salt and cholesterol:phospholipid ratios decrease. Conversely, as the rate of secretion of bile salts decreases, bile becomes more saturated with cholesterol, despite the fact that the rate of secretion of cholesterol is reduced.

Thus, one possible explanation for the increased cholesterol saturation observed in patients with cholesterol gallstones is reduced secretion of bile salts due to reduced flux of bile salts in the enterohepatic circulation. Reduced circulation of bile salts would be expected in conditions associated with excessive losses from the intestine, such as regional enteritis, ileectomy, or treatment with resins (e.g., cholestyramine) that bind bile salts. Indeed, it appears that these conditions are associated with an increased saturation of cholesterol in bile and with an increased risk of gallstones.[291, 292] However, increased biliary cholesterol saturation occurs only with severe malabsorption of bile salts; with milder degrees of bile salt wasting, synthesis of bile salts may increase sufficiently to compensate for losses and maintain a normal rate of secretion of bile salts.[293]

Reduced secretion of bile salts also might occur if modest losses of bile salts are inadequately replaced. Vlahcevic and associates[294, 295] found that cholesterol supersaturation of bile in many patients with cholesterol gallstones was

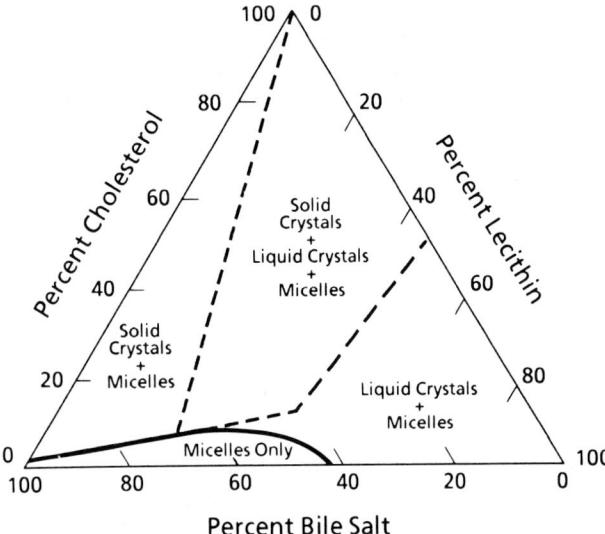

Figure 57–4. Triangular coordinate plot illustrating physical states at equilibrium of lipids in model aqueous solutions of bile salt, lecithin, and cholesterol, at a total lipid concentration of 10 g/dl. Each point within plot is defined by the relative proportion (percentage by weight) of each lipid component. (Modified from Carey MC, Small DM, the *Journal of Clinical Investigation*, 1978, 61:998, by copyright permission of the American Society for Clinical Investigation.)

associated with decreased size of the bile salt pool, a finding subsequently confirmed by others.[296, 297] Because the rate of bile salt synthesis was normal in the face of a doubling of fractional turnover rate, the authors postulated that a defect in regulation of bile salt synthesis, possibly related to oversensitive feedback inhibition of cholesterol 7α-hydroxylase, could account for the decreased bile salt pool.[10] Subsequent data[298] suggested that expansion of the bile salt pool via oral administration of bile acids might reverse this defect, increase biliary bile salt secretion, lower biliary cholesterol saturation, and prevent cholesterol crystal precipitation. Although later shown to be incorrect in several particulars,[299–301] this formulation was a key step in the development of the first successful medical therapy for gallstone dissolution (see below).

It soon became apparent that reduced bile acid pool size could not account for all cases of cholesterol gallstones. Shaffer and Small[302] reported that bile acid pool size and secretion rate were reduced in a group of non-obese subjects; however, in obese patients, both these authors and Bennion and Grundy[303] found that the bile salt pool size and secretion rates were normal. In these obese patients, the supersaturation of bile with cholesterol resulted instead from an absolute increase in secretion of cholesterol into bile. Absolute increases in secretion of cholesterol were noted subsequently in patients following treatment with estrogen or during pregnancy,[304–308] and following treatment with certain hypolipidemic medications such as clofibrate.[293, 309, 310] All of the aforementioned are established risk factors for cholesterol gallstone disease.[292] Thus, at least in some gallstone patients, the normal relation between bile salt secretion and biliary cholesterol secretion appears to be altered such that the rate of biliary cholesterol secretion for any given rate of bile salt secretion is increased; that is, the curve relating biliary cholesterol to bile salt output is shifted upward. The metabolic basis for this abnormality remains unclear. In experimental animals, diets rich in cholesterol[113, 118, 311] or deficient in essential fatty acids[81] may markedly increase the content of cholesterol in bile and lead to formation of gallstones. However, in humans diet does not appear to be a major determinant of cholesterol saturation in the bile.[312–315]

The rate of secretion of cholesterol into bile may be determined in part by the rate of synthesis of cholesterol in the liver. The rate of total body synthesis of cholesterol in obese subjects is greater than that in lean controls,[316–318] as are the biliary cholesterol saturation and the incidence of cholesterol gallstones.[292, 302, 303, 319] In some studies, the activity of the rate-limiting enzyme of cholesterol synthesis (HMG CoA reductase) has been reported to be elevated in the livers of patients with cholesterol gallstones.[320, 321] The activity of this enzyme is suppressed by administration of chenodeoxycholic acid (CDCA),[322] a treatment that also reduces biliary cholesterol secretion.[301] HMG CoA reductase is probably not suppressed by ursodeoxycholate,[322–325] another bile salt that suppresses biliary cholesterol secretion;[326, 327] conversely, treatment with deoxycholic acid suppressed HMG CoA reductase but failed to reduce the biliary cholesterol saturation index.[325, 328]

Recent studies by Duane et al.[329, 330] indicate that treatment of human subjects with simvastatin, an inhibitor of HMG CoA reductase, reduced the cholesterol saturation of bile by a mean of 20 per cent without altering bile acid pool composition. Other studies suggest that impaired metabolism of cholesterol along pathways that lead to cholesterol esters or bile acids may cause cholesterol to accumulate in the hepatocyte and lead to greater excretion of cholesterol into bile. Stone et al.[331] and Bellentani et al.[332] have found that in rats inhibition of acyl CoA:cholesterol acyltransferase (ACAT), the enzyme that catalyzes cholesterol esterification, is associated with increased secretion of cholesterol into bile. In studies of Pima Indians in the southwestern United States,[295, 297, 333, 334] a population with a marked genetic predisposition to formation of cholesterol gallstones,[335] decreased bile acid pool size and increased biliary secretion of cholesterol were found. Because bile acid synthesis is a principal pathway for elimination of cholesterol, Grundy et al.[297] suggested that this combination of defects may reflect a primary deficiency in the rate-limiting enzyme of bile acid synthesis, cholesterol 7α-hydroxylase.

Based on these and other data, it has been proposed that a critical regulatory pool of hepatic free cholesterol may be rate-determining for secretion of cholesterol into bile.[286, 331, 332, 336–338] Theoretically, the size of this pool would be determined by the balance of inputs (dietary cholesterol, intestinal absorption, de novo synthesis) and outputs (esterification, lipoprotein secretion, bile acid synthesis, biliary cholesterol secretion). Increased secretion of biliary cholesterol would result from expansion of this pool, either via increased inputs or decreased output along alternative pathways. The molecular mechanism by which increased secretion of cholesterol occurs is unclear; although conceptually useful, this model remains unproven.

An additional factor of potential importance in the coupling of bile salt and cholesterol secretion is the composition of the bile salt pool. Carulli and colleagues[339, 340] have shown, in short-term human studies, that the potency of different bile salts in promoting biliary secretion of cholesterol and phospholipid increases with increasing hydrophobicity. Since more hydrophobic bile salts are also more efficient in solubilization of cholesterol in micelles,[341] the net effect of these changes on biliary cholesterol saturation may be difficult to predict. However, it appears that the *chronic* effect of feeding different bile acids differs substantially from the *acute* effect. For example, chronic feeding of either ursodeoxycholate or chenodeoxycholate leads to an absolute reduction in secretion of cholesterol into bile,[342] even though ursodeoxycholate is strongly hydrophilic and chenodeoxycholate is hydrophobic.[341] These findings suggest that long-term effects of these bile acids may be due to such factors as suppression of HMG CoA reductase, suppression of bile acid synthesis, or stimulation of intestinal absorption of cholesterol.[322]

MECHANISM OF SECRETION OF CHOLESTEROL AND PHOSPHOLIPID INTO BILE
(See also Chap. 13)

Despite its obvious importance, the mechanism by which cholesterol is secreted into bile remains a mystery. Physiologic studies have defined several of the salient features of biliary lipid secretion that must be explained: (1) Biliary secretion of cholesterol and phospholipid is linked to secretion of bile salts in a non-linear manner.[286, 331, 332, 336–338] (2) Nearly all of the phospholipid secreted into bile is newly synthesized within the hepatocyte,[343] whereas much or most of the cholesterol secreted into bile is delivered to the hepatocyte by lipoproteins.[344, 345] (3) Essentially all of biliary phospholipid is phosphatidylcholine;[346, 347] in contrast, hepatocellular membranes contain substantial amounts of sphyingomyelin, phosphatidylethanolamine, and other phospholipids.[348–350] (4) Compared to hepatocellu-

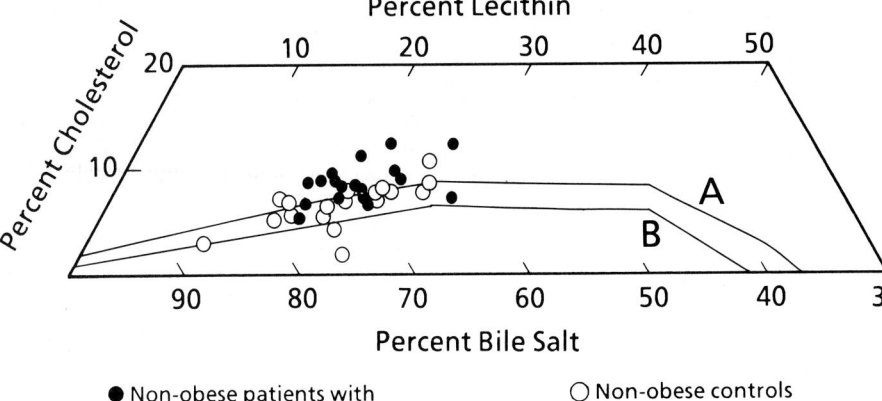

Figure 57–5. Gallbladder lipid composition in non-obese patients with and without cholesterol gallstones. The limits of micellar cholesterol solubility at equilibrium in model solutions containing total lipid concentrations of 20 per cent (comparable to maximally concentrated gallbladder bile) and 2.5 per cent (comparable to hepatic ductular bile) are depicted by lines A and B, respectively. *See* text for discussion. (Modified from Carey MC, Small DM. *The Journal of Clinical Investigation,* 1978, 61:998, by copyright permission of the American Society for Clinical Investigation.)

lar membranes, bile is enriched with selected molecular species of phosphatidylcholine.[351–353] (5) Various organic anions such as bilirubin or ampicillin selectively suppress secretion of cholesterol into bile.[354–356]

One of the most straightforward models of biliary lipid secretion is that proposed in 1972 by Hardison and Apter,[357] who hypothesized that biliary secretion of phospholipid and cholesterol occurs via formation of micelles. In its simplest form, the micellar model proposes that bile salts are actively concentrated, either within the hepatocyte or in the canalicular lumen, until their critical micellar concentration is exceeded; the bile salts then extract cholesterol and phospholipid from the surrounding membranes to form mixed micelles, which are carried via the bile ducts to the gallbladder.[358] This model is supported by the finding that a non-micelle-forming bile salt, dehydrocholate, caused little increase in biliary cholesterol and phospholipid secretion.[357] However, the micellar model fails to explain a number of important findings. Of particular note is the fact that the increase in cholesterol and phospholipid secretion caused by bile salts was greatest at low rates of bile salt secretion and diminished substantially at high rates of bile salt secretion.

More recent data suggest that cholesterol and phospholipid are secreted into bile in the form of discrete membranous vesicles. In the presence of high concentrations of bile salts secreted via a canalicular "pump," these vesicles may then dissolve rapidly to form mixed micelles. This "vesicular model" of biliary lipid secretion is suggested by the finding[359–362] that colchicine, a microtubule poison that blocks cellular translocation of vesicles, inhibits biliary lipid secretion in isolated perfused livers. It is consistent with kinetic studies of radiolabeled lipids demonstrating that the specific activity of phospholipid in bile exceeds the specific activity in the canalicular membrane.[348] Vesicles have been visualized by electron microscopy in the pericanalicular cytoplasm of the hepatocyte[363, 364] and in hepatic bile[365, 366] and have been isolated from bile samples (see following section).

A weakness of the vesicular theory of bile secretion has been the difficulty in explaining how bile acids might regulate this process. Recent data by Crawford and associates[361, 362] indicate that in addition to being secreted by an active transport system at the canalicular membrane, bile salts also may enter bile in association with phospholipid-cholesterol vesicles. It is known that bile salts may partition into membranous structures in the form of reverse

micelles,[367] perhaps in the process displacing cholesterol. Lamri and co-workers[369] have shown that bile salts are concentrated within hepatocytes in vesicles in the Golgi apparatus, where biliary vesicles presumably originate. Sakisaka and associates[364] recently demonstrated increased transcytotic vesicular transport associated with addition of bile acids to isolated hepatocyte couplets. If incorporation of bile salt into a nascent vesicle in the endoplasmic reticulum somehow expedites assembly, translocation, or secretion of the vesicle into bile, this could explain why increased bile salt fluxes are associated with increased biliary lipid secretion.

The micellar and vesicular theories of biliary lipid secretion are not mutually exclusive, and it is possible that both pathways contribute. Indeed, the data of Pattinson and Chapman[370] suggest that vesicular secretion of lipids may predominate at low rates of bile salt secretion, whereas micellar lipid secretion may predominate during bile salt–induced choleresis. If micelles are relatively poor in cholesterol compared to vesicles,[17, 183] then selective stimulation of micellar lipid secretion during bile salt–induced choleresis could explain the non-linearity of the linkage between bile salt and cholesterol secretion. Moreover, the composition of intracellular membranes at the site of assembly of secretory vesicles could change with changes in the hepatic free cholesterol pool, and this might explain the absolute increase in cholesterol secretion associated with obesity or with estrogen administration.

SUPERSATURATION OF BILE: THE METASTABLE STATE

The thermodynamic model provides an elegant explanation for gallstone disease. Nonetheless, it was clear from the first that this straightforward model was an oversimplification. Holzbach and colleagues[371] and others[160, 372, 373] found that a large fraction of normal individuals have gallbladder bile that by the criteria of Admirand and Small[7] is supersaturated with cholesterol; nonetheless, no cholesterol crystals were observed in the bile of these patients, even after days to weeks. This indicated either that the *thermodynamic* limits of micellar cholesterol solubility were different from those originally proposed (either because of technical problems with determination of these limits or because of confounding effects of other biliary components such as bilirubin, mucus, and proteins) or that the *kinetics* of precipitation were extremely slow. Subsequent studies suggested that both are true.

An even more striking observation was the finding that the concentration of cholesterol in human hepatic bile almost always exceeds the limits of solubility in micelles, even in normal individuals (Fig. 57–5).[8] This reflects the fact that hepatic bile is relatively dilute (total lipid concentration approximately 2 g/dl). The solubilities of cholesterol and lecithin in mixed micelles increase dramatically as water is removed from the system.[8, 374] Thus, removal of water in the gallbladder (to concentrations averaging 10 g/dl) markedly enhances the solubility of cholesterol in micelles. The concentrating function of the gallbladder therefore traditionally has been viewed as a mechanism by which cholesterol stone formation is prevented.[8, 13]

In 1978, 10 years after the original paper of Admirand and Small, Carey and Small[8] re-evaluated the maximum solubility of cholesterol as micelles in model systems of lecithin, bile salt, and water. They found that when supersaturated solutions were prepared by heating with excess cholesterol and then cooled, there was a region just above the thermodynamic saturation boundary in which precipitation of cholesterol crystals was very slow, requiring hours to days. They referred to such slowly equilibrating supersaturated solutions as *metastable*. However, they noted that hepatic and gallbladder bile of many normal human subjects had cholesterol concentrations in excess even of the metastable limit as calculated from model solutions, but nonetheless cholesterol crystals failed to form. Carey and Small[8] concluded that additional factors in bile must inhibit nucleation of cholesterol crystals to enhance metastability of supersaturated bile. The existence of such nucleation factors soon was graphically demonstrated by Holan et al.[20] The role of nucleating and anti-nucleating factors has now become a major area of gallstone research. Factors involved in cholesterol crystal nucleation are discussed more extensively in a subsequent section.

NON-MICELLAR CARRIERS OF CHOLESTEROL IN BILE

Many of the paradoxical and puzzling findings cited in the preceding sections may have been resolved recently with a major conceptual advance in the field of biliary lipids: namely, the discovery that micelles are not the only major cholesterol carrier in normal bile.[375] Although large (up to 5 microns) liquid crystals have long been recognized in bile,[276] until just a few years ago it was generally believed that the only quantitatively important lipid aggregates in bile were lecithin-cholesterol-bile salt micelles.[183] This view underwent drastic revision with the finding by Somjen and Gilat[376, 377] of small (70–100 nm) unilamellar vesicles in bile. This finding has since been confirmed by several groups[182, 275, 365, 370, 378–385] using a variety of complementary methods.

The concept that vesicles are important carriers of cholesterol in normal bile initially met with skepticism because the existence of vesicles was thought to be incompatible with predictions from physicochemical studies of model bile solutions. Indeed, Admirand and Small's studies[7] suggested that, in human gallbladder bile at equilibrium, the only phases present should be micelles and, in gallstone patients, cholesterol crystals. However, there was an implicit assumption in this formulation that equilibrium conditions were relevant. The demonstration of metastable cholesterol saturation made it clear that at least in some circumstances this assumption was incorrect. Vesicles are abundant in hepatic bile of all species studied to date, and, as discussed above, it is probable that exocytic secretion of phospholipid-cholesterol vesicles by the canalicular membrane of the hepatocyte is a major mode of entry of phospholipid and cholesterol into bile.[17, 28, 183, 382] It is generally presumed that canalicular bile is relatively dilute compared to gallbladder bile, and in dilute or bile salt–poor solutions, vesicles are relatively stable. In most species, however, vesicles normally are transitory. In species such as rat or dog, whose rates of secretion of cholesterol and phospholipid secretion are low relative to bile acids, vesicles are found in newly secreted hepatic bile but dissolve completely into mixed micelles within 30 minutes.[17, 386] The rate of dissolution is enhanced by concentration of bile in the gallbladder.

Human bile differs from that of most other species in having a high concentration of cholesterol and phospholipid relative to bile salts.[2] Because of this, it appears that vesicles in human bile do not always dissolve completely, even in the gallbladder. Instead, they may undergo remodeling (Fig. 57–6). In model bile with lipid composition simulating human bile, addition of modest micellar concentrations of bile salts to cholesterol:phospholipid vesicles initially leads to rapid dissolution of some vesicles to form mixed micelles.[28, 381, 386] Because micelles solubilize phospholipid much more effectively than they do cholesterol,[17, 183] the remaining vesicles rapidly become enriched with cholesterol. As a consequence, new or remodeled unilamellar vesicles may appear and may evolve via fusion into larger, multilamellar vesicles (liquid crystals) (Fig. 57–7).[17, 27, 28, 183] The new or remodeled vesicles and liquid crystals that form under these circumstances differ substantially in composition from the original secretory vesicle, in that they contain as high as a 2:1 molar ratio of cholesterol to phospholipid. These cholesterol-rich multilamellar vesicles probably are identical to the liquid crystals initially described by Holzbach and colleagues in biles of humans or cholesterol-fed prairie dogs[276, 387] and may also be related to novel lamellar structures recently described by Somjen et al.,[388] which appear to contain a major fraction of the cholesterol in human bile.

Phospholipid bilayers such as membranes and vesicles at equilibrium ordinarily can support no more than a 1:1 cholesterol-to-phospholipid ratio.[4, 275] Thus, these cholesterol-rich vesicles are unstable and eventually will lose their excess cholesterol either by transfer to less saturated vesicles or micelles or by precipitation as crystals of cholesterol monohydrate. However, experimentally this is a slow process. It appears that the metastability of cholesterol-supersaturated bile is a consequence of the slowness with which cholesterol precipitates from these cholesterol-rich vesicles.[275, 384]

The physical chemistry of these transformations has been graphically summarized by Carey and Cohen.[17] As bile is concentrated by the gallbladder, progressive translocation of vesicular lipids into micelles occurs, and the cholesterol content of the remaining vesicles increases. Depending on the ratios of the four components, four outcomes are possible: (1) if bile salts are present in sufficient excess, all cholesterol and phospholipid may be solubilized in simple and mixed micelles; (2) if the cholesterol:phospholipid ratio of the enriched vesicles remains sufficiently low (probably less than 1), a stable two-phase system of micelles and vesicles may result; (3) if cholesterol enrichment of vesicles leads to a cholesterol:phospholipid ratio much in excess of 1, then precipitation of a third phase, cholesterol monohydrate crystals, may be favored;

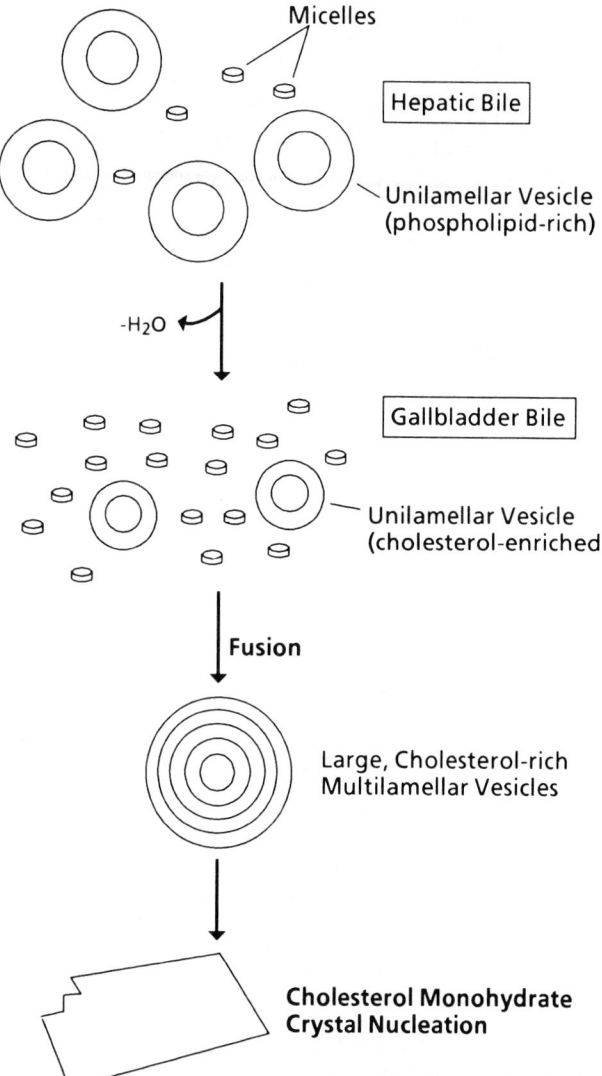

Figure 57–6. Concentration of bile leads to net transfer of phospholipid and cholesterol from vesicles to micelles. Phospholipids are transferred more efficiently than cholesterol, leading to cholesterol enrichment of the remaining (remodeled) vesicles. Aggregation of these cholesterol-rich vesicles to form multilamellar liquid crystals may be followed by precipitation of excess cholesterol as solid crystals of cholesterol monohydrate.

or (4) if the system contains adequate bile salts and a relatively low ratio of phospholipid to cholesterol, the cholesterol-rich vesicles will disappear by micellar solubilization as their cholesterol nucleates, leaving behind a two-phase system of micelles and cholesterol monohydrate crystals.

If the above sequence of events is correct, then concentration of bile by the gallbladder is necessary for formation of cholesterol-rich vesicles and nucleation of cholesterol crystals. As Carey and Cahalane[389] have stated, ". . . Only in the gallbladder does supersaturated bile become truly lithogenic in the gallstone patient." This suggests that treatments that prevent the concentration of micelle-forming bile salts in the gallbladder may prevent cholesterol enrichment of vesicles and may thereby be of value in preventing or dissolving cholesterol gallstones. This novel hypothesis runs counter to previous dogma based solely on consideration of *micellar* cholesterol solubilizing capacity (which increases with increasing concentrations of micelle-forming bile salts) and offers a plethora of new possibilities for medical therapy of gallstones. One practical example of this may relate to the therapeutic benefit of hydrophilic bile salts such as ursodeoxycholate as agents for gallstone dissolution. Hydrophilic bile salts are poor micellar solubilizers of biliary cholesterol and phospholipid.[17, 341, 374, 390–393] When ursodeoxycholate-rich bile is concentrated in the gallbladder, there is less cholesterol enrichment of vesicles, the liquid crystalline vesicular phase is stabilized, and precipitation of cholesterol crystals is inhibited. Corrigan et al.[394] and Carey and colleagues[390, 395–397] have demonstrated that ursodeoxycholate enrichment of bile prevents cholesterol crystallization, promotes liquid crystal formation, and enhances transfer of cholesterol from solid crystalline (gallstone) to liquid crystalline aggregates; the same may also be true for other hydrophilic bile salts.[398] The mechanisms by which ursodeoxycholate contributes to gallstone dissolution are discussed in a subsequent section.

NUCLEATION AND CRYSTAL GROWTH

HOMOGENEOUS AND HETEROGENEOUS NUCLEATION

Nucleation involves the aggregation of molecules into a critical cluster. When the aggregation rate exceeds the dissociation rate,[399] nucleation occurs. Two types of nucleation processes are recognized: homogeneous and heterogeneous. Homogeneous nucleation refers to crystallization in the absence of foreign material; heterogeneous nucleation refers to crystallization on a foreign surface, such as a protein, a bacterium, or even a corroded copper wire.[400] The occurrence of homogeneous nucleation generally requires a very high degree of supersaturation; many critical clusters form spontaneously and simultaneously, resulting in large numbers of small crystals. Heterogeneous nucleation, on the other hand, occurs at lower saturation indices and involves larger particles with relatively large surface areas. Homogeneous nucleation of cholesterol has been described in model bile solutions.[24] Small[130] has noted that, since very high degrees of cholesterol supersaturation (> 300 per cent) are required for homogeneous nucleation, it is highly likely that nucleation of cholesterol in bile is a heterogeneous process. Similar considerations appear to apply to calcium nucleation. At present, therefore, it seems likely that gallstones result from *heterogeneous nucleation processes* (for both cholesterol and calcium), followed by crystal growth on retained nuclei.

EVENTS IN NUCLEATION OF CHOLESTEROL

Holzbach and Halpern and their colleagues,[28, 182, 385] in recent elegant studies using video-enhanced differential contrast microscopy[401] in native bile and model bile solutions, have presented convincing evidence that vesicle aggregation is a key precursor to cholesterol nucleation. The following sequence was observed in supersaturated human bile: First, small unilamellar vesicles (70–100 nm) formed de novo, followed by the appearance of vesicle aggregates up to about 5000 nm in diameter. Aggregates enlarged and fused to form multivesicular and multilamellar liquid crystalline agglomerates that had a globular appearance with characteristic "Maltese cross" birefringence by polarized microscopy.[276] This was followed by the appearance of cholesterol monohydrate crystals within fields of clustered vesicles. The order of events and the association of solid

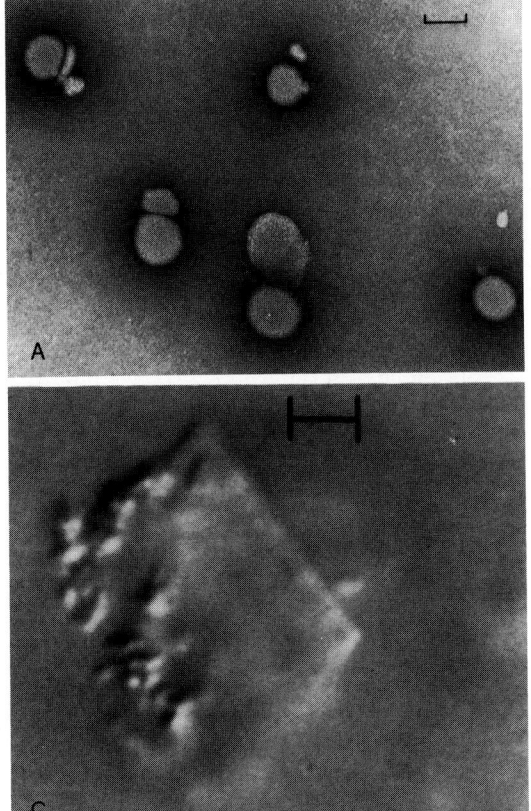
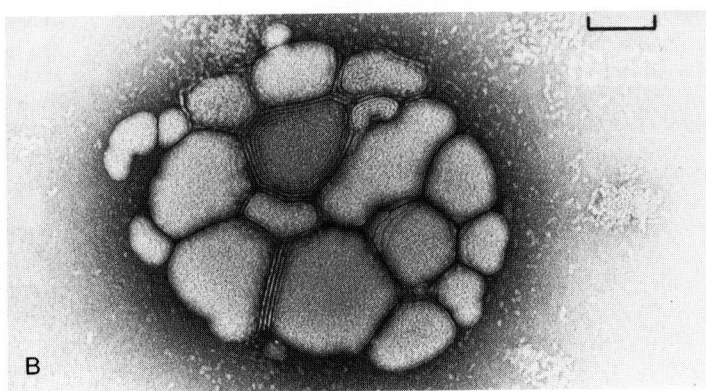

Figure 57–7. *A* and *B*, Electron micrographs of human bile showing unilamellar vesicles (*A*) and an aggregate of multilamellar vesicles (*B*). *C*, Video-enhanced contrast–differential interference contrast microscopic image of cholesterol-supersaturated gallbladder bile showing clustered vesicles on the surface of an emerging crystal of cholesterol monohydrate (bar = 2500 nm). (Photos courtesy of Dr. R. T. Holzbach; from Halpern Z, et al. Gastroenterology 90:875, 1986, with permission.)

cholesterol crystals with fields of clustered vesicles strongly suggest that cholesterol nucleation occurs from aggregated vesicles. The possibility was noted that vesicles may serve as a surface for nucleation as well as a source of cholesterol for the nucleation process. Harvey et al.[402] have recently shown that cholesterol nucleates from vesicular fractions, whereas nucleation from micellar fractions was slow or did not occur at all. Lee et al.[403] have demonstrated that further crystal growth occurs from unilamellar vesicles supersaturated with cholesterol, but not from micelles.

If cholesterol nucleation involves vesicle fusion and occurs by a heterogeneous process, two questions immediately arise: (1) What causes vesicles to fuse (aggregate)? and (2) What is the foreign surface on which nucleation occurs? Vesicle fusion is thermodynamically favored but ordinarily is a slow process. Whereas a number of proteins and proteolytic cleavage products have been found to be "fusogenic,"[183] of particular interest is the finding by Kibe et al.[182] that free Ca^{2+} ions, at concentrations encountered in bile, are fusogenic and promote nucleation of cholesterol monohydrate crystals in vesicle-containing model bile solutions composed of cholesterol, egg lecithin, and taurocholate. Ca^{2+} ions also have been shown to induce fusion of pure phospholipid vesicles.[404] Regarding the second question, since cholesterol nucleation occurs in the mucin gel in various animal models of sludge and stones, and in human sludge, a strong case can be made for mucin as a nucleating protein. This view has been expressed by Lamont,[75, 132] and Smith and Lamont.[128, 405] Mucin glycoproteins have been found to accelerate cholesterol nucleation in model bile solutions[406, 407] and in human bile.[408] Mucin contains hydrophobic domains that can bind both lipids and bilirubin,[407, 409, 410] and hydrophilic domains that can bind calcium.[186] These properties make mucin a strong candidate as a nucleating protein. However, binding alone is not equivalent to nucleation. Many proteins bind calcium, for example, but do not promote nucleation; indeed, some have anti-nucleating properties. While vesicles may have, in and of themselves, surfaces suitable for cholesterol nucleation, this does not explain why all cholesterol stones contain calcium and pigment in their centers.

It has been proposed[32, 40, 62, 70, 130, 174–176, 194, 411] that calcium salts may serve as a nidus (foreign surface) for cholesterol crystallization from bile. This hypothesis considers cholesterol nucleation to involve two steps: (1) nucleation of calcium salts (mainly calcium bilirubinate and $CaCO_3$) to form a nidus; and (2) nucleation of cholesterol monohydrate and subsequent crystal growth on this nidus. According to this view, gallstone formation is another example of biomineralization with calcium salts, consistent with the paradigm of gallstones as a spectrum of calcium-containing rocks. In this scheme, mucin is visualized as the large matrix or scaffolding protein in which the nucleation reactions occur. It does not, however, exclude mucus as a nucleating protein, particularly since some biomineralization processes appear to be "matrix-mediated."[412–414] Mucin-induced precipitation of $CaCO_3$ has been described.[162, 415] On the other hand, it is possible that mucin serves *only* as a matrix protein, in which calcium salt nucleation occurs on relatively small, acidic "regulatory proteins" similar to phosphophoryns in the dentin of teeth.[414, 416, 417] These regulatory proteins bind to large, structural (matrix) proteins.

It is well recognized that calcium salts can serve as a nidus for cholesterol nucleation and crystal growth[264, 418, 419] and that cholesterol can serve as a suitable surface for calcium nucleation. (As noted above, surface calcification of cholesterol stones is frequently observed.) Thus, Craven[264] has noted that, with the intervention of a transition layer of hydrogen-bonded water molecules, a microcrystal of either substance (i.e., calcium or cholesterol) may serve as a nucleus for growth of the other. It is apparent that much work remains to be done on nucleation reactions in mucin matrix gels before we will understand the conception of a gallstone.

PRO-NUCLEATING AND ANTI-NUCLEATING FACTORS

In a landmark study in 1979, Holan et al.[20] found that the appearance of cholesterol monohydrate crystals in bile is greatly accelerated in patients with cholesterol gallstones, compared with control patients without stones (Fig. 57–8). By defining "nucleation time" as the time required for microscopically visible cholesterol crystals to appear, a clear separation of patients with and without stones was obtained, with nucleation times of 3 days and 15 days, respectively. These findings were soon confirmed in other laboratories.[266, 420] At present, cholesterol nucleation times provide the sharpest discrimination available for distinguishing bile samples from gallstone patients from those without stones.

Subsequent studies have shown that samples of gallbladder bile from patients with cholesterol stones contain potent nucleating proteins.[22, 408, 421, 422] The nucleation-promoting factor was heat-labile and passed an ultrafiltration membrane with a nominal cut-off of 300 kd.[408] A pro-nucleating glycoprotein (130 kd) has also been found in human T-tube bile.[423] Although mucin is known to accelerate cholesterol nucleation (see above), the accelerated nucleation times observed in patients with cholesterol stones do not appear to be due to mucin, since similarly accelerated values persisted after removal of all mucin from bile.[408] In recent studies by Harvey et al.,[424] cholesterol nucleation times were not related to mucin concentrations in gallbladder bile, and it appears unlikely that mucin is responsible for the rapid in vitro nucleation times observed in bile from patients with cholesterol gallstones.[424, 425]

At present, it is not clear whether the rapid cholesterol nucleation times observed in bile samples from patients with cholesterol gallstones are due to the presence of pro-nucleating factors or to deficiency in anti-nucleating factors,

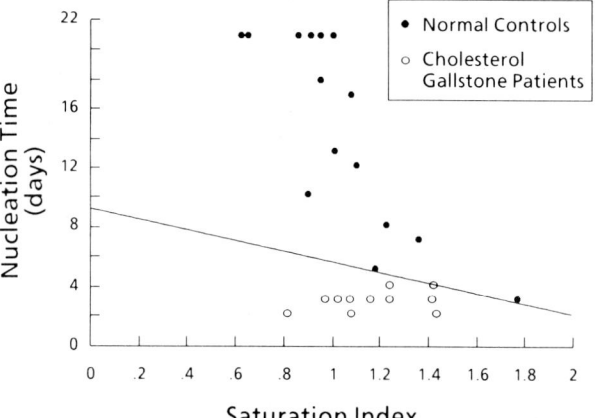

Figure 57–8. The time required for cholesterol crystals to nucleate from gallbladder bile (nucleation time) discriminates more clearly between normal individuals and those with cholesterol gallstones than does the cholesterol saturation index. The solid line indicates the discriminant function that provides the best separation between the two groups. (Modified from Holan KR et al. Gastroenterology 77:611, 1979, with permission.)

or to both of these. The presence of anti-nucleating proteins in normal bile has recently been demonstrated by Kibe et al.,[426] who found that apolipoproteins A-1 and A-2, at concentrations encountered in human bile, markedly prolong nucleation of cholesterol monohydrate crystals when added to supersaturated model bile solutions. Apolipoprotein A-3 and other serum proteins did not show this effect. As noted by Holzbach,[183] further studies are needed to determine the nature, origin, and secretory physiology of both pro- and anti-nucleating factors in bile. In a proposed scheme for cholesterol stone formation (see below), we will consider the pro-nucleating/anti-nucleating *ratio* to be the critical factor, without specifying whether it involves an increase in numerator, decrease in denominator, or both of these.[427]

For calcium, it is equally clear that there are substances in bile, almost certainly proteins, with potent anti-nucleating properties for both calcium phosphate[428] and carbonate.[227, 429, 430] Indeed, such anti-nucleating proteins have been described in many biologic systems involving stone formation or biomineralization processes, including urine,[431–437] saliva,[417, 438–441] pancreas,[442–449] bone,[450] coccoliths,[451] and mollusk shells.[452] Such anti-nucleating proteins are generally small and acidic. It is therefore noteworthy that Shimizu et al.[453] have recently isolated a 12-kd acidic protein from human cholesterol gallstones, which was also present in bile and which inhibited precipitation of $CaCO_3$. In view of the marked metastability observed with $CaCO_3$ (above), it seems clear that anti-nucleating proteins normally play a critical role in preventing calcium nucleation and/or crystal growth in bile, just as they do in other biologic systems.

The molecular mechanisms, conformational states, and so forth that impart anti-nucleating properties remain undefined. Of particular interest are "antifreeze" peptides and glycopeptides in cold-water fishes. These peptides appear to prevent growth of ice crystals by a process of adsorption of the peptide to an existing ice crystal to form a lattice match between polar (OH and COOH) groups on the peptide and oxygens in the ice lattice.[454] It seems likely that "anti-nucleating" proteins in bile may, in fact, be inhibitors of crystal growth by a process of adsorption to existing nuclei; whether this involves such an elegantly structured arrangement as that of antifreeze peptides remains to be seen. Thus, at present, the term "anti-nucleating" is operationally defined, since most nuclei are too small to be seen with existing instruments. If adsorption to existing crystals proves to be the mechanism of action in bile, then a revision of the term "anti-nucleating" will be required, since what will be meant is "anti–crystal growth" factors. At present, the terms *crystallizing* and *anti-crystallizing*, rather than *nucleating* and *anti-nucleating* may be more rigorously correct. Nucleation and crystal growth should be clearly distinguished, if possible, because they may involve different factors and mechanisms. Thus, nucleation of cholesterol and calcium probably occurs in rather tightly constrained regions involving specific domains of nucleating proteins, whereas inhibition of crystal growth may be more nonspecific, involving relatively large hydrophobic and/or hydrophilic domains of adsorbed proteins and peptides.

With the exception of apolipoproteins A-1 and A-2 (noted above), the nature of nucleating and anti-nucleating proteins and their modes of entry into bile are unknown. There are many questions: for example, are such proteins normally present in bile, or do they represent proteolytic cleavage products? If they are intact proteins that are present normally, what causes an imbalance between pro-nucleating and anti-nucleating factors? If they are proteolytic cleavage products, what produces such cleavage? Are these proteins secreted by the liver, the bile ducts, the gallbladder, or all of these? What is the physiology (or pathophysiology) of this secretion? What is the surface charge (zeta potential) on vesicles and how do they enter a negatively charged gel? What are the time-constants for cholesterol and calcium nucleation, and how do they relate to the degree of supersaturation at the locus of nucleation? These and many other questions require future study. It is anticipated that, in the next few years, important new insights will emerge regarding the chemistry and physiology of vesicles (formation, translocation into bile, aggregation, relative role in cholesterol transport, etc.), as well as the nucleation of both cholesterol and calcium in bile.

GALLSTONE GROWTH

While precipitation of crystals is a necessary step in the development of gallstones, it may not be sufficient. For gallstones to cause clinical symptoms, they must attain a size sufficient to produce mechanical injury to the gallbladder or obstruction of the biliary tree at the level of the cystic duct or the papilla of Vater. Growth of stones may occur in two ways: (1) progressive enlargement of individual crystals or stones by deposition of additional insoluble precipitate at the bile/stone interface, or (2) fusion of individual crystals or stones to form a larger agglomerate. There is evidence that both patterns of growth contribute to enlargement of gallstones.[108, 118, 455]

A striking feature of gallstones is the relative homogeneity of the type of stone found in a given gallbladder. In the majority of cases, a gallbladder containing cholesterol stones will contain no pigment stones, and a gallbladder containing pigment stones will contain no cholesterol stones. Yet hundreds of stones may be present in a given gallbladder. This not only suggests that cholesterol and pigment stones have fundamentally different mechanisms of pathogenesis, but also suggests that nuclei form in "litters"—that is, at multiple sites in the mucin matrix gel. This has been well documented in animal models of stones and sludge, as noted above. One does not find a pigment stone in a cholesterol stone litter. The situation may be analogous to hail formation in a cloud. Depending on factors within the cloud (moisture content, temperature, updrafts, etc.) most of the hail falls to the ground. This is equivalent to the emptying of mucus, containing crystals and nascent stones, from the gallbladder. Residual nuclei may remain in the cloud, or gallbladder, and serve as seeds on which subsequent crystal deposition occurs. In many systems, it is well recognized that precipitation from supersaturated solutions occurs preferentially on existing nuclei, so that only one or many stones may develop, depending on the number of residual nuclei. Once stones are present, they will grow preferentially, so that it may be impossible for a new litter of stones to develop even if a supersaturated state is sustained.[11, 456, 457] Does recurrence represent new nuclei, or is it a result of new crystal growth on old residual seeds? This interesting question merits further study and has relevance to the problem of gallstone recurrence.

THE ROLE OF THE GALLBLADDER

The gallbladder has three types of functions: absorptive, secretory, and motor. All are of importance in the pathogenesis of gallstones.

ABSORPTIVE FUNCTIONS

Active Na-Cl transport by the gallbladder epithelium is the driving force for the concentration of bile.[458-463] Water is passively absorbed in response to the osmotic force generated by solute absorption. In fully concentrated bile, the total bile salt concentration may exceed 300 mM in both humans and dogs. In this process, the concentrations of various monomeric bile salts remain essentially constant at their critical micellar concentrations; the increase in bile salts (BS) reflects a corresponding increase in the micellar fraction, so that gallbladder contents remain isosmotic with plasma. In addition to absorption of Na^+, Cl^-, and H_2O, absorption of calcium from canine gallbladder has recently been demonstrated.[464] It is suggested that as much as 50 to 80 per cent of calcium presented to the gallbladder from duct bile may be reabsorbed. This may play an important role in maintaining free $[Ca^{2+}]$ at relatively low levels, thus increasing calcium salt solubility in gallbladder bile.[465]

Concentration of bile affects both calcium and cholesterol solubilities. Thus, as noted above, free $[Ca^{2+}]$ increases in proportion to [BS]. This would lead to a corresponding decrease in calcium salt solubilities, were it not for the fact that pH declines (see below). For cholesterol, solubility in the micellar fraction is increased,[8, 466] but the stability of phospholipid-cholesterol vesicles is greatly decreased[28, 183] by concentration of bile. Since nucleation appears to occur by vesicular rather than micellar mechanisms, the net effect of bile concentration is an increased tendency to nucleate cholesterol. Support for vesicular-mediated nucleation lies in the fact that gallstones tend to develop in the gallbladder, where bile salt concentrations are maximal (i.e., where micellar solubilization of cholesterol tends to be maximal). In recent studies in our laboratory, concentrating ability (as assessed by bile salt concentrations) in patients with gallstones was similar to that observed in patients without stones,[467] so that no defect in micellar solubilization could be predicted on the basis of concentrations of available micellar bile salt. The effects of bile concentration on cholesterol solubility are complicated by the fact that biliary lipid composition may change in the gallbladder, owing to reabsorption of cholesterol, phospholipid, fatty acids,[468-470] and perhaps bile salts,[471] particularly if there is mucosal injury.[472] In addition, as noted by Cussler et al.,[473] there may be inhomogeneities in composition near the epithelial surface, owing to water flux. Clearly, more information on vesicle aggregation and cholesterol nucleation in the microenvironment of the mucus gel is needed.

Although the contents of the gallbladder are thought of as a homogeneous mixture, this is a gross simplification. Radiologists frequently observe a thin layer of floating gallstones at oral cholecystography, indicating that a stable density gradient may be maintained within the fasting gallbladder, at least in the presence of iopanoic acid. Thureborn[474] and others[475-477] have indicated that physical stratification of the lipid components of bile may occur normally within the gallbladder. The importance of these inhomogeneities in the pathogenesis of gallstones is unknown.

SECRETORY FUNCTIONS

The gallbladder epithelial cell exports at least two important products to the lumen: glycoproteins and H^+ ions. The secretion of mucin glycoproteins was considered in a previous section (see Mucus—Chemistry and Physiology). It is not known whether the gallbladder also secretes other proteins having nucleating and/or anti-nucleating properties, but this seems highly likely.

Acidification of bile by the gallbladder has been recognized for over 70 years. In 1924, Drury et al. wrote:[478] "To our surprise, (canine) bladder bile proved frankly acid to litmus in a large proportion of instances, whereas liver bile was nearly always somewhat alkaline, and usually markedly so. The literature showed that the difference had already been noticed by Okada[479] for the dog (in 1915), and by Neilson and Meyer[480] for the rabbit." Until recently, it was generally held that this acidification was due to reabsorption of bicarbonate ions.[461, 462] In the past few years, however, it has become apparent that the gallbladder epithelium secretes H^+ ions, apparently by apical Na^+/H^+ exchange,[481–483] and that this may be the major mechanism of bile acidification. Evidence for H^+ secretion now exists in at least five species: *Necturus*,[481, 482] rabbits,[484–488] guinea pigs,[483, 487] dogs,[489] and humans.[490, 491]

Of these five species, only human beings have a substantial incidence of gallstones. In view of the adverse effects of alkaline bile on calcium solubility, this suggests that acidification may be defective in patients with gallstones. Recent studies indicate that this is the case; bile pH was found to be significantly elevated in 38 of 40 patients with all types of gallstones.[492] The defect appeared to be selective, since concentrating ability in these same patients was intact.[467] As a result of the acidification defect, concentrations of $[HCO_3^-]$ and $[CO_3^{2-}]$ in the bile remained significantly elevated, so that 82 per cent of gallstone-containing biles were supersaturated with $CaCO_3$, whereas none of 13 control patients had supersaturated biles.[204] These studies, which require confirmation, provide a thermodynamic basis for the frequently observed surface calcification of cholesterol stones.

It was believed that the observed defect in acidification was due to excessive buffering of secreted H^+ ions, most likely by mucin glycoproteins.[491] If so, this would represent a heretofore unrecognized and highly undesirable effect of mucin hypersecretion—buffering of secreted H^+ ions, resulting in relative alkalinization of bile and in highly significant reduction in calcium carbonate and calcium bilirubinate solubilities. Such alkalinization in the mucus gel might promote calcium salt nucleation.

MOTOR FUNCTION

Gallbladder motility, as a factor in the pathogenesis of gallstones, has been studied for decades, and it now seems clear that there are multiple, complex, and variable effects on biliary lipid composition and cholesterol solubility. A consideration of these is beyond our scope here (see refs. 493–495 for reviews). All investigators would probably agree that residence time in the gallbladder is a key factor in gallstone pathogenesis. It is a key factor on a priori grounds, as noted in Figure 57–1. Thus, cholesterol and/or calcium nuclei must be retained in the gallbladder in order for crystal growth to occur. At some point in the growth process, the developing stone becomes sufficiently large that it can no longer be evacuated through the cystic duct. The time interval between nucleation and some undefined level of maturity of the stone constitutes a "window" in which proper emptying is crucial. In terms of gallstone pathogenesis, therefore, the question is not whether gallbladder emptying is impaired in patients with gallstones, but whether it is impaired *before* the development of stones

or during the window of time. In at least two animal models of gallstone disease, it is clear that defects in gallbladder emptying precede development of stones. Thus, in 1977, Gurll et al.[496] noted gallbladder stasis in prairie dogs prior to the appearance of stones. In subsequent studies by Pitt et al.[497] and Doty and colleagues,[498] the defect appeared to result from increased resistance at the level of the cystic duct; gallbladder compliance was normal. The increase in cystic duct resistance appeared to be due to agglomerates of mucus and cholesterol crystals, which blocked outflow.[166] Administration of cholecystokinin octapeptide prevented gallbladder stasis and reduced the incidence of gallstones by 50 per cent. In other studies, the increases in cystic duct resistance, stasis, and gallstones were prevented by salicylate administration[499] or by periodic emptying of the gallbladder.[500]

More recently, Li et al.[167] have reported that muscle contractility in the gallbladder of the prairie dog is decreased prior to the development of stones. Similarly, in studies of both prairie dogs and Richardson ground squirrels, Fridhandler et al.[116] have found that isometric tensions of in vitro gallbladder muscle, in response to cholecystokinin and other stimuli, were significantly reduced in cholesterol-fed animals prior to appearance of stones; the magnitude of the defect increased with stone development. Thus, in rodents at least, there appear to be defects in gallbladder muscle contractility prior to the development of stones. This defect is apparently compounded by the presence of viscous agglomerates of mucin and cholesterol, which physically impede outflow.

Defective emptying of the gallbladder during prolonged fasting is believed to reflect decreased stimulation by cholecystokinin.[501–505] TPN appears to be associated with an increased incidence of acalculous cholecystitis, sludge, and gallstones,[504–509] and the importance of gallbladder stasis in the generation of biliary sludge, particularly in patients receiving TPN, has been emphasized by several investigators.[125, 126, 166, 495, 498, 502, 506, 510–517] The problem with TPN is complicated by the fact that it may also produce cholestasis and other liver abnormalities,[518–526] including alteration in the composition of biliary lipids.[527] Nevertheless, there is no doubt that defective emptying of the gallbladder is important in the generation of biliary sludge, as noted by Holzbach.[495] Brugge et al.[513] have reported that gallbladder emptying in patients with cholesterol crystals in bile was only about one half that seen in patients without crystals. Thus, in both man and animals, stasis of gallbladder contents appears to play a major role in the pathogenesis of gallstones. The mechanism of the motor defects remains undefined; further work is needed, both in vitro and in vivo. It is of interest that patients with somatostatinomas appear to have a high incidence of gallstones; somatostatin is a potent inhibitor of gallbladder emptying in man.[528]

Beginning at puberty, the incidence of gallstones in females is more than twice that in males,[529, 530] and the incidence of gallstones is increased in pregnancy.[292, 306, 308, 531, 532] In view of these facts, the effects of estrogens on gallbladder motility have long been of interest. In 1927, Mann and Higgins[533] noted defective gallbladder emptying in pregnant dogs, gophers, and guinea pigs; defective emptying in human pregnancy is now well recognized.[308, 532, 534] With the use of contraceptive steroids, which are believed by many[306, 308, 532, 534] but not all investigators[305, 535] to increase the incidence of gallstones, no alterations in gallbladder motility have been found.[532, 534] These agents, however, do have an adverse effect on biliary lipid composition.[306, 307]

In the absence of pregnancy, studies of gallbladder

motility in patients with gallstones have yielded conflicting results. In some studies, impaired emptying has been noted,[536-538] whereas in others it has not.[454, 539-542] Pomeranz and Shaffer[543] have noted defective emptying following cholecystokinin administration in a subgroup of patients with gallstones (43 per cent of total patients studied). This observation is similar to that noted by Roslyn et al.[514] in the prairie dog and by Zhu et al.[476] in in vitro studies of human gallbladder mucosal strips. It is possible that the disturbances in motor function in some patients are too subtle to be detected, although this may improve with new techniques.[544, 545] Lanzini et al.[546] have reported frequent alternations in absolute gallbladder storage and emptying, in which the gallbladder is more analogous to a bellows than to a pump.

We believe that thinking should be directed toward the concept of *chemical stasis* (i.e., stasis in the mucin gel overlying the mucosa), since this gel appears to be the locus of nucleation and growth of a stone. Emptying of bulk phase contents may have little relation to emptying of this gel. Mucus does not easily drain through a small aperture. It may require a vigorous "squeeze" by the gallbladder to accomplish effective emptying of mucus, particularly since it may often require the overcoming of gravity. A gallbladder containing mature, trapped stones would not appear to be an ideal setting for study of this problem, although the presence of stones per se has been found to decrease contractility only about 20 per cent in guinea pig.[547] For mucus retention, it seems reasonable to assume that residual volume in the gallbladder is a factor of key importance.

Finally, it should be noted that the presence of a flaccid or poorly contracting gallbladder does not necessarily mean that gallstones will develop. In patients with celiac disease, for example, Low-Beer et al.[548, 549] have noted marked abnormalities in gallbladder motor function, yet these patients do not appear to have an increased risk of gallstones. Also, although the incidence of gallstones increases with age,[529, 530] aging appears to have little effect on the kinetics of gallbladder emptying.[550, 551] These findings emphasize the importance of considering gallstones as requiring a cascade, or constellation, of events in their formation.

MODEL OF PRESENT CONCEPTS OF GALLSTONE PATHOGENESIS

The constellation of factors that seem to be necessary for formation of cholesterol gallstones is illustrated in Figure 57–9. Mucus hypersecretion is listed first, but this does not necessarily have a temporal connotation; supersaturation of bile with cholesterol may precede mucus hypersecretion. Beyond this point, however, there is a temporal cascade of events. In the presence of a metastable (supersaturated) state, concentration of bile by the gallbladder is believed to produce a more or less progressive instability of phospholipid-cholesterol vesicles. If there is an increase in the ratios of pro-nucleating/anti-nucleating factors, or of pro-fusion/anti-fusion factors for vesicles, then vesicles aggregate and thermodynamic instability increases. This is followed by nucleation of cholesterol monohydrate crystals. If the nucleation occurs by a heterogeneous process, a suitable surface is required. Precisely what surfaces may be involved remains speculative; candidate surfaces are calcium salts (crystalline or possibly anhydrous), mucin matrix protein, specific nucleating proteins, and the surface of vesicles. As yet, however, possible homogeneous nucleation of cholesterol has not been rigorously excluded.

Following nucleation, cholesterol monohydrate crystals remain embedded in the mucin matrix gel, along with calcium bilirubinate (± calcium carbonate). If bile remains supersaturated with cholesterol (persistently or perhaps intermittently), and if nuclei are retained in the gallbladder, the result is progressive crystal growth and gallstone formation. Note that thermodynamic factors, kinetic factors, and time (stasis) are all involved, as was noted in Figure 57–1.

An analogous diagram can be constructed for the formation of calcium salt ("pigment") stones. It is not known whether vesicles are involved in calcium salt nucleation, but it is possible. Based on studies of other biologic systems, nucleation of calcium salts likely occurs on specific small, acidic,"regulatory" proteins, as discussed above.

THERAPEUTIC DISSOLUTION OF GALLSTONES

From 1880, when Langenbuch performed the first cholecystectomy,[552] until the advent of chenodeoxycholic acid therapy in the 1970s, gallbladder removal was considered the only effective treatment for gallstones. Because cholecystectomy was curative and safe, there was little impetus to study mechanisms of gallstone formation and to search for other modalities of therapy. Gallstones were treated as a straightforward surgical problem, and scientific investigation of their pathogenesis languished. Nonetheless, the possibility that gallstones might be amenable to medical dissolution had been suggested as early as 1896, when Naunyn[553] observed that human cholesterol gallstones surgically inserted into the gallbladder of a dog (a species whose bile is unsaturated with cholesterol) frequently dissolved within weeks to months. When the relationship between bile salts, phospholipids, and cholesterol in bile was clarified, it became possible to propose rational medical approaches to dissolve gallstones.

Although in principle all kinds of gallstones should be amenable to dissolution, most of the discussion that follows deals with cholesterol gallstones. To date, no effective medical therapy exists for calcium gallstones. Therapy of gallstones via extracorporeal shock wave lithotripsy (Chap. 61) or via endoscopic or percutaneous extraction (Chap. 60) will not be reviewed here.

PRINCIPLES OF GALLSTONE DISSOLUTION

Thermodynamic considerations dictate that stones cannot dissolve unless the surrounding medium is capable of solubilizing their crystalline components. Thus, *desaturation of bile is a prerequisite for dissolution of gallstones.* Desaturation may be achieved by enhancing solubilizing factors (e.g., bile salts and/or phospholipid, monooctanoin, or methyl tert-butyl ether for cholesterol stones; calcium chelators for calcium stones) or by reducing the concentration of the crystallizing components (cholesterol, calcium, and/or calcium-sensitive anions) in bile. The rate at which stones dissolve depend on the degree of unsaturation of bile, and also on a variety of kinetic factors, such as stirring of the bile and surface:volume ratio of the stones, which are very different from the kinetic factors involved in stone formation. Once stones have dissolved, their recurrence may be prevented by the thermodynamic approach of maintaining desaturated bile; alternatively, manipulation of kinetic factors, time factors, or the mucin gel matrix may

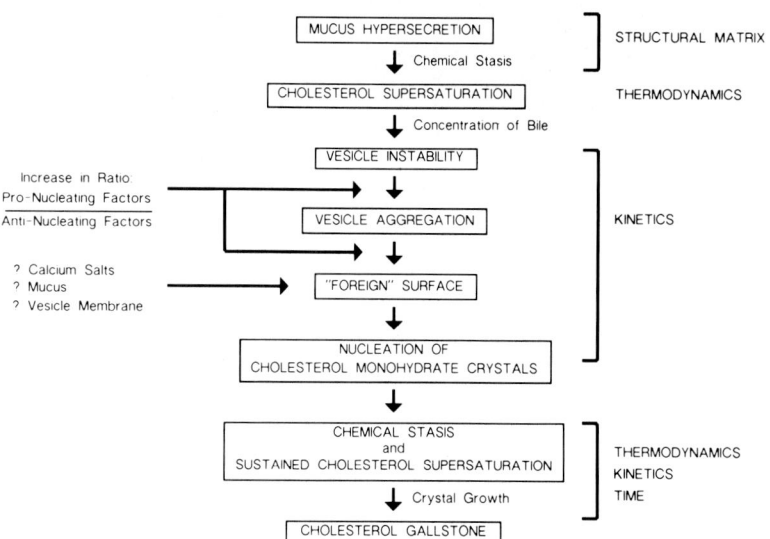

Figure 57–9. Summary of the constellation of factors required for formation of cholesterol gallstones (see text for discussion).

suffice to prevent stone recurrence even if bile should again become supersaturated.

Carey and associates[554] and others have published several important studies identifying a multitude of kinetic factors of importance in gallstone dissolution by bile acids.[390, 394, 396, 397, 555–560] The factors involved in the process of crystal dissolution are described by the Noyes-Nernst equation:[561, 562]

$$r = KA \, \Delta \, C_1$$

where "r" represents the dissolution rate (mass of crystalline substance dissolved per unit of time); K is a dissolution rate constant (mass transfer coefficient), A is the surface area of interface between the solid phase cholesterol and the solution, and ΔC_1 is the difference between the maximal solubility and actual concentration of the crystal-forming substance in the solution. It is apparent that the dissolution rate will be rapid if factors on the right side of the equation are large.

Removal of cholesterol from a gallstone by a micelle involves three steps: (1) diffusion of a cholesterol-poor micelle to the aqueous:crystalline interface, (2) transfer of cholesterol from stone to micelle, and (3) diffusion of the cholesterol-enriched micelle away from the interface. The rate at which these events occur is summarized in the dissolution rate constant K, which is influenced by a number of factors. The most important of these is adequacy of mixing. In an unstirred or stagnant solution, a gradient of micellar cholesterol concentration would be expected to develop near the gallstone surface. The existence of this gradient can lead to flow currents around the gallstone, a phenomenon termed *free convection*.[397] Stagnation may be reduced or eliminated by physical mixing or "stirring." In a poorly stirred solution, the rate of dissolution appears to be limited by diffusion of micelles to and from the interface. Conversely, in a well-stirred solution, dissolution appears to be limited by events occurring at the interface.[390]

The effects of stagnation can be reduced or eliminated by stirring, shaking, or other modalities that enhance mixing. Stirring has limited application in the process of gallstone dissolution after bile acid feeding, though it may be

enhanced somewhat by manipulations that increase the frequency of gallbladder contraction. Stirring may be prevented by the mucin gel surrounding the gallstone, and suppression of mucin secretion or reduction of mucus viscosity might thereby accelerate gallstone dissolution. Stirring appears to be very important in patients treated with methyl tert-butyl ether, in whom turbulence induced by rapid infusion/withdrawal appears to be a factor affecting the rate of cholesterol solubilization.[563]

The factor ΔC_1 is influenced by any factor that affects cholesterol solubility. With regard to micellar solubility of cholesterol, this variable can be altered in a favorable direction by (1) increasing the concentration of bile salts, (2) enriching the bile salt pool with more potent micelle-forming bile salts, (3) reducing biliary cholesterol concentration, (4) increasing ionic strength, or (5) concentrating bile. Bulk phase solubility of cholesterol is minimal in water, but may be enhanced tremendously by addition of a potent cholesterol solvent such as methyl tert-butyl ether.

Under some circumstances, cholesterol also can be removed from a gallstone through formation of a *liquid crystalline phase* at the gallstone surface. This liquid crystalline phase may be the physical equivalent of the vesicular phase in bile (discussed previously), and its formation is thermodynamically favored by those conditions that favor persistence of phospholipid-rich biliary vesicles. Thus the formation of a liquid crystalline phase is favored by dilution of bile, reduction of biliary bile salt concentration, enrichment of the bile salt pool with poor micelle-forming bile salts such as ursodeoxycholate, or increase in biliary lecithin concentration.[17] At present it is not clear whether this liquid crystalline phase results from direct interaction between pre-existing vesicles and the gallstone surface or whether new bilayers form at the interface from phospholipid deposited by micelles. Once formed, liquid crystals dissociate rapidly from the gallstone and have the effect of reducing interfacial resistance to dissolution.[390, 554]

The area factor A in the Noyes-Nernst equation refers to the interfacial surface available for dissolution. For a given volume of stone, dissolution will occur more quickly if the surface area is large. Since surface is proportional to radius squared, whereas volume is proportional to radius cubed, the surface:volume ratio is much more favorable for the dissolution of multiple small stones than for a single large stone. Physical treatments that fragment stones, such as extracorporeal shock wave lithotripsy, derive their benefit at least in part from markedly increasing the surface area available for dissolution.[564, 565]

BILE ACID THERAPY OF CHOLESTEROL GALLSTONES

Scientific Basis of Bile Acid Therapy

Following the early finding that patients with gallstones exhibited a decreased bile acid pool size, Vlahcevic et al.[294] proposed that oral administration of bile acids could lead to an increase in the size of the bile acid pool and stimulate bile acid and lecithin secretion, which would improve the cholesterol solubilizing capacity of bile and might allow gallstone dissolution. In the early stages of developing strategies for medical therapy of cholesterol gallstones, it was thought that *all* bile acids might be equally effective in dissolving stones. This assumption was soon proved wrong. Thistle and Schoenfield[566] showed that administration of CDCA decreased the cholesterol saturation of bile, and Danzinger et al.[567, 568] and Thistle and Hoffman[569] demonstrated that long-term administration of CDCA expanded the CDCA pool, desaturated bile, and eventually led in some cases to gallstone dissolution. However, surprisingly, the other two major bile acids in humans—cholic and deoxycholic acids—were ineffective at reducing cholesterol saturation of bile and did not cause dissolution of cholesterol gallstones, despite the fact that both expanded the bile acid pool and both effectively dissolve cholesterol in vitro.[299, 301, 328] Measurements of the size of the bile acid pool and kinetic studies demonstrated that augmentation of the bile acid pool occurred after feeding of deoxycholic and cholic acids as well as after administration of CDCA; yet the predicted reduction of cholesterol saturation of bile occurred only after CDCA feeding.[567] In investigating the reason for these differences, a second surprising finding was noted. Despite the fact that it expanded the bile salt pool, CDCA caused a *reduction* in biliary cholesterol secretion. This appears to be the major mechanism by which CDCA decreases cholesterol saturation of bile.[326, 327, 570, 571] In contrast, cholic acid increased biliary cholesterol secretion and consequently did not change cholesterol saturation of bile in spite of marked augmentation of the size of the bile acid pool.[571]

Soon after the beneficial effects of CDCA on gallstone dissolution were recognized, Makino and Shginozaky[572] reported that ursodeoxycholic acid (UDCA), the 7β-epimer of CDCA and a major bile acid in bears, was also effective in gallstone dissolution. The administration of UDCA expanded the bile salt pool but, like CDCA, caused a reduction of biliary cholesterol secretion.[326, 327] Thus, contrary to earlier predictions, augmentation of the bile acid pool, per se, probably plays a minor role in gallstone dissolution during bile acid therapy.

The mechanisms by which these two bile acids of vastly differing physicochemical properties (CDCA is hydrophobic and a good detergent, whereas UDCA is more hydrophilic and a much poorer micelle-former) reduce biliary cholesterol secretion remain uncertain. In general, bile acids could affect hepatic cholesterol fluxes at the level of the intestines by influencing cholesterol absorption, at the level of the sinusoidal membrane by up- or down-regulating hepatic uptake of lipoprotein cholesterol, at the level of the hepatocyte by suppressing or stimulating various pathways of hepatic cholesterol metabolism (synthesis, esterification, degradation), and/or by direct effects on the mechanisms controlling secretion of cholesterol into bile.

The literature in these areas is contradictory. CDCA apparently suppresses 3-hydroxy-3-methylglutaryl coenzyme A reductase (HMG-CoA reductase) activity. It has been suggested that decreased synthesis of cholesterol may decrease cholesterol secretion into bile.[320, 573] However, several studies in rats and humans indicate that only 15 to 20 per cent of biliary cholesterol is derived from newly synthesized cholesterol.[574-576] Moreover, in elegant experiments by Turley and Dietschy[338] 1000-fold variations in the rates of cholesterol synthesis did not alter the magnitude of biliary secretion of cholesterol. Nevertheless under some circumstances, synthesis of cholesterol may be an important determinant of biliary secretion of cholesterol. For example, Kempen et al.[577] and Pandak and colleagues[578] have shown that bolus doses of HMG CoA reductase inhibitors profoundly reduce biliary cholesterol secretion in the rat. More recently, administration of HMG CoA reductase inhibitors to patients with hypercholesterolemia resulted in a significant reduction of the cholesterol saturation index of bile,[329, 330] presumably secondary to decreased secretion of cholesterol into bile. The mechanism by which UDCA reduces biliary cholesterol secretion is also not clear. In contrast to CDCA, UDCA probably does not inhibit synthesis of cholesterol or bile acids.[323, 325] However, UDCA apparently reduces intestinal absorption of cholesterol, which in turn may reduce the transport of cholesterol from the hepatocytes and into the bile.[579]

As discussed above, the mechanisms of gallstone dissolution are different for CDCA and UDCA. CDCA desaturates bile and permits transfer of cholesterol from solid crystals to micelles. In contrast, UDCA, a poorer detergent, promotes removal of cholesterol via formation of liquid crystals.[390, 394, 396] Dissolution of cholesterol gallstones after UDCA administration can take place without a significant change in cholesterol saturation of the micellar phase of bile. Thus, the cholesterol saturation index, which is determined only by the micellar cholesterol solubilizing capacity of bile, does not necessarily reflect the cholelitholytic potential of hydrophilic bile salts such as UDCA.[580]

Patient Selection

Symptoms

Because gallstone dissolution with bile acids is a slow process and is not always successful, it would be difficult to justify were it not for the fact that the natural history of gallstones is relatively benign. Gracie and Ransohoff noted in over 20 years of follow-up of a cohort of employees at the University of Michigan that clinically asymptomatic ("silent") stones caused pain or other complications requiring surgery in only 20 per cent of the subjects.[581] On a larger scale, similar conclusions were derived from two prospective studies in Italy.[582, 583] Based on these data, it appears that patients with silent stones may not require either surgical or medical therapy.

In a formal risk-benefit analysis, Ransohoff et al.[584] concluded that expectant management of gallstones is superior to cholecystectomy in patients with silent gallstones, both in terms of cost and expected morbidity/mortality. Once symptoms have occurred, recurrence of symptoms is frequent; one study of patients with symptomatic gallstones showed 32 per cent and 64 per cent recurrence of symptoms at 12 and 24 months, respectively.[585] However, life-threatening complications of cholelithiasis were rare. It is this group of intermittently symptomatic patients who should be the prime candidates for medical therapy.

Risk Factors

One of the simplest means of treating gallstones medically would be to eliminate risk factors associated with increased biliary solute saturation. A number of risk factors/diseases predisposing to cholesterol gallstones are associated with increased cholesterol saturation of bile, including female sex,[251, 582] age,[586] racial or ethnic group,[335] obesity,[302] and rapid weight loss,[587] and certain medications such as clofibrate[310] and estrogens.[304, 306] Of these, only obesity and medications are readily subject to therapeutic intervention. Even treatment of obesity poses difficulties because rapid weight loss is associated with a transient increase in cholesterol saturation, possible related to mobilization of stored cholesterol from adipose tissues.[587]

Black pigment stones are found more commonly in patients with hemolytic anemia[245] and cirrhosis.[588] The pathogenetic mechanisms are less well defined than those of cholesterol gallstones, but the triggering factors for their formation are related to increased turnover of heme leading to increased secretion of bilirubin into bile.[589]

Brown pigment stones form in patients with chronic bacterial colonization of bile. The bacteria secrete enzymes that catalyze deconjugation of bilirubin and lysis of phospholipids, leading to subsequent deposition of calcium bilirubinate and calcium palmitate. Treatment of brown pigment stones includes adequate drainage to minimize bacterial overgrowth and elimination of foreign bodies such as sutures, which provide a protected environment for bacterial proliferation.

Stone Composition

CDCA and UDCA treatments will lead to desaturation of bile with cholesterol and dissolution of cholesterol stones; however, these agents are of no demonstrated value in dissolution of calcium salts. Therefore, it is of great importance to select the appropriate patients in order to maximize the beneficial effects. Unfortunately, no single test or combination of tests can predict with absolute accuracy the presence of cholesterol gallstones. However, several useful clues are available.

1. *Radiolucency* usually, but not always, indicates cholesterol gallstones. This criterion alone will diagnose cholesterol gallstones incorrectly about 25 per cent of the time.[590, 591] More precise discrimination is obtained with computerized tomography, although this modality is less sensitive for diagnosis of small stones. Calcified gallstones sometimes can be seen on plain films of the abdomen.[591, 592] Extensive calcification of gallstones is a contraindication to therapy with bile acids.

2. *Buoyancy* (flotation) is another important discriminatory factor. Floating stones observed on oral cholecystography have been shown to be nearly pure cholesterol gallstones. With this type of stone, maximal dissolution rates of >70 per cent can be expected.[593, 594]

3. Presence of *cholesterol microcrystals* in bile, in the absence of calcium carbonate crystals, is a reasonably sensitive and specific indicator of cholesterol gallstone disease.[266] However, this approach requires duodenal intuba-

tion for bile collection.[595] It appears to offer little advantage over less invasive diagnostic methods in selection of patients for gallstone dissolution therapy.

4. Certain *stone surface characteristics* are helpful. Large stones with irregular surface or stones with calcified rims tend to resist dissolution with bile acids.[594]

Recently, a multivariate model for non-invasive assessment of gallstone composition has been developed. This model will accurately predict gallstone composition in about 90 per cent of cases.[596] Some examples of different stone types are illustrated in Figure 57–10.

Other Factors

Non-visualized gallbladder on oral cholecystography suggests chronic inflammation with poor gallbladder concentrating capability and/or poor mixing of hepatic with gallbladder bile. For that reason, gallbladder non-visualization traditionally has been a contraindication for bile acid therapy.[594] As discussed previously, it now appears that concentration of bile may actually enhance cholesterol precipitation by causing cholesterol enrichment of vesicles; thus, this contraindication may merit re-examination. If non-visualization of the gallbladder results from poor mixing of newly secreted hepatic bile with gallbladder contents, then stasis may be an important problem, and gallstone dissolution may be expected to fail for kinetic reasons.

Other factors such as the weight, number, and size of gallstones also may play a role in determining the odds for (or against) gallstone dissolution. Obese patients have been found to be resistant to gallstone dissolution with fixed doses of bile acids; however, this resistance disappears if dosage is adjusted on the basis of total body weight.[594] The time required for complete dissolution is a function of the mass of stones present in the gallbladder. In addition, as predicted from the Noyes-Nernst equation, individual large stones (diameter of 2 cm or larger) are expected to be more resistant to therapy than multiple smaller stones because the surface:volume ratio is relatively low.

Safety and Efficacy of Bile Salt Therapy

Chenodeoxycholic Acid (CDCA)

Initial studies in a small number of patients showed that administration of CDCA will result in gallstone dissolution.[568, 593] CDCA feeding causes rapid expansion of CDCA pool (at the expense of other bile acids), marked suppression of cholic acid synthesis, reduction of biliary cholesterol secretion, and when given in appropriate doses, desaturation of bile.

The effectiveness and safety of CDCA was evaluated in the late 1970s in a large prospective randomized clinical trial in the United States. In the National Cooperative Gallstone Study (NCGS) three groups of patients were studied: those receiving a "high" dose of CDCA (700 mg/day), a "low" dose (350 mg/day), and a placebo. All patients enrolled into this study were treated for 24 months. The results of these studies were disappointing, as complete dissolution occurred in only 13.5 per cent of patients receiving a high dose of CDCA for two years. In subgroups of patients (thin patients, multiple stones, floating stones) the total and partial dissolution ranged between 42 and 57 per cent.[594]

In contrast, studies of gallstone dissolution conducted in Great Britain and elsewhere yielded better results, with

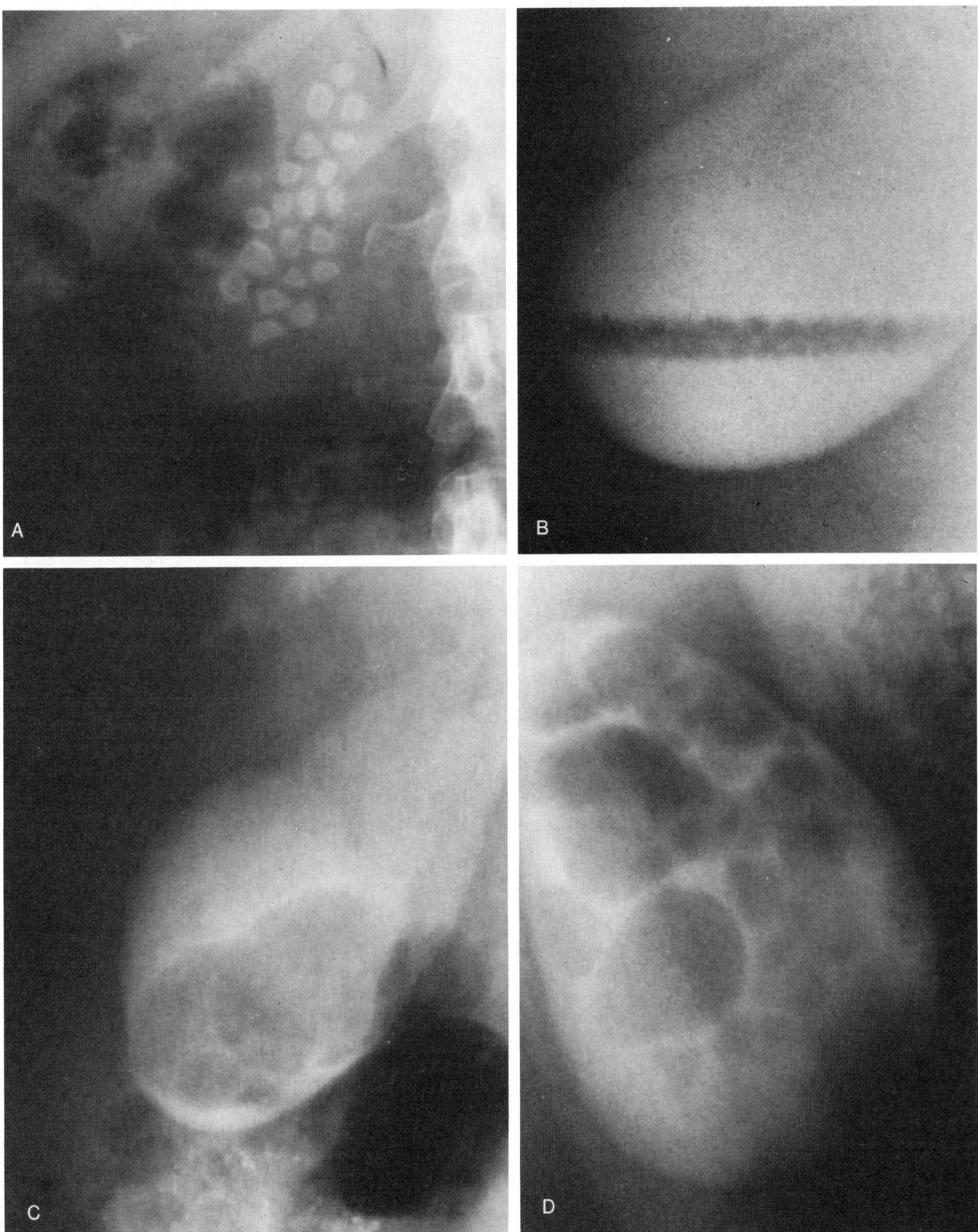

Figure 57–10. Gallstones visualized by oral cholecystography and suggested medical therapy. *A*, Multiple calcified gallstones in a nonvisualized gallbladder, these are not amenable to current non-surgical therapy. *B*, Numerous small gallstones floating in bile, forming a horizontal layer in a well-opacified gallbladder: optimal candidate for oral bile acid therapy. *C*, Two large, discrete radiolucent stones in a well-visualized gallbladder: solvent dissolution with methyl tert-butyl ether (MTBE) *or* extracorporeal shock wave lithotripsy (ESWL) with subsequent bile acid therapy should be considered. *D*, Multiple small and large radiolucent gallstones in a well-visualized gallbladder: preferred medical therapy would be solvent dissolution with MTBE.

success in gallstone dissolution ranging between 38 and 76 per cent.[597-602] If CDCA was given at night and if this regimen was coupled with low cholesterol diet, the complete dissolution of gallstones within 12 months was approximately 75 per cent.[600, 601] The major difference in design between the NCGS and British studies was that in the latter the doses of CDCA were greater. It is now clear that the dose of CDCA necessary to desaturate the bile is approximately 13 to 16 mg/kg/day.[597] Only a small fraction of patients in the NCGS received doses in this range; in most cases, the dosage was much lower. Those on the low dose regimen (375 mg/day) received an average 4.5 mg/kg/day; patients on the high dose regimen (750 mg/day) received an average of 9.5 mg/kg/day.[594] These doses were clearly inadequate to predictably desaturate the bile and are the major reason for the low dissolution rates. A retrospective statistical analysis of those patients in the NCGS who received 14 to 16 mg/kg/day of CDCA suggested that the dissolution rates of patients with floating stones were as high as 70 per cent. A review of all available data suggests that a maximum figure for gallstone dissolution with CDCA should have been between 50 and 60 per cent.[603]

The potential toxicity of CDCA has been a concern, since this primary bile acid is metabolized into lithocholic acid by the intestinal bacteria. Lithocholate was previously reported to be associated with hepatotoxicity,[604-606] and CDCA itself is toxic to cell membranes.[607-609] Long-term administration of CDCA is relatively safe; however, several side effects should be considered as predictable consequences of CDCA therapy.

1. Extensive hepatotoxicity of CDCA and/or combination of CDCA and its metabolite lithocholate has been described in a number of animal species.[610-612] In humans, however, the hepatotoxicity tends to be mild and transient.[594] Mild to moderate elevation of liver tests occurs in about 3 per cent of patients treated with CDCA. The exact mechanism by which CDCA causes elevation of liver tests in humans is uncertain. Careful light and electron microscopy studies[613-615] failed to exhibit any significant microscopic alteration of the liver.

2. Diarrhea occurs in a large percentage of patients and is the most troublesome side effect. It is caused by the known propensity of CDCA to induce secretion of water and electrolytes in the colon.[616] In the NCGS, the frequency of diarrhea was dose-related. Patients on high doses had an incidence of 49 per cent, whereas for those on the low dose, the incidence was 22 per cent. Temporary reduction of the dose resulted in the improvement of symptoms; there was no need to discontinue therapy in any of the patients. However, at the desirable dose levels of CDCA (15 mg/kg/day), diarrhea becomes a significant problem and may necessitate cessation of therapy.

3. Plasma cholesterol levels increase by about 10 per cent on high doses of CDCA; the increase occurs almost entirely in the low-density lipoprotein fraction. This is not surprising, since CDCA inhibits bile acid synthesis and reduces biliary cholesterol secretion and therefore blocks the two major routes for elimination of cholesterol from the body.[594] Although not a major concern in short-term therapy, there is a theoretical risk that long-term therapy with chenodeoxycholic acid could be associated with increased morbidity and mortality related to atherosclerosis.

The cost of CDCA has been calculated to be about $2,000 for two years (i.e., significantly lower than surgery). However, this figure does not include the cost of long-term follow-up. The failure to dissolve gallstones and potential gallstone recurrence must also be considered.

Ursodeoxycholic Acid (UDCA)

Extensive experience has also been gathered with UDCA mainly in European controlled trials and several smaller studies in the United States.[617-622] The general consensus from all these studies was that UDCA treatment can lead to dissolution of gallstones and that the effectiveness of UDCA is comparable to that of CDCA.[623] Lower doses of UDCA are required to dissolve gallstones compared to CDCA, and the time necessary to accomplish dissolution is shorter. The optimal dose of UDCA for the dissolution of gallstones appears to be about 8 mg/kg/day.[622]

UDCA was approved by the U.S. Food and Drug Administration for general use as a gallstone dissolving agent in October 1988. It is marketed in the United States under the trade name *Actigall*. Because of its lower toxicity, UDCA appears preferable to CDCA for treatment of gallstones. Unfortunately it may be significantly more expensive. Long-term administration of UDCA has many advantages over CDCA, since its use is not associated with any significant side effects such as hepatotoxicity, diarrhea, or elevation of plasma cholesterol.[623] It appears that many aspects of bile salt toxicity increase markedly with increasing hydrophobicity, and this may be the explanation for the low toxicity of UDCA (a hydrophilic bile acid). The possibility that other hydrophilic bile salts may be safe and effective in treatment of gallstones is currently under active investigation.

One complication that may be more frequent with UDCA than with CDCA treatment is surface calcification of gallstones. Although the incidence is less than 5 per cent, when it occurs it appears to prevent further gallstone dissolution.[178] Although the reason for this effect is unknown, it is possible that glycoursodeoxycholate in the presence of calcium may precipitate at the stone surface.[397] It has been suggested that calcification secondary to use of UDCA may be preventable by use of taurine conjugates of UDCA, rather than free bile acid. However, definitive information on this has not been available. The problem of surface calcification may in part be circumvented by lithotripsy (see Chapter 61).

Combination Therapy (CDCA and UDCA)

In several recent studies, a combination of CDCA (7.5 mg/kg/day) and UDCA (6.5 mg/kg/day) was used.[580, 624-626] The combination of the two drugs apparently is not more efficacious than either alone, but the side effects observed with CDCA are reduced and the cost of the combination is less than that of UDCA alone.[626] Almost complete absence of side effects of CDCA when used conjointly with UDCA is partly secondary to the reduced dosage. Some studies have also suggested that UDCA may have a "hepatoprotective" effect against toxicity of more hydrophobic bile salts.[627]

CONTACT SOLVENT DISSOLUTION

Monooctanoin

The monoglyceride monooctanoin (Capmul) is an organic solvent with excellent cholesterol solubilizing properties,[628] which does not lead to hepatic duct inflammation in primate models.[629] Monooctanoin is significantly more effective than cholate or heparin in dissolving cholesterol gallstones (Fig. 57–11).[630] Cholesterol gallstones bathed or

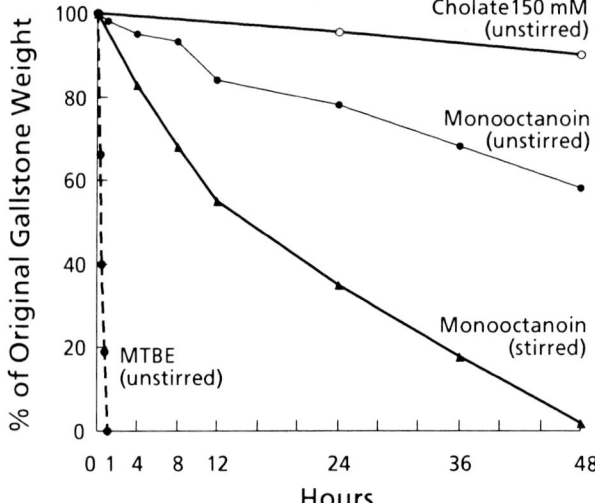

Figure 57–11. Relative rate of dissolution (approximate) of cholesterol gallstones in vitro in methyl tert-butyl ether (MTBE), monooctanoin, and 150 mM sodium taurocholate. The order of efficacy is MTBE > monooctanoin > sodium taurocholate. The rate of stone dissolution in MTBE is about three orders of magnitude faster than in taurocholate. Dissolution can be accelerated in vitro by mechanical stirring. (Composite figure from data presented.) (Thistle JL, et al. Gastroenterology 78:1016, 1980; and Allen MJ et al. Gastroenterology 89:1097, 1985, with permission.)

immersed in monooctanoin dissolve over a period of days to weeks. Clinically, monooctanoin has been infused continuously via T-tubes or transhepatic catheters to dissolve retained common bile duct stones post cholecystectomy. Average time required for dissolution is about five days. Several studies have shown that successful dissolution averages 50 to 80 per cent with monooctanoin infused at a rate of 3 to 5 ml/hour for 3 to 7 days.[630–634]

Monooctanoin has numerous side effects, both local and systemic. The local effects usually occur as a result of rapid emptying of monooctanoin into the duodenum and include nausea, vomiting, abdominal crampy pain, and diarrhea. Systemic effects can occur as a result of extravasation through the liver parenchyma. Respiratory distress and anoxia are common systemic manifestations that mandate discontinuation of therapy. With the wide availability of endoscopic sphincterotomy for gallstone retrieval, and the advent of both extracorporeal and contact lithotripsy, the use of monooctanoin is rarely indicated.

Methyl Tert-Butyl Ether (MTBE)

MTBE is an aliphatic hydrocarbon with a boiling point of 55°C, which allows it to remain liquid at body temperature.[635] It is malodorous and potentially explosive. Cholesterol is highly soluble in MTBE. In vitro, MTBE dissolves cholesterol gallstones within minutes, whereas monooctanoin requires hours, and a 100-mM solution of taurocholate requires days to weeks (see Fig. 57–11).

Allen et al.[636] demonstrated that MTBE infusion into the dog gallbladder results in a rapid dissolution of implanted cholesterol gallstones. MTBE was tolerated well, with very few side effects. Thistle and colleagues[637–639] subsequently pioneered the use of MTBE for gallstone dissolution in humans. The instillation-withdrawal of MTBE was carried out via a percutaneous transhepatic catheter positioned in the gallbladder under fluoroscopic or ultrasound guidance, using only local anaesthesia and mild sedation.

Initial studies in humans reported complete or near-complete dissolution of gallstones in greater than 90 per cent of cases in an average of 7 hours,[637, 638] without major discomfort or complications. A small amount of residual debris was commonly observed on gallbladder ultrasonography following gallstone dissolution.

Side effects of MTBE included mild anesthesia, nausea, vomiting, and occasional slight elevation of liver enzymes. These symptoms appear to relate to overfilling of the gallbladder; MTBE that escapes from the gallbladder may cause topical damage to the duodenum and may be absorbed systemically. Accidental infusion of MTBE into the liver parenchyma and/or a blood vessel would be potentially hazardous because of the lipid solubilizing capacity of MTBE. A recent report noted acute renal failure following treatment with MTBE.[640] Nonetheless, serious complications have been remarkably infrequent.

In initial studies, filling and emptying of the gallbladder with MTBE was accomplished manually. It is expected that, in the future, automated infusion-withdrawal systems will simplify the procedure. These automated systems will require safeguards against overfilling of the gallbladder in order to prevent systemic absorption of MTBE.

In summary, medical treatment of gallstones with MTBE is relatively rapid (hours), effective (near-complete dissolution of > 90 per cent of uncalcified stones), and reasonably safe in the hands of an experienced physician. The major potential indication for this therapeutic modality is treatment of patients with symptomatic cholesterol gallstones who prefer a nonsurgical approach or for whom surgery is contraindicated. It appears to be effective with all cholesterol stones regardless of size, shape, or number. Its risks are those of transhepatic gallbladder puncture (bile leak, hemorrhage) and of systemic absorption of MTBE. The effectiveness, safety, and relative benefits of this approach will be tested soon in multicenter prospective trials.

GALLSTONE RECURRENCE

Following successful dissolution of gallstones with CDCA or UDCA, and when bile acid therapy is discontinued, biliary cholesterol saturation rapidly returns to the pretreatment level.[641–643] Persistence of biliary supersaturation is also the norm in patients whose stones are eliminated via solvent dissolution or lithotripsy. This appears to be inevitable, although in a few cases it may be preventable theoretically by risk factor intervention such as dietary correction of obesity or cessation of estrogen therapy. It is not surprising that the observed recurrence rate following bile acid dissolution of stones is about 50 per cent in five years,[641, 642, 644] with the most rapid recurrence occurring during the first two years. Only occasional patients become symptomatic during this follow-up period, and it is unknown whether such recurrent stones require treatment. Stone growth is a slow process and it may take 10 to 20 years for these stones to become large enough to become symptomatic. Recurrent stones in patients who have previously exhibited complete dissolution generally dissolve rapidly during a subsequent course of bile acid therapy.[641, 645, 646]

Interestingly, the rate of gallstone recurrence seems to fall off after the first two to three years. About 50 per cent of patients following gallstone dissolution fail to have recurrence within five years. This represents an interesting group of patients who to date have not been adequately studied. Clearly, in many patients the "lithogenic state" is episodic. It appears that factors other than biliary cholesterol saturation must be invoked to explain the failure of stones to recur in these individuals.

GALLSTONE PREVENTION

In certain populations, one may anticipate a high risk of cholesterol gallstone formation over months to years. These include patients who have undergone successful gallstone dissolution therapy, patients undergoing rapid weight loss, and patients in genetically high-risk groups such as Pima Indians. For these groups, the development of safe and inexpensive treatments to prevent gallstone formation is an important goal. With the anticipated proliferation of medical gallstone therapy over the next decade, the need for therapies to prevent gallstone recurrence will become increasingly apparent.[647]

The most straightforward approach to prevention of gallstones is bile acid therapy. This thermodynamic approach eliminates stone formation by desaturating bile. Both UDCA and CDCA are effective in prevention of gallstone recurrence. Unfortunately, they are effective only so long as bile is unsaturated with cholesterol. Thus, low-dose prophylactic therapy with these agents appears to be ineffective.[648, 649] The long-term consequences of bile acid therapy are not known, and the expense of a lifetime of bile acid therapy would be substantial.

An intensive search is currently under way for modalities of therapy that address the other aspects of gallstone pathogenesis illustrated in Figure 57–1—kinetics, time, and the mucin matrix. As discussed previously, studies in the prairie dog suggest that suppression of mucin secretion via treatment with inhibitors of prostaglandin synthesis can prevent gallstone formation. Data on this approach in humans have been limited. A prospective study by Schoenfield and colleagues[587] in patients undergoing rapid weight loss failed to demonstrate prevention of gallstones by aspirin treatment, although there was a trend suggestive of slight benefit. Retrospective analysis of a European gallstone prevention trial[650] suggested that gallstone recurrence was very rare in patients who were receiving nonsteroidal anti-inflammatory agents for unrelated problems.

With the recent advances in understanding of gallstone pathogenesis and the expected explosion in clinical gallstone dissolution therapy, we anticipate an intensive effort to develop better modalities for gallstone prevention over the next decade.

MEDICAL THERAPY OF CALCIUM STONES

In theory, calcium (pigment) gallstones can be prevented by a reduction in the load of unconjugated bilirubin in bile or by a decrease in ionized calcium. Leuschner et al.[651, 652] and others[653] have attempted to dissolve pigmented stones by direct infusion of monooctanoin and a solution containing EDTA, ursodeoxycholate, and cholate. Some beneficial effect was observed, but results were not convincing. In part the poor results may have been due to inherently slow kinetics of calcium dissolution. Ostrow[76] has found evidence that the bilirubin in black pigment stones is present in the form of large, insoluble, covalently linked polymers. If this is the case, then at least the pigment component of black pigment stones may prove to be refractory to all forms of dissolution therapy. Therapy of calcium-containing stones remains in its infancy.

STRATEGY FOR MANAGEMENT OF GALLSTONES

A suggested algorithm for management of gallstones is shown in Figure 57–12. Based on the available data, about 30 per cent of patients with radiologic evidence of gallstones have symptoms attributable to gallstones. The great majority of gallstone bearers (70 per cent) have asymptomatic (silent) stones.[654] Thus, the majority of gallstone patients can be managed expectantly with no specific therapy. Among those patients with symptoms attributable to gallstones, approximately 70 per cent in the United States have radiolucent gallstones and therefore are candidates for current modalities of nonsurgical therapy. At present, there is no available medical therapy for the remaining 30 per cent of patients with calcified stones, and these patients must be treated surgically.

A non-functioning gallbladder generally is considered a contraindication for medical therapy of gallstones, although (as discussed above) the rationale for this assertion has been questioned. In 30 per cent of patients with radiolucent stones, the gallbladder fails to be visualized by oral cholecystography; at present it is recommended that these patients be managed surgically. In addition, patients presenting with complications of gallstone disease such as acute cholecystitis, cholangitis, or pancreatitis probably should undergo curative surgery if their medical condition permits.

The next consideration in assessing suitability for medical therapy is the size and number of gallstones. Gallstones with a diameter of less than 15 mm represent 35 per cent, whereas those with a diameter of more than 15 mm are present in 65 per cent of cases. Bile acid therapy is most successful in therapy of stones < 15 mm in diameter (i.e., 35 per cent of cases). Lithotripsy is most suitable for stones ranging in size between 6 and 30 mm (i.e., 80 per cent of the time). This modality is not suitable for small stones (less than 6 mm in size). MTBE is suitable for treatment of gallstones of all sizes, thereby including the vast majority of patients (approximately 90 per cent).

The choice between surgical and medical therapy is a difficult one that must weigh the risks and benefits of each approach. Surgery is curative, whereas medical therapy may be associated with recurrences of stones. Medical therapy to prevent recurrence or eliminate recurrent stones is currently less than ideal, but substantial improvements may be expected. The risks of surgery are small in healthy, young adults, but those risks are immediate, and they increase substantially with age or coexisting morbid conditions. Surgical risks also vary substantially with the skill of the surgeon. Newer modalities such as MTBE dissolution and extracorporeal shock wave lithotripsy are not yet widely available and involve unknown risks. Patient preferences also must be taken into account. No one approach can be suitable for all patients, and the algorithm shown in Figure 57–12 must be tailored to the individual circumstances.

SUMMARY

We have attempted to give a review of recent developments in gallstone pathogenesis and dissolution and to place them in perspective with the older literature. Gallstones are one of the most common serious human ailments. While much progress has been made since Rains' treatise in 1964,[655] there is still much to be learned. Gallstone formation involves some very difficult areas of organic and inorganic chemistry, but it is anticipated that, in the next

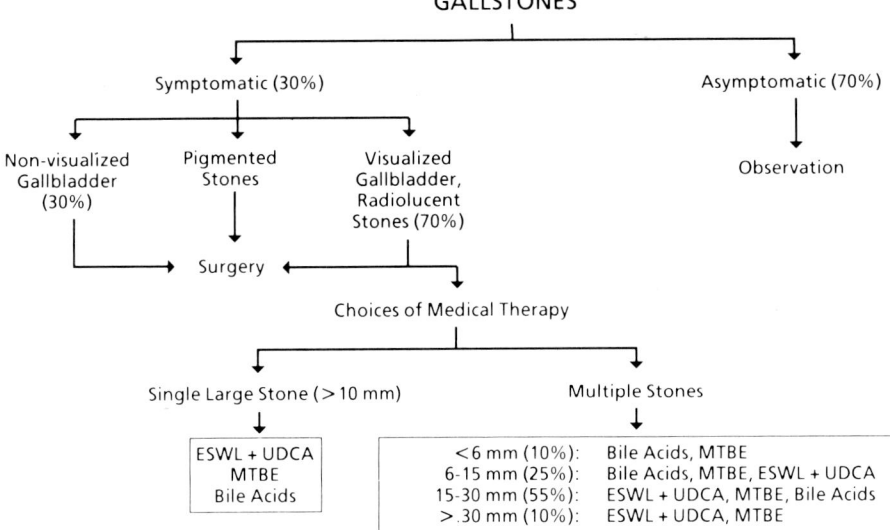

Figure 57–12. Proposed algorithm for medical management of patients with gallbladder stones (see text for discussion). MTBE = methyl tert-butyl ether solvent dissolution; ESWL + UDCA = extracorporeal shockwave lithotripsy followed by oral ursodeoxycholic acid.

few years, important new insights will emerge regarding nucleating and anti-nucleating factors in bile, the chemistry and physiology of vesicles, the derangements that lead to cholesterol and calcium nucleation and subsequent crystal growth, and the pathophysiology of gallbladder stasis. Inevitably studies of gallstone pathogenesis will also bring new insights into the chemistry of bile and the mechanisms of bile formation.

A model for the constellation of events that appear to be necessary for gallstone formation involves four requisite features: (1) Matrix gel formation, (2) presence of a supersaturated state for cholesterol and/or calcium, (3) nucleation, and (4) crystal growth (time). Each of these is believed to be crucial; gallstones do not develop simply because bile is supersaturated with either cholesterol or calcium. Their formation reflects defects in four broad but discrete areas, each of which is essential.

Several areas offer promise of therapeutic solutions, based on current understanding of gallstone pathogenesis. It may be possible to prevent gallstones by preventing mucus secretion; if the mucin viscoelastic gel provides the environment in which gallstones nucleate and grow, then pharmacologic inhibition of mucin secretion may effectively block stone formation. It may become possible temporarily to render bile unsaturated with calcium by administration of "prodrugs" that become calcium chelators upon secretion into bile. This might be useful in the treatment, and possibly prevention, of pigment stones and, if the calcium "seed" hypothesis is correct, might also prevent cholesterol nucleation and cholesterol gallstone formation. Pharmacologic manipulation of vesicle formation, cholesterol transport, and vesicle fusion may provide means of preventing cholesterol nucleation. Similarly, alteration of gallbladder motor function for prevention of stasis may have an important impact on prevention of gallstones in certain target populations. Elucidation of the structural requirements for nucleation and for inhibition of nucleation and crystal growth may eventually lead to new modes of therapy. Recent years have seen rapid advances in our understanding of the physicochemical and physiologic factors contributing to gallstone formation. The decades to come hold great promise for development of new modalities for prevention and treatment of gallstone disease.

REFERENCES

1. Cannon WB. Organization for physiological homeostasis. Physiol Rev 9:399, 1929.
2. Hofmann AF. Bile, bile acids, and gallstones: will new knowledge bring new power? Am J Radiol 151:5, 1988.
3. Small DM, Bourges MC, Dervichian DG. The biophysics of lipidic associations. I. The ternary systems lecithin–bile salt–water. Biochim Biophys Acta 125:563, 1966.
4. Bourges M, Small DM, Dervichian DG. Biophysics of lipidic associations. II. The ternary systems cholesterol-lecithin-water. Biochim Biophys Acta 137:157, 1967.
5. Bourges M, Small DM, Dervichian DG. Biophysics of lipid association. III. The quaternary systems lecithin–bile salt–cholesterol–water. Biochim Biophys Acta 144:189, 1967.
6. Small DM, Bourges M, Dervichian D. Ternary and quaternary aqueous systems containing bile salt, lecithin, and cholesterol. Nature (London) 211:816, 1966.
7. Admirand WH, Small DM. The physicochemical basis of cholesterol gallstone formation in man. J Clin Invest 47:1043, 1968.
8. Carey MC, Small DM. The physical chemistry of cholesterol solubility in bile: relationship to gallstone formation and dissolution in man. J Clin Invest 61:998, 1978.
9. Carey MC. Critical tables for calculating the cholesterol saturation of native bile. J Lipid Res 19:945, 1978.
10. Swell L, Gregory DH, Vlahcevic ZR. Current concepts of the pathogenesis of cholesterol gallstones. Med Clin North Am 58:1449, 1974.
11. Small DM. The formation of gallstones. Adv Intern Med 16:243, 1970.
12. Small DM, Dowling RH, Redinger RN. The enterohepatic circulation of bile salts. Arch Intern Med 130:552, 1972.
13. Carey MC, Small DM. Micelle formation by bile salts. Physical-chemical and thermodynamic considerations. Arch Intern Med 130:506, 1972.
14. Dowling RH, Mack E, Small DM. Primate biliary physiology. IV. Biliary lipid secretion and bile composition after acute and chronic interruption of the enterohepatic circulation in the Rhesus monkey. J Clin Invest 50:1917, 1971.
15. Shaffer EA, Small DM. Gallstone disease: Pathogenesis and management. Curr Prob Surg 13:1, 1976.
16. Strasberg SM, Redinger RN, Small DM, et al. The effect of elevated biliary tract pressure on biliary lipid metabolism and bile flow in nonhuman primates. J Lab Clin Med 99:342, 1982.
17. Carey MC, Cohen DE. Biliary transport of cholesterol in vesicles, micelles and liquid crystals. In: Paumgartner G, Stiehl A, Gerok W, eds. Bile Acids and the Liver. Lancaster, MTP Press, 1987:287.
18. Carey MC, Cahalane MJ. Whither biliary sludge? Gastroenterology 95:508, 1988.
19. Northfield TC, Hofmann AF. Biliary lipid output during three meals and an overnight fast. I. Relationship to bile acid pool size and cholesterol saturation of bile in gallstone and control subjects. Gut 16:1, 1975.
20. Holan KR, Holzbach RT, Hermann RE, et al. Nucleation time: a key factor in the pathogenesis of cholesterol gallstone disease. Gastroenterology 77:611, 1979.

21. Hofmann AF, Grundy SM, Lachin JM, et al. Pretreatment biliary lipid composition in white patients with radiolucent gallstones in the National Cooperative Gallstone Study. Gastroenterology 83:738, 1982.

22. Burnstein MJ, Ilson RG, Petrunka CN, et al. Evidence for a potent nucleating factor in the gallbladder bile of patients with cholesterol gallstones. Gastroenterology 85:801, 1983.

23. Bernhoft RA, Pellegrini CA, Broderick WC, et al. Pigment sludge and stone formation in the acutely ligated dog gallbladder. Gastroenterology 85:1166, 1983.

24. Toor EW, Evans DF, Cussler EL. The nucleation of cholesterol monohydrate crystals in model bile solution. In: Fisher MM, Goresky CA, Shaffer EA, et al., eds. Gallstones. New York, Plenum Press, 1979:169.

25. Henisch HK. Crystal Growth in Gels. University Park, Pa., Penn State Univ Press, 1979.

26. Ohki S. Physicochemical factors underlying lipid membrane fusion. In: Sowers AE, ed. Cell Fusion. New York, Plenum Press, 1987:331.

27. Schurtenberger P, Mazer N, Kaenzig W. Micelle to vesicle transition in aqueous solutions of bile salt and lecithin. J Phys Chem 89:1042, 1985.

28. Holzbach RT, Halpern Z, Dudley MA, et al. Biliary vesicle aggregation and cholesterol crystal nucleation: evidence for a coupled relationship. In: Paumgartner G, Stiehl A, Gerok W, eds. Bile Acids and the Liver. Lancaster, MTP Press, 1987:301.

29. Kienzle H-F, Radtke J. Lokalisation und verteilung von calciumsalzen in gallensteinen. Langenbecks Arch Chir 353:171, 1980.

30. Malet PF, Williamson CE, Trotman BW, et al. Composition of pigmented centers of cholesterol gallstones. Hepatology 6:477, 1986.

31. Bills PM, Lewis D. A structural study of gallstones. Gut 16:630, 1975.

32. Wosiewitz U. Scanning electron microscopy in gallstone research. Scanning Electr Microsc 1:419, 1983.

33. Ruiz de Aguiar A, Medina Nuñez JA, Lopez Domingo MI, et al. Calcium carbonate in cholesterol gallstones. J Hepatol 6:71, 1988.

34. Malet PF, Takabayashi A, Trotman BW, et al. Black and brown pigment gallstones differ in microstructure and microcomposition. Hepatology 2:227, 1984.

35. Wolpers C. Morphologie der Gallensteine. Leber Magen Darm 4:43, 1974.

36. Pitchumoni CS, Viswanathan KV, Moore EW. Analysis and localization of elements in human cholesterol gallstones: Calcium and other elements are present in the central (nidus) region. Gastroenterology 92:1764, 1987.

37. Bogren H, Larsson K. On the pigment in biliary calculi. Scand J Clin Lab Invest 15:569, 1963.

38. Sutor DJ, Wilkie LI. The crystalline salts of calcium bilirubinate in human gallstones. Clin Sci Mol Med 53:101, 1977.

39. Malet PF, Dabezies MA, Huang G, et al. Quantitative infrared spectroscopy of common bile duct gallstones. Gastroenterology 94:1217, 1988.

40. Been JM, Bills PM, Lewis D. Microstructure of gallstones. Gastroenterology 76:548, 1979.

41. Suzuki N. On bilirubin metal complex compounds in relation to black pigments of gallstones. Tohoku J Exp Med 90:195, 1966.

42. Soloway RD, Trotman BW, Maddrey WC, et al. Pigment gallstone composition in patients with hemolysis or infection/stasis. Dig Dis Sci 31:454, 1986.

43. Black BE, Carr SH, Ohkubo H, et al. Equilibrium swelling of pigment gallstones: Evidence for network polymer structure. Biopolymers 21:601, 1982.

44. Rege RV, Webster CC, Ostrow JD, et al. Validation of infrared spectroscopy for assessment of vinyl polymers of bile-pigment gallstones. Biochem J 224:871, 1984.

45. Trotman BW, Morris TA III, Sanchez HM, et al. Pigment vs. cholesterol cholelithiasis. Identification and quantification by infrared spectroscopy. Gastroenterology 72:495, 1977.

46. Suzuki N, Nakamura Y, Sato T. Infrared absorption spectroscopy of pure pigment gallstones. Tohoku J Exp Med 116:259, 1975.

47. Burnett W, Dwyer KR, Kennard CH. Black pigment or polybilirubinate gallstones: composition and formation. Ann Surg 193:331, 1981.

48. Bogren H. The composition and structure of human gallstones. Acta Radiol 226 (Suppl.):1, 1964.

49. Bogren H, Larsson K. Crystalline components of biliary calculi. Scand J Clin Lab Invest 15:457, 1963.

50. Sutor DJ, Wooley SE. The sequential deposition of crystalline material in gallstones: Evidence for changing gallbladder bile composition during the growth of some stones. Gut 15:130, 1974.

51. Bogren H. The role of cholecystitis in the precipitation of calcium carbonate in human gall stones. Acta Chir Scand 131:329, 1966.

52. Juniper K Jr. Biliary tract studies II. The significance of biliary crystals. Gastroenterology 32:175, 1957.

53. Juniper K Jr. Biliary tract studies I. X-ray diffraction analysis of gallstones: correlation with occurrence of microspheroliths in bile. Am J Med 20:383, 1956.

54. Lagergren C. Calcium carbonate precipitation in the pancreas, gall stones and urinary calculi. Acta Chir Scand 124:320, 1962.

55. Sutor DJ, Cowie AGA, Clark CG. Some observations on gallstones and bile composition. Br J Surg 64:44, 1976.

56. Sutor DJ, Wooley SE. X-ray diffraction studies of the composition of gallstones from English and Australian patients. Gut 10:681, 1969.

57. Soloway RD, Fayusal EB, Trotman BW, et al. Water content of gallstones: location and contribution to a hypothesis concerning stone structure. Hepatology 2:223, 1982.

58. Womack N, Zeppa R, Irvin G. The anatomy of gallstones. Ann Surg 157:670, 1963.

59. Zilm KW, Grant DM, Englert E Jr, et al. The use of solid 13C nuclear magnetic resonance for the characterization of cholesterol and bilirubin pigment composition of human gallstones. Biochem Biophys Res Commun 93:857, 1980.

60. Nakayama F. Quantitative microanalysis of gallstones. J Lab Clin Med 72:602, 1969.

61. Malet PF, Weston NE, Trotman BW, et al. Cyclic deposition of calcium salts during growth of cholesterol gallstones. Scanning Electr Microsc 2:775, 1985.

62. Been JM, Bills PM, Lewis D. Electron probe microanalysis in the study of gallstones. Gut 18:836, 1977.

63. Burnett W, Dwyer KR, Kennard CHL, et al. Transition metal ions in human gallstones. Bioinorganic Chem 9:345, 1978.

64. Rovsing T. Zur Beleuchtung und Wertschatzung Nauyns und anderer Infektionstheorien bezuglich der Pathogenese der Gallensteinkrankheit. Weitere Beitrage zur Pathogenese der Gallensteinkrankheit. Acta Chir Scand 56:207, 1924.

65. Womack NA. The development of gallstones. Surg Gynecol Obstet 133:937, 1971.

66. Suzuki N, Toyoda M. On infrared absorption spectra of bilirubin and calcium bilirubinate. Tohoku J Exp Med 88:353, 1966.

67. Duvaldestin P, Mahu JL, Metreau JM, et al. Possible role of defect in hepatic bilirubin glucuronidation in the initiation of cholesterol gallstones. Gut 21:650, 1980.

68. Wosiewitz U. Limy bile and radiopaque, calcified gallstones: A combined analytical, radiographic and micromorphologic examination. Pathol Res Pract 167:273, 1980.

69. Trotman BW, Ostrow JD, Soloway RD. Pigment vs cholesterol cholelithiasis: Comparison of stone and bile composition. Am J Dig Dis 19:585, 1974.

70. Moore EW. The role of calcium in the pathogenesis of gallstones: Ca^{++} electrode studies of model bile salt solutions and other biologic systems. Hepatology 4:228S, 1984.

71. Smith BF, Lamont JT. Mucin-bilirubin complex in human cholesterol gallstones. Hepatology 3:822, 1983 (Abstract).

72. Sutor DJ, Wilkie LI. Calcium in bile and calcium salts in gallstones. Clin Chim Acta 79:119, 1977.

73. Cowie AGA, Sutor DJ, Wooley SE, et al. The calcium palmitate gallstone. Br J Surg 60:16, 1973.

74. Sutor DJ. Calcium palmitate and α-palmitic acid in gallstones. Gut 11:618, 1970.

75. Lamont JT, Ventola AS, Trotman BW, et al. Mucin glycoprotein content of human pigment gallstones. Hepatology 3:377, 1983.

76. Ohkubo H, Ostrow JD, Carr SH, et al. Polymer networks in pigment and cholesterol gallstones assessed by equilibrium swelling and infrared spectroscopy. Gastroenterology 87:805, 1984.

77. Wosiewitz U, Schroebler S. "Polymer pigments" in human gallstones. Naturwissenschaft 65:162, 1978.

78. Mok YI, Druffel RM, Rampal WM. Dating gallstones from atmospheric radiocarbon produced by nuclear bomb explosions. N Engl J Med 314:1075, 1986.

79. Gurll NJ, DenBesten L. Animal models of human cholesterol gallstone disease. Lab Anim Sci 28:428, 1978.

80. Rege RV, Nahrwold DL. Animal models of pigment gallstone disease. J Lab Clin Med 110:381, 1987.

81. Dam H, Christensen F. Alimentary production of gallstones in hamsters. Acta Pathol Microbiol Scand 30:236, 1952.

82. Bergman F, Van der Linden W. Influence of D-thyroxine on gallstone formation in hamsters. Acta Chir Scand 129:547, 1964.

83. Bergman F, Van der Linden W. Further studies on the influence of thyroxine on gallstone formation in hamsters. Acta Chir Scand 131:319, 1966.

84. Bergman F, Juul AH, Van der Linden W. The effect of liver toxins on gallstone formation in Syrian hamsters. Acta Hepatosplenol 18:215, 1971.

85. Hashimoto K. Experimental studies on gallstones in hamsters. Arch Jpn Chir 35:981, 1966.

86. Bergman F, Van der Linden W. Liver morphology and gallstone formation in hamsters and mice treated with chenodeoxycholic acid. Acta Pathol Microbiol Scand 81:213, 1973.

87. Palmer RH. Gallstones produced experimentally by lithocholic acid in rats. Science 148:1339, 1965.

88. Palmer RH, Hruban Z. Production of bile duct hyperplasia and gallstones by lithocholic acid. J Clin Invest 45:1255, 1966.

89. Freston JW, Bouchier IAD, Newman J. Biliary mucous substances in dihydrocholesterol-induced cholelithiasis. Gastroenterology 57:670, 1969.

90. Hofmann AF, Bokkenheuser V, Hirsch RL, et al. Experimental cholelithiasis in the rabbit induced by cholestanol feeding: effect of neomycin treatment on bile composition and gallstone formation. J Lipid Res 9:244, 1968.

91. Hofmann AF, Mosbach EH. Identification of allodeoxycholic acid as the major component of gallstones induced in the rabbit by 5α-cholestan-3β-ol. J Biol Chem 239:2813, 1964.

92. Lee SP. Oleic acid–induced cholelithiasis in rabbits. Am J Pathol 124:18, 1986.

93. Lee SP, Scott AJ. Dihydrocholesterol-induced gallstones in the rabbit: Evidence for bile acid injury to cell membrane. Br J Exp Pathol 60:231, 1979.

94. Carlisle VF, Tasman-Jones C. Prevention of gallstone formation in rabbits by the oral administration of kanamycin. Surg Gynecol Obstet 144:195, 1977.

95. Borgman R. Gallstone formation in rabbits as affected by dietary fat and protein. Am J Vet Res 26:1167, 1965.

96. Truskett PG, Shi ECP, Rose M, et al. Model of TPN-associated hepatobiliary dysfunction in the young pig. Br J Surg 74:639, 1987.

97. Scott AJ. Lincomycin-induced cholecystitis and gallstones in guinea pigs. Gastroenterology 71:814, 1976.

98. Lee SP, Scott AJ. Further observations in lincomycin-induced cholelithiasis in guinea pigs. J Pathol 131:117, 1980.

99. Brotschi EA, LaMorte WW, Williams LF Jr. Effect of dietary cholesterol and indomethacin on cholelithiasis and gallbladder motility in the guinea pig. Dig Dis Sci 29:1050, 1984.

100. LaMorte WW, Brotschi EA, Scott TE, et al. Pigment gallstone formation in the cholesterol-fed guinea pig. Hepatology 5:21, 1985.

101. Jenkins SA. Biliary lipids, bile acids and gallstone formation in the hypovitaminotic C guinea pig. Br J Nutr 40:317, 1978.

102. Caldwell FT Jr, Levitsky K. Role of the gallbladder in the formation of gallstones. Surg Forum 17:353, 1966.

103. Caldwell FT Jr, Levitsky K, Rosenberg B. Dietary production and dissolution of cholesterol gallstones in the mouse. Am J Physiol 209:473, 1965.

104. Trotman BW, Bernstein SE, Bovie KE, et al. Studies on the pathogenesis of pigment gallstones in hemolytic anemia: Description and characteristics of a mouse model. J Clin Invest 65:1301, 1980.

105. Trotman BW, Bernstein SE, Balistreri WF, et al. Hemolysis-induced gallstones in mice: Increased unconjugated bilirubin in hepatic bile predisposes to gallstone formation. Gastroenterology 81:232, 1981.

106. Trotman BW, Bernstein SE, Balistreri WF, et al. Interaction of hemolytic anemia and genotype on hemolysis-induced gallstone formation in mice. Gastroenterology 84:719, 1983.

107. Trotman BW, Bongiovanni MB, Kahn MJ, et al. A morphologic study of the liver and gallbladder in hemolysis-induced gallstone disease in mice. Hepatology 2:863, 1982.

108. Osuga T, Portman OW, Mitamura K, et al. A morphologic study of gallstone development in the squirrel monkey. Lab Invest 30:486, 1974.

109. Englert E, Harmon CG, Wales E. Gallstones induced by normal foodstuffs in dogs. Nature 224:280, 1969.

110. Englert E, Harmon CG, Freston JW, et al. Studies on the pathogenesis of diet-induced dog gallstones. Dig Dis Sci 22:305, 1977.

111. Howell JH, Marsh ME, Theil ES, et al. Hepatic microsomal activities of cholesterol 7α-hydroxylase and 3-hydroxy-3-methylglutaryl-CoA reductase in prairie dog. An animal model for cholesterol gallstone disease. Biochim Biophys Acta 753:32, 1983.

112. Lee SP, Carey MC, Lamont JT. Aspirin prevention of cholesterol gallstone formation in prairie dogs. Science 211:1429, 1981.

113. Brenneman DW, Connor WE, Forker EL, et al. The formation of abnormal bile and cholesterol gallstones from dietary cholesterol in the prairie dog. J Clin Invest 51:1495, 1972.

114. Hutton SW, Sievert CE Jr, Vennes JA, et al. The effect of sphincterotomy on gallstone formation in the prairie dog. Gastroenterology 81:663, 1981.

115. Hutton SW, Sievert CE Jr, Vennes JA, et al. Inhibition of gallstone formation by sphincterotomy in the prairie dog: reversal by atropine. Gastroenterology 82:1308, 1982.

116. Fridhandler TM, Davison JS, Shaffer EA. Defective gallbladder contractility in the ground squirrel and prairie dog during the early stages of cholesterol gallstone formation. Gastroenterology 85:830, 1983.

117. Pemsingh RS, MacPherson BR, Scott GW. Morphological observations on the gallbladder and ground squirrels fed a lithogenic diet. J Pathol 152:127, 1987.

118. MacPherson BR, Pemsingh RS, Scott GW. Experimental cholelithiasis in the ground squirrel. Lab Invest 56:138, 1987.

119. Allen B, Bernhorft R, Blanckaert N, et al. Sludge is calcium bilirubinate associated with bile stasis. Am J Surg 141:51, 1981.

120. Lee SP, Nicholls JF. Nature and composition of biliary sludge. Gastroenterology 90:677, 1986.

121. Lee SP, Maher K, Nicholls JF. Origin and fate of biliary sludge. Gastroenterology 94:170, 1988.

122. Conrad MR, Jones RO, Dietchy J. Significance of low level echoes within the gallbladder. Am J Radiol 132:967, 1979.

123. Filly RA, Allen B, Minton MJ, et al. In vitro investigation of the origin of echoes within biliary sludge. J Clin Ultrasound 8:193, 1980.

124. Bolondi L, Gaini S, Testa S, et al. Gallbladder sludge formation during prolonged fasting after gastrointestinal tract surgery. Gut 26:734, 1985.

125. Messing B, Bories C, Kunstlinger F, et al. Does total parenteral nutrition induce gallbladder sludge formation and lithiasis? Gastroenterology 84:1012, 1983.

126. Gafa M, Sarli L, Miselli A, et al. Sludge and microlithiasis of the biliary tract after total gastrectomy and postoperative total parenteral nutrition. Surg Gynecol Obstet 165:413, 1987.

127. Smith BF, Lamont JT. Identification of gallbladder mucin-bilirubin complex in human cholesterol gallstone matrix. J Clin Invest 76:439, 1985.

128. Smith BF, Lamont JT, Small DM. Editorial: The sequence of events in gallstone formation. Lab Invest 56:125, 1987.

129. Conter RL, Roslyn JJ, Pitt HA, et al. Carbohydrate diet–induced calcium bilirubinate sludge and pigment gallstones in the prairie dog. J Surg Res 40:580, 1986.

130. Small DM. Cholesterol nucleation and growth in gallstone formation. N Engl J Med 302:1305, 1980.

131. Small DM. The staging of cholesterol gallstones with respect to nucleation and growth. Part I. Staging of cholesterol gallstone disease. In: Paumgartner G, Stiehl A, Gerok W, eds. Bile Acids and Lipids (Falk Symposium 29). Lancaster, MTP Press, 1981:291.

132. Lamont JT, Smith BF, Moore JRL. Role of gallbladder mucin in pathophysiology of gallstones. Hepatology 4:51S, 1984.

133. Lamont JT. Structure and function of gastrointestinal mucus. Viewpoints Dig Dis 17 No. 2:1, 1985.

134. Creeth JM. Constituents of mucus and their separation. Br Med Bull 34:17, 1978.

135. Carlson DM. Chemistry and biosynthesis of mucin glycoproteins. In: Elstein M, Parke DV, eds. Mucus in Health and Disease. Plenum Press, New York 1976:251.

136. Forstner JF. Intestinal mucins in health and disease. Digestion 17:234, 1978.

137. Allen A, Mantle M, Pearson JP. The structure and properties of mucus glycoproteins. In: Sturgess JM, ed. Perspectives in Cystic Fibrosis. Canadian Cystic Fibrosis Foundation, Toronto, 1980:102.

138. Allen A. Structure and function of gastrointestinal mucus. In: Johnson LR, ed. Physiology of the Gastrointestinal Tract, New York, Raven Press, 1981:617.

139. Lamont JT, Ventola AS. Purification, composition and some properties of colonic epithelial mucin glycoproteins. Biochim Biophys Acta 626:234, 1980.

140. Allen A. Structure of gastrointestinal mucus glycoproteins and the viscous and gel-forming properties of mucus. Br Med Bull 34:28, 1978.

141. Pearson JP, Kowa R, Taylor W, et al. A 70,000 molecular weight protein isolated from purified pig gastric mucus glycoprotein by reduction of disulphide bridges and its implication of the polymeric structure. Biochem J 197:155, 1981.

142. Pearson JP, Kaura J, Taylor W, et al. The composition of polymeric structure of mucus glycoprotein from human gallbladder bile. Biochim Biophys Acta 706:221, 1982.

143. Wahlin T, Bloom GD, Danielsson A. Effect of cholecystokinin-pancreozymin (CCK-PZ) on glycoprotein secretion from mouse gallbladder epithelium. Cell Tissue Res 171:425, 1976.

144. Lee SP. The mechanism of mucus secretion by the gallbladder epithelium. Br J Exp Pathol 61:117, 1980.

145. Lamont JT, Turner BS, DeBenedetto D, et al. Arachidonic acid stimulates mucin secretion in prairie dog gallbladder: organ culture studies. Am J Physiol 245:G92, 1983.

146. Smithson KW, Miller DB, Jacobs LR, et al. Intestinal diffusion barrier: unstirred water layer or membrane surface mucous coat? Science 214:1241, 1981.

147. Heatley NG. Mucosubstance as a barrier to diffusion. Gastroenterology 37:313, 1959.

148. Pfeiffer CJ. Experimental analysis of hydrogen ion diffusion in gastrointestinal mucus glycoprotein. Am J Physiol 240(3):G176, 1981.

149. Moore EW. Physiology of Intestinal Water and Electrolyte Absorption. Baltimore, Milner-Fenwick, 1976:1.

150. Wahlin T, Bloom GD, Carlsoo B. Histochemical observations with the light and the electron microscope on the mucosubstances of the normal mouse gallbladder epithelial cells. Histochemistry 42:119, 1974.

151. Moore JRL, Turner BS, Lamont JT. Hydrocortisone inhibits mucin

secretion from guinea pig gallbladder. Am J Physiol 247:G427, 1984.

152. LaMorte WW, Booker ML, Scott TE, et al. Increases in gallbladder prostaglandin synthesis before the formation of cholesterol gallstones. Surgery 98:445, 1985.

153. Cantafora A, Angelico M, DiBiase A, et al. Structure of biliary phosphatidyl choline in cholesterol gallstone patients. Lipids 16:589, 1981.

154. Ahlberg J, Curstedt T, Einarsson K, et al. Molecular species of biliary phosphatidylcholine in gallstone patients: The influence of treatment with cholic acid and chenodeoxycholic acid. J Lipid Res 22:404, 1981.

155. Weiser HB, Gray GR. Colloidal phenomena in gallstones. J Pediatr Surg 36:286, 1932.

156. Meckel von Helmsbach JH. Microgeologie. Ueber die Concremente in thierischen Organismus. In: Billroth T, ed. Berlin, Reimer, 1856.

157. Kleeberg J. Experimental studies on colloid-chemical mechanism of gallstone formation. Gastroenterologia 80:313, 1953.

158. Kleeberg J. Further physico-chemical studies in model gallstone formation: role of dehydration. Gastroenterologia 85:271, 1956.

159. Liesegang RE. Spezielle Methoden der Diffusion in Gallerten. Handbuch Biol Arbeitsmethoden 3:33, 1929.

160. Nakayama F, Van der Linden W. Bile from gallbladder harbouring gallstone: can it indicate stone formation? Acta Chir Scand 136:605, 1970.

161. Bouchier IAD, Cooperband SR, El Kodsi BM. Mucous substances and viscosity of normal and pathological human bile. Gastroenterology 49:343, 1966.

162. Maki T, Matsushiro T, Suzuki N, et al. Role of sulfated glycoprotein in gallstone formation. Surg Gynecol Obstet 132:846, 1971.

163. Lee SP, Lim TH, Scott AJ. Carbohydrate moieties of glycoproteins in human hepatic and gallbladder bile, gallbladder mucosa and gallstones. Clin Sci Mol Med 56:533, 1979.

164. Lee SP. Hypersecretion of mucus glycoprotein by the gallbladder epithelium in experimental cholelithiasis. J Pathol 134:199, 1981.

165. Lee SP, Scott AJ. The evolution of morphologic changes in the gallbladder before stone formation in mice fed a cholesterol-cholic acid diet. Am J Pathol 108:1, 1982.

166. Doty JE, Pitt HA, Kuchenbecker SL, et al. Role of gallbladder mucus in the pathogenesis of cholesterol gallstones. Am J Surg 145:54, 1983.

167. Li YF, Moody FG, Weisbrodt NW, et al. Gallbladder contractility and mucus secretion after cholesterol feeding in the prairie dog. Surgery 100:900, 1986.

168. Lamont JT, Turner BS, Bernstein SE, et al. Gallbladder mucin secretion in mice with hemolytic anemia and pigment gallstones. Hepatology 3:198, 1983.

169. Sutor DJ, Wooley SE. The organic matrix of gallstones. Gut 15:487, 1974.

170. Schrager J, Oates MDG, Rosbottom A. The isolation and partial characterization of the principal biliary glycoprotein. Digestion 6:338, 1972.

171. Ross JW Jr. Calcium-selective electrode with liquid ion-exchanger. Science 156:1378, 1967.

172. Moore EW. Studies with ion-exchange calcium electrodes: some applications in biomedical research and clinical medicine. In: Durst R, ed. Ion Exchange Electrodes. Washington, DC: Natl. Bureau of Standards, 1969:215.

173. Kretsinger RH. A comparison of the roles of calcium in biomineralization and in cytosolic signalling. In: Westbroek P, De Jong EW, eds. Biomineralization and Biological Metal Accumulation. Dordrecht, Netherlands: D. Reidel, 1983:123.

174. Williamson BWA, Percy-Robb IW. The interactions of calcium ions with glycocholate micelles in aqueous solutions. Biochem J 181:61, 1979.

175. Moore EW, Celic L, Ostrow JD. Interactions between ionized calcium and sodium taurocholate: Bile salts are important buffers for prevention of calcium-containing gallstones. Gastroenterology 83:1079, 1982.

176. Williamson BWA, Anderson JL, Percy-Robb IW. Cholesterol gallstone pathogenesis: morphology of cholesterol nucleation on calcium salt crystals. Gut 26:A561, 1985 (Abstract).

177. Whiting MJ, Jarvinen V, Watts J McK. Chemical composition of gallstones resistant to dissolution therapy with chenodeoxycholic acid. Gut 21:1077, 1981.

178. Bateson MC, Bouchier IAD, Trash DB, et al. Calcification of radiolucent gallstones during treatment with ursodeoxycholic acid. Br Med J 283:645, 1981.

179. Harada S, Hisatsugu T. Studies on calcified structure in human cholesterol gallstones. Fukuoka Acta Med (Fukuoka Igaku Zasshi) 70:732, 1979.

180. Schoenfield LJ, Lachin JW. The National Cooperative Gallstone Steering Committee: A controlled trial of the efficacy and safety of

181. Frabboni R, Bazzoli F, Mazzella G, et al. Acquired gallstone calcification during cholelitholytic treatment with chenodeoxycholic, ursodeoxycholic, and tauroursodeoxycholic acids. Hepatology 5:1004, 1985.

182. Kibe A, Dudley MA, Halpern Z, et al. Factors affecting cholesterol monohydrate crystal nucleation time in model systems of supersaturated bile. J Lipid Res 26:1102, 1985.

183. Holzbach RT. Recent progress in understanding cholesterol crystal nucleation as a precursor to human gallstone formation. Hepatology 6:1403, 1986.

184. Berenson MM, Cardinal JR. Calcium accelerates cholesterol phase transitions in analog bile. Experientia 41:1328, 1985.

185. Toor EW, Cussler EL, Evans DF. Cholesterol microcrystal growth in bile. Clin Res 25:320, 1977.

186. Forstner JF, Forstner GG. Calcium binding to intestinal goblet cell mucin. Biochim Biophys Acta 336:283, 1975.

187. Jones CA, Hofmann AF, Mysels KJ, et al. The effect of calcium and sodium ion concentration on the properties of dilute aqueous solutions of glycine conjugated bile salts: Phase behavior and solubility products of the calcium salts of the common glycine conjugated bile acids. J Colloid Interface Sci 114:452, 1986.

188. Moore EW, Ostrow JD. Interactions of calcium with bile acids in vitro studied with the calcium electrode. Gastroenterology 77:A28, 1979 (Abstract).

189. Ostrow JD, Celic L, Moore EW. Binding of calcium to glycocholate: Studies with the calcium electrode: Bile salts are important buffers for prevention of calcium-containing gallstones. Gastroenterology 86:1335, 1984 (Abstract).

190. Moore EW. Role of calcium in the pathogenesis of gallstones with an hypothesis of structural requirements for Ca^{++}-binding to proteins and bile acids. In: Barbara L, Dowling RH, Hofmann AF, eds. Recent Advances in Bile Acid Research. New York, Raven Press, 1985:109.

191. Moore EW, Ostrow JD, Hofmann AF. Pathogenesis of calcium-containing gallstones: A unifying hypothesis on the structural requirements for Ca^{++}-binding by bile salts. Gastroenterology 88:1679, 1985 (Abstract).

192. Geller D, Ostrow JD, Moore EW, et al. Binding of calcium by bile salts as assessed by perturbation of the equilibrium solubility of calcium oxalate monohydrate. Hepatology 5:1050, 1985 (Abstract).

193. Mukidjam E, Barnes S, Elgavish GA. NMR studies of the binding of sodium and calcium ions to the bile salts glycocholate and taurocholate in dilute solutions, as probed by the paramagnetic lanthanide dysprosium. J Am Chem Soc 108:7082, 1986.

194. Williamson BWA, Percy-Robb IW. Contribution of biliary lipids to calcium binding in bile. Gastroenterology 78:696, 1980.

195. Rajagopalan N, Lindenbaum S. The binding of Ca^{2+} to taurine- and glycine-conjugated bile salts micelles. Biochim Biophys Acta 711:66, 1982.

196. Gleeson D, Murphy GM, Dowling RH. Calcium (Ca) binding by bile acids (BS's) +/− phospholipids (PL's): in vitro studies using a calcium ion electrode. Gastroenterology 88:1661, 1985 (Abstract).

197. Glasstone S, Lewis D. Elements of Physical Chemistry, 2nd Ed. Princeton, Van Nostrand, 1960:258.

198. Harned HS, Owen BB. The Physical Chemistry of Electrolytic Solutions. New York, Reinhold, 1963:10.

199. Robinson RA, Stokes RH. Electrolyte Solutions. London, Butterworths, 1959:438.

200. Moore EW, Ross JW Jr. NaCl and $CaCl_2$ activity coefficients in mixed aqueous solutions. J Appl Physiol 20:1332, 1965.

201. Moore EW, Dietschy JM. Na and K activity coefficients in bile and bile salts determined with glass electrodes. Am J Physiol 206:1111, 1964.

202. Moore EW. Hydrogen and cation analysis in biological fluids in vitro. In: Eisenman G, ed. Glass Electrodes for Hydrogen and Cations: Principles and Practice. New York, Marcel Dekker, 1967:412.

203. Moore EW. Ionized calcium in normal sera, ultrafiltrates and whole blood determined by ion-exchange electrodes. J Clin Invest 49:318, 1970.

204. Shiffman ML, Moore EW. Defective acidification leads to $CaCO_3$ supersaturation of gallbladder bile in patients with all types of gallstones. Gastroenterology 94:591, 1988 (Abstract).

205. Moore EW. Defective acidification leads to $CaCO_3$ supersaturation of gallbladder bile in patients with all types of gallstones. In: Paumgartner G, Stiehl A, Gerok W, eds. Trends in Bile Acid Research. Lancaster, MTP Press, 1988. In press.

206. Rege RV, Moore EW, Nahrwold DL. Pathogenesis of calcium-containing gallstones: Relationship of total calcium and free ionized Ca^{++} in canine gallbladder and duct bile. Surg Forum 36:132, 1985.

207. Dawes LG, Moore EW, Rege RV. Gibbs-Donnan equilibrium is the

major determinant of free Ca^{++} in canine bile. Gastroenterology 94:A534, 1988.

208. Dawes LG, Rege RV, Moore EW. Bile salts, bilirubin and carbonate: The binders of calcium. Hepatology 8:1258, 1988 (Abstract).

209. Sutor DJ, Wilkie LI, Jackson MJ. Ionized calcium in pathological human bile. J Clin Pathol 33:86, 1980.

210. Moore EW, Verine HJ. Pancreatic calcification: Formation constants of $CaHCO_3$ and $CaCO_3$ complexes determined with Ca^{2+} electrode. Am J Physiol 241:G182, 1981.

211. Shimizu S, Rege RV, Webster CC, et al. High-affinity binding of ionized calcium (Ca^{2+}) by conjugated bilirubin. Hepatology 7:1110, 1987.

212. Sutor DJ, Wilkie LI. Inorganic phosphorus in human bile. Clin Chim Acta 77:31, 1977.

213. Osborne CV, Moore EW. Studies with ion-exchange calcium electrodes: Binding of calcium by purified crystalline human albumin. Clin Res 22:476, 1976 (Abstract).

214. Moore EW. The binding of calcium to albumin in normal human serum: A unique ion-protein interaction—The "clam effect." J Clin Invest 53:54a, 1974 (Abstract).

215. Moore EW, Verine HJ. Pancreatic calcification and stone formation: a thermodynamic model of calcium in pancreatic juice. Am J Physiol 252(15):G707, 1987.

216. Cummings SA, Hofmann AF. Physiologic determinants of biliary calcium secretion in the dog. Gastroenterology 87:664, 1984.

217. Moore EW, Rasmusen H, Shiffman ML. Pathogenesis of calcium-containing gallstones: All biliary calcium in guinea pig is accounted for by passive entry from plasma. Gastroenterology 90:1748, 1986 (Abstract).

218. Dawes LG, Moore EW, Rege RV. Biliary calcium secretion in the dog is passive and bile flow–dependent. Gastroenterology 94:533, 1988 (Abstract).

219. Moore EW, Gleeson D, Murphy GM, et al. Biliary calcium secretion in man: A test of the computer model in bile salt–depleted subjects. Hepatology 5:994, 1985.

220. Bills PM. The precipitation of calcium carbonate polymorphs in vitro at 37 degrees C. Calcif Tissue Int 37:174, 1985.

221. Moore EW, Verine HJ. Pathogenesis of pancreatic and biliary $CaCO_3$ lithiasis: The solubility product (K'sp) of calcite determined with the Ca^{++} electrode. J Lab Clin Med 106:611, 1985.

222. Broman AA, Hastings AB. Solubility of aragonite in salt solutions. J Biol Chem 119:241, 1931.

223. Rege RV, Moore EW. Pathogenesis of calcium-containing gallstones: Canine ductular bile, but not gallbladder bile, is supersaturated with calcium carbonate. J Clin Invest 77:21, 1986.

224. Winchester D, Rege RV, Moore EW. Calcium saturation of bile: Canine common duct bile is always supersaturated with calcium carbonate ($CaCO_3$). Hepatology 6:1153, 1986 (Abstract).

225. Shiffman ML, Carithers RC Jr, Mendez-Picon G, et al. Duct bile is supersaturated with $CaCO_3$ in man. Implications for the pathogenesis of gallstone formation. Hepatology 7:1101, 1987 (Abstract).

226. Moore EW, Zimmerman MJ. Pancreatic ionized and total calcium secretion: A test of the thermodynamic calcium model for pancreatic lithogenicity. Gastroenterology 82:1134, 1982 (Abstract).

227. Dawes LG, Ostrow JD, Shimizu S, et al. Inhibition of $CaCO_3$ precipitation by canine gallbladder bile. Gastroenterology 94:534, 1988 (Abstract).

228. Ostrow JD, Celic L, Mukerjee P. Molecular and micellar associations in the pH-dependent stable and metastable dissolution of unconjugated bilirubin by bile salts. J Lipid Res 29:335, 1988.

229. Ostrow JD, Celic L. Apparent solubility products (K'sp) of the calcium salts of unconjugated bilirubin indicate supersaturation of human gallbladder bile with $Ca(HB)_2$, but not CaB. Hepatology 7:1111, 1987 (Abstract).

230. Moore EW. The regulation of ionized calcium, $[Ca^{++}]$, in bile: Taurocholate induces powerful Gibbs-Donnan effects in vitro. Gastroenterology 94:A572, 1988.

231. Rege RV, Lee MJ, Moore EW. The Gibbs-Donnan equilibrium: Its effect on the distribution of calcium (Ca^{++}) across rabbit gallbladder epithelium. Gastroenterology 90:1761, 1986 (Abstract).

232. Dietschy JM, Moore EW. Diffusion potentials and potassium distribution across the gallbladder wall. J Clin Invest 43:1551, 1964.

233. Moore EW, Dawes LG, Rege RV. The Gibbs-Donnan equilibrium and the distribution of K^+ between bile and plasma in canine common duct and gallbladder bile. Gastroenterology 94:A572, 1988.

234. Boyer JL, Elias E, Layden TJ. The paracellular pathway and bile formation. Yale J Biol Med 52:61, 1979.

235. Moore EW. Bile salt osmosity: A key factor in bile acid–dependent flow in the biliary tract. Hepatology 6:1158, 1986 (Abstract).

236. Selle JG, Altemeier WA, Fullen WD, et al. Cholelithiasis in hyperparathyroidism. Arch Surg 105:369, 1972.

237. Werner S, Hjern B, Sjoberg HE. Primary hyperparathyroidism. Acta Chir Scand 140:618, 1974.

238. Funk C, Ammann R, Binswanger U, et al. Cholelithiasis beim primaren Hyperparathyreoidismus. Schweiz Med Wochenschr 104:1060, 1974.

239. Brunner H, Rothmund M. Primarer hyperparathyreoidismu, pankreatitis und cholelithiasis. Dtsch Med Wochenschr 98:426, 1973.

240. Weens HS. Cholelithiasis in sickle cell anemia. Adv Intern Med 22:182, 1945.

241. Jordan RA. Cholelithiasis in sickle cell disease. Gastroenterology 33:952, 1957.

242. Cameron JL, Maddrey WC, Zuidema GD. Biliary tract disease in sickle cell anemia: surgical considerations. Ann Surg 174:702, 1971.

243. Lachman BS, Lazerson J, Starshak RJ, et al. The prevalence of cholelithiasis in sickle cell disease as diagnosed by ultrasound and cholecystography. Pediatrics 64:601, 1979.

244. Sarnaik S, Corbett DP, Whittenn CF. Incidence of cholelithiasis in sickle cell anemia using the ultrasonic gray-scale technique. J Pediatr 96:1005, 1980.

245. Bates GC, Brown CH. Incidence of gallbladder disease in chronic hemolytic anemia (spherocytosis). Gastroenterology 21:104, 1952.

246. Boonyapisit ST, Trotman BW, Ostrow JD. Unconjugated bilirubin and the hydrolysis of conjugated bilirubin in gallbladder bile of patients with cholelithiasis. Gastroenterology 74:70, 1978.

247. Maki T. Pathogenesis of calcium bilirubinate gallstones: Role of E. coli, β-glucuronidase and coagulation by inorganic ions, polyelectrolytes and agitation. Ann Surg 164:90, 1966.

248. Tabata M, Nakayama F. Bacteria and gallstones: etiologic significance. Dig Dis Sci 26:218, 1981.

249. Ho KJ. Human β-glucuronidase: Studies on the effects of pH and bile acids in regard to its role in the pathogenesis of cholelithiasis. Biochim Biophys Acta 827:197, 1985.

250. Ho KJ, Hsu SC, Chen JS, et al. Human biliary β-glucuronidase: correlation of its activity with deconjugation of bilirubin in the bile. Eur J Clin Invest 16:361, 1986.

251. Sjodahl R, Tagesson C, Wetterfors J. On the pathogenesis of acute cholecystitis. Surg Gynecol Obstet 146:199, 1978.

252. Mead JF, Alfin-Slater RB, Howton DR, et al. Lipids: Chemistry, Biochemistry and Nutrition, New York, Plenum Press, 1986.

253. De Fourcroy M. De la substance feuilletée et cristalline contenue dans les calculs biliares et de la nature des concretions cystiques cristalisées. Ann Chim 3:242, 1789.

254. Chevreul M. Examen des graisses d'homme, de mouton, de boeuf, de jaguar et d'oie. Ann Chim Physique 2:339, 1816.

255. Chevreul M. Sur plusieurs corps gras, et particulierment sur leur combinaisons avec les alcalis. Ann Chim 95:5, 1815.

256. Berthelot M. Sur plusiers alcools nouveaux. Combinaisons des acides avec la cholesterine, l'ethal, le camphre de Borneo et la meconine. Ann Chim Physique 56:51, 1859.

257. Diels O, Abderhalden E. Zur Kenntniss des Cholesterins. Chem Ber 37:3092, 1904.

258. Gill JF Jr, Kennelly PJ, Rodwell VW. Control mechanisms in sterol uptake and biosynthesis. In: Danielsson H, Sjovall J, eds. Sterols and Bile Acids. New York, Elsevier, 1985:41.

259. Chapman D, Kramers MTC, Restall CJ. Cholesterol and biomembrane structures. In: Danielsson H, Sjovall J, eds. Sterols and Bile Acids. New York, Elsevier, 1985:151.

260. Small DM. Lipid classification based on interactions with water. In: Small DM, ed. Handbook of Lipid Research. IV. The Physical Chemistry of Lipids. New York, Plenum Press, 1986:89.

261. Small DM. Sterols and sterol esters. In: Small DM, ed. Handbook of Lipid Research. IV. The Physical Chemistry of Lipids. New York, Plenum Press, 1986:395.

262. Renshaw PF, Janoff AS, Miller KW. On the nature of dilute aqueous cholesterol suspensions. J Lipid Res 24:47, 1983.

263. Lange Y. Molecular dynamics of bilayer lipids. In: Small DM, ed. Handbook of Lipid Research. IV. The Physical Chemistry of Lipids. New York, Plenum Press, 1986:523.

264. Craven BM. Crystal structure of cholesterol monohydrate. Nature 260:727, 1967.

265. Whiting MJ, Down RHL, Watts J McK. Biliary crystals and granules, the cholesterol saturation index, and the prediction of gallstone type. Surg Gastroenterol 1:17, 1982.

266. Sedaghat A, Grundy SM. Cholesterol crystals and the formation of cholesterol gallstones. N Engl J Med 302:1274, 1980.

267. Moore B, Parker WH. On the functions of the bile as a solvent. Proc R Soc Lond Biol 68:64, 1901.

268. Isaksson B. On the lipid constituents of bile from human gallbladder containing cholesterol gallstones. Acta Soc Med Upsal 59:277, 1954.

269. Isaksson B. On the dissolving power of lecithin and bile salts for cholesterol in human bladder bile. Acta Soc Med Upsal 59:296, 1954.

270. Carey MC, Small DM. The characteristics of mixed micellar solutions with particular reference to bile. Am J Med 49:590, 1970.

271. Small DM. Phospholipids. In: Small DM, ed. Handbook of Lipid Research. IV. The Physical Chemistry of Lipids. New York, Plenum Press, 1986:475.
272. van der Meer W. Physical aspects of membrane fluidity. In: Shinitzky M, ed. Physiology of Membrane Fluidity, Vol. 1. Boca Raton: CRC Press, 1984:53.
273. Huang C-H. A structural model for the cholesterol phosphatidylcholine complexes in bilayer membranes. Lipids 12:348, 1977.
274. Cooper RA, Strauss JF III. Regulation of cell membrane cholesterol. In: Shinitzky M, ed. Physiology of Membrane Fluidity, Vol. 1. Boca Raton: CRC Press, 1984:74.
275. Collins JJ, Phillips MC. The stability and structure of cholesterol-rich codispersions of cholesterol and phosphatidylcholine. J Lipid Res 23:291, 1982.
276. Olszewski M, Holzbach RT, Saupe A, et al. Liquid crystals in human bile. Nature 242:336, 1973.
277. Thomas PJ, Hofmann AF. A simple calculation of the lithogenic index of the bile: expressing lipid composition on rectangular coordinates. Gastroenterology 65:698, 1973.
278. Metzger AL, Heymsfield S, Grundy SM. The lithogenic index—a numerical expression for the relative lithogenicity of bile. Gastroenterology 62:499, 1972.
279. Gregory DH, Vlahcevic ZR, Swell L. Editorial: Determination of the cholesterol saturation of human bile and its relevance to gallstone formation. Am J Dig Dis 19:268, 1974.
280. Swell L, Bell CC Jr, Gregory DH, et al. The cholesterol saturation index of human bile. Am J Dig Dis 19:261, 1974.
281. Kuroki S, Cohen BI, Carey MC, et al. Rapid computation with the personal computer of the percent cholesterol saturation of bile samples. J Lipid Res 27:442, 1986.
282. Vlahcevic ZR, Bell CC Jr, Swell L. Significance of the liver in the production of lithogenic bile in man. Gastroenterology 59:62, 1970.
283. Small DM, Rapo S. Source of abnormal bile in patients with cholesterol gallstones. N Engl J Med 283:53, 1970.
284. Grundy SM, Duane WC, Adler RD. Biliary lipid outputs in young women with cholesterol gallstones. Metabolism 23:67, 1974.
285. Kay RE, Entenman C. Stimulation of taurocholate synthesis and biliary excretion of lipids. Am J Physiol 200:855, 1961.
286. Schersten T, Nilsson S, Cahlin E, et al. Relationship between the biliary excretion of bile acids and the excretion of water, lecithin and cholesterol in man. Eur J Clin Invest 1:242, 1971.
287. Wagner CI, Trotman BW, Soloway RD. Kinetic analysis of biliary lipid secretion in man and dog. J Clin Invest 57:473, 1976.
288. Lindblad L, Lundholm K, Schersten T. Influence of cholic and chenodeoxycholic acid on biliary cholesterol secretion in man. Eur J Clin Invest 7:383, 1977.
289. Mazer NA, Carey MC. Mathematical model of biliary lipid secretion: a quantitative analysis of physiological and biochemical data from man and other species. J Lipid Res 25:932, 1984.
290. Carey MC, Mazer NA. Biliary lipid secretion in health and in cholesterol gallstone disease. Hepatology 4:31S, 1984.
291. Heaton KW, Read AE. Gall stones in patients with disorders of the terminal ileum and disturbed bile salt metabolism. Br Med J 3:494, 1969.
292. Bennion L, Grundy SM. Risk factors for the development of cholelithiasis in man. N Engl J Med 299:1161, 1978.
293. Grundy SM, Mok HYI. Colestipol, clofibrate and phytosterols in combined therapy of hyperlipidemia. J Lab Clin Med 89:354, 1977.
294. Vlahcevic ZR, Cooper-Bell C Jr, Buhac I, et al. Diminished bile acid pool size in patients with gallstones. Gastroenterology 59:165, 1970.
295. Vlahcevic ZR, Bell CC Jr, Gregory DH, et al. Relationship of bile acid pool size to the formation of lithogenic bile in female Indians of the Southwest. Gastroenterology 62:73, 1972.
296. Hepner GW, Quarfordt SH. Kinetics of cholesterol and bile acids in patients with cholesterol cholelithiasis. Gastroenterology 69:318, 1975.
297. Grundy SM, Metzger AL, Adler RD. Mechanisms of lithogenic bile formation in American Indian women with cholesterol gallstones. J Clin Invest 51:3026, 1972.
298. Bell CC Jr, Vlahcevic ZR, Swell L. Alterations in the lipids of human hepatic bile after the oral administration of bile salts. Surg Gynecol Obstet 132:36, 1971.
299. Thistle JL, Schoenfield LJ. Induced alterations in composition of bile of persons having cholelithiasis. Gastroenterology 61:488, 1971.
300. Mok HYI, von Bergmann K, Grundy SM. Kinetics of the enterohepatic circulation during fasting: biliary lipid secretion and gallbladder storage. Gastroenterology 78:1023, 1980.
301. LaRusso NF, Hoffman NE, Hofmann AF, et al. Effect of primary bile acid ingestion on bile acid metabolism and biliary lipid secretion in gallstone patients. Gastroenterology 69:1301, 1975.
302. Shaffer EA, Small DM. Biliary lipid secretion in cholesterol gallstone disease. The effects of cholecystectomy and obesity. J Clin Invest 59:828, 1977.

303. Bennion LJ, Grundy SM. Effects of obesity and caloric intake on biliary lipid composition in man. J Clin Invest 45:996, 1975.
304. Tritapepe R, Di Padova C, Zerin M, et al. Lithogenic bile after conjugated estrogen. N Engl J Med 295:961, 1972.
305. Wingrave SJ, Kay CR. Oral contraceptives and gallbladder disease. Lancet 2:957, 1982.
306. Kern F Jr, Everson GT, DeMark B, et al. Biliary lipids, bile acids, and gallbladder function in the human female: effects of contraceptive steroids. J Lab Clin Med 99:798, 1982.
307. Bennion LJ, Ginsberg RL, Garnick MB, et al. Effects of oral contraceptives on the gallbladder bile of normal women. N Engl J Med 294:189, 1976.
308. Kern F Jr, Erfling W, Simon FR, et al. Effect of estrogens on the liver. Gastroenterology 75:512, 1978.
309. Grundy SM, Ahrens EH Jr, Salen G, et al. Mechanisms of action of clofibrate on cholesterol metabolism in patients with hyperlipidemia. J Lipid Res 13:531, 1972.
310. Pertsemlidis D, Panveliwatta D, Ahrens EH. Effects of clofibrate and of an estrogen-progestin combination on fasting biliary lipids and cholic acid kinetics. Gastroenterology 66:565, 1974.
311. Meyer PD, DenBesten L, Gurll WJ. Effects of cholesterol gallstone induction on gallbladder function and bile salt pool size in the prairie dog model. Surgery 83:599, 1978.
312. DenBesten L, Connor WE, Bell S. The effect of dietary cholesterol on the composition of human bile in healthy subjects. Z Ernahrungswiss 10:178, 1971.
313. Sarles H, Hauton J, Planche NE, et al. Diet, cholesterol gallstones, and composition of the bile. Am J Dig Dis 15:251, 1970.
314. Sarles H, Crotte C, Gerolami A. Influence of cholestyramine, bile salt, and cholesterol feeding on the lipid composition of hepatic bile in man. Gastroenterology 5:603, 1970.
315. Lee DWT, Gilmore CJ, Bonorris G, et al. Effect of dietary cholesterol on biliary lipids in patients with gallstones and normal subjects. Am J Clin Nutr 42:414, 1985.
316. Miettinen TA. Cholesterol production in obesity. Circulation 44:842, 1971.
317. Nestel PJ, Schreibman PH, Ahrens EH. Cholesterol metabolism in human obesity. J Clin Invest 52:2389, 1973.
318. Leijd B. Cholesterol and bile acid metabolism in obesity. Clin Sci 59:203, 1980.
319. Barbara L, Sama C, Morselli-Labate AM, et al. A population study on the prevalence of gallstone disease: The Sirmione study. Hepatology 7:913, 1987.
320. Coyne MJ, Bonorris GG, Goldstein LI, et al. Effect of chenodeoxycholic acid and phenobarbital on the rate-limiting enzymes of hepatic cholesterol and bile acid synthesis in patients with gallstones. J Lab Clin Med 87:281, 1976.
321. Salen G, Nicolau G, Shefer S, et al. Hepatic cholesterol metabolism in patients with gallstones. Gastroenterology 69:676, 1975.
322. Tint GS, Salen G, Shefer S. Effect of ursodeoxycholic acid and chenodeoxycholic acid on cholesterol and bile acid metabolism. Gastroenterology 91:1007, 1986.
323. Angelin B, Ewerth S, Einarsson K. Ursodeoxycholic acid treatment in cholesterol gallstone disease: effects on hepatic 3-hydroxy-3-methylglutaryl coenzyme A reductase activity, biliary lipid composition, and plasma lipid levels. J Lipid Res 24:461, 1983.
324. Carulli N, Ponz de Leon M, Zironi F, et al. Hepatic cholesterol and bile acid metabolism in subjects with gallstones: comparative effects of short-term feeding of chenodeoxycholic and ursodeoxycholic acid. J Lipid Res 21:35, 1980.
325. Heuman DM, Vlahcevic ZR, Bailey ML, et al. Regulation of bile acid synthesis. II. Effect of bile acid feeding on enzymes regulating hepatic cholesterol and bile acid synthesis in the rat. Hepatology 8:892, 1988.
326. Nilsell K, Angelin B, Leijd B, et al. Comparative effects of ursodeoxycholic acid and chenodeoxycholic acid on bile acid kinetics and biliary lipid secretion in humans. Gastroenterology 85:1248, 1983.
327. von Bergmann K, Epple-Gutsfeld M, Leiss O. Differences in the effects of chenodeoxycholic and ursodeoxycholic acid on biliary lipid secretion and bile acid synthesis in patients with gallstones. Gastroenterology 87:136, 1984.
328. LaRusso NF, Szczepanik PA, Hofmann AF. Effect of deoxycholic acid ingestion on bile acid metabolism and biliary lipid secretion in normal subjects. Gastroenterology 72:132, 1977.
329. Gebhard RL, Hunninghake DB, Duane WC. Simvastatin, an inhibitor of HMG CoA reductase, lowers cholesterol saturation index of gallbladder bile in man. Gastroenterology 94:A537, 1988 (Abstract).
330. Duane WC, Hunninghake DB, Freeman ML, et al. Simvastatin, a competitive inhibitor of HMG-CoA reductase, lowers cholesterol saturation index of gallbladder bile. Hepatology 8:1147, 1988.
331. Stone BG, Erickson SK, Craig WY, et al. Regulation of rat biliary cholesterol secretion by agents that alter intrahepatic cholesterol metabolism. Evidence for a distinct biliary precursor pool. J Clin Invest 76:1773, 1985.

332. Bellentani S, Hardison WG, Manenti F. Mechanisms of liver adaptation to prolonged selective biliary obstruction (SBO) in the rat. J Hepatol 1:525, 1985.

333. Swell L, Bell CC Jr, Vlahcevic ZR. Relationship of bile acid pool size to the formation of lithogenic bile in female Indians of the Southwest. Gastroenterology 61:716, 1971.

334. Bell CC Jr, McCormick WC 3d, Gregory DH, et al. Relationship of bile acid pool size to the formation of lithogenous bile in male Indians of the Southwest. Surg Gynecol Obstet 134:473, 1972.

335. Sampliner RE, Bennet PH, Commers LJ. Gallbladder disease in Pima Indians: demonstration of high prevalence and early onset by cholecystography. N Engl J Med 283:1358, 1970.

336. Godfrey, PP, Warner MJ. and Coleman R. Enzymes and proteins in bile. Variations in output in rat cannula bile during and after depletion of the bile-salt pool. Biochem J 196:11, 1981.

337. Turley SD, Spady DK, Dietschy JM. Alteration of the degree of biliary cholesterol saturation in the hamster and rat by manipulation of the pools of preformed and newly synthesized cholesterol. Gastroenterology 84:253, 1983.

338. Turley SD, Dietschy JM. Regulation of biliary cholesterol output in the rat: dissociation from the rate of hepatic cholesterol synthesis, the size of the hepatic cholesteryl ester pool, and the hepatic uptake of chylomicron cholesterol. J Lipid Res 20:923, 1979.

339. Carulli N, Loria P, Bertolotti M, et al. Effects of acute changes of bile acid pool composition on biliary lipid secretion. J Clin Invest 74:614, 1984.

340. Loria P, Carulli N, Medici G, et al. Effect of ursocholic acid on bile lipid secretion and composition. Gastroenterology 90:865, 1986.

341. Armstrong MJ, Carey MC. The hydrophobic-hydrophilic balance of bile salts. Inverse correlation between reverse-phase high performance liquid chromatographic mobilities and micellar cholesterol-solubilizing capacities. J Lipid Res 23:70, 1982.

342. Lanzini A, Northfield TC. Effect of ursodeoxycholic acid on biliary lipid coupling and on cholesterol absorption during fasting and eating in subjects with cholesterol gallstones. Gastroenterology 95:408, 1988.

343. Cronholm T, Curstedt T, Sjovall J. Origin of biliary phosphatidylcholines studied by coenzyme labelling with [1,1-^{2}H]ethanol. Biochim Biophys Acta 753:276, 1983.

344. Robins SJ, Fasulo JM, Collins MA, et al. Evidence for separate pathways of transport of newly synthesized and preformed cholesterol into bile. J Biol Chem 260:6511, 1985.

345. Robins SJ, Brunengraber H. Origin of biliary cholesterol and lecithin in the rat: contribution of new synthesis and preformed hepatic stores. J Lipid Res 23:604, 1982.

346. Spitzer HL, Kyriakides EC, Balint JA. Bile phospholipids in various species. Nature 204:288. 1964.

347. Nilsson S. Synthesis and secretion of biliary phospholipids in man. Acta Chir Scand 405(Suppl.):1, 1970.

348. Swell L, Bell CC Jr, Entenman C. Bile acids and lipid metabolism. III. Influence of bile acids on phospholipids in liver and bile of the isolated perfused dog liver. Biochim Biophys Acta 164:278, 1968.

349. Swell L, Entenman C, Leong GF, et al. Bile acids and lipid metabolism. IV. Influence of bile acids on biliary and liver organelle phospholipids. Am J Physiol 215:1390, 1968.

350. Zilversmit DB, Van Handel E. The origin of bile lecithin and the use of bile to determine plasma lecithin turnover rates. Arch Biochem Biophys 73:224, 1958.

351. Robins SJ, Armstrong MJ. Biliary lecithin secretion. II. Effects of dietary choline and biliary lecithin synthesis. Gastroenterology 70:397, 1976.

352. Patton GM, Fasulo JM, Robins SJ. Separation of phospholipids and individual molecular species of phospholipids by high-performance liquid chromatography. J Lipid Res 23:190, 1982.

353. Robins SJ, Patton GM. Separation of phospholipid molecular species by high-performance liquid chromatography: potentials for use in metabolic studies. J Lipid Res 27:131, 1986.

354. Apstein MD, Russo AR. Ampicillin inhibits biliary cholesterol secretion. Dig Dis Sci 30:253, 1985.

355. Apstein MD. Inhibition of biliary phospholipid and cholesterol secretion by bilirubin in the Sprague-Dawley and Gunn rat. Gastroenterology 87:634, 1984.

356. Apstein MD, Robins SJ. Effect of organic anions on biliary lipids in the rat. Gastroenterology 83:1120, 1982.

357. Hardison WG, Apter JT. Micellar theory of biliary cholesterol excretion. Am J Physiol 222:61, 1972.

358. Swell L, Gregory DH, Vlahcevic ZR. Current concepts of the pathogenesis of cholesterol gallstones. Med Clin North Am 58:1449, 1974.

359. Gregory DH, Vlahcevic ZR, Schatzki P, et al. Mechanism of secretion of biliary lipids. I. Role of bile canalicular and microsomal membranes in the synthesis and transport of biliary lecithin and cholesterol. J Clin Invest 55:105, 1975.

360. Barnwell SG, Lowe PJ, Coleman R. The effects of colchicine on secretion into bile of bile salts, phospholipids, cholesterol and plasma membrane enzymes: bile salts are secreted unaccompanied by phospholipids and cholesterol. Biochem J 220:723, 1984.

361. Crawford JM, Gollan JL. Hepatocyte cotransport of taurocholate and bilirubin glucuronides: role of microtubules. Am J Physiol 255:G121, 1988.

362. Crawford JM, Berken CA, Gollan JL. Role of the hepatocyte microtubular system in the excretion of bile salts and biliary lipid: implications for intracellular vesicular transport. J Lipid Res 29:144, 1988.

363. Jones AL, Schmucker DL, Mooney JS, et al. Alterations in hepatic pericanalicular cytoplasm during enhanced bile secretory activity. Lab Invest 40:512, 1979.

364. Sakisaka S, Ng OC, Boyer JL. Tubulovesicular transcytotic pathway in isolated rat hepatocyte couplets in culture. Gastroenterology 95:793, 1988.

365. Halpern Z, Dudley MA, Lynn MP, et al. Rapid vesicle formation and aggregation in abnormal human bile. A time-lapse video-enhanced contrast microscopy study. Gastroenterology 90:875, 1986.

366. Somjen GJ, Marikovsky Y, Lelkes P, et al. Cholesterol-phospholipid vesicles in human bile: an ultrastructural study. Biochim Biophys Acta 879:14, 1986.

367. Carey MC. Measurement of the physical-chemical properties of bile salt solutions. In: Barbara L, Dowling RH, Hofmann AF, et al., eds. Bile Acids in Gastroenterology. Lancaster, MTP Press, 1983:19.

368. Gewirtz DA, Randolph JK, Goldman ID. Induction of taurocholate release from isolated rat hepatocytes in suspension by α-adrenergic agents and vasopressin: implications for control of bile salt secretion. Hepatology 4:205, 1984.

369. Lamri Y, Roda A, Dumont M, et al. Immunoperoxidase localization of bile salts in rat liver cells. Evidence for a role of the Golgi apparatus in bile salt transport. J Clin Invest 82:1173, 1988.

370. Pattinson NR, Chapman BA. Distribution of biliary cholesterol between mixed micelles and non-micelles in relation to fasting and feeding in humans. Gastroenterology 91:697, 1986.

371. Holzbach RT, Marsh M, Olszewski M, et al. Cholesterol solubility in bile: Evidence that supersaturated bile is frequent in healthy man. J Clin Invest 52:1467, 1973.

372. Dam H, Kruse I, Prange I, et al. Studies on human bile. III. Composition of duodenal bile from healthy young volunteers compared with composition of bladder bile from surgical patients with and without uncomplicated gallstone disease. Z Ernalrungswiss 10:160, 1971.

373. Mackay C, Crook JN, Smith DC, et al. The composition of hepatic and gallbladder bile in patients with gallstones. Gut 13:759, 1972.

374. Carey MC, Ko G. The importance of total lipid concentration in determining cholesterol solubility in bile and the development of critical tables for calculating percent cholesterol saturation, with a correction factor for ursodeoxycholate-rich bile. In: Paumgartner G, Stiehl A, Gerok, W, eds. Biological Effects of Bile Acids. Boston, MTP Press, 1979:299.

375. Somjen GJ, Gilat T. Changing concepts of cholesterol solubility in bile. Gastroenterology 91:772, 1986.

376. Somjen GJ, Gilat T. A non-micellar mode of cholesterol transport in human bile. FEBS Lett 156:265, 1983.

377. Somjen GJ, Gilat T. Contribution of vesicular and micellar carriers to cholesterol transport in human bile. J Lipid Res 26:699, 1985.

378. Holzbach RT. Metastability behavior of supersaturated bile. Hepatology 4:155S, 1984.

379. McLean LR, Phillips MC. Cholesterol transfer from small and large unilamellar vesicles. Biochim Biophys Acta 776:21, 1984.

380. McLean LR, Phillips MC. Kinetics of phosphatidylcholine and lysophosphatidylcholine exchange between unilamellar vesicles. Biochemistry 23:4624, 1984.

381. Mazer NA, Carey MC. Quasi-elastic light-scattering studies of aqueous biliary lipid systems. Cholesterol solubilization and precipitation in model bile solutions. Biochemistry 22:426, 1983.

382. Cohen DE, Angelico M, Carey MC. Evidence for vesicular secretion of biliary lipids and their transformation into mixed micelles in native bile. Gastroenterology 90:1786, 1986.

383. Holzbach RT. Factors influencing cholesterol nucleation in bile. Hepatology 4:173S, 1984.

384. Pattinson NR. Solubilisation of cholesterol in human bile. FEBS Lett 181:339, 1985.

385. Halpern Z, Dudley MA, Lynn MP, et al. Vesicle aggregation in model systems of supersaturated bile: relation to crystal nucleation and lipid composition of the vesicular phase. J Lipid Res 27:295, 1986.

386. Mazer NA, Schurtenberger P, Carey MC, et al. Quasi-elastic light scattering studies of native hepatic bile from the dog: comparison with aggregative behavior of model biliary lipid systems. Biochemistry 23:1994, 1984.

387. Holzbach RT, Marsh M. Transient liquid crystals in human bile analogues. Mol Cryst Liq Cryst 28:217, 1975.

388. Somjen GJ, Marikowsky Y, Wachtel E, et al. Identification and separation of phospholipid lamellae—a cholesterol carrier in human bile. Presented at the 10th International Bile Acid Meeting, Freiburg, W. Germany, 1988.
389. Carey MC, Cahalane MJ. The enterohepatic circulation. In: Arias I, Popper H, Schachter D, et al., eds. The Liver: Biology and Pathobiology. New York, Raven Press, 1988:573.
390. Salvioli G, Igimi H, Carey MC. Cholesterol gallstone dissolution in bile: dissolution kinetics of crystalline cholesterol monohydrate by conjugated chenodeoxycholate—lecithin and ursodeoxycholate—lecithin mixtures. Dissimilar phase equilibria and dissolution mechanisms. J Lipid Res 24:701, 1983.
391. Lindenbaum S, Rajagopalan N. Kinetics and thermodynamics of dissolution of lecithin by bile salts. Hepatology 4:124S, 1984.
392. Rajagopalan N, Lindenbaum S. Kinetics and thermodynamics of the formation of mixed micelles of egg phosphatidylcholine and bile salts. J Lipid Res 25:135, 1984.
393. Salvioli G, Lugli R, Pradelli JM. Effects of bile salts on membranes. In: Calandra S, Carulli N, Salvioli G, eds. Liver and Lipid Metabolism. New York, Elsevier Science Publishers, 1984:163.
394. Corrigan OI, Su CC, Higuchi WI, et al. Mesophase formation during cholesterol dissolution in ursodeoxycholic-lecithin solutions: new mechanism for gallstone dissolution in humans. J Pharm Sci 69:869, 1980.
395. Carey MC, Montet JC, Phillips MC, et al. Thermodynamic and molecular basis for dissimilar cholesterol solubilizing capacities by micellar solutions of bile salts: cases of sodium chenodeoxycholate and sodium ursodeoxycholate and their glycine and taurine conjugates. Biochemistry 20:3637, 1981.
396. Park YH, Igimi H, Carey MC. Dissolution of human cholesterol gallstones in simulated chenodeoxycholate-rich and ursodeoxycholate-rich biles: an in vitro study of dissolution rates and mechanisms. Gastroenterology 87:150, 1984.
397. Igimi H, Carey MC. Cholesterol gallstone dissolution in bile: dissolution kinetics of crystalline cholesterol (anhydrate and monohydrate) with chenodeoxycholate, ursodeoxycholate and their glycine and taurine conjugates. J Lipid Res 22:254, 1981.
398. Leighton LS, Carey MC. Bile salt hydrophilicity determines whether the physical state of native hepatic bile is predominantly vesicular or micellar. Gastroenterology 86:1157, 1984.
399. Walton AG. The Formation and Properties of Precipitates, Vol. 23. New York, R. E. Krieger, 1979.
400. Morse LJ, Millin J. Gallstone formation secondary to a foreign body. N Engl J Med 284:590, 1971.
401. Kachar B, Evans DF, Ninham BW. Video-enhanced differential interference contrast microscopy: a new tool for the study of association colloids and prebiotic assemblies. J Colloid Interface Sci 100:287, 1984.
402. Harvey PRC, Somjen G, Lichtenberg MS, et al. Nucleation of cholesterol from vesicles isolated from bile of patients with and without cholesterol gallstones. Biochim Biophys Acta 921:198, 1987.
403. Lee SP, Park HZ, Madani H, et al. Partial characterization of a nonmicellar system of cholesterol solubilization in bile. Am J Physiol 252:G374, 1987.
404. Papahadjopoulos D, Vail WJ, Pangborn WA, et al. Studies on membrane fusion. II. Induction of fusion in pure phospholipid membranes by calcium ions and other divalent metals. Biochim Biophys Acta 448:265, 1976.
405. Smith BF, Lamont JT. The central issue of cholesterol gallstones. Hepatology 6:529, 1986.
406. Levy PF, Smith BF, Lamont JT. Human gallbladder mucin accelerates nucleation of cholesterol in model bile. Gastroenterology 87:270, 1984.
407. Smith BF. Human gallbladder mucin binds biliary lipids and promotes cholesterol crystal nucleation in model bile. J Lipid Res 28:1088, 1987.
408. Gallinger S, Taylor RD, Harvey PRC, et al. Effect of mucous glycoprotein on nucleation time of human bile. Gastroenterology 89:648, 1985.
409. Smith BF, Lamont JT. Bovine gallbladder mucin binds bilirubin in vitro. Gastroenterology 85:707, 1983.
410. Smith BF, Lamont JT. Hydrophobic binding properties of bovine gallbladder mucin. J Biol Chem 259:12170, 1984.
411. Ostrow JD, Dever TJ, Gallo D. Determinants of the solubility of unconjugated bilirubin in bile. Relationship to pigment gallstones. In: Berk PD, Berlin NI, eds. Chemistry and Physiology of Bile Pigments. Washington, D.C.:NIH-DHEW Fogarty Int. Conf. Proc., 1977:404.
412. Lowenstam HA, Weiner S. Mineralization by organisms and the evolution of biomineralization. In: Westbroek P, De Jong EW, eds. Biomineralization and Biological Metal Accumulation. Dordrecht, Netherlands: D. Reidel, 1983:191.
413. Krampitz G, Drolshagen H, Hausle J, Hof-Irmscher K. Organic matrices of mollusc shells. In: Westbroek P, De Jong EW, eds.

Biomineralization and Biological Metal Accumulation. Dordrecht, Netherlands: D. Reidel, 1983:231.
414. Veis A, Sabsay B. Bone and tooth formation. In: Westbroek P, De Jong EW, eds. Biomineralization and Biological Metal Accumulation. Dordrecht, Holland:D. Reidel, 1983:273.
415. Nagashima H, Suzuki N, Yosizawa Z. Coagulating effect of calcium carbonate on sulfated glycoproteins isolated from pathological human bile. Tohoku J Exp Med 113:159, 1974.
416. Lee SL, Veis A, Glonek T. Dentin phosphoprotein: an extracellular calcium-binding protein. Biochemistry 16:2971, 1977.
417. Termine JD, Eanes ED, Conn KM. Phosphoprotein modulation of apatite crystallization. Calcif Tissue Int 31:247, 1980.
418. Lonsdale K. Epitaxy as a growth factor in urinary calculi and gallstones. Nature (London) 217:56, 1968.
419. Westbroek P, De Jong EW. Biomineralization and Biological Metal Accumulation: Biological and Geological. Dordrecht, Netherlands: D. Reidel, 1982:1.
420. Gollish SH, Burnstein MJ, Ilson RG, et al. Nucleation of cholesterol monohydrate crystals from hepatic and gallbladder bile of patients with cholesterol gall stones. Gut 24:836, 1983.
421. Gallinger S, Harvey PRC, Petrunka CN, et al. Biliary proteins and the nucleation defect in cholesterol cholelithiasis. Gastroenterology 92:867, 1987.
422. Groen AK, Stout JPJ, Drapers J, et al. Isolation of cholesterol nucleation activating activity in gallbladder bile. J Hepatol 3:S59, 1986.
423. Groen AK, Stout JPJ, Drapers JAG, et al. Cholesterol nucleation-influencing activity in T-tube bile. Hepatology 8:347, 1988.
424. Harvey PRC, Rupar CA, Gallinger S, et al. Quantitative and qualitative comparison of gallbladder mucus glycoprotein from patients with and without gallstones. Gut 27:374, 1986.
425. Whiting MJ, Watts J McK. Cholesterol gallstone pathogenesis: a study of potential nucleating agents for cholesterol crystal formation in bile. Clin Sci 68:589, 1985.
426. Kibe A, Holzbach RT, LaRusso NF, et al. Inhibition of cholesterol crystal formation by apolipoproteins in supersaturated model bile. Science 225:514, 1984.
427. Groen AK, Drapers JAG, Tytgat GNJ. Cholesterol nucleation and gallstone formation. J Hepatol 6:383, 1988.
428. Sutor DJ, Percival JM. Presence or absence of inhibitors of crystal growth in bile. I. Effect of bile on the formation of calcium phosphate, a constituent of gallstones. Gut 17:506, 1976.
429. Sutor DJ, Percival JM. The effect of bile on the crystallization of calcium carbonate, a constituent of gallstones. Clin Chim Acta 89:479, 1978.
430. Sciarretta G, Ligabue A, Garuti G, et al. Inhibitory activity of gallbladder bile on calcium carbonate crystallization in vitro. Scand J Gastroenterol 19:626, 1984.
431. Robertson WG. Physical chemical aspects of calcium stone formation in the urinary tract. In: Fleisch H, Robertson WG, Smith LH, et al, eds. Urolithiasis Research. New York, Plenum Press, 1976:25.
432. Ito H, Coe FL. Acidic peptide and polyribonucleotide crystal growth inhibitors in human urine. Am J Physiol 233(5):F455, 1977.
433. Coe FL, Margolis HC, Deutsch LH, et al. Urinary macromolecular crystal growth inhibitors in calcium nephrolithiasis. Miner Electrolyte Metab 3:268, 1980.
434. Nakagawa Y, Abram V, Kezdy FJ, et al. Purification and characterization of the principal inhibitor of calcium oxalate monohydrate crystal growth in human urine. J Biol Chem 258:2594, 1983.
435. Nancollas GH. The mechanism of formation of renal stone crystals. Proc Eur Dialysis Transplant Assoc 20:386, 1983.
436. Van Arsdalen KN. Pathogenesis of renal calculi. Urol Radiol 6:65, 1984.
437. Nakagawa Y, Abram V, Parks JH, et al. Urine glycoprotein crystal growth inhibitors. J Clin Invest 76:1455, 1985.
438. Gron P, Hay DI. Inhibition of calcium phosphate precipitation by human salivary secretions. Arch Oral Biol 21:201, 1976.
439. Schlesinger DH, Hay DI. Complete covalent structure of statherin, a tyrosine-rich acid peptide which inhibits calcium phosphate precipitation from human parotid saliva. J Biol Chem 252:1689, 1977.
440. Moreno EC, Varughese K, Hay DI. Effect of human salivary proteins on the precipitation kinetics of calcium phosphate. Calcif Tissue Int 28:7, 1979.
441. Hay DI, Schluckebier SK, Moreno EC. Saturation of human salivary secretions with respect to calcite and inhibition of calcium carbonate precipitation by salivary constituents. Calcif Tissue Int 39:151, 1986.
442. De Caro A, Lohse J, Sarles H. Characterization of a protein isolated from pancreatic calculi of men suffering from chronic calcifying pancreatitis. Biochem Biophys Res Commun 87:1176, 1979.
443. De Caro A, Multigner L, Verine H. Identification of two major proteins of bovine pancreatic stones as immunoreactive forms of trypsinogen. Biochem J 205:543, 1982.
444. Multigner L, Delano AD, Lomardo D, et al. A phosphoprotein which

inhibits calcium carbonate precipitation from human pancreatic juice. Biochem Biophys Res Commun 110:69, 1983.

445. DeCaro A, Multigner L, Lafont H, et al. The molecular characteristics of a human pancreatic acidic phosphoprotein that inhibits calcium carbonate crystal growth. Biochem J 222:669, 1984.

446. Montalto G, Bonicel J, Multigner L, et al. Partial amino acid sequence of human pancreatic stone protein, a novel pancreatic secretory protein. Biochem J 238:227, 1986.

447. Multigner L, Sarles H, Lombardo D, et al. Pancreatic stone protein. II. Implication in stone formation during the course of chronic calcifying pancreatitis. Gastroenterology 89:387, 1985.

448. Giorgi D, Bernard JP, DeCaro A, et al. Pancreatic stone protein. I. Evidence that it is encoded by a pancreatic messenger ribonucleic acid. Gastroenterology 89:381, 1985.

449. Figarella C, Guy-Crotte O, Barthe C, et al. Les proteines pancreatiques humaines à l'état normal et pathologique. Gastroenterol Clin Biol 11:891, 1987.

450. Price PA, Otsuka AS, Poser JW, et al. Characterization of a carboxy-glutamic acid–containing protein from bone. Proc Natl Acad Sci USA 73:1447, 1976.

451. Borman AH, De Jong EW, Huizinga M, et al. The role of CaCO₃ crystallization of an acid Ca²⁺-binding polysaccharide associated with coccoliths of Emiliania huxleyi. Eur J Biochem 129:179, 1982.

452. Wheeler AP, George JW, Evans CA. Control of calcium carbonate nucleation and crystal growth by soluble matrix of oyster shell. Science 212:1397, 1981.

453. Shimizu S, Sabsay B, Veis JD, et al. A 12 kDa acidic protein from cholesterol gallstones inhibits precipitation of calcium carbonate and is present in human bile. Hepatology 8:1257, 1988 (Abstract).

454. De Vries AL. Antifreeze peptides and glycopeptides in cold-water fishes. Annu Rev Physiol 45:245, 1983.

455. Osuga T, Mitamura K, Miyagava S, et al. A scanning electron microscopic study of gallstone development in man. Lab Invest 31:696, 1974.

456. Smallwood RA, Jablonski P, Watts J McK. Intermittent secretion of abnormal bile in patients with cholesterol gallstones. Br Med J 4:263, 1972.

457. Antsaklis G, Lewin MR, Sutor DJ, et al. Gallbladder function, cholesterol stones, and bile composition. Gut 16:937, 1975.

458. Frizzell RA, Dugas MC, Schultz SG. Sodium chloride transport by rabbit gallbladder. J Gen Physiol 65:769, 1975.

459. Diamond JM. Transport of salt and water in rabbit and guinea pig gallbladder. J Gen Physiol 48:1, 1964.

460. Wheeler HO. Concentrating function of the gallbladder. Am J Med 51:588, 1971.

461. Diamond JM. Transport mechanisms in the gallbladder. In: Code CF, ed. Handbook of Physiology: Alimentary Canal. Washington, D.C.:American Physiological Society, 1968:2451.

462. Rose RC. Absorptive functions of the gallbladder. In: Johnson LR, ed. Physiology of the Gastrointestinal Tract. New York, Raven Press, 1981:1021.

463. Wood JR, Svanvik J. Gallbladder water and electrolyte transport and its regulation. Gut 24:579, 1983.

464. Rege RV, Nahrwold DL, Moore EW. Absorption of biliary calcium from the canine gallbladder: Protection against the formation of calcium-containing gallstones. J Lab Clin Med 110:381, 1987.

465. Palmer RH. Editorial: The odyssey of a calcium ion: Live in the biliary tract. J Lab Clin Med 110:375, 1987.

466. Nakayama F. Cholesterol holding capacity of bile in relationship to gallstone formation. Clin Chim Acta 14:171, 1966.

467. Shiffman ML, Moore EW. Gallbladder mucosal function in patients with cholelithiasis: Dissociation between concentrating ability and H⁺ ion secretion. Gastroenterology 92:1775, 1987 (Abstract).

468. Neiderhiser DH, Harmon CK, Roth HP. Absorption of cholesterol by the gallbladder. J Lipid Res 17:117, 1976.

469. Neiderhiser DH, Pineda FM, Hejduk LJ, et al. Absorption of oleic acid by the guinea pig gallbladder. J Lab Clin Med 77:985, 1971.

470. Neiderhiser DH, Morningstar WA, Roth HP. Absorption of lecithin and lysolecithin by the gallbladder. J Lab Clin Med 82:891, 1973.

471. Ostrow JD. Absorption by the gallbladder of bile salts, sulfobromophthalein, and iodipamide. J Lab Clin Med 74:482, 1969.

472. Ostrow JD. Absorption of organic compounds by the injured gallbladder. J Lab Clin Med 78:255, 1971.

473. Cussler EL, Evans DF, De Palma RG. A model for gallbladder function and cholesterol gallstone formation. Proc Natl Acad Sci USA 67:400, 1970.

474. Thureborn E. On the stratification of human bile and its importance for the solubility of cholesterol. Gastroenterology 50:775, 1966.

475. Tera H. Stratification of human gallbladder bile in vivo. Acta Chir Scand 256(Suppl.):1, 1960.

476. Zhu X-G, Greeley GH Jr, Newman J, et al. Correlation of in vitro measurements of contractility of the gallbladder with in vivo ultrasonographic findings in patients with gallstones. Surg Gynecol Obstet 161:470, 1985.

477. Nakayama F, Van der Linden W. Stratification of bile in gallbladder and gallstone formation. Surg Gynecol Obstet 141:587, 1975.

478. Drury DR, McMaster PD, Rous P. Observations on some causes of gallstone formation. III. The relation of the reaction of the bile to experimental cholelithiasis. J Exp Med 39:403, 1924.

479. Okada S. On the reaction of bile. J Physiol (Lond) 50:114, 1915.

480. Neilson NM, Meyer KF. The reaction and physiology of the hepatic duct and cystic bile of various laboratory animals. J Infect Dis 28:510, 1921.

481. Weinman SA, Reuss L. Na⁺/H⁺ exchange at the apical membrane of Necturus gallbladder: Extracellular and intracellular pH studies. J Gen Physiol 80:299, 1982.

482. Weinman SA, Reuss L. Na⁺/H⁺ exchange and Na⁺ entry across the apical membrane of Necturus gallbladder. J Gen Physiol 83:801, 1984.

483. Petersen KU, Wehner F, Winterhager JM. Na/H exchange at the apical membrane of guinea-pig gallbladder epithelium: properties and inhibition by cyclic AMP. Pflugers Arch 405(Suppl.1):S115, 1985.

484. Whitlock RT, Wheeler HO. Hydrogen ion transport by isolated rabbit gallbladder. Am J Physiol 217:310, 1969.

485. Cremaschi D, Henin S, Meyer G. Stimulation by HCO₃⁻ of Na⁺ transport in rabbit gallbladder. J Membr Biol 47:145, 1979.

486. Cremaschi D, Meyer G, Bermano S, et al. Different sodium chloride cotransport systems in the apical membrane of rabbit gallbladder epithelial cells. J Membr Biol 73:227, 1983.

487. Heintz K, Petersen KV, Wood JR. Effects of bicarbonate on fluid and electrolyte transport by guinea pig and rabbit gallbladder: Stimulation of absorption. J Membr Biol 62:175, 1981.

488. Sullivan B, Berndt WO. Transport by isolated rabbit gallbladders in bicarbonate-buffered solutions. Am J Physiol 225(4):845, 1973.

489. Rege RV, Moore EW. Evidence for H⁺ secretion by the canine gallbladder. Gastroenterology 92:281, 1987.

490. Moore EW, Shiffman ML. Evidence for H⁺ secretion by the human gallbladder in vivo. Gastroenterology 94:A573, 1988 (Abstract).

491. Shiffman ML, Moore EW. H⁺ ion secretion by the human gallbladder in patients with and without gallstones. Hepatology 8:1223, 1988 (Abstract).

492. Shiffman ML, Moore EW. Acidification of gallbladder bile is defective in patients with all types of gallstones. Gastroenterology 94:A591, 1988 (Abstract).

493. Shaffer EA. The role of the gallbladder in gallstone formation. In: Fisher MM, Goresky CA, Shaffer EA, eds. Gallstones. New York, Plenum Press, 1979:223.

494. LaMorte WW, Schoetz DJ Jr, Birkett DH, et al. The role of the gallbladder in the pathogenesis of cholesterol gallstones. Gastroenterology 77:580, 1979.

495. Holzbach RT. Gallbladder stasis: consequence of long-term parenteral hyperalimentation and risk factor for cholelithiasis. Gastroenterology 84:1055, 1983.

496. Gurll NJ, Meyer PD, DenBesten L. Effect of cholesterol crystals on gallbladder function in cholelithiasis. Surg Forum 28:412, 1977.

497. Pitt HA, Doty JE, DenBesten L, et al. Stasis before gallstone formation: Altered gallbladder compliance or cystic duct resistance? Am J Surg 143:144, 1982.

498. Doty JE, Pitt HA, Kuchenbecker SL, et al. Impaired gallbladder emptying before gallstone formation in the prairie dog. Gastroenterology 85:168, 1983.

499. Kuckenbecker SL, Doty JE, Pitt HA, et al. Salicylate prevents gallbladder stasis and cholesterol gallstones in the prairie dog. Surg Forum 32:154, 1981.

500. Roslyn JJ, DenBesten L, Thompson JC. Effects of periodic emptying of gallbladder on gallbladder function and formation of cholesterol gallstones. Surg Forum 30:403, 1979.

501. Glenn F, Wantz GE. Acute cholecystitis following the surgical treatment of unrelated disease. Surg Gynecol Obstet 102:145, 1956.

502. Gullick GD. A roentgenologic study of gallbladder evacuation following nonbiliary tract surgery. Ann Surg 151:403, 1960.

503. Long TN, Heimbach DM, Carrico CJ. Acalculous cholecystitis in critically ill patients. Am J Surg 136:31, 1978.

504. Petersen SR, Sheldon GF. Acute acalculous cholecystitis: a complication of hyperalimentation. Am J Surg 138:814, 1979.

505. Billeaud C, Cadier L, Demarquez JL, et al. Gallbladder and biliary tract detected by echotomography in children on total parenteral nutrition. JPEN J Parenter Enteral Nutr 4:560, 1980.

506. Anderson JL. Acalculous cholecystitis—a possible complication of parenteral hyperalimentation. Report of a case. Med Ann DC 41:448, 1972.

507. Scher KS, Sarap MD, Jaggers RL. Acute acalculous cholecystitis complicating aortic aneurysm repair. Surg Gynecol Obstet 163:475, 1986.

508. Messing B, De Oliveira FJ, Galian A, et al. Cholestase au cours de la nutrition parenterale totale: mise en evidence des facteurs favorisants; association à une lithiase vésiculaire. Gastroenterol Clin Biol 6:740, 1982.

509. Whitington PF, Black DD. Cholelithiasis in premature infants treated with parenteral nutrition and furosemide. J Pediatr 97:647, 1980.

510. Doty JE, Pitt HA, Porter-Fink V, et al. The effect of intravenous fat and total parenteral nutrition on biliary physiology. JPEN J Parenter Enteral Nutr 8:263, 1984.

511. Doty JF, Pitt A, Porter-Fink V, et al. The pathophysiology of gallbladder disease induced by total parenteral nutrition. Gastroenterology 82:1046, 1982 (Abstract).

512. Roslyn JJ, Pitt HA, Man LL, et al. Gallbladder disease in patients on long-term total parenteral nutrition. Gastroenterology 84:148, 1983.

513. Brugge WR, Brand DL, Atkins JL, et al. Gallbladder dyskinesia in chronic acalculous cholecystitis. Dig Dis Sci 31:461, 1986.

514. Roslyn JJ, DenBesten L, Pitt HA, et al. Effects of cholecystokinin on gallbladder stasis and cholesterol gallstone formation. J Surg Res 30:200, 1981.

515. Cano N, Cicero F, Ranieri F, et al. Ultrasonographic study of gallbladder motility during total parenteral nutrition. Gastroenterology 91:313, 1986.

516. Matos C, Avni EF, Van Gansbeke D, et al. Total parenteral nutrition (TPN) and gallbladder diseases in neonates. Sonographic assessment. J Ultrasound Med 6:243, 1987.

517. Doty JE, Pitt HA, Porter-Fink V, et al. Cholecystokinin prophylaxis of parenteral nutrition-induced gallbladder disease. Ann Surg 201:76, 1985.

518. Sheldon GF, Petersen SR, Sanders R. Hepatic dysfunction during hyperalimentation. Arch Surg 113:504, 1978.

519. Lindor KD, Fleming CR, Abrams A, et al. Liver function values in adults receiving total parenteral nutrition. JAMA 241:2398, 1979.

520. Wagner WH, Lowry AC, Silberman H. Similar liver function abnormalities occur in patients receiving glucose-based and lipid-based parenteral nutrition. Am J Gastroenterol 78:199, 1983.

521. Farrell MK, Balistreri WF, Suchy FJ. Serum-sulfated lithocholate as an indicator of cholestasis during parenteral nutrition in infants and children. J Parenter Enteral Nutr 6:30, 1982.

522. Cooper A, Betts JM, Pereira GR, et al. Taurine deficiency in the severe hepatic dysfunction complicating total parenteral nutrition. J Ped Surg 19:462, 1984.

523. Whitington PF. Cholestasis associated with total parenteral nutrition in infants. Hepatology 5:693, 1985.

524. Latham PS, Menkes E, Phillips MJ, et al. Hyperalimentation-associated jaundice: an example of a serum factor inducing cholestasis in rats. J Clin Nutr 41:61, 1985.

525. Baker AL, Rosenberg IH. Hepatic complications of total parenteral nutrition. Am J Med 82:489, 1987.

526. Stanko RT, Nathan G, Mendelow H, et al. Development of hepatic cholestasis and fibrosis in patients with massive loss of intestine supported by prolonged parenteral nutrition. Gastroenterology 92:197, 1987.

527. Gimmon Z, Kelley RE, Simko V. Total parenteral nutrition induces increased bile lithogenicity in rat. J Surg Res 32:256, 1982.

528. Fisher RS, Rock E, Levin G, et al. Effects of somatostatin on gallbladder emptying. Gastroenterology 92:885, 1987.

529. Zahor A, Sternby NH, Kagan A, et al. Frequency of cholelithiasis in Prague and Malmö—an autopsy study. Scand J Gastroenterol 9:3, 1974.

530. Newman HF, Northup JD. Collective review: the autopsy incidence of gallstones. Int Abst Surg 109:1, 1959.

531. Friedman GD, Kannel WB, Dawber TR. The epidemiology of gallbladder disease: observation in the Framingham study. J Chronic Dis 19:273, 1966.

532. Braverman DZ, Johnson ML, Kern FK Jr. Effects of pregnancy and contraception steroids on gallbladder function. N Engl J Med 302:362, 1980.

533. Mann FC, Higgins GM. Effect of pregnancy on emptying of the gallbladder. Arch Surg 15:522, 1927.

534. Everson GT, McKinley C, Lawson M, et al. Gallbladder function in the human female: Effect of the ovulatory cycle, pregnancy, and contraceptive steroids. Gastroenterology 82:711, 1982.

535. Bateson MC. Oral contraceptives and gallstones. Lancet 1:1115, 1988.

536. Forgacs IC, Maisey MN, Murphy GM, et al. Influence of gallstones and ursodeoxycholic acid therapy on gallbladder emptying. Gastroenterology 87:299, 1984.

537. Sunderland GT, Sutherland CG, Carter DC. Gallbladder motility in the presence of gallstones. Gut 28:A1360, 1987 (Abstract).

538. Kishk SMA, Darweesh RMA, Dodds WJ, et al. Sonographic evaluation of resting gallbladder volume and postprandial emptying in patients with gallstones. Am J Radiol 148:875, 1987.

539. Maudgal DP, Kupfer RM, Zentler-Munro PL, et al. Postprandial gallbladder emptying in patients with gallstones. Br Med J 280:141, 1980.

540. von Bergmann K, Mok HYI, Grundy SM. Distribution of the bile acid pool in the fasting state in man. Gastroenterology 71:934, 1976 (Abstract).

541. Mok HYI, Grundy SM. Gallbladder storage function in subjects with gallstones. Gastroenterology 74:1162, 1978 (Abstract).

542. Van Berge Henegouwen GP, Hofmann AF. Nocturnal gallbladder storage and emptying in gallstone patients and healthy subjects. Gastroenterology 75:879, 1978.

543. Pomeranz IS, Shaffer EA. Abnormal gallbladder emptying in a subgroup of patients with gallstones. Gastroenterology 88:787, 1985.

544. Everson GT, Braverman DZ, Johnson ML, et al. A critical evaluation of real-time ultrasonography for the study of gallbladder volume and contraction. Gastroenterology 79:40, 1980.

545. Krishnamurthy GT, Bobba VR, Kingston E. Radionuclide ejection fraction: A technique for quantitative analysis of motor function of the human gallbladder. Gastroenterology 80:482, 1981.

546. Lanzini A, Jazrawi RP, Northfield TC. Simultaneous quantitative measurements of absolute gallbladder storage and emptying during fasting and eating in humans. Gastroenterology 92:852, 1987.

547. Pomeranz IS, Davison JS, Shaffer EA. The effects of prosthetic gallstones on gallbladder function and bile composition. J Surg Res 41:47, 1986.

548. Low-Beer TS, Heaton ST, Heaton KW, et al. Gallbladder inertia and sluggish enterohepatic circulation of bile-salts in coeliac disease. Lancet 2:991, 1971.

549. Low-Beer TS, Harry RF, Davies ER, et al. Abnormalities in serum cholecystokinin and gallbladder-emptying in coeliac disease. N Engl J Med 292:961, 1975.

550. Khalil T, Walker JP, Wiener I, et al. Effect of aging on gallbladder contraction and release of cholecystokinin-33 in humans. Surgery 98:423, 1985.

551. Sacchetti G, Mandelli V, Roncoroni L, et al. Influence of age and sex on gallbladder emptying induced by a fatty meal in normal subjects. Am J Roentgenol Rad Ther Nucl Med 119:40, 1973.

552. Traverso LW. Carl Langenbuch and the first cholecystectomy. Am J Surg 132:81, 1976.

553. Naunyn B. Treatise on Cholelithiasis. London, New Sydenham Society, 1896.

554. Carey MC, Park Y-H, Igimi H, et al. Factors affecting speed of gallstone dissolution during litholytic therapy. In: Paumgartner G, Stiehl A, Gerok W, eds. Falk Symposium 42. Enterohepatic Circulation of Bile Acids and Sterol Metabolism. Boston, MTP Press, 1986:321.

555. Tao JC, Cussler EL, Evans DF. Accelerating gallstone dissolution. Proc Natl Acad Sci USA 71:3917, 1974.

556. Kwan KH, Higuchi WI, Molokhia AM, et al. Dissolution behavior of cholesterol in simulated bile. I. Influence of bile acid type and concentration, bile acid-lecithin ratio and added electrolytes. J Pharm Sci 66:1094, 1977.

557. Kwan KH, Higuchi WI, Molokhia AM, et al. Cholesterol gallstone dissolution rate acceleration. I. Exploratory investigation. J Pharm Sci 68:1105, 1977.

558. Patel DC, Higuchi WI. Mechanism of cholesterol gallstone dissolution. II. Correlation between the effects of the alkyl amines as cholesterol gallstone dissolution rate accelerates and the degree of binding of alkyl amines to the bile acid micelles. J Colloid Interface Sci 74:211, 1980.

559. Patel DC, Oncley JL, Higuchi WI. Mechanism of cholesterol gallstone dissolution. III. Electrophoretic studies showing the correlation between the bile micellar charge and the effects of alkylamines as cholesterol gallstone dissolution rates accelerate. J Colloid Interface Sci 74:220, 1980.

560. Higuchi WI, Su CC, Park J-Y, et al. Mechanism of cholesterol gallstone dissolution. IV. Analysis of the kinetics of cholesterol monohydrated dissolution in taurocholate/lecithin solutions by the Mazer, Benedek and Carey model. J Phys Chem 85:127, 1981.

561. Noyes AA, Whitney WR. The rate of solution of solid substances in their own solutions. J Am Chem Soc 19:930, 1897.

562. Nernst W. Theorie der Reaktionsgeschwindigkeit in heterogenen Systemen. Z Physikal Chem 47:52, 1904.

563. Thistle JL, Nelson PE, May GR. Dissolution of cholesterol gallbladder stones using methyl-tert-butyl ether. Gastroenterology 90:1775, 1986.

564. Ferrucci JT. Gallstone ESWL—The first 175 patients. Am J Roentgenol Rad Ther Nucl Med 150:1231, 1988.

565. Neubrand M, Sauerbruch T, Stellaard F, et al. In vitro cholesterol gallstone dissolution after fragmentation with shock waves. Digestion 34:51, 1986.

566. Thistle JL, Schoenfield LJ. Lithogenic bile among young Indian women: lithogenic potential decrease with chenodeoxycholic acid. N Engl J Med 284:177, 1971.

567. Danzinger RG, Hofmann AF, Thistle JL, et al. Effect of oral chenodeoxycholic acid on bile acid kinetics and biliary lipid composition in women with cholelithiasis. J Clin Invest 52:2809, 1973.

568. Danzinger RG, Hofmann AF, Schoenfield LJ, et al. Dissolution of cholesterol gallstones by chenodeoxycholic acid. N Engl J Med 286:1, 1972.

569. Thistle JL, Hofmann AF. Efficacy and specificity of chenodeoxycholic acid therapy for dissolving gallstones. N Engl J Med 289:655, 1973.
570. Northfield TC, LaRusso NF, Hofmann AF, et al. Biliary lipid output during three meals and an overnight fast. II. Effect of chenodeoxycholic acid treatment in gallstone patients. Gut 16:12, 1975.
571. Einarsson K, Grundy SM. Effects of feeding cholic acid and chenodeoxycholic acid on cholesterol absorption and hepatic secretion of biliary lipids. J Lipid Res 21:23, 1980.
572. Makino I, Shginozaky K. Dissolution of cholesterol gallstones by ursodeoxycholic acid. Jpn J Gastroenterol 72:690, 1975.
573. Schoenfield LJ, Bonorris GG, Ganz P. Induced alterations in the rate limiting enzymes of hepatic cholesterol and bile acid synthesis in the hamster. J Lab Clin Med 82:858, 1973.
574. Long TT III, Jakoi L, Stevens R, et al. The sources of rat biliary cholesterol and bile acid. J Lipid Res 19:872, 1978.
575. Turley SD, Dietschy JM. The contribution of newly synthesized cholesterol to biliary cholesterol in the rat. J Biol Chem 256:2438, 1981.
576. Schwartz CC, Berman M, Vlahcevic ZR, et al. Multicompartmental analysis of cholesterol metabolism in man. I. Characterization of the hepatic bile acid and biliary cholesterol precursor sites. J Clin Invest 61:408, 1978.
577. Kempen HJ, de Lange J, Vos Van Holstein MP, et al. Effect of ML-236B (compactin) on biliary excretion of bile salts and lipids, and on bile flow, in the rat. Biochim Biophys Acta 794:435, 1984.
578. Pandak WM, Heuman DM, Hylemon PB, et al. Mevinolinic acid, the active metabolite of lovastatin, acutely suppresses bile acid synthesis and cholesterol 7α-hydroxylase activity in the bile fistula rat. Gastroenterology 94:A580, 1988 (Abstract).
579. Hardison WG, Grundy SM. Effect of ursodeoxycholate and its taurine conjugate on bile acid synthesis and cholesterol absorption. Gastroenterology 87:130, 1984.
580. Roehrkasse R, Fromm H, Malavolti M, et al. Gallstone dissolution treatment with a combination of chenodeoxycholic and ursodeoxycholic acids. Dig Dis Sci 31:1032, 1986.
581. Gracie WA, Ransohoff DF. The natural history of silent gallstones: the innocent gallstone is not a myth. N Engl J Med 307:798, 1982.
582. Barbara LF. The Progretto Simione. Epidemiology of gallstone disease. The Simione study. In: Capocaccia L, Ricci G, Angelico F, et al., eds. Epidemiology and Prevention of Gallstone Disease. Lancaster, MTP Press, 1984:23.
583. Capocaccia L. The Grepco Group. Clinical symptoms and gallstone disease: Lessons from a population study. In: Capocaccia L, Ricci G, Angelico F, et al., eds. Epidemiology and Prevention of Gallstone Disease. Lancaster, MTP Press, 1984:153.
584. Ransohoff DF, Gracie WA, Wolfenson LB, et al. Prophylactic cholecystectomy or expectant management for silent gallstones: a decision analysis to assess survival. Adv Intern Med 99:199, 1983.
585. Thistle JL, Cleary PA, Lachin JM, et al. The natural history of cholelithiasis: The national cooperative gallstone study. Ann Intern Med 101:171, 1984.
586. Einarsson KG, Nilsell K, Leijd B, et al. Influence of age on secretion of cholesterol and synthesis of bile acids by the liver. N Engl J Med 313:277, 1985.
587. Schoenfield LJ, Chopra R, Sheinbaum R, et al. Formation and prevention of gallstones during loss of weight in obese persons. In: Paumgartner G, Stiehl A, Gerok W, eds. Bile Acids and the Liver. Falk Symposium 45. Lancaster, MTP Press, 1987:229.
588. Nicholas P, Rinaudo PA, Conn HO. Increased incidence of cholelithiasis in Laennec's cirrhosis: A postmortem evaluation of pathogenesis. Gastroenterology 63:112, 1972.
589. Trotman BW. Formation of pigment gallstones. In: Cohen S, Soloway RD, eds. Gallstones. New York, Churchill Livingstone, 1985:299.
590. Trotman BW, Patella EJ, Soloway RD, et al. Evaluation of radiographic lucency or opaqueness of gallstones as a means of identifying cholesterol or pigment stones. Gastroenterology 68:1563, 1975.
591. Schwartz JS. Identification of patients for gallbladder stone dissolution. In: Cohen S, Soloway RD, eds. Gallstones. New York, Churchill Livingstone, 1985:179.
592. Sarva RP, Farivar S, Fromm H, et al. Study of the sensitivity and specificity of computerized tomography in the detection of calcified gallstones which appear radiolucent by conventional roentgenography. Gastrointest Radiol 6:165, 1981.
593. Thistle JL, Hofmann AF, Ott BJ, et al. Chenotherapy for gallstone dissolution. I. Efficacy and safety. JAMA 239:1041, 1978.
594. Schoenfield LJ, Lachin JM, The Steering Committee, et al. Chenodiol (chenodeoxycholic acid) for dissolution of gallstones: The National Cooperative Gallstone Study. A controlled study of efficacy and safety. Ann Intern Med 95:257, 1981.
595. Ros E, Navarros S, Fernandez I, et al. Utility of biliary microscopy for the prediction of the chemical composition of gallstones and the outcome of dissolution therapy with ursodeoxycholic acid. Gastroenterology 91:703, 1986.
596. Dolgrin SM, Schwartz JS, Kressel HY, et al. Identification of patients with cholesterol or pigment gallstones by discriminant analysis of radiographic features. N Engl J Med 304:808, 1981.
597. Mok HYI, Bell GD, Dowling RH. Effects of different doses of chenodeoxycholic acid on bile lipid composition and on frequency of side-effects in patients with gallstones. Lancet 2:253, 1974.
598. Iser JH, Dowling RH, Mok HYI, et al. Chenodeoxycholic acid treatment of gallstones: a follow-up report and analysis of factors influencing response to therapy. N Engl J Med 293:378, 1975.
599. Maton PN, Iser JH, Reuben A, et al. Outcome of chenodeoxycholic acid (CDCA) treatment in 125 patients with radiolucent gallstones. Factors influencing efficacy, withdrawal, symptoms and side effects and post-dissolution recurrence. Medicine (Baltimore) 61:86, 1982.
600. Maudgal DP, Bird R, Northfield TC. Optimal timing of doses of chenic acid in patients with gallstones. Br Med J 1:922, 1979.
601. Maudgal DP, Kupfer RM, Northfield TC. Factors affecting gallstone dissolution rate during chenic acid therapy. Gut 24:7, 1983.
602. Maudgal DP, Bird R, Blackwood WS, et al. Low-cholesterol diet: enhancement of effect of CDCA in patients with gallstones. Br Med J 2:851, 1978.
603. Hofmann AF. Medical treatment of cholesterol gallstones by bile desaturating agents. Hepatology 4:1995, 1984.
604. King JE, Schoenfield LJ. Lithocholic acid, cholestasis, and liver disease. Mayo Clin Proc 47:725, 1972.
605. Palmer RH. Bile acids, liver injury, and liver disease. Arch Intern Med 130:606, 1972.
606. Layden TJ, Schwarz J, Boyer JL. Scanning electron microscopy of the rat liver. Studies of the effect of taurolithocholate and other models of cholestasis. Gastroenterology 69:724, 1975.
607. Miyai K, Javitt NB, Gochman N, et al. Hepatotoxicity of bile acids in rabbits: ursodeoxycholic acid is less toxic than chenodeoxycholic acid. Lab Invest 46:428, 1982.
608. Carey MC. Physical-chemical methods for determining bilirubin solubilities in simulated bile systems. Hepatology 4:223S, 1984.
609. Scholmerich J, Becher MS, Schmidt K. Influence of hydroxylation and conjugation of bile salts on their membrane damaging properties. Studies on isolated hepatocytes and lipid membrane vesicles. Hepatology 4:661, 1984.
610. Sarva RP, Fromm H, Farivar S, et al. Comparisons of the effects between ursodeoxycholic acid and chenodeoxycholic acids on liver function and structure and on bile acid composition in the rhesus monkey. Gastroenterology 79:629, 1980.
611. Bazzoli F, Roda A, Fromm H, et al. Relationship between serum and biliary bile acids as an indicator of chenodeoxycholic and ursodeoxycholic acid–induced hepatotoxicity in the rhesus monkey. Dig Dis Sci 27:417, 1982.
612. Marks JW, Pearlman SBJ, Varady GGB, et al. Sulfation of lithocholate as a possible modifier of chenodeoxycholic acid–induced elevations of serum transaminase in patients with gallstones. J Clin Invest 68:1190, 1981.
613. Fisher RL, Anderson DW, Boyer JL, et al. A prospective morphologic evaluation of hepatic toxicity of chenodeoxycholic acid in patients with cholelithiasis: The National Cooperative Gallstone Study. Hepatology 2:187, 1982.
614. Fromm H, Holtz-Slomczy KM, Zobi H. Studies of liver function and structure in patients with gallstones before and during treatment with chenodeoxycholic acid. Acta Hepatogastroenterol 22:359, 1975.
615. Phillips MJ, Fisher RL, Anderson DW, et al. Ultrastructural evidence of intrahepatic cholestasis before and after chenodeoxycholic acid therapy in patients with cholelithiasis: The National Cooperative Gallstone Study. Hepatology 3:209, 1983.
616. Mekhjian HS, Phillips SF, Hofmann AF. Colonic secretion of water and electrolytes induced by bile acids: Perfusion studies in man. J Clin Invest 50:1569, 1971.
617. Maton PN, Murphy GM, Dowling RH. Ursodeoxycholic acid treatment of gallstones: dose response study of possible mechanisms of action. Lancet 2:1297, 1977.
618. Kutz C, Schulte A. Effectiveness of ursodeoxycholic acid in gallstone dissolution. Gastroenterology 73:632, 1977.
619. Stiehl A, Czygan P, Kommerell B, et al. Ursodeoxycholic acid versus chenodeoxycholic acid: comparison of their effects on bile acid and bile lipid composition in patients with cholesterol gallstones. Gastroenterology 75:1016, 1978.
620. Roda E, Bazzoli F, Morselli LA, et al. Ursodeoxycholic acid vs. chenodeoxycholic acid as cholesterol gallstone-dissolving agents: a comparative randomized study. Hepatology 2:804, 1982.
621. Fromm H, Roat JW, Gonzalez V, et al. Comparative efficacy and side effects of ursodeoxycholic and chenodeoxycholic acids in dissolving gallstones. Gastroenterology 85:1257, 1983.
622. Erlinger S, Lego A, Husson JM, et al. Franco-Belgian cooperative study of ursodeoxycholic acid in the medical dissolution of gallstones: A double-blind, randomized dose-response study, and comparison with chenodeoxycholic acid. Hepatology 4:308, 1984.

623. Fromm H. Gallstone dissolution and the cholesterol–bile acid–lipoprotein axis. Propitious effects of ursodeoxycholic acid. Gastroenterology 87:229, 1984.
624. Stiehl A, Raedsch R, Czygan P, et al. Effects of biliary bile acid composition on biliary cholesterol saturation in gallstone patients treated with chenodeoxycholic acid and/or ursodeoxycholic acid. Gastroenterology 79:1192, 1980.
625. Podda M, Zuin M, Diogurardi ML, et al. A combination of chenodeoxycholic acid and ursodeoxycholic acid is more effective than either alone in reducing biliary cholesterol saturation. Hepatology 2:334, 1982.
626. Podda M, Zuin M, Battezat PM. Non-surgical treatment of gallstones: cheno- vs. ursodeoxycholic acid. In: Northfield T, Jazrawi R, Zentler-Munro P, eds. Bile Acids in Health and Disease. Boston, Dordrecht Kluwer, 1988:187.
627. Kitani K, Ohta M, Kanai S. Tauroursodeoxycholate prevents biliary protein excretion induced by other bile salts in the rat. Am J Physiol 248:G407, 1985.
628. Flynn GL, Shah Y, Prakongpan S, et al. Observations on the solubility of cholesterol in organic solvents. J Pharm Sci 68:109, 1979.
629. Mack EA, Saito C, Goldfarb S, et al. A new agent for gallstone dissolution: experimental and clinical evaluation. Surg Forum 29:438, 1978.
630. Velasco N, Brasheto I, Osendes A, et al. Treatment of retained common bile duct stones: a prospective controlled study comparing monooctanoin and heparin. World J Surg 138:271, 1982.
631. Thistle JL, Carlson GL, Hofmann AF, et al. Monooctanoin, a dissolution agent for retained cholesterol bile duct stones: physical properties and clinical application. Gastroenterology 78:1016, 1980.
632. Hofmann AF, Schmack B, Thistle JL, et al. Clinical experience with monooctanoin for dissolution of bile duct stones. Dig Dis Sci 26:954, 1981.
633. Leuschner V, Wurbs D, Landgraf H, et al. Dissolution of biliary duct stones with monooctanoin. Lancet 2:103, 1979.
634. Steinhausen RM, Pertsemlides D. Monooctanoin dissolution of retained biliary stones in high-risk patients. Am J Gastroenterol 78:756, 1983.
635. Allen MJ, Borody TJ, Thistle JL. In vitro dissolution of cholesterol gallstones: a study of factors influencing rate and comparison of solvents. Gastroenterology 89:1097, 1985.
636. Allen MJ, Borody TJ, Bugliosi TF, et al. Cholelitholysis using methyl tertiary butyl ether. Gastroenterology 88:122, 1985.
637. Allen MJ, Borody TJ, Bugliosi TF, et al. Rapid dissolution of gallstones in humans using methyl tert-butyl ether. N Engl J Med 312:217, 1985.
638. Thistle JL, Nelson PE, May GR. Dissolution of cholesterol gallbladder stones (CGS) using methyl tert-butyl ether (MTBE). Gastroenterology 90:1775, 1986 (Abstract).
639. Gonzaga RAF, Lima FR, Carneiro S, et al. Dissolution of gallstones by methyl tert-butyl ether. N Engl J Med 313:385, 1985.
640. Savolainen H. Renal failure during dissolution of gallstones by methylbutyl ether. Lancet 2:515, 1988.
641. Dowling RH, Gleeson D, Ruppin DC, et al. British/Belgian Gallstone Study Group: Gallstone recurrence and post-dissolution management. In: Paumgartner G, Stiehl A, Gerok W, eds. Enterohepatic Circulation of Bile Acids and Sterol Metabolism. Lancaster, MTP Press, 1985:361.
642. Ruppin DC, Dowling RH. Is recurrence inevitable after gallstone dissolution by bile acid treatment?. Lancet 1:181, 1982.
643. Thistle JL, Pu PYI, Hofmann AF, et al. Prompt return of bile to supersaturated state followed by stone recurrence after discontinuation of chenodeoxycholic acid therapy. Gastroenterology 66:789, 1974.
644. Richardson SC. On the probability of gallstone recurrence. J Hepatol 4:390, 1987.
645. Lanzini A, Jazrawi RP, Kupfer DM, et al. Gallstone recurrence after medical dissolution—an overestimated threat?. J Hepatol 3:241, 1986.
646. Iser JH, Murphy GM, Dowling RH. Speed of change in biliary lipids and bile acids with chenodeoxycholic acid—is intermittent therapy feasible? Gut 18:7, 1977.
647. Grundy S, Kalser SC. Highlights of the meeting on prevention of gallstones. Hepatology 7:946, 1987.
648. Marks JW, Lan SP, The Steering Committee, et al. Low-dose chenodiol to prevent gallstone recurrence after dissolution therapy. Ann Intern Med 100:376, 1984.
649. Periz-Aguilar F, Breto M, Alfonso V, et al. Gallstone recurrence following cessation of dissolving treatment and during prophylactic administration of either low dose chenodeoxycholic acid or medium dose ursodeoxycholic acid. J Hepatol 1:S305, 1985.
650. Hood K, Gleeson D, Ruppin D, et al. Can gallstone recurrence be prevented? The British/Belgian Post-dissolution Trial. Gastroenterology 94:548, 1988 (Abstract).
651. Leuschner V, Baumgartner H. Gallstone dissolution in the biliary tract: in vitro investigations on inhibiting factors and special dissolution agents. Am J Gastroenterol 77:222, 1982.
652. Leuschner U, Girkenfeld G, Frenk H, et al. Dissolution of human pigment stones by EDTA solvents containing N-acetylcysteine and taurochoic and taurochenodeoxycholic acid. Hepatology 7:1139, 1987 (Abstract).
653. Petersen BT, Peine CJ, Felmlee JP, et al. Dissolution of radioopaque cholesterol gallstone in vitro with and without prior shock wave lithotripsy. Hepatology 7:1140, 1987 (Abstract).
654. Attili AF. Natural history and prevention. In: Bateson M, ed. Gallstone Disease and Management. Lancaster, MTP Press, 1986:57.
655. Rains AJH. Gallstones, Causes and Treatment, Springfield, Ill.: Charles C Thomas, 1964.

58

Gallbladder Disease

Philip S. Barie, M.D., F.A.C.S. • *Ira M. Jacobson, M.D.*

Symptomatic gallbladder disease accounts for substantial morbidity, mortality, and economic losses. Ten to 15 per cent of the population may be affected, which means that more than 20 million people in the United States harbor gallstones. Although gallstones do not inevitably cause disease, it has been estimated that as many as 515,000 biliary tract operations are performed annually in the United States for symptoms or complications of gallstones.[1] Glenn estimated that the direct cost of providing medical care for calculous biliary tract disease consumes 2.5 per cent of annual health care expenditures. Economic losses from disability or lost productivity during recovery from surgery or complications are incalculably higher.

EPIDEMIOLOGY OF GALLSTONES

Risk factors associated with cholelithiasis are given in Table 58–1. Both cholesterol and pigment stones become increasingly prevalent with advancing age. Cholesterol

TABLE 58–1. RISK FACTORS FOR CHOLELITHIASIS

Increasing age
Female sex
Ethnic background (highest in Pima Indians)
Obesity
Drugs (clofibrate, estrogens)
Prolonged total parenteral nutrition
Ileal disease (e.g., Crohn's disease)
Ileal resection or jejunoileal bypass
Chronic hemolysis
Cirrhosis

stones are more common in women, although the difference in prevalence between sexes decreases with increasing age. Pregnancy is thought to contribute to the female preponderance of cholesterol stones, as it is associated with increased cholesterol saturation of bile and impaired emptying of the gallbladder.[2] Increased cholesterol saturation of bile occurs with administration of exogenous estrogens, and oral contraceptives have been associated with cholelithiasis in several studies,[3] as have estrogens in men with prostate cancer.[4] However, studies of oral contraceptives have not invariably demonstrated this association.[5]

The prevalence of gallstones differs among ethnic groups. American Indians have the highest reported prevalence, with nearly 90 per cent of Pima Indian women older than 65 years of age having gallstones.[6] The following incidences have been found among other groups studied in the United States, in decreasing frequency: Mexican Americans (14 per cent of women), whites (9 per cent of women), and blacks (5 per cent of women). The relatively high frequency among Mexican Americans has been attributed to the genetic influence of partial American Indian ancestry.[7, 8]

Obesity is one of the best recognized risk factors for cholelithiasis. This has been attributed to an increase in biliary cholesterol secretion relative to bile acid and lecithin secretion.[9] When jejunoileal bypass was performed for obesity, there was a high incidence of cholesterol gallstones because of diminished ileal absorption of bile acids.[10] A diminished bile acid pool, with the resultant formation of bile supersaturated with cholesterol, is similarly responsible for the excess prevalence of gallstones in patients who have undergone ileal resection or those who have Crohn's disease of the ileum. Other systemic diseases are associated with an increased prevalence of pigment, rather than cholesterol, gallstones. These diseases include chronic hemolytic anemias, such as sickle cell disease, thalassemia, and cirrhosis. In addition, the gallstones that have been reported to develop in patients on long-term total parenteral nutrition appear to be composed predominantly of calcium bilirubinate.[11]

NATURAL HISTORY OF GALLSTONE DISEASE

Gallstones are often identified incidentally during evaluation of other disorders. The question of therapy for asymptomatic patients is an important issue. Until recently, recommendations for cholecystectomy in patients with asymptomatic disease were widespread, based on data suggesting that there was a 50 per cent chance of symptoms developing within a few years in asymptomatic patients.[12, 13] These data are considered now to be inaccurate. Recent data in truly asymptomatic patients indicate that the likelihood of symptoms developing is about 2 per cent/year.[14, 15] After 10 to 15 years, there may be little additional risk.

Moreover, in the rare instance that serious complications develop, symptoms that were present prior to the acute problem can be identified 90 per cent of the time.[15] Data from the National Cooperative Gallstone Study (NCGS) also indicate that asymptomatic gallstones uncommonly cause subsequent symptoms. Thistle and colleagues required that the patients entered in the NCGS be asymptomatic for three months prior to entry.[16] Biliary symptoms developed within two years in 13 per cent of placebo-treated patients. However, placebo-treated patients in whom biliary symptoms developed were also more likely to have had symptoms during the 12 months prior to the 3-month asymptomatic period.

With little likelihood of symptoms developing in the previously asymptomatic patient, but also with little inherent risk from elective cholecystectomy, the benefits that might be derived from prophylactic cholecystectomy require careful examination. Decision analysis by Ransohoff and colleagues failed to show an improvement in long-term survival from cholecystectomy unless operative mortality was reduced to zero, and even then there was only a minuscule increase in life expectancy at an enormous additional cost.[17] Since the operative mortality rate from elective cholecystectomy can never be zero, there seems little advantage to aggressive surgical management of a disease that is benign in the vast majority of cases. Even if one considers that gallstones are a premalignant lesion, these analyses are not altered because of the rarity of carcinoma of the gallbladder.[18]

Certain populations with especially high risk for complications from gallstones do benefit from prophylactic cholecystectomy. This procedure may be justified in American Indians, for example, because of the high likelihood of gallbladder carcinoma in these patients.[19] Likewise, patients with calcified (porcelain) gallbladders are at substantial risk for carcinoma and should undergo cholecystectomy.[20] It also has been suggested that patients with cholelithiasis associated with sickle cell disease should undergo prophylactic surgery because of the very high morbidity from sickle cell crisis after emergency gallbladder surgery.[21] The relative risk in diabetic patients remains controversial. Patients with diabetes mellitus have increased morbidity from complications of cholecystitis,[22, 23] and perhaps slightly increased mortality.[24, 25] However, symptoms are no more likely to develop in asymptomatic diabetic patients than in nondiabetic patients with gallstones, and the data suggesting an increased mortality rate are not clear-cut in diabetic patients with gallstones.[23, 26, 27] Many surgeons believe that symptomatic diabetic patients should undergo elective surgery, since the likelihood of later morbidity is substantial.

In contrast to cholelithiasis, asymptomatic choledocholithiasis is more likely to be dangerous, and expectant management cannot be justified. Although there is little prospective data on the natural history of asymptomatic choledocholithiasis, autopsy data suggest that common duct stones are a contributing cause of death in about 50 per cent of cases of choledocholithiasis found at autopsy.[28]

Episodic pain, or biliary colic, accounts for three quarters of presenting symptoms in patients with symptomatic gallstones. The symptoms are sufficiently typical that a diagnosis of gallbladder disease can often be made from historic information alone. This is fortunate, since findings on physical examination in patients with mild symptoms are generally lacking. The pain characteristically begins 15 to 60 min, or more, after a meal and is associated with ingestion of fatty foods in many patients. The pain is felt maximally in the epigastrium and right upper quadrant but may be present anywhere in the abdomen or precordium. The pain radiates, usually to the back, in more than half of patients. Some patients have simultaneous nausea or vomiting. One or more dyspeptic symptoms, such as belching, excessive flatus, bloating, or early satiety, are present in more than 80 per cent of patients,[29] but these symptoms are nonspecific and of little diagnostic value in themselves. Once symptoms develop, strong consideration should be given to surgical intervention, since the operative mortality rate is tenfold greater for emergency biliary surgery.[30]

The pathologic features of chronic cholecystitis are notable for their lack of correlation with antecedent symptoms. Since biliary colic is caused by transient cystic duct obstruction without an inflammatory response, patients with prominent symptoms may have a gallbladder that appears only mildly abnormal on pathologic examination. Histologically, the gallbladder wall is fibrotic but minimally thickened. There is a mononuclear cell infiltrate, but the mucosa is intact. Bacteria can be cultured from gallbladder bile in about 30 per cent of patients.

RADIOGRAPHIC DIAGNOSIS OF GALLBLADDER DISEASE

Plain abdominal radiographs are of little value for evaluating gallbladder disease. Only 15 per cent of gallstones are calcified and therefore visible (Figs. 58–1 and 58–2). Unless abdominal x-ray films are obtained during evaluation of an acute abdominal process, they are seldom indicated. Oral cholecystography (Fig. 58–3) was once the technique of choice in the diagnosis of gallbladder stones. Gallstones are identified as radiolucencies within an opacified gallbladder. Alternatively, failure to visualize the gallbladder after double-dose ingestion of contrast tablets is a highly reliable indicator of gallbladder disease, provided that the serum bilirubin level is less than 2 mg/dl and vomiting or diarrhea does not impair absorption of the contrast material. However, its accuracy of 95 per cent was slightly surpassed by the advent of real-time ultrasonography (Figs. 58–4 and 58–5), the accuracy of which ranges from 96 to 98 per cent.[31] The slightly greater accuracy of sonography, principally because of enhanced detection of very small stones, combined with the lack of exposure to radiation or the need to ingest and then excrete contrast material into the gallbladder, has made it the initial modality of choice in most circumstances (see also Chap. 26).

Patients with symptoms suggestive of biliary colic in whom cholelithiasis has been shown to exist by ultrasonography and who are considered suitable surgical candidates require no further preoperative imaging studies of the biliary system when cholecystitis or jaundice is lacking. However, oral cholecystography is sometimes needed because of its ability to provide information about the composition of gallstones and gallbladder function or for identification of noncalculous causes of gallbladder symptoms such as adenomyomatosis (Fig. 58–6). Oral cholecystography is most often required in patients for whom oral dissolution therapy or other nonsurgical alternatives are being considered (see Chaps. 57 and 61). Cheno- or ursodeoxycholic acids, for example, are contraindicated in patients with gallbladders that do not function on oral cholecystography. Rarely, abnormal gallbladder contraction on oral cholecystography, in response to a test meal of a lipid emulsion, may supplement the sonographic finding of cho-

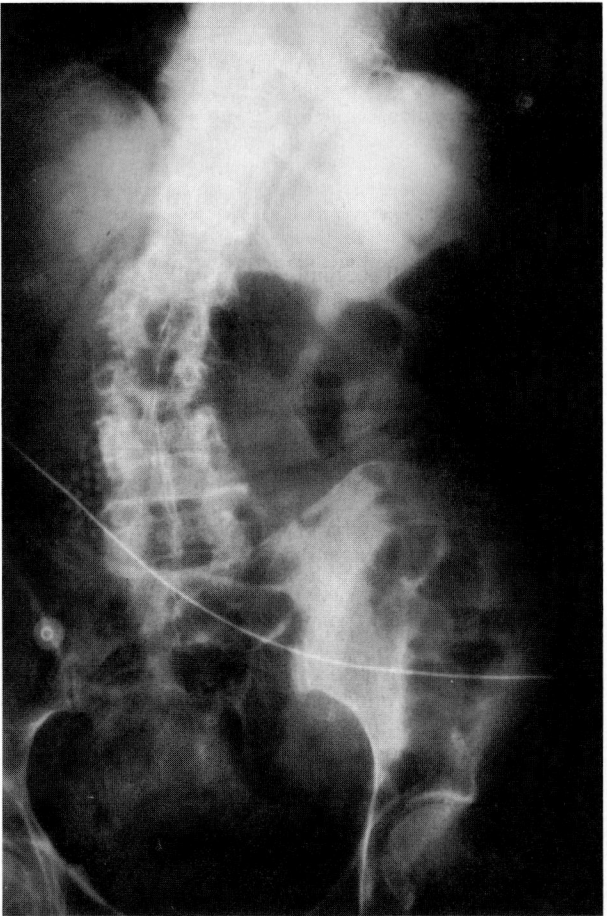

Figure 58–1. A plain abdominal radiograph was taken in an elderly patient with scoliosis who presented with severe, generalized abdominal pain. The multiple circular radiopacities at the level of the fourth and fifth lumbar vertebrae, just at the edge of the vertebral bodies to the patient's right, represent multiple gallstones. Immediate radiographic identification of gallstones may greatly simplify diagnosis, but only 15 per cent of gallstones (those containing calcium bilirubinate) are radiopaque. Moreover, the identification of gallstones does not confirm whether the gallbladder pathologic picture is symptomatic.

lelithiasis by enhancing the clinician's suspicion that a patient's symptoms are related to the gallbladder.

INTRAOPERATIVE MANAGEMENT OF GALLBLADDER DISEASE

With proper assessment of risk and careful preoperative preparation, cholecystectomy is a safe operation. Although emergency operation for complications,[1] advanced age,[32, 33] and the presence of hepatic cirrhosis all increase operative risk,[34, 35] cholecystectomy is now performed with an overall operative mortality of less than 1 per cent.[1] This is particularly true for elective cholecystectomy in good-risk patients who are less than 50 years of age, in whom the mortality rate is approximately 0.2 per cent. Cardiovascular complications are the leading cause of death; pulmonary complications are the leading cause of morbidity.[36]

Cholecystectomy is generally performed through a right subcostal (Kocher) incision and may be accomplished safely by either of two techniques. Before the dissection is begun, operative exposure must be optimal. The falciform ligament is divided to facilitate exposure, and the other

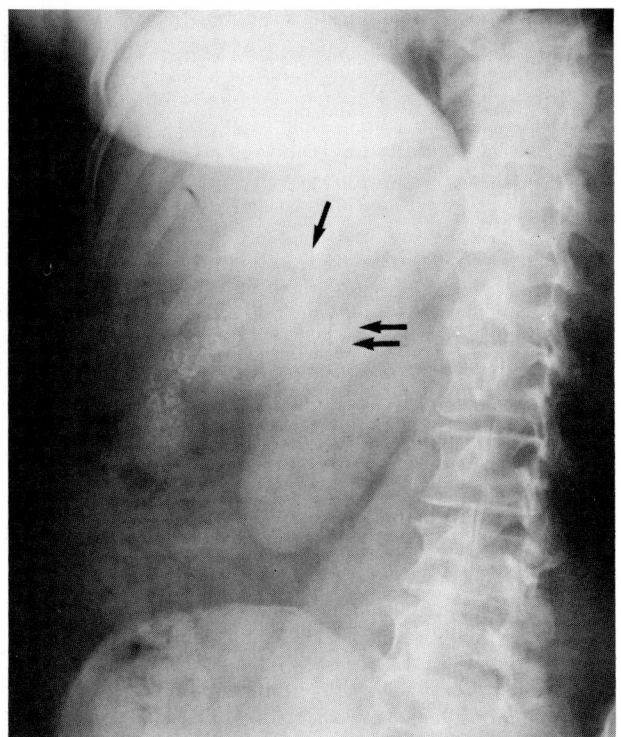

Figure 58–2. This abdominal radiograph was obtained in an otherwise asymptomatic patient prior to an intravenous pyelogram for the evaluation of microscopic hematuria. Numerous calcified gallstones were identified within the gallbladder, cystic duct (*single arrow*), and common bile duct (*double arrows*). Cholecystectomy and common duct exploration were performed.

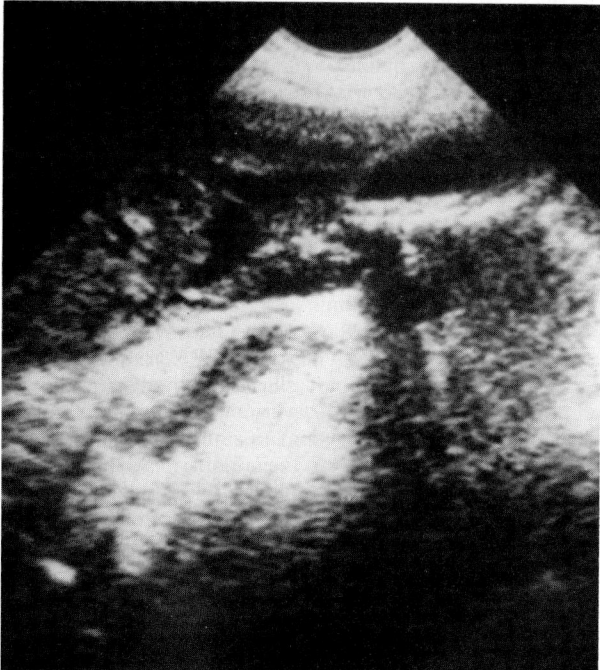

Figure 58–4. Ultrasound of the gallbladder, showing the organ in sagittal section in the upper right portion. Although the layering of echogenic material within the gallbladder is strongly suggestive of cholelithiasis, the diagnosis is confirmed by the echo-poor areas projecting downward from the gallbladder. This posterior acoustic shadowing is pathognomonic for cholelithiasis. No conclusions can be drawn regarding gallbladder function or the presence of acute cholecystitis.

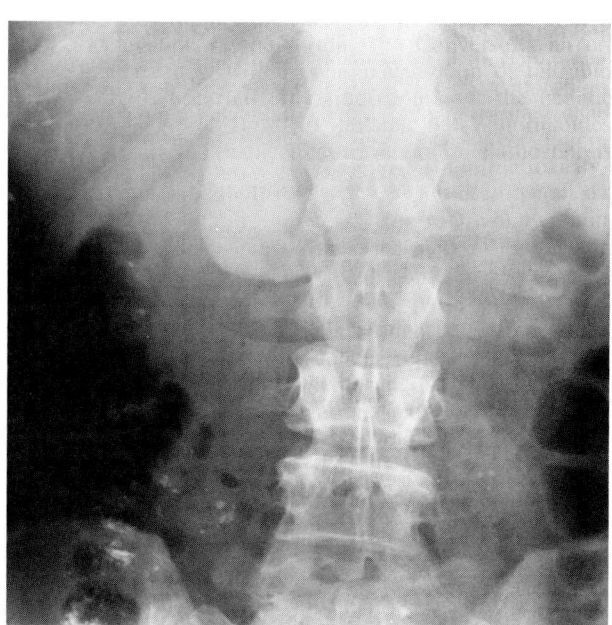

Figure 58–3. An oral cholecystogram was performed for episodic postprandial right upper quadrant abdominal pain. Three gallstones can be seen clustered within the lumen of the opacified gallbladder in this view.

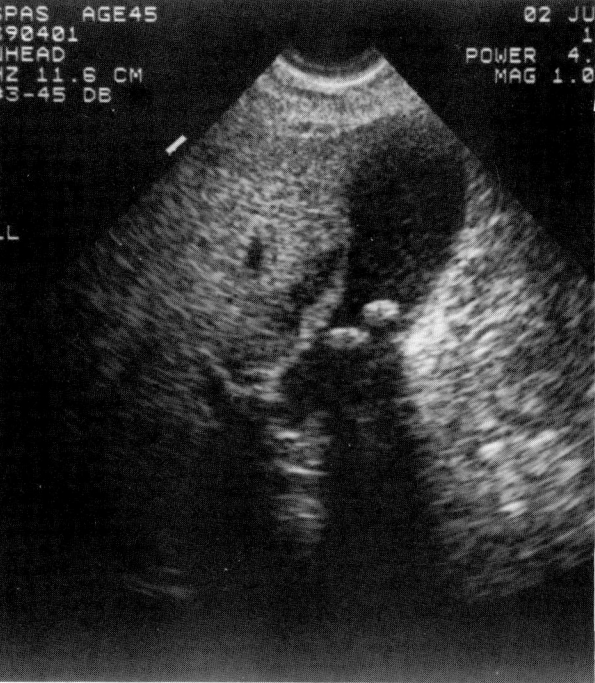

Figure 58–5. Ultrasound of the gallbladder with the transducer passed obliquely over the organ. Two echogenic foci (gallstones) are clearly seen within the gallbladder lumen, and the requisite posterior acoustic shadowing is well demonstrated. Moreover, an echo-dense (*white*) area just to the right of the gallstones represents thickening of the gallbladder wall. Identification of a thickened gallbladder wall or a fluid collection in the gallbladder bed is consistent with acute cholecystitis.

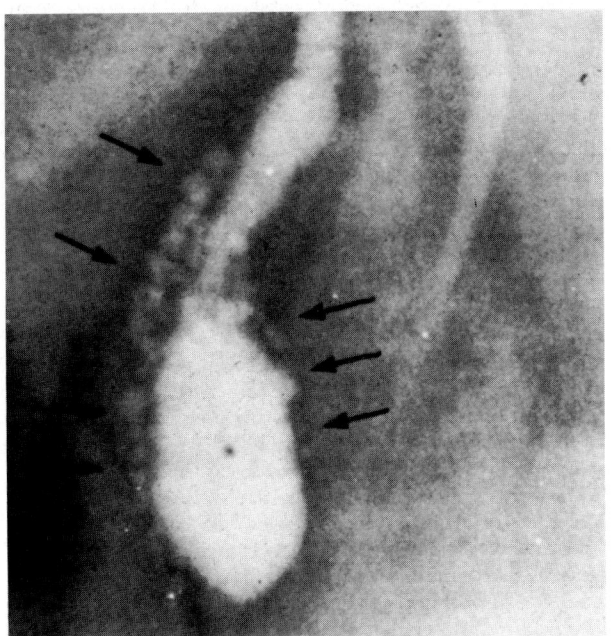

Figure 58–6. This oral cholecystogram was performed in a patient who presented with upper abdominal pain, nausea, and vomiting. There is diffuse involvement of the wall of the gallbladder with Rokitansky-Aschoff sinuses (*arrows*), which is pathognomonic for adenomyomatosis. A portion of normal common bile duct can be seen in the upper right of the figure. (Photograph courtesy of A. F. Govoni, M.D., Department of Radiology, Cornell University Medical College.)

abdominal viscera are palpated. The vacuum between the diaphragm and the right hepatic lobe is broken by palpation, bringing the liver to an inferior position. Adhesions between the gallbladder and adjacent organs are lysed, and the organs are packed away from the field with moist pads. Placement of retractors completes the exposure. With this exposure, the gallbladder can be palpated. With a finger placed through the foramen of Winslow, the distal common bile duct can be inspected for size and palpated for stones. The duodenum and pancreatic head should also be palpated to exclude the presence of tumor or distal calculus. The peritoneum overlying the triangle of Calot in the hepato-duodenal ligament is then incised, and the cystic duct and artery are isolated by blunt dissection.

Some surgeons divide the cystic duct and artery at this point, dissecting the gallbladder up from the undersurface of the liver. Most surgeons prefer to occlude the cystic duct and artery temporarily after isolation and then dissect the gallbladder from the fundus downward toward the infundibulum. In this manner, nothing is divided until the hilar anatomy has been defined precisely. The serious morbidity associated with operative injury to the common bile duct makes it imperative that the highly variable anatomy in this region be identified with precision.[37] Careful attention to hemostasis is also critical, since most inadvertent injuries to the duct occur during blind clamping to control hemorrhage.

When the dissection is nearing completion, division of the cystic artery facilitates exposure of the cystic duct and its junction with the common hepatic duct. At this point, the cystic duct can be divided and ligated within 1 cm of the confluence of the ducts. The cystic duct stump is then cultured. At this point, the operation can be concluded. Recent data suggest that neither nasogastric tubes nor subhepatic drains need be placed routinely in elective cholecystectomy.

Before transection of the cystic duct, it may be advisable to perform an intraoperative cholangiogram by placing a small catheter into the common duct via an incision in the cystic duct just proximal to the proposed point of transection (Fig. 58–7). Diluted radiographic contrast material (usually Hypaque in a final concentration of 25 per cent) is injected under minimal pressure, with care to avoid introducing air bubbles, and a radiograph is taken. Routine operative cholangiography has been advocated,[38] but it remains controversial.[39] Cholangiography as a matter of routine has been recommended as a way to eliminate the problem of retained common duct stones that are missed during cholecystectomy. However, the procedure has an extremely low yield in certain situations, for example, in patients with large solitary stones or very small-caliber cystic ducts, and it provides misleading information (usually false-positive) in 4 per cent of cases.[40] Routine use of this technique does not reduce the incidence of retained common duct stones to less than about 2 per cent.[41] Rather than serving as a routine screening test for occult common duct stones, cystic duct cholangiography is best used to determine which patients with relative indications for common duct exploration should undergo the procedure.[39, 42]

Refinements in the absolute and relative indications for common duct exploration have greatly increased the therapeutic yield of duct exploration. Using these criteria (Table 58–2), an indication for operative cholangiography exists in about 25 per cent of cholecystectomy cases. The selective use of cholangiography has decreased the incidence of common duct exploration and substantially increased the likelihood of positive findings on exploration to more than 60 per cent.[43] Since common duct exploration carries a higher mortality rate (2.7 per cent) than does elective cholecystectomy,[44] the information provided by cystic duct cholangiography can be of great value.

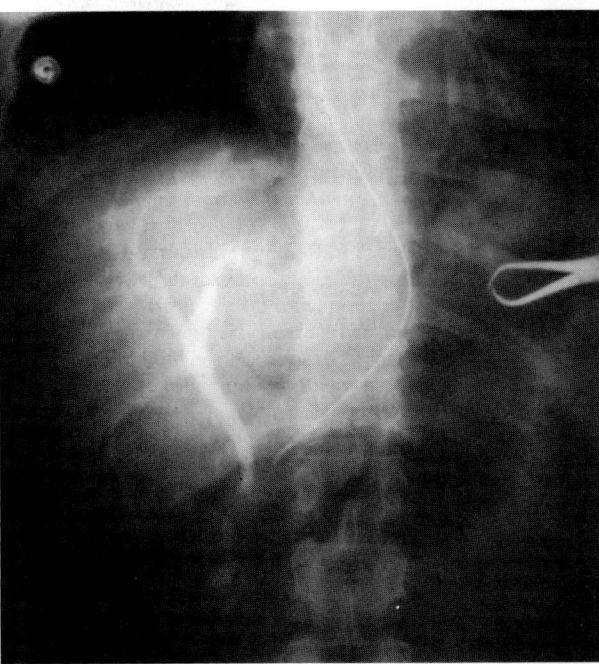

Figure 58–7. This intraoperative cholangiogram of the cystic duct was performed during a cholecystectomy for biliary pancreatitis. A nasogastric tube courses downward from above. The cholangiocatheter enters the patient's cystic duct from the lower left of the photograph. The common bile duct is of normal caliber. The common hepatic duct and intrahepatic radicles are adequately visualized. However, minimal contrast material enters the duodenum. A meniscus in the distal duct identifies a common duct stone.

EXPLORATION OF THE COMMON BILE DUCT

Once an indication for common duct exploration has been established during elective cholecystectomy, the problem should be addressed as soon as the cystic duct has been transected. A longitudinal choledochotomy is made in the supraduodenal portion of the common duct for a distance of 2 cm.[44, 45] Bile from the common duct is cultured separately. Spillage is prevented with pads and suction. The duct is then gently explored with specialized instruments, including stone forceps and malleable spoons. If a distal impacted stone is suspected, mobilization of the duodenum and pancreatic head by the Kocher maneuver will improve exposure. Passage of dilators through the sphincter of Oddi is no longer recommended, as injury to the sphincter or pancreatitis may result.[45, 46] Catheter irrigation will often yield stones or debris, and palpation of the catheter in the distal duodenum will confirm that the distal duct is not obstructed. The Fogarty balloon–tipped biliary catheter is particularly useful for retrieval of intrahepatic or impacted distal stones,[47] although it must also be used with care to avoid the serious complication of perforation of the common duct.

Historically, there has been a 10 per cent incidence of retained common duct stones following common duct exploration. However, the increasing use of choledochoscopy for direct visualization of intraductal pathologic features has decreased the incidence of retained stones to less than 2 per cent.[48] In addition to decreasing the incidence of retained common duct stones after exploration of the common duct, these techniques have made it much easier to identify and remove impacted distal stones via the choledochotomy. As a consequence, surgical duodenotomy and sphincterotomy for stone removal are now rarely required.

Before the common duct is closed, a decision must be made regarding the type of duct drainage to be employed. Strictures are prone to occur if the choledochotomy incision is closed primarily, so duct drainage is almost universally employed. For routine choledochotomies, the common duct is closed with absorbable suture material over a T-tube, and another cholangiogram is performed by injecting contrast through the T-tube. If accessible calculi are recognized when the x-ray films are repeated and the patient is stable, the choledochotomy incision should be reopened for retrieval of the stones. If not, a closed suction drain is placed in the subhepatic space, and the operation is completed. Another T-tube cholangiogram is performed between seven and ten days postoperatively to check again for retained stones (Fig. 58–8). If the study is again normal, the T-tube is removed and the patient is discharged. If calculi are identified, the patient is discharged with the tube in place,

TABLE 58–2. INDICATIONS FOR COMMON BILE DUCT EXPLORATION

Absolute	Relative*
Palpable abnormality in the common bile duct	Dilation of the common duct (12 mm or greater diameter)
Suppurative cholangitis (see Chap. 59)	Multiple small stones in the gallbladder
Jaundice with duct dilation at the time of operation	Cystic duct diameter 5 mm or greater
	History of pancreatitis
	History of jaundice

*Relative indications for common duct exploration constitute absolute indications for cystic duct cholangiography.

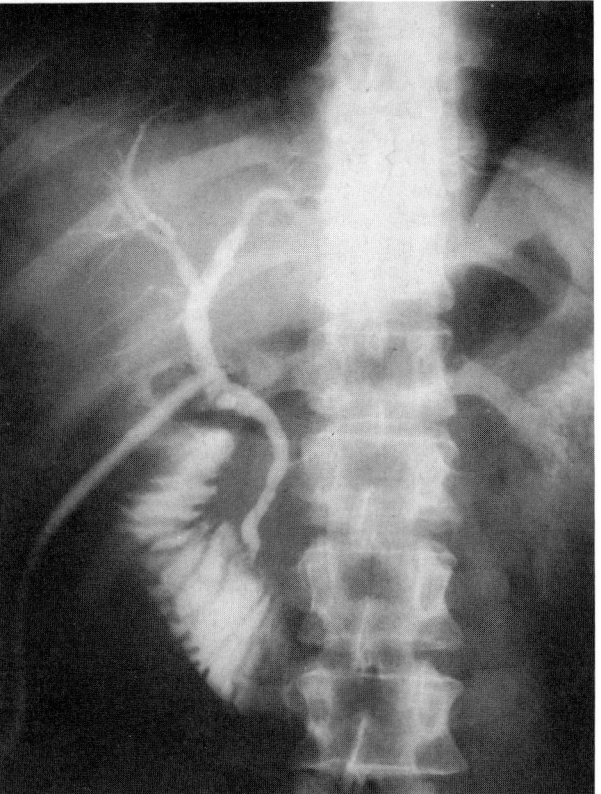

Figure 58–8. A normal T-tube cholangiogram was performed ten days postoperatively on the patient depicted in Figure 58–7, with excellent visualization of the biliary tree and duodenum.

and he or she returns again in about six weeks for stone extraction via the T-tube tract (see Chap. 60).

The need may exist for a surgical drainage procedure other than placement of a T-tube, for example, a choledochoduodenostomy or transduodenal sphincteroplasty.[49, 50] General indications for additional drainage in gallstone disease include reoperation for recurrent (primary) choledocholithiasis or intrahepatic or impacted periampullary stones, which cannot be retrieved at surgery. Occasionally, there will be so many stones that the surgeon cannot be sure all have been removed despite diligent attempts. If the duct is suitably dilated so that the resulting stoma will be at least 2 cm in diameter, side-to-side choledochoduodenostomy using the original choledochotomy is easier and often less hazardous than transduodenal sphincteroplasty. Transduodenal sphincteroplasty is generally reserved for duct drainage when a common duct of normal caliber is encountered and is found unsuitable for anastomosis. Rarely, stenosis of the ampulla of Vater will be diagnosed intraoperatively by the failure of radiopaque contrast material to pass from the common duct into the duodenum during cholangiography. This condition is also treated with sphincteroplasty.

CHOLECYSTECTOMY IN SPECIAL CIRCUMSTANCES

Incidental Cholecystectomy

Although the natural history of asymptomatic gallstones may be so benign that it precludes mandatory surgical intervention, gallstones discovered incidentally at laparotomy for another condition behave quite differently. Despite their asymptomatic course until the time of laparotomy, gallstones knowingly left behind appear to produce subsequent symptoms at a far greater rate. Among patients undergoing gastric exclusion surgery for morbid obesity, 29 per cent required cholecystectomy within three years.[51] In another study, 50 per cent of patients who were operated on for various types of unrelated intra-abdominal pathologic conditions had biliary tract symptoms within six months postoperatively if gallstones were identified intraoperatively but cholecystectomy was not performed.[52]

Cholecystectomy may be performed safely in conjunction with other intra-abdominal procedures.[53, 54] The high incidence of symptomatic gallstone disease following laparotomy, especially in patients undergoing surgery for morbid obesity, has led to the recommendation that cholelithiasis discovered incidentally at laparotomy be treated by cholecystectomy.[55] The identification of cholelithiasis by gallbladder palpation is imprecise. Identification of small gallstones in a fasted, distended gallbladder at laparotomy may be impossible without vigorous palpation, which carries the risk of pushing a stone into the common duct. Intraoperative ultrasound, although a suitable approach, is available in relatively few centers. It is unclear whether certain groups of high-risk patients should be screened preoperatively with ultrasound. Preoperative gallbladder sonography could be considered in patients undergoing surgery for complications of regional enteritis or before operation in obese or diabetic patients.[55]

Cholecystectomy and Hepatic Cirrhosis

Gallstones (usually pigmented) are present in approximately 25 per cent of patients with cirrhosis.[56] Several recent investigations have noted that biliary tract surgery in cirrhotic patients is associated with very high morbidity and mortality,[34, 35, 57] principally from hemorrhagic complications. The mortality rate may exceed 80 per cent in cirrhotic patients with prolonged prothrombin times.[34]

Cholecystectomy should be undertaken in cirrhotic patients only for severe symptoms, and only then with the expectation of substantial bleeding from the gallbladder bed. An alternative surgical approach worth considering in these difficult situations is subtotal cholecystectomy, in which only the peritoneal portion of the gallbladder is removed.[57] The posterior wall of the gallbladder is not dissected from the liver, and the cut edge of the liver is oversewn with a continuous suture, since the cystic artery is not ligated. The residual gallbladder mucosa is cauterized; the cystic duct can be ligated from within the neck of the gallbladder. Dangerous dissection in the triangle of Calot in the presence of portal hypertension is thus avoided. Although not appropriate for the otherwise healthy individual, this technique has considerable merit for this difficult problem of cholecystectomy in the cirrhotic patient.

NONSURGICAL TREATMENT OF GALLBLADDER STONES

The development of nonsurgical approaches to the treatment of gallstones is in evolution. The bile acids chenodeoxycholic acid and ursodeoxycholic acid were the first widely available alternatives to surgery, and they retain a role in the therapy of selected patients. Their use is discussed in Chapter 57. Other solvents, such as methyl tert-butyl ether, which is instilled directly into the gallbladder after percutaneous puncture of the organ, has stimulated recent interest.[58] The development of extracorporeal shock-wave lithotripsy for gallstones was perhaps an inevitable corollary of the proven success of this technique in the treatment of kidney stones. This mode of therapy is discussed in Chapter 61.

ACUTE CHOLECYSTITIS

Acute cholecystitis complicates the course of symptomatic gallstones in 10 to 20 per cent of patients.[1] The majority of patients have had prior biliary symptoms. Despite the frequency of the disease, the cause is not well understood, perhaps because the development of acute cholecystitis is multifactorial. Acute cholecystitis can result from bacterial infection or ischemia. The majority of cases are caused by stasis following obstruction of the cystic duct, usually by a gallstone. The overall mortality rate from acute cholecystitis is about 5 per cent. However, in elderly patients and possibly in diabetic patients, the mortality rate is higher, 10 and 6.5 to 7.9 per cent, respectively.[22, 25, 59]

In the usual circumstance, the diagnosis of acute cholecystitis is apparent on clinical grounds. The disease is most common in older women, although men are by no means spared. The pain typically is constant and localizes in the right subcostal region, although epigastric pain may predominate in early stages. Radiation of the pain is usually not a prominent complaint. Physical findings are more variable, although right upper quadrant tenderness is common. Signs of the irritation, other than involuntary guarding, are encountered uncommonly unless perforation has occurred. A tender, palpable gallbladder, although present in only 20 per cent of patients, is virtually pathognomonic of acute cholecystitis in the presence of typical symptoms.

Leukocytosis is very common, and abnormalities of liver function tests can also occur. Mild elevations of transaminase or alkaline phosphatase levels may occur even when there are no common duct stones, although the incidence of common duct stones accompanying acute cholecystitis is higher than in chronic cholecystitis.[60] Patients are seldom jaundiced, although the serum bilirubin level may rise as high as 5 mg/dl without implicating choledocholithiasis by necessity.[61] Serum amylase levels are commonly elevated to a mild degree. The differential diagnosis of acute cholecystitis includes a number of possibilities. Acute pancreatitis must always be considered, in part because of the hyperamylasemia but also because acute cholecystitis sometimes accompanies acute pancreatitis. Perforated gastroduodenal ulcers, right-sided nephroureterolithiasis, acute hepatitis, or hepatic congestion from right-sided cardiac failure may mimic cholecystitis, as may hepatic lesions, such as abscess or primary or metastatic tumors. It may also be difficult to distinguish diaphragmatic myocardial infarction on clinical grounds. Most commonly, however, acute cholecystitis is mistaken for acute appendicitis. A ptotic or distended gallbladder may extend well down into the pelvis, or confusion may be caused by a highly placed appendix, as in partial malrotation of the midgut. In the occasional jaundiced patient with advanced disease, cholangitis may be difficult to distinguish from acute cholecystitis. This distinction is of vital importance, since cholangitis carries a much higher risk of morbidity and mortality than does acute cholecystitis.

Obstruction of the cystic duct is nearly always present in patients with suspected acute cholecystitis. The accuracy of sonography in diagnosing cholelithiasis remains high, but cholescintigraphy with technetium-99m iminodiacetic acid (DISIDA) compounds is superior for the assessment of obstruction of the cystic duct and the presence of acute cholecystitis (Figs. 58–9 through 58–11). Sonographic signs, such as thickening of the wall of the gallbladder, pericholecystic fluid, or gallbladder distention, are less sensitive or specific than cholescintigraphy in most cases of acute cholecystitis. The usual diagnostic error with ultrasonography is of the false-negative type. By contrast, gallbladder visualization on cholescintigraphy excludes the diagnosis of acute cholecystitis with a reliability in the range of 98 to 100 per cent. Lack of visualization of the gallbladder by scintigraphy is nearly equally predictive of the disease. The incidence of false-positive results is only 4 to 5 per cent.[62] Virtually all diagnostic errors with cholescintigraphy are false-positive and involve the failure of a normal gallbladder to become visible. This can occur because the patient has eaten a meal recently, which leads to contraction of the gallbladder, or because of distention and stasis of the gallbladder secondary to a prolonged fast. The availability and accuracy of cholescintigraphy have rendered intravenous cholangiography obsolete.

The progression of events from obstruction of the cystic duct to acute cholecystitis is not entirely clear. Obstruction of the cystic duct does not progress to cholecystitis in some patients; acute cholecystitis without evidence of gallstones or cystic duct obstruction (acalculous cholecystitis) develops

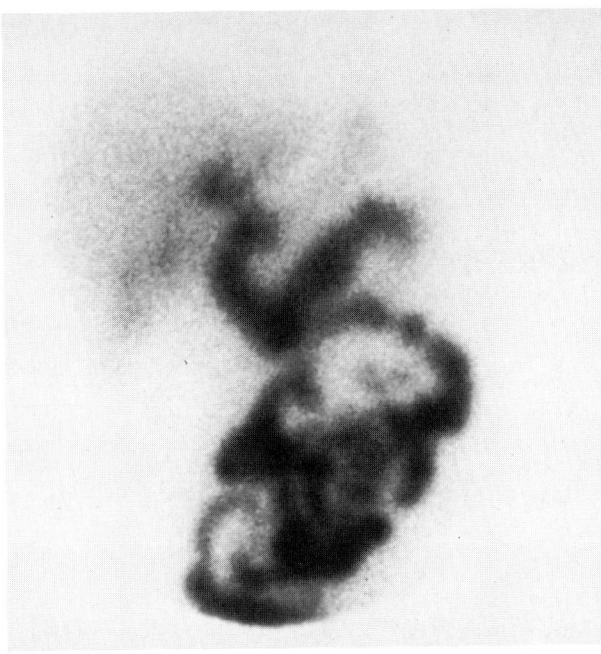

Figure 58–10. This positive DISIDA scan was obtained four hours after intravenous injection of the radioactive tracer in the patient whose sonogram is shown in Figure 58–4. Contrast is disappearing from the liver and biliary tree but is clearly within the duodenum and much of the small intestine. The faintly increased uptake beneath the right lobe of the liver does not represent gallbladder, but hyperemia in the gallbladder bed and adjacent liver. When the gallbladder cannot be visualized after four hours, DISIDA scans are 90 per cent reliable for the diagnosis of acute cholecystitis. Continuing the study for up to 24 hours increases the overall accuracy to 98 per cent in the usual patient.

in about 5 per cent of patients. The presumed sequence of events has recently been summarized by Pellegrini and Way.[63] Cystic duct occlusion in the presence of saturated bile activates inflammatory mediators, including prostaglandins, which are present in high concentrations in the wall of the gallbladder in acute cholecystitis. Prostaglandin E_1 stimulates the mucosa of the gallbladder to secrete and not absorb water,[64] thereby possibly mediating the gallbladder distention seen in acute cholecystitis. As the gallbladder distends with mucus, and luminal pressures increase, gallbladder perfusion is impaired with resultant necrosis or perforation. Inhibition of prostaglandin synthesis by indomethacin relieves the pain of acute cholecystitis in humans.[65]

High concentrations of bile acids have been implicated as initiators of the inflammatory response,[66] since these substances decrease transepithelial transport of water. Lithogenic bile may also play a role in the pathogenesis of acute cholecystitis. Gallbladder mucosa becomes inflamed when exposed to lithogenic bile, particularly if cholesterol crystals are present. It has been suggested that cholesterol crystals may injure gallbladder mucosa directly.[67] Lysolecithin, the product of the action of phospholipase A_2 on lecithin, has also been implicated. Phospholipase A_2 may be released from damaged gallbladder epithelium,[68] leading to increased lysolecithin in bile and resultant disruption of cell membranes in patients with cholecystitis.[69]

Bacterial infection appears to play a secondary role in the pathogenesis of acute cholecystitis. Bacteria can be cultured from gallbladder bile in only one half of patients,[70] although primary biliary infection with *Clostridium* species, *Salmonella typhi*, or *Escherichia coli* may occasionally cause acute acalculous infections.[63] Infection is not an important factor in the development of cholecystitis; suppurative

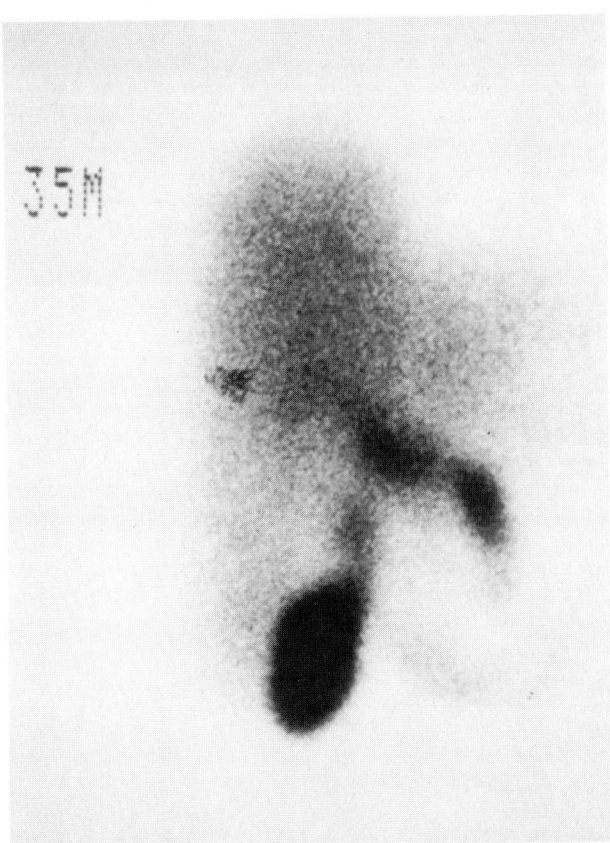

Figure 58–9. Radionuclide hepatobiliary scanning performed 35 minutes after the injection of a Technetium-99m (^{99m}Tc)-labeled iminodiacetic acid derivative (DISIDA) shows rapid uptake and excretion by the liver. Contrast material in the extrahepatic bile ducts and duodenum is readily apparent. The area of intense radioactivity beneath the liver represents concentration of radionuclide within the gallbladder, indicating that the cystic duct is patent. This is a normal scan.

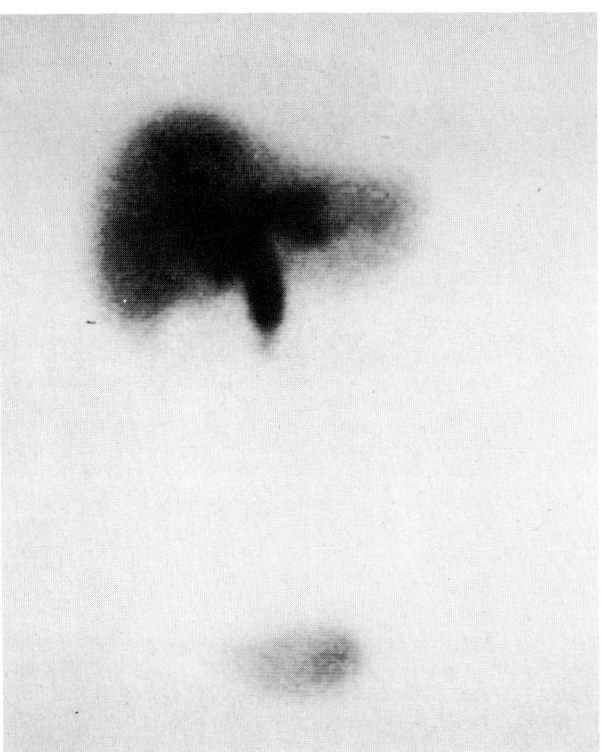

Figure 58–11. This DISIDA scan fails to show the gallbladder, but it also fails to show the duodenum. Additionally, the intra- and extrahepatic biliary radicles are unusually prominent, suggesting dilation secondary to obstruction of the distal common duct. The diagnosis of acute cholecystitis cannot be made reliably from this study. Normal filling of the gallbladder may not occur in the setting of increased pressure in the common duct caused by distal obstruction, even if the cystic duct is patent. The contrast material at the bottom of the figure is in the urinary bladder.

complications produce much of the morbidity and mortality in the disease. Edema of the gallbladder wall from venous and lymphatic outflow obstruction develops early in acute cholecystitis after the stone becomes impacted in the cystic duct. If the stone dislodges, the attack may be brief and self-limited, but if the gallbladder remains obstructed, the subsequent possible development of ischemia or secondary infection will determine the severity of the disease. The severity of the symptoms may not correlate with the severity of the gallbladder pathology, particularly in diabetic patients and the elderly. In these patients, gangrene of the gallbladder may develop rapidly and lead to perforation, even with minimal symptoms. Gallbladder ischemia, the antecedent of perforation in acute cholecystitis, appears to be mediated, as mentioned already, by large increases in intralumenal pressure caused by production of an active secretory state in response to inflammation. Gallbladder blood flow, particularly to mucosa, drops dramatically as gallbladder pressure increases.[64] Although the cystic artery usually remains patent and the gallbladder is hyperemic,[71] thromboses of small vessels do occur. This is perhaps why diabetic patients, with pre-existing small vessel disease, are particularly prone to gallbladder perforation.

TREATMENT OF ACUTE CHOLECYSTITIS

Increasingly, treatment of acute cholecystitis is considered to be surgical unless circumstances preclude surgery. The patient is admitted to the hospital, and a nasogastric tube is placed for decompression of the upper gastrointes-

tinal tract. Fluid resuscitation with a balanced saline solution is important, particularly if the disease process has been complicated by prerenal azotemia or hemoconcentration. Antibiotic therapy is a mainstay of treatment and is usually started before corroborative tests have been completed. The choice of antibiotic in acute cholecystitis is predicated on known or suspected pathogens; the microflora are very similar to those outlined for cholangitis in Chapter 59. Since coliform organisms predominate, single-agent therapy with a first- or second-generation cephalosporin may suffice. However, in elderly patients, diabetic patients, or patients with advanced disease, specific coverage against enterococci, *Pseudomonas*, and anaerobes should be considered. Because of these considerations, combination therapy with penicillin and an aminoglycoside is often employed.[64, 72] Recent evidence suggests that single-agent therapy with a broad-spectrum penicillin such as piperacillin is as effective as the combination of ampicillin and tobramycin for therapy of acute cholecystitis.[72] Once diagnostic tests have been completed and supportive therapy has been started, the proper time to perform surgery must be determined.

Traditionally, cholecystectomy has been performed either six to eight weeks following successful medical management of the acute attack or within 48 hours of the onset of the acute attack. Recent data from four randomized, prospective trials that included more than 400 patients and compared early and delayed surgery, indicate that early surgery is preferable.[73–76] Early surgery reduced the total hospital stay by nine days and was not associated with either mortality or operative injury to the common duct.[73–76] Early edema may actually accentuate tissue planes, thereby facilitating safe dissection. Moreover, planned delayed surgery was associated with a noncompliance rate of nearly 20 per cent—that is, patients refused surgery after the acute attack subsided.

Early surgery should be undertaken in any patient with proven acute cholecystitis who is within 48 hours of the onset of the attack and who has no serious concomitant illness contraindicating surgery. Any patient with evidence of suppurative complications should undergo surgery as soon as possible. About 60 per cent of patients will meet these criteria.[63] Early surgery in these patients may interdict the course of the disease and decrease the incidence of infectious complications. The principal indication for delayed surgery is illness of more than two days' duration at the time of presentation in patients with no signs of suppurative complications. The inflammatory reaction may be sufficiently established in these patients that dissection planes are obscured. Interval surgery, though sometimes arduous, may be safer to perform. Approximately two thirds of these patients will respond to initial nonoperative management.[63] One has to be alert to increasing pain, fever, leukocytosis, enlargement of a palpable mass, or the development of systemic toxicity from sepsis in these patients, all of which may mandate early surgery.

Surgical Management of Acute Cholecystitis

The principles of safe surgery in acute cholecystitis are the same as for elective operations for chronic disease, although certain modifications apply. Aspiration of the gallbladder by trocar facilitates handling of the organ and provides material for cultures. Operative cholangiography is more liberally employed during operations for acute disease because of the increased incidence (15 to 20 per cent) of choledocholithiasis in acute cholecystitis and because cholangiography may provide an anatomic "road map" for safe dissection when anatomy might be obscured.[60] Cholecystectomy can be performed in 85 to 90 per cent of cases of acute cholecystitis.[77] Occasionally, the dissection is so difficult that the gallbladder cannot be removed with safety. Cholecystostomy is an important option in the management of these patients. More importantly, cholecystostomy may be a lifesaving procedure for elderly patients or others who are unstable.[77] The gallbladder may be exposed using local anesthesia if desired. The gallbladder is decompressed and evacuated as with cholecystectomy, and a Malecot catheter is inserted into the gallbladder via a separate incision. Usually, the gallbladder is then sutured to the anterior abdominal wall. If the gallbladder is necrotic, partial cholecystectomy with closure of the gallbladder over the drainage tube will also achieve control. As with cholecystectomy for acute cholecystitis, drainage of the gallbladder bed is essential. The operative mortality rate for cholecystostomy is about 15 per cent and reflects not only the seriously ill patient population for whom the operation is generally reserved but also perhaps that severe cholecystitis may be mistaken for cholangitis and that cholecystostomy cannot be relied upon to drain the common duct.[78] If any possibility of cholangitis exists, the common duct should be drained directly by choledochotomy and placement of a T-tube.

Cholangiography is performed approximately one week after surgery to determine the presence of residual calculi (Fig. 58–12). Ordinarily, interval cholecystectomy is performed about six weeks after cholecystostomy. However, symptoms will recur in only about 50 per cent of patients if the gallbladder is left in place, so a clinical decision to defer further surgery may sometimes be made in elderly or high risk patients.

Occasional reports of ultrasound-guided percutaneous transhepatic cholecystostomy have appeared,[79] but the technique has disadvantages that limit its utility. The catheters tend to occlude with debris, so effective prolonged drainage may be problematic. Also, persistent symptoms from bile leakage around an unsecured catheter or an additional overlooked pathologic condition such as a pericholecystic abscess may occur. Currently, percutaneous drainage of acute cholecystitis should be reserved for highly selected patients.

COMPLICATIONS OF ACUTE CHOLECYSTITIS

Although it is certainly a complication of gallstone disease, acute cholecystitis is sometimes further complicated by a number of processes that account for much of the morbidity and mortality associated with the disease (Table 58–3). The incidence of choledocholithiasis in patients with acute cholecystitis is between 15 and 20 per cent, in contrast to the presence of common duct stones in 9 per cent of patients undergoing surgery for chronic disease. However, rather than being a direct result of the acute inflammatory process, the increased incidence may reflect the longstanding disease that is present in most patients with acute cholecystitis.

When cystic duct obstruction does not immediately result in infection or ischemia, hydrops of the gallbladder develops. In hydrops, bile pigments are absorbed, and the gallbladder contents become a clear viscous fluid. However, with persistent undrained obstruction, gallbladder bile will become purulent. This suppurative cholecystitis, or empyema of the gallbladder, may behave like an intra-abdominal abscess with rapid progression of symptoms. This complication may be more common in diabetic patients.[63] Fry and colleagues reviewed 34 patients with empyema,[80] of whom 32 were treated with cholecystectomy and 2 by cholecystostomy. Fifty-one complications developed in 17 of the patients. Infection was prominent as a complicating factor: 34 per cent of patients had pneumonia, 24 per cent postoperative wound infection, and 12 per cent an intra-abdominal abscess.

Gallbladder ischemia contributes significantly to the production of complicated acute cholecystitis. In addition to the rare circumstances of torsion or infarction of the gallbladder,[81] necrosis is a common result of progressive edema and thrombosis of small vessels in acute cholecystitis. When necrosis occurs and surgery is not promptly undertaken, perforation of the gallbladder may follow.

Gallbladder perforation occurs in about 10 per cent of patients with acute cholecystitis,[82] with an overall mortality

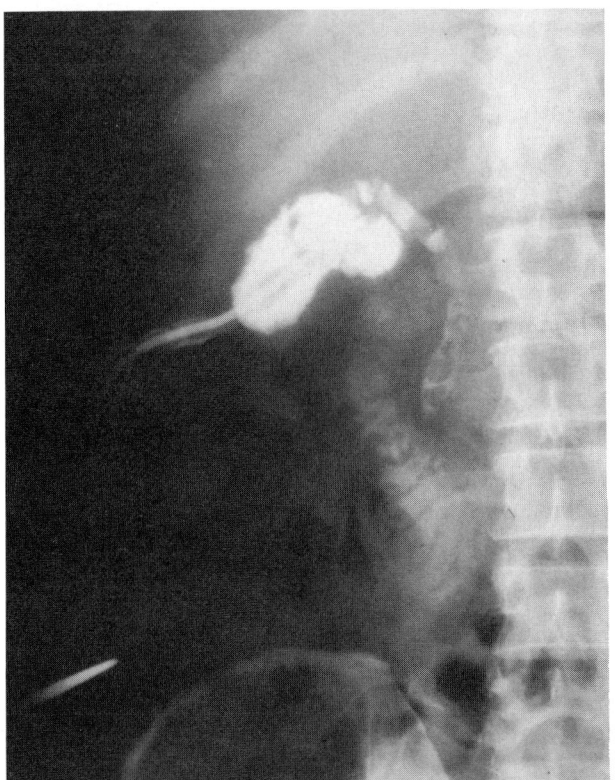

Figure 58–12. Contrast injection through a cholecystostomy tube placed for acute cholecystitis in an unstable, septic patient is depicted. Multiple common duct stones are apparent. The cystic duct was patent in this patient. The failure to visualize the common hepatic duct is of no concern. Common duct injury does not occur, since no hilar dissection is performed with this rapid, minimally invasive solution to a life-threatening clinical situation.

TABLE 58–3. INTRA-ABDOMINAL COMPLICATIONS OF ACUTE CHOLECYSTITIS

Empyema
Infarction
Perforation
  Generalized peritonitis
  Subhepatic abscess
Biliary-enteric fistula
  Mechanical bowel obstruction (gallstone ileus) from cholecystoduodenal or cholecystogastric fistulae
  Bacterial cholangitis, from cholecystocolic fistulae

rate of 15 to 20 per cent. Perforation results in local contamination of the subhepatic space with abscess formation in about one half of the affected patients. Free perforation with resultant generalized peritonitis occurs in an additional 30 to 35 per cent of cases and accounts for the overall high mortality rate in gallbladder perforation. The mortality rate is 40 per cent in this subgroup of patients. A major contribution to the high mortality rate in these patients is the difficulty and common failure to make the diagnosis prior to operation. The remaining 15 to 20 per cent of patients undergo perforation into the gastrointestinal tract, causing a biliary-enteric fistula. Perforation into the hepatic parenchyma with resulting liver abscess occurs occasionally.

Biliary fistulae are rare, but gallstones account for more than 90 per cent of cases.[83] In a review of 11,808 patients with nonmalignant biliary tract disease who underwent surgery at The New York Hospital from 1932 to 1978, the incidence of biliary-enteric fistula was 0.9 per cent. The ratio of males to females was 2.3:1.[84] The vast majority of patients had antecedent symptoms. Biliary-enteric fistulae usually result from repeated attacks of cholecystitis. The gallbladder becomes adherent to a surrounding viscus as a result of inflammation; the processes of ischemia and perforation promote erosion of the gallstone through both walls and into the lumen of the adjacent viscus.[85] Overall, nearly 90 per cent of internal biliary fistulae arise from the gallbladder.[86] Most commonly, fistulae are cholecystoduodenal (75 per cent),[87, 88] with cholecystocolic (15 per cent) and cholecystogastric (5 per cent) fistulae also being encountered.[87] In Asian countries, where pigment stones predominate and the incidence of choledocholithiasis is higher, choledochoenteric fistulae predominate. Choledochoduodenal fistulae may be present in 15 per cent of Asian patients with common duct stones,[89] but in western patients, penetration of a posterior duodenal ulcer is the cause of choledochoduodenal fistula formation in 80 per cent of patients.[90] Other, rarer fistulae, including those to the bronchus, urinary tract, and female genital tract, and fistulae to multiple organs have also been reported.[91] The overall incidence appears to be decreasing, perhaps because of the clear advantages to early surgery for acute cholecystitis. The overall mortality rate remains approximately 15 per cent, in part because of the large numbers of elderly, poor-risk patients who are afflicted.

The majority of biliary-enteric fistulae are not diagnosed preoperatively (Fig. 58–12). Certain symptoms are worthy of consideration, including volume depletion and hyponatremia, diarrhea, intestinal obstruction, and symptoms of cholangitis. Large losses of bile, as with bile peritonitis or an external biliary fistula, may result in massive losses of sodium. As the fluid and electrolyte abnormalities progress, metabolic acidosis and prerenal azotemia may supervene.

Cholangitis is unusual with fistulae in the upper gastrointestinal tract, but it complicates about one half of cases of cholecystocolic fistula. This predilection is explained by both the large numbers of bacteria in feces and the relatively small caliber of cholecystocolic fistulae. Diarrhea is commonly associated with colonic fistulae as well. Bile is strongly cathartic, and bile that bypasses the reabsorptive mechanisms in the terminal ileum may produce profound diarrhea. However, the most dramatic presentation of biliary-enteric fistula is intestinal obstruction resulting from an impacted stone.

Intestinal obstruction from gallstones, or gallstone ileus, is the presenting sign in about 15 per cent of patients with biliary-enteric fistula (Fig. 58–13). The point of obstruction is usually the terminal ileum, although jejunum and gastric outlet obstruction (Bouveret's syndrome) are reported occasionally.[92] The diagnosis may be difficult to make before obstruction is complete, because symptoms may be vague and intermittent as the stone traverses the small intestine. Once the diagnosis (usually of intestinal obstruction without regard for the possibility of gallstones) has been made, delaying surgery, except for prompt resuscitation of the patient, is pointless because gallstones almost never pass beyond the point of obstruction.

Operative strategies for biliary-enteric fistulae are numerous, and the approach to a patient must be individualized. Much controversy centers around whether the primary pathologic condition in the biliary tract should also be addressed at the initial operation. When considering operation for intestinal obstruction from gallstones, the answer to this question generally is no. Affected patients often are so unstable that the goal of surgery is solely to relieve the obstruction. This generally can be accomplished by enterotomy and extraction of the stone without resection. It is important to examine the entire intestine, however, since more than one gallstone is present within the intestine in 10 per cent of patients. The principal argument for simultaneous cholecystectomy is prevention of recurrent gallstone ileus, but this occurs in only four per cent of patients. In fact, in patients with gallstone ileus, the gallbladder seldom contains additional stones, and cholangitis is uncommon. It has been argued convincingly that an aggressive

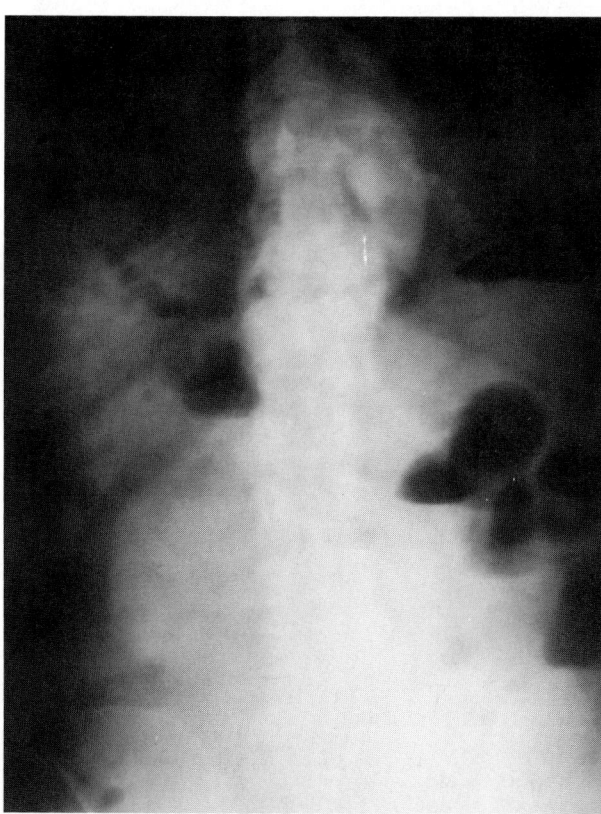

Figure 58–13. This abdominal radiograph was obtained from an elderly woman with a three-day history of lethargy, abdominal pain, and vomiting. Mechanical small intestinal obstruction was diagnosed from the dilated small bowel loops with differential air-fluid levels present in the left upper quadrant. A linear, branching radiolucency in the right upper quadrant represents pneumobilia. This x-ray film is pathognomonic for gallstone ileus or distal small bowel obstruction secondary to an intraluminal gallstone usually following a cholecystoduodenal fistula.

policy of simultaneous cholecystectomy adds morbidity and mortality beyond that caused by recurrent disease.[93]

Elective operations for biliary fistula must be undertaken with the knowledge that choledocholithiasis is common in these cases. Accordingly, all operations must include choledochal decompression. Ideally, dissection and isolation of the primary components of the fistula are followed by careful closure of the intestinal opening, cholecystectomy, and common duct exploration. As with other biliary tract procedures, cholecystostomy and placement of a T-tube in the common bile duct may be advisable if the dissection will be hazardous or prolonged in a poor-risk patient. Extra effort should be made to dismantle cholecystocolic fistulae because of the high rate of cholangitis in this setting. The surgeon must also be aware of the possibility of a fistula between the gallbladder and the common duct resulting from an impacted gallstone. When this leads to obstructive jaundice (Mirizzi's syndrome) or to formation of a fistula,[94, 95] the possibility of operative injury to the common duct increases unless particular care is taken.

ACALCULOUS CHOLECYSTITIS

About five per cent of patients with acute cholecystitis do not have gallstones. The entity of acalculous cholecystitis warrants separate consideration because particular groups of patients are commonly afflicted, diagnosis may be very difficult, and the mortality rate is much higher than for acute cholecystitis in general. About 50 per cent of children with acute cholecystitis have acalculous disease,[96] but it is more common in adults. Acalculous cholecystitis is most likely to occur in adults who are critically ill or who have recently undergone stress in the form of severe trauma,[97] burns,[98] or recent major surgery.[99–101]

Bile stasis and increased lithogenicity of bile have been implicated in the pathophysiology of acalculous disease,[102] as with acute cholecystitis associated with gallstones (see earlier discussion). Similarly, the ability of increased lysolecithin in bile to alter the permeability of the gallbladder wall to water and protein has been proposed as a mechanism.[103] However, an intrinsic biliary pathologic condition

may not be the sole explanation. Bile stasis induced by lack of gallbladder contraction during total parenteral nutrition may also contribute to the problem.[104] Mechanisms separate from biliary physiology may also be important. There is an association between acute acalculous cholecystitis and circulating activated coagulation factors in experimental animals.[105]

Primary infectious processes of the gallbladder may explain some cases of acalculous cholecystitis, for example, emphysematous cholecystitis. This is a rare, rapidly progressive, and often fatal disease in which gas bubbles appear in the inflamed tissue. The organism is *Clostridium* in 45 per cent of patients and *Escherichia coli* in one third of patients. Anaerobic streptococci occasionally are identified as the causative agent. The disease preferentially attacks males; about 20 per cent of patients also have diabetes mellitus. Thirty per cent of cases of emphysematous cholecystitis are acalculous.

Overall, the mortality rate of acute acalculous cholecystitis is as high as 30 to 50 per cent,[106] in part because the disease progresses rapidly in these often critically ill patients and in part because the diagnosis can be exceedingly difficult to make. Frequently, these patients are on ventilator support in the intensive care unit or have altered mentation as a result of their underlying severe illness and cannot be examined reliably. Patients seldom will have a palpable, tender right upper quadrant mass. Often, the diagnosis may be considered only after signs of sepsis are present, such as an increasing fluid requirement, sudden carbohydrate intolerance from peripheral insulin resistance, or unexplained fever or thrombocytopenia. Alternately, the abnormality may be elevated bilirubin or alkaline phosphatase levels from cholestasis. The differential diagnosis of cholestasis in these patients usually includes fatty liver secondary to excess carbohydrate in intravenous nutrition, drug toxicity, and sepsis. The disease is sufficiently common and devastating that acute acalculous cholecystitis belongs in the differential diagnosis of every patient with sepsis in the postoperative or post-traumatic period.

The diagnostic confusion is compounded by the limitations of conventional studies in this disease. Most of the diagnostic errors from sonography and cholescintigraphy

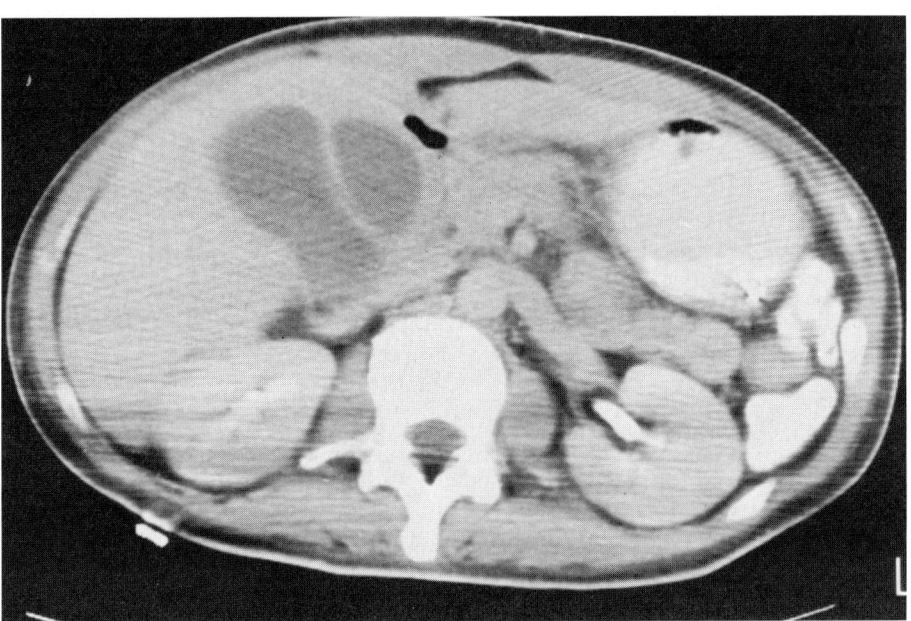

Figure 58–14. CT scan through the gallbladder two weeks following hospitalization for multiple fractures of the pelvis and lower extremities. The scan shows a dilated gallbladder with a thickened wall as well as a fluid collection surrounding the gallbladder in the subhepatic space. A perforated gallbladder with a subhepatic abscess was treated with cholecystectomy and drainage.

occur in the acalculous form of the disease.[107-109] The overall accuracy of cholescintigraphic (DISIDA) scans in acalculous disease may be as low as 40 per cent,[110] leading many to conclude that sonography should be undertaken initially. Good quality ultrasound examinations may be obtained at the bedside, which is a distinct advantage in the critically ill patient. The ultrasound findings of a gallbladder wall thickness of at least 3.5 mm, or the presence of a pericholecystic fluid collection, must be present to confirm the diagnosis of acute acalculous cholecystitis, since gallstones are not present by definition. Computed tomography (CT) (Fig. 58–14) may also be of value, although transport to the CT facility may be precluded in the unstable patient.

Once the diagnosis has been made, operation should be undertaken promptly. The disease progresses so rapidly that it is unlikely that antibiotic therapy alone will interdict the course of the disease. Perforation, gangrene, empyema, and cholecystitis are all more common in acalculous disease, and one or more is present in more than 50 per cent of cases. Cholecystectomy is the treatment of choice.

OTHER CAUSES OF SYMPTOMATIC GALLBLADDER DISEASE

On occasion, patients with pain resembling biliary colic cannot be proved to have gallstones. Diagnostic possibilities in these patients include the so-called hyperplastic cholecystoses, benign tumors, and syndromes of gallbladder dysmotility (biliary dyskinesia).

The two most common abnormalities of the gallbladder, other than cholelithiasis, are probably the hyperplastic cholecystoses known as cholesterolosis (see Fig. 58–12) and adenomyomatosis. Patients with cholesterolosis have deposits of cholesterol esters in submucosal macrophages, creating a yellow reticular pattern on the gallbladder mucosa. The usual normal levels of serum and bile cholesterol and the lack of cholesterol gallstones in many patients imply that the pathogenesis of cholesterolosis and cholesterol gallstone formation are different.[111-113] Cholesterol polyps occur in about 20 per cent of cases of cholesterolosis.[111] Unlike gallstones, cholesterol polyps appear as fixed radiographic defects on oral cholecystography (Fig. 58–15). Microscopic analysis of bile for cholesterol crystals has been proposed as a diagnostic adjunct in the diagnosis of cholesterolosis.[114-116] Positive findings are highly predictive of an abnormal gallbladder pathologic condition, which may include cholesterolosis, cholelithiasis, or chronic cholecystitis, or varying combinations of these.[114-116] Relief of pain after cholecystectomy usually occurs even when cholesterolosis is unaccompanied by cholelithiasis.[117]

The other common hyperplastic cholecystosis is adenomyomatosis, in which there is epithelial proliferation with muscular hypertrophy and mucosal diverticuli called Rokitansky-Aschoff sinuses. This condition may affect the gallbladder locally, particularly in the fundus, or diffusely.[118-120] On oral cholecystography, there are small collections of contrast in the sinuses, adjacent to the lumen of the gallbladder.[120] Sometimes the gallbladder appears to be divided into two compartments by a septum that lies in the transverse axis of the gallbladder. Although other diseases of the gallbladder often occur concomitantly,[118, 119] isolated adenomyomatosis appears capable of causing symptoms that are relieved after cholecystectomy,[118-120] as it did in eight of nine patients in one series.[118]

Benign tumors of the gallbladder are unusual and are seldom diagnosed preoperatively. The vast majority are

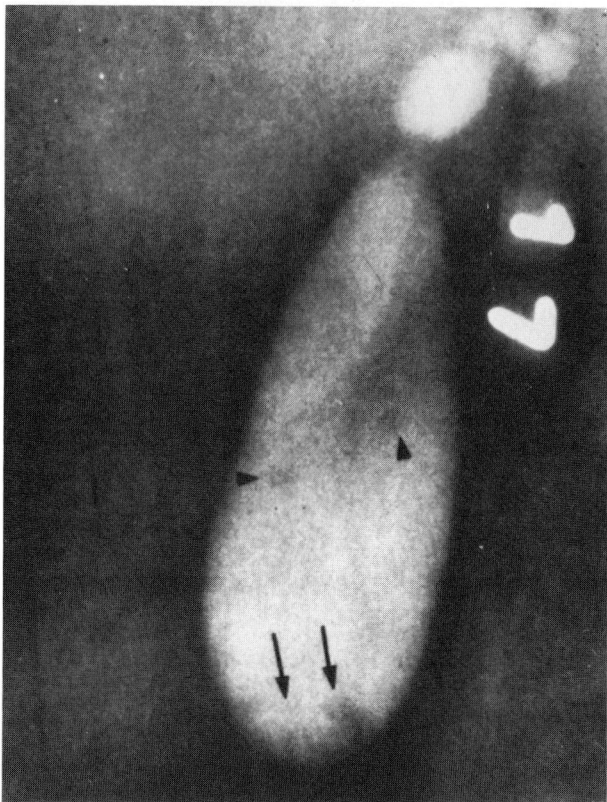

Figure 58–15. This oral cholecystogram was performed in a patient with a history of right upper quadrant pain and nausea of many years' duration. The gallbladder is normally opacified (arrows), and both fixed (*arrowheads*) and movable lucencies are demonstrated. The presence of cholesterolosis (fixed lesions) and gallstones was confirmed by cholecystectomy. (Photograph courtesy of A. F. Govoni, M.D., Department of Radiology, Cornell University Medical College.)

adenomata.[121] Benign tumors of the supporting tissues of the gallbladder are rare and usually incidental findings.[118] However, an association between symptoms and granular cell myoblastomata has been reported.[122, 123] Adenomatous hyperplasia of the gallbladder, distinct from adenomyomatosis, has been established as an additional cause of biliary symptoms and abnormalities on cholecystography.[124]

The term *biliary dyskinesia* has been used to describe patients who do not have structural abnormalities of the gallbladder demonstrable by conventional tests and who have biliary symptoms associated with disordered motility. Cholecystography accompanied by the administration of cholecystokinin has been used in the diagnosis of this syndrome. Studies have been characterized by nonuniform diagnostic criteria, including reproduction of pain, variable degrees of contraction and emptying, and spasm. Although several authors have concluded that an abnormal test result is highly predictive of a good response to cholecystectomy, other studies have failed to demonstrate predictably good results.[125, 126]

The difficulty with diagnostic precision in patients without demonstrable cholelithiasis leads to occasional uncertainty in the formulation of management plans for patients with biliary pain. In the presence of substantial symptoms for which no other cause is apparent, surgery appears to be justifiable when one of the hyperplastic cholecystoses is found; cholecystectomy for cholesterolosis is supported particularly well (see earlier discussion). Patients with frequent or protracted symptoms associated with a benign tumor of the gallbladder should also undergo cholecystectomy.[122] The most difficult group consists of those patients with typical biliary symptoms and normal studies. Cholecystokinin cholecystography is considered useful in some centers, but its efficacy remains unproved. Although such patients may occasionally prove to have abnormalities such as cholesterolosis or chronic cholecystitis, any decision to operate on such patients must be based on the conviction that other problems, including irritable bowel syndrome, are not responsible and only after the patient understands that the outcome of surgery is uncertain.

CARCINOMA OF THE GALLBLADDER

Carcinoma of the gallbladder, as a general rule, is curable only when discovered incidentally after cholecystectomy for calculous disease. Gallstones of both major classes of composition have been associated with carcinoma. The incidence of carcinoma clearly increases with advancing age and with gallstones greater than 3 cm in diameter.[127, 128] Calcified (porcelain) gallbladders pose substantial risk for the development of carcinoma, with a reported incidence of 22 per cent,[20] in comparison with an identified incidence of carcinoma in cholecystectomy specimens (removed for symptomatic or complicated cholelithiasis) of approximately 3 per cent.[20, 129]

The vast majority of gallbladder cancers are adenocarcinomata, but squamous tumors and carcinomata with mixed elements may occur. Gallbladder adenomata may be premalignant lesions, since the predilection for malignancy increases with increasing size. In one report, none of 18 adenomata smaller than 10 mm that were discovered in cholecystectomy specimens harbored carcinoma, whereas all of those greater than 15 mm contained malignant tumor.[130]

Most patients have symptoms (presumably from cholelithiasis). When considered in the context of possible surgical cure, the common presenting symptoms and signs of gallbladder carcinoma (pain, weight loss, hepatomegaly, right upper quadrant mass) are irrelevant, since gallbladder carcinomata that are large enough to cause symptoms are rarely, if ever, curable.[131] With rare exceptions, patients surgically cured of gallbladder carcinoma are successfully treated only because small carcinomata were found incidentally during cholecystectomy for gallstone disease. Virtually all of the diagnostic modalities employed for gallstone disease have been tried, without success, to improve the diagnosis of carcinoma. There is usually little point to surgery in those patients with strong evidence of gallbladder carcinoma, unless it is to palliate biliary or gastrointestinal obstruction. In such cases, biopsy by percutaneous techniques should be used for histologic confirmation.

Gallbladder carcinomata are locally aggressive despite being histologically well differentiated in the vast majority of cases. Tumors may arise anywhere in the gallbladder, and the gallbladder typically is contracted and thickened when involved by scirrhous carcinoma. The surgeon's first indication of the presence of carcinoma may be dense adhesions to surrounding viscera or the lack of a dissection plane in the gallbladder bed. Localized perforation occurs in about 10 per cent of cases and may be either into an adjacent hollow viscus or freely within the peritoneum, resulting in a pericholecystic abscess.[132] Spread to regional nodes or distant sites occurs late in the course of the disease. Lymphatic metastasis is first to cystic and common duct nodes in the porta hepatitis and then to retroduodenal nodes and the celiac axis.[133] Direct extension into liver is the most common visceral organ involvement, occurring in more than one half of cases.[131] Invasion of bile ducts, duodenum, stomach, colon, vena cava, and right kidney may also occur. Intraductal spread of tumor has been reported occasionally with papillary tumors. Metastases to distant organs are unusual. Peritoneal seeding is much less common than with primary carcinoma of the bile duct.

At surgery, the most common finding is that the tumor is beyond the limits of resection. Only about 25 per cent of these lesions (including in situ lesions discovered on pathologic examination) are resectable for cure.[131] Cholecystectomy is the operation most often performed for resectable gallbladder carcinoma, although the operation may be extended to include a regional lymphadenectomy, partial hepatectomy, or en bloc resection of adjacent involved viscera. It is difficult to discern whether these extended procedures are warranted. On theoretic grounds, a rationale for lymphadenectomy and resection of a margin of normal liver can be developed, since distant spread occurs late in the disease. This approach has widespread appeal among surgeons, although supportive data are inconclusive.[134–136] Details of pathologic findings and operative technique are often scant in available reports, and controlled trials of various operations have not been performed.

Wedge resection of the liver may be appropriate in selected cases in which the tumor appears confined to the gallbladder or has only microscopic transmural extension.[137] Major hepatic resection hardly seems justified, since mean survival is only four months, and overall one-year survival is less than 10 per cent. The major operative mortality rate for extended operations exceeds 20 per cent in collected series, whereas five-year survival is 4 per cent.[138] Among all patients resected with curative intent, five-year survival is less than 15 per cent.[131] Moreover, virtually all (92 to 95 per cent) of the five-year survivors are treated with cholecystectomy alone, strongly suggesting that eradication of very early disease rather than aggressive local control dictates survival.[131] Even localized disease resected for cure by cholecystectomy does not guarantee long-term survival, with the five-year cumulative survival rate reported to be as low as 25 to 33 per cent,[138, 139] although localized papillary carcinomata are prognostically favorable.

Adjunctive therapy has had, at best, a limited impact on this disease. The tendency of gallbladder cancer to invade locally but not metastasize widely has led to interest in radiation therapy. The experience with radiotherapy is limited, but it may provide useful palliation for jaundice. In one series, radiation therapy resulted in a doubling of the mean survival time to approximately 10 months,[140] although only two patients who survived more than five years have been reported.[141, 142] The use of intraoperative or locally delivered radiation with agents such as iridium may improve results. Currently available chemotherapeutic agents have no influence on gallbladder carcinoma.

Despite this dismal outlook, prophylactic cholecystectomy for the purpose of preventing gallbladder cancer cannot be justified, because the incidence of the disease is too low and the operative mortality rate cannot be zero.[143] Exceptions to this rule include patients with calcified gallbladders and possibly good-risk patients with large stones.[55] Even in elderly women with gallstones, however, the risk of death from cholecystectomy is as great or greater than the risk of death from gallbladder carcinoma; therefore, the operative risk cannot be justified.[55]

POSTCHOLECYSTECTOMY SYNDROMES

The vast majority of patients with biliary calculi are cured following cholecystectomy or exploration of the common duct. About 5 per cent of patients will have persistent or recurrent symptoms.[144] It can be extremely difficult to diagnose the cause of these symptoms.

The potential causes of symptoms following cholecystectomy are numerous and are not all related to the biliary tree. From the outset, it is essential to remember that symptoms mimicking biliary pain may be caused by peptic ulceration, hiatal hernia with gastroesophageal reflux, or other nonbiliary sources. The patient with postcholecystectomy symptoms usually complains of dyspepsia or upper abdominal pain, although the patient may present with related disease, for example, persistent or recurrent jaundice, pancreatitis, and cholangitis.[145, 146] Once extrabiliary causes of symptoms are excluded, further diagnostic studies are appropriately focused on the biliary tree and pancreas. The differential diagnosis is extensive and includes recurrent or retained calculi in the cystic duct or common bile duct. Other possible causes include operative injury to the biliary tree and simultaneous lesions missed when stones were identified at surgery. For example, ampullary or cholangiocarcinoma may coexist with common duct stones and may be unrecognized at surgery. Similarly, coexistent primary hepatocellular processes resulting from longstanding intermittent obstruction such as primary biliary cirrhosis could explain persistent jaundice following choledocholithotomy. Disorders of the sphincter of Oddi have drawn increasing attention as a source of symptoms in patients following cholecystectomy. The role of endoscopic retrograde cholangiopancreatography and sphincter of Oddi manometry in the diagnosis and treatment of these patients is discussed in Chapter 60.

REFERENCES

1. Glenn F. Trends in surgical treatment of calculous disease of the biliary tract. Surg Gynecol Obstet 140:877, 1975.
2. Kern F. Epidemiology and natural history of gallstones. Semin Liver Dis 3:87, 1983.
3. Boston Collaborative Drug Surveillance Program: Oral contraceptives and venous thromboembolic disease, surgically confirmed gallbladder disease, and breast tumors. Lancet 1:1399, 1973.
4. Grundy SM, Kalser SC. Highlights of the meeting on prevention of gallstones. Hepatology 7:946, 1987.
5. Royal College of General Practitioners' Oral Contraceptive Study: Oral contraceptives and gallbladder disease. Lancet 1:957, 1982.
6. Sampliner RE, Bennett PH, Comess LJ, et al. Gallbladder disease in Pima Indians: demonstration of high prevalence and early onset by cholecystography. N Engl J Med 1979:1358, 1970.
7. Diehl AK, Stern MP, Ostrower VS, et al. Prevalence of clinical gallbladder disease in Mexican-American, Anglo and Black women. South Med J 73:438, 1980.
8. Freeman JB, Meyer PD, Printen KJ, et al. Analysis of gallbladder bile in morbid obesity. Am J Surg 129:163, 1975.
9. Mabee TM, Meyer P, DenBesten L, et al. The mechanism of increased gallstone formation in obese human subjects. Surgery 79:460, 1976.
10. Faloun WW, Rubulis A, Knipp J, et al. Fecal fat, bile acid, and sterol excretion and biliary lipid changes in jejunoileostomy patients. Am J Clin Nutr 30:21, 1977.
11. Roslyn JJ, Berquist WE, Pitt HA, et al. Increased risk of gallstones in children on total parenteral nutrition. Pediatrics 71:784, 1983.
12. Lund J. Surgical indications in cholelithiasis: prophylactic cholecystectomy elucidated on the basis of long-term followup on 526 non-operated cases. Ann Surg 151:153, 1960.
13. Wenckert A, Robertson B. The natural course of gallstone disease: eleven year review of 781 nonoperated cases. Gastroenterology 50:376, 1966.
14. Gracie WA, Ransohoff DF. The natural history of silent gallstones. The innocent gallstone is not a myth. N Engl J Med 307:798, 1982.
15. McSherry CK, Ferstenberg H, Calhoun WF, et al. The natural history of diagnosed gallstone disease in symptomatic and asymptomatic patients. Ann Surg 202:59, 1985.
16. Thistle JL, Cleary PA, Lachin JM, et al. The natural history of cholelithiasis: the National Cooperative Gallstone Study. Ann Intern Med 101:171, 1984.
17. Ransohoff DF, Gracie WA, Wolfenson LB, et al. Prophylactic cholecystectomy or expectant management for silent gallstones. A decision analysis to assess survival. Ann Intern Med 99:199, 1983.
18. Strauch GO. Primary carcinoma of the gallbladder. Surgery 47:368, 1960.
19. Weiss KM, Ferrell RE, Hanis CL, et al. Genetics and epidemiology of gallbladder disease in New World native peoples. Am J Hum Genet 36:1259, 1984.
20. Polk HC. Carcinoma and the calcified gallbladder. Gastroenterology 50:582, 1966.
21. Stephens CG, Scott RB. Cholelithiasis in sickle cell anemia. Surgical or medical management. Arch Intern Med 140:648, 1980.
22. Ransohoff DF, Miller GL, Forsythe SB, et al. Outcome of acute cholecystitis in patients with diabetes mellitus. Ann Intern Med 106:829, 1987.
23. Hickman MS, Schwesinger WH, Page CP. Acute cholecystitis in the diabetic. Arch Surg 123:409, 1988.
24. Mundth E. Cholecystitis and diabetes mellitus. N Engl J Med 267:642, 1962.
25. Sandler RS, Maule WF, Baltus ME. Factors associated with postoperative complications in diabetes following biliary tract surgery. Gastroenterology 91:157, 1986.
26. Turrill F, McCarron M, Mikkelson W. Gallstones and diabetes: an ominous association. Am J Surg 102:184, 1961.
27. Walsh DB, Eckhauser FE, Ramsburgh SR. Risk associated with diabetes mellitus in patients undergoing gallbladder surgery. Surgery 91:254, 1982.
28. Bateson MC, Bouchier IAD. Prevalence of gallstones in Dundee: a necropsy study. Br Med J 4:4271, 1975.
29. Johnson AG. Cholecystectomy and gallstone dyspepsia. Clinical and physiological study of a symptom complex. Ann Roy Coll Surg Engl 56:69, 1975.
30. Glenn F, McSherry CK, Dineen P. Morbidity of surgical treatment for nonmalignant biliary tract disease. Surg Gynecol Obstet 126:15, 1968.
31. Cooperberg PL, Burhenne HJ. Real-time ultrasonography: diagnostic technique of choice in calculus gallbladder disease. N Engl J Med 302:1277, 1980.
32. Huber DF, Martin EW, Cooperman M. Cholecystectomy in elderly patients. Am J Surg 146:719, 1983.
33. Sullivan DM, Hood TR, Griffen WO Jr. Biliary tract surgery in the elderly. Am J Surg 143:218, 1982.
34. Aranha GV, Sontag SJ, Greenlee HB. Cholecystectomy in cirrhotic patients: a formidable operation. Am J Surg 143:55, 1982.
35. Schwartz SI. Biliary tract surgery and cirrhosis: a critical combination. Surgery 90:577, 1981.
36. Stelzer MH, Steiger E, Rosato FE. Mortality following cholecystectomy. Surg Gynecol Obstet 130:64, 1970.
37. Way LW, Bernhoft RA, Thomas MJ. Biliary stricture. Surg Clin North Am 61:963, 1981.
38. Salzstein EC, Evan SV, Mann RW. Routine operative cholangiography. Arch Surg 107:289, 1973.
39. Gerber A. A requiem for the routine operative cholangiogram. Surg Gynecol Obstet 163:363, 1986.
40. Stark ME, Coughry CW. Routine operative cholangiography with cholecystectomy. Surg Gynecol Obstet 151:657, 1980.
41. Duff JH, Salvian AG, Finley R. The incidence of secondary common bile duct exploration. Surg Gynecol Obstet 139:723, 1974.
42. Mills JL, Beck DE, Harford FJ. Routine operative cholangiography. Surg Gynecol Obstet 161:343, 1985.
43. Kakos GS, Tompkins RK, Turnipseed W, et al. Operative cholangiography during routine cholecystectomy. Arch Surg 104:484, 1972.
44. Glenn F. Choledochotomy in nonmalignant disease of the biliary tract. Surg Gynecol Obstet 124:974, 1967.
45. Morgenstern L. Exploration of the common bile duct for stones. In: Way LW, Pellegrini CA, eds. Surgery of the Gallbladder and Bile Ducts. Philadelphia, WB Saunders, 1987:351.
46. Heimbach DM, White TT. Immediate and long-term effects of instrumental dilation of the sphincter of Oddi. Surg Gynecol Obstet 148:79, 1979.
47. Fogarty TJ, Krippaehne WW, Dennis DL, et al. Evaluation of an improved operative technique in common duct surgery. Am J Surg 116:177, 1968.
48. Kappes SK, Adams MB, Wilson SD. Intraoperative biliary endoscopy. Mandatory for all common duct explorations. Arch Surg 117:603, 1982.
49. Stuart M, Hoerr SO. Late results of side to side choledochoduodenostomy for benign disorders. A twenty year comparative study. Am J Surg 123:67, 1972.

50. Jones SA, Smith U. A reappraisal of sphincteroplasty (not sphincterotomy). Surgery 71:565, 1972.
51. Amaral JF, Thompson WR. Gallbladder disease in the morbidly obese. Am J Surg 149:551, 1985.
52. Thompson JS, Philben VJ, Hodgson PE. Operative management of incidental cholelithiasis. Am J Surg 148:821, 1984.
53. Ouriel K, Ricotta JJ, Adams JT. Management of choledocholithiasis in patients with abdominal aortic aneurysm. Surgery 198:717, 1983.
54. Kovalcik PJ, Burrell MJ, Old WJ. Cholecystectomy concomitant with other intraabdominal operations. Arch Surg 118:1059, 1983.
55. Tompkins RK, Doty JE. Modern management of biliary tract stone disease. In: Mannick JA, Cameron JL, Jordan GL, eds. Advances in Surgery, Vol. 20. Chicago, Yearbook Medical, 1987:279.
56. Nicholas P, Rinaudo PA, Conn HO. Increased incidence of cholelithiasis in Laennec's cirrhosis. Gastroenterology 63:112, 1972.
57. Bornham PC, Terblanche J. Subtotal cholecystectomy: for the difficult gallbladder in portal hypertension and cholecystitis. Surgery 98:1, 1985.
58. Allen MJ, Bowdy TJ, Bagliosi TF, et al. Rapid dissolution of gallstones by methyl tert-butyl ether. Preliminary observations. N Engl J Med 312:217, 1985.
59. Glenn F. Surgical management of acute cholecystitis in patients 65 years of age and older. Ann Surg 183:56, 1981.
60. Pitluk HC, Beal JM. Choledocholithiasis associated with acute cholecystitis. Arch Surg 114:887, 1979.
61. Jarvinen H. Abnormal liver function tests in acute cholecystitis; the predicting of common duct stones. Ann Clin Res 10:323, 1978.
62. Weissman HS, Berkowitz D, Fox MS, et al. The role of technetium-99m iminodiacetic acid (IDA) cholescintigraphy in acute acalculous cholecystitis. Radiology 146:177, 1983.
63. Pellegrini CA, Way LW. Acute cholangitis. In: Way LW, Pellegrini CA, eds. Surgery of the Gallbladder and Bile Ducts. Philadelphia, WB Saunders, 1987:251.
64. Csendes A, Sepulveda A. Intraluminal gallbladder pressure measurements in patients with chronic or acute cholecystitis. Am J Surg 139:383, 1980.
65. Thornell E, Kral JG, Jansson R, et al. Inhibition of prostaglandin systhesis as a treatment for biliary pain. Lancet 1:584, 1979.
66. Thomas CG Jr, Womack NA. Acute cholecystitis, its pathogenesis and repair. Arch Surg 64:590, 1952.
67. Roslyn JJ, DenBesten L, Thompson JE Jr, et al. Roles of lithogenic bile and cystic duct occlusion in the pathogenesis of acute cholecystitis. Am J Surg 140:126, 1980.
68. Sjodahl R, Wetterfors J. Lysolecithin and lecithin in the gallbladder wall and bile: their possible roles in the pathogenesis of acute cholecystitis. Scand J Gastroenterol 9:525, 1975.
69. Sjodahl R, Tagesson C, Wetterfors J. On the pathogenesis of acute cholecystitis. Surg Gynecol Obstet 146:199, 1978.
70. Claesson B, Holmlund D, Matzch T. Biliary microflora in acute cholecystitis and the clinical implications. Acta Chir Scand 150:229, 1984.
71. Rosch J, Groleman JH Jr, Steckel RJ. Arteriography in the diagnosis of gallbladder disease. Radiology 92:1485, 1969.
72. Muller EL, Pitt HA, Thompson JE Jr, et al. Antibiotics in infections of the biliary tract. Surg Gynecol Obstet 165:285, 1987.
73. Jarvinen HJ, Hastbacka J. Early cholecystectomy for acute cholecystitis. A prospective randomized study. Ann Surg 191:501, 1980.
74. Lahitnen I, Alhava EM, Auke S. Acute cholecystitis treated by early and delayed surgery. A controlled clinical trial. Scand J Gastroenterol 13:673, 1978.
75. McArthur P, Cuschieri A, Sells RA, et al. Controlled clinical trial comparing early with interval cholecystectomy for acute cholecystitis. Br J Surg 62:850, 1975.
76. van der Linden W, Sunzel H. Early versus delayed operation for acute cholecystitis: a controlled clinical trial. Am J Surg 120:7, 1970.
77. Glenn F. Cholecystostomy in the high-risk patient with biliary tract disease. Ann Surg 185:185, 1977.
78. Gagic N, Frey CF. The results of cholecystectomy for the treatment of acute cholecystitis. Am J Surg 141:366, 1981.
79. Eggermont AM, Lameris JS, Jeeker J. Ultrasound-guided percutaneous transhepatic cholecystostomy for acute acalculous cholecystitis. Arch Surg 120:1354, 1985.
80. Fry DE, Cox RA, Harbrecht PJ. Empyema of the gallbladder: a complication in the natural history of acute cholecystitis. Am J Surg 141:366, 1981.
81. Wetstein L, Atkiss M, Aufses AH Jr. Acute torsion of the gallbladder: review of the literature and report of a case. Am Surg 42:138, 1976.
82. Strohl EL, Diffenbaugh WG, Baker JH, et al. Gangrene and perforation of the gallbladder. Int Abstr Surg 114:1, 1962.
83. Piedad OH, Wels PB. Spontaneous internal biliary fistula: obstructive and nonobstructive types. Twenty-year review of 55 cases. Ann Surg 175:75, 1972.
84. Glenn F, Reed C, Grafe WR. Biliary-enteric fistula. Surg Gynecol Obstet 153:693, 1981.
85. Glenn F, Mannix H. Biliary-enteric fistula. Surg Gynecol Obstet 105:693, 1957.
86. Hicken NF, Coray QB. Spontaneous gastrointestinal biliary fistulas. Surg Gynecol Obstet 82:723, 1946.
87. Alberti-Flor JJ, Hernandez M, Dunn GGD, et al. Cholecystoduodenal fistula. Am J Gastroenterol 80:95, 1985.
88. Karotin L. Spontaneous internal biliary fistula. Med Ann Dist Columbia 27:623, 1981.
89. Urakami Y, Kishi S. Endoscopic fistulotomy (EFT) for parapapillary choledochoduodenal fistula. Endoscopy 10:289, 1978.
90. Hoppenstein JM, Mendoza CB, Watke AL. Choledochoduodenal fistula due to perforating duodenal ulcer disease. Am Surg 173:145, 1971.
91. Pangan JC, Estrada R, Rosales R. Cholecystoduodenocolic fistula with recurrent gallstone ileus. Arch Surg 119:1201, 1984.
92. Cooper SG, Sherman SB, Steinhardt JE, et al. Bouveret's syndrome. Diagnostic considerations. JAMA 258:26, 1987.
93. Kasahara Y, Umemora H, Shiraha S. Gallstone ileus. Review of 112 patients in the Japanese literature. Am J Surg 140:437, 1980.
94. Mirizzi PL. Sindrone del conducto hepatico. J Int Chir 8:731, 1948.
95. McSherry CK, Feirstenberg H, Virshop M. The Mirizzi syndrome: suggested classification and surgical therapy. Surg Gastroenterol 1:219, 1982.
96. Pieretti R, Auldist AW, Stephens CA. Acute cholecystitis in children. Surg Gynecol Obstet 140:16, 1975.
97. Flanebaum L, Majerns TC, Cox EF. Acute post-traumatic acalculous cholecystitis. Am J Surg 150:252, 1985.
98. McDermott MW, Scudamore LH, Boileau LO, et al. Acalculous cholecystitis: its role as a complication of major burn injury. Can J Surg 28:529, 1985.
99. Ottinger LW. Acute cholecystitis as a postoperative complication. Ann Surg 184:162, 1976.
100. Leitman IM, Paull DE, Barie PS, et al. Intraabdominal complications of cardiopulmonary bypass surgery. Surg Gynecol Obstet 165:251, 1987.
101. Glenn F, Becker CG. Acute acalculous cholecystitis. An increasing entity. Ann Surg 193:131, 1982.
102. Deitch EA, Engel JM. Acute acalculous cholecystitis. Am J Surg 142:290, 1981.
103. Heuman R, Norrby S, Sjodahl R. Altered gallbladder bile composition in gallstone disease. Relation to gallbladder wall permeability. Scand J Gastroenterol 15:581, 1980.
104. Petersen SR, Sheldon GF. Acute acalculous cholecystitis. A complication of hyperalimentation. Am J Surg 138:814, 1979.
105. Becker CG, Dubin T, Glenn F. Induction of acute cholecystitis by activation of factor XII. J Exp Med 51:81, 1980.
106. Ullman M, Hasselgren PO, Tveit E. Posttraumatic and postoperative acute acalculous cholecystitis. Acta Chir Scand 150:507, 1984.
107. Shuman WP, Rogers JV, Rudd TG, et al. Low sensitivity of sonography and cholecystography in acalculous cholecystitis. Am J Roentgenol 142:531, 1984.
108. Ramanna L, Brachman MB, Tanasescu DE, et al. Cholescintigraphy in acute acalculous cholecystitis. Am J Gastroenterol 79:650, 1984.
109. Weissman HS, Freeman LM. Section II. The biliary tract. In: Freeman LM, ed. Freeman and Johnson's Clinical Radionuclide Imaging, 3rd ed. Orlando, Grune & Stratton, 1984:879.
110. Mirvis SE, Vainright JR, Nelson AW, et al. The diagnosis of acute acalculous cholecystitis: a comparison of sonography, scintigraphy, and CT. AJR 147:1476, 1986.
111. Holzbach RT, Marsh M, Tang P. Cholesterolosis: physical-chemical characteristics of human diet-induced canine lesions. Exp Mol Pathol 27:324, 1977.
112. Tilvis RS, Aro J, Strandberg TE, et al. Lipid composition of bile and gallbladder mucosa in patients with acalculous cholesterolosis. Gastroenterology 82:607, 1982.
113. Lindstrom CG. Frequency of gallstone disease in a well-defined Swedish population. A prospective necropsy study in Malmo. Scand J Gastroenterol 12:341, 1977.
114. Burnstein MJ, Vassa KP, Strasberg SM. Results of combined biliary drainage and cholecystokinin cholecystography in 81 patients with normal oral cholecystograms. Ann Surg 196:627, 1982.
115. Freeman JB, Cohen WN, DenBesten L. Cholecystokinin cholecystrography and analysis of duodenal bile in the investigation of pain in the right upper quadrant of patients without gallstones. Surg Gynecol Obstet 140:371, 1975.
116. Sigman HH, Goldberg N, Niloff PH, et al. Use of biliary drainage in diagnosis of biliary tract disease. Am J Gastroenterol 67:439, 1977.
117. Salmenkivi K. Cholesterolosis of the gallbladder, a clinical study based on 269 cholecystectomies. Acta Chir Scand (Suppl) 324:1, 1964.
118. Meguid MM, Aun F, Bradford ML. Adenomyomatosis of the gallbladder. Am J Surg 147:260, 1984.
119. Woodard BH. Adenomyomatous hyperplasia of the human gallbladder. South Med J 75:533, 1982.
120. Berk RN, van der Vegt JH, Lichtenstein JE. The hyperplastic chole-

cystoses: cholesterolosis and adenomyomatosis. Radiology 146:593, 1983.

121. Christensen AH, Ishak KG. Benign tumors and pseudotumors of the gallbladder. Report of 180 cases. Arch Pathol 90:423, 1970.
122. Nahrwold DL. Benign tumors and pseudotumors of the biliary tract. In: Way LW, Pellegrini CA, eds. Surgery of the Gallbladder and Bile Ducts. Philadelphia, WB Saunders, 1987:459.
123. Reul GJ Jr, Rubio PA, Berkmen NL. Granular cell myoblastoma of the cystic duct. Am J Surg 129:583, 1975.
124. Elfving G, Lehtonen T, Teir H. Clinical significance of primary hyperplasia of gallbladder mucosa. Ann Surg 165:61, 1967.
125. Berk RN. Oral cholecystography, IV cholangiography. In: Way LW, Pellegrini CA, eds. Surgery of the Gallbladder and Bile Ducts. Philadelphia, WB Saunders, 1987:121.
126. Dunn FH, Christensen ED, Reynolds J, et al. Cholecystokinin cholecystography. JAMA 228:997, 1974.
127. Weiss KM, Hanis CL. All "silent" gallstones are not silent. N Engl J Med 310:657, 1984.
128. Diehl AK. Gallstone size and the risk of gallbladder cancer. JAMA 250:2323, 1983.
129. Moossa AR, Anganost M, Hall AW, et al. The continuing challenge of gallbladder cancer. Am J Surg 130:57, 1975.
130. Kozuka S, Tsubone M, Yasui I, et al. Relation of adenocarcinoma to carcinoma of the gallbladder. Cancer 50:2226, 1982.
131. Vaittinen E. Carcinoma of the gallbladder. A study of 390 cases diagnosed in Finland 1953–1967. Ann Chir Gynecol (Suppl) 168:7, 1970.
132. Arminski TC. Primary carcinoma of the gallbladder. Cancer 2:379, 1949.
133. Fahim RB, McDonald JR, Richards JC, et al. Carcinoma of the gallbladder. Ann Surg 156:114, 1962.

134. Hamrick RE, Liner FJ, Hastings PR, et al. Primary carcinoma of the gallbladder. Ann Surg 195:270, 1982.
135. Kelly TR, Chamberlain TR. Carcinoma of the gallbladder. Am J Surg 143:737, 1982.
136. Wanebo HJ, Castle WN, Fechner RE. Is carcinoma of the gallbladder a curable lesion? Ann Surg 195:270, 1982.
137. Adson MA. Carcinoma of the gallbladder. Surg Clin North Am 53:1202, 1973.
138. Foster J. Carcinoma of the gallbladder. In: Way LW, Pelligrini CA, eds. Surgery of the Gallbladder and Bile Ducts. Philadelphia, WB Saunders, 1987:471.
139. Hart J, Modan B. Factors affecting survival of patients with gallbladder neoplasms. Arch Intern Med 129:931, 1972.
140. Hanna SS, Rider WD. Carcinoma of the gallbladder or extrahepatic bile ducts: the role of radiotherapy. Can Med Assoc J 129:931, 1978.
141. Del Regato JA, Spjut HJ. Cancer: diagnosis, treatment and prognosis, 5th ed. St. Louis, CV Mosby, 1977.
142. Smoron GL. Radiation therapy of carcinoma of the gallbladder and biliary tract. Cancer 40:1422, 1977.
143. Richard PF, Cantin J. Primary carcinoma of the gallbladder. Study of 108 cases. Can J Surg 19:27, 1976.
144. Bodvall B. The post-cholecystectomy syndrome. Clin Gastroenterol 2:103, 1973.
145. Blumgart LH, Carachi R, Imrie CW, et al. Diagnosis and management of postcholecystectomy symptoms: the place of endoscopy and retrograde cholangiopancreatography. Br J Surg 64:809, 1977.
146. Hunt DR, Blumgart LH. Endoscopic abnormalities in patients with postcholecystectomy symptoms. Surg Gastroenterol 1:155, 1981.

59

Diseases of the Bile Ducts

Ira M. Jacobson, M.D. • Philip S. Barie, M.D., F.A.C.S.

ABBREVIATIONS

CT = computed tomography
ERCP = endoscopic retrograde cholangiopancreatography
PTC = percutaneous transhepatic cholangiography

The ultimate expression of diseases that affect the bile ducts is jaundice. Although biliary tract disease can occur without the development of hyperbilirubinemia, evaluations of the diagnostic approach to patients with biliary obstruction have usually centered on jaundiced patients.[1-3] The clinician can usually form a correct impression of whether a jaundiced patient has parenchymal or obstructive disease by history and physical examination, supplemented by routine biochemical tests (Table 59–1).[4] If biliary obstruction is suspected, the two primary diagnostic modalities used for confirmation are sonography (Fig. 59–1) and computed tomographic scanning. Each of these techniques detects bile duct dilation in obstruction in more than 90 per cent of cases, with sonography slightly more sensitive. Computed tomography (CT) appears to be more accurate in defining the level and cause of obstruction, particularly with respect to malignancy.[5, 6] Obstruction in the absence

TABLE 59–1. CLINICAL CLUES IN THE DISTINCTION BETWEEN PARENCHYMAL AND OBSTRUCTIVE CAUSES OF JAUNDICE

Feature	Predictive Value
Age	Obstruction more likely in elderly patients
Pain	More common in obstructive disease
High fever	Favors obstruction and secondary cholangitis
Prolonged symptoms (anorexia, weight loss)	Suggests malignancy with obstruction
Exposure to hepatotoxic drugs	Favors hepatocellular disease or intrahepatic cholestasis
Alkaline phosphatase > three times normal	Favors obstructive disease or intrahepatic cholestasis
Aminotransferases > ten times normal	Favors hepatocellular disease but can occur in acute obstruction

of duct dilation on sonography or CT is usually associated with stones rather than tumors.[3, 7] In patients with malignant diseases, CT is better for delineation of the extent of disease, visualization of the pancreas, and the detection of metastases. Despite the common recommendation that sonography be performed as the initial imaging study in virtually all patients with suspected obstruction because of

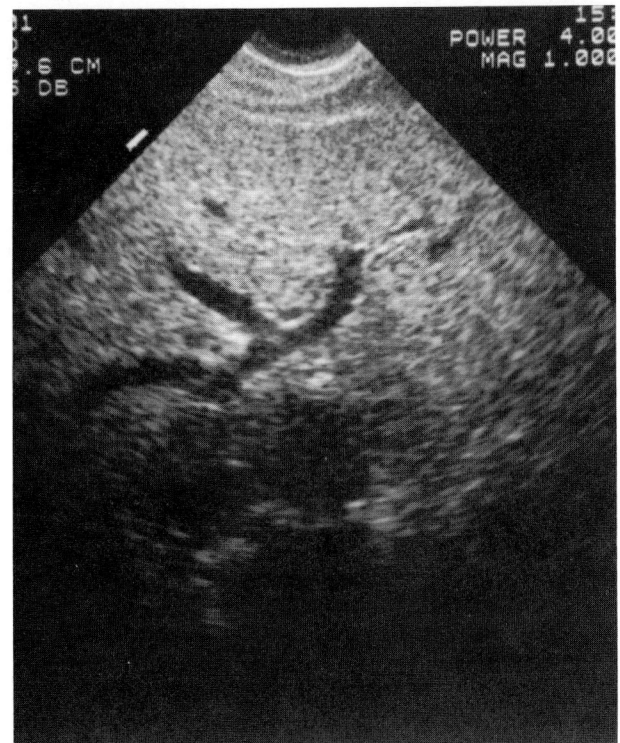

Figure 59–1. Ultrasonography of the left hepatic lobe in a patient presenting with jaundice, showing dilated intrahepatic bile ducts. Ultrasonography is generally considered the initial diagnostic study in the jaundiced patient because of its particular sensitivity for identifying and quantitating dilation of the biliary tree. Ultrasonography can estimate bile duct diameter within 0.5 mm, which is superior to computed tomographic scanning for this purpose.

lower expense and the lack of ionizing radiation,[1] CT is the preferred test for the evaluation of patients with malignant biliary obstruction, especially if a pancreatic neoplasm is suspected. CT also is more sensitive than sonography for the detection of choledocholithiasis, with detection rates for sonography reported from 13 to 75 per cent (Fig. 59–2)[5, 8–10] and for CT as high as 80 to 90 per cent.[11, 12] The sensitivity of CT is substantially greater for calcium bilirubinate than for cholesterol stones. In practice, both sonography and CT are often obtained in patients with obstructive jaundice before more invasive procedures are undertaken.

Direct visualization of the biliary tree by cholangiography may be required for both diagnosis and treatment. Cholangiography is of value in determining whether obstruction is present and in distinguishing between benign and malignant causes of obstruction when these issues are unresolved after noninvasive imaging tests. Cholangiography also provides precise information about the level and length of biliary strictures, and occasionally, diagnostic cytologic or biopsy material is obtained. However, in certain circumstances, surgery can be performed solely on the basis of noninvasive studies. For example, a patient with cholelithiasis and choledocholithiasis demonstrated by sonography or CT can proceed directly to cholecystectomy and common duct exploration. In this situation, intraoperative cholangiography or choledochoscopy can provide additional information so that preoperative contrast studies are unnecessary.

The choice of cholangiographic techniques is between percutaneous transhepatic cholangiography (PTC) and endoscopic retrograde cholangiopancreatography (ERCP). Visualization of the biliary tree by PTC approaches 100 per

cent when the ducts are dilated but falls to 70 to 80 per cent with ducts of normal caliber.[13] The biliary tree is successfully visualized by ERCP in 85 to 90 per cent of cases, and success is only slightly more likely when the ducts are dilated.[14] The frequency of successful visualization by ERCP, however, is much more dependent on the experience of the operator than is PTC, especially if the ducts are dilated. Complications of PTC include bleeding, bile peritonitis, and cholangitis. ERCP may cause pancreatitis and cholangitis. These procedures have important therapeutic applications, including placement of stents across obstructed ducts, dilation of strictures, and endoscopic sphincterotomy for removal of common duct stones. Because ERCP provides visualization of the pancreatic duct and the ampulla of Vater, affords the opportunity to remove stones if choledocholithiasis is found, and is somewhat less invasive than PTC, it is the procedure of choice in most patients with obstructive jaundice who need cholangiography. A randomized study concluded that ERCP yielded a specific diagnosis in obstructive jaundice more often than did PTC.[15] When ERCP fails, PTC is the ready alternative. PTC should be performed initially in patients with suspected proximal obstruction—for example, suspected tumors at the hilum of the liver. In these patients, PTC provides better delineation of the proximal extent of the tumor, which is critical for planning the surgical approach. Moreover, although some expert endoscopists are frequently successful in inserting biliary stents into these patients,[16] it is more difficult than with distal strictures.[17]

CHOLEDOCHOLITHIASIS

The spectrum of illness produced by common duct stones ranges from pain and jaundice to biliary pancreatitis and suppurative cholangitis. Overall, about 9 per cent of patients undergoing cholecystectomy for chronic cholecystitis have common duct stones.[18] The incidence of common duct stones increases both with advancing age and as the

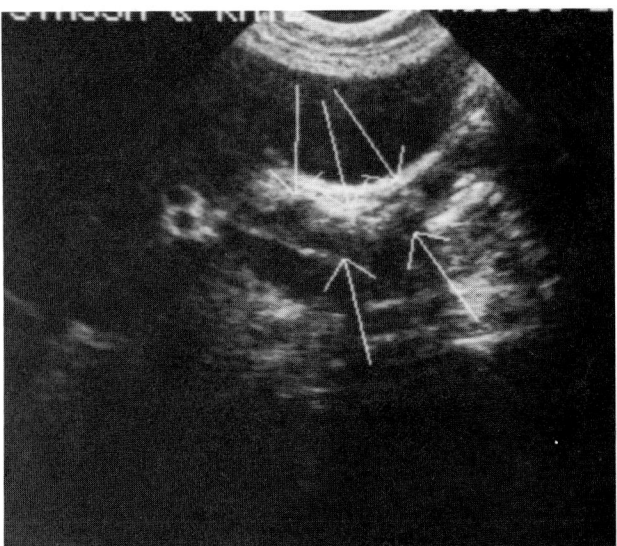

Figure 59–2. Biliary ultrasound study in a patient with jaundice and biliary colic. The common duct is visualized in longitudinal section and measures approximately 1.6 cm in diameter. Numerous echogenic densities within the bile duct lumen are identified by the arrows. Since there is also posterior acoustic shadowing, the study is diagnostic for choledocholithiasis, which was confirmed at laparotomy. Although common duct stones were readily apparent on this study, computed tomography is superior to ultrasound for this purpose.

duration of symptoms prior to surgery increases. In addition, common duct stones may be discovered after cholecystectomy at intervals ranging from several days postoperatively, in which case they are clearly retained, to many decades, in which case they are more likely to be stones that have formed de novo. Since the vast majority of common duct stones are secondary to gallbladder disease and are managed concurrently during gallbladder surgery, the operative management of uncomplicated choledocholithiasis is described in the chapter on gallbladder disease (Chap. 58).

The frequency with which common duct stones originate in the gallbladder or, alternatively, de novo in the duct has been assessed in terms of stone composition. Bernhoft and coworkers divided stones into those containing more or less than 50 per cent cholesterol by weight, calling them cholesterol and pigment stones, respectively.[19] Pigment stones can be characterized as black pigment stones, which contain derivatives of polymerized bilirubin, and brown pigment stones, containing calcium bilirubinate. The latter stones are soft, easily crushed, orange to dark brown, and are often referred to as "earthy."[19–22] Several lines of evidence indicate that primary formation of stones does occur in the bile ducts and that brown pigment stones usually are formed. Such stones are often the ones found in patients with biliary strictures or markedly dilated ducts in which stasis is likely to be present.[19] Patients with the syndrome of Oriental cholangiohepatitis, who have intrahepatic and extrahepatic duct calculi, have brown pigment stones. These stones are thought to form through the effect of bacterial β-glucuronidase on conjugated bilirubin. This reaction yields free bilirubin, which is relatively insoluble, leading to stone formation.[23] Moreover, when common duct stones are present early after cholecystectomy, they are usually composed predominantly of cholesterol.[24] Therefore, cholesterol stones in the duct usually are attributed to a gallbladder origin, and brown stones are attributed to de novo formation. Black pigment stones do not have the strong relationship to bacteria in the bile that calcium bilirubinate stones demonstrate and are most commonly of gallbladder origin.[23, 25]

Choledocholithiasis is associated with diverse clinical presentations. Patients with common duct stones may have a history of transient episodes of recurrent, mild pain, or they may be severely ill with cholangitis or pancreatitis in the absence of any prior history of biliary tract disease or symptoms. The pain of uncomplicated choledocholithiasis is often similar to that associated with cholelithiasis; as such, its greatest intensity may be felt either in the epigastrium or the right upper quadrant. When it radiates to the back, the pain tends to be described as going around the right side, in contrast to the pain of pancreatitis, which is predominant in the epigastrium and "bores through" to the back. Some episodes of pain may be accompanied by jaundice; occasionally, patients or family members may recall a yellow tinge in the eyes that accompanied an episode of pain occurring weeks before. Occasionally, jaundice may be the predominant manifestation of choledocholithiasis in the absence of pain. This latter presentation is especially likely in elderly or mentally impaired patients. Jaundice is usually transient but may be progressive and deep, similar to the picture more commonly associated with malignant biliary obstruction. The presence of fever signifies that cholangitis has complicated the situation.

CHOLANGITIS

Cholangitis refers to any inflammatory process involving the bile ducts but most commonly describes a bacterial infection. Clinical cholangitis—that is, systemic toxicity resulting from infection in the common bile duct—does not occur unless there are bacteria in the biliary tree and intraductal pressure is sufficiently elevated to cause the reflux of bacteria or endotoxin into the blood.[26] Obstruction plays a key role by both increasing intraductal pressure and promoting bacterial overgrowth as a result of bile stasis. The presence of a foreign body such as a gallstone or parasite within the biliary tree may readily cause obstruction and may thereby promote the development of cholangitis. Other diseases less commonly associated with cholangitis include choledochal cysts and neoplastic obstruction, either by primary carcinomas of the bile duct, pancreas, or ampulla. Iatrogenic conditions have also been associated with the development of cholangitis, notably obstruction caused by operative injury to the bile duct with resultant stricture[27] or reflux of gastrointestinal contents into the biliary tree via a transduodenal sphincteroplasty or other type of biliary-enteric anastomosis.[28] Cholangitis in these latter situations is rare unless there is coincident biliary tract obstruction.

The assumption that the source of the biliary bacteria in this disease is ascension of bacteria from the duodenum[29] has led to the widespread use of the term *ascending* cholangitis to describe these syndromes. Substantial evidence now exists, however, that other portals of entry for biliary bacteria may be more important (see later). The term *suppurative* cholangitis has come to denote a rapidly progressive and highly lethal form of cholangitis despite the recognition that there is considerable overlap in the degree of symptomatology and the presence or absence of purulent bile in the common duct. Despite these misnomers, this terminology is widely used and understood and so will serve as the basis of this discussion.

Bile is normally sterile, but cultures of gallbladder bile are positive in up to one half of patients with cholecystitis,[30] and most patients with common duct stones have positive bile cultures.[29–31] The pathways by which bacteria reach the biliary tree remain unclear. The five potential routes include ascension from the duodenum, by gastrointestinal and biliary lymphatics, by the hepatic artery, by the portal vein, and from a chronically infected gallbladder.[26] Evidence for the ascending route is indirect. Although clinical and experimental evidence of reflux with normal sphincter function is lacking, when the sphincter mechanism has been surgically bypassed or destroyed, recurrent cholangitis may occasionally result.[28] Similarly, cholangitis is rare in complete neoplastic obstruction of the common duct.[32] Evidence regarding the role of the periductal lymphatics and the portal vein in the pathogenesis of cholangitis was provided by Dineen,[33] who noted that bacteria introduced into duodenal lymphatics are recovered from bile in insignificant numbers because the predominant direction of lymph flow in the porta hepatis is toward duodenal and celiac lymph nodes. However, bacteria in portal venous blood can be recovered from bile in large numbers, particularly if bile flow is obstructed.[33] Portal venous blood is normally sterile in humans; however, the incidence of portal bacteremia during acute cholangitis may be more than twice as high as in systemic venous blood.[34] Evidence also suggests that infection may descend the biliary tree from a chronically infected gallbladder,[35] since gallbladder and common duct bile almost always yield the same organism in a given patient.

The clinical presentation of ascending cholangitis is quite variable and crosses a wide spectrum of severity of illness. The classic description of Charcot's triad of intermittent fever and chills, jaundice, and abdominal pain is well recognized as typical of cholangitis.[36] Unfortunately, Charcot's triad is present in as few as 60 per cent of cases,[37] with jaundice the most likely of the three to be absent (about 20 per cent of the time).[37] It is the absence of jaundice that makes the diagnosis difficult to establish in the patient with fever, chills, and abdominal pain. In contrast, the absence of either fever or pain (each about 10 per cent) in a jaundiced patient will be unlikely to divert attention away from the biliary tract.

Acute cholecystitis is often the most difficult disease process to distinguish from cholangitis. Acute hepatitis, liver abscess, and acute pancreatitis also must be considered. The patient with cholangitis, in contrast to one with cholecystitis, is more likely to have chills and less likely to have severe pain or marked tenderness in the right upper quadrant. Although some patients with acute cholecystitis may have elevation of serum bilirubin up to 5 mg/dl,[38] a total bilirubin level over 5 mg/dl is far more common with cholangitis.[37] Similarly, other liver chemistries may be elevated in both conditions,[38] but as with bilirubin, marked elevations favor the diagnosis of cholangitis. The key to diagnosis is an awareness that cholangitis may manifest as a mild and self-limited or as a life-threatening illness.

The life-threatening form of the illness (suppurative cholangitis), in which an often moribund patient presents in septic shock, has justifiably earned its reputation as a true emergency. Reynolds and Dargan added altered mental status and hypotension to Charcot's triad;[39] the so-called Reynolds's pentad is now considered pathognomonic for suppurative cholangitis. Although traditionally considered to reflect biliary obstruction with "pus under pressure" in the common bile duct, not all patients with suppurative cholangitis have purulent bile, and pus in the common duct does not always result in Reynolds's pentad.[40] However, the association is sufficiently common and the clinical syndrome of sufficient gravity to mandate that all syndromes of cholangitis be considered serious. A number of studies have attempted to define the criteria that differentiate suppurative cholangitis from its less severe form.[40–42] In general, fever greater than 40°C (104°F), hypotension, rebound tenderness, marked leukocytosis (greater than 20,000/mm³), and serum bilirubin levels in excess of 9 mg/dl may help identify critical cases of cholangitis.

Radiographic corroboration of the diagnosis can be difficult to achieve. Plain abdominal x-ray films are seldom abnormal, and the abnormalities tend to be nonspecific for biliary tract disease, such as ileus.[37] Hepatobiliary scintigraphy is much less helpful than it is in the diagnosis of cholecystitis because of its inability to precisely define biliary tract anatomy.[43] Ultrasound (see Fig. 59–1) and CT are more helpful in that they identify dilated bile ducts in most patients with biliary obstruction and may give additional information about the site or cause of obstruction.[5–7] The diagnosis of acute cholangitis usually rests on clinical and biochemical criteria with supportive evidence provided by sonography, CT scanning, or both. The differentiation between suppurative cholangitis and its less severe forms is often based solely on appropriate responses to fluid and antibiotic therapy within the first few hours following the diagnosis. In particular, hypotension that does not respond to fluid administration promptly and durably is a genuine emergency warranting urgent biliary decompression.[26] This period is undoubtedly critical, since failure to respond initially defines a subgroup of patients with suppurative cholangitis with an overall mortality of 40 per cent as opposed to mortality of about 10 per cent for less severe forms of cholangitis.

TREATMENT OF CHOLANGITIS

Therapy for cholangitis must be individualized because of the spectrum of severity of illness. Virtually all patients will require hydration with a balanced salt solution, such as Ringer's lactate solution. Since many patients are elderly, monitoring of volume support with a central venous or pulmonary artery catheter, as appropriate, should be considered early in the course of the illness. All patients should have nasogastric and urinary bladder catheters placed. Prophylaxis against sepsis-induced upper gastrointestinal hemorrhage is strongly recommended. Antibiotic therapy (see later) is initiated promptly on an empiric basis, but any patient failing to respond to these measures within 24 hours should be considered for immediate biliary decompression. In particular, use or even consideration of vasopressor support of hypotension suggests that the patient should undergo emergency decompression of the common bile duct. If surgery is indicated, the operating room is a suitable environment in which to conduct the patient's resuscitation, and delay in transport to the operating room on the grounds that initial resuscitation has not been completed cannot be justified.

The majority of patients (about 70 per cent) with cholangitis will respond appropriately to antibiotics and intravenous fluids.[40] Empiric antibiotic therapy is based on information obtained from other studies in which cultures of blood and bile were obtained (Table 59–2). Whereas bile cultures are ultimately positive in more than 90 per cent of patients with cholangitis, blood cultures are positive in only about 40 per cent of patients.[37, 40, 44] The correlation between organisms in blood and bile is poor because bile cultures are usually polymicrobial, whereas blood cultures are generally positive for a single organism.

Coliform organisms, Escherichia coli and Klebsiella pneumoniae, are the most common organisms causing cholangitis. E. coli is recovered from up to 60 per cent, Klebsiella from about 40 per cent of patients.[37, 40, 44] These two organisms combined account for as much as 70 per cent of positive bile cultures and as much as 85 per cent of positive blood cultures.[37] Streptococcus faecalis (enterococcus) is the third most commonly isolated organism in studies such as these, accounting for 30 per cent of bile isolates. Whereas enterococcus seldom causes bacteremia, arguments that enterococci can be pathogenic in biliary tract

TABLE 59–2. BACTERIOLOGY OF CHOLANGITIS

	Saik[44]	Saharia[37]	Boey[40]
Bile Cultures			
% Positive	93	100	92
% Polymicrobial	61	60	48
Organisms (%)			
Escherichia coli	65	74	58
Klebsiella pneumoniae	50	40	35
Streptococcus faecalis	27	31	18
Pseudomonas	15	?	22
Blood Cultures			
% Positive	47	40	44
Organisms (%)			
E. coli	53	45	39
K. pneumoniae	47	40	7
S. faecalis	12	5	—
Bacteroides fragilis	6	5	—
Pseudomonas	18	—	7

sepsis appear justified, and therapy should be tailored accordingly.[45] Anaerobes are increasingly recognized as important pathogens in cholangitis.[42] Anaerobic species, in particular *Bacteroides fragilis* and, occasionally, species of *Clostridium*, may be isolated in as many as 10 per cent of cases.

There is no consensus regarding the primacy of one particular antibiotic or combination of antibiotics in cholangitis. Based on current data, rational empiric therapy should include coverage of enteric gram-negative organisms, enterococci, and anaerobes. Historically, the combination of penicillin and an aminoglycoside was recommended[40, 42] and was effective in up to 90 per cent of cases.[42] This regimen did not allow for the importance of *B. fragilis* in the pathogenesis of cholangitis but was an excellent choice for activity against coliforms and synergistic activity against enterococci. Addition of effective therapy against *Bacteroides* with clindamycin or metronidazole to an aminoglycoside would be an appropriate modification of this historically effective regimen. Third-generation cephalosporins appear to be unsuitable for biliary tract sepsis. Not only do these drugs have generally poor activity against enterococci but they (except moxalactam) also appear effective against less than 50 per cent of *Bacteroides* isolates. The recent introduction of broad-spectrum acylureido penicillins such as piperacillin may prove to be a rational alternative, since these agents combine excellent activity against enterococci, anaerobes, and coliforms. The current practice of the authors is to begin piperacillin and tobramycin therapy in all non–penicillin-allergic patients with cholangitis, pending the results of cultures. Newer antibiotics with extremely broad antibacterial spectra, such as imipenem, may prove eventually to be suitable for single-agent therapy of suppurative cholangitis, although there is currently insufficient data to make this determination. Any diagnostic or therapeutic manipulation of the biliary tract, even beyond the initial 10- to 14-day course of antibiotics, must be covered appropriately.

If the patient responds promptly to systemic antibiotics, additional diagnostic studies may be warranted to adequately define biliary anatomy. Precise anatomic definition can be accomplished with either PTC or ERCP.[46] ERCP is preferable to PTC as the initial procedure, because it obviates the risk of bleeding and bile leak from puncture of the liver and affords the opportunity to perform sphincterotomy and stone extraction if stones are discovered (see later).

SURGICAL MANAGEMENT

The surgical approach to decompression depends on the urgency of the procedure and on biliary anatomy. Cholecystectomy and common duct exploration will be required in most patients except those with cholangitis secondary to retained or recurrent choledocholithaisis following cholecystectomy. Intraoperative bile cultures should be taken despite prior antibiotic therapy as a guide to management of possible postoperative infections, such as subhepatic abscess. In addition to common duct exploration, a biliary "bypass" procedure such as transduodenal sphincteroplasty or choledochoduodenostomy may be indicated if stones cannot be extracted—for example, when multiple stones remain in the intrahepatic biliary radicles on intraoperative cholangiography or when primary common duct stones are the cause of the cholangitis.[47] Choledochoduodenostomy is the preferred biliary bypass procedure if technically feasible. In properly selected patients, failure of the choledochoduodenostomy caused by stricture formation or the "sump syndrome" (the presence of inspissated food in the distal duct between the anastomosis and the ampulla) should be negligible.[48, 49] When the duct is of insufficient caliber (less than 2 cm in diameter) to allow construction of a choledochoduodenostomy, transduodenal sphincterotomy is suitable.[50]

The principles of surgical decompression for suppurative cholangitis are completely different, since the goal is to achieve only decompression in an extremely unstable patient. Adequate decompression with minimal surgery is extremely important. At surgery, incision of the distended common duct will result in the release of pus under considerable pressure, often with immediate improvement in the patient's condition. Minimal manipulation of the bile duct should be carried out because of the risk of further bacteremia, but readily encountered stones should be removed. A T-tube of sufficient size (16 French) to allow extraction of residual stones with a Dormia basket a few weeks later (Figs. 59–3 and 59–4) is inserted into the common duct, and the operation is terminated. Cholecystostomy alone is inadequate in cholangitis, because the thick pus in the common duct cannot flow into the gallbladder through the cystic duct and is associated with extremely high mortality.[51] This also highlights the need to distinguish cholangitis from acute cholecystitis, since cholecystostomy alone may occasionally be lifesaving in acute cholecystitis. Proper surgical decompression as dictated by the individual circumstances cannot be overemphasized, since inadequate surgical drainage may explain half of the overall mortality from suppurative cholangitis.[37]

An alternative to surgery is the extraction of bile duct stones (Fig. 59–5) or in some acutely ill patients, insertion of a drainage tube alone after endoscopic sphincterotomy. Anecdotal data support the potential efficacy of ERCP in patients with acute cholangitis.[52, 53] A single retrospective study suggested a lower mortality in patients treated endoscopically than those treated surgically.[52] However, no randomized controlled trials have been reported, and ERCP cannot yet be considered the procedure of choice in all patients with cholangitis. In addition, in acutely ill patients the risk of ERCP is increased in the presence of hypotension or in a setting that is not conducive to careful monitoring of blood pressure, respiratory status, and electrocardiographic data. ERCP should not be considered if not readily available within the same time frame as surgery if urgent decompression is indicated.

If ERCP and sphincterotomy are performed, cholecystectomy may proceed electively at a later date. In selected patients, the gallbladder may be left in place if the patient's presenting illness was thought to be caused by choledocholithiasis alone. This approach appears to be associated with a low incidence of subsequent cholecystitis or biliary pain severe enough to require cholecystectomy (e.g., 5 to 20 per cent during 3- to 5-year follow-up periods).[54, 55] The risk that cholecystectomy may be required later is low enough to be considered potentially acceptable in elderly patients or those with medical conditions posing a high operative risk (see Chap. 58).

RECURRENT PYOGENIC CHOLANGITIS

Recurrent pyogenic cholangitis, described by Cook and colleagues in 1954,[56] is commonly known as Oriental cholangiohepatitis because of the striking association of this disease with inhabitants of and immigrants from countries in the Asian Pacific Basin.[57] The disease occurs after repeated episodes of cholangitis from gallstone-induced biliary obstruction, typically from impacted intrahepatic stones. Consequently, the pathologic changes are most marked in the intrahepatic ducts, with patchy stenosis and dilation serving to entrap stones within the liver. The duct walls become thickened and fibrotic, and secondary biliary cirrhosis may develop after repeated infections.[57] The extrahepatic ducts are also typically affected by dilation and fibrosis. It has been suggested that the intrahepatic calculi are secondary to congenital biliary stricture associated with cystic dilatation of the common bile duct.[58] Previous hy-

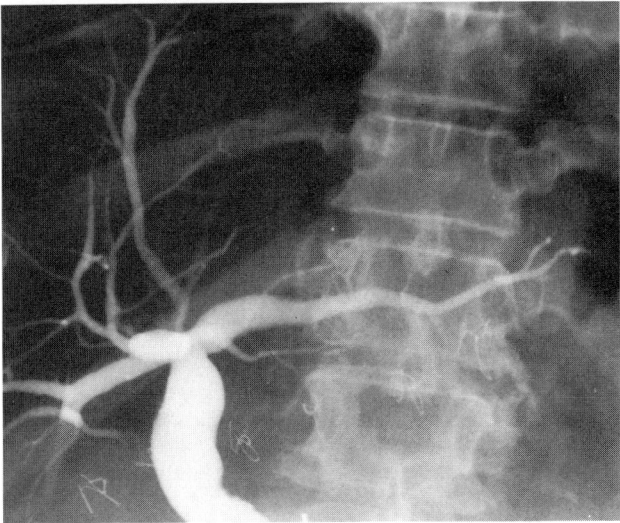

Figure 59–4. Careful cholangiography of the intrahepatic ducts excluded residual intrahepatic choledocholithiasis in the same patient depicted in Figure 59–3.

potheses about the pathogenesis of the syndrome include parasitic infestation of the biliary tract with *Ascaris lumbricoides* or *Clonorchis sinensis*. This theory was based on the finding that the stones typical of the disease sometimes harbor parasites on microscopic section.[59] The presence of parasites however is not a consistent finding, and they are unlikely to be a primary cause of this disease. Another contributing factor is that many patients with intrahepatic calculi have colonization of the bile with *E. coli* that contain a β-glucuronidase that deconjugates bilirubin glucuronides to form precipitates of bilirubin.[23]

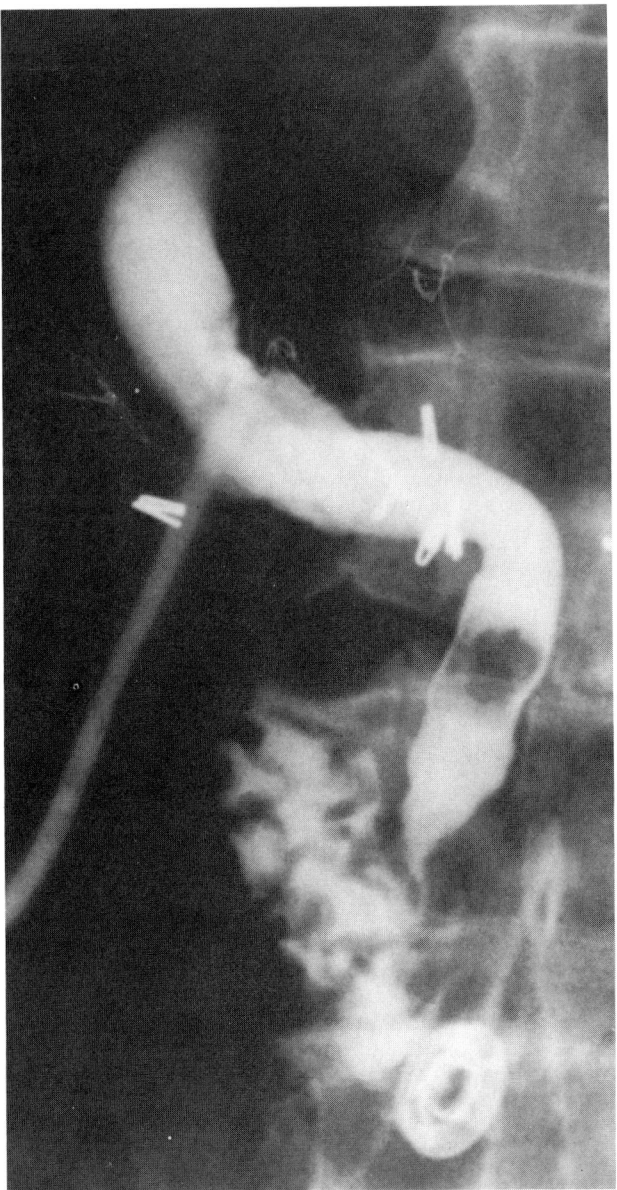

Figure 59–3. This T-tube cholangiogram shows a very large (15 mm) retained stone in the distal portion of the dilated common duct. Retained stones of this size are difficult to manage, since they are larger than can be retrieved intact via either Dormia basket or endoscopic papillotomy. In this case, a steerable, crushing forceps was used to fragment the stone within the common duct, thereby allowing easy removal of the fragments. Particular care must be taken when resorting to this technique, since fragments of retained stone may also give rise to obstructive jaundice, cholangitis, or pancreatitis.

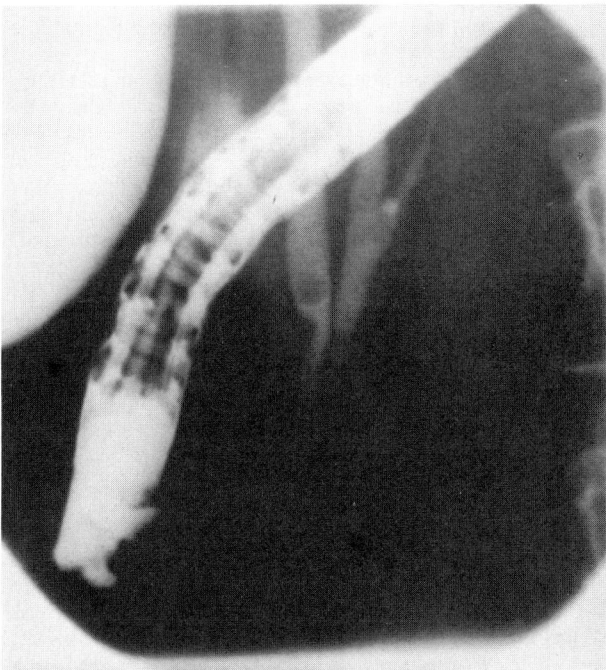

Figure 59–5. This radiograph was obtained during endoscopic retrograde cholangiopancreatography (ERCP). The side-viewing endoscope dominates the roentgenogram, passing obliquely downward from the upper right. Contrast material introduced via catheter through the ampulla of Vater revealed both the common bile duct and both pancreatic ducts with a single injection, which is indicative of a common channel. The round lucency present in the distal common bile is a single, nonimpacted common duct stone, which was retrieved after endoscopic papillotomy.

The first attack may begin mildly and insidiously with low-grade fevers and barely perceptible jaundice, which then subsides spontaneously. However, the hallmark of this illness is attacks that increase in frequency and severity. Ultimately, without intervention, the process develops features of suppurative cholangitis. When the patient seeks medical attention, there may be hepatomegaly as well as splenomegaly if portal vein thrombosis has occurred. Jaundice and leukocytosis are present but generally not to the degree seen in common forms of cholangitis. The gallbladder is often palpable when distal common duct obstruction is a feature of the disease. Acute pancreatitis is a common accompaniment (12 per cent) of recurrent pyogenic cholangitis.[60]

In addition to pancreatitis, complicating features of the disease include peritonitis from perforation of the gallbladder, liver abscess, biliary-enteric fistula, gram-negative bacteremia, and portal vein thrombosis. Rarely, hepatic vein thrombosis occurs that can lead to septic embolization of the pulmonary circulation.[61]

Therapy, in addition to supportive measures and appropriate antibiotics, is directed toward surgical biliary decompression. The microbiology of recurrent pyogenic cholangitis is identical to that of ascending cholangitis, with the exception of frequent superimposed parasitism in this disease. In addition to choledochotomy and drainage, cholecystectomy or cholecystostomy is performed if there is perforation, gallstones, or empyema of the gallbladder. Operative cholangiography or choledochoscopy may greatly assist the search for residual intrahepatic stones. Transduodenal sphincteroplasty may be indicated if common bile duct dilation extends to the ampulla. If there are no intrahepatic stones or strictures, sphincteroplasty may render as much as 85 per cent of patients permanently symptom-free.[62] Roux-en-Y choledochojejunostomy is indicated for dilation of the common duct above the duodenum. Using this approach, excellent results can be anticipated in about 70 per cent of patients.[63]

The presence of intrahepatic stones in about 25 per cent of patients poses special management problems.[64] For unclear reasons, the majority of these stones are confined to the left hepatic ductal system. This form of disease frequently is refractory to medical therapy, and a left hepatic lobectomy often is necessary. If stones are also confined in the right ductal system, a transhepatic approach to the right hepatic duct is performed for the purpose of right lobar decompression. Dissection in the interlobar fissure will encounter the bifurcation of the common hepatic duct, and choledochotomy above the stenosis can be performed. Stones are rarely found only in the right ductal system, making right hepatic lobectomy a rarely performed operation for this disorder.[64]

BILIARY PANCREATITIS

Gallstones and alcohol are by far the commonest causes of pancreatitis, with gallstones responsible for roughly half of cases in many areas.[65–68] The first direct implication of gallstones in the pathogenesis of pancreatitis in humans was made in 1900 by Opie,[69] who identified an impacted stone in the ampulla of Vater in a patient who died of pancreatitis. Based on this observation and later experiments in animals, Opie proposed the "common channel theory." He suggested that the impaction of an ampullary stone produced reflux of bile into the pancreatic duct, thereby giving rise to pancreatitis in patients in whom the common bile duct

and the pancreatic duct joined before entering the duodenum. The ability of impacted stones to cause pancreatitis has remained uncontested, but hypertension in the pancreatic duct, rather than reflux of bile or duodenal contents, is now considered the likeliest initiator of inflammation.[70]

Evidence for the gallstone migration theory of pancreatitis has developed along several lines. Gallstones can be identified in the stool within ten days of the attack of pancreatitis in roughly 90 per cent of patients with pancreatitis and cholelithiasis.[71, 72] In contrast, the chance of finding gallstones in stool is less than 10 per cent in patients with cholelithiasis but without pancreatitis.[71] Moreover, studies have shown repeatedly that the incidence of choledocholithiasis or of stones impacted at the ampulla of Vater at surgery decreases as the time interval between pancreatitis and surgery increases, presumably because the stones have passed prior to operation.[50, 73] For example, Armstrong and co-workers found common duct stones in all patients operated on within 48 hours of the onset of pancreatitis[73] and in 66 per cent of patients operated on within three to seven days after the attack. When surgery was delayed beyond 7 days, however, the incidence of choledocholithiasis decreased to 23 per cent within 21 days and 11 per cent after that. Impacted stones have been found in as many as 62[74] to 75[75] per cent of patients operated on within 48 hours of the onset of pancreatitis, but the incidence of stone impaction decreases with time.[73] Even when a low incidence of ampullary stone impaction was found in one surgical report, a substantial number of patients had gallstones in the duodenum, suggesting recent passage, and ampullary edema with acute inflammation of the distal common bile duct was present in the majority.[50] Although even transient impaction can doubtless cause pancreatitis, such observations leave open the possibility of an additional contribution of ampullary edema, perhaps with spasm, to the pathogenesis of biliary pancreatitis. Endoscopic observations provide similar support for the gallstone migration theory of biliary pancreatitis. In a randomized trial of early ERCP versus conservative treatment, Neoptolemos and colleagues found stones in the common bile duct in 50 per cent of patients with suspected biliary pancreatitis who underwent ERCP within 72 hours of admission but in only 12 per cent of patients undergoing surgery before discharge but who had not undergone endoscopy early in their course.[76] Thus, choledocholithiasis appears to be a transient phenomenon in many patients with pancreatitis.

In most cases, the stones that migrate through the ampulla and cause pancreatitis are small.[71, 72, 75, 77, 78] Houssin and associates underscored the importance of microlithiasis (stones 3 mm or smaller) in the pathogenesis of pancreatitis by finding that 22 per cent of their patients with microlithiasis had pancreatitis prior to cholecystectomy, a fourfold greater than expected incidence.[77] Also, patients with gallstone pancreatitis tend to have larger numbers of gallstones in their gallbladders, even though the aggregate weight of the stones is less than concurrent controls with cholelithiasis.[78] The relationship of cystic duct diameter to stone size may be important. Studies involving perfusion of resected gallbladders suggest higher flow rates through the cystic ducts of gallbladders from patients with pancreatitis, suggesting larger cystic duct diameter.[78] The combination of small stones and low resistance to flow in the cystic duct may increase the risk of biliary pancreatitis. In some patients, however, the primary source of stones is the common bile duct rather than the gallbladder. Following cholecystectomy, residual or recurrent common duct stones can give rise to pancreatitis even when pancreatitis was not the original indication for surgery.[79]

Many patients pass gallstones into the duodenum without developing pancreatitis. It has been suggested that differences in ampullary physiology may predispose some patients with cholelithiasis to the development of pancreatitis. Impaction may be more frequent in patients with high basal pressure in the sphincter of Oddi,[80] failure of the sphincter to relax in response to physiologic stimuli, or both.[81] The true role of such disturbances and the question of whether they are primary abnormalities or secondary to ampullary fibrosis following the passage of gallstones are unresolved issues.

The clinical features and prognosis of acute biliary pancreatitis may be indistinguishable from other forms of pancreatitis, and general support of these patients is identical regardless of the etiology. The reader is referred to standard reviews of acute pancreatitis for diagnostic criteria.[82] A possible biliary etiology should be excluded promptly in all patients with pancreatitis. Discussion herein centers upon the diagnosis of associated biliary tract disease. Some patients will have histories suggestive of gallstones because of prior biliary symptoms, and in a few patients, the diagnosis of cholelithiasis may already have been made. Patients with biliary pancreatitis are more frequently jaundiced or have a history of jaundice in comparison with patients with alcoholic pancreatitis. Serum levels of alkaline phosphatase, aspartate aminotransferase (AST), alanine aminotransferase (ALT), bilirubin, and amylase are higher in gallstone pancreatitis than in alcoholic pancreatitis,[83, 84] although considerable overlap in these values limits their utility.

Ultrasonography is recommended for all patients with the first attack of pancreatitis because of its sensitivity in the detection of cholelithiasis.[85] Identification of cholelithiasis is usually considered evidence that pancreatitis is biliary in origin. However, the absence of gallbladder stones on sonography does not preclude choledocholithiasis as the cause of pancreatitis. As discussed earlier, sonography is less accurate for choledocholithiasis than for cholelithiasis. CT is superior to sonography in the detection of choledocholithiasis but is generally not necessary for this purpose in nonalcoholic patients with gallbladder stones demonstrated sonographically. The causative common duct stone may no longer be in the biliary tract even if imaging studies are performed early. A CT scan may be helpful when the diagnosis of pancreatitis is in doubt, since it provides superior visualization of the pancreas in comparison with sonography. The CT scan may also provide prognostic information. For example, Ranson and colleagues demonstrated that the likelihood of pancreatic abscess formation was 17 per cent when one peripancreatic fluid collection was noted in conjunction with pancreatic inflammation on CT scan. The incidence of abscess formation increased to 61 per cent when two or more fluid collections were identified.[86]

When cholelithiasis is identified but there is still a question of etiology, as in the alcoholic patient, there are few additional tests with sufficient specificity to be helpful. Screening of the stools will yield gallstones over 85 per cent of the time,[71] but it is cumbersome and may take days. Biliary scanning with ^{99m}Tc-labeled iminodiacetic acid derivatives during acute pancreatitis has been recommended,[87] since the gallbladder can be visualized less often in patients with biliary pancreatitis (53.5 per cent) than in those with other forms of pancreatitis (76 per cent).[55] This difference is insufficient to allow conclusions to be drawn from this study in an individual patient. Moreover, reliance on this modality substitutes one diagnostic problem for another,

since acute cholecystitis, the leading cause of a nonvisualized gallbladder, may manifest simultaneously with acute pancreatitis in about 5 per cent of patients with biliary pancreatitis.[87] The identification of simultaneous acute cholecystitis and acute pancreatitis may be difficult in this setting but is important, since surgery for acute cholecystitis (see Chap. 58) may be required sooner than is otherwise optimal in acute biliary pancreatitis. Direct cholangiography, both percutaneous[88] and by retrograde cannulation methods,[89] also may reveal otherwise undetectable stones. These invasive tests are generally not recommended for diagnostic purposes alone in the acute setting, but as discussed below, ERCP may have a therapeutic role in selected patients.

MANAGEMENT OF ASSOCIATED BILIARY TRACT PATHOLOGY IN PATIENTS WITH PANCREATITIS

The long-term course of the patient following biliary pancreatitis is profoundly influenced by whether or not cholelithiasis is treated. Pancreatitis may recur in as many as two thirds of patients within six months of the initial attack, unless the biliary tract pathology is eradicated.[65, 72] The majority of these recurrences occur within the first six weeks following the initial attack[74, 90] and may be severe or fatal.[74, 91] However, less than 5 per cent of patients develop recurrent pancreatitis following adequate surgical therapy for the biliary tract disease.[79] Generally, the patients who develop recurrent pancreatitis following cholecystectomy and common duct exploration (if indicated) do so because of residual or recurrent common duct stones.

Since improved outcome in biliary pancreatitis is clearly associated with proper surgical management of calculous biliary tract disease, the pertinent issue is not whether a surgical procedure should be performed but whether it should be performed promptly (at the height of an acute attack) or after the patient's condition has stabilized for a few days. Corollary questions include whether or not early surgical intervention will help stabilize the acutely ill, unstable patient and whether endoscopic papillotomy is an acceptable way to decompress the common duct in the critically ill patient. Because of the high recurrence rate for pancreatitis in the six-week period following the attack, waiting for this interval of time, once popularly recommended, has largely been discarded.[82]

Most surgical authorities agree that the optimal time for surgical intervention in acute biliary pancreatitis is five to seven days after the onset of the attack, after the pancreatitis has subsided.[66, 75, 82, 91–94]

Some authors argue that surgery should be performed within 48 hours of the onset of the attack.[85, 95] Arguments for very early surgical intervention in biliary pancreatitis are based on the hypothesis that the duration of stone impaction may dictate the extent of pancreatic necrosis and that early disimpaction will favorably influence the course of the disease. There is evidence, for example, that biliary pancreatitis in humans may progress from early, edematous pancreatitis to hemorrhagic necrosis.[67] Whether all cases of pancreatic necrosis are preceded by a milder, edematous form of the disease is less clear but probable on the basis of available evidence. Acosta and co-workers suggested that prolonged stone impaction promotes pancreatic necrosis,[75] since impaction of less than 24 hours duration never caused necrosis, whereas stones impacted for 72 to 96 hours were associated with necrosis in 5 of 6 patients. Stone and associates also noted only edematous pancreatitis in patients operated on within 24 hours.[50] Further indirect evidence that pancreatitis may be mild and reversible if impaction is transient is that late complications of pancreatitis, particularly pancreatic pseudocysts and abscesses, are unusual when the patency of the pancreatic duct is restored promptly.[50, 76] However, about 85 per cent of patients with biliary pancreatitis respond promptly to the usual resuscitative measures of intravascular volume repletion, nasogastric intubation, and analgesia and improve without any additional intervention. The decreasing incidence of choledocholithiasis at surgery with respect to the time interval before surgery indicates that most patients with biliary pancreatitis and impacted stones will spontaneously disimpact and do not require immediate duct decompression.[92]

Other concerns regarding early surgery have been raised. Pancreatic fistula and abscess formation have been reported after transduodenal sphincteroplasty in the setting of acute pancreatitis,[93] and biliary tract surgery is known occasionally to cause or exacerbate pancreatitis.[96] Moreover, it is not proven that early surgery improves the outcome of biliary pancreatitis. Acosta and colleagues found that patients undergoing common duct exploration (with transduodenal sphincteroplasty if necessary) within the first 48 hours of the onset of the attack had a mortality rate of 3 per cent compared with patients operated on later, in whom the mortality rate was 16 per cent.[95] However, severity-of-illness data were not provided, so it is impossible to determine the comparability of these patient groups. Stone and co-workers randomized 70 patients to surgery within 72 hours or 3 months after recovery, with 36 of the patients comprising the early surgery group.[50] All patients underwent a transduodenal sphincteroplasty, even though impacted stones were found in only 6 per cent of the early operation group. Early operation was associated with equally low mortality (3 per cent versus 6 per cent) leading Stone to recommend this aggressive early approach. Others have raised questions regarding this approach,[85] since few of Stone's patients had impacted stones and overall mortality among his 70 patients was only 4 per cent, suggesting that this study may have been conducted in a population of patients who were not very ill. Most of these patients might have recovered without early sphincteroplasty in view of the fact that none of the patients randomized to surgery three months later failed initial nonoperative management. Several studies in fact suggest that mortality may be increased when surgical intervention occurs early. Ranson reported 23 per cent mortality in 22 patients operated on early as opposed to no mortality among 58 patients operated upon after the pancreatitis had subsided.[92] Similarly, Kelly reported a mortality rate of 12 per cent for surgery within 48 hours, versus no mortality for surgery performed after 5 to 7 days of medical therapy.[74] Both of these authors recommend the more conservative approach, based on their data, although these two studies were not randomized and the decision to operate was based on a number of factors, including clinical deterioration and lack of response to nonoperative therapy. Patient selection for operation based on these factors could result in early surgery in the sickest of the patients. This was the case in the Kelly series, in which an attempt to defer surgery was made in all patients, and early operation was undertaken only in the 14 per cent of patients who failed to improve. However, 13 of the 22 patients undergoing early surgery in Ranson's series had mild pancreatitis, according to his own well-accepted severity criteria (Table 59–3),[90] and operative mortality was not limited to those with severe disease.[92] None of the 14 patients with severe pancreatitis who underwent surgery on

TABLE 59–3. SEVERITY CRITERIA IN ACUTE PANCREATITIS

Criteria	Value
On Admission	
Age	Over 55 years
Glucose	Over 200 mg/dl
WBC	Over 16,000 mm³
LDH	Over 700 I.U.
AST	Over 250 I.U.
During First 48 Hours	
Calcium	Below 8 mg/dl
BUN	Up more than 5 mg/dl
Hematocrit	Down more than 10 percentage points
Base deficit	Over 4 mEq/l
Pa$_{O_2}$	Below 60 mmHg
Fluid sequestration	More than 6 L of crystalloid

Source: Modified from Ranson JHC, et al. Surg Gynecol Obstet 139:69, 1974. By permission of SURGERY, GYNECOLOGY, OBSTETRICS.
The presence of three or more positive criteria denotes severe pancreatitis.

a delayed basis died. It is unproven that the increased surgical mortality noted by Kelly[75] and Ranson[92] was due to the performance of surgery rather than the severity of the disease process itself. Although some data exist to show that mortality from pancreatitis is not increased by laparotomy,[97] Ranson and associates demonstrated that operation results in a two- to fourfold increase in the incidence of pancreatic abscess formation, perhaps by inoculating nonviable tissues with bacteria and thus promoting the suppurative complications associated with a high mortality.[90]

The conclusions that can be drawn from these four surgical studies are that most patients with biliary pancreatitis will improve spontaneously, that early biliary tract decompression does not improve the already excellent prognosis of mild pancreatitis, and that early surgery is hazardous in patients with severe disease.[50, 75, 92, 95] Aggressive early surgery in all patients with biliary pancreatitis would result in many patients with mild, self-limited disease undergoing common duct decompression or transduodenal sphincteroplasty when cholecystectomy (with a normal cystic duct cholangiogram—see Chap. 58) at a later time would be sufficient. On the other hand, about 15 per cent of patients with biliary pancreatitis are refractory to nonoperative supportive measures.[85] Mortality may be 50 per cent or greater in this subpopulation of patients, who account for most of the mortality in series of biliary pancreatitis. It is in this group of patients that the question of prompt biliary decompression is critical. Randomized, prospective trials of patients with objectively determined severe pancreatitis are needed to determine when and which patients should undergo prompt decompression.

Endoscopic sphincterotomy of the sphincter of Oddi has been evaluated as a way to restore patency of the ampulla without laparotomy in high-risk patients (Fig. 59–5).[89, 98] Acute pancreatitis was considered at one time to be a contraindication to ERCP because of fears of worsening the pancreatitis as a result of procedure-related ampullary edema, the injection of hypertonic contrast medium into the pancreatic duct, hemorrhage,[99] or increased risk of infection.[88, 92] These concerns have proved to be unfounded. The morbidity of papillotomy in patients with pancreatitis is no greater than that generally associated with the procedure.[76, 100] Several authors have reported that symptoms and signs of pancreatitis have subsided rapidly after endoscopic sphincterotomy.[89, 98] Safrany and Cotton reported successful extraction of stones from the common bile duct in 11 patients, 6 of whom had impacted distal stones.[89] Others have also reported successful disimpaction of stones.[98] As with conventional surgical intervention, the most aggressive possible extrapolation of this experience is that all patients with biliary pancreatitis should undergo prompt ERCP. A randomized, prospective series of 70 patients, 20 of whom had severe pancreatitis, examined this approach in comparison with nonoperative supportive measures.[76] This study failed to demonstrate a significant difference in outcome in patients wih mild pancreatitis. Even in those with severe disease, there was no advantage to urgent ERCP, although the subgroup with severe disease was too small for meaningful statistical analysis. Expansion of this study, with accrual of larger numbers of patients, confirmed the absence of significant benefit from ERCP and sphincterotomy in those patients with mild pancreatitis. However, the study showed for the first time significant reductions in complications (24 per cent versus 61 per cent), hospitalization time (9.5 days versus 17.0 days), and a trend toward reduced mortality, in patients with severe pancreatitis who underwent ERCP within 72 hours.[101] Currently, the same conclusions regarding the value of urgent duct decompression for biliary pancreatitis can be drawn for endoscopic sphincterotomy as for laparotomy. Patients with mild disease do not require decompression, because they will improve spontaneously, and subsequent deterioration, late complications, and mortality are rare.[74, 90, 92, 96]

Endoscopic decompression in patients with severe disease appears promising. At the present time, urgent ERCP should be considered for patients with severe pancreatitis suspected to be biliary, especially if the patient fails to improve during the initial 24-hour observation period. As definitive therapy, endoscopic sphincterotomy occupies a central role in patients who have had a cholecystectomy. Considerations regarding sphincterotomy with the gallbladder in situ are similar to those discussed previously for patients with cholangitis.

DISEASES OF THE SPHINCTER OF ODDI

The motor properties of the sphincter of Oddi give it an important role in the regulation of bile flow. It is generally accepted that alterations in the function of the sphincter of Oddi can produce illness. The end-point in the evaluation of patients with suspected disease of the sphincter of Oddi is the decision whether or not to ablate the sphincter by endoscopic or surgical techniques in an attempt to relieve the patient's symptoms. The major challenge in this area has been the development of criteria that reliably establish the diagnosis of sphincter of Oddi disease and predict a good response to sphincterotomy.

SPHINCTER OF ODDI FUNCTION

Manometric recordings of the sphincter of Oddi through a duodenoscope have contributed to our understanding of the function of this structure.[102] Pressure measurements are taken with a low-compliance system using a catheter with three ports near the tip separated by 2-mm intervals for separate recordings (Fig. 59–6). Basal pressure is about 15 mmHg higher than duodenal pressure and 5 mmHg higher than pressure in the common bile duct. The sphincter contracts four to five times per minute, as manifested by phasic pressure waves on manometric recordings. The direction of peristalsis can be determined by comparing

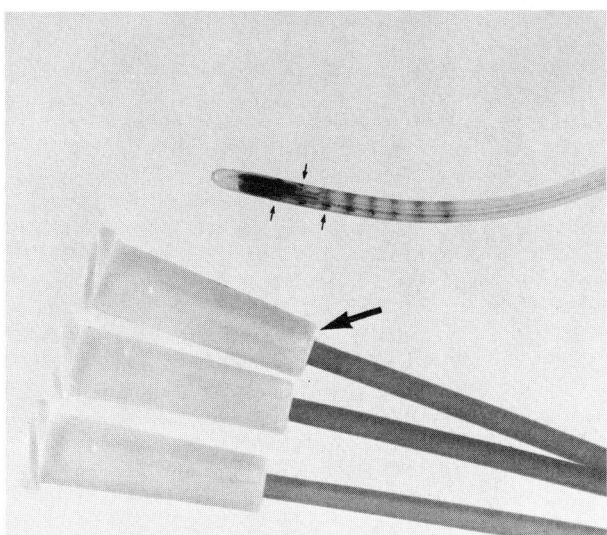

Figure 59–6. Triple-lumen catheter used for sphincter of Oddi manometry. The three distal orifices (small arrows) are 2 mm apart and attach to the manometer by individual connectors.

the timing of each contraction from each port. The majority of contractions propagate antegrade, but some simultaneous or retrograde contractions also occur.[102]

The sphincter of Oddi can be affected by at least two types of disorders. The first is fixed stenosis resulting from inflammation and fibrosis, most commonly related to prior instrumentation or the passage of stones. The pathology found in some but not all patients with suspected ampullary stenosis (inability to pass 3-mm probes through the ampulla) is inflammation and fibrosis.[103–106] The absence of histologic abnormalities in some patients, along with data from manometric studies, supports the concept that a second group of patients with sphincter of Oddi disease have a motility disorder rather than a fixed anatomic abnormality. The term sphincter of Oddi dysfunction has been proposed to describe both types of disorder.[102]

CLINICAL PRESENTATION OF SPHINCTER OF ODDI DYSFUNCTION

It has long been recognized that, following cholecystectomy, patients may complain of right upper quadrant or epigastric pain resembling their symptoms prior to surgery. It is important in all patients with the so-called postcholecystectomy syndrome to exclude such entities as peptic ulcer disease, esophageal reflux, and functional bowel disease, the latter being particularly difficult to rule out.[107] The presence of transient or constant abnormalities in liver tests lends support to a biliary origin for the patient's symptoms. Noninvasive imaging studies such as sonography or CT and endoscopic retrograde cholangiography often fail to demonstrate common duct stones or strictures. It is in such patients that interest has centered on the papilla and the sphincter of Oddi. Although the presence of the gallbladder does not preclude sphincteric disease, it is possible that the reservoir function of the gallbladder prevents pressure changes within the duct that might otherwise result in symptoms.

ASSESSMENT OF SPHINCTER OF ODDI FUNCTION

Prior to the advent of ERCP and sphincter of Oddi manometry, the morphine-prostigmine test sometimes was used in the diagnosis of sphincter dysfunction. In this test, reproduction of pain and elevations of amylase, lipase, or liver enzymes were sought after administration of these agents. Despite the initial interest in this test, several reports have questioned its accuracy.[108–111]

One of the earliest ERCP criteria proposed as a measure of papillary stenosis was the degree of difficulty in cannulating the papilla. Although individual endoscopists may find this useful on the basis of their own experience, there is no published correlation between ease of cannulation and manometric or surgical findings. Objective markers include (1) ductal dilation in the absence of stones or supraduodenal bile duct strictures and (2) persistence of contrast in the bile ducts more than 45 minutes after injection. When these findings are present in a patient with biliary pain and elevated liver enzymes on at least two occasions, sphincter of Oddi manometry almost always reveals elevated basal pressures.[102] Geenen and colleagues have designated such patients as having "definite" sphincter of Oddi dysfunction, whereas patients with one or two of the above criteria (delayed drainage, dilated ducts, abnormal liver tests) have "presumptive" dysfunction, and patients with biliary pain alone are said to have "possible" dysfunction.[102]

Several types of motility disturbances of the sphincter of Oddi have been described: (1) elevated basal pressure (30 mmHg or more above duodenal pressure), (2) paradoxical response to cholecystokinin with an elevation in sphincter pressure compared with the usual reduction, (3) predominance of retrograde contractions, and (4) *tachyoddia*, a term adopted to describe abnormally frequent sphincter of Oddi contractions (more than 10 per minute).[102, 112, 113] In a study of 32 patients with suspected sphincter of Oddi dysfunction, there were 6 patients with pain, elevated liver enzymes, and duct dilation; 4 patients with pain and enzyme elevations alone; and 22 patients with pain and duct dilatation but normal enzymes. In only seven patients sphincter of Oddi manometry was normal, but none of those seven patients met all three criteria. An excess of retrograde contractions was the most common abnormality, but the frequencies of the four types of motility disturbance were nearly equal.[112]

Biliary scintigraphy has been proposed as a noninvasive tool in the diagnosis of sphincter of Oddi dysfunction.[114–116] Studies have varied in their definition of sphincter dysfunction, but abnormalities in the rate of colloidal flow into the duodenum have been correlated with elevated sphincter pressures,[114] inability to pass a 3-mm dilator through the ampulla intraoperatively,[115] and ERCP findings of duct dilation or delayed emptying. Therefore, biliary scintigraphy may be of supplementary value in the noninvasive assessment of patients with sphincter of Oddi dysfunction.

TREATMENT OF SPHINCTER OF ODDI DYSFUNCTION

Geenen and co-workers have found that patients with "definitive" sphincter of Oddi dysfunction, as defined earlier, almost always have elevated basal sphincter pressures and have a favorable clinical response to endoscopic sphincterotomy in over 90 per cent of cases. Therefore, in these patients sphincter of Oddi manometry is not essential before sphincterotomy.[102] In contrast, nearly 40 per cent of patients with "presumptive" dysfunction had normal basal sphincter pressures. Patients with presumptive dysfunction were randomized in a blinded study to sphincterotomy versus sham

sphincterotomy. Of those with elevated basal sphincter pressures, sphincterotomy relieved pain in 91 per cent after one year compared with only 25 per cent of the patients who had the sham procedure. In contrast, of patients with normal basal sphincter pressures, true and sham sphincterotomy were associated with pain relief in 42 and 33 per cent of cases, respectively, an insignificant difference (see also Chap. 60). Patients with elevated sphincter pressures who crossed over from the sham group to true sphincterotomy at one year usually improved, and pain relief persisted for at least four years.[117] On the basis of their experience, Geenen and co-workers consider sphincter of Oddi manometry important in patients with "presumptive" dysfunction.[102, 117]

Sphincter of Oddi manometry is not widely available because of several limitations. It is a difficult technique that requires an endoscopist with a mastery of ERCP as well as additional expertise in manometry. Patients cannot be given narcotics or atropine, and glucagon must be avoided for at least ten minutes before manometric recordings are made, even if used for the preceding ERCP. Compounding these technical considerations is the failure of other groups to demonstrate that sphincter of Oddi manometry is of special value, because criteria such as dilated ducts and delayed drainage were at least as accurate in predicting a favorable response to sphincterotomy.[110, 118] Finally, despite a trend toward the performance of endoscopic sphincterotomy in these patients, endoscopic and surgical sphincterotomy have not been compared in controlled trials, nor has the role of surgical sphincterotomy combined with transampullary septectomy[105] been definitively established, even in patients with suspected sphincter of Oddi dysfunction who present with pancreatitis.

The decision to perform a sphincterotomy for biliary pain attributed to sphincter of Oddi dysfunction is best made in the patient with frequent or severe symptoms and substantial objective support (biochemical, radiographic, manometric, or any combination of these) for the diagnosis. Enthusiasm for the procedure must be tempered by experience suggesting that the morbidity and mortality are higher when sphincterotomy is performed for sphincter of Oddi dysfunction than when it is performed for choledocholithiasis.[119]

CARCINOMA OF THE EXTRAHEPATIC BILE DUCTS

Malignant neoplasms of the extrahepatic biliary tree are unusual, which is fortunate because current therapy is of limited benefit. The single most important aspect to consider both diagnostically and therapeutically is the location of the tumor, since this will dictate both the presenting symptoms and signs and the operative and postoperative management. Of all bile duct neoplasms, 20 per cent occur proximally at or near the bifurcation of the common hepatic duct, whereas about 30 per cent arise in the distal common hepatic duct or proximal common duct as defined by the location of the cystic duct. Half of the lesions develop in the distal common duct. Experience with choledochoscopy suggests that some extrahepatic bile duct carcinomas may be multicentric, a phenomenon recognized for some time with tumors of the intrahepatic ducts.[120]

Although rare in the Western Hemisphere, the large numbers of bile duct carcinomas associated with liver fluke infestation (*Clonorchis sinensis*, *Opisthorchis felineus*, and *O. viverrini*) in Asian countries makes such infestation the most common causative factor worldwide.[120] Bismuth and Malt have hypothesized that the inflammatory response to the parasites may promote secretion of carcinogens in bile. These carcinomas also have been associated with ulcerative colitis.[121] The incidence of bile duct tumors in patients with ulcerative colitis is approximately 0.4 per cent.[122] This association is further strengthened by the observation that coexistent ulcerative colitis may be present in as much as 8 per cent of patients with bile duct carcinomas (see Chap. 52).[122] Other conditions associated with the development of bile duct tumors are congenital choledochal cysts[123-125] and sclerosing cholangitis. It is unclear whether sclerosing cholangitis is a premalignant lesion or whether the usually present inflammatory bowel disease predisposes the patient to the development of both lesions.

Biliary carcinomas can present difficult diagnostic problems since the presenting symptoms may mimic benign diseases. Clinical presentations occur relatively late in the course of the disease since jaundice, the most common presenting sign, will not develop until a major duct is completely obstructed.[126] Pain from local invasion of hepatic parenchyma or rarely from distant metastases also is a late finding. All of these mechanisms make early detection difficult. Uncommonly, pruritus may precede clinical jaundice, and tender hepatomegaly may develop as obstruction progresses.[127] Fever and pain with jaundice are also unusual unless the bile duct carcinoma is associated with sclerosing cholangitis. Essentially, the diagnostic evaluation of these cases is the same as for other cases of obstructive jaundice. In addition to liver chemistries, ultrasonography should be obtained.[128] Sonography will reliably identify dilated ducts in the presence of obstruction, although occasional patients with early obstruction may present with normal-caliber ducts. Once the presence of obstruction has been established, the anatomic site and nature of the obstruction can be obtained by PTC or ERCP. ERCP also is indicated when obstructive jaundice is suspected despite normal bile ducts revealed by ultrasonography. PTC is the preferred diagnostic method when imaging studies suggest a proximal lesion, since only studies from above can determine the proximal extent of the obstruction.[127] This information is essential for surgical planning.

Preoperative information is necessary because the extrahepatic bile ducts vary considerably in length, course, and in relation to one another, making it difficult to determine the pathologic anatomy by inspection at surgery. Lessions commonly spread locally by direct extension either within the duct lumen (which may be nearly impossible to identify at laparotomy) or with extraductal involvement of surrounding organs, including liver, portal vein, hepatic artery, duodenum, and head of the pancreas. Extension of tumor through the duct wall, leading to submucosal spread and regional lymph node metastases in the porta hepatis and celiac axis occur early because of the extensive network of lymphatics in duct walls. Lymph node metastasis can be identified in 40 to 45 per cent of surgical and autopsy specimens.[129, 130] When regional metastases occur, periportal involvement is twice as likely as celiac involvement.[129] In later stages, metastases to distant peritoneal surfaces may occur in as much as 10 per cent of patients. The difficulty in managing these tumors is highlighted by observations that the entire extrahepatic biliary system may be involved diffusely with tumor in up to 15 per cent of cases,[129, 131] undoubtedly because of the propensity of these tumors to spread submucosally. There also is evidence that certain of these tumors may be multicentric in origin.[132]

Intra-abdominal metastasis by peritoneal implantation is quite common late in the disease, perhaps because more effective local palliation now allows death from metastatic disease rather than from hepatic failure from unrelieved biliary obstruction. At the time of initial exploration, however, peritoneal metastases are identified in less than 10 per cent of cases.[130, 133]

The key to therapy of malignant tumors of the bile ducts is the quality of palliation that can be achieved, since the prognosis for these tumors is poor. Besides the notorious propensity of these tumors to present late in the course of the disease, they also have a propensity for local invasion of several unresectable vital structures in the liver hilum. Long-term survivals of three or four years are unusual, seldom more than 15 per cent in reported series.[133, 134] These results might be even less favorable except for the occasional but well-recognized patient with an indolent tumor, who may survive for years even if suitable palliation cannot be achieved. Occasional reports of long-term survival of 30 per cent or more with resectable lesions at the bifurcation are seen,[135] but these cases are atypical. Lesions of the mid-common duct are associated with a comparably poor outlook. For anatomic reasons, lesions of the distal common duct are more often resectable for cure, with survival rates of 30 per cent reported.[129, 136] The vast majority of these tumors are well-differentiated adenocarcinomas, with epidermoid and mesenchymal tumors being extremely unusual. About one third are associated with fibrosis and are called scirrhous carcinomas; patients with papillary lesions may have a better prognosis.

Preoperative evaluation is critical since cholangiocarcinoma can be exceedingly difficult to identify at surgery.[120] Local lesions are usually identifiable, but the differentiation between diffuse benign (sclerosing cholangitis) and malignant lesions may be impossible at surgery. Biopsy specimens of sufficient size for adequate histopathologic assessment increase the risk of postoperative biliary fistula. In addition, malignant tumors may be so well differentiated that a diagnosis of malignancy cannot be made on frozen section. Tumors at the bifurcation of the common hepatic duct may be very difficult to identify.[137] The surgeon is aided by the knowledge that in the absence of an iatrogenic biliary stricture from prior surgery, the only two lesions that occur at the bifurcation are sclerosing cholangitis and carcinoma. If sclerosing cholangitis can be excluded by proximal cholangiography, the surgeon may then perform a hilar dissection to assess resectability. Palliative resection should be accomplished if possible, since a Roux-en-Y hepaticojejunostomy is clearly the best form of palliation, and resection may facilitate this anastomosis. If resection cannot be achieved, anastomosis to the left hepatic duct at the base of the falciform ligament is technically feasible and affords good palliation even if right-lobe drainage is completely obstructed.[138]

Lesions arising in the common duct are easier to evaluate surgically than those in the hepatic ducts. The tumor is accessible, and the dilated proximal bile duct can be visualized and dissected distally for precise definition of the point of obstruction. Resection can be accomplished if the hepatic artery and portal vein are spared by tumor; otherwise hepaticojejunostomy is performed.

Distal common duct tumors are evaluated for resection by pancreaticoduodenectomy (Whipple's procedure). It may be difficult to distinguish between pancreatic or ampullary adenocarcinoma, but the distinction is worthwhile, since resection for distal cholangiocarcinoma is justifiable even with local nodal metastases because of the relatively favorable prognosis, which contrasts sharply with the poor prognosis of pancreatic carcinoma. Thus, operative evaluation is designed to exclude hepatic metastases, or nodal metastases beyond the limits of resection, as well as the obvious contraindication to resection posed by local invasion. Unfortunately, as with tumors in all duct locations, about one half of resections with curative intent prove to be palliative resections because the presence of tumor at the margins of resection is evident on permanent section.[139]

For unresectable tumors, when suitable palliation by biliary enteric anastomosis cannot be accomplished, tube drainage in the form of intraluminal stents may be helpful. The best form of palliation of this kind appears to be the U-tube, as described by Terblanche and associates.[140] Placed at operation, these tubes emerge from the bile duct through liver parenchyma proximally and the wall of the common duct distal to the obstruction, with both ends brought through the skin. Tubes placed in this manner will not dislodge and can be changed percutaneously. The tubes usually are of 16 French caliber. They occlude from debris every 6 to 18 months, but are readily exchanged. Experience has accumulated with stents placed percutaneously or endoscopically, but these techniques have not been compared with surgical placement of U-tubes for palliation of cholangiocarcinoma.

Adjunctive measures to surgical decompression are probably of limited benefit. There has been little enthusiasm for external beam radiation therapy. Cholangiocarcinoma is radioresistant, and the limited data available show no improvement in survival after external beam therapy.[135] Newer techniques of transcatheter irradiation and intraoperative radiation are causing a reassessment of radiation therapy. The results of transcatheter irradiation are preliminary but do offer some encouragement. Generally, the best results (temporary reduction in tumor size in up to 80 per cent of patients) are achieved when 2000 to 2500 rad is given by external beam, followed in three to five weeks by transcatheter boost techniques with [192][Ir] iridium.[141] The liver parenchyma and bile ducts develop fibrosis at radiation doses in excess of 3000 rad[142] so that prolonged stenting, even with successful palliation, is essential. Despite these possible advances, firm evidence of improved survival is lacking. Cholangiocarcinoma is minimally responsive to chemotherapy as well. Based on very limited experience, mitomycin-C appears to be the best single agent, with a partial response rate of 30 to 40 per cent, either alone or in combination with 5-fluorouracil and doxorubicin (Adriamycin).[135, 143, 144]

BILIARY CYSTS AND BILE DUCT NEOPLASIA

Cysts of the biliary tract (see also Chapter 52) are generally considered to be congenital, although data suggest that a small percentage of bile duct cysts may be acquired.[145] The origin of malformations of the bile ducts resulting in cystic dilation is obscure, and symptoms from these lesions are dependent on the degree to which the cysts are in direct continuity with the biliary system. Since dilation of the major extrahepatic or intrahepatic bile ducts has been described in conjunction with lesions involving only the terminal intralobular ducts (congenital hepatic fibrosis) or noncommunicating parenchymal cysts (polycystic liver disease), it is possible that all of these lesions may share a common causality.

Morphologic variants of choledochal cyst can be identified throughout the entire length of the biliary tree.[146] Saccular (in children) or fusiform dilation of the entire extrahepatic biliary system (Alonso Lej type I) is by far the most common variant, representing about 95 per cent of cases. The fusiform variant in adults is associated commonly with choledocholithiasis. Saccular dilations projecting from the side of the common bile duct (Alonso Lej type II) are uncommon, representing about 4 per cent of cases. Choledochocele, a rare variant consisting of localized dilation of the intrapancreatic common duct, accounts for the remainder of cases (Alonso Lej type III). About 25 per cent of these patients also have a variable degree of cystic dilation of their intrahepatic ducts.

An anomalous junction between the pancreatic and bile ducts above the level of the papilla of Vater has been found in a large number of patients with choledochal cysts.[147–149] A popular concept is that pancreatic juice, free from the regulatory effects of the sphincter mechanisms normally present within the ampulla of Vater, refluxes freely into the bile duct, leading to chronic inflammation and eventual cystic dilation. High amylase levels observed in the cystic fluid are consistent with this hypothesis.[150] Also consistent is that intraoperative biliary manometry in a group of children with choledochal cysts failed to demonstrate a high pressure zone analogous to that within the sphincter of Oddi in the area of the pancreaticobiliary junction.[150] Long-standing damage from pancreatic reflux may ultimately result in malignant transformation of the biliary epithelium, accounting for the high incidence of adenocarcinoma within choledochal cysts.

Caroli's disease consists of multiple congenital saccular dilations of the intrahepatic bile ducts. Since it is now recognized that dilation of intrahepatic radicals may accompany cystic disease of the extrahepatic biliary system, the designation of Caroli's disease should be reserved for patients with cystic disease confined to the intrahepatic system.

Patients with choledochal cysts usually present with intermittent symptoms that include fever, abdominal pain, vomiting, and jaundice. A mass in the right upper quadrant may be palpable; this is more common in children.[149] Some patients present with symptoms suggestive of pancreatitis accompanied by hyperamylasemia.[151] Variceal hemorrhage has been reported in patients with secondary biliary cirrhosis.[151]

Surgical decompression of choledochal cysts is important for a number of reasons. Patients with untreated disease will experience recurrent attacks of biliary tract sepsis, even when these anomalies have been asymptomatic throughout childhood and adolescence. At operation, the connection between the pancreatic and bile ducts must be severed to prevent continued reflux of pancreatic fluid into the bile duct. If possible, cystic malformations should be resected because of the increased risk of cholangiocarcinoma. Some investigators have considered this a weak association, since choledochal cysts are rare and cholangiocarcinoma does not usually develop. However, there is a twentyfold increased incidence of cholangiocarcinoma in patients with choledochal cysts compared with the general population, and concern is justified.[124] Primary resection is not always feasible, usually as a result of either the extent of the abnormality or, more likely, the intensive inflammatory reaction between the cyst and surrounding structures. It may be necessary to resort to a drainage procedure in the presence of portal hypertension as well. If primary excision cannot be accomplished, Roux-en-Y choledochojejunostomy with cholecystectomy is the treatment of choice. Since primary excision also usually requires Roux-en-Y reconstruction of the biliary tract, long-term complications related to the reconstruction may occur in both groups. The complications include recurrent cholangitis, anastomotic stricture, progression of residual biliary tract disease, and occasional symptomatic fat malabsorption. Surgically treatable Caroli's disease may occur with abdominal pain and fever at any time after birth, but the average age at manifestation is 22 years. Cholelithiasis, cholangitis, and liver abscess formation are common manifestations. Surgical removal of stones and drainage of infected bile can afford temporary palliation, but definitive control usually is impossible because of the multiple intrahepatic dilations and strictures. Rarely, Caroli's disease may be confined to the left lobe of the liver, allowing for significant palliation by left hepatic lobectomy.[123-125]

PRIMARY SCLEROSING CHOLANGITIS

This disease is characterized by chronic fibrosing inflammation of the bile ducts that usually affects both the extrahepatic and intrahepatic ducts.[152] It is associated in nearly 75 per cent of cases with ulcerative colitis. The term *primary* is used to distinguish this disease from the biliary strictures that may result from operative injury or choledocholithiasis.

Since the advent of endoscopic retrograde cholangiography, recognition of this disorder has increased. It now appears likely that "pericholangitis" associated with ulcerative colitis is actually the intrahepatic histologic expression of sclerosing cholangitis.[153] Sclerosing cholangitis in fact is the commonest form of hepatobiliary disease associated with ulcerative colitis. Sclerosing cholangitis is, on the other hand, unusual in patients with Crohn's disease, including Crohn's colitis.[153, 154]

The disease is most prevalent in persons under 50 years of age, with a male to female ratio of about 3:1.[152] The diagnosis is being made increasingly in patients with ulcerative colitis and asymptomatic elevations of serum alkaline phosphatase. The earliest symptoms are pruritus and fatigue. Acute cholangitis is said to be unusual in some studies[152] but was a presenting feature in 45 per cent of the patients treated at the Royal Free Hospital.[155]

The most consistent biochemical feature is an elevated alkaline phosphatase, although this is not invariable;[156] modest aminotransferase elevations are present in most patients. Hyperbilirubinemia frequently is noted at the time of presentation. No autoantibodies are found consistently.

At present, the diagnosis usually is made by ERCP, which reveals diffusely distributed strictures often producing a "beaded" appearance to the bile ducts. In the Mayo Clinic series, both intra- and extrahepatic duct involvement was nearly universal; the authors believe that involvement of intrahepatic ducts alone is not a distinct clinical variant but an early stage in the evolution of the disease.[152] Involvement of the pancreatic duct has been noted in 8 to 50 per cent of patients.[157, 158] Clincally or radiographically significant gallbladder involvement is unusual, but edema, inflammation, and fibrosis have been described, and papillary hyperplasia of the gallbladder mucosa appears to be frequent.[159] The common histologic abnormalities in the liver include portal inflammation and bile duct proliferation, diminished bile ducts, periductal fibrosis, piecemeal necrosis, and Kupffer cell hyperplasia.[155] Hepatic copper stores are nearly always elevated, with the degree of elevation related to the duration of the disease.[160] However, a pathogenic role for copper in the progression of this disease has not been demonstrated.

Primary sclerosing cholangitis is a progressive disease that culminates in death from cirrhosis and portal hypertension. However, the course in any individual patient is unpredictable, and long periods of stability can occur.

No medical therapy has a proven effect on the course of this disease, despite anecdotal reports involving corticosteriods and immunosuppressive agents.[152] Because of the copper overload that occurs, penicillamine was administered in a randomized trial; despite effective copper mobilization, no favorable effect on disease progression or survival was seen.[161] Low-dose methotrexate treatment resulted in dramatic improvement in two patients, leading Kaplan and co-workers to initiate a prospective, randomized trial.[162] Proctocolectomy in patients with ulcerative colitis has not improved the outcome or delayed progression of the biliary tract disease. Biliary surgery is possible only in limited circumstances but is occasionally performed when a biliary enteric (usually by Roux-en-Y) anastomosis proximal to a dominant stricture appears likely to improve biliary drainage. Cameron and associates reported improvement in jaundice after resection of the hepatic bifurcation, bilateral dilation and stenting of the hepatic ducts, and bilateral hepaticojejunostomies.[163] With the advent of liver transplantation, however, there has been a trend toward the avoidance of palliative surgical procedures that might make subsequent hepatic transplantation difficult or impossible, especially in younger patients.[164]

REFERENCES

1. Scharschmidt BF, Goldberg HI, Schmid R. Current concepts in diagnosis: approach to the patient with cholestatic jaundice. N Engl J Med 308:1515, 1983.
2. Matzen P, Malchow-Miller A, Brun B, et al. Ultrasonography, computed tomography and cholescintigraphy in suspected obstructive jaundice—a prospective comparative study. Gastroenterology 84:1492, 1983.
3. Goldberg HI, Filly RA, Korolkin M, et al. Capability of CT body scanning and ultrasonography to demonstrate the status of the biliary ductal system in patients with jaundice. Radiology 129:731, 1978.
4. Martin WB, Apostolakos PC, Roazen H. Clinical versus actuarial prediction in the differential diagnosis of jaundice. A study of the relative accuracy of predictions made by clinicians and by a statistically derived formula in differentiating parenchymal and obstructive jaundice. Am J Med Sci 240:571, 1960.
5. Baron RL, Pedrosa CS, Casanova R, et al. Computed tomography in obstructive jaundice. Part I. The level of obstruction. Radiology 139:627, 1981.
6. Pedrosa CS, Casanova R, Lezana AH, et al. Computed tomography in obstructive jaundice. Part II. The cause of obstruction. Radiology 139:635, 1981.
7. Baron RL, Stanley RJ, Lee JKT, et al. A prospective comparison of biliary obstruction using computed tomography and ultrasonography. Radiology 145:91, 1982.
8. Cronan JJ, Mueller PR, Simeone JF, et al. Prospective diagnosis of choledocholithiasis. Radiology 146:467, 1983.
9. Laing F, Jeffrey RB Jr, Wing VW. Improved visualization of choledocholithiasis by sonography. Am J Roentgenol 143:949, 1984.
10. Laing FC, Jeffrey RB Jr. Choledocholithiasis and cystic duct obstruction: difficult ultrasonographic diagnosis. Radiology 146:475, 1983.
11. Baron RL, Stanley RJ, Lee JKT, et al. Computed tomographic findings of biliary obstruction. Radiology 140:1673, 1983.
12. Jeffrey RB, Federle MP, Laing FC, et al. Computed tomography of choledocholithiasis. Radiology 140:1179, 1983.
13. Lintott DJ. Percutaneous transhepatic cholangiography. Clin Gastroenterol 14:373, 1985.
14. Cotton PB. Direct choledochography and related diagnostic methods. Part I. Direct choledochoscopy. Clin Gastrenterol 12:101, 1983.
15. Matzen P, Malchow-Moller A, Lejerstofte J, et al. Endoscopic retrograde cholangiography in patients with obstructive jaundice: a randomized study. Scand J Gastroenterol 17:731, 1982.
16. Speer AG, Cotton PB, Dineen LP. Endoscopic shunts in malignant hilar strictures—results in 70 patients. Gastrointest Endosc 32:156, 1986.

17. Stoker J, Dees J, Blankenstein M, et al. Results of endoscopic stenting in malignant stricture of the biliary tract. Gut 26:A1135, 1985.
18. Glenn F. Choledochotomy in non-malignant disease of the biliary tract. Surg Gynecol Obstet 124:974, 1967.
19. Bernhoft RA, Pellegrini CA, Motson RW, et al. Composition and morphological and clinical features of common duct stones. Am J Surg 148:77, 1984.
20. Maki T, Matsushiro T, Suzuki N. Clarification of the nomenclature of pigment gallstones. Am J Surg 14:302, 1982.
21. Ostrow JD. Bilirubin solubility and the etiology of pigment gallstones. In: Okuda A, Nakayama F, Wong J, eds. Intrahepatic Calculi. New York, Alan R. Liss, 1984:53.
22. Suzuki N, Takahashi W, Sato T. Types and chemical composition of intrahepatic stones. In: Okuda A, Nakayama F, Wong J, eds. Intrahepatic Calculi. New York, Alan R. Liss, 1984:71.
23. Tabata M, Nakayama F. Bacteria and gallstones—etiological significance. Dig Dis Sci 26:218, 1981.
24. Way LA, Malet PF, Huang G, et al. The postcholestectomy interval influences the composition of common bile duct gallstones. Hepatology 2:743, 1982.
25. Neoptolemos JP, Hoffman AF, Moussa AF. Chemical composition of stones in the biliary tree. Br J Surg 73:515, 1986.
26. Pitt HA, Cameron JL. Acute cholangitis. In: Way LW, Pellegrini CA, eds. Surgery of the Gallbladder and Bile Ducts. Philadelphia, WB Saunders, 1987:295.
27. Way LW, Bernhoft RA, Thomas MJ. Biliary stricture. Surg Clin North Am 61:963, 1981.
28. Blumgart LH, Carachi R, Imrie CW. Diagnosis and management of post cholecystectomy symptoms: the place of endoscopy and retrograde choledochopancreatography. Br J Surg 64:809, 1977.
29. Edlund YA, Moustedt BO, Ouchterlong O. Bacteriological investigation of the biliary system and liver in biliary tract disease correlated to clinical data and microstructure of the gallbladder and liver. Acta Chir Scand 46:461, 1959.
30. Flemma RJ, Flint IM, Osterhout S, et al. Bacteriologic studies of biliary tract infection. Ann Surg 166:563, 1967.
31. Keighley MRB, Flinn R, Alexander-Williams J. Multivariant analysis of clinical and operative findings associated with biliary sepsis. Br J Surg 63:528, 1976.
32. O'Connor MJ, Schwartz ML, McQuarrie DG, et al. Cholangitis due to malignant obstruction to biliary outflow. Ann Surg 193:341, 1981.
33. Dineen P. The importance of the route of infection in experimental biliary obstruction. Surg Gynecol Obstet 119:1001, 1964.
34. Ong GB. A study of recurrent pyogenic cholangitis. Arch Surg 84:63, 1962.
35. Scott AJ, Kahn GA. Origin of bacteria in common duct bile. Lancet 2:790, 1967.
36. Charcot JM. Lecons sur les maladies du foie des voies biliaires et des veins. Paris. Faculte de Médecine de Paris. Recueillies et publiées par Bouneville et Sénestre, 1877.
37. Saharia PC, Cameron JL. Clinical management of cholangitis. Surg Gynecol Obstet 142:369, 1976.
38. Raine PAM, Gunn AA. Acute choleystitis. Br J Surg 62:697, 1975.
39. Reynolds BM, Dargan EL. Acute obstructive cholangitis. A distinct clinical syndrome. Ann Surg 150:299, 1959.
40. Boey JH, Way LW. Acute cholangitis. Ann Surg 191:264, 1980.
41. Andrew DJ, Johnson SE. Acute suppurative cholangitis. A medical and surgical emergency. Am J Gastroenterol 54:141, 1970.
42. Pitt HA, Postier RG, Cameron JL. Consequences of preoperative cholangitis and its treatment on the outcome of surgery for choledocholithiasis. Surgery 94:447, 1983.
43. Rosenthal L, Shaffer ER, Lisboner R, et al. Diagnosis of hepatobiliary disease by 99mTc Hida cholescintigraphy. Radiology 126:467, 1978.
44. Saik RP, Greenburg AG, Farris JM, et al. Spectrum of cholangitis. Am J Surg 130:143, 1975.
45. Jones WG, Barie PS. Enterococcal infections in surgical patients. Influence of enterococci on mortality from bacteremia and the role of antienterococcal therapy. Infect Surg. (In press.)
46. Davis JL, Milligan FD, Cameron JL. Septic complications following endoscopic retrograde cholangiopancreatography. Surg Gynecol Obstet 140:365, 1975.
47. Johnson AG, Rains AJH. Prevention and treatment of recurrent bile duct stones by choledochoduodenostomy. World J Surg 2:487, 1978.
48. DeAlmeida AM, Cruz AG, Aldeia FJ. Side-to-side choledochoduodenostomy in the management of choledocholithiasis and associated disease. Facts and fiction. Am J Surg 147:253, 1984.
49. Kraus MA, Wilson SD. Choledochoduodenostomy. Importance of common duct size and occurrence of cholangitis. Arch Surg 115:1212, 1978.
50. Stone HH, Fabian TC, Dunlop WE. Gallstone pancreatitis: biliary pathology in relation to time of operation. Ann Surg 194:305, 1981.
51. Glenn F, Moody FC. Acute obstructive suppurative cholangitis. Surg Gynecol Obstet 113:265, 1961.
52. Leese T, Neptolemos JP, Barer AR, et al. Management of acute cholangitis and the impact of endoscopic sphincterotomy. Br J Surg 73:988, 1986.
53. Siegel JH, Ramsey WH, Pillano W. Endoscopic management of 947 patients with cholangitis—proven safety and efficacy. Gastrointest Endosc 32:154, 1986.
54. Escourrou J, Cordova JA, Lagorthes F, et al. Early and late complications after endoscopic sphincterotomy for biliary lithiasis with and without gallbladder "in situ." Gut 25:598, 1984.
55. Neoptolemos JP, Carr-Locke DL, Fraser I, et al. The management of common bile duct calculi by endoscopic sphincterotomy in patients with gallbladder in situ. Br J Surg 71:69, 1984.
56. Cook J, Hou PC, Ho HC, et al. Recurrent pyogenic cholangitis. Br J Surg 42:188, 1954.
57. Chou ST, Chan CW. Recurrent pyogenic cholangitis: a necropsy study. Pathology 12:415, 1980.
58. Matsumoto M, Fujii H, Yoshioku M, et al. Biliary strictures as a cause of primary intrahepatic bile duct stones. World J Surg 10:867, 1986.
59. Teoh TB. A study of gallstones and included worms in recurrent pyogenic cholangitis. J Pathol Bacteriol 86:123, 1963.
60. Ong GB, Adisehiah M, Leong CH. Acute pancreatitis associated with recurrent pyogenic cholangitis. Br J Surg 58:891, 1971.
61. Lai KS, McFadzean AJS, Yeung R. Microembolic pulmonary hypertension in pyogenic cholangitis. Br Med J 1:22, 1968.
62. Choi TK, Wong J, Lau KH, et al. Late result of sphincteroplasty in the treatment of primary cholangitis. Arch Surg 116:1173, 1981.
63. Choi TK, Wong J, Ong GB. Choledochojejunostomy in the treatment of primary cholangitis. Surg Gynecol Obstet 155:43, 1982.
64. Choi TK, Wong J, Ong GB. The surgical management of primary intrahepatic stones. Br J Surg 69:86, 1982.
65. Frey CF. Gallstone pancreatitis. Surg Clin North Am 61:923, 1981.
66. Martin JK, Van Heerden JA, Bess MA. Surgical management of acute pancreatitis. Mayo Clin Proc 59:259, 1984.
67. Becker V. Pathological anatomy and pathogenesis of acute pancreatitis. World J Surg 5:303, 1981.
68. Mercadier M. Surgical treatment of acute pancreatitis: tactics, techniques, and results. World J Surg 5:393, 1981.
69. Opie EL. The relationships of cholelithiasis to disease of the pancreas and fat necrosis. Johns Hopkins Hosp Bull XII 118:19, 1901.
70. Steer ML, Meldolesi J. The cell biology of experimental pancreatitis. N Engl J Med 316:144, 1987.
71. Acosta JM, Ledesma CL. Gallstone migration as a cause of acute pancreatitis. N Engl J Med 290:484, 1974.
72. Kelly TR. Gallstone pancreatitis. Arch Surg 109:294, 1974.
73. Armstrong CP, Taylor TV, Jeajock J, et al. The biliary tract in patients with acute gallstone pancreatitis. Br J Surg 72:551, 1985.
74. Kelly TR. Gallstone pancreatitis. The timing of surgery. Surgery 88:345, 1980.
75. Acosta JM, Pellegrini CA, Skinner DB. Etiology and pathogenesis of acute biliary pancreatitis. Surgery 88:118, 1980.
76. Neoptolemos JP, London N, Slater ND, et al. A prospective study of ERCP and endoscopic sphincterotomy in the diagnosis and treatment of gallstone acute pancreatitis. Arch Surg 121:697, 1986.
77. Houssin D, Castain D, Lemoine J, et al. Microlithiasis of the gallbladder. Surg Gynecol Obstet 157:20, 1983.
78. McMahon MJ, Shefta JR. Physical characteristics of gallstones and the calibre of the cystic duct in patients with acute pancreatitis. Br J Surg 67:6, 1980.
79. Kelly TR, Swaney PE. Gallstone pancreatitis: the second time around. Surgery 92:577, 1982.
80. Guelrud M, Mendoza S, Vicent S, et al. Pressures in the sphincter of Oddi in patients with gallstones, common duct stones, and recurrent pancreatitis. J Clin Gastroenterol 5:37, 1983.
81. Cuschieri A, Cumming JGR, Wood RAB, et al. Evidence for sphincter dysfunction in patients with gallstone-associated pancreatitis: effect of ceruletide in patients undergoing cholecystectomy for gallbladder disease and gallstone-associated pancreas. Br J Surg 71:885, 1984.
82. Warshaw AL, Richter JM. A practical approach to pancreatitis. Curr Probl Surg 21:1, 1984.
83. Blamey SL, Osborne DH, Gilmour WH, et al. The early identification of patients with gallstone pancreatitis using clinical and biochemical factors only. Ann Surg 198:574, 1983.
84. Neoptolemos JP, Hall JW, Finlay DF, et al. The urgent diagnosis of gallstones in acute pancreatitis: a prospective study of three methods. Br J Surg 71:230, 1984.
85. Pelligrini CA. Biliary pancreatitis. In: Way LW, Pelligrini CF, eds. Surgery of the Gallbladder and Bile Ducts. Philadelphia, WB Saunders, 1987:315.
86. Ranson JHC, Balthasar E, Caccavale R, et al. Computed tomography and the prediction of pancreatic abscess in acute pancreatitis. Ann Surg 201:656, 1985.

87. Mackie CR, Wood AB, Preece PE, et al. Surgical pathology at early elective operation for suspected acute gallstone pancreatitis: preliminary report of a prospective clinical trial. Br J Surg 72:179, 1985.

88. Coppa GF, Le Fleur R, Ranson JHC. The role of Chiba-needle cholangiography in the diagnosis of possible acute pancreatitis with cholelithiasis. Ann Surg 193:393, 1981.

89. Safrany L, Cotton PB. A preliminary report: urgent duodenoscopic sphincterotomy for acute gallstone pancreatitis. Surgery 89:424, 1981.

90. Ranson JHC, Rifkin RM, Roses DF, et al. Prognostic signs and the role of operative management in acute pancreatitis. Surg Gynecol Obstet 139:69, 1974.

91. Mayer AD, McMahon MJ, Benson EA, et al. Operation upon the biliary tract in patients with acute pancreatitis: aims, indications and timing. Ann R Coll Surg Engl 66:179, 1984.

92. Ranson JHC. The timing of biliary surgery in acute pancreatitis. Ann Surg 189:654, 1979.

93. Welch JP, White CE. Acute pancreatitis of biliary origin: is urgent operation necessary? Am J Surg 143:120, 1982.

94. Glenn F, Frey C. Re-evaluation of the treatment of pancreatitis associated with biliary tract disease. Ann Surg 160:723, 1964.

95. Acosta JM, Rossi R, Galli MR, et al. Early surgery for acute gallstone pancreatitis: evaluation of a systematic approach. Surgery 83:367, 1978.

96. Ranson JHC. Acute pancreatitis. In: Schwartz SI, Ellis H, eds. Maingot's Abdominal Operations. Norwalk, Conn.: Appleton-Century-Crofts, 1985:2061.

97. Trapnell JE, Anderson MC. Role of early laparotomy in acute pancreatitis. Ann Surg 165:49, 1967.

98. Rosseland AR, Solhaug JH. Early or delayed endoscopic papillotomy in gallstone pancreatitis. Ann Surg 199:165, 1984.

99. Roesch W, Demling L. Endoscopic management of pancreatitis. Surg Clin North Am 61:923, 1981.

100. Neoptolemos JP, Harvey MH, Slate ND, et al. Abdominal wall bile staining and "biliscrotum" after retroperitoneal perforation following endoscopic sphincterotomy. Br J Surg 71:684, 1984.

101. Neoptolemos JP, Carr-Locke DL, London NJ, et al. Controlled trial of urgent endoscopic retrograde cholangiopancreatography and endoscopic sphincterotomy versus conservative treatment for acute pancreatitis due to gallstones. Lancet 2:979, 1986.

102. Geenen J, Hogan W, Dodds WJ. Sphincter of Oddi. In: Sivak MV Jr, ed. Gastroenterologic Endoscopy. Philadelphia, WB Saunders, 1987:735.

103. Acosta JM, Cavantos F, Nardi GL, et al. Fibrosis of the papilla of Vater. Surg Gynecol Obstet 124:787, 1987.

104. Gage TB, Lober PH, Imanoglu K, et al. Stenosis of the sphincter of Oddi: a clinical review of 50 cases. Surgery 48:304, 1960.

105. Moody FG, Becker JM, Potts JR. Transduodenal sphincteroplasty and transampullary septectomy for post cholecystectomy pain. Ann Surg 197:627, 1983.

106. Moody FG, Berenson MM, McClosky D. Transampullary septectomy for postcholecystectomy pain. Ann Surg 186:415, 1977.

107. Moody FG. The postcholecystectomy syndrome. In Moody FG, Carey LC, Johns RS, et al. Surgical Treatment of Digestive Disease. Chicago, Year Book Medical Publishers, 1986:296.

108. Aronchik CA, Long WB, Soloway RD. Endoscopic biliary manometry and a modified morphine-prostigmine test as predictors of clinical response in biliary dyskinesia. Gastrointest Endosc 30:140, 1984. (Abstract.)

109. LoGuidice JA, Geenen JE, Hogan WJ, et al. Efficacy of the morphine-prostigmine test for evaluating patients with suspected biliary stenosis. Dig Dis Sci 24:455, 1979.

110. Roberts-Thompson IC, Toouli J. Is endoscopic sphincterotomy for disabling biliary-type pain after cholecystectomy effective? Gastrointest Endosc 31:370, 1985.

111. Steinberg WM, Salvato RF, Toskes PP. The morphine-prostigmine provocative test—is it useful for making clinical decisions? Gastroenterology 78:728, 1980.

112. Toouli J, Roberts-Thomson K, Dent J, Lee J. Manometric disorders in patients with suspected sphincter of Oddi dysfunction. Gastroenterology 88:1243, 1985.

113. Venu RP, Geenen JE. Diagnosis and treatment of diseases of the papilla. Clin Gastroenterol 15:439, 1986.

114. Lee RGL, Gregg JA, Koroshetz AM. Sphincter of Oddi stenosis: diagnosis using hepatobiliary scintigraphy and endoscopic manometry. Radiology 156:793, 1985.

115. Shaffer EA, Hershfield NB, Logan K, et al. Cholescintigraphic detection of the sphincter of Oddi: effect of papillotomy. Gastroenterology 90:726, 1986.

116. Zeman RK, Burrell MI, Dobbins J, et al. Postcholecystectomy syndrome: evaluation using biliary scintigraphy and endoscopic retrograde cholangiopancreatography. Radiology 156:787, 1985.

117. Geenen JE, Hogan WJ, Dodds WJ, et al. The efficacy of endoscopic sphincterotomy after cholecystectomy in patients with sphincter-of-Oddi dysfunction. N Engl J Med 320:82, 1989.

118. Thatcher BS, Sivak MV Jr, Tedesco FJ, et al. Endoscopic sphincterotomy for suspected dysfunction of the sphincter of Oddi. Gastrointest Endosc 33:91, 1987.

119. Classen M. Endoscopic papillotomy—new indications, short- and long-term results. Clin Gastroenterol 15:457, 1986.

120. Bismuth H, Malt RA. Carcinoma of the biliary tract. N Engl J Med 301:704, 1979.

121. Levin B, Riddell RH, Kissner JB. Management of precancerous lesions of the gastroentestinal tract. Clin Gastroenterol 5:827, 1976.

122. Ross AP, Braasch JW. Ulcerative colitis and carcinoma of the proximal bile duct. Gut 14:94, 1973.

123. Dayton MT, Longmire WP Jr, Tompkins RK. Caroli's disease: a premalignant condition? Am J Surg 145:41, 1983.

124. Todani T, Watanabe Y, Narusue M, et al. Congenital bile duct cysts: classification, operative procedures, and review of 37 cases including cancer arising from choledochal cysts. Am J Surg 134:263, 1977.

125. Tsuchiya R, Harada N, Ito T, et al. Malignant tumors in choledochal cysts. Ann Surg 186:22, 1977.

126. Wanebo HJ, Grunes OF. Cancer of the bile duct. The occult malignancy. Am J Surg 130:262, 1975.

127. Mercadier M. Carcinoma of the bile duct. In: Way LW, Pellegrini CA, eds. Surgery of the Gallbladder and Bile Ducts. Philadelphia, WB Saunders, 1987:487.

128. Subramanyam BR, Raghaventira BN, Balthazar EJ, et al. Ultrasonic features of cholangiocarcinoma. J Ultrasound Med 3:405, 1984.

129. Warren KW, Choe DS, Plaza J, Pelihan M. Results of radical resection for periampullary cancer. Ann Surg 181:534, 1975.

130. Kopelson G, Harisiadis L, Tretter P. The role of radiation therapy in cancer of the extrahepatic biliary system: an analysis of thirteen patients and review of the literature of the effectiveness of surgery, chemotherapy and radiotherapy. Int J Radiat Oncol Biol Phys 2:883, 1977.

131. Braasch JW, Warren KW, Kune GA. Malignant neoplasms of the bile ducts. Surg Clin North Am 47:627, 1967.

132. Tompkins RK, Johnson J, Storm FK. Operative endoscopy in the management of biliary neoplasms. Am J Surg 132:174, 1976.

133. Warren KW, Mountain JD, Lloyd-Jones W. Malignant tumors of the bile ducts. Br J Surg 59:501, 1972.

134. Longmire WP, McArthur MS, Bastomis EA, Hiolt J. Carcinoma of the extrahepatic biliary tract. Ann Surg 178:333, 1973.

135. Cady BS, MacDonald JS, Gunderson LL. Cancer of the hepatobiliary system. In: DeVita VT, Hellman S, Rosenberg SA, eds. Cancer: Principles and Practice of Oncology. Philadelphia, JB Lippincott, 1985:741.

136. Aston SJ, Longmire WP. Pancreaticoduodenal resection. Arch Surg 106:813, 1973.

137. Klatskin G. Adenocarcinoma of the hepatic duct at its bifurcation within the porta hepatis. An unusual tumor with distinctive clinical and pathological features. Am J Med 38:241, 1965.

138. Dudley SE, Adson MA. Biliary decompression in hilar obstruction. Arch Surg 114:579, 1979.

139. Iwaski Y, Ohto M, Todoroki T, et al. Treatment of carcinoma of the biliary system. Surg Gynecol Obstet 144:219, 1977.

140. Terblanche J, Saunders SJ, Louw JH. Prolonged palliation in carcinoma of the main hepatic duct junction. Surgery 71:720, 1972.

141. Herskovic A, Heaston D, Engler MJ, et al. Irradiation of biliary carcinomas. Radiology 131:219, 1981.

142. Todorki T, Iwasaki Y, Okamura T, et al. Intraoperative radiotherapy for advanced carcinoma of the biliary system. Cancer 46:2179, 1980.

143. Falkson G, MacIntyre JM, Moertel CG. Eastern Cooperative Oncology Group experience with chemotherapy for inoperable gallbladder and bile duct cancer. Cancer 54:965, 1984.

144. Smith GW, Bukowski RM, Hewlett JS, et al. Hepatic artery infusion of 5-fluorouracil and mitomycin-C in cholangiocarcinoma and gallbladder carcinoma. Cancer 54:1513, 1984.

145. Flanigan DF. Biliary cysts. Ann Surg 182:635, 1975.

146. Alonso-Lej F, Rever WB, Persagno DJ. Congenital choledochal cyst, with a report of two and an analysis of 94 cases. Surg Gynecol Obstet Intl Abstr Surg 108:1, 1959.

147. Jonas JZ, Babbitt DP, Starshak RJ, et al. Anatomic observations and etiologies and surgical considerations in choledochal cyst. J Pediatr Surg 14:315, 1979.

148. Okada A, Oguchi Y, Kamata S, et al. Common channel syndrome-diagnosis with endoscopic retrograde cholangiopancreatography and surgical management. Surgery 93:634, 1983.

149. Ono J, Sakoda K, Akita H. Surgical aspects of cystic dilatation of the bile duct. Ann Surg 195:203, 1982.

150. Iwai N, Tokiwa K, Tsuto T, et al. Biliary manometry in choledochal cyst with abdominal choledochopancreatico ductal junction. J Pediatr Surg 21:873, 1986.

151. Nagorney DM, McIlrath DC, Adson MA. Choledochal cysts in adults: clinical management. Surgery 96:656, 1984.
152. La Russo DF, Wiesner RH, Ludwig J, et al. Primary sclerosing cholangitis. N Engl J Med 310:899, 1984.
153. Wee A, Ludwig J. Pericholangitis in chronic ulcerative colitis: primary sclerosing cholangitis of the bile ducts? Ann Intern Med 102:581, 1985.
154. Dew MJ, Thompson H, Allain RN. The spectrum of hepatic dysfunction in inflammatory bowel disease. Q J Med 48:113, 1979.
155. Chapman RWG, Marborgh BA, Rhodes JM, et al. Primary sclerosing cholangitis: a review of its clinical features, cholangiography and hepatic histology. Gut 21:870, 1980.
156. Wiesner RH, LaRusso NF. Primary sclerosing cholangitis with normal levels of serum alkaline phosphatase. Hepatology 5:1053, 1985. (Abstract.)
157. MacCarty RL, LaRusso NF, Wiesner RH, et al. Primary sclerosing cholangitis: findings on cholangiography and pancreatography. Radiology 149:39, 1983.
158. Muller EL, Miyamoto T, Pitt HA, et al. Anatomy of the choledocho-pancreatic duct junction in primary sclerosing cholangitis. Surgery 97:21, 1985.
159. Lefkowitch JH. Primary sclerosing cholangitis. Arch Intern Med 142:1157, 1982.
160. Gross JB Jr, Ludwig J, Wiesner RH, et al. Abnormalities in tests of copper metabolism in primary sclerosing cholangitis. Gastroenterology 89:272, 1985.
161. LaRusso N, Wiesner R, Ludwig J, et al. Randomized trial of penicillamine in primary sclerosing cholangitis. Hepatology 6:1205, 1986.
162. Kaplan MM, Arona S, Pincus SH. Primary sclerosing cholangitis and low-dose oral pulse methotrexate therapy: clinical and histologic response. Ann Intern Med 106:231, 1987.
163. Cameron JL, Gayler BW, Herlong HF, et al. Biliary reconstruction with Silastic transhepatic stents. Surgery 94:324, 1983.
164. National Institutes of Health Consensus Development Conference Statement: Liver Transplantation. June 20–23, 1983. Hepatology 4:107S, 1984.

60

Nonsurgical Treatment of Biliary Tract Disease

Ira M. Jacobson, M.D.

In the past 15 years, radiologic and endoscopic techniques have provided alternatives to surgery in the treatment of benign and malignant diseases of the biliary tract. Experience with some techniques, such as endoscopic sphincterotomy for stones in the common duct of the patient who has had a cholecystectomy, has been sufficiently favorable that the procedure has been adopted in the absence of randomized, controlled comparisons with surgery. Numerous unresolved issues in the nonsurgical treatment of diseases of the biliary tract remain, however, and the role of nonsurgical procedures is undergoing clarification and expansion as additional data emerge and the technology is refined. Given the importance of endoscopic sphincterotomy in the nonsurgical management of these patients, this technique is reviewed in some detail.

SPHINCTEROTOMY

STANDARD TECHNIQUE

Endoscopic sphincterotomy is performed most effectively and safely by endoscopists with considerable prior experience in diagnostic endoscopic retrograde cholangiopancreatography (ERCP). Whereas ERCP is performed by injecting contrast into a catheter that has been inserted through a side-viewing duodenoscope into the papilla of Vater, sphincterotomy requires a special catheter, or

sphincterotome, containing a wire coursing through its length and emerging a short distance from the tip (Fig. 60–1). The sphincterotome is connected to a diathermy machine.

Following diagnostic ERCP, sphincterotomy is performed in the following manner. The sphincterotome is inserted deeply into the bile duct. Its position in the bile duct must be confirmed fluoroscopically to be certain that the pancreatic duct has not been entered. After cannulation of the bile duct has been confirmed, the sphincterotome is withdrawn slowly until only a short length of the wire is inside the duct. The sphincterotome is then bowed moderately, so that the wire is applied in apposition to the roof of the papilla. When the sphincterotome is positioned correctly, the wire should be oriented at an 11- to 12-o'clock position in the endoscopist's field of view. A blended coagulating and cutting current is used to incise the intraduodenal portion of the common bile duct in short increments. If too much of the wire is inside the duct, there is less control over the speed and length of the incision. The usual length of a completed endoscopic sphincterotomy is in the range of 10 to 15 mm. The length of the incision is individualized according to the size of the stone to be removed and the length of the intramural portion of the common bile duct. Although many stones, especially those under 10 mm in diameter, can pass spontaneously after sphincterotomy, attempts are usually made to extract all but the smallest stones with a basket or balloon catheter. The choice of extraction technique varies with the endoscopist. Balloons are easier to use and avoid completely the small possibility of impaction of a basket with an entrapped stone that is too large to pass through the

The author wishes to thank Thomas A. Sos, M.D., Department of Radiology, New York Hospital-Cornell Medical Center, for his review of the manuscript.

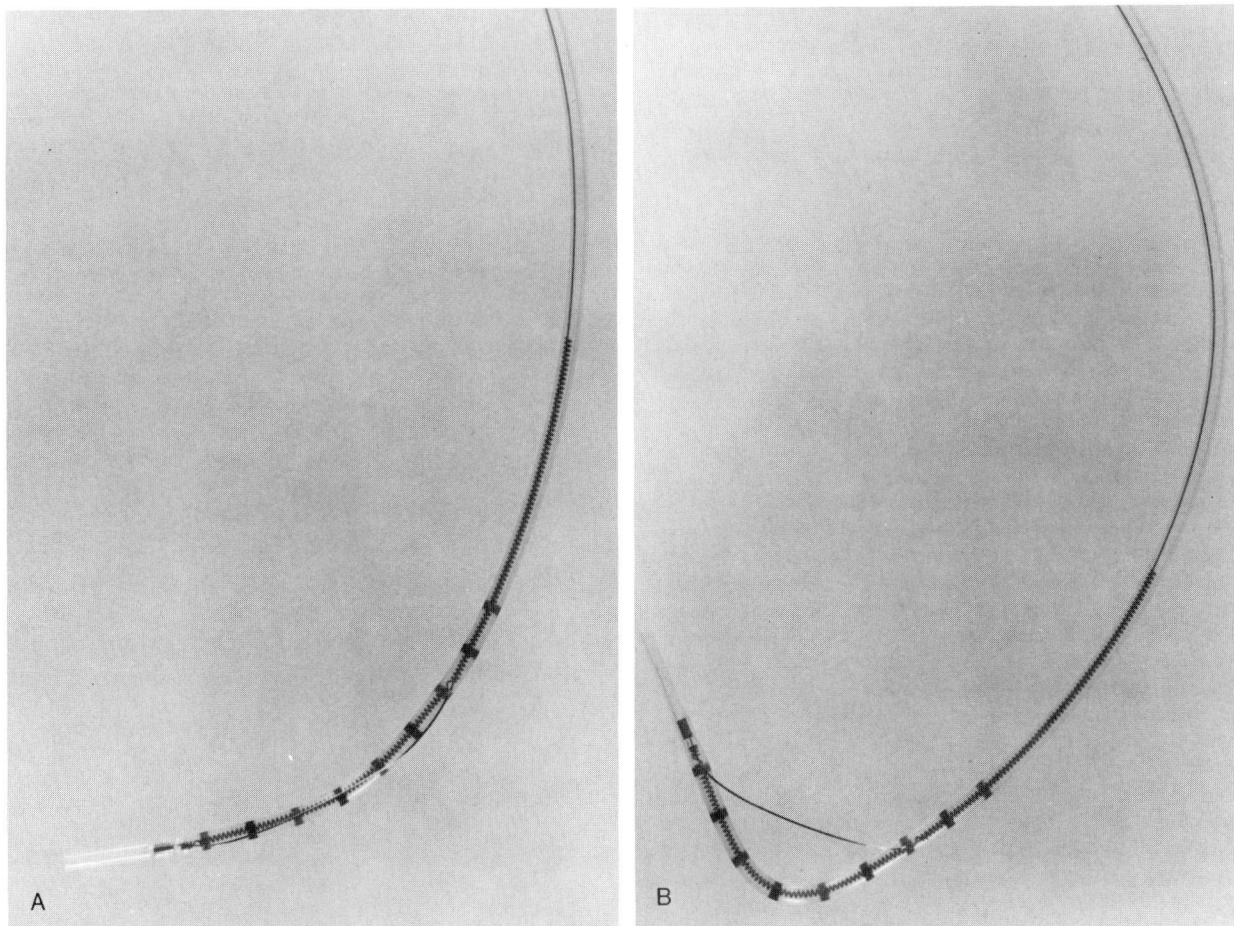

Figure 60–1. *A,* A sphincterotome with wire in the "relaxed" position, parallel to the catheter. The wire is held in this position as the sphincterotome is inserted into the bile duct. *B,* Sphincterotomy is performed with the wire in the "bowed" position.

sphincterotomy incision (Fig. 60–2). Balloons also are useful for estimating the size of the sphincterotomy incision. However, they are more fragile and expensive than baskets and are less useful when stones are present in a markedly dilated duct. In this instance, stones can slip proximally past the balloon. Extracted stones are usually left in the duodenum and allowed to pass spontaneously (Fig. 60–3). Occasionally, extraction of stones immediately after sphincterotomy can be difficult because there is a large number of stones or because of edema or the small amount of bleeding that can occur after the procedure. Extraction of stones in this setting may be easier if several days are allowed to pass and a second endoscopy is then performed. The likelihood of spontaneous passage of stones that have not been extracted immediately after sphincterotomy depends upon their size, the size of the sphincterotomy, and the size and configuration of the distal bile duct. If there is any doubt that a residual stone will pass spontaneously, a nasobiliary tube is placed in the common bile duct to ensure adequate drainage, thereby reducing the risk of cholangitis, and to permit convenient follow-up cholangiography (Fig. 60–4). If, after several days, cholangiography via the nasobiliary tube reveals that the stone (or stones) is still present, repeated attempts at extraction are necessary. Approaches to the management of unextractable stones are discussed later.

Endoscopic sphincterotomy can be performed successfully by experienced endoscopists in more than 90 per cent of patients, and clearance of the bile duct is accomplished

successfully in roughly 90 per cent of patients who have had a sphincterotomy.[1–3] Failures of the technique are related to inability to cannulate the bile duct, inability to insert the sphincterotome to the necessary depth even after successful cannulation, and failure to extract large stones after a successful sphincterotomy.

VARIATIONS IN SPHINCTEROTOMY TECHNIQUE

Variations in technique used when deep cannulation with the standard sphincterotome is impossible have been described. One such variation is the performance of a so-called precut. In standard sphincterotomes, the wire exits the catheter several centimeters above the tip and reenters it in such a way that a short length of the tip contains no wire, serving as a "lead" for cannulation. In precut instruments, on the other hand, the wire is attached at the extreme tip of the catheter and is used to incise through the papilla until sufficient access to the bile duct is attained to permit deep cannulation and completion of a standard sphincterotomy.[4] It is usually agreed that the risk of pancreatitis is greater with this technique because of the less controlled nature of the incision.[5] This was not the case, however, in a recent study in which a needle-knife precut instrument was used by a highly experienced group.[6] A second alternative when the bile duct cannot be cannulated with the standard sphincterotome is the performance of a fistulotomy, in which cutting into the bile duct is performed

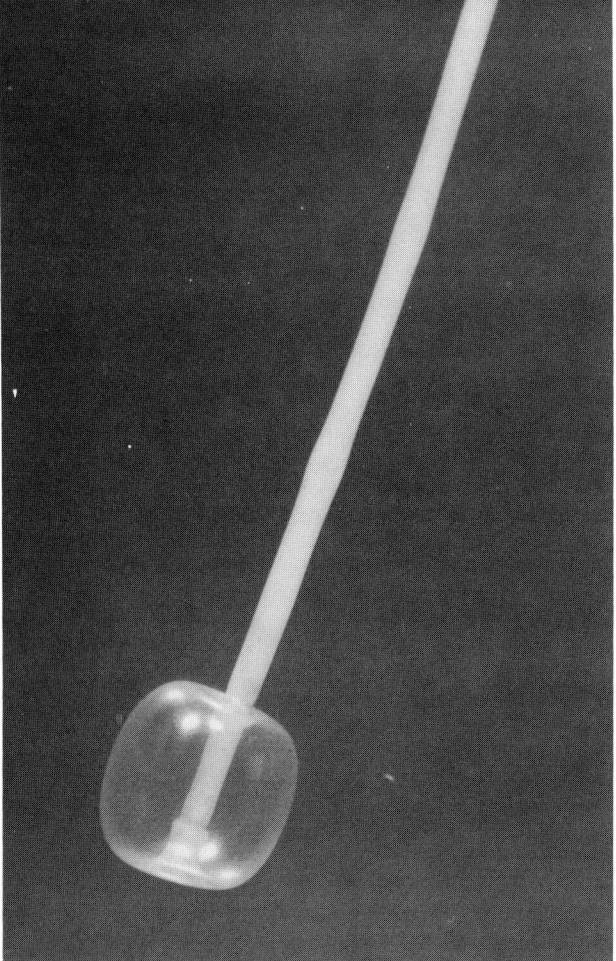

Figure 60–2. A balloon catheter, with balloon inflated, used to extract stones from the bile duct after sphincterotomy.

through the roof of the papilla, superior to the orifice, until the bile duct is reached, rather than through the orifice itself.[7, 8] This technique is most applicable when there is a prominent intraduodenal segment of bile duct, manifested by a longitudinal bulge extending up from the papillary orifice in a cephalad direction. Precuts and fistulotomies have been used predominantly by highly experienced endoscopists. There are relatively few published critical evaluations of the indications, technique, success rates, and risks of these alternatives to conventional sphincterotomy.

Still another variation, when deep insertion of the sphincterotome proves impossible, is the transhepatic insertion of guidewires or baskets to facilitate retrograde cannulation of the common duct.[5, 9, 10] In this approach, involving a collaborative effort between the endoscopist and interventional radiologist, a basket is extruded through the papilla, and the sphincterotome is pulled up into the bile duct within the basket. Alternatively, a guidewire can be advanced through the papilla and pulled up the channel of the endoscope with a snare so that the ends of the wire protrude from the skin at the site of percutaneous entry and from the endoscope, respectively. A sphincterotome capable of fitting over a guidewire then can be advanced through the endoscope and up the bile duct.[11]

One of the major technical challenges to the biliary endoscopist is the patient with a partial gastrectomy and Billroth II anastomosis, which is considered by some to be

a relative contraindication to the endoscopic approach to the bile ducts.[1] However, many endoscopists make the attempt before resorting to surgery, especially in high-risk patients, and success in over two thirds of patients has been reported by several groups.[12–16] Use of a forward-viewing endoscope or various modified types of sphincterotomes or a combination of these may enhance the success rate and safety of sphincterotomy in these patients.

COMPLICATIONS OF SPHINCTEROTOMY (Table 60–1)

The major complications of sphincterotomy are, in roughly decreasing order of frequency, hemorrhage, pancreatitis, cholangitis, and perforation. Impaction of baskets containing large stones unextractable through the sphincterotomy incision and gallstone ileus, caused by very large stones, have also been reported. The problem of basket impaction should be eliminated with the availability of mechanical lithotripsy baskets. The overall incidence of complications is 5 to 10 per cent, and the mortality rate is approximately 1 per cent.[2, 17–19]

Brisk bleeding is related to cutting through a branch of the gastroduodenal artery that runs anterior to the bile duct, unusually close to the papilla. Use of a Doppler probe has been suggested as a means of detecting such vessels prior to sphincterotomy, but this has not been tested widely. Life-threatening bleeding usually requires surgery, although endoscopically applied cautery and angiographic embolization of the gastroduodenal artery have been used.

Pancreatitis after endoscopic sphincterotomy may be related to damage to the orifice of the pancreatic duct but may also occur as a result of papillary manipulation or injection of contrast during the diagnostic part of the procedure. Management of patients with procedure-related pancreatitis is similar to that of pancreatitis from other causes—that is, withholding of oral feedings and use of nasogastric suction and intravenous hydration. There may be a rationale for antibiotics in these patients because of the injection of contaminated material into the pancreatic duct during ERCP, but the usefulness of antibiotics in this setting is not established. In severe pancreatitis, serial CT scans may be helpful in detecting the development of pseudocysts or abscesses.

When cholangitis occurs, it usually is related to impaction of a stone that is too large to pass through the sphincterotomy incision. Placement of a nasobiliary tube usually prevents this complication and is recommended whenever there is doubt that a retained stone will pass spontaneously through the distal duct or sphincterotomy incision.

When perforation occurs after endoscopic sphincterotomy, it is retroperitoneal rather than intraperitoneal. A common symptom is pain in the back. CT scanning of the abdomen may be helpful in patients in whom it is difficult to distinguish pancreatitis from perforation. Initial treatment with nasogastric suction and antibiotics may obviate the need for operation in some patients.[19–21] The success of conservative treatment may depend in part on rapid recognition of the complication.

Recurrent stones or stenosis of the ampulla or both occur in about 4 to 8 per cent of patients after sphincterotomy.[2, 22, 23] Most sphincterotomies appear to decrease in size with time but remain patent. For example, Geenen and coworkers showed that the mean size of their sphincterotomies decreased from about 11 to 6 mm during a two-

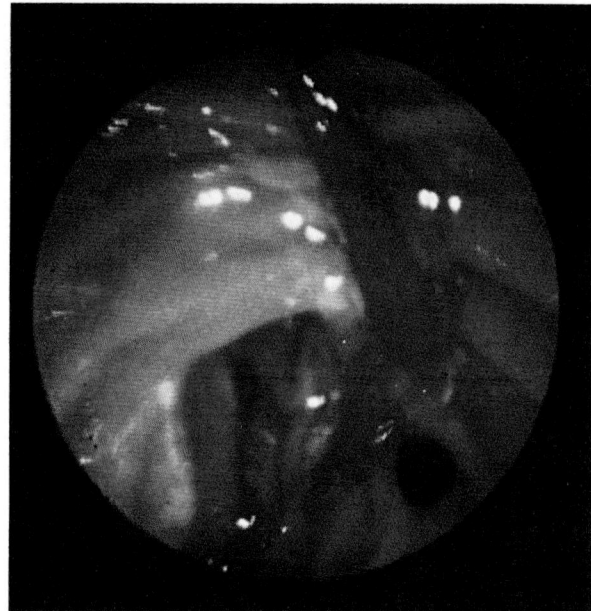

Figure 60–3. A black pigment stone has been extracted from the bile duct with a balloon catheter and left in the duodenum to pass spontaneously.

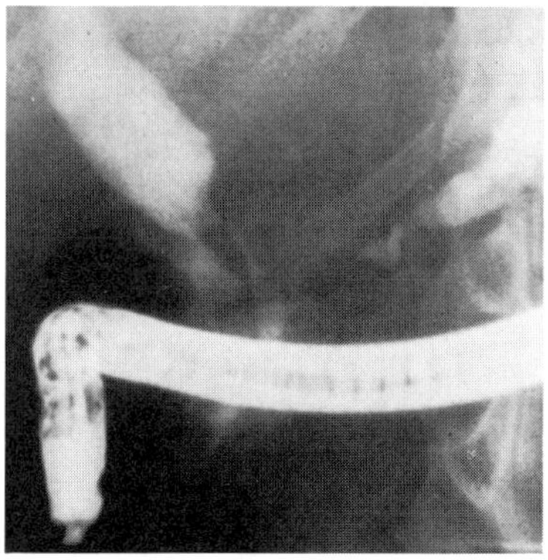

Figure 60–11*A*

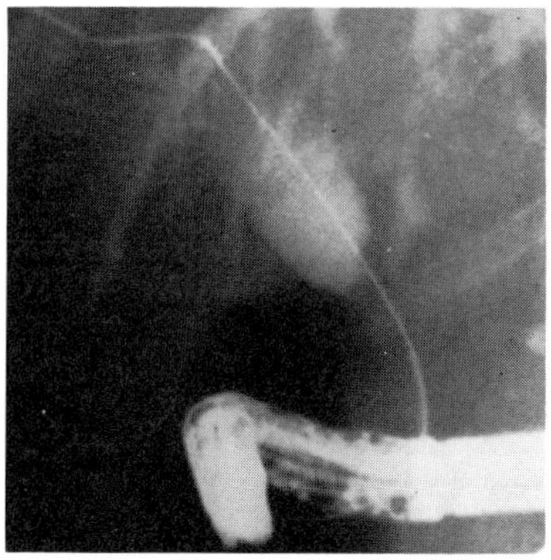

Figure 60–11*B*

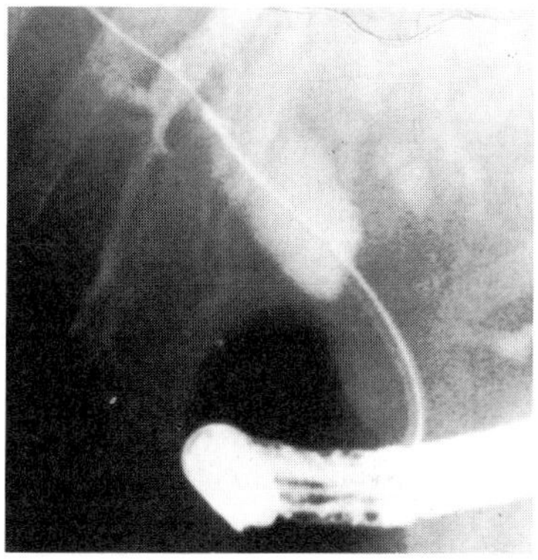

Figure 60–11*C*

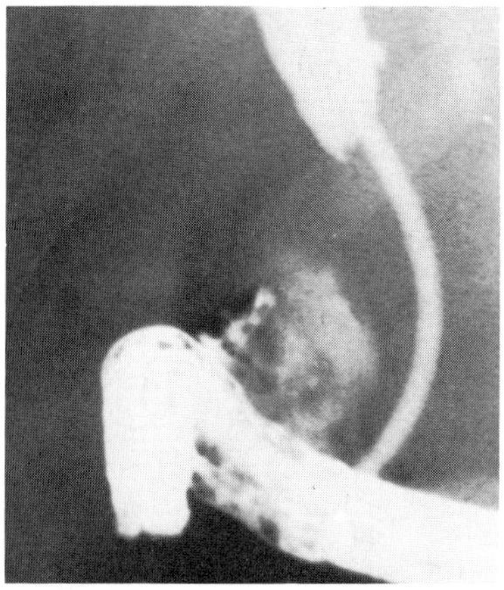

Figure 60–11*D*

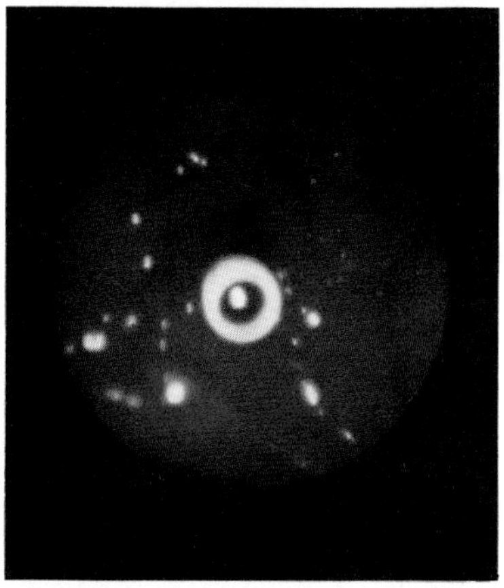

Figure 60–11*E*

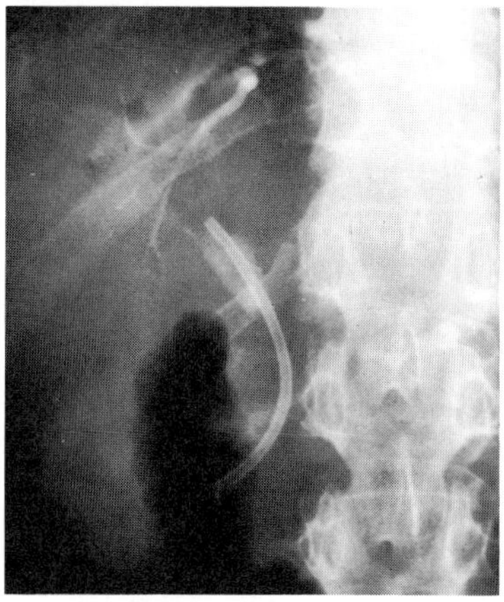

Figure 60–11*F*

Figure 60–11. *A,* ERCP in a patient with carcinoma of the head of the pancreas. There are strictures of the head of the pancreatic duct and distal bile duct (double-duct sign). *B,* A guidewire has been advanced through the bile duct stricture into the right hepatic duct system. *C,* A 6-French catheter has been advanced over the guidewire through the stricture. *D,* A biliary endoprosthesis is being pushed through the stricture over the 6-French inner catheter. *E,* When the endoprosthesis is advanced to its final position, the inner catheter and guidewire are withdrawn. About 1 cm of the stent protrudes from the papilla. *F,* Radiograph of endoprosthesis in final position after withdrawal of endoscope. Note rapid drainage of contrast from bile ducts.

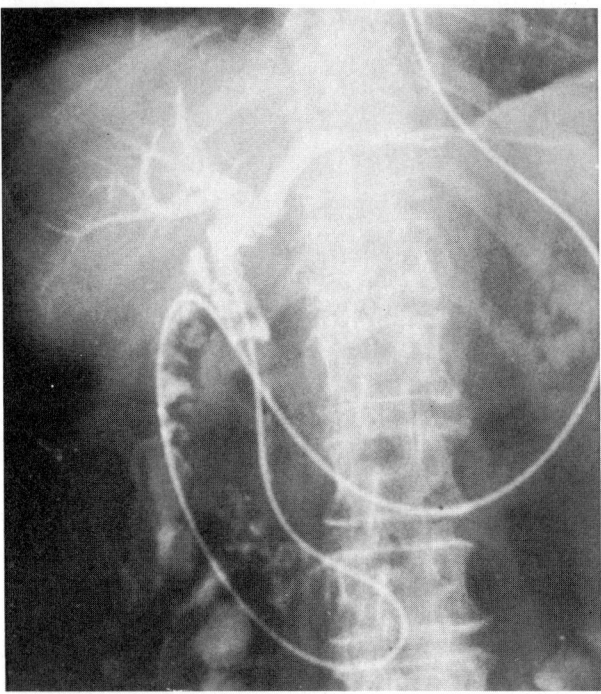

Figure 60–4. Nasobiliary tube with tip above two retained stones that could not be extracted after sphincterotomy. The larger stone is manifested as a "meniscus sign" at the bottom of the column of contrast in the bile duct. The tube ensures continued biliary drainage despite retention of stones.

year period. They supplemented their observations with manometric studies demonstrating that during the same follow-up period, basal sphincter of Oddi pressure was not restored.[24] Bacterial contamination of the bile is common but is unassociated with cholangitis in the presence of a patent orifice.

CHOLEDOCHOLITHIASIS

Endoscopic sphincterotomy is the cornerstone of nonoperative treatment for choledocholithiasis in patients without a T-tube.[25, 26] No controlled trials have compared surgery with endoscopic sphincterotomy in postcholecystectomy patients, but the latter approach offers unequivocal reductions in recovery time, duration of hospitalization, and cost.

The mortality rate for endoscopic sphincterotomy is about 1 per cent in most series.[1] Mortality rates for choledochotomy or choledochoduodenostomy in surgical series are in the range of 0 to 7.4 per cent.[27–35] The true significance of this difference in mortality is uncertain, however. Mortality in surgical series is dependent on age[29, 35] and on severity of illness. In the series reported by McSherry and Glenn, for example, mortality was 2.1 per cent for choledocholithotomy in postcholecystectomy patients but only 1.2 per cent if patients with pancreatitis or cholangitis were excluded.[35] Similarly, in the series of Lygidakis, mortality

TABLE 60–1. COMPLICATIONS OF ENDOSCOPIC SPHINCTEROTOMY

Hemorrhage
Pancreatitis
Retroduodenal perforation
Cholangitis
Impacted basket
Gallstone ileus

was 2.2 per cent (2 of 90 patients), but the two patients who died in this series had bacterial cholangitis.[30] On the other hand, figures for the morbidity and mortality of endoscopic sphincterotomy apply to patients who have been at least as ill and elderly as those in surgical series.[1] It seems likely, therefore, that there indeed is a difference in mortality between endoscopic sphincterotomy and surgery. This difference is small or perhaps nonexistent in young and otherwise healthy patients but increases with age and other systemic diseases.

APPROACHES TO UNEXTRACTABLE STONES

Intense interest centers on the development of nonoperative approaches for removing large common bile duct stones that have proved to be unextractable after endoscopic sphincterotomy. The methods that have been proposed for this purpose include the following:

1. Mono-octanoin can dissolve cholesterol-rich stones in the bile duct when infused through a nasobiliary tube or T-tube. It succeeds in at most 50 per cent of patients, and to be successful, treatment usually requires at least one to two weeks of infusion. Common side effects are vomiting, diarrhea, and abdominal cramps. Less often, duodenal ulceration may occur.[36, 37] In the largest series, complete dissolution of the stones occurred 26 per cent of the time. Partial dissolution, permitting extraction of the stones via percutaneous or endoscopic approaches, was observed in an additional 29 per cent of patients.[38] Among the reasons for the limited efficacy of mono-octanoin is that many stones in the bile duct are composed predominantly of bilirubin rather than cholesterol.

2. Mechanical lithotripsy can be performed with specially designed crushing baskets. Success rates of 90 per cent have been reported.[39]

3. Electrohydraulic lithotripsy, in which hydraulic pressure waves capable of fragmenting stones are generated by a spark, has been demonstrated to be feasible in vitro and in animals.[40, 41] Preliminary data indicate that it is a successful technique in humans,[41–44] but it is still an investigational procedure.

4. Shock wave lithotripsy holds promise for the treatment of large bile duct stones and on a much larger scale, gallbladder stones (see Chap. 61).[45]

5. Stent placement with double-pigtail endoprostheses appears to provide good biliary drainage in the presence of large retained stones unextractable after sphincterotomy (Fig. 60–5). Adequate drainage persists in these patients beyond the time the stents would be expected to have become clogged. Presumably, the stent provides space around the stones through which the bile drains.[46] In one study, of 17 patients treated by stent insertion 2 had successful endoscopic extraction of stones at a later date, 5 died of nonbiliary causes, 2 required surgery for recurrent biliary symptoms, and 8 were alive and well from 24 to 59 months later (median 39 months). Ursodeoxycholic acid did not dissolve ductal stones in any of these patients.[47] The use of stents for unextractable bile duct stones is most appropriate for poor surgical candidates. The use of this approach can be expected to decline as lithotripsy techniques are refined.

6. Gallstone lithotripsy with lasers has been accomplished in vitro with tunable dye lasers,[48] and in vivo, via the endoscopic approach, with neodymium-yttrium aluminum garnet (YAG) laser.[49]

Extensive clinical experience with these techniques will

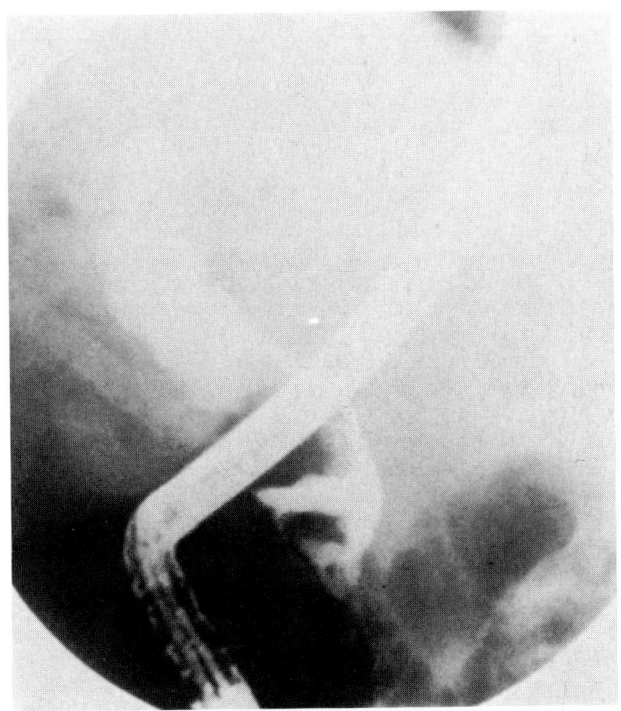
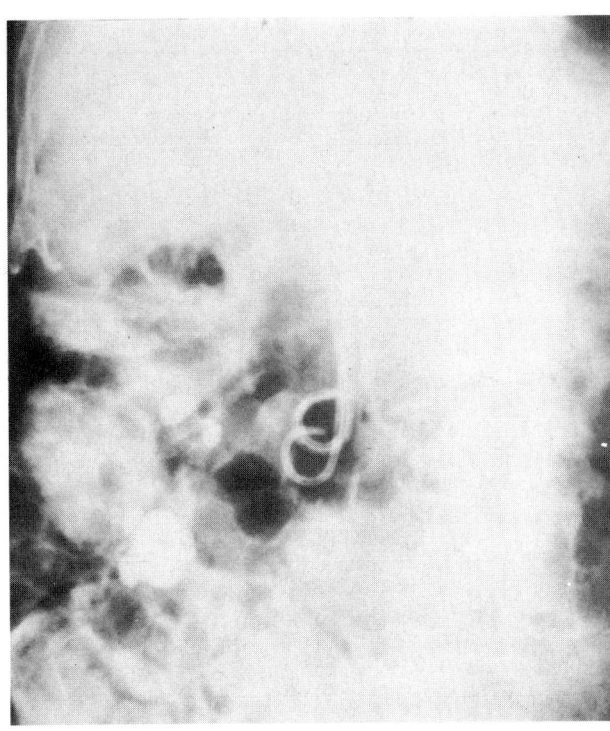

A   B

Figure 60–5. *A,* Endoscopic retrograde cholangiogram in an 87-year-old woman with recent cholangitis showing two stones, the larger approximately 2 cm in diameter. *B,* Extraction of the larger stone after sphincterotomy was not possible. Therefore, two endoprostheses, each 8 French, were left in the duct to ensure adequate biliary drainage. The pigtail shape of the end of each stent prevents migration (though straight stents have recently also been shown not to migrate).[47] This patient has been followed for over two years without further illness related to the biliary tract.

be needed to determine their relative merits. Until one (or more) technique of lithotripsy or dissolution is further refined and available on a widespread scale, surgery will continue to be important in the treatment of patients with large common duct stones.

SPHINCTEROTOMY WITH INTACT GALLBLADDER

A substantial proportion of patients currently undergoing endoscopic sphincterotomy for common duct stones have intact gallbladders. Sphincterotomy in this setting is sometimes related to an urgent indication for the procedure—for example, cholangitis or biliary pancreatitis—and is followed by surgery when the patient's condition improves. Increasingly, however, sphincterotomy is offered as the only therapy to patients who are elderly or are poor surgical candidates when the presenting illness is caused by stones in the duct rather than those in the gallbladder. Experience with these patients indicates that only 5 to 20 per cent require cholecystectomy during the first few years following sphincterotomy; half or more of these patients will have surgery for biliary pain rather than for acute cholecystitis (Table 60–2).[50–52] Further studies of these patients are needed, but available data have led to widespread acceptance of this approach in many elderly or high-risk patients.

An unresolved issue is whether preoperative endoscopic sphincterotomy should be performed in patients with known stones in the bile duct when cholecystectomy is planned. Since choledochotomy adds to the morbidity and mortality of cholecystectomy, it has been suggested that sphincterotomy plus cholecystectomy would compare favorably with cholecystectomy and exploration of the common bile duct in terms of risk and overall duration of hospitalization.[53] A randomized study of preoperative endoscopic sphincterotomy versus surgery alone demonstrated a trend, albeit statistically insignificant, toward greater morbidity and mortality in the patients treated by sphincterotomy followed by cholecystectomy. The overall rate of major complications in this group was 16.4 per cent and the mortality rate, 3.6 per cent, compared with 13.6 per cent and 1.7 per cent in the group treated by surgery alone.[54] These data do not support the use of preoperative sphincterotomy. Preoperative sphincterotomy may still be appropriate in some patients, however, such as those with an intercurrent illness that can be expected to improve before cholecystectomy.[54] Another situation in which preoperative sphincterotomy may be justified is in the patient with known gallbladder stones undergoing ERCP to evaluate unexplained jaundice. If choledocholithiasis is discovered in this setting, sphincterotomy is probably warranted if the bile duct can be cannulated readily with a standard sphincterotome and multiple or unusually large stones are not present.

URGENT INDICATIONS FOR SPHINCTEROTOMY

Most patients with acute cholangitis can be managed initially with intravenous antibiotics followed by definitive correction of the underlying problem on an elective basis. However, patients with severe or suppurative disease require drainage of the biliary system to prevent overwhelming sepsis. Mortality rates for urgent surgery tend to be high (e.g., 30 to 40 per cent) in this group of very ill patients.[55, 56] Nonoperative biliary drainage may represent an alternative, potentially less morbid approach to the management of such patients. However, when ERCP is

TABLE 60–2. LONG-TERM FOLLOW-UP AFTER SPHINCTEROTOMY WITH INTACT GALLBLADDERS

Author	No. of Patients	Follow-up Period	Illnesses from Biliary Disease	No. with Cholecystectomy
Escourrou[50]	130	6–66 months (mean 22 months)	8 cholecystitis 5 cholangitis 2 restenosis 1 gallbladder cancer	8 (6.2%)
Rosseland[51]	66	Up to 8 years	11 cholecystitis 3 biliary pain	13 (20%) (2 were incidental)
Cotton[52]	118	2–9 years (median 40 months)	6 biliary pain	6 (5.1%) (6 others had elective cholecystectomy during initial hospitalization)

performed in this situation, it is important to avoid injection of excessive contrast material and protracted instrumentation of the bile duct. If common duct stones cannot be extracted quickly after sphincterotomy, a drain should be placed and further maneuvers deferred until the patient's condition improves. No controlled trials have been conducted, but anecdotal experience[57, 58] and a retrospective comparison of early endoscopic drainage versus surgical drainage[59] suggest that mortality is significantly lower with immediate endoscopic drainage. This issue warrants further study.

Most patients with pancreatitis secondary to a stone in the bile duct improve with conservative therapy alone, and many pass their stones spontaneously. On the other hand, several centers have reported dramatic improvement in patients with biliary pancreatitis after sphincterotomy and extraction of stones from the bile duct in the acute setting.[60, 61] In a multicenter study in France, the mortality of 1.7 per cent, which was related to bleeding after sphincterotomy, was thought to compare favorably with the anticipated mortality from biliary pancreatitis.[62] The most important study of this issue was a prospective, randomized trial of ERCP and sphincterotomy versus conventional treatment for acute biliary pancreatitis conducted in Leicester, England. In patients with pancreatitis predicted to be severe, on the basis of modified Glasgow criteria, but not in patients with predicted mild disease, there was a significant reduction in the frequency of complications (e.g., pseudocysts, cardiovascular, pulmonary, and renal failure) and length of hospital stay. Mortality also was reduced, but not to the point of statistical significance.[63] As in patients with acute cholangitis, it appears that urgent ERCP in patients with biliary pancreatitis will be useful in some cases. There are insufficient data to warrant its performance in all patients with the disease.

EXTRACTION OF BILE DUCT STONES THROUGH T-TUBE TRACTS

Following exploration of the common bile duct, a T-tube is left in the duct postoperatively and a T-tube cholangiogram is obtained from seven to ten days after surgery. Retained stones have been reported to be discovered postoperatively in 4 to 15 per cent of patients who have undergone common duct exploration, usually in ducts within which stones were found intraoperatively.[64–66] Intraoperative choledochoscopy has been reported to be associated with rates of stone retention of about 2 per cent in some series.[67–70] When retained stones are discovered on a T-tube cholangiogram, percutaneous extraction can be attempted through the T-tube tract, using a basket, a procedure developed initially by Burhenne.[71]

When it is decided to remove the stone via the tract

created by a T-tube, there is usually a waiting period of four to six weeks to allow the tract to develop a fibrous wall. Most patients or their families can be taught to manage the tube and drainage bag at home during this interval. The patient then returns to the hospital, and a preliminary cholangiogram is obtained. Following this, a steerable catheter is advanced to the region of the stone, and a basket is introduced through the catheter (Fig. 60–6). The reader is referred to more detailed reviews for further descriptions of the technical details.[72, 73] In centers with experience with more than 100 cases, success in clearing the common duct using this technique ranges from 78 to 95 per cent.[72–75] The procedure is more difficult when the T-tube is small, there are multiple stones, the stones are impacted in the distal common duct, or the T-tube is positioned anteriorly rather than laterally.[72, 73] More than one session may be required to achieve removal of all stones.

A complication rate of 5 per cent has been reported with this technique. Morbidity most often is due to cholangitis, pancreatitis, and perforation of the tract. The latter complication is rarely a serious problem. The mortality rate is reported to be less than 0.1 per cent and has been related to severe pancreatitis.[72]

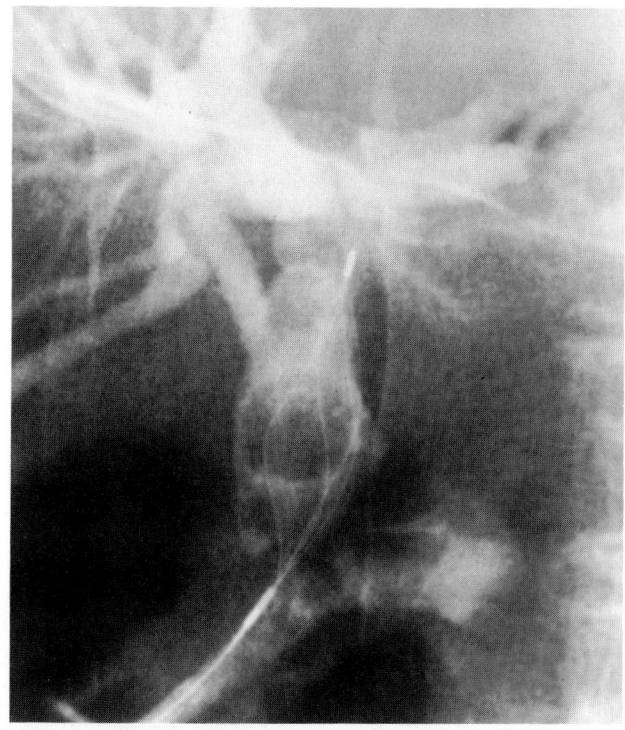

Figure 60–6. A basket introduced into the bile duct through a T-tube tract in position to entrap a common duct stone. (Courtesy of Thomas A. Sos, M.D.)

Endoscopic sphincterotomy can obviate the need to await maturation of the T-tube tract in patients with retained stones. In a series of patients with retained stones and T-tubes in place, the morbidity and success rate for sphincterotomy were similar to reported figures from patients without T-tubes.[76] Occasionally, stones proximal to the T-tube can be difficult to extract even after sphincterotomy has been performed successfully, and the tube must be pulled to allow the endoscopist access to the stones. However, because the success rate for removal of stones via the T-tube tract compares favorably with sphincterotomy and the complication rate for approaching the stone via the drainage tract is lower, the preferred treatment plan is to await maturation of the T-tube tract and to attempt percutaneous extraction of stones in these patients. If for some reason the surgeon or patient finds the waiting period unacceptable, or if factors associated with an anticipated low likelihood of success are present (discussed earlier), sphincterotomy can be performed without further delay. In addition, sphincterotomy should be performed if multiple stones are present and a permanent drainage procedure is indicated but surgery was performed under conditions precluding such a procedure in the operating room (for example, sepsis, inflammation, or scarring).

When cholecystostomy tubes are placed in patients who cannot undergo cholecystectomy at the initial operation (e.g., patients with empyema of the gallbladder) and in whom subsequent surgery poses a high risk, stones can be removed from the gallbladder or, in some centers, occasionally from the common duct through the drainage tract by techniques analogous to those used with T-tube tracts. When common duct stones are to be extracted, the cystic duct must be dilated first with balloon catheters.[72]

SPHINCTER OF ODDI DYSFUNCTION ("PAPILLARY STENOSIS") (See Also Chap. 59)

Occasionally, patients who have undergone cholecystectomy subsequently present with abdominal pain that is similar to the pain before surgery or with pain consistent with biliary tract disease. Elevations in liver enzymes or dilated ducts on imaging studies may add further evidence for the existence of biliary disease. Much interest centers on the frequency with which such patients suffer from a disorder of the sphincter of Oddi in the absence of stones in the bile duct. It is generally agreed that in the absence of common duct stones, biliary symptoms can arise from disease at the level of the papilla. Some affected patients may have fixed stenosis of the papilla due to fibrosis. Others may have a motility disorder without demonstrable histologic changes. The term *sphincter of Oddi dysfunction* is commonly used to collectively describe these disorders.

Clinical criteria for sphincter of Oddi dysfunction used by Geenen and co-workers include biliary-type pain (especially in postcholecystectomy patients), elevated liver enzymes on two or more occasions, a dilated bile duct, and drainage of contrast from the bile duct that is delayed beyond 45 minutes after injection (Table 60–3). Patients who meet all of these criteria nearly always have relief of pain after endoscopic sphincterotomy, and sphincter of Oddi manometry is not considered an essential diagnostic test in them.[77] However, patients with biliary pain who meet one or two of the other criteria do not respond to sphincterotomy with the same degree of uniformity. Manometry of the sphincter of Oddi may be useful for reaching therapeutic decisions in this group. Controlled trials, in

TABLE 60–3. CLINICAL CRITERIA DEVELOPED AT THE MEDICAL COLLEGE OF WISCONSIN FOR SPHINCTER OF ODDI DYSFUNCTION

Biliary-type pain
Elevation in bilirubin and/or alkaline phosphatase (twice normal values) on at least two occasions
Dilated common bile duct (over 12 mm)
Delayed drainage of contrast from the common bile duct after ERCP (over 45 minutes)

Source: Geneen JE, et al. In: Gastroenterologic Endoscopy. WB Saunders, 1987, with permission.
"Definitive" sphincter of Oddi dysfunction: all four criteria.
"Presumptive" sphincter of Oddi dysfunction: biliary pain plus one or two others.

which patients were randomized to treatment with real versus sham sphincterotomy at the time of ERCP, indicated that elevated basal sphincter of Oddi pressure was strongly associated with a favorable response to sphincterotomy in such patients (Table 60–4). Pain relief persisted to the end of the 4-year follow-up period. Conversely, patients with similar symptoms but normal basal sphincter of Oddi pressures do not respond well to sphincterotomy. Thus, in these investigators' hands, sphincter of Oddi manometry has emerged as a useful tool in formulating therapeutic decisions in this difficult group of patients.[78, 79] Basal sphincter of Oddi pressure has been less helpful in other units in predicting response to sphincterotomy, and the superiority of manometry to such criteria as delayed drainage or duct dilation at ERCP is not uniformly accepted.[80, 81] The reasons for these discordant observations are unclear.

It is generally thought that endoscopic sphincterotomy for sphincter of Oddi disease is associated with greater morbidity and mortality[2] and a higher incidence of subsequent papillary stenosis[22] than it is when choledocholithiasis is the indication. In a series from Germany, mortality was 2 per cent, compared with 1 per cent when sphincterotomy was performed to treat choledocholithiasis.[17] In the absence of a clear consensus on criteria for the performance of sphincterotomy in these patients, this increment of risk only reinforces the need for additional data and for careful selection of patients on an individual basis.

BILIARY OBSTRUCTION SECONDARY TO MALIGNANT DISEASE

Percutaneous transhepatic drainage of the biliary system by passage of a stent into the duodenum is a logical extension of percutaneous transhepatic cholangiography. In this approach, a cholangiogram is first obtained with a 22-gauge needle, as in standard transhepatic cholangiography. A guidewire is then introduced into a branch of the right hepatic biliary tree and passed across the point of obstruction into the duodenum. The left lobe can be decompressed instead of or in addition to the right lobe in

TABLE 60–4. RESULTS OF ENDOSCOPIC SPHINCTEROTOMY (ES) IN PATIENTS WITH SUSPECTED SPHINCTER OF ODDI (SO) DYSFUNCTION

Basal SO Pressure	Group	Pain Relief at One Year (%)
>30 mmHg (high)	ES	91
<30 mmHg	Sham	25
(normal)	ES	42
	Sham	33

Source: Geneen JE, et al. Gastroenterology 92:1401, 1987, with permission.

patients with obstruction of the hilum or left hepatic duct.[82] When drainage of the left duct is necessary, it can be approached through the right ducts or by direct subxiphoid puncture. A biliary drainage catheter with multiple side-holes is passed over the guidewire and through the stricture so that one end of the catheter emerges from the skin and the other is in the duodenum. If, during the initial session, the guidewire cannot be made to traverse the stricture readily, the system is left to external drainage (Fig. 60–7); some radiologists routinely avoid attempts to traverse the stricture during the initial session. One or two subsequent sessions are needed to insert an indwelling stent of maximal size (usually 10 to 14 French), because the tract through the liver must be established in graded stages. Two types of stents are used. One is an external-internal stent with its external and internal ends outside the patient and distal to the stricture, respectively (Fig. 60–8). The external end is capped, and the patient is instructed on the care of the skin, and of the stent by periodic flushing. The other type of stent is completely internalized, without an external port (i.e., a biliary endoprosthesis) (Fig. 60–9). Because endo-prostheses lack external access, some interventional radiologists reserve them for patients in whom an anticipated short life span makes it unlikely that repeated exchanges of the stent will be required. Others recommend endo-prostheses for "all patients with malignant biliary obstruction in whom placement of an endoprosthesis is technically feasible."[83]

Major acute complications of transhepatic stenting occur in 5 to 10 per cent of patients[84–86] and are listed in Table 60–2. In the series of Mueller and colleagues,[85] 2 of 200 patients died from bleeding related to multiple hepatic punctures.[85] One additional patient died as a result of pneumothorax and bilious pleural effusion. In a larger series of 300 cases from the same institution, there were 7 deaths that could be related to the procedure.[84] Similar mortality figures have been reported elsewhere.[87, 88] Transient fever is more common than frank sepsis. Rates for acute complications are similar when endoprostheses are inserted.[89–93]

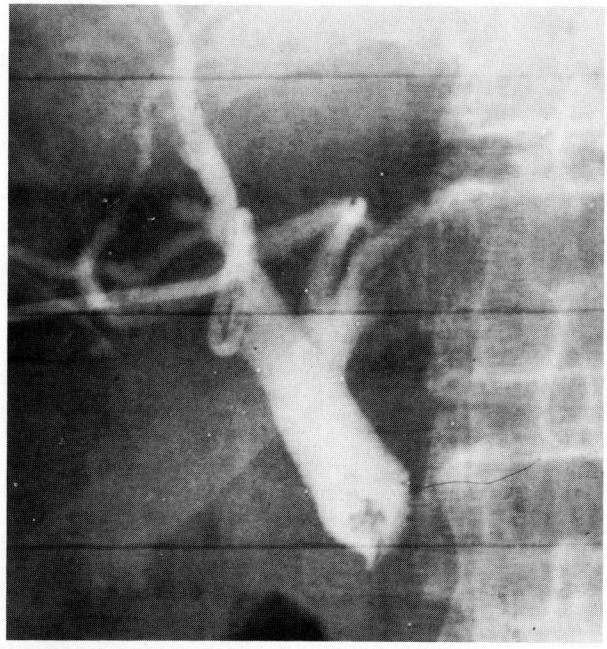

Figure 60–7. An "accordion"-type percutaneous external drain. The end is designed to avoid dislodgment of the tube. (Courtesy of Thomas A. Sos, M.D.)

Experienced radiologists are successful in catheterizing the dilated biliary tract in at least 95 per cent of patients. Internal drainage can be established in the great majority of these patients. Partial or complete normalization of levels in serum bilirubin occurs in up to 90 per cent of patients.[84, 86] Success rates for insertion of endoprostheses range from 82 to 88 per cent.[89–93] The most important late complication in patients with stents is occlusion of the stent, which may manifest as recurrent jaundice, cholangitis, or both. In patients with external-internal stents, the risk of this problem may be reduced by routine flushing of the catheter with saline.[83] Some groups perform periodic exchanges of external-internal stents on an outpatient basis. Less frequent long-term complications include dislodgment of the catheter when endoprostheses are used,[94] skin infections, and (rarely) growth of malignant tumor along the catheter tract with externalized tubes.

Nasobiliary tubes are unsuitable for long-term drainage. Therefore, the endoscopic approach to stent placement in patients with biliary obstruction caused by malignant tumors has centered almost from the outset on the use of endoprostheses.[95, 96] Initially, the diameter of these stents was limited by the 2.8-mm channel within standard duodenoscopes. Accordingly, the stents were 5 to 7 French in diameter. With the development of duodenoscopes with larger channels (3.7 or 3.8 mm), 10-French stents became feasible,[97] and more recently a duodenoscope with a 4.2-mm channel has permitted the placement of 12-French stents.[98] Large stents were considered desirable because single stents of smaller caliber become clogged relatively easily, leading to recurrent jaundice or cholangitis.[99–102] Although it has been suggested that multiple small stents are safe and effective,[18] no formal studies comparing the merits of multiple small stents versus single large ones have been reported, and there is a decided preference in favor of large-caliber stents among biliary endoscopists. Flow rates are higher and time to occlusion longer with large stents than with small ones. Because of higher flow rates and greater ease of insertion, straight stents are preferred to the pigtail stents that were used initially (Fig. 60–10).[103, 104]

Placement of an endoprosthesis is preceded by ERCP. A small sphincterotomy is made by most endoscopists to facilitate insertion of the stent. Fluoroscopy is essential to placement of the stent, which is pushed into the bile duct until its proximal end is above the stricture and its distal end protrudes from the papilla about 1 cm into the duodenum. The stents come in various lengths and are chosen according to the location and length of the patient's stricture. The sequence of events in the insertion of stents endoscopically is shown in Figure 60–11 (see p. 1551). Some endoscopists perform the initial ERCP with a standard 2.8mm channel endoscope and then switch to the large-channel endoscope to insert the stent. Others use the large-channel instrument for the entire procedure. Because standard catheters and sphincterotomes are more difficult to manipulate in large channels, the use of a biliary cannulation sleeve of large diameter through which standard accessories can be introduced has been suggested in order to facilitate the use of a single large-channel duodenoscope for the entire procedure.[105]

Experienced endoscopists report success rates of 85 to 90 per cent for placement of stents.[100–102, 106] There is widespread agreement that in patients with proximal tumors, especially at the hilum of the liver, placement of stents is technically more difficult than through the strictures in the distal duct.[107] As with percutaneous stents, successful place-

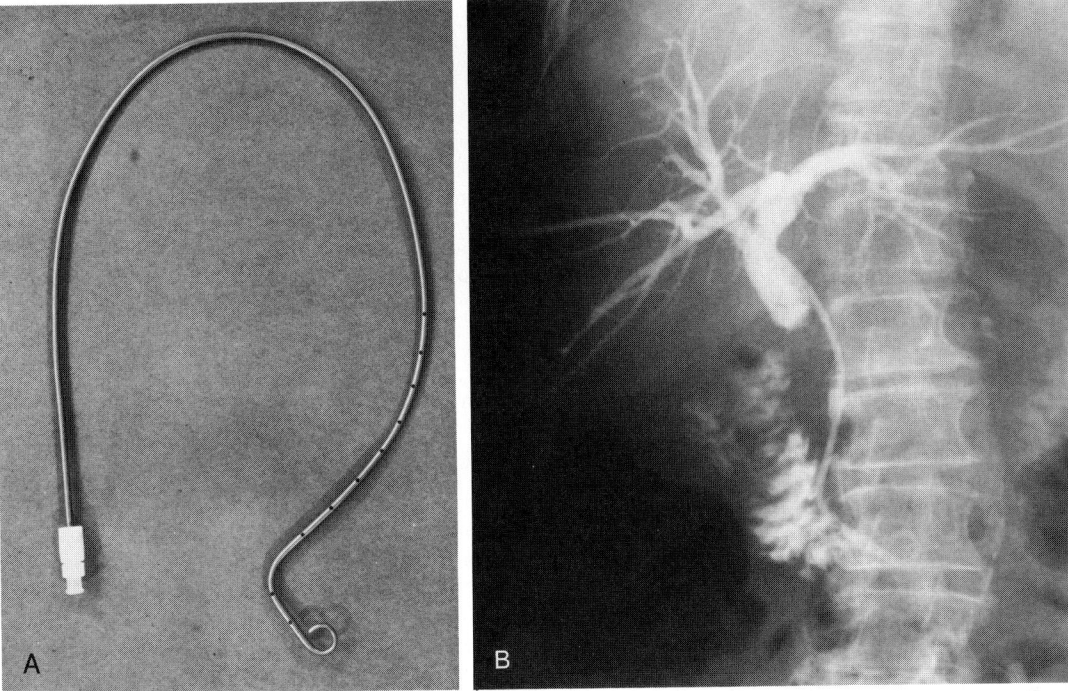

Figure 60–8. *A,* Ring-type external-internal stent. *B,* The external-internal stent has been placed across a malignant stricture into the duodenum. (Courtesy of Thomas A. Sos, M.D.)

ment usually, but not invariably, leads to partial or complete normalization of serum bilirubin.

Tumors of the ampulla account for relatively few of the patients presenting for long-term nonsurgical drainage. These tumors are less common than those arising from the pancreas, and when they do occur, there is a higher chance of cure with pancreaticoduodenectomy. In patients with

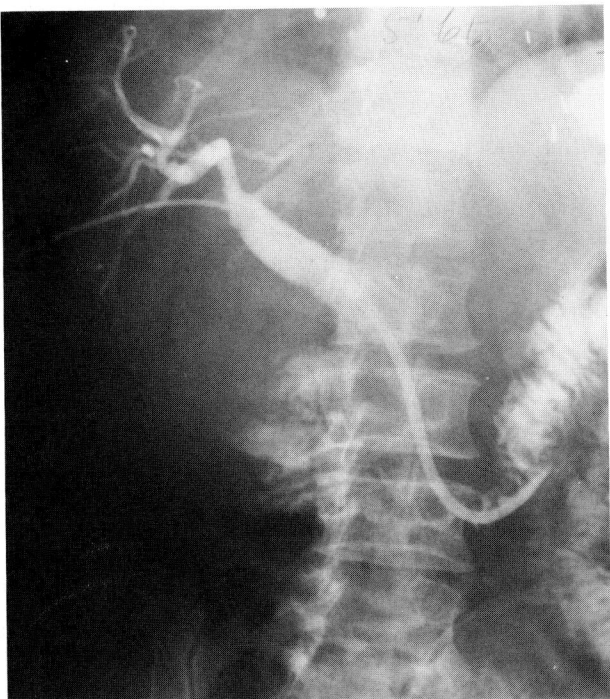

Figure 60–9. An endoprosthesis placed percutaneously through a malignant biliary stricture. The external drain placed initially, seen at left, is still in position. (Courtesy of Thomas A. Sos, M.D.)

ampullary tumors that are inoperable, the choice is between placement of a stent or sphincterotomy. The latter approach is preferred in some centers, especially in Europe.[108]

Stenting of tumors in the hilum of the liver presents a mechanical challenge, and results in drainage of only one lobe of the liver if a single stent is inserted. This may result in sufficient drainage to effect a fall in serum bilirubin, but the risk of cholangitis in the undrained lobe has been perceived to be high and is therefore thought to mandate placement of stents in both lobes.[100, 109, 110] On the other hand, in a series of 70 patients with malignant hilar strictures at the Middlesex Hospital, 46 of 54 patients with single stents had a fall in serum bilirubin. Eight developed early cholangitis, but in long-term followup only two were thought to have developed cholangitis in undrained segments of the liver.[111] This issue therefore requires further clarification.

Cholangitis is the most common complication of endoscopic stent placement. Although sphincterotomy is usually performed to facilitate insertion of the stent, the incision when made for this indication is small, and the risks of bleeding and perforation are correspondingly low. In Amsterdam, in a group of over 200 patients with pancreatic cancer in whom 10-French stents were placed, the overall complication rate was 10.5 per cent and the mortality, 2 per cent.[102] In New York, in another group of 277 patients with pancreatic cancer, 20 per cent had transient fever and 3 per cent had cholangitis with sepsis. The incidence of infection decreased as stents of increasingly large caliber were inserted (from 7 through 12 French). Bleeding, perforation, and pancreatitis each occurred in 1 per cent or less of patients.[106]

As with transhepatic stents, the major long-term problem after endoscopic insertion is occlusion of the stent. In the series of patients from Amsterdam with pancreatic cancer, 10-French stents were placed. Jaundice recurred in 37.5 per cent of patients; in 21 per cent, the stent was

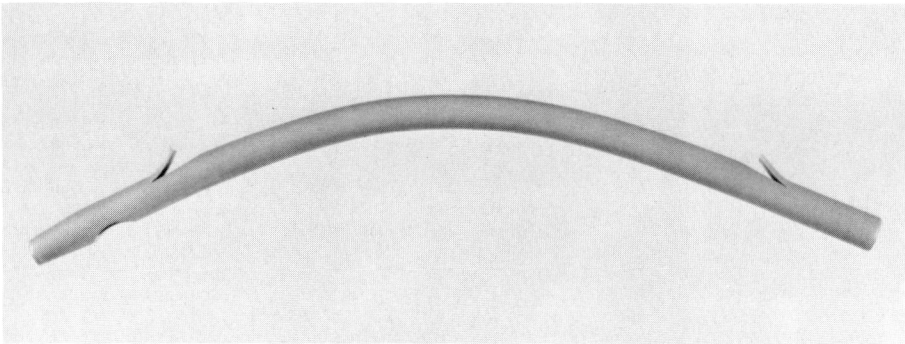

Figure 60–10. A straight stent intended for endoscopic placement across malignant biliary strictures. The flaps at either end are designed to prevent migration.

found to be clogged after it was removed. The stents in the remaining patients may also have been clogged, but these patients were in "near-terminal condition" and not investigated further. The mean time to stent occlusion was five months (range 8 to 419 days).[102] In the New York series, 30 per cent of the 10-French stents occluded within three months and 70 per cent within six months.[106] No occlusions were reported with 12-French stents in this initial study, but further follow-up data suggested that the life span of these stents was longer than that of narrower stents. The mean duration of patency was 190 days for 12-French stents and 150 days for 9- to 10-French stents.[112]

Comparisons between the methods for palliation of malignant biliary obstruction are hindered by a paucity of comparative data from controlled studies. Two points are generally accepted, however. First, the patient with a potentially curable lesion should have surgery if the operative risk is acceptable. If the disease is unresectable at laparotomy, a biliary bypass should be performed. Second, there is little to suggest that stents are preferable to surgery in incurable patients with respect to long-term survival.[106, 113] The issue is how to provide relief of malignant biliary obstruction with the least procedure-related morbidity, mortality, cost, and total time spent in the hospital.

Perhaps the ideal way to address these questions would be a multicenter, randomized three-armed study comparing surgery and the two techniques for stenting. In the absence of such a study, the only controlled trials available are those from single centers comparing two of the three treatment modalities. The first prospective, randomized trial of transhepatic stents versus surgery for pancreatic cancer, reported from Cape Town, showed similar rates of successful insertion, complications, and 30-day morbidity. Survival was not significantly different between the two groups, but there was a favorable trend in 30-day survival in the patients receiving stents. A shorter median initial hospitalization in the group that was stented was offset later by the greater need for readmission caused by blocked stents and gastric outlet obstruction.[114] A controlled trial of transhepatic versus endoscopic stents at the Middlesex Hospital revealed slightly better biliary drainage in the endoscopic group and a higher complication rate in the percutaneous group. This was the first prospective, controlled trial to demonstrate a higher morbidity with the percutaneous approach. It should be noted that the Middlesex study involved a highly proficient group of endoscopists and that the rates for successful transhepatic insertion and drainage of 76 per cent and 61 per cent, respectively, were lower than reported in several other series. Also, the rate of complications for transhepatic stent insertion, 67 per cent, was high. Complications were rigorously defined and included occurrences such as intraperi-

toneal bile discovered at autopsy or by sonography that have not been included as complications in other series. Even if this is taken into consideration, it is notable that 30-day mortality was lower in the group in whom stents were placed endoscopically and that the authors attributed the difference in mortality (15 per cent versus 33 per cent) at least in part to complications related to the percutaneous procedure.[115] Finally, in a randomized study of stents placed endoscopically versus surgical biliary bypass in patients with unresectable carcinoma of the pancreas, there was a trend, not reaching statistical significance, toward a higher 30-day mortality in the operated group (9 per cent versus 20 per cent). Both initial and total hospital times were significantly less in the stented group.[116]

On the basis of presently available information, it seems reasonable to conclude that stenting is a viable alternative to surgery in patients with malignant biliary obstruction and unresectable tumors and that when stenting is chosen, the endoscopic approach should be the initial one. The transhepatic approach should be reserved for patients in whom the endoscopic approach fails. Some endoscopists, however, may prefer the transhepatic approach initially in patients with tumors at the hilum of the liver.

The most important contraindication to biliary stenting is duodenal obstruction by the tumor, in which case surgery with biliary bypass and gastroenterostomy should be performed.

PREOPERATIVE BILIARY DRAINAGE

A potential indication for nonoperative drainage of the biliary tract, distinct from long-term palliation, is in the preoperative care of patients for whom surgery is ultimately planned. A variety of clinical and experimental observations led to the notion that postoperative morbidity and mortality could be reduced by providing biliary drainage preoperatively.[117–119] Decreases in postoperative sepsis and renal failure were particularly prominent among the proposed advantages of preoperative biliary decompression.

The soundness of this belief initially appeared to be supported by several retrospective or uncontrolled studies demonstrating favorable effects on postoperative mobidity, mortality, or both when the biliary tract was drained preoperatively by the percutaneous route.[120–123] However, three prospective, randomized, controlled trials in which percutaneous drainage was performed for a mean of 11 to 18 days prior to surgery failed to demonstrate any salutory effects.[124–126] Moreover, costs of hospitalization and time in hospital were increased significantly in the patients drained preoperatively.[124] In one of the three randomized studies,[125] half the patients who died after laparotomy preceded by biliary drainage had technically difficult operations attributed to dislodgement of catheters, bile leakage, or both. Nevertheless, there is no definite indication in these randomized studies that the preoperative drainage approach would have emerged as superior in terms of postoperative morbidity and mortality if the complications of the drainage itself are discounted.

BENIGN STRICTURES OF THE BILE DUCT

Radiologists and endoscopists have acquired some experience with Gruntzig-type balloon dilation for benign postoperative strictures of the bile duct and for stenotic choledochoenterostomies.[127-131] High rates of success have been reported in the short term. Mueller and colleagues reported a patency rate of 67 per cent at three years after percutaneous dilation of strictures.[130] Several sessions over a period of months may be required to permit inflation with the largest available balloons. It is unclear how often it is necessary to place a stent in a duct that has just been dilated with a balloon. This course is advocated by some on the basis of high recurrence rates with balloon dilation alone.[131] Conversely, at least one endoscopic group considers stenting to be effective in its own right, with efficacy extending past the time of stent clogging or removal, and reserves dilation for patients in whom stents cannot be passed initially.[132] The role of nonoperative treatment for biliary strictures and the standardization of technique will require further study.

Combinations of balloon dilation and stents have also been used in patients with primary sclerosing cholangitis.[130, 133] This approach would appear to have its greatest potential effect in patients with dominant extrahepatic duct strictures. Favorable short-term responses have been reported even with dilation of multiple strictures.

Recent data from small numbers of patients suggest that balloon dilation of the papilla in patients with stenosis may not be as effective in producing clinical improvement or decreases in sphincter of Oddi pressures as sphincterotomy and may be associated with a substantial risk of pancreatitis.[134]

REFERENCES

1. Cotton PB. Endoscopic management of bile duct stones (apples and oranges). Gut 25:587, 1984.
2. Classen M. Endoscopic papillotomy—new indications, short and long-term results. Clin Gastroenterol 15:457, 1986.
3. Silvis SE. Current status of endoscopic sphincterotomy. Am J Gastroenterol 79:731, 1984.
4. Siegel JH. Precut papillotomy: a method to improve success of ERCP and papillotomy. Endoscopy 12:130, 1980.
5. Tanaka M, Matsumoto S, Ikeda S, et al. Endoscopic sphincterotomy in patients with difficult cannulation: use of an antegrade guide. Endoscopy 18:87, 1986.
6. Huibregtse K, Katon RM, Tytgat GNJ. Precut papillotomy via fine needle-knife papillotome: a safe and effective technique. Gastrointest Endosc 32:403, 1986.
7. Zimmon DS. New bile duct interventions: critiques and caveats. Gastrointest Endosc 32:425, 1986.
8. Kozarek RA, Sanowski RA. Endoscopic choledochoduodenostomy. Gastrointest Endosc 29:119, 1983.
9. Shorvon PJ, Cotton PB, Mason RR, et al. Percutaneous transhepatic assistance for duodenoscopic sphincterotomy. Gut 26:1373, 1986.
10. Long W, Ring E. Endoscopic sphincterotomy assisted by catheterization antegrade. Gastrointest Endosc 30:36, 1984.
11. Cohen H, Quinn M. Antegrade assistance for retrograde sphincterotomy using a new sphincterotome. Gastrointest Endosc 32:405, 1986.
12. Rosseland AR, Osnes M, Krause A. Endoscopic sphincterotomy in patients with Billroth II gastrectomy. Endoscopy 13:19, 1981.
13. Siegel JH, Yatto RP. ERCP and endoscopic papillotomy in patients with a Billroth II gastrectomy: report of a method. Gastrointest Endosc 29:116, 1983.
14. Safrany L, Neuhaus B, Portocarrero G, et al. Endoscopic sphincterotomy in patients with Billroth II gastrectomy. Endoscopy 12:16, 1980.
15. Forbes A, Cotton PB. ERCP and sphincterotomy after Billroth II gastrectomy. Gut 25:971, 1984.
16. Osnes M, Rosseland AR, Aabakken L. Endoscopic retrograde cholangiography in patients with a previous Billroth II resection. Gut 27:1193, 1986.
17. Haagenmuller F, Classen M. Therapeutic endoscopic and percutaneous procedures for biliary disorders. In: Popper H, Schaffner F, eds. Progress in Liver Diseases, Vol. 8, New York, Grune & Stratton, 1982:299.
18. Geenen JE, Vennes JA, Silvis SE. Resume of a seminar on endoscopic retrograde cholangiopancreatography. Gastrointest Endosc 27:31, 1981.
19. Leese T, Neoptolemos JP, Carr-Locke DL. Successes, failures, early complications and their management following endoscopic sphincterotomy: results in 394 consecutive patients from a single center. Br J Surg 72:215, 1985.
20. Dunham F, Bourgeois N, Gelin M, et al. Retroperitoneal perforations following endoscopic sphincterotomy, clinical course and management. Endoscopy 14:92, 1982.
21. Sarr MG, Fishman EK, Mulligan FD. Pancreatitis or duodenal perforation after peri-Vaterian therapeutic endoscopic procedures: diagnosis, differentiation and management. Surgery 100:461, 1986.
22. Ell C, Geocze S, Riemann JF. Successful endoscopic treatment of extensive papillary stenosis six years after endoscopic sphincterotomy. Endoscopy 16:246, 1984.
23. Hawes R, Vallon AG, Holton JM, et al. Long-term follow-up after duodenoscopic sphincterotomy (DS) for choledocholithiasis in patients with prior cholecystectomy. Gastrointestinal Endoscopy 33:157, 1987. (Abstract.)
24. Geenen JE, Toouli J, Hogan WJ, et al. Endoscopic sphincterotomy: follow-up evaluation of effects on the sphincter of Oddi. Gastroenterology 87:754, 1984.
25. Classen M, Demling L. Endoskopische Sphinkterotomie der papilla Vateri. Dtsch Med Wochenschr 99:496, 1974.
26. Kawai K, Akasaka Y, Murakami K, et al. Endoscopic sphincterotomy of the ampulla of Vater. Gastrointest Endosc 20:148, 1974.
27. Girard RM, Legros G. Retained and recurrent bile duct stones. Surgical or non-surgical removal. Ann Surg 193:150, 1981.
28. de Almeida AM, Cruz AG, Aldeia FJ. Side-to-side choledochoduodenostomy in the management of choledocholithiasis and associated disease: facts and fiction. Am J Surg 147:253, 1984.
29. McSherry CK, Glenn F. The incidence and causes of death following surgery for non-malignant biliary tract disease. Ann Surg 191:271, 1980.
30. Lygidakis NJ. Surgical approaches to recurrent choledocholithiasis. Am J Surg 145:633, 1983.
31. Schein CJ, Gliedman ML. Choledochoduodenostomy as an adjunct to choledocholithotomy. Surg Gynecol Obstet 146:25, 1978.
32. Moesgaard F, Nielsen ML, Pedersen T, et al. Protective choledochoduodenostomy in multiple common duct stones in the aged. Surg Gynecol Obstet 154:232, 1982.
33. Doyle PJ, Ward-McQuaid JN, McEwen-Smith A. The value of routine pre-operative cholangiography—a report of 4000 cholecystectomies. Br J Surg 69:617, 1982.
34. Vellacott KD, Powell PH. Exploration of the common bile duct: a comparative study. Br J Surg 66:389, 1979.
35. Glenn F. Trends in surgical management of calculus disease of the biliary tract. Surg Gynecol Obstet 140:877, 1975.
36. Venu RP, Geenen JE, Toouli J, et al. Gallstone dissolution using mono-octanoin infusion through an endoscopically placed nasobiliary catheter. Am J Gastroenterol 77:287, 1982.
37. Schmack B. Dissolution of bile duct stones. Endoscopy 15:186, 1983.
38. Palmer KR, Hoffman AF. Intraductal mono-octanoin for the direct dissolution of bile duct stones: experience in 343 patients. Gut 27:196, 1986.
39. Riemann JF, Demling L. Lithotripsy of bile duct stones. Endoscopy 15:191, 1983.
40. Harrison J, Morris DL, Haynes J, et al. Electrohydraulic lithotripsy of gallstones—in vitro and animal studies. Gut 28:267, 1987.
41. Tanaka M, Yushimoto H, Ikeda S, et al. Two approaches for electrohydraulic lithotripsy in common bile duct. Surgery 98:313, 1985.
42. Burhenne HJ. Electrohydraulic fragmentation of retained common duct stones. Radiology 117:721, 1975.
43. Koch H, Stolze N, Waly V. Endoscopic lithotripsy in the common bile duct. Endoscopy 9:95, 1977.
44. Silvis SE, Siegel JE, Hughes R, et al. Use of electrohydraulic lithotripsy

to fracture common bile duct stones. Gastrointest Endosc 32:155, 1986. (Abstract.)

45. Sauerbruch T, Delius M, Paumgartner G. Fragmentation of gallstones by extracorporeal shock waves. N Engl J Med 314:818, 1986.

46. Siegel JH, Yatto RP. Biliary endoprosthesis for the management of retained common bile duct stones. Am J Gastroenterol 79:50, 1984.

47. Cotton PB, Forbes A, Leung JWC. Endoscopic stenting for long-term treatment of large bile duct stones: 2- to 5-year follow-up. Gastrointest Endosc 33:411, 1987.

48. Nishioka NS, Levins PC, Murray SC, et al. Fragmentation of biliary calculi with tunable dye lasers. Gastroenterology 93:250, 1987.

49. Lux G, Ell C, Hochberger J, et al. The first successful endoscopic retrograde laser lithotripsy of common bile duct stones in man using a pulsed neodynium-YAG laser. Endoscopy 18:144, 1986.

50. Escourrou J, Cordova JA, Lagorthes F, et al. Early and late complications after endoscopic sphincterotomy for biliary lithiasis with and without the gallbladder "in situ." Gut 25:598, 1984.

51. Rosseland AR, Solhaug JH. Primary endoscopic papillotomy (EPT) in patients with stones in the common bile duct and the gallbladder in situ: a 5–8 year follow-up study. World J Surg 12:111, 1988.

52. Cotton PB. Two to nine year follow-up after sphincterotomy for stones in patients with gallbladders. Gastrointest Endosc 32:157, 1986.

53. Siegel JH, Ramsey WH, Pullano W. Cost effectiveness of two interventional endoscopic biliary procedures: Does anyone really care? Gastrointest Endosc 32:181, 1986. (Abstract.)

54. Neoptolemos JP, Carr-Locke DL, Fossard DP. Prospective randomized study of preoperative endoscopic sphincterotomy versus surgery alone for common bile duct stones. Br Med J 294:470, 1987.

55. Boey JH, Way LW. Acute cholangitis. Ann Surg 191:264, 1980.

56. Andrew DJ, Johnson SE. Acute suppurative cholangitis. A medical and surgical emergency. Am J Gastroenterol 54:141, 1970.

57. Gogel HK, Runyon BA, Volpicelli NA, et al. Acute suppurative obstructive cholangitis due to stones: treatment by urgent endoscopic sphincterotomy. Gastrointest Endosc 33:210, 1987.

58. Leung JWC, Chung SCS, Li AKC. Is there a role for urgent endoscopic drainage in acute suppurative cholangitis? Gastrointest Endosc 33:157, 1987. (Abstract.)

59. Leese T, Neoptolemos JP, Baker AR, et al. Management of acute cholangitis and the impact of endoscopic sphincterotomy. Br J Surg 73:988, 1986.

60. Safrany L, Cotton PB. A preliminary report. Urgent duodenoscopic sphincterotomy for acute gallstone-related pancreatitis. Surgery 89:424, 1981.

61. Rosseland AR, Solhaug JH. Early or delayed endoscopic papillotomy in gallstone pancreatitis. Ann Surg 199:165, 1984.

62. Escourrou J, Ligoury C, Boyer J, et al. Emergency and endoscopic sphincterotomy in acute biliary pancreatitis: results of a multicenter study. Gastrointest Endosc 33:187, 1987. (Abstract.)

63. Neoptolemos JP, Carr-Locke DL, London NJ, et al: Controlled trial of urgent endoscopic retrograde cholangio-pancreatography and endoscopic sphincterotomy versus conservative treatment for acute pancreatitis due to gallstones. Lancet 2:979, 1988.

64. Glenn F. Retained calculi within the biliary ductal system. Ann Surg 179:528, 1974.

65. Way LW, Admirand WH, Dunphy JE. Management of choledocholithiasis. Ann Surg 176:347, 1972.

66. Heuman R, Smeds S, Hellgren E, et al. Evaluation of factors affecting the incidence of retained calculi in the bile ducts. Acta Chir Scand 148:185, 1982.

67. Bauer JJ, Sulky BA, Gelernt KM, et al. Experience with the flexible fiberoptic choledochoscope. Ann Surg 194:161, 1981.

68. Kappes SK, Adams MB, Wilson SD. Intraoperative biliary endoscopy: mandatory for all common duct operations? Arch Surg 117:603, 1982.

69. Yap PC, Atacodor M, Yap AG, et al. Choledochoscopy as a complementary procedure to operative cholangiography in biliary surgery. Am J Surg 140:648, 1980.

70. Nora PF, Berci G, Dorazio RA, et al. Operative choledochoscopy: results of a prospective study in several institutions. Am J Surg 133:105, 1977.

71. Burhenne HJ. The technique of biliary duct stone extraction: experience with 126 cases. Radiology 113:567, 1974.

72. Mason RR. Percutaneous extraction of retained gallstones. Clin Gastroenterol 14:403, 1985.

73. Ferrucci JT Jr, Butch RJ, Mueller PR. Biliary stone removal. In: Ferrucci JT Jr, Wittenberg J, Mueller PR, et al, eds. Interventional Radiology of the Abdomen, 2nd ed. Baltimore, Williams & Wilkins, 1985:298.

74. Garrow DG. The removal of retained biliary tract stones: report of 105 cases. Br J Surg 50:777, 1977.

75. Burhenne HJ. Percutaneous extraction of retained biliary tract stones: 661 patients. Am J Roentgenol 134:888, 1980.

76. O'Doherty DP, Neoptolemos JP, Carr-Locke DL. Endoscopic sphinc-

terotomy for retained common bile duct stones in patients with T-tubes in situ in the early postoperative period. Br J Surg 73:454, 1986.

77. Geenen JE, Hogan WJ, Dodds WJ. Sphincter of Oddi. In: Sivak MV Jr. Gastroenterologic Endoscopy. Philadelphia, WB Saunders, 1987:735.

78. Geenen J, Hogan W, Toouli J, et al. A prospective randomized study of the efficacy of endoscopic sphincterotomy for patients with presumptive sphincter of Oddi dysfunction. Gastroenterology 86:1086, 1983. (Abstract.)

79. Geenen JE, Hogan WJ, Dodds WJ, et al: The efficacy of endoscopic sphincterotomy after cholecystectomy in patients with sphincter-of-Oddi dysfunction. N Engl J Med 32:82, 1989.

80. Roberts-Thompson IC, Toouli J. Is endoscopic sphincterotomy for disabling biliary-type pain after cholecystectomy effective? Gastrointest Endosc 31:370, 1985.

81. Thatcher BS, Sivak MV Jr, Tedesco FJ, et al. Endoscopic sphincterotomy for suspected dysfunction of the sphincter of Oddi. Gastrointest Endosc 33:91, 1987.

82. Mueller PR, Ferrucci JT Jr, van Sonnenberg E, et al. Obstruction of the left hepatic duct: diagnosis and treatment by selective fine-needle cholangiography and percutaneous biliary drainage. Radiology 145:297, 1982.

83. Pogany AC, Kerlan RK Jr, Ring EJ. Percutaneous biliary drainage. Clin Gastroenterol 14:387, 1985.

84. Mueller PR, Butch RJ, Bonnel D. Percutaneous biliary drainage: results and complications. In: Ferrucci JT Jr, Wittenberg J, Mueller PR, et al, eds. Interventional Radiology of the Abdomen, 2nd ed. Baltimore, Williams & Wilkins, 1985:250.

85. Mueller PR, van Sonnenberg E, Ferrucci JT Jr. Percutaneous biliary drainage: technical and catheter-related problems in 200 procedures. Am J Roentgenol 138:17, 1982.

86. Nakayama T, Ikeda A, Okuda K. Percutaneous transhepatic drainage of the biliary tract: technique and results in 104 cases. Gastroenterology 74:554, 1978.

87. Hamlin JA, Friedman M, Stein MG, et al. Percutaneous biliary drainage: complications of 118 consecutive catheterizations. Radiology 158:199, 1986.

88. Carrasco CH, Zornoza J, Bechtel WJ. Malignant biliary obstruction: complications of percutaneous biliary drainage. Radiology 152:343, 1984.

89. Dooley JS, Dick R, George P, et al. Percutaneous transhepatic endoprosthesis for bile duct obstruction: complications and results. Gastroenterology 86:905, 1984.

90. Burcharth F, Jensen LI, Olesen K. Endoprosthesis for internal drainage of the biliary tract: technique and results in 48 cases. Gastroenterology 77:133, 1979.

91. Riemann JF. Complications of percutaneous bile drainage. In: Classen M, Geenen J, Kawai K, eds. Nonsurgical Biliary Drainage. New York, Springer-Verlag, 1984:29.

92. Burcharth F, Efsen F, Christiaansen LA, et al. Nonsurgical internal biliary drainage by endoprosthesis. Surg Gynecol Obstet 153:857, 1981.

93. Pereiros RU, Rheingold OJ, Hutton D, et al. Relief of malignant obstructive jaundice by percutaneous insertion of a permanent prosthesis in the biliary tree. Ann Intern Med 39:589, 1978.

94. Coons HG, Carey PH. Large-bore, long biliary endoprostheses (biliary stents) for improved drainage. Radiology 148:89, 1983.

95. Soehendra N, Reijnders-Frederix V. Palliative bile duct drainage. A new endoscopic method of introducing a transpapillary drain. Endoscopy 12:8, 1980.

96. Laurence BH, Cotton PB. Decompression of malignant biliary obstruction by duodenscopic intubation of the bile duct. Br Med J 280:522, 1980.

97. Huibregtse K, Tytgat GNJ. Palliative treatment of obstructive jaundice by transpapillary introduction of large-bore bile duct endoprostheses. Experience in 45 patients. Gut 23:371, 1982.

98. Siegel JH, Pullano W, Kodsi B, et al: Optimal palliation of malignant bile duct obstruction: experience with endoscopic 12 French prostheses. Endoscopy 20:137, 1988.

99. Siegel JH. Improved biliary decompression with large-caliber endoscopic prostheses. Gastrointest Endosc 30:21, 1984.

100. Haagenmuller F. Results of endoscopic bilioduodenal drainage in malignant bile duct stenosis. In: Classen M, Geenen JE, Kawai K, eds. Nonsurgical biliary drainage, New York, Springer-Verlag, 1984:93.

101. Cotton PB. Endoscopic methods for relief of malignant obstructive jaundice. World J Surg 8:854, 1984.

102. Huibregste K, Katon RM, Coene PP, et al. Endoscopic palliative treatment in pancreatic cancer. Gastrointest Endosc 32:334, 1986.

103. Leung JWC, Del Farero G, Cotton PB. Endoscopic biliary prosthesis: a comparison of materials. Gastrointest Endosc 31:93, 1985.

104. Speer AG, Leung JWC, Yin TP, et al. Ten–French gauge straight biliary stents perform significantly better than 8–French gauge pigtail stents. Gastrointest Endosc 31:140, 1985. (Abstract.)

105. Cunningham JT, Cotton PB, Speer AG. A biliary cannulation sleeve. Gastrointest Endosc 32:407, 1986.

106. Siegel JH, Snady H. The significance of endoscopically placed prostheses in the management of biliary obstruction due to carcinoma of the pancreas: results of nonoperative decompression in 277 patients. Am J Gastroenterol 81:634, 1986.

107. Stoker J, Dees J, Blankenstein M van, Nux GAJJ. Results of endoscopic stenting in malignant stricture of the biliary tract. Gut 26:A1135, 1985.

108. Leung JWC, Emery R, Cotton PB. Management of malignant obstructive jaundice at the Middlesex Hospital. Br J Surg 70:584, 1983.

109. Huibregtse K. Techniques of endoscopic bile drainage. In: Classen M, Geenen J, Kawai K, eds. Nonoperative biliary drainage. New York, Springer-Verlag, 1984:69.

110. Tytgat GNJ, Huibregtse K, Bartelsman JFWM, et al. Endoscopic palliative therapy of gastrointestinal and biliary tumors with prostheses. Clin Gastroenterol 15:249, 1986.

111. Speer AG, Cotton PB, Dineen LP. Endoscopic stents in malignant hilar strictures—results in 70 patients. Gastrointest Endosc 32:156, 1986. (Abstract.)

112. Siegel JH, Pullano W, Cooperman A. Carcinoma of the pancreas: endotherapy as primary care. Gastrointest Endosc 33:159, 1987. (Abstract.)

113. Cotton PB. Endoscopic biliary stents—trick or treatment? Gastrointest Endosc 32:364, 1986. (Editorial.)

114. Bornman PC, Harriet-Jones EP, Tobias R, et al. Prospective controlled trial of transhepatic biliary endoprosthesis versus bypass surgery for incurable carcinoma of the pancreas. Lancet 1:69, 1986.

115. Speer AG, Cotton PB, Russell RCG, et al. Randomized trial of endoscopic versus percutaneous stent insertion in malignant obstructive jaundice. Lancet 2:57, 1987.

116. Shepherd HA, Royle G, Ross APR, et al: Endoscopic biliary endoprostheses in the palliation of malignant obstruction of the distal common bile duct: a randomized trial. Br J Surg 75:1166, 1988.

117. Koyuma K, Takagi Y, Ito K, et al. Experimental and clinical studies on the effect of biliary drainage in obstructive jaundice. Am J Surg 142:293, 1981.

118. Blumgart LH. Biliary tract obstruction: new approaches to old problems. Am J Surg 135:19, 1978.

119. Pitt HA, Cameron JL, Postier RG, et al. Factors affecting mortality in biliary tract surgery. Am J Surg 141:66, 1981.

120. Nakayama T, Ikeda A, Okuda K. Percutaneous transhepatic drainage of the biliary tract—technique and results in 104 cases. Gastroenterology 74:554, 1978.

121. Denning DA, Ellison EC, Carey LC. Preoperative percutaneous transhepatic biliary decompression lowers operative morbidity in patients with obstructive jaundice. Am J Surg 141:61, 1981.

122. Norlander A, Kalin B, Sundblad R. Effect of percutaneous transhepatic drainage upon liver function and postoperative mortality. Surg Gynecol Obstet 144:161, 1982.

123. Gundry SR, Strodel WE, Knol JA, et al. Efficacy of preoperative biliary tract decompression in patients with obstructive jaundice. Arch Surg 119:703, 1984.

124. Hatfield ARW, Tobias R, Terblanche J, et al. Preoperative external biliary drainage in obstructive jaundice: a prospective controlled clinical trial. Lancet 2:896, 1982.

125. McPherson GAD, Benjamin IS, Hodgson HJF, et al. Preoperative percutaneous biliary drainage: the results of a controlled trial. Br J Surg 71:371, 1984.

126. Pitt HA, Gomes AS, Lois JF, et al. Does preoperative percutaneous biliary drainage reduce operative risk or increase hospital cost? Ann Surg 201:545, 1985.

127. Geenen JE. Balloon dilatation of the bile duct strictures. In: Classen M, Geenen J, Kawai K, eds. Nonsurgical Biliary Drainage. New York, Springer-Verlag, 1984:105.

128. Siegel JH, Guelrud M. Endoscopic cholangiopancreatography: hydrostatic balloon dilatation in the bile duct and pancreas. Gastrointest Endosc 29:99, 1983.

129. Foutch PG, Sivak MV Jr. Therapeutic endoscopic balloon dilatation of the extraheptic biliary ducts. Am J Gastroenterol 80:575, 1985.

130. Mueller PR, van Sonnenberg E, Ferrucci JT Jr, et al. Biliary stricture dilatation: multicenter review of clinical management in 73 patients. Radiology 160:17, 1986.

131. Salomonowitz E, Castaneda-Zuniga WR, Lund G, et al. Balloon dilatation of biliary strictures. Radiology 151:613, 1984.

132. Huibregtse K, Katon RM, Tytgat GNJ. Endoscopic treatment of postoperative biliary strictures. Endoscopy 18:133, 1986.

133. May GR, Bender CE, LaRusso NF, et al. Nonoperative management of dominant strictures in primary sclerosing cholangitis. Am J Roentgenol 145:1061, 1985.

134. Bader M, Geenen JE, Hogan WJ, et al. Endoscopic balloon dilatation of the sphincter of Oddi in patients with suspected biliary dyskinesia: results of a prospective randomized trial. Gastrointest Endosc 32:158, 1986. (Abstract.)

61

Extracorporeal Shock Wave Lithotripsy of Gallstones

Gustav Paumgartner, M.D. • Tilman Sauerbruch, M.D.

Shock wave lithotripsy of kidney stones became a standard procedure soon after its introduction in 1980.[1] The same principle had been tested for the destruction of gallstones in animal experiments by Brendel and Enders[2] in 1983 and had for the first time been applied to patients by Sauerbruch and co-workers in 1986.[3] By 1989, more than 3000 patients with gallstones had been treated in different centers throughout the world by this novel technique. Extracorporeal shock wave lithotripsy of gallstones may now be regarded as a rapidly evolving new technology in medicine. In the United States it is still restricted to investigational programs, since gallstone lithotripters have not been approved by the Food and Drug Administration at this time.

PHYSICAL AND BIOLOGICAL ASPECTS OF SHOCK WAVES

Shock waves are pressure waves that obey the laws of acoustics. Unlike sound waves or conventional diagnostic or therapeutic ultrasound waves, they are not a sinusoidally varying alternating compression and rarefaction of the medium through which they travel. The pressure wave form

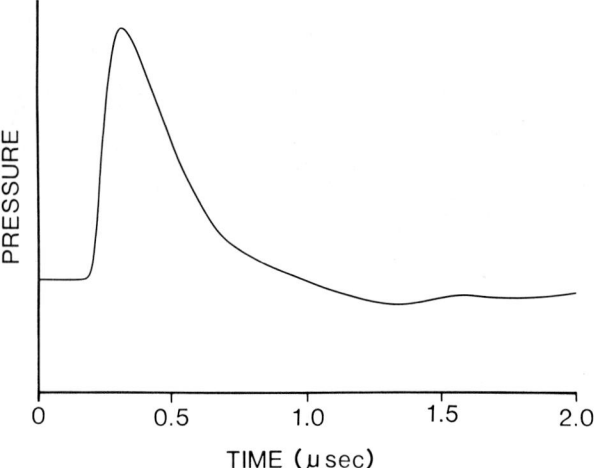

Figure 61–1. Pressure wave form measured at the focus of the Dornier lithotripter MPL 9000 using a polyvinylidene fluoride (PVDF) membrane hydrophone needle probe.

is highly distorted from the normal representation of a sinusoidally varying pressure. This distortion of an acoustic wave occurs when the pressure and density locally become so high that the relationship between pressure and density becomes nonlinear and the speed of sound increases as the pressure rises.[4, 5] Shock waves are characterized by a positive pressure pulse with an extremely short rise time, which is in the order of nanoseconds, and a slower pressure decline. The total positive pressure pulse duration is less than 1 μsec (Fig. 61–1). The positive pressure pulse is followed by a negative pressure pulse of much lower amplitude and longer duration.[5]

Shock waves can be generated by different principles. In the currently available lithotripters, an underwater spark discharge, piezoelectric crystals, and electromagnetic membranes are used (Table 61–1). For medical purposes, only focused shock waves are used. Focusing of shock waves creates high pressures (up to about 1000 bar) in a small volume. Depending on the principle used for shock wave generation, the shock waves are focused with one of the following devices: An ellipsoidal metal reflector is used when the shock waves are generated by underwater spark discharge. In order to focus piezoelectrically generated shock waves, several thousand piezoelectric crystals are mounted on a spherical dish. Acoustic lenses are used to focus electromagnetically generated shock waves. The focal volume is defined as the space in which pressures of at least 50 per cent of the maximum pressure occur. In the more advanced lithotripters, the length and width of the focal volume range from 9 to 90 mm and from 3 to 15 mm, respectively.[6] This design keeps shock wave–induced tissue

TABLE 61–1. PRINCIPLES OF SHOCK WAVE GENERATION AND FOCUSING EMPLOYED IN VARIOUS LITHOTRIPTER DESIGNS

Shock Wave Generation	Focusing	Manufacturers
Underwater spark discharge	Ellipsoidal reflector	Dornier, Direx, Medstone, Northgate, Technomed
Piezoelectric crystals	Shaped array	EDAP, Wolf
Electromagnetic membrane	Acoustic lens	Siemens

injury outside this zone to a minimum. Tissues particularly susceptible to shock wave damage are the lungs, where rupture of alveoli may occur. In the liver, gallbladder, and kidney, no major tissue damage has been observed provided a certain dose limit is not exceeded. Minor tissue damage and hematuria can occur if the kidney is exposed to focused shock waves. In the skin, at the site of shock wave entry, petechiae can be caused. Tissue injury depends not only on the energy of the single shock wave pulse but also on the cumulative energy applied during treatment.

In all three types of lithotripters, the shock wave source is under water. The shock waves travel through water with little loss of energy. They are transmitted into the body by a compressible bag filled with water that is interfaced with the skin by an ultrasonic coupling gel or by various types of water basins. The shock waves travel practically unimpeded through the body's soft tissues. When they hit the stone, there is a change of acoustical impedance at the anterior and posterior surfaces of the stone. Accordingly, compressive and tensile forces act on the stone. Most importantly, cavitation phenomena occur on the stone's surface. These effects of shock waves result in stone fragmentation.

The physicochemical characteristics of gallstones that facilitate fragmentation by shock waves have not been defined. The ease with which stones are fragmented cannot be predicted from chemical composition.[7] Size of stones and characteristics of their structure, which are still poorly defined, appear to be important determinants for fragmentability by shock waves.

GALLBLADDER STONES

INDICATIONS FOR EXTRACORPOREAL SHOCK WAVE LITHOTRIPSY

The major selection criteria for shock-wave lithotripsy at present are derived from the first large series, in which a combination of lithotripsy and bile acid dissolution therapy was employed.[8, 9] These criteria may undergo modification as experience increases, the method proves to be safe, and early second treatments can be considered (Table 61–2).

Patients with asymptomatic gallbladder stones should not undergo prophylactic shock wave lithotripsy.[10] This recommendation is based on studies of the natural history of gallstone disease, which show that asymptomatic cholelithiasis is a benign disease that in general does not warrant intervention by presently available treatments.[11, 12] Therefore, patients considered for shock wave lithotripsy should be symptomatic—that is, they must have had one or more episodes of acute biliary pain, conventionally misnamed colic. Acute biliary pain is characterized by epigastric or right upper quadrant pain lasting more than 15 minutes but less than five hours.[10]

The stones should consist predominantly of cholesterol—that is, they must be radiolucent or should have a low density by computed tomography. Experience shows that not all retained fragments are discharged from the gallbladder and that such fragments must be dissolved by adjuvant litholytic therapy. Further selection criteria can be derived from the early results of shock wave lithotripsy of gallbladder stones.[9] These studies show that the success rate, defined as complete disappearance of fragments, decreases with an increase in stone size and number and also with stone calcification. Therefore, single stones should be

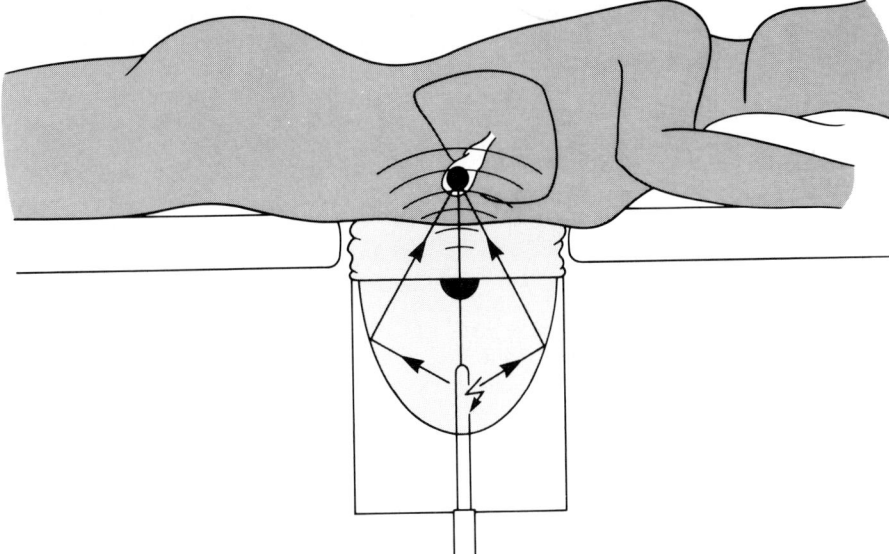

Figure 61-2. Schematic illustration of Dornier lithotripter MPL 9000 and positioning of the patient for treatment of gallbladder stone. The shock waves are generated by underwater spark discharge at the first focus of an ellipsoidal reflector. The stone is positioned at the second (remote) focus. Coupling of the shock wave generator to the skin is achieved by a compressible bag filled with water. An in-line ultrasound transducer is used for targeting.

less than 30 mm in diameter (corresponding to a stone volume of about 14 cc) and multiple stones should exceed neither three in number nor a total stone volume of about 14 ml. It has been shown that stones with calcified rims can be fragmented, but the time required for complete disappearance of stones is longer, more retreatments are needed, or both.[13]

Patency of the cystic duct is required for both passage and dissolution of fragments. This must be documented prior to lithotripsy either by oral cholecystography[9] or by ultrasonography and stimulation of gallbladder contraction.[14]

The complete list of inclusion and exclusion criteria is given in Table 61-2. Patients with complications of gallstone disease such as acute cholecystitis, cholangitis, acute biliary pancreatitis, or biliary obstruction should not undergo extracorporeal shock wave lithotripsy.[8] Extracorporeal shock wave lithotripsy of a gallbladder stone should not be considered if a bile duct stone is present, unless the bile duct stone can be removed endoscopically or by shock wave lithotripsy prior to the treatment of the gallbladder stone.

Because of the risk of hematoma, patients with coagulopathy or those receiving medication with anticoagulant effects must be excluded. Pregnancy must be ruled out by a laboratory test.

TABLE 61-2. SELECTION OF PATIENTS WITH GALLBLADDER STONES FOR EXTRACORPOREAL SHOCK WAVE LITHOTRIPSY

Inclusion Criteria

History of biliary pain
Solitary radiolucent stone with a diameter up to 30 mm or 2 to 3 radiolucent stones with similar total stone volume
Gallbladder visualization on oral cholecystography
Clear detection of stone(s) by ultrasound and positioning in the shock wave focus possible

Exclusion Criteria

Acute cholecystitis or cholangitis
Biliary obstruction or bile duct stone
Acute pancreatitis
Coagulopathy or current medication with anticoagulant effects
Vascular aneurysms in the shock wave path
Pregnancy

PROCEDURE

The most important aspects of the procedure are stone imaging, positioning of the patient, targeting, monitoring of the process of fragmentation, and if necessary, relief of pain. For imaging of gallbladder stones, ultrasonography has been far superior to fluoroscopy. Consequently, lithotripters for gallbladder stones should be equipped with ultrasound. An outline scanner can be used to locate the gallbladder and the stone. For exact targeting, however, an in-line scanner in the axis of the shock wave beam is preferable. Inaccuracies in targeting that result from different paths and diffraction of ultrasound and shock waves by tissue layers can thus be eliminated. Lithotripters with a small focal volume, especially, must be equipped with an accurate targeting system.

In general, patients are treated in the prone position (Fig. 61-2).[8, 15] In this position, the stone is close to the surface of the skin and the shock waves reach the stone from the ventral side. If there are floating stones or fragments, the supine position can be more advantageous.

Pain during shock wave application is closely related to the shock wave energy used and especially to the shock-wave pressure applied to the skin. With several lithotripters, mainly of the piezoelectric type, energies that produce pain are not reached. The more powerful lithotripters that use the spark gap principle for shock wave generation, such as the Dornier lithotripter MPL 9000, operate over a wider range of shock wave energies. If higher energies are used for spark discharge, they usually cause pain, and the intravenous administration of an analgesic or sedoanalgesic is needed.[16] Such high energies are mainly necessary for large stones. With the MPL 9000, about half of all procedures require analgesics and the rest are performed without any medication.

ADJUVANT THERAPY

It cannot be expected that all stone fragments be spontaneously discharged from the gallbladder. In fact, many patients with gallstones have a motility defect of the gallbladder that may have contributed to the retention of cholesterol crystals and microliths during stone formation.[17-22] Therefore, in all published studies, extracorporeal shock wave lithotripsy has been combined with oral bile salt therapy in order to dissolve remaining stone fragments.[3, 9, 14, 23-25] The exact role of adjuvant bile acid therapy is now being evaluated in prospective trials.

Most groups[9, 14, 23-25] have used a combination of ursodeoxycholic and chenodeoxycholic acids as suggested in the first report on shock wave lithotripsy of gallbladder stones.[3] Monotherapy with ursodeoxycholic acid is an alternative. The combination of ursodeoxycholic and chenodeoxycholic acids at reduced dose has been chosen because of reports that at full dosage of ursodeoxycholic acid, which is practically free of side effects, stone calcification is more frequent than with chenodeoxycholic acid, which at full dosage often causes diarrhea and elevation of serum transaminase activity. In addition, there is evidence that the combination leads to more rapid dissolution of small stones.[26] This may be explained by the fact that the two bile acids have somewhat different mechanisms of action, so that their effects may therefore be additive.

Dissolution of stone fragments by methyl *tert*-butyl ether is being explored as an alternative adjuvant therapy for patients with very large stone burdens.[27] This therapy must however still be regarded as investigational.

RESULTS OF EXTRACORPOREAL SHOCK WAVE LITHOTRIPSY

Although the initial fragmentation of the stone is of critical importance for the outcome, complete disappearance of all stone fragments and the time required for it are the most important criteria for evaluating the efficacy of extracorporeal shock wave lithotripsy. Disintegration of stones is of value only if successful clearance of fragments can be achieved either by spontaneous passage or by dissolution (Fig. 61–3). Both fragmentation efficacy and efficacy of stone clearance depend not only on the size, number, and type of stones but also on the lithotripter used and on the energy and number of shock waves applied. They may also be influenced by the compliance of the patient with bile acid therapy. With the Dornier lithotripter MPL 9000, a spark-gap instrument, fragmentation, defined as reduction of stone size by more than 50 per cent, was achieved in 94 per cent to 98 per cent of patients.[9, 23] In 75 per cent of patients, fragments were less than 3 mm in diameter.[9] Other instruments have been used in only relatively small numbers of patients.[14, 24, 25] With the Wolf Piezolith 2200/2300, initial fragmentation has been achieved in 88 per cent of patients.[14, 25] In one of these studies,[25] the mean maximal diameter of the largest fragment after the first lithotripsy was 4.3 mm.

Results of stone clearance after a longer period of observation are available from two studies using a lithotripter with spark-gap shock wave generation and targeting by an in-line ultrasound scanner.[9, 23] Sackmann and colleagues achieved complete stone clearance in 48 per cent of all patients at 2 to 4 months, in 63 per cent at 4 to 8 months, in 78 per cent at 8 to 12 months, and in 91 per cent at 12 to 18 months.[9] Results of Greiner and associates, who used the same type of lithotripter, have been somewhat less favorable.[23] This may be explained by a less rigid selection of patients. Ponchon and co-workers,[24] who also used a lithotripter with a spark-gap shock wave generator but used an out-line ultrasound scanner for targeting, reported 53 per cent of patients free of stones at six months after lithotripsy. In the studies of Hood and associates[25] and Ell and colleagues,[14] who used the piezoelectric principle for shock wave generation (Wolf Piezolith 2200/2300), the patients have not been followed long enough to permit a valid comparison with the studies using spark-gap lithotripters. Within two and four months after lithotripsy, 28 and 46 per cent, respectively, of the patients of Ell's group were free of stones.[14] Stone size and number, commonly referred to as stone burden of the gallbladder, are important determinants of the time required for complete stone disappearance. Small solitary stones disappear earlier than do large solitary stones. Thus, solitary stones with a diameter up to 20 mm disappeared in 69 per cent of patients after 2 to 4 months and in 86 per cent after 8 to 12 months. The corresponding figures for large solitary stones were 29 and 81 per cent and for multiple stones, 17 and 40 per cent.[9]

The less favorable results in patients with very large and multiple stones can be explained by the presence of larger fragments after lithotripsy.[9] This appears to be related to the difficulty in identifying residual stones or fragments during lithotripsy treatment after disintegration of the first stone. The same difficulty arises when many relatively large fragments have been created during lithotripsy of a very large stone. Fragmentation of the first stone or a very large stone produces a cloud of fragments in which remaining stones or larger fragments can be hidden. The disintegration of the latter is often less complete and results in larger residual fragments. A longer period of adjuvant bile acid therapy is necessary for dissolution of these remaining calculi.

In patients who are eligible for medical dissolution of

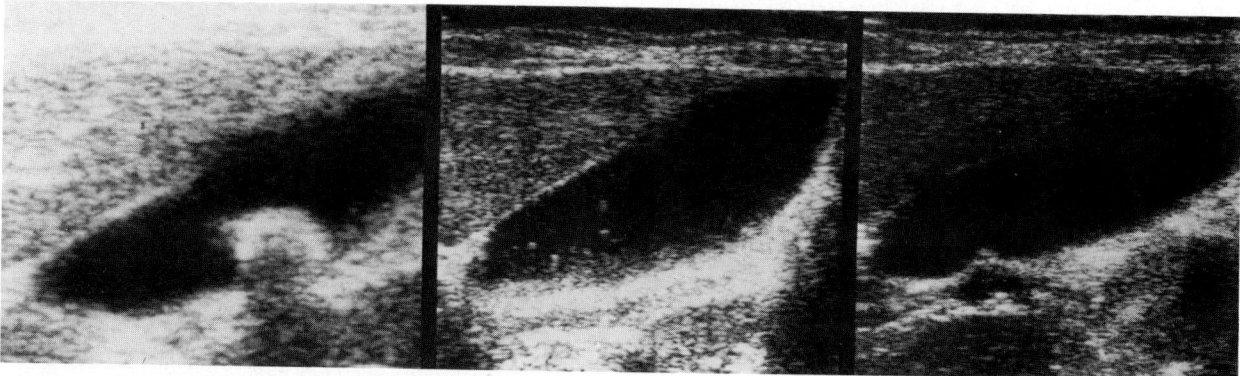

Figure 61–3. Ultrasonogram of a gallbladder with a single stone before (A), one day after (B), and six weeks after (C) extracorporeal shock wave lithotripsy. One day after treatment, multiple small fragments are visible that had disappeared six weeks after lithotripsy and adjuvant litholytic therapy with a combination of ursodeoxycholic and chenodeoxycholic acids.

their gallstones, the combination of shock wave lithotripsy and bile acid therapy achieves complete stone disappearance in a much shorter time and in a higher percentage of patients than does bile acid therapy alone. Stones that fulfill the generally accepted inclusion criteria for dissolution by oral bile acid therapy (radiolucent stones with a diameter of 5 to 15 mm) had completely disappeared in 74 and 94 per cent of patients within 6 and 12 months, respectively, after shock wave and bile acid therapy.[9] The corresponding values reported for litholytic therapy alone are 17 and 36 per cent, respectively.[26]

Results in patients with stones exhibiting a calcified rim have been less favorable.[13] Four to eight months after shock wave lithotripsy, complete stone clearance was observed in only 16 per cent of the patients. Twelve to 18 months after shock wave lithotripsy, this percentage rose to 62 per cent but still stayed far behind the results obtained with radiolucent stones free of calcification. These rather disappointing results are to be expected, since only part of the fragments are susceptible to dissolution by bile acids, and disappearance of the fragments from the gallbladder depends largely on their passage. In the treatment of calcified stones, it therefore is of utmost importance to achieve very small fragments, ideally smaller than 2 to 3 mm in diameter. An early second treatment may be the solution in all those instances previously discussed in which too large fragments delay the achievement of final success. New strategies for the handling of these patients are presently being evaluated. They may considerably influence the success rate of shock wave treatment and may also modify the criteria for patient selection.

Complications directly related to shock wave treatment have been minimal. Sackmann and co-workers observed petechiae of the skin at the site of shock wave entry in 14 per cent of patients.[9] Three per cent of patients had transient gross hematuria. Ell and associates have reported a thickening of the gallbladder wall, detected by ultrasound on the day after shock wave treatment, in 6 per cent of the patients.[14] No hematoma in liver, kidneys, lungs, or other organs could be detected by ultrasound or computed tomography. There were no elevations of transaminases, alkaline phosphatase, γ-glutamine transpeptidase, or bilirubin.[9]

Shock wave treatment had no short-term or long-term effects on parameters of gallbladder motility such as fasting volume, contraction, percentage of emptying, and residual volume, as assessed by cholecystokinin infusion and ultrasonography.[22]

About one third of all patients treated by extracorporeal shock wave lithotripsy had one or more episodes of biliary pain related to the presence of stone fragments. These symptoms disappeared once the gallbladder was free of calculi. This percentage of patients experiencing episodes of pain after lithotripsy appears acceptable if one considers that all patients have been symptomatic before treatment. About 1 to 3 per cent of the patients develop mild pancreatitis.[9, 14, 23] These events are also not directly related to the application of shock waves. They usually occur weeks to months after lithotripsy and in only some of these patients who still harbor fragments in their gallbladders. Only rarely is endoscopic sphincterotomy necessary to remove prepapillary stone fragments from the common bile duct.[9, 14] Cystic duct obstruction with subsequent cholecystitis has been reported by Greiner and colleagues in 2 per cent of the patients.[23] Elective cholecystectomy has been necessary in only a small percentage of patients. In one of the largest studies, it has been performed without mortality

in about 1 per cent of patients because of insufficient stone fragmentation within an investigation period of about two years.[28] No emergency operations have been necessary in this study during the same time period.

All treatments of gallstones that leave the gallbladder in place are associated with the risk of stone recurrence. After successful dissolution of gallbladder stones by oral bile acid therapy, stone recurrence has been observed in 30 to 50 per cent of the patients within a time period of three to five years.[29, 30] Thereafter, the risk of recurrence may be low. The rate of stone recurrence may be somewhat higher in patients who have had multiple stones than in those who have had single stones.[31, 32] First results of a post–fragmentation-dissolution study suggest that stone recurrence within the first year after successful shock wave lithotripsy and stone clearance is about 10 per cent.[33] This rate is similar to that observed within the first year after medical dissolution of gallstones.[29, 30]

BILE DUCT STONES

Stones in the bile ducts may cause symptoms and complications such as obstructive jaundice, cholangitis, and pancreatitis. Therefore, removal of these stones is generally recommended. In cholecystectomized patients as well as in high-risk patients, endoscopic sphincterotomy with removal of the stones in general is preferred to open surgery with choledochotomy.[34] Yet in some cases, the anatomy of the bile ducts in relation to the size of the stones may prevent successful extraction of the calculi by endoscopic means. Several measures have been reported to overcome this problem: direct electrohydraulic- or laser-induced lithotripsy,[35–38] mechanical lithotripsy with a specially constructed Dormia basket,[39] or dissolution of the stones by direct application of solvents.[40–42] In addition, some centers favor the placement of stents to permit drainage of bile in the presence of stones.[43] The percentage of patients requiring these additional measures after endoscopic sphincterotomy is in the range of 10 per cent.[34, 43]

Although all these adjuvant procedures have been reported to be successful in selected cases, disadvantages have to be considered. Stones may resist mechanical lithotripsy because the forces that can be applied are insufficient for shattering the stone or because the basket cannot be placed around the calculus. In laser lithotripsy or electrohydraulic lithotripsy, sufficient contact of the tip of the probe with the stone is crucial to obtain stone fragmentation as well as to avoid bile duct injury. Direct lithotripsy by laser beams or electrohydraulic shock waves often require additional devices such as a basket to hold the stone[35, 36] or the use of a choledochofiberscope.[44] This may render the procedure technically demanding and sometimes impossible, particularly in patients with intrahepatic stones. Chemical treatment of the stones in the biliary tree by direct application of solvents is less subject to these shortcomings, but it is time consuming (average time several days to two weeks), and the success rate (partial or complete dissolution) does not exceed 50 per cent.

First observations,[3, 45] which have been substantiated by a prospective multicenter trial,[46] suggest that extracorporeal shock wave lithotripsy of bile duct stones may become the procedure of choice in patients with bile duct stones that are refractory to routine endoscopic measures and to mechanical lithotripsy.

TABLE 61–3. SELECTION OF PATIENTS WITH BILE DUCT STONES FOR EXTRACORPOREAL SHOCK WAVE LITHOTRIPSY

Inclusion Criteria

Failure of routine endoscopic measures and mechanical lithotripsy
Access to the bile ducts (nasobiliary tube or transhepatic catheter)
Orifice of the common bile duct in the intestine large enough for spontaneous passage or extraction of fragments
Positioning of stone(s) in the shock wave focus possible

Exclusion Criteria

Coagulopathy or current medication with anticoagulant effects
Lung tissue, vascular aneurysms, or bowel loops in the shock wave path

INDICATIONS FOR EXTRACORPOREAL SHOCK WAVE LITHOTRIPSY

Basically, all patients with bile duct stones in whom endoscopic measures, including mechanical lithotripsy, have failed are candidates for extracorporeal shock wave lithotripsy. Fragmentation of the stones in these patients often is more coarse than fragmentation of gallbladder stones. There are several explanations for this observation. In general, total stone burden is larger, the structure of the stones is less crystalline, and the percentage of impacted stones is high. Since bile duct stones and the fragments after extracorporeal shock wave lithotripsy must be visualized by fluoroscopy after instillation of contrast medium and must be extracted from the bile ducts in a high percentage of the patients, access to the biliary tree is necessary, via either a percutaneous transhepatic catheter or a nasobiliary tube. As with any patient undergoing extracorporeal shock wave lithotripsy, the coagulation parameters must be in the normal range because of the risk of hematoma. In order to avoid tissue damage, there should be no lung tissue or vascular aneuryms in the shock wave path. To avoid absorption or reflection of the shock waves, no gas-filled bowel loops should be interposed between the shock wave source and the stone (Table 61–3).

PROCEDURE

Shock wave lithotripsy of bile duct stones differs from that of gallbladder stones with respect to stone location and shock wave entry (Fig. 61–4). When the shock waves are applied ventrally, common bile duct stones may be shadowed by gas-filled intestine. Therefore, an entry from the back is preferable, at least in the case of extrahepatic bile duct stones. Fluoroscopy is necessary, because location and fragmentation of these stones cannot be monitored accurately enough by ultrasound. For the treatment of bile duct stones, most centers therefore use kidney lithotripters with a radiographic system. Especially for large bile duct stones, lithotripters with a large focal volume are preferable. If the first session of shock wave lithotripsy fails, which occurs in about 20 per cent of patients, it can be repeated with about a 50 per cent chance of success.[46] The best time interval between the first and the second treatments appears to be about one week. Since septic complications immediately following shock wave lithotripsy of biliary stones have been reported, prophylactic administration of antibiotics has been recommended.[46] Patients with septic cholangitis should be adequately drained by a nasobiliary tube or a transhepatic catheter and should then be treated electively if possible.

RESULTS OF EXTRACORPOREAL SHOCK WAVE LITHOTRIPSY

In an uncontrolled multicenter trial,[46] 113 patients with bile duct stones in whom routine endoscopic procedures for removal of the calculi had failed were treated by

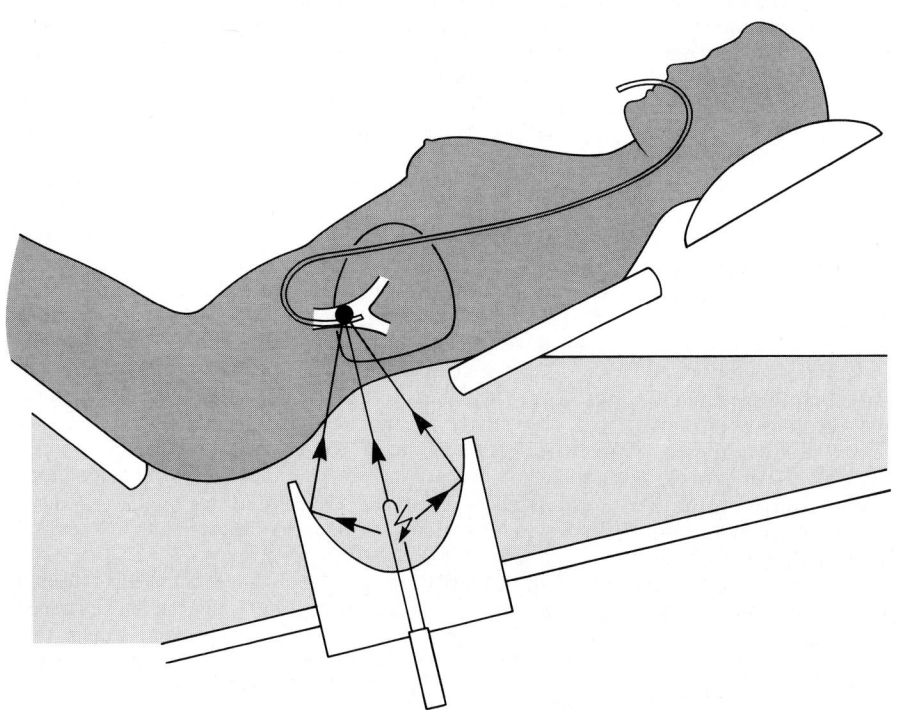

Figure 61–4. Schematic illustration of Dornier lithotripter HM3 and positioning of the patient for treatment of bile duct stone. The shock waves are generated by underwater spark discharge at the first focus of an ellipsoidal reflector. The stone is positioned at the second (remote) focus. The shock waves are introduced into the body by using a water bath into which the patient is partially immersed. The bile ducts and the stone are visualized after instillation of contrast medium via a nasobiliary tube employing a two-dimensional radiographic system that is used for targeting.

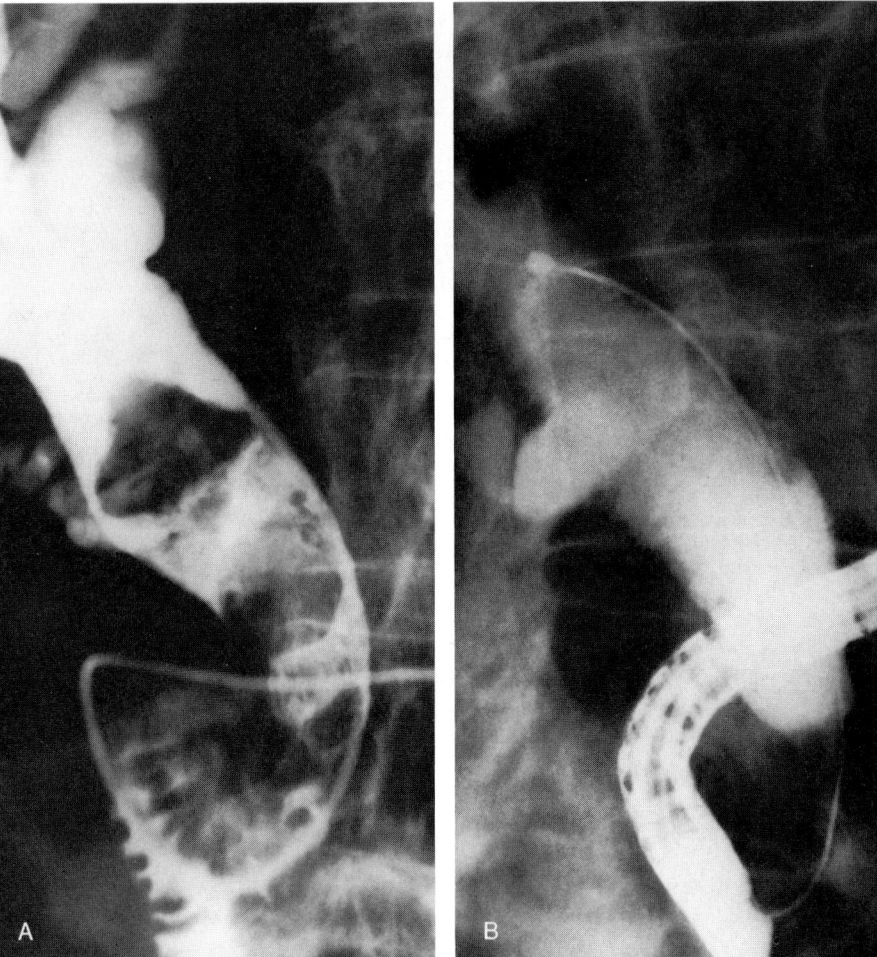

Figure 61–5. Retrograde cholangiogram showing the common bile duct with multiple large stones before (A) and one day after (B) extracorporeal shock wave lithotripsy when fragments had been removed using a Dormia basket.

extracorporeal shock wave lithotripsy. These patients represented 8 per cent of all those referred to the participating centers for endoscopic extraction of their stones. Sixteen per cent of these patients required more than one treatment. The overall fragmentation rate was 91 per cent, and complete stone clearance from the bile ducts was obtained in 86 per cent of the 113 patients (Fig. 61–5). In about 75 per cent of the patients in whom the stone could be disintegrated, the fragments had to be extracted by endoscopy. Most of the patients were treated with the Dornier kidney lithotripter HM3 (shock wave generation by spark discharge) with a capacitance of 80 nF. This lithotripter has a large focal volume, with a length of about 9 cm and a width of about 1.5 cm. Most of the patients received general anesthesia during treatment.

Preliminary reports on the use of the Siemens lithotripter (electromagnetic shock wave generation) also indicate that a high percentage of bile duct stones that are not amenable to routine endoscopic measures can successfully be treated by extracorporeal shock waves.[47]

Mild and mostly transient hemobilia induced by shock wave lithotripsy occurs in less than 10 per cent of the patients. Further complications directly caused by the shock waves may be hematoma of the liver and the skin and macrohematuria. These findings are probably caused by damage of small vessels of the tissue lying in the shock wave path. If patients have normal coagulation parameters, these tissue alterations rarely are of clinical relevance. Despite the close vicinity of pancreatic tissue to the shock

wave focus in patients with prepapillary stones, only one mild attack of pancreatitis after shock wave lithotripsy has been observed in 113 patients. When lithotripters with a large focal volume and an electrohydraulic shock wave source are used, some patients may have arrhythmias during treatment. Therefore, adequate ECG monitoring is of importance. It should also be kept in mind that pacemakers can be disturbed by the shock wave field.

Extracorporeal shock wave lithotripsy of bile duct stones is an adjuvant procedure to interventional endoscopic measures for extraction of stones from the biliary tree. The number of patients who require adjuvant extracorporeal shock wave lithotripsy is small, but in this group, the treatment is highly beneficial. Although reports of controlled trials are not available, side effects, complications, and mortality are probably lower than with surgery.

REFERENCES

1. Chaussy C, Brendel W, Schmiedt E. Extracorporeally induced destruction of kidney stones by shock waves. Lancet 2:1265, 1980.
2. Brendel W, Enders G. Shock waves for gallstones: animal studies. Lancet 1:1054, 1983.
3. Sauerbruch T, Delius M, Paumgartner G, et al. Fragmentation of gallstones by extracorporeal shock waves. N Engl J Med 314:818, 1986.
4. Ison KT. Physical and technical introduction to lithotripsy. In: Coptcoat MJ, Miller RA, Wickham JEA, eds. Lithotripsy II. London, BDI, 1987:7.
5. Coleman AJ, Saunders JE. Comparison of extracorporeal shock-wave

lithotripters. In: Coptcoat MJ, Miller RA, Wickham JEA, eds. Lithotripsy II. London, BDI, 1987:121.

6. Sauerbruch T, Sackmann M, Holl J, et al. Stosswellenlithotripsie von Gallensteinen. Dtsch Med Wochenschr 113:1401, 1988.

7. Schachler R, Sauerbruch T, Wosiewitz U, et al. Fragmentation of gallstones using extracorporeal shock waves: An in vitro study. Hepatology 8:925, 1988.

8. Paumgartner G. Fragmentation of gallstones by extracorporeal shock waves. Semin Liver Dis 7:317, 1987.

9. Sackmann M, Delius M, Sauerbruch T, et al. Shock-wave lithotripsy of gallbladder stones: the first 175 patients. N Engl J Med 318:393, 1988.

10. Paumgartner G, Carr-Locke DL, Roda E, et al. Biliary stones: non-surgical therapeutic approach. Gastroenterol Int 1:17, 1988.

11. Gracie WA, Ransohoff DF. The natural history of silent gallstones: the innocent gallstone is not a myth. N Engl J Med 307:798, 1982.

12. Ransohoff DF, Gracie WA, Wolfenson LB, et al. Prophylactic cholecystectomy or expectant management for persons with silent gallstones: a decision analysis to assess survival. Ann Intern Med 99:199, 1983.

13. Sackmann M, Sauerbruch T, Holl J, et al. Results of ESWL in gallbladder stones with radiopaque rim compared to radiolucent calculi. J Hepatol 7:S74, 1988. (Abstract.)

14. Ell C, Kerzel W, Heyder N, et al. Piezoelektrische Lithotripsie von Gallensteinen. Dtsch Med Wohenschr 113:1503, 1988.

15. Sackmann M, Sauerbruch T, Holl J, et al. Gallstone treatment by extracorporeal shock-wave lithotripsy. J Hepatol 7:283, 1988.

16. Sackmann M, Weber W, Delius M, et al. Extracorporeal shock-wave lithotripsy of gallstones without general anesthesia: first clinical experience. Ann Intern Med 107:347, 1987.

17. Shaffer EA, McOrmond P, Duggan H. Quantitative cholescintigraphy: assessment of gallbladder filling and emptying and duodenogastric reflux. Gastroenterology 79:899, 1980.

18. Fisher RS, Stelzer F, Rock E, et al. Abnormal gallbladder emptying in patients with gallstones. Dig Dis Sci 27:1019, 1982.

19. Forgacs IC, Maisey MN, Murphy GM, et al. Influence of gallstones and ursodeoxycholic acid therapy on gallbladder emptying. Gastroenterology 87:299, 1987.

20. Pomeranz IS, Shaffer EA. Abnormal gallbladder emptying in a subgroup of patients with gallstones. Gastroenterology 88:787, 1985.

21. Sylwestrowicz TA, Shaffer EA. Gallbladder function during gallstone dissolution. Effect of bile acid therapy in patients with gallstones. Gastroenterology 95:740, 1988.

22. Spengler U, Sackmann M, Sauerbruch T, et al. Gallbladder motility before and after extracorporeal shock wave lithotripsy. Gastroenterology (In press.)

23. Greiner L, Wenzel H, Jakobeit C. Biliaere Stowellen-Lithotripsie. Fragmentation und Lyse—ein neues Verfahren. Dtsch Med Wochenschr 112:1893, 1987.

24. Ponchon T, Martin X, Mestas JL, et al. Extracorporeal lithotripsy of gallstones. Lancet 2:448, 1987.

25. Hood KA, Keightley A, Dowling RH, et al. Piezo-ceramic lithotripsy of gallbladder stones: initial experience in 38 patients. Lancet 1:1322, 1988.

26. Podda M, Zuin M, Battezzati PM, et al. Efficacy and safety of a combination of chenodeoxycholic acid and ursodeoxycholic acid for gallstone dissolution: a comparison with ursodeoxycholic acid alone. Gastroenterology 96:222, 1989.

27. Thistle JL. Direct-contact dissolution of gallstones. Semin Liver Dis 7:311, 1987.

28. Teichmann RK, Sauerbruch T, Sackmann M, et al. Surgical intervention following fragmentation of gallstones by extracorporeal shock waves. World J Surg. (In press.)

29. Lanzini A, Jazrawi RP, Kupfer RM, et al. Gallstone recurrence after medical dissolution. An overestimated threat? J Hepatol 3:241, 1986.

30. O'Donnell LDJ, Heaton KW. Recurrence and re-recurrence of gall stones after medical dissolution: a long-term follow-up. Gut 29:655, 1988.

31. Villanova N, Bazzoli F, Frabboni R, et al. Gallstone recurrence after successful oral bile acid treatment: a three-year follow-up and evaluation of long-term postdissolution treatment. Gastroenterology 92:1787, 1987. (Abstract.)

32. Hood K, Gleeson D, Ruppin D, et al. Can gallstone recurrence be prevented? The British/Belgian post-dissolution trial. Gastroenterology 94:A548, 1988. (Abstract.)

33. Sackmann M, Ippisch E, Sauerbruch T, et al. Early gallstone recurrence after successful shock-wave therapy. Hepatology 8:1221, 1988. (Abstract.)

34. Cotton PB. Endoscopic management of bile duct stones (apples and oranges). Gut 25:587, 1984.

35. Frimberger E, Kuehner W, Weingart J, et al. Eine neue Methode der elektrohydraulischen Cholelithotripsie (Lithoklasie). Dtsch Med Wochenschr 107:213, 1982.

36. Koch H, Stolte M, Walz V. Endoscopic lithotripsy in the common bile duct. Endoscopy 9:95, 1977.

37. Lear JL, Ring EA, Macoviak, et al. Percutaneous transhepatic electro-hydraulic lithotripsy. Radiology 150:589, 1984.

38. Ell C, Lux G, Hochberger J, et al. Laserlithotripsy of common bile duct stones. Gut 29:746, 1988.

39. Riemann JF, Seuberth K, Demling L. Clinical application of a new mechanical lithotriptor for smashing common bile duct stones. Endoscopy 14:226, 1982.

40. Leuschner U, Wurbs D, Baumgärtel H, et al. Alternating treatment of common bile duct stones with a modified glyceryl-1-monooctanoate preparation and a bile acid–EDTA solution by nasobiliary tube. Scand J Gastroenterol 16:497, 1981.

41. Thistle JL, Carlson GL, Hofmann AF, et al. Monooctanoin, a dissolution agent for retained cholesterol bile duct stones: physical properties and clinical application. Gastroenterology 78:1016, 1980.

42. Neoptolemos JP, Hofmann AF, Moossa AR. Chemical treatment of stones in the biliary tree. Br J Surg 73:515, 1986.

43. Cotton PB, Forbes A, Leung JWC, et al. Endoscopic stenting for long-term treatment of large bile duct stones: 2- to 5-year follow-up. Gastrointest Endosc 33:411, 1987.

44. Hwang MH, Lee HH, Lin J, et al. Transcholecystic endoscopic choledocholithotripsy: successful management of retained common bile duct stone. Endoscopy 19:24, 1987.

45. Sauerbruch T, Holl J, Sackmann M, et al. Treatment of bile duct stones by extracorporeal shock waves. Semin Ultrasound CT MR 8:155, 1987.

46. Sauerbruch T, Stern M. The Study Group for Shock Wave Lithotripsy. Fragmentation of bile duct stones by extracorporeal shock waves. A new approach to biliary calculi after failure of routine endoscopic measures. Gastroenterology 96:146, 1989.

47. Staritz M, Floth A, Rambow A, et al. Shock-wave lithotripsy of gallstones with second-generation device without conventional water-bath. Lancet 2:155, 1987. (Letter.)

INDEX

Note: Page numbers in *italics* refer to illustrations;
page numbers followed by (t) refer to tables.

Endocytosis, receptor-mediated, 137–172, *138*, *163*. See also *Receptor(s)*.
  acidification in, 144–145, 314
Endoplasmic reticulum, 18, *19*, *20*, 21
  protein glycosylation in, 128, *129*
  smooth, phenobarbital-induced hypertrophy of, 21, *21*
Endoplasmic reticulum membrane, translocation of secretory proteins across, 128
Endoscopic retrograde cholangiopancreatography, 684–685, *685*, 1533
  in biliary pancreatitis, 1541
  in cholangitis, 1536
  in extrahepatic bile duct atresia, 1374
Endoscopic sphincterotomy, 1548–1550, *1549*
  complications of, 1550, 1552, 1552(t)
  in biliary pancreatitis, 1540, 1541
  in choledocholithiasis, 1552
  in patient with intact gallbladder, 1553, 1554(t)
  in sphincter of Oddi dysfunction, 1555, 1555(t)
  urgent indications for, 1553–1554
Endosomes, *148*
Endothelial sinusoidal lining cells, 14, *15*
Endothelialitis, hepatic, 714, *717*
Endotoxin, and renal failure in cirrhosis, 507
  in liver disease, 1122–1123, 1135
End-stage liver disease, chronic, 1462, 1462(t)
  causes of, 1460(t)
  transplantation for, 1460–1465
End-to-side mesocaval shunt, portal circulation following, *603*
End-to-side portacaval shunt, 603
  portal circulation following, *603*
End-to-side splenorenal shunt, portal circulation following, *603*, 605
Energy metabolism, liver function and, 65. See also *Hepatic metabolism* and specific fuels, e.g., *Glucose.*
Enflurane, liver disease induced by, 766, 881–882
  metabolism of, 882, *882*
Entactin (nidogen), 428
Entamoeba histolytica infection, and hepatic abscess formation, 668, 669, 1061–1064, *1062*, *1063*, 1065(t), 1067
Enterically transmitted non-A, non-B hepatitis, 930–931, 968
  vs. other viral hepatitides, 969(t)
Enterohepatic circulation, *45*
  of bile acids, 341–364, *348*
    factors affecting, 350, 352
    gallbladder's role in, 361–362
    in infants, 364–365
    interruption of, abnormal bile acid metabolism associated with, 366–367
    intestine's role in, 363–364
    liver's role in, 352–360
    pathophysiology of, 365–368
    physiology of, 341–364
    portal circulation and, 364
  of drugs, 241
  of folate, 541, *541*
    effects of alcohol on, 541, *541*
Enteropathy, choleretic, abnormal bile acid metabolism in, 366–367
Environmental toxins, liver disease induced by, 791–814, 792(t), 1159. See also *Hepatotoxin(s).*
Enzyme(s), catalytic function of, in alcohol metabolism, 824–829, *828*
  in bile acid metabolism by gut bacteria, *357*
  in bile acid synthesis, 352, 354(t)
  in heme biosynthesis, *379*, 381–384, 382(t)
  copper in, 1252, 1253
  deficiencies of, and disorders of metabolism, 1353(t)
    of carbohydrates, 1301–1311
    of lipids, 1328, 1331
    of tyrosine, 1323(t)

Enzyme(s) *(Continued)*
  deficiencies of, and glycogen storage diseases, 1311–1322
    and porphyrias, *379*, *398*, *407*
  degradation of extracellular matrix by, 433
  drug-metabolizing, induction of, 220–222, 221(t)
  gluconeogenic, 73(t). See also *Gluconeogenesis.*
    distribution of, in hepatic lobule, 76
  glycolytic, 73(t). See also *Glycolysis.*
    distribution of, in hepatic lobule, 76
  heme-degrading, *258*, 258–259
  in bile, 325, 346
  lysosomal, in bile, 325
  microsomal, oxidation of alcohol by, 825
  plasma membrane, *332*
    in bile, 325
  serum levels of, in liver disease, 654, *654*, *655*, 658, 659, *659*, 660
Enzyme activity, in pregnancy, 1440, *1440*
  mechanisms regulating, *112*
Epidemic non-A, non-B hepatitis. See *Enterically transmitted non-A, non-B hepatitis.*
Epidermal growth factor, 58
  binding of, *165*, 168
Epidermal growth factor receptor, 140(t), *143*, 167–170
Epinephrine, effects of, on hepatic blood flow, 39, *40*
Epithelioid granuloma, 1098, *1099*
Epithelioid hemangioendothelioma, of liver, 1228
Epoxide hyrolase, 213
Epping jaundice, 803
Erythema, palmar, in pregnancy, 1440
Erythritol, in studies of hepatocellular transport, 315, *317*
Erythrocyte. See *Red blood cell(s).*
Erythrocyte sedimentation rate, in primary biliary cirrhosis, 1164(t), 1168
Erythrocytosis, in hepatocellular carcinoma, 1209
Erythromycin, liver disease induced by, 768–769
Erythropoiesis, pathologic, and hyperbilirubinemia, 271
Erythropoietic coproporphyria, 396
Erythropoietic porphyria(s), 395(t), 395–396
  congenital, 395–396
Escherichia coli infection, liver dysfunction in, 1092
Esophageal transection, for bleeding varices, 602
Esophageal variceal bleeding, 594–609
  and prognosis, in alcoholic cirrhosis, 851, *852*
  as complication of peritoneovenous shunt, 631
  balloon tamponade for, 597–598
  cause of, 594–595
  diagnosis of, 595
  in primary biliary cirrhosis, 1184, 1195
  injection sclerotherapy for, 599–601, 600(t), 601(t)
    complications associated with, 599–600, 600(t)
  ligation for, 602
  medical management of, 596–597
  portal-systemic shunt for, 602–609, 606(t), *607*, 607(t)
  portal vein–azygos vein disconnection for, 602
  portal venous pressure in, 577, *578*, 595
  portal-systemic shunt for, 602–609, 606(t), *607*, 607(t)
  prevention of, injection sclerotherapy in, 600–601, 601(t)
    propranolol in, 598–599, 599(t)
  somatostatin for, 597
  transection for, 602
  transhepatic thrombosis for, 601–602
  vasopressin for, 596–597, 597(t)
Esophageal variceal pressure, 578
Esophageal varices, 575, *575*, 595
Esterase, 211, 213
Esterification, of bilirubin, 255, 266
  of cholesterol, by lecithin-cholesterol acyltransferase, *103*, 103–104, *104*, *105*
Estrogen, *517*, 517–518
  liver disease induced by, 777–779, 1229, 1443

Fulminant hepatic failure *(Continued)*
encephalopathy in, 464–467, 472. See also *Encephalopathy, hepatic.*
fatty infiltration of hepatocytes in, 462, *463*
hepatocellular necrosis in, 462, *463*
hypoglycemia in, 470, 476
hypotension in, 469, 477–478, 535
hypoxemia in, 536
in infants, 483, 483(t)
in pregnancy, 483
increased intracranial pressure in, 467, 467(t)
infections causing, 461, 461(t). See also *Fulminant viral hepatitis.*
lactic acidosis in, 535–536
L-dopa for, 482
liver disease after, 473
liver hypoxia and ischemia causing, 461(t), 461–462
liver regeneration in, 472
management of, 475–483
natural history and course of, 472–473, 481, *481*
pancreatitis in, 470–471
pathogenesis of, 464
pathology of, 462
portal hypertension in, 471
prognosis in, 473–474
prostaglandins for, 482
pulmonary edema in, 469,536
recovery from, 473
renal failure in, 470, 477
sepsis in, 471, 477
severity of, indices of, 473–474
temporary hepatic support for, 479–482, 480(t)
toxins causing, 461, 461(t)
transplantation for, 482, 1463
trends in research into, 483–484
type I, 462, 462(t), *463*
type II, 462, 462(t), *463*
ventilatory defects in, 469, 477
Fulminant viral hepatitis, 464, 971
diagnosis of, 482
Fulminant viral hepatitis A, 464
Fulminant viral hepatitis B, 464
chronic hepatitis delta virus infection and, 918
Fungal infection, and primary biliary cirrhosis, 1159
dissemination of, to liver, 1110
drugs for, hepatotoxicity of, 770

GABA receptor, *454*, 455
in hepatic encephalopathy, 455, 466
GABA-ergic neurotransmitter system, 455
in hepatic encephalopathy, 455–456, 466
Galactitol, accumulations of, in transferase-deficiency galactosemia, 1307, 1308, 1309
Galactokinase-deficiency galactosemia, 1311
Galactose, conversion of, to glucose, *78*, *1306*
Galactose breath tests, 648
results of, in liver disease, 648, *649*
Galactose elimination tests, 648
Galactose-free diet, 1310
Galactose metabolism, 78, *78*, *1306*, *1308*
disorder(s) of, 1305–1311
transferase-deficiency galactosemia as, 1306–1311, 1307(t), 1353(t)
Galactosemia, galactokinase-deficiency, 1311
transferase-deficiency, 1306–1311, 1307(t), 1353(t)
uridine diphosphate galactose-epimerase deficiency, 1311
Gallbladder, 26, 326–327
adenocarcinoma of, *680*, 1529
adenoma of, 1528
adenomyomatosis of, *678*, *1520*, 1528

Gallbladder *(Continued)*
and circulation of bile acids, 361–362. See also *Enterohepatic circulation, of bile acids.*
calcification of wall of, *676*
carcinoma of, *680*, 1529
cholesterolosis of, 1528, *1528*
development of, 6, 7
emptying of, 327, 362
filling of, 326–327
gallstones in, extracorporeal shock-wave lithotripsy for, 1562–1565, *1563*, 1563(t), *1564*
inflammation of. See *Cholecystitis.*
mucosa of, 26, *27*
intercellular spaces in, and transport, 327, *328*, *329*
nonopacification of, on cholecystography, 678, 678(t)
porcelain, 675
radiographic examination of, 675, 1518. See also *Cholecystography.*
resection of, 1518, 1520
cholangiography during and after, 1520, *1520*, 1521, *1521*
exploration of common bile duct at, 1521
extraction of retained gallstones after, 685–686, *686*, *1554*, 1554–1555
for acute cholecystitis, 1524, 1535
for carcinoma, 1529
for cholelithiasis, 1520
incidental, 1521–1522
in patient with cirrhosis, 1522
symptoms occurring after, 1530
response of, to cholecystokinin, 362
role of, in bile formation, 326–327
scintigraphic evaluation of, 681. See also *Radionuclide scanning.*
transport in, intercellular spaces in mucosa and, 327, *328*, *329*
ultrasonographic examination of, 679–681, 1518. See also *Ultrasonography.*
vasculature of, 26, *28*
Gallbladder bile, conversion of hepatic bile to, 326, *326*, *362*, 362
Gallbladder disease, 1516–1530
cholecystectomy for, 1518, 1520, 1524, 1525, 1529
cholangiography during and after, 1520, *1520*, 1521, *1521*
exploration of common bile duct at, 1521
in patient with cirrhosis, 1522
symptoms occurring after, 1530
inflammatory. See *Cholecystitis.*
neoplastic, benign, 1528
malignant, *680*, 1529
radiographic examination for, 675, 1518. See also *Cholecystography.*
scintigraphic examination for, 681. See also *Radionuclide scanning.*
symptoms of, in conditions other than cholelithiasis, 1528–1529
ultrasonographic diagnosis of, 679–681, 1518. See also *Ultrasonography.*
Gallbladder function, absorptive, 1495
motor, 1496–1497
secretory, 1495–1496
Gallstone(s), 1480, 1482, 1495. See also *Gallstone disease.*
and pancreatitis, 1538
bile acid dissolution of, 1499–1500, 1502
black, 272, 1500
brown, 272, 1500
calcium in, 1482, 1484, 1486
chenodeoxycholic acid for, 1499, 1500, 1502
cholesterol, 1481, 1482, 1487
abnormal bile acid metabolism associated with, 366
contact solvent dissolution of, 1502–1503
dissolution of 1497–1505
recurrence of cholelithiasis following, 1503
extracorporeal shock-wave destruction of, 1561–1567, *1563*, 1563(t), *1566*, 1566(t)
results of, *1564*, 1564–1565, 1567, *1567*

Gallstones *(Continued)*
  in bile duct, extracorporeal shock-wave lithotripsy for, 1565–
      1567, *1566*, 1566(t), *1567*
    percutaneous extraction of, after cholecystetomy, 685–686,
      686, *1554*, 1554–1555
  in common bile duct, 1533–1534, *1533*, *1537*
    endoscopic sphincterotomy for, 1552
    unextractable, 1552, *1553*
  in gallbladder, extracorporeal shock-wave lithotripsy for, 1562–
      1565, *1563*, 1563(t), *1564*
  methyl tert-butyl ether for, 1503, *1503*
  mono-octanoin for, 1502–1503, *1503*
  on cholecystography, *677*, 678, 1518, *1519*
  on plain radiography, 1518, *1518*, *1519*
  on ultrasonography, 680, *680*, 681, 1518, *1519*
  pigment, 272, 1482, 1504
    hemolytic disorders and, 272
  prevention of, 1504
  recurrence of, after dissolution therapy, 1503
  types of, therapy choices based on, *1501*, 1504, *1505*
  unextractable, in common bile duct, 1552, *1553*
  urodeoxycholic acid for, 1499, 1502
Gallstone disease. See also *Gallstone(s).*
  and cholecystitis, 1522
  and pancreatitis, 1538
  animal models of, 1482
  bile acid therapy for, 1499–1500, 1502
  biliary sludge and, 1482–1483
  chenodeoxycholic acid for, 1499, 1500, 1502
  cholecystectomy for, 1520
  cholecystitis in, 1522
  cholecystographic findings in, *677*, 678, 1518, *1519*
  contact solvents used for, 1502–1503
  dissolution therapy for, 1497–1505
    recurrence of cholelithiasis following, 1503
  epidemiology of, 1516–1517
  extracorporeal shock-wave lithotripsy for, 1561–1567, *1563*,
      1563(t), *1566*, 1566(t)
    results of, *1564*, 1564–1565, *1567*, 1567
  in Crohn's disease, 1154
  in cystic fibrosis, 1340
  in pregnancy, 1443
  in premature infants, 1384
  in primary biliary cirrhosis, 1184, 1195
  in protoporphyria, *393*
  in sickle cell anemia, 1426–1427
  in Wilson's disease, 1258
  methyl tert-butyl ether for, 1503, *1503*
  mono-octanoin for, 1502–1503, *1503*
  mucus hypersecretion and, 1483–1484
  natural history of, 1517–1518
  nonsurgical management of, 1497–1505, 1522
  oral contraceptive use and, 779
  pathogenesis of, 1481, *1482*, 1497, *1498*
  prevention of, 1504
  radiographic diagnosis of, 1518, *1518*, *1519*
  recurrence of, after dissolution therapy, 1503
  risk factors for, 1517(t)
  types of, therapy choices based on, *1501*, 1504, *1505*
  ultrasonographic findings in, 680, *680*, 681, 1518, *1519*
  ursodeoxycholic acid for, 1499, 1502
Gallstone ileus, 1526, *1526*
Gamma-amino acid neurotransmitter system, 455
  in hepatic encephalopathy, 455–456, 466
Gamma-aminobutyric acid receptor, *454*, 455
  in hepatic encephalopathy, 455, 466
Gamma-glutamyl transferase, isoenzymes of, in hepatocellular
    carcinoma, 1211
Gamma-glutamyl transpeptidase, 658–659
  serum levels of, in liver disease, 659, *659*
Gammopathy, monoclonal, remission of, in viral hepatitis, 987–
    988

Gangrene, gaseous, liver dysfunction in, 1091
Gap junctions, between hepatocytes, 22, *304*, 306
Gas gangrene, liver dysfunction in, 1091
Gastric varices. See also *Esophageal varices.*
  in patient with splenic vein thrombosis, 585, *586*
Gastrin, vasoactive potency of, 35
Gastritis, hemorrhagic, in portal hypertension, 595–596
Gastrointestinal tract, radiographic evaluation of, for gallbladder
    disease, 675
Gauche conformation, of acyl chains of phospholipids, 831
Gautier classification, of extrahepatic bile duct atresia, 1357,
    1358–1359
Genetic hemochromatosis, 1277–1292, *1282*, 1285(t)
  diagnosis of, 1287–1290, 1288(t), 1290(t)
  mechanisms of cellular injury in, *1279*, 1279–1280
  phlebotomy for, *1291*, 1291–1292
Genome, hepadnavirus, 895, *896*, 897–899
  replication of, *897*, 899–900
Gianotti's disease (papular acrodermatitis), in child with viral
    hepatitis, 983–984
Giant cells, in hepatic granuloma, 1098–1099, *1100*
  parenchymal, conditions associated with, 1388(t)
  in neonatal hepatitis, *1385*, 1387, *1387*
Giant hepatic mitochondria, 714, *717*
  alcohol-induced, 830, *830*
Gibbs-Donnan forces, 1486
Gilbert's syndrome, 282–285
  bilirubin production in, *256*, 284
  reduced hepatic clearance of bilirubin in, *256*, 284
  unconjugated hyperbilirubinemia in, *279*, 285
Glisson's capsule, 4
Globulin, corticosteroid-binding, 515
  sex hormone–binding, 516
  thyroxine-binding, in hepatocellular carcinoma, 527
Glomerulonephritis, in chronic active hepatitis, 1037
  in viral hepatitis, 982–983
Glucagon, vasoactive potency of, 36, *37*
Glucagon and insulin therapy, for alcoholic hepatitis, 854
α-1,4Glucanglycosyl transferase deficiency (type IV glycogeno-
    sis), 1321–1323, 1353(t)
Glucokinase, in liver cells, 71
  phosphorylation of glucose by, 70, *70*
Gluconeogenesis, effects of alcohol on, 836–837, *837*
  enzymes of, 73(t)
    distribution of, in hepatic lobule, 76
  glycolysis and, reciprocal regulation of, 75–76, *76*
  one-way reactions in, 69, *70*
  substrates for, 83
    quantitative aspects of, 85
  zonation of liver function and, 76
Glucose, conversion of galactose to, *78*, *1306*
  effects of, on aminolevulinic acid synthase, 388–389
  levels of, in sinusoidal blood, hepatic response to, 66, 70
  metabolism of, alterations in, in viral hepatitis, 968
    in liver, *74*
    in pathways other than synthesis of glycogen, 74
    in pentose pathway, 76, *77*
    separation of degradative and synthetic pathways for, 68
    vs. metabolism of fructose, 77
  phosphorylation of, by glucokinase, 70, *70*
    by hexokinase, 70, *70*
  production and release of, in type I glycogen storage disease,
    1316
  synthesis of. See *Gluconeogenesis.*
  utilization of, by liver, 69–71
    in fasted state, 66, *68*, 84–85
    in fed state, 66, *67*
    in postabsorptive state, 66, *67*
Glucose effect, 388–389
Glucose feedings, for type I glycogenosis, 1317, 1318
Glucosephosphatase deficiency (type I glycogenosis), 1312–1318,
    1353(t), *1813*

Reticuloendothelial cell dysfunction, 539–540
Retinoids, liver disease induced by, 782
Retinol, *183*. See also *Vitamin A*.
Retrograde cholangiopancreatography, endoscopic, 684–685, *685*, 1533
   in biliary pancreatitis, 1541
   in cholangitis, 1536
   in extrahepatic bile duct atresia, 1374
Reye's syndrome, 1434–1435, *1434*, 1434(t)
Rheumatoid arthritis, liver disease in, 1430
   vs. HBsAg-positive arthritis, 981(t)
Ribonucleic acid, messenger, translation of, 125, 127, *127*
Ribophorins, 128
Richner-Hanhart syndrome (persistent tyrosinemia), 1323(t), 1325
Rifampin, liver disease induced by, 772
Right ventricular failure, liver in, 1416–1417, 1416(t), 1417(t)
Ring, Kayser-Fleischer, in Wilson's disease, *1259*, 1259–1260
RNA, messenger, translation of, 125, 127, *127*
Ro 15-1788 (flumazenil), for hepatic encephalopathy, 455, 455(t), 466, 482
   in rabbits, *466*
Rocky Mountain spotted fever, liver dysfunction in, 1096
Rodent liver. See *Rat liver* and *Mouse liver*.
Rokitansky-Aschoff crypts, 26, *28*
Rose bengal sodium iodine-131, test for excretion of, in cholestasis, 1374
Rosette, hepatocyte, 718, *720*
Rotor's syndrome, 288–289
   coproporphyrinuria in, 288, 414
Rupture, hepatic, in pregnancy, 1452
   of hepatic amebic abscess, into chest, 1064

Salicylates, liver disease induced by, 1430
   Reye's syndrome in patients using, 1434–1435
Salmonella species, infection by, liver dysfunction in, 1092–1093
Salt, bile. See *Bile* and *Bile acid(s)*.
Sarcoid granuloma, hepatic, 1102, *1103*, 1105–1106
   laboratory findings in, 1102(t)
Sarcoidosis, hepatic, 1102, *1103*, 1105–1106, *1106*
   laboratory findings in, 1102(t)
   portal hypertension in, 588
Sarcoma, undifferentiated (embryonal), of liver, 1228
Sawaguchi operation, for extrahepatic bile duct atresia, *1376*
Scan-directed biopsy, 704–705
Scheuer staging, of primary biliary cirrhosis, 1169(t)
Schistosomiasis, hepatic, 1067(t), 1072–1074, 1083(t), 1110–1111, *1111*, *1112*
   portal hypertension in, 587, 1074
Scintigraphy. See *Radionuclide scanning*.
Scintiphotosplenoportography, 576
Scirrhous hepatocellular carcinoma, 1216
Scleroderma, primary biliary cirrhosis associated with, 1176, 1430–1431
Sclerosing cholangitis, primary. See *Primary sclerosing cholangitis*.
Sclerosing hyaline necrosis, of liver, *857*, 857–858, *858*
Sclerotherapy, for esophageal variceal bleeding, 599–601, 600(t), 601(t)
   complications associated with, 599–600, 600(t)
Screening, for genetic hemochromatosis, 1290, 1290(t)
   for hepatocellular carcinoma, 948–949
Secondary bile acids, 342, *344*
Secondary iron overload, 1273, 1283, 1292
Secondary micelles, 345
Secondary porphyrinuria, 413–414
Secondary syphilis, 1093–1094
   liver dysfunction in, 1094
Secretin, effect of, on bile ducts, 326
   vasoactive potency of, 36, *37*

Secretory cell, constitutive, 132
   hepatocyte as, 132
      vs. nonhepatic secretory cells, 303, *304*
   regulated, 132
Secretory protein, cotranslational and post-translational modifications of, 128–129
   glycosylation of, 128–129, *129*
      vitamin A in, 185, *185*
   intracellular degradation of, 131
   intracellular movement of, Golgi complex in, 130, *130*
   proteolytic modifications of, 128
   synthesis and segregation of, *127*, 127–128
   translocation of, across endoplasmic reticulum membrane, 128
Seizures, drugs for, hepatotoxicity of, 766–768
   in acute intermittent porphyria, 403
Selective portal-systemic shunt, 604
   portal circulation following, *605*
   vs. nonselective portal-systemic shunt, 607, 607(t)
Selenium, deficiency of, and primary biliary cirrhosis, 1160
   liver disease induced by, 812
Self-aggregation, of bile salts, 343, 345
   and critical micellar concentration, 345
Semisynthetic penicillins, liver disease induced by, 768
Senecio. See *Pyrrolizidine*.
Sengstaken-Blakemore tube, balloon tamponade of varices with, 598
Sepsis, as complication of peritoneovenous shunt, 631
   in fulminant hepatic failure, 471, 477
   jaundice accompanying, 883, 1090
   liver dysfunction in, 1089–1090
Septa, fibrous, in primary biliary cirrhosis, 714, *717*, 1172, *1173*
Serotonin, vasoactive potency of, 39
Serum sickness–like syndrome, in viral hepatitis, 981
Sex hormone(s). See also specific hormones, e.g., *Estrogen*.
   hepatic handling of, shunting due to liver disease and, 524, *524*
Sex hormone–binding globulin, 516
Sex hormone–related liver disease, 519–520
Sexual dimorphism, of liver function, 519, 519(t)
Shigellosis, liver dysfunction in, 1093
Shock, intraoperative, and ischemic hepatitis, 883–884
Shock liver, 1421
Shock wave(s), 1561–1562, *1562*, 1562(t)
Shock-wave lithotripsy, extracorporeal, 1561–1567, *1563*, 1563(t), *1566*, 1566(t)
   results of, 1564–1655, *1564*, 1567, *1567*
Shunt, cholehepatic, 321, 342
   coronary-caval, 604
      portal circulation following, *605*
   intrapulmonary, in chronic liver disease, 533
   mesocaval, 603–604
      end-to-side, portal circulation following, *603*
   peritoneovenous, 629
      complication(s) of, 630–631, 631(t)
         disseminated intravascular coagulation as, 560, 630–631
      effects of, 629–630, 630(t)
      for cirrhotic ascites, 501, 631
      for hepatorenal syndrome, 509
   portacaval, 603
      effects of, 604–605
         on availability of drugs normally efficiently extracted by liver, 238, *238*
      emergency, 605–606
      end-to-side, 603
         portal circulation following, *603*
      for bleeding esophageal varices, 603, 606, 607(t)
      for hepatorenal syndrome, 509
      portal circulation following, *603*
      side-to-side, 603
         portal circulation following, *603*
   portal-pulmonary, in chronic liver disease, 533–534
   portal-systemic, 603–604